DISTINCTIVE FEATURES

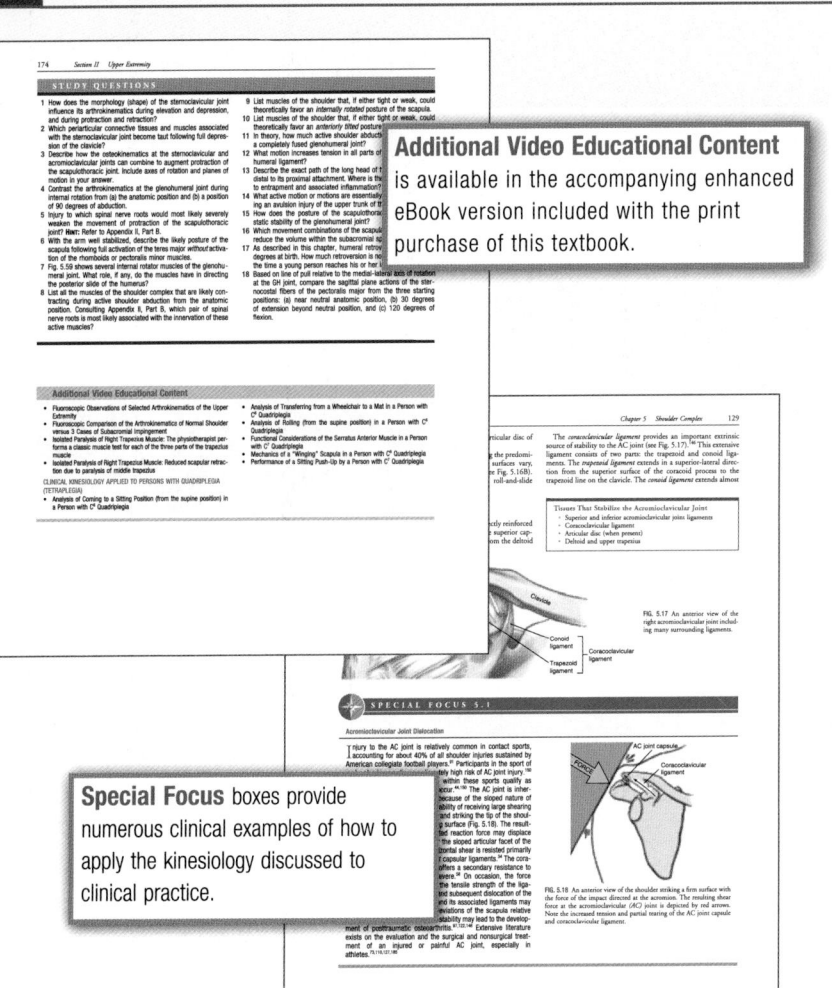

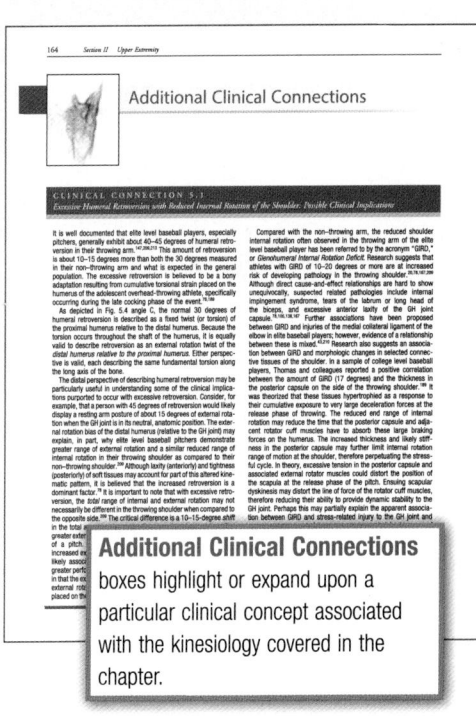

Additional Video Educational Content is available in the accompanying enhanced eBook version included with the print purchase of this textbook.

Additional Clinical Connections boxes highlight or expand upon a particular clinical concept associated with the kinesiology covered in the chapter.

Special Focus boxes provide numerous clinical examples of how to apply the kinesiology discussed to clinical practice.

Study Questions designed to challenge the reader to review or reinforce the main concepts contained within the chapter. Detailed answers provided by the author in the enhanced eBook will serve as an extension of the learning process.

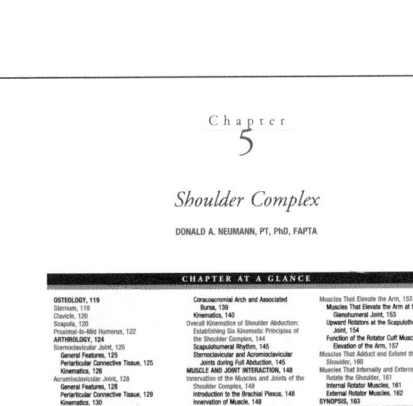

Chapter at a Glance boxes list the important topics that will be explored in the chapter.

References demonstrate the extensive evidence-based approach of this textbook.

NEUMANN'S
KINESIOLOGY OF THE
MUSCULOSKELETAL
SYSTEM

Donald A. Neumann, PT, PhD, FAPTA

Professor Emeritus
Department of Physical Therapy and Exercise Science
Marquette University
Milwaukee, Wisconsin

Primary Artwork by

Elisabeth Roen Kelly, BSc, BMC

Fourth Edition

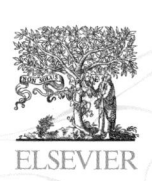

ELSEVIER

Elsevier
3251 Riverport Lane
St. Louis, Missouri 63043

NEUMANN'S KINESIOLOGY OF THE MUSCULOSKELETAL SYSTEM,
FOURTH EDITION

ISBN: 978-0-323-71859-2

Previous editions copyrighted 2017, 2010, and 2002.

Senior Content Strategist: Lauren Willis
Content Development Manager: Danielle M. Frazier
Publishing Services Manager: Julie Eddy
Project Manager: Becky Langdon
Design Direction: Amy Buxton

Printed in India

Last digit is the print number: 9 8 7 6 5 4 3 2 1

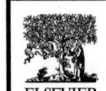

Working together
to grow libraries in
developing countries

www.elsevier.com • www.bookaid.org

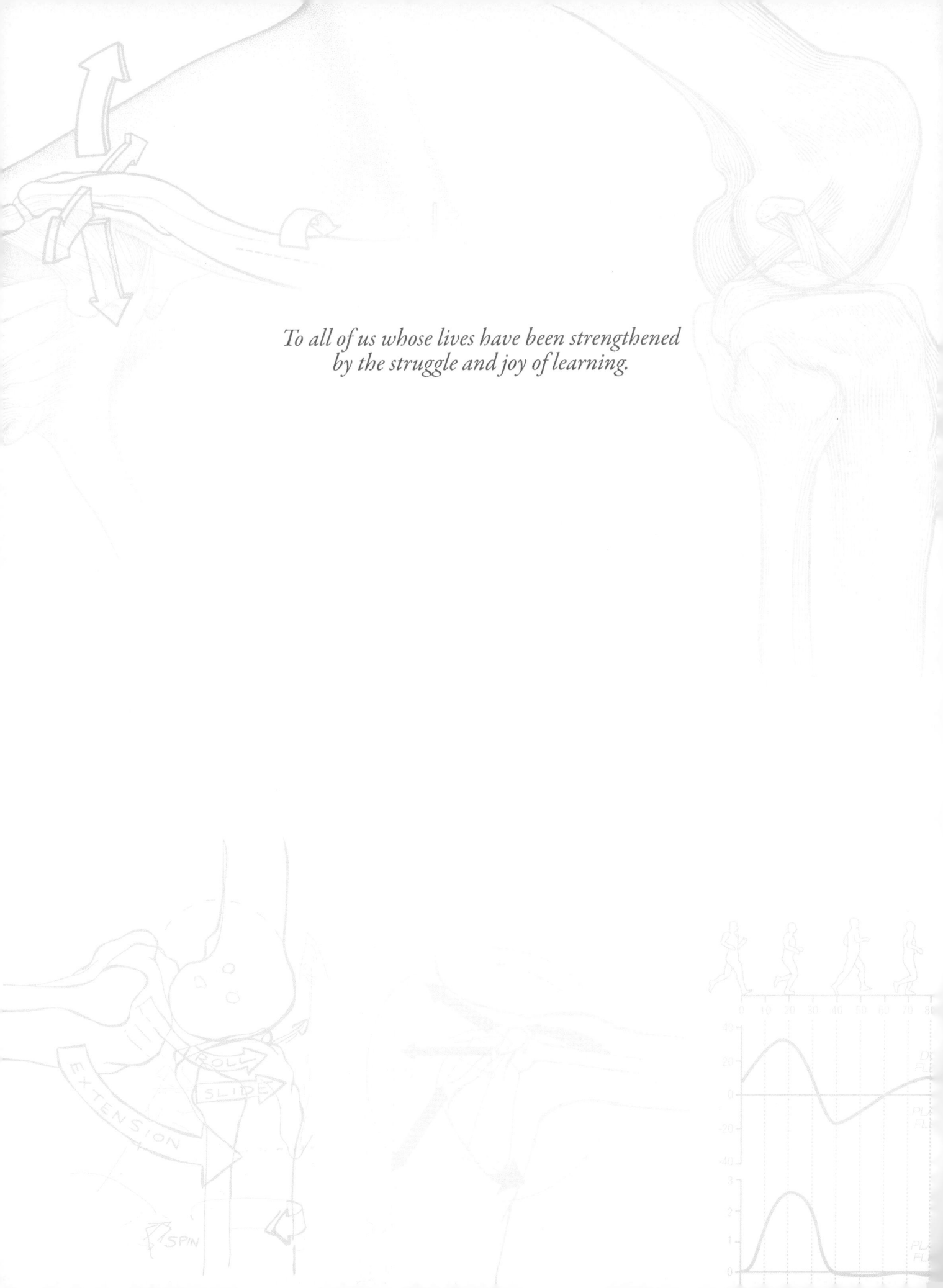

*To all of us whose lives have been strengthened
by the struggle and joy of learning.*

ABOUT THE AUTHOR

Donald A. Neumann, PT, PhD, FAPTA

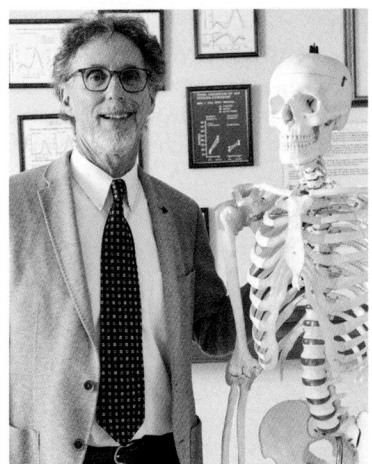

Don was born in New York City, the oldest of five siblings. He is the son of Charles J. and Elizabeth ("Betty") Neumann. Charles was a meteorologist and world-renowned hurricane forecaster who lived with polio the last 65 years of his life, which he contracted flying as a "hurricane hunter" for the U.S. Navy in the early 1950s. Don grew up in Miami, Florida, the location of the United States Weather Bureau. Today, Don's mother, Betty, lives near Ocala, Florida.

Soon after graduating from high school, Don was involved in a serious motorcycle accident. After receiving extensive physical therapy, Don chose physical therapy as his lifelong career. In 1972, he started his study and practice of physical therapy by earning a 2-year degree from Miami Dade Community College as a physical therapist assistant. In 1976, Don graduated with a Bachelor of Science degree in physical therapy from the University of Florida. He went on to practice as a physical therapist at Woodrow Wilson Rehabilitation Center in Virginia, where he specialized in the rehabilitation of patients with spinal cord injuries. In 1980, Don attended the University of Iowa, where he earned his Master's degree in science education and a PhD in exercise science.

In 1986, Dr. Neumann started his academic career as a teacher, writer, and researcher in the Physical Therapy Department at Marquette University. His teaching efforts concentrated on kinesiology as it relates to physical therapy. Don remained clinically active as a physical therapist on a part-time basis for 20 years, working primarily in the area of rehabilitation after spinal cord injury, outpatient orthopedics, and geriatrics. Currently, Dr. Neumann is Professor Emeritus within the Physical Therapy Department, College of Health Sciences, Marquette University, where he remains involved with teaching, mentoring, and other scholarly pursuits.

In addition to receiving several prestigious teaching, research, writing, and service awards from the American Physical Therapy Association (APTA), Dr. Neumann received a *Teacher of the Year Award* at Marquette University in 1994, and in 2006, he was named by the Carnegie Foundation as *Wisconsin's College Professor of the Year*. Over the years, Dr. Neumann's research and teaching projects have been funded by the National Arthritis Foundation and the Paralyzed Veterans of America. He has published extensively on methods to protect the arthritic or painful hip from damaging forces. Don has extensive anatomic dissection experience and has authored the 41st through 43rd editions of the "Pelvis and Hip" chapter in *Gray's Anatomy* (Elsevier).

Dr. Neumann has received multiple Fulbright Scholarships to teach kinesiology to physiotherapists in Lithuania (2002), Hungary (2005 and 2006), Japan (2009 and 2010), and Ireland (2022). In 2007, Don received an honorary doctorate from the Lithuanian Sports Academy, located in Kaunas, Lithuania. In 2015, Don received the *International Service Award in Education* from the World Confederation of Physical Therapy (WCPT) in Singapore. Don also served as an associate editor for the *Journal of Orthopaedic & Sports Physical Therapy* from 2002 to 2015.

Don lives with his wife Brenda and their family dog in Wisconsin. His son Donald Jr. ("Donnie"), stepdaughter Megann, and their families also live in Wisconsin. Don has three grandsons: Jack, Ben, and Cole.

Outside of work, Don enjoys playing the guitar, exercising, being in the mountains, volunteering, and paying close attention to the weather.

About the Illustrations

The collection of art in this edition has continued to evolve since the first edition published in 2002. The overwhelming majority of the approximately 700 illustrations are original, produced over the course of compiling the four editions of this text. The illustrations were first conceptualized by Dr. Neumann and then meticulously rendered primarily through the unique talents of Elisabeth Roen Kelly. Dr. Neumann states, "The artwork really drove the direction of much of my writing. I needed to thoroughly understand a particular kinesiologic concept at its most essential level to effectively explain to Elisabeth what needed to be illustrated. In this way, the artwork kept me honest; I wrote only what I truly understood."

Dr. Neumann and Ms. Kelly produced three primary forms of artwork for this text. Elisabeth depicted the anatomy of bones, joints, and muscles by hand, creating very detailed pen-and-ink drawings (Fig. 1). These drawings started with a series of pencil sketches, often based on anatomic specimens carefully dissected by Dr. Neumann. The pen-and-ink medium was chosen to give the material an organic, classic feeling.

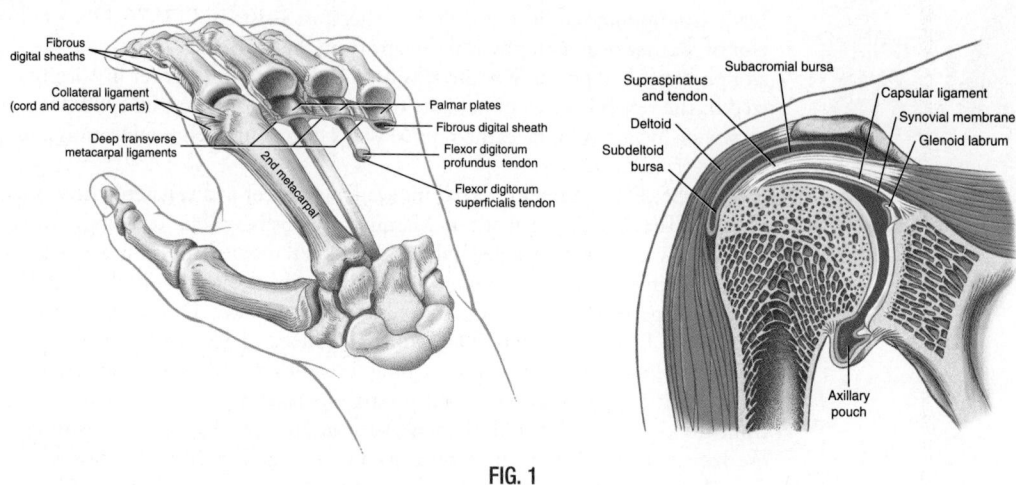

FIG. 1

The second form of art used a layering of artistic media, integrated with the use of software (Fig. 2). Neumann and Kelly often started with a photograph that was transformed into a simplified image of a person performing a particular movement. Images of bones, joints, and muscles were then electronically embedded within the human outline. Overlaying various biomechanical images further enhanced the resultant illustration. The final design displayed specific and often complex biomechanical concepts in a relatively simple manner, while preserving human form and expression.

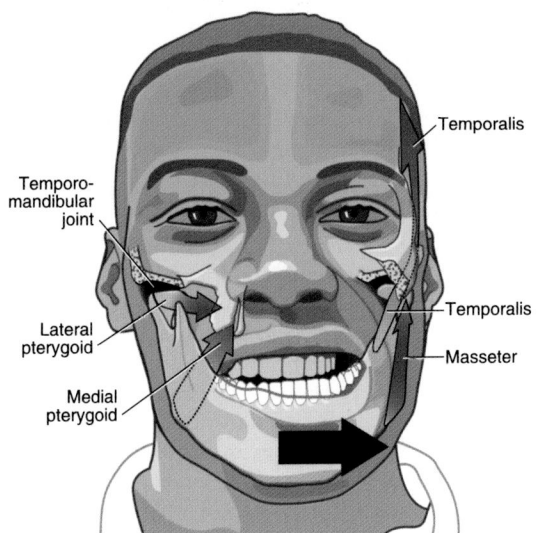
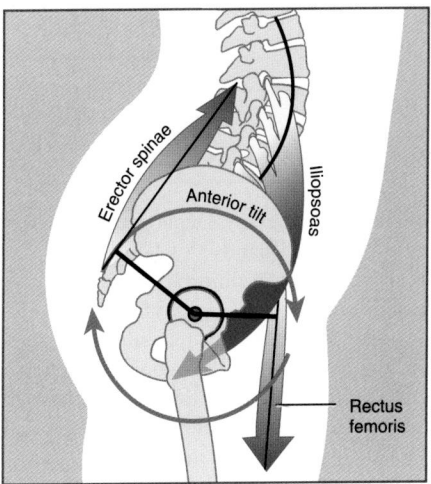

FIG. 2

A third form of art was later developed by Neumann and Kelly (Fig. 3). With the help of software, prepared anatomic specimens were rendered to a textured three-dimensional shape. The depth and anatomic precision of these images provide important insight into the associated kinesiology. Dr. Neumann feels that "good art is universally inspiring and transcends language—it is a fundamental element of my teaching."

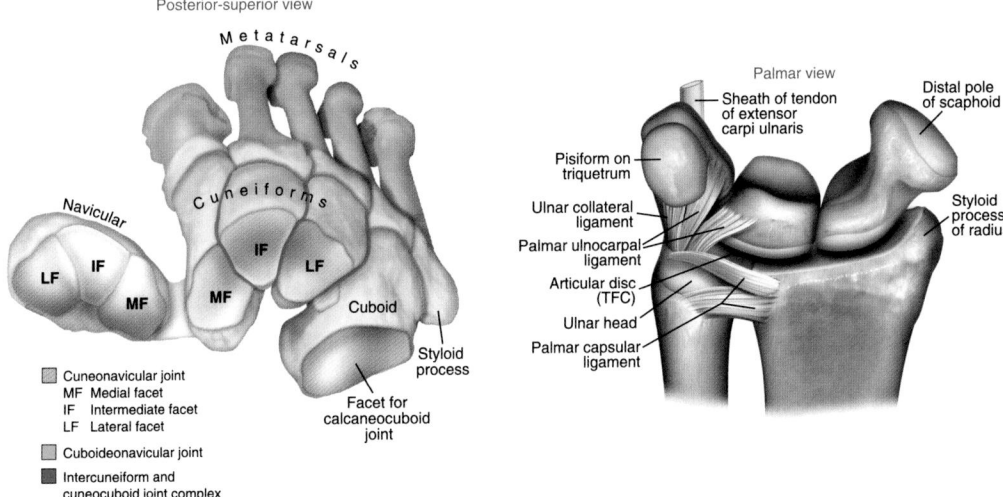

FIG. 3

ABOUT THE CONTRIBUTORS

Peter R. Blanpied, PT, PhD

Professor Emeritus, Physical Therapy Department, University of Rhode Island, Kingston, Rhode Island

Dr. Blanpied received his basic training at Ithaca College, graduating with a Bachelor of Science degree in physical therapy in 1979. After practicing clinically in acute, adult rehabilitation, and sports settings, he returned to school and in 1982 completed an advanced Master of Science degree in physical therapy from the University of North Carolina, specializing in musculoskeletal therapeutics. In 1989, he received a PhD from the University of Iowa. Before retiring, he served on the faculty at the University of Rhode Island, teaching in the areas of biomechanics, research, and musculoskeletal therapeutics. In addition to continuing clinical practice, he was active in funded and unfunded research and is the author of many peer-reviewed research articles as well as national and international professional research presentations. He lives in West Kingston, Rhode Island, with his wife Carol (also a physical therapist) and enjoys traveling, hiking, snowshoeing, and fishing.

Bryan C. Heiderscheit, PT, PhD, FAPTA

Professor, Department of Orthopedics and Rehabilitation, University of Wisconsin, Madison, Wisconsin

Dr. Heiderscheit received a Bachelor of Science degree in physical therapy from the University of Wisconsin-La Crosse and a PhD in biomechanics from the University of Massachusetts in Amherst. He is the Frederick Gaenslen Professor of Orthopedics and the vice chair of research for the Department of Orthopedics and Rehabilitation. He has been on the faculty at the University of Wisconsin since 2003, where he previously taught tissue and joint mechanics and the kinesiology of walking and running within the Doctor of Physical Therapy Program. As the founding director of the UW Health Sports Medicine Runners' Clinic, Dr. Heiderscheit has an active clinic practice focusing on individuals with running-related injuries. He is the director of the Badger Athletic Performance program with UW Athletics and the co-director of the UW Neuromuscular Biomechanics Laboratory. Dr. Heiderscheit's research is aimed at understanding and enhancing the clinical management of orthopedic conditions, with particular focus on sports-related injuries. Support for his research includes the National Institutes of Health, NFL, NBA, and GE Healthcare. He is an active member of the American Physical Therapy Association, previously serving on the Executive Committee of the American Academy of Sports Physical Therapy and past senior editor for the *Journal of Orthopaedic & Sports Physical Therapy*.

Sandra K. Hunter, PhD, FACSM

Professor, Exercise Science Program, Marquette University, Milwaukee, Wisconsin

Dr. Hunter received a Bachelor of Education degree in physical education and health from the University of Sydney (Australia), a Graduate Diploma in human movement science from Wollongong University (Australia), and a PhD in exercise and sport science (exercise physiology) from The University of Sydney, where her research focused on neuromuscular function with aging and strength training. Dr. Hunter moved to Boulder, Colorado, in 1999 to take a position as a postdoctoral research associate in the Neurophysiology of Movement Laboratory directed by Dr. Roger Enoka. She has been a faculty member in the Exercise Science Program in the Department of Physical Therapy at Marquette University since 2003, where her primary area of teaching is applied, rehabilitative, and exercise physiology and research methods. In addition, Dr. Hunter is Director of the Athletic and Human Performance Research Center at Marquette University. Hunter's own research program focuses on understanding the mechanisms of (1) neuromuscular fatigue and muscle function with aging and in clinical populations, (2) the protective effects of exercise training, and (3) for the sex differences in athletic performance. She is the author of several book chapters, many peer-reviewed research articles, and national and international research presentations. Dr. Hunter has received research funding from the National Institutes of Health (NIH), including the National Institute of Aging as well as from many other funding sources. She is a fellow of the American College of Sports Medicine (FACSM). Dr. Hunter has editorial responsibilities for several journals including as Editor-in-Chief of *Exercise and Sports Science Reviews*, and Associate Editor of *Medicine and Science in Sports and Exercise*. In her free time, Sandra enjoys traveling, camping, hiking, cycling, with her family and participating in triathlons.

Lauren K. Sara, PT, DPT, PhD

Postdoctoral Research Fellow, Boston University, Boston, Massachusetts

Dr. Sara received degrees in biomechanical engineering (Bachelor of Science, 2010), physical therapy (Doctorate of Physical Therapy, 2012), and exercise and rehabilitation sciences (PhD, 2021) from Marquette University. During her undergraduate, professional, and graduate studies, Lauren was recognized for her academic achievement, scholarship, and service by the Jesuit National Honor Society, the National Biomedical Engineering Honor Society (Alpha Eta Mu Beta), the Department of Physical Therapy (Mary Pat Murray Award), and the Foundation for Physical Therapy Research. Additional clinical and research training include an orthopedic physical therapy residency at the University of Chicago Hospital (2014-2015), a postdoctoral research fellowship at Harvard Medical School (2021-2022), and a postdoctoral research fellowship at Boston University (2022-2023). Lauren enjoys cooking with her husband, dancing with her kids, and traveling to see family and friends. She lives with her husband (Brian), two children (Adrienne and William), and dog (Scout) in Massachusetts.

Jonathon (Jack) W. Senefeld, PhD

Assistant Professor, Department of Kinesiology and Community Health, University of Illinois Urbana-Champaign, Urbana, Illinois

Dr. Senefeld received a Bachelor of Science degree in exercise physiology from Marquette University and a PhD in clinical and translational rehabilitation health sciences, also from Marquette University. Dr. Senefeld completed a post-doctoral research fellowship at Mayo Clinic in Human and Integrative Physiology and Clinical Pharmacology, directed by Dr. Michael Joyner. He has been a faculty member at the University of Illinois flagship campus in Urbana-Champaign since 2023, where his primary teaching is applied exercise physiology and cardiovascular physiology. Dr. Senefeld's primary research is centered on advancing the understanding of nonpharmacological interventions (such as exercise) to mitigate the detrimental effects of human aging and metabolic diseases. Beginning with the coronavirus disease 2019 (COVID-19) pandemic, Dr. Senefeld's research program also focuses on understanding passive antibody administration for treatment of infectious diseases, particularly among patients who are immunocompromised. His research was an important component of the scientific evidence considered by the U.S. Food and Drug Administration in the decision to issue an emergency-use authorization for convalescent plasma in the treatment of patients with COVID-19. His research is primarily supported by the National Institutes of Health (NIH). In his free time, Dr. Senefeld enjoys running, bicycling, and spending time with family. He lives in Illinois with his wife Carly, their son Jameson, and daughter Margaret.

Guy G. Simoneau, PT, PhD, FAPTA

Professor, Department of Physical Therapy, Marquette University, Milwaukee, Wisconsin

Dr. Simoneau received a Bachelor of Science degree in physiotherapy from the Université de Montréal, Canada, a Master of Science degree in physical education (sports medicine) from the University of Illinois at Urbana-Champaign, Illinois, and a PhD in exercise and sports science (locomotion studies) from The Pennsylvania State University, State College, Pennsylvania, where he focused much of his work on the study of gait, running, and posture. Dr. Simoneau has been a faculty member in the Department of Physical Therapy at Marquette University since 1992. His primary area of teaching is orthopedic and sports physical therapy. His research and teaching efforts have been recognized through several national awards from the American Physical Therapy Association, and he was the recipient of the 2019 World Confederation for Physical Therapy International Service Award for Education. In 2007, Guy received an honorary doctorate from the Lithuanian Academy of Physical Education, Kaunas, Lithuania. He also had the honor of being a Fulbright Scholar in Nepal in 2014 (Kathmandu University School of Medical Sciences – Dhulikhel Hospital; 5 months) and in Brazil in 2022 (Universidade Federal de Minas Gerais, Belo Horizonte; 4 months). Dr. Simoneau is editor-in-chief emeritus for the *Journal of Orthopaedic & Sports Physical Therapy*. In his free time, Guy enjoys traveling and hiking.

Past Contributors

The following three individuals deserve strong recognition for their prior contributions to Section I of this textbook. Their intellect and creativity have made an indelible impact on this part of the textbook. Thank you all.

David A. Brown, PT, PhD, FAPTA (Chapter 3)
Deborah A. Nawoczenski, PT, PhD (Chapter 4)
A. Joseph Threlkeld, PT, PhD (Chapter 2)

SUBJECT MATTER CONSULTANTS

Paul D. Andrew, PT, PhD
Ibaraki-ken, Japan

Brent F. Bode, PT, MPT, OCS
Marquette University
Department of Physical Therapy
Milwaukee, WI (USA)

Eugene R. Boeglin, DPT, OCS, CHT
Beth Israel Deaconess Medical Center
Chestnut Hill, MA (USA)

Yoko Bourne, PT, MSc
CDI College, Rehabilitation Assistant program
Edmonton, Alberta, Canada

Paula R. Camargo, PT, PhD
Department of Physical Therapy
Universidade Federal de São Carlos
São Carlos, SP, Brazil

Jordan Cannon, PhD
Department of Kinesiology and Health Sciences
University of Waterloo
Waterloo, Ontario, Canada

Bryan C. Heiderscheit, PT, PhD, FAPTA
Department of Orthopedics and Rehabilitation
University of Wisconsin-Madison
Madison, WI (USA)

Nicole A. Hoover, MS, OTR/L, CHT
Department of Rehabilitation Sciences
University of Wisconsin- Milwaukee
Milwaukee, WI (USA)

Teresa A. Jeardeau, OTR/L, CHT
Mayo School of Health Sciences
Mayo Clinic Rochester
Rochester, MN (USA)

Michael R. Karegeannes, PT, MHSc, LAT, CFC
Freedom Physical Therapy Services
Fox Point, WI (USA)

Jeremy Karman, PT, OCS
Aurora Sports Health
Milwaukee, WI (USA)

Linda J. Klein, OTR, CHT
Hand to Shoulder Specialists of Wisconsin
Milwaukee, WI (USA)

Yuta Koshino, PT, PhD
Faculty of Health Sciences, Hokkaido University
Sapporo, Japan

Paolo Leone, PT, DO
Torino, Italy

Kathleen Lukaszewicz, PT, PhD
Department of Physical Therapy
Marquette University
Milwaukee, WI (USA)

Philip Malloy, PT, Ph.D.
Department of Physical Therapy
Arcadia University
Glenside, PA (USA)

Ailish Malone, CORU Registered Physiotherapist (Ireland), PhD, MISCP
School of Physiotherapy
Royal College of Surgeons in Ireland University of Medicine and Health
   Sciences
Dublin, Ireland

Jon D. Marion, OTR, CHT
Hand and Upper Extremity Rehabilitation
Vanderbilt University Medical Center
Nashville, TN (USA)

Brenda L. Neumann, OTR, BCB-PMD
Consultant/Pelvic Floor Specialist
Marquette University
Milwaukee, WI (USA)

Anne Pleva, PT, DPT, PCS
Marquette University
Department of Physical Therapy
Milwaukee, WI (USA)

Ann K. Porretto-Loehrke, PT, DPT, CHT, COMT
Hand to Shoulder Center of Wisconsin
Appleton, WI (USA)

Jodi Sandvik, DSC, PT, SCS, ATC
Program in Physical Therapy
Trine University
Fort Wayne, IN (USA)

Lauren K. Sara, PT, DPT, PhD, OCS
BURRT T32 Post-doctoral Research Fellow
Chobanian & Avedisian School of Medicine, Section of Rheumatology
& College of Health & Rehabilitation Sciences, Dept. of Physical Therapy
Boston University
Boston, MA (USA)

Guy G. Simoneau, PT, PhD, FAPTA
Department of Physical Therapy and Program in Exercise Science
Marquette University
Milwaukee, WI (USA)

Kristi A. Streeter, PhD
Department of Physical Therapy
Marquette University
Milwaukee, WI (USA)

Mariko K. Usuba, PT, PhD
Tsukuba University of Technology
Tsukuba, Ibaraki, Japan

Adam Wielechowski, PT, DPT, OCS, FAAOMPT
University of Illinois at Chicago
Department of Physical Therapy
Chicago, IL (USA)

Jeffrey J. Wilkens, PT, DPT, OCS
Marquette University
Department of Physical Therapy
Milwaukee, WI (USA)

David Williams, MPT, PhD, ATC
Physical Therapy Program
University of Iowa
Iowa City, IA (USA)

PREFACE

I am pleased to introduce the fourth edition of *Neumann's Kinesiology of the Musculoskeletal System*. I am proud to state that the third edition has been published in 10 languages and used extensively around the world. The fourth edition continues to develop based on the enthusiastic feedback from teachers and students, as well as the increasing body of research literature. Each of the approximately 3000 references cited in the fourth edition has been carefully selected to support the science and clinical relevance behind the material described throughout this textbook. Extensive effort has been made to include topics that may improve the ability of the practitioner to address mechanical-based changes in movement that may occur across a person's lifespan, whether in the context of rehabilitation, recreation, or promotion of health and wellness.

The popularity of the illustrations created in the first three editions have stimulated the creation of more illustrations. As in the previous editions, the descriptive art, coupled with the evidence-based and clinically relevant text, drives the educational mission of this textbook.

Instructional elements used in the third edition (Study Questions, Special Focus boxes, and Additional Clinical Connections) have been expanded. This fourth edition provides Educational eContent, including a more extensive set of videos, images, and other material. Components of these materials have been used in the classroom to successfully teach kinesiology for over 35 years. Hopefully, teachers and students will appreciate the list of Additional Video Educational Content located at the end of Chapters 5–16. This content expands on the highly visual approach used to teach kinesiology, and includes videos of fluoroscopy of joint movement, cadaver dissections, short lectures by the author, special teaching models, examples of persons displaying abnormal kinesiology, methods which persons with spinal cord injury learn to perform certain movements despite varying levels of paralysis, visual EMG-based display of activated muscles, and more. In addition, several new electronic videos (and images) have been integrated directly into the substance of several chapters. For example, Chapters 15 and 16 allow access to unique video material of animated skeletons walking and running, alongside graphs detailing certain kinetic and kinematics. All video and other electronic educational media in the fourth edition is easily viewable on a computer or mobile devices in the enhanced eBook version included with the print purchase of this textbook.

Naturally, I used the previous editions of the text to teach my students at Marquette University. The close working relationship among the students, textbook, and I generated many practical ways to improve the writing, the organization or flow of topics, and the clarity of images. Many improvements in both the text and the illustrations are a result of the feedback I have received from my own students, as well as from other students and instructors around the United States and in other countries. As the fourth edition finds its way into the classrooms of universities and colleges, I look forward to receiving continued feedback and suggestions on improving this work.

Background

Kinesiology is the study of human movement, typically pursued within the context of sport, art, medicine, and health. To varying degrees, *Neumann's Kinesiology of the Musculoskeletal System* relates to all four areas. This textbook is primarily intended, however, to provide the kinesiologic foundations for the practice of physical rehabilitation, which strives to optimize functional movement of the human body following injury, disease, or other detriment in mobility. Although the subject of kinesiology is presented worldwide from many different perspectives, my contributing authors and I have focused primarily on the mechanical and physiologic interactions between the muscles and joints of the body. These interactions are described for normal movement and, in the case of disease, trauma, or otherwise altered musculoskeletal tissues, for abnormal movement. I hope that this textbook provides a valuable educational resource for a wide range of health- and medical-related professions, both for students and for clinicians.

Approach

This textbook places a major emphasis on the anatomic detail of the musculoskeletal system. By applying a few principles of physics and physiology to a sound anatomic background, the reader should be able to mentally transform a static anatomic image into a dynamic, three-dimensional, and relatively predictable movement. The illustrations created for *Neumann's Kinesiology of the Musculoskeletal System* are designed to encourage this mental transformation. This approach to kinesiology reduces the need for rote memorization and favors reasoning based on mechanical analysis, which can assist students and clinicians in developing proper evaluation, diagnosis, and treatment related to dysfunction of the musculoskeletal system.

This textbook represents the synthesis of over 45 years of experience as a physical therapist. This experience includes a blend of clinical research, anatomical dissection, and teaching activities that are related, in one form or another, to kinesiology. Although I was unaware of it at the time, my work on this textbook began the day I prepared my first kinesiology lecture as a brand-new college professor at Marquette University in 1986. Since then, I have had the good fortune of being exposed to intelligent and passionate students. Their desire to learn has continually fueled my ambition and love for teaching. As a way to encourage my students to listen actively rather than just to transcribe my lectures, I developed an extensive set of kinesiology lecture notes. Year after year, my notes evolved, forming the blueprints of the first edition of the text. Now, over 20 years later, I, along with several contributing coauthors, present the fourth edition of this text.

Organization

The organization of this textbook reflects the overall plan of study used in my kinesiology courses as well as other courses in our curriculum at Marquette University. The textbook contains 16 chapters, divided into 4 major sections. *Section I* provides the essential topics of kinesiology, including an introduction to terminology and basic concepts, a review of basic structure and function of the musculoskeletal system, and an introduction to biomechanical and quantitative aspects of kinesiology. *Sections II* through *IV* present the specific anatomic details and kinesiology of the three major regions of the body. *Section II* focuses entirely on the upper extremity, from the shoulder to the hand. *Section III* covers the kinesiology of the axial skeleton, which includes the head, trunk, and spine. A special chapter is included within this section on the kinesiology of mastication and ventilation. *Section IV* presents the kinesiology of the lower extremity, from the hip to the foot. The final two chapters in this section, "Kinesiology of Walking" and "Kinesiology of Running," functionally integrate and reinforce much of the kinesiology of the lower extremity.

This textbook is specifically designed primarily for the purpose of *teaching*. To that end, concepts are presented in layers, starting with Section I, which lays much of the scientific foundation for chapters contained in Sections II through IV. The material covered in these chapters is also presented layer by layer. Most chapters begin with *osteology*—the study of the morphology and subsequent function of bones. This is followed by *arthrology*—the study of the anatomy and the function of the joints, including the associated periarticular connective tissues. Included in this study is a thorough description of the regional kinematics.

The most extensive component of most chapters in Sections II through IV highlights the *muscle and joint interactions*. This topic begins by describing the muscles within a region, including a summary of the innervations to muscles and joints. Once the anatomy and physical orientation of the muscles are established, the mechanical interplay between the muscles and the joints is discussed. Topics presented include: strength and movement potential of muscles; muscular-produced forces imposed on joints; intermuscular and interjoint synergies; important functional roles of muscles in movement, posture, and stability; and the functional relationships that exist between the muscles and underlying joints. Multiple examples are provided throughout each chapter on how disease, trauma, or advanced age may cause reduced function or adaptations within the musculoskeletal system. This information sets the foundation for understanding many of the evaluations and treatments used in most clinical situations to treat persons with musculoskeletal as well as neuromuscular disorders, across the lifespan.

Distinctive Features

Key features of the fourth edition include the following:
- Full-color illustrations
- Special Focus boxes
- Chapter at a Glance boxes
- Additional Clinical Connections following most chapters
- Study Questions
- Evidence-based approach, based on 3000 references
- Appendices that contain detailed information on muscle attachments, innervations, cross-sectional areas, and much more
- Additional Video Educational Content
- Web-based videos, images, and tables that are referred to directly from the text material
- Highly specialized videos in Chapters 15 and 16 of skeletal figures walking and running alongside graphs detailing certain kinetics and kinematics

Educational eContent
A wealth of resources is provided to enhance both teaching and learning, as follows:

For the Instructor, the Evolve website (http://evolve.elsevier.com/Neumann) contains the following resources:

- **Image Collection:** All of the textbook's artwork is reproduced online for download into PowerPoint or other presentations.
- **Laboratory Study Guide:** Teaching material developed by the author based on more than 35 years of teaching. The teaching "labs" coincide with the material in most chapters (Chapters 5–14).
- **Practical Teaching Tips:** Practical suggestions for teaching selected concepts of biomechanical principles.

For the Student and Instructor, visit Elsevier eBooks+ (eBooks.Health.Elsevier.com) for the following resources included with print purchase:

- **Video Educational Content:** Dozens of videos were compiled and used by the authors to reinforce or highlight kinesiologic concepts presented in the text. These videos include videofluoroscopy of joint movements, cadaver dissections, short lectures or demonstrations of teaching models designed by the author, functional analysis of persons with partial paralysis, and other concepts related to clinical kinesiology.
- **Answers to Study Questions:** Detailed answers to the Study Questions provide reinforcement for the material covered in the textbook
- **Answers to Clinically Related Biomechanical Problems Posed in Chapter 4**
- **References with Links to Medline Abstracts:** Medline links to the references found in the textbook provide evidence-based support for the material.

Acknowledgments

Once again, I welcome this opportunity to acknowledge many people who have provided me with kind and thoughtful assistance throughout the evolution of this textbook to its fourth edition. I am sure that I have inadvertently overlooked some people and, for that, I apologize.

The best place to start with my offering of thanks is with my immediate family, especially my wife Brenda, who, in her charming and unselfish style, supported me emotionally and physically during all four editions. I thank my son Donnie and stepdaughter Megann and their children for their patience and understanding. I also thank my caring parents, Betty and Charlie Neumann, for the many opportunities they have provided me throughout my life. I am not sure what I would do without my mother's sustaining sense of humor and kindness and father's lessons on perseverance.

Many persons significantly influenced the realization of this project. Foremost, I wish to thank Elisabeth Roen Kelly, the primary medical illustrator of the text, for her years of dedication, incredible talent, and uncompromisingly high standard of excellence. I also extend a thank you to the Elsevier staff and affiliates for their patience or perseverance, in particular Lauren Willis, Danielle Frazier, and Becky Langdon.

I wish to express my sincere gratitude to Drs. Lawrence Pan, (the late) Richard Jensen, and Allison Hyngstrom, past and current directors of the Department of Physical Therapy at Marquette

University, as well as Drs. Jack Brooks and William Cullinan, past and present deans, respectively, of the College of Health Sciences at Marquette University. These individuals all, in different ways, unselfishly provided me with the opportunity and freedom to fulfill a dream.

I am also indebted to the following men and women who contributed chapters or co-authored work in this fourth edition: Peter R. Blanpied, Sandra K. Hunter, Bryan C. Heiderscheit, Guy G. Simoneau, Lauren K. Sara, and Jonathon W. Senefeld. These talented individuals provided an essential depth and breadth to this textbook. I am also grateful to the many persons who served as subject matter consultants, who did so without financial remuneration. These reviewers are listed elsewhere.

Several people at Marquette University provided me with invaluable technical and research assistance. I thank Dan Johnson, Chief Photographer, not only for his 30-year friendship but also for much of the photography contained in this book. I am also grateful to the talents of Gary Bargholz and John Blandino, and other members of the Instructional Media Center, for their talents in producing many of my book and teaching-related video projects. I also wish to thank Ljudmila ("Milly") Mursec, Martha Gilmore Jermé, Alissa Fial, and other fine librarians at Raynor Library for their important help with my research.

Many persons affiliated directly or indirectly with Marquette University helped with a wide range of activities throughout the evolution of this textbook. This help included proofreading, tracking down research papers, listening, verifying references or clinical concepts, posing for or supplying photographs, taking or providing x-rays or MRIs, and providing clerical and other valuable assistance. For this help, I am grateful to Mitch Adams, Michael Branda, Kelly Brush, Allison Budreck, Therese Casey, Allison Czaplewski, Sarah D'Astice, Albojay Deacon, Santana Deacon, Caress Dean, Kerry Donahue, Rebecca Eagleeye, Kevin Eckert, Kim Fowler, Jessica Fuentes, Gregg Fuhrman, Marybeth Geiser, Matt Giordanelli, Jacki Green, Savannah Gutsch, Barbara Haines, Douglas Heckenkamp, Lisa Hribar, Erika Jacobson, Tia Jandrin, Clare Kennedy, Michael Kiely, Davin Kimura, Kristin Kipp, Courtney Kruggel, Stephanie Lamon, Michelle Lanouette, Thomas Lechner, Jesse Lee, John Levene, Ryan Lifka, Lorna Loughran, Brenda L. Neumann, Jessica Niles, Christopher Melkovitz, Melissa Merriman, Carl Meyer, Liz Meyer, Preston Michelson, Alicia Nowack, Samuel O'Melia, Rebecca Palarz, Ellen Perkins, Anne Pleva, Grace Pitzen, Gregory Rajala, Rachel Sand, Janet Schuh, Robert Seeds, Jonathon Senefeld, Elizabeth Shanahan, Bethany Shutko, Jeff Sischo, Pamela Swiderski, Michelle Treml, Stacy Weineke, Andy Weyer, Sidney White, and Brian Zamzow.

I am very fortunate to have this forum to acknowledge those who have made a significant, positive impact on my professional life. In a sense, the spirit of these persons is interwoven within all four editions. I acknowledge Shep Barish for first inspiring me to teach kinesiology; Martha Wroe for serving as a role model for my practice of physical therapy; Claudette Finley for providing me with a rich foundation in human anatomy; Gary Soderberg for his overall mentorship and firm dedication to principle; Thomas Cook for showing me that all this can be fun; Mary Pat Murray for setting such high standards for kinesiology education at Marquette University; Paul Andrew for his continued lessons (or "scoldings") on the importance of succinct and clear writing; and Guy Simoneau for constantly reminding me what an enduring work ethic can accomplish.

I wish to acknowledge several special people who have influenced this project in ways that are difficult to describe. These people include family, old and new friends, professional colleagues, and, in many cases, a combination thereof. I thank the following people for their sense of humor or adventure, their loyalty, and their intense dedication to their own goals and beliefs, and for their tolerance and understanding of mine. For this I thank my four siblings, Chip, Suzan, Nancy, and Barbara; as well as Brenda Neumann, Tad Hardee, David Eastwold, Darrell Bennett, Diane Slaughter, Joseph Berman, Bob Myers, Robert and Kim Morecraft, Guy Simoneau, my special WWRC friends from Fishersville, Va, and the Mehlos family, especially Harvey, for always asking "How's the book coming?" I wish to thank two special colleagues and friends, Tony Hornung and Jeremy Karman, two physical therapists who assisted me with teaching kinesiology at Marquette University for several decades. They both help keep the class vibrant, fun, and clinically relevant.

Finally, I want to thank my past students for making my job so rewarding.

DAN

CONTENTS

VIDEO CONTENTS

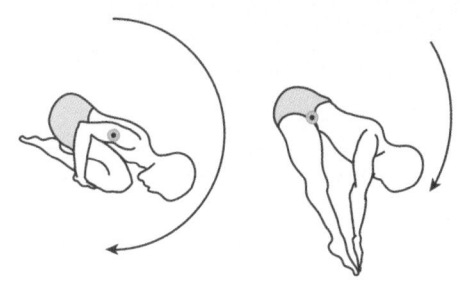

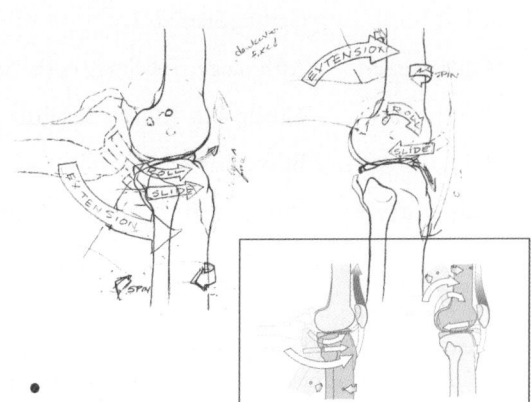

Section

I

Essential Topics
of Kinesiology

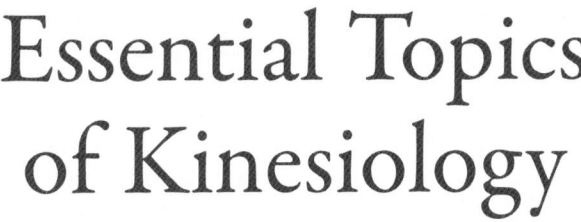

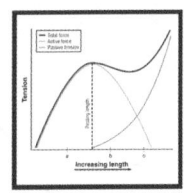

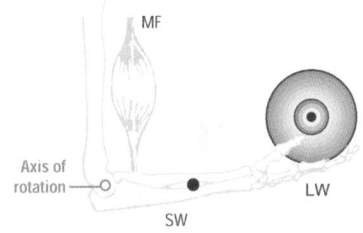

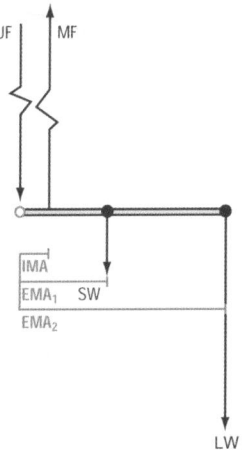

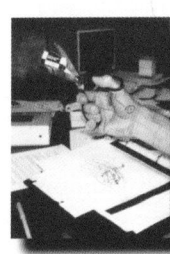

Section I

Essential Topics of Kinesiology

Section I is divided into four chapters, each describing a different topic related to kinesiology. This section provides the background for the more specific kinesiologic discussions of the various regions of the body (Sections II to IV). Chapter 1 provides introductory terminology and biomechanical concepts related to kinesiology. A glossary of important kinesiologic terms with definitions is located at the end of Chapter 1. Chapter 2 presents the basic anatomic, histologic, and functional aspects of human joints—the pivot points for movement of the body. Chapter 3 reviews the basic anatomic and functional aspects of skeletal muscle—the source that produces active movement and stabilization of the skeletal system. More detailed discussion and quantitative analysis of many of the biomechanical principles introduced in Chapter 1 are provided in Chapter 4.

ADDITIONAL CLINICAL CONNECTIONS

Additional Clinical Connections are included at the end of Chapter 4. This feature is intended to highlight or expand on particular clinical concepts associated with the kinesiology covered in the chapter.

STUDY QUESTIONS

Study Questions are included at the end of each chapter and within Chapter 4. These questions are designed to challenge the reader to review or reinforce some of the main concepts contained within the chapter. The process of answering these questions is an effective way for students to prepare for examinations. The answers to the questions are available in the accompanying enhanced eBook version included with the print purchase of this textbook. Visit Elsevier eBooks+ (eBooks.Health.Elsevier.com) to access this content.

C h a p t e r

1

Getting Started

DONALD A. NEUMANN, PT, PhD, FAPTA

WHAT IS KINESIOLOGY?

The origins of the word *kinesiology* are from the Greek *kinesis,* to move, and *logy,* to study. *Neumann's Kinesiology of the Musculoskel-etal System* serves as a guide to the study of movement by focusing on the anatomic and biomechanical interactions within the muscu-loskeletal system. The beauty and complexity of these interactions have been captured by many great artists, such as Michelangelo Buonarroti (1475–1564) and Leonardo da Vinci (1452–1519). Their work likely inspired the creation of the classic text *Tabulae Sceleti et Musculorum Corporis Humani,* published in 1747 by the anatomist Bernhard Siegfried Albinus (1697–1770). A sample of this work is presented in Fig. 1.1.

The primary intent of this textbook is to provide students and clini-cians with a literature-based foundation for understanding kinesiol-ogy, with a focus on the musculoskeletal system. Discussions are presented on expected movement mechanics and those that deviate from the expected, which may interfere with a person's potential for effective and pain-free movement. A sound understanding of kinesiol-ogy allows for the development of a rational evaluation, a precise diag-nosis, and an effective treatment for virtually any dysfunction involving the musculoskeletal system. Such an understanding enhances the ability of the practitioner to effectively address the mechanical-based changes in movement across a person's lifespan, whether in the context of rehabilitation, recreation, or promotion of health and wellness.

This text of kinesiology borrows heavily from three bodies of knowledge: anatomy, biomechanics, and physiology. *Anatomy* is the science of the shape and structure of the human body and its parts. *Biomechanics* is a discipline that uses principles of physics to quan-titatively study how forces interact within a living body. *Physiology* is the biologic study of living organisms. This textbook interweaves an extensive review of musculoskeletal anatomy with selected prin-ciples of biomechanics and physiology. Such an approach allows the kinesiologic functions of the musculoskeletal system to be reasoned rather than purely memorized.

OVERALL PLAN OF THIS TEXTBOOK

This text is divided into four sections. *Section I: Essential Topics of Kinesiology* includes Chapters 1 to 4. To get the reader started, Chapter 1 provides many of the fundamental concepts and terminology related to kinesiology. A glossary is provided at the end of Chapter 1 with definitions of these fundamental concepts and terms. Chapters 2 to 4 describe the necessary background regarding the mechanics of joints, physiology of muscle, and principles of biomechanics.

The material presented in Section I sets forth the kinesiologic foundation for the more anatomic- and regional-based chapters included in Sections II to IV. Section II (Chapters 5–8) describes the kinesiology related to the upper extremity;

3

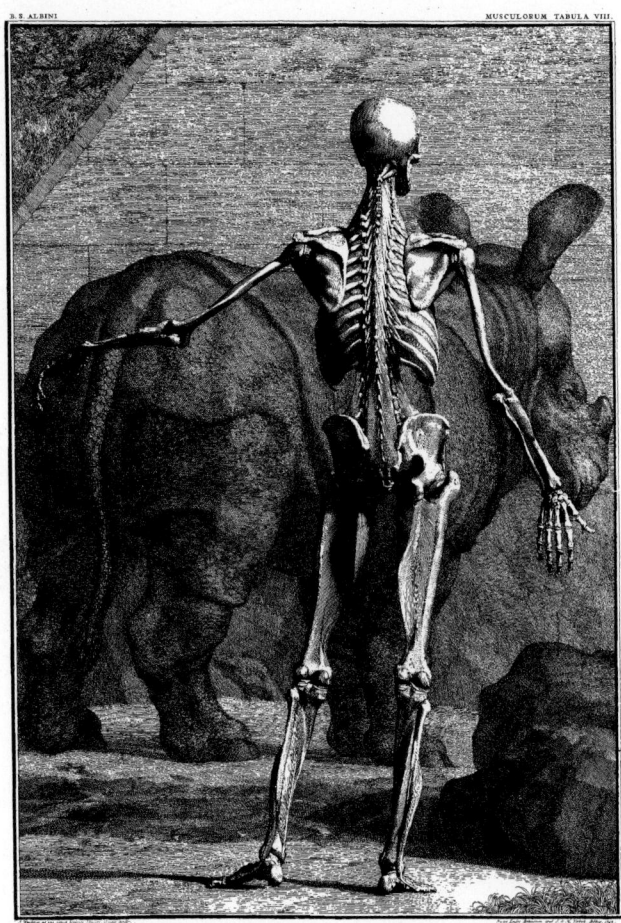

FIG. 1.1 An illustration from the anatomy text *Tabulae Sceleti et Musculorum Corporis Humani* (1747) by Bernhard Siegfried Albinus.

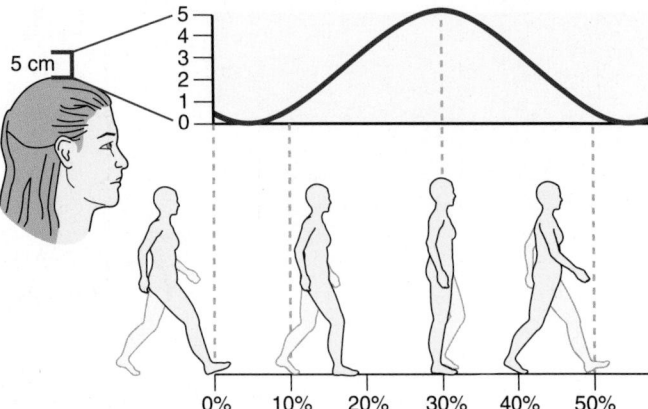

FIG. 1.2 A point on the top of the head is shown translating upward and downward in a curvilinear fashion during walking. The horizontal axis of the graph shows the percentage of completion of one entire gait (walking) cycle.

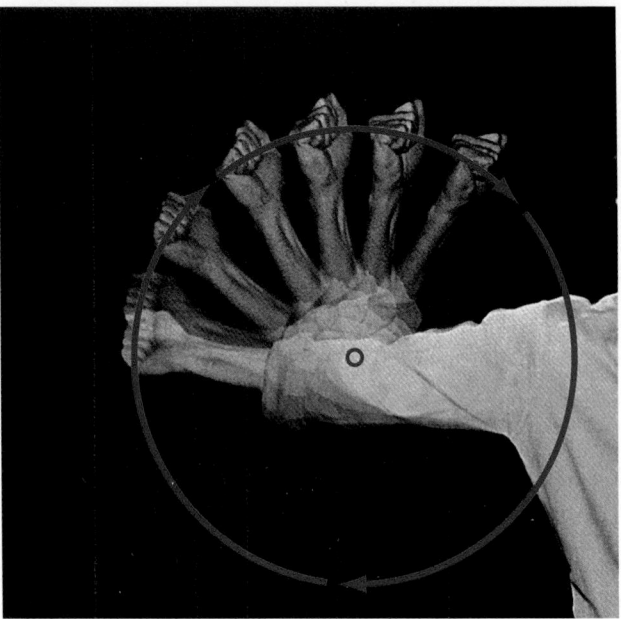

FIG. 1.3 With a stroboscopic flash, a camera is able to capture the rotation of the forearm around the elbow. If not for the anatomic constraints of the elbow, the forearm could, in theory, rotate 360 degrees around an axis of rotation located at the elbow *(open circle).*

Section III (Chapters 9–11) covers the kinesiology primarily involving the axial skeleton and trunk; finally, Section IV (Chapters 12–16) presents the kinesiology of the lower extremity, including a pair of closing chapters that focus on walking and running.

KINEMATICS

Kinematics is a branch of biomechanics that describes the *motion* of a body, without regard to the forces or torques that may produce the motion. In biomechanics, the term *body* is used rather loosely to describe the entire body, or any of its parts or segments, such as individual bones or regions. In general, there are two types of motions: translation and rotation.

Translation Compared with Rotation

Translation describes a linear motion in which all parts of a rigid body move parallel to and in the same direction as every other part of the body. Translation can occur in either a *straight line (rectilinear)* or a *curved line (curvilinear).* During walking, for example, a point on the head moves in a general curvilinear manner (Fig. 1.2).

Rotation, in contrast to translation, describes a motion in which an assumed rigid body moves in a circular path around some pivot point. As a result, all points in the body simultaneously rotate in the same angular direction (e.g., clockwise and counterclockwise) across the same number of degrees.

Movement of the human body as a whole is often described as a translation of the body's *center of mass,* located generally just anterior to the sacrum. Although a person's center of mass translates through space, it is powered by muscles that *rotate* the limbs. The fact that limbs rotate can be appreciated by watching the path created by a fist while the elbow is flexing (Fig. 1.3). (It is customary in kinesiology to use the phrases "rotation of a joint" and "rotation of a bone" interchangeably.)

The pivot point for angular motion of the body or body parts is called the *axis of rotation.* The axis is the point where motion of the rotating body is zero. For most movements of the limbs or trunk, the axis of rotation is located within or very near the structure of the joint.

Movement of the body, regardless of translation or rotation, can be described as active or passive. *Active movements* are caused by stimulated muscle, such as when bending the elbow to drink a glass of water. *Passive movements,* in contrast, are caused by sources other

TABLE 1.1 Common Conversions between Units of Kinematic Measurements

SI Units	English Units
1 meter (m) = 3.28 feet (ft)	1 ft = 0.305 m
1 m = 39.37 inches (in)	1 in = 0.0254 m
1 centimeter (cm) = 0.39 in	1 in = 2.54 cm
1 m = 1.09 yards (yd)	1 yd = 0.91 m
1 kilometer (km) = 0.62 miles (mi)	1 mi = 1.61 km
1 degree = 0.0174 radians (rad)	1 rad = 57.3 degrees

than active muscle contraction, such as a push or pull from another person, the pull of gravity, tension in stretched connective tissues, and so forth.

The primary variables related to kinematics are position, velocity, and acceleration. Specific units of measurement are needed to indicate the quantity of these variables. Units of meters or feet are used for translation, and degrees or radians are used for rotation. In most situations, *Neumann's Kinesiology of the Musculoskeletal System* uses the *International System of Units,* adopted in 1960. This system is abbreviated *SI,* for Système International d'Unités, the French name. This system of units is widely accepted in many journals related to kinesiology, medicine, and rehabilitation. The kinematic conversions between the more common SI units and other measurement units are listed in Table 1.1. Additional units of measurements are described in Chapter 4.

Osteokinematics

PLANES OF MOTION

Osteokinematics describes the *motion of bones* relative to the three cardinal (principal) planes of the body: sagittal, frontal, and horizontal. These planes of motion are depicted in the context of a person standing in the *anatomic position* as in Fig. 1.4. The *sagittal plane* runs parallel to the sagittal suture of the skull, dividing the body into right and left halves; the *frontal plane* runs parallel to the coronal suture of the skull, dividing the body into front and back halves. The *horizontal* (or *transverse*) *plane* courses parallel to the horizon and divides the body into upper and lower halves. A sample of the terms used to describe the different osteokinematic patterns is shown in Table 1.2. More specific terms are defined in Chapters 5 to 14, the body region-specific chapters in this book.

AXIS OF ROTATION

Bones rotate around a joint in a plane that is perpendicular to an *axis of rotation.* As a rough estimation, the axis (or pivot point) can be assumed to pass through the convex member of the joint. The shoulder, for example, allows movement in all three planes and therefore has three axes of rotation (Fig. 1.5). Although the three orthogonal axes are depicted as stationary, in reality, as in all joints, each axis shifts slightly throughout the range of motion. The axis of rotation would remain stationary only if the convex member of a joint were a perfect sphere, articulating with a perfectly reciprocally shaped concave member. The convex members of most joints, like the humeral head at the shoulder, are imperfect spheres with changing surface curvatures. The issue of a migrating axis of rotation is discussed further in Chapter 2.

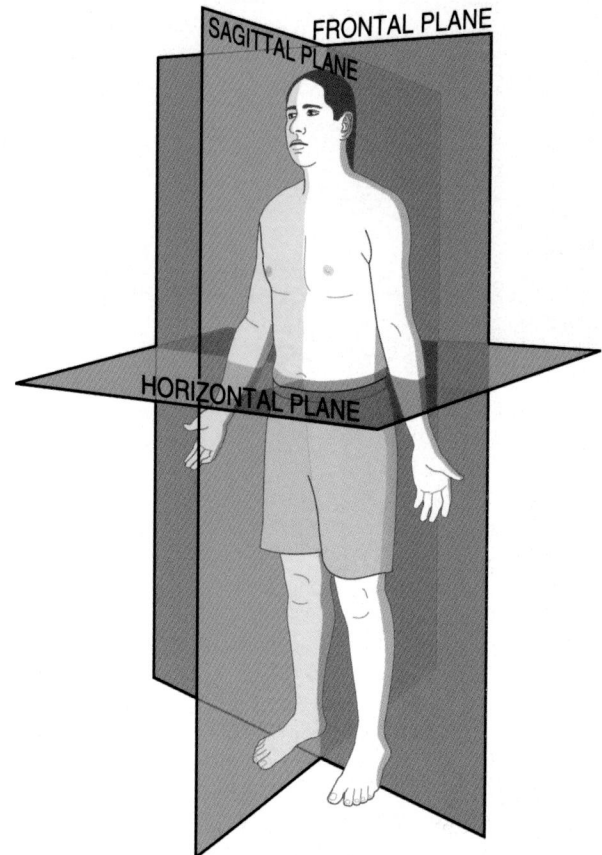

FIG. 1.4 The three cardinal planes of the body are shown while a person is standing in the anatomic position.

TABLE 1.2 A Sample of Common Osteokinematic Terms*

Plane	Common Terms
Sagittal plane	Flexion and extension Dorsiflexion and plantar flexion Forward and backward bending
Frontal plane	Abduction and adduction Lateral flexion Ulnar and radial deviation Eversion and inversion
Horizontal plane	Internal (medial) and external (lateral) rotation Axial rotation

*Many of the terms are specific to a particular region of the body. The thumb, for example, uses different terminology.

DEGREES OF FREEDOM

Degrees of freedom are the number of planes of movement that are under volitional control at a joint. A joint can have up to three degrees of angular freedom, corresponding to the three cardinal planes. As depicted in Fig. 1.5, for example, the shoulder has three degrees of angular freedom, one for each plane. The wrist allows only two degrees of freedom (rotation within sagittal and frontal planes), and the elbow allows just one (within the sagittal plane).

Unless specified differently throughout this text, the term "degrees of freedom" indicates the number of volitionally controlled *planes of angular motion* at a joint. From a strict engineering

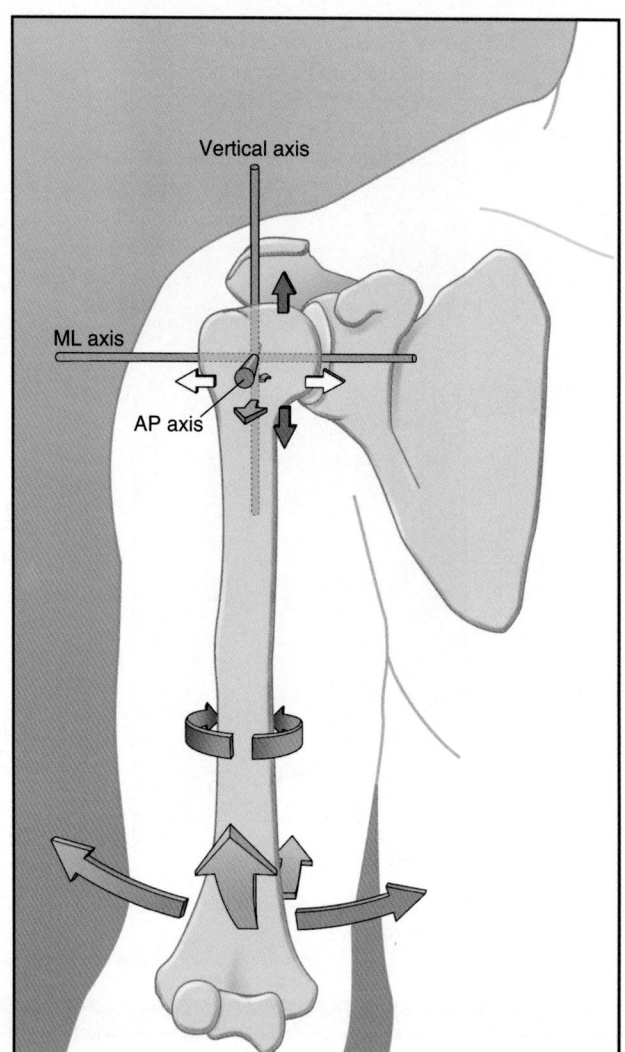

FIG. 1.5 The right glenohumeral (shoulder) joint highlights three orthogonal axes of rotation and associated planes of angular motion: flexion and extension *(green curved arrows)* occur around a medial-lateral *(ML)* axis of rotation; abduction and adduction *(purple curved arrows)* occur around an anterior-posterior *(AP)* axis of rotation; and internal rotation and external rotation *(blue curved arrows)* occur around a vertical axis of rotation. Each axis of rotation is color-coded with its associated plane of movement. The short, straight arrows shown parallel to each axis represent the slight translation potential of the humerus relative to the scapula. This illustration shows both angular and translational degrees of freedom.

perspective, however, degrees of freedom apply to translational (linear) as well as angular movements. All synovial joints in the body possess at least some translation, driven actively by muscle or passively because of the natural laxity within the structure of the joint. The slight passive translations that occur in most joints are referred to as *accessory movements* (or joint "play") and are commonly defined in three linear directions. From the anatomic position, the spatial orientation and direction of accessory movements can be described relative to the three axes of rotation. In the relaxed glenohumeral joint, for example, the humerus can be passively translated slightly: anterior-posteriorly, medial-laterally, and superior-inferiorly (see short, straight arrows near proximal humerus in Fig. 1.5). At many joints, the amount of translation is used clinically to test the health of the joint. Excessive translation of a bone relative to the joint may indicate ligamentous injury or abnormal laxity. In contrast, a significant reduction in translation

(accessory movements) may indicate pathologic stiffness within the surrounding periarticular connective tissues. Abnormal translation within a joint typically affects the quality of the active movements, potentially causing increased intra-articular microtrauma.

OSTEOKINEMATICS: A MATTER OF PERSPECTIVE

In general, the articulation of two or more bony or limb segments constitutes a joint. Movement at a joint can, therefore, be considered from two perspectives: (1) the proximal segment can rotate against the relatively fixed distal segment, and (2) the distal segment can rotate against the relatively fixed proximal segment. (In reality, both perspectives can and often do occur simultaneously; although for ease of discussion and analysis, this situation is often omitted within this text.) The two kinematic perspectives are shown for knee flexion in Fig. 1.6. A term such as *knee flexion,* for example, describes only the *relative motion* between the thigh and leg. It does not describe which of the two segments is actually rotating. Often, to be clear, it is necessary to state the bone that is considered the rotating segment. As in Fig. 1.6, for example, the terms *tibial-on-femoral movement* and *femoral-on-tibial movement* adequately describe the osteokinematics.

Most routine movements performed by the upper extremities involve distal-on-proximal segment kinematics. This reflects the need to bring objects held by the hand either toward or away from the body. The proximal segment of a joint in the upper extremity is usually stabilized by muscles, gravity, or its inertia, whereas the distal, relatively unconstrained segment rotates.

Feeding oneself and throwing a ball are common examples of distal-on-proximal segment kinematics employed by the upper extremities. The upper extremities are certainly capable of performing proximal-on-distal segment kinematics, such as flexing and extending the elbows while one performs a pull-up.

The lower extremities routinely perform both proximal-on-distal *and* distal-on-proximal segment kinematics. These kinematics reflect, in part, the two primary phases of walking: the *stance phase,* when the limb is planted on the ground under the load of body weight, and the *swing phase,* when the limb is advancing forward. Many other activities, in addition to walking, use both kinematic strategies. Flexing the knee in preparation to kick a ball, for example, is a type of distal-on-proximal segment kinematics (see Fig. 1.6A). Descending into a squat position, in contrast, is an example of proximal-on-distal segment kinematics (see Fig. 1.6B). In the latter example, a relatively large demand is placed on the quadriceps muscle of the knee to control the gradual descent of the body.

The terms *open* and *closed kinematic chains* are frequently used in the physical rehabilitation literature and clinics to describe the concept of relative segment kinematics. A *kinematic chain* refers to a series of articulated segmented links, such as the connected pelvis, thigh, leg, and foot of the lower extremity. The terms "open" and "closed" are typically used to indicate whether the distal end of an extremity is fixed to the ground or some other immovable object. An *open kinematic chain* describes a situation in which the distal segment of a kinematic chain, such as the foot in the lower limb, is *not fixed* to the ground or another immovable object. The distal segment, therefore, is free to move (see Fig. 1.6A). A *closed kinematic chain* describes a situation in which the distal segment of the kinematic chain is *fixed* to the ground or another immovable object. In this case, the proximal segment is most free to move (see Fig. 1.6B). These terms are often employed to describe methods of applying resistive exercise to muscles. Although the terms can be used to describe movement at any joint region in the body, their usage is especially prevalent within knee rehabilitation literature.[12,14,18]

Knee flexion

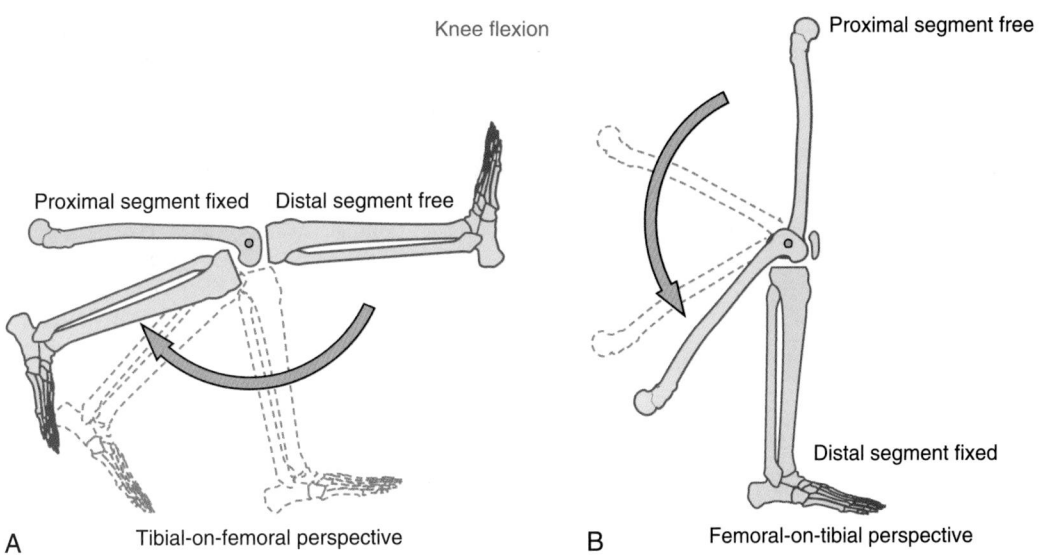

Proximal segment fixed   **Distal segment free**

Proximal segment free

Distal segment fixed

A   Tibial-on-femoral perspective

B   Femoral-on-tibial perspective

FIG. 1.6 Sagittal plane osteokinematics at the knee show an example of (A) distal-on-proximal segment kinematics and (B) proximal-on-distal segment kinematics. The axis of rotation is shown as a circle at the knee.

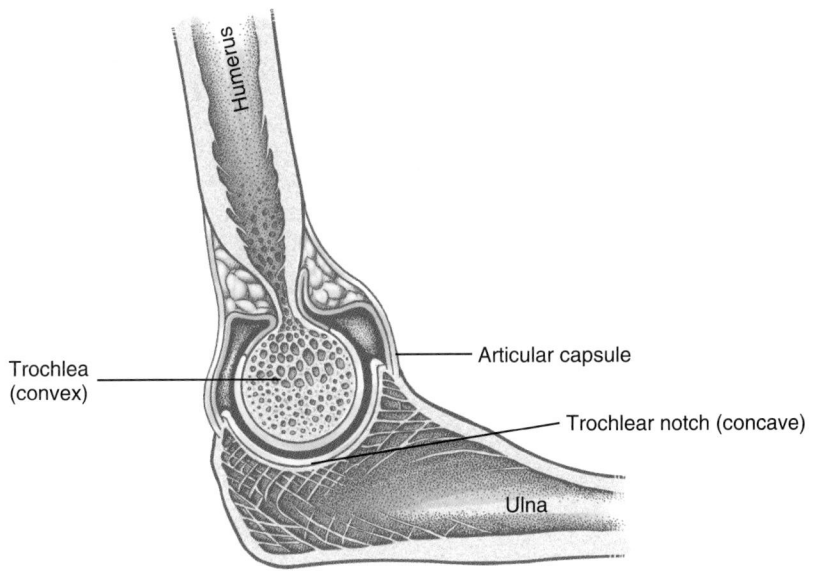

Humerus

Trochlea
(convex)

Articular capsule

Trochlear notch (concave)

Ulna

FIG. 1.7 The humero-ulnar joint at the elbow is an example of a convex-concave relationship between two articular surfaces. The trochlea of the humerus is convex, and the trochlear notch of the ulna is concave.

Although very convenient terminology, the terms *open* and *closed kinematic chains* may be ambiguous. From a strict engineering perspective, the terms apply more to the *kinematic interdependence* of a series of connected rigid links, which is not the same as the previous definitions given here. From this engineering perspective, the chain is "closed" if *both ends* are fixed to a common object, much like a closed circuit. In this case, movement of any one link requires a kinematic adjustment of one or more of the other links within the chain.

"Opening" the chain by disconnecting one end from its fixed attachment interrupts this kinematic interdependence. This more precise terminology does not apply universally across all health-related and engineering disciplines. Performing a one-legged partial squat, for example, is often referred to clinically as the movement of a closed kinematic chain. It could be argued, however, that this is a movement of an open kinematic chain because the contralateral leg

is not fixed to the ground (i.e., the circuit formed by the total body is open). To avoid confusion across professional disciplines, this text uses the terms *open* and *closed kinematic chains* sparingly, and the preference is to explicitly state which segment (proximal or distal) is considered fixed and which is considered free.

Arthrokinematics

TYPICAL JOINT MORPHOLOGY

Arthrokinematics describes the motion that occurs *between the articular surfaces* of joints. As described further in Chapter 2, the shapes of the articular surfaces of joints range from flat to curved. Most joint surfaces, however, are at least slightly curved, with one surface being relatively convex and one relatively concave (Fig. 1.7).

For most articulations, the convex-concave relationship improves congruency (fit), increases the surface area for dissipating contact forces, and helps guide the motion between the bones.

FUNDAMENTAL MOVEMENTS BETWEEN JOINT SURFACES

Three fundamental movements exist between curved joint surfaces: roll, slide, and spin. These movements occur as a convex surface moves on a concave surface, and vice versa (Fig. 1.8). Although other terms are used, these are useful for visualizing the relative movements that occur within a joint. The terms are formally defined in Table 1.3.

Roll-and-Slide Movements

Rotation of a bone often occurs as a result of one bone's articular surface rolling against another bone's articular surface.

Convex-on-concave arthrokinematics

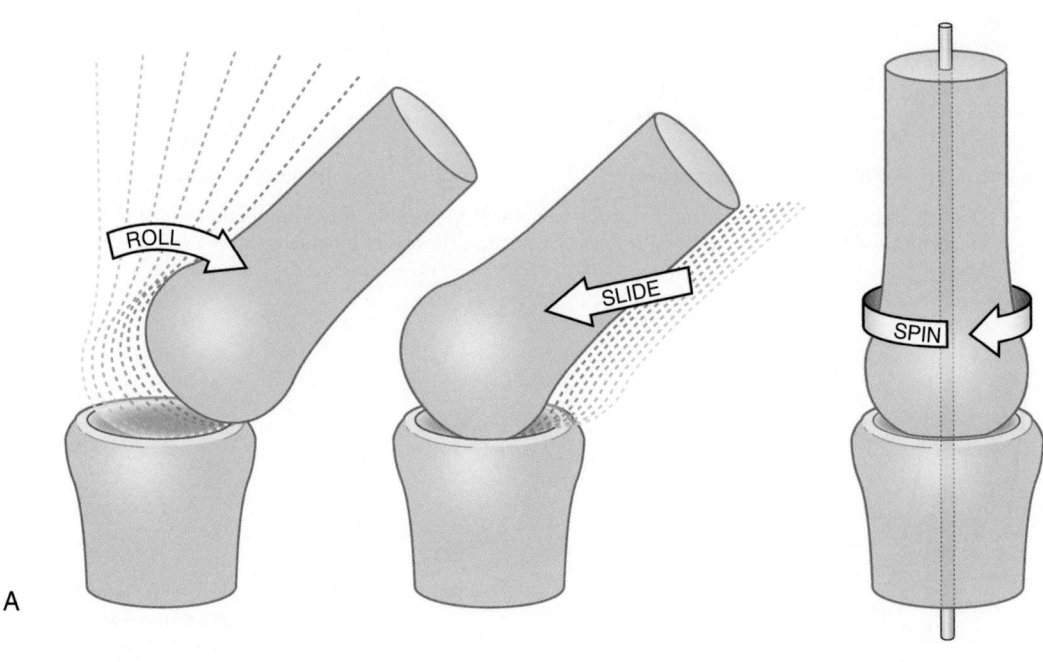

Concave-on-convex arthrokinematics

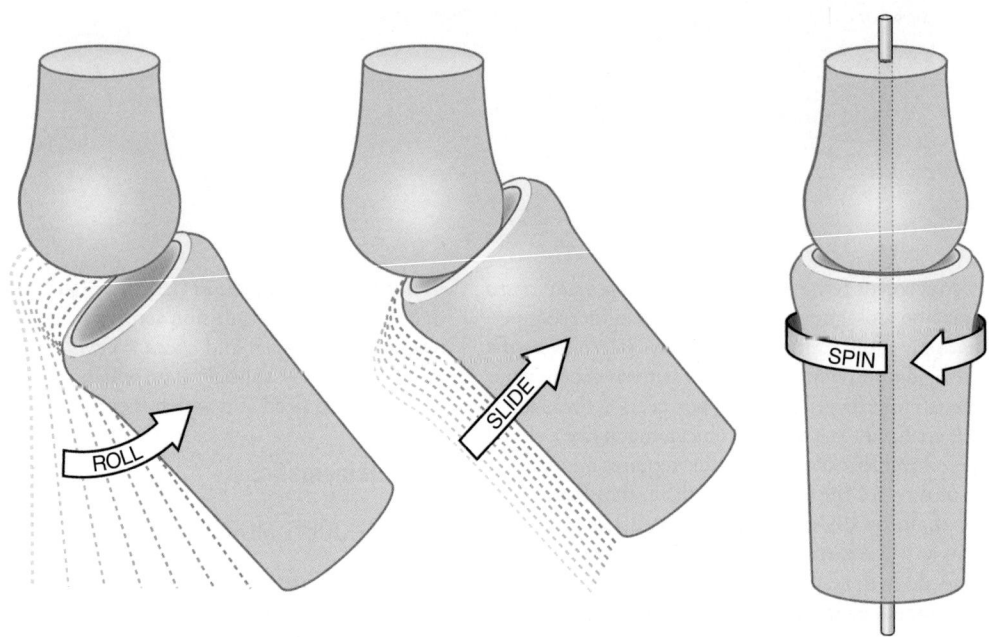

FIG. 1.8 Three fundamental arthrokinematics that occur between curved joint surfaces: roll, slide, and spin. (A) Convex-on-concave movement. (B) Concave-on-convex movement.

TABLE 1.3	Three Fundamental Arthrokinematics: Roll, Slide, and Spin	
Movement	**Definition**	**Analogy**
Roll*	*Multiple points* along one rotating articular surface contact *multiple points* on another articular surface.	A tire rotating across a stretch of pavement
Slide†	A *single point* on one articular surface contacts *multiple points* on another articular surface.	A nonrotating tire skidding across a stretch of icy pavement
Spin	A *single point* on one articular surface rotates on a *single point* on another articular surface.	A toy top rotating on one spot on the floor

*Also termed *rock*.
†Also termed *glide*.

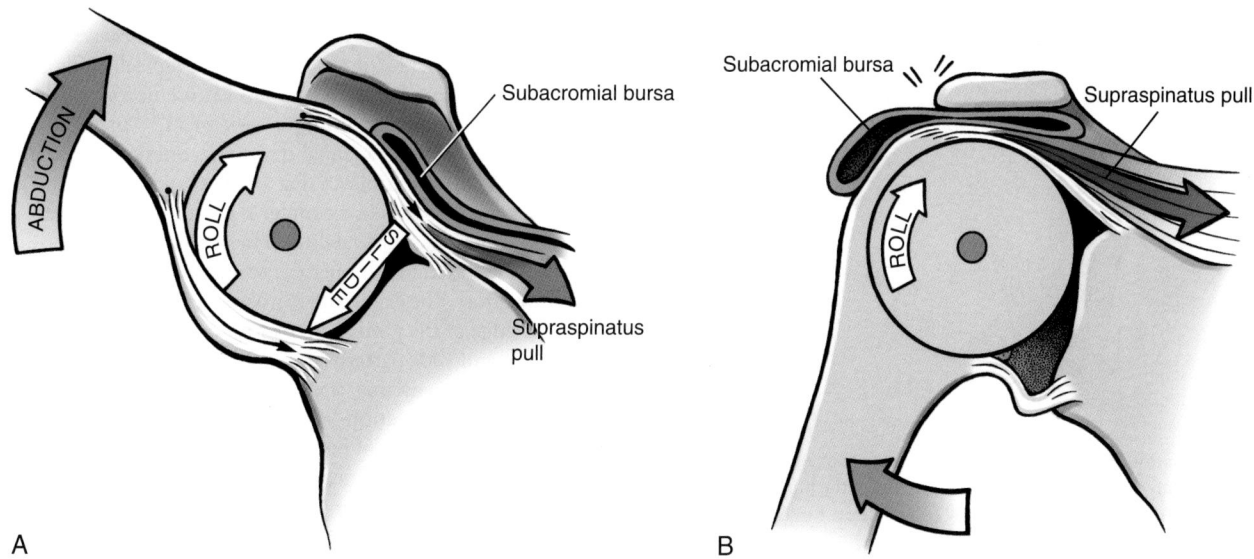

FIG. 1.9 Arthrokinematics at the glenohumeral joint during abduction. The glenoid fossa is concave, and the humeral head is convex. (A) Roll-and-slide arthrokinematics typical of a convex articular surface moving on a relatively stationary concave articular surface. (B) Consequences of a roll occurring without a sufficient offsetting slide.

The motion is shown for a convex-on-concave surface movement at the glenohumeral joint in Fig. 1.9A. The contracting supraspinatus muscle rolls the convex humeral head against the slight concavity of the glenoid fossa. In essence, the roll directs the osteokinematic path of the abducting shaft of the humerus.

A rolling convex surface typically involves a concurrent, oppositely directed slide. As shown in Fig. 1.9A, the inferior-directed *slide* of the humeral head offsets most of the potential superior migration of the rolling humeral head. The offsetting roll-and-slide kinematics are analogous to a tire on a car that is spinning on a sheet of ice. The potential for the tire to rotate forward on the icy pavement is offset by a continuous sliding of the tire in the opposite direction to the intended rotation. A classic pathologic example of a convex surface rolling *without* an offsetting slide is shown in Fig. 1.9B. The humeral head translates upward and impinges on the delicate tissues in the subacromial space. The migration alters the relative location of the axis of rotation, which may alter the effectiveness of the muscles that cross the glenohumeral joint.

As shown in Fig. 1.9A, the concurrent roll-and-slide motion maximizes the angular displacement of the abducting humerus

and minimizes the net translation between joint surfaces. This mechanism is particularly important in joints in which the articular surface area of the convex member exceeds that of the concave member.

Spin

Another primary way that a bone rotates is by *spinning* its articular surface against the articular surface of another bone. This occurs, for example, as the radius of the forearm spins against the capitulum of the humerus during pronation of the forearm (Fig. 1.10). Another example is internal and external rotation of the 90-degree abducted glenohumeral joint. Spinning is the primary mechanism for joint rotation when the longitudinal axis of the moving bone intersects the surface of its articular mate at right angles.

Motions That Combine Roll-and-Slide and Spin Arthrokinematics

Several joints throughout the body combine roll-and-slide with spin arthrokinematics. A classic example of this combination occurs during flexion and extension of the knee. As shown during femoral-on-tibial knee extension (Fig. 1.11A), the femur spins slightly internally as the femoral condyle rolls and slides relative to the fixed (stationary) tibia. These arthrokinematics are also shown as the tibia extends relative to the fixed femur in Fig. 1.11B. In the knee, the spinning motion that occurs with flexion and extension occurs automatically and is mechanically linked to the primary motion of

extension. As described in Chapter 13, the obligatory spinning rotation is based on the shape of the articular surfaces at the knee. The conjunct rotation helps to securely lock the knee joint when fully extended.

PREDICTING AN ARTHROKINEMATIC PATTERN BASED ON JOINT MORPHOLOGY

As previously stated, most articular surfaces of bones are either convex or concave. Depending on which bone is moving, a convex surface may rotate on a concave surface or vice versa (compare Fig. 1.11A with Fig. 1.11B). Each scenario presents a different roll-and-slide arthrokinematic pattern. As depicted in Figs. 1.11A and 1.9A for the shoulder, during a *convex-on-concave movement,* the convex surface rolls and slides in *opposite directions.* As previously described, the contradirectional slide offsets much of the translation tendency inherent to the rolling convex surface. During a *concave-on-convex movement,* as depicted in Fig. 1.11B, the concave surface typically rolls and slides in *similar directions.* These two axioms are useful for visualizing the arthrokinematic patterns during a movement.[11] In addition, they serve as a basis for some manual therapy techniques. External forces may be applied by the clinician that assist or guide the natural arthrokinematics at the joint. For example, in certain circumstances, glenohumeral abduction can be facilitated by applying an inferior-directed force at the proximal humerus, simultaneously with an active-abduction effort. The expected arthrokinematic patterns are based on the knowledge of the joint surface morphology.

The roll-and-slide patterns described earlier provide a conceptual framework for predicting the most likely arthrokinematics for a typical movement situation.[11] The actual arthrokinematics may vary based on a combination of factors, including the radius of curvature of the convexity, health, age, and stability of the joint, specific arc of motion, and the overriding capsular, muscular, and gravitational forces associated with the movement.[15]

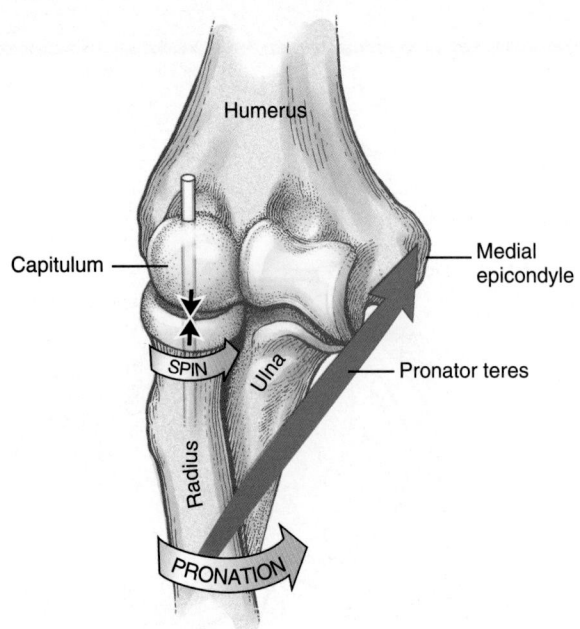

FIG. 1.10 Pronation of the forearm shows an example of a spinning motion between the head of the radius and the capitulum of the humerus. The pair of opposed short black arrows indicates compression forces between the head of the radius and the capitulum.

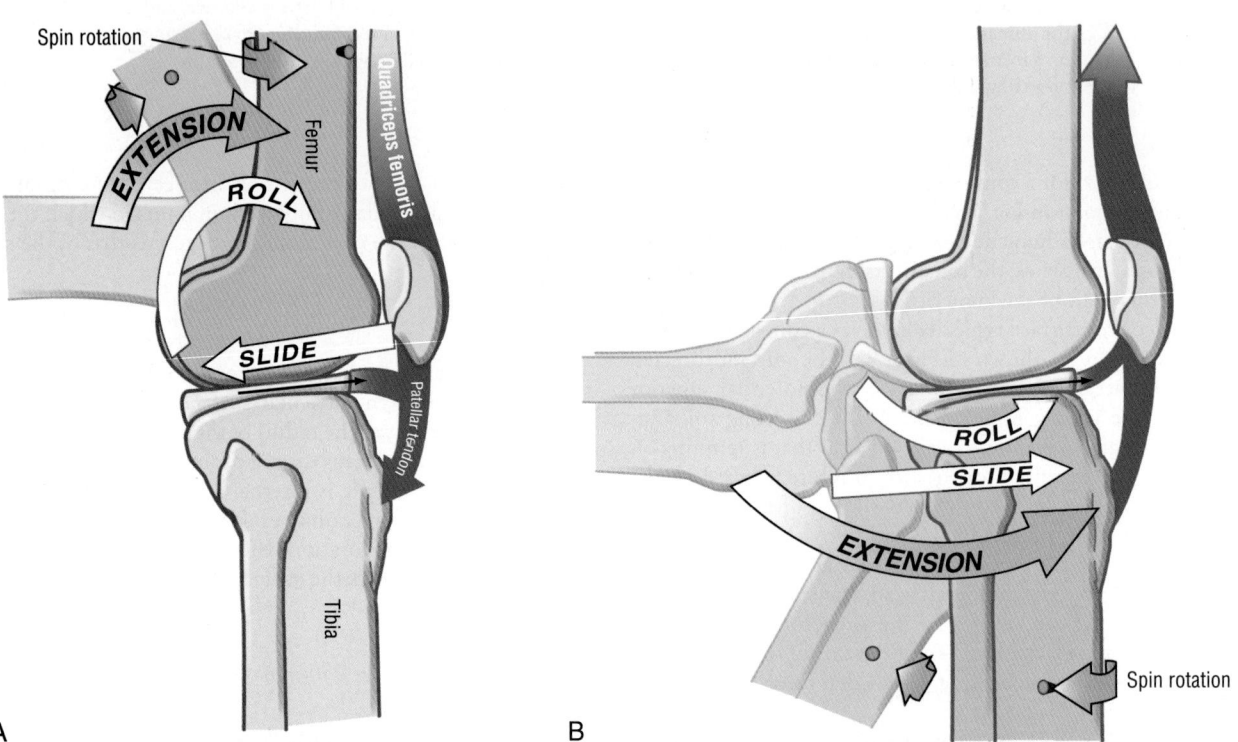

FIG. 1.11 Extension of the knee demonstrates a combination of roll-and-slide with spin arthrokinematics. The femoral condyle is convex, and the tibial plateau is slightly concave. (A) Femoral-on-tibial (knee) extension. (B) Tibial-on-femoral (knee) extension.

> **Expected Arthrokinematic Patterns During Movement**
>
> • For a *convex-on-concave* surface movement, the convex member rolls and slides in *opposite* directions.
> • For a *concave-on-convex* surface movement, the concave member rolls and slides in *similar* directions.

CLOSE-PACKED AND LOOSE-PACKED POSITIONS AT A JOINT

Within most joints, the pair of articular surfaces "fits" best in only one position, usually in or near the end range of a motion. This position of maximal congruency is referred to as the joint's *close-packed position.*[16] In this position, most ligaments and parts of the capsule are pulled taut, providing an element of natural stability to the joint. Accessory movements are typically minimal in a joint's close-packed position.

For many joints in the lower extremity, the close-packed position is associated with a habitual function. At the knee, for example, the close-packed position includes full extension—a position that is typically approached while standing. The combined effect of maximal joint congruity and stretched ligaments helps to provide transarticular stability to the knee.

All positions other than a joint's close-packed position are referred to as the joint's *loose-packed positions* (also referred to as *open-packed* positions). In these positions, the ligaments and capsule are relatively slackened, allowing an increase in accessory movements. The joint is generally least congruent near its midrange. In the lower extremity, the loose-packed positions of the hip and knee include some flexion, and the ankle is biased toward plantar flexion. These loose-packed positions are not typically used during standing but frequently are preferred by the patient during long periods of immobilization, such as prolonged bed rest. Accordingly, common positions of joint "tightness" in the lower limb due to prolonged bed rest are often biased toward to the joints' loose-packed positions.

KINETICS

Kinetics is a branch of the study of mechanics that describes the effect of forces on the body. Although the topic of kinetics is introduced here, a more detailed and mathematical approach to this subject matter is provided in Chapter 4.

From a kinesiologic perspective, a *force* can be considered as a push or pull that can produce, arrest, or modify movement. Forces therefore provide the ultimate impetus for movement and stabilization of the body. As described by Newton's second law, the quantity of a force (F) can be measured by the product of the mass (m) that receives the push or pull, multiplied by the acceleration (a) of the mass. The formula $F = ma$ shows that, given a constant mass, a force is directly proportional to the acceleration of the mass: measuring the force yields the acceleration of the body, and vice versa. A net force is zero when the acceleration of the mass is zero.

The standard international unit of force is the *newton (N)*: $1\text{ N} = 1\text{ kg} \times 1\text{ m/sec}^2$. The English equivalent of the newton is the pound (lb): $1\text{ lb} = 1\text{ slug} \times 1\text{ ft/sec}^2$ ($4.448\text{ N} = 1\text{ lb}$).

Musculoskeletal Forces

EFFECT OF FORCES ON THE MUSCULOSKELETAL SYSTEM: INTRODUCTORY CONCEPTS AND TERMINOLOGY

A force that acts on the body is often referred to generically as a *load.* Forces or loads that move, fixate, or otherwise stabilize the body also

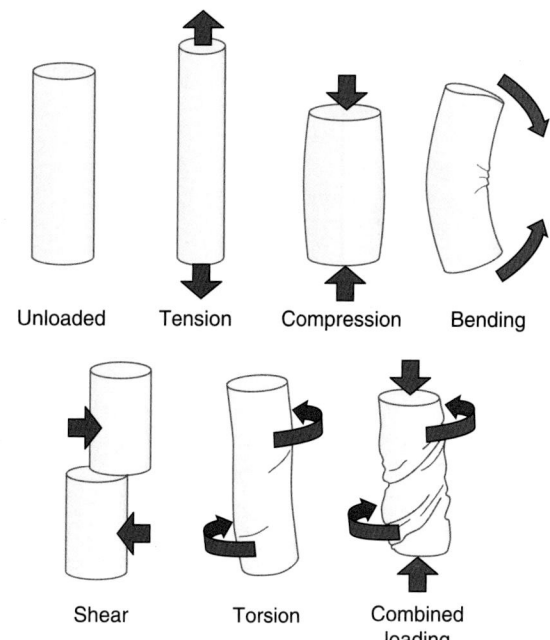

Unloaded   Tension   Compression   Bending

Shear   Torsion   Combined loading

FIG. 1.12 The manner by which forces or loads are most frequently applied to the musculoskeletal system is shown. The combined loading of torsion and compression is also illustrated.

 **SPECIAL FOCUS 1.1**

Body Weight Compared with Body Mass

A kilogram (kg) is a unit of *mass* that indicates the relative number of particles within an object. Strictly speaking, therefore, a kilogram is a measure of mass, not weight. Under the influence of gravity, however, a 1-kg mass *weighs* about 9.8 N (2.2 lb). This is the result of gravity acting to accelerate the 1-kg mass toward the center of the Earth at a rate of about 9.8 m/sec². Very often, however, the weight of a body is expressed in kilograms. The assumption is that the acceleration resulting from gravity acting on the body is constant and, for practical purposes, ignored. Technically, however, the weight of a person varies inversely with the square of the distance between the mass of the person and the center of the Earth. A person on the summit of Mt. Everest at 29,031 ft (8848 m), for example, weighs slightly less than a person with identical mass at sea level. The acceleration resulting from gravity on Mt. Everest is 9.782 m/sec² compared with 9.806 m/sec² at sea level.

have the potential to deform and injure the body. The loads most frequently applied to the musculoskeletal system are illustrated in Fig. 1.12. (See the glossary at the end of this chapter for formal definitions.) Healthy tissues are typically able to partially resist changes in their structure and shape. The force that stretches a healthy ligament, for example, is met by an intrinsic tension generated within the elongated (stretched) tissue. Any tissue weakened by disease, trauma, or prolonged disuse may not be able to adequately resist the application of the loads depicted in Fig. 1.12. The proximal femur weakened by osteoporosis, for example, may fracture from the

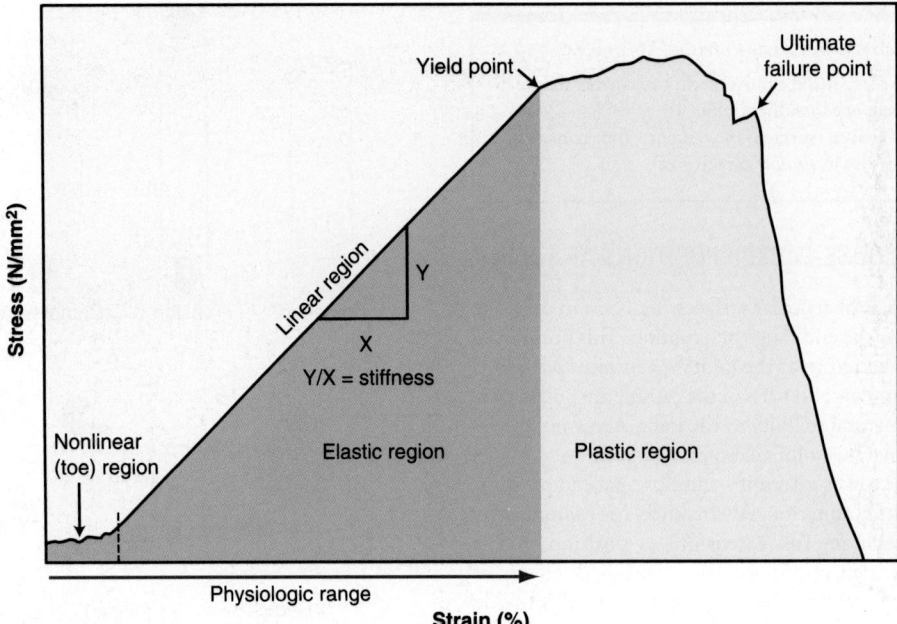

FIG. 1.13 The stress-strain relationship of an excised ligament that has been stretched to a point of mechanical failure (disruption).

impact of a fall secondary to *compression or torsion (twisting), shearing,* or *bending* of the neck of the femur. Fracture may also occur in a severely osteoporotic hip after a very strong muscle contraction.

The ability of periarticular connective tissues to accept and disperse loads is an important topic of research within physical rehabilitation, manual therapy, and orthopedic medicine. Clinicians and scientists are very interested in how variables such as aging, trauma, altered activity or weight-bearing levels, or prolonged immobilization affect the load-accepting functions of periarticular connective tissues. One laboratory-based method of measuring the ability of a connective tissue to tolerate a load is to plot the force required to deform an excised tissue. This type of experiment is typically performed using animal or human cadaver specimens. Fig. 1.13 shows a theoretical graph of the tension generated by a generic ligament (or tendon) that has been stretched to a point of mechanical failure. The vertical (Y) axis of the graph is labeled *stress,* a term that quantifies the internal resistance generated as the ligament resists deformation. (Stress, as used in this context, is the ratio of the force applied to a tissue relative to the cross-sectional area of that tissue. The units of stress are therefore expressed as N/m^2.) The horizontal (X) axis is labeled *strain,* which, in this case, is the percent increase in a tissue's stretched length relative to its original, preexperimental length. (A similar procedure may be performed by *compressing* rather than stretching an excised slice of cartilage or bone, for example, and then plotting the amount of stress produced within the tissue.) Note in Fig. 1.13 that under a relatively slight strain (stretch), the ligament experiences only a small amount of stress due to the applied tension. This *nonlinear* or "toe" region of the graph reflects the fact that the collagen fibers within the tissue are initially wavy or *crimped* and must be drawn taut before significant tension is measured. Further elongation, however, shows a *linear relationship* between stress and strain. The ratio of the stress (Y) caused by an applied strain (X) in the ligament is a measure of its *stiffness* (often referred to as *Young's modulus*). All normal connective tissues within the musculoskeletal system exhibit some degree of stiffness. The clinical term "tightness" often implies a pathologic condition or a sensation of abnormally

high stiffness, although the sensation of tightness does not always imply a stiffer tissue.[17]

The initial nonlinear and subsequent linear regions of the curve shown in Fig. 1.13 are often referred to as the *elastic region.* Ligaments, for example, are routinely strained within the lower limits of their elastic region. The anterior cruciate ligament, for example, is strained about 3%–4% during common activities such as climbing stairs, pedaling a stationary bicycle, or squatting.[6,7] It is important to note that a healthy and relatively young ligament that is strained within the elastic zone returns to its original length (or shape) once the deforming force is removed. The area under the curve (in darker blue) represents *elastic deformation energy.* Most of the energy used to deform the tissue is released when the force is removed. Even in a static sense, elastic energy has an important function within joints. When stretched even a moderate amount into the elastic zone, ligaments and other connective tissues perform important joint stabilization functions.

A tissue that is elongated beyond its physiologic range eventually reaches its *yield point.* At this point, increased strain results in only marginally increased stress (tension). This physical behavior of an overstretched (or overcompressed) tissue is known as *plasticity.* The overstrained tissue has experienced *plastic deformation.* At this point, microscopic failure has occurred, and the tissue remains permanently deformed. The area under this region of the curve (in lighter blue) represents *plastic deformation energy.* Unlike elastic deformation energy, plastic energy is not recoverable in its entirety, even when the deforming force is removed. As elongation continues, the ligament eventually reaches its *ultimate failure point,* the point when the tissue partially or completely separates and loses its ability to hold any level of tension. The ultimate failure point of the anterior cruciate ligament (ACL), for example, occurs at strain lengths of 11%–19%.[10,3]

The graph in Fig. 1.13 does not indicate the variable of *time* of load application. Tissues in which the physical properties associated with the stress-strain curve change as a function of time are considered *viscoelastic.* Most tissues within the musculoskeletal system demonstrate at least some degree of viscoelasticity. One phenomenon of viscoelastic material is creep. As demonstrated by the tree

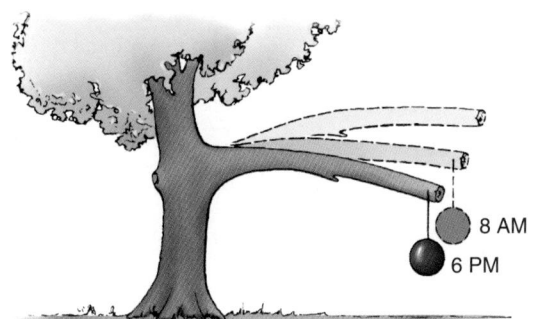

FIG. 1.14 The branch of the tree is demonstrating a time-dependent property of creep associated with a *viscoelastic material.* Hanging a load on the branch at 8 AM creates an immediate deformation. By 6 PM, the load has caused additional deformation in the branch. (From Panjabi MM, White AA: *Biomechanics in the musculoskeletal system,* New York, 2001, Churchill Livingstone.)

branch in Fig. 1.14, *creep* describes a progressive strain of a material when exposed to a constant load over time. The phenomenon of creep helps to explain why a person is taller in the morning than at night. The constant compression caused by body weight on the spine throughout the day literally squeezes a small amount of fluid out of the intervertebral discs. The fluid is reabsorbed at night while the sleeping person is in a non–weight-bearing position.

Another way to view how time makes a difference in viscoelasticity is to change the *rate* at which a tissue is loaded. In general, the slope of a stress-strain relationship when placed under tension or compression increases throughout its elastic range as the rate of the loading increases. The rate-sensitivity nature of viscoelastic connective tissues may protect surrounding structures within the musculoskeletal system. Articular cartilage in the knee, for example, becomes stiffer as the rate of compression increases, such as during running. The increased stiffness affords greater protection to the underlying bone at a time when forces acting on the joint are greatest.

SPECIAL FOCUS 1.2

Productive Antagonism: The Body's Ability to Convert Passive Tension into Useful Work

A stretched or elongated tissue within the body generally produces tension (i.e., a resistance force that opposes the stretch). In pathologic cases this tension may be abnormally large, thereby interfering with functional mobility. However, even relatively low levels of tension produced by stretched connective tissues (including muscle) can perform useful functions, and several such examples are provided throughout this textbook. This phenomenon is called *productive antagonism* and is demonstrated for a pair of muscles in the simplified model in Fig. 1.15. As shown by the figure on the left, part of the energy produced by active contraction of muscle *A* is transferred and stored as elastic energy in the stretched connective tissues within the antagonist muscle *B.* The elastic energy is released as muscle *B* actively contracts to

drive the nail into the board (right illustration). Part of the contractile energy produced by muscle *B* is used to stretch muscle *A,* and the cycle is repeated.

This transfer and storage of energy between opposing muscles is useful for overall metabolic efficiency. This phenomenon is often expressed in different ways by multiarticular muscles (i.e., muscles that cross several joints). Consider the rectus femoris, a muscle that flexes the hip and extends the knee. During the upward phase of jumping, for example, the rectus femoris contracts to extend the knee. At the same time, the extending hip stretches the active rectus femoris across the front of the hip. As a consequence, the overall shortening of the rectus femoris is minimized, which helps preserve useful passive tension within the muscle.

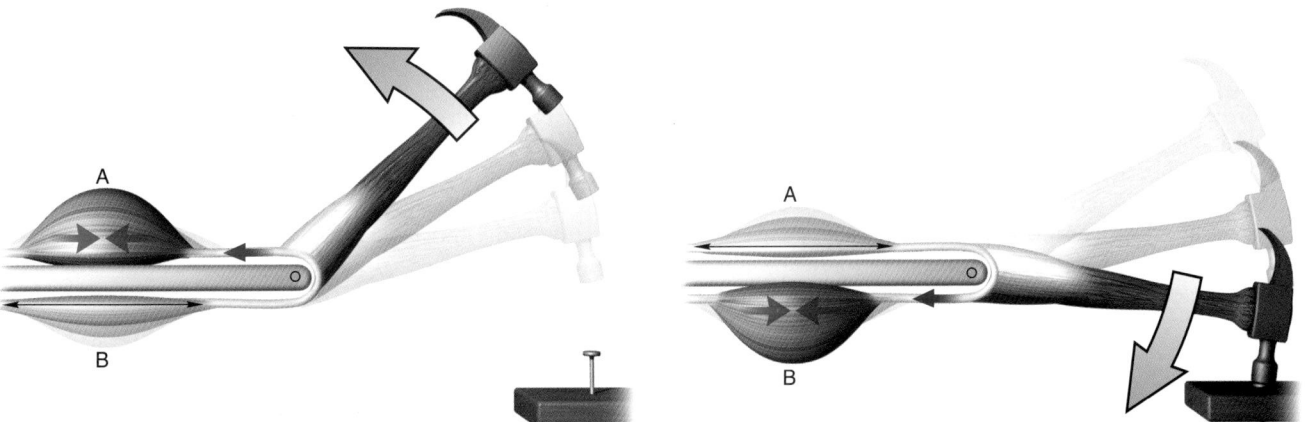

FIG. 1.15 A simplified model showing a pair of opposed muscles surrounding a joint. In the left illustration, muscle *A* is contracting to provide the force needed to lift the hammer in preparation to strike the nail. In the right illustration, muscle *B* is contracting, driving the hammer against the nail while simultaneously stretching muscle *A.* (Redrawn from Brand PW: *Clinical biomechanics of the hand,* St Louis, 1985, Mosby.)

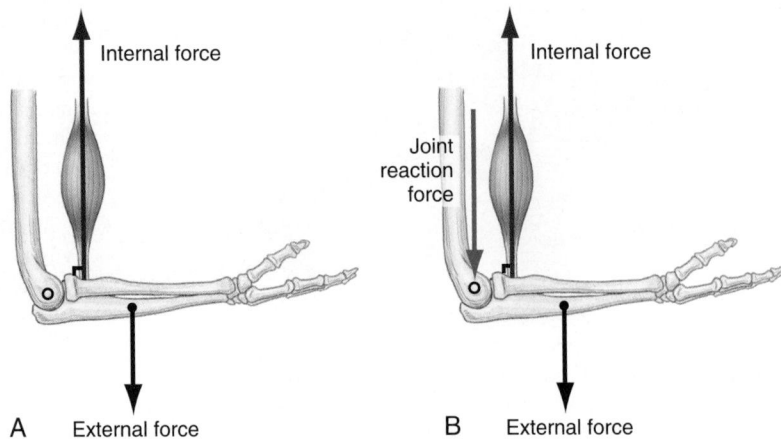

FIG. 1.16 A sagittal plane view of the elbow joint and associated bones. (A) Internal (muscle) and external (gravitational) forces are shown both acting vertically, but each in a different direction. The two vectors have different magnitudes and different points of application to the forearm. (B) Joint reaction force is added to prevent the forearm from accelerating upward. (Vectors are drawn to relative scale.)

In summary, similar to building materials such as steel, concrete, and fiberglass, the periarticular connective tissues within the human body possess unique physical properties when loaded or strained. In engineering terms, these physical properties are formally referred to as *material properties.* The topic of material properties of periarticular connective tissues (such as stress, strain, stiffness, plastic deformation, ultimate failure load, and creep) are frequently addressed in the research literature.[2,4,5,9,13] Although much of the data on this topic are from animal or cadaver research, they do provide insight into many aspects of patient care, including understanding mechanisms of injury, improving the design of orthopedic surgery, and judging the potential effectiveness of certain forms of physical therapy, such as prolonged stretching or application of heat to induce greater tissue extensibility.

INTERNAL AND EXTERNAL FORCES

As a matter of convenience, the forces that act on the musculoskeletal system can be divided into two sets: internal and external. *Internal forces* are produced from structures located *within* the body. These forces may be "active" or "passive." Active forces are generated by stimulated muscle, generally but not necessarily under volitional control. Passive forces, in contrast, are typically generated by tension in stretched periarticular connective tissues, including the intramuscular connective tissues, ligaments, and joint capsules. Active forces produced by muscles are typically the largest of all internal forces.

External forces are produced by forces acting from *outside* the body. These forces usually originate from either *gravity* pulling on the mass of a body segment or an external load, such as that of luggage, "free" weights, or *physical contact,* such as that applied by a therapist against the limb of a patient. Fig. 1.16A shows an opposing pair of internal and external forces: an internal force (muscle) pulling the forearm, and an external (gravitational) force pulling on the center of mass of the forearm. Each force is depicted by an arrow that represents a vector. By definition, a *vector* is a quantity that is completely described by its magnitude and its direction.

(Quantities such as mass and speed are scalars, not vectors. A scalar is a quantity that is completely specified by its magnitude and has no direction.)

To completely describe a vector in a biomechanical analysis, its magnitude, spatial orientation, direction, and point of application must be known. The forces depicted in Fig. 1.16A indicate these four factors.

1. The *magnitude* of the force vectors is indicated by the length of the shaft of the arrow.
2. The *spatial orientation* of the force vectors is indicated by the position of the shaft of the arrows. Both forces are oriented vertically, often referred to as the Y axis (further described in Chapter 4). The orientation of a force can also be described by the angle formed between the shaft of the arrow and a reference coordinate system.
3. The *direction* of the force vectors is indicated by the arrowhead. In the example depicted in Fig. 1.16A, the internal force acts upward, typically described in a *positive* Y sense; the external force acts downward in a *negative* Y sense. Throughout this text, the direction and spatial orientation of a muscle force and gravity are referred to as their *line of force* and *line of gravity,* respectively.
4. The *point of application* of the vectors is where the base of the vector arrow contacts the part of the body. The point of application of the muscle (internal) force is where the muscle inserts into the bone. The *angle-of-insertion* describes the angle formed between a tendon of a muscle and the long axis of the bone into which it inserts. In Fig. 1.16A, the angle-of-insertion is 90 degrees. The angle-of-insertion changes as the elbow rotates into flexion or extension. The point of application of the external force depends on whether the force is the result of gravity, or the result of a resistance applied by physical contact. Gravity acts on the *center of mass* of the body segment (see Fig. 1.16A, dot at the forearm). The point of application of a resistance generated from physical contact can occur anywhere on the body.

Factors Required to Completely Describe a Vector in Most Simple Biomechanical Analyses
- Magnitude
- Spatial orientation
- Direction
- Point of application

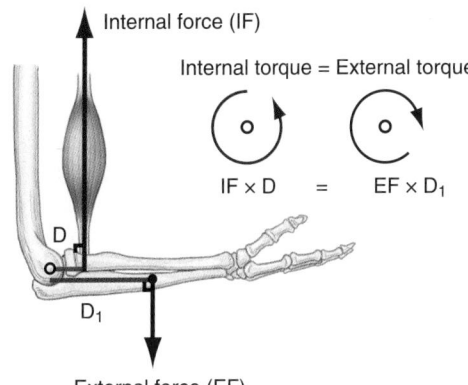

FIG. 1.17 The balance of internal and external torques acting in the sagittal plane around the axis of rotation at the elbow *(small circle)* is shown. The *internal torque* is the product of the internal force multiplied by the internal moment arm *(D)*. The internal torque has the potential to rotate the forearm in a counterclockwise direction. The *external torque* is the product of the external force (gravity) and the external moment arm *(D₁)*. The external torque has the potential to rotate the forearm in a clockwise direction. The internal and external torques are equal, demonstrating a condition of static rotary equilibrium. (Vectors are drawn to relative scale.)

As a push or a pull, all forces acting on the body cause a potential translation of the segment. The direction of the translation depends on the net effect of all the applied forces. In Fig. 1.16A, because the muscle force is three times greater than the weight of the forearm, the net effect of both forces would accelerate the forearm vertically upward. In reality, however, the forearm is typically prevented from accelerating upward by a *joint reaction force* produced between the surfaces of the joint. As depicted in Fig. 1.16B, the distal end of the humerus is pushing *down* with a reaction force (shown in blue) against the proximal end of the forearm. The magnitude of the joint reaction force is equal to the difference between the muscle force and external force. As a result, the sum of all vertical forces acting on the forearm is balanced, and net acceleration of the forearm in the vertical direction is zero. The system is, therefore, in *static linear equilibrium.*

Musculoskeletal Torques

Forces exerted on the body can have two outcomes. First, as depicted in Fig. 1.16A, forces can potentially *translate* a body segment. Second, the forces, if applied at some distance perpendicular to the axis of rotation, have a potential to produce a *rotation* of the joint. The perpendicular distance between the axis of rotation of the joint and the force is called a *moment (or lever) arm*. The product of a force and its moment arm produces a *torque* or a moment. A torque can be considered as a rotatory equivalent to a force. A force acting without a moment arm can push and pull an object generally in a linear fashion, whereas a torque rotates an object around an axis of rotation. This distinction is a fundamental concept in the study of kinesiology.

A torque is described as occurring around a joint in a plane perpendicular to a given axis of rotation. Fig. 1.17 shows the torques produced within the sagittal plane by the internal and external forces introduced in Fig. 1.16. The *internal torque* is defined as the product of the internal force (muscle) and the internal moment arm. The *internal moment arm* (see *D* in Fig. 1.17) is the perpendicular distance between the axis of rotation and the internal force. As depicted in Fig. 1.17, the internal torque has the potential to rotate the forearm around the elbow joint in a counterclockwise, or flexion, direction. (Other conventions for describing rotation direction are explored in Chapter 4.)

The *external torque* is defined as the product of the external force (such as gravity) and the external moment arm. The *external moment arm* (see *D₁* in Fig. 1.17) is the perpendicular distance between the axis of rotation and the external force. The external torque has the potential to rotate the forearm around the elbow joint in a clockwise, or extension, direction. Because the magnitudes of the opposing internal and external torques are assumed to be equal in Fig. 1.17, no rotation occurs around the joint. This condition is referred to as *static rotary equilibrium*.

The human body typically produces or receives torques repeatedly in one form or another. Muscles generate internal torques constantly throughout the day, to unscrew a cap from a jar, advance the lower limb while walking, or propel a wheelchair. Manual contact forces received from the environment, in addition to gravity, are typically converted to external torques across joints. Internal and external torques are constantly "competing" for dominance across joints—the more dominant torque is reflected by the direction of movement or position of the joints at any given time throughout the body.

Torques are involved in most therapeutic situations with patients, especially when physical exercise or strength assessment is involved. A person's "strength" is the product of their muscles' force and, equally important, the internal moment arm: the perpendicular distance between the muscle's line of force and the axis of rotation. *Leverage* describes the relative moment arm length possessed by a particular force. As explained further in Chapter 4, the length of a muscle's moment arm, and hence leverage, changes constantly throughout a range of motion. This partially explains why a person is naturally stronger in certain parts of a joint's range of motion.

Clinicians frequently apply manual resistance against their patients or clients as a means to assess, facilitate, and challenge a particular muscle activity. The *force* applied against a patient's extremity is often performed with the intent of producing an external *torque* against the patient's musculoskeletal system. A clinician can challenge a particular muscle group by applying an external torque by way of a small manual force exerted a great distance from the joint, or a large manual force exerted close to the joint. Because torque is the *product* of a resistance force and its moment arm, either means can produce the same external torque against the patient. Modifying the force and external moment arm variables allows different strategies to be employed based on the strength and skill of the clinician.

Muscle-Produced Torques Across a Joint: An Essential Concept in Kinesiology

How muscles produce torques across joints is one of the most important (and often difficult) concepts to understand in kinesiology. A simple analogy between a muscle's potential to produce a torque (i.e., rotation) and the action of a force attempting to swing open a door can be used to help understand this concept.

The essential mechanics in both scenarios are surprisingly similar. This analogy is described with the assistance of Fig. 1.18A–B.

Fig. 1.18A shows top and side views of a door mounted on a vertical hinge (depicted in blue). Horizontally applied forces

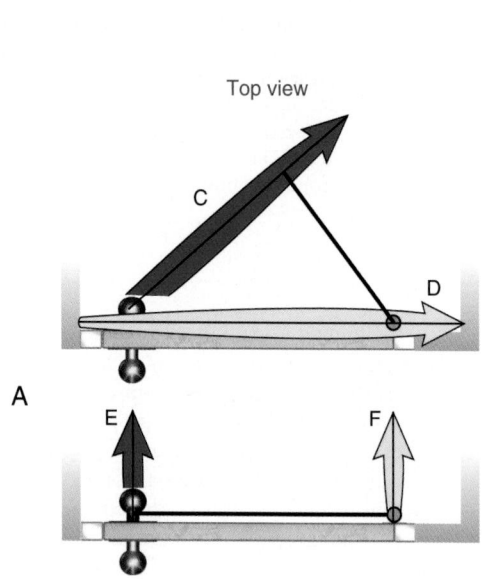
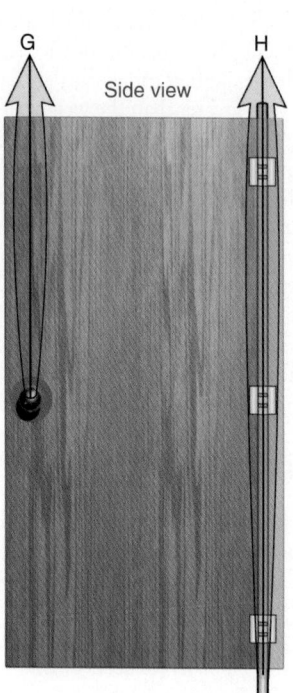
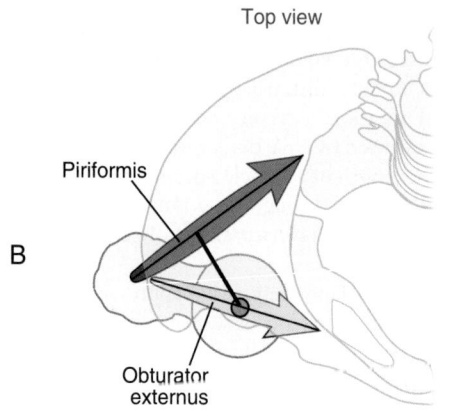
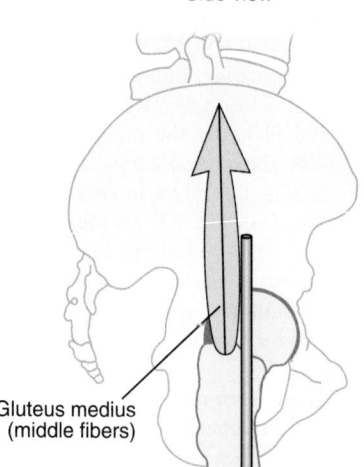

FIG. 1.18 Mechanical analogy depicting the fundamental mechanics of how a force can be converted into a torque. (A) Six manually applied forces are indicated *(colored arrows),* each attempting to rotate the door in the horizontal plane. The vertical hinge of the door is shown in blue. The moment arms available to two of the forces (on the left) are indicated by dark black lines, originating at the hinge. (B) Three muscle-produced forces are depicted *(colored arrows),* each attempting to rotate the femur (hip) in the horizontal plane. The axes of rotation are shown in blue, and the moment arm as a dark black line. As described in the text, for similar reasons, only a selected number of forces is actually capable of generating a torque that can rotate either the door or the hip. For the sake of this analogy, the magnitude of all forces is assumed to be the same.

Muscle-Produced Torques Across a Joint: An Essential Concept in Kinesiology—*cont'd*

(*C* to *F*) represent different attempts at manually pulling open the door. *Although all forces are assumed equal,* only forces *C* and *E* (applied at the doorknob) are actually capable of rotating the door. This holds true because only these forces meet the basic requirements of producing a torque: (1) each force is applied in a plane *perpendicular* to the given axis of rotation (door hinge in this case), and (2) each force is associated with a *moment arm* distance (dark black line originating at the hinge). In this example, the torque is the product of the pulling force times its moment arm. Force *E* will produce a greater torque than force *C* because it has the longer moment arm (or greater leverage). Nevertheless, forces *C* and *E* both satisfy the requirement to produce a torque in the horizontal plane.

Forces *D* and *F,* however, cannot produce a torque within the horizontal plane and therefore are not able to rotate the door, regardless of their magnitude. Although this may seem intuitively obvious based on everyone's experience closing or opening doors, the actual mechanical reasoning may not be so clear. Forces *D* and *F* are directed *through* the axis of rotation (the hinge in this case) and, therefore, have a moment arm distance of zero. Any force multiplied by a moment arm of zero produces zero torque, or zero rotation. Although these forces may compress or distract the hinge, they will not rotate the door.

Forces *G* and *H,* shown at the right in Fig. 1.18A, also cannot rotate the door. Any force that runs *parallel* with an axis of rotation cannot produce an associated torque. A torque can be generated only by a force that is applied *perpendicular to a given axis of rotation.* Forces *G* and *H,* therefore, possess no ability to produce a torque in the horizontal plane.

To complete this analogy, Fig. 1.18B shows two views of the hip joint along with three selected muscles. In this example the muscles are depicted as producing forces in attempt to rotate the femur within the horizontal plane. (The muscle forces in these illustrations are analogous to the manual forces applied to the door.) The axis of rotation at the hip, like the hinge on the door, is in a vertical direction (shown in blue). As will be explained, even though all the muscles are assumed to produce an identical force,

only one is capable of actually rotating the femur (i.e., producing a torque).

The force vectors illustrated on the left side of Fig. 1.18B represent the lines of force of two hip muscles that are predominantly aligned in the horizontal plane: the piriformis and obturator externus. The piriformis can produce an external rotation torque within the horizontal plane for the same reasons given for the analogous force *C* applied to the door (Fig. 1.18A). Both forces are applied in a plane perpendicular to the axis of rotation, and each possesses an associated moment arm distance (depicted as the dark line). In sharp contrast, however, the obturator externus muscle *cannot* produce a torque in the horizontal plane. This muscle force (as with the analogous force *D* acting on the door) passes directly *through* the vertical axis of rotation. Although the muscle force will compress the joint surfaces, it will not rotate the joint, at least not in the horizontal plane. As will be described in Chapter 12, which studies the hip, changing the rotational position of the joint often creates a moment arm distance for a muscle. In this case, the obturator externus likely generates external rotation torque at the hip, although relatively small.

The final component of this analogy is illustrated on the right of Fig. 1.18B. The middle fibers of the gluteus medius are shown attempting to rotate the femur in the horizontal plane around a vertical axis of rotation (depicted as a blue pin). Because the muscle force acts essentially *parallel* with the vertical axis of rotation (like forces *G* and *H* acting on the door), it is incapable of generating a torque in the horizontal plane. This same muscle, however, is very capable of generating torque in other planes, especially the frontal.

To summarize, a muscle can produce a torque (or rotation) at a joint only provided it (1) produces a force in a plane perpendicular to the axis of rotation of interest, and (2) acts with an associated moment arm distance greater than zero. Stated from a different perspective, an active muscle is *incapable* of producing a torque if the force either *pierces or parallels* the associated axis of rotation. This applies to all axes of rotation that may exist at a joint: vertical, anterior-posterior (AP), or medial-lateral (ML). These principles will be revisited many times throughout this textbook

Muscle and Joint Interaction

The term *muscle and joint interaction* refers to the overall effect that a muscle force may have on a joint. A force produced by a muscle that has a moment arm causes a torque, and a potential to rotate the joint. A force produced by a muscle that lacks a moment arm cannot cause a torque or a rotation. The muscle force is still important, however, because it usually provides a source of stability and sensory information to the joint.

TYPES OF MUSCLE ACTIVATION

A muscle is considered activated when it is stimulated by the nervous system. Once activated, a muscle produces a force in one of three ways: isometric, concentric, and eccentric. The physiology of the three types of muscle activation is described in greater detail in Chapter 3 and briefly summarized subsequently.

Isometric activation occurs when a muscle is producing a pulling force while maintaining a constant length. This type of activation is

Three types of muscle activation

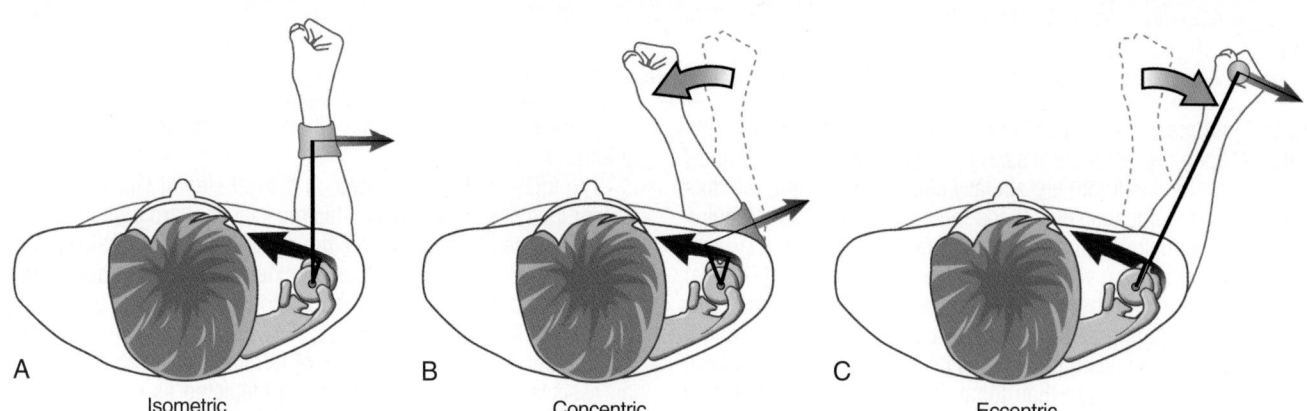

FIG. 1.19 Three types of muscle activation are shown as the pectoralis major produces a force in an attempt to internally rotate the shoulder (glenohumeral) joint. In each of the three illustrations, the internal torque is assumed to be the same: the product of a constant level of muscle force *(red)* times its internal moment arm. The external torque is the product of the external force applied throughout the arm *(gray)* and its external moment arm. Note that the external moment arm, and therefore the external torque, is different in each illustration. (A) Isometric activation is shown as the internal torque matches the external torque. (B) Concentric activation is shown as the internal torque exceeds the external torque. (C) Eccentric activation is shown as the external torque exceeds the internal torque. The axis of rotation is vertical and depicted in blue through the humeral head. All moment arms are shown as thick black lines, originating at the axis of rotation piercing the glenohumeral joint. (Vectors are not drawn to scale.)

apparent by the origin of the word *isometric* (from the Greek *isos,* equal, and *metron,* measure or length). During an isometric activation, the internal torque produced within a given plane at a joint is equal to the external torque; hence, there is no muscle shortening or rotation at the joint (Fig. 1.19A).

Concentric activation occurs as a muscle produces a pulling force as it contracts (shortens) (see Fig. 1.19B). Literally, *concentric* means "coming to the center." During a concentric activation, the internal torque at the joint exceeds the opposing external torque. This is evident as the contracting muscle creates a rotation of the joint in the direction of the pull of the activated muscle.

Eccentric activation, in contrast, occurs as a muscle produces a pulling force as it is being elongated by another more dominant force. The word *eccentric* literally means "away from the center." During an eccentric activation, the external torque around the joint exceeds the internal torque. In this case, the joint rotates in the direction dictated by the relatively larger external torque, such as that produced by the handheld external force in Fig. 1.19C. Many common activities employ eccentric activations of muscle. Slowly lowering a cup of water to a table, for example, is caused by the pull of gravity on the forearm and water. The activated biceps slowly elongates to control the descent. The triceps muscle, although considered as an elbow "extensor," is most likely inactive during this particular process.

The term *contraction* is often used synonymously with *activation,* regardless of whether the muscle is actually shortening, lengthening, or remaining at a constant length. The term *contract* literally means to be *drawn together;* this term, however, can be confusing when describing either an isometric or an eccentric activation. Technically, contraction of a muscle occurs during a concentric activation only.

MUSCLE ACTION AT A JOINT

A *muscle action* at a joint is defined as the potential for a muscle to cause a torque in a particular rotation direction and plane. The

actual naming of a muscle's action is based on an established nomenclature, such as flexion or extension in the sagittal plane, abduction or adduction in the frontal plane, and so forth. The terms *muscle action* and *joint action* are used interchangeably throughout this text, depending on the context of the discussion. If the action is associated with a nonisometric muscle activation, the resulting osteokinematics may involve distal-on-proximal segment kinematics, or vice versa, depending on which of the segments comprising the joint is least constrained.

The study of kinesiology allows one to determine the action of a muscle without relying purely on memory. Suppose the student desires to determine the actions of the *posterior deltoid* at the glenohumeral (shoulder) joint. In this particular analysis, two assumptions are made. First, it is assumed that the humerus is the freest segment of the joint, and that the scapula is fixed, although the reverse assumption could have been made. Second, it is assumed that the body is in the anatomic position at the time of the muscle activation.

The first step in the analysis is to determine the planes of rotary motion (degrees of freedom) allowed at the joint. In this case, the glenohumeral joint allows rotation in all three planes (see Fig. 1.5). It is therefore theoretically possible that *any* muscle crossing the shoulder can express an action in up to three planes. Fig. 1.20A shows the potential for the posterior deltoid to rotate the humerus in the frontal plane. The axis of rotation passes in an anterior-posterior direction through the humeral head. In the anatomic position, the line of force of the posterior deltoid passes inferior to the axis of rotation. By assuming that the scapula is stable, a contracting posterior deltoid would rotate the humerus toward adduction, with strength equal to the product of the muscle force multiplied by its internal moment arm (shown as the dark line from the axis). This same logic is next applied to determine the muscle's action in the horizontal and sagittal planes. As depicted in Fig. 1.20B–C, it is apparent that the muscle is also an external (lateral) rotator and an extensor of the glenohumeral joint. As will be described throughout

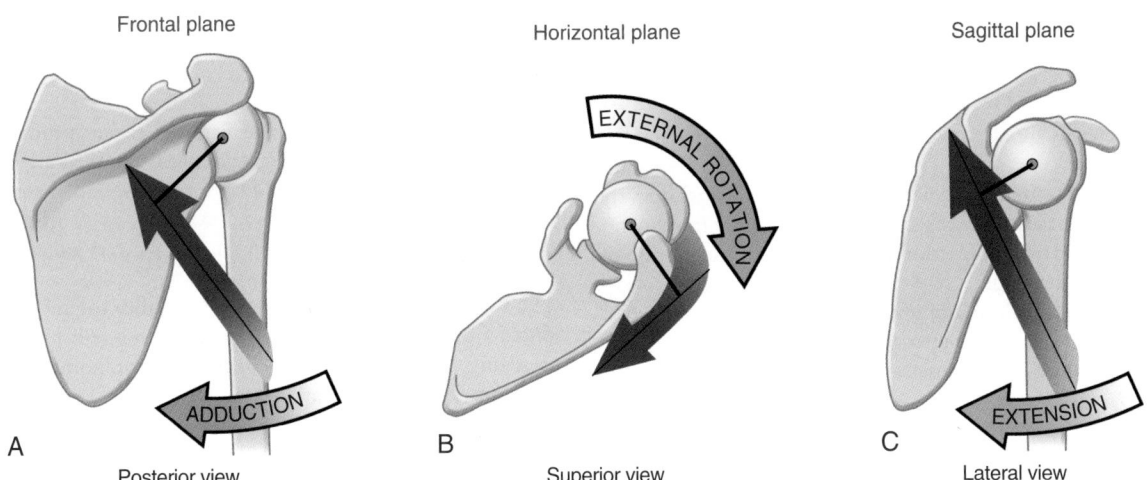

FIG. 1.20 The multiple actions of the posterior deltoid are shown at the glenohumeral joint. (A) Adduction in the frontal plane. (B) External rotation in the horizontal plane. (C) Extension in the sagittal plane. The internal moment arm is shown extending from the axis of rotation (small circle through humeral head) to a perpendicular intersection with the muscle's line of force.

this text, it is common for a muscle that crosses a joint with at least two degrees of freedom to express multiple actions. A particular action may not be possible, however, if the muscle either lacks a moment arm or does not produce a force in the associated plane.

Determining the potential action (or actions) of a muscle is a central theme in the study of kinesiology. This skill is the basis for a clinician being able to evaluate a specific muscle for weakness, tightness, guarding, or source of pain, and responding with an appropriate intervention.

The logic presented within the context of Fig. 1.20 can be used to determine the action of *any* muscle in the body, at any joint. If available, an articulated skeleton model and a piece of string (or thin elastic material) that mimics the line of force of a muscle are helpful

in applying this logic. This exercise is particularly helpful when analyzing a muscle whose action switches depending on the position of the joint. One such muscle is the posterior deltoid. From the anatomic position the posterior deltoid is an *adductor* of the glenohumeral joint (previously depicted in Fig. 1.20A). If the arm is lifted (abducted) well overhead, however, the line of force of the muscle shifts just to the *superior* side of the axis of rotation. As a consequence, the posterior deltoid actively abducts the shoulder. The example shows how one muscle can have opposite actions depending on the position of the joint at the time of muscle activation. It is important, therefore, to establish a reference position for the joint when analyzing the actions of a muscle. One common reference position is the anatomic position (see Fig. 1.4). Unless otherwise

---

SPECIAL FOCUS 1.4

A Simple but Useful Axiom of Kinesiology

Typically, a contracting muscle with adequate leverage will cause a rotation of the bones around a joint. The expected direction of the rotation, or "muscle action," is traditionally defined by the anticipated movement of the *distal* bony segment of the joint relative to the proximal segment. Consider, for example, the contracting biceps brachii as it flexes the elbow to bring the hand to the mouth. This standard definition of muscle action assumes that the distal segment is less constrained, or less fixed, than the proximal segment.

Perhaps a more inclusive way to consider the effect of a muscle contraction is to use the axiom that a contracting muscle moves the *freest segment of the joint.* Factors that determine the freest segment include some combination of inertia, external resistance, passive tension, or activation of other muscles. Using this axiom can be very enlightening when evaluating human movement, especially when it appears abnormal. Assume that, for example, you observe a person performing active shoulder abduction, and you note an accompanying and obviously abnormal and distorted movement of the scapula. The abnormal scapular movement may

be caused by a contraction of the middle deltoid (which attaches to the scapula) without adequate stabilization provided by an axial-scapular muscle. With weakness of a muscle such as the serratus anterior, for example, contraction of the deltoid causes the *scapula* to be the freest segment of the glenohumeral joint (shoulder segment), not the humerus. Using the traditional assumption that a contracting middle deltoid only abducts the arm (i.e., moves the distal segment of the joint), the identification of axial-scapular muscle weakness may have been overlooked. Although distal-on-proximal segment movement is typically the desired outcome of deltoid activation, this scenario only occurs when the scapula is restrained from moving by activation of other muscles, leaving the humerus as the "freest" segment.

Although this axiom may appear overly simplistic, it can provide useful clinical clues for understanding the pathomechanic origin of certain abnormal movements or postures. Furthermore, the axiom allows the student of kinesiology to understand the large possibilities of actions available to muscles even in the healthy state; *either* segment of a joint is equally likely to move following a muscle contraction.

specified, the actions of muscles described throughout Sections II to IV in this text assume that the joint is in the anatomic position.

Terminology Related to the Actions of Muscles

The following terms are often used when the actions of muscles are described:

- The *agonist* is the muscle or muscle group that is most directly related to the initiation and execution of a particular movement. For example, the tibialis anterior is the agonist for the motion of dorsiflexion of the ankle.
- The *antagonist* is the muscle or muscle group that is considered to have the opposite action of a particular agonist. For example, the gastrocnemius and soleus muscles are considered the antagonists to the tibialis anterior.
- Muscles are considered *synergists* when they cooperate during the execution of a particular movement. Actually, most meaningful movements of the body involve multiple muscles acting as synergists. Consider, for example, the flexor carpi ulnaris and flexor carpi radialis muscles during flexion of the wrist. The muscles act synergistically because they cooperate to flex the wrist. Each muscle, however, must neutralize the other's tendency to move the wrist in a side-to-side (radial and ulnar deviation) fashion. Paralysis of one of the muscles significantly affects the overall action of the other.

Another example of muscle synergy is described as a muscular force-couple. A muscular *force-couple* is formed when two or more muscles simultaneously produce forces in different linear directions, although the resulting torques act in the same rotary direction. A familiar analogy of a force-couple occurs between the two hands while turning the steering wheel of a car. Rotating the steering wheel to the right, for example, can occur by the action of the right hand pulling down and the left hand pulling up on the wheel. Although the hands are producing forces in different linear directions, they cause a torque on the steering wheel in the same rotary direction. The hip flexor and low back extensor muscles, for example, form a force-couple to rotate the pelvis in the sagittal plane around the hip joints (Fig. 1.21).

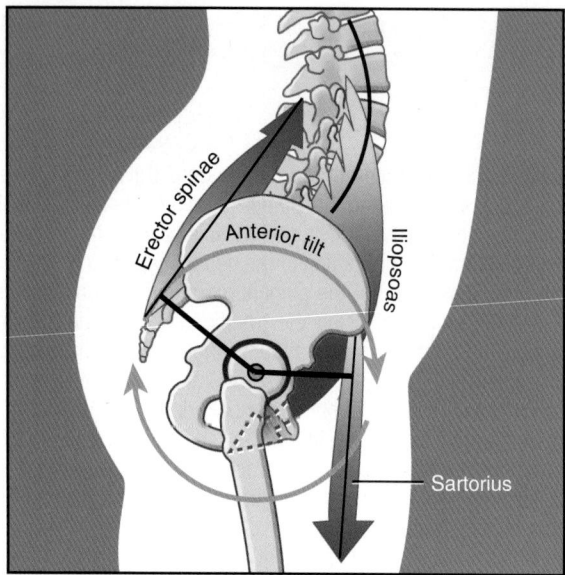

FIG. 1.21 Side view of the force-couple formed between two representative hip flexor muscles (sartorius and iliopsoas) and back extensor muscles (erector spinae) as they contract to tilt the pelvis in an anterior direction. The internal moment arms used by the muscles are indicated by the black lines. The axis of rotation runs through both hip joints.

Musculoskeletal Levers

THREE CLASSES OF LEVERS

Within the body, internal and external forces produce torques through a system of bony levers. Generically speaking, a lever is a simple machine consisting of a rigid rod suspended across a pivot point. The seesaw is a classic example of a first-class lever (Fig. 1.22). One function of a lever is to convert a linear force into a rotary torque. As shown in the seesaw in Fig. 1.22, a 672-N (about 150-lb) man sitting 0.91 m (about 3 ft) from the pivot point produces a torque that balances a boy weighing half his weight who is sitting twice the distance from the pivot point. In Fig. 1.22, the opposing torques are equal $(BW_m \times D = BW_b \times D_1)$: the lever system is balanced and in equilibrium. As indicated, the boy has the greatest leverage $(D_1 > D)$. An important underlying concept of the lever is that with unequal moment arm lengths, the opposing torques can balance each other only if the opposing forces (or body weights in the preceding figure) are of different magnitudes.

The most dominant forces involved with musculoskeletal levers are those produced by muscle, gravity, and physical contact within the environment. The pivot point, or fulcrum, is located at the joint. As with the seesaw, the internal and external torques within the musculoskeletal system may be equal, such as during an isometric activation; or, more often, one of the two opposing torques dominates, resulting in movement at the joint.

Levers are classified as either *first, second,* or *third class* (see inset in Fig. 1.22).

First-Class Lever

As depicted in Fig. 1.22, the first-class lever has its axis of rotation positioned *between* the opposing forces. An example of a first-class lever in the human body is the head-and-neck extensor muscles that control the posture of the head in the sagittal plane (see Fig. 1.23A). As in the seesaw example, the head is held in equilibrium when the product of the muscle force (MF) multiplied by the internal moment arm (IMA) equals the product of head weight (HW) multiplied by its external moment arm (EMA). In first-class levers, the internal and external forces typically act in similar linear directions, although they produce torques in opposing rotary directions.

Second-Class Lever

A second-class lever always has two features. First, its axis of rotation is located at one end of a bone. Second, the muscle, or internal force, possesses greater leverage than the external force. Second-class levers are very rare in the musculoskeletal system. Although likely an oversimplification, the classic example is the calf muscles producing the torque needed to stand on tiptoes (see Fig. 1.23B). The axis of rotation for this action is assumed to act through the metatarsophalangeal joints. Based on this assumption, the internal moment arm used by the calf muscles greatly exceeds the external moment arm used by body weight.

Third-Class Lever

As in the second-class lever, the third-class lever has its axis of rotation located at one end of a bone. The elbow flexor muscles use a third-class lever to produce the flexion torque required to support a weight in the hand (see Fig. 1.23C). Unlike with the

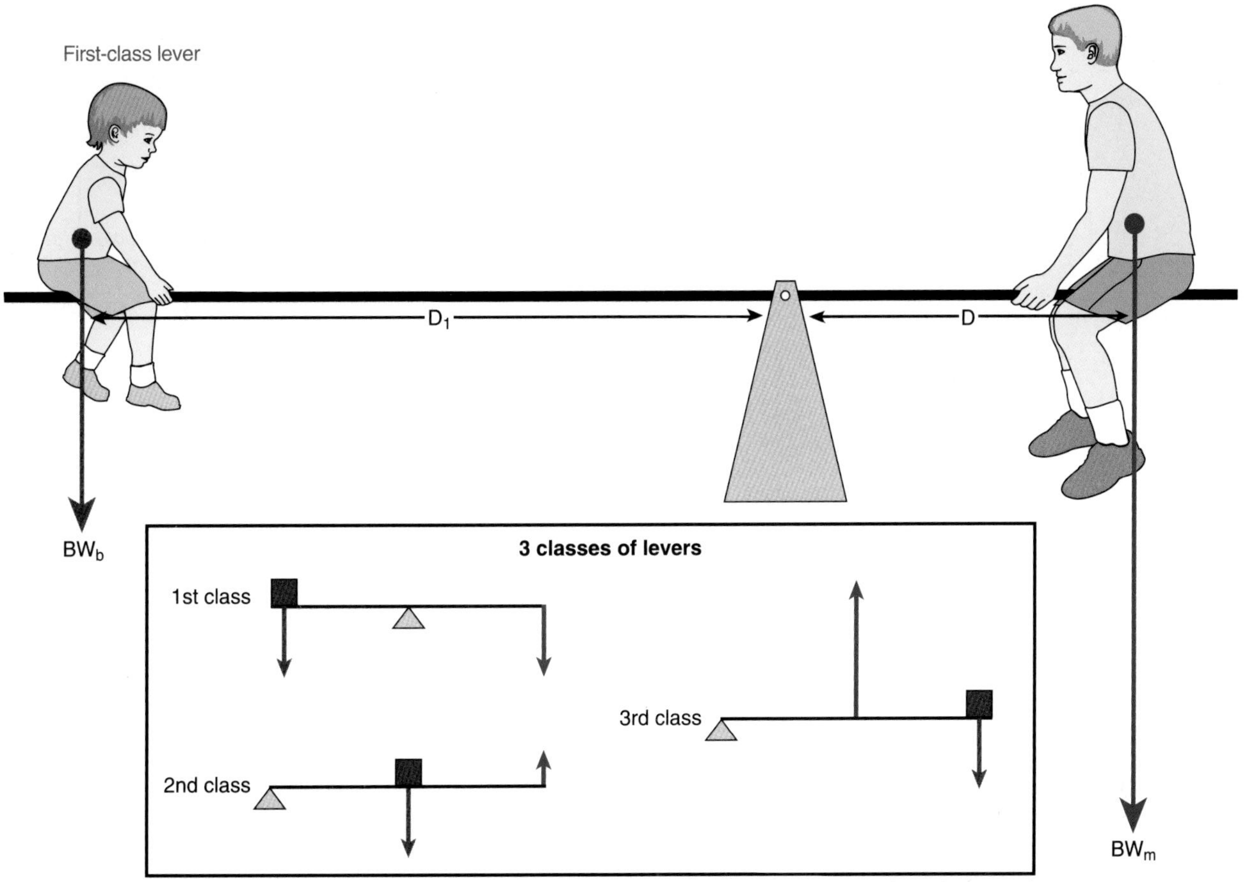

First-class lever

FIG. 1.22 A seesaw is shown as a typical first-class lever. The body weight of the man *(BW_m)* is 672 N (about 150 lb). He is sitting 0.91 m (about 3 ft) from the pivot point (man's moment arm = D). The body weight of the boy *(BW_b)* is only 336 N (about 75 lb). He is sitting 1.82 m (about 6 ft) from the pivot point (boy's moment arm = D_1). The seesaw is balanced because the clockwise torque produced by the man is equal in magnitude to the counterclockwise torque produced by the boy: 672 N × 0.91 m = 336 N × 1.82 m. The inset compares the three classes of levers. In each lever the opposing forces may be considered as an internal force (such as a muscle pull depicted in red) and an external force or load (depicted in gray). The axis of rotation or pivot point is indicated as a wedge. (Force vectors are drawn to scale.)

second-class lever, the external weight supported by a third-class lever *always* has greater leverage than the muscle force. *The third-class lever is the most common lever used by the musculoskeletal system.*

MECHANICAL ADVANTAGE

The *mechanical advantage* (MA) of a musculoskeletal lever can be defined as the ratio of the internal moment arm to the external moment arm. Depending on the location of the axis of rotation, the first-class lever can have an MA equal to, less than, or greater than 1. Second-class levers always have an MA greater than 1. As depicted in the boxes associated with Fig. 1.23A–B, lever systems with an MA greater than 1 are able to balance the torque equilibrium equation by an internal (muscle) force that is *less than* the external force. Third-class levers always have an MA less than 1. As depicted in Fig. 1.23C, to balance the torque equilibrium equation, the muscle must produce a force much *greater than* the opposing external force.

The majority of muscles throughout the musculoskeletal system function with an MA of much *less than 1.* Consider, for example, the biceps at the elbow, the quadriceps at the knee, and the

supraspinatus and deltoid at the shoulder. Each of these muscles attaches to bone relatively close to the joint's axis of rotation. The external forces that oppose the action of the muscles typically exert their influence considerably *distal* to the joint, such as at the hand or the foot. Consider the force demands placed on the supraspinatus and deltoid muscles to maintain the shoulder abducted to 90 degrees while an external weight of 35.6 N (8 lb) is held in the hand. For the sake of this example, assume that the muscles have an internal moment arm of 2.5 cm (about 1 in) and that the center of mass of the external weight has an external moment arm of 50 cm (about 20 in). (For simplicity, the weight of the limb is ignored.) In theory, the 1/20 MA requires that the muscle would have to produce 711.7 N (160 lb) of force, or *20 times* the weight of the external load! (Mathematically stated, the relationship between the muscle force and external load is based on the *inverse* of the MA.) As a general principle, most skeletal muscles produce forces several times larger than the external loads that oppose them. Typically, depending on the shape of the muscle and configuration of the joint, a large percentage of the muscle force produces large compression or shear forces across the joint surfaces. These *myogenic* (muscular-produced) forces are most responsible for the amount and direction of the joint reaction force.

First-class lever

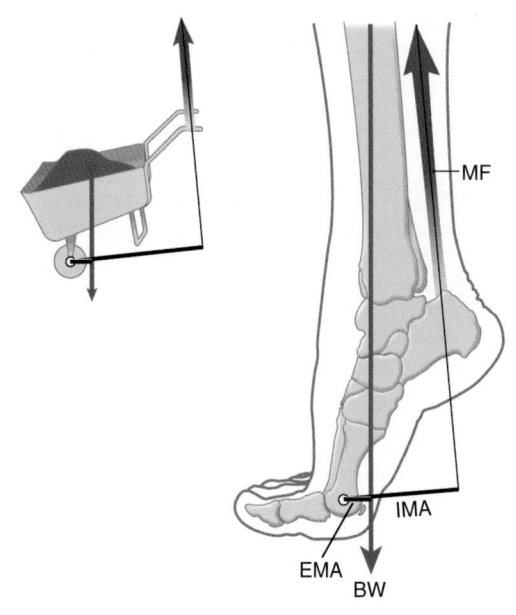

Data for first-class lever:
Muscle force (MF) = unknown
Head weight (HW) = 46.7 N (10.5 lbs)
Internal moment arm (IMA) = 4 cm
External moment arm (EMA) = 3.2 cm
Mechanical advantage = 1.25

$MF \times IMA = HW \times EMA$
$MF = \dfrac{HW \times EMA}{IMA}$
$MF = \dfrac{46.7\ N \times 3.2\ cm}{4\ cm}$
$MF = 37.4\ N\ (8.4\ lbs)$

A

Second-class lever

Data for second-class lever:
Muscle force (MF) = unknown
Body weight (BW) = 667 N (150 lbs)
Internal moment arm (IMA) = 12 cm
External moment arm (EMA) = 3 cm
Mechanical advantage = 4

$MF \times IMA = BW \times EMA$
$MF = \dfrac{BW \times EMA}{IMA}$
$MF = \dfrac{667\ N \times 3\ cm}{12\ cm}$
$MF = 166.8\ N\ (37.5\ lbs)$

B

Third-class lever

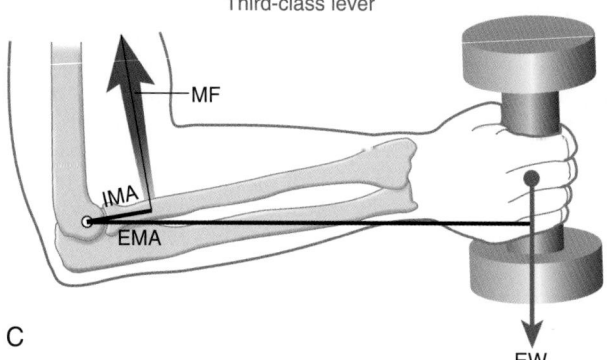

Data for third-class lever:
Muscle force (MF) = unknown
External weight (EW) = 66.7 N (15 lbs)
Internal moment arm (IMA) = 5 cm
External moment arm (EMA) = 35 cm
Mechanical advantage = 0.143

$MF \times IMA = EW \times EMA$
$MF = \dfrac{EW \times EMA}{IMA}$
$MF = \dfrac{66.7\ N \times 35\ cm}{5\ cm}$
$MF = 467\ N\ (105\ lbs)$

C

FIG. 1.23 Anatomic examples are shown of first-class (A), second-class (B), and third-class (C) levers. (The vectors are not drawn to scale.) The data contained in the boxes to the right show how to calculate the muscle force required to maintain static rotary equilibrium. Note that the mechanical advantage is indicated in each box. The muscle activation *(depicted in red)* is isometric in each case, with no movement occurring at the joint.

SPECIAL FOCUS 1.5

Mechanical Advantage: A Closer Look at the Torque Equilibrium Equation

As stated, the mechanical advantage (MA) of a musculoskeletal lever can be defined as the ratio of its internal and external moment arms.

- First-class levers may have an MA less than 1, equal to 1, or greater than 1.
- Second-class levers always have an MA greater than 1.
- Third-class levers always have an MA less than 1.

The mathematic expression of MA is derived from the balance of torque equation:

$$MF \times IMA = EF \times EMA \qquad \text{(Eq. 1.1)}$$

where
MF = Muscle force
EF = External force
IMA = Internal moment arm
EMA = External moment arm
Eq. 1.1 can be rearranged as follows:

$$IMA/EMA = EF/MF \qquad \text{(Eq. 1.2)}$$

- In some first-class levers, IMA/EMA = 1; the torque equation is balanced only when MF = EF.
- In some first-class and all second-class levers, IMA/EMA > 1; the torque equation is balanced only when MF is less than EF.
- In some first-class and all third-class levers, IMA/EMA < 1; the torque equation is balanced only when MF is greater than EF.

As indicated by Eq. 1.2, MA can also be expressed by the ratio of external force to muscle force (EF/MF). Although this is correct, this text uses the convention of defining a muscle-and-joint's MA as the ratio of its internal-to-external moment arms (IMA/EMA).

The Trade-Off Between Force and Distance

As previously described, most muscles are obligated to produce a force much greater than the resistance applied by the external load. At first thought, this design may appear biomechanically flawed. The design is absolutely necessary, however, when considering the many functional movements that require large displacement and velocity of the more distal points of the extremities.

To explain further, consider that *work* is the product of force and the distance through which it is applied. In addition to converting a force to a torque, a musculoskeletal lever converts the work of a contracting muscle to the work of a rotating bone and external load. The MA of a particular musculoskeletal lever dictates *how* the work is to be performed. Because work is the product of force and distance, it can be performed through *either* a relatively large force exerted over a short distance or a small force exerted over a large distance. Consider the small mechanical advantage of 1/20 described earlier for the supraspinatus and deltoid muscles. This MA implies that the muscle must produce a force 20 times greater than the weight of the external load. What must also be considered, however, is that the muscles need to contract only 5% (1/20) the distance that the center of mass of the load would be raised by the abduction action.

A very short contraction distance (excursion) of the muscles produces a much larger vertical displacement of the load. When considering the element of *time* in this example, the muscles produce a relatively large force at a relatively slow contraction *velocity*. The mechanical benefit, however, is that a lighter external load can be lifted at a much faster velocity.

In summary, most muscle and joint systems in the body function with an MA of much less than 1. This being the case, the distance and velocity of the load displacement will always exceed that of the muscle contraction. (This arrangement is functionally advantageous because muscles are only physiologically capable of generating useful forces over a short distance.) Obtaining a high linear velocity of the distal end of the extremities is a necessity for generating large contact forces against the environment. These high forces can be used to rapidly accelerate objects held in the hand, such as a tennis racket, or to accelerate the limbs purely as an expression of art and athleticism, such as dance. Regardless of the nature of the movement, muscle-and-joint systems that operate with an MA of less than 1 must pay a force "penalty" by generating relatively large internal forces, even for seemingly low-load activities. Periarticular tissues, such as articular cartilage, fat pads, and bursa, must partially absorb or dissipate these large myogenic forces. In the absence of such protection, joints may partially degenerate and become painful and chronically inflamed. This presentation is often the hallmark of osteoarthritis.

SYNOPSIS

The human body moves primarily through rotations of its limbs and trunk. Two useful terms that describe these movements are osteokinematics and arthrokinematics. *Osteokinematics* describes movement of the limbs or trunk in one of the three cardinal planes, each occurring around an associated axis of rotation. Osteokinematic descriptors, such as internal rotation or extension, facilitate the study of these movements. *Arthrokinematics* are the movements that occur between the articular surfaces of joints. The wide acceptance of arthrokinematic descriptors such as roll, slide, and spin, for example, has improved the ability of clinicians and students to conceptualize movements that occur at joints. Such terminology is particularly useful when treating disorders that affect the mechanical coordination of kinematics occurring *between* joint surfaces. The strong association between arthrokinematics and articular morphology has stimulated the growth of the topic of arthrology: the study of the structure and function of joints and their surrounding connective tissues. This topic is explored in Chapter 2.

Whereas *kinematics* refers to the *motion* of bones and joints, *kinetics* refers to the *forces* that cause or arrest the motion. Muscles produce the forces that propel the body into motion. A fundamental concept presented in this chapter is an appreciation of how a muscle force acting in a linear direction produces a torque around a joint. An internal torque is the angular expression of a muscle force, with a magnitude that equals the product of the muscle force times its moment arm; both variables are equally important when one considers the strength of a muscle action.

Also important to the study of kinesiology is the understanding of how an external torque affects a joint. An external torque is defined as the product of an external force (such as gravity or physical contact) times its associated moment arm. Ultimately, movement and posture are based on the instantaneous interaction *between* internal and external torques—the prevailing direction and extent of which are determined by the more dominant torque.

Surgically Altering a Muscle's Mechanical Advantage

A surgeon may perform a muscle-tendon transfer operation as a means to partially restore the loss of internal torque at a joint.[1,8] Consider, for example, complete paralysis of the elbow flexor muscles after poliomyelitis. Such a paralysis can have profound functional consequences, especially if it occurs bilaterally. One approach to restoring elbow flexion is to surgically reroute the fully innervated triceps tendon to the anterior side of the elbow (Fig. 1.24). The triceps, now passing anteriorly to the medial-lateral axis of rotation at the elbow, becomes a flexor instead of an extensor. The length of the internal moment arm for the flexion action can be exaggerated, if desired, by increasing the perpendicular distance between the transferred tendon and the axis of rotation. By increasing the muscle's mechanical advantage (MA), the activated muscle produces a *greater torque per level of muscle force.* This may be a beneficial outcome, depending on the specific circumstances of the patient.

An important mechanical trade-off exists whenever a muscle's MA is surgically increased. Although a greater torque is produced per level of muscle force, a given amount of muscle shortening results in a *reduced angular displacement of the joint.* As a result, a full muscle contraction may produce an ample torque, but the joint may not complete its full range of motion. In essence, the active range of motion "lags" behind the muscle contraction. The reduced displacement and velocity of the distal segment of the joint may have negative functional consequences. This mechanical trade-off needs to be considered before the muscle's internal moment arm is surgically enhanced. Often, the greater torque potential gained by increasing the moment arm functionally "outweighs" the loss of the speed and distance of the movement.

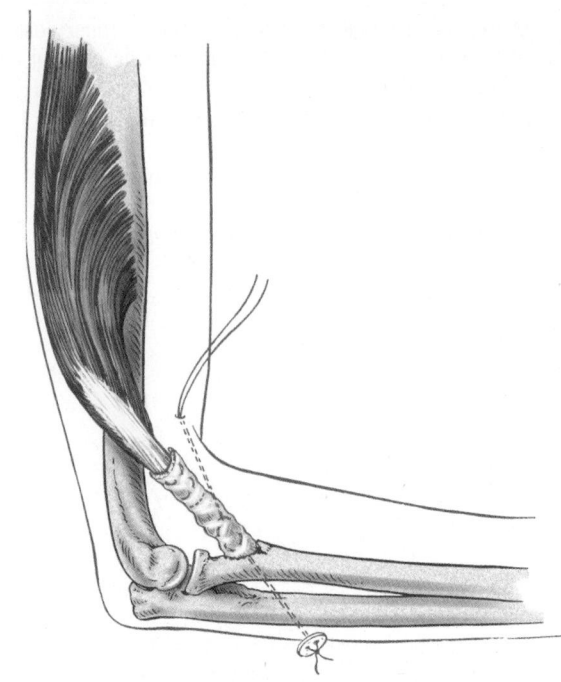

FIG. 1.24 An anterior transfer of the triceps tendon after paralysis of the elbow flexor muscles. The triceps tendon is elongated by a graft of fascia. (From Bunnell S: Restoring flexion to the paralytic elbow, *J Bone Joint Surg Am* 33:566, 1951.)

Most muscles in the body act through a skeletal lever system with a mechanical advantage of much less than 1. This design favors a relatively high speed and large displacement of the distal end of the extremities. This so-called biomechanical "advantage" is at the expense of a muscle force that is usually much *larger* than the combined weight of the limb and supported external load. The obligatory large muscle forces are usually directed across the articular surfaces of joints and on to bone and are most often described in terms of compression and shear. In order for these forces to be physiologically tolerated over a lifetime, the articular ends of most bones are relatively large, thereby increasing their surface area as a means to reduce peak contact pressure. Additional protection is provided through the presence of a sponge-like, relatively absorbent subchondral bone located just deep to articular cartilage. These features are essential for the dissipation of forces that would otherwise cause degeneration, possibly leading to osteoarthritis.

The study of kinesiology pays strict attention to the actions of individual muscles and their unique lines of force relative to the joints' axes of rotation. Once this is understood, the focus of study typically shifts to understanding how multiple muscles cooperate to control complex movements, often across multiple joints. Muscles act synergistically with one another for many reasons. Muscular interactions may serve to stabilize proximal attachment sites, neutralize unwanted secondary or tertiary actions, or simply augment the power, strength, or control of a particular movement. When muscle function is disrupted by disease or injury, the lack of such synergy is often responsible for the pathomechanics of a movement. Consider, for example, the consequences of paralysis or weakness of a selected few muscles within a functional muscle group. Even the healthy unaffected muscles (when acting in relative isolation) have a dominant role in an abnormal movement pattern. The resulting kinetic imbalance across the region can lead to certain compensatory movements or postures, possibly causing deformity and reduced function. Understanding how muscles interact normally is a prerequisite to comprehending the overall pathomechanics of the region. Such an understanding serves as the foundation for designing effective therapeutic interventions, aimed at restoring or maximizing function.

Kinesiology is the study of human motion, studied both in healthy, ideal conditions and in those conditions affected by trauma, disease, or disuse. To facilitate this study, this textbook focuses heavily on the structure and function of the musculoskeletal system. A strong emphasis is placed on the interactions between the forces and tensions created by muscles, gravity, and connective tissues that surround the joints. This chapter has helped to establish a foundation of many of the basic concepts and terminology used throughout this textbook.

GLOSSARY

Acceleration: change in velocity of a body over time, expressed in linear (m/sec²) and angular (degrees/sec²) terms.

Accessory Movements: slight, passive, nonvolitional movements allowed in most joints (also called *joint play*).

Active Force: push or pull generated by stimulated muscle.

Active Movement: motion caused by stimulated muscle.

Agonist Muscle: muscle or muscle group that is most directly related to the initiation and execution of a particular movement.

Anatomic Position: the generally agreed upon reference position of the body used to describe the location and movement of its parts. In this position, a person is standing fully upright and looking forward, with arms resting by the side, forearms fully supinated, and fingers extended.

Angle-of-Insertion: angle formed between a tendon of a muscle and the long axis of the bone into which it inserts.

Antagonist Muscle: muscle or muscle group that has the action opposite to a particular agonist muscle.

Arthrokinematics: motions of roll, slide, and spin that occur between curved articular surfaces of joints.

Axial Rotation: angular motion of an object in a direction perpendicular to its longitudinal axis; often used to describe a motion in the horizontal plane.

Axis of Rotation: an imaginary line extending through a joint around which rotation occurs (also called the *pivot point* or the *center of rotation*).

Bending: effect of a force that deforms a material at right angles to its long axis. A bent tissue is compressed on its concave side and placed under tension on its convex side. A bending moment is a quantitative measure of a bend. Similar to a torque, a bending moment is the product of the bending force and the perpendicular distance between the force and the axis of rotation of the bend.

Center of Mass: point at the exact center of an object's mass (also referred to as *center of gravity* when considering the weight of the mass).

Close-Packed Position: unique position of most joints of the body where the articular surfaces are most congruent and the ligaments are maximally taut.

Compliance: the inverse of stiffness.

Compression: a perpendicularly applied force that pushes one surface directly against another.

Concentric Activation: process by which an activated muscle shortens as it produces a pulling force.

Creep: a progressive strain of a material when exposed to a constant load over time.

Degrees of Freedom: number of planes of movement that are under volitional control at a joint. A joint can have up to three degrees of translation and three degrees of rotation.

Displacement: change in the linear or angular position of an object.

Distal-on-Proximal Segment Kinematics: type of movement in which the distal segment of a joint rotates relative to a fixed proximal segment (also called *an open kinematic chain*).

Distraction: a force, applied perpendicularly to the contact surface, that pushes or pulls one object directly away from another.

Eccentric Activation: process by which an activated muscle produces a pulling force while simultaneously being elongated by another more dominant force.

Elasticity: property of a material demonstrated by its ability to return to its original length after the removal of a deforming force.

External Force: push or pull produced by sources located *outside* the body. These typically include gravity and physical contact applied against the body.

External Moment Arm: perpendicular distance between an axis of rotation and the external force.

External Torque: product of an external force and its external moment arm (also called *external moment*).

Force: a push or a pull that produces, arrests, or modifies a motion.

Force-Couple: two or more muscles acting in different linear directions but producing a torque in the same rotary direction.

Friction: resistance to movement between two contacting surfaces.

Gravity: force resulting from potential acceleration of a body toward the center of the Earth.

Internal Force: push or pull produced by a structure located within the body. Most often, *internal force* refers to the force produced by an active muscle.

Internal Moment Arm: perpendicular distance between the axis of rotation and the internal (muscle) force.

Internal Torque: product of an internal force and its internal moment arm.

Isometric Activation: process by which an activated muscle maintains a constant length as it produces a pulling force.

Joint Reaction Force: force that exists at a joint, developed in reaction to the net effect of internal and external forces. The joint reaction force includes contact forces between joint surfaces, as well as forces from any periarticular structure.

Kinematics: branch of mechanics that describes the motion of a body, without regard to the forces or torques that may produce the motion.

Kinematic Chain: series of articulated segmented links, such as the pelvis, thigh, leg, and foot.

Kinetics: branch of mechanics that describes the effect of forces and torques on the body.

Leverage: relative moment arm length possessed by a particular force.

Line of Force: direction and orientation of a muscle's force.

Line of Gravity: direction and orientation of the gravitational pull on a body.

Load: general term that describes the application of a force to a body.

Longitudinal Axis: axis that extends within and parallel to a long bone or body segment.

Loose-Packed Positions: positions of most synovial joints of the body in which the articular surfaces are least congruent and the ligaments are slackened (also referred to as *open-packed positions*).

Mass: quantity of matter in an object.

Mechanical Advantage: ratio of the internal moment arm to the external moment arm.

Moment Arm: perpendicular distance between an axis of rotation and the line of force.

Muscle Action: potential of a muscle to produce a torque within a particular plane of motion and rotation direction (also called *joint action* when referring specifically to a muscle's potential to rotate a joint). Terms that describe a muscle action are flexion, extension, pronation, supination, and so forth.

Osteokinematics: motion of bones relative to the three cardinal, or principal, planes.

Passive Force: push or pull generated by sources other than stimulated muscle, such as tension in stretched periarticular connective tissues, physical contact, and so forth.

Passive Movement: motion produced by a source other than activated muscle.

Plasticity: property of a material demonstrated by remaining permanently deformed after the removal of a force.

Pressure: force divided by a surface area.

Productive Antagonism: phenomenon in which relatively low-level tension within stretched connective tissues performs a useful function.

Proximal-on-Distal Segment Kinematics: type of movement in which the proximal segment of a joint rotates relative to a fixed distal segment (also referred to as a *closed kinematic chain*).

Roll: arthrokinematic term that describes when multiple points on one rotating articular surface contact multiple points on another articular surface.

Rotation: angular motion in which a rigid body moves in a circular path around a pivot point or an axis of rotation.

Scalar: quantity, such as speed, work, or temperature that is completely described by its magnitude and has no direction.

Segment: any part of a body or limb.

Shear: a force produced as two compressed objects slide past each other in opposite directions (like the action of two blades on a pair of scissors).

Shock Absorption: the act of dissipating a force.

Slide: arthrokinematic term describing when a single point on one articular surface contacts multiple points on another articular surface (also called *glide*).

Spin: arthrokinematic term describing when a single point on one articular surface rotates on a single point on another articular surface (like a top).

Static Linear Equilibrium: state of a body at rest in which the sum of all forces is equal to zero.

Static Rotary Equilibrium: state of a body at rest in which the sum of all torques is equal to zero.

Stiffness: ratio of stress (force per unit area) to strain (percent elongation) within an elastic material, or N/m^2 (also referred to as *Young's modulus* or *modulus of elasticity*).

Strain: ratio of a tissue's deformed length to its original length. As it is a measure of relative length change, it has no units.

Stress: a tissue's resistance to deformation, equal to the force applied to the tissue divided by its cross-sectional area; stress is an intrinsic material property. (The term "stress" is often used informally to describe generalized physical trauma or overload of a tissue.)

Synergists: two or more muscles that cooperate to execute a particular movement.

Tension: a force that pulls apart or separates a material (also called a *distraction force*).

Torque: a force multiplied by its moment arm; tends to rotate a body or segment around an axis of rotation.

Torsion: application of a force that twists a material around its longitudinal axis.

Translation: linear motion in which all parts of a rigid body move parallel to and in the same direction as every other point in the body.

Ultimate Failure Point: length at which a tissue structurally fails and loses its ability to hold a load.

Vector: quantity, such as velocity or force that is completely described by its magnitude and direction.

Velocity: change in position of a body over time, expressed in linear (m/sec) and angular (degrees/sec) terms.

Viscoelasticity: property of a material expressed by a changing stress-strain relationship as a function of time.

Weight: gravitational force acting on a mass.

REFERENCES

1. Brand PW: *Clinical biomechanics of the hand*, St Louis, 1985, Mosby.
2. Busscher I, van Dieen JH, van der Veen AJ, et al.: The effects of creep and recovery on the in vitro biomechanical characteristics of human multi-level thoracolumbar spinal segments, *Clin Biomech* 26(5):438–444, 2011.
3. Butler DL, Guan Y, Kay MD, et al.: Location-dependent variations in the material properties of the anterior cruciate ligament, *J Biomech* 25(5):511–518, 1992.
4. Cannon J, Cambridge EDJ, McGill SM: Increased core stability is associated with reduced knee valgus during single-leg landing tasks: investigating lumbar spine and hip joint rotational stiffness, *J Biomech* 116:110240, 2021.
5. Englander ZA, Garrett WE, Spritzer CE, et al.: In Vivo attachment site to attachment site length and strain of the ACL and its bundles during the full gait cycle measured by MRI and high-speed biplanar radiography, *J Biomech* 98:109443, 2020.
6. Escamilla RF, MacLeod TD, Wilk KE, et al.: Anterior cruciate ligament strain and tensile forces for weight-bearing and non-weight-bearing exercises: a guide to exercise selection, *J Orthop Sports Phys Ther* 42(3):208–220, 2012.
7. Fleming BC, Beynnon BD, Renstrom PA, et al.: The strain behavior of the anterior cruciate ligament during bicycling. An in vivo study, *Am J Sports Med* 26:109–118, 1998.
8. Kirby DJ, Merkow DB, Catalano WL, et al.: A brief history of tendon transfer and, specifically, the opposition tendon transfer, *Bull Hosp Jt Dis* 80(2):186–189, 2022.
9. Knaus KR, Handsfield GG, Blemker SS: A 3D model of the soleus reveals effects of aponeuroses morphology and material properties on complex muscle fascicle behavior, *J Biomech* 130:110877, 2022.
10. Lipps DB, Wojtys EM, Ashton-Miller JA: Anterior cruciate ligament fatigue failures in knees subjected to repeated simulated pivot landings, *Am J Sports Med* 41(5):1058–1066, 2013.
11. Neumann DA: Arthrokinematics: flawed or just misinterpreted? *J Orthop Sports Phys Ther* 34:428–429, 2012.
12. Noehren B, Snyder-Mackler L: Who's afraid of the big bad wolf? open-chain exercises after anterior cruciate ligament reconstruction, *J Orthop Sports Phys Ther* 50(9):473–475, 2020.
13. Olesen AT, Malchow-Møller L, Bendixen RD, et al.: Intramuscular connective tissue content and mechanical properties: Influence of aging and physical activity in mice, *Exp Gerontol* 166:111893, 2022.
14. Perriman A, Leahy E, Semciw AI: The effect of open-versus closed-kinetic-chain exercises on anterior tibial laxity, strength, and function following anterior cruciate ligament reconstruction: a systematic review and meta-analysis, *J Orthop Sports Phys Ther* 48(7):552–566, 2018.
15. Scarvell JM, Hribar N, Galvin CR, et al.: Analysis of kneeling by medical imaging shows the femur moves back to the posterior rim of the tibial plateau, prompting review of the concave-convex rule, *Phys Ther* 99(3):311–318, 2019.
16. Standring S: *Gray's anatomy: the anatomical basis of clinical practice*, ed 42, St Louis, 2021, Elsevier.
17. Wiesinger HP, Seynnes OR, Kösters A, et al.: Mechanical and material tendon properties in patients with proximal patellar tendinopathy, *Front Physiol* 11:704, 2020.
18. Wilk KE, Arrigo CA, Bagwell MS, et al.: Considerations with open kinetic chain knee extension exercise following ACL reconstruction, *Int J Sports Phys Ther* 16(1):282–284, 2021.

STUDY QUESTIONS

1. Contrast the fundamental difference between *kinematics* and *kinetics*.
2. Describe a particular movement of the body or body segment that incorporates both *translation* and *rotation* kinematics.
3. Note the accessory movements at your metacarpophalangeal joint of your index finger in full flexion and in full extension. Which position has greater accessory movements? Which position (flexion or extension) would you assume is the joint's close-packed position?
4. Fig. 1.8 depicts the three fundamental movements between joint surfaces for both convex-on-concave and concave-on-convex arthrokinematics. Using a skeleton or an image of a skeleton, cite an example of a specific movement at a joint that matches each of these six situations. NOTE: Examples may include *combinations* of roll-and-slide.
5. Provide examples of how the six forces depicted in Fig. 1.12 could naturally occur at either the disc or spinal cord associated with the junction of the fifth and sixth cervical vertebrae.
6. Contrast the fundamental differences between *force* and *torque*. Use each term to describe a particular aspect of a muscle's contraction relative to a joint.
7. Define and contrast *internal torque* and *external torque*.
8. The elbow model in Fig. 1.17 is assumed to be in static equilibrium. While maintaining this equilibrium, how would a change in the variables EF, D_1, or D independently affect the required amount of internal force (IF)? How can a change in these variables "protect" an arthritic joint from unnecessarily large joint reaction forces?
9. Slowly lowering a book to the table uses an eccentric activation of the elbow flexor muscles. Explain how changing the speed at which you lower the book can affect the type of activation (e.g., eccentric, concentric) and choice of muscle.
10. Assume a surgeon performs a tendon transfer surgery to increase the internal moment arm of a particular muscle relative to a joint. Are there potential negative biomechanical consequences of increasing the muscle's moment arm (leverage) too far? If so, please explain.
11. Describe a possible pathologic situation in which the inferior-directed joint reaction force (JFR) depicted Fig. 1.16B is *not* able to be generated by the distal humerus.
12. What is the difference between force and pressure? How could these differences apply to protecting the skin of a patient with a spinal cord injury and reduced sensation?
13. Describe the difference between mass and weight.
14. Most muscle and joint systems within the body function as *third-class levers. Cite a biomechanic or physiologic reason for this design.
15. Assume a patient developed adhesions with marked increased stiffness in the posterior capsular ligaments of his knee. How would this change in tissue property affect full *passive* range of motion at the joint?

Answers to the study questions can be found in the accompanying enhanced eBook version included with the print purchase of this textbook.

Arthrology: The Study of the Structure and Function of Human Joints

LAUREN K. SARA, PT, DPT, PhD
DONALD A. NEUMANN, PT, PhD, FAPTA

Arthrology is the study of the classification, structure, and function of joints. "*Joint*" refers to the junction or pivot point between two or more bones. Movement of the body occurs primarily through rotation of bones around individual joints; therefore, understanding a joint and its periarticular connective tissues is foundational to the study of kinesiology. Joints also transfer and disperse internal and external forces. Long-term immobilization, trauma, disease, and aging all affect the structure and ultimate function of joints. These factors also significantly influence the quality and quantity of human movement.

This chapter focuses on the anatomic structure and function of joints, including the role of periarticular connective tissues in promoting stability and mobility of joints. The chapters contained in Sections II to IV of this text describe the specific anatomy and detailed function of the individual joints throughout the body. This information is a prerequisite for understanding impairments of joints as well as for selecting the most effective rehabilitation interventions and preventative measures for persons with joint dysfunction.

CLASSIFICATION OF JOINTS BASED ON MOVEMENT POTENTIAL

One method to classify joints focuses primarily on their movement potential. Based on this scheme, two major types of joints exist within the body: *synarthroses* and *diarthroses* (Fig. 2.1).

Synarthroses

A *synarthrosis* is a junction between bones that allows relatively slight to essentially no movement. Synarthrodial joints are described

Classification of joints

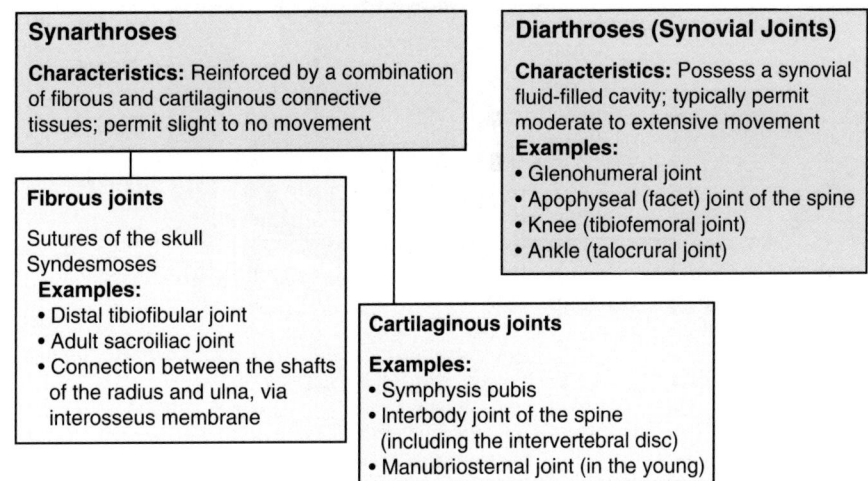

FIG. 2.1 A classification scheme for describing two main types of articulations found in the musculoskeletal system. Synarthrodial joints can be further classified as either fibrous or cartilaginous.

as *fibrous* or *cartilaginous.* This classification is based on the dominant type of periarticular connective tissue that reinforces the articulation.[132]

As the name implies, *fibrous joints* are stabilized by fibrous connective tissues. These relatively rigid joints are further categorized as either sutures, referring to the sutures of the skull, or syndesmoses. A syndesmosis is reinforced by either fibrous cords, a dense fibrous membrane, or an interosseus ligament. Examples of a syndesmosis include the distal tibiofibular joint, adult sacroiliac joint, and the membranous junction between the shafts of the radius and ulna.

While *cartilaginous joints* are also limited in their movement potential, they are often less rigid than fibrous joints. They are stabilized by varying forms of fibrocartilage or hyaline cartilage and are occasionally supported by ligaments. Cartilaginous joints generally exist in the midline of the body, such as the symphysis pubis, the interbody joints of the spine, and, in the young, the manubriosternal joint.

Synarthrodial joints are well supported by periarticular connective tissues. As a rule, this anatomic arrangement limits movement and provides functional stability to the articulation or region. With aging, some synarthrodial joints, such as the sacroiliac joints, naturally become more rigid as their supporting tissues partially ossify. Ossification further limits the movement in these joints, thereby enhancing their ability to stabilize across a region in the growing adult.

Diarthroses: Synovial Joints

A *diarthrosis* is an articulation that typically allows moderate to extensive motion. These joints also possess a synovial fluid–filled cavity. Because of this feature, diarthrodial joints are frequently referred to as *synovial joints.* Most joints within the musculoskeletal system are synovial joints.

Diarthrodial, or synovial, joints are specialized for movement and always exhibit seven elements (Fig. 2.2). *Articular cartilage*

covers the articular surfaces of bones. The joint is enclosed by connective tissues that form the *joint capsule* (also referred to as the articular capsule). The joint capsule is composed of two histologically distinct layers. The external, or fibrous, layer is composed of dense connective tissue. This part of the joint capsule provides support between the bones and containment of the joint contents. The internal layer of the joint capsule consists of a *synovial membrane,* which averages 3 to 10 cell layers thick. The cells within this specialized connective tissue manufacture a *synovial fluid* that is usually clear or pale yellow, with a slightly viscous consistency.[132] The synovial fluid contains many of the proteins found in blood plasma, including hyaluronan and other lubricating glycoproteins.[132,157] The synovial fluid coats the articular surfaces of the joint. This fluid reduces the friction between the joint surfaces as well as provides nourishment to the articular cartilage.

Ligaments are connective tissues that attach between bones, thereby protecting the joint from excessive movement. The thickness of ligaments differs considerably depending on the functional demands placed on the joint. Most ligaments can be described as either capsular or extracapsular. Capsular ligaments are usually thickenings of the articular capsule, such as the glenohumeral ligaments and deeper parts of the medial (tibial) collateral ligament of the knee. Capsular ligaments typically consist of a broad sheet of fibers that, when pulled taut, resist movements in two or often three planes. Most extracapsular ligaments are more cordlike and may be partially or completely separate from the joint capsule. Consider, for example, the lateral (fibular) collateral ligament of the knee or the alar ligament of the craniocervical region. These more discrete ligaments are usually oriented in a specific manner to optimally resist movement in just one or two planes.

Small *blood vessels* (i.e., capillaries) penetrate the joint capsule, usually as deep as the junction of the fibrous layer of the joint capsule and the adjacent synovial membrane. *Sensory nerves* also supply the external layer of the capsule and ligaments with receptors for pain and proprioception.

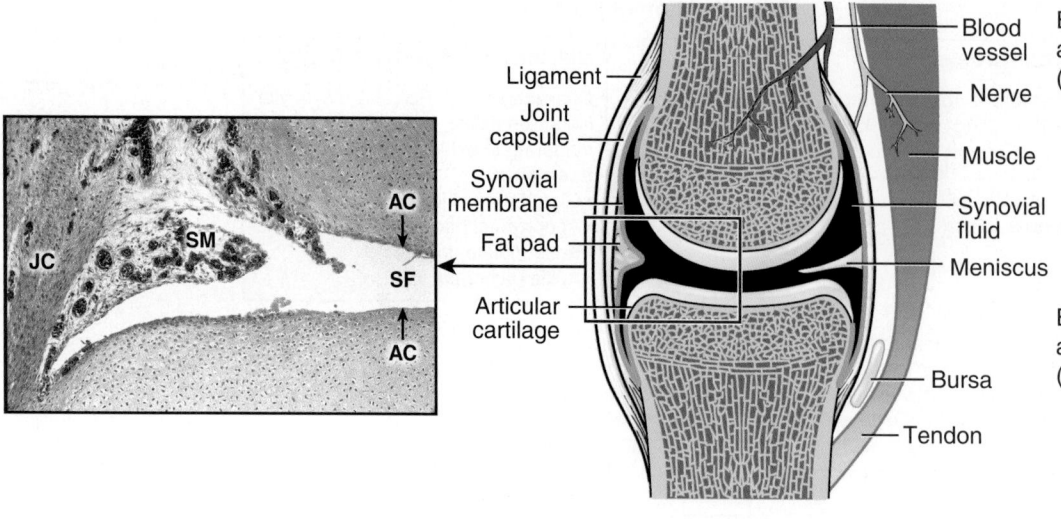

Blood vessel
Ligament
Nerve
Joint capsule
Muscle
Synovial membrane
Synovial fluid
Fat pad
Meniscus
Articular cartilage
Bursa
Tendon

Elements ALWAYS associated with diarthrodial (synovial) joints
• Articular cartilage
• Joint (articular) capsule
• Synovial membrane
• Synovial fluid
• Ligaments
• Blood vessels
• Sensory nerves

Elements SOMETIMES associated with diarthrodial (synovial) joints
• Intra-articular discs or menisci
• Peripheral labra
• Fat pads
• Bursae
• Synovial plicae

FIG. 2.2 Elements associated with a generic diarthrodial (synovial) joint. Note that a peripheral labrum and plica are not included in the illustration. The inset (left) is a section of a human fetal joint as viewed through a microscope and represents the tissues depicted in the boxed region of the main illustration. Highlighted in this image are the joint capsule *(JC)*, synovial membrane *(SM)*, synovial fluid *(SF)*, and articular cartilage surfaces *(AC)*. (Inset from Standring S: *Gray's anatomy: the anatomical basis of clinical practice,* ed 42, St Louis, 2020, Elsevier.)

There are additional elements that appear in only some synovial joints, which accommodate the wide spectrum of joint shapes and functional demands (see Fig. 2.2). *Intra-articular discs,* or *menisci,* are pads of fibrocartilage imposed between articular surfaces. These structures increase articular congruency and improve force dispersion. Intra-articular discs and menisci are found in several joints of the body (see box below).

Intra-articular Discs (Menisci) Found in Several Synovial Joints of the Body
• Tibiofemoral (knee)
• Distal radio-ulnar
• Sternoclavicular
• Acromioclavicular
• Temporomandibular
• Apophyseal (variable)

A *peripheral labrum* of fibrocartilage extends from the bony rims of the glenoid fossa of the shoulder and the acetabulum of the hip. These specialized structures deepen the concave member of these joints and support and thicken the attachment of the joint capsule. *Fat pads* may reinforce the internal aspects of the capsule as well as fill nonarticulating joint spaces (i.e., recesses) formed by incongruent bony contours. In doing so, fat pads reduce the volume of synovial fluid necessary for proper joint function. They are variable in size and positioned within the substance of the joint capsule, often interposed between the fibrous layer and the synovial membrane. If these fat pads become enlarged or inflamed, they may alter the mechanics of the joint. Fat pads are most prominent in the elbow and the knee joints.

Bursae often form adjacent to fat pads. A bursa is an extension or outpouching of the synovial membrane of a diarthrodial joint. Bursae are filled with synovial fluid and usually exist in areas of potential stress. Like fat pads, bursae help absorb force and protect periarticular connective tissues, including bone. The subacromial bursa in the shoulder, for example, is located between the undersurface of the acromion of the scapula and the head of the humerus.[64] The bursa may become inflamed because of repetitive compression between the humerus and the acromion. This condition is frequently referred to as *subacromial bursitis.*

Synovial plicae (i.e., synovial folds, synovial redundancies, or synovial fringes) are slack, overlapped pleats of tissue composed of the innermost layers of the joint capsule. They occur normally in joints with large capsular surface areas such as the knee and elbow. Plicae increase synovial surface area and allow full joint motion without undue tension on the synovial lining. If these folds are too extensive or become thickened or adherent because of inflammation, they can produce pain and altered joint mechanics. The plicae of the knee are further described in Chapter 13.

CLASSIFICATION OF SYNOVIAL JOINTS BASED ON MECHANICAL ANALOGY

Thus far in this chapter, joints have been classified into two broad categories based primarily on movement potential. Because an in-depth understanding of synovial joints is so crucial to an understanding of the mechanics of movement, they are here further classified using an analogy to familiar mechanical objects or shapes (Table 2.1).

A *hinge joint* is generally analogous to the hinge of a door, formed by a central pin surrounded by a larger hollow cylinder (Fig. 2.3A). Angular motion at hinge joints occurs primarily in a plane perpendicular to the hinge, or axis of rotation. The humero-ulnar joint is a clear example of a hinge joint (see Fig. 2.3B). As in all synovial joints, slight translation (i.e., sliding) is allowed in addition to the rotation. Although the mechanical similarity is less complete, the interphalangeal joints of the digits are also classified as hinge joints.

TABLE 2.1 Classification of Synovial Joints Based on Mechanical Analogy

	Primary Angular Motions	Mechanical Analogy	Anatomic Examples
Hinge joint	Flexion and extension only	Door hinge	Humero-ulnar joint Interphalangeal joint
Pivot joint	Spinning of one member around a single axis of rotation	Doorknob	Humeroradial joint Atlanto-axial joint
Ellipsoid joint	Biplanar motion (flexion-extension and abduction-adduction)	Flattened convex ellipsoid paired with a concave trough	Radiocarpal joint
Ball-and-socket joint	Triplanar motion (flexion-extension, abduction-adduction, and internal-external rotation)	Spherical convex surface paired with a concave cup	Glenohumeral joint Coxofemoral (hip) joint
Plane joint	Typical motions include slide (translation) or combined slide and rotation	Relatively flat surfaces apposing each other, like a book on a table	Intercarpal or intertarsal joints Carpometacarpal joints of digits II–V (often called modified plane joints)
Saddle joint	Biplanar motion; spin between bones is possible but may be limited by the interlocking nature of the joint	Each member has a reciprocally curved concave and convex surface oriented at right angles to the other, like a horse rider and a saddle	Carpometacarpal joint of the thumb Sternoclavicular joint
Condyloid joint	Biplanar motion; either flexion-extension and abduction-adduction, or flexion-extension and axial rotation (internal-external rotation)	Mostly spherical convex surface that is enlarged in one dimension like a knuckle; paired with a shallow concave cup	Metacarpophalangeal joint Tibiofemoral (knee) joint

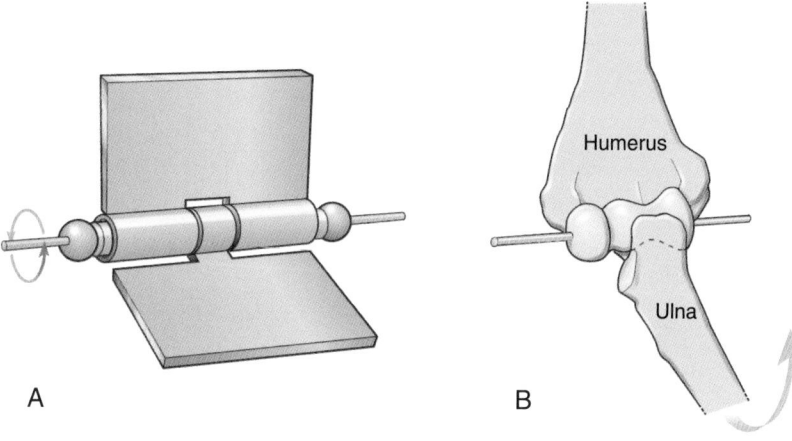

FIG. 2.3 A hinge joint (A) is illustrated as analogous to the humero-ulnar joint (B). The axis of rotation (i.e., pivot point) is represented by the pin.

A *pivot joint* is formed by a central pin surrounded by a larger cylinder. Unlike a hinge, the mobile member of a pivot joint is oriented parallel to the axis of rotation. This mechanical orientation produces the primary angular motion of spin, like a doorknob's spin around a central axis (Fig. 2.4A). Two examples of pivot joints are the humeroradial joint, shown in Fig. 2.4B, and the atlanto-axial joint in the craniocervical region.

An *ellipsoid joint* has one partner with a convex elongated surface in one dimension that is mated with a similarly elongated concave surface on the second partner (Fig. 2.5A). The elliptic mating surfaces restrict the spin between the two surfaces but allow biplanar motions, usually defined as flexion-extension and abduction-adduction. The radiocarpal joint is an example of an ellipsoid joint (see Fig. 2.5B). The flattened convex member of the joint (i.e., carpal bones) limits the spin within the matching concavity (i.e., distal radius).

A *ball-and-socket joint* has a spherical convex surface that is paired with a cuplike socket (Fig. 2.6A). Unlike the ellipsoid joint, this joint provides motion in three planes because the symmetry of curves of its two mating surfaces allows spin without potential dislocation. Ball-and-socket joints within the body include the glenohumeral joint and the hip joint (Fig. 2.6B). As will be described further in Chapter 5, most of the concavity of the glenohumeral joint is formed not only by the glenoid fossa, but also by the surrounding muscle, labrum, joint capsule, and capsular ligaments.

A *plane joint* is the pairing of two flat or minimally curved surfaces. Movements combine sliding and some rotation of one partner with respect to the other, much as a book can slide or rotate across a tabletop (Fig. 2.7A). Because plane joints lack a definitive axis of rotation, they are typically not described in terms of degrees of freedom. As depicted in Fig. 2.7B, the carpometacarpal joints within

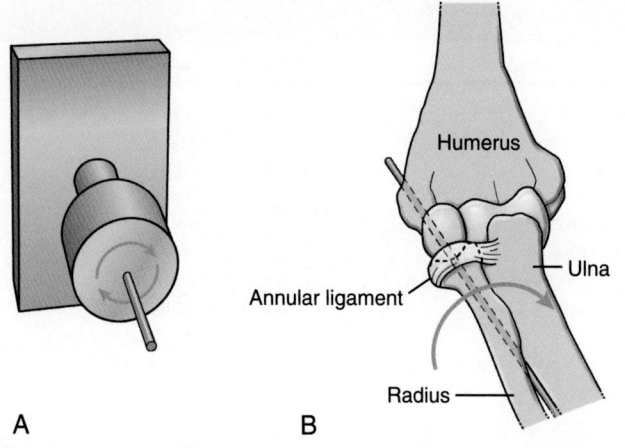

FIG. 2.4 A pivot joint (A) is shown as analogous to the humeroradial joint (B). The axis of rotation is represented by the pin, extending through the capitulum of the humerus.

digits II to V are often considered plane—or modified plane—joints. Many intercarpal and intertarsal joints are also considered plane joints. The forces that cause or restrict movement between the bones are supplied by tension in muscles or ligaments.

Each partner of a *saddle joint* has two surfaces: one surface is concave, and the other is convex. These surfaces are oriented at approximate right angles to each other and are reciprocally curved. The shape of a saddle joint is best visualized using the analogy of a horse's saddle and rider (Fig. 2.8A). From front to back, the saddle presents a concave surface reaching from the saddle pommel in front to the cantle (the raised, curved part) in back. From side to side, the saddle is convex, stretching from one stirrup across the back of the horse to the other stirrup. The rider has reciprocal convex and concave curves to complement the shape of the saddle. The carpometacarpal joint of the thumb is the clearest example of a saddle joint (see Fig. 2.8B). The reciprocal, interlocking nature of this joint allows ample motion in two planes but limited spin between the trapezium and the first metacarpal.

FIG. 2.5 An ellipsoid joint (A) is shown as analogous to the radiocarpal joint (wrist) (B). The two axes of rotation are shown by the intersecting pins.

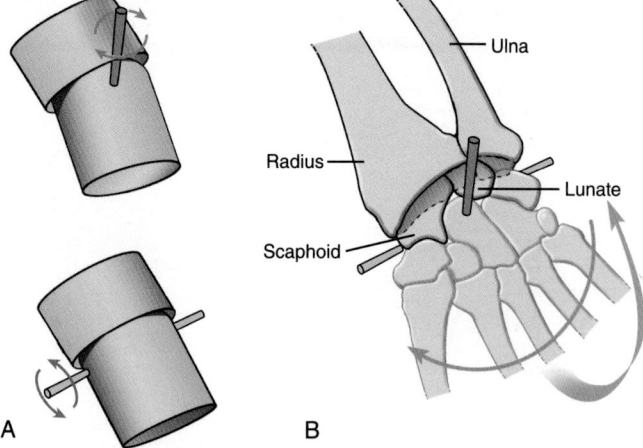

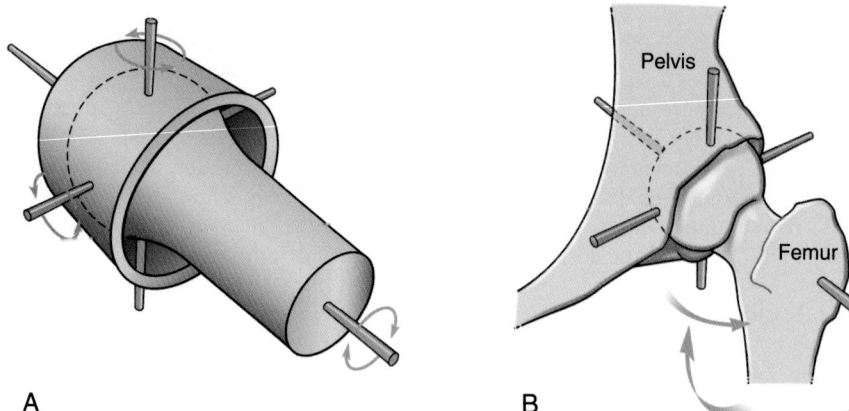

FIG. 2.6 A ball-and-socket articulation (A) is drawn as analogous to the hip joint (B). The three axes of rotation are represented by the three intersecting pins.

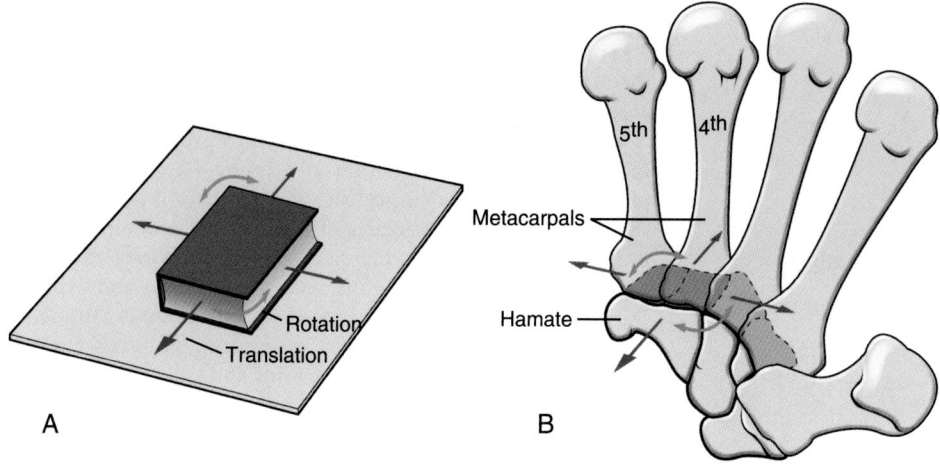

FIG. 2.7 A plane joint is formed by the opposition of two flat or slightly curved surfaces. The book moving on the tabletop (A) is depicted as analogous to the combined slide and rotation at the carpometacarpal joints of digits II–V (B).

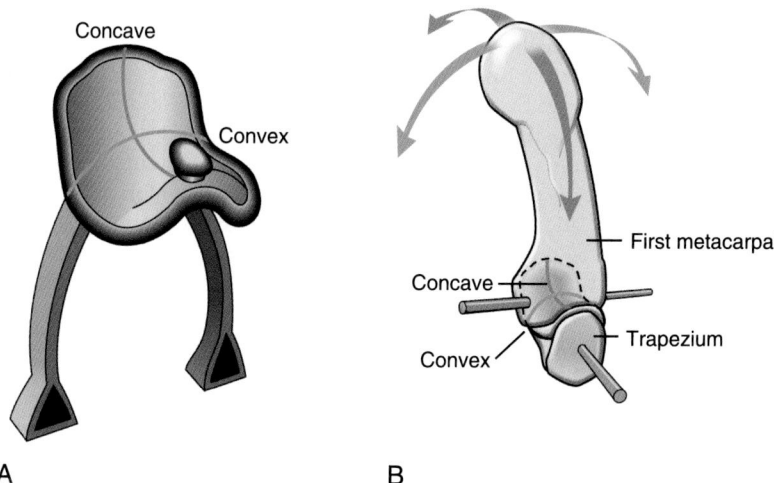

FIG. 2.8 A saddle joint (A) is illustrated as analogous to the carpometacarpal joint of the thumb (B). The saddle in (A) represents the trapezium bone. The rider, if present, would represent the base of the thumb's metacarpal. The two axes of rotation are shown in (B).

A *condyloid joint* is much like a ball-and-socket articulation except that the concave member of the joint is relatively shallow (Fig. 2.9A). Condyloid joints usually allow two degrees of freedom. Ligaments or bony incongruities often restrain the third degree. Examples of condyloid joints include the knees (see Fig. 2.9B) and the atlanto-occipital joints (i.e., articulation between the occipital condyles and the first cervical vertebra). The metacarpophalangeal joint of the finger is another example of a condyloid joint. The root of the word *condyle* actually means "knuckle."

The kinematics at condyloid joints vary by joint structure. At the knee, for example, the femoral condyles fit within the slight concavity provided by the tibial plateau and menisci. This articulation allows flexion-extension and axial rotation (i.e., spin). Abduction-adduction, however, is restricted primarily by ligaments. The metacarpophalangeal joints, in contrast, allow flexion-extension and abduction-adduction, while restricting axial rotation.

Simplifying the Classification of Synovial Joints: Ovoid and Saddle Joints

It is often difficult to classify synovial joints based on analogy to mechanics alone. The metacarpophalangeal joint (condyloid) and

the glenohumeral joint (ball-and-socket), for example, have similar shapes but differ considerably in the relative magnitude of movement and overall function. Joints always display subtle variations that make simple mechanical descriptions less applicable. A good example of the difference between mechanical classification and true function is seen in the gentle undulations that characterize the intercarpal and intertarsal joints. Several of these joints produce complex multiplanar movements that are inconsistent with their simple "planar" mechanical classification. To circumvent this difficulty, a simplified classification scheme recognizes only two articular forms: the ovoid joint and the saddle joint (Fig. 2.10).

An *ovoid joint* has paired mating surfaces that are imperfectly spherical, or egg-shaped, with changing surface curvature. In each case the articular surface of one bone is convex and that of the other is concave. Most joints in the body fit this scheme. A *saddle joint* has been previously described. Each member presents paired convex and concave surfaces oriented at approximately 90 degrees to each other.

Essentially all synovial joints of the body, with the notable exception of planar joints, can be categorized under this scheme. This simplified classification system is functionally associated with the arthrokinematics of roll, slide, or spin (see Chapter 1).

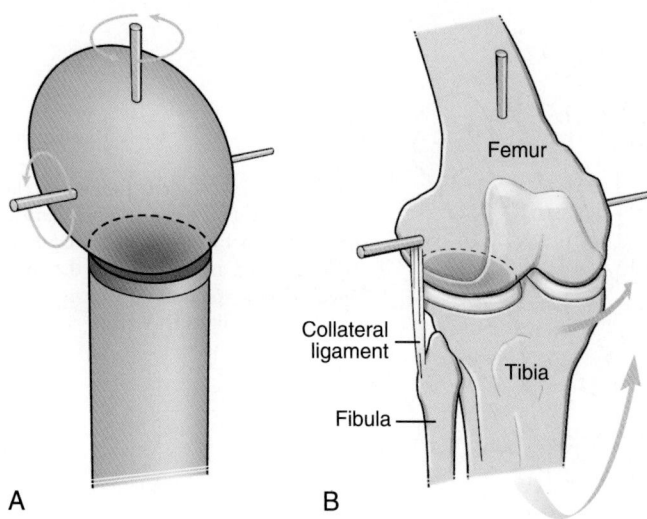

FIG. 2.9 A condyloid joint (A) is analogous to the tibiofemoral (knee) joint (B). The two axes of rotation are shown by the pins. The potential frontal plane motion at the knee is blocked by tension in the collateral ligament.

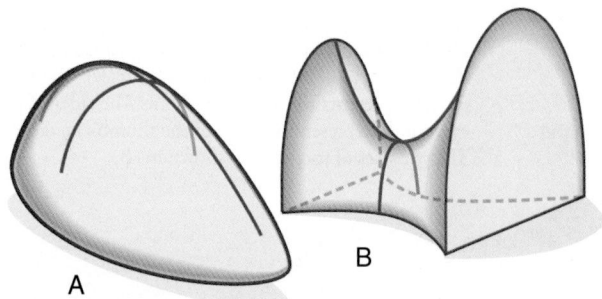

FIG. 2.10 Two fundamental shapes of joint surfaces found in the body. (A) The egg-shaped *ovoid surface* represents a characteristic of most synovial joints of the body (e.g., hip joint, radiocarpal joint, knee joint, metacarpophalangeal joint). The diagram shows only the convex member of the joint. A reciprocally shaped concave member would complete the pair of ovoid articulating surfaces. (B) The *saddle surface* is the second basic type of joint surface, having one convex surface intersecting one concave surface. The paired articulating surface of the other half of the joint would be turned so that a concave surface is mated to a convex surface of the partner.

AXIS OF ROTATION

In the analogy of a door hinge (see Fig. 2.3A), the axis of rotation (i.e., the pin through the hinge) is *fixed* because it remains stationary as the door opens and closes. With the axis of rotation fixed, all points on the door experience equal degrees of rotation. In anatomic joints, however, the axis of rotation is rarely, if ever, fixed during bony rotation. Determining the exact position of the axis of rotation in anatomic joints is, therefore, not a simple task. A method of estimating the position of the axis of rotation in anatomic joints is shown in Fig. 2.11A. The intersection of the two perpendicular lines bisecting a to a′ and b to b′ defines the *instantaneous axis of rotation* for the 90-degree arc of knee flexion. The word *instantaneous* indicates that the location of the axis holds true only for the specified arc of motion. The smaller the angular range used to calculate the instantaneous axis, the more accurate the estimate. If a series of line drawings is made for a sequence of small angular arcs of motion, the location of the instantaneous axes can be plotted for each portion

within the arc of motion. The resulting path of the serial locations of the instantaneous axes of rotation is referred to as an *evolute* (Fig. 2.11B). The path of the evolute is longer and more complex when the mating joint surfaces are less congruent or have greater differences in their radii of curvature, such as in the knee.

A series of radiographs can be used to precisely identify the instantaneous axis of rotation at a joint. This method is not practical in ordinary clinical situations, where it is often necessary to make simple estimates of a joint's axis of rotation. These estimates are necessary when performing *goniometry,* measuring torque around a joint, or constructing prostheses and orthoses. For these applications, an *average axis of rotation* is assumed to occur throughout the entire arc of motion. This axis typically pierces the *convex* member of the joint and is located using anatomic landmarks.

HISTOLOGIC ORGANIZATION OF PERIARTICULAR CONNECTIVE TISSUES

The human body, despite its anatomic complexity, can be organized into just four primary types of tissue: muscle, nerve, epithelium, and connective tissue. Connective tissue, a derivative of the mesoderm, forms the basic structure of joints. The following section provides an overview of the histologic organization of the different kinds of connective tissues that form capsule, ligament, tendon, articular cartilage, and fibrocartilage. Throughout this textbook, these tissues are referred to as *periarticular connective tissues.* Bone is a very specialized form of connective tissue closely related to joints and is briefly reviewed later in this chapter.

Very generally, the fundamental materials that comprise all connective tissues in the body are *fibrous proteins, ground substance,* and *cells.* Even structures that are apparently as different as the capsule of the spleen, a fat pad, bone, and articular cartilage are made of these same fundamental materials. Each of these structures, however, consists of a unique composition, proportion, and arrangement of fibrous proteins, ground substance, and cells. The specific combination of these materials reflects the structures' unique mechanical or physiologic functions. The following section describes the basic biological materials that form periarticular connective tissues.

Fundamental Biologic Materials That Form Periarticular Connective Tissues

1. Fibrous Proteins
   - Collagen (types I and II)
   - Elastin
2. Ground Substance
   - Glycosaminoglycans
   - Water
   - Solutes
3. Cells (Fibroblasts and Chondrocytes)

Fibrous Proteins

Collagen and elastin fibrous proteins are present in varying proportions in all periarticular connective tissues. Collagen is the most ubiquitous protein in the body, accounting for 20% to 25% of all proteins.[38] At the most basic level, collagen consists of amino acids wound in a triple helical fashion. These spiraled molecular threads, called *tropocollagen,* are placed together in a strand, several of which

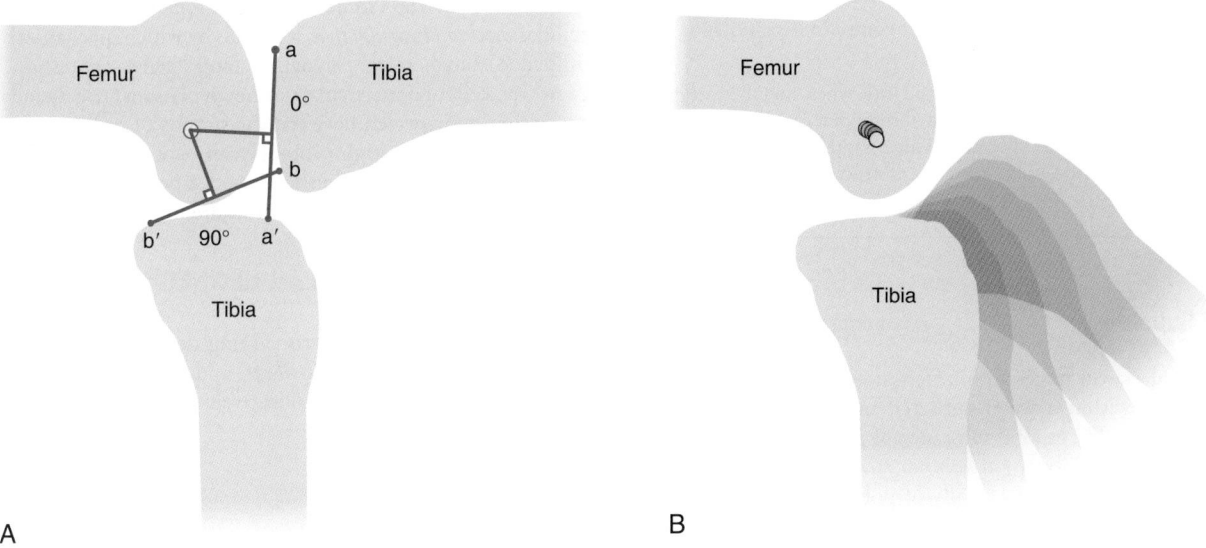

A

B

FIG. 2.11 A method for determining the instantaneous axis of rotation for 90 degrees of knee flexion (A). With images retraced from a radiograph, two points (*a* and *b*) are identified on the proximal surface of the tibia. With the position of the femur held stationary, the same two points are again identified following 90 degrees of flexion (*a'* and *b'*). Lines are then drawn connecting *a* to *a'*, and *b* to *b'*. Next, two perpendicular lines are drawn from the midpoint of lines *a* to *a'* and *b* to *b'*. The point of intersection of these two perpendicular lines identifies the instantaneous axis of rotation for the 90-degree arc of motion. This same method can be repeated for many smaller arcs of motion, resulting in several axes of rotation located in slightly different locations, ultimately forming the "evolute" (B). At the knee, the average axis of rotation is oriented in the medial-lateral direction, generally through the lateral epicondyle of the femur.

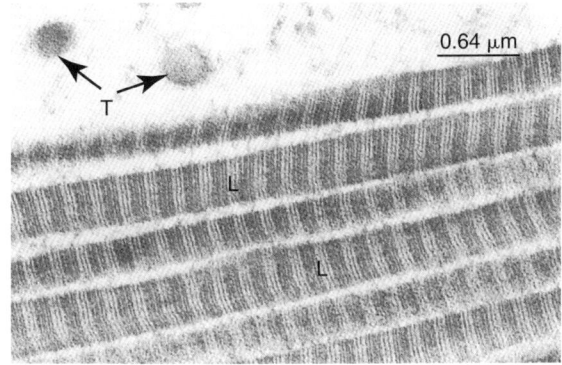

FIG. 2.12 Type I collagen fibers as viewed from a two-dimensional electron microscope (magnification × 32,000). Fibers are shown in longitudinal *(L)* and transverse *(T)* sections. The individual collagen fibrils display a characteristic cross-banding appearance. (From Young B, Lowe JS, Stevens A, et al: *Wheater's functional histology: a text and colour atlas,* ed 6, London, 2014, Churchill Livingstone.)

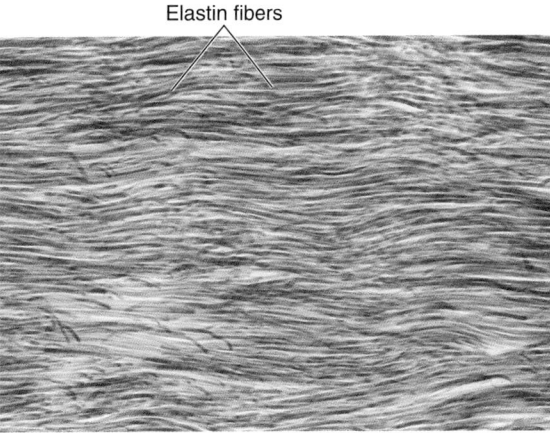

FIG. 2.13 Note dark-stained elastin fibers within the ground substance of a sample of fibrous connective tissue. (From Gartner L, Hiatt J: *Color textbook of histology,* ed 3, Philadelphia, 2007, Saunders.)

are cross-linked into ropelike *fibrils.* A collagen fibril may be 20 to 200 nm in diameter.[157] Many fibrils interconnect to form bundles or *fibers.* Twenty-eight specific types of collagen have been described based primarily on their amino acid sequences.[100,126] However, just two types make up the majority of collagen found in periarticular connective tissues: type I and type II.[157] *Type I collagen* consists of thick fibers that minimally elongate (i.e., minimally stretch) when placed under tension. Being relatively stiff and strong, type I collagen is ideal for binding and supporting the articulations between bones. Type I collagen is, therefore, the primary protein found in ligaments and fibrous joint capsules. This type of collagen also makes up the parallel fibrous bundles that comprise tendons—the structures that transmit forces between muscle and bone. Fig. 2.12 shows a high resolution and magnified image of type I collagen fibrils.

Type II collagen fibers are typically much thinner than type I fibers and possess less tensile strength. These fibers provide a framework for maintaining the general shape and consistency of more complex structures, such as hyaline cartilage. Type II collagen still provides internal strength to the tissue in which it resides.

In addition to collagen, periarticular connective tissues have varying amounts of *elastin fibers* (Fig. 2.13). These protein fibers are composed of a netlike interweaving of small fibrils that resist tensile (stretching) forces but have more "give" when elongated. Tissues with a high proportion of elastin readily return to their original shape after being greatly deformed. This property is useful in structures such as hyaline or elastic cartilage and certain spinal ligaments (such as the ligamentum flavum, which helps realign the vertebrae to their original position after bending forward).

Two Predominant Types of Collagen Found in Periarticular Connective Tissues

Type I: thick, rugged fibers that elongate little when stretched; comprise ligaments, tendons, fascia, and fibrous joint capsules

Type II: thinner than type I fibers; provide a framework for maintaining the general shape and consistency of structures, such as hyaline cartilage

---

Ground Substance

Collagen and elastin fibers within periarticular connective tissues are embedded within a water-saturated matrix or gel known as *ground substance.* The ground substance of periarticular connective tissues consists primarily of *glycosaminoglycans* (GAGs), *water,* and *solutes.*[98,132] The GAGs are a family of polysaccharides, which are polymers of repeating monosaccharides. GAGs confer physical resilience to the ground substance. Fig. 2.14A depicts individual GAG chains attached to a core protein, forming a large complex *proteoglycan side unit.* Structurally, each proteoglycan side unit resembles a bottle brush—the wire stem of the brush being the core protein, and the three-dimensionally arranged bristles being the GAG chains. Many proteoglycan side units, in turn, are bonded to a central hyaluronan (hyaluronic acid), forming a *large proteoglycan complex* (Fig. 2.14B).[38,51,132,157] Fig. 2.14C shows a stylized illustration of the ground substance within articular cartilage.

Because the GAGs are highly negatively charged, the individual chains (or bristles on the brush) repel one another, greatly increasing three-dimensional volume of the proteoglycan complex (Fig. 2.14C). The negatively charged GAGs also make the proteoglycan complexes extremely hydrophilic, able to capture water equivalent to 50 times their weight.[51] The ability of proteoglycans to imbibe and hold water is essential to the function of ground substance for two reasons: (1) it provides a fluid medium for diffusion of nutrients within the matrix, and (2) it causes the tissue to swell. Swelling is limited by the embedded and entangled network of collagen (and elastin) fibers within the ground substance (see Fig. 2.14C). As such, water and other positive ions confer a unique mechanical property to the tissue: the interaction between the restraining fibers and the swelling proteoglycans provides a turgid, semifluid structure that resists compression, much like a water-filled mattress. The tissue shown in Fig. 2.14 depicts the ground substance that is unique to articular cartilage. This important tissue provides an ideal surface covering for joints and is capable of dispersing millions of repetitive forces that likely affect joints throughout a lifetime.[87,141]

Cells

Fibroblasts are the primary cells within most connective tissues, including ligaments, tendons, and joint capsules. *Chondrocytes* are the primary cells within hyaline articular cartilage and fibrocartilage.[132] Both types of cells are responsible for synthesizing the specialized ground substance and fibrous proteins unique to a tissue, as well as for conducting maintenance and repair. In contrast to muscle cells, fibroblasts and chondrocytes do not confer significant mechanical properties on the tissue.

Damaged or aged components of periarticular connective tissues are constantly being removed, as new components are manufactured and remodeled. The extent and type of remodeling is influenced by cellular *mechanotransduction,* a process by which mechanical stimuli influence biochemical signaling and gene expression.[46,50,147] However, cells of periarticular connective tissues are generally sparse and either interspersed between the strands of fibers or embedded deeply in regions of high proteoglycan content. This sparseness of cells in conjunction with limited blood supply can result in poor or incomplete healing of damaged or injured joint tissues.

TYPES OF PERIARTICULAR CONNECTIVE TISSUES

Three types of tissues exist to varying degrees in all joints: *dense connective tissue, articular cartilage,* and *fibrocartilage* (Table 2.2). These tissues are referred to collectively within this chapter as periarticular connective tissues.

Dense Connective Tissue

Dense connective tissue includes most of the nonmuscular "soft tissues" surrounding a joint: the fibrous (external) layer of the joint capsule, ligaments, and tendons. These tissues have few cells (fibroblasts), relatively low to moderate proportions of proteoglycan and elastin, and an abundance of tightly packed type I collagen fibers. As with most periarticular connective tissues, ligaments, tendons, and capsules possess a limited blood supply; therefore, they have a relatively low metabolism. When physically loaded or stressed, however, the metabolism of these tissues can increase, often as a means of functionally adapting to physical stimuli.[78,121,144,153] Such adaptation has been well documented at the histologic level in tendons.[76] Strain placed on fibroblasts within the ground substance is believed to stimulate increased synthesis of collagen and GAGs, which can alter the tissue's structure and thereby modify its material properties, such as its stiffness or ultimate failure point.[53,56,75,111]

Dense connective tissues have been classically described as having two subsets—irregular and regular—based on the spatial orientation of the collagen fibers.[70,132] The fibrous layer of the capsule surrounding a joint is considered *irregular* dense connective tissue because of its irregular and often haphazard orientation of collagen fibers within the ground substance. This type of tissue is well suited to resist tensile forces from multiple directions, such as what is often required by the spiraled nature of the joint capsules at the glenohumeral or hip joints. Ligaments and tendons are considered *regular* dense connective tissue because of the more orderly or near-parallel orientation of their collagen fibers. The collagen fibers in most ligaments function most effectively when they are stretched nearly parallel to the long axis of the ligament. After the initial slack is pulled tight, the tissues provide immediate tension that restricts excessive (and potentially damaging) motion between bony partners.

When trauma, disease, or excessive strain produce laxity in the joint capsules or ligaments, muscles take on a more dominant role in restraining joint movement. However, when a joint's supporting structures are unnaturally loose, muscles are an imperfect solution: even if the surrounding musculature is strong, there is still potential for loss of joint stability. Compared with ligaments, muscles are slower to supply force because of reaction time and the electromechanical delay necessary to build active force. Also, muscle forces typically have a less than ideal alignment for restraining undesirable joint movements and, therefore, cannot always provide an optimal stabilizing force. Thus it is perhaps unsurprising that loss in ligamentous integrity hastens cartilage degeneration.[39]

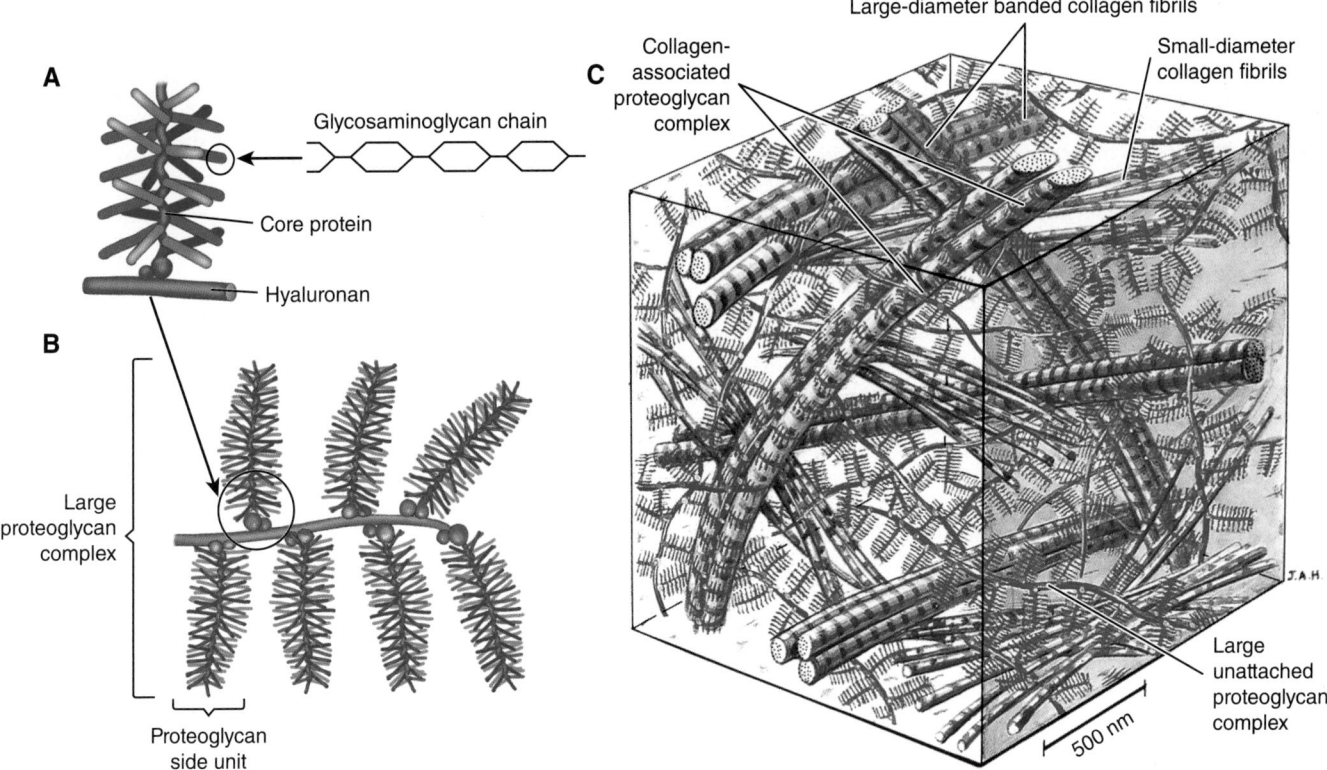

A
Glycosaminoglycan chain
Core protein
Hyaluronan

B
Large proteoglycan complex
Proteoglycan side unit

C
Collagen-associated proteoglycan complex
Large-diameter banded collagen fibrils
Small-diameter collagen fibrils
Large unattached proteoglycan complex
500 nm

FIG. 2.14 Histologic organization of the ground substance of (hyaline) articular cartilage. (A) Repeating monosaccharide units constitute a glycosaminoglycan chain (GAG). Many GAG chains attach to a core protein, which makes up a proteoglycan side unit. (B) The basic structure of a large proteoglycan complex, made up of many proteoglycan side units. (C) The three-dimensional image shows the ground substance, which includes large quantities of proteoglycan complexes interwoven within collagen fibers. Not depicted in the ground substance are interspersed cells (chondrocytes). In healthy tissue, water occupies much of the space between the proteoglycan complexes and fibers. (From Standring S: *Gray's anatomy: the anatomical basis of clinical practice,* ed 42, St Louis, 2020, Elsevier.)

TABLE 2.2 Three Main Types of Periarticular Connective Tissues

Type	Histologic Consistency	Primary Function	Clinical Correlate
Dense connective tissue Ligaments Fibrous layer of the joint capsule Tendons	High proportion of parallel to slightly wavy type I collagen fibers; relatively low elastin content Sparsely populated fibroblasts Relatively low to moderate proteoglycan content	Resists tension Ligaments and joint capsules protect and bind the joint Tendons transfer forces between muscle and bone	Repeated sprains of the lateral collateral ligament of the ankle may lead to chronic joint instability and potential posttraumatic osteoarthritis
Articular cartilage (specialized hyaline cartilage)	High proportion of type II collagen fibers Sparsely to moderately populated chondrocytes Relatively high proteoglycan content	Distributes and absorbs joint forces (compression and shear) Reduces joint friction	During early stages of osteoarthritis, proteoglycans are lost from the ground substance, reducing the ability of the tissue to absorb water. The cartilage, therefore, loses its load attenuation property, leaving the subchondral bone vulnerable to damaging stresses
Fibrocartilage Menisci (e.g., knee) Labra (e.g., hip) Discs (e.g., intervertebral, temporomandibular joint)	High proportion of multidirectional type I collagen fibers Sparsely to moderately populated fibroblasts and chondrocytes Relatively moderate proteoglycan content (depending on the structure)	Supports and mechanically stabilizes joints Dissipates loads across multiple planes Guides complex arthrokinematics	Torn or degenerated disc in the temporomandibular joint may increase stress on the adjacent bone, leading to degeneration, abnormal joint sounds, reduced jaw movements, and pain

Tendons are equipped to transfer large tensile loads between an activated muscle and the bone (or other connective tissue) into which it inserts. The type I collagen fibers within tendons provide high tensile strength once they are fully elongated. Fig. 2.15 illustrates a microscopic image of a tendon *(T)* as it inserts into bone *(B)*. Note the near-parallel arranged collagen fibers, many of which are blending with the collagen of the periosteum. Some collagen fibers can be seen extending deeper into the bone material, often referred to as *Sharpey's fibers (SF)*.

Although structurally strong, tendons experience varying amounts of elongation when subjected to high tensile forces. The human Achilles tendon, for example, elongates up to 8% of its resting length after a maximal contraction of the calf muscle.[74] This elastic property provides a mechanism to store and release energy during walking or jumping.[68,145] The property also allows the Achilles tendon to partially dissipate large or rapidly produced tensile force, which may offer some protection against injury.[76] Though well-adapted for dissipating and propagating loads, tendons are susceptible to injury when repeatedly overstressed or as a result of high-energy trauma. Chronic overuse can lead to development of tendinopathy, while trauma can lead to tendon rupture or avulsion.[19,75]

Articular Cartilage

Articular cartilage is a specialized type of hyaline cartilage that forms the load-bearing surface of joints. Its unique structure (described later) serves to simultaneously reduce friction and dissipate joint loads.[129]

Chondrocytes of various shapes are located within different layers or zones of articular cartilage (Fig. 2.16A). These cells are bathed and nourished by nutrients contained within synovial fluid. Nourishment is facilitated by the "milking" action of articular surface deformation during intermittent joint loading. The chondrocytes are surrounded

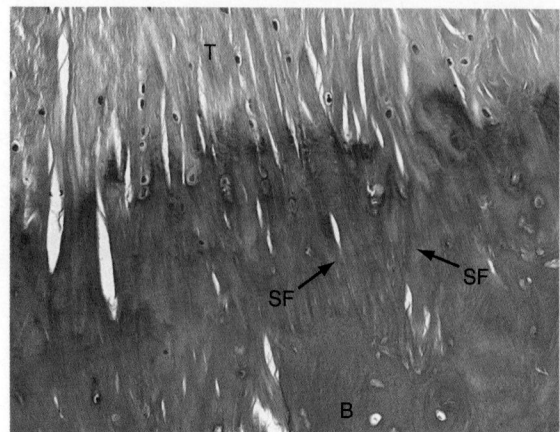

FIG. 2.15 Light microscopic image of the collagen fibers of a tendon *(T)* blending with the collagen of the periosteum of a bone (pink-to-blue transition). Note the deeper collagen fibers known as *Sharpey's fibers (SF)* extending well into the bone tissue *(B)*. (Hematoxylin-eosin stain; × 280.) (From Young B, Lowe JS, Stevens A, et al: *Wheater's functional histology: a text and colour atlas,* ed 6, London, 2014, Churchill Livingstone.)

by predominantly type II collagen fibers. These fibers are arranged within the ground substance to form a restraining network or "scaffolding" that adds structural stability to the tissue (see Fig. 2.16B).[98] The deepest fibers in the calcified zone are firmly anchored to the subchondral bone. These fibers are linked to the vertically oriented fibers in the adjacent deep zone, which in turn are linked to the obliquely oriented fibers of the middle zone and finally to the transversely oriented fibers of the superficial tangential zone. The series of chemically interlinked fibers forms a netlike fibrous structure that

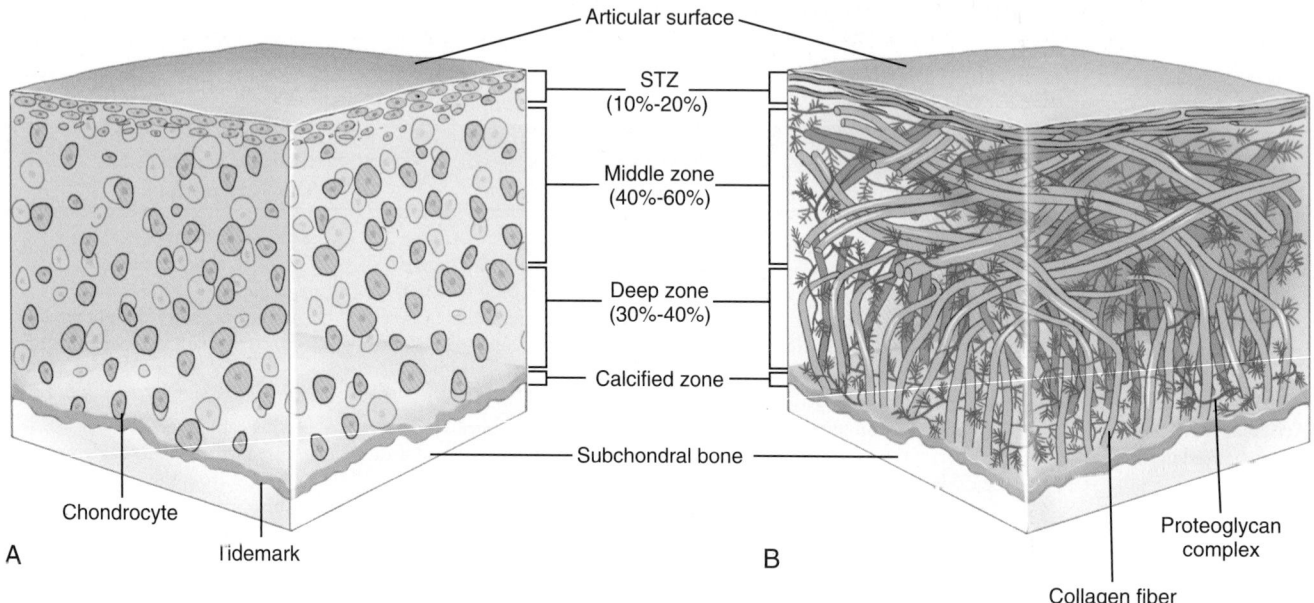

FIG. 2.16 A highly diagrammatic depiction of the cellular (A) and ground substance (B) constituents within articular cartilage, displayed as separate illustrations for clarity. (A) The distribution of the cells (chondrocytes) is shown throughout the articular cartilage. The flattened chondrocytes near the articular surface are within the *superficial tangential zone (STZ)* and are oriented parallel to the joint surface. The STZ comprises about 10% to 20% of the articular cartilage thickness. The cells are more rounded in the *middle zone* and *deep zones.* A region of calcified cartilage *(calcified zone)* joins the deep zone with the underlying subchondral bone. The edge of the calcified zone that abuts the deep zone is known as the *tidemark* and forms a diffusion barrier between the articular cartilage and the underlying bone. Nutrients and gases must, therefore, pass from the synovial fluid through all the layers of articular cartilage to nourish the chondrocytes, including those in the deep zone. (B) The organization of the *collagen fibers* in articular cartilage is shown within the ground substance. In the STZ, collagen is oriented nearly parallel to the articular surface, forming a fibrous grain that helps resist abrasion of the joint surface. The fibers become less tangential and more obliquely oriented in the *middle zone,* finally becoming almost perpendicular to the articular surface in the *deep zone.* The deepest fibers are anchored into the calcified zone to help tie the cartilage to the underlying subchondral bone. Proteoglycan complexes are also present throughout the ground substance.

entraps the large proteoglycan complexes beneath the articular surface. The large amounts of proteoglycans, in turn, attract water, which provides a unique element of rigidity to articular cartilage. This rigidity increases the ability of cartilage to adequately withstand loads.

Articular cartilage distributes and disperses compressive forces to the subchondral bone. It also reduces friction between joint surfaces. The coefficient of friction between two surfaces covered by articular cartilage and wet with synovial fluid is extremely low, ranging from 0.005 to 0.02 in the human knee, for example. This is 5 to 20 times lower and more slippery than ice on ice, which

has a coefficient of friction of 0.1. Therefore the forces of normal weight-bearing activities are reduced to a load level that typically can be absorbed without damaging the skeletal system.

The thickness of articular cartilage ranges from approximately 1 to 4 mm in most human joints and depends, in part, on joint congruity between articular surfaces.[58,122] In relatively congruent joints with large contact areas, such as the talocrural joint in the ankle, thinner cartilage—which deforms minimally—is sufficient to distribute joint stresses. However, in joints with lesser congruence between articulating bones (such as the tibiofemoral joint in the

SPECIAL FOCUS 2.1

Fasciae, the Fascial System and Myofascial Chains

Fasciae are broad sheets of connective tissue that surround, support and physically link the muscles, some joints, and the viscera of the body. As such, they are not exclusively periarticular connective tissue. However, some fasciae are intimately related to a joint and its functioning, aiding in joint stability and serving as a connection between muscles and other periarticular connective tissues.[6,90,49]

Fasciae are arranged in layers of dense connective tissue, usually interspersed with loose connective tissue.[133] The dense connective tissue layers contain large proportions of type I collagen in varied orientations, which confers the tissue with high, multidirectional tensile strength. The loose connective tissue layers enable gliding between the dense layers.

Fasciae can facilitate force transmission by providing a physical link between muscles, tendon, and bone and by optimizing the length-tension relationships of surrounding muscles. These anatomic and biomechanical associations have been demonstrated through cadaveric studies, finite element modeling, and animal models.[48,71,90,158] For example, there is evidence that activation of one muscle may result in measurable force changes in a neighboring muscle—regardless of whether that muscle is an agonist or antagonist.[48,71] Furthermore, in humans, myofascial force transmission can be appreciated following complete tenotomy of the flexor carpi ulnaris in children with cerebral palsy: even without its distal insertion, activation of the flexor carpi ulnaris can still produce wrist flexion.[26] In addition, properties of fascia (such as thickness and stiffness) are correlated with joint range of motion and passive torque production, both local and remote to the fascial region of interest.[36,150,152]

Though long assumed to be aneural, researchers have discovered potential roles for fascia in proprioception and pain, based on the presence and density of nerve fibers and corpuscles.[32,63] Similarly, despite long-held beliefs that fasciae are inert and noncontractile, researchers have demonstrated the ability to elicit *contraction* in isolated rat fascial tissues using pharmacologic stimulants.[118] The amount of contractility correlated with the density of myofibroblasts in the fascia. Although more research is needed in this area, these findings suggest that fascia likely has a more direct and relevant role in movement, proprioception, and pain than traditionally believed.[32,63,118]

Fasciae can be separated into superficial and deep components. Deep fascia (or fascia profunda) is of particular relevance to the musculoskeletal system. Deep fascia encases all skeletal muscles in the body. It is continuous with the connective tissues that surround muscle fibers (endomysium), muscle fiber bundles

(perimysium), individual muscles (epimysium), and muscle compartments (intermuscular septa).[134] Through these and the connections with tendon, ligament, and joint capsule, fasciae provide a interconnectedness throughout the musculoskeletal system, enabling coordination between whole muscles, located either in parallel or in series with one another.[151]

The continuity between fascia and muscle may prove relevant for whole-body function, such as in cellular signaling and biomechanical force transmission.[1,161] Accordingly, some researchers have defined a new, purposively global term: *the fascial system.* This system encompasses the full spectrum of soft connective tissues that give the body its functional structure and whose tissues possess similar biochemical, histologic, and biomechanical properties.[132] These include any soft, collagen-containing connective tissues of the body: adipose tissue, ligaments, membranes, joint capsules, tendons, connective tissues surrounding muscles, bones and peripheral vessels, and all layers of fascia. The phrase *fascial system* is meant to reflect the interdependent, collaborative nature of these tissues on human function.[135]

Discussing fasciae within the context of a fascial system may improve our understanding of human movement from a whole-body lens. For example, instead of viewing a muscle's action as an isolated event, the fascial system allows us to integrate individual muscle actions into movements occurring across multiple joints or across regions of the body. The ability of fascia to impart forces in distant regions of the body is based on the concept of *myofascial chains.* Myofascial chains are linkages of muscle, fascia, and other fibrous connective tissues that cross multiple joint regions.[113] They are defined by their anatomic structure, namely the uninterrupted connections between consecutive soft tissues. The degree to which these forces are functionally relevant has yet to be determined.[71,161]

Understanding the anatomy and physiology of myofascial chains may improve our understanding of not only movement, but also disease and rehabilitation. Such an understanding may help explain some of the purported benefits of several manual-based therapeutic interventions whose mechanism of action are not well understood.[14] In a similar way, myofascial chains may be, in part, responsible for the benefits seen when interventions are applied to neighboring joints, as opposed to (or in addition to) those provided directly to the injured joint.[161] Finally, understanding myofascial chains may assist in understanding nuances of referred pain, of myofascial pain syndromes, and of age-related changes in joint range of motion.[149]

knee), thicker articular cartilage is advantageous: thicker articular cartilage deforms to a greater extent, which serves to increase joint contact area and reduce stresses experienced by the joint.[122]

Thickness of articular cartilage varies as a function of loading. In the short term, articular cartilage thickness fluctuates with the amount of time spent weight-bearing. For example, thickness is greater in the morning following bed rest compared with the end of the day following prolonged weight-bearing. Articular cartilage thickness also decreases following a walk.[23,61] These changes are the result of cartilage compression, not of tissue remodeling, and are reversible within minutes to hours. However, long-term changes in articular cartilage thickness can also occur. Though seemingly paradoxical, both disuse and excessive magnitudes of loading can cause thinning of articular cartilage, which in turn could expose subchondral bone to excessive loads and potentially serve as a trigger for degenerative changes.[95,129,142] Disuse results in decreased nourishment of the cartilage, while excessive loading triggers inflammatory pathways, both eventually leading to articular cartilage thinning. Fortunately, there is evidence that exercise may serve to mitigate—or even potentially reverse—some of these changes. For example, in animal models, moderate-dose exercise results in hypertrophy and improved tissue composition of the articular cartilage—findings that are consistent with the exercise-induced adaptations seen in other connective tissues in humans.[10,16,47,137] However, human subjects research is needed to know whether these same exercise-induced adaptations occur in the articular cartilage of humans.

Articular cartilage is both avascular and aneural. Unlike most hyaline cartilage throughout the body, articular cartilage lacks a perichondrium. Perichondrium—like periosteum on bone—is a layer of connective tissue that covers most cartilage. It contains blood vessels and a ready supply of primitive cells that maintain and repair underlying tissue. These are advantages not available to articular cartilage. Importantly, while the absence of a perichondrium negatively affects maintenance and repair, this tradeoff allows the opposing surfaces of articular cartilage to form ideal load-bearing surfaces.

As explained earlier, the absence of a perichondrium on articular cartilage has the negative consequence of eliminating a ready source of primitive fibroblasts used for repair. Even though articular cartilage is capable of normal maintenance and replenishment of its matrix, significant damage to adult articular cartilage is often repaired poorly or not at all. Neural ingrowth and angiogenesis (i.e., new growth of nerves and blood vessels into the tissue) have been identified in damaged articular cartilage, perhaps an attempt by the tissue to compensate for its limited healing potential.[136,138] Unfortunately, these changes are part of an abnormal joint remodeling process and may come at a price; instead of promoting healthy remodeling, these micro vessels may actually contribute to pain and further degradation of the articular cartilage.[47,136,138]

When articular cartilage becomes damaged, the subchondral bone loses its primary source of mechanical protection and becomes subjected to high and damaging stress. The combination of degenerated or denuded articular cartilage and stressed subchondral bone are key factors in the often-disabling condition of osteoarthritis (described later in this chapter). When severe, painful, and uncontrolled, the articular components of the arthritic or otherwise damaged joint may be replaced through arthroplastic surgery (arthroplasty stems from Greek roots *arthro,* joint; and *plasty,* formed or molded). One of the most common joints to receive total component arthroplasty is the hip. Materials vary but typically involve some combination of ceramics, metal-based alloy, and poly-ethylene (plastic).[82]

Fibrocartilage

As its name implies, fibrocartilage is a mixture of dense connective tissue and articular cartilage (Fig. 2.17). As such, fibrocartilage provides the resilience and shock absorption of articular cartilage and the tensile strength of ligaments and tendons. Dense bundles of type I collagen exist along with moderate amounts of proteoglycans. Depending on the tissue, fibrocartilage has varying numbers of chondrocytes and fibroblasts, located within a dense and often multidirectional collagen network.[38]

Fibrocartilage forms much of the substance of the intervertebral discs, the labra associated with the hip and shoulder, and the discs located within the pubic symphysis, temporomandibular joint, and some joints of the extremities (e.g., the menisci of the knee). These structures help support and stabilize the joints, guide complex arthrokinematics, and help dissipate forces. Fibrocartilage is also found in some ligaments and tendons, especially at the point of insertion into bone.[132,157] The dense interwoven collagen fibers of fibrocartilage allow the tissue to resist multidirectional tensile, shear, and compressive forces. Fibrocartilage is, therefore, an ideal tissue to dissipate loads.

Like articular cartilage, fibrocartilage typically lacks a perichondrium.[38] Fibrocartilage is also largely aneural. It, therefore, does not produce pain or participate in proprioception, although some neural receptors may be found at the periphery where fibrocartilage abuts a ligament or joint capsule. Most fibrocartilaginous tissues have a limited blood supply and are largely dependent on diffusion of nutrients from synovial fluid or from adjacent blood vessels. As in articular cartilage, neural and vascular ingrowth can occur in degenerated regions of fibrocartilage,[62] likely an attempt at tissue repair following injury. Otherwise, in healthy fibrocartilaginous discs, the diffusion of nutrients and the removal of metabolic wastes are assisted by the "milking" action of intermittent weightbearing. This principle is readily apparent in adult intervertebral discs that are insufficiently nourished when the spine is held

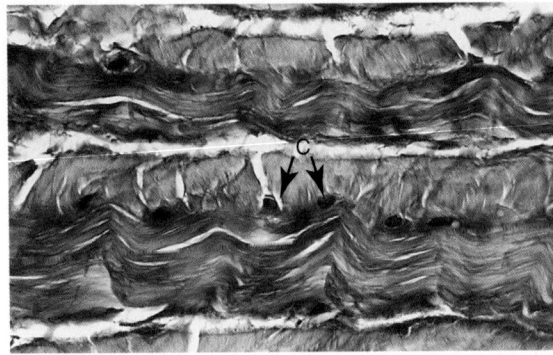

FIG. 2.17 Photograph of a light microscopic image of fibrocartilage. (Hematoxylin-eosin and Alcian blue stain; × 320.) Note the alternating layers of hyaline cartilage matrix and thick collagen fibers. These layers are oriented in the direction of stress imposed on the tissues. Observe the pair of chondrocytes *(C)* located between a layer of collagen and hyaline cartilage. (From Young B, Lowe JS, Stevens A, et al: *Wheater's functional histology: a text and colour atlas,* ed 6, London, 2014, Churchill Livingstone.)

in fixed postures for extended periods. Without proper nutrition, the discs may partially degenerate and lose part of their protective function.[9,103]

A direct blood supply penetrates the outer rim of some fibrocartilaginous structures where they attach to joint capsules or ligaments, such as menisci in the knee or intervertebral discs. In adult joints, some repair of damaged fibrocartilage can occur near the vascularized periphery, such as the outer one-third of menisci of the knee and the outermost lamellae of intervertebral discs. The innermost regions of fibrocartilage structures, much like articular cartilage, demonstrate poor or negligible healing because of the lack of a ready source of undifferentiated fibroblastic cells.[17,93]

SPECIAL FOCUS 2.2

A Brief Overview of Sensory Innervation of Joints

Joint proprioception is the ability to sense the static or dynamic position of a joint or limb. This sensory awareness, which is essential to normal movement, is dependent on sensory nerve fibers embedded in the skin, muscles, and periarticular connective tissues. The sensors, or "afferent" joint receptors associated with a particular set of nerve fibers, are often referred to as *mechanoreceptors* based on their ability to respond to mechanical stimuli, such as stretch or touch. Four primary types of mechanoreceptors have been described in the context of joint innervation (Table 2.3).[35,112] Other mechanoreceptors have also been described, such as Meissner's corpuscles and Merkel cells. Meissner's corpuscles are found in the skin and detect movement across the skin (often referred to as light touch).[160] Merkel cells are found in skin and hair follicles, and they respond to pressure, convey information regarding texture and object shape, and modulate the sensation of itch that can arise from light touch.[33] Merkel cells and Meissner's corpuscles can provide indirect information regarding joint position with movement of the skin or hair surrounding a joint;[84] however, these are not commonly included as primary joint proprioception end organs.

Conflicting evidence exists on ways to classify mechanoreceptors in general, as well as how they each contribute to joint proprioception.[34,91,108] Advances in tissue staining techniques, specifically in immunohistochemical analysis, however, have enabled more specific identification of nerve tissues in the human body—something that was previously made difficult by techniques that lacked the ability to selectively stain vascular, reticular, and nerve fibers. This has enabled a greater appreciation of the distribution and relative importance of mechanoreceptors within joints.[112] For example, ligaments with few mechanoreceptors likely have a greater role in stabilizing the joint whereas those with a greater number of mechanoreceptors likely contribute a greater degree to proprioception. Sensory innervation of ligaments can also influence neuromuscular activity: through reflex pathways, they can either promote or inhibit muscle activity, thereby indirectly influencing myogenic stability.[43,115] Joint innervation and its role in proprioception may prove to be a valuable consideration in the prevention and treatment of ligamentous injury or instability.[85]

TABLE 2.3 Summary of Naming and Basic Information for Selected Joint Sensory Receptors			
Receptor Type*/Name	**Location**	**Characteristics**	**Function**
Type I /Ruffini	Fibrous joint capsule, especially superficial layers	Slow-adapting, low threshold	Provide feedback regarding static joint position and joint acceleration; sensitive to tensile forces
Type II/Pacini	Fibrous joint capsule, especially its deeper layers, and articular fat pads	Fast-adapting, low threshold	Provide feedback regarding joint acceleration; sensitive to compressive forces
Type III/Golgi-like	Ligaments	Slow-adapting, high threshold	Active at the extremes of joint motion; provide feedback regarding tissue deformation
Type IV/Free nerve endings	Capsular ligaments, fat pads, intramuscular connective tissues	High threshold; these may be either fast- or slow-adapting	Signal presence of noxious, chemical, mechanical, and inflammatory stimuli

*The receptor types described here are based on the morphology and neurophysiological traits of each receptor and are consistent with the classification scheme first developed in 1967 by Freeman and Wyke.[35,43] This naming system is distinct from the classification scheme often used for other sensory nerve receptors, such as for muscle (Chapter 3), which is solely based on the diameter of nerve fibers.

BONE

Bone is a specialized connective tissue, sharing several fundamental histologic characteristics with other periarticular connective tissues. Bone tissue consists of a highly cross-linked type I collagen, cells (such as osteoblasts), and a hard ground substance rich in mineral salts. The proteoglycans within the ground substance contain glycoproteins (such as osteocalcin) that strongly bind to calcium- and phosphorous-rich mineral salts—*calcium hydroxyapatite* $(Ca_{10}[PO_4]_6[OH]_2)$.[157]

Bone gives rigid support to the body and provides the muscles with a system of levers. The outer cortex of the long bones of the adult skeleton has a shaft composed of thick, *compact bone* (Fig. 2.18). The ends of long bones, however, are formed of a thinner layer of compact bone that surrounds a network of *cancellous bone*. Bones of the adult axial skeleton, such as the vertebral bodies, possess an outer shell of relatively thick compact bone that is filled with a supporting core of cancellous bone. As described earlier, articular cartilage covers the diarthrodial articular surfaces of all bones throughout the musculoskeletal system.

Bone formation occurs in two main stages: primary and secondary osteogenesis. The primary stage is more rapid and less organized, resulting in bone with a woven appearance (aptly named "woven bone"). Woven bone is observed during embryonic development and in response to pathology in adult bones. Secondary osteogenesis involves remodeling of woven bone into lamellar bone (often referred to as "secondary bone"). This bone is highly organized and develops more slowly. Lamellar bone is the main bone of the adult skeleton and is described later.

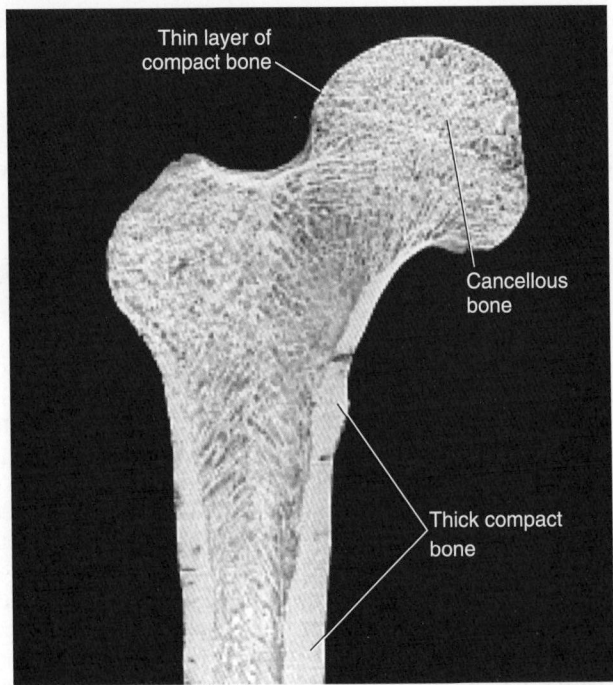

FIG. 2.18 A cross-section showing the internal architecture of the proximal femur. Note the thicker areas of compact bone around the shaft and the lattice like cancellous bone occupying most of the medullary region. (From Neumann DA: *An arthritis home study course: the synovial joint: anatomy, function, and dysfunction,* LaCrosse, WI, 1998, Orthopedic Section of the American Physical Therapy Association.)

SPECIAL FOCUS 2.3

Laws of Bone Remodeling

Bone is a very dynamic tissue, constantly altering its shape, strength, and density in response to external forces.[20,37,101] Two prominent concepts define the relationships between external forces and bone remodeling: *The Hueter-Volkmann Law* and *Wolff's Law.* These concepts are credited to three German surgeons: Carl Hueter (1838–1882), Richard Von Volkmann (1830–1889), and Julius Wolff (1839–1902). These laws are seemingly in contradiction to one another, yet deal with two different conditions: that of the skeletally immature and the skeletally mature.

The Hueter-Volkmann Law states that bone growth *in the skeletally immature* is inhibited in regions exposed to high stress and stimulated in regions of low stress.[25,81] This can be appreciated in the progression of frontal plane curvatures in idiopathic scoliosis: vertebral bodies are exposed to increased stress ipsilateral to the concavity and decreased stress ipsilateral to the convexity of the scoliotic curve. As adolescents with scoliosis continue to grow, bone growth in the spinal column is stimulated along the convexity and inhibited along the concavity, thereby amplifying the lateral bend component of the scoliotic deformity.

Wolff's law, in contrast, refers to the relationship between external forces and bone remodeling in the skeletally mature. Loosely translated, Wolff's law states that "bone is laid down in areas of high stress and reabsorbed in areas of low stress." This simple axiom has many clinical applications. A deteriorated and dehydrated intervertebral disc, for example, may be unable to

protect the underlying bone from stress. According to Wolff's law, bone responds to stress by synthesizing more bone. Bone "spurs" or osteophytes may form if the response is excessive. Occasionally osteophytes can block motion or compress an adjacent spinal nerve root, causing pain in the corresponding extremity or weakness in associated muscles.

Wolff's law can also explain the *loss* of bone and its reduced strength after chronic unloading. For example, bone mineral density in persons with spinal cord injury rapidly declines, likely caused by the unloading of bone stemming from the paralysis.[30,31,80] Reduced bone density can place the bones of the person with a spinal cord injury at a higher risk for fracture. Fractures are not uncommon, occurring from trauma such as falling out of a wheelchair, during daily activities such as performing "self" range-of-motion exercises to the lower extremities, or during a transfer between a bathtub and chair. In an effort to reduce the magnitude of bone loss after spinal cord injury, electrical stimulation of the paralyzed limb muscles may be used.[123] The forces produced by the stimulated muscle are transferred across the bone with the goal of preventing fractures in persons with chronic paralysis after a spinal cord injury. Additional research is needed to determine the feasibility and long-term benefits of using electrical stimulation as a regular part of rehabilitation for individuals with a spinal cord injury.[125]

The structural subunit of compact bone is the *osteon* (also known as *the Haversian system),* which organizes the collagen fibers and mineralized ground substance into a unique series of concentric spirals that form *lamellae* (Fig. 2.19).[132,157] This infrastructure, made rigid by the calcium phosphate crystals, allows cortical bone to accept tremendous compressive loads. The osteoblasts eventually become surrounded by their secreted ground substance and become confined within narrow lacunae (i.e., spaces) positioned between the lamellae of the osteon.[98] (The confined osteoblasts are technically referred to as *osteocytes.)* Because bone deforms very little, blood vessels (and some accompanying sensory nerve fibers) can pass into its substance from the outer periosteal and the inner endosteal surfaces. The blood vessels can then turn to travel along the long axis of the bone in tunnels formed by *Haversian canals* (which reside in the center of the osteons; see Fig. 2.19). This system allows a rich source of blood to reach the cells deep within the cortex. Furthermore, the connective tissue comprising the periosteum and endosteum of bone is also richly vascularized, as well as innervated with sensory receptors for pressure and pain.

Bone is a very dynamic tissue. Osteoblasts are constantly synthesizing ground substance and collagen as well as orchestrating the deposition of mineral salts. Remodeling occurs in response to forces applied through physical activity and in response to hormonal influences that regulate systemic calcium balance. The large-scale removal of bone is carried out by osteoclasts—specialized cells that originate from within the bone marrow. Primitive fibroblasts essential for the repair of fractured bone originate from the periosteum and endosteum and from the perivascular tissues that are woven throughout the bone's vascular canals. Of the tissues involved with joints, bone has by far the best capacity for remodeling, repair, and regeneration.

Bone demonstrates its greatest strength when compressed along the long axis of its shaft. This loads the Haversian systems longitudinally, which is comparable to compressing a straw along its long axis. The ends of long bones receive multidirectional compressive forces through the weight-bearing surfaces of articular cartilage. Stresses are spread to the subjacent subchondral bone and then into the network of cancellous bone, which in turn acts as a series of struts to redirect the forces into the long axis of the compact bone of the shaft. This structural arrangement redirects forces for absorption and transmission by taking advantage of bone's unique architectural design.

In summary, in contrast to periarticular connective tissues, bone has a rich blood supply coupled with a very dynamic metabolism. This allows bone to constantly remodel in response to physical stress. A rich blood supply also affords bone with a good potential for healing after fracture.

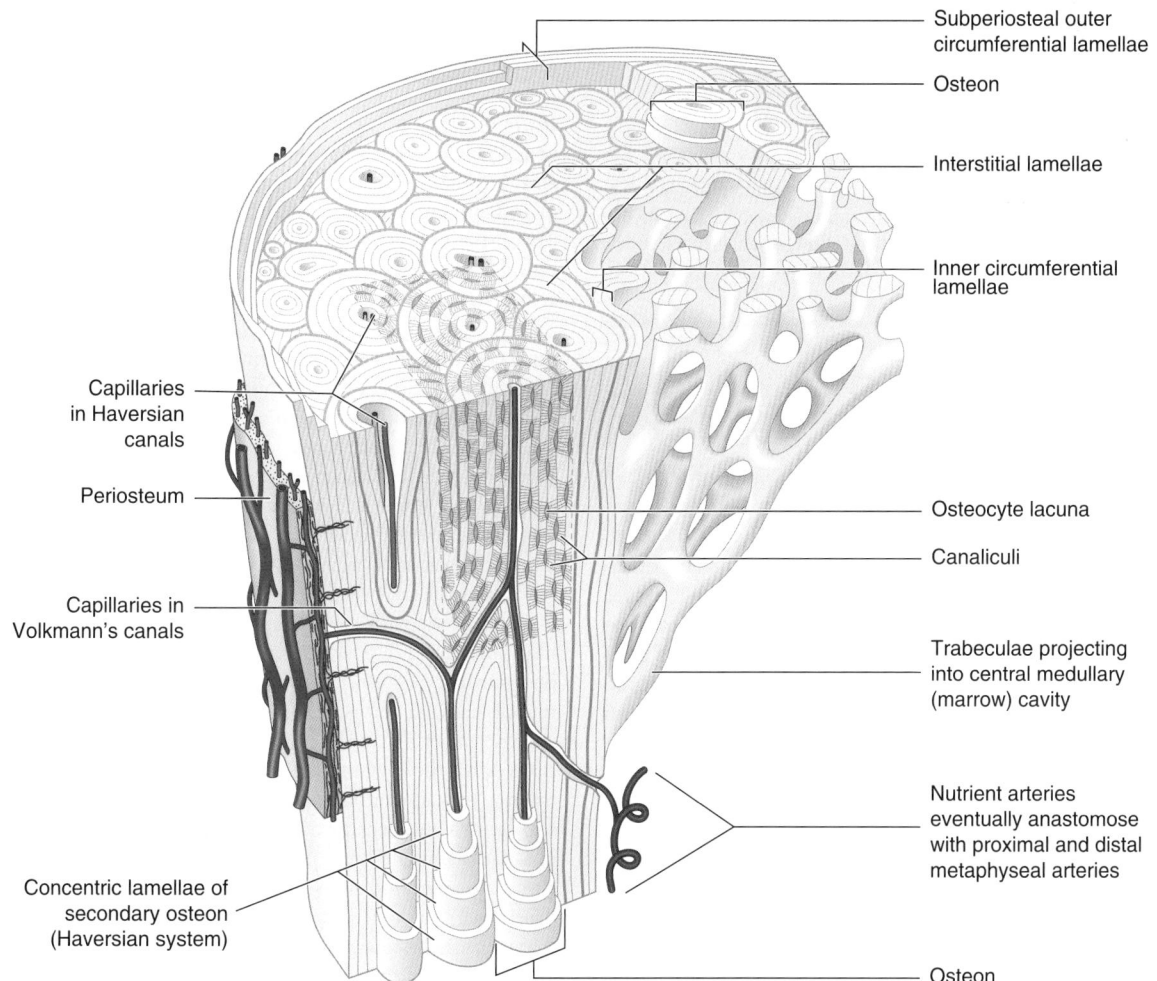

FIG. 2.19 The ultrastructure of compact bone. Note the concentric lamellae that make up a single osteon (also known as a Haversian system). (From Standring S: *Gray's anatomy: the anatomical basis of clinical practice,* ed 42, St. Louis, 2020, Elsevier.)

Osteochondritis Dissecans: An Example of Intra-articular Trauma

Osteochondritis dissecans is an example of an intra-articular injury that involves fracture through the articular cartilage and subchondral bone (Fig. 2.20). Osteochondritis dissecans is not a disease but rather a condition wherein the articular cartilage and subchondral bone become detached from the joint surface. This condition occurs most often in adolescent males and is either the result of repetitive trauma or a secondary response to joint injury, especially if there is insufficient blood flow during the healing process.[96,159] As with many articular injuries, osteochondritis dissecans may be associated with eventual development of posttraumatic osteoarthritis, whether due to an unfavorable biomechanical environment or caused by impaired or altered joint healing.[45]

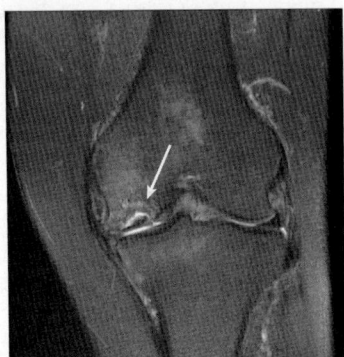

FIG. 2.20 A coronal, T2-weighted magnetic resonance image of a left knee with osteochondritis dissecans. The bright white (*arrow*) at the medial aspect of the knee joint shows the detachment of the articular cartilage and subchondral bone from the superior aspect of the tibiofemoral joint surface.

THE EFFECTS OF ALTERED ACTIVITY, ADVANCED AGE, AND DISEASE ON JOINT STRUCTURE AND FUNCTION

Some Effects of Immobilization on the Strength of Periarticular Connective Tissue and Bone

The amount and arrangement of the fibrous proteins, ground substance, and water that constitute periarticular connective tissues are influenced by physical activity.[20,52,60,154] At a normal level of physical activity, the composition of the tissues is typically strong enough to adequately resist the natural range of forces imposed on the musculoskeletal system. A joint immobilized for an extended period demonstrates marked changes in the structure and function of its associated connective tissues. The mechanical strength of the tissue is reduced in accordance with the decreased forces of the immobilized condition. This is a normal response to an abnormal condition. Placing a body part in a cast and confining a person to a bed are examples in which immobilization can dramatically reduce the level of force imposed on the musculoskeletal system.

The rate of decline of periarticular connective tissue strength is somewhat dependent on the normal metabolic activity of the specific tissue.[13,76] For example, in a period of weeks, chronic

immobilization can produce a marked decrease in tensile strength of the ligaments of the knee.[94,154] The earliest biochemical markers of this remodeling can be detected within days after immobilization.[44,88] Even after the cessation of the immobilization and after the completion of an extended postimmobilization exercise program, the ligaments continue to have lower tensile strength than ligaments that were never subjected to immobilization.[44,154] Other tissues such as bone and articular cartilage also show a loss of mass, volume, and strength after immobilization.[20,42,54,57] The results from experimental studies imply that tissues can rapidly lose strength in response to reduced loading. Full recovery of strength after restoration of loading is much slower and often incomplete.

Immobilizing a joint for an extended period is often necessary to limit pain and promote healing after an injury, such as a fractured bone. Clinical judgment is required to balance the potential negative effects of the immobilization with the need to promote healing. The maintenance of maximal tissue strength around joints requires judicious use of immobilization and, when feasible, a relatively quick return to loading and early rehabilitative intervention.

Brief Overview of Joint Trauma and Pathology

Trauma to periarticular connective tissues can occur from a single overwhelming event (acute trauma) or in response to an accumulation of lesser injuries over an extended period (chronic trauma).

ACUTE TRAUMA

Acute trauma often produces detectable structural damage. A torn or severely stretched ligament or joint capsule, for example, causes an acute inflammatory reaction, which involves a predictable cascade of inflammatory mediators and inflammation-induced pain.[117,127] This entire process relies heavily upon appropriate intercellular communication, something that is accomplished through a network of cell-signaling molecules known as cytokines.[18]

Cytokines are released as part of a normal immune response to injury or infection. *Pro*-inflammatory cytokines promote and maintain inflammation and contribute to joint pain through their action on pain fibers. Inflammation and the inflammatory pain processes that ensue constitute a normal, healthy response to acute trauma. However, the persistence of pro-inflammatory cytokines represents a pathologic state.[117] For example, pro-inflammatory cytokines are implicated in the production and perpetuation of chronic joint pain in conditions such as arthritis, tendinopathy, and patellofemoral pain syndrome.[116,119,120]

Consistent with a pro-inflammatory response to acute trauma, high-intensity physical exercise can also increase circulation of pro-inflammatory cytokines. This is likely a result of exercise-induced muscle damage and is an important consideration when prescribing exercise, particularly for persons with chronic inflammatory conditions or for those who initiate exercise too quickly following an acute trauma. In stark contrast, however, both acute (i.e., a single bout) and regular or consistent physical exercise can increase circulating levels of anti-inflammatory cytokines.[117] Anti-inflammatory cytokines contribute to an overall anti-inflammatory state within the body, thereby protecting the body against low-grade inflammation associated with many chronic, systemic diseases.[105] The precise exercise parameters (e.g., exercise intensity, duration, and mode) required to elicit an optimal cytokine response is, as yet, undetermined. However, it seems that moderate intensity exercise may be the best compromise between high and low intensities, simultaneously minimizing exercise-induced muscle damage and maximizing the anti-inflammatory cytokine cascade.[4] Exercise *frequency* is also key: consistent or regular exercise lends itself to a self-protective, anti-inflammatory phenotype, while physical *in*activity may lead to a pro-inflammatory phenotype.[4,117] Greater understanding of exercise-induced cytokine production may prove useful in optimizing exercise prescription, especially in postoperative phases of rehabilitation or in persons with chronic disease.

Inflammation and damage to periarticular connective tissues may limit a joint's ability to restrain the natural extremes of motion, resulting in structural instability of the joint. Joints most frequently affected by acute traumatic instability are typically associated with the longest external moment arms of the skeleton and, therefore, are exposed to high external torques. For this reason, the tibiofemoral, talocrural, and glenohumeral joints are frequently subjected to acute ligament damage with resultant instability.

Acute trauma can also result in intra-articular fractures involving articular cartilage and subchondral bone. Careful reduction or realignment of the fractured fragments helps to restore congruity to the joint and thereby facilitate smooth, low-friction sliding functions of articular surfaces. However, this does not guarantee recovery of function; while bone has excellent healing potential, the repair of fractured articular cartilage is often incomplete. This can result in mechanically compromised regions of a joint surface that are prone to further injury or degeneration. Inadequate articular cartilage strength in conjunction with focal increases in stress can lead to chronic conditions such as posttraumatic osteoarthritis.[3] As such, efforts are ongoing to establish optimal interventions for cartilage restoration. Surgical interventions have evolved from microfracture and abrasion chondroplasty in the mid-1900s to autologous chondrocyte implantation, mesenchymal stem cell implantation, and matrix-assisted autologous chondrocyte transplantation in the late 1900s and early 2000s.[5,27,66] Despite these advancements, there are still no perfect solutions for articular cartilage damage, and future successes will likely rely upon a combination of prevention efforts and nonsurgical interventions.[66]

The repair of damaged fibrocartilaginous joint structures depends on the proximity and adequacy of blood supply. A tear of the outermost region of the meniscus of the knee adjacent to blood vessels embedded within the joint capsule may completely heal.[114] In contrast, tears of the innermost circumference of a meniscus do not typically heal. This is also the case in the inner lamellae of the adult intervertebral disc, which does not have the capacity to heal after significant damage.[9,40,41]

CHRONIC TRAUMA

Chronic trauma is often classified as a type of "overuse syndrome," reflecting an accumulation of unrepaired, relatively minor damage. Chronically damaged joint capsules and ligaments gradually lose their restraining functions, leading to instability of the joint and potentially further damage. This instability may be masked by activation of local muscles, which can serve as relatively effective—albeit energy-consumptive—stabilizers of joints. In this case the instability becomes apparent only when the muscles are fatigued or when the speed or magnitude of an external perturbation exceeds neuromuscular capabilities. Though joint stability may be improved through local "muscle guarding," the associated increased and unnecessarily large myogenic load on the joint may, over time, cause further cumulative damage. With or without muscle guarding, however, recurrent joint instability may progressively lead to excessive wear on the joint. The surfaces of articular cartilage and fibrocartilage may become fragmented, with a

concurrent loss of proteoglycans and subsequent lowered resistance to compressive and shear forces.[28] Early stages of degeneration often demonstrate a roughened or "fibrillated" surface of the articular cartilage.[7] A fibrillated region of articular cartilage may later develop cracks, or clefts, that extend from the surface into the middle or deepest layers of the tissue. These changes reduce the shock absorption quality of the tissue.

OSTEOARTHRITIS AND RHEUMATOID ARTHRITIS

Two disease states that commonly cause joint dysfunction are osteoarthritis (OA) and rheumatoid arthritis (RA). *Osteoarthritis* is characterized by a gradual erosion of articular cartilage, persistent pain, and inflammation.[16,47,59] Though articular cartilage and subchondral bone receive the most attention, OA is a pathology that can affect all elements of the joint (including ligaments, synovium, and joint capsule).[47,95] As erosion of articular cartilage progresses, the underlying subchondral bone becomes more mineralized and, in severe cases, becomes the weight-bearing surface when the articular cartilage is completely worn. As the disease progresses, the fibrous joint capsule and synovium become distended and thickened and ligamentous damage can occur.[39,69] The severely involved joint may be completely unstable and dislocate or may fuse, allowing no motion. Interestingly, the relationship between magnitude of joint damage and patient-reported pain levels has not been well established.[155]

Although the frequency of OA increases with age, this does not mean that advanced aging universally *causes* OA. The association may be partially due to years of habitual and perhaps specific joint loading patterns that exceed the stress tolerance of the articular cartilage—a scenario that may or may not be associated with previous trauma.[92,104] Consider, for example, a habitual loading pattern associated with increased genu varus (i.e., a bow-legged position) during walking. Over the years, the increased loading of the medial tibial plateau may trigger or predispose the medial compartment of the tibiofemoral joint to excessive wear and ultimately OA (see Chapter 13).

Mechanical abnormalities are among the most common risk factors for OA.[95] Altered mechanical loading can occur as a result of trauma, chronic overuse, atypical joint morphology, and obesity. Posttraumatic OA may affect any synovial joint that has been exposed to a trauma of sufficient severity or chronicity.[146] In a similar manner, joint morphology can be a risk factor for OA. For example, abnormal morphology of the femur and acetabulum can cause repeated impingement within the hip joint, which can lead to hip OA.[11] Biological sex and genetic factors can also increase the risk of OA. Familial OA, for example, affects the joints of the hand and is more frequent in women. Finally, some cases of OA occur in the absence of a known cause. Idiopathic OA affects only one or a few joints, particularly those that are subjected to the highest weight-bearing loads: hip, knee, and lumbar spine.

Rheumatoid arthritis typically differs markedly from OA, because it is a systemic, autoimmune connective tissue disorder with a strong, systemic inflammatory component. An accurate diagnosis of this disorder is contingent upon joint involvement, serologic results, and symptom duration, with the involvement of multiple joints as a prominent characteristic of RA.[2] The joint dysfunction is manifested by significant inflammation of the capsule, synovium, and synovial fluid. The articular cartilage is exposed to an enzymatic process that can rapidly erode the articular surface. The joint capsule is distended by the recurrent swelling and inflammation, often causing marked joint instability and pain. Interestingly, levels of B-cell activating factor, a cytokine mediator, have been found to be elevated in RA and in other autoimmune diseases, influencing immune responses and oscillating with the level of disease activity. This suggests possible applications of B-cell activating factor antagonists in the pharmacologic management of RA; however, further research and development are required.[148]

A Brief Look at Some Effects of Advanced Aging on Periarticular Connective Tissue and Bone

Reaching an advanced age is associated with histologic changes in periarticular connective tissues and bone that, in turn, may produce mechanical changes in joint function.[72,79] It is often not possible to separate the effects of aging in humans from the effects of reduced physical activity or immobilization. At a fundamental level, the physiologic effects of all three variables are remarkably similar.

The rate and process by which tissue ages is highly individualized and can be modified, positively or negatively, by the types and frequency of activities and by a host of medical, hormonal, genetic and nutritional factors.[20,72,102] In the broadest sense, aging is accompanied by a slowing of the rate of fibrous protein and proteoglycan replacement and repair in all periarticular connective tissues and bone.[8,65,77,128] Tissues, therefore, lose their ability to restrain and optimally disperse forces produced at the joint. The effects of microtrauma over the years can accumulate to produce subclinical damage that may progress to a structural failure or a measurable change in mechanical properties. Such a scenario may also explain the apparent association between OA and aging. Another clinical example of this phenomenon is the age-related deterioration of the ligaments and articular capsule associated with the glenohumeral joint. Reduced structural support provided by these tissues may eventually culminate in tendonitis or tears in the rotator cuff muscles.

The *glycosaminoglycan* (GAG) molecules produced by aging cells in connective tissues are fewer in number and smaller in size than those produced by young cells.[29,65,89,106,130] This reduced concentration of GAGs (and hence proteoglycans) reduces the water-binding capacity of the extracellular matrix. More specifically, less proteoglycan content reduces the ability of the nucleus to attract and retain water, thereby limiting the ability of connective tissue to effectively absorb and transfer loads.[24] Aged articular cartilage, for example, contains less water and is less able to attenuate and distribute imposed forces on subchondral bone. These age-related changes, particularly when combined with either over- or underloading, may serve as precursors to osteoarthritis.[16,47]

Collagen fibers within poorly hydrated ligaments lack the ability to slide across one another with ease. As a result, fibers within ligaments do not align themselves with the imposed forces as readily, hampering the ability of the tissue to maximally resist a rapidly applied force. The likelihood of adhesions forming between previously mobile tissue planes is increased, thus promoting range-of-motion restrictions in aging joints.[12,139,140]

Interestingly, tendons have been shown to become *less* stiff (or more compliant) with aging and with chronic unloading.[73,97] A significant increase in compliance may reduce the mechanical efficiency and speed of transferring muscle force to bone. Consequently, muscles may become less able to optimally stabilize a joint. The specific mechanisms causing reduced stiffness (or greater compliance)

Work in recent decades has uncovered the importance of gene sequences and genetic variation on many human diseases. While much remains to be discovered, a role for genetics in disease susceptibility is well established, including for musculoskeletal diseases.[22,55]

Genetic advances have implications for diagnostics and pharmacologic interventions (i.e., gene therapy). However, genetic code cannot be modified through conservative interventions. Instead, conservative interventions have the potential to influence gene expression through *epigenetics.*

Epigenetics refers to the processes that modulate gene expression. In brief, the same genetic code can be expressed differently based on changes in the gene structure (a process known as folding) or the accessibility of specific regions of DNA (such as through DNA methylation or acetylation of histones).[15,86] Changes in gene structure and accessibility are the result of our environment, both in the literal and figurative sense. Diet and exercise, for example, have the potential to influence epigenetics.[109]

Of course, it is well-established that exercise and physical activity have substantial benefits for overall health. However, greater understanding of the epigenetic processes that mediate improvements in health and wellness may lead to more targeted interventions for rehabilitation. For example, such knowledge may guide a clinician when selecting dosages of cardiovascular exercise or strength-training for a patient with fibromyalgia.[107] While more research is needed, it is clear that rehabilitation experts are well-poised to influence health and wellness through a greater understanding of epigenetics.[124]

are unknown, but data suggests these differ between males and females.[102] Such changes may explain age- and sex-associated differences in the frequency of tendon overuse injuries, known as "tendinopathies."

Bone becomes weaker with aging, a result of decreased osteoblastic activity and reduced differentiation of bone marrow stem cells.[20,67,99] Age-related changes in bone metabolism contribute to osteoporosis and to slower healing of fractures in persons of advanced age. Osteoporosis is a condition that results in thinning of both trabecular and compact bone in males and females. The altered metabolism of bone—and cartilage—is sex-specific, though, which may explain sex differences in bone and joint pathologies, such as osteoporosis and osteoarthritis.[21,131,156]

Fortunately, many of the potentially negative physiologic effects of aging periarticular connective tissues and bone can be mitigated, to an extent, through physical activity and resistance training.[76,79,83,110,143] These responses serve as the basis for many of the physical rehabilitation principles used in the treatment of persons of advanced age.

SYNOPSIS

Joints provide the foundation of musculoskeletal motion and permit the stability and dispersion of forces between segments of the body. Several classification schemes exist to categorize joints and to allow discussion of their mechanical and kinematic characteristics. Motions of anatomic joints are often complex because of their asymmetric shapes and incongruent surfaces. The axes of rotation are often estimated for purposes of clinical measurement, such as goniometry.

The function and resilience of joints are determined by the architecture and the types of tissues that make up the joints. All periarticular connective tissues (and bone) share a fundamentally similar histologic organization. Each tissue contains cells, a ground substance or matrix, and fibrous proteins. The extent and proportion of these components vary considerably based on the primary functional demand imposed on the tissue. Joint capsules, ligaments, fasciae, and tendons are designed to resist tension in multiple or single directions. Articular cartilage is extraordinarily suited to resist compression and shear within joints and, in the presence of synovial fluid, provides a remarkably smooth interface for joint movement. Fibrocartilage shares structural and functional characteristics of dense connective tissues and articular cartilage. The fibrocartilaginous menisci at the knee, for example, must resist large compressive forces from the surrounding large muscles and tolerate the multidirectional shearing stress created by the sliding arthrokinematics within the joint. Bone is a highly specialized connective tissue, designed to support the body and its limbs and to provide a series of levers for the muscles to move the body.

The ability to repair damaged joint tissues is strongly related to the presence of a direct blood supply and the availability of progenitor cells. The functional health and longevity of joints are also affected by age, loading, immobilization, trauma, and certain disease states.

REFERENCES

1. Adstrum S, Hedley G, Schleip R, et al.: Defining the fascial system, *J Bodyw Mov Ther* 21:173–177, 2017. https://doi.org/10.1016/j.jbmt.2016.11.003.
2. Aletaha D, Neogi T, Silman AJ, et al.: 2010 Rheumatoid arthritis classification criteria, *Arthritis Rheum* 62:2569–2581, 2010.
3. Anderson DD, Chubinskaya S, Guilak F, et al.: Posttraumatic osteoarthritis: improved understanding and opportunities for early intervention [Review], *J Orthop Res* 29(6):802–809, 2011.
4. Antunes BM, Campos EZ, Dos Santos RVT, et al.: Anti-inflammatory response to acute exercise is related with intensity and physical fitness, *J Cell Biochem* 120:5333–5342, 2019. https://doi.org/10.1002/jcb.27810.
5. Armiento AR, Stoddart MJ, Alini M, et al.: Biomaterials for articular cartilage tissue engineering: learning from biology, *Acta Biomater* 65:1–20, 2018. https://doi.org/10.1016/j.actbio.2017.11.021.
6. Ashby K, Yilmaz E, Mathkour M, et al.: Ligaments stabilizing the sacrum and sacroiliac joint: a comprehensive review, *Neurosurg Rev* 45:357–364, 2022. https://doi.org/10.1007/s10143-021-01625-y.
7. Bae WC, Wong VW, Hwang J, et al.: Wear-lines and split-lines of human patellar cartilage: relation to tensile biomechanical properties, *Osteoarthritis Cartilage* 16:841–845, 2008.
8. Bauge C, Boumediene K: Use of adult stem cells for cartilage tissue engineering: current status and future developments, *Stem Cells Int Epub* 2015:1–14, 2015, https://doi.org/10.1155/2015/438026.
9. Beattie PF: Current understanding of lumbar intervertebral disc degeneration: a review with emphasis upon etiology, pathophysiology, and lumbar magnetic resonance imaging findings, *J Orthop Sports Phys Ther* 38:329–340, 2008.
10. Beaulieu ML, DeClercq MG, Rietberg NT, et al.: The anterior cruciate ligament can become hypertrophied in response to mechanical loading: a magnetic resonance imaging study in elite athletes, *Am J Sports Med* 49:2371–2378, 2021. https://doi.org/10.1177/03635465211012354.
11. Beck M, Kalhor M, Leunig M, et al.: Hip morphology influences the pattern of damage to the acetabular cartilage: Femoroacetabular impingement as a cause of early osteoarthritis of the hip, *J Bone Joint Surg Br* 87:1012–1018, 2005. https://doi.org/10.1302/0301-620X.87B7.15203.
12. Begg RK, Sparrow WA: Aging effects on knee and ankle joint angles at key events and phases of the gait cycle, *J Med Eng Technol* 30:382–389, 2006.
13. Benjamin M, Kaiser E, Milz S: Structure-function relationships in tendons: a review, *J Anat* 212(3):211–228, 2008.
14. Bialosky JE, Beneciuk JM, Bishop MD, et al.: Unraveling the mechanisms of manual therapy: modeling an approach, *J Orthop Sports Phys Ther* 48:8–18, 2018. https://doi.org/10.2519/jospt.2018.7476.
15. Bonev B, Cavalli G: Organization and function of the 3D genome, *Nat Rev Genet* 17:661–678, 2016. https://doi.org/10.1038/nrg.2016.112.
16. Bricca A, Juhl CB, Grodzinsky AJ, et al.: Impact of a daily exercise dose on knee joint cartilage - a systematic review and meta-analysis of randomized controlled trials in healthy animals, *Osteoarthritis Cartilage* 25:1223–1237, 2017. https://doi.org/10.1016/j.joca.2017.03.009.
17. Buckwalter JA, Brown TD: Joint injury, repair, and remodeling: roles in post-traumatic osteoarthritis, *Clin Orthop Relat Res* 423:7–16, 2004.
18. Butterfield TA, Best TM, Merrick MA: The dual roles of neutrophils and macrophages in inflammation: a critical balance between tissue damage and repair, *J Athl Train* 41:457–465, 2006.
19. Capogna B, Strauss E, Konda S, et al.: Distal patellar tendon avulsion in association with high-energy knee trauma: a case series and review of the literature, *Knee* 24:468–476, 2017. https://doi.org/10.1016/j.knee.2016.10.020.
20. Chen JS, Cameron ID, Cumming RG, et al.: Effect of age-related chronic immobility on markers of bone turnover, *J Bone Miner Res* 21:324–331, 2006.
21. Choi KH, Lee JH, Lee DG: Sex-related differences in bone metabolism in osteoporosis observational study, *Medicine (Baltim)* 100:e26153, 2021. https://doi.org/10.1097/MD.0000000000026153.
22. Claussnitzer M, Cho JH, Collins R, et al.: A brief history of human disease genetics, *Nature* 577:179–189, 2020. https://doi.org/10.1038/s41586-019-1879-7.
23. Coleman JL, Widmyer MR, Leddy HA, et al.: Diurnal variations in articular cartilage thickness and strain in the human knee, *J Biomech* 46:541–547, 2013. https://doi.org/10.1016/j.jbiomech.2012.09.013.
24. Cortes DH, Han WM, Smith LJ, et al.: Mechanical properties of the extra-fibrillar matrix of human annulus fibrosus are location and age dependent, *J Orthop Res* 31(11):1725–1732, 2013.
25. D'Andrea CR, Alfraihat A, Singh A, et al.: Part 1. Review and meta-analysis of studies on modulation of longitudinal bone growth and growth plate activity: a macro-scale perspective, *J Orthop Res* 39:907–918, 2021. https://doi.org/10.1002/jor.24976.
26. de Bruin M, Smeulders MJ, Kreulen M: Flexor carpi ulnaris tenotomy alone does not eliminate its contribution to wrist torque, *Clin Biomech* 26:725–728, 2011. https://doi.org/10.1016/j.clinbiomech.2011.03.007.
27. Deng Z, Jin J, Zhao J, et al.: Cartilage defect treatments: with or without cells? Mesenchymal stem cells or chondrocytes? Traditional or matrix-assisted? A systematic review and meta-analyses [Review], *Stem Cells Int* 2016:9201492, 2016.
28. Ding C, Cicuttini F, Scott F, et al.: Association between age and knee structural change: a cross sectional MRI based study, *Ann Rheum Dis* 64:549–555, 2005.
29. Dudhia J: Aggrecan, aging and assembly in articular cartilage, *Cell Mol Life Sci* 62:2241–2256, 2005.
30. Dudley-Javoroski S, Saha PK, Liang G, et al.: High dose compressive loads attenuate bone mineral loss in humans with spinal cord injury, *Osteoporos Int* 23(9):2335–2346, 2012.
31. Dudley-Javoroski S, Shields RK: Active-resisted stance modulates regional bone mineral density in humans with spinal cord injury, *J Spinal Cord Med* 36(3):191–199, 2013.
32. Fede C, Petrelli L, Guidolin D, et al.: Evidence of a new hidden neural network into deep fasciae, *Sci Rep* 11:12623, 2021. https://doi.org/10.1038/s41598-021-92194-z.
33. Feng J, Luo J, Yang P, et al.: Piezo2 channel-Merkel cell signaling modulates the conversion of touch to itch, *Science* 360:530–533, 2018. https://doi.org/10.1126/science.aar5703.
34. Ferrell WR, Gandevia SC, McCloskey DI: The role of joint receptors in human kinaesthesia when intramuscular receptors cannot contribute, *J Physiol* 386:63–71, 1987.
35. Freeman MA, Wyke B: The innervation of the ankle joint: an anatomical and histological study in the cat, *J Anat* 101:505–532, 1967.
36. Freitas SR, Vaz JR, Bruno PM, et al.: Stretching effects: high-intensity & moderate-duration vs. Low-intensity & long-duration, *Int J Sports Med* 37:239–244, 2016. https://doi.org/10.1055/s-0035-1548946.
37. Frost HM: A: 2003 update of bone physiology and Wolff's Law for clinicians, *Angle Orthod* 74:3–15, 2004.
38. Gartner LP, Lee LM: *J: Gartner & Hiatt's atlas and text of histology*, ed 8, Philadelphia, 2022, Wolters Kluwer, Inc.
39. Gersing AS, Schwaiger BJ, Nevitt MC, et al.: Anterior cruciate ligament abnormalities are associated

with accelerated progression of knee joint degeneration in knees with and without structural knee joint abnormalities: 96-month data from the osteoarthritis initiative, *Osteoarthritis Cartilage* 29:995–1005, 2021. https://doi.org/10.1016/j.joca.2021.03.011.

40. Gregory DE, Bae WC, Sah RL, et al.: Disc degeneration reduces the delamination strength of the annulus fibrosis in the rabbit anular disc puncture model, *Spine J* 14(7):1265–1271, 2014.

41. Grunhagen T, Wilde G, Soukane DM, et al.: Nutrient supply and intervertebral disc metabolism, *J Bone Joint Surg Am* 88(Suppl 2):30–35, 2006.

42. Haapala J, Arokoski J, Pirttimaki J, et al.: Incomplete restoration of immobilization induced softening of young beagle knee articular cartilage after 50-week remobilization, *Int J Sports Med* 21:76–81, 2000.

43. Hagert E, Lluch A, Rein S: The role of proprioception and neuromuscular stability in carpal instabilities, *J Hand Surg Eur Vol* 41:94–101, 2016. https://doi.org/10.1177/1753193415590390.

44. Hayashi K: Biomechanical studies of the remodeling of knee joint tendons and ligaments, *J Biomech* 29:707–716, 1996.

45. Heijink A, Gomoll AH, Madry H, et al.: Biomechanical considerations in the pathogenesis of osteoarthritis of the knee, *Knee Surg Sports Traumatol Arthrosc* 20:423–435, 2012.

46. Hoffman BD, Grashoff C, Schwartz MA: Dynamic molecular processes mediate cellular mechanotransduction, *Nature* 475:316–323, 2011. https://doi.org/10.1038/nature10316.

47. Hu Y, Chen X, Wang S, et al.: Subchondral bone microenvironment in osteoarthritis and pain, *Bone Res* 9:20, 2021. https://doi.org/10.1038/s41413-021-00147-z.

48. Huijing PA, Baan GC: Myofascial force transmission via extramuscular pathways occurs between antagonistic muscles, *Cells Tissues Organs* 188:400–414, 2008. https://doi.org/10.1159/000118097.

49. Hutchinson LA, Lichtwark GA, Willy RW, et al.: The iliotibial band: a complex structure with versatile functions, *Sports Med* 52:995–1008, 2022. https://doi.org/10.1007/s40279-021-01634-3.

50. Ingber DE: Cellular mechanotransduction: putting all the pieces together again, *FASEB J* 20:811–827, 2006. https://doi.org/10.1096/fj.05-5424rev.

51. Iozzo RV, Schaefer L: Proteoglycan form and function: a comprehensive nomenclature of proteoglycans, *Matrix Biol* 42:11–55, 2015.

52. Jeong S, Lee DY, Choi DS, et al.: Acute effect of heel-drop exercise with varying ranges of motion on the gastrocnemius aponeurosis-tendon's mechanical properties, *J Electromyogr Kinesiol* 24(3):375–379, 2014.

53. Kjaer M, Magnusson P, Krogsgaard M, et al.: Extracellular matrix adaptation of tendon and skeletal muscle to exercise, *J Anat* 208:445–450, 2006.

54. Klein GL: *Disruption of bone and skeletal muscle in severe burns*, Bone Res Epub, 2015.

55. Koromani F, Alonso N, Alves I, et al.: The "GEnomics of musculo skeletal traits TranslatiOnal NEtwork": origins, rationale, organization, and prospects, *Front Endocrinol* 12:709815, 2021. https://doi.org/10.3389/fendo.2021.709815.

56. Kubo Y, Hoffmann B, Goltz K, et al.: Different frequency of cyclic tensile strain relates to anabolic/catabolic conditions consistent with immunohistochemical staining intensity in tenocytes, *Int J Mol Sci* 21, 2020. https://doi.org/10.3390/ijms21031082.

57. Kunz RI, Coradini JG, Silva LI, et al.: Effects of immobilization on the ankle joint in Wistar rats, *Braz J Med Biol Res* 47(10):842–849, 2014.

58. Kurrat HJ, Oberlander W: The thickness of the cartilage in the hip joint, *J Anat* 126:145–155, 1978.

59. Kuttapitiya A, Assi L, Laing K, et al.: Microarray analysis of bone marrow lesions in osteoarthritis demonstrates upregulation of genes implicated in osteochondral turnover, neurogenesis and inflammation, *Ann Rheum Dis* 76:1764–1773, 2017. https://doi.org/10.1136/annrheumdis-2017-211396.

60. Lacourpaille L, Nordez A, Hug F, et al.: Time-course effect of exercise-induced muscle damage on localized muscle mechanical properties assessed using elastography, *Acta Physiol* 211(1):135–146, 2014.

61. Lad NK, Liu B, Ganapathy PK, et al.: Effect of normal gait on in vivo tibiofemoral cartilage strains, *J Biomech* 49:2870–2876, 2016. https://doi.org/10.1016/j.jbiomech.2016.06.025.

62. Lama P, Le Maitre CL, Harding IJ, et al.: Nerves and blood vessels in degenerated intervertebral discs are confined to physically disrupted tissue, *J Anat* 233:86–97, 2018. https://doi.org/10.1111/joa.12817.

63. Langevin HM: Fascia mobility, proprioception, and myofascial pain, *Life* 11, 2021. https://doi.org/10.3390/life11070668.

64. Lanham NS, Swindell HW, Levine WN: The subacromial bursa: current concepts review, *JBJS Rev* 9, 2021. https://doi.org/10.2106/JBJS.RVW.21.00110.

65. Laureano PE, Oliveira KD, Aro AA, et al.: Structure and composition of arytenoids cartilage of the bullfrog (*Lithobates catesbeianus*) during maturation and aging, *Micron* 77:16–24, 2015.

66. Lee DH, Kim SJ, Kim SA, et al.: Past, present, and future of cartilage restoration: from localized defect to arthritis, *Knee Surg Relat Res* 34:1, 2022. https://doi.org/10.1186/s43019-022-00132-8.

67. Li CJ, Cheng P, Liang MK, et al.: MicroRNA-188 regulates age-related switch between osteoblasts and adipocyte differentiation, *J Clin Invest* 125(4):1509–1522, 2015.

68. Lichtwark GA, Wilson AM: Interactions between the human gastrocnemius muscle and the Achilles tendon during incline, level and decline locomotion, *J Exp Biol* 209(21):4379–4388, 2006.

69. Loeser RF: Aging and osteoarthritis, *Curr Opin Rheumatol* 23:492–496, 2011.

70. Lowe J, Anderson P, Anderson S: *Stevens & Lowe's human histology*, ed 5, Philadelphia, 2018, Elsevier.

71. Maas H, Sandercock TG: Force transmission between synergistic skeletal muscles through connective tissue linkages, *J Biomed Biotechnol* 2010:575672, 2010. https://doi.org/10.1155/2010/575672.

72. Madej W, van Caam A, Blaney Davidson EN, et al.: *Ageing is associated with reduction of mechanically-induced activation of Smad2/3P signaling in articular cartilage*, Osteoarthritis Cartilage Epub, 2015.

73. Maganaris CN, Reeves ND, Rittweger J, et al.: Adaptive response of human tendon to paralysis, *Muscle Nerve* 33:85–92, 2006.

74. Magnusson SP, Hansen P, Aagaard P, et al.: Differential strain patterns of the human gastrocnemius aponeurosis and free tendon, in vivo, *Acta Physiol Scand* 177:185–195, 2003.

75. Magnusson SP, Kjaer M: The impact of loading, unloading, ageing and injury on the human tendon, *J Physiol* 597:1283–1298, 2019. https://doi.org/10.1113/JP275450.

76. Magnusson SP, Narici MV, Maganaris CN, et al.: Human tendon behaviour and adaptation, in vivo, *J Physiol* 586:71–81, 2008.

77. Martin JA, Brown TD, Heiner AD, et al.: Chondrocyte senescence, joint loading and osteoarthritis, *Clin Orthop Relat Res* 427(Suppl):S96–S103, 2004.

78. Matsuzaki T, Yoshida S, Kojima S, et al.: Influence of ROM exercise on the joint components during immobilization, *J Phys Ther Sci* 25(12):1547–1551, 2013.

79. McCarthy MM, Hannafin JA: The mature athlete: aging tendon and ligament, *Sports Health* 6(1):41–48, 2014.

80. McHenry CL, Shields RK: A biomechanical analysis of exercise in standing, supine, and seated positions: implications for individuals with spinal cord injury, *J Spinal Cord Med* 35(3):140–147, 2012.

81. Mehlman CT, Araghi A, Roy DR: Hyphenated history: the Hueter-Volkmann law, *Am J Orthop (Belle Mead NJ)* 26:798–800, 1997.

82. Mihalko WM, Haider H, Kurtz S, et al.: New materials for hip and knee joint replacement: what's hip and what's in kneed? *J Orthop Res* 38:1436–1444, 2020. https://doi.org/10.1002/jor.24750.

83. Mikesky AE, Mazzuca SA, Brandt KD, et al.: Effects of strength training on the incidence and progression of knee osteoarthritis, *Arthritis Rheum* 55:690–699, 2006.

84. Mildren RL, Hare CM, Bent LR: Cutaneous afferent feedback from the posterior ankle contributes to proprioception, *Neurosci Lett* 636:145–150, 2017. https://doi.org/10.1016/j.neulet.2016.10.058.

85. Mohammadi F, Roozdar A: Effects of fatigue due to contraction of evertor muscles on the ankle joint position sense in male soccer players, *Am J Sports Med* 38:824–828, 2010.

86. Moore LD, Le T, Fan G: DNA methylation and its basic function, *Neuropsychopharmacology* 38:23–38, 2013. https://doi.org/10.1038/npp.2012.112.

87. Mosher TJ, Liu Y, Torok CM: Functional cartilage MRI T2 mapping: evaluating the effect of age and training on knee cartilage response to running, *Osteoarthritis Cartilage* 18:358–364, 2010.

88. Muller FJ, Setton LA, Manicourt DH, et al.: Centrifugal and biochemical comparison of proteoglycan aggregates from articular cartilage in experimental joint disuse and joint instability, *J Orthop Res* 12:498–508, 1994.

89. Muller-Lutz A, Schleich C, Pentang G, et al.: *Age-dependency of glycosaminoglycan content in lumbar discs: a 3t gagCEST study*, J Magn Reson Imaging Epub, 2015.

90. Neumann DA, Garceau LR: A proposed novel function of the psoas minor revealed through cadaver dissection, *Clin Anat* 28:243–252, 2015. https://doi.org/10.1002/ca.22467.

91. Newton RA: Joint receptor contributions to reflexive and kinesthetic responses, *Phys Ther* 62:22–29, 1982.

92. Nielsen AW, Klose-Jensen R, Hartlev LB, et al.: Age-related histological changes in calcified cartilage and subchondral bone in femoral heads from healthy humans, *Bone* 129:115037, 2019. https://doi.org/10.1016/j.bone.2019.115037.

93. Noyes FR, Heckmann TP, Barber-Westin SD: Meniscus repair and transplantation: a comprehensive update [Review], *J Orthop Sports Phys Ther* 42(3):274–290, 2012.

94. Noyes FR: Functional properties of knee ligaments and alterations induced by immobilization: a correlative biomechanical and histological study in primates, *Clin Orthop Relat Res* 123:210–242, 1977.

95. Occhetta P, Mainardi A, Votta E, et al.: Hyperphysiological compression of articular cartilage induces an osteoarthritic phenotype in a cartilage-on-a-chip model, *Nat Biomed Eng* 3:545–557, 2019. https://doi.org/10.1038/s41551-019-0406-3.

96. Olstad K, Ekman S, Carlson CS: *An update on the pathogenesis of osteochondrosis*, Vet Pathol Epub, 2015.

97. Onambele GL, Narici MV, Maganaris CN: Calf muscle-tendon properties and postural balance in old age, *J Appl Physiol* 100:2048–2056, 2006.

98. Ovalle WK, Nahirney PC: *Netter's essential histology*, ed 3, Philadelphia, 2020, Elsevier.

99. Panwar P, Lamour G, Mackenzie NC, et al.: Changes in structural-mechanical properties and degradability of collagen during ageing-associated modifications, *J Biol Chem Epub*, 2015.

100. Patil VA, Masters KS: Engineered collagen matrices, *Bioeng (Basel)* 7:163, 2020. https://doi.org/10.3390/bioengineering7040163.

101. Pearson OM, Lieberman DE: The aging of Wolff's "law": ontogeny and responses to mechanical loading in cortical bone, *Am J Phys Anthropol* 39(Suppl):63–99, 2004.

102. Pease LI, Clegg PD, Proctor CJ, et al.: Cross platform analysis of transcriptomic data identifies ageing has distinct and opposite effects on tendon in males and females, *Sci Rep* 7:14443, 2017. https://doi.org/10.1038/s41598-017-14650-z.

103. Peng BG: Pathophysiology, diagnosis, and treatment of discogenic low back pain, *World J Orthop* 4(2):42–52, 2013.

104. Peters AE, Akhtar R, Comerford EJ, et al.: The effect of ageing and osteoarthritis on the mechanical properties of cartilage and bone in the human knee joint, *Sci Rep* 8:5931, 2018. https://doi.org/10.1038/s41598-018-24258-6.

105. Petersen AM, Pedersen BK: The anti-inflammatory effect of exercise, *J Appl Physiol* 98:1154–1162, 2005. https://doi.org/10.1152/japplphysiol.00164.2004.

106. Podichetty VK: The aging spine: the role of inflammatory mediators in intervertebral disc degeneration, *Cell Mol Biol* 53:4–18, 2007.

107. Polli A, Nijs J, Ickmans K, et al.: Linking lifestyle factors to complex pain states: 3 reasons why understanding epigenetics may improve the delivery of patient-centered care, *J Orthop Sports Phys Ther* 49:683–687, 2019. https://doi.org/10.2519/jospt.2019.0612.

108. Proske U, Gandevia SC: The kinaesthetic senses, *J Physiol* 587:4139–4146, 2009.

109. Quach A, Levine ME, Tanaka T, et al.: Epigenetic clock analysis of diet, exercise, education, and lifestyle factors, *Aging (Albany NY)* 9:419–446, 2017. https://doi.org/10.18632/aging.101168.

110. Racunica TL, Teichtahl AJ, Wang Y, et al.: Effect of physical activity on articular knee joint structures in community-based adults, *Arthritis Rheum* 57:1261–1268, 2007.

111. Reeves ND, Maganaris CN, Narici MV: Effect of strength training on human patella tendon mechanical properties of older individuals, *J Physiol* 548:971–981, 2003. https://doi.org/10.1113/jphysiol.2002.035576.

112. Rein S, Hagert E, Hanisch U, et al.: Immunohistochemical analysis of sensory nerve endings in ankle ligaments: a cadaver study, *Cells Tissues Organs* 197:64–76, 2013.

113. Richter P: Myofascial chains: a review of different models. 2012. In Schleip R, Findley T, L C, et al.: *Fascia. The tensional network of the human body*, ed 1, Edinburgh, 2012, Churchill Livingstone, pp 123–131.

114. Rubman MH, Noyes FR, Barber-Westin SD: Arthroscopic repair of meniscal tears that extend into the avascular zone. A review of 198 single and complex tears, *Am J Sports Med* 26:87–95, 1998.

115. Salva-Coll G, Garcia-Elias M, Hagert E: Scapholunate instability: proprioception and neuromuscular control, *J Wrist Surg* 2:136–140, 2013. https://doi.org/10.1055/s-0033-1341960.

116. Schaible H-G, von Segond Banchet G, Boettger MK, et al.: The role of proinflammatory cytokines in the generation and maintenance of joint pain, *Ann N Y Acad Sci* 1193:60–69, 2010.

117. Scheffer DDL, Latini A: Exercise-induced immune system response: anti-inflammatory status on peripheral and central organs, *Biochim Biophys Acta, Mol Basis Dis* 1866:165823, 2020. https://doi.org/10.1016/j.bbadis.2020.165823.

118. Schleip R, Gabbiani G, Wilke J, et al.: Fascia is able to actively contract and may thereby influence musculoskeletal dynamics: a histochemical and mechanographic investigation, *Front Physiol* 10:336, 2019. https://doi.org/10.3389/fphys.2019.00336.

119. Schulze-Tanzil G, Al-Sadi O, Wiegand E, et al.: The role of pro-inflammatory and immunoregulatory cytokines in tendon healing and rupture: new insights, *Scand J Med Sci Sports* 21:337–351, 2011. https://doi.org/10.1111/j.1600-0838.2010.01265.x.

120. Servodio Iammarrone C, Cadossi M, Sambri A, et al.: Is there a role of pulsed electromagnetic fields in management of patellofemoral pain syndrome? Randomized controlled study at one year follow-up, *Bioelectromagnetics* 37:81–88, 2016. https://doi.org/10.1002/bem.21953.

121. Setton LA, Chen J: Cell mechanics and mechanobiology in the intervertebral disc, *Spine* 29:2710–2723, 2004.

122. Shepherd DE, Seedhom BB: Thickness of human articular cartilage in joints of the lower limb, *Ann Rheum Dis* 58:27–34, 1999. https://doi.org/10.1136/ard.58.1.27.

123. Shields RK, Dudley-Javoroski S, Law LA: Electrically induced muscle contractions influence bone density decline after spinal cord injury, *Spine* 31:548–553, 2006.

124. Shields RK, Dudley-Javoroski S: Epigenetics and the international classification of functioning, disability and health model: bridging nature, nurture, and patient-centered population health, *Phys Ther* 102, 2022. https://doi.org/10.1093/ptj/pzab247.

125. Shields RK, Dudley-Javoroski S: Musculoskeletal adaptations in chronic spinal cord injury: effects of long-term soleus electrical stimulation training, *Neurorehabil Neural Repair* 21:169–179, 2007.

126. Shoulders MD, Raines RT: Collagen structure and stability, *Annu Rev Biochem* 78:929–958, 2009.

127. Shubayev VI, Kato K, Myers RR: Cytokines in pain. In Kruger L, Light AR, editors: *Translational pain research: from mouse to man. Frontiers in neuroscience*, Boca Raton (FL), 2010, CRC Press/Taylor & Francis.

128. Smith K, Rennie MJ: New approaches and recent results concerning human-tissue collagen synthesis, *Curr Opin Clin Nutr Metab Care* 10:582–590, 2007.

129. Sophia Fox AJ, Bedi A, Rodeo SA: The basic science of articular cartilage: structure, composition, and function, *Sports Health* 1:461–468, 2009. https://doi.org/10.1177/1941738109350438.

130. Squires GR, Okouneff S, Ionescu M, et al.: The pathobiology of focal lesion development in aging human articular cartilage and molecular matrix changes characteristic of osteoarthritis, *Arthritis Rheum* 48:1261–1270, 2003.

131. Srikanth VK, Fryer JL, Zhai G, et al.: A meta-analysis of sex differences prevalence, incidence and severity of osteoarthritis, *Osteoarthritis Cartilage* 13:769–781, 2005. https://doi.org/10.1016/j.joca.2005.04.014.

132. Standring S: *Gray's anatomy: the anatomical basis of clinical practice*, ed 42, St Louis, 2020, Elsevier.

133. Stecco C, Pirri C, Fede C, et al.: Fascial or muscle stretching? A narrative review, *Appl Sci* 11:307, 2020. https://doi.org/10.3390/app11010307.

134. Stecco C, Porzionato A, Lancerotto L, et al.: Histological study of the deep fasciae of the limbs, *J Bodyw Mov Ther* 12:225–230, 2008. https://doi.org/10.1016/j.jbmt.2008.04.041.

135. Stecco C, Schleip R: A fascia and the fascial system, *J Body Mov Ther* 20:139–140, 2016. https://doi.org/10.1016/j.jbmt.2015.11.012.

136. Suri S, Gill SE, Massena de Camin S, et al.: Neurovascular invasion at the osteochondral junction and in osteophytes in osteoarthritis, *Ann Rheum Dis* 66:1423–1428, 2007. https://doi.org/10.1136/ard.2006.063354.

137. Svensson RB, Heinemeier KM, Couppe C, et al.: Effect of aging and exercise on the tendon, *J Appl Physiol* 121:1237–1246, 2016. https://doi.org/10.1152/japplphysiol.00328.2016.

138. Szadek KM, Hoogland PV, Zuurmond WW, et al.: Possible nociceptive structures in the sacroiliac joint cartilage: an immunohistochemical study, *Clin Anat* 23(2):192–198, 2010.

139. Thornton GM, Lemmex DB, Ono Y, et al.: *Aging affects mechanical properties and lubricin/PRG4 gene expression in normal ligaments*, J Biomech Epub, 2015.

140. Troke M, Moore AP, Maillardet FJ, et al.: A normative database of lumbar spine ranges of motion, *Man Ther* 10:198–206, 2005.

141. Van GA, Roosen P, Almqvist KF, et al.: Effects of in-vivo exercise on ankle cartilage deformation and recovery in healthy volunteers: an experimental study, *Osteoarthritis Cartilage* 19:1123–1131, 2011.

142. Vincent TL, Wann AKT: Mechanoadaptation: articular cartilage through thick and thin, *J Physiol* 597:1271–1281, 2019. https://doi.org/10.1113/JP275451.

143. von Stengel S, Kemmler W, Kalender WA, et al.: Differential effects of strength versus power training on bone mineral density in postmenopausal women: a 2-year longitudinal study, *Br J Sports Med* 41:649–655, 2007.

144. Wackerhage H, Rennie MJ: How nutrition and exercise maintain the human musculoskeletal mass, *J Anat* 208:451–458, 2006.

145. Wade L, Lichtwark G, Farris DJ: Movement strategies for countermovement jumping are potentially influenced by elastic energy stored and released from tendons, *Sci Rep* 8:1–11, 2018. https://doi.org/10.1038/s41598-018-20387-0.

146. Wang LJ, Zeng N, Yan ZP, et al.: Post-traumatic osteoarthritis following ACL injury, *Arthritis Res Ther* 22:57, 2020. https://doi.org/10.1186/s13075-020-02156-5.

147. Wang N: Review of cellular mechanotransduction, *J Phys D Appl Phys* 50, 2017. https://doi.org/10.1088/1361-6463/aa6e18.

148. Wei F, Chang Y, Wei W: The role of BAFF in the progression of rheumatoid arthritis, *Cytokine* 76(2):537–44, 2015.

149. Wilke J, Krause F, Vogt L, et al.: What is evidence-based about myofascial chains: a systematic review, *Arch Phys Med Rehabil* 97:454–461, 2016. https://doi.org/10.1016/j.apmr.2015.07.023.

150. Wilke J, Macchi V, De Caro R, et al.: Fascia thickness, aging and flexibility: is there an association? *J Anat* 234:43–49, 2019. https://doi.org/10.1111/joa.12902.

151. Wilke J, Schleip R, Yucesoy CA, et al.: Not merely a protective packing organ? A review of fascia and its force transmission capacity, *J Appl Physiol* 124:234–244, 2018. https://doi.org/10.1152/japplphysiol.00565.2017.

152. Wilke J, Vogt L, Niederer D, et al.: Is remote stretching based on myofascial chains as effective as local exercise? A randomised-controlled trial, *J Sports Sci* 35:2021–2027, 2017. https://doi.org/10.1080/02640414.2016.1251606.

153. Woo SL, Abramowitch SD, Kilger R, et al.: Biomechanics of knee ligaments: injury, healing, and repair, *J Biomech* 39:1–20, 2006.

154. Woo SL, Gomez MA, Sites TJ, et al.: The biomechanical and morphological changes in the medial collateral ligament of the rabbit after immobilization and remobilization, *J Bone Joint Surg Am* 69:1200–1211, 1987.

155. Woolf CJ: Central sensitization: implications for the diagnosis and treatment of pain, *Pain* 152:S2–S15, 2011.

156. Yang Y, You X, Cohen JD, et al.: Sex differences in osteoarthritis pathogenesis: a comprehensive study based on bioinformatics, *Med Sci Monit* 26:e923331, 2020. https://doi.org/10.12659/MSM.923331.

157. Young B, O'Dowd G, Woodford P: *Wheater's functional histology: a text and colour atlas*, ed 6, Philadelphia, 2013, Churchill Livingstone.

158. Yucesoy CA, Koopman BH, Grootenboer HJ, et al.: Extramuscular myofascial force transmission alters substantially the acute effects of surgical aponeurotomy: Assessment by finite element modeling, *Biomech Model Mechanobiol* 7:175–189, 2008. https://doi.org/10.1007/s10237-007-0084-z.

159. Zanon G, Di Vico G, Marullo M: Osteochondritis dissecans of the knee, *Joints* 2:29–36, 2014.

160. Zimmerman A, Bai L, Ginty DD: The gentle touch receptors of mammalian skin, *Science* 346(6212):950–954, 2014.

161. Zugel M, Maganaris CN, Wilke J, et al.: Fascial tissue research in sports medicine: from molecules to tissue adaptation, injury and diagnostics: consensus statement, *Br J Sports Med* 52:1497, 2018. https://doi.org/10.1136/bjsports-2018-099308.

STUDY QUESTIONS

1. Describe the morphologic differences between ovoid and saddle joints. Provide an anatomic example of each type of joint.
2. Cite the major distinguishing structural and functional differences between a synarthrodial and a diarthrodial (synovial) joint.
3. Intra-articular discs (or menisci) are sometimes found in diarthrodial joints. Name three joints in the body that contain intra-articular discs. Describe the most likely function(s) of these structures at these joints.
4. List the four primary types of tissues that exist throughout the body.
5. Which of the joints illustrated in Figs. 2.3 through 2.9 have (a) the greatest and (b) the least degrees of freedom?
6. Cite the major functional differences between type I collagen and elastin. Cite tissues that contain a high proportion of each protein.
7. What is the difference between an *evolute* and an *instantaneous axis of rotation?* Cite one biomechanical or practical consequence of a joint that possesses a significantly large, although normal, evolute.
8. Define (a) perichondrium and (b) periosteum. What is the primary function of these tissues?
9. Describe the fundamental mechanism used by articular cartilage to repeatedly disperse compression forces across joints.
10. Describe the primary reasons why bone possesses a far superior healing potential than articular cartilage.
11. Wolff's Law and the Hueter-Volkmann Law describe the relationships between external loading and bone formation. Describe the relationships and explain how these two seemingly opposing laws can coexist?
12. Describe two natural effects of advanced aging on periarticular connective tissues. In extreme cases, how could these changes manifest themselves clinically?
13. List three histologic features that are common to articular cartilage, tendon, and bone.
14. Briefly contrast osteoarthritis and rheumatoid arthritis.
15. List three structures *always* found in synovial joints. Cite common pathologies that may affect these structures, and comment on the nature of the resulting impairment.
16. What is the function of synovial fluid?
17. Persons who repeatedly sprain their ankles often show signs of reduced ankle proprioception. Describe a possible association between these clinical issues.

Answers to the study questions are available in the accompanying enhanced eBook version included with the print purchase of this textbook.

Chapter

3

Muscle: The Primary Stabilizer and Mover of the Skeletal System

JONATHON W. SENEFELD, PhD

SANDRA K. HUNTER, PhD, FACSM

DONALD A. NEUMANN, PT, PhD, FAPTA

CHAPTER AT A GLANCE

Stable posture results from a balance of competing forces. Movement, in contrast, occurs when competing forces are unbalanced. Force generated by muscles is the primary means for controlling the intricate balance between posture and movement. This chapter examines the role of muscle and tendon in generating, modulating, storing, and transmitting force; these functions are necessary to stabilize and/or move skeletal structures. Specifically, this chapter investigates the following:

• How muscle stabilizes bones by generating an appropriate amount of force at a given muscle length. Muscles generate force passively (i.e., by a muscle's resistance to stretch) and, to a much greater extent, actively (e.g., by active contraction).

• The ways in which muscle modulates or controls force so that bones move smoothly and forcefully. Normal movement is highly regulated and refined, regardless of the infinite environmental constraints imposed on a given task.

• The use of electromyography (EMG) in the study of kinesiology.

• Basic mechanisms of muscle fatigue.

• Adaptations of muscle attributable to strength training, immobilization, and advanced age.

This approach enables the student of kinesiology to understand the multiple roles of muscles in controlling the postures and movements that are used in daily tasks. In addition, the clinician also has the information needed to form clinical diagnoses about muscular impairments and adaptations that interfere or assist with functional activities. This understanding can lead to the judicious application of interventions to improve a person's functional abilities.

MUSCLE AS A SKELETAL STABILIZER: GENERATING AN APPROPRIATE AMOUNT OF FORCE AT A GIVEN LENGTH

Bones support the human body as it interacts with the environment. Although many tissues that attach to the skeleton support the body, only muscle can adapt to both immediate (acute) and repeated, long-term (chronic) external forces that can destabilize the body. Muscle tissue is ideally suited for this function because it is coupled to both the external environment and the internal control mechanisms provided by the nervous system. Under the fine control of the nervous system, muscle generates the force required to stabilize skeletal structures under a remarkably wide range of conditions. For example, muscle exerts fine control to stabilize fingers manipulating a tiny scalpel during eye surgery. Muscles also generate large forces during the final seconds of a "dead-lift" weightlifting task.

Understanding the special role of muscle in generating stabilizing forces begins with an introduction of the muscle fiber and the sarcomere. This topic is followed by discussion of how muscle morphology and muscle-tendon architecture affect the range of forces transferred to bone. The function of muscle is explored with regard to how it produces *passive tension* from being elongated (or stretched) or to how it generates *active force* as it is stimulated, or "activated," by the nervous system. The relation between muscle force and length and how this relation influences the isometric torque generated about a joint are then examined. Box 3.1 lists a summary of the major concepts addressed in this section.

Introduction to the Structural Organization of Skeletal Muscle

Whole muscles throughout the body, such as the biceps brachii or gastrocnemius, consist of many individual *muscle fibers,* ranging in thickness from about 10 to 100 μm and in length from about 1 to 30 cm.[157] The structural relationship between a muscle fiber and the muscle belly is shown in Fig. 3.1. Each muscle fiber is an individual cell with multiple nuclei. Contraction or shortening of the individual muscle fiber is ultimately responsible for contraction of the whole muscle.

BOX 3.1   Major Concepts: Muscle as a Skeletal Stabilizer

- Introduction to the structural organization of skeletal muscle
- Extracellular connective tissues within muscle
- Muscle morphology
- Muscle architecture: physiologic cross-sectional area and pennation angle
- Passive length-tension curve
- Parallel and series elastic components of muscle and tendon
- Elastic and viscoelastic properties of muscle
- Active length-tension curve
- Histologic structure of the muscle fiber
- Sliding filament theory
- Total length-tension curve: summation of the active and passive forces
- Isometric force and the internal torque–joint angle curve
- Mechanical and physiologic properties affecting the internal torque–joint angle curve

---

The fundamental unit within each muscle fiber is known as the *sarcomere.* Because the sarcomeres are aligned in series throughout each muscle fiber, the shortening of sarcomeres produces a corresponding shortening of the entire fiber. For this reason, the sarcomere is considered the ultimate force generator within muscle. Although the structure and function of the sarcomere are described in more detail later in the chapter, it is important to understand that muscle contains proteins that may be classified as either contractile or noncontractile. *Contractile proteins* within the sarcomere, such as actin and myosin, interact to shorten the muscle fiber and generate an active force. (For this reason, the contractile proteins are also referred to as "active" proteins.) *Noncontractile proteins,* conversely, constitute much of both the cytoskeleton within muscle fibers and supportive infrastructure between fibers. These noncontractile proteins are often referred to as "structural proteins" because of their role in supporting the structure of the muscle fibers. Although structural proteins do not directly create contraction of the muscle fiber, they play an important secondary role in the generation and transmission of force. For example, structural proteins such as the abundant and large *titin* molecule provides passive tension within the muscle fiber, whereas *desmin* stabilizes the alignment of adjacent sarcomeres.[62,90,110,114] In general, structural proteins (1) generate passive tension when stretched, (2) provide internal and external support and alignment of the muscle fiber, and (3) help transfer active forces throughout the muscle. These concepts are further explained in upcoming sections of the chapter.

In addition to active and structural proteins introduced in the previous paragraph, a whole muscle consists of an extensive set of *extracellular connective tissues,* composed mostly of collagen and some elastin.[46] Along with the structural proteins, these extracellular connective tissues are classified as noncontractile tissues, providing structural support and elasticity to the muscle.

Extracellular connective tissues within muscle are separated into three anatomic divisions: epimysium, perimysium, and endomysium. Fig. 3.1 shows these tissues as they surround the various components of muscle—from the muscle belly to the individual muscle fibers. The *epimysium* is a tough structure that surrounds the entire surface of the muscle belly and separates it from other muscles. In essence, the epimysium gives form to the muscle belly. The epimysium contains tightly woven bundles of collagen fibers that resist stretch. The *perimysium* lies within the epimysium and divides muscle into fascicles (i.e., groups of fibers) that provide a conduit for blood vessels and nerves. The perimysium, like epimysium, is tough, relatively thick, and resistive to stretch. The *endomysium* surrounds individual muscle fibers, immediately external to the sarcolemma (cell membrane). The endomysium represents the location of the metabolic exchange between muscle fibers and capillaries.[137] This delicate tissue is composed of a relatively dense meshwork of collagen fibers that is partly connected to the perimysium. Through lateral connections from the muscle fiber, the endomysium transfers part of the muscle's contractile force to the tendon.

Muscle fibers may be of varying length, some extending from tendon to tendon and others only a fraction of this distance. Extracellular connective tissues help interconnect individual muscle fibers and therefore help transmit contractile forces throughout the entire length of the muscle.[87] Although the three sets of connective tissues are described as separate entities, they are interwoven as a continuous band of tissue. This arrangement confers strength, support, and

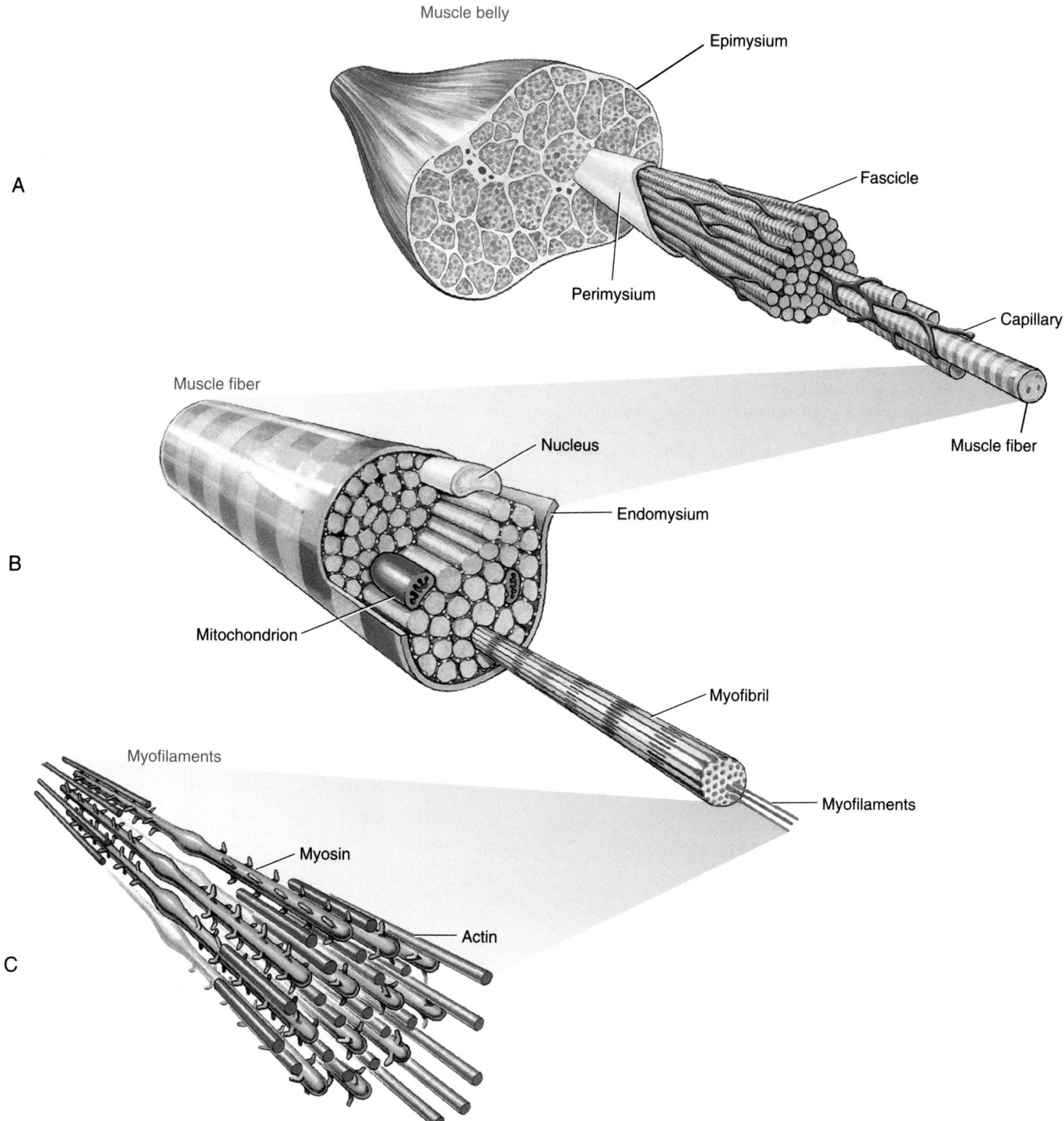

FIGURE 3.1 Basic components of muscle are shown, from the belly to the individual contractile, or active, proteins (myofilaments). Three sets of connective tissues are also depicted. (A) The muscle belly is enclosed by the *epimysium;* individual fascicles (groups of fibers) are surrounded by the *perimysium.* (B) Each muscle fiber is surrounded by the *endomysium.* Each *myofibril* within the muscle fibers contains many myofilaments. (C) The myofilaments consist of the contractile proteins actin and myosin. (Modified from Standring S: *Gray's anatomy: the anatomical basis of clinical practice,* ed 41, New York, 2015, Churchill Livingstone.)

elasticity to the whole muscle. Box 3.2 provides a summary of the functions of extracellular connective tissues within muscle.

Muscle Morphology

Muscle morphology describes the basic shape of a whole muscle. Muscles have many shapes, which influence their ultimate function (Fig. 3.2). Two of the most common shapes are fusiform and pennate

---

BOX 3.2 Summary of the Functions of Extracellular Connective Tissues within Muscle

- Provides gross structure and shape to muscle
- Serves as a conduit for blood vessels and nerves
- Generates passive tension, most notably when the muscle is stretched to its near-maximal length
- Temporarily stores energy and assists muscle to regain shape after it is stretched
- Transmits contractile force to the tendon and ultimately across the joint

---

(from the Latin *penna,* meaning feather). *Fusiform muscles,* such as the biceps brachii, have fibers running parallel to one another and to a central tendon. *Pennate* muscles, in contrast, possess fibers that approach their central tendon obliquely. For reasons described in the next section, pennate muscles contain a larger number of fibers within a given area and therefore generate relatively large forces.[1] Most muscles are considered pennate and may be further classified as unipennate, bipennate, or multipennate, depending on the number of similarly angled sets of fibers that attach to the central tendon.

Muscle Architecture

This section describes two important architectural features of a muscle: *physiologic cross-sectional area* and *pennation angle.* These features have a strong influence on the amount of force that is transmitted through the muscle and its tendon, and ultimately to the skeleton.

The *physiologic cross-sectional area* of a whole muscle reflects the number of active proteins available to generate active force. The physiologic cross-sectional area of a fusiform muscle is determined by cutting through its muscle belly, or by dividing the muscle's overall volume by its length.[107] The physiologic

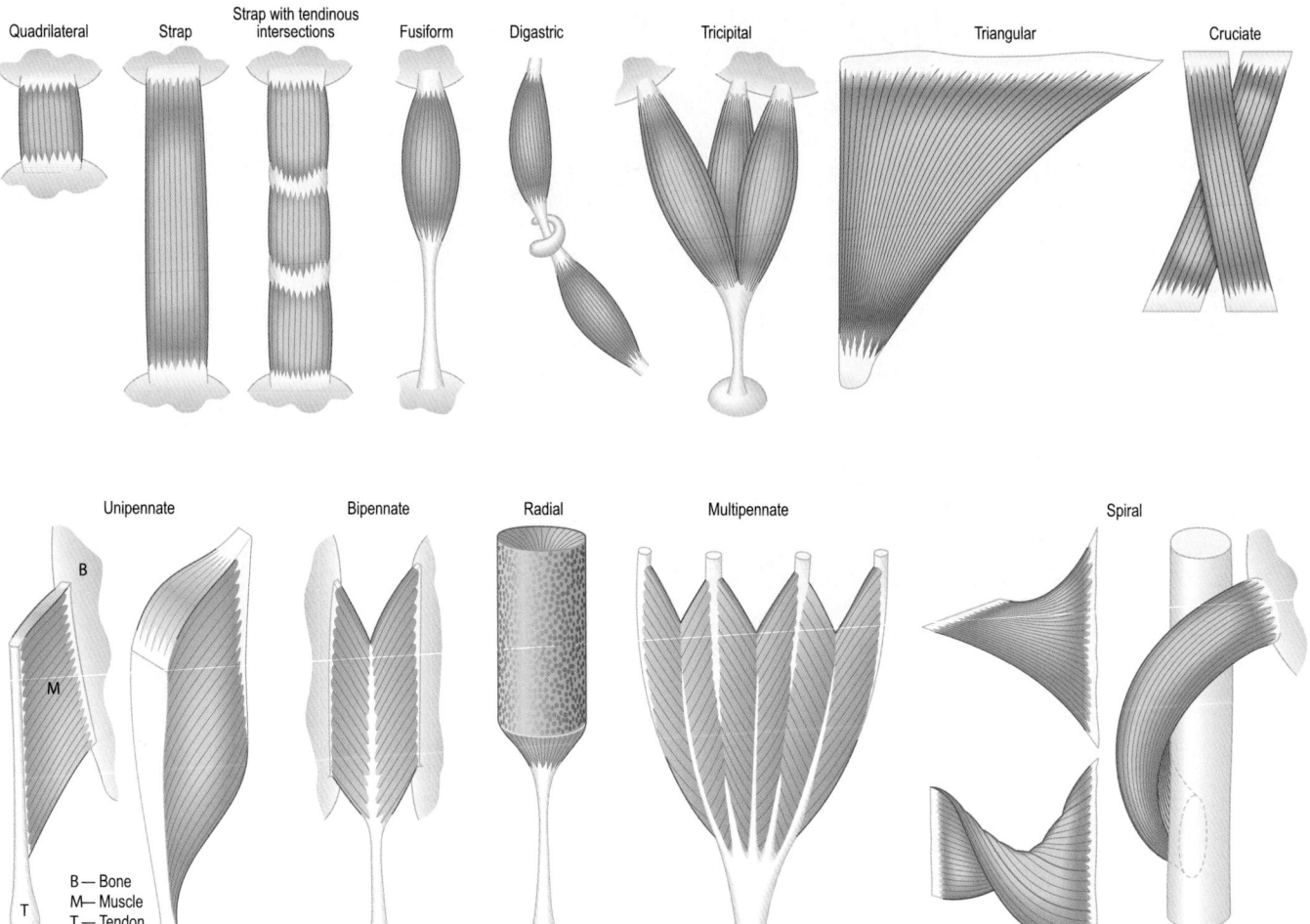

FIGURE 3.2 Morphologic "shapes" of muscle based on their general form and fascicular architecture. The varying shapes are based on dissimilar fiber orientations relative to the tendon and the direction of pull. (Modified from Standring S: *Gray's anatomy: the anatomical basis of clinical practice,* ed 42, St. Louis, 2021, Elsevier.)

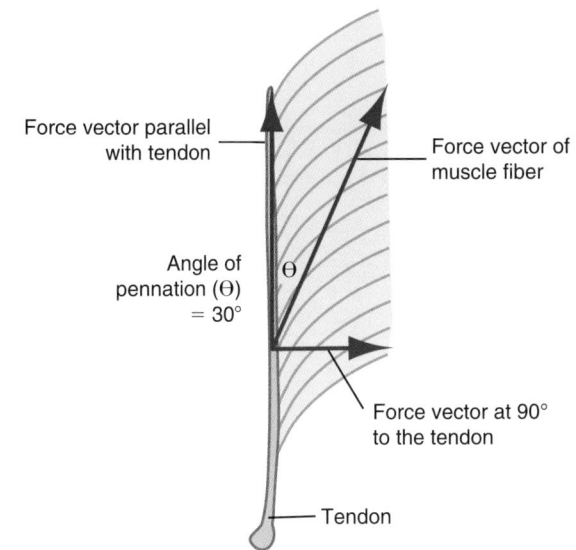

FIGURE 3.3 Unipennate muscle is shown with its muscle fibers oriented at a 30-degree pennation angle (θ).

cross-sectional area, typically expressed in square centimeters or millimeters, represents the sum of the cross-sectional areas of all muscle fibers within the muscle. Assuming full activation, the *maximal force potential of a muscle is proportional to the sum of the cross-sectional area of all its fibers.* In normal conditions, therefore, a thicker muscle generates greater force than a thinner muscle of similar morphology. Measuring the physiologic cross-sectional area of a fusiform muscle is relatively straight-forward because the fibers are primarily parallel. Caution needs to be used, however, when measuring the physiologic cross-section of pennate muscles, because fibers can be at different pennation angles relative to one another. For physiologic cross-sectional area to be measured accurately, the cross-section must be made perpendicular to each of the muscle fibers. The physiologic cross-sectional areas of selected muscles in the human body are listed in Appendixes II and IV.

Pennation angle refers to the angle of orientation between the muscle fibers and tendon (Fig. 3.3). If muscle fibers attach parallel to the tendon, the pennation angle is defined as 0 degrees. In this case all the force generated by the muscle fibers is transmitted to the tendon and across a joint. If, however, the pennation angle is greater than 0 degrees (i.e., oblique to the tendon), then only a portion of the force produced by the muscle fiber is transmitted longitudinally through the tendon. Theoretically, a muscle with a pennation angle of 0 degrees transmits 100% of its contractile force through the tendon, whereas the same muscle with a pennation angle of 30 degrees transmits 87% of its force through the tendon. (The cosine of 30 degrees is 0.87.) Most human muscles have pennation angles that range from 0 to 30 degrees.[87]

In general, pennate muscles produce greater maximal force than fusiform muscles of similar volume. By orienting fibers obliquely to the central tendon, a pennate muscle can fit more fibers into a given area of muscle. This space-saving strategy provides pennate muscles with a relatively large physiologic cross-sectional area and hence a relatively large capability for generating high force. Consider, for example, the multipennate gastrocnemius muscle, which must generate very large forces during jumping.

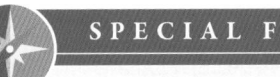

SPECIAL FOCUS 3.1

Estimating the Maximal Force Potential of Muscle

Specific force of skeletal muscle is defined as the maximal amount of active *force* produced *per unit physiologic cross-sectional area* and is typically expressed in units such as newtons per square meter (N/m^2) or pounds per square inch (lb/in^2). The specific force of human muscle is difficult to estimate, but studies indicate values between 15 and 60 N/cm^2 or, commonly, between 30 and 45 N/cm^2 (about 43–65 lb/in^2).[33,88,107] This large variability likely reflects the technical difficulty in measuring a person's true physiologic cross-sectional area, in addition to differences in fiber type composition across persons and muscles.[52] Generally, a muscle with a higher proportion of *fast twitch* fibers will have a slightly higher specific force than a muscle with a higher proportion of *slow twitch* fibers.

The fact that the maximal force generated by a healthy muscle is reasonably correlated with its cross-sectional area is a simple but very informative concept. Consider, for example, a quadriceps muscle in a healthy, well-developed man, with a physiologic cross-sectional area of 180 cm^2. Assuming for the purpose of this example a specific force of 30 N/cm^2, the muscle would be expected to exert a maximal force of about 5400 N (180 cm^2 × 30 N/cm^2), or about 1214 lb.[25] Consider, in contrast, the much smaller adductor pollicis muscle in the hand—a muscle that has a similar estimated specific force as the quadriceps muscle. Because an average-sized adductor pollicis has a physiologic cross-sectional area of only about 2.5 cm^2, this muscle is estimated to be capable of producing only about 75 N (17 lb) of contractile force.

The striking difference in maximal force potential in the two aforementioned muscles is not surprising considering their very different functional roles. Normally the demands on the quadriceps are large—these muscles are used routinely to lift or support much of the weight of the body against gravity. The architecture of the quadriceps muscle significantly affects the amount of force that is transmitted through its tendon and ultimately across the knee. Assuming the quadriceps has an average pennation angle of about 30 degrees, the maximal force expected to be transmitted through the tendon and across the knee would be about 4676 N (cosine 30 degrees × 5400 N), or 1051 lb. Although the magnitude of this force may seem implausible, it is actually within reason. Expressing this force in terms of *torque* may be more meaningful for the clinician who regularly works with strength-testing devices that measure knee extension strength. Assuming the quadriceps has a knee extensor moment arm of 4 cm, the best estimate of the maximal knee extensor torque would be about 187 Nm (0.04 m × 4676 N)—a value that certainly falls within the range reported in the literature for an adult healthy male.[25,44,157]

The reduced transfer of force from the pennate fiber to the tendon, because of the relatively large pennation angle, is small compared with the large force potential gained in physiologic cross-sectional area. As shown in Fig. 3.3, a pennation angle of 30 degrees still enables the fibers to transfer 87% of their force through to the long axis of the tendon.

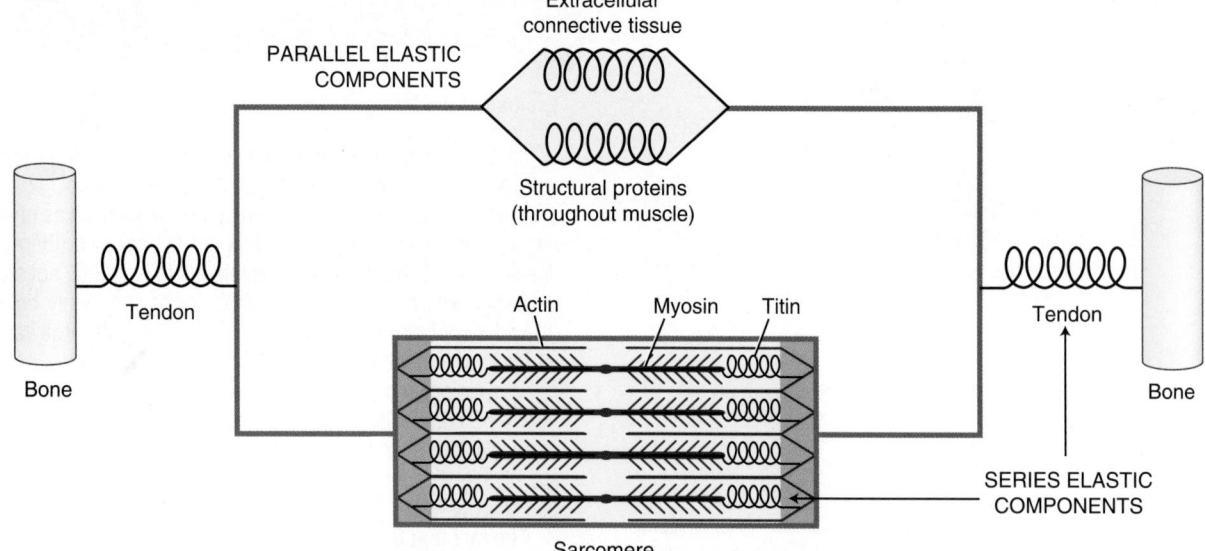

FIGURE 3.4 A diagrammatic model of a whole muscle attaching between two bones, depicting noncontractile elements (such as extracellular connective tissues and the dominant protein titin) and contractile elements (such as actin and myosin). The model depicts the noncontractile elements as coiled springs and differentiates the noncontractile elements as either series or parallel elastic components. *Series elastic components* (aligned in series with the contractile components) are illustrated by the tendon and the structural protein titin, shown within the sarcomere. The *parallel elastic components* (aligned in parallel with the contractile components) are represented by extracellular connective tissues (such as perimysium) and other structural proteins located throughout the muscle.

Muscle and Tendon: Generation of Force

PASSIVE LENGTH-TENSION CURVE

On stimulation from the nervous system, the contractile (active) proteins within the sarcomeres cause a contraction or shortening of the entire muscle. These proteins—most notably actin and myosin—are physically supported by structural proteins and a network of other noncontractile extracellular connective tissues, namely, the epimysium, perimysium, and endomysium. For functional rather than anatomic purposes, these noncontractile tissues have been described as parallel and series elastic components of muscle (Fig. 3.4). *Series elastic components* are tissues attached in series (i.e., end-to-end) with the active proteins. Examples of these tissues are the tendon and large structural proteins, such as titin. The *parallel elastic components,* in contrast, are tissues that surround or lie in parallel with the active proteins. These noncontractile tissues include the extracellular connective tissues (such as the perimysium) and a family of other structural proteins that surround and support the muscle fiber.

Stretching a whole muscle by rotating a joint elongates both the parallel and the series elastic components, generating a springlike resistance, or stiffness, within the muscle. The resistance is referred to as *passive tension* because it does not depend on active or volitional contraction. The concept of parallel and serial elastic components is a very simplified description of the anatomy; however, it is useful to explain the levels of resistance generated by a stretched muscle.

When the parallel and series elastic components are elongated within a muscle, a generalized *passive length-tension curve* is generated (Fig. 3.5). The passive length-tension curve is similar to that obtained by stretching a rubber band and resembles the shape of an exponential mathematical function. The passive elements within the muscle begin generating passive tension after a *critical length* at which all the relaxed (i.e., slack) tissue has been brought to an initial level

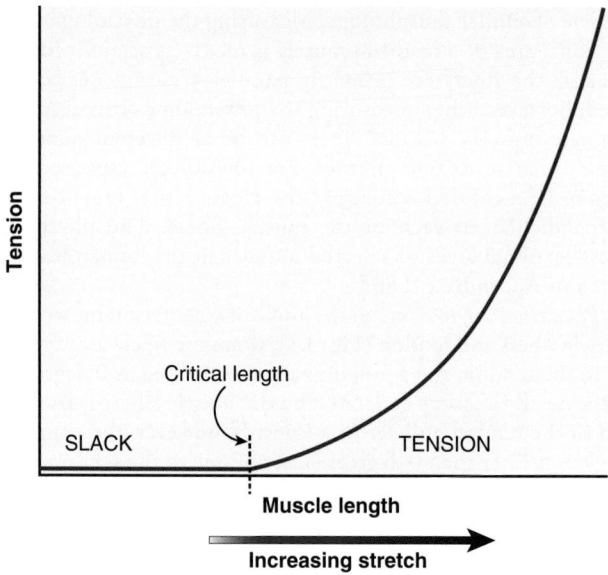

FIGURE 3.5 A generalized passive length-tension curve is represented. As a muscle is progressively stretched, the tissue is slack during the muscle's initial shortened length until it reaches a critical length at which it begins to generate passive tension. Beyond this critical length, the tension progressively increases as an exponential function.

of tension. After this critical length has been reached, tension progressively increases until the muscle reaches levels of very high stiffness. At even higher tension, the tissue eventually ruptures, or fails.

The passive tension in a stretched healthy muscle is attributed to the elastic forces produced by noncontractile elements, such as extracellular connective tissues, the tendon, and structural proteins. These tissues demonstrate different stiffness characteristics. When a muscle is only slightly or moderately stretched, structural proteins (in particular titin[57,81,90]) contribute most of the passive tension within the muscle. When a muscle is more extensively stretched, however, the extracellular connective tissues—especially those that compose the tendon—contribute much of the passive tension.[55]

The simple passive length-tension curve represents an important part of the overall force-generating capability of the musculotendinous unit.[86] This capability is especially important at very long lengths where muscle fibers begin to lose their active force-generating capability because there is limited overlap among the active proteins (i.e., actin and myosin) that generate force. The steepness (or slope) of the exponential increase of the passive length-tension curve varies among muscles, depending on the specific muscle architecture and amount and type of supporting connective tissue.

Passive tension within stretched muscles serves many useful purposes, such as moving or stabilizing a joint against the forces of gravity, physical contact, or other activated muscles. Consider, for example, the passive elongation of the calf muscles and Achilles tendon at the end of the stance phase of fast-paced walking, just before the push off phase. This passive tension assists with the transmission of muscular force through the foot and to the ground, thereby helping to initiate the propulsion phase of walking.[74,93] Although passive tension within stretched muscles is typically useful, its functional effectiveness at times is limited because of (1) the delayed mechanical responsiveness of the tissue to rapidly changing external forces and (2) the significant amount of lengthening that must occur before the tissue can generate meaningful passive tension.

Stretched muscle tissue exhibits the property of elasticity, as it temporarily stores a fraction of the energy used to generate the muscle stretch.[124] This stored energy, when released, can sustain or augment the force potential of a muscle, significantly improving its overall metabolic efficiency.[74,124] A stretched muscle also exhibits viscoelastic properties (see Chapter 1) because its passive resistance (stiffness) increases with increased velocity of stretch. Properties of both elasticity and viscoelasticity are important components of plyometric exercise.

Although the stored energy in a moderately stretched muscle may be relatively small compared with the full force potential of the muscle, stored energy may also help prevent a muscle from being damaged during maximal elongation.[94] Elasticity therefore can serve as a damping mechanism that can protect the structural components of the muscle and tendon.

ACTIVE LENGTH-TENSION CURVE

This section of the chapter describes how a muscle generates active force. Active force is produced by an *activated* muscle fiber, that is, one that is being stimulated by the nervous system to contract. As diagrammed in Fig. 3.4, both active force and passive tension are ultimately transmitted to the bones that constitute the joint.

Muscle fibers are composed of many tiny strands called *myofibrils* (see Fig. 3.1). *Myofibrils* contain the contractile (active) proteins of the muscle fiber and have a distinctive structure. Each myofibril is 1 to 2 μm in diameter and consists of many *myofilaments*. The two most important myofilaments within the myofibril are the proteins *actin* and *myosin*. As will be described, muscle contraction involves a complex physiologic and mechanical interaction primarily between these two proteins. The patterned organization of these myofilaments produces the characteristic banded appearance of the myofibril as seen by viewing two adjacent fibers under the microscope (Fig. 3.6). The repeating functional subunits of the myofibril are the sarcomeres (Fig. 3.7). The dark band within a single sarcomere, also called the *A band,* correspond to the presence of *myosin*—thick filaments. Myosin also contains projections, called *myosin*

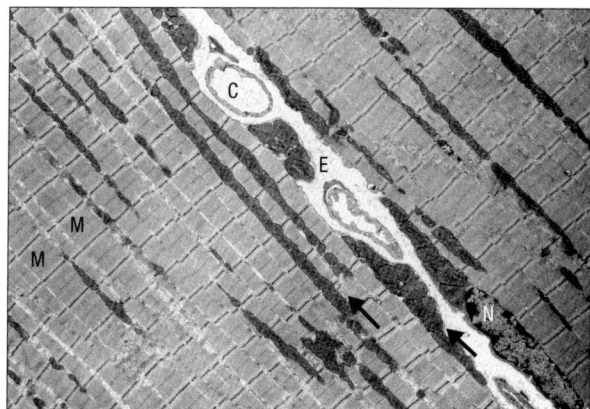

FIGURE 3.6 Electron micrograph of parts of two adjacent muscle fibers demonstrates the regularly banded organization of skeletal muscle. Note the many myofibrils (M) within a muscle fiber. The Z-discs, repeating dark transverse lines across each myofibril, define individual sarcomeres. This micrograph illustrates the size of a sarcomere relative to endomysium (E), capillaries (C), nucleus (N), and mitochondria *(identified by arrows).* (Courtesy of Professor Hans Hoppeler, Institute of Anatomy, University of Bern, Switzerland.)

heads, which are arranged in pairs (Fig. 3.8). The light bands, also called *I bands,* contain *actin*—thin filaments (see Fig. 3.7). In a resting or relaxed muscle fiber, actin filaments partially overlap the myosin filaments. Under an electron microscope, a more complex pattern is revealed that consists of an H band, M line, and Z discs (defined in Table 3.1). Actin and myosin are aligned within the sarcomere with the help of structural proteins, providing mechanical stability to the fiber during contraction and stretch.[81,90,152] By way of the structural proteins and the endomysium, myofibrils ultimately connect with the tendon. This elegant connective web, formed between the proteins and connective tissues, allows forces to be distributed longitudinally and laterally within a muscle.[102,153]

As described earlier, the sarcomere is the fundamental active force generator within the muscle fiber. Understanding the contractile events that take place in an individual sarcomere provides the basis for understanding the contraction process across the entire muscle. The contraction process is remarkably similar from one sarcomere to another, and the simultaneous shortening of many sarcomeres creates movement. The model for describing active force generation within the sarcomere is called the *sliding filament hypothesis* and was developed independently by Hugh Huxley[73] and Andrew Huxley[72] (no relation) in the 1950s. In this model, active force is generated as actin filaments slide past myosin filaments, pulling the Z discs within a sarcomere closer together and narrowing the H band. This action results in a progressively increasing overlap of the actin

TABLE 3.1	Defined Regions within a Sarcomere
Region	**Description**
A band	Dark bands caused by the presence of thick myosin myofilaments
I band	Light bands caused by the presence of thin actin myofilaments
H band	Region within A band where actin and myosin do not overlap
M line	Midregion thickening of myosin myofilaments in the center of the H band
Z disc	Connecting points between successive sarcomeres; Z discs help anchor the thin actin myofilaments

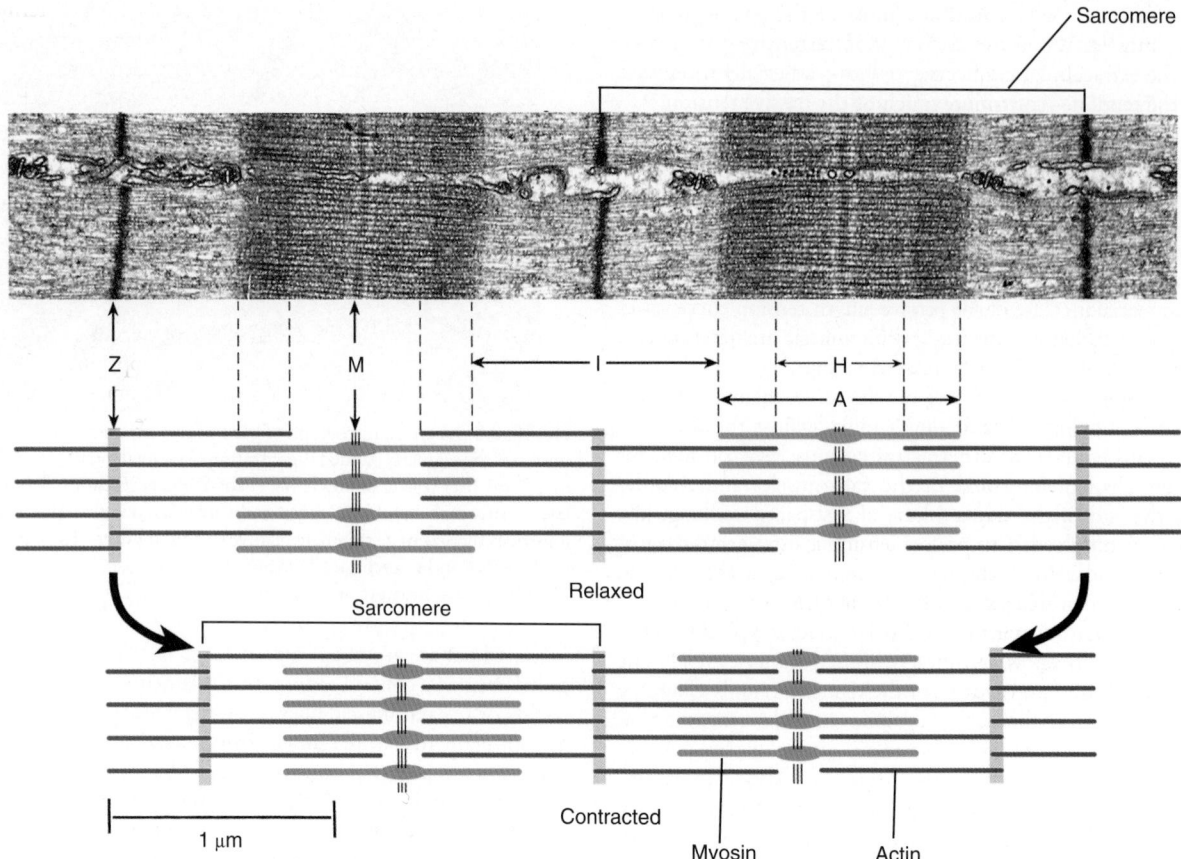

FIGURE 3.7 On top are electron micrographs of two full sarcomeres within a myofibril. The illustrations below show relaxed and contracted myofibrils, indicating the position of the thick (myosin) and thin (actin) filaments. Detail of the regular, banded organization of the myofibril shows the position of the A band, I band, H band, M line, and Z discs. Relaxed and contracted states are shown to illustrate the changes that occur during shortening of the sarcomere. (Modified from Standring S: *Gray's anatomy: the anatomical basis of clinical practice,* ed 42, St. Louis, 2021, Elsevier. Photographs by Brenda Russell, Department of Physiology and Biophysics, University of Illinois at Chicago. Original art by Lesley Skeates.)

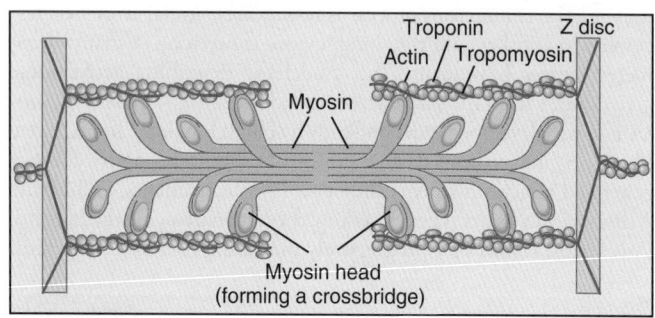

FIGURE 3.8 Detailed illustration of a sarcomere showing the crossbridge structure formed by the myosin heads and their attachment to the actin filaments. Note that the actin filament also contains the proteins troponin and tropomyosin. Troponin is responsible for exposing the actin filament to the myosin head, thereby allowing crossbridge formation. (From Levy MN, Koeppen BM, Stanton BA: *Berne and Levy principles of physiology,* ed 4, St Louis, 2006, Mosby.)

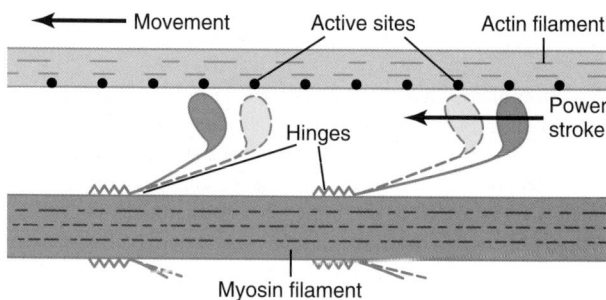

FIGURE 3.9 The sliding filament action showing myosin heads attaching and then releasing from the actin filament. This process is known as *crossbridge cycling.* Contractile force is generated during the power stroke of each crossbridge cycle. (From Hall JE & Hall ME: *Guyton & Hall textbook of medical physiology,* ed 14, Philadelphia, 2021, Elsevier.)

and myosin filaments, which, in effect, produces a shortening of each sarcomere, although the active proteins themselves do not actually shorten (Fig. 3.9). Each myosin head attaches to an adjacent actin filament, forming a *crossbridge*. The amount of force generated within each sarcomere therefore depends on the number of simultaneously formed crossbridges. The greater the number of crossbridges formed, the greater the force generated within the sarcomere.

As a consequence of the arrangement between the actin and myosin within a sarcomere, the amount of active force depends, in part, on the instantaneous *length* of the muscle fiber. A change in muscle fiber length—from either active contraction or passive elongation—alters the amount of overlap between actin and myosin, and thus the number of potential crossbridges.[49] The active length-tension curve for a sarcomere is presented in Fig. 3.10. The ideal *resting length* of a muscle fiber (or individual sarcomere) is the length that allows the greatest number of potential crossbridges and therefore the greatest potential force. As the sarcomere is lengthened or shortened from its resting length, the number of potential crossbridges decreases so that lesser amounts of active force are generated, even under conditions of full activation or effort. The resulting active length-tension curve is described by an inverted U-shape with its peak at the ideal resting length.

The term *length-force* relationship is more appropriate for considering the terminology established in this text (see definitions of force and tension in the glossary of Chapter 1). The phrase *length-tension* is used, however, because of its wide acceptance in the physiology literature.

SUMMATION OF ACTIVE FORCE AND PASSIVE TENSION: THE TOTAL LENGTH-TENSION CURVE

The active length-tension curve, when combined with the passive length-tension curve, yields the *total* length-tension curve of muscle. The combination of active force and passive tension allows for a large range of muscle forces over a wide range of muscle lengths. Consider the total length-tension curve for the muscle shown in Fig. 3.11. At shortened lengths *(a)*, below active resting length and below the

length that generates passive tension, active force determines the force-generating capability of the muscle. The force-generating capacity continues to rise as the muscle is lengthened (stretched) toward its resting length. As the muscle fiber is stretched beyond its resting length *(b)*, passive tension begins to contribute to total muscle force so that the decrement in active force is offset by increased passive tension, effectively "flattening" this portion of the total length-tension curve. This "flattened" portion of the passive length-tension curve helps muscle maintain high levels of force even as the muscle is stretched to a point at which active force generation is compromised. As the muscle fiber is further stretched *(c)*, passive tension dominates the curve so that connective tissues are subjected to near-maximal force. High levels of passive tension are most apparent in muscles that are stretched across multiple joints. For example, as the wrist is actively and fully extended, the fingers passively flex slightly because of the stretch placed on the finger flexor muscles as they cross the front of the wrist. The amount of passive tension depends, in part, on the natural stiffness of the muscle. The shape of the total muscle length-tension curve therefore can vary considerably between muscles of different structure and function.[8]

Isometric Muscle Force: Development of the Internal Torque–Joint Angle Curve

As defined in Chapter 1, isometric activation of a muscle produces force without a significant change in its length. This occurs naturally when the joint over which an activated muscle crosses is constrained from movement. Constraint often occurs from a force produced by an antagonistic muscle or an external source. Isometrically produced forces provide necessary stability to the joints and body as a whole. Isometrically produced force from a given muscle reflects a summation of length-dependent active force and passive tension.

Maximal isometric force of a muscle is often used as a general indicator of a muscle's peak strength and can indicate neuromuscular recovery after injury as well as the readiness of an athlete to return to a certain occupation or level of sporting activity. In typical clinical

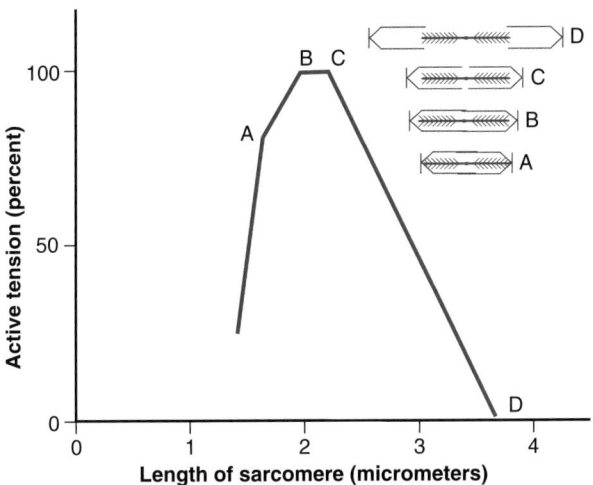

FIGURE 3.10 Active length-tension curve of a sarcomere represented at four specified sarcomere lengths (upper right, *A* through *D*). Actin filaments (A) overlap so that the number of crossbridges is reduced. In *B* and *C*, actin and myosin filaments are positioned to allow an optimal number of crossbridges. In *D*, actin filaments are positioned out of the range of the myosin heads so that no crossbridges are formed. (Modified from Gordon AM, Huxley AF, Julian FJ: The length-tension diagram of single vertebrate striated muscle fibers. *J Physiol* 171:28P, 1964.)

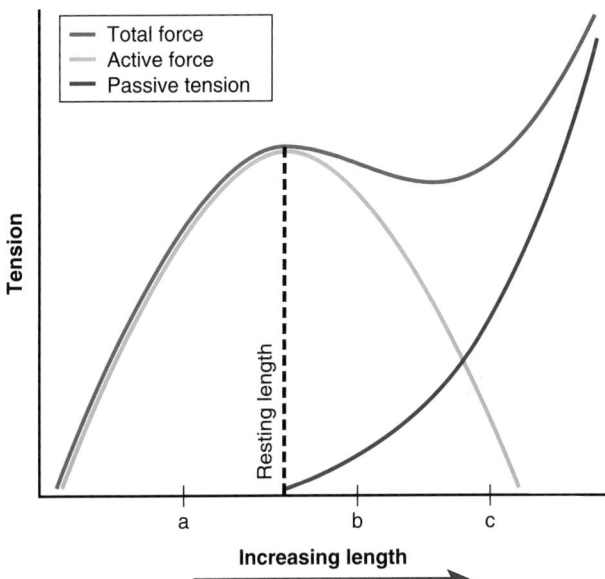

FIGURE 3.11 Idealized total length-tension curve for a typical muscle. At shortened lengths *(a)*, force is generated actively. As the muscle fiber is stretched beyond its resting length *(b)*, passive tension begins to contribute to the total force. In *(c)* the muscle is further stretched, and passive tension accounts for most of the total force.

settings, it is not possible to directly measure length or force of maximally activated muscle. However, a muscle's internal *torque* generation can be measured isometrically at several joint angles. Fig. 3.12 shows the internal torque relative to the joint angle (so-called "torque-angle curve") of two muscle groups under isometric, maximal-effort conditions. (The torque-angle curve is the rotational analog to the total length-tension curve of a muscle group.) The isometric internal torque potential of a muscle group can be determined by asking an individual to produce a maximal-effort contraction against a known external torque. As described in Chapter 4, an external torque can be determined by using an external force-sensing device (dynamometer) at a known distance from the joint's axis of rotation. Because the measurement is performed during an isometric activation, the value of the internal torque is assumed to be equal to that of the external torque. When a maximal-strength test is performed in conjunction with considerable encouragement provided by the tester, most healthy adults can achieve near-maximal activation of their muscle.[4] Near-maximal activation is not always possible, however, in persons with pathologic conditions or with trauma affecting their neuromuscular system.

The shape of a maximal-effort torque-angle curve is specific to each muscle group (compare Fig. 3.12A with Fig. 3.12B). The shape of each curve can yield important information about the physiologic and mechanical factors that determine the muscle groups' torque potential. Consider the two factors shown in Fig. 3.13, muscle length and moment arm. First, muscle *length* changes as the joint angle changes. The biceps brachii, for example, is longer in elbow extension than in elbow flexion. As previously described, a muscle's force output—in both active and passive terms—is highly dependent on muscle length. Second, the changing joint angle alters the length of the muscle's moment arm, or *leverage*. For a given muscle force, a progressively longer moment arm contributes to a greater torque. Because both muscle length and moment arm are altered simultaneously by rotation of the joint, it is not always possible to know which factor is more influential in determining the shape of the torque-angle curve. A change in either variable—physiologic or mechanical—alters the clinical expression of a muscular-produced internal torque. Several clinically related examples are listed in Table 3.3.

SPECIAL FOCUS 3.2

Muscle Proteins: An Expanding Area of Study for Muscle Physiologists

Thus far, this chapter has focused primarily on the active proteins of actin and myosin within the sarcomere. More advanced study of this topic, however, reveals a far more complicated picture. Myosin, for example, is further classified into *heavy chain* or *light chain* proteins, with differing functions. The light chain myosin appears to have a more regulatory role in the contraction process, as do the proteins *tropomyosin* and *troponin*. Furthermore, other proteins serve an important structural or supportive role within or between the sarcomeres. The importance of these noncontractile proteins has been realized in recent decades. The information contained in Table 3.2 is intended primarily as background material and summarizes the most likely function of the more commonly studied muscle proteins. The interested reader may consult other sources for more detailed discussions on this topic.[16,22]

TABLE 3.2 Summary of Functions of Selected Muscle Proteins

Proteins	Function
Active: Contractile	
Myosin heavy chain (several isoforms)	Molecular motor for muscle contraction—binds with actin to generate contraction force
Actin	Binds with myosin to translate force and shorten the sarcomere
Active: Regulatory	
Tropomyosin	Regulates the interaction between actin and myosin; stabilizes actin filament
Troponin (several isoforms)	Influences the position of tropomyosin; binds with calcium ions
Myosin light chain (several isoforms for slow and fast light chains)	Influences the contraction velocity of the sarcomere; modulates the kinetics of crossbridge cycling
Structural	
Nebulin	Anchors actin to Z discs
Titin	Stabilizes the position of myosin within the sarcomere. Acts as a large molecular "spring" that confers elasticity to the sarcomere, helping it recoil after being stretched
Desmin	Helps to stabilize the longitudinal and lateral alignment of adjacent sarcomeres
Vimentin	Helps maintain periodicity of Z discs
Skelemin	Helps stabilize the position of M lines
Dystrophin	Provides structural stability to the cytoskeleton and sarcolemma of the muscle fiber
Integrins	Stabilizes the cytoskeleton of the muscle fiber

Adapted from Caiozzo VJ: The muscular system: structural and functional plasticity. In Farrell PA, Joyner MJ, Caiozzo VJ, editors: *ACSM's advanced exercise physiology*, ed 2, Baltimore, 2012, Lippincott Williams & Wilkins.

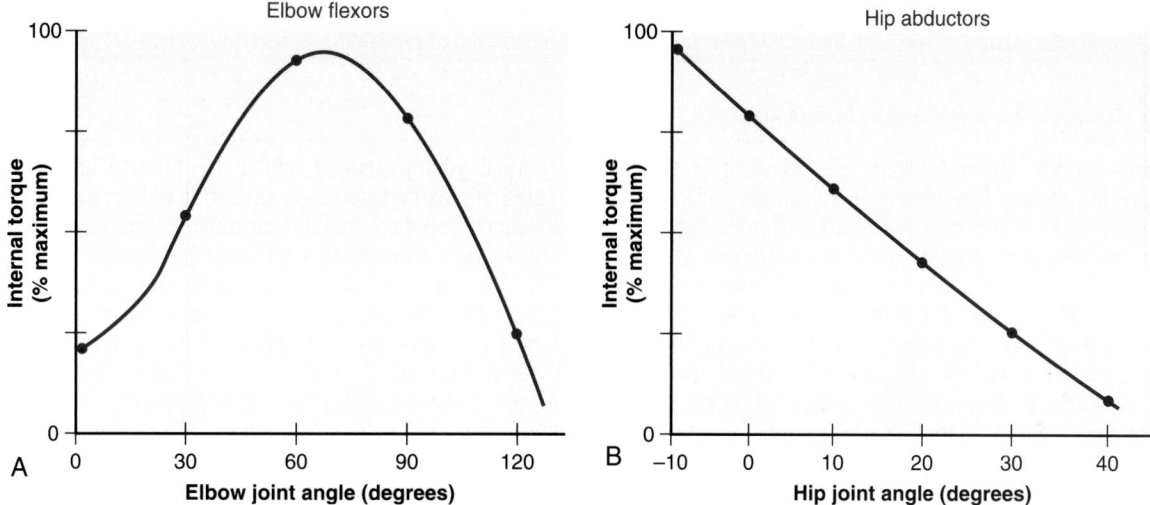

FIGURE 3.12 Internal torque in relation to joint angle of two muscle groups under isometric, maximal-effort conditions. The shapes of the curves are different for each muscle group. (A) Internal torque of the elbow flexors is greatest at an angle of about 75 degrees of flexion. (B) Internal torque of the hip abductors is greatest at a frontal plane angle of about −10 degrees (i.e., 10 degrees of adduction).

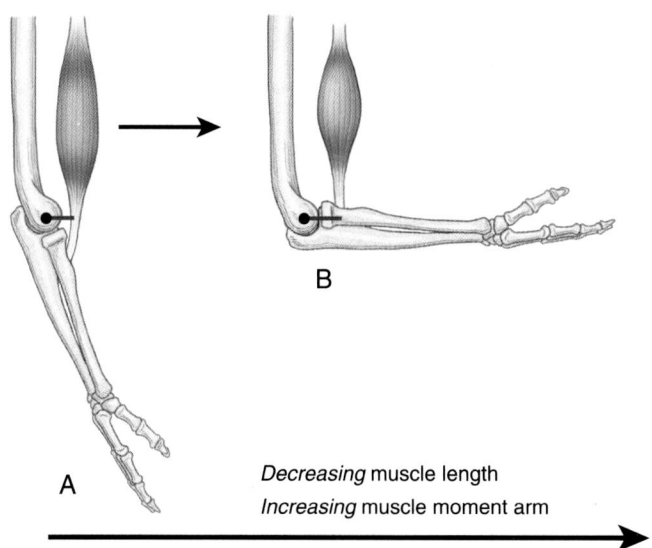

Decreasing muscle length
Increasing muscle moment arm

FIGURE 3.13 A change in joint angle following movement typically alters both muscle length and moment arm, thereby impacting maximal-effort torque such as, for example, the biceps brachii acting to flex the elbow. (A) Muscle is at its near-greatest length, and muscle moment arm *(brown line)* is at its near-shortest length. (B) Muscle length is shortened, and muscle moment arm length is greatest.

The shape of a muscle group's torque-angle curve relates to the functional demands placed on the muscles and the joint. Each muscle group, therefore, has a unique isometric torque-angle curve. For the elbow flexors, for example, the maximal internal torque potential is *greatest* in the midranges of elbow motion and *least* near full extension and full flexion (see Fig. 3.12A). Not coincidentally, in the upright position the external torque caused by gravity acting on the forearm and hand-held objects is also greatest in the midranges of elbow motion and least at the extremes of elbow motion.

For the hip abductor muscles, the internal torque potential is greatest near neutral (0 degrees of abduction) (see Fig. 3.12B). This hip joint angle coincides with the approximate angle at which the hip abductor muscles are most needed for frontal plane stability in the single-limb support phase of walking. Large amounts of hip abduction torque are rarely functionally required in a position of maximal hip abduction. The torque-angle curve of the hip

abductors depends primarily on muscle length, as shown by the linear reduction of maximal torque produced at progressively greater abduction angles of the hip (see Fig. 3.12B). Regardless of the muscle group, however, the combination of high total muscle force (based on muscle length) and great leverage (based on moment arm length) results in the greatest relative internal torque.

In summary, the magnitude of isometric torque differs considerably based on the angle of the joint at the time of activation, even with maximal effort. Accordingly, it is important that clinical measurements of isometric torque include the joint angle so that future comparisons are valid. The testing of isometric strength at different joint angles enables the characterization of the functional range of a muscle's strength. This information may be required to determine the suitability of a person for a certain task in the workplace, especially if the task requires a critical internal torque to be produced at certain joint angles.

Method of Measuring Maximal Voluntary Muscle Activation

In normal clinical strength-testing situations, it is difficult to know for certain if a person is maximally activating a given muscle, even when maximal effort and good health are assumed. In laboratory settings, *maximal voluntary activation* can be assessed by applying a brief electrical stimulus to the motor nerve or directly over the skin of a muscle while the person is attempting a maximal voluntary contraction. Any increase in measured force during the voluntary effort that immediately follows the electrical stimulus indicates that not all the muscle fibers were volitionally activated. This technique is known as the *interpolated stimulus technique.*[43,134] The magnitude of voluntary activation is typically expressed as a percent of a muscle's maximal activation potential.

Most young, healthy adults are able to achieve 90% to 100% of maximal isometric activation of the elbow flexor, knee extensor, and ankle dorsiflexor muscle groups, although these values vary considerably between individuals and trials.[43,48] The average level of maximal voluntary activation can also vary among muscle groups.[43] Lower levels of maximal voluntary activation have been reported in muscles after trauma or disease, such as in the hamstring muscle after strain injury[15] or the quadriceps muscle after anterior cruciate ligament injury,[45] or in the diaphragm muscle in persons with asthma.[3] Persons with multiple sclerosis have been shown to generate only 86% of maximal voluntary activation of their dorsiflexor muscles, compared with 96% maximal voluntary activation in a healthy control group.[109]

TABLE 3.3 Clinical Examples and Consequences of Changes in Mechanical or Physiologic Variables That Influence the Production of Internal Torque			
Changed Variable	**Clinical Example**	**Effect on Internal Torque**	**Possible Clinical Consequence**
Mechanical: Increased internal moment arm	Surgical displacement of greater trochanter to increase the internal moment arm of hip abductor muscles	Decrease in the amount of muscle force required to produce a given level of hip abduction torque	Decreased hip abductor force can reduce the force generated across an unstable or a painful hip joint; considered a means of "protecting" a joint from damaging forces
Mechanical: Decreased internal moment arm	Patellectomy after severe fracture of the patella	Increase in the amount of quadriceps force required to produce a given level of knee extension torque	Increased force needed to extend the knee may increase the wear on the articular surfaces of the knee joint
Physiologic: Decreased muscle activation	Damage to the deep portion of the fibular nerve	Decreased strength in the dorsiflexor muscles	Reduced ability to walk safely
Physiologic: Decreased muscle length at the time of neural activation	Damage to the radial nerve with paralysis of wrist extensor muscles	Decreased strength in wrist extensor muscles causing the finger flexor muscles to flex the wrist during grasping	Ineffective grasp because of overcontracted (shortened) finger flexor muscles

MUSCLE AS A SKELETAL MOVER: FORCE MODULATION

The previous sections considered how an isometrically activated muscle can stabilize the skeletal system; the next section considers how muscles actively regulate forces while changing lengths, which is necessary to move the skeletal system in a highly controlled fashion.

Modulating Force through Concentric or Eccentric Activation: Introduction to the Force-Velocity Relationship of Muscle

As introduced in Chapter 1, the nervous system stimulates a muscle to generate or resist a force, which can be classified as *concentric, eccentric,* or *isometric* activation. During concentric activation, the muscle shortens (contracts). This occurs when the

internal (muscle) torque exceeds the external (load) torque. During eccentric activation, the external torque exceeds the internal torque; the muscle is driven by the nervous system to contract but is elongated in response to a larger force, usually from an external source or from an antagonist muscle. During an isometric activation, the length of the muscle remains nearly constant, as the internal and external torques are equally matched.

During concentric and eccentric activations, a very specific relationship exists between a muscle's maximal force output and its velocity of contraction (or elongation). During concentric activation, for example, the muscle contracts at a maximal velocity when the load is negligible (Fig. 3.14). As the load increases, the maximal contraction velocity of the muscle decreases. At some point, a very large load results in a contraction velocity of zero (i.e., the isometric state). Eccentric activation may be considered separately from concentric activation. With eccentric activation, a load that barely exceeds the isometric force level

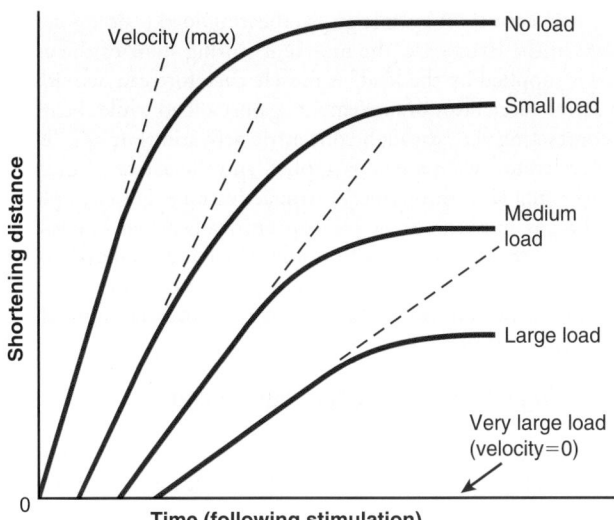

FIGURE 3.14 Relation between muscle load (external resistance) and maximal shortening (contraction) velocity. The maximal shortening velocity is equal to the slope (or mathematical derivative) of the dashed lines. Without an external load, a muscle can shorten at a high velocity. As the load on the muscle progressively increases, the maximal shortening velocity of the muscle decreases. Eventually, with a very large external load, the muscle is incapable of shortening and the velocity is zero. (Redrawn from McComas AJ: *Skeletal muscle: form and function,* Champaign, IL, 1996, Human Kinetics.)

causes the muscle to lengthen slowly. Speed of lengthening increases as a greater load is applied. There is a maximal load that the muscle cannot resist, and beyond this load level the muscle uncontrollably lengthens.

FORCE-VELOCITY CURVE

The relationship between the velocity of a muscle's change in length and its maximal force output is often expressed by the *force-velocity curve* depicted in Fig. 3.15. This curve is shown during concentric, isometric, and eccentric activations, expressed with the force on the vertical axis and with the shortening and lengthening velocity of the muscle on the horizontal axis. This force-velocity curve demonstrates several important points about the physiology of muscle. During a maximal-effort *concentric* activation, the amount of muscle force produced is *inversely proportional* to the velocity of muscle shortening. This relationship was first described by physiologist and Nobel Laureate A.V. Hill in 1938 in the skeletal muscle of frog and is similar to that in humans.[58,59] The reduced force-generating capacity of muscle at higher velocities of contraction results primarily from the inherent limitation in the speed of attachment and reattachment of the crossbridges. At higher velocities of contraction, the number of attached crossbridges at any given time is less than that when the muscle is contracting slowly. At a contraction velocity of zero (i.e., the isometric state), a maximal number of attached crossbridges exists within a given sarcomere at any given instant. For this reason, a muscle produces greater force isometrically than at any speed of shortening.

The underlying physiology behind the force-velocity relationship of *eccentrically active muscle* is different from that of concentric muscle activation. During a maximal-effort eccentric activation, the muscle force is, to a point, *directly proportional* to the velocity of the

muscle lengthening. For most individuals, however, the curve reaches a zero slope at lower lengthening velocities than that depicted in the theoretical curve of Fig. 3.15. Although the reason is not completely understood, most humans (especially untrained) are unable to maximally activate their muscles eccentrically, especially at high velocities.[28] This may be a protective mechanism to guard against potential muscle damage produced by excessively large forces.

The clinical expression of a force-velocity relationship of muscle is often expressed by a *torque-joint angular velocity relationship*. This type of data can be derived through *isokinetic dynamometry* (see Chapter 4). Fig. 3.16 shows the peak torque generated by the knee extensor and flexor muscles of healthy men, across a range of muscle shortening and lengthening velocities. Although the two muscle groups produce different amplitudes of peak torque, each exhibits similar characteristics: maximal-effort torques decrease with increasing

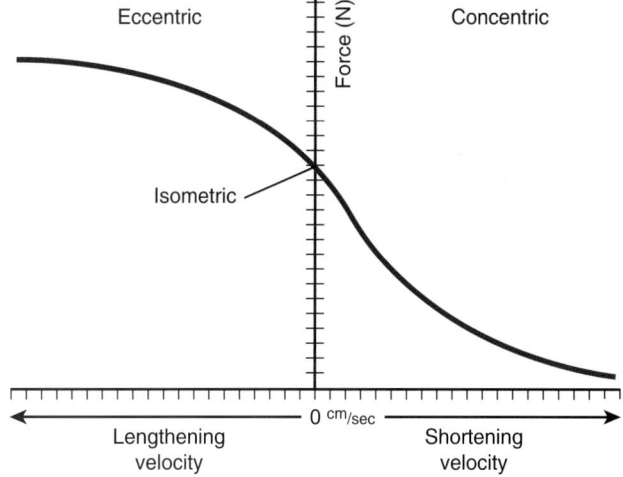

FIGURE 3.15 Theoretical relationship between force and velocity of muscle shortening or lengthening during maximal-effort muscle activation. Concentric (muscle-shortening) activation is shown on the right, and eccentric (muscle-lengthening) activation on the left. Isometric activation occurs at a velocity of zero.

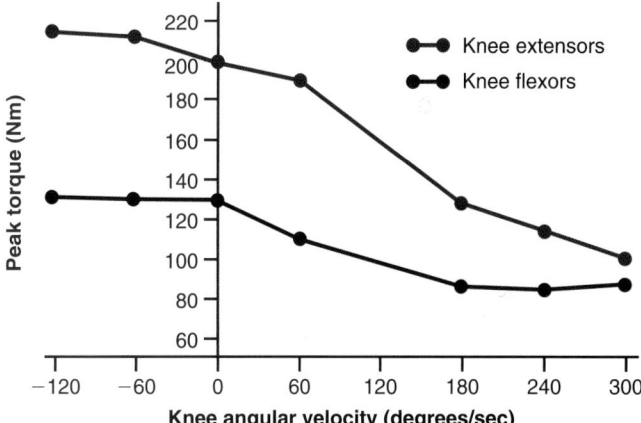

FIGURE 3.16 Peak torque generated by the knee extensor and flexor muscles. Positive velocities denote concentric activation, and negative velocities denote eccentric activation. Data are from 64 untrained, healthy men. (Data from Horstmann T, Maschmann J, Mayer F, et al: The influence of age on isokinetic torque of the upper and lower leg musculature in sedentary men, *Int J Sports Med* 20:362, 1999.)

velocity of muscle contraction (shortening) and maximal-effort torques increase (to a point) with increasing velocity of muscle lengthening.

The shape of the force-velocity curves shown in Figs. 3.15 and 3.16 reflects that muscles can produce greater force during eccentric activation than during isometric or any velocity of concentric activation. Although the reasons are not well understood, the higher forces produced during eccentric activation result, in part, from (1) a greater average force produced per crossbridge, as each crossbridge is pulled apart and detached,[91] (2) a more rapid reattachment phase of crossbridge formation, and (3) passive tension produced by the viscoelastic properties of the stretched parallel and serial elastic components of the muscle. Also, emerging theories propose that the structural protein *titin,* the largest known protein in the human body, binds with calcium to functional increase the resistance to elongation.[56] Indirect evidence for increased passive tension during eccentric contractions is the well-known phenomenon of *delayed onset muscle soreness* which is common after heavy bouts of eccentric muscle-based exercise, especially in untrained persons.[61] One partial explanation for this characteristic soreness is based on strain-related injury to the forcefully (and rapidly) stretched muscle, which includes the myofibrils, cytoskeleton of the sarcomere, and extracellular connective tissues.[120]

The functional role of eccentrically active muscles is important to the metabolic and neurologic "efficiency" of movement.[61] Eccentrically activated muscle stores energy when stretched, and the energy is used as the muscle begins to shorten. In addition, the ratio of electromyographic amplitude and oxygen consumption per force level is less for eccentrically activated muscle than for similar absolute workloads performed with concentric activation.[29] The mechanisms responsible for this efficiency are closely related to the factors cited in the previous paragraph for why greater forces are produced through eccentric activation compared with noneccentric activation. The metabolic cost and electromyographic activity are less because, in part, a comparable task performed with eccentric activation requires slightly fewer active muscle fibers.

POWER AND WORK: ADDITIONAL CONCEPTS RELATED TO THE FORCE-VELOCITY RELATIONSHIP OF MUSCLE

The inverse relation between a muscle's maximal force potential and its shortening velocity is related to the concept of power. *Power,* or the rate of work, can be expressed as a product of force and contraction velocity. Power of a muscle contraction is therefore related to the area under the force-velocity curve. A constant power output of a muscle can be sustained by increasing the load (resistance) while proportionately decreasing the contraction velocity, or vice versa. This is similar in concept to switching gears while riding a bicycle. Of note, peak power of a muscle contraction is achieved at about one-third of maximal contraction velocity.[154] Similarly, peak power when riding a bicycle is generally achieved with an intermediate gear that enables the cyclist to apply large forces to the foot pedals at a velocity corresponding to about one-third of the cyclist's maximal leg speed.

A muscle performing a concentric activation against a load is doing *positive work* on the load. In contrast, a muscle undergoing eccentric activation against an overbearing load is doing *negative work.* In the latter case, the muscle is storing some of the energy that is supplied by the load. A muscle therefore can act either as an active accelerator of movement against a load while the muscle is contracting (i.e., through concentric activation) or as a "brake" or decelerator when a load is applied and the activated muscle is lengthening (i.e., through eccentric activation). For example, the quadriceps muscles are active concentrically when one ascends stairs and lifts the weight of the body, which is considered positive work. Negative work, however, is performed by these muscles as they lower the body down the stairs in a controlled fashion, during eccentric activation.

Activating Muscle via the Nervous System

This chapter has thus far examined several important mechanisms underlying the generation of muscle force. Of utmost importance, however, is that muscle is excited by impulses generated from within the nervous system, specifically by *alpha motor neurons,* with their cell bodies located in the ventral (anterior) horn of the spinal cord. Each alpha motor neuron has an axon that extends from the spinal cord and connects with multiple muscle fibers located throughout a whole muscle. The single alpha motor neuron together with its entire family of innervated muscle fibers is called a *motor unit* (Fig. 3.17). Excitation of alpha motor neurons arises from many sources, including cortical descending neurons, spinal interneurons, and other afferent (sensory) neurons. Each source can activate an alpha motor neuron by first *recruiting* a particular motor neuron and then by driving it to higher rates of sequential activation—a process called *rate coding.* The process of rate coding provides a finely controlled mechanism of smoothly increasing muscle force. Recruitment and rate coding are the two primary strategies employed by the nervous system to activate motor neurons. The spatial arrangement of motor units throughout a muscle and the strategies available to activate motor neurons allow for the production of very small forces involving only a few motor units, or very large forces involving most of the motor units within the muscle. Because motor units are distributed across an entire muscle, the forces from the activated fibers summate across the entire muscle and are then transmitted to the tendon and across the joint.

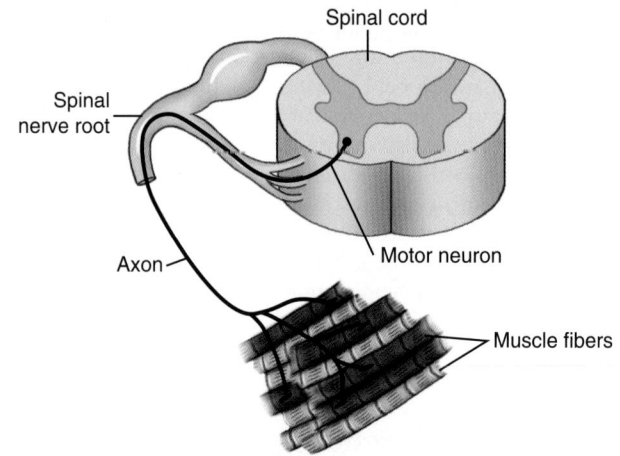

FIGURE 3.17 A motor unit consists of the (alpha) motor neuron and the muscle fibers it innervates.

SPECIAL FOCUS 3.4

Combining the Length-Tension and Force-Velocity Relationships

Although a muscle's length-tension and force-velocity relationships are described separately, in reality, both are in effect simultaneously. At any given time, an active muscle is functioning at a specific length and at a specific contraction velocity, including isometric. It is useful, therefore, to conceptualize a plot that represents the three-dimensional relationship among muscle force, length, and contraction velocity (Fig. 3.18). The plot does not, however, include the

passive length-tension component of muscle. The plot shows, for example, that a muscle contracting at a high velocity at its shortened length produces relatively low force levels, even with maximal effort. In contrast, a muscle contracting at a low (near-isometric) velocity at a longer length (e.g., near its optimal muscle length) theoretically produces a substantially greater active force.

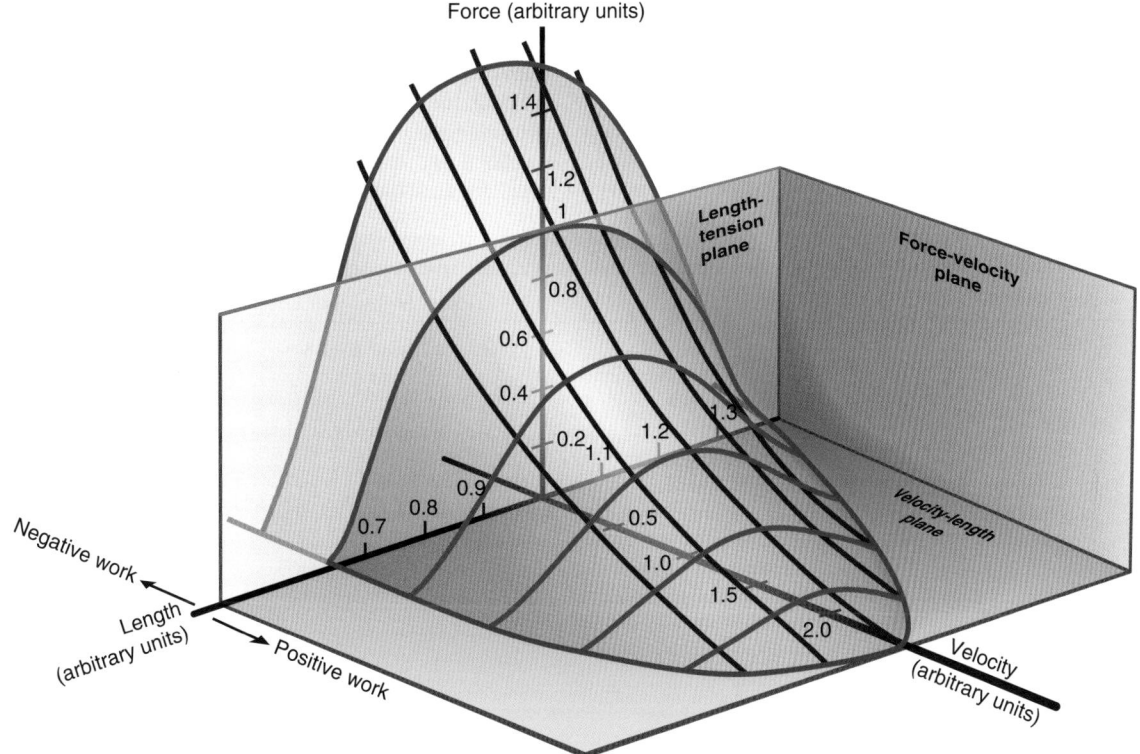

FIGURE 3.18 A theoretical plot representing the three-dimensional relationships among muscle force, muscle length, and muscle contraction velocity during a maximal effort. Positive power is associated with concentric muscle activation, and negative power is associated with eccentric muscle activation. Power can be expressed as muscle force multiplied by muscle contraction velocity. (Redrawn and modified from Winter DA: *Biomechanics and motor control of human movement,* ed 2, New York, 1990, John Wiley & Sons.)

RECRUITMENT

Recruitment of muscle refers to the initial activation of specific motor neurons that causes activation of their associated muscle fibers. The nervous system recruits a motor unit by altering the voltage potential across the membrane of the cell of the alpha motor neuron. This process involves a net summation of competing inhibitory and excitatory inputs. At a critical voltage, ions flow across the cell membrane and produce an electrical signal known as an *action*

potential. The action potential is propagated down the axon of the alpha motor neuron to the motor endplate at the neuromuscular junction. Once the muscle fiber is activated, a muscle contraction (also called a *twitch*) occurs, and a small amount of force is generated. Through recruitment of more motor neurons, more muscle fibers are activated, and therefore more force is generated within the whole muscle.

The muscle fibers associated with each motor unit normally share similar contractile characteristics and are distributed within a region

Appreciating the Complexity of the Term "Innervation" of Skeletal Muscle

Muscles are stimulated to contract through an outflow of *efferent* signals emanating from the central nervous system. Once stimulated, muscles generate force by one of two basic mechanisms: either contracting or resisting being pulled apart. The resulting force is refined through a continuous source of *afferent,* or sensory, feedback that helps orchestrate the amount, timing, and precision of movement.

This Special Focus is intended to reinforce the notion that quality active movement relies as much on sensory innervation as it does motor innervation. As a muscle generates movement, the central nervous system receives a near simultaneous array of afferent impulses from a wide variety of locations. These afferent impulses can initiate from the eyes, semicircular canals of the ears, soles of the feet, as well as from receptors located in activated muscles and adjacent mechanoreceptors in the skin and periarticular connective tissues. The importance of sensory feedback during movement is evident when observing the reduced quality of movement

in persons with pathology primarily involving the sensory system. In the healthy state, muscle innervation encompasses *both* the afferent and the efferent components of neurologic signaling, to and from the central nervous system, across multiple peripheral and central locations.

Table 3.4 lists one of several ways to classify sensory receptors located in skeletal muscle. Most receptors signal the nervous system of changes in stretch and force in muscle and its tendon. The nervous system responds by adjusting the relative excitability of the motor units in the agonist or antagonist muscles. Furthermore, muscle receptors detect changes in the mechanical pressure as well as the local metabolic environment, thereby guiding changes in cardiovascular output and excitability of the motor neuron pool. The information included in Table 3.4 may help clarify an often confusing and overlapping nomenclature system of sensory receptors and their nerves in general. This information may be useful for additional study and reading in this area.

TABLE 3.4   Summary of the Naming and Basic Information of Selected Sensory Receptors in Skeletal Muscle

Group*	Sensory Receptor	Function	Primary Stimulus of Receptor	Comments
Ia	Muscle spindle (primary)	Increases excitability of agonist muscle; decreases excitability of antagonist muscle	Rate of muscle stretch	Most responsible for tendon tap reflex
Ib	Golgi tendon organ (GTO)	Decreases excitability of agonist muscle; increases excitability of antagonist muscle	Muscle-tendon force	Stimulated throughout a wide range of forces
II	Muscle spindle (secondary)	Increases excitability of agonist muscle; decreases excitability of antagonist muscle	Muscle stretch	Present in nearly all muscles, except the tongue
III	Mechanoreceptor	Increases cardiovascular and ventilatory output; inhibits central motor drive	Change of intramuscular pressure	Influences excitation of the motor neuron pool during exercise
IV	Metaboreceptor	As cell above	Change of muscular metabolism	As cell above

*The Roman numerals designate the classification of the nerve fiber associated with a particular receptor. Groups are ranked on the basis of relative nerve fiber diameter and conduction velocity. (Group I has the largest diameter and fastest conduction velocity.)

of a muscle. Although each whole muscle may contain a few hundred motor units, each axon within a given motor unit may innervate 5 to 2000 muscle fibers.[32] Muscles that require fine motor control and generate relatively low forces, such as those that control movement of the eye or digits of the hand, are usually associated with smaller-sized motor units. Typically, these motor units have a small number of muscle fibers innervated per axon (i.e., possess a *low innervation ratio*). In contrast, muscles used to control less-refined movements involving the production of larger forces are generally associated with larger-sized motor units. These motor units tend to innervate a relatively large number of muscle fibers per axon (i.e., possess a *high innervation ratio*).[32] Any given whole muscle, regardless of its functional role, possesses motor units with a wide variation of innervation ratios.

The size of the motor neuron influences the order in which it is recruited by the nervous system. Smaller neurons are recruited *before* the larger motor neurons (Fig. 3.19). This principle is called

the *Henneman Size Principle,* first experimentally demonstrated and developed by Elwood Henneman in the late 1950s.[54] The Size Principle accounts for much of the orderly recruitment of motor units, specified by size, which allows for smooth and controlled increments in force development.

Muscle fibers innervated by small motor neurons have *twitch responses* that are relatively long in duration ("slow twitch") and small in amplitude. Motor units associated with these fibers have been classified as *S* (for slow) because of the slower contractile characteristics of the muscle fibers. The associated fibers are referred to as *SO* fibers, indicating their slow and oxidative histochemical profile. Fibers associated with slow (S) motor units are relatively *fatigue resistant* (i.e., experience little loss of force during a sustained activation). Consequently, a muscle such as the soleus (which makes continuous and often small adjustments in the postural sway of the body over the foot) has a relatively large proportion of SO fibers.[76]

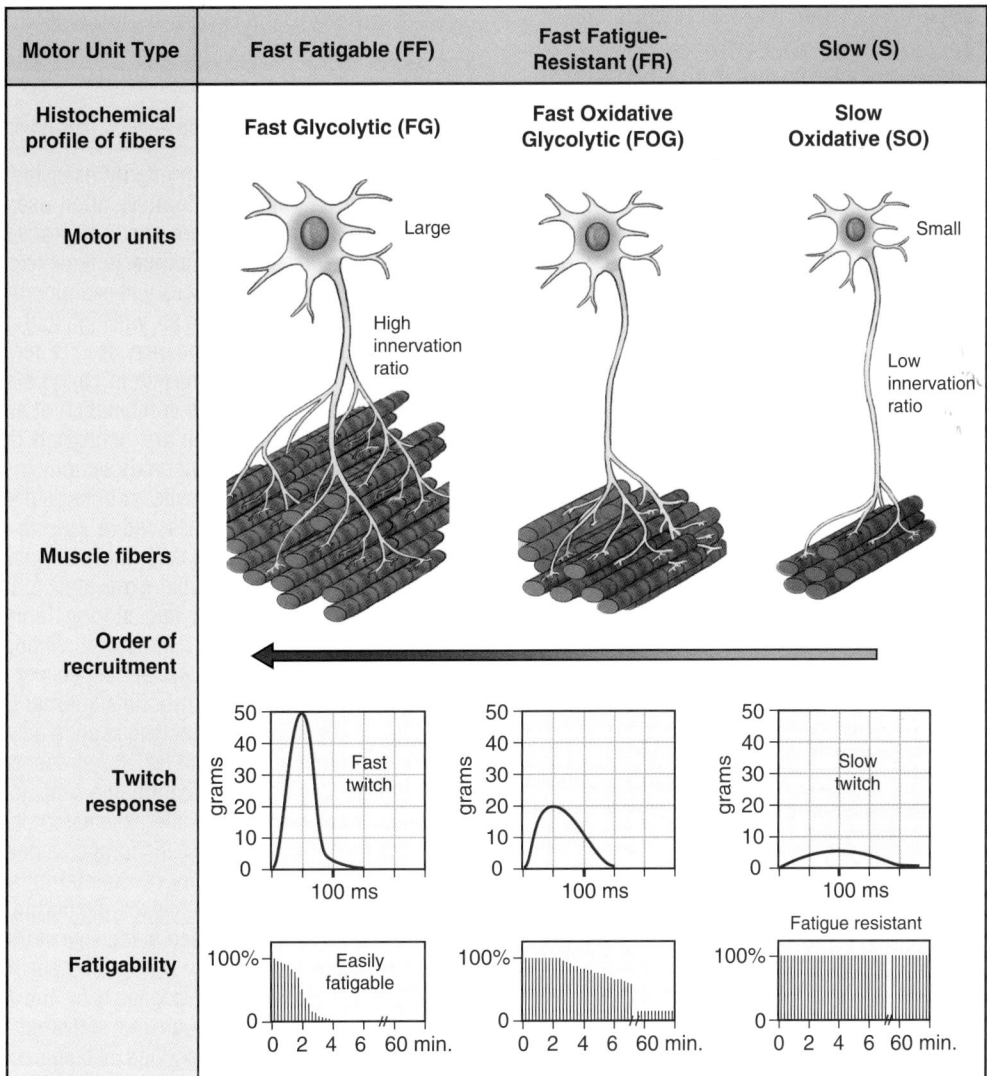

Motor Unit Type	Fast Fatigable (FF)	Fast Fatigue-Resistant (FR)	Slow (S)
Histochemical profile of fibers	Fast Glycolytic (FG)	Fast Oxidative Glycolytic (FOG)	Slow Oxidative (SO)
Motor units	Large / High innervation ratio		Small / Low innervation ratio
Muscle fibers			
Order of recruitment	⟵		
Twitch response	Fast twitch		Slow twitch
Fatigability	Easily fatigable		Fatigue resistant

FIGURE 3.19 Classification of motor unit types from muscle fibers based on histochemical profile, size, and twitch (contractile) characteristics. A theoretical continuum of differing contractile and morphologic characteristics is shown for each of the three motor unit types. It is important to note that the range of any single characteristic may vary considerably within any given motor unit (either within or between whole muscles).

This slow fiber type allows "postural muscles" such as the soleus to sustain low levels of force over a long duration.

In contrast, muscle fibers associated with larger motor neurons have twitch responses that are relatively brief ("fast twitch") and higher in amplitude. Motor units associated with these fibers are classified as *FF* (fast and easily fatigable). The associated fibers are classified as *FG,* indicating their fast twitch, glycolytic histochemical profile. These fibers are easily fatigable. The larger FF motor units are generally recruited *after* the smaller SO motor units, when very large forces are required.

Fig. 3.19 shows, in a diagrammatic fashion, the existence of a spectrum of intermediate motor units that have physiologic and histochemical profiles somewhere between "slow" and "fast fatigable." The more "intermediate" motor units are classified as *FR* (fast fatigue-resistant). The fibers are referred to as *FOG* fibers, indicating the utilization of oxidative and glycolytic energy sources.

The arrangement of the motor unit types depicted in Fig. 3.19 allows for a broad continuum of physiologic responses from skeletal muscle. The smaller (slower) recruited motor units are typically recruited early during a movement and generate relatively low muscle forces that can be sustained over a relatively long time. The contractile characteristics associated with the muscle fibers are ideal for the control of fine or smoothly graded low-intensity contractions. Larger (faster) motor units are recruited after the smaller motor units and add successively greater forces of shorter duration. Through this spectrum, the nervous system can activate muscle fibers that sustain stable postures over a long period of time and, when needed, produce large, short-duration bursts of force for more impulsive movements.

RATE CODING

After a specific motor neuron has been recruited, the force produced by the associated muscle fibers is primarily modulated by the discharge rate of action potentials. This process is referred to as *rate coding.* Although a single action potential in a skeletal muscle fiber persists for several milliseconds (ms), the resulting muscle fiber *twitch* (isolated contraction) may last for as long as 130 ms to 300 ms in a slow twitch fiber. When a motor unit is first recruited, it will discharge (or spike) at about 10 action potentials per second, or 10 Hz.

(The average discharge rate of an action potential is represented as a frequency [Hz], or by its reciprocal, the *interspike interval;* 10 Hz is equivalent to an interspike interval of 100 ms.) With increased excitation, the discharge rate may increase to about 50 Hz (20 ms interspike interval) during a high-force contraction, although this is usually sustained for only a brief period.[32] Because the twitch duration is often longer than the interval between discharges of action potentials, it is possible for several subsequent action potentials to occur during the initial twitch. If a muscle fiber can relax completely before the subsequent action potential, the second fiber twitch generates a force about equal to that of the first twitch (Fig. 3.20A). If the next action potential arrives before the preceding twitch has relaxed, however, the muscle twitches summate and generate an even greater peak force. Furthermore, if the next action potential arrives closer to the peak force level of the initial twitch, the force is even greater.

A set of repeating action potentials that each activates the muscle fiber before the relaxation of the previous twitch generates a series of summated mechanical twitches, referred to as an *unfused tetanus* (Fig. 3.20A). As the time interval between activation of successive twitches shortens, the unfused tetanus generates greater force until the successive peaks and valleys of mechanical twitches fuse into a single, stable level of muscle force, termed *fused tetanus.* Fused tetanus represents the greatest force level that is possible for a single muscle fiber. Motor units activated at high rates therefore can generate greater overall force than the same number of motor units activated at lower rates.

The mechanics of the single muscle fiber twitch and fused tetanus were described earlier in the context of a single muscle fiber. A similar phenomenon, however, can be demonstrated at the level of a whole muscle in a healthy person (Fig. 3.20B). Although the strength of a contraction is much greater at the whole muscle level compared with a single fiber, the overall relationship between the force (or torque in this case) and frequency is similar. This relationship is not specific to just skeletal muscle, which, interestingly, was first described in the cardiac muscle of a frog in the 1870s.[121] The relationship between the force and the frequency at which a motor unit is activated is curvilinear in shape, with a steep rise in force at low to moderate frequencies of activation, followed by a force plateau at high frequencies (usually by about 50 Hz for whole human muscle). The precise force-frequency relationship however, depends on the duration of each twitch. A slow motor unit, for example, that generates a muscle twitch of a long duration will reach a fused tetanus at a lower frequency than a fast motor unit.

The mechanisms of recruitment and rate coding of the motor unit operate simultaneously during the increase in muscle force. The prevailing strategy (recruitment or rate coding) is highly specific to the demands and type of motor task. For example, motor unit recruitment during eccentric activation is different from that during concentric activation. During an eccentric activation, a relatively large force is generated per crossbridge. Consequently, the number of motor units recruited is less than that for the same force produced during a concentric activation. Thus a concentric activation requires the recruitment of a larger number of motor units to produce the same force as an eccentric activation. Furthermore, rate coding is particularly important in production of a rapid force, especially in the early stages of an isometric activation. The rate coding may drive some motor units to discharge action potentials in quick succession (double discharges) to further increase force development. Double discharges occur when a motor unit discharges an action potential within about 20 ms of the previous discharge—that is, at or more than 50 Hz, which is the upper limit of regular motor unit discharge rate in humans.[32] Regardless of the specific strategy used to volitionally increase force, the order of recruitment from small to larger motor units is still maintained.

SPECIAL FOCUS 3.6

"Muscle" or "Musculotendinous Unit": Which tells the fuller story?

Although this chapter primarily uses the concise term of "muscle," research literature often uses the term "musculotendinous unit" to more accurately account for the passive mechanisms used by a muscle to develop, store, and use force.[82,154] This Special Focus will examine the term musculotendinous unit and, in doing so, will highlight a means by which skeletal muscle stores and recycles its force. As described throughout this chapter, muscle is capable of producing and absorbing forces through a combination of active and passive mechanisms. Active forces are generated by the sarcomere after stimulation from the nervous system. In addition to these active forces, the semielastic structural proteins and intramuscular connective tissues within muscle produce passive tension, primarily by resisting the elongation of the entire muscle. These noncontractile-generated forces are essential for efficiently transferring and storing force within muscle. The tendon of a muscle—a structural continuum of the intramuscular connective tissues—is especially important in the storing and recycling of a muscle's internal force, particularly during rapid and rhythmic activities such as running. Thus the term musculotendinous unit (MTU) represents the entire muscle, which contains both contractile and noncontractile elements, such as its tendon and associated connective tissues. Conceptually, the term MTU encourages a deeper appreciation of the physiologic versatility of skeletal muscle. To illustrate, consider the action of the flexor digitorum brevis MTU (an intrinsic muscle located deep in the sole of the foot) during the push off phase of walking. During this part of the gait cycle, the toes are pushed into extension by the floor as the heel lifts off the ground. Although the activated flexor digitorum brevis (FDB) is typically described as being eccentrically active at this time, this may not tell the full story. Analysis has shown that although the FDB MTU is indeed lengthening as the toes are pushed into extension, the active muscle fibers are in a near *isometric* state.[78] Because the muscle is maintaining a nearly constant length, much of the overall lengthening of the MTU occurs from elongation (stretch) of its *multiple tendons.* This mechanism allows the MTU to store energy elastically for other subsequent events of the relatively strenuous push off phase. Similar such phenomena have been shown for other muscles of the foot during the stance phase of walking, including the tibialis posterior, tibialis anterior, and gastrocnemius-soleus complex—muscles that have relatively long and elastic tendons, apparently well suited for this function.[82,95,96,154] This and related topics will be described in more detail in chapters associated with the ankle and foot and the kinesiology of walking and running.

For matters of brevity, this textbook most often uses the term muscle rather than the term musculotendinous unit. Nevertheless, the use of the term muscle implies the entire organ: muscle fibers and associated connective tissues, including the tendon. This perspective allows for a richer appreciation of the energetics of skeletal muscle, including concepts associated with the MTU's "total" length-tension and force-velocity relationships.

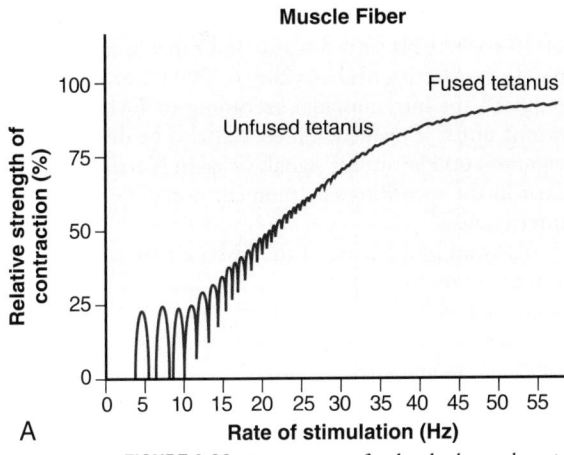

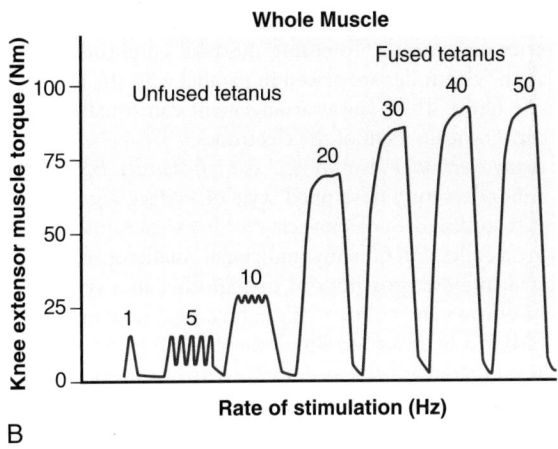

FIGURE 3.20 Summation of individual muscle twitches (contractions) recorded over a wide range of electrical stimulation frequencies. Plot in (A) shows theoretical data from a single muscle fiber. Plot in (B) shows actual knee extension torque data from seven electrical stimulations each of a different frequency applied to the quadriceps in a healthy 23-year-old man. Note that at low frequencies of stimulation (< 5 Hz), the initial twitch is relaxed before the next twitch can summate. At progressively higher frequencies, the twitches summate to generate higher force levels until a fused tetanus occurs. (A from Hall JE: *Guyton & Hall textbook of medical physiology,* ed 13, Philadelphia, 2016, Saunders.)

INTRODUCTION TO ELECTROMYOGRAPHY

Electromyography (EMG) is the science of recording and interpreting the electrical activity that emanates from activated skeletal muscle. EMG is one of the most important research tools used in the field of kinesiology. On careful and skillful analysis, it is possible for the clinician and researcher to determine the timing and magnitude of activation of several muscles, both superficial and deep, during simple or relatively complex functional movements. Especially over the last half-century, EMG studies have provided great insight into the specific actions of muscles. While EMG remains the gold standard for recording muscle activity, other less common technologies are available to record muscle activity, including mechanomyography and ultrasound imaging. In brief, *mechanomyography* records the mechanical vibrations generated by active muscle fibers through an external electronic condenser microphone secured over the muscle.[144] *Ultrasound imaging* uses an external probe placed on the skin over the region of an active muscle to record the deformations or displacements that occur within the muscle.[14,39] Ultrasound imaging is often used to indirectly access and visualize the activation of deeper muscles of the trunk. This technique is often used as an assessment tool to determine the effectiveness of certain exercises aimed at improving the strength and control of key muscles of the trunk and spine in persons with low back pain.[83,146,150]

Although EMG is also an important tool for the diagnosis and treatment of certain neuromuscular pathologic conditions or impairments (e.g., peripheral neuropathy and amyotrophic lateral sclerosis), this chapter focuses on its use in the study of the kinesiology of the musculoskeletal system. EMG studies are regularly cited throughout this text, primarily to support a muscle's action or synergistic function during a movement or task. EMG research can also help explain or justify a wide range of other kinesiologic and pathokinesiologic phenomena, encompassing topics related to the fatigue of muscle, motor learning and control, biofeedback, protection of damaged or unstable joints, locomotion, rehabilitation techniques, ergonomics, and sport and recreation.[26,35,100] For this reason the reader needs to understand the basic technique, use, and limitations of EMG in the study of kinesiology.

Recording of Electromyography

When a motor neuron is activated, the electrical impulse travels along the axon until it arrives at the motor endplates, and then it propagates in both directions away from the motor endplate along the length of the muscle fibers. The electrical signal that propagates along each muscle fiber is called the *motor unit action potential.* Electrodes can measure the sum of the change in electrical activity (represented as voltage measurement) associated with all action potentials involved with the activated muscle fibers.[35,37] The EMG signal is often referred to as a *raw* or *interference EMG* signal. The EMG signal can be detected before the actual generation of force by a muscle, commonly referred to as an *electromechanical delay.* The delay is short, typically lasting between 40 and 60 ms.[11] EMG signals can be sensed by indwelling electrodes (fine wires inserted into the muscle) or by surface electrodes (placed on the skin overlying the muscle).

EMG recording electrodes are often connected to a cable that attaches directly to signal-processing hardware. More recent technical developments allow EMG signals to be reliably recorded using wireless systems. Wireless systems are usually desired for monitoring and recording muscle activity from long distances from the subject or patient, or during activities in which the cabling may disrupt freedom of movement. Wireless surface EMG signals are transmitted to a recording computer by radio frequency waves and therefore are more susceptible to electrical interference than when direct cable attachments are used to transmit the EMG signal.

The choice of electrodes depends on the situation and purpose of the EMG recording. *Surface electrodes* are used most often because they are easy to apply, are noninvasive, and can detect signals from a relatively large area overlying the muscle. A common electrode arrangement involves the placement of two surface electrodes over the muscle (each approximately 4–8 mm in diameter), side by side, on the skin overlying the muscle belly of interest. An additional reference (ground) electrode is placed over a bony area that has no muscle directly underneath. To ensure maximal amplitude of the EMG signal, the electrodes are placed in parallel with the long axis of the muscle fibers. This typical arrangement can usually detect action potentials within 2 cm of the electrodes.[36,101]

Linear array electrodes also known as *high density EMG electrodes* are a more recently developed style of surface sensors that cover a large recording area of a muscle.[34,38] In essence, linear array electrodes are a collection of many traditional smaller surface electrodes aligned in close proximity to one another in a systematic arrangement of rows and columns (i.e., arrays) to allow numerous signals of EMG to be recorded simultaneously. The arrangement and size can vary from as little as 8 small recording areas in 1 row to as many as 128 very small recording areas arranged in multiple columns and rows. These arrangements can detect many action potentials over a large portion of the muscle. Through a complex mathematical analysis, the raw EMG signals from the multiple pairs and combinations of array electrodes can be decomposed into individual waveforms and extracted to represent the activity of single motor units.[98] The individual motor units can be tracked across the array electrodes to quantify properties of the motor unit, including recruitment of the motor unit as well as its conduction velocity and discharge rate.[35,36] Although linear array electrodes are ideal for the study of individual motor units, they are primarily limited to superficial muscles. They do however provide insight into the behavior of single motor units in healthy and clinical populations[106,115,130] that were previously only accessible with fine wire and needle electrodes.

Fine wire electrodes inserted directly into the muscle permit a more specific region of a muscle to be monitored, as well as those deeper muscles not easily accessible through the use of surface electrodes, such as the brachialis, tibialis posterior, and transversus abdominis. Although the recording area is much smaller, fine wire electrodes can also discriminate single action potentials produced by one or a few motor units. Inserting fine wire electrodes into human muscle requires a relatively high level of technical skill and appropriate training before its safe implementation.

The voltage of the raw EMG signal is generally only a few millivolts, and therefore the signal can easily be distorted by other electrical sources caused by movement of electrodes and cables, adjacent or distant active muscles, and electromagnetic radiation from the surrounding environment. Several strategies can be used to minimize unwanted electrical artifact (often referred to as "noise"), including using the bipolar and ground electrode configuration described previously. This arrangement minimizes common electrical artifact detected by both electrodes, a method electromyographers often refer to as "common mode rejection."[33,100]

Other strategies for reducing unwanted electrical artifact include adequate skin preparation and proper electrical shielding of the recording environment. Electrical signals can also be preamplified at the electrode site. This boost of the EMG signal at the electrode site reduces artifact produced by movement of the electrode cables, which is a special concern when EMG is monitored during dynamic activities such as walking or running.[136] *Filtering* of the EMG signal can reduce certain interfering electrical signals by restricting the frequency range of the recorded EMG. A *band-pass filter* involves the combination of a high-pass filter (frequencies below a specified frequency are blocked, and higher frequencies are allowed to pass) and a low-pass filter (frequencies above a specified frequency are blocked, and lower frequencies are allowed

to pass). A typical band-pass filter for surface EMG retains signals of 10 to 500 Hz and discards the other frequencies.[99] Broader band-pass filtering of about 200 to 2000 Hz or even greater is often required for intramuscular recording of EMG to extract single motor units. If needed, a filter can also be designed to eliminate common 60 Hz current signals (used in North America) that may exist in the recording environment because of ambient electrical interference.

To avoid losing parts of the EMG signal, it is essential that the sampling rate be at least twice the rate of the highest frequency contained within the EMG signal. For example, using a band-pass filter set at 10 to 500 Hz ideally requires a sampling rate of at least 1000 Hz (samples per second).[99]

Analysis and Normalization of Electromyography

EMG can provide valuable insight into the actions of muscles, particularly when combined with additional data such as time, joint kinematics and kinetics, external forces, or additional data derived from biomechanical modeling.[12,143] In many kinesiologic analyses, the timing and amplitude of the EMG signal are of great interest. Consider, for example, the potential relevance of studying the normal *timing* or sequencing of activation of the muscles associated with stabilization of the vertebral column. A delay or inhibition of the activation of a muscle such as the transversus abdominis or lumbar multifidus, for example, may suggest a cause for instability in the lower spine. Treatments can therefore be directed to concentrate on activities that specifically recruit and challenge these muscles.[60,111] Measuring the relative timing or order of muscle activation with EMG can be performed visually on a digital chart recorder or data acquisition system, or by more quantitative descriptive or mathematical or statistical methods.

Assessing the demands placed on a muscle is usually determined by the relative *amplitude* of the EMG signal. Greater amplitude of EMG is generally assumed to indicate greater intensity of muscle activation and, in certain cases, greater relative muscle force. Fig. 3.21A–B depicts a force generated by the isometric activation of an elbow flexor muscle producing a bipolar raw (interference) EMG signal. The raw EMG signal is a voltage that fluctuates on either side of zero and therefore often needs to be mathematically manipulated to serve as a useful quantitative measurement of muscle activation. One such method is called *full-wave rectification,* which converts the raw signal to positive voltages, resulting in the absolute value of the EMG (see Fig. 3.21C). The amplitude of the rectified EMG signal can be determined by averaging a sample of data collected over a specified time of activation. Furthermore, the rectified signal may be electronically filtered or *smoothed,* a process that flattens its "peaks and valleys" (see Fig. 3.21D). This smoothed signal is often referred to as a "linear envelope," which can be quantified as a "moving average," specified over a certain time frame or other event. Although not depicted in Fig. 3.21, the smoothed signal may also be *integrated,* a mathematical process that calculates the area under the (voltage-time) curve. This process allows for cumulative EMG quantification over a fixed period of time.

An alternative analysis for representing the raw EMG amplitude is to calculate the root mean squared *(RMS)* value over a period of time, which correlates with the standard deviation of the voltage relative to zero.[36] This mathematical analysis involves squaring the signal (to ensure a completely positive signal), averaging, and then calculating the square root. EMG voltages mathematically treated

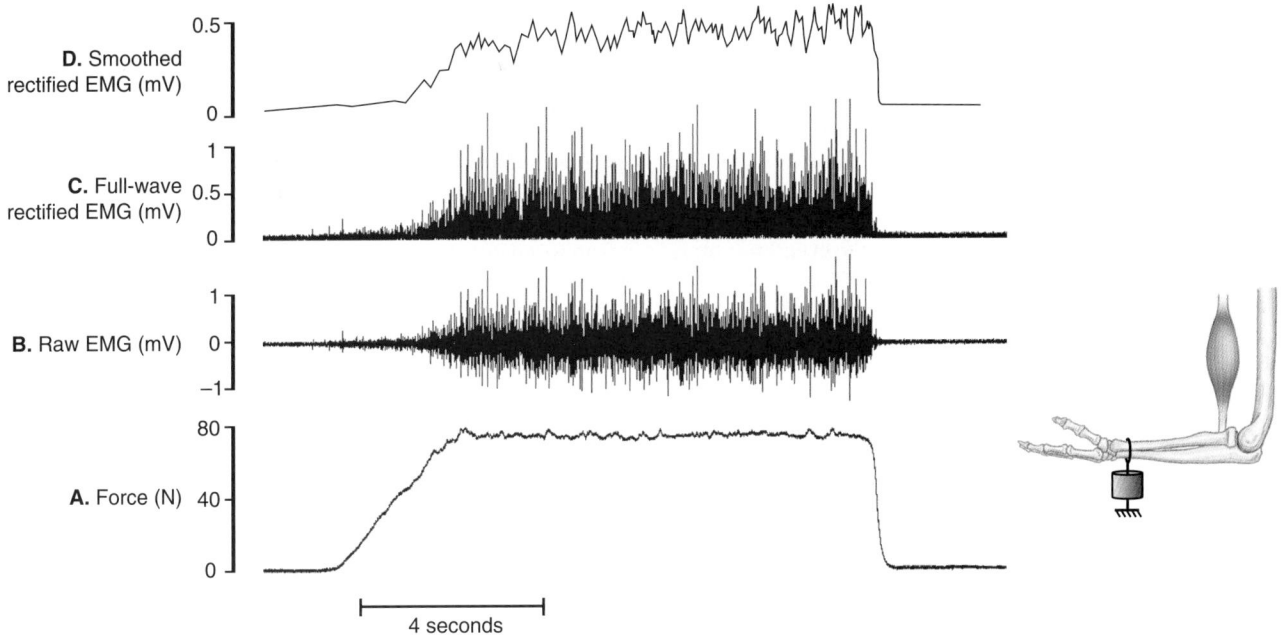

FIGURE 3.21 Diagram depicting several ways to process EMG signals caused by an isometric activation of the elbow flexor muscles at a submaximal effort performed by a young healthy woman. An external force produced by activation of the elbow flexor muscles is held at 80 N for about 10 seconds (A). The EMG signal is recorded as a raw signal (B), then is processed by full-wave rectification (C), and finally is filtered and smoothed to remove the higher frequencies (D).

by any of the techniques described can also be used in biofeedback devices, such as visual meters or audio signals, or to trigger other devices, such as electrical stimulators, to activate a muscle at a preset threshold of voluntary contraction.

When the magnitude of a processed EMG signal is compared between different muscles, days, or conditions, it is often necessary that the signal be *normalized* to some common reference signal. Expressing EMG amplitude in absolute voltage may produce meaningless data in some kinesiologic studies, especially when one is attempting to average data across different subjects and muscles. This is especially true when EMG data are collected across several sessions, requiring that the recording electrodes be reapplied. Even with the same muscular effort, absolute voltage will vary according to the choice of recording electrode (including size), skin condition, and exact site of electrode placement. One common method of normalizing EMG involves referencing the signal produced by an activated muscle to that produced by the same muscle during a *maximal voluntary isometric contraction* (MVIC). Meaningful comparisons can then be made on the *relative* amplitude or intensity of muscle activation across different subjects or days, expressed as a percent of MVIC.[20,66] Alternatively, instead of using an MVIC as a reference signal, some electromyographers use the electrical response evoked from electrical stimulation of the muscle (i.e., M wave) for analysis.[158] or the rate of increase in the EMG from initial activation.[21] Also, a muscle's activation level can be referenced to some other meaningful reference task that does not involve maximal effort.[66,108]

Electromyographic Amplitude during Muscular Activation

To avoid the misinterpretation of EMG as it relates to a muscle's action or overall function, it is essential to understand the physiologic and technical factors that influence the amplitude of the EMG signal.[151]

The amplitude of the EMG signal is generally proportional to the number and discharge rate of active motor units within the recording area of the EMG electrodes. These same factors also contribute to the force generated by a muscle. It is often tempting, therefore, to use a muscle's relative EMG magnitude as a measure of its relative *force* production. Although a generalized positive relationship may be assumed between these two variables during an isometric activation,[66] it cannot be assumed during all forms of nonisometric activations.[50,112] This caveat is based on several and often simultaneous factors, both physiologic and technical.

Physiologically, the EMG amplitude during a nonisometric activation can be influenced by the muscle's *length-tension* and *force-velocity* relationships. Consider the following two extreme hypothetic examples. Muscle A produces 30% of maximal force via a high-velocity *eccentric* activation, across a muscle length that favors the production of relatively large active and passive forces. Muscle B, in contrast, produces an equivalent submaximal force via a high-velocity *concentric* activation, across a muscle length that favors the production of relatively small active and passive forces. Based on the combined influences of the muscle's length-tension and force-velocity relationships (depicted in Figs. 3.11 and 3.15), Muscle A is assumed to operate at a relative *physiologic advantage* for producing force. Muscle A therefore requires fewer motor units to be recruited than Muscle B. EMG levels would therefore be less for the movement performed by Muscle A, although both muscles may be producing equivalent submaximal forces. In this extreme and hypothetic example, the EMG magnitude could not be used to reliably compare the relative forces produced by these two muscles.

Consider also that when an activated muscle is lengthening or shortening, the muscle fibers (the source for the electrical signal of EMG) change their spatial orientation to the recording electrodes. The EMG signal therefore may represent a compilation of several action potentials from different regions of a muscle or even from different muscles during the range of motion. This can alter the voltage signal recorded by the electrodes with a nonproportional change in the muscle force.

Other technical factors potentially affecting the magnitude of an EMG signal during movement are listed in the following box. A detailed discussion of this topic can be found elsewhere.[35,36,37,101]

Technical Factors That May Affect the Magnitude of the EMG Signal

- Electrode configuration and size
- Range and type of filtering of the frequency content of the signal
- Magnitude of "cross-talk" from nearby muscles
- Location of the electrodes relative to the motor unit endplates
- Orientation of the electrodes relative to the muscle fiber

Throughout this textbook, EMG studies are cited that have compared average EMG amplitudes across different muscles from different subjects. Depending on the experimental design and technique (including appropriate normalization), specifics of the movement, and type and speed of the muscles' activation, it may be appropriate to assume that a greater relative amplitude of an EMG signal from a muscle is associated with a greater relative contractile force. In general, the confidence of this assumption is greatest when two muscles are compared while performing isometric activations. Confidence is less, however, when muscles are compared while performing movement that requires eccentric and concentric activations or when muscles are fatigued (see later in this chapter).

In closing, although it may not be possible to predict the relative force in all muscles based on EMG amplitude, the amplitude (or timing) of the activation still provides very useful clues into the muscle's kinesiologic role in a given action. These clues are often reinforced through the analysis of other kinetic and kinematic variables, such as those provided by goniometers, accelerometers, video or other optical sensors, strain gauges, and force plates (see Chapter 4).

SPECIAL FOCUS 3.7

"Fiber Typing"—A Long History of Classification Nomenclature

As described in Fig. 3.19, three types of motor units are recognized: slow (S), fast fatigue-resistant (FR), and fast fatigable (FF) motor units. Most muscle fibers associated with a given motor unit are physiologically similar and therefore have similar functional characteristics.

Over the years, researchers have attempted to identify via biopsy and histochemical or biochemical analysis muscle fibers that are physiologically associated with each of the main types of motor units. This process is referred to as "fiber typing." Several techniques of fiber typing have evolved over the last 50 to 60 years, three of which are highlighted in Table 3.5. The first method analyzed the histochemical profile of the fibers based on their relative *oxidative or glycolytic metabolism*. This system, as previously described in this chapter, conveniently links the contractile characteristics of the fibers with the classification nomenclature of the motor units (compare columns 1 and 2 in Table 3.5). This original method was developed from studies of animal motor units by Edgerton and colleagues in the 1960s, and later refined in the early 1970s.[116]

In 1970, Brooke and Kaiser[13] designed a technique of fiber typing human muscles. This technique studied the histochemical profile of fibers based on the activity of the enzyme *myosin ATPase*

(column 3 in Table 3.5). The relative activity of this enzyme allowed the fast twitch (type II) fibers to be differentiated from the slow twitch (type I) fibers. In human muscle, the faster type II fibers can be furthered classified as type IIA and type IIX. (Note that type IIX in humans was originally identified as type IIB until in more recent years, when the molecular composition of the myosin was truly identified as described subsequently.)

Until the early 1990s, histochemical techniques performed on cross-sections of muscle fibers were the dominant method for fiber typing human muscles. Biochemical analysis of protein molecules soon developed that allowed portions of muscle or single fibers to be analyzed based on the proportion of structurally similar isoforms of *myosin (heavy chain)*—a primary active (contractile) protein within the sarcomere. At least three isoforms of this myosin heavy chain (MHC) protein have been identified in humans: MHC I, MHC IIA, and MHC IIX (column 4 in Table 3.5). The dominant isoform found within a fiber is correlated with several of its mechanical properties, including maximal rate of shortening and force development, and force-velocity characteristics.[129] This technique, currently considered the "gold standard" for fiber typing, is well correlated with the myosin ATPase histochemistry.[129,138]

TABLE 3.5 A Comparison of Three Methods of Fiber Typing Skeletal Muscle

Motor Unit Types	Histochemical Profile of Fibers Based on Relative Oxidative or Glycolytic Metabolism	Histochemical Profile of Fibers Based on Relative Activity of Myosin ATPase	Molecular Profile of Fibers Based on the Dominance of an Isoform of Myosin Heavy Chain (MHC)
Slow (S)	Slow oxidative (SO)	Type I (low activity)	MHC I
Fast fatigue-resistant (FR)	Fast oxidative glycolytic (FOG)	Type IIA (high activity)	MHC IIA
Fast fatigable (FF)	Fast glycolytic (FG)	Type IIX (high activity)	MHC IIX

CAUSES OF MUSCLE FATIGUE IN HEALTHY PERSONS

Muscle fatigue is classically defined as an exercise-induced decline in maximal voluntary muscle force or power, despite maximal effort.[30,31,79] Muscle fatigue can define the limits of human performance during athletic endeavors, ergonomic tasks, physical training, and rehabilitation. Understanding muscle fatigue is very important to the clinician because it is the basis of neuromuscular overload and adaptation that is necessary for rehabilitation and training of the neuromuscular system. Even in healthy persons, muscle fatigue occurs during and after a sustained physical effort. Normally muscle fatigue is reversible with rest and should not be confused with being chronically "tired" or with muscle weakness that persists even with ample rest.[30] Although muscle fatigue is a normal response to sustained physical effort, excessive or chronic muscle fatigue or tiredness is not normal and is often a symptom of an underlying neuromuscular disorder or disease.[30]

In the healthy person, muscle fatigue can be subtle, especially during the performance of tasks involving prolonged, submaximal levels of effort.[135] This is apparent in Fig. 3.22 (top panel), as a healthy person is instructed to perform a series of isometric elbow flexion contractions at a 50% submaximal effort, with every sixth effort (indicated by the arrows) being a maximal (100%) effort.[64] As observed in the figure, the magnitude of force produced by the maximal efforts gradually declines, although the person is still able to successfully generate the 50% level of maximal force. Continued performance of this repetitive submaximal effort, however, would eventually result in a decline in muscle force well below the 50% target level. Thus while muscle fatigue is often measured as reduction in the maximal force or power of a muscle group, it can also be quantified as the time to failure of a given submaximal task.[31] Of interest, as evident in Fig. 3.22 (bottom panel), the amplitude of the EMG signal gradually *increases* throughout the repeated submaximal efforts held at the constant force. This increased EMG signal reflects the recruitment of additional larger motor units as the muscle fibers within the active motor units lose their maximal force-generating capability and concurrently cease or reduce their discharge rates.[123] This recruitment strategy is an attempt at maintaining a relatively stable force output.

In contrast to the submaximal efforts depicted in Fig. 3.22, a sustained muscle contraction at *maximal* effort results in a much more rapid rate of decline in maximal force. In this case EMG amplitude *declines* as muscle force declines. This reduced EMG activity reflects a cessation or slowing of the discharge rate of the fatiguing motor units. Because all motor units are presumably active during the initial stages of the maximal effort, there are no other motor units in reserve to compensate for the decline in muscle force, as is the case with prolonged submaximal efforts.

The magnitude or rate of muscle fatigue is specific to the performance of the task, including the duration of the rest-work cycle.[31] A muscle that is rapidly fatigued by high-intensity and short-duration exercise can recover after a rest of only several minutes. In contrast, a muscle that is fatigued by low-intensity, long-duration exercise usually requires a much longer time to recover its force-generating capacity. Furthermore, the *type of activation* influences muscle fatigue. A muscle that is repeatedly activated eccentrically will exhibit less muscle fatigue than when activated concentrically at the same velocity and under the same external load.[10] The relative fatigue-resistant nature of eccentric activation reflects the greater force generated per crossbridge and therefore the lower recruitment of motor units for a given submaximal load. Caution is required, however, when eccentric activation is employed as the primary rehabilitative training tool in a muscle that is unaccustomed to this type of activation. Delayed onset of muscle soreness (DOMS) experienced after repeated eccentric activations is usually more severe than after bouts of concentric or isometric activations.[119] DOMS tends to peak 24 to 72 hours after the bout of exercise and is ultimately caused by disruption of the sarcomeres and damage to the cytoskeleton within and around the fiber.[19,120]

From a clinical perspective, it is important to understand that muscle fatigue in healthy persons may differ based on the age and sex of the person.[7,70,71,79] Women, for example, are usually less fatigable than men for exercise involving isometric and slow-to-moderate velocity concentric activation when the relative intensity is similar across sexes.[70] The mechanism for this sex-related difference occurs because women usually possess a greater proportion of type I (slow twitch) fibers than men; therefore their muscle is more fatigue resistant.[70] Muscle fatigue can also differ markedly between young and older adults,[65,79] although this age-related difference will depend on whether the task involves isometric activation or fast dynamic contractions. For muscle activated isometrically, older adults are usually *less* fatigable than young adults due to age-related differences in fiber type proportions (see section below titled "Changes in Muscle with Advanced Age").[7] For muscle repeatedly

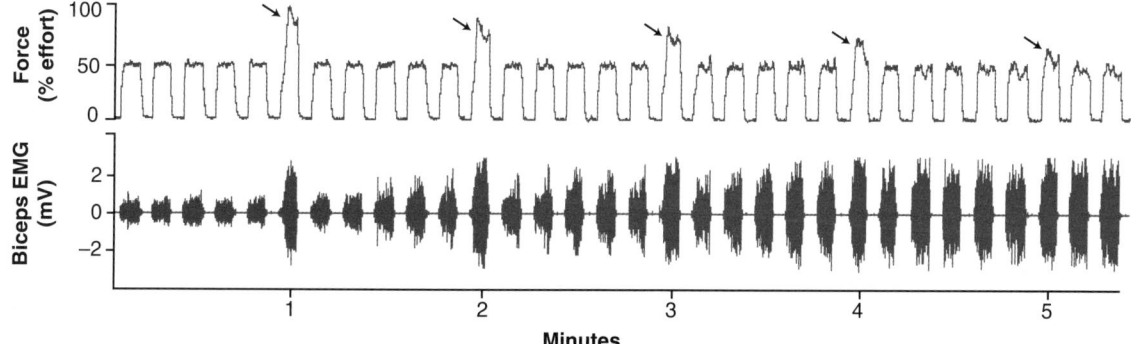

FIGURE 3.22 Isometric force of the elbow flexor muscles sustained intermittently (6 seconds on and 4 seconds off) at a magnitude 50% of initial maximal force. A maximal (100%) effort is performed every sixth effort (at 1-minute intervals) and is indicated by the small arrows in the top panel. The bottom panel shows the raw EMG signal recorded from the biceps brachii during the fatiguing task. (Data from Hunter SK, Critchlow A, Shin IS, et al: Men are more fatigable than strength-matched women when performing intermittent submaximal contractions, *J Appl Physiol* 96:2125, 2004.)

activated concentrically at fast velocities, older adults are usually *more* fatigable than young adults.[131,142] For the clinician who is prescribing rehabilitation exercises that result in fatiguing exercise of limb muscles to young and older men and women, these task and population differences in muscle fatigue are important considerations.

There are several proposed mechanisms to explain the exact causes of muscle fatigue. These mechanisms may be located at all points within and between the activation of the motor cortex and the sarcomere.[31,43,79,140] Mechanisms may occur in the muscle or at the neuromuscular junction (often referred to as *muscular or peripheral mechanisms*). Alternatively, mechanisms may occur in the nervous system (often referred to as *neural or central mechanisms*). The distinction between muscular and neural mechanisms is not always clear. As an example, Group IV afferents within muscle respond to the local metabolic byproducts associated with muscle fatigue. Activation of these neurons in a fatiguing muscle can inhibit the discharge rate of the associated motor neurons,[5,97] paradoxically further reducing the force output of the fatigued muscle. In this example, the reason for the loss in force in the fatiguing muscle can be partially explained by both muscular and neural mechanisms.

Many mechanisms of muscle fatigue in healthy persons are associated with the muscle itself. The mechanisms that limit force or power, however, depend on the task itself and which region of the neuromuscular system is most stressed (muscle or nervous system or both). These mechanisms can be investigated by measuring the reduction in muscle force produced by electrical stimulation, which is independent of the central nervous system and voluntary effort.[43,70,79] These and other tests suggest that several muscular mechanisms may be responsible for muscle fatigue (see list in the following box).[79]

Possible Muscular Mechanisms Contributing to Muscle Fatigue

- Reduced excitability at the neuromuscular junction
- Reduced excitability at the sarcolemma
- Changes in excitation-contraction coupling because of reduced sensitivity and availability of intracellular calcium
- Changes in contractile mechanics, including a slowing of crossbridge cycling and ATPase efficiency
- Reduced energy source (metabolic origin)
- Reduced blood flow and oxygen supply

Several mechanisms of muscle fatigue have been proposed that involve the nervous system—that is, regions proximal to the neuromuscular junction.[43,145] These neural mechanisms typically involve reduced excitatory input to supraspinal centers or a net decline in excitatory input to alpha motor neurons.[43] As a consequence, in healthy persons activation of the pool of motor neurons is reduced and muscle force declines. Persons with pathology involving the nervous system such as multiple sclerosis or stroke may experience even greater muscle fatigue than healthy adults because of delays or blocks in the conduction of central neural impulses.[133]

In closing, considerable research is required to better understand the mechanisms of muscle fatigue among both healthy and clinical populations, and how these relate to limitations of athletic performance and during daily tasks. For the therapist and exercise training specialist, muscle fatigue coupled with adequate recovery is used as a training stimulus to enhance performance. Thus optimizing recovery from fatiguing exercise is an area that requires further attention. Lastly, how muscle fatigue varies across different tasks and patient populations will provide the therapist with a more individualized

and effective approach to rehabilitation.[160] Clarity in these areas will benefit virtually any rehabilitation procedure that involves physical effort from the patient or client, irrespective of whether there is an underlying pathologic process.

CHANGES IN MUSCLE WITH STRENGTH TRAINING, REDUCED USE, AND ADVANCED AGE

Changes in Muscle with Strength Training

The healthy neuromuscular system shows a remarkable ability to accommodate to different external demands or environmental stimuli. Such plasticity is evident in the robust and almost immediate alteration in the structure and function of the neuromuscular system after strength training. *Strength,* in the context of this chapter, refers to the maximal force or power produced by a muscle or muscle group during a maximal voluntary effort.

Repeated sessions of activating a muscle with progressively greater resistance will result in increased strength and hypertrophy.[80,159] Strength gains are commonly quantified by a *one-repetition maximum,* or 1 RM. By definition, 1 RM is the maximal load that can be lifted *once* as a muscle contracts through the joint's full or near-full range of motion. (For safety and practical reasons, formulas have been developed that allow a person's 1 RM strength to be determined by lifting a reduced load with a larger number of repetitions.[159]) The amount of resistance employed during strength training is often specified as a multiple of 1 RM; for example, the term *3 RM* is the maximal load that can be lifted through a joint's full range of motion three times, and so on.

General Recommendations for Resistance Training

- *High-resistance training* involves a progressive increase in the magnitude of the load from within the 3 to 12 RM range, performed over three bouts per exercise session.
- *Low-resistance training* involves lifting a lighter load equivalent to at least 15 RM, usually performed over three bouts per exercise session.

Note that these guidelines are general. The program details vary among patients and clients and depend on specific goals of the training or rehabilitation. More detailed guidelines can be obtained from other sources.[80,89,159]

Increases in muscle strength from training are specific to the type and intensity of the exercise program. For example, high-resistance training involving concentric and eccentric activations performed three times a week for a 12-week period has been shown to increase 1 RM strength by 30% to 40%.[68] (On average, this represents an increase of about 1% of strength per day of training.) The same dynamic training regimen employing concentric and eccentric activations, however, resulted in only a 10% increase in *isometric* strength.[68] These results suggest that, in general, most strength-training programs should involve a component of eccentric activation. Because eccentric activations produce greater force per unit of muscle, this form of training can be more effective in promoting muscle hypertrophy than the same training using isometric and concentric activations.[125]

As expected, gains in 1 RM strength from low-resistance training are less than those for high-resistance training, but gains in muscle endurance can be greater.

One of the most dramatic responses to strength training is hypertrophy of muscle.[1,80,125,132] Hypertrophy results from increased protein synthesis within muscle fibers and therefore an increase in the physiologic cross-sectional area of the whole muscle. The protein synthesis results in sarcomeres being added in *parallel* within the muscle fiber, thereby partially explaining the increased contraction force. An increase in the number of sarcomeres in *series* (i.e., end-to-end) is not a primary mechanism of hypertrophy in skeletal muscle.[53] Serial addition of sarcomeres within a fiber, in contrast, results in an increase in the speed of contraction of the muscle fiber.[88] Increased pennation angles in hypertrophied muscles have also been demonstrated, perhaps as a way to accommodate the larger amounts of contractile proteins.[1,77] Increased cross-sectional area in human muscle is primarily a result of fiber hypertrophy, with limited evidence of an increase in the actual number of fibers (hyperplasia). Staron and colleagues showed that the cross-sectional area of muscle increases as much as 30% in young adults after 20 weeks of high-resistance strength training, with increases in fiber size detected after only 6 weeks.[138] Although training causes hypertrophy in all exercised muscle fibers, it is usually greatest in the fast twitch (type II) fibers.[68,138,156] It has been proposed that increased strength in muscle may also be the result of an increase in the protein filament *desmin* (reviewed in Table 3.2), which is believed to help transfer forces within and between muscle fibers.[156]

While much is known about skeletal muscle hypertrophy associated with exercise training, recent advances in technology have enabled more in-depth study of the biologic steps that contribute to the increased protein synthesis leading to hypertrophy. New research focused on "omics" (genomics,[84] epigenomics,[155] and proteomics[47]) is characterizing the changes in gene regulation, transcription, and translation associated with exercise training with a goal of providing more precise exercise prescription that may optimize individual responses to exercise training— an approach often referred to as *precision physical therapy*.[155]

Strength gains from resistance training are also caused by adaptations within the nervous system.[18,27,42,75] Neural influences are especially evident during the first few training sessions. Some of the adaptations include an increased area of activity within the cortex of the brain during a motor task (as shown by functional magnetic resonance imaging), increased supraspinal motor drive, increased motor neuron excitability, and greater discharge frequency of motor units coupled with a decrease in neural inhibition at both spinal and supraspinal levels.[18,27] Perhaps the most convincing evidence of a neurogenic basis for strength training is documented increases in muscle strength through imagery training[161] or increases in the strength or control of the (non-exercised) muscles located *contralateral* to the exercised muscles.[17] In general, strength gains are often greater than what can be attributed to hypertrophy alone.[27] Although most of the neural adaptations cause greater activation of the agonist muscles, evidence suggests that training can result in *less* activation of the antagonist muscles.[42] The reduced force from opposing muscles would result in a greater net force produced by the agonist muscles.

Strength gains from resistance training may be enhanced with supplementary methods that can be applied during training, such as blood flow restriction training. *Blood flow restriction training* generally incorporates a moderate external pressure that occludes venous outflow while maintaining arterial inflow to the exercising muscle, thus contributing to a greater oxidative and metabolic stress on the muscle without increasing the external load.[113,117] The greater oxidative and metabolic stressors associated with blood flow restriction contribute to greater adaptations to training, such as increased skeletal muscle hypertrophy and capillarization.[117] Notably, blood flow restriction training should *not* be considered as

a surrogate training method but rather as a method to enhance the effects of resistance training particularly, during rehabilitation after musculoskeletal injury. Despite evidence in young healthy populations, the effectiveness of blood flow restriction training to enhance strength in older adults and clinical populations, and the involved mechanisms, are not fully understood.

Some of these concepts outlined earlier can be used by the clinician when more traditional methods of strength training are unsuccessful. This is especially relevant in persons with neurologic or neuromuscular pathologies who cannot tolerate the physical rigor of a strength-training regimen. Imagery training, for example, may be effective in very early stages of recovery of an injured limb after a stroke, when use of the affected limb is otherwise limited. Ultimately, the most effective method of strengthening a weakened muscle involves specific and adequate progressive overload to evoke changes not only in the nervous system but also in the structure of the muscle.

Changes in Muscle with Reduced Use

Trauma that requires a person's limb or joint to be rigidly immobilized for many weeks significantly reduces the use of the associated muscles. Periods of reduced muscle use (or disuse) also occur as a person confined to bed rest recovers from an illness or disease. These periods of reduced muscle activity lead to atrophy and usually marked reductions in strength, even in the first few weeks of inactivity.[2,23,118,149] The loss in strength can occur early, up to 3% to 6% per day in the first week alone.[6] After only 10 days of immobilization, healthy individuals can experience up to a 40% decrease of initial 1 RM strength.[147] Reduced strength after immobilization is usually twice that of the muscle atrophy—a 20% reduction in fiber cross-sectional area is associated with a 40% decline in strength. These relatively early changes suggest some neurologic basis for the reduced strength, in addition to the loss in the muscle's contractile proteins.

Protein synthesis is reduced in all muscle fiber types within a chronically immobilized limb[2] but most notably in the slow twitch (type I) fibers.[118] Because slow twitch fibers are used so frequently throughout most routine daily activities, they are subjected to greater *relative* disuse when the limb is immobilized compared with fast twitch fibers. As a consequence, whole muscles of immobilized limbs tend to experience a relative transformation toward faster twitch characteristics,[51] and this shift can occur as early as 3 weeks after the onset of immobilization.[63]

The neuromuscular changes following prolonged immobilization of a limb depend on several factors. The loss of strength is greatest when the muscle is maintained in its shortened position.[41,88] The greater slack placed on muscle fibers immobilized in a shortened length may specifically promote degradation of contractile proteins. Furthermore, "postural" muscles and some single-joint muscles show a more rapid atrophy than other muscles within a chronically immobilized limb. These muscles include the soleus, vastus medialis, vastus intermedius, and multifidus.[88] In the lower extremity, the knee extensors generally demonstrate greater disuse atrophy and relative loss in strength than the knee flexor (hamstring) muscles.[105] The propensity for disuse atrophy in the quadriceps may be a concern when stability of the partially flexed knee is required, such as when a person is transferring to and from a chair, bed, or commode.

Resistive exercise can reverse or mitigate many of the changes that occur with chronic immobilization of a limb. A strengthening program incorporating eccentric activation demonstrates the greatest gains in strength and increases in fiber size.[63] Because the fibers associated with the smaller motor units are more prone to atrophy, a rehabilitation program should incorporate low-intensity, long-duration muscle activations early in the exercise program as a means to target these muscle fibers.

Changes in Muscle with Advanced Age

Even in healthy persons, reaching an advanced age is associated with reduced strength, speed of muscle contraction and muscle power.[65] Although these changes can be subtle, they can be striking in very old age.[142] Because of the relative rapid loss in the speed of muscle contraction, aged persons typically show greater loss in power (product of force and velocity) than in peak force and strength alone.[9,65,139]

Although changes are highly variable across different muscles and persons, in general, healthy aged persons experience an approximate 10% per decade decline in peak strength after 60 years of age, with a more rapid decline after 75 years of age.[67,103] Loss in strength and power is generally more pronounced in the muscles of the lower limb, such as the quadriceps,[67,92] compared with the upper limb. Lower-limb weakness can interfere with functions required for independent living, such as safely walking, or rising from a chair.[139] Such age-related decrements in muscle strength and power are often accelerated in very old adults (> 80 years), sedentary older adults or those with underlying pathology.[67,142]

The primary cause of reduced strength and power in healthy aged persons is a loss in muscle tissue with advanced age, known as *sarcopenia*.[24,104] Sarcopenia may be dramatic, with a marked loss of muscle tissue and an infiltration of excessive amounts of connective tissue and intramuscular fat (compare muscles in Fig. 3.23) and loss of physical function.[139] The causes of sarcopenia are not fully understood and may be associated with the normal biologic processes of aging (such as programmed cell death—"apoptosis") or changes in physical activity, nutrition, and hormone levels.[105,122]

Sarcopenia occurs through a reduction in the actual number of muscle fibers as well as a decrease in size (atrophy) of all existing fibers.[122,141] Loss in the number of fibers and number of motor units (as shown in Fig 3.24) is caused by a gradual demise of the associated alpha motor neurons.[85,148] Although the proportional *number* of type II and type I fibers is usually maintained in healthy older adults, there is a greater atrophy of the type II fast fibers.[68,122] The result of these age-related changes is a greater proportional *volume* of muscle that expresses type I (slow twitch) characteristics compared with young adults, which explains in part why whole muscles in aged adults take longer to contract and to relax and ultimately are less forceful and powerful.[24,141] Although a more sedentary lifestyle will accelerate these changes in muscle morphology, even the active older adult will experience these alterations to varying degrees. This phenomenon is apparent when excised cross-sections of stained muscle fibers of a young and a relatively older person are compared (Fig. 3.25). The cross-section of the older muscle in Fig. 3.25B shows all fibers are smaller compared with the young muscle, especially the type II (fast twitch) fibers. The muscle sample obtained from the older person in Fig. 3.25B demonstrates a greater proportional number of type I (slow twitch) fibers than in the younger person, although this is not always typical in healthy older adults.[68,122] The typical net result of sarcopenia is a similar reduction in the proportional number of type I and type II muscle fibers, and a greater reduction in the relative size of type II muscle fibers.[141]

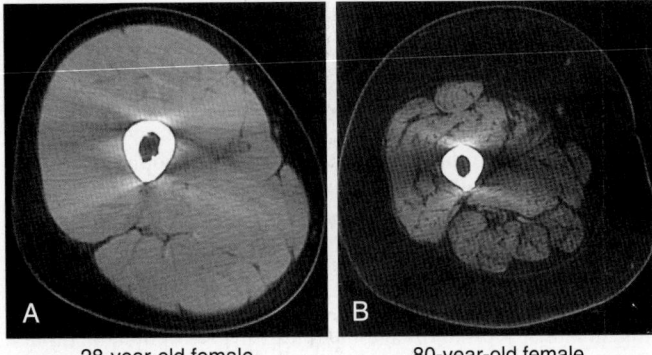

28-year-old female   80-year-old female

FIGURE 3.23 Computed tomographic image showing a cross-section of the muscles in the midthigh region of (A) a healthy 28-year-old woman and (B) a healthy but sedentary 80-year-old woman. The image of the older woman's thigh shows comparably less muscle mass, and more adipose and other intramuscular connective tissues.

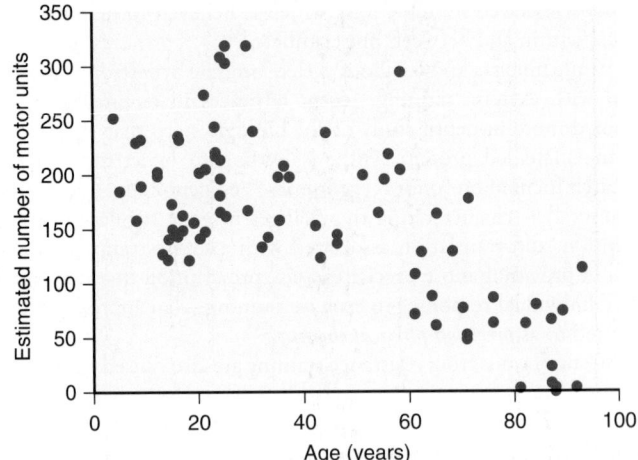

FIGURE 3.24 Estimated number of functional motor units associated with the extensor digitorum brevis of healthy human subjects across the lifespan from age 3 to 96 years. (Redrawn from Campbell MJ, McComas AJ, Petito F: Physiological changes in ageing muscles, *Journal of Neurology, Neurosurgery, and Psychiatry* 36:174-182, 1973.)

Sarcopenia in aged persons explains most but not all of the loss in strength and power production. Loss of force with maximal effort may also involve a reduced ability of the nervous system to maximally activate the available muscle fibers.[69,127] When given sufficient practice, some older adults can learn to activate their available muscle to a greater level, nearly equivalent to that in younger adults.[126] Clinically, this may be an important consideration during initial assessment of the strength of an older individual.

The age-related alterations in muscle morphology can have marked effects on the ability of some older adults to effectively perform daily tasks. Fortunately, however, age in itself does not drastically alter the *plasticity* of the neuromuscular system, until likely an advanced age of 85 years or older. Strength and power training can theoretically compensate for some but certainly not all the loss in strength and power in older adults.[40,128] Resistive exercise, if performed safely and appropriately, can be very helpful in maintaining the critical level of muscle force and power required for the performance of the basic activities of daily living.

27-year-old female   67-year-old female

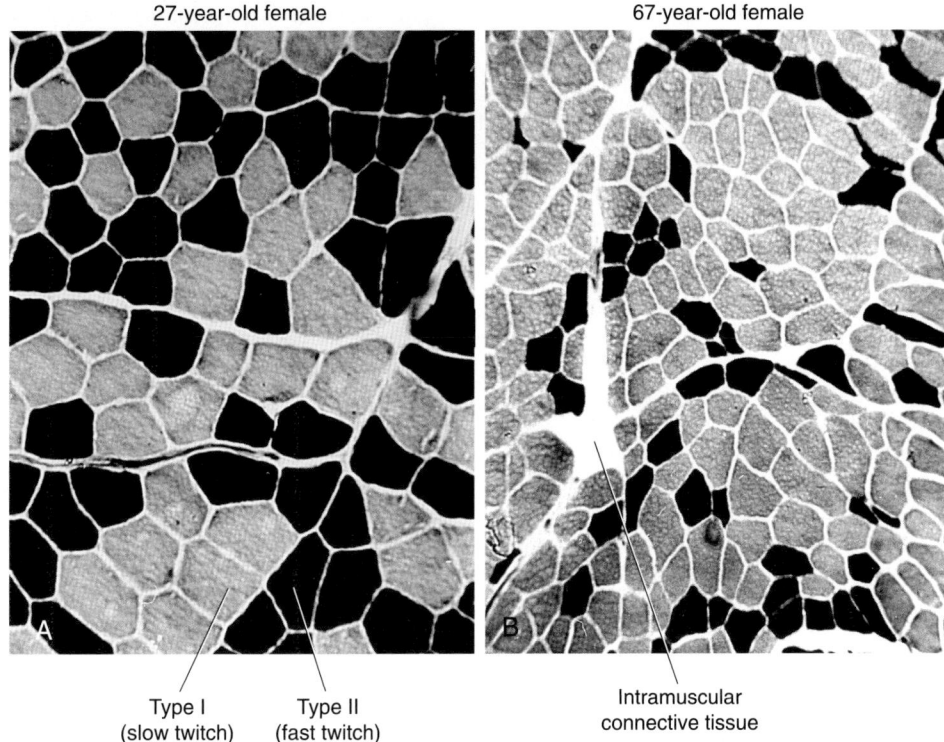

Type I   Type II
(slow twitch)   (fast twitch)

Intramuscular
connective tissue

FIGURE 3.25 Cross-section of human muscle fibers from the vastus lateralis of (A) a healthy 27-year-old woman and (B) a healthy 67-year-old woman. The images are printed to similar scales. The fibers were histochemically stained for myosin ATPase activity to show the distribution of type I (slow twitch) fibers that stained light, and type II (fast twitch) fibers that stained dark. (During the histochemical analysis procedures, the fibers were preincubated at pH 10.3.) Note the following in the older muscle: the reduced cross-sectional areas of the fibers, most notably the type II fibers, and greater intramuscular connective tissue.

SYNOPSIS

Skeletal muscle provides the primary forces that stabilize and move the bones and joints of the body. After activation by the nervous system via action potentials, muscles produce force by either contracting or resisting elongation. The contractile proteins of actin and myosin play a key role in driving this active process—referred to as the *sliding-filament hypothesis*. More recently appreciated is the important supportive and structural role of the noncontractile proteins. Proteins such as titin and desmin, for example, contribute to passive tension and provide elasticity, alignment, and stability to the sarcomeres and hence the whole muscle fiber. Furthermore, extracellular connective tissues surround individual and groups of muscle fibers, ultimately encasing the entire muscle belly before blending with the tendon and attaching to bone.

As described in Chapter 1, a muscle's action and ultimate function is based on its line of force relative to the axis of rotation at the joint. Chapter 3 focuses more on mechanisms responsible for the generation of the force. Ultimately, these mechanisms are governed by the nervous system but also by the unique morphology (shape) and overall architecture of the individual muscles. Each individual muscle in the body has a unique form and therefore unique function. A small fusiform muscle such as the lumbrical in the hand, for example, generates only a small force because of its small cross-sectional area. Because this muscle is well endowed with sensory receptors, it excels in providing the nervous system with proprioception. The larger gastrocnemius muscle, in contrast, produces large forces because of its larger cross-sectional area, resulting in part from the pennation arrangement of its fibers. A large force is required

from this calf muscle to lift or propel the entire body during activities such as jumping and climbing.

Regardless of the shape or architecture of a muscle, the forces ultimately transferred through the tendon and to the bone are produced by a combination of active and passive mechanisms. Active mechanisms are typically under volitional control, based primarily on the interaction between actin and myosin. Passive mechanisms, in contrast, are based more on the inherent stiffness characteristics of the muscle, collectively attributable to the structural proteins and all connective tissues including those that constitute the tendon. Although relatively small within a muscle's midrange of movement, passive tension can be very large at the more extremes of the range, especially for muscles that cross multiple joints. Some passive tension produced in response to a muscle stretch is normal and performs useful physiologic functions, such as stabilizing the joint and protecting it from stretch-related injury. Excessive passive tension, however, is abnormal and can restrict the optimal postural alignment of the body as a whole, as well as reduce the ease and fluidity of movement. Increased stiffness in muscle can occur as a result of trauma or disease within the musculoskeletal system. In addition, excessive passive tension (or stiffness) within muscle may result from abnormal levels of involuntary activation by the nervous system. This impairment is often referred to as *spasticity* or *rigidity* and is typically associated with injury or disease of the central nervous system.

Two of the most important clinically related principles of muscle physiology are the length-tension and force-velocity relationships. These basic principles, although originally formulated using isolated muscle fibers in the animal model, need to be applied clinically to whole muscles of patients or clients. The very relevant length-tension relationship of a single muscle fiber is expressed clinically as a torque–joint angle relationship of the whole muscle or muscle group, where torque is functionally analogous to force, and joint angle to length. The elbow flexor muscles, for example, produce their greatest elbow flexion torque near a 90-degree elbow joint angle. This joint angle corresponds approximately to where the biceps brachii has its greatest moment arm (leverage) as a flexor but also approximately to the length at which this muscle produces its greatest force based on the action-myosin overlap of its individual fibers. Even with maximal effort, peak elbow flexion torque drops considerably at full elbow extension or at full flexion because of these same leverage and physiologic factors.

In addition, a muscle's force-velocity relationship needs to be appreciated clinically within the scope of the muscle's torque–joint angular velocity relationship. For reasons described in this chapter, a muscle activated at a high joint angular velocity via eccentric activation produces greater force than any speed of concentric activation, including isometric. This principle can have important clinical implications, often physiologically linked to the muscle's length-tension relationship. Paralysis of proximal muscles, for example, often causes functional weakness in more distal but otherwise healthy muscles. Failure of proximal muscles to adequately stabilize the skeleton can cause a situation in which the more distal muscle is obligated to contract to an overly shortened length, at a quicker velocity than normal. This is evident, for example, by a weakened grasp after paralysis of the wrist extensor muscles. This and other kinesiologic examples are described in greater detail throughout this textbook.

The concept of the motor unit is an important premise behind much of the discussion of this chapter. A motor unit is a single cell body (located in the spinal cord), its axon, and all innervated muscle fibers. Because all the fibers within a given motor unit maximally contract on stimulation of the cell body, a finite amount of force is generated from each motor unit. Forces are increased across the entire muscle through the recruitment of additional motor units. In addition, motor units can increase their force output by discharging at faster rates. The processes of recruitment and rate coding allow motor units to finely control the gradation of forces across the entire muscle.

Considerations for collecting, processing, and normalizing EMG data were introduced in this chapter. When interpreted correctly, the EMG signal can provide very useful information on the timing, level of activation, and ultimate function of muscles. Information obtained from EMG is often analyzed in conjunction with anatomic, biomechanical, kinetic, and kinematic data; these analyses serve as the foundation for much of the kinesiology described throughout this text.

This chapter concludes with a broad overview of selected topics that have important relevance to clinical practice. These topics include causes of muscle fatigue and the changes that occur in muscles with strength training, reduced use, and aging. Inducing fatigue within muscle is often necessary for effective neuromuscular adaptation during training and rehabilitation in healthy and clinical populations. Consequently, understanding the adaptation of muscle and its function to strength training, and in contrast to reduced use and aging, will aid the therapist in prescribing optimal therapies for rehabilitation to patient populations.

REFERENCES

1. Aagaard P, Andersen JL, Dyhre-Poulsen P, et al.: A mechanism for increased contractile strength of human pennate muscle in response to strength training: changes in muscle architecture, *J Physiol* 534:613–623, 2001.
2. Adams GR, Caiozzo VJ, Baldwin KM: Skeletal muscle unweighting: spaceflight and ground-based models, *J Appl Physiol* 95:218–2201, 2003.
3. Allen GM, McKenzie DK, Gandevia SC, et al.: Reduced voluntary drive to breathe in asthmatic subjects, *Respir Physiol* 93:29–40, 1993.
4. Allen GM, McKenzie DK, Gandevia SC: Twitch interpolation of the elbow flexor muscles at high forces, *Muscle Nerve* 21:318–328, 1998.
5. Amann M, Wan HY, Thurston TS, et al.: On the influence of group III/IV muscle afferent feedback on endurance exercise performance, 48(4):209–216, 2020.
6. Appell HJ: Muscular atrophy following immobilisation, a review, *Sports Med* 10:42–58, 1990.
7. Avin KG, Frey Law LA: Age-related differences in muscle fatigue vary by contraction type: a meta-analysis, *Phys Ther* 91:1153–1165, 2011.
8. Baratta RV, Solomonow M, Best R, et al.: Isotonic length/force models of nine different skeletal muscles, *Med Biol Eng Comput* 31:449–458, 1993.
9. Bassey EJ, Fiatarone MA, O'Neill EF, et al.: Leg extensor power and functional performance in very old men and women, *Clin Sci* 82:321–327, 1992.
10. Baudry S, Klass M, Pasquet B, et al.: Age-related fatigability of the ankle dorsiflexor muscles during concentric and eccentric contractions, *Eur J Appl Physiol* 100:515–525, 2006.
11. Begovic H, et al.: Detection of the electromechanical delay and its components during voluntary isometric contraction of the quadriceps femoris muscle, *Front Physiol* 5:494, 2014.

12. Brandon SC, Graham RB, Almosnino S, et al.: Interpreting principal components in biomechanics: representative extremes and single component reconstruction, *J Electromyogr Kinesiol* 23:1304–1310, 2013.
13. Brooke MH, Kaiser KK: Muscle fiber types: how many and what kind? *Arch Neurol* 23:369–379, 1970.
14. Brown SH, McGill SM: A comparison of ultrasound and electromyography measures of force and activation to examine the mechanics of abdominal wall contraction, *Clin Biomech* 25:115–123, 2010.
15. Buhmann R, Trajano GS, Kerr G, et al.: Voluntary activation and reflex responses after hamstring strain injury, *Med Sci Sports Exerc* 52(9):1862–1869, 2020.
16. Caiozzo VJ: The muscular system: structural and functional plasticity. In Farrell PA, Joyner MJ, Caiozzo VJ, editors: *ACSM's advanced exercise physiology*, ed 2, Baltimore, 2012, Lippincott Williams & Wilkins.
17. Carroll TJ, Herbert RD, Munn J, et al.: Contralateral effects of unilateral strength training: evidence and possible mechanisms, *J Appl Physiol* 101:1514–1522, 2006.
18. Carroll TJ, Selvanayagam VS, Riek S, et al.: Neural adaptations to strength training: moving beyond transcranial magnetic stimulation and reflex studies, *Acta Physiol (Oxf)* 202:119–140, 2011.
19. Chen TC, Lin KY, Chen HL, et al.: Comparison in eccentric exercise-induced muscle damage among four limb muscles, *Eur J Appl Physiol* 111:211–223, 2011.
20. Deering RE, Senefeld JW, Pashibin T, et al.: Muscle function and fatigability of trunk flexors in males and females, *Biol Sex Differ* 8:12, 2017.
21. Delgadillo JD, Sundberg CW, Kwon M, et al.: Fatigability of the knee extensor muscles during high-load fast and low-load slow resistance exercise in young and older adults, *Exp Gerontol* 154:111546, 2021.
22. Dillon EL, Soman KY, Wiktorowicz JE, et al.: Proteomic investigation of human skeletal muscle before and after 70 days of head down bed rest with or

without exercise and testosterone countermeasures, *PLoS One* 14(6):e0217690, 2019.
23. Dirks ML, Wall BT, van de Valk B, et al.: One week of bed rest leads to substantial muscle atrophy and Induces whole-body insulin resistance in the absence of skeletal muscle lipid accumulation, *Diabetes* 65(10):2862–2875, 2016.
24. Doherty TJ: Invited review: aging and sarcopenia, *J Appl Physiol* 95:1717–1727, 2003.
25. Domire ZJ, et al.: An examination of possible quadriceps force at the time of anterior cruciate ligament injury during landing: a simulation study, *J Biomech* 44(8):1630–1632, 2011.
26. Drost G, Stegeman DF, van Engelen BG, et al.: Clinical applications of high-density surface EMG: a systematic review, *J Electromyogr Kinesiol* 16:586–602, 2006.
27. Duchateau J, Enoka RM: Neural adaptations with chronic activity patterns in able-bodied humans, *Am J Phys Med Rehabil* 81:S17–S27, 2002.
28. Duchateau J, Enoka RM: Neural control of lengthening contractions, *J Exp Biol* 219(2):197–204, 2016.
29. Duchateau J, Enoka RM: Neural control of shortening and lengthening contractions: influence of task constraints, *J Physiol* 586:5853–5864, 2008.
30. Enoka RM, Almuklass AM, Alenazy M, et al.: Distinguishing between fatigue and fatigability in multiple sclerosis, *Neurorehabil Neural Repair*, 2021.
31. Enoka RM, Duchateau J: Muscle fatigue: what, why and how it influences muscle function, *J Physiol* 586:11–23, 2008.
32. Enoka RM, Fuglevand AJ: Motor unit physiology: some unresolved issues, *Muscle Nerve* 24(4–17), 2001.
33. Enoka RM: *Neuromechanics of human movement*, ed 5, Champaign, Ill, 2015, Human Kinetics.
34. Enoka RM: Physiological validation of the decomposition of surface EMG signals, *J Electromyogr Kinesiol* 46:70–83, 2019.

35. Farina D, et al.: The extraction of neural strategies from the surface EMG: an update, *J Appl Physiol* 117(11):1215–1230, 2014.

36. Farina D, Holobar A, Merletti R, et al.: Decoding the neural drive to muscles from the surface electromyogram, *Clin Neurophysiol* 121:1616–1623, 2010.

37. Farina D, Merletti R, Enoka RM: The extraction of neural strategies from the surface EMG, *J Appl Physiol* 96:1486–1496, 2004.

38. Farina D, Negro F, Muceli S, et al.: Principles of motor unit physiology evolve with advances in technology, *Physiology (Bethesda)* 31(2):83–94, 2016.

39. Ferreira PH, Ferreira ML, Hodges PW: Changes in recruitment of the abdominal muscles in people with low back pain: ultrasound measurement of muscle activity, *Spine (Phila Pa 1976)* 29(22):2560–2566, 2004.

40. Fiatarone MA, O'Neill EF, Ryan ND, et al.: Exercise training and nutritional supplementation for physical frailty in very elderly people, *N Engl J Med* 330:1769–1775, 1994.

41. Fournier M, Roy RR, Perham H, et al.: Is limb immobilization a model of muscle disuse? *Exp Neurol* 80:147–156, 1983.

42. Gabriel DA, Kamen G, Frost G: Neural adaptations to resistive exercise: mechanisms and recommendations for training practices, *Sports Med* 36:133–149, 2006.

43. Gandevia SC: Spinal and supraspinal factors in human muscle fatigue, *Physiol Rev* 81:1725–1789, 2001.

44. Ghena DR, Kurth AL, Thomas M, et al.: Torque characteristics of the quadriceps and hamstring muscles during concentric and eccentric loading, *J Orthop Sports Phys Ther* 14:149–154, 1991.

45. Giles LS, et al.: Does quadriceps atrophy exist in individuals with patellofemoral pain? A systematic literature review with meta-analysis, *J Orthop Sports Phys Ther* 43(11):766–776, 2013.

46. Gillies AR, Lieber RL: Structure and function of the skeletal muscle extracellular matrix, *Muscle Nerve* 44:318–331, 2011.

47. Gonzalez-Freire M, Semba RD, Ubaida-Mohien C, et al.: The human skeletal muscle proteome project: a reappraisal of the current literature, *J Cachexia Sarcopenia Muscle* 8:5–18, 2017.

48. Goodall S, Romer LM, Ross EZ: Voluntary activation of human knee extensors measured using transcranial magnetic stimulation, *Exp Physiol* 94:995–1004, 2009.

49. Gordon AM, Huxley AF, Julian FJ: The variation in isometric tension with sarcomere length in vertebrate muscle fibres, *J Physiol* 184:170–192, 1966.

50. Graves AE, Kornatz KW, Enoka RM: Older adults use a unique strategy to lift inertial loads with the elbow flexor muscles, *J Neurophysiol* 83:2030–2039, 2000.

51. Haggmark T, Eriksson E: Cylinder or mobile cast brace after knee ligament surgery. A clinical analysis and morphologic and enzymatic studies of changes in the quadriceps muscle, *Am J Sports Med* 7:48–56, 1979.

52. Haizlip KM, Harrison BC, Leinwand LA: Sex-based differences in skeletal muscle kinetics and fiber-type composition, *Physiology (Bethesda)* 30:30–39, 2015.

53. Haun CT, Vann CG, Roberts BM, et al.: A critical evaluation of the biological construct skeletal muscle hypertrophy: size matters but so does the measurement, *Front Physiol* 10:247, 2019.

54. Henneman E, Mendell L: Functional organization of motoneuron pool and its inputs. In Brookhart JM, Mountcastle VB, Brooks VB, editors: *Handbook of physiology* (vol 2). Bethesda, 1981, American Physiological Society.

55. Herbert RB, Gandevia SC: The passive mechanical properties of muscle, *J Appl Physiol* 126:1442–1444, 2019.

56. Herzog W, Schappacher G, DuVall M, et al.: Residual force enhancement following eccentric contractions: a new mechanism involving titin, *Physiology (Bethesda)* 31(4):300–312, 2016.

57. Herzog W: The multiple roles of titin in muscle contraction and force production, *Biophys Rev* 10:1187–1199, 2018.

58. Hill A: *The first and last experiments in muscle mechanics*, New York, 1970, Cambridge University Press.

59. Hill A: The heat of shortening and the dynamic constraints of muscle, *Proc R Soc Lond B Biol Sci* 126:136–195, 1938.

60. Hodges PW, Richardson CA: Contraction of the abdominal muscles associated with movement of the lower limb, *Phys Ther* 77:132, 1997.

61. Hody S, Croisier JL, Bury T, et al.: Eccentric muscle contractions: risks and benefits, *Front Physiol* 10:536, 2019.

62. Horowits R, Kempner ES, Bisher ME, et al.: A physiological role for titin and nebulin in skeletal muscle, *Nature* 323:160–164, 1986.

63. Hortobagyi T, Dempsey L, Fraser D, et al.: Changes in muscle strength, muscle fibre size and myofibrillar gene expression after immobilization and retraining in humans, *J Physiol* 524:293–304, 2000.

64. Hunter SK, Critchlow A, Shin IS, et al.: Men are more fatigable than strength-matched women when performing intermittent submaximal contractions, *J Appl Physiol* 96:2125–2132, 2004.

65. Hunter SK, Pereira HM, Keenan KG: The aging neuromuscular system and motor performance, *J Appl Physiol* 121(4):982–995, 2016.

66. Hunter SK, Ryan DL, Ortega JD, et al.: Task differences with the same load torque alter the endurance time of submaximal fatiguing contractions in humans, *J Neurophysiol* 88:3087–3096, 2002.

67. Hunter SK, Thompson MW, Adams RD: Relationships among age-associated strength changes and physical activity level, limb dominance, and muscle group in women, *J Gerontol A Biol Sci Med Sci* 55:B264–B273, 2000.

68. Hunter SK, Thompson MW, Ruell PA, et al.: Human skeletal sarcoplasmic reticulum Ca2+ uptake and muscle function with aging and strength training, *J Appl Physiol* 86:1858–1865, 1999.

69. Hunter SK, Todd G, Butler JE, et al.: Recovery from supraspinal fatigue is slowed in old adults after fatiguing maximal isometric contractions, *J Appl Physiol* 105:1199–1209, 2008.

70. Hunter SK: The relevance of sex differences in performance fatigability, *Med Sci Sports Exerc* 48(11):2247–2256, 2016.

71. Hunter SK: Performance fatigability: mechanisms and task specificity, *Cold Spring Harb Perspect Med* 8(7):a029728, 2018.

72. Huxley AF, Niedergerke R: Structural changes in muscle during contraction: interference microscopy of living muscle fibres, *Nature* 173:971–973, 1954.

73. Huxley H, Hanson J: Changes in the cross-striations of muscle during contraction and stretch and their structural interpretation, *Nature* 173:973–976, 1954.

74. Ishikawa M, Komi PV, Grey MJ, et al.: Muscle-tendon interaction and elastic energy usage in human walking, *J Appl Physiol* 99:603–608, 2005.

75. Jenkins NDM, Miramonti AA, Hill EC, et al.: Greater neural adaptations following high- vs. Low-load resistance training, *Front Physiol* 8:331, 2017.

76. Johnson MA, Polgar J, Weightman D, et al.: Data on the distribution of fibre types in thirty-six human muscles. An autopsy study, *J Neurol Sci* 18:111–129, 1973.

77. Kawakami Y, Abe T, Fukunaga T: Muscle-fiber pennation angles are greater in hypertrophied than in normal muscles, *J Appl Physiol* 74:2740–2744, 1993.

78. Kelly LA, Farris DJ, Cresswell AG, et al.: Intrinsic foot muscles contribute to elastic energy storage and return in the human foot, *J Appl Physiol* 126(1):231–238, 2019.

79. Kent-Braun JA, Fitts RH, Christie A: Skeletal muscle fatigue, *Compr Physiol* 2:997–1044, 2012.

80. Kraemer WJ, Ratamess NA: Fundamentals of resistance training: progression and exercise prescription, *Med Sci Sports Exerc* 36:674–688, 2004.

81. Labeit S, Kolmerer B: Titins: giant proteins in charge of muscle ultrastructure and elasticity, *Science* 270:293–296, 1995.

82. Lai A, Lichtwark GA, Schache AG, et al.: In vivo behavior of the human soleus muscle with increasing walking and running speeds, *J Appl Physiol* 118(10):1266–1275, 2015.

83. Lee DH, Hong SK, Lee YS, et al.: Is abdominal hollowing exercise using real-time ultrasound imaging feedback helpful for selective strengthening of the transversus abdominis muscle? A prospective, randomized, parallel-group, comparative study, *Medicine (Baltim)* 97(27):e11369, 2018.

84. Leońska-Duniec A, Ahmetov II , Zmijewski P: Genetic variants influencing effectiveness of exercise training programmes in obesity - an overview of human studies, *Biol Sport* 33(3):207–214, 2016.

85. Lexell J, Taylor CC, Sjostrom M: What is the cause of the ageing atrophy? Total number, size and proportion of different fiber types studied in whole vastus lateralis muscle from 15- to 83-year-old men, *J Neurol Sci* 84:275–294, 1988.

86. Lieber RL, Binder-Markey BI: Biochemical and structural basis of the passive mechanical properties of whole skeletal muscle, *J Physiol* 599(16):3809–3823, 2021.

87. Lieber RL, Friden J: Clinical significance of skeletal muscle architecture, *Clin Orthop Relat Res* 383:140–151, 2001.

88. Lieber RL: *Skeletal muscle structure, function and plasticity*, ed 3, Baltimore, 2010, Lippincott Williams & Wilkins.

89. Liguori G: *ACSM's guidelines for exercise testing and prescription*, ed 11, Philadelphia, PA, 2022, Wolters Kluwer.

90. Linke WA, Freundt JK: Titin as a force-generating muscle protein under regulatory control, *J Appl Physiol* 126:1474–1482, 2019.

91. Lombardi V, Piazzesi G: The contractile response during steady lengthening of stimulated frog muscle fibres, *J Physiol* 431:141–171, 1990.

92. Lynch NA, Metter EJ, Lindle RS, et al.: Muscle quality. I. Age-associated differences between arm and leg muscle groups, *J Appl Physiol* 86:188–194, 1999.

93. Maganaris CN, Paul JP: Tensile properties of the in vivo human gastrocnemius tendon, *J Biomech* 35:1639–1646, 2002.

94. Magnusson SP, Narici MV, Maganaris CN, et al.: Human tendon behaviour and adaptation, in vivo, *J Physiol* 586:71–81, 2008.

95. Maharaj JN, Cresswell AG, Lichtwark GA: Subtalar joint pronation and energy absorption requirements during walking are related to tibialis posterior tendinous tissue strain, *Sci Rep* 7(1):17958, 2017.

96. Maharaj JN, Cresswell AG, Lichtwark GA: Tibialis anterior tendinous tissue plays a key role in energy absorption during human walking, *J Exp Biol* 222(Pt 11):04, 2019.

97. Martin PG, Smith JL, Butler JE, et al.: Fatigue-sensitive afferents inhibit extensor but not flexor motoneurons in humans, *J Neurosci* 26:4796–4802, 2006.

98. Merletti R, Farina D, Gazzoni M: The linear electrode array: a useful tool with many applications, *J Electromyogr Kinesiol* 13:37–47, 2003.

99. Merletti R, Hermens HJ: Detection and conditioning of the surface EMG signal. In Merletti R, Parker P, editors: *Electromyography: physiology, engineering and noninvasive applications*, Piscataway, NJ, 2004, IEEE Press, Wiley-Interscience.

100. Merletti R, Parker P: *Electromyography: physiology, engineering and noninvasive applications*, Piscataway, NJ, 2004, IEEE Press, Wiley-Interscience.

101. Merletti R, Rainoldi A, Farina D: Surface electromyography for noninvasive characterization of muscle, *Exerc Sport Sci Rev* 29:20–25, 2001.

102. Monti RJ, Roy RR, Hodgson JA, et al.: Transmission of forces within mammalian skeletal muscles, *J Biomech* 32:371–380, 1999.

103. Narici MV, Bordini M, Cerretelli P: Effect of aging on human adductor pollicis muscle function, *J Appl Physiol* 71:1277–1281, 1991.

104. Narici MV, Maffulli N: Sarcopenia: characteristics, mechanisms and functional significance, *Br Med Bull* 95:139–159, 2010.

105. Narici MV, Maganaris CN: Plasticity of the muscle-tendon complex with disuse and aging, *Exerc Sport Sci Rev* 35:126–134, 2007.

106. Negro F, Bathon KE, Nguyen JN, et al.: Impaired firing behavior of individually tracked paretic motor units during fatiguing contractions of the dorsiflexors and functional implications post stroke, *Front Neurol* 11:540893, 2020.

107. Neumann DA, Garceau LR: A proposed novel function of the psoas minor revealed through cadaver dissection, *Clin Anat* 28:243–252, 2015.

108. Neumann DA: An electromyographic study of the hip abductor muscles as subjects with a hip prosthesis walked with different methods of using a cane and carrying a load, *Phys Ther* 79:1163, 1999.

109. Ng AV, Miller RG, Gelinas D, et al.: Functional relationships of central and peripheral muscle alterations in multiple sclerosis, *Muscle Nerve* 29:843–852, 2004.

110. Nishikawa KC, Monroy JA, Uyeno TE, et al.: Is titin a 'winding filament'? A new twist on muscle contraction, *Proc Biol Sci* 279:981–990, 2012.

111. Okubo Y, Kaneoka K, Imai A, et al.: Electromyographic analysis of transversus abdominis and lumbar multifidus using wire electrodes during lumbar stabilization exercises, *J Orthop Sports Phys Ther* 40:743–750, 2010.

112. Pasquet B, Carpentier A, Duchateau J, et al.: Muscle fatigue during concentric and eccentric contractions, *Muscle Nerve* 23:1727–1735, 2000.

113. Patterson SD, Hughes L, Warmington S, et al.: Blood flow restriction exercise: considerations of methodology, application, and safety, *Front Physiol* 10:533, 2019.

114. Paulin D, Li Z: Desmin: a major intermediate filament protein essential for the structural integrity and function of muscle, *Exp Cell Res* 301(1):1–7, 2004.

115. Pereira HM, Schlinder-DeLap B, Keenan KG, et al.: Oscillations in neural drive and age-related reductions in force steadiness with a cognitive challenge, *J Appl Physiol* 126(4):1056–1065, 2019.

116. Peter JB, Barnard RJ, Edgerton VR, et al.: Metabolic profiles of three fiber types of skeletal muscle in Guinea pigs and rabbits, *Biochemistry* 11:2627–2633, 1972.

117. Pignanelli C, Christiansen D, Burr JF: Blood flow restriction training and the high-performance athlete: science to application, *J Appl Physiol* 130(4):1163–1170, 2021.

118. Ploutz-Snyder L, Bloomfield S, Smith SM, et al.: Effects of sex and gender on adaptation to space: musculoskeletal health, *J Womens Health* 23:963–966, 2014.

119. Prasartwuth O, Taylor JL, Gandevia SC: Maximal force, voluntary activation and muscle soreness after eccentric damage to human elbow flexor muscles, *J Physiol* 567:337–348, 2005.

120. Proske U, Morgan DL: Muscle damage from eccentric exercise: mechanism, mechanical signs, adaptation and clinical applications, *J Physiol* 537:333–345, 2001.

121. Puglisi JL, Negroni JA, Chen-Izu Y, et al.: The force-frequency relationship: insights from mathematical modeling, *Adv Physiol Educ* 37:28–34, 2013.

122. Reeves ND, Narici MV, Maganaris CN: Myotendinous plasticity to ageing and resistance exercise in humans, *Exp Physiol* 91:483–498, 2006.

123. Riley ZA, Maerz AH, Litsey JC, et al.: Motor unit recruitment in human biceps brachii during sustained voluntary contractions, *J Physiol* 586:2183–2193, 2008.

124. Roberts TJ: Contribution of elastic tissues to the mechanics and energetics of muscle function during movement, *J Exp Biol* 219(Pt 2):266–275, 2016.

125. Roig M, O'Brien K, Kirk G, et al.: The effects of eccentric versus concentric resistance training on muscle strength and mass in healthy adults: a systematic review with meta-analyses, *Br J Sports Med* 43:556–568, 2009.

126. Rozand V, Senefeld JW, Hassanlouei H, et al.: Voluntary activation and variability during maximal dynamic contractions with aging, *Eur J Appl Physiol* 117(12):2493–2507, 2017.

127. Rozand V, Sundberg CW, Hunter SK, et al.: Age-related deficits in voluntary activation: a systematic review and meta-analysis, *Med Sci Sports Exerc* 52(3):549–560, 2020.

128. Schaun GZ, Bamman MM, Alberton CL: High-velocity resistance training as a tool to improve functional performance and muscle power in older adults, *Exp Gerontol* 156:111593, 2021.

129. Schiaffino S, Reggiani C: Fiber types in mammalian skeletal muscles, *Physiol Rev* 91:1447–1531, 2011.

130. Senefeld JW, Keenan KG, Ryan KS, et al.: Greater fatigability and motor unit discharge variability in human type 2 diabetes, *Physiol Rep* 8(13):e14503, 2020.

131. Senefeld JW, Yoon T, Hunter SK: Age differences in dynamic fatigability and variability of arm and leg muscles: Associations with physical function, *Exp Gerontol* 87(A):74–83, 2017.

132. Seynnes OR, de Boer M, Narici MV: Early skeletal muscle hypertrophy and architectural changes in response to high-intensity resistance training, *J Appl Physiol* 102:368–373, 2007.

133. Sheean GL, Murray NM, Rothwell JC, et al.: An electrophysiological study of the mechanism of fatigue in multiple sclerosis, *Brain* 120:299–315, 1997.

134. Shield A, Zhou S: Assessing voluntary muscle activation with the twitch interpolation technique, *Sports Med* 34:253–267, 2004.

135. Smith JL, Martin PG, Gandevia SC, et al.: Sustained contraction at very low forces produces prominent supraspinal fatigue in human elbow flexor muscles, *J Appl Physiol* 103:560–568, 2007.

136. Soderberg GL, Knutson LM: A guide for use and interpretation of kinesiologic electromyographic data, *Phys Ther* 80:485–498, 2000.

137. Standring S, Ellis H, Healy JC: *Gray's anatomy: the anatomical basis of clinical practice*, ed 41, New York, 2015, Churchill Livingstone.

138. Staron RS, Leonardi MJ, Karapondo DL, et al.: Strength and skeletal muscle adaptations in heavy-resistance-trained women after detraining and retraining, *J Appl Physiol* 70:631–640, 1991.

139. Suetta C, Haddock B, Alcazar J, et al.: The Copenhagen Sarcopenia Study: lean mass, strength, power, and physical function in a Danish cohort aged 20-93 years, *J Cachexia Sarcopenia Muscle* 10(6):1316–1329, 2019.

140. Sundberg CW, Fitts RH: Bioenergetic basis of skeletal muscle fatigue, *Curr Opin Physiol* 10:118–127, 2019.

141. Sundberg CW, Hunter SK, Trappe SW, et al.: Effects of elevated H^+ and P_i on the contractile mechanics of skeletal muscle fibres from young and old men: implications for muscle fatigue in humans, *J Physiol* 596(17):3993–4015, 2018.

142. Sundberg CW, Kuplic A, Hassanlouei H, et al.: Mechanisms for the age-related increase in fatigability of the knee extensors in old and very old adults, *J Appl Physiol* 125(1):146–158, 2018.

143. Sutherland DH: The evolution of clinical gait analysis part l: kinesiological EMG, *Gait Posture* 14:61–70, 2001.

144. Tarata MT: Mechanomyography versus electromyography, in monitoring the muscular fatigue, *Biomed Eng Online* 2:3, 2003.

145. Taylor JL, Todd G, Gandevia SC: Evidence for a supraspinal contribution to human muscle fatigue, *Clin Exp Pharmacol Physiol* 33:400–405, 2006.

146. Teyhen DS, Rieger JL, Westrick RB, et al.: Changes in deep abdominal muscle thickness during common trunk-strengthening exercises using ultrasound imaging, *J Orthop Sports Phys Ther* 38:596–605, 2008.

147. Thom JM, Thompson MW, Ruell PA, et al.: Effect of 10-day cast immobilization on sarcoplasmic reticulum calcium regulation in humans, *Acta Physiol Scand* 172:141–147, 2001.

148. Tomlinson BE, Irving D: The numbers of limb motor neurons in the human lumbosacral cord throughout life, *J Neurol Sci* 34:213–219, 1977.

149. Trappe S, Costill D, Gallagher P, et al.: Exercise in space: human skeletal muscle after 6 months aboard the International Space Station, *J Appl Physiol* 106(4):1159–1168, 2009.

150. Vasseljen O, Dahl HH, Mork PJ, et al.: Muscle activity onset in the lumbar multifidus muscle recorded simultaneously by ultrasound imaging and intramuscular electromyography, *Clin Biomech (Bristol, Avon)* 21:905–913, 2006.

151. Vigotsky AD, Halperin I, Lehman GJ, et al.: Interpreting signal amplitudes in surface electromyography studies in sport and rehabilitation sciences, *Front Physiol* 8:985, 2018.

152. Wang K, McCarter R, Wright J, et al.: Viscoelasticity of the sarcomere matrix of skeletal muscles. The titin-myosin composite filament is a dual-stage molecular spring, *Biophys J* 64:1161–1177, 1993.

153. Willingham TB, Kim Y, Lindberg E, et al.: The unified myofibrillar matrix for force generation in muscle, *Nat Commun* 11:3722, 2020.

154. Wilson A, Lichtwark G: The anatomical arrangement of muscle and tendon enhances limb versatility and locomotor performance, *Philos Trans R Soc Lond B Biol Sci* 366(1570):1540–1553, 2011.

155. Woelfel JR, Dudley-Javoroski S, Shields RK: Precision physical therapy: exercise, the epigenome, and the heritability of environmentally modified traits, *Phys Ther* 98(11):946–952, 2018.

156. Woolstenhulme MT, Conlee RK, Drummond MJ, et al.: Temporal response of desmin and dystrophin proteins to progressive resistance exercise in human skeletal muscle, *J Appl Physiol* 100:1876–1882, 2006.

157. Yamaguchi G, Sawa A, Moran D: A survey of human musculotendon actuator parameters. In Winters JW, Woo S-LY, editors: *Multiple muscle systems: biomechanics and movement organization*, New York, 1990, Springer-Verlag.

158. Yoon T, Doyel R, Widule C, et al.: Sex differences with aging in the fatigability of dynamic contractions, *Exp Gerontol* 70:1–10, 2015.

159. Zatsiorsky VM, Kraemer WJ, Fry AC: *Science and practice of strength training*, ed 3, Champaign, Ill, 2021, Human Kinetics.

160. Zijdewind I, Hyngstrom A, Hunter SK: Editorial: fatigability and motor performance in special and clinical populations, *Front Physiol* 11:570861, 2020.

161. Zijdewind I, Toering ST, Bessem B, et al.: Effects of imagery motor training on torque production of ankle plantar flexor muscles, *Muscle Nerve* 28:168–173, 2003.

STUDY QUESTIONS

1. What functional purpose does pennation architecture serve within a muscle?
2. What tissues within a muscle are most responsible for the shape of the whole muscle's (a) passive, (b) active, and (c) total length-tension curve?
3. How does an activated muscle generate force without an actual shortening of its myofilaments?
4. The duration of a single action potential can be as brief as 10 ms as it propagates along the muscle fiber. With such a short duration, how can a muscle develop and sustain a state of fused tetanus?
5. Define muscle fatigue. Explain how electromyographic (EMG) amplitude can be used to detect the onset of muscle fatigue in a prolonged submaximal-effort muscle contraction.
6. What factors limit the ability of a muscle's EMG amplitude to be predictive of its relative force output in a freely activated muscle?
7. What are some methods used to minimize unwanted "electrical noise" during collection of EMG signals?
8. Define physiologic cross-sectional area.
9. Explain why internal torque produced by a muscle during isometric activation changes with a change in joint angle.
10. Consider the plot depicted in Fig. 3.16.
    a. Explain possible reasons why the peak torque of the knee extensor muscles exceeds that of the knee flexor muscles, regardless of the velocity of muscle activation.
    b. Describe possible physiologic reasons for the nearly 40% reduction in peak torque of the knee extensor muscles at contraction velocities of 60 to 240 degrees/sec.
11. Describe the two fundamental strategies used by the nervous system to gradually increase muscle force.
12. Define motor unit. What is the Henneman Size Principle?
13. Describe how it is physiologically possible for a person to demonstrate clinically measurable increases in muscle strength before signs of muscle hypertrophy.
14. Explain how an otherwise healthy muscle within an immobilized limb can experience a relative shift toward faster twitch characteristics.
15. What is the primary cause of reduced strength in healthy, aged persons?
16. What are the primary functional consequences of adding sarcomeres in (a) parallel or (b) in series within the muscle fiber?
17. Explain the anatomic and functional differences between efferent and afferent innervation of skeletal muscle. Describe a likely consequence of a disease that affects either the efferent or afferent innervation specifically to skeletal muscle.
18. Explain how it is physiologically possible and beneficial for an entire musculotendinous unit (MTU) to elongate as its embedded muscle fibers are simultaneously isometrically active.

Answers to the study questions are available in the accompanying enhanced eBook version included with the print purchase of this textbook.

Chapter

4

Biomechanical Principles for Understanding Movement

LAUREN K. SARA, PT, DPT, PhD

PETER R. BLANPIED, PT, PhD

DONALD A. NEUMANN, PT, PhD, FAPTA

CHAPTER AT A GLANCE

A thorough understanding of human movement and posture is necessary for a wide variety of applications. Whether for rehabilitation, surgery, ergonomics, orthotics and prosthetics, athletic performance, or advising in compensatory strategies, optimal musculoskeletal assessment and intervention depend on accurate analyses and descriptions of human movement. But human movement is less straightforward than it seems, frequently being influenced by a dynamic interplay of environmental, psychological, and physiological factors. Most often, analyzing complex movements is simplified by assuming the body behaves as a series of rigid body segments. This is followed by a basic evaluation of forces acting from within and outside of the body and studying the effects of these forces on the rigid segments. Newton's laws of motion help explain the relationships between forces, their effects on individual joints, and the outcomes for the entire body. Even at a basic level of analysis, this information can be used to understand mechanisms of injury and to guide treatment decisions.

For example, a simple planar force analysis during a straight leg raise exercise provides estimates of hip muscle and joint forces, which can guide exercise prescription for clinical diagnoses as varied as iliopsoas tendinopathy, hip arthritis, and stroke. These force estimates are advantageous when balancing the needs for muscle strengthening, symptom control, and disease management in clinical populations.

In daily practice, clinicians rarely perform the more complex computations described in this chapter to define movement and posture. However, understanding the conceptual framework of the computations, appreciating the magnitude of forces that exist within the body, and applying the concepts contained in this chapter are essential to understanding rehabilitation techniques and principles, whether for the elite athlete, a young child with cerebral palsy, or an older adult patient with neurodegenerative disease. Such understanding makes clinical work interesting and provides a flexible, varied, and rich source of treatment ideas.

UNDERLYING PRINCIPLES OF BIOMECHANICS

Biomechanics applies the principles of mechanics to biological systems, considering questions of force, mass, and motion from smaller scale (such as cellular mechanics) to larger scale applications (such as system-level or whole-body mechanics). In the seventeenth century, Sir Isaac Newton observed that forces were related to mass and motion in a very predictable way. His *Philosophiae Naturalis Principia Mathematica* (1687) provided the basic laws and principles of mechanics that form the cornerstone for the study and understanding of human movement. These laws, referred to as the *law of inertia,* the *law of acceleration,* and the *law of action-reaction,* are collectively known as the *laws of motion* and form the framework from which advanced motion analysis techniques are derived.

Newton's Laws of Motion

This chapter uses Newton's laws of motion to introduce relationships between forces applied to the body and the consequences of those forces on human motion and posture. Newton's laws are described for both linear and rotational (angular) motion (see ahead Table 4.1). Throughout the chapter, the term *body* is used when elaborating on the concepts related to the laws of motion and the methods of quantitative analysis. This term may be used interchangeably with the entire human body, a segment or part of the body (such as the forearm segment), or an object (such as a weight that is being lifted). In most cases, the term *body* is used to simplify descriptions of biomechanical concepts.

NEWTON'S FIRST LAW: LAW OF INERTIA

Newton's first law states that a body remains at rest or at a constant linear velocity except when compelled by an external force to change its state. This means that a *force* is required to start, stop, decelerate, accelerate, or alter the direction of *linear motion.* The application of Newton's first law to *rotational motion* states that a body remains at rest or at a constant angular velocity around an axis of rotation unless compelled by an external *torque* to change its state. This means that a torque is required to start, stop, reduce, accelerate, or alter the direction of rotational motion. Whether the motion is linear or rotational, Newton's first law describes the case in which a body is in equilibrium. A body is in *static equilibrium* when its linear and rotational velocities are zero—the body is not moving. Conversely, the body is in *dynamic equilibrium* when its linear and/or rotational velocity is constant but *not* zero—the body is moving but at a constant speed. In all cases of equilibrium, the linear and rotational accelerations of the body are zero.

Newton's first law is also called the law of inertia. *Inertia* is an object's resistance to a change in its motion. The word inertia is derived from the same Latin word as the word inert (*iners,* meaning "idle" or "sluggish"), which means "sluggish in action or motion." In essence, inertia describes how sluggish, or resistant to motion, a body is. The inertia of a body is directly proportional to its *mass* (i.e., the amount of matter constituting the body). The concept is quite intuitive: more energy is required to speed up or slow down a 7-kg dumbbell compared with a 5-kg dumbbell.

Each body has a point, called the *center of mass,* about which its mass is evenly distributed in all directions. The center of mass

of a body is equivalent to its *center of gravity* in a uniform gravitational field. The center of gravity is the point about which the effects of gravity are completely balanced. The center of mass of the human body in the anatomic position lies just anterior to the second sacral vertebra, but the exact position of the center of mass will change as a person changes his or her body position.

Each body segment, such as the arm or trunk, also has a defined center of mass. In the lower extremity, for example, the major segments include the thigh, shank (lower leg), and foot. Fig. 4.1 shows the center of mass of these segments in a sprinter, indicated by black circles. The location of the center of mass remains relatively stationary within the segment, with only very small variations caused by dynamic changes in the shape of activated muscle. In contrast, the location of the center of mass of the *entire* lower extremity can change substantially with a change in spatial configuration of the segments (compare red circles in Fig. 4.1). As shown for the left (flexed) lower extremity, the specific configuration of the segments can displace the center of mass of the lower limb *outside* the body. Additional information regarding the center of mass of body segments is discussed later in this chapter under the section titled Anthropometry.

The *mass moment of inertia* of a body is a quantity that indicates its resistance to a change in *angular velocity.* Unlike inertia, its linear counterpart, the mass moment of inertia depends not only on the mass of the body but also on the distribution of its mass with respect to an axis of rotation. Mass moment of inertia is often indicated by I and is expressed in units of kilogram-meters squared [kg-m^2]. Because most human motion is angular rather than linear, the concept of mass moment of inertia is particularly relevant and important to kinesiology. Consider again the two positions of the lower extremities in Fig. 4.1. Within each segment, the individual centers of mass of the thigh, shank, and foot are in the same location in both lower extremities. However, due to differing degrees of knee flexion, the

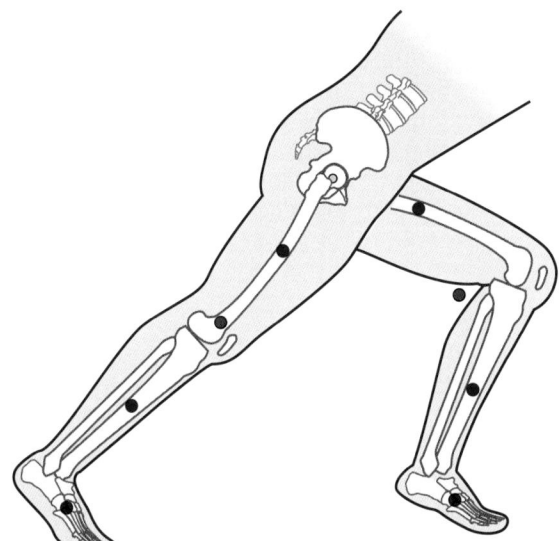

FIGURE 4.1 Lower extremities of a sprinter are illustrated, showing the centers of mass for the thigh, shank (lower leg), and foot segments as black circles. The center of mass for each lower extremity is shown as a red circle. The center of mass of the sprinter's left lower extremity exists outside of the body. The axis of rotation of the right hip is indicated by the smaller green circle.

TABLE 4.1 Newton's Laws: Linear and Rotational Applications

Linear Application	Rotational Application
First Law of Inertia	
A body remains at rest or at a constant linear velocity except when compelled by an external force to change its state.	A body remains at rest or at a constant angular velocity around an axis of rotation unless compelled by an external torque to change its state.
Second Law of Acceleration	
The linear acceleration of a body is directly proportional to the force causing it, takes place in the same direction in which the force acts, and is inversely proportional to the mass of the body.	The angular acceleration of a body is directly proportional to the torque causing it, takes place in the same rotary direction in which the torque acts, and is inversely proportional to the mass moment of inertia of the body.
Third Law of Action-Reaction	
For every force there is an equal and opposite directed force.	For every torque there is an equal and opposite directed torque.

Key Terms Associated with Newton's First Law
- Static equilibrium
- Dynamic equilibrium
- Inertia
- Mass
- Center of mass (gravity)
- Mass moment of inertia

---

distances between the hip joint and the centers of mass of the shank and foot segments have changed. Consequently, the mass moment of inertia of the entire limb changes, leaving the extended (and "longer") right lower extremity with a greater mass moment of inertia than the flexed ("shorter") left. The change in mass moment of inertia can also be conceptualized using the center of mass of the entire lower extremity (depicted by the red circles in Fig. 4.1): as the right knee extends, the center of mass of the entire right lower extremity moves farther from the hip. As a result, mass moment of inertia, which is the product

of mass and distance squared, increases (see Special Focus 4.1 for further explanation). Understand that the inertial resistance to angular acceleration of the limb applies even in the absence of gravity. For example, consider the positions of the lower limb in Fig. 4.1 but with the person on their side in a "gravity eliminated" position. Because of changes in the mass moment of inertia, less muscular effort will be required to flex the hip with the knee flexed than with the knee extended.

The ability to actively change an entire limb's mass moment of inertia can profoundly affect the forces and torques necessary for movement. For example, during the swing phase of running, the entire lower limb functionally shortens by the combined movements of knee flexion and ankle dorsiflexion (as in the left lower extremity in Fig. 4.1). The lower limb's reduced mass moment of inertia reduces the torque required by the hip muscles to accelerate and decelerate the limb during the swing phase. In contrast, running with the knees held nearly extended throughout the swing phase would increase both the mass moment of inertia and the torque required of the hip muscles.

Mass moment of inertia is also a relevant consideration in rehabilitation settings. Consider, for example, the design of a prosthesis for someone with a lower limb amputation. The use of lighter components in the prosthetic foot not only reduces the overall mass (and weight) of the prosthesis, but also results in a change in the distribution of mass to a more proximal location in the leg. As a result, less resistance is imposed on the residual limb during the swing phase of gait, which reduces the energy requirements for the person with an amputation. In a similar way, footwear choices can influence torque and energy requirements. Consider how the mass moment of inertia—and thus the torques required in gait—differ when wearing a lightweight tennis shoe compared with a steel-toed work boot.

Athletes often attempt to control the mass moment of inertia of their entire body by altering the position of their individual body segments relative to the axis of rotation. This is particularly advantageous due to conservation of angular momentum, which states that the total momentum of a closed system remains unchanged if no external torque acts on it. So, by changing mass moment of inertia, they can manipulate their angular velocities. This concept is well illustrated by divers who reduce their moment of inertia to successfully complete multiple somersaults while in the air (Fig. 4.2A). The athlete can assume an extreme "tuck" position by placing the head near the knees and holding the arms and legs tightly together, thereby bringing each segment's center of

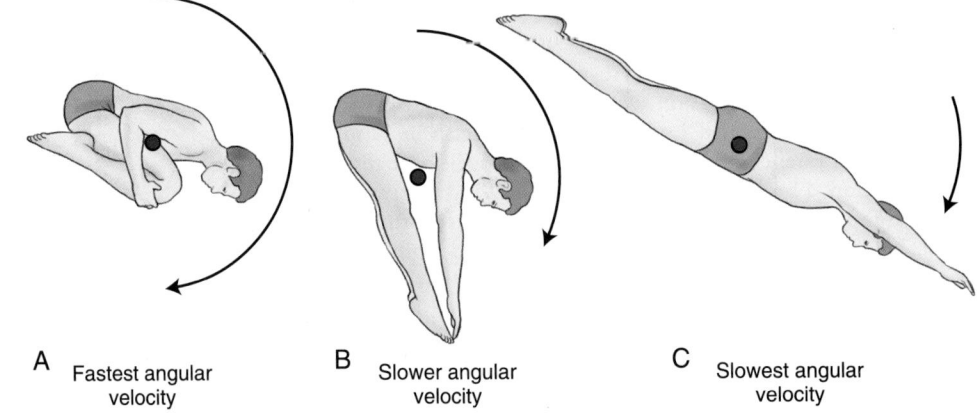

FIGURE 4.2 A diver illustrates an example of how the mass moment of inertia around a medial-lateral axis *(red circle)* can be altered through changes in position of the extremities. In position A, the diver decreases the mass moment of inertia, which increases the angular velocity of the spin. In positions B and C, the extremities are positioned progressively farther from the axis, and the angular velocity is progressively slower.

A   Fastest angular velocity

B   Slower angular velocity

C   Slowest angular velocity

mass closer to the axis of rotation. Reducing the body's mass moment of inertia results in increased angular velocity. Conversely, the athlete could slow the rotation by assuming a "pike" (see Fig. 4.2B) position, which increases the body's mass moment of inertia, or assuming a "layout" position (see Fig. 4.2C), which maximizes the body's mass moment of inertia and greatly slows the body's angular velocity.

NEWTON'S SECOND LAW: LAW OF ACCELERATION

Force (Torque)-Acceleration Relationship

Newton's second law states that the linear acceleration of a body is directly proportional to the force causing it, takes place in the same direction in which the force acts, and is inversely proportional to the mass of the body. Note the reference to "direction" in that statement; force and acceleration are vector quantities, meaning that they have both magnitude *and* direction. Mass, a scalar quantity, has only magnitude. Going forward, vector quantities are denoted by bold-face font.

Newton's second law generates an equation that relates force ($\mathbf{F}$), mass (m), and acceleration ($\mathbf{a}$) (Eq. 4.1). Conceptually, Eq. 4.1 defines a *force-acceleration relationship*. Considered a cause-and-effect relationship, the left side of the equation, force ($\mathbf{F}$), can be regarded as a cause because it represents a push or pull exerted on a body; the right side, $m \times \mathbf{a}$, represents the effect of the push or pull. In this equation, $\Sigma\mathbf{F}$ designates the sum of, or net, forces acting on a body. If the sum of the forces acting on a body is zero (i.e., $\Sigma\mathbf{F} = 0$), acceleration is also zero and the body is in linear equilibrium. As previously discussed, this case is described by Newton's first law. If, however, the net force produces acceleration, the body will accelerate in the direction of the resultant force. In this case, the body is no longer in equilibrium.

Newton's Second Law of Linear Motion Quantifying a Force

$$\Sigma\mathbf{F} = m \times \mathbf{a} \qquad \text{(Eq. 4.1)}$$

Force is measured in newtons, where 1 newton (N) = 1 kg-m/sec.^{2}

The rotary or angular counterpart to Newton's second law states that a *torque* will cause an *angular acceleration* of a body around an *axis of rotation*. Furthermore, the angular acceleration of a body is directly proportional to the torque causing it, takes place in the same *rotary* direction in which the torque acts, and is inversely proportional to the *mass moment of inertia* of the body. (The previously shown italicized words denote the essential differences between the linear and angular counterparts of this law.) For the rotary condition, Newton's second law generates an equation that relates the torque (τ), mass moment of inertia (I), and angular acceleration (α) (Eq. 4.2). In this equation, $\Sigma\tau$ designates the sum of, or net, torques acting to rotate a body. (Although the terms *torque,* moment, and moment of force are used interchangeably in biomechanics literature, this textbook uses the term torque almost exclusively. The terms moment and moment of force allude to the relationship between torque, moment arm, and force, as defined in Chapter 1.)

Conceptually, Eq. 4.2 defines a *torque–angular acceleration relationship*. Within the musculoskeletal system, the primary torque producers are muscles. A contracting biceps brachii muscle, for example, produces a net internal flexion torque at the elbow. Neglecting external influences such as gravity, the angular acceleration of the rotating forearm is proportional to the

internal torque (i.e., the product of the muscle force and its internal moment arm) but is inversely proportional to the mass moment of inertia of the forearm-and-hand segment. Given a constant internal torque, the forearm-and-hand segment with the smaller mass moment of inertia will achieve a greater angular acceleration than one with a larger mass moment of inertia. (A smaller mass moment of inertia can be achieved by moving a cuff weight from the wrist to the midforearm, for example.) Recall that the inertial resistance to angular acceleration of the forearm-and-hand segment is independent of gravity; moving the arm into a gravity-lessened position will not affect the mass moment of inertia.

Newton's Second Law of Rotary Motion Quantifying a Torque

$$\Sigma\tau = I \times \alpha \qquad \text{(Eq. 4.2)}$$

Torque is expressed in newton-meters, where 1 Nm = 1 kg-m^2 × radians/sec.^{2}

Impulse-Momentum Relationship

Momentum is the product of mass and velocity (Eq. 4.3). Momentum describes the quantity of motion possessed by a body. It is generally represented by the letter "p" and has units of kilogram-meters per second (kg-m/sec). Additional relationships can be derived from Newton's second law through the broadening and rearranging of Eqs. 4.1 and 4.2. Acceleration, for example, is the rate of change of velocity ($\Delta v / \Delta t$). Substituting this expression for linear acceleration in Eq. 4.1 results in Eq. 4.4. Eq. 4.4 can be further rearranged to Eq. 4.5, which defines the linear *impulse-momentum relationship*.

Equations for Linear Impulse, Momentum, and the Impulse-Momentum Relationship

Momentum	$\mathbf{p} = m \times \mathbf{v}$	(Eq. 4.3)
Impulse	$\mathbf{J} = \Delta\mathbf{p}$	
	$a = \Delta v / \Delta t$	
	$F = m \times \Delta v / \Delta t$	(Eq. 4.4)
Impulse-Momentum Relationship	$F \times \Delta t = m \times \Delta v$	(Eq. 4.5)

Momentum is expressed in kilogram-meters per second (kg-m/s).

Impulse ($\mathbf{J}$) is simply the change in momentum ($\Delta\omega/\Delta\mathbf{p}$), as indicated in the box. As such, it can be understood as either the product of mass and change in velocity (as in the right side of Eq. 4.5) or as a force applied over a period of time (as in the left side of Eq. 4.5). Impulse and momentum are vector quantities.

Application of a linear impulse leads to a change in linear momentum. Consider, for example, the linear momentum of a moving car. The application of an impulse can be used to stop the vehicle; in other words, applying a force over a given time can reduce the velocity of the car, and thus its momentum, to zero. The magnitudes of force and time will vary depending on the situation. During an emergency stop, for example, a very large brake force is applied for a short time to produce a rapid change in momentum. A more gradual stop can be completed by applying a smaller brake force over a longer period of time. Both conditions would result in the same magnitude of impulse, and thus the same change in momentum. However, less brake force for the same time, or the same brake force

SPECIAL FOCUS 4.1

The Functional Relevance and Mathematics of Mass Moment of Inertia

Mass moment of inertia (*I*) is formally defined in the following equation, in which *n* indicates the number of particles in a body, m_i is the mass of each particle in the body, and r_i is the distance of each particle to the axis of rotation.

Mass Moment of Inertia

$$I = \sum_{i=1}^{n} m_i r_i^2 \qquad \text{(Eq. 4.6)}$$

Force is measured in newtons, where 1 newton (N) = 1 kg-m/sec².

Eq. 4.6 can be used to illustrate how the placement of the grip applied to a baseball bat dramatically affects its mass moment of inertia and, therefore, the ease or difficulty in swinging the bat. The bat illustrated in Fig. 4.3 is simplified into six point-masses (m_1 to m_6), ranging from 0.1 to 0.225 kg, each located 0.135 m from another. During a swing, the bat rotates about an axis of rotation near the proximal end of the bat (the knob). If the bat is not sized correctly for the batter, the batter will often "choke up" by shifting his or her grip away from the knob (toward the fat end of the bat). For simplicity, the axis of rotation is assumed to be either Y_1 (red line), if the batter's hands are near the knob of the bat, or Y_2 (blue line), if the batter is choking up on the handle.

The following calculations demonstrate how the distribution of mass particles, relative to an axis of rotation, dramatically affects the mass moment of inertia of the rotating bat. The mass moment of inertia of the bat is determined separately for the two conditions (i.e., Y_1 versus Y_2 as the axis of rotation) using Eq. 4.6 and substituting known values. The important point here is that the mass particles are distributed differently around the two axes. As seen in the calculations, when Y_2 is the axis of rotation, the moment of inertia is 58% of the moment of inertia when Y_1 is the considered axis. The reason for the reduced moment of inertia is that the point-masses m_2 through m_6 are closer to the Y_2 axis. The distance is particularly significant mathematically, considering that the mass moment of inertia of each point is related to the *square* of the distance to the axis.

This is functionally relevant because the batter could achieve the same angular acceleration with 58% less torque. Or, for the same torque, the bat would accelerate 1.72 times as fast. This is a significant functional advantage gained by choking up on the bat; the bat is easier to swing, although its mass and weight have not changed. Of course, there's a tradeoff; linear acceleration at any point along the length of the bat increases at farther distances from the axis of rotation. So, assuming all other variables are the same (masses of the ball and bat, angular velocities of the bat, and initial velocity of the ball), the tip of the functionally longer bat (the one rotating about Y_1) will experience higher linear acceleration, thereby resulting in a higher final velocity of the baseball.

$$I = \sum_{i=1}^{n} m_i r_i^2$$
$$= m_1 (r_1)^2 + m_2 (r_2)^2 + m_3 (r_3)^2 + m_4 (r_4)^2 + m_5 (r_5)^2 + m_6 (r_6)^2$$

Y_1 Axis of Rotation

$$I = 0.1 \text{ kg} (0.0 \text{ m})^2 + 0.1 \text{ kg} (0.135 \text{ m})^2 + 0.1 \text{ kg} (0.270 \text{ m})^2 +$$
$$0.15 \text{ kg} (0.405 \text{ m})^2 + 0.175 \text{ kg} (0.54 \text{ m})^2 + 0.225 \text{ kg} (0.675 \text{ m})^2$$
$$= 0.187 \text{ kg} \bullet \text{m}^2$$

Y_2 Axis of Rotation

$$I = 0.1 \text{ kg} (0.135 \text{ m})^2 + 0.1 \text{ kg} (0.0 \text{ m})^2 + 0.1 \text{ kg} (0.135 \text{ m})^2$$
$$+ 0.15 \text{ kg} (0.270 \text{ m})^2 + 0.175 \text{ kg} (0.405 \text{ m})^2 + 0.225 \text{ kg} (0.54 \text{ m})^2$$
$$= 0.109 \text{ kg} \bullet \text{m}^2$$

Consider another illustration of the relevance of mass moment of inertia, this time as it relates to gait. Patients with ataxia often have poor coordination and instability when walking. To address gait instability, one intervention involves placement of cuff weights around the ankles during gait training sessions.[47] Mass moment of inertia helps explain why this works: adding weight far from the axis of rotation dramatically increases the mass moment of inertia of the lower extremities. Put simply, the legs become more resistant to motion. Thus the addition of cuff weights can minimize the magnitude of unwanted movement caused by central nervous system dysfunction.

The mass moments of inertia of human body segments are more difficult to determine than for the baseball bat, although they are based on the same mathematic principle. Much of the difficulty stems from the fact that segments in the human body are made up of different tissues (such as bone, muscle, fat, and skin) of nonuniform densities. Values for the mass moment of inertia for each body segment have been estimated from cadaver studies, mathematic modeling, and various imaging techniques.[9,14]

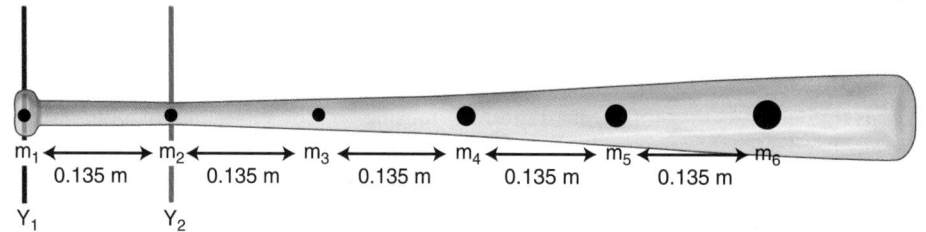

FIGURE 4.3 A baseball bat is shown with a potential to rotate around two separate axes of rotation (Y_1, Y_2). The set of calculations associated with each axis of rotation shows how the distribution of mass relative to the axis of rotation affects the mass moment of inertia. The bat is assumed to consist of six mass points (m_1 to m_6), ranging from 0.1 to 0.225 kg, located at equal distances from one another.

for even less time, would result in a smaller impulse of insufficient magnitude to stop the moving vehicle.

The impulse-momentum relationship provides another perspective from which to study human performance and gain insight into injury mechanisms. The human body, for example, can utilize various structures and mechanisms to reduce peak forces, essentially by manipulating the time variable (Δt). When landing from a jump, peak joint forces can be reduced if the impact of the landing is prolonged (greater Δt), such as through a lower level and prolonged eccentric activation of muscles crossing the hip, knee, and ankle joints. During normal gait, the plantar fat pad on the plantar surface of the calcaneus) provides cushioning between the foot and ground. The fat pad increases the time over which a change in momentum is experienced, thereby reducing the force experienced deep to the fat pad (see Eq. 4.4). Running footwear often augments this function with shock-absorbing outsoles to further cushion the impact of the foot on the ground. Bicycle helmets, rubber or spring flooring, and protective padding are additional examples of equipment designs intended to reduce injuries by increasing *duration* to minimize peak force of the impact.

Momentum, impulse, and the impulse-momentum relationship similarly apply to rotary conditions. Rotational momentum is the product of mass moment of inertia and angular velocity (Eq. 4.7). Like the substitutions and rearrangements for the linear relationship, the angular relationship can be expressed by substitution and rearrangement of Eq. 4.2. Substituting $\Delta \omega / \Delta t$ (rate of change in angular velocity) for α (angular acceleration) results in Eq. 4.8. Eq. 4.8 can be rearranged to Eq. 4.9—the angular equivalent of the impulse-momentum relationship. Angular momentum and angular impulse are vector quantities.

Equations for Rotary Impulse, Momentum, and the Impulse-Momentum Relationship		
Momentum	$p = I \times \omega$	(Eq. 4.7)
Impulse	$J = \Delta p$	
	$\alpha = \Delta \omega / \Delta t$	(Eq. 4.8)
	$\tau = I \times \Delta \omega / \Delta t$	
Impulse-Momentum Relationship	$\tau \times \Delta t = I \times \Delta \omega$	(Eq. 4.9)
Angular momentum is expressed in kg-m²/s.		

Application of an angular impulse (torque multiplied by time) leads to a change in angular momentum (mass moment of inertia multiplied by a change in angular velocity).

SPECIAL FOCUS 4.2

A Closer Look at the Impulse-Momentum Relationship

As impulse is the product of force and its time of application, it can also be represented graphically as the area under a force-time curve. Fig. 4.4 displays a force-time curve of the horizontal component of the anterior-posterior shear force applied by the ground against the foot *(ground reaction force)* as an individual runs across a force plate embedded in the floor. The curve is biphasic: the posterior-directed impulse during initial floor contact is negative, and the anterior-directed impulse during propulsion is positive. If the two impulses (i.e., areas under the curves) are equal, the net impulse is zero, and there is no change in the momentum of the system. In this example, however, the posterior-directed impulse is greater than that of the anterior, indicating that the runner's forward momentum is decreasing.

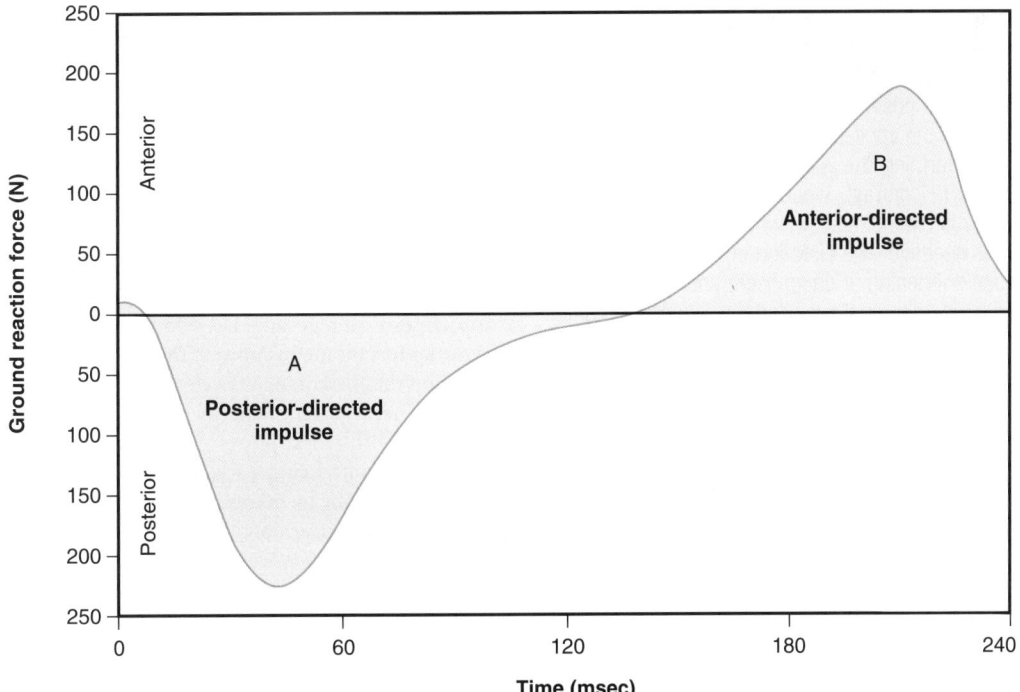

FIGURE 4.4 Graphic representation of the areas under a force-time curve showing the (A) posterior-directed and (B) anterior-directed impulses of the horizontal component of the ground reaction force while running.

Work-Energy Relationship

To this point, Newton's second law has been described using (1) the force (torque)-acceleration relationship (Eqs. 4.1 and 4.2) and (2) the impulse-momentum relationship (Eqs. 4.5 and 4.9). Newton's second law can also be restated to provide a *work-energy relationship*. This third approach can be used to study human movement by analyzing the extent to which work causes a change in an object's energy. Work occurs when a force or torque results in some linear or angular displacement. *Work (W)* is a scalar quantity, having only magnitude. In a linear sense, work is equal to the product of the magnitude of *force* (F) applied against an object and the *linear displacement(s)* of the object in the direction of the applied force (Eq. 4.10). If no movement occurs in the direction of the applied force, no mechanical work is done. Like the linear case, angular work can be defined as the product of the magnitude of *torque* (τ) applied against the object and the *angular displacement* (θ) of the object in the direction of the applied torque (see equation box). Work is expressed in joules (J). One joule is equivalent to one newton of force applied over a one-meter distance (linear work) or one newton-meter of torque applied over one radian (angular work). Work can be either positive or negative, a designation that depends on the direction of displacement compared with the application direction of force (or torque). If they are the same, work is positive; if displacement occurs in a direction opposite to force application, work is negative.

SPECIAL FOCUS 4.3

Positive Work, Negative Work, and Isometric "Work"

As described, work is found by multiplying an applied force by the object's displacement. Work can occur in the same direction or opposite to the direction of the applied force. Consider, for example, the force applied by the contracting elbow flexor muscles to flex the elbow and bring the hand to the mouth. In a linear sense, the work is the product of the muscles' contractile force and the distance the muscles shorten. In an angular sense, rotary work is the product of torque applied by the elbow flexors and the amount of flexion (in radians) occurring at the elbow. In this scenario, the work is positive: the rotation of the forearm is in the same direction as the applied torque. In addition, the elbow flexors, which are performing the work, are shortening through concentric activation. In contrast, when the elbow flexors are active, but the elbow is extending (e.g., when slowly lowering a weight), the work is negative. The direction of muscle activation (which would cause shortening, if unopposed) and the direction of displacement (i.e., lengthening) are occurring opposite to one another. Eccentric activation, then, is considered negative work: the rotation is in a direction opposite to the applied torque and change in muscle length is opposite to the muscle force. The final scenario is when the elbow flexors are active, but no movement is taking place, as when a muscle is active isometrically. In this case, even though considerable metabolic energy may be expended, no mechanical work is being performed.

Energy (a scalar quantity) exists in two forms: potential energy and kinetic energy. *Potential energy* is a function of the height of the object's center of mass within a gravitational field (Eq. 4.11). Similar to momentum, *kinetic energy* is influenced by the object's mass and velocity, regardless of the influence of gravity (Eq. 4.12). An object's angular kinetic energy is related to its mass moment of inertia (I) and its angular velocity.

Relationships between Work (*W*), Potential Energy (*PE*), and Kinetic Energy (*KE*)

$$where\ d = linear\ displacement,\ \theta = angular\ displacement,$$
$$g = gravity,\ and\ h = height$$

$$W_{linear} = F \times d$$
$$W_{angular} = \tau \times \theta \qquad \text{(Eq. 4.10)}$$

$$PE = m \times g \times h \qquad \text{(Eq. 4.11)}$$

$$KE_{linear} = \tfrac{1}{2}\,m \times v^2 \qquad \text{(Eq. 4.12)}$$

$$KE_{angular} = \tfrac{1}{2}\,I \times \omega^2$$

$$W = KE_{final} - KE_{initial} + PE_{final} - PE_{initial} \qquad \text{(Eq. 4.13)}$$

(angular or linear)

Just as the impulse-momentum relationship describes the change in momentum caused by a force applied over a given *time,* the work-energy relationship describes the change in kinetic energy caused by a force applied over a given *displacement* (Eq. 4.13). The example described earlier can illustrate the similarity in these concepts. The kinetic energy of an object, such as a moving car, is changed by the application of a force over a displacement. When a quick change in kinetic energy is required (e.g., for an emergency stop), a very large brake force is applied over a short displacement. Less brake force for the same displacement or the same brake force applied for less displacement results in a smaller change in kinetic energy.

The work-energy relationship does not consider the *time* over which the forces or torques are applied. Yet in most daily activities, it is often the rate of work that is important. The *rate of work* (or the amount of work done in a period of time) is defined as *power.* The ability of muscles to generate adequate power is often critical to the success of movement, whether for completing basic functional mobility tasks or for optimizing athletic performance.[15,19,30,40] Muscular power, for example, is necessary to overcome gravity in a sit-to-stand transfer. It is also key to winning a rebound on the basketball court.

Power (P) is work (*W*) divided by time, or the rate of performing work (Eq. 4.14). Similar to work, power is a scalar quantity, having magnitude but not direction. Because work is the product of the magnitude of force (*F*) and displacement (*d*), the rate of work can be restated in Eq. 4.15 as the product of force (*F*) and velocity (*v*). Angular power, using the angular analogs of force and linear velocity, is the product of the magnitudes of torque (τ) and angular velocity (ω) (Eq. 4.16). Angular power is often used as a clinical measure of muscle performance. The mechanical power produced by the quadriceps, for example, is equal to the internal torque produced by the muscle multiplied by the angular velocity of knee extension. This can be expressed as either average power (the net torque and average angular velocity over a specified window of time) or instantaneous power (the torque at a given instant, multiplied by the instantaneous velocity). Power is often used to designate the net transfer of energy between active muscles and external loads. As with work, power can be described as either positive or negative, despite being a scalar quantity. *Positive power* reflects the rate of work done by *concentrically active muscles* against an external load. *Negative power*, in contrast, reflects the rate of work done by *eccentrically active muscles* against a more dominant external load.

Equations for Power

$$P = W/t \qquad \text{(Eq. 4.14)}$$

$$W = F \times d,\ v = d/t$$

$$P = F \times v \qquad \text{(Eq. 4.15)}$$

$$P_{angular} = \tau \times \omega \qquad \text{(Eq. 4.16)}$$

Power is expressed in watts (W) or J/s

TABLE 4.2 Physical Measurements Associated with Newton's Second Law

Physical Measurement	Linear Application		Conversion English → SI Units*	Rotational Application	
	Definition	Units		Definition	Units
Distance	Linear displacement	Meter (m)	ft × 0.305 = m	Angular displacement	Degrees†
Velocity	Rate of linear displacement	Meters per second (m/sec)	ft/sec × 0.305 = m/sec	Rate of angular displacement	Degrees/sec
Acceleration	Rate of change in linear velocity	m/sec²	ft/sec² × 0.305 = m/sec²	Rate of change in angular velocity	Degrees/sec²
Mass	Quantity of matter in an object; influences the object's resistance to a change in linear velocity	Kilogram (kg)	lbm‡ × 0.454 = kg	Not applicable	
Mass moment of inertia	Not applicable		lbm-ft² × 0.042 = kg-m²	Quantity and distribution of matter around an object's axis of rotation; influences an object's resistance to a change in angular velocity	kg-m²
Force	A push or pull; mass times linear acceleration	Newton (N) = kg-m/sec²	lb × 4.448 = N	Not applicable	
Torque	Not applicable		ft-lb × 1.356 = Nm	A force times a moment arm; mass moment of inertia times angular acceleration	Newton-meter (Nm)
Impulse	Force times time	N-sec	lb-sec × 4.448 = N-sec ft-lb-sec × 1.356 = Nm-sec	Torque times time	Nm-sec
Momentum	Mass times linear velocity	kg-m/sec	lbm-ft/sec × 0.138 = kg-m/sec lbm-ft²/sec × 0.042 = kg-m²/sec	Mass moment of inertia times angular velocity	kg-m²/sec
Work	Force times linear displacement	Joule (J)	lb-ft × 1.356 = J	Torque times angular displacement	Joules (J)
Average power	Rate of linear work	Watt (W) = J/sec	lb-ft/sec × 1.356 = W	Rate of angular work	Watts (W) = J/sec

*To convert from English units to SI units, multiply the English value by the corresponding number in the table cell. To convert from SI units to English units, divide by that number. If two equations are in the cell, the upper equation is used to convert the linear measure, and the lower equation is used to convert the angular measure.

†Radians, which are unitless, may be used instead of degrees (1 radian ≈ 57.3 degrees).

‡The English unit of a mass is a pound-mass (lbm) or slug.

Table 4.2 summarizes the definitions and units needed to describe many of the physical measurements related to Newton's second law.

NEWTON'S THIRD LAW: LAW OF ACTION-REACTION

Newton's third law of motion states that for every action there is an equal and opposite reaction. Every effect that one body exerts on another is counteracted by an effect that the second body exerts on the first. The two bodies interact simultaneously, and the consequence is specified by Newton's law of acceleration ($\Sigma F = m \times a$). Each body experiences a different effect, and that effect depends on its mass. For example, a person who falls off the roof of a second-story building exerts a force on the ground, and the ground exerts an equal and opposite force on the person. Because of the huge discrepancies in mass between the earth and the person, the effect, or acceleration experienced by the person, is much greater than the effect "experienced" by the ground. As a result, the person may sustain significant injury.

Another application of Newton's law of action-reaction is the *ground reaction force*. When walking or standing, the foot produces a force against the ground. In accordance with Newton's third law, the ground generates a ground reaction force of equal magnitude in the opposite direction (Fig. 4.5). The ground reaction force changes in magnitude, direction, and point of application on the foot throughout the stance period of gait. Newton's third law also has an angular equivalent. For example, during an isometric exercise, the internal and external torques are equal and in opposite rotary directions.

FOUNDATIONS OF MOVEMENT ANALYSIS

The previous section describes the nature of the cause-and-effect relationships between force and motion as outlined by Newton's laws. This section focuses on the steps and conventions used to formally analyze movement. Special attention is paid to the analyses of internal and external forces and torques and the explanation of how these variables affect the body and its joints. This section should prepare the reader to follow the mathematic solutions to three sample problems introduced later in the chapter.

Anthropometry

Anthropometry is derived from the Greek root *anthropos*, man, + *metron*, measure. In the context of human movement analysis, anthropometry may be broadly defined as the measurement of certain physical features of the human body, such as length, mass, weight, volume, density, center of gravity, and mass moment of inertia. Knowledge of these parameters is often essential to conducting kinematic and kinetic analyses for both normal and pathologic motion. Variables

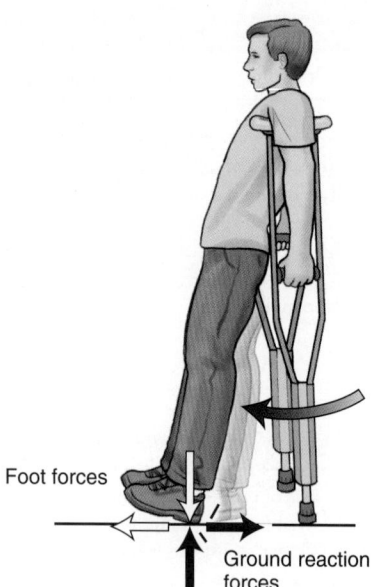

Foot forces

Ground reaction forces

FIGURE 4.5 The action of the forces produced between the ground and foot are illustrated during the contact phase of the "swing-through" method of crutch-assisted walking. The action of the foot forces *(white arrows)* is counteracted by the ground reaction forces *(black arrows)*. If the horizontal component of the ground reaction force (caused by friction) is less than the horizontal component of the foot force, the foot will slide forward on the floor according to Newton's second law: $F = m \times a$.

such as mass and mass moment of inertia of individual limb segments, for example, are needed to determine the inertial properties that muscles must overcome to generate movement. Anthropometric information is also valuable in the design of work environments, furniture, tools, sports and exercise equipment, and in strength testing.

Much of the information pertaining to center of gravity and mass moment of inertia of individual body segments has been derived from cadaver studies.[6,9] Other methods for deriving anthropometric data include mathematic modeling and imaging techniques, such as computed tomography and magnetic resonance imaging. Table I.2 in Part B of Appendix I contains anthropometric data on body segments, including their proportional weights and locations of center of gravity.

Free Body Diagram

The analysis of movement requires consideration of all forces that act on the body. Before any analysis, a *free body diagram* can be constructed to facilitate solving biomechanical problems. A free body diagram is a "snapshot" that represents the interaction between a body and its environment, where "interactions" are quantified as all forces and moments acting on the body. Typically, the components of the free body diagram are assumed to be rigid to simplify calculations. The body under consideration may be a single rigid segment, such as the foot, or it may be several segments, such as the head, arms, and trunk. When the body consists of several segments, these are assumed to be rigidly connected as a single rigid system.

A free body diagram requires that all relevant forces acting on the system are carefully drawn. These forces may be produced by muscle, gravity (as reflected in the weight of the segment), fluid, air resistance, friction, joint reaction forces, and ground reaction forces. Arrows are used to indicate force vectors.

A free body diagram is configured based on the intended purpose of the analysis. Consider the example presented in Fig. 4.6. In this example, the free body diagram represents the shank-and-foot at initial heel contact during walking. The free body diagram involves figuratively "cutting through" the desired joint(s) to isolate or "free"

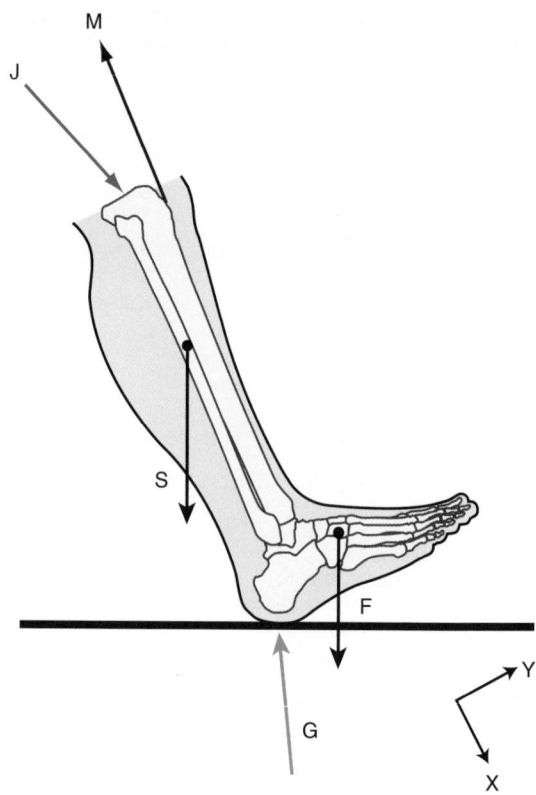

FIGURE 4.6 Free body diagram of the shank-and-foot at the instant of heel contact during walking. The segment is isolated by figuratively "cutting through" the knee joint. Relevant forces are drawn in as shown. The *xy*-coordinate reference frame is placed so the *x*-axis is parallel with the shank.

the body of interest. In the example presented in Fig. 4.6, the knee joint was separated to isolate the shank-and-foot segment. The effects of active muscle force are usually distinguished from the effects of other soft tissues, such as passive tension created in stretched joint capsule and ligaments. Although the contribution of individual muscles acting across a joint may be determined, a single resultant muscle force (**M**) vector is often used to represent the sum of all individual muscle forces. Other forces external to the system can be added to the diagram, which may include the ground reaction force (**G**) and the weights of the shank-and-foot segments (**S** and **F**). As specified by Newton's third law, the ground reaction force is equal and opposite to the force developed by the foot striking the earth.

An additional force is identified in Fig. 4.6: the *joint reaction force* (**J**). This force includes joint contact forces as well as the net or cumulative effect of all other forces transmitted from one segment to another. Much like ground reaction forces, joint reaction forces are the equal and opposite forces that develop "in reaction" to other forces, such as those produced by activation of muscle, by passive tension in stretched periarticular connective tissues, and by gravity (body weight). As will be discussed, the free body diagram is completed by defining an *xy*-coordinate reference frame and writing the governing equations of motion.

Reducing joint reaction force is often a major focus of musculoskeletal interventions, with the goal of reducing pain and preventing further joint injury or degeneration. This would be particularly relevant for diagnoses such as intra-articular fracture and osteoarthritis. Frequently, treatments are directed toward reducing joint forces through changes in the magnitude of muscle activity and their activation patterns or through a reduction in the weight transmitted through a joint. Consider the patient with osteoarthritis of the hip joint as an example. The magnitude of the hip's joint reaction force may be reduced by decreasing walking velocity, thereby lessening the magnitude of muscle activation. Highly cushioned shoes may be recommended to reduce impact forces. In addition, a cane may be

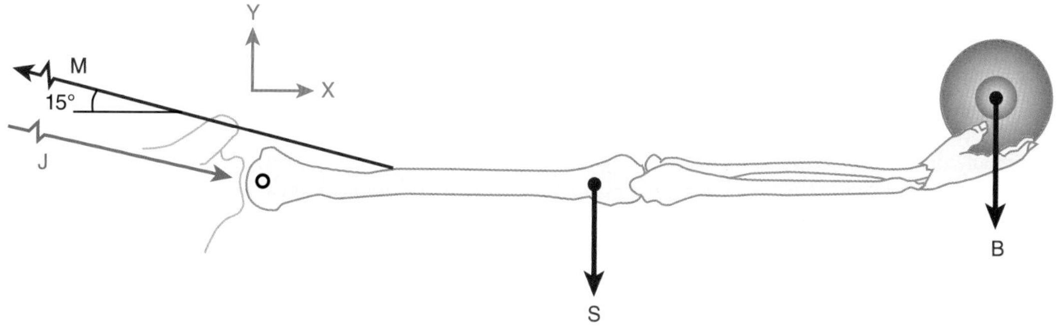

FIGURE 4.7 A frontal plane depiction of a free body diagram isolating the system as a right arm and ball combination (Step I, outlined in *orange*). The axis of rotation is shown as an open black circle at the glenohumeral joint. The *xy*-coordinate reference frame (Step II, shown in *green*) is placed so the *x*-axis is parallel with the upper extremity. Resultant shoulder abductor muscle force (M), segment weight (S), and ball weight (B) are shown in red (Step III). Glenohumeral joint reaction force (J) is shown in blue (Step IV). (Modified from LeVeau BF: *Williams & Lissner's biomechanics of human motion,* ed 3, Philadelphia, 1992, Saunders.)

used to reduce forces through the hip joint.[2,22,29] If obesity is a factor, a weight-reduction program may be recommended.

STEPS FOR CONSTRUCTING THE FREE BODY DIAGRAM

Solving problems related to human movement requires the identification of (1) the purpose of the analysis, (2) the free body of interest, and (3) all the forces that act on that body. The following example presents steps to assist with construction of a free body diagram.

Consider the situation in which an individual is holding a weight out to the side, as shown in Fig. 4.7. This free body is assumed to be in static equilibrium, which means that the sum of all forces and the sum of all torques acting on the body are equal to zero. One purpose of the analysis might be to determine how much muscle force is required by the glenohumeral joint abductor muscles (M) to keep the arm abducted to 90 degrees; another purpose might be to determine the magnitude of the glenohumeral joint reaction force (J) during this same activity.

Step I of constructing the free body diagram is to identify and isolate the free body under consideration. In this example, the glenohumeral joint was "cut through," and the free body, outlined in orange, is the combination of the entire arm and the resistance (exercise ball weight).

Step II involves defining a coordinate reference frame that allows the position and movement of a body to be defined with respect to a known point, location, or axis (see Fig. 4.7, *green xy*-coordinate reference frame). More detail on establishing a reference frame is discussed ahead.

Step III involves identification and inclusion of all relevant forces that act on the free body (shown in red in Fig. 4.7). Internal force in this analysis is limited to those produced only by activated muscle (M). External forces include the force of gravity on the mass of the exercise ball (B), as well as the force of gravity on the arm segment (S). Although not relevant to Fig. 4.7, other examples of external forces could include forces applied by clinicians, cables, resistance bands, the ground, air resistance, and orthotics. Other examples of internal forces could include the passive tension produced by a stretched inert tissue, such as ligament or skin, or the passive tension produced by an inactive, stretched muscle. The forces are drawn on the figure while specifying their approximate point of application and spatial orientation. For example, vector S acts at the center of gravity of the upper extremity, a location determined by using anthropometric data, such as those presented in Table I.2 in Part B of Appendix I.

The direction of the muscle force (M) is drawn to correspond to the line of muscle pull. Because of the assumption of static equilibrium, the torque generated by the active muscle should be in a rotary direction opposite to the torque generated by external forces. In this example, the torque produced by the external forces, S and B, tends

to rotate the arm in a clockwise, −*z*-direction, which corresponds to adduction. The line of force of M, therefore, in combination with its moment arm, creates a torque in a counterclockwise, +*z*-direction, which corresponds to abduction. (The convention of using + *z* or −*z* to designate rotation direction is described later.)

Step IV of the procedure is to draw the joint reaction force (J). This is shown in blue in Fig. 4.7. In this example, the relevant joint reaction force is at the glenohumeral articulation. Initially, the direction of the joint reaction force may not be known. As explained later, it is typically drawn in a direction *opposite* to the pull of the dominant muscle force. The precise direction of J can be determined after static analysis is carried out and unknown variables are calculated.

Step V involves writing the three governing equations required to solve two-dimensional (2D) static equilibrium problems encountered in this chapter. These equations specify that the net torque and forces are equal to zero: $\Sigma \text{Torque}_z = 0$; $\Sigma \text{Force}_x = 0$; $\Sigma \text{Force}_y = 0$. These equations are explained later in the chapter.

Steps in Constructing the Free Body Diagram

Step I: Identify and isolate the free body under consideration.
Step II: Establish a coordinate reference frame.
Step III: Draw the internal (muscular) and external forces that act on the system.
Step IV: Draw the joint reaction force.
Step V: Write the governing equations of motion.

SPATIAL REFERENCE FRAMES

To accurately describe motion or solve for unknown forces, a spatial reference frame needs to be established. This reference allows the position and direction of movement of a body, a segment, or an object to be defined with respect to some known point, location, or segment's axis of rotation. If a reference frame is not identified, it becomes very difficult to interpret and compare measurements in clinical and research settings.

A spatial reference frame is arbitrarily established and may be placed inside or outside the body. Reference frames used to describe position or motion may be considered either relative or global. A *relative reference frame* describes the position of one limb segment with respect to an adjacent segment, such as the foot relative to the leg, the forearm relative to the upper arm, or the trunk relative to the thigh. A measurement is made by comparing motion of an anatomic landmark or coordinates between segments of interest. Goniometry provides one example of a relative reference frame used in clinical practice. Elbow joint range of motion, for example, describes a measurement using a relative reference frame defined by the long axes of the upper arm and forearm segments, with an axis of rotation through the elbow.

Relative reference frames, however, lack the information needed to define motion with respect to a fixed point or location in space. To analyze motion with respect to the ground, direction of gravity, or another type of externally defined reference frame in space, a *global (laboratory) reference frame* must be defined. Excessive anterior or lateral deviations of the trunk during gait are examples of a measurement made with respect to a global reference frame. In these examples, the position of the trunk is measured with respect to an external vertical reference.

Whether motion is measured via a relative or global reference frame, the location of a point or segment in space can be specified using a coordinate reference frame. In laboratory-based human movement analysis, the *Cartesian coordinate system* is most frequently employed. The Cartesian system uses coordinates for locating a point on a plane in 2D space by identifying the distance of the point from each of two intersecting lines, or in three-dimensional (3D) space by the distance from each of three planes intersecting at a point. A 2D coordinate reference frame is defined by two imaginary axes arranged perpendicular to each other *with the arrowheads pointed in positive directions.* The two axes (labeled, for example, *x* and *y*) may be oriented in any manner that facilitates quantitative solutions (compare Figs. 4.6 and 4.7, for example). A 2D reference frame is frequently used when the motion being described is predominantly planar (i.e., in one plane), such as knee flexion and extension during gait.

SPECIAL FOCUS 4.4

The "Right-Hand Rule": A Convention for Describing Spatial Orientation of a Three-Dimensional Coordinate Reference Frame

When a Cartesian coordinate system is set up, the direction or orientation of the orthogonal axes is not arbitrary. A convention must be used to facilitate the sharing of research from different laboratories throughout the worldwide scientific community. Using Fig. 4.7 as an example, the *x* and *y* axes are in the plane of the page or, relative to the subject, parallel with the frontal plane. (For consistency, this textbook typically orients the *xy*-axes so that the *x*-axis is parallel with the body segment of interest. While helpful for teaching the concepts and techniques, it is not mandatory to set up the axes in this manner.) A third axis, the *z*-axis, must be defined. Although not drawn in the figure, the *z*-axis is oriented perpendicular to the *xy*-plane. By convention, the directions of the arrowheads shown on the *xy*-coordinate reference frame indicate the positive directions. As shown in Fig. 4.7, positive *x* direction is to the right and positive *y* direction is upward. The right-hand rule can be used to define the direction (+ or −) of the *z*-axis. The *right-hand rule* can be performed by laying the ulnar border of your *right* hand along the *x*-axis, with the straight fingers pointing in a + *x* direction (toward the ball on the model). Your hand should be positioned along the *x*-axis so that when your fingers flex, they curl from the + *x* direction toward the + *y* direction. Your extended thumb is pointing *out of the page,* thereby defining the direction of the + *z*-axis.[10] By necessity, the −*z*-axis is oriented perpendicularly *into the page.* An alternate application of the right-hand rule is to configure your thumb in the + *x* direction with the index finger (second digit) in the + *y* direction. Flex the middle finger (third digit) until it is perpendicular to the palmer surface of the hand. The middle finger will point in the + *z* direction. The benefit of the right-hand rule is that only two axes ever need to be defined and shown; use of the right-hand rule allows the third axis to be completely described.

In most cases, human motion occurs in more than one plane. To fully describe this type of motion, a 3D coordinate reference frame is necessary. A 3D reference frame typically has three perpendicular (or orthogonal) axes. These are most commonly labeled *x*, *y*, and *z*. As with the 2D system, the arrowheads point in positive directions. A universal convention for orienting this triplanar coordinate system in space utilizes the *right-hand rule.* This rule is used throughout most quantitative biomechanical studies (see Special Focus 4.4).

Throughout most of this textbook, the terminology used to describe linear direction within planes (such as the direction of a muscle force or an axis of rotation around a joint) is less formal than that dictated by the right-hand rule. As described in Chapter 1, linear direction in space is loosely described relative to the human body standing in the anatomic position, using terms such as *anterior-posterior, medial-lateral,* and *vertical.* Although useful for most qualitative or anatomic-based descriptions, this convention is not well suited for quantitative analyses, such as those introduced later in this chapter. In these cases, the Cartesian coordinate system is used, and the orientation of its 3D axes is designated by the right-hand rule.

Angular motion and torques are often described as occurring in a plane around a perpendicular axis of rotation. In most kinesiologic literature, a segment's rotation direction is typically described by terms such as *flexion* and *extension* and, to a lesser extent, by *clockwise* or *counterclockwise rotation.* Such a system is adequate for most clinical analysis and is used throughout this textbook. More formal, quantitative analysis, however, may be necessary to designate the direction of angular motion and torques. Such a system is based on the 3D Cartesian coordinate reference frame and uses another form of the *right-hand rule,* as described in Special Focus 4.5.

SPECIAL FOCUS 4.5

Another Use of the "Right-Hand Rule": Determining the Direction of Angular Motion and Torque

The right-hand rule can also be used to define the *rotation direction* of angular motion and torque. Consider once again the coordinate reference frame depicted in Fig. 4.7. This reference frame indicates that the path of humeral motion (abduction) is in the *xy*- (frontal) plane, around a perpendicular anterior-posterior axis (or, as described in Special Focus 4.4, the *z*-axis). Using references such as clockwise and counterclockwise could result in confusion; standing in front of or behind the person in Fig. 4.7, for example, would result in different descriptions of the direction of torque. Instead, the direction of a torque vector is defined to exist along its axis of rotation. The right-hand rule is again applied to Fig. 4.7, this time to determine the positive and negative rotation directions. Begin by aligning the ulnar side of your right hand parallel with the arm segment of the model, so that flexing your fingers curls them in the rotation path of shoulder abduction. The direction of your extended thumb points in the + *z* direction, indicating abduction is a + *z* rotation. Shoulder adduction is in a -*z* direction. In a similar way, force **M**, produced by the shoulder abductor muscles, generates a positive (+ *z*) torque, whereas the shoulder adductor muscles (not shown) generate a negative (-*z*) torque. With the coordinate reference frame oriented as shown, the shoulder abductors will always generate a positive (+ *z*) torque, regardless of concentric action (associated with a positive rotation direction), or eccentric action (associated with a negative rotation direction).

The quantitative analyses described in this chapter focus on movements that are restricted to two dimensions. Analyzing movement within three dimensions is more complicated but does provide a more comprehensive profile of human movement. There are excellent references available that describe techniques for conducting 3D analysis, some of which are provided at the end of the chapter.[35,43]

Forces and Torques

Forces are vector quantities. As such, there is value in both their magnitudes and directions, and they can be considered in isolation or in combination with many other forces. For example, several forces can be combined into a single resultant force, represented by a single vector. Adding forces together uses processes called *vector composition*. Alternatively, a single force may be resolved or "decomposed" into two or more forces, the combination of which has the exact effect of the original force. The process of decomposing a single force into its components is termed *vector resolution*. The analysis of vectors using the processes of composition and resolution provides the means of understanding how forces rotate or translate body segments and subsequently cause rotation, compression, shear, or distraction at the joint surfaces. These analyses can provide insight into many pathomechanical and treatment scenarios.

GRAPHICAL AND MATHEMATICAL METHODS OF FORCE ANALYSIS

Composition and resolution of forces can be accomplished using either graphical or mathematical methods of analysis. The graphic method of force analysis represents force vectors as arrows and is performed by aligning them in a tip-to-tail fashion. The length of the arrows must be precisely scaled to the magnitudes of the forces, and the orientations and directions of the arrows must match the forces exactly. The mathematical approach includes either the simple

addition and subtraction of vectors or, in some cases, right-angle trigonometry.

The trigonometric method does not require the same precision of drawing and often provides more accurate results. This method uses rectangular components and right-angle trigonometry to determine magnitudes and angles of forces. Common trigonometric functions are reviewed in Appendix I, Part A.

Proficiency in these techniques is needed to represent and subsequently calculate muscle and joint forces. Both graphic and trigonometric methods are explained here, but the remainder of the chapter will use only the trigonometric method.

Composition of Forces

Two or more forces are collinear if they share a common line of force. Vector composition allows several collinear forces to be simply combined graphically as a single *resultant force* (Fig. 4.8). In Fig. 4.8A, the weight of the shank-and-foot segments (**S**) and the exercise weight (**W**) are added graphically by means of a ruler and a scale factor determined for the vectors. In this example, **S** and **W** act downward, so the resultant force (**R**) also acts downward and has the tendency to distract (pull apart) the knee joint. **R** is found graphically by aligning the tail of **W** to the tip of **S**. The resultant force **R** is depicted by the blue arrow that starts at the tail of **S** and ends at the tip of **W**. Fig. 4.8B illustrates a cervical traction device that employs a weighted pulley system, acting upward, opposite to the force of gravity acting on the head (**H**). Graphically, the tail of **H** is aligned to the tip of **T** (representing the traction force), and the resultant vector (**R**) starts at the tail of **T** and ends at the tip of **H**. The upward direction of **R** (in *blue*) indicates a net upward distraction force on the head and neck.

The collinear forces depicted in Fig. 4.8 can also be combined by simply adding the force magnitudes of the vectors while paying attention to their directions. In Fig. 4.8A, **S** and **W** are collinear and both act entirely in a $-y$ direction. As indicated by the boxed equation, the result, which also acts in a y direction, is found by

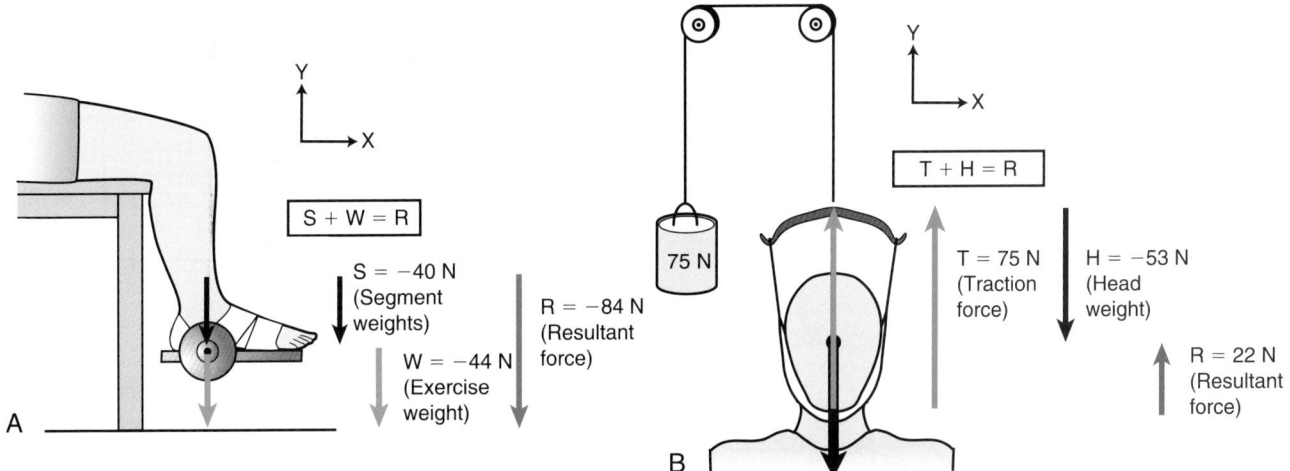

FIGURE 4.8 Vector composition of collinear forces. (A) Two force vectors are acting on the knee: the weight of the shank-and-foot segment (S) and the exercise weight (W) applied at the ankle. These forces are added to determine the resultant force (R). The xy-coordinate frame indicates + y as upward; the negative sign assigned to the forces indicates a downward pull. (B) The weight of the head (H) and the traction force (T) act along the same line but in opposite directions. R is the algebraic sum of these vectors.

adding the magnitudes of the collinear forces. In Fig. 4.8B, the forces are collinear but acting in opposite directions (**T** acting in a + *y* direction; **H** acting in a −*y* direction). Adding the two magnitudes while heeding their directions results in a 22-N force acting in a + *y* direction (**R**). In this example, a collinear traction force of at least 53 N would be needed to offset the weight of the head. Using less force would result in no actual distraction (separation) of the cervical vertebrae, though it may still provide a therapeutic benefit.

Forces acting on a body can be coplanar (in the same plane) without being collinear. In such a case, the individual force vectors may be composed graphically using the *polygon method.* Fig. 4.9 illustrates how the polygon method can be applied to a frontal plane model to estimate the joint reaction force on a prosthetic hip while the subject is standing on one limb. With the arrows drawn in proportion to their magnitude and in the correct orientation, the vectors of body weight (**W**) and hip abductor muscle force (**M**) are added in a tip-to-tail fashion (see Fig. 4.9B). The combined effect of **W** and **M** is determined by placing the tail of vector **M** to the tip of vector **W**. Completing the polygon yields the resultant force (**R**) starting at the tail of **W** and traveling to the tip of **M**, thus encompassing both the

magnitude and direction of the resultant force (see Fig. 4.9B). Note that **R** is equal in magnitude, but opposite in direction, to the prosthetic hip joint reaction force (**J**) depicted in Fig. 4.9A. An excessively large joint reaction force may, over time, contribute to premature loosening of the hip prosthesis.

A *parallelogram* can also be constructed to determine the resultant of two coplanar but noncollinear forces. Instead of placing the force vectors tip to tail, as discussed in the previous example, the resultant vector can be found by drawing a parallelogram based on the magnitude and direction of the two component force vectors. The diagonal of the parallelogram, drawn from the tips of the two component vectors to the tails of their parallel vectors, becomes the resultant vector. As with all graphical techniques of vector analysis, practice is required to accurately draw the size and orientation of the associated force vectors. Fig. 4.10 provides an illustration of the parallelogram method used to combine several component vectors into one resultant vector. The component force vectors, F_1 and F_2 (black solid arrows), are generated by the pull of the flexor digitorum superficialis and profundus as they pass palmar (anterior) to the metacarpophalangeal joint. The diagonal, originating at the intersection of F_1 and F_2, represents the resultant force (**R**) (see Fig. 4.10, thick red arrow). Because of the directions of F_1 and F_2, the resultant force tends to raise the tendons away from the joint in a palmar direction. Clinically, this phenomenon is described as a *bowstringing force* because of the tendons' resemblance to drawing back a bowstring in archery. Normally, the bowstringing force is resisted by forces developed in the flexor pulley and collateral ligaments (see force **P** in *blue* in Fig. 4.10). In severe cases of rheumatoid arthritis, however, the bowstringing force may eventually rupture the ligaments and dislocate the metacarpophalangeal joints.

As explained earlier, two or more forces applied to a segment can be combined into a single resultant force. The magnitude of the resultant force is considered equal to the sum of the component vectors. The resultant force can be determined graphically as summarized in the following box.

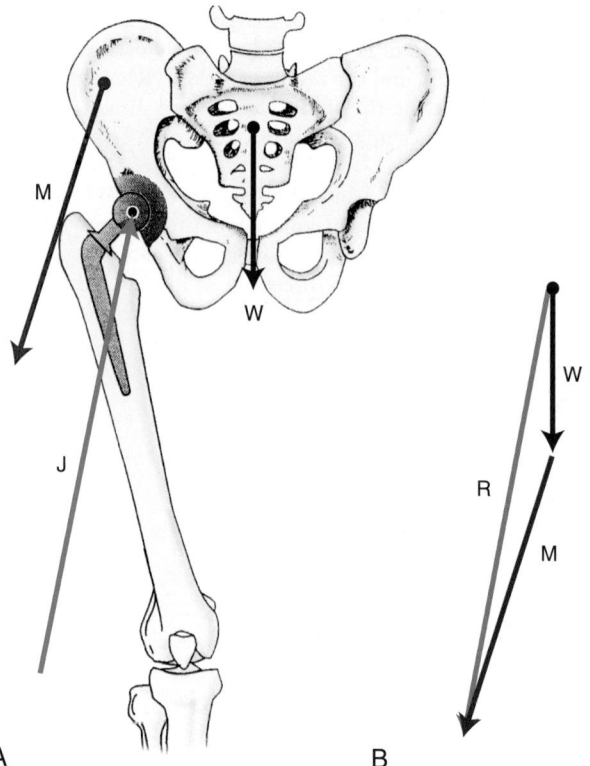

Summary of How to Graphically Compose Force Vectors

- Collinear force vectors can be combined by simple addition or subtraction (see Fig. 4.8).
- Nonparallel, coplanar force vectors can be composed by using the polygon (tip-to-tail) method (see Fig. 4.9) or the parallelogram method (see Fig. 4.10).

FIGURE 4.9 (A) Three forces are shown acting on a pelvis that is involved in single-limb standing over a right prosthetic hip joint. The forces are hip abductor muscle force (M), body weight (W), and prosthetic hip joint reaction force (J). (B) The polygon (or tip-to-tail) method is used to determine the magnitude and direction of the resultant force (R), based on the magnitude and direction of M and W. J in (A) is equal in magnitude and opposite in direction to R in (B). (Redrawn from Neumann DA: Hip abductor muscle activity in persons who walk with a hip prosthesis while using a cane and carrying a load. *Phys Ther* 79:1163, 1999.)

Resolution of Forces

The previous section describes vector composition, a method of replacing multiple coplanar forces acting on a body with a single resultant force. In many clinical situations, however, knowledge of the effect of the *individual components* that produce the resultant force may be more relevant to understanding the effect of these forces on motion and joint loading, as well as for developing specific treatment strategies. *Vector resolution* is the process of replacing a single force with two or more forces that, when combined, are equivalent to the original force.

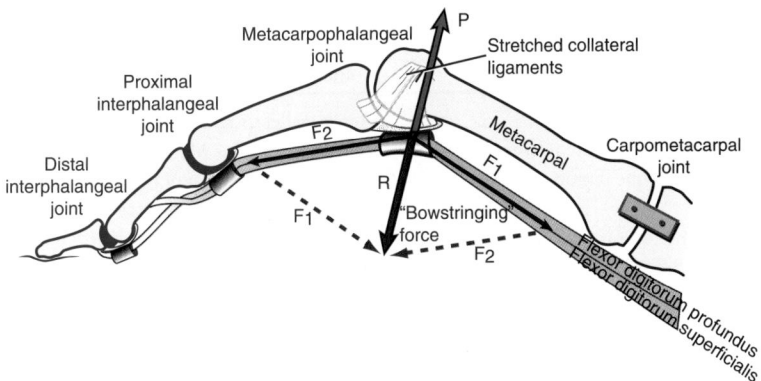

FIGURE 4.10 Parallelogram method is used to illustrate the effect of two force vectors (F$_1$ and F$_2$) produced by contraction of the flexor digitorum superficialis and profundus muscles across the metacarpophalangeal *(MCP)* joint. The resultant force (R) vector creates a bowstringing force resisted by the flexor pulley and collateral ligaments (force P in *blue*) at the MCP joint.

One of the most useful applications of the resolution of forces involves the description and calculation of the rectangular components of a muscle force. As depicted in Fig. 4.11, the rectangular components of the muscle force are shown at right angles to each other and are referred to as the *x-* and *y*-components (M_x and M_y). (The *x*-axis is set to be parallel to the long axis of the segment, with positive directed distally.) In the elbow model depicted in Fig. 4.11, the *x-component* represents the component of the muscle force that is directed *parallel* to the forearm. The effect of this force component is to either compress and stabilize the joint or to distract (i.e., separate) the segments forming the joint. When defined in this manner, the *x*-component of a muscle force does *not* produce a torque; it passes through the axis of rotation and thus has no moment arm (see Fig. 4.11, M_x). In the model depicted in Fig. 4.11, the *y-component* represents the component of the muscle force that acts *perpendicularly* to the long axis of the segment. Because of the internal moment arm associated with this force component (see Chapter 1), M_y produces a + *z*-direction torque about the mediolateral axis of rotation. Therefore M_y has the potential to cause angular displacement (i.e., rotation) of the forearm around the elbow joint. In this example, the M_y component may also create a shear force at the humeroradial joint because of its tendency to cause translation of the radius in the + *y* direction.

For the purposes of this chapter, anatomic joints will be considered as frictionless hinge or pin joints with a stationary axis of rotation, allowing rotation in only one plane. Although even the simplest joint in the body is far more complex, this approach simplifies the teaching and learning of concepts in this chapter. For example, if the *x*-component of the muscle force (M_x) is directed *toward* the elbow joint, as in Fig. 4.11, it may be assumed that the muscle force causes compression of the radial head against the capitulum of the humerus. The *y*-component of the muscle force (M_y in Fig. 4.11) tends to move the forearm in the +*y* direction (in this case upward and slightly posteriorly). These forces are opposed by oppositely directed joint reaction forces (not shown in Fig. 4.11). Table 4.3 summarizes the characteristics of the *x-* and *y*- components of a muscle force, as illustrated in Fig. 4.11.

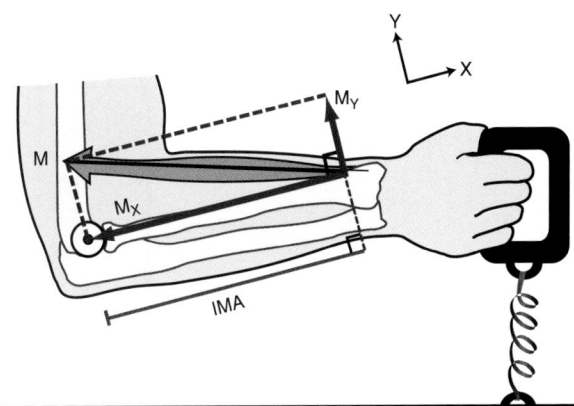

FIGURE 4.11 The muscle force (M) produced by the brachioradialis is represented as the hypotenuse (diagonal) of the rectangle. The *x*-component (M_x) and the *y*-component (M_y) are also indicated. The internal moment arm (IMA) is the perpendicular distance between the axis of rotation *(red circle)* and M_y. The *xy*-coordinate reference frame is placed so the *x*-axis is parallel with the body segment of interest; the thin black arrowheads point toward positive directions.

CONTRASTING INTERNAL VERSUS EXTERNAL FORCES AND TORQUES

The previously described examples of resolving forces into *x-* and *y*-components focused on the forces and torques produced by muscle. As described in Chapter 1, muscles, by definition, produce internal forces and torques. The resolution of forces into *x-* and *y*-components can also be applied to *external forces* acting on the human body, such as those from gravity, physical contact, external loads, elastic bands, and manual resistance as applied by a clinician. In the presence of an external moment arm, external forces produce an *external torque*. In a condition of rotatory equilibrium, the external torque acts relative to the joint's axis of rotation in a rotary direction opposite to the net internal torque.

TABLE 4.3 Typical Characteristics of *x*- and *y*-components of a Muscle Force*

y-component of Muscle Force	*x*-component of Muscle Force
Acts perpendicular to a bony segment.	Acts parallel to a bony segment.
Often indicated as $\mathbf{M}_y$, depending on the choice of the reference system.	Often indicated as $\mathbf{M}_x$, depending on the choice of the reference system.
Can cause translation of the bone and/or torque if moment arm > 0.	Can cause translation of the bone. Often does not cause a torque because the chosen reference system reduces the moment arm to zero.
In a simple hinge joint model, $\mathbf{M}_y$ creates a shear force between the articulating surfaces. (In reality, $\mathbf{M}_y$ can create shear, compressive, and distractive forces depending on the anatomic complexity of the joint surfaces.)	In a simple hinge joint model, $\mathbf{M}_x$ creates a compression or distraction force between the articulating surfaces. (In reality, $\mathbf{M}_x$ can create shear, compressive, and distractive forces depending on the anatomic complexity of the joint surfaces.)

*as illustrated in Fig. 4.11

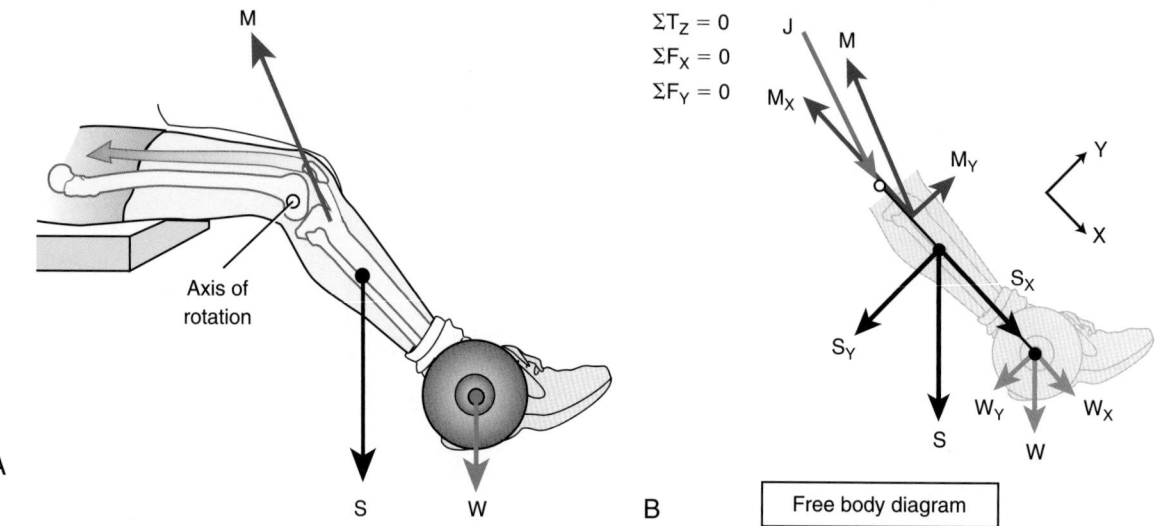

FIGURE 4.12 Resolution of internal forces *(red)* and external forces *(black and green)* for an individual performing an isometric knee extension exercise. (A) The following resultant force vectors are depicted: muscle force (M) of the knee extensors; shank-and-foot segment weight (S); and exercise weight (W) applied at the ankle. (B) The free body diagram shows the forces resolved into their *x*- and *y*-components. The joint reaction force (J) is also shown *(blue)*. In both panels A and B, the open circles mark the medial-lateral axis of rotation at the knee. (Vectors are not drawn to scale.) Observe that the *xy*-coordinate reference frame is set so the *x*-direction is parallel to the shank segment; thin black arrowheads point toward the positive direction.

Fig. 4.12 demonstrates vector resolution for both internal and external forces during an isometric knee extension exercise. Three forces are represented in Fig. 4.12A: the *internal* knee extensor muscle force (**M**), the *external* shank-and-foot segment weight (**S**), and the *external* exercise weight (**W**) applied at the ankle. Forces **S** and **W** act at the center of their respective masses.

Fig. 4.12B shows the free body diagram of the exercise performed in Fig. 4.12A, with **M**, **S**, and **W** resolved into their *x*- and *y*-components. Assuming static rotary and linear equilibrium, the governing torque (**T**) and force (**F**) equations listed to the left of the figure may be used to solve for unknown variables. This will be addressed in the final section of the chapter.

INFLUENCE OF CHANGING THE ANGLE OF THE JOINT

The relative magnitudes of the *x*- and *y*-components of internal and external forces depend on the position of the limb segment. First, consider how the change in angular position of a joint alters the *angle-of-insertion* of the muscle (see glossary, Chapter 1). Fig. 4.13 shows the constant magnitude biceps muscle force (**M**) at four

different angles of the elbow joint, each with a different angle-of-insertion to the forearm (designated as α in each of the four parts of the figure). In this example, the angle-of-insertion is drawn as the angle between the resultant muscle force and its $\mathbf{M}_x$ component. It could also be drawn as the angle between the resultant muscle force and the resultant internal moment arm vector. Both versions result in identical solutions assuming the appropriate trigonometric function is used.

Each angle-of-insertion in Fig. 4.13 results in a different combination of $\mathbf{M}_x$ and $\mathbf{M}_y$ force components. The $\mathbf{M}_x$ component results in a compression force if it is directed *toward* the elbow, as in Fig. 4.13A, or distraction force if it is directed *away from* the elbow as in Fig. 4.13C,D. By acting with an internal moment arm (brown line labeled IMA), the $\mathbf{M}_y$ components in Fig. 4.13A–D generate a + *z* torque (in this example, a counterclockwise, flexion torque) at the elbow.

As shown in Fig. 4.13A, a relatively small angle-of-insertion of 20 degrees favors a relatively large *x*-component force; in this case, a larger percentage of the total muscle force is directed toward compression of the elbow joint. Because the angle-of-insertion is

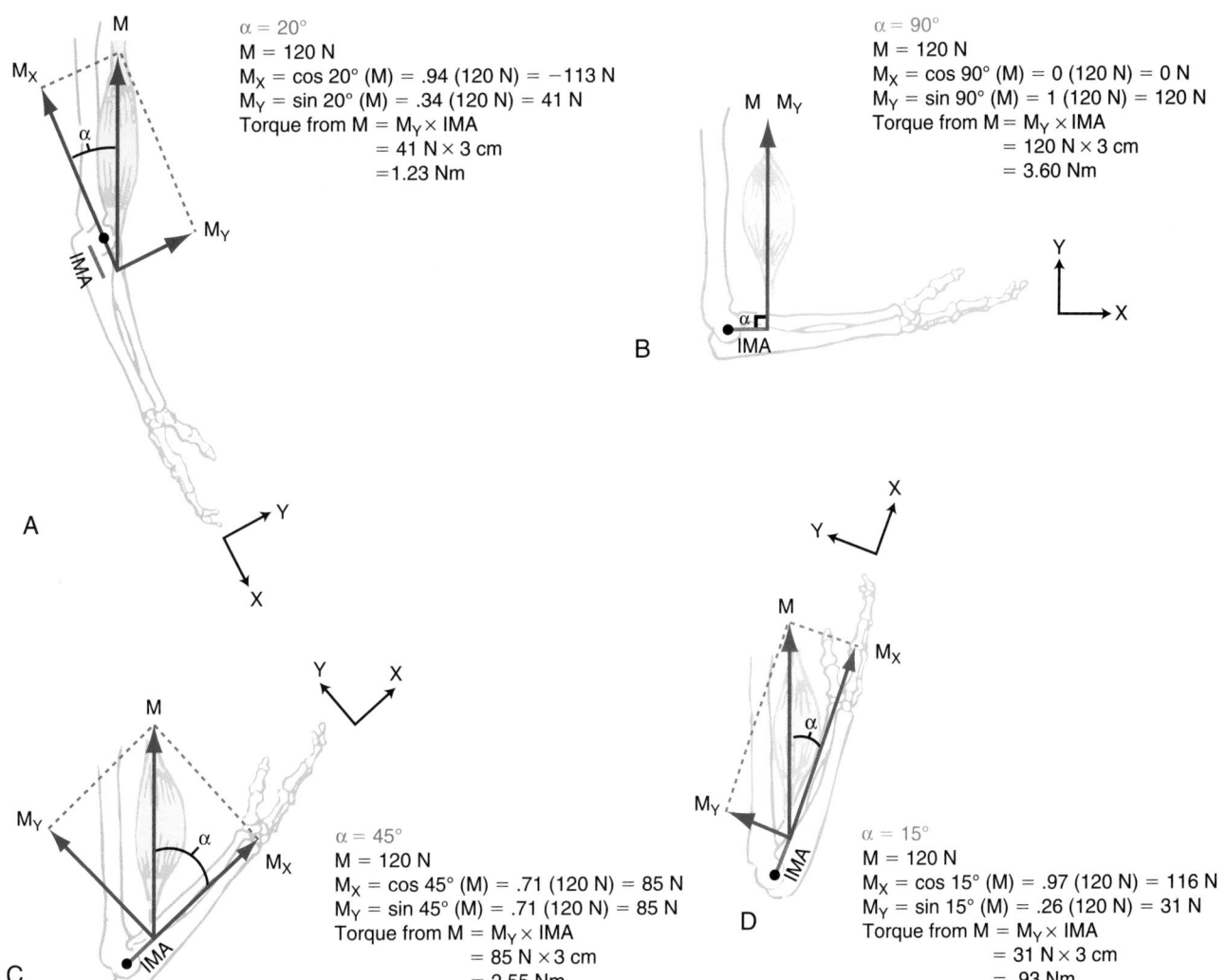

FIGURE 4.13 Changing the angle of the elbow joint alters the angle-of-insertion of the muscle to the forearm. These changes, in turn, alter the magnitude of the *x*- (M_x) and y- (M_y) components of the biceps muscle force (M). Using trigonometric functions, the magnitudes of M_x and M_y can be found for each position: (A) angle-of-insertion of 20 degrees; (B) angle-of-insertion of 90 degrees; (C) angle-of-insertion of 45 degrees; and (D) angle-of-insertion of 15 degrees. Although the magnitude of M is assumed to be constant (120 N), the changing magnitude of M_y alters the internal torque significantly throughout the range of motion. The internal moment arm (IMA) is drawn as a brown line extending from the axis of rotation *(black dot)* to the point of application of M and remains constant throughout panels A to D. Note that the *xy*-coordinate reference frame is set so the *x*-direction is always parallel to the forearm segment; thin black arrowheads point toward the positive direction. (Modified from LeVeau BF: *Williams & Lissner's biomechanics of human motion,* ed 3, Philadelphia, 1992, Saunders.)

less than 45 degrees in Fig. 4.13A, the magnitude of the M_x component exceeds the magnitude of the M_y component. When the angle-of-insertion of the muscle is 90 degrees (see Fig. 4.13B), 100% of **M** is in the *y*-direction and available to produce an elbow flexion torque. At an angle-of-insertion of 45 degrees (see Fig. 4.13C), the M_x and M_y components have equal magnitude, with each about 70% of **M**. In Fig. 4.13C,D, the angle-of-insertion (shown to the right of **M** as α) produces an M_x component that is directed *away from* the joint, thereby producing a distracting or separating force on the joint.

In Fig. 4.13A–D, the internal torque is always in a + *z* direction and is the product of M_y and the internal moment arm (**IMA**). Even though the magnitude of **M** is assumed to remain constant throughout the range of motion, the change in M_y (resulting from changes in angle-of-insertion) produces differing magnitudes of internal torque. Note that the + *z* (flexion) torque ranges from 0.93 Nm at near full elbow flexion to 3.60 Nm at 90 degrees of elbow flexion—a near fourfold difference. This concept helps explain why people have greater strength (torque) in certain parts of the joint's range of motion. The torque-generating capabilities of the muscle depend not only on the angle-of-insertion, and subsequent magnitude of M_y, but also on other physiologic factors, discussed in Chapter 3. These include muscle length, type of activation (i.e., isometric, concentric, or eccentric), and velocity of shortening or elongation of the activated muscle.

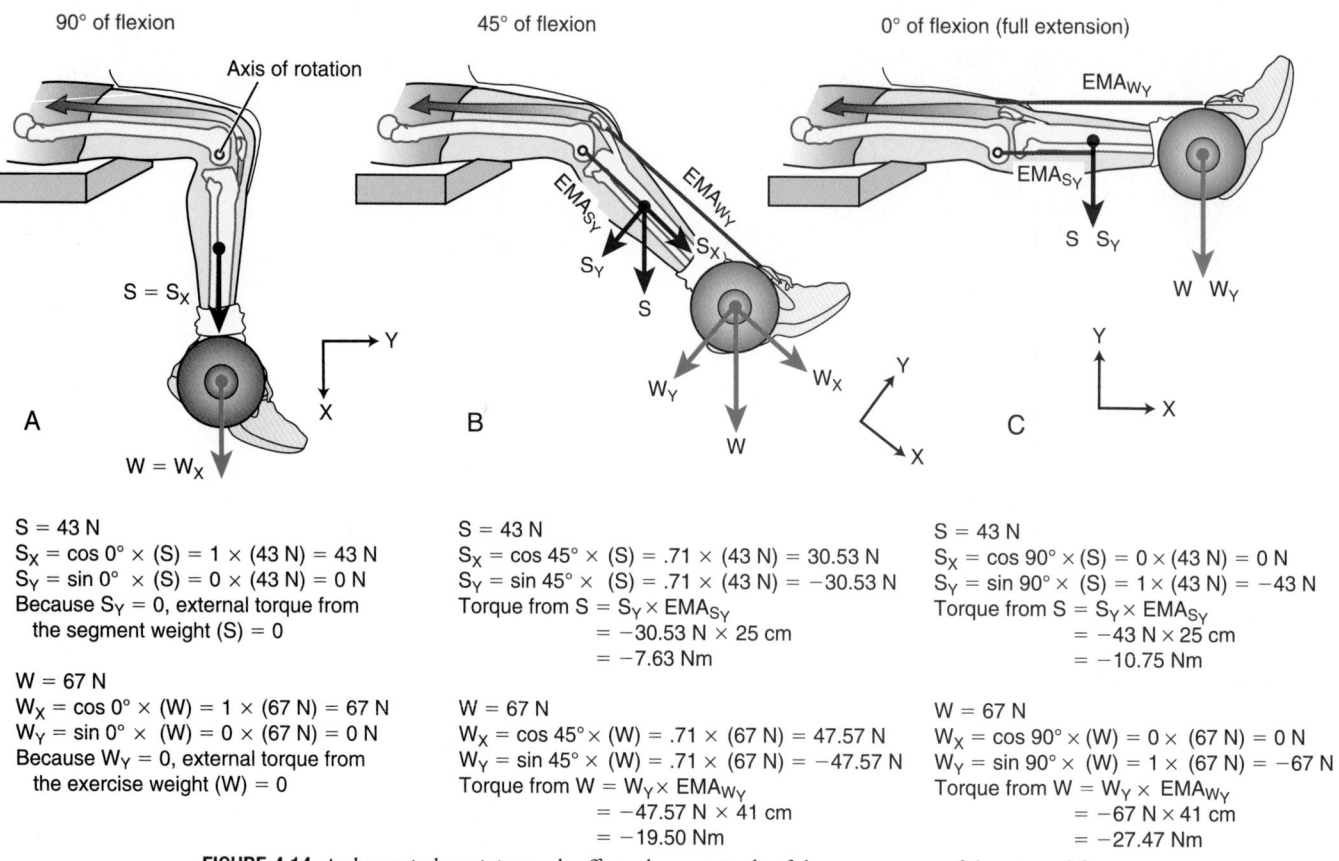

90° of flexion

S = 43 N
$S_X = \cos 0° \times (S) = 1 \times (43\ N) = 43\ N$
$S_Y = \sin 0° \times (S) = 0 \times (43\ N) = 0\ N$
Because $S_Y = 0$, external torque from
the segment weight (S) = 0

W = 67 N
$W_X = \cos 0° \times (W) = 1 \times (67\ N) = 67\ N$
$W_Y = \sin 0° \times (W) = 0 \times (67\ N) = 0\ N$
Because $W_Y = 0$, external torque from
the exercise weight (W) = 0

45° of flexion

S = 43 N
$S_X = \cos 45° \times (S) = .71 \times (43\ N) = 30.53\ N$
$S_Y = \sin 45° \times (S) = .71 \times (43\ N) = -30.53\ N$
$\begin{aligned} \text{Torque from S} &= S_Y \times EMA_{S_Y} \\ &= -30.53\ N \times 25\ cm \\ &= -7.63\ Nm \end{aligned}$

W = 67 N
$W_X = \cos 45° \times (W) = .71 \times (67\ N) = 47.57\ N$
$W_Y = \sin 45° \times (W) = .71 \times (67\ N) = -47.57\ N$
$\begin{aligned} \text{Torque from W} &= W_Y \times EMA_{W_Y} \\ &= -47.57\ N \times 41\ cm \\ &= -19.50\ Nm \end{aligned}$

0° of flexion (full extension)

S = 43 N
$S_X = \cos 90° \times (S) = 0 \times (43\ N) = 0\ N$
$S_Y = \sin 90° \times (S) = 1 \times (43\ N) = -43\ N$
$\begin{aligned} \text{Torque from S} &= S_Y \times EMA_{S_Y} \\ &= -43\ N \times 25\ cm \\ &= -10.75\ Nm \end{aligned}$

W = 67 N
$W_X = \cos 90° \times (W) = 0 \times (67\ N) = 0\ N$
$W_Y = \sin 90° \times (W) = 1 \times (67\ N) = -67\ N$
$\begin{aligned} \text{Torque from W} &= W_Y \times EMA_{W_Y} \\ &= -67\ N \times 41\ cm \\ &= -27.47\ Nm \end{aligned}$

FIGURE 4.14 A change in knee joint angle affects the magnitude of the components of the external forces generated by the shank-and-foot segment weight *(S)* and exercise weight *(W)*. In A, all of W and S act in the + *x*-direction and have no external moment arms to produce a sagittal plane external torque at the knee. In B and C, S_y and W_y act in a −*y*-direction, and each possesses an external moment arm (**EMA**$_{S_y}$ refers to the external moment arm for S_y; **EMA**$_{W_y}$ refers to the external moment arm for W_y). Different external torques are generated at each of the three knee angles. The *xy*-coordinate reference frame is set so the *x*-direction is parallel to the shank segment; thin black arrowheads point toward the positive direction.

Changes in joint angle also affect the amount of external or "resistance" torque encountered during an exercise. Returning to the example of the isometric knee extension exercise, Fig. 4.14 shows how a change in knee joint angle affects the *y*-component of the external forces **S** and **W**. The external torque generated by gravity on the segment (**S**) and the exercise weight (**W**) is equal to the product of the external moment arm (brown line labeled EMA in parts B and C) and the *y*-component of the external forces (S_y and W_y). In Fig. 4.14A, no external torque exists in the sagittal plane because **S** and **W** force vectors are entirely in the + *x* direction (S_y and $W_y = 0$). The **S** and **W** vectors are directed through the knee's axis of rotation and therefore have no external moment arm. Because these external forces are pointed in the + *x* direction, they tend to distract the joint. Parts B and C of Fig. 4.14 show how a greater external torque is generated with the knee fully extended (in C) compared with the knee flexed 45 degrees (in B). Although the magnitudes of the external forces, **S** and **W**, are the same in all three cases, the −*z*-directed (flexion) external torque is greatest when the knee is in full extension. *As a general principle,* the external torque around a joint is greatest when the resultant external force vector intersects the bone or body segment at a *right angle* (as in Fig. 4.14C). When free weights are used, for example, external torque is generated by gravity acting vertically. Resistance torque from the weight is therefore greatest when the body segment is positioned horizontally. Alternatively, with use of a cable attached to a column of stacked weights, resistance torque

from the cable is greatest in the position where the cable acts at a right angle to the segment. Unless the lines of force for the cable and gravity are collinear, the body positions corresponding to peak external torque will differ. Resistive elastic bands and tubes present further complications: resistance torque from elastic materials varies with the angle of the force vector (i.e., spatial orientation of the elastic material) *and* the amount of stretch in the material, and both factors vary through a range of motion.[39,42]

COMPARING TWO METHODS FOR DETERMINING TORQUE AROUND A JOINT

In the context of kinesiology, a torque is the effect of a force tending to rotate a body segment around a joint's axis of rotation. *Torque is the rotary equivalent of a force.* Mathematically, torque is the product of a force and its perpendicular moment arm. It is usually expressed in units of newton-meters (Nm). Torque is a vector quantity, having both magnitude and direction.

Two methods for determining torque yield identical mathematic solutions. Understanding both methods provides valuable insight into the concept of torque, especially how it relates to clinical kinesiology. The methods apply to both internal and external torque, assuming that the system in question is in rotational equilibrium (i.e., net angular acceleration around the joint is zero).

Internal Torque

Two methods for determining internal torque are illustrated in Fig. 4.15. To calculate torque, the associated force and moment arm must intersect each other at a 90-degree angle. As force and moment arm are both vectors (both having magnitude and direction), vector resolution can be used for either the force or the moment arm. Both approaches will yield the same result. For example, Method 1 calculates the internal torque as the product of M_y and its perpendicular internal moment arm (IMA_{M_y}). Method 2 uses the entire muscle force (M) in its calculation, rather than resolving it into rectangular components. Instead, the moment arm (IMA_{M_y}) must be resolved into its rectangular components so that the associated force and moment arm intersect each other at a 90-degree angle. Therefore in Method 2, internal torque is calculated as the product of the muscle force (the whole force, not a component) and IMA_M (i.e., the internal moment arm that extends perpendicularly between the axis of rotation and the line of action of M). Methods 1 and 2 both satisfy the definition of a torque (i.e., the product of a force and its associated moment arm), and they result in equivalent internal torques.

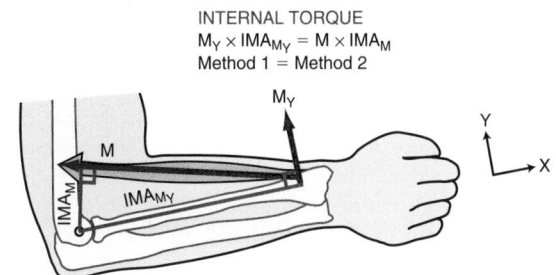

INTERNAL TORQUE
$M_Y \times IMA_{M_Y} = M \times IMA_M$
Method 1 = Method 2

FIGURE 4.15 The internal (muscle-produced) flexion torque at the elbow can be determined using two different methods. Method 1 calculates torque as the product of the *y*-component of the muscle force (M_y) times its internal moment arm (IMA_{M_y}). Method 2 calculates torque as the product of the entire force of the muscle (M) times its internal moment arm (IMA_M). Both expressions yield equivalent internal torques. The axis of rotation is depicted as the open black circle at the elbow. The *xy*-coordinate reference frame is set so the positive *x*-direction is parallel to the forearm segment.

SPECIAL FOCUS 4.6

Designing Resistive Exercises to Optimally Match External and Internal Torque Potentials

The concept of altering the angle of a joint is frequently used in exercise programs to adjust the magnitude of resistance experienced by the patient or client. It is often desirable to design an exercise program so that *the external torque matches the internal torque potential* of the muscle or muscle group. Consider a person performing a "bicep curl" exercise, shown in Fig. 4.16A. With the elbow flexed to 90 degrees, both the internal and the external torque potentials are greatest, because the products of each resultant force (**M** and **W**) and their moment arms (*IMA* and *EMA*) are maximal. At this elbow position, the internal and external torque potentials are maximal as well as optimally matched. As the elbow position is altered in Fig. 4.16B, the external torque remains the same; however, the angle-of-insertion of the muscle is different, requiring a much larger muscle force, **M**, to produce the same internal + *z*-directed torque. Note the *y*-component of the muscle force (M_y) in Fig. 4.16B has the same magnitude as the muscle force **M** in Fig. 4.16A. A person with significant weakness of the elbow flexor muscle may have difficulty holding an object in position B but may have no difficulty holding the same object in position A.

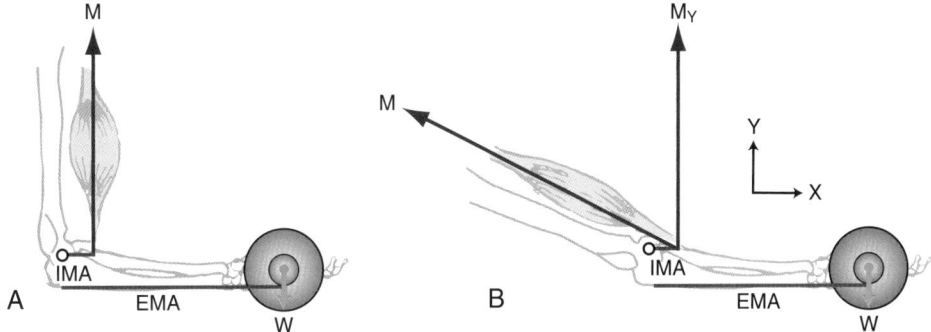

FIGURE 4.16 Changing the angle of elbow flexion can alter both internal and external torque potential. (A) The 90-degree position of the elbow maximizes the potential for both the internal and the external torque. (B) With the forearm horizontal and the elbow closer to extension, the external torque remains maximal, but the overall biceps force (M) must increase substantially to yield sufficient M_y force to support the weight. *EMA,* external moment arm; *IMA,* internal moment arm; *M,* muscle force; *M_Y,* Y component of the muscle force; *W,* exercise weight.

External Torque

Fig. 4.17 shows an external torque applied to the elbow through an elastic resistance band (depicted in *green* as **R**). The weight of the body segment is ignored in this example. As with internal torque, the associated external force and external moment arm must intersect each other at a 90-degree angle. Method 1 determines external torque as the product of the *y*-component of **R** ($\mathbf{R}_y$) times its perpendicular external moment arm, $\mathbf{EMA}_{R_y}$. Method 2 uses the product of the band's entire resistive force (**R**) and its perpendicular external moment arm ($\mathbf{EMA}_R$). Method 1 utilizes vector resolution for the force vector, while Method 2 utilizes vector resolution for the moment arm vector. As with internal torque, both methods yield the same external torque and satisfy the definition of a torque (i.e., the product of a force and its associated moment arm).

MANUALLY APPLYING EXTERNAL TORQUES DURING EXERCISE AND STRENGTH TESTING

External or resistance torques are often applied manually during an exercise program. For example, if a patient is beginning a knee rehabilitation program to strengthen the quadriceps muscle, the clinician may initially apply manual resistance to the knee extensors at the midtibial region. As the patient's knee strength increases, the clinician can exert a greater force at the midtibial region, or the same force near the ankle.

Because external torque is the product of a force (resistance) and an associated external moment arm, an equivalent external torque can be applied by a relatively short external moment arm and a large external force, or a long external moment arm and a smaller external force. The knee extension resistance exercise depicted in Fig. 4.18 shows that the same external torque (15 Nm) can be generated by two combinations of external forces and moment arms. Note that the resistance force applied to the leg is greater when applied closer to the axis of rotation (as in Fig. 4.18A) and lesser when applied farther from the axis of rotation (as in Fig. 4.18B). A higher contact force (applied more proximally) may be uncomfortable for the patient, a factor that warrants consideration when applying resistance. Additionally, a larger external moment arm, as shown in Fig. 4.18B, may be necessary if the clinician chooses to manually challenge a muscle group as potentially forceful as the quadriceps. Even when using a long external moment arm, however, clinicians may be unable to provide enough torque to maximally resist large and strong muscle groups.[25]

A handheld dynamometer is a device used to manually measure the maximal isometric strength of certain muscle groups. This device directly measures the force generated between the device and

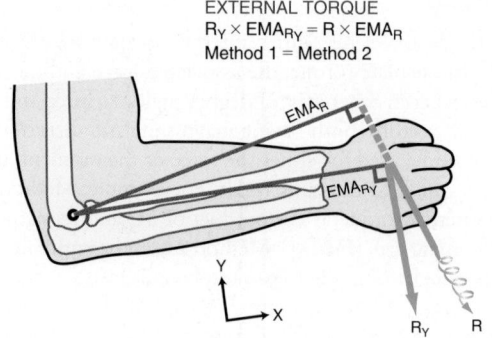

EXTERNAL TORQUE
$R_Y \times EMA_{R_Y} = R \times EMA_R$
Method 1 = Method 2

FIGURE 4.17 An external torque is applied to the elbow through a resistance generated by tension in a cable (R). The weight of the body segment is ignored. The external torque can be determined using two different methods. Method 1 uses the product of the *y*-component of the resistance (R_y) times its external moment arm (EMA_{R_y}). Method 2 calculates torque as the product of the entire force of the resistance (R) times its external moment arm (EMA_R). Both expressions yield equivalent external torques. The axis of rotation is depicted as the open black circle at the elbow. The *xy*-coordinate reference frame is set so the positive *x*-direction is parallel to the forearm segment.

the limb during a maximal-effort muscle contraction. Fig. 4.19 shows this device used to measure the maximal-effort, isometric elbow extension torque in an adult woman. The external force (**R**) measured by the dynamometer is in response to the internal force generated by the elbow extensor muscles (**E**). Because the test is performed isometrically, the measured external torque (**R** × **EMA**) will be equal in magnitude but opposite in direction to the actively generated internal torque (**E** × **IMA**). If the clinician is documenting external *force* (as indicated by the dial on the dynamometer), he or she needs to pay close attention to the position of the dynamometer relative to the person's limb. Changing the external moment arm of the device will alter the external force reading. This is shown by comparing the two placements of the dynamometer in parts A and B of Fig. 4.19. The same elbow extension internal force (**E**) will result in two different external force readings (**R**). The longer external moment arm used in Fig. 4.19A results in a lower external force than the shorter external moment arm used in Fig. 4.19B. On repeated testing, such as before and after a strengthening program, the force dynamometer must be positioned with the exact same external moment arm to enable valid strength comparisons between pre- and poststrengthening timepoints. Documenting external *torques* rather than forces does not require the external moment arm to be identical during testing sessions. However, the external moment arm needs to be measured each time to allow conversion

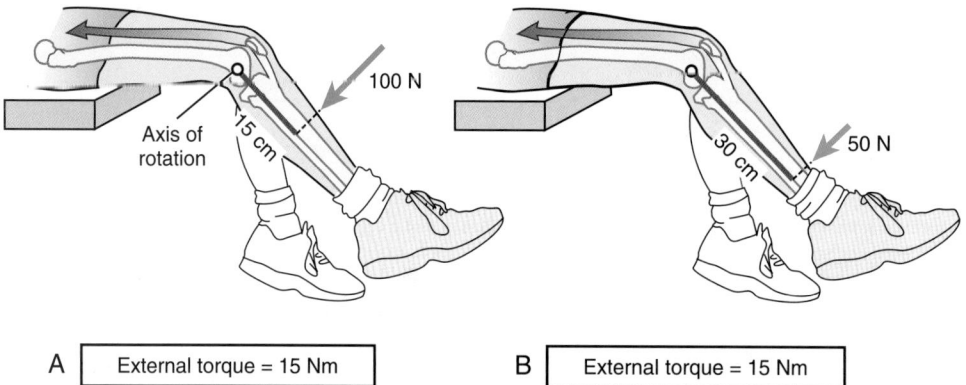

A — External torque = 15 Nm   B — External torque = 15 Nm

FIGURE 4.18 The same external torque (15 Nm) is applied against the quadriceps muscle by using a relatively large resistance (100 N) and small external moment arm (A), or a relatively small resistance (50 N) and large external moment arm (B). The external moment arms are indicated by the brown lines that extend from the medial-lateral axis of rotation at the knee.

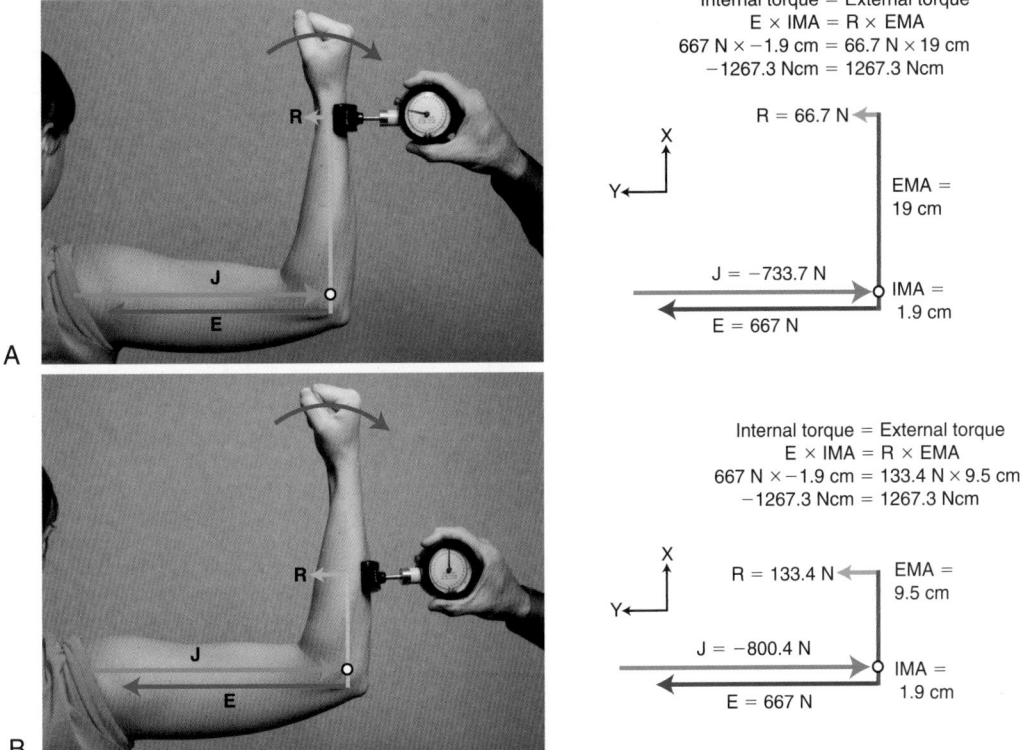

FIGURE 4.19 A dynamometer is used to measure the maximal, isometric strength of the elbow extensor muscles. The external moment arm (EMA) is the distance between the axis of rotation *(open circle)* and the point of external force (R) measured by the dynamometer. The different placement of the device on the limb creates a different EMA in parts A and B. The elbow extension force (E) is the same in both panels A and B, as is the internal moment arm (IMA). Thus the internal torques in panels A and B *(depicted as curved red lines)* are equivalent. Despite differences in external force and moment arm, internal torques are equal in magnitude but opposite in direction to the external torques generated by the product of R and EMA. The joint reaction force (J), shown in blue, is equal but opposite in direction to the sum of R + E. The distal application of the measuring device shown in part A results in a longer EMA and a lower external force reading. Because R is less, J is also less. The more proximal application of the device in part B results in a shorter EMA, a higher external force reading, and a greater J. Vectors are drawn to approximate scale. (The *xy*-coordinate reference frame is set so the *x*-direction is parallel to the forearm; *thin black arrowheads* point in positive directions. Based on conventions described in the next section [summarized in Box 4.1], the internal moment arm is assigned a negative number. This, in turn, appropriately assigns opposite rotational directions to the opposing torques.)

of external force (as measured by the force dynamometer) to external torque (the product of the external force and the external moment arm).

Note, also, that although the elbow extension internal force and torque are the same in Fig. 4.19A,B, the joint reaction force (**J**) and external force (**R**) are higher in Fig. 4.19B. Consequently, the contact pressure between the force dynamometer pad and the patient's skin is higher and could potentially cause discomfort. In some cases, the discomfort could be great enough to reduce the amount of internal torque the patient is willing to develop, thereby influencing a maximal strength assessment. In addition, larger joint reaction force could be detrimental to compromised articular cartilage.

PROBLEM-SOLVING IN BIOMECHANICS

In the previous sections, concepts were introduced that provide the framework for quantitative methods of biomechanical analysis. Many approaches are applied when solving problems in biomechanics. These approaches can be employed to assess (1) the effect of a force at an instant in time *(force-acceleration relationship)*; (2) the effect of a force applied over an interval of time *(impulse-momentum*

relationship); and (3) the application of a force that causes an object to move through some distance *(work-energy relationship)*. The approach selected depends on the objective of the analysis. The subsequent sections in this chapter are directed toward the analysis of forces or torques at one instant in time, or the *force (torque)-acceleration approach*.

When considering forces and acceleration at an instant in time, two situations can be defined. In the first case, the object is either stationary or moving at a constant velocity. As a result, the effects of the forces cancel and there is no acceleration. This is the situation described previously as equilibrium and is analyzed using a branch of mechanics known as *statics*. In the second situation, the system is subjected to unbalanced forces or torques. As a result, linear and/or angular accelerations are occurring; acceleration is not zero. In this situation, the system is *not* in equilibrium, and analysis requires using a branch of mechanics known as *dynamics*. Static analysis is the simpler approach to problem solving in biomechanics and is the focus of this chapter. A full appreciation of the biomechanics of normal and abnormal motion, including most treatment techniques, is facilitated through learning the components of these mathematic analyses. For example, recommendations for treatment of articular cartilage disorders should consider variables that influence compressive joint reaction forces. In contrast, ligament reconstruction grafts, which often require a period of protective loading, should consider variables that influence distractive joint reaction forces (and translational forces) that would otherwise strain the healing ligament. Such tasks can be safely accomplished while strengthening muscles if the magnitude and direction of muscle and joint forces are considered.

Static Analysis

Biomechanical studies often utilize the assumption of static equilibrium to simplify analyses of human movement. In static analyses, acceleration is assumed to be zero. This places the system in a state of equilibrium with its environment. Consequently, the sum of forces and the sum of torques acting on the system are zero. While individual forces and torques can be nonzero, they are completely balanced by the forces and torques acting in the opposing directions. Similarly, because linear and angular acceleration are equal to zero, the inertial effect of the mass and moment of inertia of the bodies can be ignored.

The force equilibrium equations (Eqs. 4.17A and 4.17B) are used for static (uniplanar) translational equilibrium. In the case of static rotational equilibrium, the sum of the torques around any axis of rotation is zero (Eq. 4.18). The equations depicted in Fig. 4.19 provide a simplified example of static rotational equilibrium about the elbow. The muscle force of the elbow extensors ($\mathbf{E}$) times the internal moment arm ($\mathbf{IMA}$) creates a potential extension (clockwise, $-z$) torque. This torque (product of $\mathbf{E}$ and $\mathbf{IMA}$) is balanced by a flexion (counterclockwise, $+z$) torque at the force transducer (product of the transducer's force ($\mathbf{R}$) and its external moment arm [$\mathbf{EMA}$]). Assuming no movement of the elbow, $\Sigma\tau_z = 0$; in other words, the opposing torques at the elbow are assumed to be equal in magnitude and opposite in direction.

Governing Equations for Static Uniplanar Analysis

Force Equilibrium Equations

$\Sigma\mathbf{F}_x = 0$ (Eq. 4.17 A)

$\Sigma\mathbf{F}_y = 0$ (Eq. 4.17 B)

Torque Equilibrium Equation

$\Sigma\tau_z = 0$ (Eq. 4.18)

SAMPLE PROBLEMS

This section introduces three practice problems and includes detailed instructions for carrying out the analyses. Additional problem-solving examples and related clinical questions are posed in the Study Questions found at the end of this chapter.

In each of the three upcoming problems, an assumption of static equilibrium is required to solve the magnitude and direction of torque, muscle force, and joint reaction force.

Box 4.1 summarizes the steps needed to solve biomechanical problems in static equilibrium and may be a helpful reference when solving problems such as these. Note that step 5 has not yet been introduced. It describes the convention used to assign direction to moment arms, which, like forces, are vector quantities.

Problem 1

Consider Fig. 4.20A, in which a person generates isometric elbow flexor muscle force at the elbow while holding a weight in the hand. Assuming equilibrium, the three unknown variables are (1) internal (muscle-produced) elbow flexion torque, (2) elbow flexor muscle force, and (3) joint reaction force at the elbow. All abbreviations and pertinent data are included in the box associated with Fig. 4.20.

BOX 4.1 Steps for Determining Muscle Force, Torque, and Joint Reaction Force

1. Draw the free body diagram, isolating the body segment(s) under consideration. Add all forces acting on the free body. Possible examples include gravity, an external load or resistance, muscle-generated forces, and joint reaction forces. Identify the axis of rotation at the center of the joint.
2. Establish an xy-reference frame that will specify the desired orientation of the x- and y-components of forces. Use arrowheads on the x and y axes to designate positive directions. To match the reference frames utilized in this text: designate the x-axis parallel with the isolated body segment (typically a long bone), positive pointing distally. The y-axis is oriented perpendicularly to the same body segment.
3. Resolve all known forces into their x- and y-components.
4. Identify the moment arms associated with the y-component of each force. The moment arm associated with a given force component is the perpendicular distance between the axis of rotation and the line of force. Note that the joint reaction force and the x-components of all forces will *not* have a moment arm, because the line of force of these forces typically passes through the axis of rotation (center of the joint).
5. Assign direction to each moment arm. By convention, moment arms are measured *from* the axis of rotation *to* the y-component of the force. If this measurement travels in a $+x$ direction, it is assigned a positive value. If the measurement travels in a $-x$ direction, it is assigned a negative value.
6. Use $\Sigma\tau_z = 0$ (Eq. 4.18) to find the unknown muscle torque and force.
7. Use $\Sigma\mathbf{F}_x = 0$ and $\Sigma\mathbf{F}_y = 0$ (Eqs. 4.17A and B) to find the x- and y-components of the unknown joint reaction force.
8. Compose x- and y-components of the joint reaction force to find the magnitude of the total joint reaction force.

Note: There are other, more elegant methods to determine torques and component forces in applications similar to the ones illustrated in this chapter. However, these methods require a working knowledge of cross products, dot products, and unit vectors, topics that are beyond the scope of this chapter.

To begin, a free body diagram and xy-reference frame are constructed (see Fig. 4.20B). At this point, the direction of the joint reaction force ($\mathbf{J}$) is unknown. However, here it is assumed to act in a direction *opposite* to the pull of muscle and is illustrated to reflect this assumption. This assumption holds true in an analysis in which the mechanical advantage of the system is less than one (i.e., when the muscle forces are greater than the external resistance forces; see Chapter 1).

Resolving Known Forces into X- and Y-Components

In the elbow position depicted in Fig. 4.20, all forces act parallel to the y-axis; there is no force acting in the x-direction. This means the magnitudes of the y-components of the forces are equal to the magnitudes of their respective force vectors, and the x-components are all zero. This situation is unique to this position, in which muscle force and gravity are vertical and the segment is positioned horizontally.

The magnitudes of the forces are determined through trigonometric functions; then the direction ($+$ or $-$) is applied.

$\mathbf{S}_y = \sin 90° \times 17\,\text{N} = -17\,\text{N}$

$\mathbf{S}_x = \cos 90° \times 17\,\text{N} = 0\,\text{N}$

$\mathbf{W}_y = \sin 90° \times 60\,\text{N} = -60\,\text{N}$

$\mathbf{W}_x = \cos 90° \times 60\,\text{N} = 0\,\text{N}$

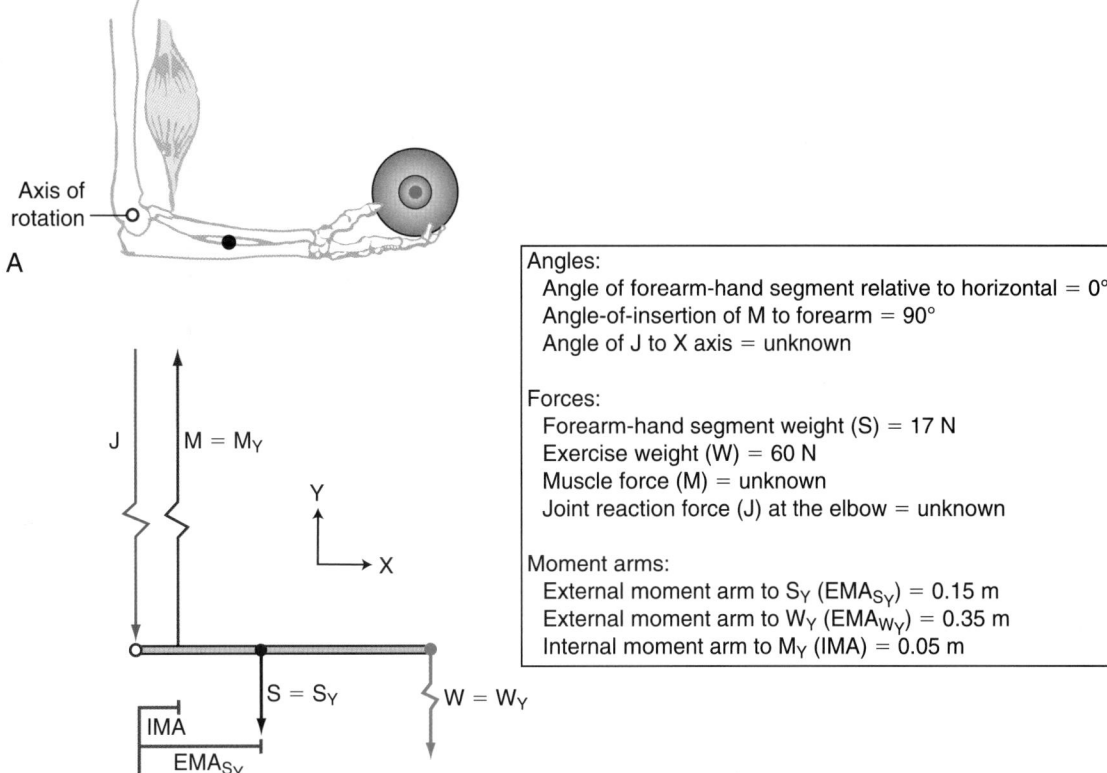

FIGURE 4.20 Problem 1. (A) An isometric elbow flexion exercise is performed against an exercise weight held in the hand. The black dot marks the segment's center of gravity; the exercise weight's center of gravity is marked by the green dot. The forearm is held in the horizontal position. (B) A free body diagram is shown of the exercise, including a box with the abbreviations and data required to solve the problem. The medial-lateral axis of rotation at the elbow is shown as an open red circle; the vectors are not drawn to scale. (The *xy*-coordinate reference frame is set so the *x*-direction is parallel to the forearm; *black arrowheads* point in positive directions.)

Note that trigonometric functions are not actually required in this problem: the full magnitude of the forces are acting in the *y*-direction, and all *x*-components are zero. Of course, if trigonometric functions are utilized, they will yield the same result.

Solving for Internal Torque and Muscle Force

The external torques originating from the weight of the forearm-hand segment (S_y) and the exercise weight (W_y) generate a $-z$ (clockwise, extension) torque about the elbow. For the system to remain in equilibrium, the elbow flexor muscles have to generate an opposing internal $+z$ (counterclockwise, flexion) torque. Summing the torques around the elbow axis allows the line-of-action of J to pass through the axis, thus making the moment arm of J equal to zero. This results in only one unknown in Eq. 4.18: the magnitude of the muscle force.

$$\Sigma\tau_z = 0 = \tau_S + \tau_W + \tau_M + \tau_J$$
$$0 = \left(S_y \times EMA_{S_y}\right) + \left(W_Y \times EMA_{W_y}\right) + \left(M_y \times IMA\right) + \left(J \times 0\,m\right)$$
$$0 = \left(-17\,N \times 0.15\,m\right) + \left(-60\,N \times 0.35\,m\right) + \left(M_y \times 0.05\,m\right) + 0\,Nm$$
$$0 = -2.55\,Nm + -21\,Nm + \left(M_y \times 0.05\,m\right) + 0\,Nm$$
$$M_y \times 0.05\,m = 23.55\,Nm$$
$$M_y = 471.00\,N = M$$

The resultant muscle (internal) force is the result of all the active muscles that flex the elbow. This type of analysis does not, however, provide information about *how* the force is distributed among the various elbow flexor muscles. This requires more sophisticated procedures, such as muscle modeling and optimization techniques, which are beyond the scope of this text.

The magnitude of the muscle force is more than six times greater than the magnitude of the external forces (i.e., forearm-hand weight and load weight). The larger force requirement can be explained by the disparity in moment arm length of the elbow flexors compared with that of the two external forces. The disparity in moment arm lengths is not unique to the elbow flexion model; rather, it is ubiquitous throughout joint regions of the body. For this reason, most muscles of the body routinely generate force many times greater than the externally applied force. The combinations of external and muscular forces often require bone and articular cartilage to absorb and transmit very large joint reaction forces, sometimes resulting from seemingly easy and nonstressful activities. The next set of calculations determines the magnitude and direction of the joint reaction force.

Solving for Joint Reaction Force

Because the joint reaction force (J) is the only remaining unknown variable depicted in Fig. 4.20B; this variable is determined by Eqs. 4.17A,B.

$$\Sigma F_x = 0 = M_x + S_x + W_x + J_x$$
$$0 = 0\,N + 0\,N + 0\,N + J_x$$
$$J_x = 0\,N$$

Because there are no x-components of the internal force or either of the two external forces, the joint reaction force does not have an x-component either.

$$\Sigma \mathbf{F}_y = 0 = \mathbf{M}_y + \mathbf{S}_y + \mathbf{W}_y + \mathbf{J}_y$$

$$0 = 471\,\text{N} + -17\,\text{N} + -60\,\text{N} + \mathbf{J}_y$$

$$\mathbf{J}_y = -394\,\text{N}$$

The negative y-component of the joint reaction force indicates that the joint force acts in a −y-direction (downward), which is consistent with the assumption made earlier.

Total joint reaction force can be found by using the Pythagorean theorem with the x- and y-components. While this step is unnecessary for problems such as this, where one of the component forces is zero, it is included here for consistency of method.

$$\mathbf{J}^2 = (\mathbf{J}_x)^2 + \left(\mathbf{J}_y\right)^2$$

$$\mathbf{J} = \sqrt{\left[(\mathbf{J}_x)^2 + \left(\mathbf{J}_y\right)^2\right]} = \sqrt{\left[(0\,\text{N})^2 + (-394.0\,\text{N})^2\right]} = 394\,\text{N}$$

Because muscle force is usually the largest force acting about a joint, the direction of the net joint reaction force often opposes the pull of the muscle. Without such a force, the muscle indicated in Fig. 4.20 would accelerate the forearm upward, resulting in an unstable joint. The joint reaction force in this case (largely supplied by the humerus pushing against the trochlear notch of the ulna) provides the required force to maintain linear static equilibrium at the elbow. As stated earlier, the joint reaction force does not produce a torque because it has no moment arm; it is assumed to act through the axis of rotation. Most often, joint reaction forces are physiologically beneficial. These forces help stabilize a joint's articulation, stimulate the formation and shape of bones of the growing child, and assist indirectly with the nourishment of articular cartilage. In some pathologic conditions, however, such as severe osteoporosis, a large joint reaction force can disrupt the structural integrity of the bone and joint.

Clinical Questions Related to Problem 1

1. Assume a patient with osteoarthritis of the elbow is holding a load similar to that depicted in Fig. 4.20. How would you respond to the question posed by a patient, "Why would my elbow be so painful from holding such a light weight?"
2. Describe a few clinical conditions in which the magnitude and direction of the joint reaction force could be biomechanically (physiologically) unhealthy for a patient.
3. Which variable is most responsible for the magnitude and direction of the joint reaction force at the elbow?
4. Assume a person with a recent elbow joint replacement surgery needs to strengthen the elbow flexor muscles. Given the isometric situation depicted in Fig. 4.20:
   a. How could the joint reaction force on the elbow be reduced while the same size exercise weight is used?
   b. How could the joint reaction force on the elbow be reduced without changing the magnitude of external torque?

Answers to the clinical questions can be found in the accompanying enhanced eBook version included with the print purchase of this textbook.

Problem 2

In Problem 1, the forearm is held horizontally, thereby orienting the internal and external forces perpendicular to the forearm. Although this presentation greatly simplifies the calculations, it does not represent a typical biomechanical situation. Problem 2 shows a more common situation, in which the forearm is held in a position other than the horizontal (Fig. 4.21A). As a result of the change in elbow angle, the angle-of-insertion of the elbow flexor muscles and the angle of application of the external forces are no longer right angles. In principle, all other aspects of this problem are identical to Problem 1. Assuming equilibrium, three unknown variables once again need to be determined: (1) the internal (muscle-produced) torque, (2) the muscle force, and (3) the joint reaction force at the elbow.

Fig. 4.21B illustrates the free body diagram of the forearm and hand segment held at 30 degrees below the horizontal (θ). The reference frame is established such that the x-axis is parallel to the forearm-hand segment with + x pointing distally. All forces acting on the system are indicated, and each is resolved into their respective x- and y-components. The angle-of-insertion of the elbow flexors to the forearm (α) is 60 degrees. All numeric data and abbreviations are listed in the box associated with Fig. 4.21.

Resolving Known Forces into X- and Y-Components

Trigonometric functions are used to determine the magnitude of composite forces. Directions (+ or −) are applied based on the established xy-coordinate reference frame:

$$\mathbf{S}_y = \cos 30° \times 17\,\text{N} = -14.72\,\text{N}$$

$$\mathbf{S}_x = \sin 30° \times 17\,\text{N} = 8.5\,\text{N}$$

$$\mathbf{W}_y = \cos 30° \times 60\,\text{N} = -51.96\,\text{N}$$

$$\mathbf{W}_x = \sin 30° \times 60\,\text{N} = 30\,\text{N}$$

Solving for Internal Torque and Muscle Force

$$\Sigma \tau_Z = 0 = \tau_S + \tau_W + \tau_M + \tau_J$$

$$0 = \left(\mathbf{S}_y \times \text{EMA}_{S_y}\right) + \left(\mathbf{W}_y \times \text{E MA}_{W_y}\right) + (\mathbf{M}_y \times \text{I MA}) + (\mathbf{J} \times 0\,\text{m})$$

$$0 = (-14.72\,\text{N} \times 0.15\,\text{m}) + (-51.96\,\text{N} \times 0.35\,\text{m}) + \left(\mathbf{M}_y \times 0.05\,\text{m}\right) + 0\,\text{Nm}$$

$$0 = -2.21\,\text{Nm} - 18.19\,\text{Nm} + \left(\mathbf{M}_y \times 0.05\,\text{m}\right)$$

$$\mathbf{M}_y \times 0.05\,\text{m} = 20.40\,\text{Nm}$$

$$\mathbf{M}_y = 408.00\,\text{N}$$

The previous calculation yielded the magnitude of $\mathbf{M}_y$, the y-component of $\mathbf{M}$, not the total muscle force $\mathbf{M}$. The total muscle force $\mathbf{M}$ is determined as follows:

$$\mathbf{M} = \mathbf{M}_y/\sin 60° = 408.00\,\text{N}/0.866 = 471.13\,\text{N}$$

The x-component of the muscle force, $\mathbf{M}_x$, can be solved as follows:

$$\mathbf{M}_x = \mathbf{M} \times \cos 60° = 471.13\,\text{N} \times 0.5 = -235.57\,\text{N}$$

The negative sign was added to indicate $\mathbf{M}_x$ is pointed in the −x direction. The correct direction can be determined either using tip-to-tail vector composition or trigonometry. In the tip-to-tail methodology, a right triangle is created using $\mathbf{M}$ as the hypotenuse. The

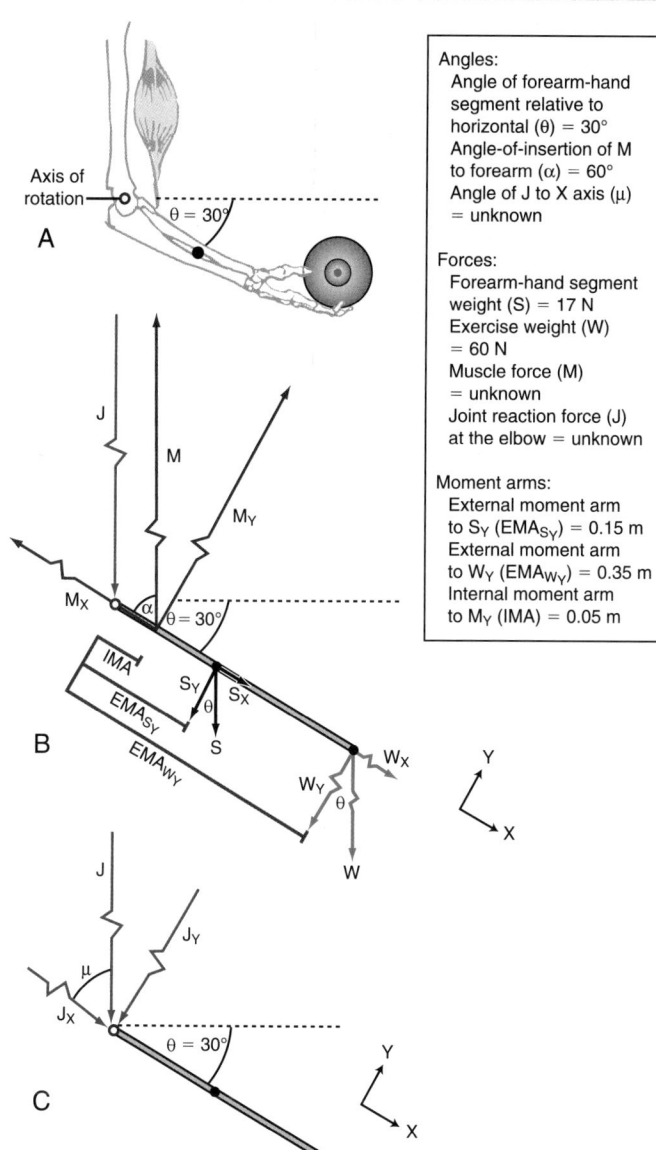

Angles:
Angle of forearm-hand segment relative to horizontal (θ) = 30°
Angle-of-insertion of M to forearm (α) = 60°
Angle of J to X axis (μ) = unknown

Forces:
Forearm-hand segment weight (S) = 17 N
Exercise weight (W) = 60 N
Muscle force (M) = unknown
Joint reaction force (J) at the elbow = unknown

Moment arms:
External moment arm to S_Y (EMA_{S_Y}) = 0.15 m
External moment arm to W_Y (EMA_{W_Y}) = 0.35 m
Internal moment arm to M_Y (IMA) = 0.05 m

The directions of J_y and J_x are assumed to act downward (toward negative y) and to the right (toward positive x). These are directions that oppose the force of the muscle. The components of the joint reaction force can be readily determined using Eqs. 4.17A,B, as follows:

$$\Sigma F_x = 0 = M_x + S_x + W_x + J_x$$
$$0 = -235.57 \text{ N} + 8.50 \text{ N} + 30 \text{ N} + J_x$$
$$J_x = 197.07 \text{ N}$$
$$\Sigma F_y = 0 = M_y + S_y + W_y + J_y$$
$$0 = 408 \text{ N} + -14.72 \text{ N} + -51.96 \text{ N} + J_y$$
$$J_y = -341.32 \text{ N}$$

As depicted in **Fig. 4.21C**, J_y and J_x act in directions that oppose the force of the muscle (**M**). This reflects the fact that muscle force, by far, is the largest of all the forces acting on the forearm-hand segment. A positive J_x indicates that the joint is under compression, whereas a negative J_y indicates that the joint is under anterior and superior shear. If J_y did not exist, the forearm would accelerate in an anterior and superior ($+ y$) direction.

The magnitude of the resultant joint force (**J**) can be determined using the Pythagorean theorem, as follows:

$$J = \sqrt{\left[\left(J_y\right)^2 + (J_x)^2\right]}$$
$$J = \sqrt{\left[(-341.3 \, N)^2 + (197.1 \, N)^2\right]}$$
$$J = 394.1 \text{ N}$$

To determine the angle between **J** and the forearm (the *x*-axis), the inverse cosine function can be used as follows:

$$Cos \, \mu = J_x/J$$
$$\mu = \cos^{-1}(197.07 \text{ N} / 394.1 \text{ N})$$
$$\mu = 60°$$

The resultant joint reaction force has a magnitude of 394.1 N and is directed toward the joint at an angle of 60 degrees to the forearm segment (i.e., the *x*-axis). It is no coincidence that the angle of approach of **J** is the same as the angle-of-insertion of the elbow flexor muscles (**M**).

Clinical Questions Related to Problem 2
1. Assume the forearm (depicted in Fig. 4.21) is held 30 degrees above rather than below the horizontal plane.
   a. Does the change in forearm angle alter the magnitude of the external torque?
   b. Can you conclude that is it "easier" to hold the forearm 30 degrees above compared with below the horizontal plane?
2. In what situation would a large force demand on the muscle be a clinical concern?
3. What would happen if, from the position depicted in Fig. 4.21A, the muscle force suddenly decreased or increased slightly, while all other variables remained unchanged?

Answers to the clinical questions can be found in the accompanying enhanced eBook version included with the print purchase of this textbook.

FIGURE 4.21 Problem 2. (A) An isometric elbow flexion exercise is performed against an identical weight as that depicted in Fig. 4.20. The forearm is held 30 degrees below the horizontal position. (B) A free body diagram is shown, including a box with the abbreviations and data required to solve the problem. The vectors are not drawn to scale. (C) The joint reaction force (J) vectors are shown in response to the biomechanics depicted in part B. The *xy*-coordinate reference frame is set so the *x*-direction is parallel to the forearm; black arrowheads point in positive directions.

adjacent and opposite sides of the triangle, M_x and M_y, must travel from the tail of **M** in an upward and leftward direction to reach the tip of **M**. In this case based on our coordinate reference frame, that means M_x is in a negative direction, while M_y is in a positive direction. (Trigonometry could also give us the correct direction: using the concept of a unit circle, the angle we would use for our trigonometry functions would actually be 120 degrees rather than 60 degrees, as **M** is 120 degrees from the $+ x$ direction. While the cosine of 60 is 0.5, the cosine of 120 is -0.5, giving us the correct direction for M_x.)

Solving for Joint Reaction Force
The joint reaction force (**J**) and its *x*- and *y*-components (J_y and J_x) are shown separately in Fig. 4.21C for clarity of the illustration.

Problem 3

In Problem 2, while the forearm was not horizontal, all resultant forces were parallel to one another. Problem 3 adds further complexity: the forearm is not horizontal, the forces are not parallel, and it utilizes a first-class (versus a third-class) lever (see Chapter 1).

Problem 3 analyzes the isometric phase of a standing triceps-strengthening exercise using resistance applied by a cable (Fig. 4.22A). The patient is maintaining a position of slight elbow flexion against the resistance cable, which is transmitting 15 pounds of force from the stack of weights. Assuming equilibrium, three unknown variables are once again to be determined using the same steps as before: (1) the internal (muscle-generated) torque, (2) the muscle force, and (3) the joint reaction force at the elbow.

Fig. 4.22B illustrates the free body diagram of the elbow held partially flexed with the forearm oriented 25 degrees from the vertical (θ). The coordinate reference frame is again established such that the x-axis is parallel to the forearm-hand segment, with +x pointed distally. All forces acting on the system are indicated, and each is resolved into their respective x- and y-components. The angle-of-insertion of the elbow extensors to the forearm (α) is 20 degrees, and the angle between the cable and the long axis of the forearm (β) is 70 degrees. All numeric data and abbreviations are listed in the box associated with Fig. 4.22.

Resolving Known Forces Into X- and Y-Components

Trigonometric functions are used to determine the magnitude of each component force. Direction (+ or −) for each component force is applied based on the established xy-coordinate reference frame.

$$S_y = \sin 25° \times 17\ N = -7.18\ N$$
$$S_x = \cos 25° \times 17\ N = 15.41\ N$$
$$C_y = \sin 70° \times 66.75\ N = 62.72\ N$$
$$C_x = \cos 70° \times 66.75\ N = -22.83\ N$$

Solving for Internal Torque and Muscle Force

This system is a first-class lever with the muscle force and external forces located on opposite sides of the elbow's mediolateral axis of rotation. The internal moment arm for M_y, **IMA**, is assigned a negative value because it travels in a negative x-direction from the axis of rotation to where it intersects M_y (review no. 5 in Box 4.1).

$$\Sigma \tau_Z = 0 = \tau_S + \tau_C + \tau_M + \tau_J$$
$$0 = (S_y \times EMA_{S_y}) + (C_y \times EMA_{C_y}) + (M_y \times IMA) + (J \times 0\ m)$$
$$0 = (-7.18\ N \times 0.18\ m) + (62.72\ N \times 0.33\ m) + (M_y \times -0.02\ m) + 0\ Nm$$
$$0 = -1.29\ Nm + 20.70\ Nm + (M_y \times -0.02\ m)$$
$$M_y \times -0.02\ m = -19.41\ Nm$$
$$M_y = 970.5\ N$$

The relatively large y-component of **M** is necessary due to the small **IMA** compared with the large external torque produced by **C**. The total muscle force, or **M**, is determined as follows:

$$M = M_y / \sin 20° = 970.5\ N / 0.34 = 2854.41\ N$$

The x-component of the muscle force, M_x can be solved as follows:

$$M_x = M \times \cos 20° = 2854.41\ N \times 0.94 = -2683.15\ N$$

The negative sign was added to indicate M_x is pointed in the −x-direction. As in problem 2, this can be determined using tip-to-tail vector composition or trigonometry. (If the latter, the angle used for the cosine function would be 160 degrees, as this is the angle between +x and **M**. The cosine of 160 is -0.94, thus giving M_x its negative direction.)

Solving for Joint Reaction Force

The joint reaction force (**J**) and its x- and y-components (J_x and J_y) are shown separately in Fig. 4.22C for the purpose of clarity. The directions of J_y and J_x are assumed to act in −y and +x directions, respectively. These directions oppose the y- and x-components of the muscle force. This assumption can be verified by determining the J_y and J_x components using Eqs. 4.17A,B.

$$\Sigma F_x = 0 = M_x + S_x + C_x + J_x$$
$$0 = -2683.15\ N + 15.41\ N + -22.83\ N + J_x$$
$$J_x = 2690.57\ N$$
$$\Sigma F_y = 0 = M_y + S_y + C_y + J_y$$
$$0 = 970.5\ N + -7.18\ N + 62.72\ N + J_y$$
$$J_y = -1026.04\ N$$

As depicted in Fig. 4.22C, J_y and J_x act in directions that oppose the force of the muscle. A positive J_x indicates that the joint is under compression, whereas a negative J_y indicates that the joint is experiencing anterior shear. If J_y did not exist, the forearm would accelerate in a +y (or approximately anterior) direction.

The magnitude of the resultant joint force (**J**) can be determined using the Pythagorean theorem:

$$J = \sqrt{\left[(J_y)^2 + (J_x)^2\right]}$$
$$J = \sqrt{\left[(-1026.04\ N)^2 + (2690.57\ N)^2\right]}$$
$$J = 2879.57\ N$$

The direction of the resultant joint force (**J**) can be expressed as its angle from the x-axis (the axis of the forearm). This can be calculated using the inverse cosine function:

$$Cos\ \mu = J_x / J$$
$$\mu = \cos^{-1}(2690.57\ N / 2879.57\ N)$$
$$\mu = 21.57°$$

The resultant joint reaction force has a magnitude of 2879.57 N and is directed toward the elbow and approximately 22 degrees from the x-axis (which corresponds to the forearm segment). The angle is almost the same as the angle-of-insertion of the muscle force (α), and the magnitude of **J** is similar to the magnitude of **M**. These similarities serve as a reminder of the dominant role of muscle in

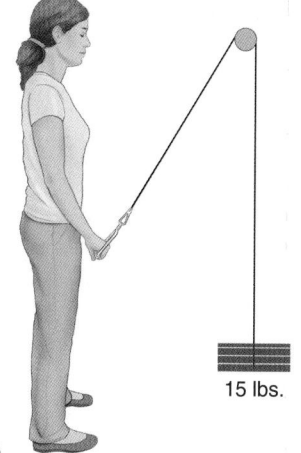

A

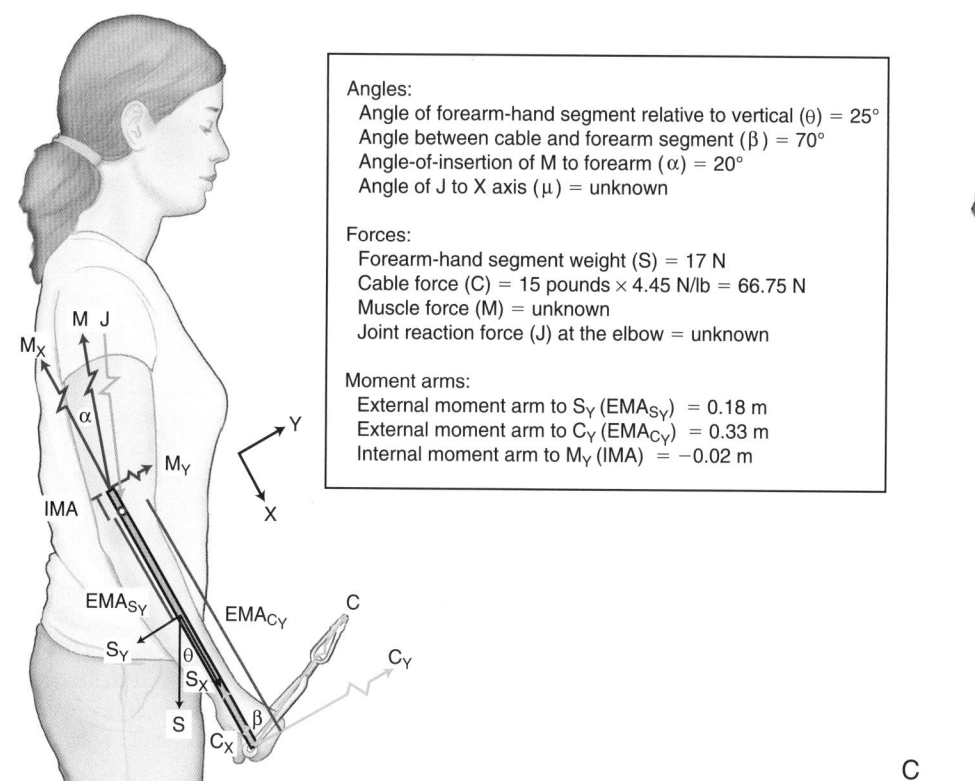

FIGURE 4.22 Problem 3. (A) A standing isometric elbow extension exercise is performed against resistance provided by a cable. The forearm is held 25 degrees from the vertical position. (B) A free body diagram is shown, including a box with the abbreviations and data required to solve the problem. The vectors are not drawn to scale. (C) The joint reaction force (J) vectors are shown in response to the biomechanics depicted in part B. (The *xy*-coordinate reference frame is set so the *x*-direction is parallel with the forearm; *black arrowheads* point in positive directions.)

Angles:
  Angle of forearm-hand segment relative to vertical (θ) = 25°
  Angle between cable and forearm segment (β) = 70°
  Angle-of-insertion of M to forearm (α) = 20°
  Angle of J to X axis (μ) = unknown

Forces:
  Forearm-hand segment weight (S) = 17 N
  Cable force (C) = 15 pounds × 4.45 N/lb = 66.75 N
  Muscle force (M) = unknown
  Joint reaction force (J) at the elbow = unknown

Moment arms:
  External moment arm to S_Y (EMA_{SY}) = 0.18 m
  External moment arm to C_Y (EMA_{CY}) = 0.33 m
  Internal moment arm to M_Y (IMA) = −0.02 m

B

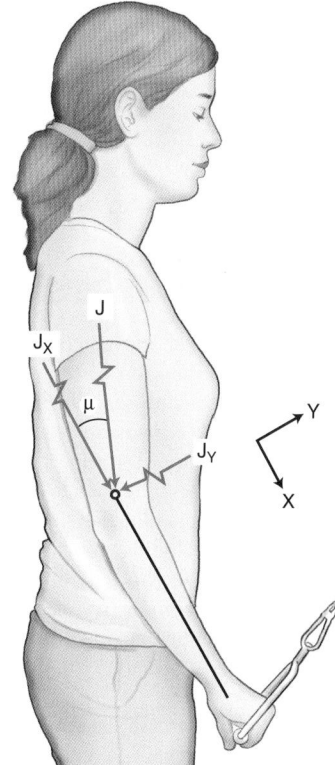

C

determining both the magnitude and the direction of the joint reaction force. Note that if the **M** and **J** vector arrows were drawn to scale with the length of **S**, they would extend far beyond the limits of the page!

Clinical Questions Related to Problem 3

1. Fig. 4.22 shows the pulley used by the resistance cable located at eye level. Assuming the subject maintains the same position of her upper extremity, what would happen to the required muscle force and components of the joint reaction force if the pulley was relocated at:
   a. Chest level?
   b. Floor level?
2. How would the exercise change if the pulley was located at floor level with the patient facing away from the pulley?
3. Note in Fig. 4.22 that the angle (β) between the force in the cable (**C**) and the forearm is 70 degrees.
   a. At what angle of β would force **C** produce the greatest external torque?

b. With the pulley at eye level, at approximately what elbow angle would force **C** produce the greatest external torque?

Answers to the clinical questions can be found in the accompanying enhanced eBook version included with the print purchase of this textbook.

Dynamic Analysis

Static analysis is the more basic approach to analyzing human movement. This form of analysis is used to evaluate forces and torques on a body when the body experiences no linear or angular acceleration. External forces that act against a body at rest can be measured directly by various instruments, such as force transducers (shown in Fig. 4.19), cable tensiometers, and force plates. Forces acting internal to the body are usually measured indirectly by knowledge of external torques and internal moment arms. This approach was highlighted in the previous three sample problems. In contrast, when a body experiences net linear or angular accelerations, a dynamic analysis must be performed.

Walking is an example of a dynamic movement caused by unbalanced forces acting on the body: body segments are constantly accelerating or decelerating, and the body is in a continual state of losing and regaining balance with each step. As such, dynamic analyses are required to calculate forces and torques produced during walking.

Solving for forces and torques under dynamic conditions requires knowledge of masses, mass moments of inertia, and linear and angular accelerations (for 2D dynamic analysis, see Eqs. 4.19A,B and 4.20). Anthropometric data provide inertial characteristics of body segments (mass, mass moment of inertia), lengths of body segments, and locations of joints' axes of rotation. Kinematic data, such as displacement, velocity, and acceleration of segments, are measured through various laboratory techniques, which are described next. This is followed by a description of the techniques commonly used to directly measure external forces, which may be used in static or dynamic analysis.

Two-Dimensional Dynamic Analyses of Force and Torque

Force Equations

$$\Sigma \mathbf{F}_x = m\mathbf{a}_x \qquad \text{(Eq. 4.19 A)}$$

$$\Sigma \mathbf{F}_y = m\mathbf{a}_y \qquad \text{(Eq. 4.19 B)}$$

Torque Equation

$$\Sigma \boldsymbol{\tau}_z = I \times \boldsymbol{\alpha}_z \qquad \text{(Eq. 4.20)}$$

KINEMATIC MEASUREMENT SYSTEMS

Detailed analysis of movement requires a careful and objective evaluation of the motion of the joints and body as a whole. This analysis most frequently includes an assessment of position, velocity, and acceleration. Kinematic analysis may be used to assess the quality and quantity of motion of the body and its segments, the results of which describe the effects of internal and external forces and torques. Kinematic analysis can be performed in a variety of environments, including sport, ergonomics, and rehabilitation. There are several methods to objectively measure human motion, including electrogoniometry, accelerometry, imaging techniques, and electromagnetic tracking devices.

Electrogoniometers

An electrogoniometer measures joint angular rotation during movement. The device typically consists of an electrical potentiometer built into the pivot point (hinge) of two rigid arms. The arms of the electrogoniometer are strapped to the body segments, such that the axis of rotation of the goniometer is approximately aligned with the joint's axis of rotation (Fig. 4.23). Rotation of a potentiometer produces output voltage, which is typically measured by a data acquisition system. Calibration factors are used to convert voltage into angular position. When combined with time data, angular velocity and acceleration can also be derived.

Although the electrogoniometer provides a fairly inexpensive and direct means of capturing joint angular displacement, it can be burdensome to wear during movement and is difficult to fit and secure over soft tissues. Uniaxial electrogoniometers are further limiting, as they can only measure range of motion in one plane. As shown in Fig. 4.23, the uniaxial electrogoniometer can measure knee flexion and extension but is unable to detect the subtle but important rotation that also can occur in the horizontal plane. In contrast, Fig. 4.24 shows a biaxial electrogoniometer, which can measure motion in two planes. In this example, sensors are attached to the subject's skin using double-sided tape.

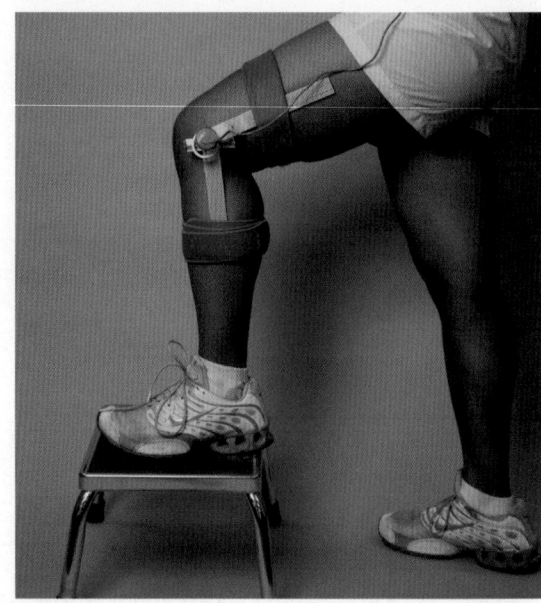

FIGURE 4.23 An electrogoniometer is shown strapped to the thigh and leg. The axis of the goniometer contains the potentiometer and is aligned over the medial-lateral axis of rotation at the knee joint. This particular instrument records only a single plane of motion at the knee.

Accelerometers

An accelerometer is a device that measures acceleration of the object to which it is attached—either an individual segment or the whole body. Linear and angular accelerometers measure accelerations either parallel to or rotating around a specific axis. Whole-body accelerometers can be used to estimate an individual's relative physical activity during daily life.[41] Multiple accelerometers can be used for 3D or multisegmental analyses, such as with electrogoniometers.[5,32] For example, by placing two accelerometers across a joint of interest, relative data from the two accelerometers enables estimation and tracking of joint position. Data from accelerometers can also be used with body segment inertial information such as mass and mass moment of inertia to estimate net internal forces ($\mathbf{F} = m \times \mathbf{a}$) and torques ($\tau = I \times \alpha$). For this reason, some researchers refer to accelerometry data as "impacts," alluding to their ability to approximate ground reaction force loading rates at time of impact.[37,38,45]

Inertial Measurement Units and Inertial Motion Capture

Inertial measurement units (IMUs) are devices that incorporate triaxial accelerometers and triaxial gyroscopes to simultaneously measure linear acceleration and angular velocity. They can also incorporate magnetometers, which, based on relative strength of the magnetic field, supply data regarding relative inclination of a body segment independent of acceleration.[3] The combination of these diverse sensor types enables more accurate measurements of linear and angular position, velocity, and acceleration compared with stand-alone accelerometers.[7,11]

Inertial motion capture systems utilize data from IMUs to quantify single joint and full body kinematics.[18] Multiple IMUs can be used in combination to evaluate and track relative joint position across an activity.[1,12,33] In fact, even a single IMU may be able to predict joint angles, although this is heavily dependent on sophisticated modeling that incorporates the specific expectations and constraints of a movement.[4] When combined with inverse dynamics or machine learning methodologies, IMUs can also be used to estimate joint kinetics during functional activities.[18,26]

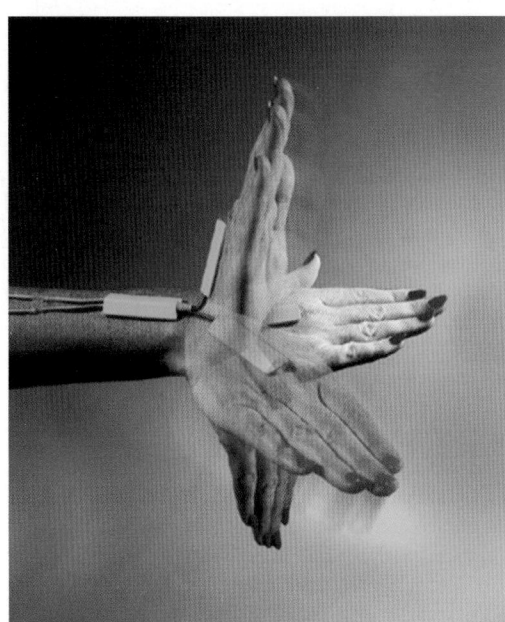

FIGURE 4.24 A biaxial electrogoniometer measuring wrist flexion and extension as well as radial and ulnar deviation. (Courtesy Biometrics, Ltd, Ladysmith, VA.)

Quantifying Movement Using Imaging Techniques

Human kinematics and kinetics are commonly evaluated using images acquired during movement tasks. While not an exhaustive list, the technology used to produce visual-based data ranges from photography and videography to optoelectronics and fluoroscopy. Unlike electrogoniometry and accelerometry, which measure movement directly from a body, image-based methods typically require additional signal conditioning, processing, and interpreting before meaningful output is obtained.

Photography is one of the oldest techniques for obtaining kinematic data. With the camera shutter held open, light from a flashing strobe can be used to track the location of reflective markers worn on the skin of a moving subject (see example in Chapter 15 and Fig. 15.3). If the frequency of the strobe light is known, displacement data can be converted to velocity and acceleration data. In addition to using a strobe as an interrupted light source, a camera can use a constant light source and take multiple film or digital exposures of a moving event.

Cinematography, the art of movie photography, was once the most popular method of recording motion. High-speed cinematography, using 16-mm film, allowed for the measurement of fast movements. With the shutter speed known, a labor-intensive, frame-by-frame digital analysis on the movement in question was performed. Digital analysis was performed on movement of anatomic landmarks or of markers worn by subjects. Two-dimensional movement analysis was performed with the aid of one camera; 3D analysis, however, required two or more cameras.

Videography refers to any form of digital video recording, spanning from high-tech laboratories utilizing reflective markers to smartphone-based applications recording joint range of motion to balance training using the Nintendo Wii.[21,23] Videography has largely replaced photography and cinematography in the study of human motion. The methods used in photography and cinematography are less practical because of the substantial time required for manually analyzing the data. Optical motion capture, a specific type of videography, has replaced these methods as the gold standard for

collecting kinematic data.[8,36] The system typically consists of one or more digital video cameras, a signal processing device, a calibration device, and a computer. The procedures involved in video-based systems typically require markers to be attached to a subject at selected anatomic landmarks. Markers are considered passive if they are not connected to another electronic device or power source. Passive markers serve as a light source by reflecting the light back to the camera (Fig. 4.25A). Two-dimensional and 3D coordinates of markers are identified in space by a computer and are then used to reconstruct the image (or stick figure) for subsequent kinematic analysis (see Fig. 4.25B). Though commonly utilized to evaluate lower extremity kinematics, optical motion capture can also be used to evaluate kinematics of the upper extremities. However, the validity and reliability for upper extremity kinematics are less well-established and the methodologies more variable.[44] Optical motion capture is often combined with floor-mounted force plates (see Kinetic Measurement Systems) to enable direct measurement of external forces. Compared with photography and videography, optical motion capture greatly diminishes the time required for data processing. However, the setup can be time-consuming, and the equipment is expensive.[24]

Markerless systems, which combine digital videography and machine learning (also known as deep neural networks), are emerging as a practical and less time-consuming approach to laboratory and clinic-based evaluations of human gait.[24,34] Markerless systems are quite versatile and are used to analyze human functional activities ranging from whole-body motion (e.g., swimming, running) to

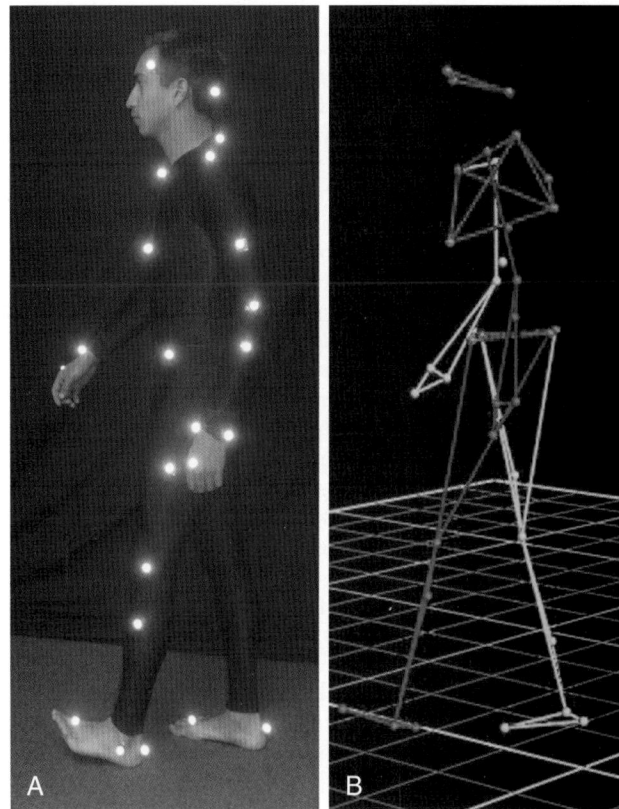

FIGURE 4.25 (A) Reflective markers are used to indicate anatomic locations for determination of joint angular displacement of a walking individual. Marker location is acquired using video-based cameras that can operate at variable sampling rates. (B) A computerized animated "stick figure" generated by data collected from the subject shown in part A. (Courtesy Vicon Motion Systems, Inc., Centennial, CO.)

smaller motor tasks (e.g., typing, reaching). Some systems allow movement to be captured outdoors and processed at a later time, whereas others can process the signal almost in real time. Another desirable feature of these and other video-based systems is that the subject is not encumbered by wires or other electronic devices.

Markerless systems have been shown to be adequately reliable for most gait analyses and yield similar data as systems that use markers, with the exception of relatively small motions and those in the horizontal plane.[34] However, it is important to note that validity of markerless systems is often determined based on the kinematics measured by optical motion capture. Although more feasible for laboratory-based comparisons, optical motion capture is not truly the gold standard for kinematic accuracy. Instead, fluoroscopy (described later) and evaluations using bone pins are more rigorous methods for accurately measuring joint-level kinematics. However, the limitations of these techniques—namely radiation exposure and invasiveness— prevent them from being practical gold standard measures with which to compare other techniques. As such, at present, it is difficult to establish the true validity of markerless systems.

Optoelectronics is another popular type of kinematic acquisition system. It uses active markers that are pulsed sequentially. The light is detected by special cameras that focus it on a semiconductor diode surface. The system enables collection of data at high sampling rates and can acquire real-time, 3D data. When combined with feedforward neural networks (a type of machine learning), optoelectronics can be used as a cost-effective way to predict kinematics and kinetics during gait.[27] These systems are limited in their ability to acquire data outside of a controlled, laboratory environment. Subjects may feel hampered by the wires that are connected to the active markers. Telemetry systems enable data to be gathered without the subjects being tethered to a power source, but these systems are vulnerable to ambient electrical interference.

Fluoroscopy is an imaging technique used to visualize movement of tissues deep to the skin. This technique utilizes a fluorescent screen to visualize otherwise-invisible x-rays. Based on variable attenuation of x-rays by different tissue types, fluoroscopy recreates images of the inner body. The compilation of these images results in a dynamic radiograph, or "moving x-ray" images, which can demonstrate joint-level kinematics with submillimeter accuracy.[13] Despite such impressive accuracy, limitations of fluoroscopy prevent its more widespread use. These include a relatively small field of view and radiation exposure. Measuring kinematics using fluoroscopy can also prove limiting: methodologies are either invasive, relying on implantable radio-opaque markers, or time-intensive, requiring manual identification of bony landmarks.[16]

Two-dimensional movement analyses require only a single fluoroscope. Three-dimensional movement analyses typically utilize biplanar fluoroscopy, or biplanar videoradiography, which relies on synchronization of images from two or more fluoroscopes. However, when combined with machine learning (such as image matching methods), single-plane fluoroscopy can estimate 3D movement with acceptable accuracy and reliability, all while exposing patients to less radiation.[17,46]

Electromagnetic Tracking Devices

Electromagnetic tracking devices measure six degrees of freedom (three rotational and three translational), providing position and orientation data during both static and dynamic activities. Small sensors are secured to the skin overlying anatomic landmarks. Position and orientation data from the sensors located within a specified operating range of the transmitter are sent to the data capture system.

One disadvantage of this system is that the transmitters and receivers can be sensitive to metal in their vicinity that distorts the electromagnetic field generated by the transmitters. Although telemetry (wireless technology) is available for these systems, most operate with wires that connect the sensors to the data capture system. The wires limit the volume of space from which motion can be recorded.

In any motion analysis system that uses skin sensors to record underlying bony movement, there is the potential for error associated with the extraneous movement of skin and soft tissue.

KINETIC MEASUREMENT SYSTEMS

Mechanical Devices

Mechanical devices measure an applied force by the amount of strain of a deformable material. Through purely mechanical means, the strain in the material causes the movement of a dial. The numeric values associated with the dial are calibrated to a known force. Some of the most common mechanical devices for measuring force include a bathroom scale, a grip strength dynamometer, and a handheld dynamometer (as shown in Fig. 4.19).

Transducers

Transducers are used to convert one form of energy into a different form of energy. For example, mechanical signals, such as force, can be converted into electrical signals, such as changes in voltage. When a known relationship exists between the input (force) and output (voltage), the output can be converted back into a meaningful value of force using calibration processes. Force transducers most commonly use piezoelectric, piezoresistive, capacitive, and strain gauge sensors. These transducers operate on the principle that an applied force deforms the transducer, resulting in predictable changes in voltage.

One of the most common devices used for collecting kinetic data during gait is the *force plate*. An example of a force plate is shown in Fig. 4.27, ahead, under the subject's forward right foot. Force plates consist of force transducers placed in each of the four corners of the plate. The transducers are sensitive to load in three orthogonal directions, thereby capturing the vertical, mediolateral, and anteroposterior vector components of a ground reaction force. The relative deformation of each transducer enables calculations of center of pressure and resultant forces. Ground reaction force data can be used in subsequent dynamic analysis.

Electromechanical Devices

A common electromechanical device used for dynamic strength assessment is the *isokinetic dynamometer*. Isokinetic dynamometers commonly have three testing modes, which hold constant either the velocity, torque, or position during testing. For example, an isokinetic device can maintain constant angular velocity of the test limb while measuring the external torque required to resist the subject's internally produced torque. The term "isokinetic" can be somewhat misleading. "Kinetic" is often inferred to mean "force" or "torque," particularly when considering the engineering fields of kinetics and dynamics, and torque does not necessarily remain constant in isokinetic dynamometry. However, the word isokinetic comes from iso- (meaning "same") and -kinetic (meaning "motion"), implying that motion is being constrained in some manner during isokinetic testing. Most often, velocity is constrained while measuring torque production. Regardless, the term "isovelocity" is increasingly being used to minimize confusion.[20]

Isokinetic dynamometers can often be configured to measure most major joint regions of the body. Most isokinetic dynamometers can measure kinetic data produced by concentric, isometric, and eccentric activation of muscles. The angular velocity is determined by the user, varying between 0 degrees/sec (isometric) and typically up to 500 degrees/sec during concentric activations. Fig. 4.26 shows a person who is exerting maximal-effort knee extension torque through a concentric contraction of the right knee extensor musculature. Isokinetic dynamometry provides an objective record of muscular kinetic data, as well as kinematic (i.e., position) data, produced during different types of muscle activation at multiple test velocities. The system also provides immediate feedback of kinetic data, which may serve as a source of feedback during training or rehabilitation.

SUMMARY

Many evaluation and treatment techniques used in rehabilitation involve the application or generation of forces and torques. A better understanding of the rationale and consequences of these techniques can be gained through the application of Newton's laws of motion and through static equilibrium or dynamic analyses. Although it is recognized that formal analyses are rarely completed in a clinic setting, principles learned from these analyses are clinically important and frequently applied.

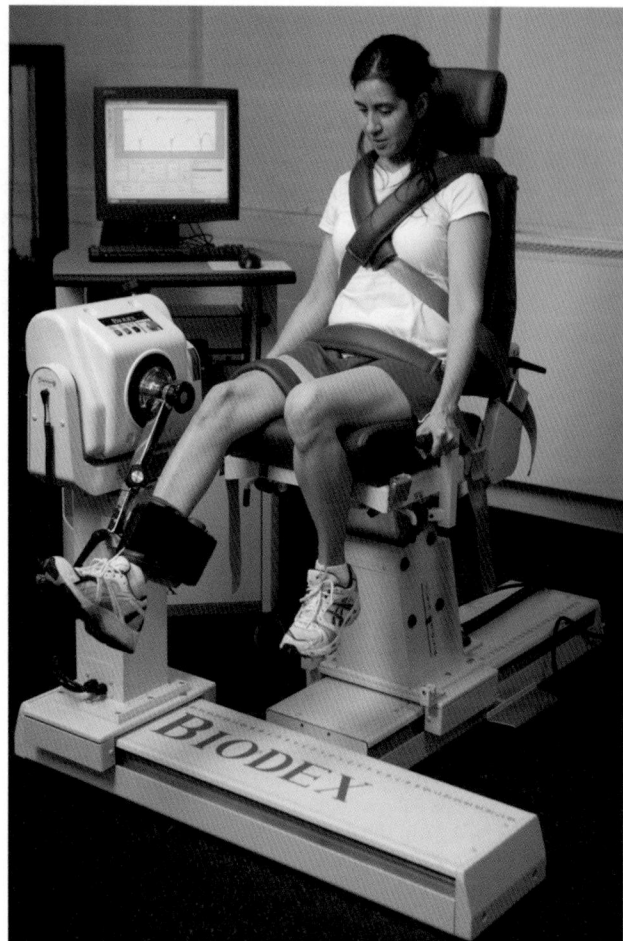

FIGURE 4.26 Isokinetic dynamometry. The subject is generating a maximal-effort knee extension torque at a joint angular velocity of 60 degrees/sec. The machine is functioning in its "concentric mode," providing resistance against the contracting right knee quadriceps muscle. Note that the medial-lateral axis of rotation of the tested knee is aligned with the axis of rotation of the dynamometer. (Courtesy Biodex Medical Systems, Shirley, NY.)

Introduction to the Inverse Dynamic Approach for Solving for Internal Forces and Torques

Joint reaction forces and muscle-produced torques during dynamic conditions are often not directly measured. Instead, an *inverse dynamic approach* is used. This approach determines internal forces and torques through knowledge of external forces and torques.[35,43] Typically, this requires measurements of ground reaction forces and kinematic data. The inverse dynamic approach seeks to answer the question: "how much internal torque was required to achieve this final position and velocity?" In this approach, position data are derived to yield velocity and acceleration (first and second derivatives, respectively), which are used to estimate joint-specific torques (or moments). From there, estimates of muscle force can be calculated.

In the inverse dynamics approach, the system under consideration is defined as a series of linked segments. Fig. 4.27A illustrates the experimental setup for investigating the forces and torques in the right lower limb during different versions of a forward lunge exercise with three different trunk and upper extremity positions. The ground reaction forces (components G_y and G_x) acting on the distal end of the segment are measured in this example by a force plate built into the floor. To simplify calculations, the subject's right lower limb is considered a linked segment model consisting of solid foot, leg, and thigh segments linked by frictionless hinges at the ankle and knee, and to the body at the hip (see Fig. 4.27B). The center of mass *(CM)* is depicted for each segment. In Fig. 4.27C the modeled segments of the right lower limb are disarticulated and the individual forces and torques (moments) are identified at each segment endpoint. The analysis on the series of links begins with the analysis *of the most distal segment,* in this case the foot. Information gathered through motion analysis techniques,

typically camera-based, serves as input data for the dynamic equations of motion (Eqs. 4.19A,B and 4.20). This information includes the position and orientation of the segments in space, the acceleration of the segments, and the segments' centers of mass. From these data, the ankle joint reaction force (components JA_y and JA_x) and the net muscle torque at the ankle joint are determined. This information is then used as input for continued analysis of the next most proximal segment, the leg. Analysis takes place until all segments or links in the model are studied.

The inverse dynamic approach relies on data from anthropometry, kinematics, and external forces. Anthropometric data—including segment masses, mass moments of inertia, and centers of mass—are often estimated from prior data sets rather than measured (or estimated) from individual subjects in a biomechanics study. The accuracy of inverse dynamic analyses also relies heavily upon accurate position data; errors in position data become magnified when calculating velocity and acceleration data. Additional assumptions of the inverse dynamic approach are included in the box.

Assumptions Made during the Inverse Dynamic Approach

- The length, mass, and center of mass of each segment remain constant and fixed during movement.
- The joints in this model are considered frictionless hinge joints.
- The mass moment of inertia of each segment is constant during the movement.

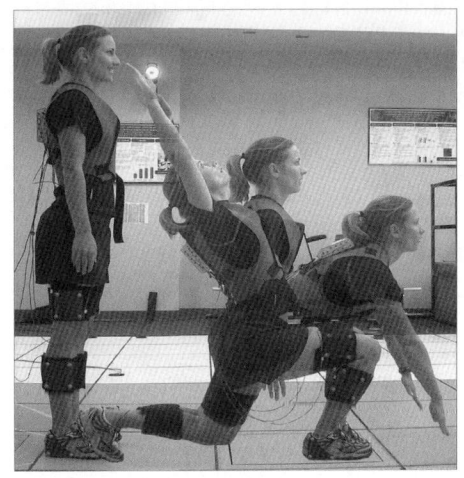
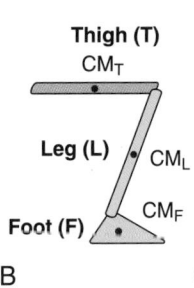
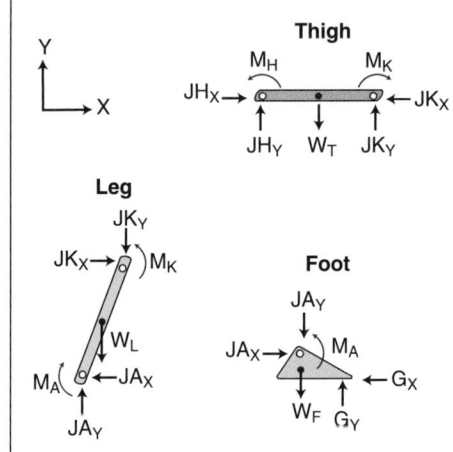

FIGURE 4.27 Example of an inverse dynamic approach to kinetic analysis of three versions of a forward lunge. (A) Photograph of the experimental setup with the subject lunging onto the force plate with her right leg. Videography-based passive reflective markers used to collect motion analysis data are visible on the lateral aspect of the subject's right shoe and on cuffs attached to her leg and thigh. (B) The link model of the lower limb is shown as consisting of three articulated segments: thigh *(T),* leg *(L),* and foot *(F).* The center of mass *(CM)* of each segment is represented as a fixed point *(red circle): CM_T, CM_L,* and *CM_F.* (C) The three link segments are disarticulated to assist with determining the internal forces and torques, beginning with the most distal foot segment. The *red curved arrows* represent torque (moment) around each axis of rotation: M_A, M_K, and M_H are moments at the ankle, knee, and hip respectively; W_F, W_L, and W_T are segment weights of foot, leg, and thigh, respectively; JA_x and JA_y, JK_x and JK_y, and JH_x and JH_y are joint reaction forces at the ankle, knee, and hip, respectively; G_x and G_y are ground reaction forces acting on the foot. The coordinate system is set up with *x* as horizontal and *y* as vertical; *arrowheads* point in positive directions. (Image in Part A borrowed from Farrokhi S, Pollard C, Souza R, et al: Trunk position influences the kinematics, kinetics, and muscle activity of the lead lower extremity during the forward lunge exercise, *J Orthop Sports Phys Ther* 38:403, 2008.)

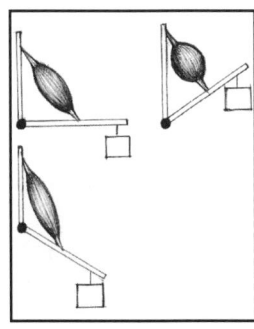

ADDITIONAL CLINICAL CONNECTIONS

CONTENTS

CLINICAL CONNECTION 4.1
A Practical Method for Estimating Relative Torque Potential Based on Leverage

Earlier in this chapter, Figs. 4.15 and 4.17 showed two methods for estimating internal and external torques. In both figures, Method 2 is considered a "shortcut" method because the resolution of the resultant forces into their component forces is unnecessary. First consider *internal torque* (see Fig. 4.15). The internal moment arm (depicted as **IMA**$_M$)—or leverage—of most muscles in the body can be qualitatively assessed by simply visualizing the shortest distance between a given whole muscle's line of force and the associated joint's axis of rotation. This experience can be practiced with the aid of a skeletal model and a piece of string that represents the resultant muscle's line of force (Fig. 4.28). As apparent in the figure, the internal moment arm (shown in brown) is greater in position *A* than in position *B;* this means that for the same biceps force, more internal torque will be generated in position *A* than in position *B.* In general, the internal moment arm of any muscle is greatest when the angle-of-insertion of the muscle is 90 degrees to the bone.

Next, consider the shortcut method for determining *external torque.* Clinically, it is often necessary to quickly compare the relative external torque generated by gravity or other external forces applied to a joint. Consider, for example, the external torque at the knee during two squat postures (see Fig. 4.29 ahead). By visualizing the external moment arm between the knee joint axis of rotation and the line of gravity from body weight, it can be readily concluded that the external torque is greater in a deep squat (A) compared with a partial squat (B). The ability to judge the relative demand placed on the muscles because of the external torque is useful in terms of protecting a joint that is painful or otherwise abnormal. For example, a person with arthritic pain between the patella and femur is often advised to limit activities that involve lowering and rising from a deep squat position. This activity places large demands on the quadriceps muscle, which increases the compressive forces on the joint surfaces.

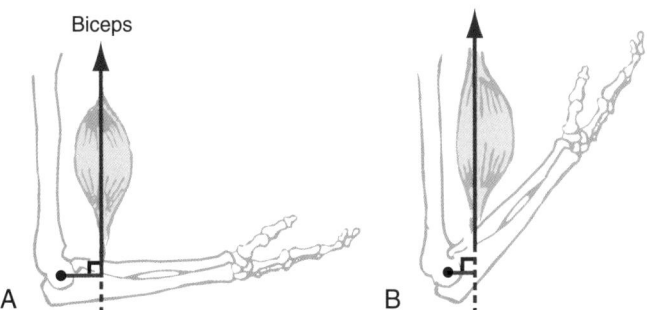

FIGURE 4.28 A piece of string can be used to mimic the line of force of the resultant force vector of an activated biceps muscle. The internal moment arm is shown as a brown line; the axis of rotation at the elbow is shown as a solid black circle. Note that the moment arm is greater when the elbow is in position A compared with position B. (Modified from LeVeau BF: *Williams & Lissner's biomechanics of human motion,* ed 3, Philadelphia, 1992, Saunders.)

ADDITIONAL CLINICAL CONNECTIONS

CLINICAL CONNECTION 4.1
A Practical Method for Estimating Relative Torque Potential Based on Leverage—cont'd

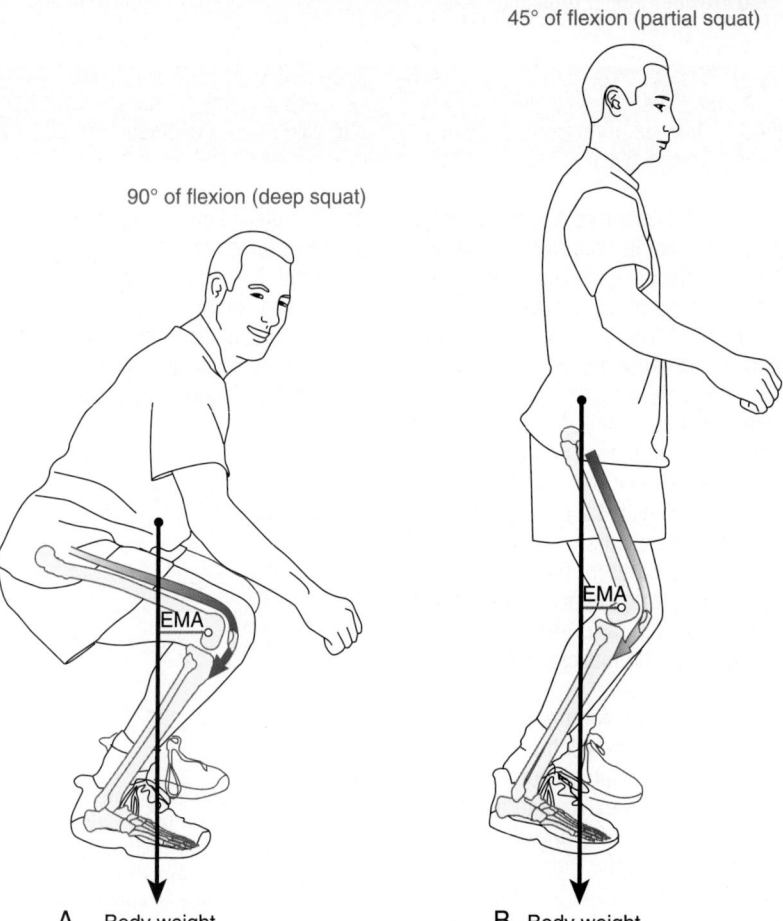

FIGURE 4.29 The depth of a squat significantly affects the magnitude of the external torque at the knee, even without changing the magnitude of external force. In panels A and B, the only external force being considered is body weight. However, the distance between the body weight force vector and the mediolateral axis of rotation at the knee (shown as an open circle) is changing. This distance is the external moment arm (EMA), here shown as a brown line originating at the axis of rotation and intersecting body weight force at a right angle. Within the sagittal plane, the relative external knee flexion torque – and thus the relative demands of the task – can be estimated by comparing the EMA between panels A and B. Such a comparison reveals panel A to be the more demanding scenario: the EMA—and thus the external torque created by identical external loads (i.e., body weight)—is greater in A than in B.

ADDITIONAL CLINICAL CONNECTIONS

CLINICAL CONNECTION 4.2
Modifying Internal Torque to Provide "Joint Protection"

Some treatments in rehabilitation medicine are directed at reducing the magnitude of force on joint surfaces during the performance of a physical activity. The purpose of such treatment is to protect a weakened or painful joint from large and potentially damaging forces. This result can be achieved by reducing the rate of movement (power), providing shock absorption (e.g., cushioned footwear), or limiting the mechanical force demands on the muscle.

Minimizing large muscular-based joint forces may be important for persons with a prosthesis (artificial joint replacement). A person with a hip replacement, for example, is often advised on ways to minimize unnecessarily large forces produced by the hip abductor muscles. Fig. 4.30 depicts a simple schematic representation of the pelvis and femur while a person with a prosthetic hip is in the single-limb support phase of gait. In order for equilibrium to be maintained within the frontal plane, the internal (counterclockwise, + z) and the external (clockwise, −z) torques around the stance hip must be balanced. As shown in both the anatomic (A) and the seesaw (B) illustrations of Fig. 4.30, the product of the body weight (**W**) times its moment arm D_1 must be equal in magnitude and opposite in direction to the hip abductor muscle force (**M**) times its moment arm (**D**): $W \times D_1 = M \times D$. Note that the external moment arm around the hip is almost twice the length of the internal

moment arm.[28,31] This disparity in moment arm lengths requires that the muscle force be almost twice the force of superincumbent body weight to maintain equilibrium. In theory, reducing excessive body weight, carrying lighter loads, or carrying loads in certain fashions can decrease the external force and/or the external moment arm and therefore decrease the external torque about the hip. Reduction of large external torques substantially decreases large force demands from the hip abductors, thereby decreasing joint reaction forces on the prosthetic hip joint.

Certain orthopedic procedures illustrate how concepts of joint protection are used in rehabilitation practice. Consider the case of severe hip osteoarthritis, which results in destruction of the femoral head and a subsequent reduced size of the femoral neck and head. The bony loss shortens the internal moment arm length (**D** in Fig. 4.30A) available to the hip abductor muscles (**M**); thus greater muscle forces are needed to maintain frontal plane equilibrium, and greater joint reaction forces result. A surgical procedure that attempts to reduce joint forces on the hip entails the relocation of the greater trochanter to a more lateral position. This procedure increases the length of the internal moment arm of the hip abductor muscles. An increase in the internal moment arm reduces the force required by the abductor muscles to generate a given torque during the single-limb support phase of gait.

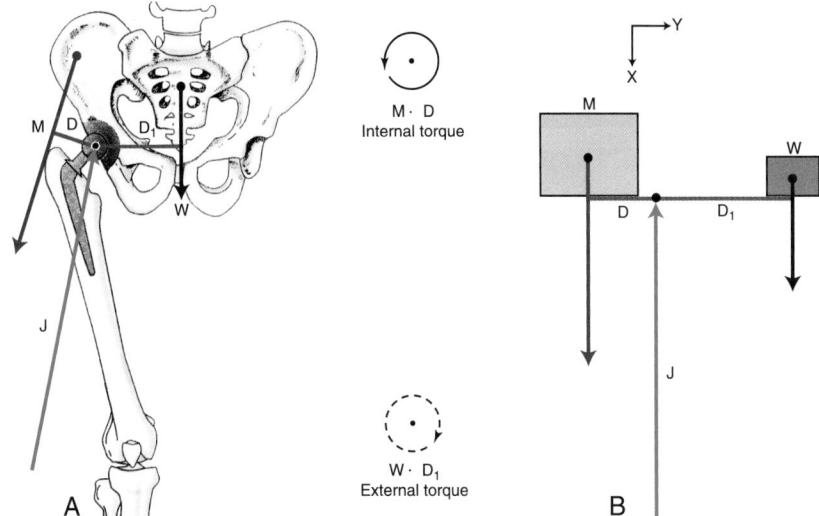

FIGURE 4.30   (A) Hip abductor muscle force (M) produces a torque necessary for the frontal plane stability of the pelvis during the right single-limb support phase of gait. Rotary stability is established, assuming static equilibrium, when the external (clockwise, −z) torque created by superincumbent body weight (W) is exactly balanced by the internal (counterclockwise, + z) torque from the hip abductor muscles (M). The counterclockwise torque is the product of M and its moment arm (D), while the clockwise torque is the product of W and its moment arm (D_1). (B) This first-class lever seesaw model simplifies the model shown in part A. The joint reaction force (J), assuming that all force vectors act vertically, is shown as an upward-directed force with a magnitude equal to the sum of the hip abductor force and superimposed body weight. The *xy*-coordinate reference frame is placed so the *x*-axis is parallel with the body weight (W); thin black arrowheads point toward the positive direction. (Modified from Neumann DA: Biomechanical analysis of selected principles of hip joint protection. *Arthritis Care Res* 2:146, 1989.)

ADDITIONAL CLINICAL CONNECTIONS

CLINICAL CONNECTION 4.3
The Influence of Antagonist Muscle Coactivation on the Clinical Measurement of Torque

When muscle strength is measured, care must be taken to encourage *activation* of the agonist muscles and relative *relaxation* of the antagonist muscles (review definitions of *agonist* and *antagonist* muscles in Chapter 1). Coactivation of antagonist muscles alters the net internal torque and decreases the ability to control or overcome external forces and torques. This concept is shown with the use of a hand-held dynamometer, similar to that previously described in Fig. 4.19. Fig. 4.31A shows the measurement of elbow extension torque with activation *only* from the agonist (elbow extensor) muscles while the antagonist elbow flexors are relaxed. In contrast, Fig. 4.31B show a maximal-effort strength test of the elbow extensors with coactivation of both the agonist (**E**) and the antagonist elbow flexor (**F**) muscles. (This situation may occur in a healthy person who is simply unable to relax the antagonist muscles or in a patient with neurologic pathology

such as Parkinson's disease or cerebral palsy.) The internal torque produced by the antagonist muscles *subtracts* from the internal torque produced by the agonist muscles. As a result, the *net* internal torque is reduced, as indicated by the reduced external force (**R**) applied against the dynamometer. Because the test condition is isometric, the measured external torque is equal in magnitude but opposite in direction to the reduced net internal torque. The important clinical point here is that even though the elbow extensor forces and torques may be equivalent in tests *A* and *B* of Fig. 4.31, the external torque measures *less* in test *B*. This scenario may give an erroneous impression of relative weakness of the agonist muscles when, in fact, they are not weak. As always, the joint reaction force (**J**) occurs in response to the sum of *all* forces across the joint and therefore will be *increased* in test *B* with antagonist activation.

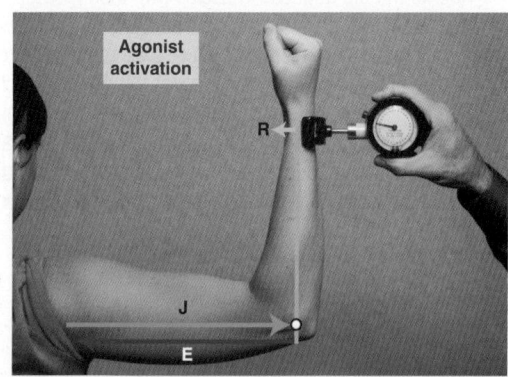

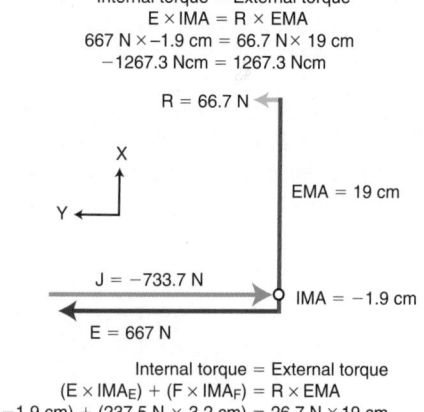

Internal torque = External torque
$E \times IMA = R \times EMA$
$667\ N \times -1.9\ cm = 66.7\ N \times 19\ cm$
$-1267.3\ Ncm = 1267.3\ Ncm$

$R = 66.7\ N$

$EMA = 19\ cm$

$J = -733.7\ N$ $IMA = -1.9\ cm$

$E = 667\ N$

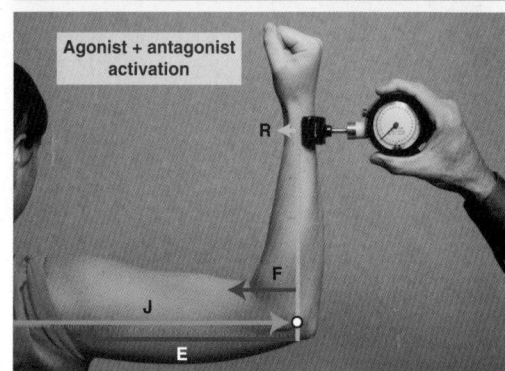

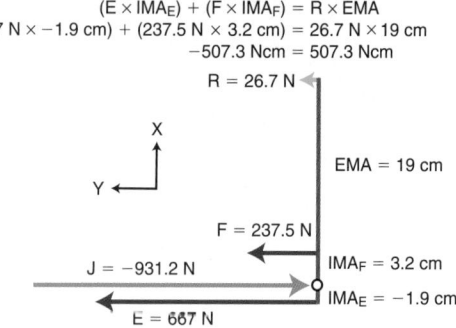

Internal torque = External torque
$(E \times IMA_E) + (F \times IMA_F) = R \times EMA$
$(667\ N \times -1.9\ cm) + (237.5\ N \times 3.2\ cm) = 26.7\ N \times 19\ cm$
$-507.3\ Ncm = 507.3\ Ncm$

$R = 26.7\ N$

$EMA = 19\ cm$

$F = 237.5\ N$

$J = -931.2\ N$ $IMA_F = 3.2\ cm$
$IMA_E = -1.9\ cm$

$E = 667\ N$

FIGURE 4.31 The influence of coactivation of the agonist (elbow extensor) and antagonist (elbow flexor) muscle groups is shown on the apparent strength (torque) of isometric elbow extension. (A) Agonist (elbow extensor) activation only, with the same conditions and abbreviations used in Fig. 4.19A. (B) Subject is simultaneously coactivating her elbow extensors and (antagonistic) elbow flexors muscles, producing a simultaneous elbow extension force (E) and an elbow flexion force (F). Because F and E generate oppositely directed torques around the elbow, the *net* elbow extension torque is reduced. Note, however, that the magnitude of the joint reaction force (J) is increased in part B. Vectors are drawn to approximate scale. Based on conventions summarized in Box 4.1, the internal moment arm used by the extensor muscles is assigned a negative number. This, in turn, assigns opposite rotational directions to the opposing internal torques. *EMA,* external moment arm; *IMA_F* and *IMA_E,* internal moment arms of the elbow flexors and extensor muscles, respectively; *R,* external force measured by the dynamometer.

REFERENCES

1. Ahmadi A, Destelle F, Unzueta L, et al.: 3D human gait reconstruction and monitoring using body-worn inertial sensors and kinematic modeling, *IEEE Sensors J* 16:8823–8831, 2016. https://doi.org/10.1109/jsen.2016.2593011.
2. Ajemian S, Thon D, Clare P, et al.: Cane-assisted gait biomechanics and electromyography after total hip arthroplasty, *Arch Phys Med Rehabil* 85:1966–1971, 2004.
3. Bonnet S, Heliot R: A magnetometer-based approach for studying human movements, *IEEE Trans Biomed Eng* 54:1353–1355, 2007. https://doi.org/10.1109/TBME.2007.890742.
4. Bonnet V, Joukov V, Kulić D, et al.: Monitoring of hip and knee joint angles using a single inertial measurement unit during lower limb rehabilitation, *IEEE Sensors J* 16:1557–1564, 2015.
5. Caldas R, Mundt M, Potthast W, et al.: A systematic review of gait analysis methods based on inertial sensors and adaptive algorithms, *Gait Posture* 57:204–210, 2017. https://doi.org/10.1016/j.gaitpost.2017.06.019.
6. Chandler R, Clauser CE, McConville JT, et al.: *Investigation of inertial properties of the human body, DTIC document*, Fort Belvoir, Va, 1975, Defense Technical Information Center.
7. Chen H, Schall Jr MC, Fethke N: Accuracy of angular displacements and velocities from inertial-based inclinometers, *Appl Ergon* 67:151–161, 2018. https://doi.org/10.1016/j.apergo.2017.09.007.
8. Cuadrado J, Michaud F, Lugrís U, et al.: Using accelerometer data to tune the parameters of an extended Kalman filter for optical motion capture: preliminary application to gait analysis, *Sensors* 21, 2021. https://doi.org/10.3390/s21020427.
9. Dempster WT: *Space requirements for the seated operator, WADC-TR-55-159*, Dayton, Ohio, 1955, Wright Patterson Air Force Base.
10. Enoka RM: *Neuromechanics of human movement*, ed 5, Champaign, Ill, 2015, Human Kinetics.
11. Fan X, Lind CM, Rhen IM, et al.: Effects of sensor types and angular velocity computational methods in field measurements of occupational upper arm and trunk postures and movements, *Sensors* 21, 2021. https://doi.org/10.3390/s21165527.
12. Favre J, Aissaoui R, Jolles BM, et al.: Functional calibration procedure for 3D knee joint angle description using inertial sensors, *J Biomech* 42:2330–2335, 2009. https://doi.org/10.1016/j.jbiomech.2009.06.025.
13. Fernandez JW, Pandy MG: Integrating modelling and experiments to assess dynamic musculoskeletal function in humans, *Exp Physiol* 91:371–382, 2006. https://doi.org/10.1113/expphysiol.2005.031047.
14. Hatze H: A mathematical model for the computational determination of parameter values of anthropomorphic segments, *J Biomech* 13:833–843, 1980.
15. Hetherington-Rauth M, Magalhaes JP, Alcazar J, et al.: Relative sit-to-stand muscle power predicts an older adult's physical independence at age 90 beyond that of relative handgrip strength, physical activity and sedentary time: a cross-sectional analysis, *Am J Phys Med Rehabil* 101(11):995–1000, 2022. https://doi.org/10.1097/PHM.0000000000001945.
16. Kessler SE, Rainbow MJ, Lichtwark GA, et al.: A direct comparison of biplanar videoradiography and optical motion capture for foot and ankle kinematics, *Front Bioeng Biotechnol* 7:199, 2019. https://doi.org/10.3389/fbioe.2019.00199.
17. Lawrence RL, Ellingson AM, Ludewig PM: Validation of single-plane fluoroscopy and 2d/3d shape-matching for quantifying shoulder complex kinematics, *Med Eng Phys* 52:69–75, 2018. https://doi.org/10.1016/j.medengphy.2017.11.005.
18. Lee CJ, Lee JK: Inertial motion capture-based wearable systems for estimation of joint kinetics: a systematic review, *Sensors* 22(7):2507, 2022. https://doi.org/10.3390/s22072507.
19. Lee KL, Oh TW, Gil YC, et al.: Correlation between muscle architecture and anaerobic power in athletes involved in different sports, *Sci Rep* 11:13332, 2021. https://doi.org/10.1038/s41598-021-92831-7.
20. Lewis MGC, Yeadon MR, King MA: The effect of accounting for biarticularity in hip flexor and hip extensor joint torque representations, *Hum Mov Sci* 57:388–399, 2018. https://doi.org/10.1016/j.humov.2017.09.016.
21. Marques-Sule E, Arnal-Gomez A, Buitrago-Jimenez G, et al.: Effectiveness of Nintendo Wii and physical therapy in functionality, balance, and daily activities in chronic stroke patients, *J Am Med Dir Assoc* 22:1073–1080, 2021. https://doi.org/10.1016/j.jamda.2021.01.076.
22. McGibbon CA, Krebs DE, Mann RW: In vivo hip pressures during cane and load-carrying gait, *Arthritis Care Res* 10:300–307, 1997.
23. Modest J, Clair B, DeMasi R, et al.: Self-measured wrist range of motion by wrist-injured and wrist-healthy study participants using a built-in iPhone feature as compared with a universal goniometer, *J Hand Ther* 32:507–514, 2019. https://doi.org/10.1016/j.jht.2018.03.004.
24. Moro M, Marchesi G, Hesse F, et al.: Markerless vs. Marker-based gait analysis: a proof of concept study, *Sensors* 22(5):2011, 2022. https://doi.org/10.3390/s22052011.
25. Mulroy SJ, Lassen KD, Chambers SH, et al.: The ability of male and female clinicians to effectively test knee extension strength using manual muscle testing, *J Orthop Sports Phys Ther* 26:192–199, 1997.
26. Mundt M, Koeppe A, David S, et al.: Estimation of gait mechanics based on simulated and measured IMU data using an artificial neural network, *Front Bioeng Biotechnol* 8:41, 2020. https://doi.org/10.3389/fbioe.2020.00041.
27. Mundt M, Koeppe A, David S, et al.: Prediction of ground reaction force and joint moments based on optical motion capture data during gait, *Med Eng Phys* 86:29–34, 2020. https://doi.org/10.1016/j.medengphy.2020.10.001.
28. Neumann DA, Soderberg GL, Cook TM: Comparison of maximal isometric hip abductor muscle torques between hip sides, *Phys Ther* 68:496–502, 1988.
29. Neumann DA: Hip abductor muscle activity as subjects with hip prostheses walk with different methods of using a cane, *Phys Ther* 78:490–501, 1998.
30. Nooijen CFJ, Muchaxo R, Liljedahl J, et al.: The relation between sprint power and road time trial performance in elite para-cyclists, *J Sci Med Sport* 24:1193–1198, 2021. https://doi.org/10.1016/j.jsams.2021.04.014.
31. Olson VL, Smidt GL, Johnston RC: The maximum torque generated by the eccentric, isometric, and concentric contractions of the hip abductor muscles, *Phys Ther* 52:149–158, 1972.
32. Papi E, Koh WS, McGregor AH: Wearable technology for spine movement assessment: a systematic review, *J Biomech* 64:186–197, 2017. https://doi.org/10.1016/j.jbiomech.2017.09.037.
33. Picerno P, Caliandro P, Iacovelli C, et al.: Upper limb joint kinematics using wearable magnetic and inertial measurement units: an anatomical calibration procedure based on bony landmark identification, *Sci Rep* 9:14449, 2019. https://doi.org/10.1038/s41598-019-50759-z.
34. Sandau M, Koblauch H, Moeslund TB, et al.: Markerless motion capture can provide reliable 3D gait kinematics in the sagittal and frontal plane, *Med Eng Phys* 36(9):1168–1175, 2014.
35. Schellenberg F, Oberhofer K, Taylor WR, et al.: Review of modelling techniques for in vivo muscle force estimation in the lower extremities during strength training, *Comput Math Methods Med* 2015:483921, 2015. https://doi.org/10.1155/2015/483921.
36. Shahabpoor E, Pavic A: Measurement of walking ground reactions in real-life environments: a systematic review of techniques and technologies, *Sensors* 17(9):2085, 2017. https://doi.org/10.3390/s17092085.
37. Sheerin KR, Besier TF, Reid D: The influence of running velocity on resultant tibial acceleration in runners, *Sports BioMech* 19:750–760, 2020. https://doi.org/10.1080/14763141.2018.1546890.
38. Sheerin KR, Reid D, Besier TF: The measurement of tibial acceleration in runners-a review of the factors that can affect tibial acceleration during running and evidence-based guidelines for its use, *Gait Posture* 67:12–24, 2019. https://doi.org/10.1016/j.gaitpost.2018.09.017.
39. Simoneau GG, Bereda SM, Sobush DC, et al.: Biomechanics of elastic resistance in therapeutic exercise programs, *J Orthop Sports Phys Ther* 31:16–24, 2001.
40. Simpkins C, Yang F: Muscle power is more important than strength in preventing falls in community-dwelling older adults, *J Biomech* 134:111018, 2022. https://doi.org/10.1016/j.jbiomech.2022.111018.
41. Steene-Johannessen J, Hansen BH, Dalene KE, et al.: Variations in accelerometry measured physical activity and sedentary time across Europe - harmonized analyses of 47,497 children and adolescents, *Int J Behav Nutr Phys Act* 17:38, 2020. https://doi.org/10.1186/s12966-020-00930-x.
42. Thomas M, Muller T, Busse MW: Quantification of tension in Thera-Band and Cando tubing at different strains and starting lengths, *J Sports Med Phys Fitness* 45:188–198, 2005.
43. Thomas SJ, Zeni JA, Winter DA: *Winter's biomechanics and motor control of human movement*, ed 5, Hoboken, NJ, 2022, John Wiley & Sons.
44. Valevicius AM, Jun PY, Hebert JS, et al.: Use of optical motion capture for the analysis of normative upper body kinematics during functional upper limb tasks: a systematic review, *J Electromyogr Kinesiol* 40:1–15, 2018. https://doi.org/10.1016/j.jelekin.2018.02.011.
45. Van den Berghe P, Six J, Gerlo J, et al.: Validity and reliability of peak tibial accelerations as real-time measure of impact loading during over-ground rearfoot running at different speeds, *J Biomech* 86:238–242, 2019. https://doi.org/10.1016/j.jbiomech.2019.01.039.
46. Zhu Z, Massimini DF, Wang G, et al.: The accuracy and repeatability of an automatic 2D-3D fluoroscopic image-model registration technique for determining shoulder joint kinematics, *Med Eng Phys* 34:1303–1309, 2012. https://doi.org/10.1016/j.medengphy.2011.12.021.
47. Zonta MB, Diaferia G, Pedroso JL, et al.: *Rehabilitation of ataxia, Movement disorders rehabilitation*, SpringerLink, 2017, pp 83–95.

STUDY QUESTIONS

1. The first set of questions expands on the concepts introduced in Special Focus 4.6. Referencing Fig. 4.16A, and assuming unchanging (submaximal) muscular effort:
   (a) Describe why internal torque would likely be reduced if the elbow were positioned in 110 degrees of flexion.
   (b) How does the external torque from gravity acting on the forearm-and-hand segment change if the elbow were to be positioned in 45 degrees of flexion?
2. The next set of questions expands on the concept of muscle coactivation introduced in Clinical Connection 4.3. Using Fig. 4.31B, what would happen to the magnitude of the external force (R) if:
   (c) F remained the same but E increased?
   (d) F remained the same but E decreased?
   (c) E remained the same but F increased?
   (d) E remained the same but F decreased?
3. How does an object's mass differ from its mass moment of inertia?
   (a) Provide an example of how the mass moment of inertia of a rotating limb could increase without an increase in its mass.
   (b) Describe a situation in which the mass moment of inertia of a rotating limb does not affect the force demands of the activated muscles.
4. Where is the approximate location of the center of mass of the human body in the anatomic position?
   (a) How would the location of the center of mass of the human body change if the arms were raised overhead?
   (b) How would the location of the center of mass of the human body change after a bilateral (transfemoral) amputation of the legs?
5. In which situation would a muscle produce a force across a joint that does not create a torque?

6. Fig. 4.29 shows two levels of external (knee flexion) torque produced by body weight. At what knee angle would the external torque at the knee:
   (a) Be reduced to zero?
   (b) Cause a flexion torque?
7. Severe arthritis of the hip can cause a bony remodeling of the femoral head and neck. In some cases, this remodeling reduces the internal moment arm of the hip abductors (D in Fig. 4.30).
   (a) In theory, while frontal plane rotary equilibrium around the right (stance) hip is maintained, how would a 50% reduction in internal moment arm affect the hip joint reaction force?
   (b) Assuming erosion of the articular surface of the femoral head, how would the reduction in internal moment arm affect the hip joint pressure?
8. Assume a person is preparing to quickly flex his hip while in a side-lying (essentially gravity-eliminated) position. What effect would keeping the knee extended have on the force requirements of the hip flexor muscles?
9. Assume the quadriceps muscle shown in Fig. 4.18A has an internal moment arm of 5 cm.
   (a) Based on the magnitude of the applied external torque, how much knee extensor muscle force is required to maintain static rotary equilibrium around the knee?
   (b) How much muscle force would be needed if the same external force (100 N) was applied 30 cm distal to the knee?
10. A therapist is helping a patient with weak quadriceps stand up from a standard chair. In preparation for this activity, the therapist often instructs the patient to bend as far forward from the hips as safely possible. How does this preparatory action likely increase the success of (or at least ease) the sit-to-stand activity?

STUDY QUESTIONS—cont'd

EXPANDED CLINICAL BIOMECHANICAL SCENARIOS
The following two sample biomechanical problems are similar to the three sample problems presented in this chapter. These problems are presented based on the assumption of static equilibrium. Selected parts of these problems require anthropometric data listed in the table in Appendix I, Part B.

11. The subject shown in Fig. 4.32 is performing a standing internal rotation exercise of the shoulder muscles against a resistance supplied by a cable attached to a wrist cuff. The exercise is based on isometric activation of the internal rotator muscles with the shoulder in 35 degrees of external rotation. The shoulder remains in neutral flexion-extension and abduction-adduction throughout the effort. Using the data provided in the box and the conversion factors in Table 4.2, determine the muscle force (M) and the joint reaction force (J) in newtons.

a) At what rotary (horizontal plane) position of the shoulder is the resistance (external) torque the greatest?

b) How can the subject's body be repositioned so that maximal resistance (external) torque occurs at (i) 70 degrees of external rotation and (ii) 30 degrees of internal rotation?

c) In previous problems encountered in this chapter, segment weight was included in the analyses of forces and torques. In this problem, does forearm-and-hand segment weight contribute to the horizontal plane torque (i.e., + z- and −z-directed torque)? Why or why not?

d) Consider the same exercise, but instead of standing, as in Fig. 4.32, assume the subject is positioned supine. How does the forearm-and-hand segment weight now contribute to + z- or −z-directed torque as the shoulder moves through complete internal and external range of motion?

Continued

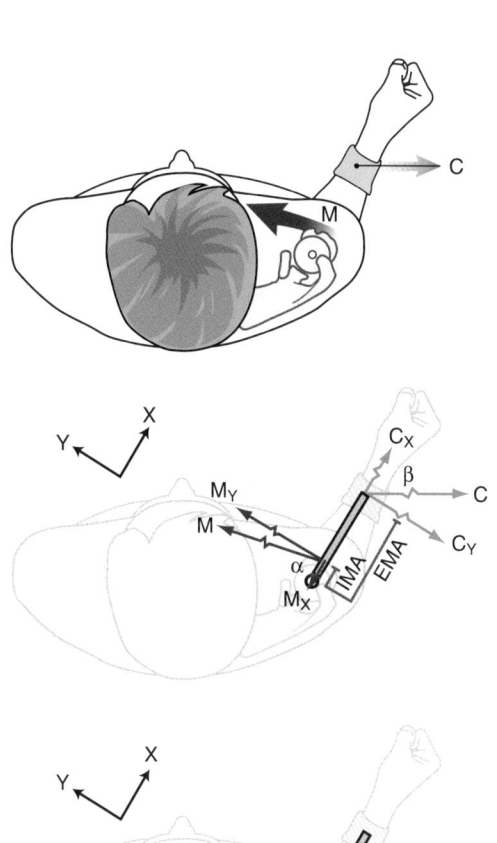

Angles:
  Angle-of-insertion of M to humerus (α) = 70°
  Angle between cable and X axis (β) = 55°
  Angle of J to X axis (μ) = unknown

Forces:
  Cable force (C) = 15 lbs
  Muscle force (M) = unknown
  Joint reaction force (J) at the shoulder = unknown

Moment arms:
  External moment arm to C_Y (EMA) = 8 inches
  Internal moment arm to M_Y (IMA) = 2.6 inches

FIGURE 4.32

STUDY QUESTIONS—cont'd

12. Fig. 4.33 is a sagittal plane view of a 180-pound subject performing shoulder flexion against the resistance supplied by an elastic band. Use the figure and data in the box to determine the muscle force (M) and the joint reaction force (J) in newtons.

This problem requires unit conversion using Table 4.2 and anthropometric information from Appendix I, Part B, Table I.2. For Table I.2, use the anthropometric data for "total arm" segment, even though this does not include the length of the hand. This "total arm" segment is referred to as the 60-cm

a) What part of the capsule of the glenohumeral joint is likely being most stressed by this exercise?

b) At what sagittal plane position of the shoulder is the external torque due to the total arm weight maximal?

c) At what sagittal plane position of the shoulder would the external moment arm of the elastic be maximal? Would this also be the position of maximal torque produced by the elastic? Why or why not?

d) While ignoring the weight of the upper limb, estimate the external torque produced in the −z(extension) direction through 0 to 180 degrees of flexion while using (a) a handheld weight of 27 N (about 6 lb) and (b) elastic force.

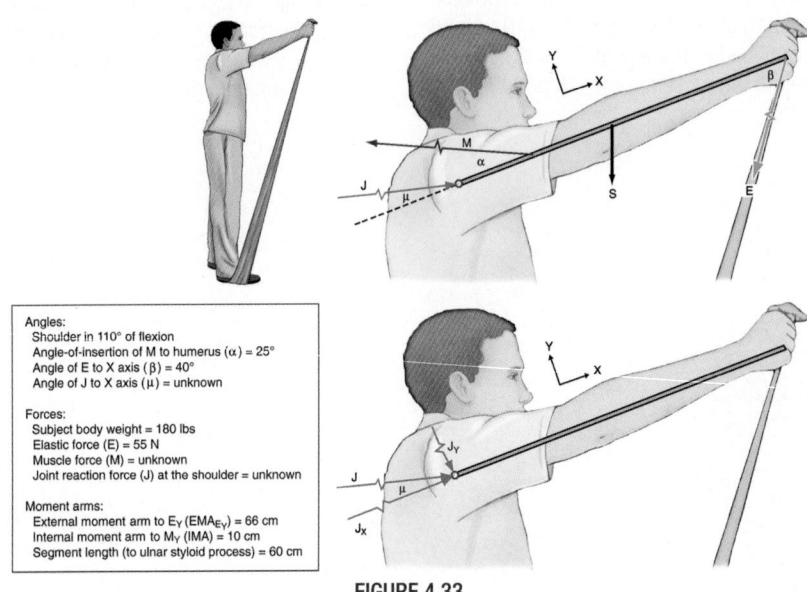

Angles:
    Shoulder in 110° of flexion
    Angle-of-insertion of M to humerus (α) = 25°
    Angle of E to X axis (β) = 40°
    Angle of J to X axis (μ) = unknown

Forces:
    Subject body weight = 180 lbs
    Elastic force (E) = 55 N
    Muscle force (M) = unknown
    Joint reaction force (J) at the shoulder = unknown

Moment arms:
    External moment arm to E_Y (EMA_{EY}) = 66 cm
    Internal moment arm to M_Y (IMA) = 10 cm
    Segment length (to ulnar styloid process) = 60 cm

FIGURE 4.33

Answers to the Study Questions can be found in the accompanying enhanced eBook version included with the print purchase of this textbook.

A P P E N D I X
I

Trigonometry Review and Anthropometric Data

Part A:
Basic Review of Right-Angle Trigonometry

Part B:
Anthropometric Data

Part A: Basic Review of Right-Angle Trigonometry

Trigonometric functions are based on the relationship that exists between the angles and sides of a right triangle. The sides of the triangle can represent distances, force magnitude, velocity, and other physical properties. Four of the common trigonometric functions used in quantitative analysis are found in Table I.1. Each trigonometric function has a specific value for a given angle. If the vectors representing two sides of a right triangle are known, the remaining side of the triangle can be determined by using the *Pythagorean theorem:* $a^2 = b^2 + c^2$, where a is the hypotenuse of the triangle. If one side and one angle other than the right angle are known, the remaining sides of the triangle can be determined by using one of the four trigonometric functions listed in the table paragraphs. Angles can be determined by knowing any two sides and using the inverse trigonometric functions (arcsine, arccosine, arctangent, and so on).

Fig. I.1 illustrates the use of trigonometry to determine the force components of the posterior deltoid muscle during its isometric activation. The angle-of-insertion (α) of the muscle with the bone is 45 degrees. Based on the chosen X-Y coordinate reference frame, the rectangular components of the muscle force (M) are designated as M_X (parallel with the arm) and M_Y (perpendicular to the arm). Given a muscle force of 200 N, M_Y and M_X can be determined as follows:

$$M_X = M \cos 45° = 200N \times 0.707 = -141.4N^*$$
$$M_Y = M \sin 45° = 200N \times 0.707 = 141.4N$$

If M_X and M_Y are known, M (hypotenuse) can be determined as follows, using the Pythagorean theorem:

$$M^2 = (M_X)^2 + (M_Y)^2$$
$$M = \sqrt{-141.4^2 + 141.4^2}$$
$$M = 200N$$

---

*The negative M_X value indicates that the force is directed *away from* the arrowhead of the X axis.

The rectangular components of *external forces,* such as those exerted by a wall pulley, by body weight, or by the clinician manually, are determined in a manner similar to that described for the muscle (internal) force.

Trigonometry can also be used to determine the magnitude of the resultant muscle force when one or more components and the angle-of-insertion (α in Fig. I.1) are known. Consider the same example as given in Fig. I.1, but now consider that the goal of the analysis is to determine the resultant muscle force of the posterior deltoid muscle if M_Y is known. As indicated in Fig. I.1, the direction (angle-of-insertion) of muscle (M) is 45 degrees relative to the X

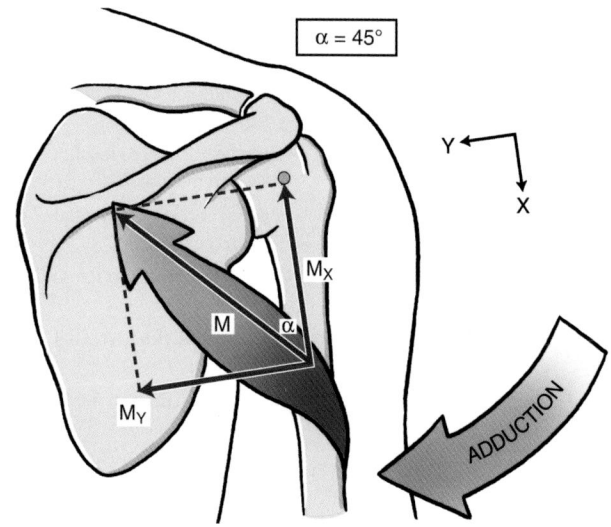

FIGURE I.1 Given the angle-of-insertion of the posterior deltoid (α = 45 degrees) and the resultant posterior deltoid muscle force (M), the two rectangular force components of the muscle force (M_X and M_Y) are determined using trigonometric relationships. The axis of rotation at the glenohumeral joint is indicated by the small circle at the head of the humerus.

TABLE I.1 Right-Angle Trigonometric Functions Commonly Used in Biomechanical Analysis

Trigonometric Function	Definition
Sine (sin) α	Side opposite/hypotenuse
Cosine (cos) α	Side adjacent/hypotenuse
Tangent (tan) α	Side opposite/side adjacent
Cotangent (cot) α	Side adjacent/side opposite

α, angle within a right triangle.

121

axis. The magnitude of the resultant muscle force (hypotenuse of the triangle) can be derived using the relationship of the rectangular components, as follows:

$$\sin 45° = M_Y/M$$
$$M = 141.4N/\sin 45°$$
$$M = 200N$$

The direction (angle-of-insertion) of M relative to the X axis can be mathematically verified by any one of several trigonometric functions, such as the inverse sine function. If only M_Y and M_X are known, the direction of M can be determined using the inverse tangent function. Note that the components of the force always have a magnitude less than the magnitude of the resultant force.

NOTE: Resultant forces can arise from any combination of positive- or negative-directed X and Y component forces. As such, unless one of the component forces is zero, *direction* cannot be described by simply assigning a positive or negative to the resultant force. For the purposes of this text, and particularly Chapter 4, the direction of the resultant force is expressed as the absolute *angle* relative to the X or Y axis of the reference frame. (Trigonometrically solved resultant forces or their angles that have a negative value may be considered positive.)

Part B: Anthropometric Data

TABLE I.2 Anthropometric Data Based on Body Segments' Weight and Center of Gravity Location in the Anatomic Position (Extremity Data are Unilateral Only)

Segment	Definition*	Segment Weight as a Percentage of Total Body Weight	Center of Gravity: Location from Proximal (or Cranial) End as a Percentage of Segment Length
Hand	Wrist axis to proximal interphalangeal (PIP) joint of third digit	0.6%	50.6%
Forearm	Elbow axis to ulnar styloid process	1.6%	43%
Upper arm	Glenohumeral axis to elbow axis	2.8%	43.6%
Forearm-and-hand	Elbow axis to ulnar styloid process	2.2%	68.2%
Total arm	Glenohumeral axis to ulnar styloid process	5%	53%
Foot	Lateral malleolus to head of second metatarsal	1.45%	50%
Shank (lower leg)	Femoral condyles to medial malleolus	4.65%	43.3%
Thigh	Greater trochanter to femoral condyles	10%	43.3%
Shank-and-foot	Femoral condyles to medial malleolus	6.1%	60.6%
Total leg	Greater trochanter to medial malleolus	16.1%	44.7%
Head-and-neck	Ear canal to C7–T1 (first rib)	8.1%	0% (at ear canal)
Trunk	Glenohumeral axis to greater trochanter	49.7%	50%
Trunk-head-and-neck	Glenohumeral axis to greater trochanter	57.8%	34%

*Even though some definitions listed in this table do not represent the endpoints of the segment, they are easily identified locations on the human. The values for segment weight and center of gravity location in this table take into consideration the discrepancy between the definition of the segment and the true endpoints. For example, the segment definition for the forearm is the same for the forearm-and-hand, but the percentages listed for the segment weight and center of gravity location of the forearm-and-hand are higher, taking into consideration the mass of the hand.

Compiled results in Winter DA: *Biomechanics and motor control of human movement,* ed 3, New York, 2005, John Wiley & Sons. Mass moments of inertia are not included in this table because the focus of this chapter is limited to static analysis.

Section
II

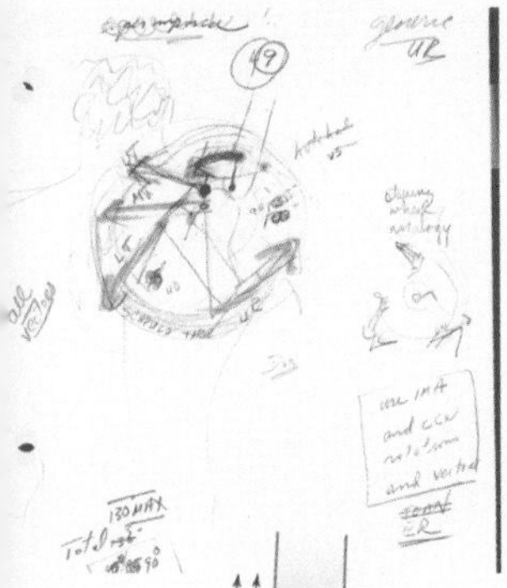

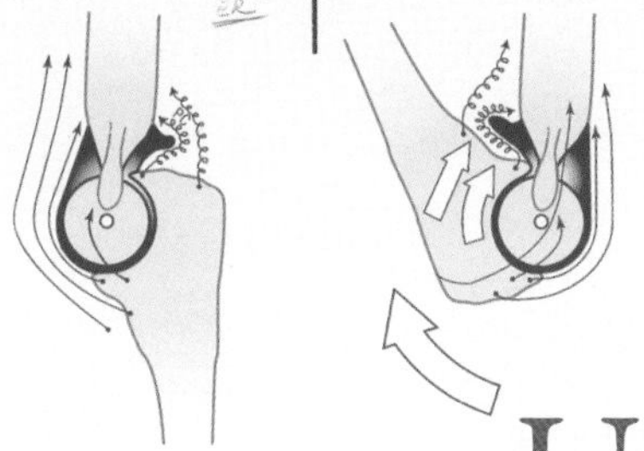

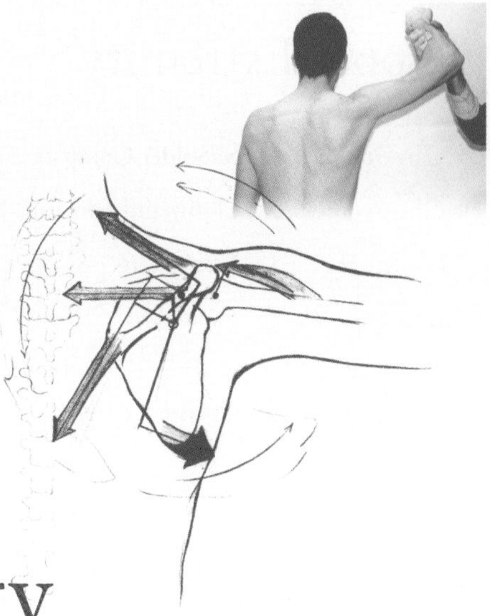

Upper Extremity

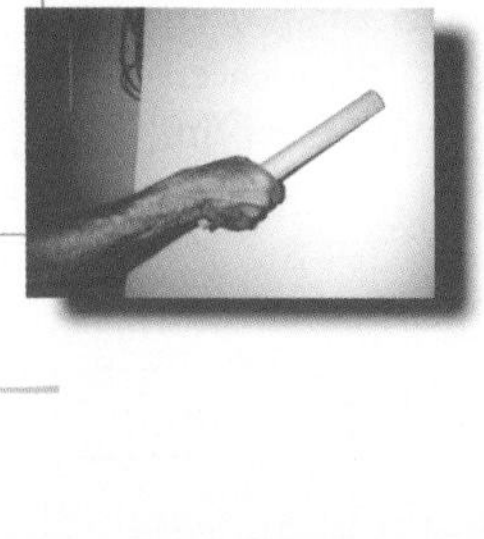

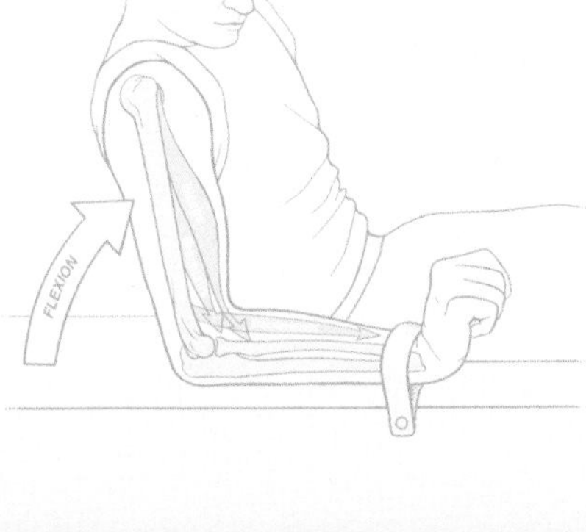

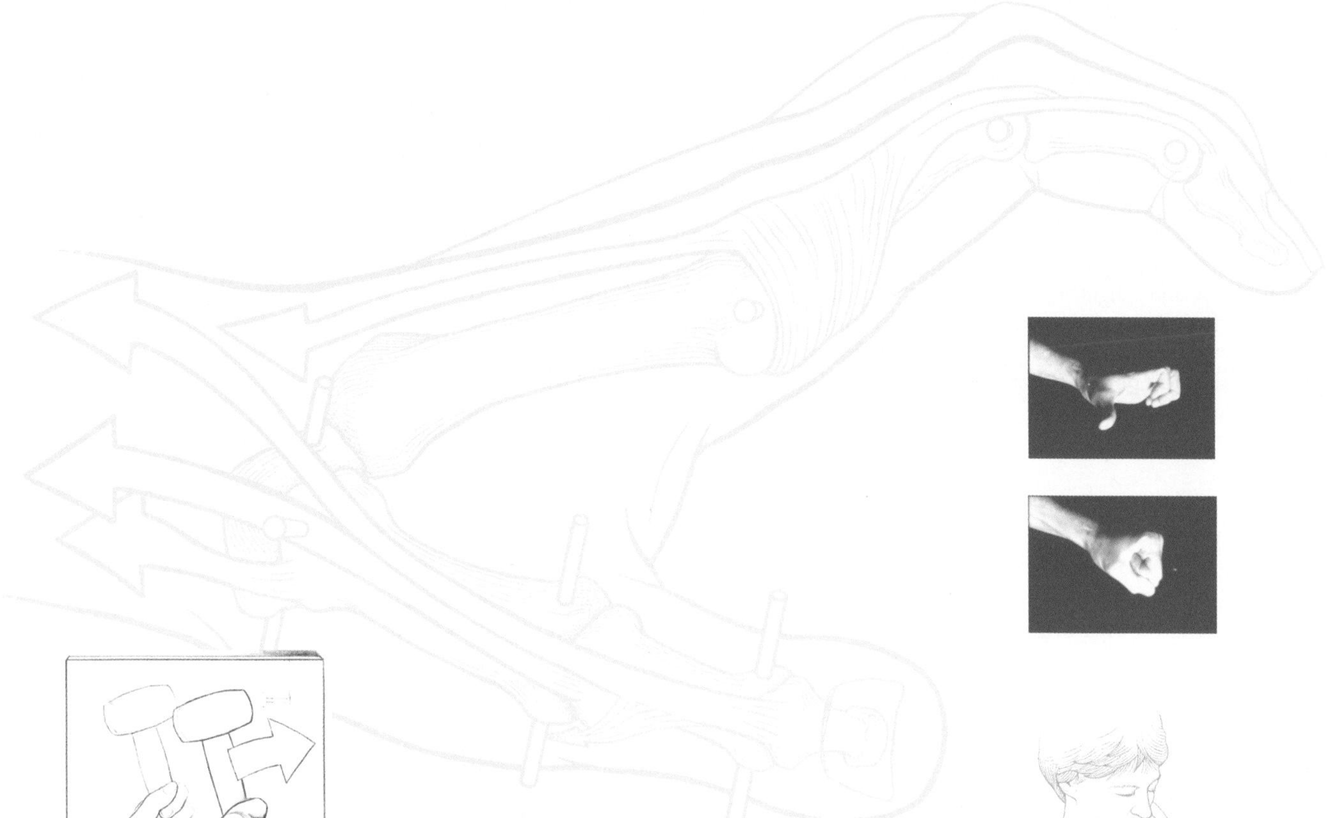

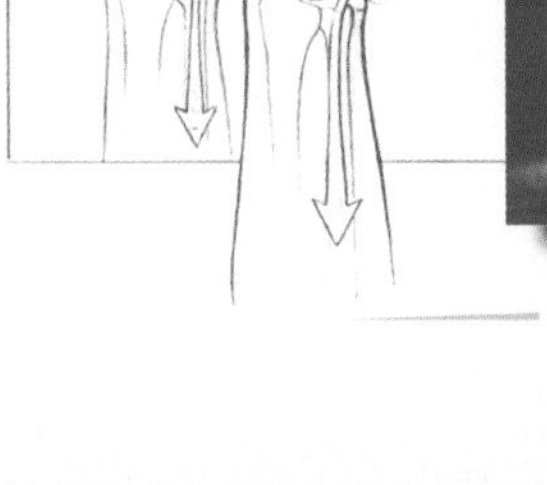

Section II

Upper Extremity

Section II is made up of four chapters, each describing the kinesiology of a major articular region within the upper extremity. Although presented as separate anatomic entities, the four regions cooperate functionally to place the hand in a position to interact with the environment most optimally. Disruption in the function of the muscles or joints of any region can greatly interfere with the capacity of the upper extremity as a whole. As described throughout Section II, impairments involving the muscles and joints of the upper extremity can significantly reduce the quality or the ease of performing many important activities related to personal care, livelihood, and recreation.

 EDUCATIONAL eCONTENT

Chapters 5-8 contain several videos and e-figures that are designed to enhance the understanding of the kinesiology presented within Section II. Material includes videos of fluoroscopy of joint movement, cadaver dissections and demonstrations, short lectures by the author, special teaching models (including a giant mechanical finger), examples of persons displaying abnormal kinesiology, methods which persons with spinal cord injury learn to perform certain movements despite varying levels of paralysis, and more.

Certain videos and e-figures relate specifically to the text material. Other materials, referred to as *additional video educational content*, are not indicated in the text, but are listed at the very end of each chapter.

How to view? The videos and e-figures are available in the accompanying enhanced eBook version included with the print purchase of this textbook. Visit Elsevier eBooks+ (eBooks.Health.Elsevier.com) to access this content.

 ADDITIONAL CLINICAL CONNECTIONS

Additional Clinical Connections are included at the end of each chapter. This feature is intended to highlight or expand on a particular clinical concept associated with the kinesiology covered in the chapter.

 STUDY QUESTIONS

Study Questions are also included at the end of each chapter. These questions are designed to challenge the reader to review or reinforce some of the main concepts contained within the chapter. The process of answering these questions is an effective way for students to prepare for examinations. The answers to the questions are available in the accompanying enhanced eBook version included with the print purchase of this textbook.

C h a p t e r

5

Shoulder Complex

DONALD A. NEUMANN, PT, PhD, FAPTA

CHAPTER AT A GLANCE

The study of the upper extremity begins with the *shoulder complex,* a set of four mechanically interrelated articulations involving the sternum, clavicle, ribs, scapula, and humerus (Fig. 5.1). These joints provide an extensive range of motion to the upper extremity, thereby increasing the ability to reach and manipulate objects. Reduced structural integrity within any single articulation can disrupt the functional fluidity and pain-free movement throughout the entire region. The muscles within the shoulder complex work in "teams" to produce highly coordinated actions that are expressed over multiple joints. The very cooperative nature among the muscles promotes versatility, control, and a wide range of active movements. Weakness or reduced activation of any single muscle, however, can disrupt the kinematic sequencing of the entire shoulder.

A thorough understanding of the musculoskeletal anatomy and mechanical basis for movement is essential for assessing and

determining the pathomechanical origins of movement impairments associated with the shoulder, as well as making informed decisions on effective treatment.

OSTEOLOGY

Sternum

The sternum consists of the manubrium, body, and xiphoid process (Fig. 5.2). The *manubrium* possesses a pair of oval-shaped *clavicular facets,* which articulate with the clavicles. The *costal facets* located on the lateral edge of the manubrium bilaterally provide attachment sites for the first two ribs. The *jugular notch* is located at the superior aspect of the manubrium, between the clavicular facets.

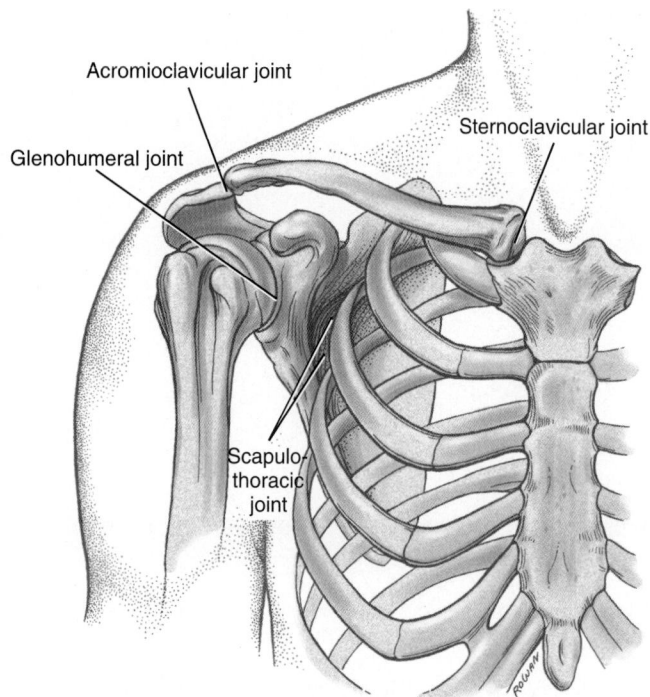

FIGURE 5.1 The joints of the right shoulder complex.

Osteologic Features of the Sternum
- Manubrium
- Clavicular facets
- Costal facets
- Jugular notch

Clavicle

A look from above reveals that the *shaft* of the clavicle is curved, with its anterior surface being generally convex medially and concave laterally (Fig. 5.3). With the arm at rest in the anatomic position, the long axis of the clavicle is oriented slightly above the horizontal plane and about 20 degrees posterior to the frontal plane (Fig. 5.4, angle A).[154] The rounded and prominent medial or *sternal end* of the clavicle articulates with the sternum (see Fig. 5.3). The *costal facet* of the clavicle (see Fig. 5.3; inferior surface) rests against the first rib. Lateral and slightly posterior to the costal facet is the distinct *costal tuberosity,* an attachment for the costoclavicular ligament.

Osteologic Features of the Clavicle
- Shaft
- Sternal end
- Costal facet
- Costal tuberosity
- Acromial end
- Acromial facet
- Conoid tubercle
- Trapezoid line

The lateral or *acromial end* of the clavicle articulates with the scapula at the oval-shaped *acromial facet* (Fig. 5.3; inferior surface).

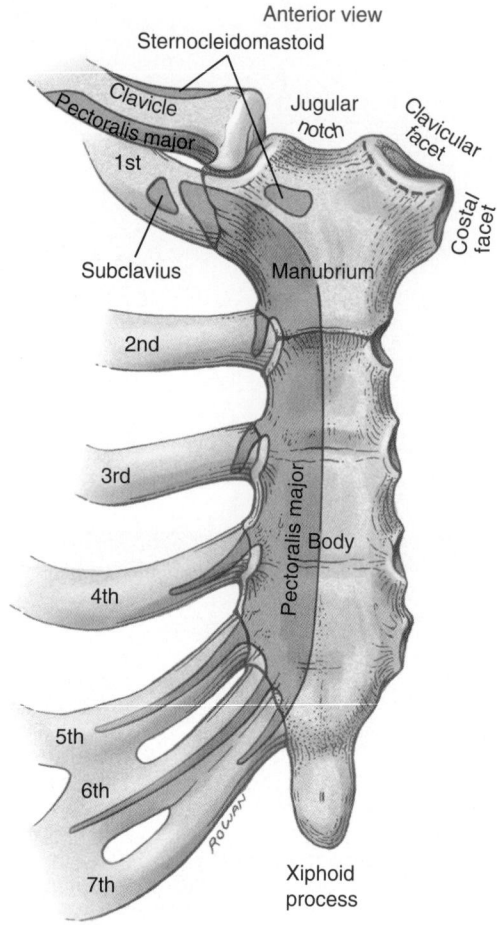

FIGURE 5.2 An anterior view of the sternum with left clavicle and ribs removed. The right side shows the first seven ribs and clavicle. The dashed line around the clavicular facet shows the attachments of the capsule at the sternoclavicular joint. Proximal attachments of muscle are shown in red.

The inferior surface of the lateral end of the clavicle is well marked by the *conoid tubercle* and the *trapezoid line*.

Scapula

The triangular-shaped scapula has three angles: *inferior, superior,* and *lateral* (see ahead Fig. 5.5). Palpation of the inferior angle provides a convenient method to follow the movement of the scapula during arm motion. The scapula also has three borders. With the arm resting by the side, the *medial border* runs almost parallel to the spinal column. The *lateral border* runs from the inferior angle to the lateral angle of the scapula. The *superior border* extends from the superior angle laterally toward the coracoid process.

The posterior surface of the scapula is separated into a *supraspinous fossa* and an *infraspinous fossa* by the prominent *spine*. The depth of the supraspinous fossa is filled by the supraspinatus muscle. The medial end of the spine diminishes in height at the *root of the spine*. In contrast, the lateral end of the spine gains considerable height and flattens into the broad and prominent *acromion* (from the Greek *akros,* meaning topmost, highest). The acromion extends in a lateral and anterior direction, forming a horizontal shelf over the glenoid fossa. The *clavicular facet* on the acromion forms part of the acromioclavicular joint (see ahead Fig. 5.16B).

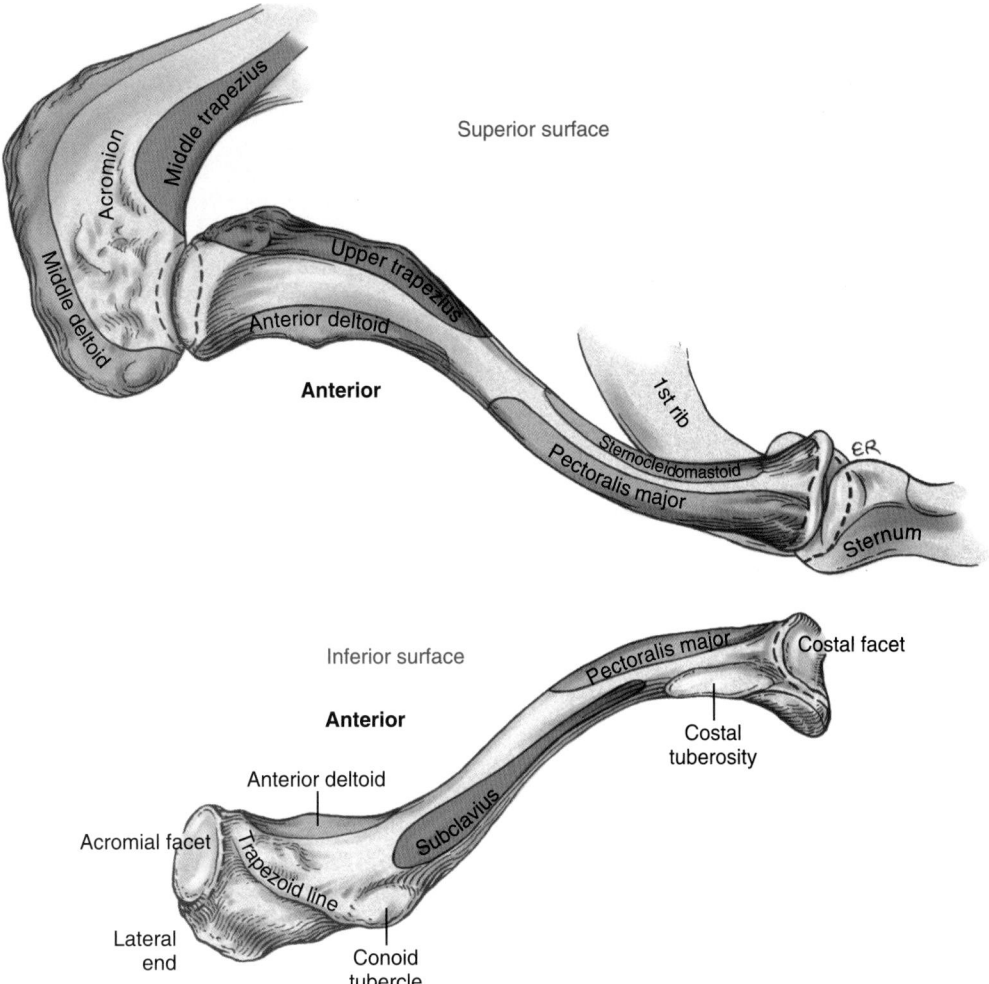

FIGURE 5.3 The superior and inferior surfaces of the right clavicle. The dashed line around the ends of the clavicle shows attachments of the joint capsule. Proximal attachments of muscles are shown in red, distal attachments in gray.

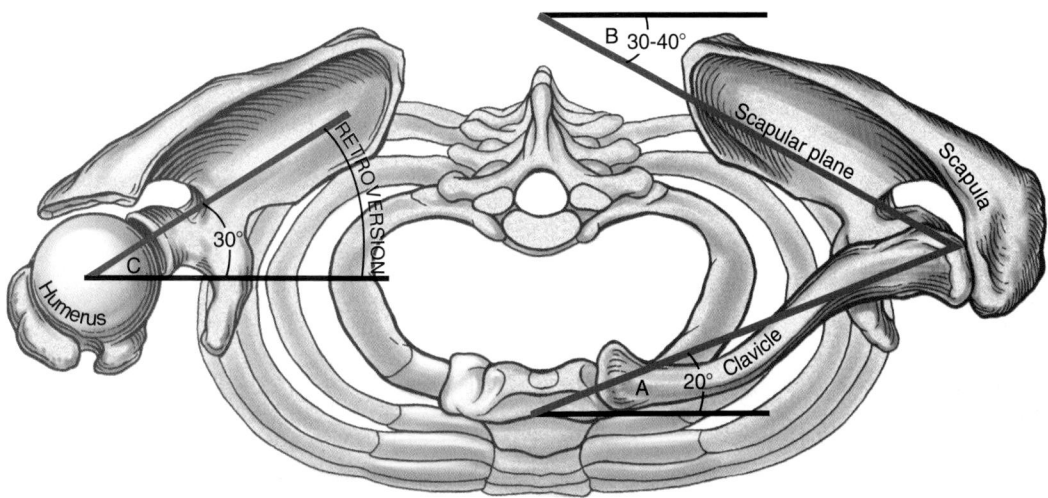

FIGURE 5.4 Superior view of both shoulders in the anatomic position. Angle A: The orientation of the clavicle deviated about 20 degrees posterior to the frontal plane. Angle B: The orientation of the scapula (scapular plane) deviated about 30 to 40 degrees anterior to the frontal plane. Angle C: Retroversion of the humeral head about 30 degrees posterior to the medial-lateral axis at the elbow. The right clavicle and acromion have been removed to expose the top of the right glenohumeral joint.

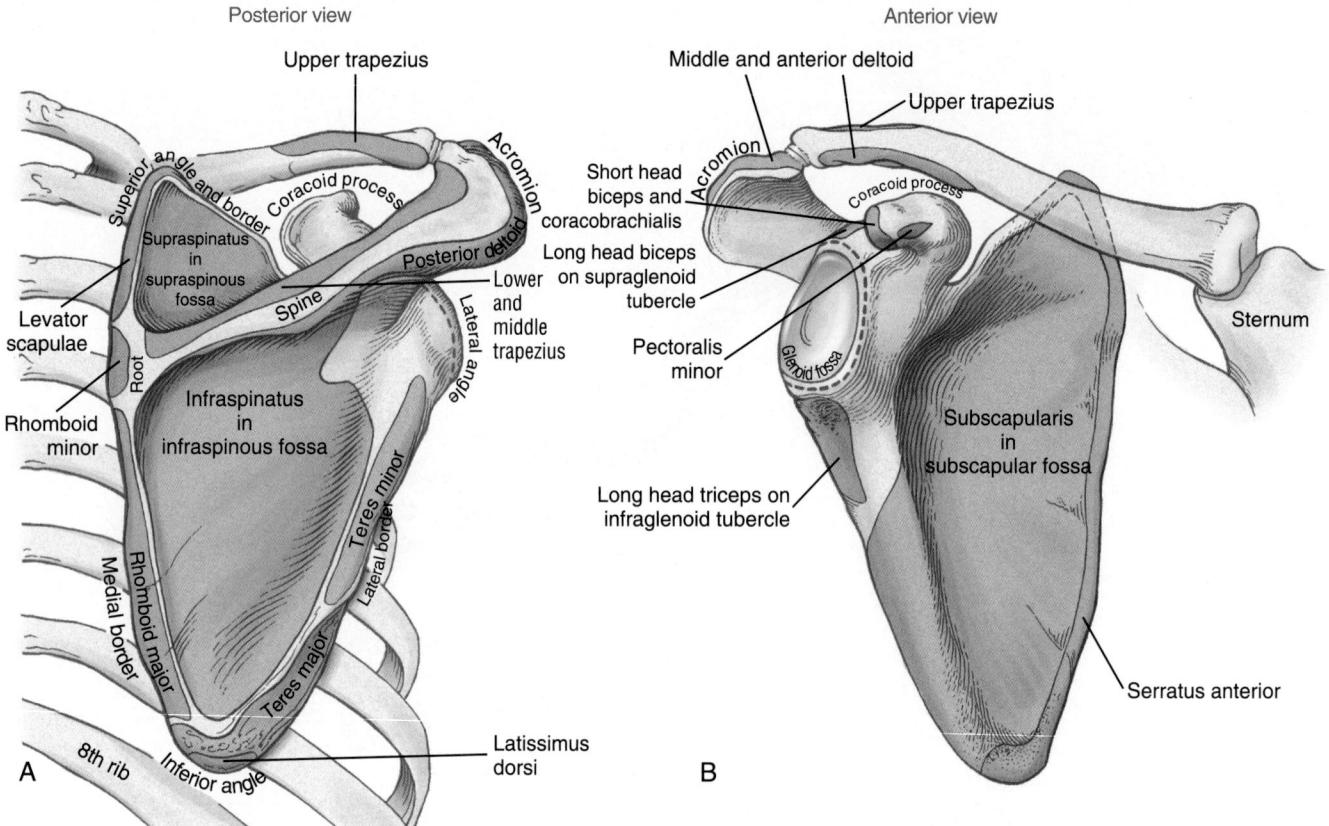

FIGURE 5.5 Posterior (A) and anterior (B) surfaces of the right scapula. Proximal attachments of muscles are shown in red, distal attachments in gray. The dashed lines show the capsular attachments around the glenohumeral joint.

Osteologic Features of the Scapula

- Angles: inferior, superior, and lateral
- Borders: medial, lateral, and superior
- Supraspinous fossa
- Infraspinous fossa
- Spine
- Root of the spine
- Acromion
- Clavicular facet
- Glenoid fossa
- Supraglenoid and infraglenoid tubercles
- Coracoid process
- Subscapular fossa

The scapula articulates with the head of the humerus at the slightly concave *glenoid fossa* (from the Greek root *glene,* socket of joint, and *eidos,* resembling) (Fig. 5.5B). The slope of the glenoid fossa is inclined upward about 4 degrees relative to a horizontal axis through the body of the scapula.[39] This inclination is highly variable, ranging from a downward inclination of 7 degrees to an upward inclination of nearly 16 degrees. At rest in the anatomic position, the scapula is typically positioned flush against the posterior-lateral surface of the thorax, with the glenoid fossa facing about 30 to 40 degrees anterior to the frontal plane (see Fig. 5.4, angle B). This orientation of the scapula is referred to as the *scapular plane.* The scapula and humerus tend to follow this plane when the arm is naturally raised overhead.

Located at the superior and inferior rim of the glenoid fossa are the *supraglenoid* and *infraglenoid tubercles.* These tubercles serve as the proximal attachments for the long head of the biceps and triceps brachii, respectively (Fig. 5.5B). Near the superior rim of the glenoid fossa is the prominent *coracoid process,* meaning "the shape of a crow's beak." The coracoid process projects sharply from the scapula, providing multiple attachments for ligaments and muscles (Fig. 5.6). The *subscapular fossa* is located on the anterior surface of the scapula (Fig. 5.5B). The concavity within the fossa is filled with the thick subscapularis muscle.

Proximal-to-Mid Humerus

The *head of the humerus,* nearly one half of a sphere, forms the convex component of the glenohumeral joint (Fig. 5.7). The head faces medially and superiorly, forming an approximate 135-degree angle of inclination with the long axis of the humeral shaft (see Fig. 5.8A). Relative to a medial-lateral axis through the elbow, the humeral head in the adult is normally rotated (or twisted) posteriorly about 30 degrees within the horizontal plane (see Fig. 5.8B). This rotation, known as *retroversion,* naturally aligns the humeral head within the scapular plane for articulation with the glenoid fossa (see Fig. 5.4, angle C). Interestingly, when an individual is less than about 4 years old, humeral retroversion is approximately 65 degrees, but it naturally "de-rotates" (decreases) to its final 30-degree adult angle by about 16 to 20 years of age.[64,127,243] Excessive torsional stress on the proximal physis (growth plate) of the humerus well prior to this age can influence the final expression of retroversion as an adult. For

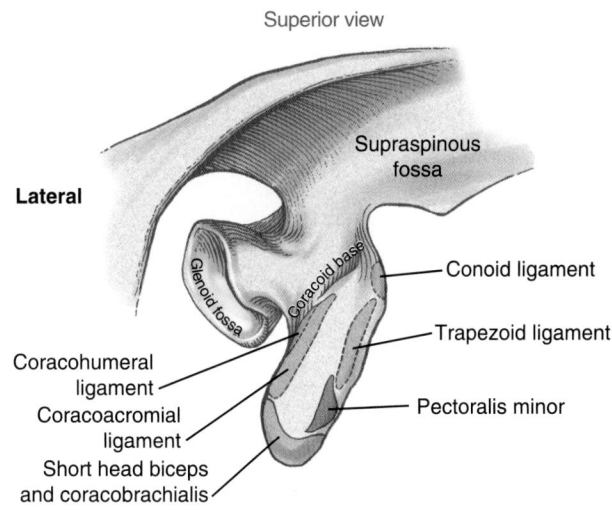

FIGURE 5.6 A close-up view of the right coracoid process seen from above. Proximal attachments of muscle are in red, distal attachments in gray. Ligamentous attachment is indicated by light blue outlined by dashed line.

example, torsional stress placed on the arms of young, elite overhead baseball pitchers secondary to repetitive external rotation *inhibits* the natural reduction of retroversion.[213,243,272] Studies consistently show that the dominant shoulder in skeletally mature, elite baseball pitchers has about 10 to 15 degrees *more* humeral retroversion than the nondominant limb.[192,249] The likelihood of these players developing excessive retroversion is believed to be greater if they started pitching before about 11 years of age.[132,243]

The *anatomic neck* of the humerus separates the smooth articular surface of the head from the proximal shaft (see Fig. 5.7A). The prominent lesser and greater tubercles surround the anterior and lateral circumference of the extreme proximal end of the humerus (Fig. 5.7B). The *lesser tubercle* projects rather sharply and anteriorly for attachment of the subscapularis. The large and rounded *greater tubercle* has *upper, middle,* and *lower facets,* marking the primary distal attachments of the supraspinatus, infraspinatus, and teres minor, respectively (see Fig. 5.7B and Fig. 5.9).

Sharp *crests* extend distally several centimeters from the anterior side of the greater and lesser tubercles. These crests receive the distal attachments of the pectoralis major and teres major (Fig. 5.7A). Between these crests is the *intertubercular (bicipital) groove,* which houses the tendon of the long head of the biceps brachii. The latissimus dorsi muscle attaches to the floor of the intertubercular groove, immediately medial to the biceps tendon. Distal and lateral to the termination of the intertubercular groove is the *deltoid tuberosity.*

> **Osteologic Features of the Proximal-to-Mid Humerus**
> - Head of the humerus
> - Anatomic neck
> - Lesser tubercle and crest
> - Greater tubercle and crest
> - Upper, middle, and lower facets on the greater tubercle
> - Intertubercular (bicipital) groove
> - Deltoid tuberosity
> - Radial (spiral) groove

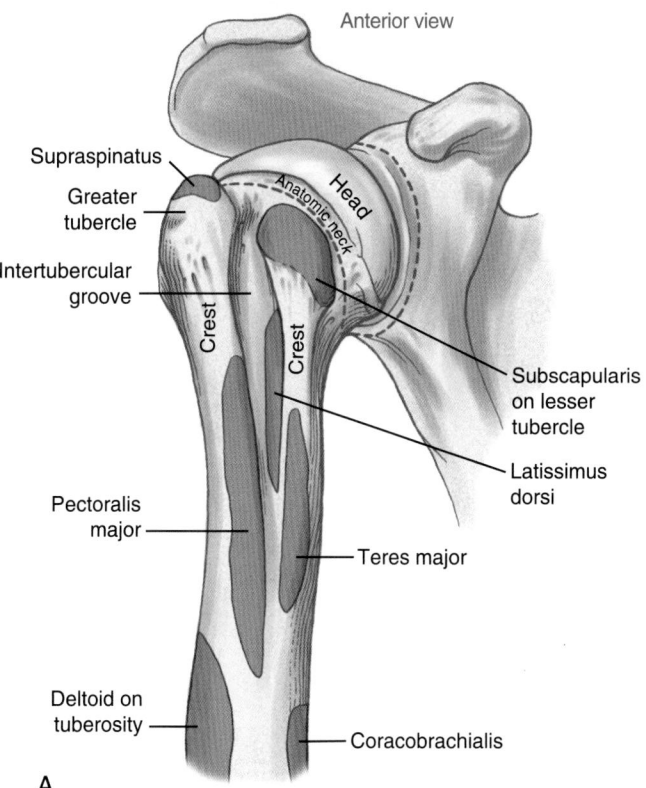

A

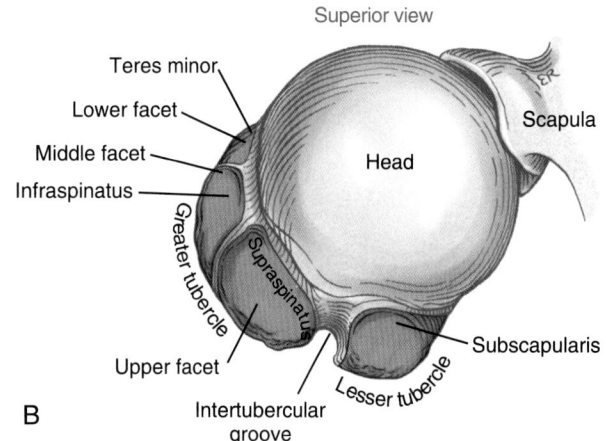

B

FIGURE 5.7 Anterior (A) and superior (B) aspects of the right humerus. The dashed line in (A) shows the capsular attachments around the glenohumeral joint. Distal attachment of muscles is shown in gray.

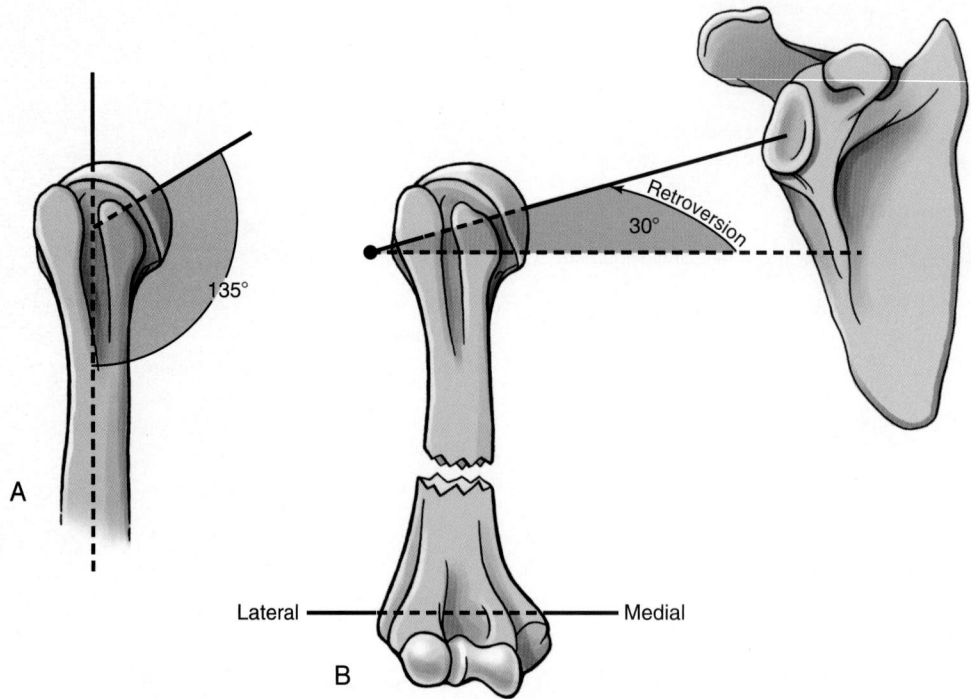

FIGURE 5.8 The right humerus showing a 135-degree "angle of inclination" between the shaft and head of the humerus in the frontal plane (A) and the retroversion of the humeral head relative to the distal humerus (B).

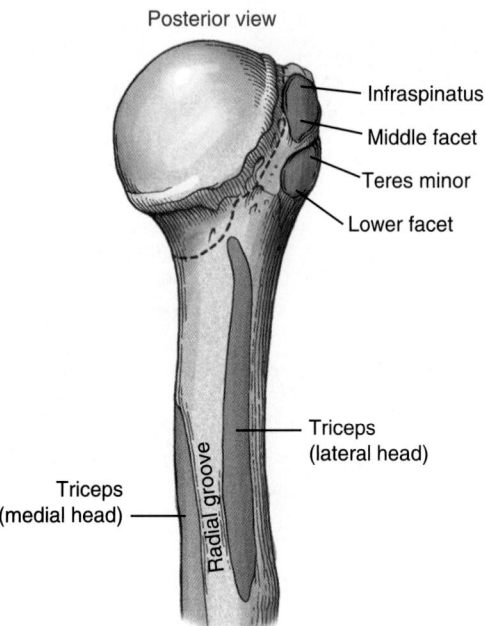

FIGURE 5.9 Posterior aspect of the right proximal humerus. Proximal attachments of muscles are in red, distal attachments in gray. The dashed line shows the capsular attachments of the glenohumeral joint.

The *radial (spiral) groove* runs obliquely across the posterior surface of the humerus. The groove separates the proximal attachments of the lateral and medial heads of the triceps (Fig. 5.9). Traveling distally, the radial nerve spirals around the posterior side of the humerus in the radial groove, heading toward the distal-lateral side of the humerus. The oblique path of the radial groove and its

contained nerve may be explained as a physical remnant of the natural de-rotation of the excessively retroverted humerus present in early life.[64]

ARTHROLOGY

The most proximal articulation within the shoulder complex is the *sternoclavicular joint* (see Fig. 5.1). The clavicle, through its attachment to the sternum, functions as a mechanical strut, or prop, holding the scapula at a relatively constant distance from the midline of the body.[35] Located at the lateral end of the clavicle is the *acromioclavicular joint* which firmly suspends the scapula from the clavicle. The anterior surface of the scapula rests snugly against the slightly curved posterior-lateral surface of the thorax, forming the *scapulothoracic joint*. This articulation is not a true anatomic joint; rather, it is an interface between bones. Movements at the scapulothoracic joint are mechanically linked to the movements at both the sternoclavicular and the acromioclavicular joints. The position of the scapula on the thorax provides a base of operation for the *glenohumeral joint,* the most distal and mobile link of the complex. The term "shoulder movement" describes the combined motions at both the glenohumeral and the scapulothoracic joints.

Four Joints within the Shoulder Complex

- Sternoclavicular
- Acromioclavicular
- Scapulothoracic
- Glenohumeral

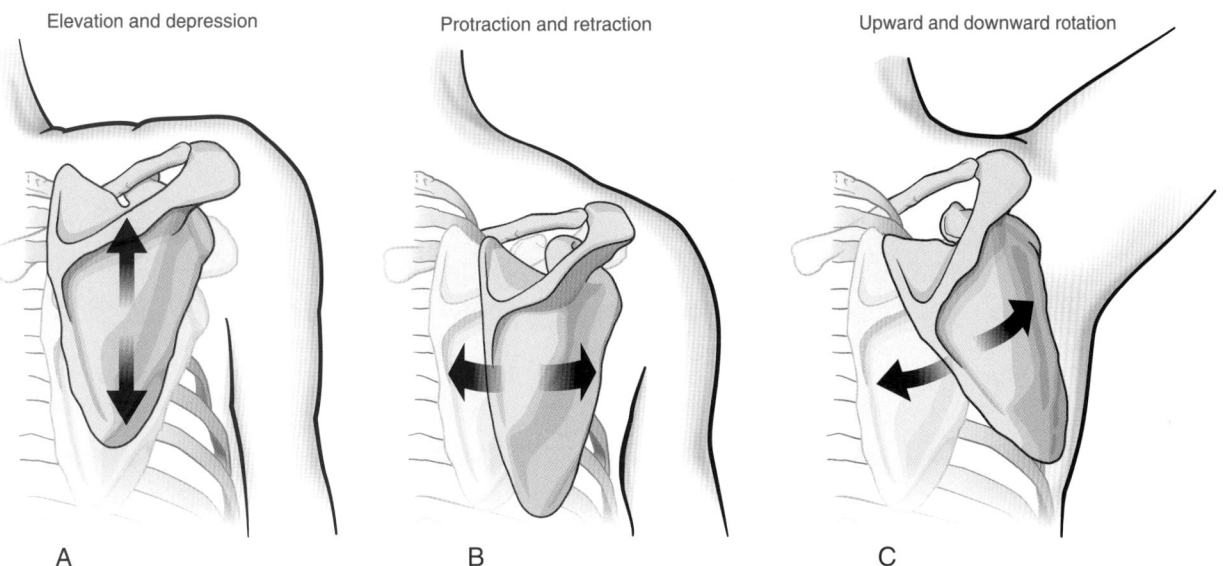

Elevation and depression   Protraction and retraction   Upward and downward rotation

A   B   C

FIGURE 5.10 Motions of the right scapulothoracic joint. (A) Elevation and depression. (B) Protraction and retraction. (C) Upward and downward rotation.

The joints of the shoulder complex function as a series of kinematic links, all cooperating to maximize the range of motion available to the upper limb. A weakened, painful, or unstable link anywhere along the chain significantly decreases the effectiveness of the entire complex and arguably the entire upper limb.

Before the kinematics of the sternoclavicular and acromioclavicular joints are described, the primary movements at the scapulothoracic joint must be defined (Fig. 5.10). These movements, defined in the box below, are elevation and depression, protraction and retraction, and upward and downward rotation. More subtle rotations of the scapula will be introduced as the chapter unfolds.

Terminology Describing the Primary Movements at the Scapulothoracic Joint

Elevation—The scapula slides superiorly on the thorax, as when "shrugging the shoulders."

Depression—From an elevated position, the scapula slides inferiorly on the thorax.

Protraction—The medial border of the scapula slides anterior-laterally on the thorax away from the midline, as when maximizing forward reach.

Retraction—The medial border of the scapula slides posterior-medially on the thorax toward the midline, as when "pinching the shoulder blades" together.

Upward rotation—The inferior angle of the scapula rotates in a superior-lateral direction, facing the glenoid fossa upward. This rotation occurs as a natural component of raising the arm upward.

Downward rotation—From an upward rotated position, the inferior angle of the scapula rotates in an inferior-medial direction. This motion occurs as a natural component of lowering the arm down to the side.

Sternoclavicular Joint

GENERAL FEATURES

The sternoclavicular (SC) joint is a complex articulation, involving the medial end of the clavicle, the clavicular facet on the sternum, and the superior border of the cartilage of the first rib (see Fig. 5.11). The SC joint functions as the *basilar joint* of the entire upper extremity, linking the appendicular skeleton with the axial skeleton. The joint thus needs to be stable enough to withstand high loads even as it allows a considerable range of shoulder movement. These seemingly paradoxical functions are accomplished through extensive periarticular connective tissues and an irregular saddle-shaped articular surface (see Fig. 5.12). Although highly variable, the medial end of the clavicle is usually convex along its longitudinal diameter and slightly concave along its transverse diameter.[233] The clavicular facet on the sternum typically is reciprocally shaped, with a slightly concave longitudinal diameter and a slightly convex transverse diameter.

PERIARTICULAR CONNECTIVE TISSUE

The SC joint is enclosed by a relatively thick capsule reinforced by *anterior* and *posterior sternoclavicular ligaments* (see Fig. 5.11). When active, muscles add further stability to the joint: anteriorly by the sternocleidomastoid, posteriorly by the sternothyroid and sternohyoid, and inferiorly by the subclavius. The *interclavicular ligament* spans the jugular notch, connecting the medial end of the right and left clavicles.

Tissues That Stabilize the Sternoclavicular Joint

- Anterior and posterior sternoclavicular joint ligaments
- Interclavicular ligament
- Costoclavicular ligament
- Articular disc
- Sternocleidomastoid, sternothyroid, sternohyoid, and subclavius muscles

---

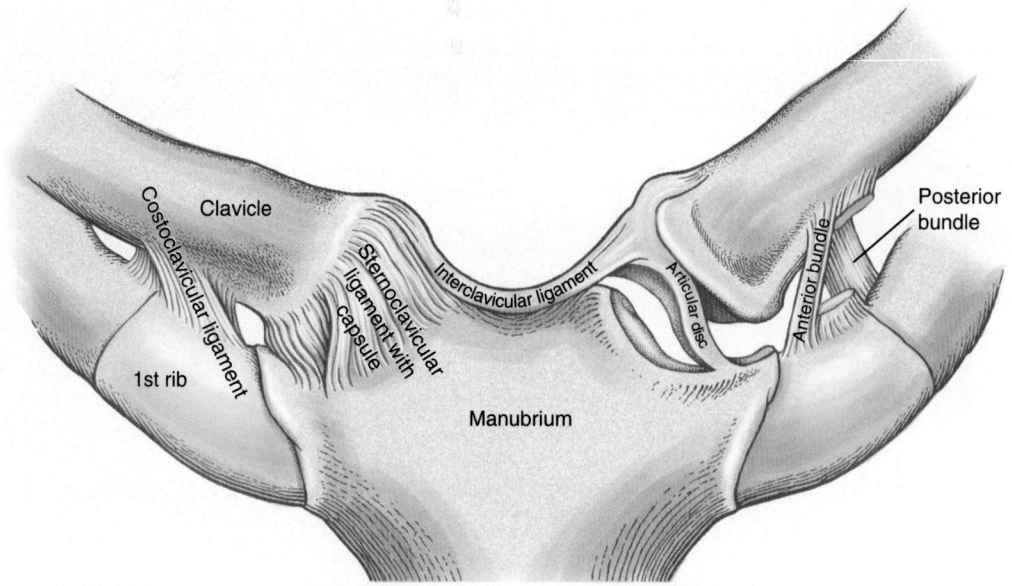

FIGURE 5.11 The sternoclavicular joints. The capsule and lateral section of the anterior bundle of the costo-clavicular ligament have been removed on the left side.

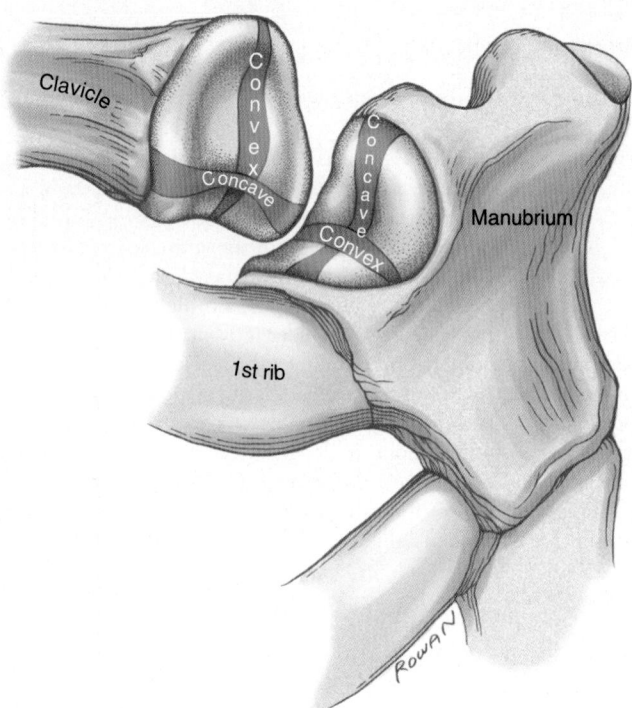

FIGURE 5.12 An anterior-lateral view of the articular surfaces of the right sternoclavicular joint. The joint has been opened up to expose its articular surfaces. The longitudinal diameters *(purple)* extend roughly in the frontal plane between superior and inferior points of the articular surfaces. The transverse diameters *(blue)* extend roughly in the horizontal plane between anterior and posterior points of the articular surfaces.

The *costoclavicular ligament* is a strong structure extending from the cartilage of the first rib to the costal tuberosity on the inferior surface of the clavicle. The ligament has two distinct fiber bundles running perpendicular to each other.[233] The anterior bundle runs obliquely in a superior and lateral direction, and the posterior bundle runs obliquely in a superior and medial direction (Fig. 5.11). The crisscrossing of fibers assists with stabilizing the joint through

all motions, except for a downward movement of the clavicle (i.e., depression).

An *articular disc* exists at the SC joint; however, the disc was found to be fully formed in only about 50% of a sample of cadaver specimens.[253] When fully formed, the disc separates the joint into distinct medial and lateral joint cavities (Fig. 5.11). Typically, the disc appears as a flattened piece of fibrocartilage that attaches inferiorly near the lateral edge of the clavicular facet and superiorly at the sternal end of the clavicle and interclavicular ligament. The remaining outer edge of the disc attaches to the internal surface of the capsule. The disc not only strengthens the articulation but functions as a shock absorber by increasing the surface area of joint contact. This absorption mechanism apparently works well because significant age-related degenerative arthritis is relatively rare at this joint.[56]

The SC joint is remarkably mechanically stable owing to the combination of periarticular connective tissues, muscles, and the interlocking of the articular surfaces. Traumatic dislocation of the SC joint is a rare orthopedic event;[222] large external forces on the clavicle often fracture the midshaft of the bone before the SC joint dislocates.

KINEMATICS

The osteokinematics of the clavicle involve rotations in three degrees of freedom about the SC joint. The clavicle can (1) elevate or depress, (2) protract or retract, or (3) rotate about the bone's longitudinal axis (Fig. 5.13). In conjunction with the acromioclavicular joint, specific combinations of these clavicular movements place the glenoid fossa of the scapula in a position to maximize its mechanical engagement with the head of the humerus. As described later in this chapter, the clavicle moves in all three degrees of freedom as the arm is raised overhead.

Elevation and Depression

Elevation and depression of the clavicle occur approximately parallel to the frontal plane, about a near anterior-posterior axis of rotation through the medial end of the clavicle (see Fig. 5.13). Maximum angles of approximately 35 to 45 degrees of elevation and 10 degrees

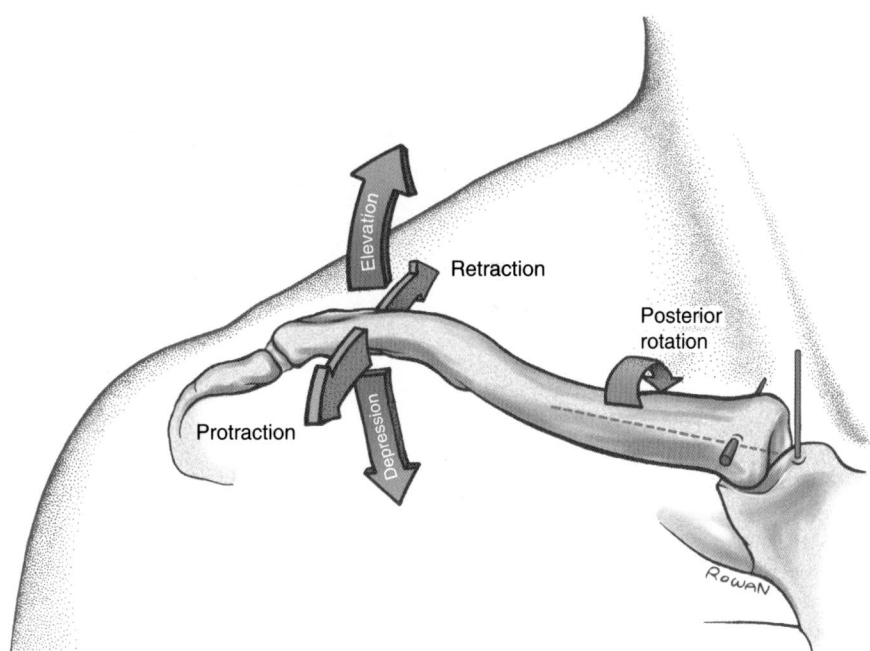

FIGURE 5.13 The osteokinematics of the right sternoclavicular joint. The motions are elevation and depression in a near frontal plane *(purple),* protraction and retraction in a near horizontal plane *(blue),* and posterior clavicular rotation in a near sagittal plane *(green).* The vertical and anterior-posterior axes of rotation are color-coded with the corresponding planes of movement. The longitudinal axis is indicated by the dashed green line.

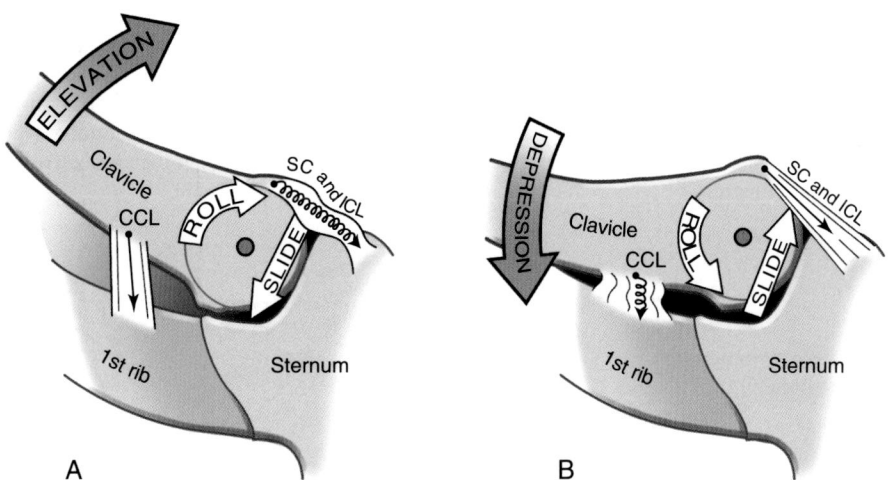

FIGURE 5.14 Anterior view of a mechanical diagram of the arthrokinematics of roll and slide during elevation (A) and depression (B) of the clavicle around the right sternoclavicular joint. The axes of rotation are shown in the anterior-posterior direction near the head of the clavicle. Stretched structures are shown as thin elongated arrows; slackened structures are shown as wavy arrows. Note in (A) that the stretched costoclavicular ligament produces a downward force in the direction of the slide. *CCL,* costoclavicular ligament; *ICL,* interclavicular ligament; *SC,* superior capsule.

of depression have been reported.[43,177] Elevation and depression of the clavicle help guide the path of movement of the scapula on the thorax.

The arthrokinematics for elevation and depression of the clavicle occur along the SC joint's longitudinal diameter (Fig. 5.12). *Elevation* of the clavicle occurs as the bone's convex articular surface rolls superiorly and simultaneously slides inferiorly on the concavity of the sternum (Fig. 5.14A). The stretched costoclavicular ligament helps limit and stabilize the elevated position of the clavicle. *Depression* of the clavicle occurs by the action of its convex surface rolling inferiorly and sliding superiorly (Fig. 5.14B). A fully depressed clavicle elongates and stretches the interclavicular ligament and the superior portion of the capsular ligaments.

Protraction and Retraction

Protraction and retraction of the clavicle occur nearly parallel to the horizontal plane, around a near vertical axis of rotation (see Fig. 5.13). (The axis of rotation is shown in Fig. 5.13 as intersecting the sternum because, by convention, the axis of rotation for a given motion intersects the *convex* member of the joint.) Maximum values of 15 to 30 degrees of motion have been reported in each direction.[43,177,235] The horizontal plane motions of the clavicle are strongly associated with protraction and retraction motions of the scapula relative to the thorax.

The arthrokinematics for protraction and retraction of the clavicle occur along the SC joint's transverse diameter (see Fig. 5.12). Retraction occurs as the concave articular surface of the clavicle rolls and slides posteriorly on the convex surface of the sternum (Fig. 5.15). The end ranges of retraction elongate the anterior bundles of the costoclavicular ligament and the anterior capsular ligaments.

The arthrokinematics of protraction around the SC joint are like those of retraction, except that they occur in an anterior direction. The extremes of protraction occur during a motion involving maximal forward reach. Excessive tightness in the posterior bundle of the costoclavicular ligament, the posterior capsular ligament of the SC joint, and the scapular retractor muscles can limit full clavicular protraction.

Axial (Longitudinal) Rotation of the Clavicle

The third degree of freedom at the SC joint is a rotation of the clavicle around the bone's longitudinal axis (see Fig. 5.13). As one raises the arm overhead (i.e., during shoulder abduction or flexion), a point on the superior aspect of the clavicle rotates *posteriorly* 20 to 35 degrees.[105,138,154,252] As the arm is returned to the side, the clavicle rotates back to its original position. The arthrokinematics of clavicular rotation involve a *spin* of its sternal end relative to the lateral surface of the articular disc.

Axial rotation of the clavicle is mechanically linked or coupled with the overall kinematics of abduction or flexion of the shoulder and cannot be independently performed with the arm resting at the side. The complex mechanics of this motion are further described later in this section on shoulder kinematics.

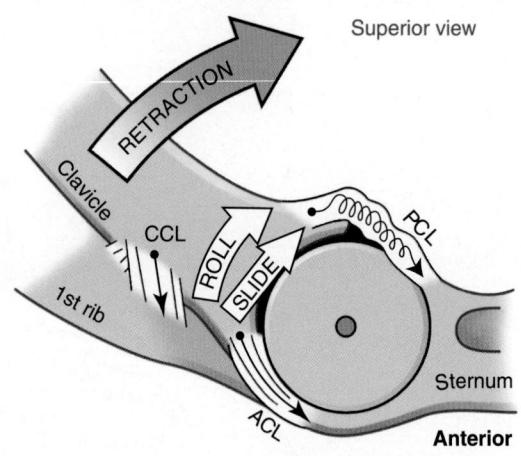

FIGURE 5.15 Superior view of a mechanical diagram of the arthrokinematics of roll and slide during retraction of the clavicle around the right sternoclavicular joint. The vertical axis of rotation is shown through the sternum. Stretched structures are shown as thin elongated arrows; slackened structure is shown as a wavy arrow. *ACL,* anterior capsular ligament; *CCL,* costoclavicular ligament; *PCL,* posterior capsular ligaments.

Acromioclavicular Joint

GENERAL FEATURES

The acromioclavicular (AC) joint is the articulation between the lateral end of the clavicle and the acromion of the scapula (Fig. 5.16A). The clavicular facet on the acromion typically faces medially and slightly superiorly, providing a point of attachment with the corresponding acromial facet on the clavicle.

The AC joint is a gliding or plane joint, reflecting the generally flat contour of the joint surfaces.[42] Joint surface shapes vary, however, from flat to slightly convex or concave (Fig. 5.16B).[233] Because of the predominance of flat joint surfaces, roll-and-slide arthrokinematics are not described here.

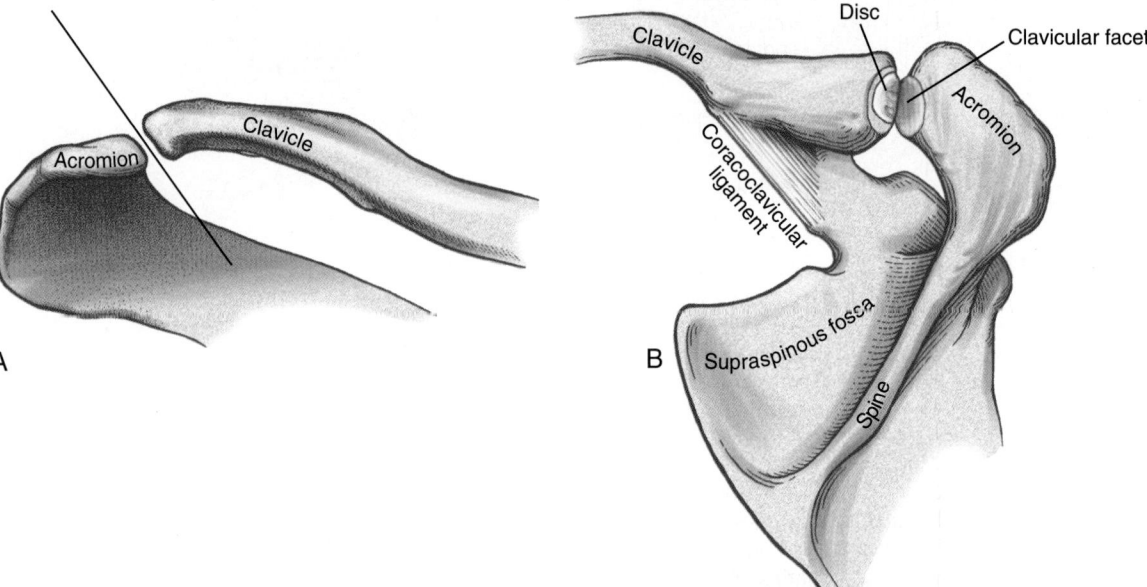

FIGURE 5.16 The right acromioclavicular joint. (A) An anterior view showing the sloping nature of the articulation. (B) A posterior view of the joint opened up, showing the clavicular facet on the acromion and the fragmented disc.

PERIARTICULAR CONNECTIVE TISSUE

The capsule of the AC joint is reinforced by *superior and inferior* ligaments (Fig. 5.17). The thicker superior ligament is reinforced through fascia from the deltoid and trapezius.[50,185,233]

The *coracoclavicular ligament* provides an important extrinsic source of stability to the AC joint (see Fig. 5.17).[188] This extensive ligament consists of two parts: the trapezoid and conoid ligaments.[233] The *trapezoid ligament* extends in a superior-lateral direction from the superior surface of the coracoid process to the trapezoid line on the clavicle. The *conoid ligament* extends almost vertically from the proximal base of the coracoid process to the conoid tubercle on the clavicle.

Tissues That Stabilize the Acromioclavicular Joint
- Acromioclavicular joint capsular ligaments
- Coracoclavicular ligament
- Deltoid and upper trapezius

Both parts of the coracoclavicular ligament are of similar length, cross-sectional area, stiffness, and tensile strength.[48] The ligament is stronger and absorbs more energy at the point of rupture than most other ligaments of the shoulder. These structural features, in conjunction with the coracoclavicular ligament's near-vertical orientation, suggest an important role in superior-inferior stabilization of the joint and in securely suspending the scapula (and upper extremity) from the clavicle.

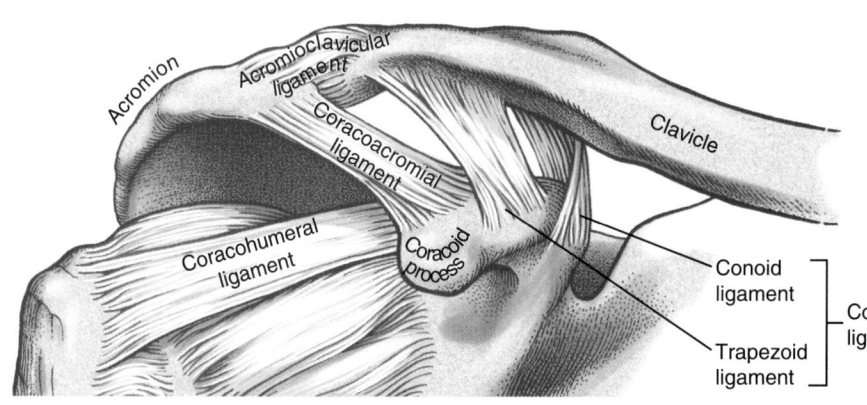

FIGURE 5.17 An anterior view of the right acromioclavicular joint including many surrounding ligaments.

SPECIAL FOCUS 5.1

Acromioclavicular Joint Dislocation

Injury to the acromioclavicular (AC) joint is relatively common in contact sports, accounting for about 40% of all shoulder injuries sustained by American collegiate football players.[111] Participants in the sport of rugby also have a disproportionately high risk of AC joint injury.[195] Although most AC joint injuries within these sports qualify as partial sprains, dislocations (or "separations") do occur.[61,195] The AC joint is inherently susceptible to dislocation in part because of the slightly sloped nature of the articulation combined with the high probability of receiving large external forces. Consider a person falling and striking the tip of the shoulder abruptly against an unyielding surface (Fig. 5.18). The resulting medially and inferiorly directed force typically displaces the acromion medially and slightly anteriorly under the sloped articular facet of the clavicle. The horizontal shear component is resisted primarily by the joint's capsular ligaments.[50] The coracoclavicular ligament, however, offers a secondary resistance to horizontal shear, especially if severe.[69] On occasion, the force applied to the scapula exceeds the tensile strength of the ligaments, resulting in their rupture and subsequent dislocation of the AC joint. Trauma to the AC joint and its associated ligaments may cause joint instability and postural deviations of the scapula, potentially leading to the development of posttraumatic osteoarthritis.[158,188] Extensive literature exists on the evaluation and the surgical and nonsurgical treatment of an injured or painful AC joint, especially in athletes.[44,49,86,146,244]

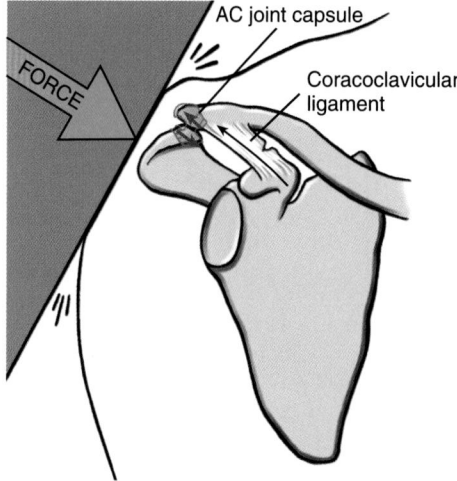

FIGURE 5.18 An anterior view of the shoulder striking a firm surface with the force of the impact directed at the acromion. The resulting shear force at the acromioclavicular *(AC)* joint is depicted by red arrows. Note the increased tension and partial tearing of the AC joint capsule and coracoclavicular ligament.

The AC joint has articular surfaces that are lined with a layer of fibrocartilage and typically includes a fragmented *articular disc.*[90] The presence of nerve fibers around the disc suggests it can be a source of pain.[190] An extensive dissection of 223 sets of AC joints reveals complete discs in only about 10% of the joints.[56] The majority of the incomplete discs are crescent-shaped and fragmented (as the disc depicted in Fig. 5.16B). A complete disc is typically present in juvenile and adolescent joints, often separating the joint cavity into medial and lateral compartments.[233] The fragmented discs typically observed in adult AC joints likely result from natural degeneration.[56]

KINEMATICS

Functions of the SC and AC joints distinctly differ. The SC joint permits extensive motion of the clavicle that helps guide the overall path of the scapula relative to the thorax. The AC joint, in contrast, permits movements of varying magnitude between the scapula and lateral end of the clavicle. The motions at the AC joint are kinesiologically important, as they optimize the mobility and fit between the scapula and thorax, and ultimately at the glenohumeral joint.

The motions of the AC joint are described by the movement of the scapula relative to the lateral end of the clavicle. Motion has been defined for 3 degrees of freedom (Fig. 5.19A). The primary, or most obvious, motions are called *upward* and *downward rotation*. Secondary motions—referred to as *rotational adjustment*

motions—fine-tune the position of the scapula, in both the horizontal and the sagittal planes. Measuring isolated motions at the AC joint can be technically complex and usually is not done in ordinary clinical situations.

Upward and Downward Rotation

Upward rotation of the scapula at the AC joint occurs as the scapula "swings upwardly" relative to the lateral end of the clavicle (see Fig. 5.19A). This motion occurs as a natural component of abduction or flexion of the shoulder. Reports vary widely, but up to 30 degrees of upward rotation at the AC joint occurs as the arm is raised fully over the head.[105,138,154,246] The motion contributes significantly to the overall upward rotation at the scapulothoracic joint.[138] Downward rotation at the AC joint returns the scapula back toward the anatomic position, a motion mechanically associated with shoulder adduction or extension.

Horizontal and Sagittal Plane "Rotational Adjustment Motions" at the Acromioclavicular Joint

Careful kinematic measurement of the AC joint during shoulder movement reveals pivoting or twisting type motions of the scapula around the lateral end of the clavicle. These so-called "rotational adjustment motions" optimally align the scapula against the external surface of the thorax, as well as add to the total amount of its motion. Rotation adjustment motions at the AC joint are described

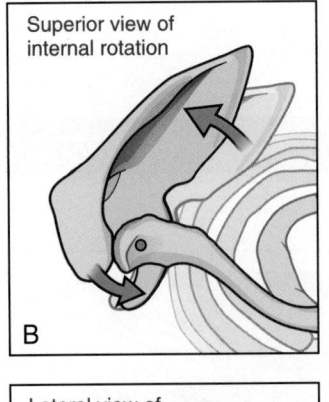
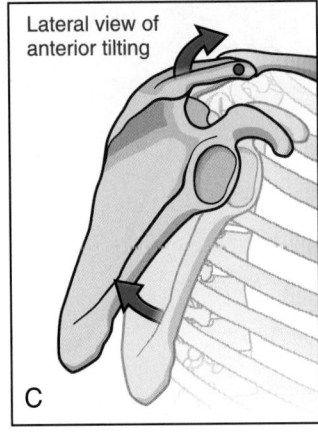
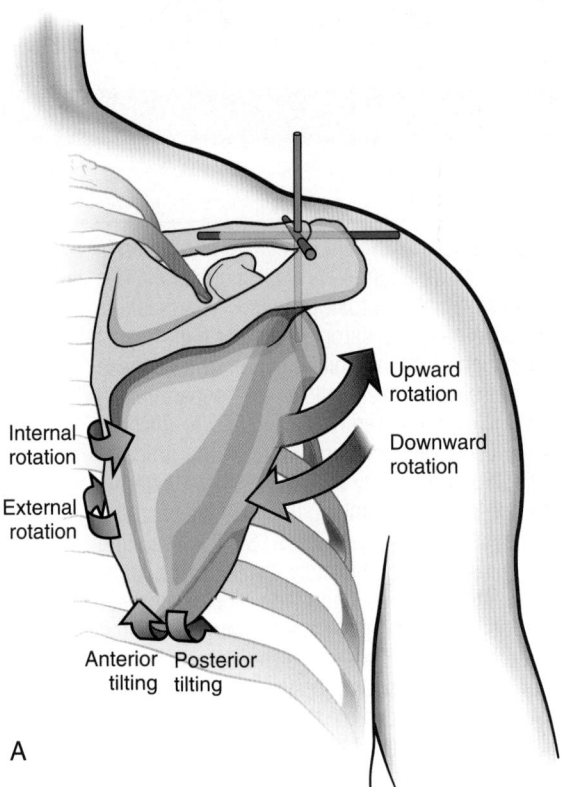

FIGURE 5.19 (A) Posterior view showing the osteokinematics of the right acromioclavicular (AC) joint. The primary motions of upward and downward rotation are shown in purple. Horizontal and sagittal plane adjustment motions, considered as secondary motions, are shown in blue and green, respectively. Note that each plane of movement is color-coded with a corresponding axis of rotation. Images (B) and (C) show examples of rotational adjustment motions at the AC joint: internal rotation during extreme scapulothoracic protraction (B), and anterior tilting during scapulothoracic elevation (C).

within horizontal and sagittal planes (blue and green arrows in Fig. 5.19A, respectively).

Horizontal plane adjustments at the AC joint occur around a near vertical axis, evident as the medial border of the scapula pivots slightly away and toward the posterior surface of the thorax. These horizontal plane motions are described as *internal* and *external rotation,* defined by the direction of rotation of the glenoid fossa. *Sagittal plane adjustments* at the AC joint occur around a near medial-lateral axis, evident as the inferior angle of the scapula pivots slightly away from or toward the posterior surface of the thorax. The terms *anterior tilting* and *posterior tilting* describe the directions of this rotation based on the direction of rotation of the glenoid fossa, *not* the inferior angle (see Fig. 5.19A).

Using relatively sophisticated technology and methods, several studies have measured the horizontal and sagittal plane adjustment motions at the AC joint during shoulder abduction or flexion. Most reports cite ranges of motion between about 5 and 20 degrees.[63,139,154,215,246] Although difficult to appreciate through simple clinical observation, these kinematics are important as they enhance the quality and quantity of movement at the scapulothoracic joint. Qualitatively, for example, during protraction of the scapulothoracic joint, the AC joint internally rotates slightly within the horizontal plane (Fig. 5.19B). This rotation helps the anterior surface of the scapula fit with the curved contour of the thorax. For similar reasons of alignment, the scapula is allowed to tilt anteriorly slightly during elevation of the scapulothoracic joint, as during "shrugging" of the shoulders (Fig. 5.19C). Without these rotational adjustments, the scapula would be obligated to follow essentially the same path of the moving clavicle, without the freedom to fine-tune its position on the thorax.

Scapulothoracic Joint

The scapulothoracic (ST) joint is not a true joint per se but rather a functional interface between the anterior surface of the scapula and the slightly spherical posterior-lateral wall of the thorax (see Fig. 5.10).[197] The two surfaces do not make direct bony contact; rather, they are separated primarily by relatively soft tissues such as the subscapularis, serratus anterior, and an interposed bursa. The relatively thick and moist "articular" surfaces reduce shear within the

articulation during movement. An audible clicking sound during scapular movements may indicate abnormal contact or alignment within the articulation, possibly from an imbalance of muscle forces, excessive thoracic kyphosis, abnormal bony shape, an osseous or soft tissue mass, or a fibrotic bursa.[189,259]

In the anatomic position, the adult scapula is usually positioned between the second and the seventh ribs, with the medial border located about 6 cm lateral to the spine. Although highly variable, the average "resting" posture of the scapula is about 10 degrees of anterior tilt, 5 to 10 degrees of upward rotation, and about 30 to 40 degrees of internal rotation—a position consistent with the previously described plane of the scapula.[154]

The movements at the ST joint are fundamental components of shoulder kinesiology. The wide range of motion available to the shoulder is due, in part, to the large movement available to the scapula. As will be described throughout this chapter, abnormal posture, movement, or control of the ST joint can significantly impact the kinematic and kinetic environment within the glenohumeral joint.

KINEMATICS

The movements of the ST joint are based on the kinematic interactions between the SC and the AC joints. Examples of these interactions (or couplings) are depicted in in Figs. 5.20 through 5.22. Greater detail on these mechanical couplings will be described as the chapter progresses. The couplings are important clinically, as motion at either the SC or AC joint can significantly influence the quality or quantity of motion of the scapula, and ultimately of the entire shoulder.

Elevation and Depression

Fig. 5.20A shows scapular elevation as a composite of SC and AC joint motion. For the most part, the motion of shrugging the shoulders is a direct result of the scapula following the path of the elevating clavicle around the SC joint (Fig. 5.20B). Slight downward rotation of the scapula at the AC joint allows the lateral border scapula to remain nearly vertical throughout the elevation (Fig. 5.20C). Additional adjustments at the AC joint help the scapula remain flush with the changing curvature of the thorax. Depression of the scapula occurs as the reverse action described for elevation.

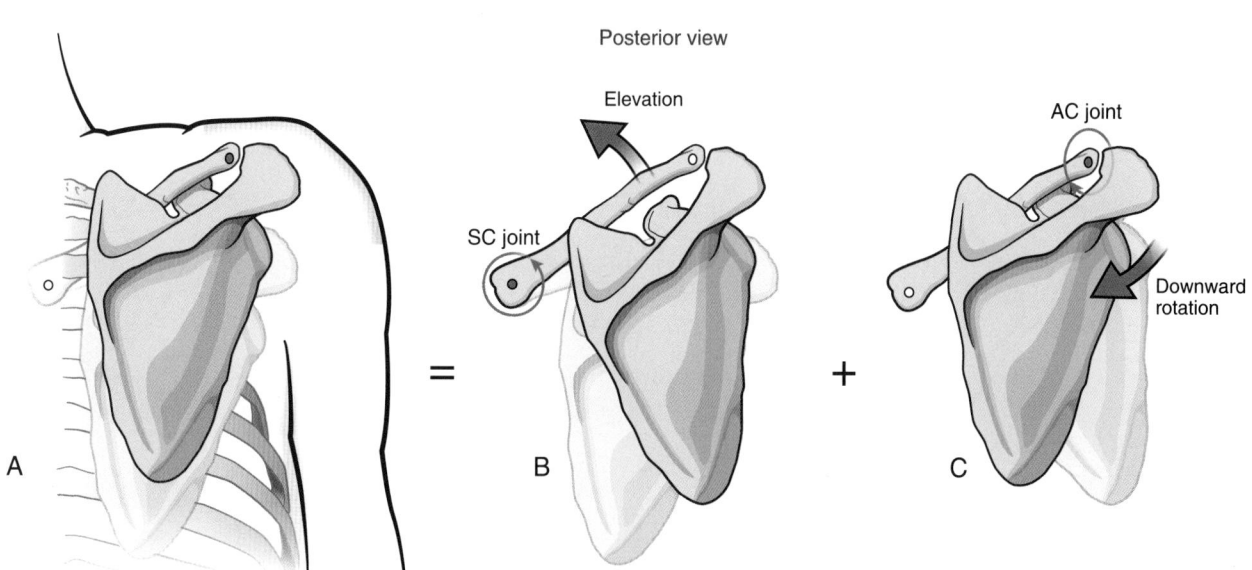

FIGURE 5.20 (A) Scapulothoracic elevation shown as a summation of (B) elevation at the sternoclavicular joint and (C) downward rotation at the acromioclavicular joint.

Protraction and Retraction

Protraction of the scapula occurs through a summation of horizontal plane rotations at both the SC and the AC joints (Fig. 5.21A). The scapula follows the general path of the protracting clavicle around the SC joint (Fig. 5.21B). The AC joint can amplify, offset, or otherwise adjust the total amount of ST protraction by contributing varying amounts of internal rotation (Fig. 5.21C). Because ST protraction occurs as a composite of motions at the SC and AC joints, a decrease in motion at one joint can be partially compensated for by an increase at the other. Consider, for example, an individual with severe degenerative arthritis and decreased motion at the AC joint. The SC joint may compensate by contributing a greater degree of protraction, thereby limiting the functional loss associated with forward reach of the upper limb.

Retraction of the scapula is similar to protraction but in a reverse direction. Retraction of the scapula is often performed in the context of pulling an object toward the body, such as pulling on a wall pulley, climbing a rope, or preparing to place the arm in a coat sleeve.

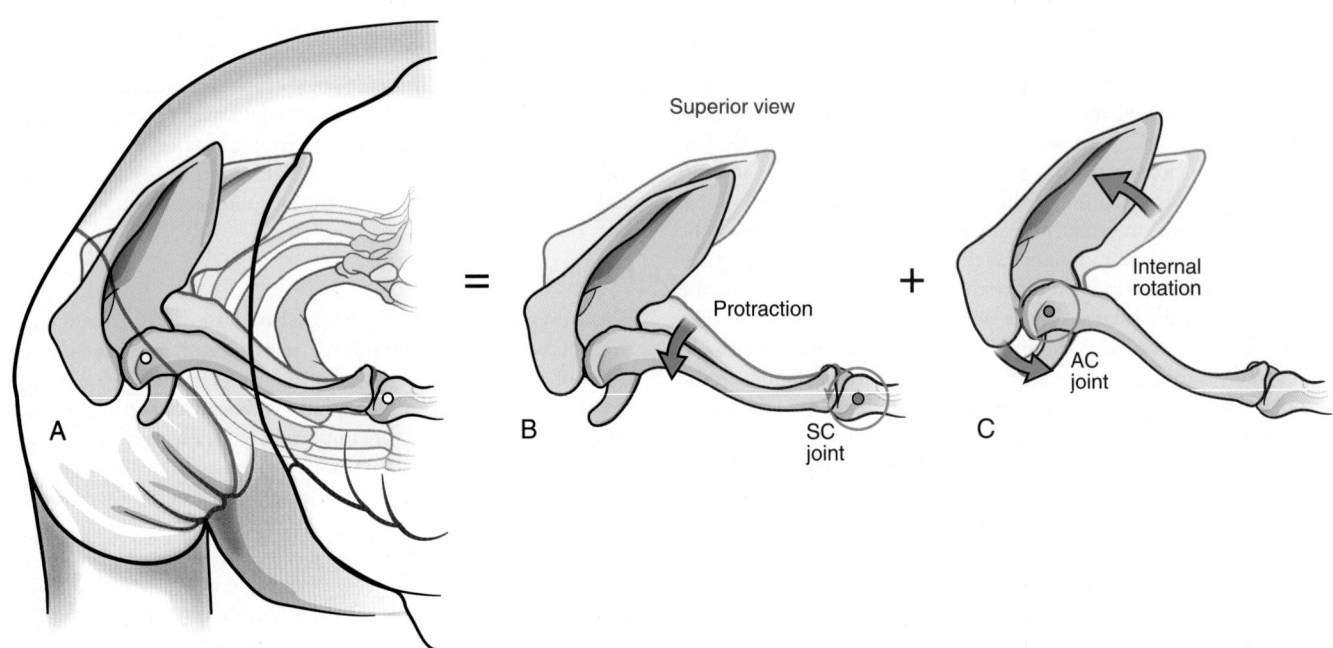

FIGURE 5.21 (A) Scapulothoracic protraction shown as a summation of (B) protraction at the sternoclavicular joint and (C) internal rotation at the acromioclavicular joint.

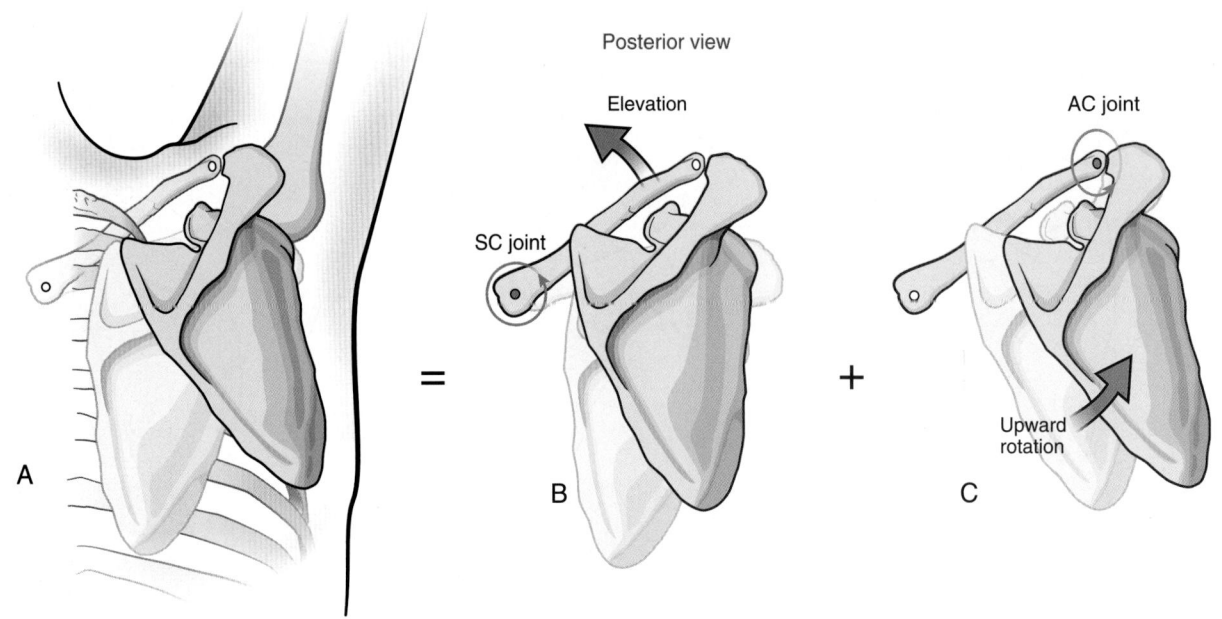

FIGURE 5.22 (A) Scapulothoracic upward rotation shown as a summation of (B) elevation of the clavicle at the sternoclavicular joint and (C) upward rotation of the scapula at the acromioclavicular joint.

Upward and Downward Rotation

Upward rotation of the ST joint is an essential part of raising the arm overhead (Fig. 5.22A). Complete upward rotation of the scapula requires kinematic contributions from *both* the SC and AC joints.[138] One of the more familiar kinematic pairings is the summation of clavicular elevation at the SC joint (Fig. 5.22B) *and* scapular upward rotation at the AC joint (Fig. 5.22C).[105,154] As will be further described, other movements at the SC and AC joints contribute to the specific position or path of scapular movement during elevation of the arm, depending on the plane, specific arc of motion, and kinematic context of the shoulder movement.[138]

Downward rotation of the scapula occurs as the arm is returned to the side from a raised position. The motion is described similarly to upward rotation, except that the clavicle depresses at the SC joint and the scapula downwardly rotates at the AC joint. The motion of downward rotation usually ends when the scapula has returned to the anatomic position.

Glenohumeral Joint

GENERAL FEATURES

The glenohumeral (GH) joint is the articulation between the relatively large convex head of the humerus and the shallow concavity of the glenoid fossa (Fig. 5.23). This joint operates in conjunction with the moving scapula to produce an extensive range of motion of the shoulder. In the anatomic position, the articular surface of the glenoid fossa is directed anterior-laterally in the scapular plane. In most people, the glenoid fossa is upwardly rotated slightly: a position dependent on the amount of fixed upward inclination of the fossa and on the degree of upward rotation of the ST joint.

In the anatomic position, the humeral head is directed medially and superiorly, as well as posteriorly because of its natural retroversion. This orientation places the head of the humerus more directly into the scapular plane and therefore directly against the face of the glenoid fossa (see Fig. 5.4, angles B and C).

The Functional Importance of Upward Rotation of the Scapulothoracic Joint

The ability to raise the arm fully overhead in a relatively pain-free and effective manner is a prerequisite for many functional activities. A fully upwardly rotated scapula is a necessary component of this movement, accounting for almost one-third of full shoulder abduction. As with all ST motions, upward rotation is mechanically linked to the motions of the SC and AC joints.

Upward rotation of the scapula while raising the arm overhead serves at least three functions. *First,* the upwardly rotated scapula projects the glenoid fossa upward and typically anterior-laterally, providing a structural base of support for the elevated humerus. *Second,* the upwardly rotated scapula preserves the optimal length-tension relationship of the abductor muscles of the glenohumeral joint, such as the middle deltoid and supraspinatus. *Third,* the upwardly rotated scapula shifts the undersurface of the acromion away from the abducted or flexed humeral head. This process may help preserve the size of the subacromial space: the space between the undersurface of the acromion and the humeral head (see Figs. 5.24 and 5.25).[117,169] A reduced subacromial space could increase the risk of compressing the residing tissues, such as the supraspinatus tendon.[78,155,170]

Altered kinematics of ST upward rotation have been associated with impairments other than subacromial impingement, particularly those related to painful and degenerative changes to the rotator cuff group.[138] The specific mechanism by which altered scapular kinematics may *cause* stress-related pathology involving the GH joint is not clear; understanding such a relationship could improve the treatment for or reduce the risk of developing painful shoulders.[13,70,138,276]

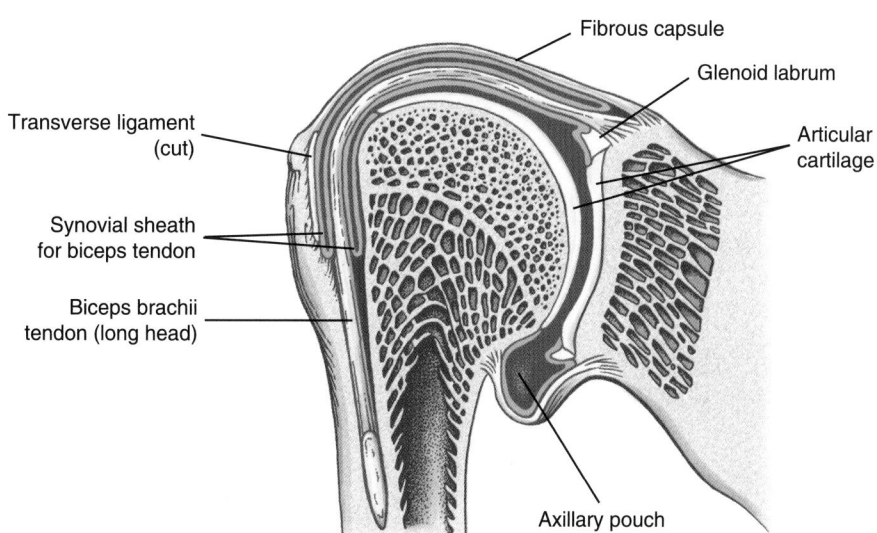

FIGURE 5.23 Anterior view of a frontal section through the right glenohumeral joint. Note the fibrous capsule, synovial membrane *(blue),* and the long head of the biceps tendon. The axillary pouch is shown as a recess in the inferior capsule.

PERIARTICULAR CONNECTIVE TISSUE AND OTHER SUPPORTING STRUCTURES

The GH joint is surrounded by a *fibrous capsule* that surrounds and isolates the joint cavity from most surrounding tissues (see Fig. 5.23). The capsule attaches along most of the rim of the glenoid fossa and extends to the anatomic neck of the humerus. Type I-IV sensory nerve receptors (see Chapter 2) have been identified in all regions of the capsule, most notably anteriorly.[116] A *synovial membrane* lines the inner wall of the joint capsule. An extension of this synovial membrane lines the intracapsular portion of the tendon of the *long head of the biceps brachii*. This synovial membrane continues to surround the biceps tendon as it exits the joint capsule and descends into the intertubercular (i.e., bicipital) groove. The head of the humerus and the glenoid fossa are both lined with *articular cartilage*.

The potential volume of space within the GH joint capsule is about twice the size of the humeral head. The loose-fitting and expandable capsule allows extensive mobility at the GH joint. This mobility is apparent by the ample passive translation normally available at the GH joint. The humeral head can typically be pulled away from the fossa a moderate distance without causing pain or trauma to the joint. In the anatomic or adducted position, the inferior portion of the capsule appears as a slackened or redundant recess called the *axillary pouch* (Fig. 5.23 and Fig. 5.24).

The fibrous capsule of the GH joint is relatively thin and is reinforced by thicker external ligaments (described later). The primary stability of the GH joint is based not only on passive tension within ligaments and other connective tissues, but also on the active forces produced by local muscles, especially the rotator cuff (subscapularis,

supraspinatus, infraspinatus, and teres minor). Unlike the capsular ligaments, which produce their greatest stabilizing tension only when stretched at relatively extreme motions, muscles generate large, active stabilizing forces at essentially any joint position. The rotator cuff muscles are considered the "dynamic" stabilizers of the GH joint because of their predominant role in maintaining articular stability during active motions.

Capsular Ligaments

The external layers of the anterior and inferior walls of the joint capsule are thickened by fibrous connective tissue known simply as the *glenohumeral capsular ligaments* (Fig. 5.24). The ligaments are composed of an intermingling of many loosely wound fiber bundles of varying lengths.[74] To generate stabilizing tensions across the joint, the inherently slack capsular ligaments must be elongated or twisted; the resulting passive tension generates mechanical support for the GH joint and limits the extremes of rotation and translation.

By surrounding and enclosing the GH articulation, the capsular ligaments also assist with sealing the joint to maintain a negative intra-articular pressure. This slight suction offers an additional source of stability.[3,106] Puncturing (or venting) the capsule equalizes the pressure on both sides, removing the slight suction force between the humeral head and the fossa. Experimental release of the pressure by piercing the capsule of cadaveric specimens significantly increases overall passive mobility within the joint, most notably in anterior-posterior directions with the joint abducted to 30 degrees.[3] This partially abducted position coincides with the approximate position where the intra-articular pressure is normally lowest (i.e., where the suction effect is the greatest).[89,106]

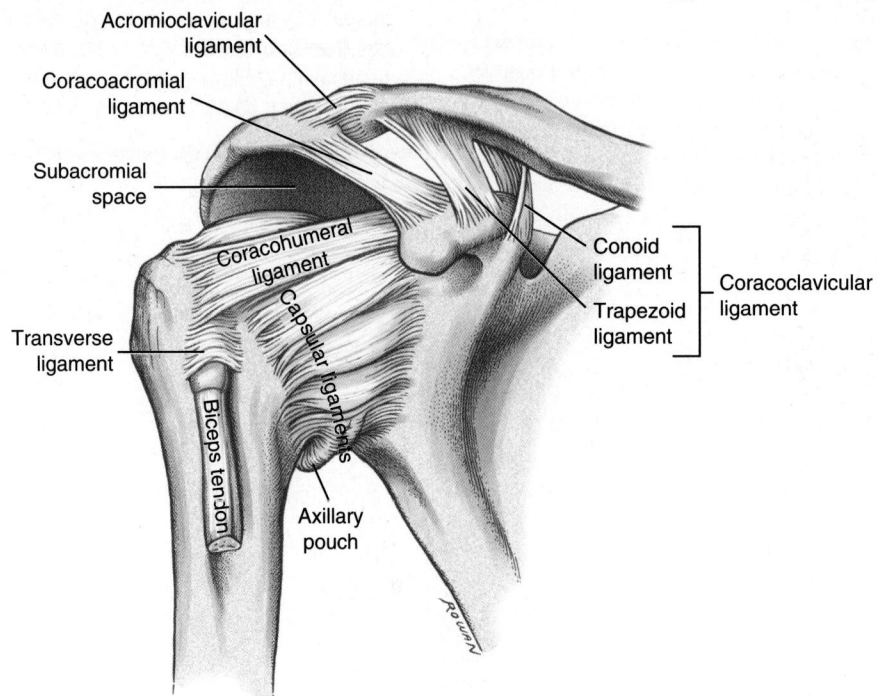

FIGURE 5.24 Anterior view of the right glenohumeral joint showing the primary ligaments.

SPECIAL FOCUS 5.3

The "Loose Fit" of the Glenohumeral Joint: An Inherent Problem of Instability

Several anatomic features of the glenohumeral (GH) joint contribute to a design that *favors mobility at the expense of stability.* The articular surface of the glenoid fossa covers only 25% to 30% of the articular surface of the humeral head during typical joint movements.[6] This size difference allows only a small part of the humeral head to contact the glenoid fossa in any given shoulder position. In a typical adult, the longitudinal diameter of the humeral head is about 1.9 times larger than the longitudinal diameter of the glenoid fossa (Fig. 5.25). The transverse diameter of the humeral head is about 2.3 times larger than the opposing transverse diameter of the glenoid fossa. The GH joint is often described as a ball-and-socket joint, although this description gives the erroneous impression that the head of the humerus fits *into* the glenoid fossa. The actual structure of the GH joint roughly resembles more that of a golf ball pressed against a coin the size of a US quarter. This bony fit offers little structural stability to the GH joint; instead, the mechanical integrity of the articulation is maintained primarily through the surrounding muscles and periarticular connective tissues.

For a host of reasons, select periarticular connective tissues or muscles may fail to adequately support and stabilize the GH joint. Such lack of support is manifested by excessive translation of the humeral head. Although some degree of laxity is normal at the GH joint, excessive laxity associated with large translations of the humeral head is generally considered as pathologic and formally referred to as *shoulder instability.* A diagnosis of shoulder instability typically means that the laxity is associated with pain, apprehension, or a lack of function.

Although GH joint instability can occur in multiple directions, most cases exhibit excessive translation anteriorly or inferiorly. In some cases, an unstable GH joint may lead to a subluxation or dislocation. *Subluxation* of the GH joint involves an incomplete or partial separation of the articular surfaces, often involving a palpable gap between the acromion and the humeral head.[41] *Dislocation* of the GH joint, in contrast, involves a more serious and complete separation of articular surfaces. Typically, a dislocated joint must be rearticulated by a special maneuver, often requiring assistance from another person. Although the terms subluxation and dislocation are intended to define distinct clinical conditions, they often describe a similar pathologic process, just expressed at different ends of a severity spectrum.[53]

Instability of the GH joint is often associated with less-than-optimal alignment and disrupted arthrokinematics, which over time can place damaging stress on the joint's periarticular connective tissues.[202] It is not always clear if shoulder instability is the result or the cause of the abnormal arthrokinematics. The pathomechanics of shoulder instability are not well understood and occupy the forefront of interest among clinicians, researchers, and surgeons.[53,162,207,231]

Ultimately, stability at the GH joint is achieved by a combination of passive and active mechanisms. *Active mechanisms* rely on the forces produced by muscle. These forces are provided primarily by the embracing and compressive nature of the rotator cuff muscle group across the GH joint. *Passive mechanisms* include (1) restraint provided by capsule, ligaments, glenoid labrum (connective tissue attaching to most of the rim of the glenoid fossa), and tendons; (2) mechanical support predicated on ST posture; and (3) negative intracapsular pressure. Because of the variability and complexity of most shoulder movements, a combination of passive and active mechanisms is typically required to ensure joint stability. This important and multifaceted topic of stability at the GH joint will be a recurring theme throughout the chapter.

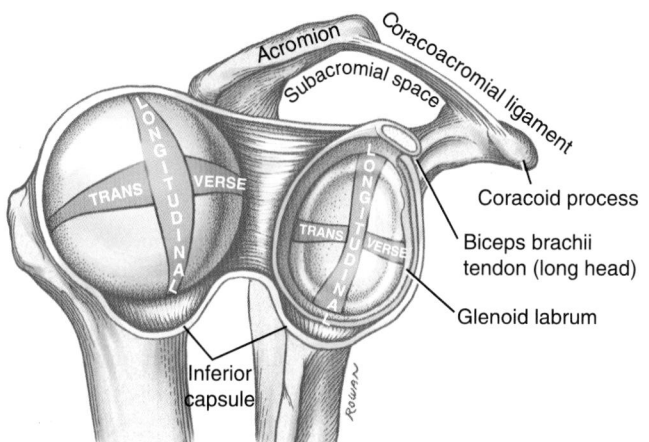

FIGURE 5.25 Side view of right glenohumeral joint with the joint opened up to expose the articular surfaces. Note the extent of the subacromial space under the coracoacromial arch. Normally this space is filled with the supraspinatus muscle and its tendon, and the subacromial bursa. The longitudinal and horizontal diameters are illustrated on both articular surfaces.

TABLE 5.1 Distal Attachments and Selected Functions of the Glenohumeral Joint's Capsular Ligaments

Ligament	Distal (Humeral) Attachments	Primary Motions Drawing Structure Taut
Superior glenohumeral ligament	Anatomic neck, superior to the lesser tubercle	External rotation in 0 degrees of abduction; inferior and anterior translations of the humeral head
Middle glenohumeral ligament	Along the anterior anatomic neck near the lesser tubercle; blends with the subscapularis tendon	External rotation in 0 and 90 degrees of abduction; anterior translation of the humeral head, especially in about 45–90 degrees of abduction
Inferior glenohumeral ligament (three parts: anterior band, posterior band, and connecting axillary pouch)	As a broad sheet to the anterior-inferior and posterior-inferior margins of the anatomic neck	Axillary pouch: 90 degrees of abduction, combined with anterior-posterior and inferior translations Anterior band: external rotation in 90 degrees of abduction; anterior translation of humeral head Posterior band: internal rotation in 0 and 90 degrees of abduction, and again in full abduction
Coracohumeral ligament	Anterior side of the greater and lesser tubercle; also blends with the superior capsule and supraspinatus and subscapularis tendons	Inferior and posterior translation of the humeral head; external rotation

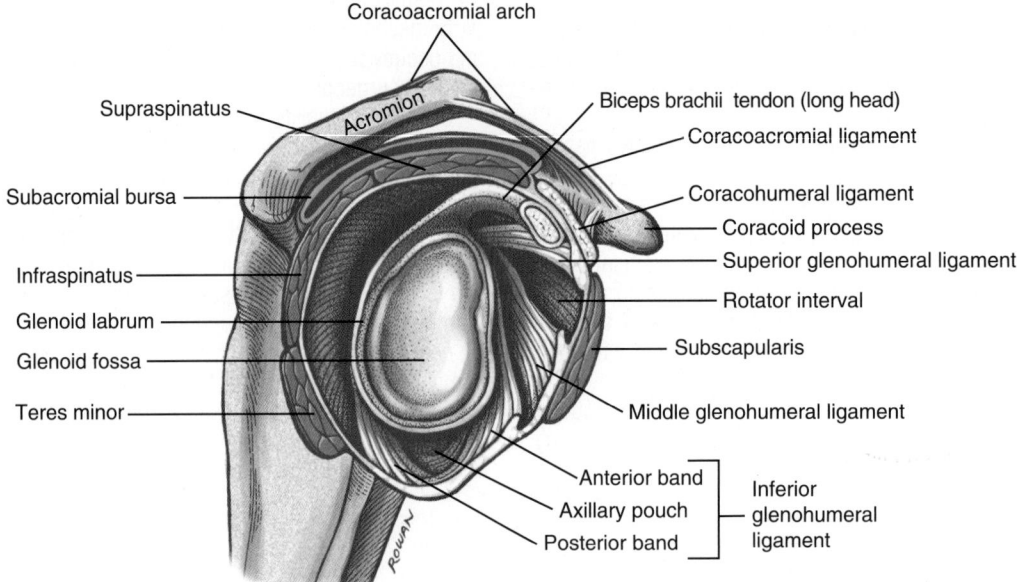

FIGURE 5.26 Lateral aspect of the internal surface of the right glenohumeral joint. The humerus has been removed to expose the capsular ligaments and the glenoid fossa. Note the prominent coracoacromial arch and underlying subacromial bursa *(blue)*. The four rotator cuff muscles are shown in red.

The following discussion describes the essential anatomy and functions of the GH joint capsular ligaments. Although a separate entity, the coracohumeral ligament will be considered with this group. The following material is essential for determining which ligament, or part of the capsule, is most responsible for restricting a particular movement. Such information assists the clinician to understand mechanisms responsible for ligamentous or capsular injury and joint instability, as well as the rationale for some methods of manual therapy and arthroscopic surgical intervention. Table 5.1 lists the distal attachments of the ligaments and a sample of motions that render each ligament taut (or stretched). Motions that most dramatically increase the stretch (length) in a ligament define its primary function. Information contained in Table 5.1 serves only as an introduction to an extensive body of literature; more detail on this topic can be found in other sources.[a]

The GH joint has three distinct capsular ligaments consisting of interlacing collagen fibers: superior, middle, and inferior ligaments.[37] These ligaments of the capsule are best visualized as discrete structures from an internal view of the GH joint (Fig. 5.26). The *superior glenohumeral ligament* has its proximal attachment near the superior rim of the glenoid fossa and adjacent glenoid labrum, just anterior to the supraglenoid tubercle and attachment of the long head of the biceps.[55] The other end of the ligament, with adjacent capsule, attaches near the anatomic neck of the humerus above the lesser tubercle. This ligament is slightly taut in and near the anatomic position, capable of resisting external rotation and inferior and anterior translations of the humeral head.[216] As the GH joint is abducted beyond 35 to 45 degrees, the superior GH ligament slackens significantly.[159,216]

The *middle glenohumeral ligament* has its proximal attachment to the anterior-superior rim of the glenoid fossa and adjacent glenoid labrum. The ligament blends with the anterior capsule and broad tendon of the subscapularis muscle, then attaches along the anterior aspect of the anatomic neck, near the lesser tubercle.[37,55,175] The middle

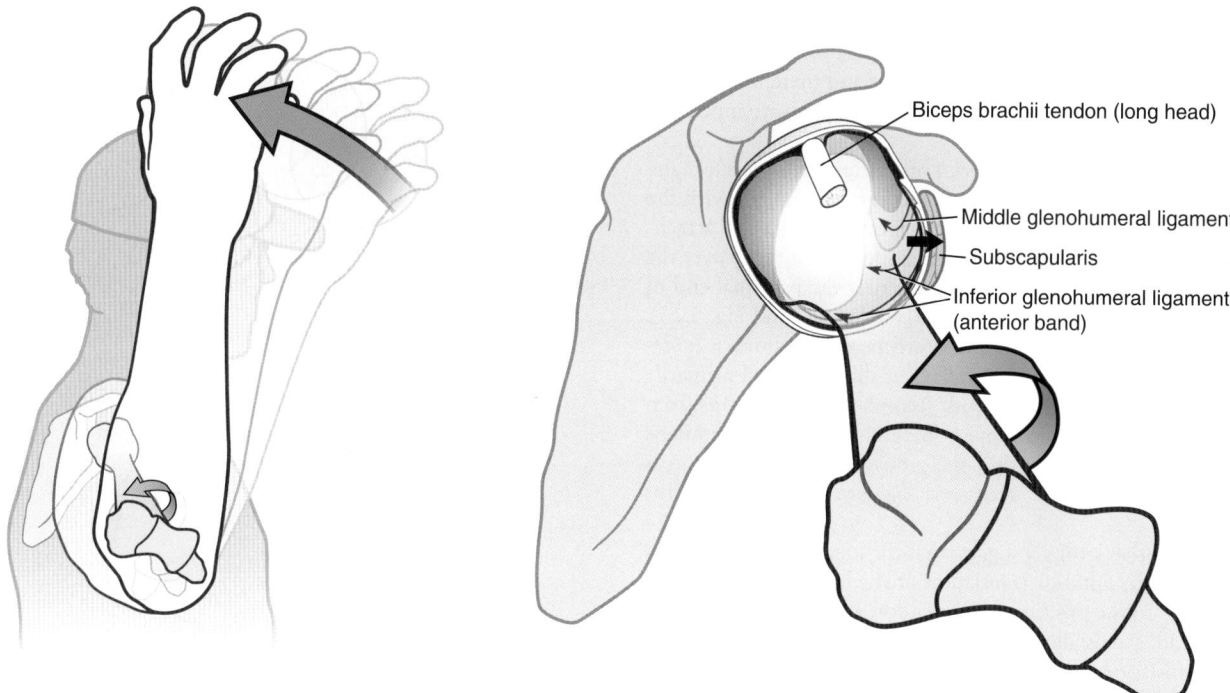

Biceps brachii tendon (long head)

Middle glenohumeral ligament

Subscapularis

Inferior glenohumeral ligament (anterior band)

FIGURE 5.27 Illustration showing a high-velocity abduction and external rotation motion of the glenohumeral joint during the cocking phase of pitching a baseball. This motion twists and elongates the middle GH ligament and anterior band of the inferior GH ligament (depicted as *thin red arrows* pointed toward the rim of the glenoid fossa). The humeral head has been removed to show the aforementioned stretched structures and glenoid fossa. This active motion tends to translate the humeral head anteriorly *(thick black arrow),* toward the anterior glenoid labrum and subscapularis muscle. Tension in the stretched ligaments and subscapularis muscle naturally resists this anterior translation.

GH ligament provides substantial anterior restraint against the humeral head, especially in a position of 45 to 90 degrees of abduction (which further stretches the ligament).[51,159,275] As expected by its location and fiber direction, the middle GH ligament is effective at limiting the end-range of external rotation, at least when tested at 0 and 90 degrees of abduction; predictably, the ligament readily slackens upon internal rotation.[159,186,216]

The well-studied and extensive *inferior glenohumeral ligament* attaches proximally along much of the anterior-inferior and posterior-inferior rim of the glenoid fossa and adjacent glenoid labrum.[37,55] Distally, the inferior GH ligament attaches as a broad sheet to the anterior-inferior and posterior-inferior margins of the anatomic neck. The hammocklike inferior capsular ligament has three separate components: an *anterior band,* a *posterior band,* and a sheet of tissue connecting these bands known as an *axillary pouch* (Fig. 5.26).[55,186] The axillary pouch and the surrounding inferior capsular ligaments generally become uniformly taut at and above about 90 degrees of abduction. Acting as a sling, the taut axillary pouch cradles the suspended humeral head as it resists inferior and anterior-posterior translations.[230,258] From this abducted position, the anterior and posterior bands become further taut at the extremes of external and internal rotation, respectively.[216,258] The anterior band—the strongest and thickest part of the entire capsule—is particularly important, as it furnishes the primary ligamentous restraint to anterior translation of the humeral head, both in an abducted and in a neutral position.[187] Forceful and dynamic activities involving *abduction* and *external rotation* specifically stress the anterior band of the inferior capsule.[159] Such stress, for example, may occur during the "cocking phase" of throwing a baseball (Fig. 5.27). Over many repetitions, this action can overstretch or tear the anterior band, thereby compromising one of the prime restraints to anterior

translation of the humeral head. Injury and increased laxity of this portion of the anterior and inferior capsule are indeed associated with recurrent anterior dislocations of the GH joint.[135,251] Once the anterior bands of the inferior capsule have been torn or made lax, recurrences of anterior dislocation may be part of a vicious cycle that can progressively damage the tissue further.

The GH joint capsule is also strengthened by the *coracohumeral ligament* (see Figs. 5.24 and 5.26). This ligament extends from the lateral border of the coracoid process to the anterior sides of the greater and lesser tubercles of the humerus, blending with the distal attachments of the superior capsule and supraspinatus and subscapularis tendons.[55,233] In the anatomic position, the coracohumeral ligament provides restraint to inferior and posterior translation and external rotation of the humeral head.[55,131,275]

Rotator Cuff Muscles and Long Head of the Biceps Brachii

As previously stated, the GH joint capsule receives significant structural reinforcement from the *rotator cuff muscles* (Fig. 5.26). The subscapularis, the thickest of the four muscles[26] partially blends with and reinforces the anterior capsule. The supraspinatus, infraspinatus, and teres minor partially blend with and reinforce the superior and posterior capsule. The four muscles form a cuff that protects and actively stabilizes the GH joint. This anatomic arrangement partially explains why the mechanical stability of the GH joint is so reliant on the innervation, strength, and motor control of the rotator cuff group. It is clinically noteworthy that, as evident in Fig. 5.26, the rotator cuff fails to cover two regions of the capsule: inferiorly, as well as in a space between the supraspinatus and subscapularis known as the *rotator (cuff) interval.*[101] The natural interval or recess within the anterior-superior region is reinforced by the tendon of the long head of the biceps, the coracohumeral ligament, and the superior and (sometimes upper parts of the) middle GH ligaments. The rotator interval is a relatively common site for anterior dislocation of the GH joint and therefore the anatomic detail is of concern to the arthroscopic surgeon attempting to reinforce the region.[270]

The *long head of the biceps brachii* originates from the supraglenoid tubercle of the scapula, where it becomes continuous with the adjacent glenoid labrum (see Fig. 5.26). From this proximal attachment, the intracapsular tendon widens as it crosses directly over the humeral head, then angulates distally to enter the proximal end of intertubercular groove of the humerus (see Fig. 5.7 and Fig. 5.23). As the deflected tendon enters the intertubercular groove, it is stabilized by a capsuloligamentous pulley (or sling), formed primarily by the coracohumeral ligament with secondary contributions from the superior capsule and upper margin of the subscapularis tendon.[196] More distally within the groove, the biceps tendon is further stabilized by the *transverse ligament* of the humerus (see Fig. 5.24).

Cadaver studies strongly suggest that the long head of the biceps naturally restricts anterior translation of the humeral head.[3,193] In addition, due to the position of the tendon across the dome of the humeral head, a musculotendinous force in the biceps can resist a superior translation of the humeral head,[119,196] a force that can help control the natural arthrokinematics of GH joint abduction.

Glenoid Labrum

The bony rim of the glenoid fossa is encircled by a triangular fibrocartilaginous ring, or lip, known as the *glenoid labrum* (see Fig. 5.26). In addition to gradually blending with the adjacent articular cartilage of the fossa, the labrum, as described earlier, serves as a proximal attachment for several ligaments, capsule, and the long head of the biceps. About 50% of the overall depth of the glenoid fossa has been attributed to the glenoid labrum.[6,99] The resulting greater depth of the cavity increases articular contact area and thus reduces contact pressure. Furthermore, in conjunction with active forces produced particularly by the rotator cuff muscles, the deepened concavity forms a secure seat for the humeral head, particularly important to dynamic stability of the GH joint.[6,119]

Tissues That Reinforce or Deepen the Glenohumeral Joint

- Joint capsule and associated GH capsular ligaments
- Coracohumeral ligament
- Rotator cuff muscles (subscapularis, supraspinatus, infraspinatus, and teres minor)
- Long head of the biceps brachii
- Glenoid labrum

SCAPULOTHORACIC POSTURE AND ITS EFFECT ON STATIC STABILITY

Normally, when one stands at rest with arms at the sides, the head of the humerus remains stable (fixed) against the glenoid fossa. This stability is referred to as *static* because it exists at rest. One passive mechanism for controlling static stability at the GH joint is based on the analogy of a ball compressed against an inclined surface (Fig. 5.28A).[14] At rest, the superior capsuloligamentous structures (SCS) provide the primary mechanical support for the humeral head. These structures include the superior capsular ligament, the coracohumeral

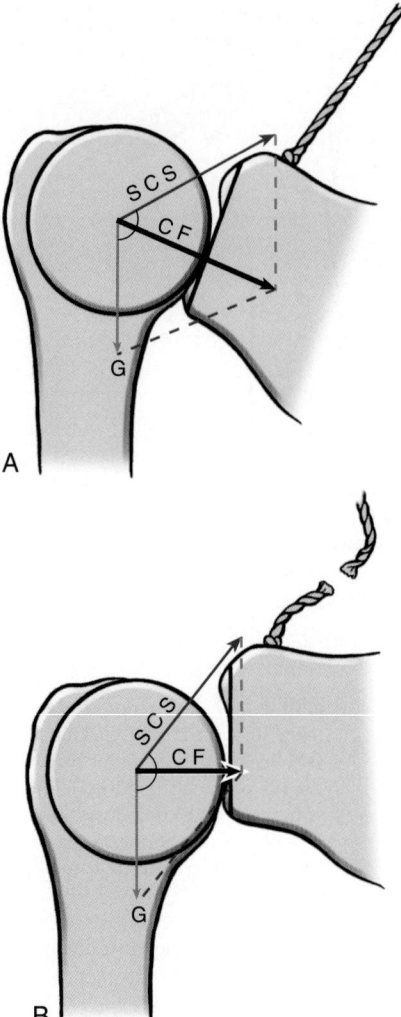

FIGURE 5.28 Scapular posture and its effect on static stability at the glenohumeral (GH) joint. (A) The rope indicates a muscular force that holds the glenoid fossa in a slightly upward-rotated position. In this position, the passive tension in the taut superior capsuloligamentous structures *(SCS)* is added to the force produced by gravity *(G),* yielding the compression force *(CF)*. The compression force applied against the slight incline of the glenoid "locks" the joint. (B) With a loss of upward rotation posture of the scapula (indicated by the cut rope), the change in angle between the *SCS* and *G* vectors reduces the magnitude of the compression force across the GH joint. As a consequence, the head of the humerus may slide down the now vertically oriented glenoid fossa. The dashed lines indicate the parallelogram method of adding force vectors. Vectors are not drawn to proper scale.

ligament, and the tendon of the supraspinatus. As depicted in Fig. 5.28A, combining the resultant SCS force vector with the force vector due to *gravity (G)* yields a compressive force (labeled CF), oriented at right angles to the surface of the glenoid fossa. The compression force stabilizes or "locks" the GH joint by firmly pushing the humeral head against the glenoid fossa, thereby resisting a gravity-induced descent of the humerus The inclined plane of the glenoid acts as a partial shelf that also offers some support for the weight of the arm.

The passive mechanism just described for static stability of the GH joint is often adequate for activities such as standing with the relatively unweighted arm hanging freely at the side. A secondary, muscular-based mechanism may be needed to ensure additional

Why the Glenoid Labrum Is So Vulnerable to Injury

Several structural and functional factors explain why the glenoid labrum is so frequently involved in shoulder pathology. First, the superior part of the glenoid labrum is only loosely attached to the adjacent glenoid rim. Furthermore, approximately 50% of the fibers of the tendon of the long head of the biceps are direct extensions of the superior glenoid labrum; the remaining 50% arise from the supraglenoid tubercle.[254] Exceedingly large or repetitive forces within the biceps tendon can partially detach the loosely secured superior labrum from its near–12 o'clock position on the glenoid rim. The relatively high incidence of superior labral tears in throwing athletes, such as baseball pitchers, can be related to the forces within the biceps during this activity. The long head of the biceps is stressed (along with the anterior and inferior capsule) during the "cocking" phase of pitching, and again as the muscle rapidly decelerates the extending shoulder and pronating forearm during the follow-through release phase of the pitch.[131] Much of this stress is transferred directly to the superior labrum. A weakening of the proximal attachment of the long head of the biceps likely limits the muscle's ability to restrain

anterior translation of the humeral head.[57] These pathomechanics may predispose the throwing athlete to anterior instability and further associated stress. Lesions or detachments of the glenoid labrum occur also along the anterior-inferior rim of the glenoid fossa.[6,181] Normally this region of the labrum is firmly attached to the anterior band of the inferior capsular ligament. As previously described, increased laxity or tears in this portion of the capsule can lead to excessive and repetitive anterior translations or recurrent anterior dislocations of the humeral head. A rapidly anteriorly translating humeral head may further stress the adjacent anterior-inferior capsule and attached glenoid labrum. The resulting frayed or partially torn labrum or adjacent capsule may create a vicious cycle of greater anterior GH joint instability and more frequent episodes of stress in this region. Conservative, nonsurgical management of a detached or torn glenoid labrum may be unsuccessful, especially in the throwing athlete with a demonstrable unstable GH joint. Surgical repair may therefore be required, followed by a specific postoperative rehabilitation program.[147,268]

stability when the upper limb encounters a more significant inferiorly oriented distractive load, such as when holding a pail of water by hand at waist level. The secondary, active source of static support is furnished primarily by the rotator cuff muscles. The overall force vector generated by much of the rotator cuff is oriented nearly horizontally, roughly parallel with the compression force generated by the passive mechanism. Isometric activation of the rotator cuff muscles effectively compresses the humeral head firmly against the shallow glenoid—a mechanism often referred to as *concavity compression*.[179] Of interest is a classic study by Basmajian and Bazant[14] that suggests that the nervous system normally recruits the more *horizontal* rotator cuff muscles (and, when needed, the posterior deltoid) as a secondary source of static stability *before* the more vertically running muscles, such as the biceps, triceps, and middle deltoid. The important stabilizing role of the rotator cuff group will be described in greater detail later in the chapter.

An underlying component of the static locking mechanism illustrated in Fig. 5.28A is that the ST posture orients the glenoid fossa slightly *upward*. Chronic downward rotation may be associated with "poor posture" or may be secondary to paralysis or weakness of certain muscles, such as the upper trapezius. Regardless of the cause, loss of the upwardly rotated position increases the angle between the force vectors created by the superior capsuloligamentous structures (SCS) and gravity (G); see Fig. 5.28B. Adding these force vectors now yields a *reduced* compressive force (CF). Gravity can pull the humerus down the face of the glenoid fossa. Over time, and if not supported by external means, the downward pull can result in plastic deformation of the superior capsuloligamentous structures. As a consequence, the inadequately supported head of the humerus may eventually sublux or dislocate inferiorly from the glenoid fossa.

CORACOACROMIAL ARCH AND ASSOCIATED BURSA

The *coracoacromial arch* is formed by the coracoacromial ligament and the acromion process of the scapula (see Fig. 5.26). The *coracoacromial ligament* attaches between the anterior margin of the acromion and the lateral border of the coracoid process.

The coracoacromial arch forms the functional "roof" of the GH joint. The space between the coracoacromial arch and the underlying humeral head was referred to earlier in the chapter as the *subacromial space*. The reported height of the subacromial space varies widely for the asymptomatic adult, but, on average, measures about 8 to 10 mm with the arm resting by the side.[72,79,182,221] This clinically relevant space is packed relatively tight with several tissues, including the supraspinatus muscle and tendon, the subacromial bursa, the long head of the biceps, and part of the superior capsule.

Multiple separate *bursa sacs* exist around the shoulder. Some of the sacs are extensions of the synovial membrane of the GH joint, such as the subscapular bursa, whereas others are separate structures. All are situated in regions where significant frictional forces develop, such as between tendons, capsule and bone, muscle and ligament, or two adjacent muscles. Two important bursa sacs are located superior to the humeral head (Fig. 5.29). The *subacromial bursa* lies within the subacromial space, above the supraspinatus muscle and below the acromion process. This bursa normally protects the relatively soft and vulnerable supraspinatus muscle and tendon from the rigid undersurface of the acromion. The *subdeltoid bursa* is a lateral extension of the subacromial bursa, limiting frictional forces between the deltoid and the underlying supraspinatus tendon and humeral head.

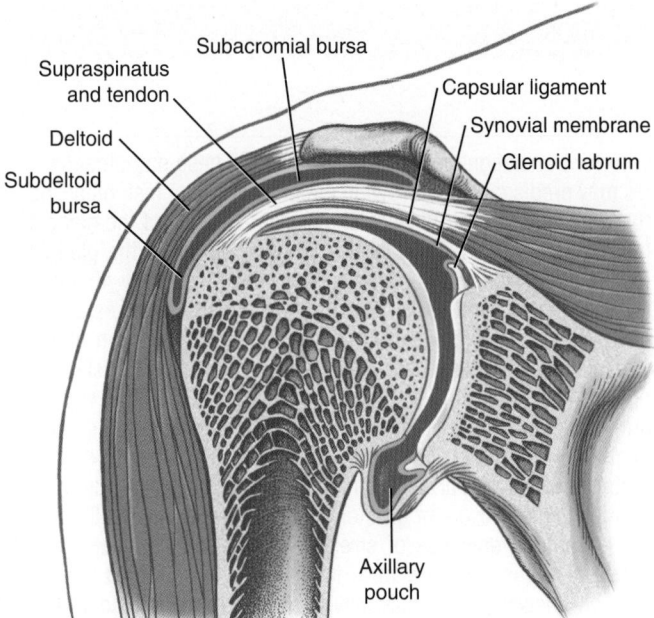

FIGURE 5.29 An anterior view of a frontal plane cross-section of the right glenohumeral joint. Note the subacromial and subdeltoid bursa within the subacromial space. Bursa and synovial lining are depicted in blue. The deltoid and supraspinatus muscles are also shown.

KINEMATICS

The GH joint rotates in all three planes and therefore possesses 3 degrees of freedom. The primary rotational movements at the GH joint are *flexion and extension, abduction and adduction,* and *internal and external rotation* (Fig. 5.30). Often, a fourth motion is defined at the GH joint: *horizontal adduction and abduction* (also called *horizontal flexion and extension,* respectively). This fourth motion is typically defined with the humerus elevated 90 degrees. This being the case, the humerus moves around a vertical axis of rotation: anteriorly during horizontal adduction and posteriorly during horizontal abduction.

Reporting motion at the GH joint uses the anatomic position as the 0-degree or neutral reference point. In the sagittal plane, for example, flexion is the motion that would rotate the humerus anteriorly from the 0-degree position. Extension, in contrast, is what would rotate of the humerus posteriorly from the 0-degree position.

Virtually any purposeful motion of the GH joint involves motion at the ST joint, including the associated movements at the SC and AC joints. The following discussion, however, focuses primarily on the isolated kinematics of the GH joint.

Abduction and Adduction

Abduction and adduction are traditionally defined as rotation of the humerus in the near frontal plane around an axis oriented in the near anterior-posterior direction (see Fig. 5.30). Normally, the healthy or typically developed person has up to about 120 degrees of abduction at the GH joint, although a range of values has been reported.[105,154] Achieving close to 180 degrees of abduction of the *shoulder,* however, requires a simultaneous approximate 60 degrees of upward rotation of the scapula; these kinematics were introduced previously in this chapter.

The arthrokinematics of abduction involve the convex head of the humerus rolling superiorly while simultaneously sliding inferiorly (Fig. 5.31). Roll-and-slide arthrokinematics occur along, or

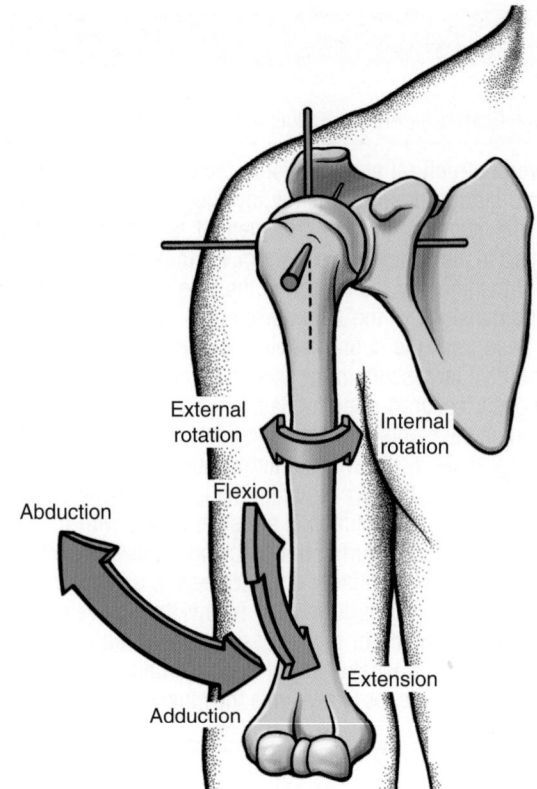

FIGURE 5.30 The osteokinematics of the glenohumeral joint includes abduction and adduction *(purple),* flexion and extension *(green),* and internal and external rotation *(blue).* Note that each axis of rotation is color-coded with its corresponding plane of movement.

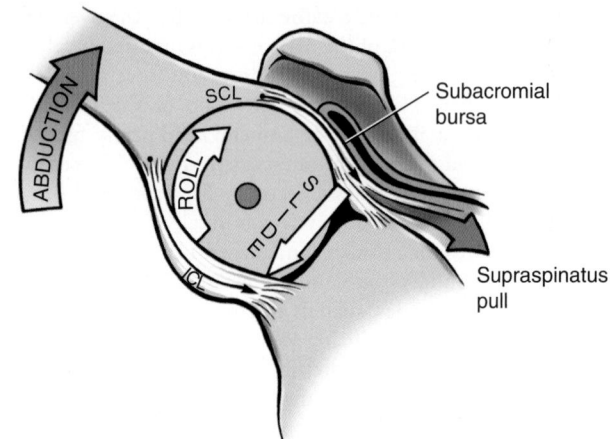

FIGURE 5.31 The arthrokinematics of the right glenohumeral joint during active abduction. The supraspinatus is shown contracting to direct the superior roll of the humeral head. The taut inferior capsular ligament *(ICL)* is shown supporting the head of the humerus like a hammock (see text). Note that the superior capsular ligament *(SCL)* remains relatively taut because of the pull from the attached contracting supraspinatus. Stretched tissues are depicted as long black arrows.

close to, the longitudinal diameter of the glenoid fossa (see Fig. 5.25). The arthrokinematics associated with adduction are like those associated with abduction but occur in reverse.

Fig. 5.31 depicts part of the tendon of the supraspinatus muscle blending with the superior capsule of the GH joint. In addition to producing abduction, the active muscular contraction pulls the superior capsule taut, thereby protecting it from being pinched

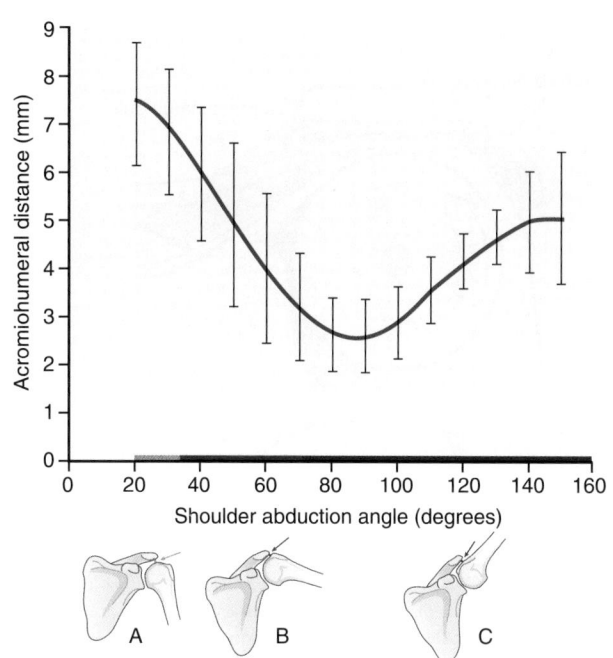

FIGURE 5.32 Means and standard deviations of the acromiohumeral distance during active shoulder abduction in the scapular plane. Data were collected from eight healthy males (mean age 30 years) seated in an upright position. The orange bar (along horizontal axis) indicates the arc of abduction where the *humeral head* is closest to the undersurface of the acromion. The red bar indicates the arc of abduction where the distal attachment of the *supraspinatus* is closest to the undersurface of the acromion. The blue bar indicates the arc of abduction where the *proximal shaft* of the humerus is closest to the undersurface of the acromion. (Shoulder abduction angle is defined as the angle between a vertical reference and the long axis of the humerus.) (Data and plot design redrawn from Giphart JE, van der Meijden OA, Millett PJ: The effects of arm elevation on the 3-dimensional acromiohumeral distance: a biplane fluoroscopy study with normative data, *J Shoulder Elbow Surg* 21[11]:1593–1600, 2012.)

between the humeral head and undersurface of the acromion process. The muscular force also provides dynamic stability to the joint. (*Dynamic stability* refers to the stability achieved while the joint is moving.) As abduction reaches about 90 degrees, the prominent humeral head gradually unfolds and stretches the axillary pouch of the inferior capsular ligament of the GH joint. The resulting tension within the inferior capsule acts as a hammock or sling, which supports the head of the humerus.[3]

The roll-and-slide arthrokinematics depicted in Fig. 5.31 are essential to the completion of full-range abduction. Recall that the longitudinal diameter of the articular surface of the humeral head is almost twice the size of the longitudinal diameter on the glenoid fossa. The arthrokinematics of abduction demonstrate how a simultaneous roll and offsetting slide allow a larger convex surface to roll over a much smaller concave surface without running out of articular surface.[184] In combination, the simultaneous roll-and-slide arthrokinematics at the GH joint and accompanying scapular kinematics influence the height and volume of the subacromial space throughout abduction.[136] A critical minimal height must be maintained to prevent undesired compression of the contents within the space. Understanding the variables that might influence the height of the subacromial space during abduction is an important area of research.[40,136,140] Giphart and colleagues used biplanar fluoroscopy to measure the acromiohumeral distance (i.e., the previously defined subacromial space) as healthy persons performed active shoulder abduction in the scapular plane, between 20 and 150 degrees.[72] As depicted in Fig. 5.32, this study showed that during shoulder abduction, the acromiohumeral distance (AHD) naturally fluctuates from about 7.5 mm at 20 degrees of abduction to its smallest distance of 2.6 mm near 85 degrees of abduction. The AHD then increases to about 5 mm at 150 degrees of abduction. As indicated by the orange shaded bar in Fig. 5.32, at about 20 to 35 degrees of abduction, the AHD is formed between the acromion and the articular surface of the humeral head. Between about 35 and 70 degrees of abduction, the AHD shifts to between the acromion and

the attachment site of the supraspinatus at the greater tubercle of the humerus (red shaded bar). This is of clinical interest because this arc of abduction may place the supraspinatus tendon at its most vulnerable position for an undesired and potentially painful compression within the subacromial space. As indicated by the blue shaded bar in Fig. 5.32, at abduction angles *greater* than about 70 degrees, the AHD shifts to between the acromion and the proximal shaft of the humerus. This region of the humerus is well distal to the "footprint" made by the supraspinatus on the upper facet of the greater tubercle. Shoulder pain during resisted abduction at shoulder angles significantly greater than 70 degrees may not necessarily stem from direct subacromial impingement on the supraspinatus tendon but rather from other stressed-related mechanisms perhaps coupled with a generalized tendinopathy of the rotator cuff.[117,137] All local tissues, inflamed or otherwise, would naturally be subjected to relatively large kinetic loads as the external moment arm (due to gravity) increases when the shoulder approaches 90 degrees of abduction. A better understanding of how the arc of shoulder abduction influences the biomechanics and spatial dimensions within the subacromial space may help with the diagnosis, evaluation, and treatment of pathology or other painful conditions suspected in this region.[40,136,140]

Clinical Relevance of Roll-and-Slide Arthrokinematics at the Glenohumeral Joint

In some pathologic conditions, the ideal roll-and-slide arthrokinematics depicted in Fig. 5.31 do not occur. Consider, for example, excessive thickening or stiffness in the inferior capsular ligament of the GH joint associated with *adhesive capsulitis*.[168] Such stiffness could limit the inferior slide of the humeral head during abduction. Without a sufficient concurrent inferior slide, the superior rolling humeral head would likely migrate upwards toward the unyielding coracoacromial arch. Theoretically, an adult-sized humeral head that is rolling up a glenoid fossa *without* a concurrent inferior slide would translate through a 10-mm subacromial space after only 22 degrees of GH joint abduction (Fig. 5.33A). The resulting excessive

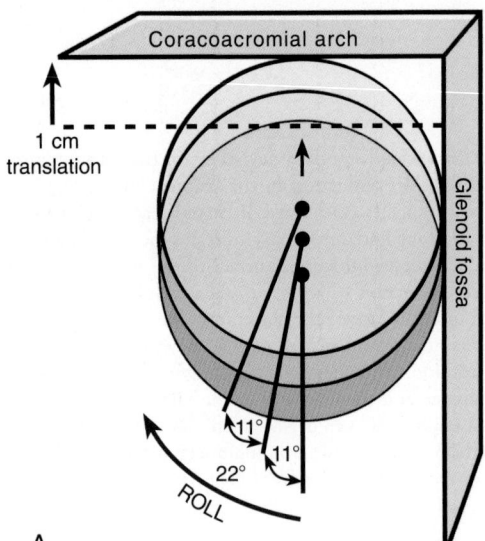
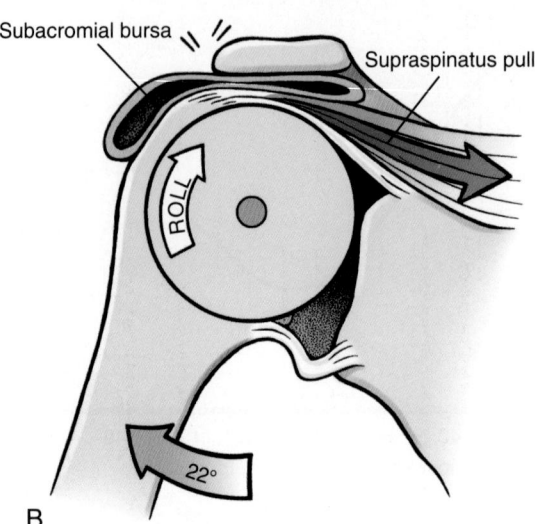

FIGURE 5.33 (A) A model of the glenohumeral joint depicting a ball the size of a typical adult humeral head rolling across a flattened (glenoid) surface. Based on the assumption that the humeral head is a sphere with a circumference of 16.3 cm, the head of the humerus would translate upward 1 cm after a superior roll (abduction) of only 22 degrees. This magnitude of translation would cause the humeral head to press against the contents of the subacromial space. (B) Anatomic representation of the model used in (A). Note that abduction *without* a concurrent inferior slide causes the humeral head to impinge against the arch and block further abduction.

superior migration of the humeral head would likely lead to excessive stress placed on the articular cartilage of the humeral head or tissues located within the subacromial space, such as the supraspinatus tendon and associated bursa (see Fig. 5.33B). Such abnormal arthrokinematics may also physically block further abduction. Although data vary, most in vivo measurements of the asymptomatic shoulder show that throughout scapular plane abduction, the center of the humeral head experiences only a few millimeters of net translation relative to the glenoid.[b] It is clear, therefore, that the concurrent inferior slide of the humeral head relative to the fossa offsets its inherent tendency to translate significantly superiorly with abduction.

In most healthy persons, the offsetting roll-and-slide arthrokinematics in conjunction with a pliable inferior capsule help maintain a sufficiently unobstructed subacromial space during abduction. In cases of excessive stiffness and reduced volume of the axillary pouch, however, the humeral head may be forced upward a considerable distance during abduction, against the delicate tissues within the subacromial space. Such unnatural and repeated compression or abrasion may damage and inflame the supraspinatus tendon, subacromial bursa, long head of the biceps tendon, or superior parts of the capsule. Over time, this repeated compression may lead to the painful condition traditionally referred to as *subacromial impingement syndrome.* Recent literature, however, has advocated use of the term *subacromial pain syndrome,* reflecting the findings that actual impingement may not always be part of the pathomechanics of this condition.[7,167]

Flexion and Extension

Flexion and extension at the GH joint are defined as a rotation of the humerus in the near sagittal plane around a near medial-lateral axis of rotation (Fig. 5.34). The arthrokinematics involve primarily a *spinning* of the humeral head relative to the glenoid fossa. As shown in Fig. 5.34, the spinning of the humeral head draws much of the surrounding capsular structures relatively taut.

At least 120 degrees of flexion can occur at the GH joint. Flexing the shoulder to nearly 180 degrees requires an accompanying upward rotation of a relatively protracted ST joint.[154] As the humerus begins to flex from the anatomic position along a near sagittal plane path, the distal attachment of the supraspinatus emerges posteriorly from underneath the acromion process. The muscle's tendon may thus become less vulnerable to impingement at low angles of elevation during flexion than during GH abduction.[141]

Full extension of the shoulder beyond the anatomic position reaches a position of about 65 degrees actively (and 80 degrees passively) behind the frontal plane. This motion stretches the capsular ligaments, causing a slight anterior tilting of the scapula. This forward tilt may enhance the extent of a backward reach.

Internal and External Rotation

From the anatomic position, internal and external rotation at the GH joint is defined as an axial rotation of the humerus in the horizontal plane (see Fig. 5.30). This rotation occurs around a vertical or longitudinal axis that runs through the shaft of the humerus. The arthrokinematics of external rotation take place over the transverse diameters of the humeral head and the glenoid fossa (see Fig. 5.25). The humeral head simultaneously rolls posteriorly and slides anteriorly on the glenoid fossa (Fig. 5.35). The arthrokinematics for internal rotation are similar, except that the directions of the roll and slide are reversed.

A simultaneous slide during internal and external rotation allows the much larger transverse diameter of the humeral head to roll over a much smaller surface area of the glenoid fossa. The importance of these anterior and posterior slides is evident by

[b]72,125,139,159,161,194,206,248

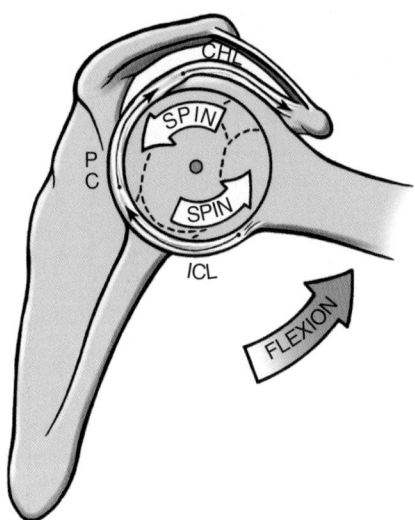

FIGURE 5.34 Side view of flexion in the near sagittal plane of the right glenohumeral joint. A point on the head of the humerus is shown spinning around a point on the glenoid fossa. Stretched structures are shown as long thin arrows. *PC,* posterior capsule; *ICL,* inferior capsular ligament; *CHL,* coracohumeral ligament.

returning to the model of the humeral head shown in Fig. 5.33A but envisioning the humeral head rolling over the glenoid fossa's transverse diameter. If, for example, external rotation of 75 degrees were to consist of a posterior roll with no concurrent anterior slide, the head would be displaced posteriorly by roughly 38 mm. This amount of translation would likely disarticulate the joint because the entire transverse diameter of the glenoid fossa is only about 25 mm (about 1 inch). Normally, however, full external rotation results in only 1 to 2 mm of posterior translation of the center of the humeral head, demonstrating that an "offsetting" anterior slide accompanies the posterior roll.[88]

From the anatomic position, about 75 to 85 degrees of internal rotation and 60 to 75 degrees of external rotation are usually possible, but much variation can be expected. In a position of 90 degrees of abduction, the external rotation range of motion usually increases to near 90 degrees, accompanying by significant elongation of the middle GH ligament and anterior band of the inferior GH ligament.[216] Regardless of the position at which these rotations occur, there is typically associated movement at the ST joint. From the anatomic position, full internal and external rotation of the shoulder includes varying amounts of scapular protraction and retraction, respectively.

 SPECIAL FOCUS 5.5

"Dynamic Centralization" of the Humeral Head: An Important Interaction between the Glenohumeral Joint Capsule and the Rotator Cuff Muscles

During virtually all volitional shoulder motions, rotator cuff muscles play an essential role in the dynamic stability of the GH joint. Activated muscle forces combine with the passive forces from stretched capsular ligaments to maintain the humeral head in proper position relative to the glenoid fossa. Dynamic stability at the GH joint relies heavily on the interaction of these forces, particularly because of the lack of bony containment of the joint. Fig. 5.35 highlights an example of a dynamic stabilizing mechanism during active *external rotation.* The infraspinatus (one of the rotator cuff muscles) is shown contracting to produce external rotation at the GH joint. Because the infraspinatus attaches partially to the posterior capsule, its active contraction limits the slack produced in this structure.[108] The resulting maintenance of tension in the posterior capsule, combined with the natural rigidity of the activated muscle, helps stabilize the posterior side of the joint during active external rotation. In the healthy shoulder, the anterior side of the joint is also stabilized during active external rotation. Passive tension within the partially overlapping and stretched subscapularis, middle GH ligament, and coracohumeral ligament adds rigidity to the anterior capsule. Forces therefore are generated on both sides of the joint during active external rotation, serving to stabilize and centralize the humeral head against the glenoid fossa.

An excessively tight GH joint capsule may interfere with the effectiveness of the centralization process just described. For example, during active external rotation (as shown in Fig. 5.35), an overly tight anterior capsule could position (or "push") the humeral head too far posteriorly. This mechanism could decentralize the humeral head, creating abnormal contact areas around the joint. Alternatively (and likely more commonly), during active internal rotation an overly tight posterior capsule can displace the humeral

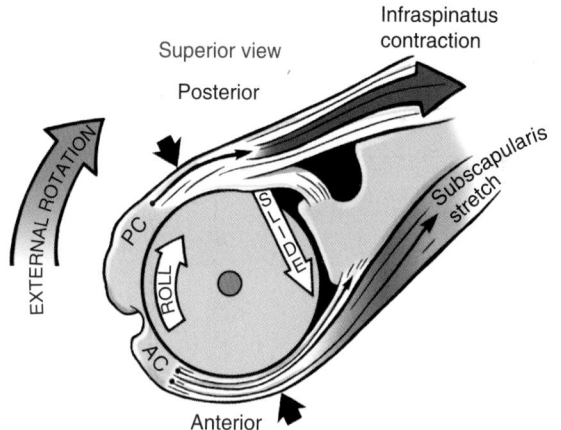

FIGURE 5.35 Superior view of roll-and-slide arthrokinematics during active external rotation of the right glenohumeral joint. The infraspinatus is shown contracting *(dark red),* causing the posterior roll of the humerus. The subscapularis muscle and anterior capsular *(AC)* structures generate passive tension from being stretched. The posterior capsule *(PC)* is pulled relatively taut because of the pull of the contracting infraspinatus muscle. The two large bold black arrows represent forces that centralize and thereby stabilize the humeral head during external rotation. Stretched tissues are depicted as *thin, elongated arrows.*

head too far anteriorly. The magnitude of the anterior displacement may partially depend on the presence of excessive laxity within the anterior capsule. Regardless, a tight posterior capsule has been associated with several shoulder impairments, including GH instability, scapular malalignment, subacromial pain, or painful impingement, both internal and external to the capsule.[107,163,172,180,211]

As with all motions of the GH joint, the specific arthrokinematics depend on the exact plane of the osteokinematics. As previously described, from the anatomic position, internal and external rotation are associated with roll-and-slide arthrokinematics. Rotation of the GH joint with the humerus abducted about 90 degrees, however, requires the humeral head to mainly spin about its center against the glenoid fossa. Visualizing the relationship between the osteokinematics and arthrokinematics at a joint provides a useful mental construct for the treatment and evaluation of patients. Some of these relationships are summarized in Table 5.2.

Overall Kinematics of Shoulder Abduction: Establishing Six Kinematic Principles of the Shoulder Complex

To this point in this chapter, the study of shoulder arthrology has focused primarily on the isolated kinematics of the various joints, or links, within the shoulder complex. The next and final discussion integrates the kinematics across multiple regions of the shoulder, with a focus on how the bones or joints interact and contribute to full active abduction. This discussion will define *six kinematic principles* related to shoulder abduction, each possessing a fundamental mechanical role in the movement. These principles are summarized in Fig. 5.36. As a visual supplement to this figure, Videos 5.1, 5.2, and 5.3 show in vivo-based computer animations (across three orthogonal views) of a heathy subject performing scapular plane

TABLE 5.2 Summary of the Kinematic Relationships at the Glenohumeral Joint

Osteokinematics	Plane of Motion/ Axis of Rotation	Arthrokinematics
Abduction and adduction	Near frontal plane/near anterior-posterior axis of rotation	Roll and slide along joint's longitudinal diameter
Internal and external rotation	Horizontal plane/vertical axis of rotation	Roll and slide along joint's transverse diameter
Flexion and extension, internal and external rotation (in 90 degrees of abduction)	Near sagittal plane/near medial-lateral axis of rotation	Primarily a spin between humeral head and glenoid fossa

abduction. These videos, constructed from data obtained from biplanar fluoroscopy,[142] should be referred to throughout the upcoming discussions.

Information used to conceive the kinematic principles is based on different technologies for measuring movements of the shoulder, which have included cadaver testing systems, in vivo-based radiography, goniometry, photography, cinematography, biplanar

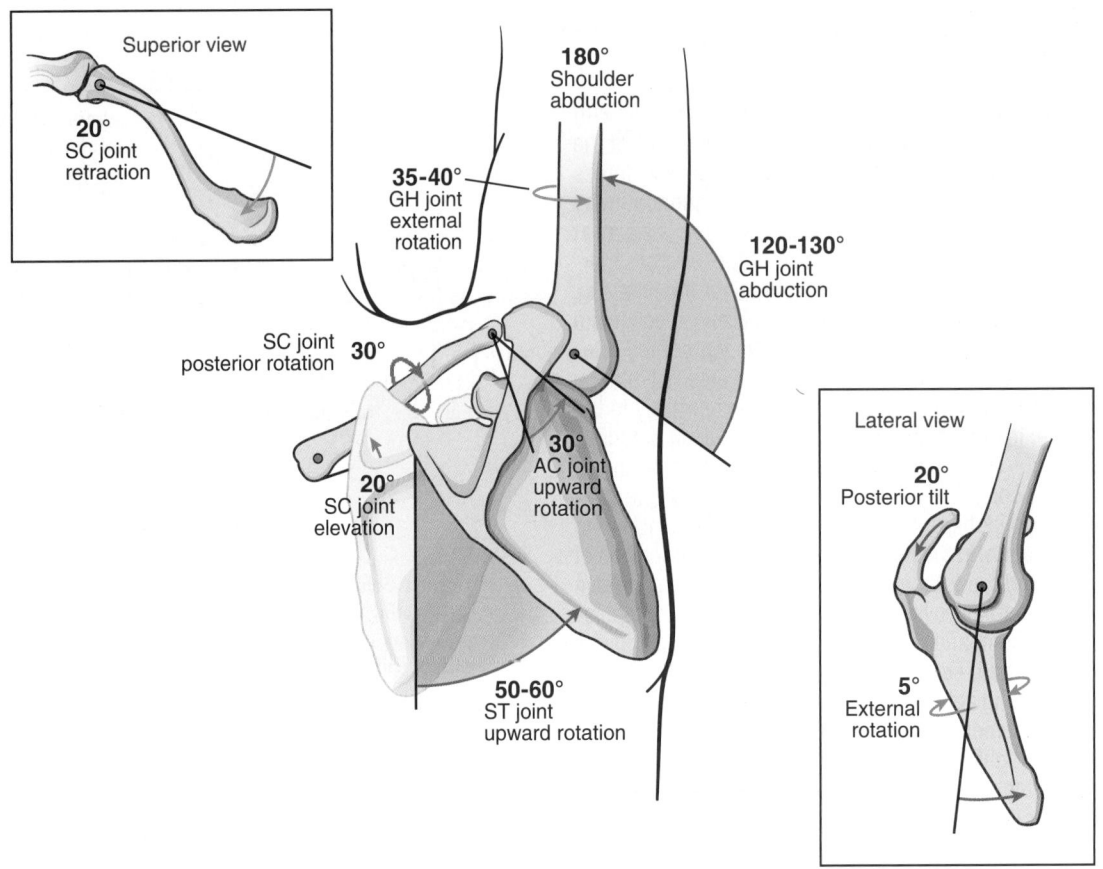

FIGURE 5.36 Posterior view of the right shoulder complex after the arm has abducted about 180 degrees. The approximate magnitudes of scapulothoracic *(ST)* joint upward rotation and glenohumeral *(GH)* joint abduction are shown shaded in purple. Additional boxes depict superior and lateral views of selected kinematics of the clavicle and scapula, respectively. All numeric values are approximations, chosen from a wide range of estimates cited in the text. *(SC,* sternoclavicular; *AC,* acromioclavicular)

radiographic or fluoroscopic imagining, magnetic resonance (MR) imaging, computed tomography (CT) scans, ultrasound, and opto-electronic, electromechanical, electromagnetic tracking devices (with skin-mounted, marker-less, or surgically implanted sensors), and inertial measurement systems. Several of these methods are used in conjunction with computer modeling.[38,72,142,178]

The term *abduction* is used loosely throughout the upcoming discussion of the six kinematic principles to imply an active movement of lifting the arm fully overhead, without necessarily specifying the exact plane of movement (e.g., scapular, frontal, near sagittal). Regardless of the specific path of abduction, raising the arm overhead in a pain-free and natural manner usually indicates optimal kinematic sequencing or coupling of the joints across the shoulder. Understanding how the multiple joints operate together informs the clinician on how impairments in one part of the shoulder complex can affect another. This understanding can serve as a foundation for effective evaluation and treatment of the shoulder.

SCAPULOHUMERAL RHYTHM

In the healthy shoulder, a natural kinematic rhythm or timing exists between GH joint abduction and ST upward rotation. This rhythm is one of the more dominant and observable kinematic relationships of shoulder abduction (Video 5.4). Inman, in his pioneering research published many decades ago, popularized the term "scapulohumeral rhythm" to explain this kinematic relationship.[105] Inman reported that after about 30 degrees of (frontal plane) abduction this rhythm remained remarkably constant, occurring at a ratio of 2:1, meaning for every 3 degrees of shoulder abduction, 2 degrees occurs by GH abduction and 1 degree by ST upward rotation. The *first kinematic principle* of shoulder abduction states that based on a generalized 2:1 scapulohumeral rhythm, a full arc of nearly 180 degrees of abduction is due to a simultaneous and approximate 120 degrees of GH joint abduction and 60 degrees of ST joint upward rotation (see two purple arcs in the main illustration of Fig. 5.36). Published scapulohumeral rhythms vary, most ranging from 1.25:1 to 2.9:1, relatively close to Inman's reported 2:1 ratio.[c] Furthermore, variations in reported scapulohumeral rhythms reflect differences in measurement technique, age of subjects, speed, direction and plane of motion, and amount of external loading. Regardless of the differing reported ratios, Inman's classic 2:1 ratio remains a simple yet valuable axiom for evaluating kinematic quality of shoulder abduction. Scapulohumeral rhythm may deviate from the usual population-based norms when pathology or pain is present. For example, a person with a significant tear in the rotator cuff is likely to use greater scapular upward rotation and less GH abduction to achieve a given amount of shoulder abduction.[125] Using greater upward rotation may be a compensation strategy intended to reduce the movement demands on a painful GH joint.

STERNOCLAVICULAR AND ACROMIOCLAVICULAR JOINTS DURING FULL ABDUCTION

As stated, upward rotation of the scapula during abduction is one of the essential components of shoulder kinematics. What dictates the overall path of the scapula, however, are the combined kinematics at the SC and AC joints.[138,150,154] The combined kinematics about these joints' near–anterior-posterior axis of rotation is visually depicted in Fig. 5.22. This figure aptly introduces the *second kinematic principle* of abduction, which states that the approximate 60 degrees of upward rotation of the scapula during full shoulder abduction involves a

simultaneous elevation of the clavicle at the SC joint combined with upward rotation of the scapula at the AC joint. Because of conflicting data and different measurement techniques, the exact contribution of each joint movement to the full excursion of scapula upward rotation is uncertain.[105,138,139,154,160] The most compelling research in this area, however, indicates that the upward rotation at the AC joint dominates the aforementioned kinematics.[138]

The *third kinematic principle* of abduction states that the clavicle *retracts* at the SC joint during full shoulder abduction. Recall that in the anatomic position the clavicle lies approximately horizontal, about 20 degrees posterior to the frontal plane (see Fig. 5.4, angle A). During shoulder abduction, the clavicle retracts another 15 to 20 degrees (see Fig. 5.36, top left inset).[72,139,164] Expectedly, the clavicle retracts a greater distance during shoulder abduction in the pure frontal plane than during abduction in the scapular plane or with flexion.[154] This difference reflects the important role of the clavicle in positioning the scapula in the desired plane of elevation of the arm.[35,150]

The *fourth kinematic principle* of abduction states that as the shoulder abducts, the upwardly rotating scapula progressively *posteriorly tilts* and, most notably in the final range of abduction, *externally rotates* (Fig. 5.36, lower right inset).[27,70] (Although scapular posterior tilting and external rotation were described previously in Fig. 5.19A for the AC joint, they may also be used to describe the overall motion of the scapula relative to the thorax.) At rest in the anatomic position, the scapula is anteriorly tilted about 10 degrees and internally rotated approximately 30 to 40 degrees (i.e., in the scapular plane; see Fig. 5.4, angle B). As shoulder abduction proceeds, the upwardly rotating scapula posteriorly tilts about 20 degrees, primarily by motion at the AC joint.[35,154] The external rotation movement of the scapula, although relatively slight and variable, naturally occurs as a *net* of the horizontal plane rotations occurring nearly simultaneously at the SC and AC joints.[118,150] Interestingly, although the scapula typically displays a slight net external rotation by the end of shoulder abduction, it typically undergoes a slight net internal rotation in earlier ranges of shoulder abduction.[27,70] By the end range of shoulder abduction, despite a net movement toward scapular external rotation, the upwardly rotated scapula remains oriented generally within or close to the scapular plane.[118] Literature describing the magnitude and pattern of the aforementioned scapular motions varies considerably, especially those concerning horizontal plane movements of the scapula. The variability in data reflects differences in shoulder pathology or impairments in the participants enrolled in studies as well as in dissimilar experimental methodologies (e.g., plane, magnitude, or direction of movement).[d]

In summary, varying amounts of posterior tilting and external rotation movements of the upwardly rotating scapula serve several useful functions during shoulder abduction. These kinematics (1) help position the scapula relatively flush with the changing curvature of the thorax, (2) orient the glenoid fossa in the specific plane of the intended elevation of the arm (i.e., scapular, frontal, or sagittal), and (3) move the coracoacromial arch *away* from the advancing (abducting) humeral head—a strategy that may reduce or minimize impingement of structures within or near the subacromial space.[154]

The *fifth kinematic principle* of abduction states that the clavicle rotates posteriorly around its own long axis (see Fig. 5.36, main illustration). This clavicular motion was described earlier as one of the primary motions of the SC joint (review in Fig. 5.13 and see Video 5.5). Studies report 20 to 35 degrees of posterior

---

[c]11,27,70,72,80,123,154,164,206,240

[d]36,67,70,77,80,150,151,154,164

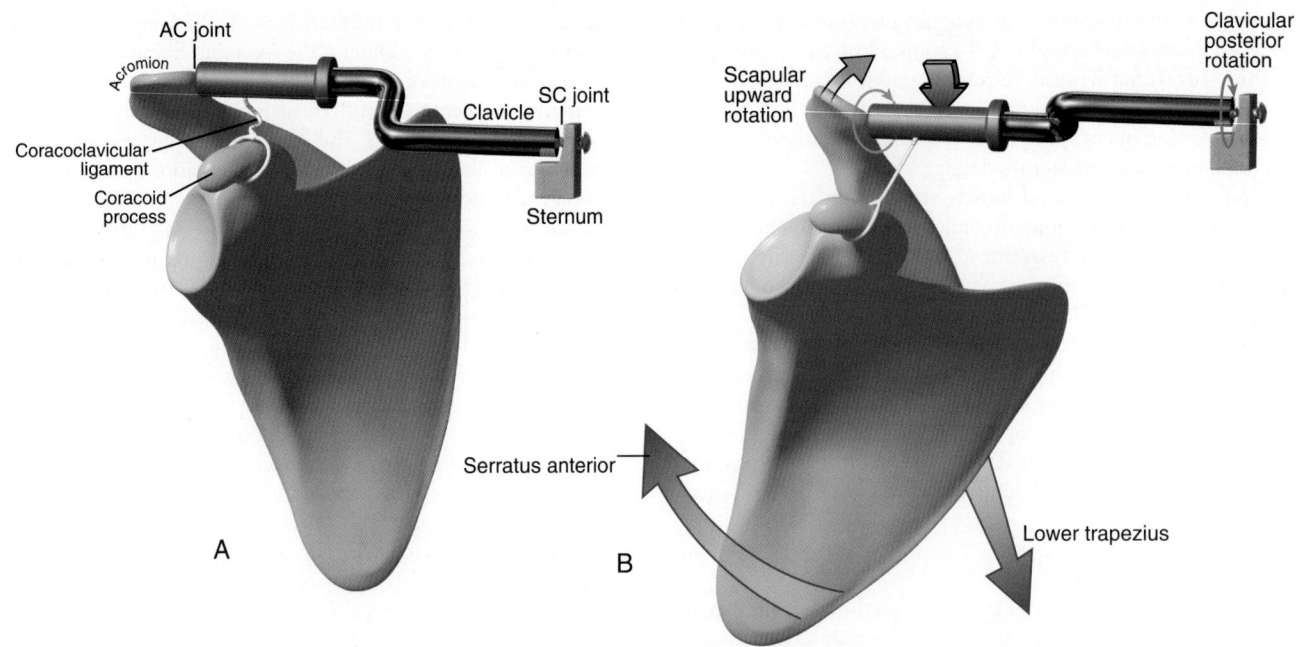

FIGURE 5.37 The mechanics of posterior rotation of the right clavicle are shown in a highly mechanical and diagrammatic fashion. (A) At rest in the anatomic position, the acromioclavicular *(AC)* and sternoclavicular *(SC)* joints are shown with the coracoclavicular ligament represented by a slackened cord. (B) As the serratus anterior and lower trapezius rotate the scapula upward, the coracoclavicular ligament is drawn taut. The tension created within the stretched ligament rotates (flips) the crank-shaped clavicle in a posterior direction. This action allows the AC joint to augment and direct the scapular plane upward rotation (see text for full description).

clavicular rotation during abduction.[105,149,154,252] An in vivo study shows that posterior rotation at the SC joint is the predominant motion of the clavicle during scapular plane abduction, occurring primarily in the middle and late ranges of shoulder abduction.[154] As will be described, the posterior rotation contributes significantly to the mechanics of upward rotation of the scapula.

The mechanism responsible for the posterior rotation of the clavicle is based on a combination of multijoint kinematics, driven by forces transferred from muscle to ligaments.[105,138,140,150,188] Fig. 5.37A shows in a highly diagrammatic fashion the relatively slackened coracoclavicular ligament while at rest in the anatomic position. At the early phases of shoulder abduction, the scapula begins to upwardly rotate at the AC joint, stretching the relatively stiff coracoclavicular ligament (see Fig. 5.37B). The inability of this ligament to significantly elongate restricts further upward rotation at this joint. The tension within the stretched ligament, however, is transferred to the conoid tubercle region of the clavicle, a point located posterior to the bone's longitudinal axis. The application of this force rotates the crank-shaped clavicle posteriorly. This rotation places the clavicular attachment of the coracoclavicular ligament closer to the coracoid process, unloading the ligament slightly and permitting the scapula to continue its final degrees of upward rotation. The posterior rotation of the clavicle also influences the specific path of the accompanying scapular movement. This influence can be appreciated by noting, from a top view, that the clavicle and scapula typically join at the AC joint at an angle roughly between 50 to 60 degrees (review Fig. 5.4A-B. By acting through the AC joint, this orientation allows the posteriorly rotating (and elevating) clavicle to help steer the glenoid fossa *forward and upward* during abduction.[138,149] These kinematics emphasize the biomechanical complexity of the upwardly rotating scapula, incorporating simultaneous and multiplanar kinematics across both the SC and AC joints, optimally positioning the glenoid fossa for the intended path of the abducting humerus.[150]

The *sixth kinematic principle* of abduction states that the humerus externally rotates at the GH joint during shoulder abduction (see Fig. 5.36, main illustration).[123,139,154] One functional benefit of this rotation is that it allows the greater tubercle of the humerus to pass posterior to the acromion process and avoid jamming against the contents within the subacromial space, such as the supraspinatus tendon.[8,140] Stokdijk and colleagues have shown differing ratios of external rotation to humeral elevation based on the specific plane of elevation.[237] Strict frontal plane abduction had a higher ratio (i.e., greater external rotation per degree of abduction) than abduction in the scapular plane. Most of the external rotation at the GH joint that accompanies full shoulder abduction occurs between 0 and about 60 to 70 degrees of shoulder abduction.[154,161]

Even though the humerus externally rotates mainly at the GH joint, the sum of humeral external rotation with respect to the trunk has other contributing influences, especially beyond 60 to 70 degrees of abduction. For example, during the last half of full scapular or frontal plane abduction, the upwardly rotating ST joint combined with posterior tilting of the scapula contributes significantly to the externally rotated position of the humerus.[5] As with virtually all movements across the shoulder, the actual position of the humerus is strongly influenced by the positioning of the more proximal joints. Being aware of these kinematic relationships can help clinicians target movement impairments in the shoulder complex and refine clinical interventions.

In closing, the six kinematic principles associated with the fully abducting shoulder are succinctly summarized in Box 5.1.

SPECIAL FOCUS 5.6

Shoulder Abduction in the Frontal Plane versus the Scapular Plane

Shoulder abduction performed strictly in the frontal plane has historically been used as a representative motion to evaluate overall shoulder function. This motion, however, is not very natural. Abducting the shoulder in the *scapular plane* (about 30–40 degrees anterior to the frontal plane) is a more natural movement and typically allows greater (or at least more comfortable) elevation of the humerus than abducting in the pure frontal plane. Furthermore, abducting in the scapular plane is less mechanically coupled to an obligatory external rotation of the humerus.[237] This can be demonstrated by the following example. Attempt to maximally abduct your shoulder in the *pure* frontal plane while consciously avoiding any accompanying external rotation. The difficulty or inability to complete the extremes of this motion results in part from the greater tubercle of the humerus compressing the contents of the subacromial space against a low point on the coracoacromial arch (Fig. 5.38A).[274] Full frontal plane abduction typically requires an accompanying

external rotation of the humerus. The external rotation ensures that the prominent greater tubercle clears the posterior edge of the undersurface of the acromion.

Next, fully abduct your arm in the *scapular* plane. This abduction movement can usually be performed with greater ease and with less external rotation, at least in the early to midranges of shoulder motion. Impingement is avoided because scapular plane abduction places the apex of the greater tubercle under a relatively high point of the coracoacromial arch (see Fig. 5.38B). Abduction in the scapular plane also allows the naturally retroverted humeral head to be oriented more directly into the glenoid fossa. The proximal and distal attachments of the supraspinatus muscle are also placed along a straight line. These mechanical differences between frontal plane and scapular plane abduction should be considered during evaluation and treatment of patients with shoulder dysfunction, particularly if subacromial impingement or supraspinatus tendinopathy are suspected.

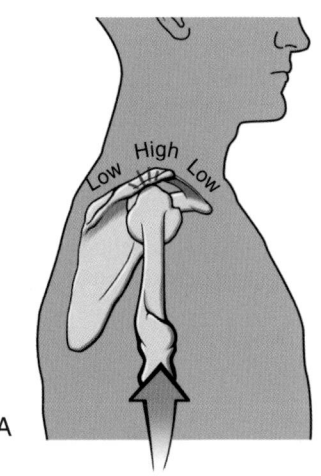

A Frontal plane abduction

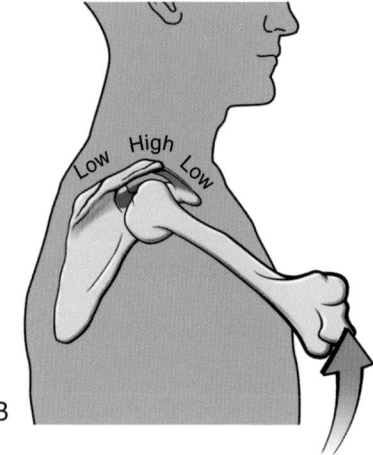

B Scapular plane abduction

FIGURE 5.38 Side view of the right glenohumeral joint comparing abduction of the humerus in (A) the true frontal plane and (B) the scapular plane. In both (A) and (B), the glenoid fossa is oriented in the scapular plane. The relative low and high points of the coracoacromial arch are also depicted. The line of force of the supraspinatus is shown in (B), coursing under the coracoacromial arch.

BOX 5.1 Six Kinematic Principles Associated with Full Abduction of the Shoulder

Principle 1: Based on a generalized 2:1 scapulohumeral rhythm, active shoulder abduction through about 180 degrees occurs due to a simultaneous 120 degrees of GH joint abduction and 60 degrees of scapulothoracic upward rotation.

Principle 2: The 60 degrees of upward rotation of the scapula during full shoulder abduction involves a simultaneous elevation of the clavicle at the sternoclavicular (SC) joint combined with upward rotation of the scapula at the acromioclavicular (AC) joint.

Principle 3: The clavicle retracts at the SC joint during shoulder abduction.

Principle 4: Throughout shoulder abduction, the upwardly rotating scapula progressively posteriorly tilts and, at the end ranges of abduction, externally rotates.

Principle 5: Throughout shoulder abduction, the clavicle posteriorly rotates around its own axis, thereby contributing to the mechanics of upward rotation of the scapula.

Principle 6: The GH joint externally rotates during shoulder abduction.

MUSCLE AND JOINT INTERACTION

Innervation of the Muscles and Joints of the Shoulder Complex

INTRODUCTION TO THE BRACHIAL PLEXUS

The upper extremity receives its innervation primarily through the brachial plexus—a consolidation of ventral rami from the C^5 to T^1 nerve roots (Fig. 5.39). The basic anatomic plan of the brachial plexus is as follows. Nerve *roots* C^5 and C^6 form the upper *trunk,* C^7 forms the middle *trunk,* and C^8 and T^1 form the lower *trunk.* Trunks course a short distance before forming anterior or posterior *subdivisions.* The subdivisions then reorganize into three *cords* (lateral, posterior, and medial), named according to their relationship to the axillary artery. The cords finally branch into named major *nerves,* such as the ulnar, median, radial, axillary, and so on.

INNERVATION OF MUSCLE

The majority of the muscles that drive the shoulder complex receive their motor innervation from two regions of the brachial plexus: (1) nerves that branch from the posterior cord, such as the axillary, subscapular, and thoracodorsal nerves, and (2) nerves that branch from more proximal segments of the brachial plexus, such as the dorsal scapular, long thoracic, pectoral, and suprascapular nerves. This information is summarized in Table 5.3. An exception to this innervation scheme is the trapezius muscle, which is innervated primarily through cranial nerve XI, with lesser motor and sensory innervation from upper cervical nerve roots.[233]

As a reference, the primary nerves and nerve roots that supply the muscles of the upper extremity are contained in Appendix II, Parts A-B, and Fig. II.2 in Part C. In addition, Appendix II, Part D and

Fig. II.3 in Part E include reference materials that may help with the clinical assessment of the motor and sensory C^5 to T^1 nerve roots.

SENSORY INNERVATION TO THE JOINTS

The SC joint receives sensory (afferent) innervation from the C^3 and C^4 nerve roots from the cervical plexus.[233] The AC and GH joints receive sensory innervation via the C^5 and C^6 nerve roots via the suprascapular, axillary, lateral pectoral, and subscapular nerves.[250]

Action of the Shoulder Muscles

Most of the muscles of the shoulder complex fall into one of two functional categories: proximal stabilizers or distal mobilizers. The proximal stabilizers are muscles that originate on the spine, ribs, and cranium and insert on the scapula and clavicle, such as trapezius or serratus anterior. The distal mobilizers are muscles that originate on the scapula and clavicle and insert on the humerus or the forearm, such as the deltoid or biceps brachii. An important recurring theme within this chapter is that optimal function of the shoulder complex requires a coordinated, kinetic interaction between and within these two sets of muscles. For reasons to be explained, understanding these interactions requires a firm knowledge of the bony attachments made and shared by these two sets of muscles. As a reference, the proximal and distal attachments and nerve supply of the muscles of the shoulder complex are listed in Appendix II, Part F. Also, as a reference, a list of cross-sectional areas of selected muscles of the shoulder are listed in Appendix II, Part G.

Muscles of the Scapulothoracic Joint

The muscles of the ST joint are categorized according to their actions as elevators or depressors, protractors or retractors, or

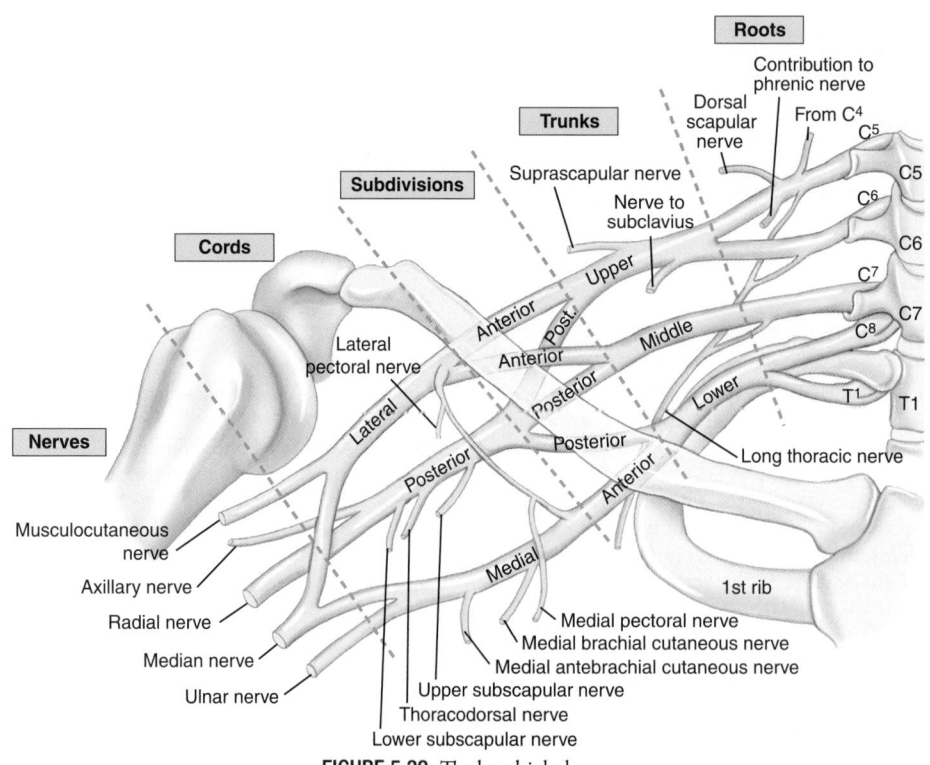

FIGURE 5.39 The brachial plexus.

TABLE 5.3 Nerves That Flow from the Brachial Plexus and Innervate the Primary Muscles of the Shoulder

Nerve	Relation to Brachial Plexus	Primary Nerve Root(s)*	Muscles Supplied
Axillary	Posterior cord	C^5, C^6	Deltoid and teres minor
Thoracodorsal (middle subscapular)	Posterior cord	C^6, C^7, C^8	Latissimus dorsi
Upper subscapular	Posterior cord	C^5, C^6	Upper fibers of subscapularis
Lower subscapular	Posterior cord	C^5, C^6	Lower fibers of subscapularis and teres major
Lateral pectoral	At or proximal to lateral cord	C^5, C^6, C^7	Pectoralis major and occasionally the pectoralis minor
Medial pectoral	At or proximal to medial cord	C^8, T^1	Pectoralis major (sternocostal head) and pectoralis minor
Suprascapular	Upper trunk	C^5, C^6	Supraspinatus and infraspinatus
Subclavian	Upper trunk	C^5, C^6	Subclavius
Dorsal scapular	C^5 nerve root	C^5	Rhomboids (major and minor); levator scapulae†
Long thoracic	Proximal to trunks	C^5, C^6, C^7	Serratus anterior

*Note: The primary spinal nerve roots that contribute to each nerve are listed.
†Also innervated by C^3 and C^4 nerve roots from the cervical plexus.

upward or downward rotators. Some muscles act on the ST joint indirectly by attaching to the clavicle or the humerus.

Muscles with Primary Actions at the Scapulothoracic Joint

ELEVATORS
- Upper trapezius
- Levator scapulae
- Rhomboids

DEPRESSORS
- Lower trapezius
- Latissimus dorsi
- Pectoralis minor
- Subclavius

PROTRACTOR
- Serratus anterior

RETRACTORS
- Middle trapezius
- Rhomboids
- Lower trapezius

UPWARD ROTATORS
- Serratus anterior
- Upper and lower trapezius

DOWNWARD ROTATORS
- Rhomboids
- Pectoralis minor

ELEVATORS

The muscles primarily responsible for elevation of the ST joint are the *upper trapezius, levator scapulae,* and, to a lesser extent, the *rhomboids* (Fig. 5.40). Functionally, these muscles support the posture of the shoulder "girdle" (scapula and clavicle) and the upper extremity. Although variable, ideal posture of the shoulder girdle incorporates a slightly elevated and relatively retracted scapula, with the glenoid fossa facing slightly upward. The upper trapezius, by attaching to the lateral end of the clavicle, provides favorable leverage around the SC joint for maintenance of this ideal posture.

Several pathologies may cause a reduced muscular support of the shoulder girdle. For example, isolated paralysis of the upper trapezius may occur from damage to the spinal accessory nerve (cranial nerve XI) or following polio (a virus affecting the cells of motor nerves). More generally, however, all the elevators of the ST joint may be weakened or paralyzed after a stroke or from a disease such as muscular dystrophy or Guillain-Barré syndrome. Regardless of the pathology, loss of muscular support of the shoulder girdle allows gravity to be the dominant force in determining the resting posture of the shoulder girdle. Such a posture typically includes excessive depression, protraction, and downward rotation of the scapula. Over time this posture can produce damaging stress on other structures located within the shoulder region.

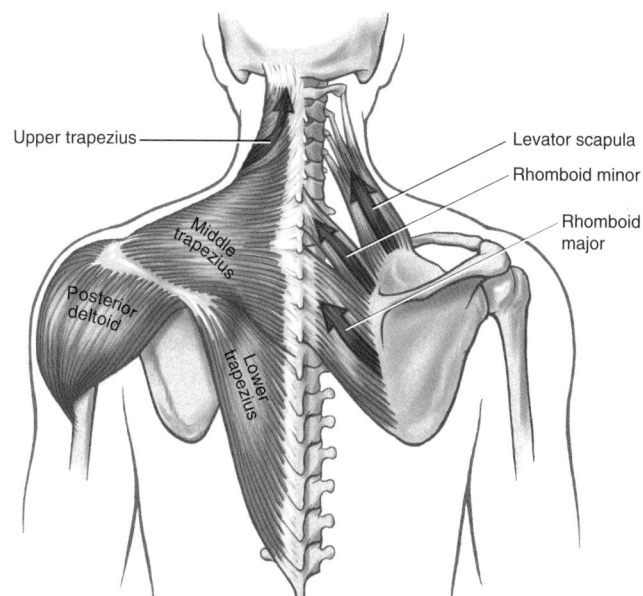

FIGURE 5.40 Posterior view showing the upper trapezius, levator scapulae, and rhomboids (shown separably as major and minor) as elevators of the scapulothoracic joint. Parts of the middle deltoid, the posterior deltoid, and the middle and lower trapezius are also illustrated.

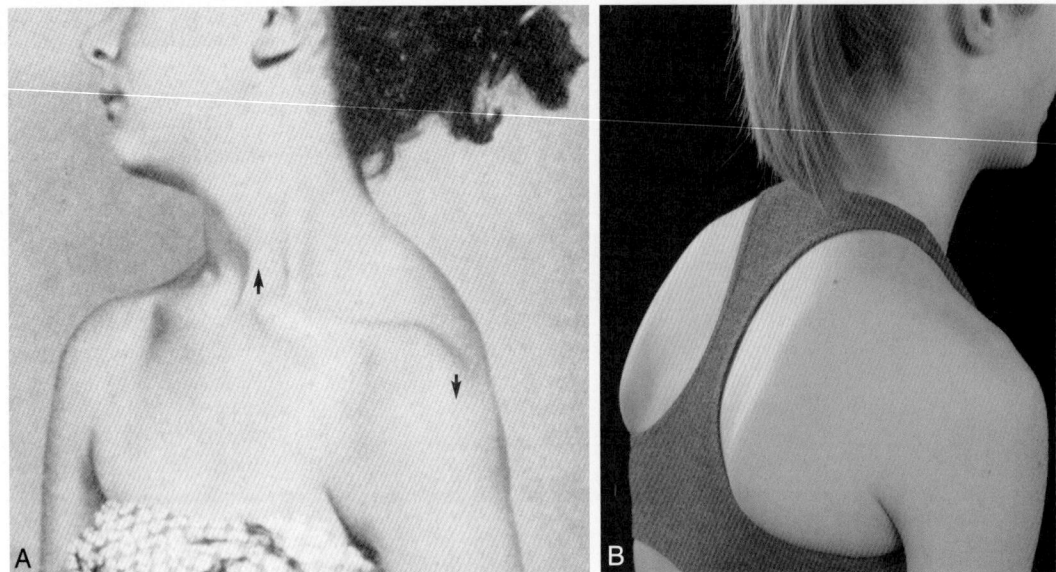

FIGURE 5.41 Examples of abnormal posture of the scapulothoracic joint. (A) Photograph of a girl with paralysis of her left upper trapezius caused by polio virus. The small arrows indicate the direction of subluxation at the sternoclavicular (SC) and glenohumeral (GH) joints. (B) Photograph of a healthy young woman with a posture of "rounded shoulders" without neurologic deficit. The prominence of the medial borders and inferior angles of the scapulae yields clues to the overall scapular posture. (A, modified from Brunnstrom S: Muscle testing around the shoulder girdle, *J Bone Joint Surg Am* 23:263, 1941.)

Fig. 5.41A shows the posture of a girl with paralysis of her left upper trapezius caused by the polio virus.[29] Over time, a depressed lateral end of the clavicle has resulted in superior dislocation of the SC joint (see arrow at medial end of clavicle in Fig. 5.41A). As the lateral end of the clavicle is lowered, the medial end is forced upward because of the fulcrum action of the underlying first rib. The depressed shaft of the clavicle may compress the subclavian vessels and part of the brachial plexus.

Another consequence of long-term paralysis of the upper trapezius is an inferior dislocation (or subluxation) of the GH joint (see arrow in Fig. 5.41A). Recall from earlier discussion that static stability of the GH joint is maintained in part by the humeral head being held firmly against the inclined plane of the glenoid fossa (see Fig. 5.28A). With long-term paralysis of the trapezius, the glenoid fossa typically loses its upwardly rotated position, allowing the humerus to slide inferiorly. The downward pull imposed by gravity on an unsupported arm may strain the capsular ligaments at the GH joint and lead to an irreversible dislocation or subluxation. This complication is often observed in persons with flaccid hemiplegia, which may necessitate a sling to support the weight of the arm.

The previous paragraphs highlight examples of abnormal scapular posturing occurring from a relatively extreme pathology involving denervation and subsequent muscular paralysis. Less extreme examples, however, may involve persons who have no history of neurologic or muscular pathology. For example, Fig. 5.41B features an otherwise healthy young woman with the classic "rounded shoulders" posture. Both scapulae are slightly depressed, downwardly rotated, and protracted. In principle, this posture can lead to similar (but usually far less damaging) biomechanical stress on the SC and GH joints as described for the girl with actual muscle paralysis. As evident by the position of the medial border and inferior angle in the subject in Fig. 5.41B, both scapulae are also slightly internally rotated and anteriorly tilted—postures hypothesized to increase the risk of impinging tissues within the subacromial space.[24,152] Abnormal scapular posture in otherwise neurologically intact persons may be caused by or associated with several factors, including generalized laxity of connective tissues; muscle tightness, control, fatigue or weakness; GH joint capsule tightness; abnormal cervicothoracic posture; or simply habit or mood.

Regardless of the underlying cause or severity of abnormal posturing of the ST joint, this phenomenon clearly affects the biomechanics of the entire shoulder complex. Clinical inspection of the shoulder should always include an analysis of the support provided by the muscles that position the ST joint. Treatment to improve abnormal ST posture can vary depending on the underlying cause. In mild cases the condition may be improved by strengthening or stretching of selected muscles, combined with improving the person's awareness of their postural fault.

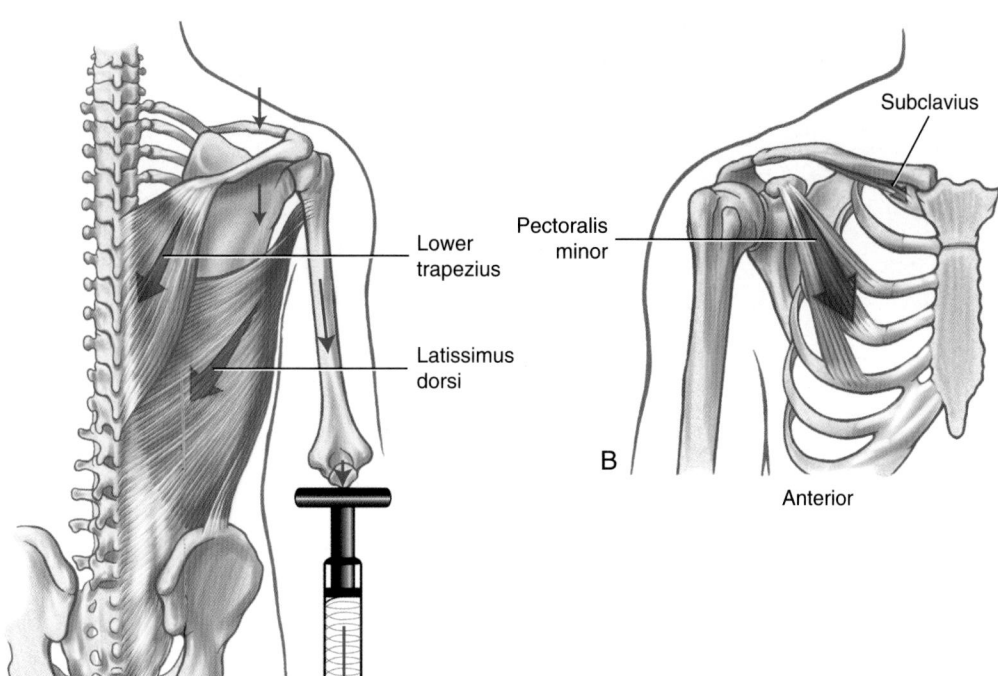

FIGURE 5.42 (A) A posterior view of the lower trapezius and the latissimus dorsi depressing the shoulder girdle (scapula and clavicle). These muscles are pulling down against the resistance provided by the spring mechanism. (B) An anterior view of the pectoralis minor and subclavius during the same activity described in (A).

DEPRESSORS

Depression of the ST joint is performed primarily by the *lower trapezius, latissimus dorsi, pectoralis minor,* and the *subclavius* (Fig. 5.42). The small subclavius muscle acts indirectly on the scapula through its inferior pull on the clavicle.[209] This muscle's near–parallel line of force with the shaft of the clavicle suggests that it produces only a small amount of depression torque on the clavicle, and that its more important function is to compress and thereby stabilize the SC joint. The lower trapezius and pectoralis minor act directly on the scapula to depress the shoulder girdle. The latissimus dorsi, however, depresses the shoulder girdle indirectly, primarily by pulling the humerus inferiorly. The force generated by the depressor muscles can be directed through the scapula and upper extremity and applied against some object, such as the spring shown in Fig. 5.42A. Such an action can increase the overall functional length of the upper extremity.

If the arm is physically blocked from being depressed, force from the depressor muscles can raise the thorax relative to the fixed scapula and arm. This action can occur only if the scapula is stabilized to a greater extent than the thorax. For example, Fig. 5.43 shows a person sitting in a wheelchair using the ST depressors to relieve the contact pressure in the tissues superficial to the ischial tuberosities. With the arm firmly held against the armrest of the wheelchair, contraction of the lower trapezius and latissimus dorsi pulls the thorax and pelvis *up* toward the fixed scapula. This is a very useful movement especially for persons with tetraplegia (quadriplegia) who lack sufficient triceps strength to lift the body weight through elbow extension. This ability to partially unload the weight of the trunk and lower body is also a very important component of transferring between a wheelchair and another surface, such as a bed.

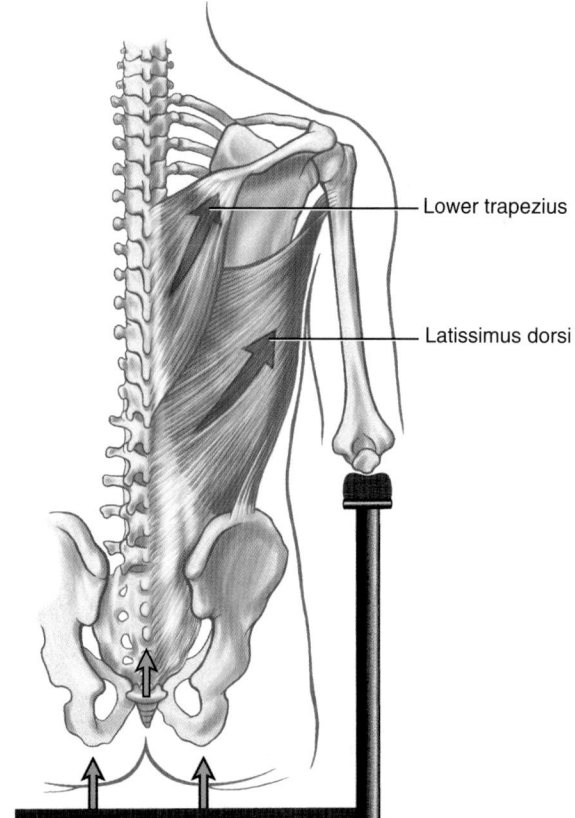

FIGURE 5.43 The lower trapezius and latissimus dorsi are shown indirectly elevating the ischial tuberosities away from the seat of the wheelchair. The contraction of these muscles lifts the pelvic-and-trunk segment up toward the fixed scapula-and-arm segment.

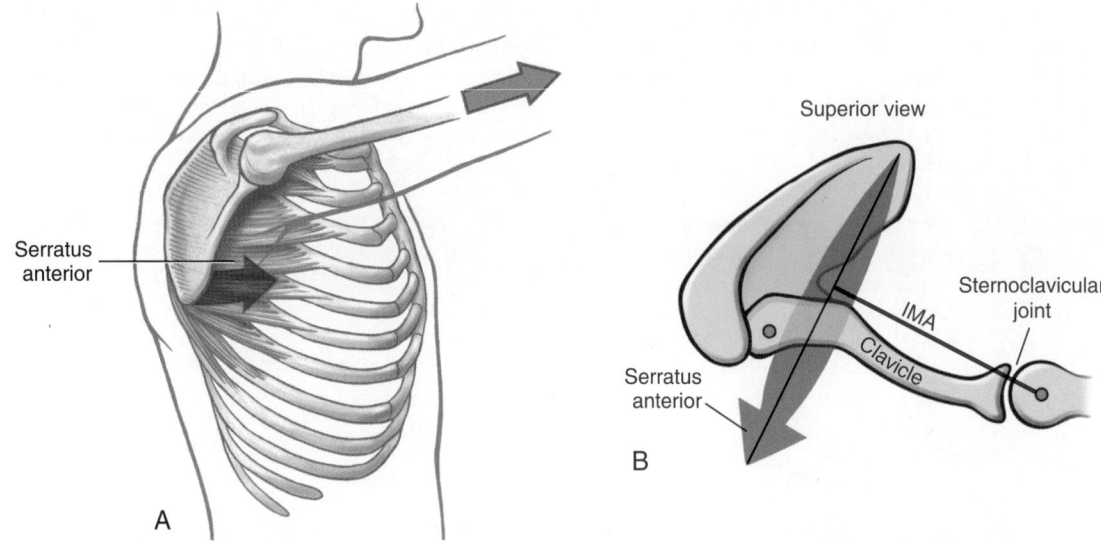

FIGURE 5.44 The right serratus anterior muscle. (A) This expansive muscle passes anterior to the scapula to attach along the entire length of its medial border. The muscle's line of force is shown protracting the scapula and arm in a forward pushing or reaching motion. The fibers that attach near the inferior angle may assist slightly with scapulothoracic depression. (B) A superior view of the right shoulder girdle showing the protraction torque produced by the serratus anterior. The strength of the protraction torque is primarily the result of the muscle force multiplied by the internal moment arm *(IMA)* originating at the vertical axis of rotation at the sternoclavicular joint. The vertical axis of rotation is also shown at the acromioclavicular joint.

PROTRACTORS

The *serratus anterior* is the prime protractor at the ST joint (Fig. 5.44A). This extensive muscle has excellent leverage for protraction around the SC joint's vertical axis of rotation (Fig. 5.44B). The force of scapular protraction is usually transferred across the GH joint and employed for forward pushing and reaching activities.[183] Persons with serratus anterior weakness have significant difficulty performing forward pushing motions, because no other muscle can provide such a direct and effective protraction force on the scapula. Although the pectoralis minor may be considered a secondary scapular protractor, its ability to generate pure ST joint protraction is relatively small. Isolated contraction (or tightness) of this muscle would likely result in an unnatural posture that combines modest scapular protraction, downward rotation, and depression, coupled with significant anterior tilt and internal rotation (apparent by observing the muscle's line of force in Fig. 5.42B). Components of this scapular posture may contribute to a reduced subacromial space.[22,23]

Another function of the serratus anterior is to amplify the final phase of the standard prone push-up. The early phase of a push-up places strong demand on the triceps and pectoralis major. After the elbows are completely extended, however, the chest can be raised farther from the floor by a deliberate protraction of both scapulae. This final component of the push-up is dominated by contraction of the serratus anterior. Bilaterally, the muscles raise the thorax *toward* the fixed and stabilized scapulae. This so-called "push-up plus" action of the serratus anterior may be visualized by rotating Fig. 5.44A 90 degrees clockwise and reversing the direction of the arrow overlying the serratus anterior. Such a movement places specific demands on the serratus anterior and therefore is often incorporated into exercises for strengthening this important muscle.[121,153,183]

RETRACTORS

Contracting synergistically, the *middle trapezius, rhomboids,* and the *lower trapezius* function as primary retractors of the scapula (Fig. 5.45). These muscles dominate the retraction kinetics based on their strong horizontal fiber direction, most notably in the middle

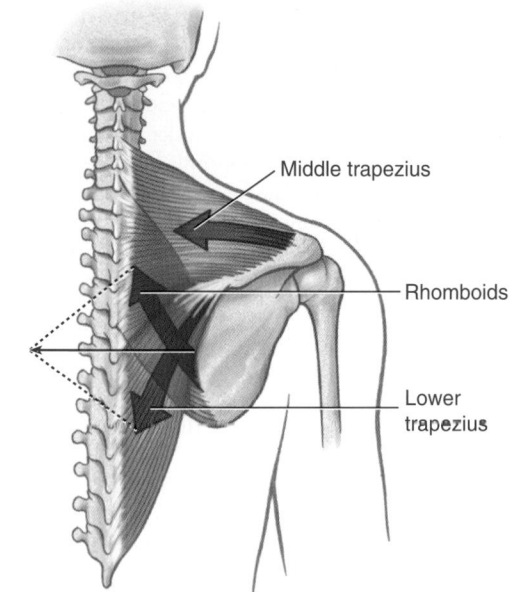

FIGURE 5.45 Posterior view of the middle trapezius, lower trapezius, and rhomboids cooperating to retract the scapulothoracic joint. The dashed lines of force of both the rhomboids and the lower trapezius combine to yield a single retraction force, shown by the thin straight arrow.

trapezius. The levator scapulae can assist with retraction, especially from a position of full protraction. The upper trapezius, particularly the lower more obliquely running fibers, may contribute a secondary means of retracting the scapula via a stable AC joint (review Fig. 5.40).[34] As a group, the retractor muscles dynamically anchor the scapula to the axial skeleton. This proximal stabilization is essential for pulling activities, such as climbing and rowing.

The rhomboids and the lower trapezius show how two muscles can share similar actions (such as retraction) but also function as direct antagonists to one another. During a vigorous retraction effort, the elevation tendency of the rhomboids is neutralized by the depression tendency of the lower trapezius. The lines of force of both muscles combine, however, to produce pure retraction (see Fig. 5.45).

Complete paralysis of the trapezius, and to a lesser extent the rhomboids, significantly reduces the retraction potential of the scapula. The scapula tends to "drift" slightly into protraction as a result of the partially unopposed protraction action of the serratus anterior muscle.[29]

UPWARD AND DOWNWARD ROTATORS

Muscles that perform upward and downward rotation of the ST joint are discussed next in the context of movement of the entire shoulder.

Muscles That Elevate the Arm

The term "elevation" of the arm describes the active movement of bringing the arm overhead without necessarily specifying the plane of the motion. Elevation of the arm is performed by muscles that can be classified into three groups: (1) muscles that elevate (i.e., abduct or flex) the humerus at the GH joint; (2) scapular muscles that control the upward rotation and associated rotational adjustment movements of the ST joint; and (3) rotator cuff muscles that control the dynamic stability and arthrokinematics at the GH joint.

Muscles Primarily Responsible for Elevation of the Arm

GLENOHUMERAL JOINT MUSCLES
- Anterior and middle deltoid
- Supraspinatus
- Coracobrachialis
- Biceps brachii

SCAPULOTHORACIC JOINT MUSCLES
- Serratus anterior
- Trapezius

ROTATOR CUFF MUSCLES
- Supraspinatus
- Infraspinatus
- Teres minor
- Subscapularis

MUSCLES THAT ELEVATE THE ARM AT THE GLENOHUMERAL JOINT

The prime muscles that abduct the GH joint are the *anterior deltoid, middle deltoid,* and *supraspinatus* (Fig. 5.46). Elevation of the arm through flexion is performed primarily by the *anterior deltoid, coracobrachialis,* and the *biceps brachii* (Fig. 5.47). The anterior deltoid and clavicular fibers of the pectoralis major function similarly as very effective horizontal adductors.[130,234]

The anterior deltoid, middle deltoid, and supraspinatus are activated at the onset of abduction, reaching a maximum level of activation generally within 60 to 120 degrees of abduction—an arc where the external torque due to the weight of the arm is relatively large.[129] The middle deltoid and supraspinatus have cross-sectional areas and average abduction moment arms that differ only by 10% to 12%.[95,100] Although varying based on the degree of humeral elevation,[91] each muscle produces significant proportions of the abduction torque at the GH joint.[100,199] With the deltoid paralyzed, the supraspinatus muscle is generally capable of fully abducting the GH joint, although

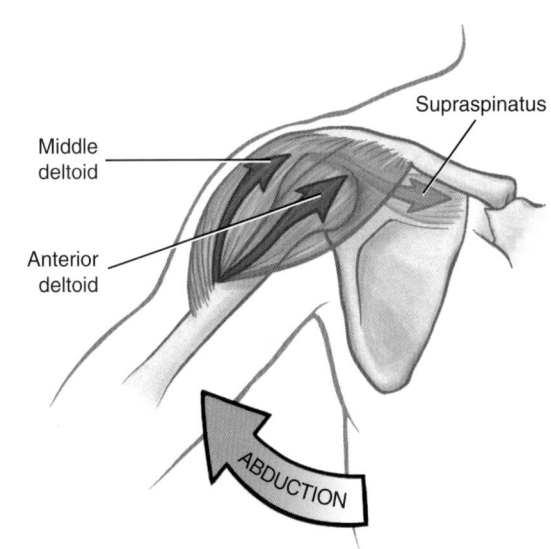

FIGURE 5.46 Anterior view showing the middle deltoid, anterior deltoid, and supraspinatus as abductors of the glenohumeral joint.

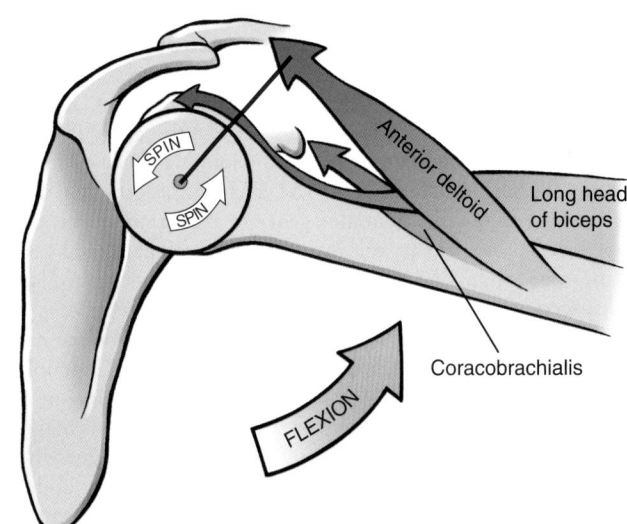

FIGURE 5.47 Lateral view of the anterior deltoid, coracobrachialis, and long head of the biceps flexing the glenohumeral joint in the pure sagittal plane. The medial-lateral axis of rotation is shown at the center of the humeral head. An internal moment arm is shown intersecting the line of force of the anterior deltoid only. The short head of the biceps is not shown.

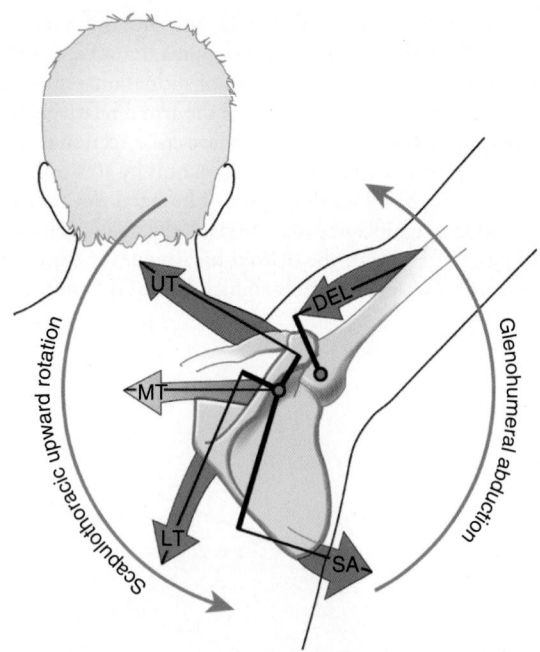

FIGURE 5.48 Posterior view of a healthy shoulder showing the muscular interaction between the scapulothoracic upward rotators and the glenohumeral abductors. Shoulder abduction requires a muscular "kinetic arc" between the humerus and the axial skeleton. Note two axes of rotation: the scapular axis, located near the acromion; and the glenohumeral joint axis, located at the humeral head. Internal moment arms for all muscles are shown as dark black lines. *DEL,* deltoid and supraspinatus; *LT,* lower trapezius; *MT,* middle trapezius; *SA,* serratus anterior; *UT,* upper trapezius.

the abduction torque is much reduced. Similarly, with the supraspinatus paralyzed or its tendon completely ruptured, full abduction is often difficult, albeit typically achievable.[218] For some persons however, especially those with complete rupture of the supraspinatus as well as damage to other rotator cuff tendons, full abduction is impossible due not only to the extensive weakness but, more importantly, to the disrupted muscular-driven arthrokinematics at the GH joint.[25] Full active abduction is normally not possible with paralysis of both the deltoid and the supraspinatus.

Research indicates that the extreme upper fibers of the infraspinatus and subscapularis muscles have limited moment arms to abduct the GH joint.[71,145] This occurs because the upper fibers of these muscles pass slightly superior to the joint's anterior-posterior axis of rotation (see ahead Figs. 5.51 and 5.52). Although these muscles have a limited potential to generate abduction torque, they nevertheless play a primary role in dynamically stabilizing and steering the joint's abducting arthrokinematics, functions described later in this section.

The muscles that actively abduct the shoulder produce relatively large compression forces across the GH joint. These joint forces reach 80% to 90% of body weight in a position of 90 degrees of abduction.[17,205,247] It is worth noting that this magnitude of compression rises to almost 130% of body weight when a load of just 2 kg is held at a position of 90 degrees of abduction.[17] The surface area at the GH joint available for accepting these muscular-based compressive forces is greatest between 60 and 120 degrees of abduction.[229] This corresponding increase in surface contact area occurring at the peak of the compression force can help maintain joint contact pressure at tolerable physiologic levels.

UPWARD ROTATORS AT THE SCAPULOTHORACIC JOINT

Upward rotation of the scapula is an essential component of elevation of the arm. The primary upward rotator muscles are the *serratus anterior* and the *upper* and *lower fibers of the trapezius* (Fig. 5.48). These muscles drive the upward rotation and furnish important rotational adjustments to the scapula. Equally important, the muscles provide stable attachments for the more distal mobilizers, such as the deltoid and rotator cuff muscles.

Trapezius and Serratus Anterior Interaction during Upward Rotation of the Scapula

The axis of rotation for scapular upward rotation is depicted in Fig. 5.48 as passing in an anterior-posterior direction through the scapula. This axis allows a convenient way to analyze the *force-couple* formed between the serratus anterior, upper trapezius, and lower trapezius to upwardly rotate the scapula.[11] This force-couple rotates the scapula in the same rotary direction as the abducting humerus. The mechanics of this force-couple is based on the force of each of the three muscles acting virtually simultaneously, not in isolation.[34,183] The pull of the lower fibers of the serratus anterior on the inferior angle of the scapula rotates the glenoid fossa upward and laterally. These fibers are the most effective upward rotators of the force-couple, primarily because of their larger moment arm for this action (Fig. 5.48). The lower trapezius upwardly rotates the scapula by an inferior-and-medial pull on the root of the spine of the scapula. The upper trapezius contributes to the force-couple only indirectly, by acting through a stable AC joint and exerting a modest superior-and-medial pull on the clavicle.[34] The muscular force-couple formed by these three muscles may be considered analogous to the mechanics of three people walking through a revolving door (e-Fig. 5.1).

Electromyographic (EMG) analysis of upward rotation of the scapula shows relatively large and consistent activation of the upper and lower trapezius and serratus anterior throughout active elevation of the arm.[12,109,261] The lower trapezius is particularly active during the later phase of shoulder abduction. The middle trapezius, a prime retractor, is also active during shoulder abduction.[12,65,242] As depicted in Fig. 5.48, the line of force of the middle trapezius runs essentially *through* the rotating scapula's axis of rotation. In this case the middle trapezius is robbed of its leverage to contribute to an upward rotation torque. This muscle, however, still contributes a needed retraction force on the scapula which, along with the rhomboids, helps neutralize the strong protraction effect of the serratus anterior. It is interesting that the serratus anterior and parts of the trapezius function simultaneously as agonists and antagonists: acting synergistically in upward rotation but opposing, and thus partially limiting, each other's strong protraction and retraction effects. The net force dominance between the two muscles during elevation of the arm helps determine the final retraction-protraction position of the upward rotated scapula. During shoulder abduction (especially in the frontal plane), the scapular retractors typically dominate the kinetics, as evident by the fact that the clavicle (and linked scapula) typically *retracts* about 20 degrees during shoulder abduction (review kinematic principle 3 in Box 5.1 and Fig. 5.36). The lower fibers of the upper trapezius may assist with retracting the scapula.[34]

In addition to the force-couple mechanics described in Fig. 5.48, the literature suggests that the serratus anterior and components of the trapezius also assist with *posteriorly tilting* and *externally rotating* the upwardly rotating scapula, most evident as the shoulder approaches full abduction (Fig. 5.49A).[118,138,150,153,183] (These subtle but important adjustment motions of the scapula were

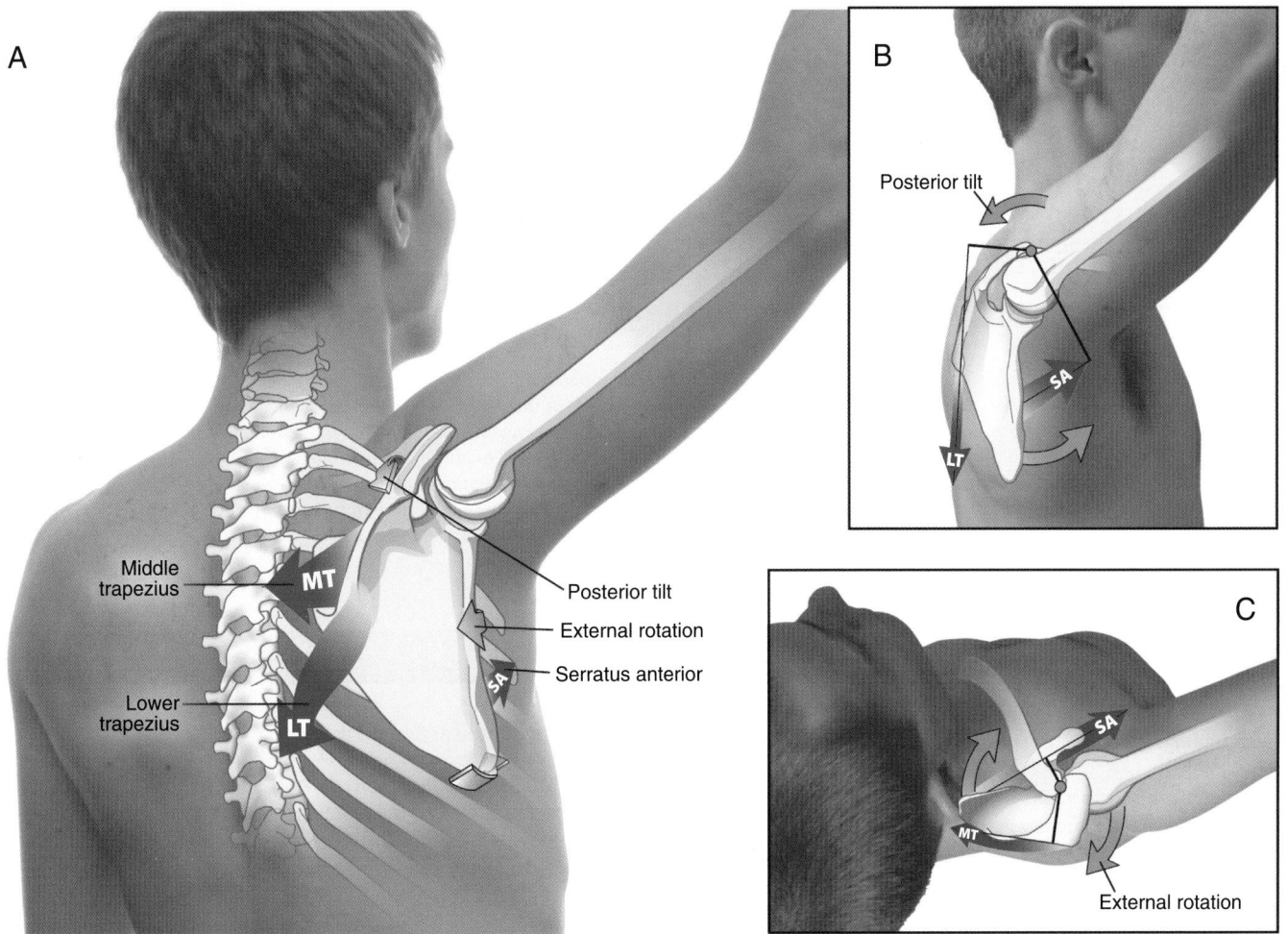

FIGURE 5.49 (A) Mechanism of actions of the serratus anterior and middle and lower trapezius muscles in controlling the adjustment motions of the upwardly rotating scapula during scapular plane abduction. (B) The serratus anterior *(SA)* and lower trapezius *(LT)* act in a force-couple to posteriorly tilt the scapula relative to the axis of rotation at the AC joint (indicated by the *green circle*). (C) The serratus anterior *(SA)* and middle trapezius *(MT)* act in a force-couple to externally rotate the scapula relative to the axis of rotation at the AC joint (indicated by the *blue circle*). Each muscle's moment arm is indicated as a dark black line, originating at the axis of rotation of the AC joint.

described earlier as the fourth kinematic principle of shoulder abduction.) Fig. 5.49B–C present a mechanical scenario of how these actions may be performed by these muscles, relative to the AC joint. As indicated in Fig. 5.49B, the lower trapezius (LT) pulls inferiorly on the scapula, as fibers of the serratus anterior (SA) pull anterior-laterally on the scapula. These simultaneous muscular actions possess the lines of force and moment arms to *posteriorly tilt* the upwardly rotating scapula (moment arms depicted as dark black lines). As indicated in Fig. 5.49C, the middle trapezius (MT) pulls medially on the scapula as fibers of the serratus anterior pull anterior-laterally on the medial border of the scapula. These simultaneous muscular actions, combined with their moment arms, could *externally rotate* the upwardly rotating scapula. This external rotation torque would also secure the medial border of the scapula firmly against the thorax.

Understanding how the axial-scapular muscles control the scapula is a prerequisite to the effective design of exercises or other efforts aimed at correcting abnormal scapular motion during abduction or flexion.[34,79,87,117,183] Such correction may optimize the effectiveness of the rotator cuff muscles at stabilizing the GH joint and, by maintaining adequate volume within the subacromial space, reduce stress on the residing tissues.

Functional Consequences of Weakness of the Upward Rotators of the Scapulothoracic Joint

Trapezius Muscle Weakness

Depending on the severity of the impairment, reduced strength or control of the trapezius can produce a wide range of disruptions in the mechanics associated with scapular upward rotation. Usually, an otherwise healthy person with isolated paralysis of the trapezius has moderate to marked difficulty in *flexing* the shoulder above the head. The action can usually be accomplished, however, provided the serratus anterior is sufficiently strong.[113] Typically, such a compensation positions the upwardly rotated scapula into excessive protraction due to the inability of the trapezius to limit the unopposed action of the dominant serratus anterior.[29] Elevation of the arm above the head strictly in the frontal plane (i.e., *pure abduction*), however, is usually very difficult, and often not achievable[113] (Video 5.6). Pure abduction of the shoulder normally demands a deliberate and strong scapular retraction force from muscles such as the middle trapezius which, in the context of this discussion, is not available. Although the rhomboids are strong scapular retractors, their involvement would produce a downward rotation force on the scapula—potentially counterproductive to the desired action of scapular upward rotation.

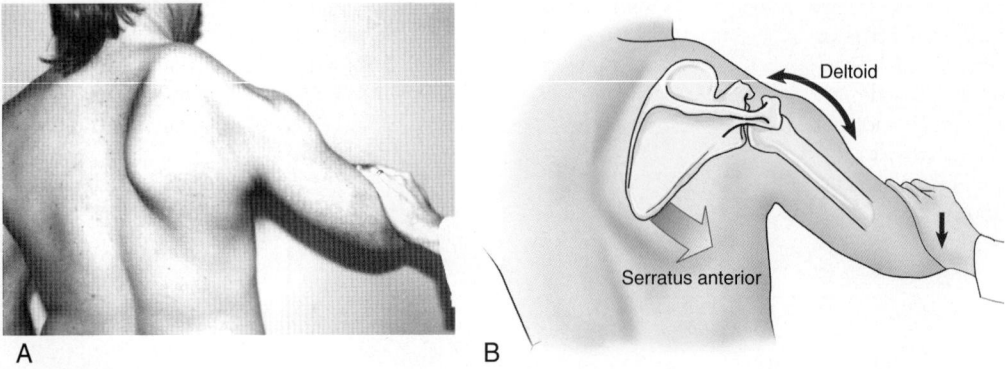

A   B

FIGURE 5.50 The pathomechanics of the right scapula after paralysis of the right serratus anterior caused by an injury of the long thoracic nerve. (A) The dominant feature of the scapula is its paradoxical downwardly rotated position, which can be exaggerated by applying resistance against the shoulder abduction effort. Note also that the scapula is abnormally anteriorly tilted and internally rotated. (B) Kinesiologic analysis of the extreme downward rotated position. Without an adequate upward rotation force from the serratus anterior *(fading arrow)*, the scapula is not properly stabilized against the thorax and cannot resist the pull of the deltoid. Subsequently the force of the deltoid *(bidirectional arrow)* causes the *combined actions* of downward rotation of the scapula and partial elevation (abduction) of the humerus.

Serratus Anterior Muscle Weakness

Weakness of the serratus anterior typically causes significant disruption in normal shoulder kinesiology. The etiology of isolated serratus anterior paralysis is often unknown, although it is often associated with trauma, overuse, or inflammation of the long thoracic nerve.[68,201,223]

As a general rule, persons with complete paralysis of the serratus anterior have great difficulty actively elevating the arm completely above the head, regardless of plane of motion. Most often it is not possible. This difficulty exists even though the trapezius and glenohumeral abductor muscles are fully innervated. Attempts at shoulder abduction, especially against resistance, typically result in limited elevation of the arm coupled with an excessively *downwardly rotated scapula* (Fig. 5.50). Normally, contraction of the serratus anterior strongly upwardly rotates the scapula, thus allowing the contracting middle deltoid and supraspinatus to rotate the humerus in the same rotary direction as the scapula (see Fig. 5.48). In cases of paralysis of the serratus anterior, however, the contracting middle deltoid and supraspinatus dominate the scapular kinetics, paradoxically rotating the scapula downward and only incompletely elevating the arm. This scenario weakens the deltoid and supraspinatus because, compared with the normal situation, these two muscles shorten too quickly (as indicated by the force-velocity relation) and shorten too much (as indicated by the length-tension relation). This reduced force potential, in conjunction with the downwardly rotated position of the scapula, reduces both the range of motion and the torque production of the elevating arm.

An analysis of the pathomechanics associated with paralysis of the serratus anterior provides a valuable lesson in the kinesiologic importance of this muscle. Normally, during elevation of the arm against gravity, the serratus anterior produces a surprisingly large upward rotation torque on the scapula, one that must *match and exceed* the downward rotation torque exerted by the active middle deltoid and supraspinatus.[36] In addition, and as described earlier in this chapter, the serratus anterior contributes a subtle but important posterior tilting and external rotation torque to the upwardly rotating scapula. These secondary actions become clear when observing a person with serratus anterior paralysis, as depicted in Fig. 5.50. In addition to the more obvious downwardly rotated position, the scapula is also slightly *anteriorly tilted* and *internally rotated* (evident by the "flaring" of the scapula's inferior angle and medial border, respectively). Such a distorted

SPECIAL FOCUS 5.7

Defining "Scapular Dyskinesis"

Scapular dyskinesis (SD) describes the abnormal positioning or movement of the scapula, regardless of cause.[117] Several examples of SD have been previously introduced, such as reduced upward rotation, excessive downward rotation, internal rotation, and anterior tilt—kinematics that may potentially increase the risk of developing subacromial or rotator cuff pain, at least in certain populations.[9,117,138,150]

SD has been associated with several pathologies involving the neuromusculoskeletal systems.[117,118,120] Examples of pathologies *directly* associated with SD are "snapping scapula" (i.e., grinding or popping of the scapula against the thorax), excessive thoracic kyphosis, tightness in the pectoralis minor, and paralysis or reduced motor control of ST muscles. Examples of *indirectly* associated pathologies are a fractured clavicle, unstable AC joint, tightened or lax ligaments at the GH joint, multidirectional GH joint instability, tightened or weakened muscles at the GH joint, subacromial pain, and degeneration of the rotator cuff muscles. Regardless of pathologic association, SD has the potential to alter the effectiveness of muscle actions and distort the arthrokinematics in the region.[16,148]

Although SD describes and highlights abnormal scapular kinematics, understanding how a particular expression or severity of SD can be used to personalize shoulder treatment remains unclear. Because of the large natural variability in scapular movement and posture, it is not uncommon that an asymptomatic person may exhibit some form of SD.[204] Furthermore, the mere presence of scapular dyskinesis alone cannot reliably predict the risk of future injury, at least in the athletic population.[96] How much therapeutic emphasis, therefore, should be placed on altering SD in an asymptomatic person? Such a question may be better addressed by continued research into the biomechanical origins of SD, and the development of a standardized, validated, and accessible measurement tool for this disorder.[58]

posture is often referred to clinically as a "winging" scapula. Such a position, if maintained, would likely cause adaptive shortening of the pectoralis minor muscle, which may further promote an anteriorly tilted, internally rotated and downwardly rotated position of the scapula.[23] The muscular imbalance scenario described for the "winging scapula" depicted in Fig. 5.50A can apply across a wide continuum of cases involving serratus anterior weakness, from simply a lack of control due to a still developing neuromuscular system, disuse muscle atrophy, and adaptive shortening of antagonist muscles, to isolated nerve injury, midlevel cervical tetraplegia, muscular dystrophy, or cerebral palsy.

It is clinically relevant that even a modest reduction in performance of the serratus anterior can disrupt the normal arthrokinematics at the shoulder. Ludewig and Cook studied a group of overhead laborers diagnosed with subacromial impingement syndrome.[152] During attempts at active abduction of the shoulder, the researchers found a relationship between *reduced* serratus anterior activation and the combined kinematics of reduced upward rotation, reduced posterior tilting, and reduced external rotation of the scapula. Reduced upward rotation, in particular, can narrow the space between the undersurface of the acromion and the distal attachment of the supraspinatus tendon, especially in abduction angles of less than 60 degrees.[137] The diminished volume can increase the risk of impingement or shearing of the supraspinatus or other tissues in the subacromial space.

FUNCTION OF THE ROTATOR CUFF MUSCLES DURING ELEVATION OF THE ARM

The rotator cuff muscles include the subscapularis, supraspinatus, infraspinatus, and teres minor (Figs. 5.51 and 5.52). These muscles are active across a wide range of routine activities, such as raising the arm overhead, lifting objects, and opening a jar.[10,129,157,261] The rotator cuff muscles are essential for regulating dynamic GH joint stability and controlling the arthrokinematics.

Regulators of Dynamic Stability at the Glenohumeral Joint
The naturally loose fit between the head of the humerus and glenoid fossa permits extensive range of motion, thereby enhancing reach of the entire limb. The surrounding joint capsule therefore must be free of thick restraining ligaments that would otherwise restrict such motion. As stated earlier in this chapter, the anatomic design of the GH joint clearly favors mobility at the expense of stability. Although all muscles that cross the GH joint provide some dynamic stability, the rotator cuff group excels in this capacity.[255] The distal attachments of the rotator cuff muscles blend directly into the joint capsule before attaching to the proximal humerus (see Figs. 5.51 and 5.52). These direct capsular attachments, combined with the muscles' overall horizontal fiber direction, creates an enclosing musculoligamentous "membrane" around the joint.[10] When activated by the nervous system, the cuff becomes relatively rigid. Nowhere else in the body do so many muscles form such an intimate structural part of a joint's periarticular structure.

An example of the dynamic stabilizing function of the rotator cuff was previously described during active external rotation (see Fig. 5.35). A similar compression-based stabilization function can be described for the entire rotator cuff for virtually all active shoulder motions. The muscles (and their attachments into the capsule) not only actively rotate the humeral head in multiple planes but also compress and centralize it firmly against the glenoid fossa.[1,218,261] Dynamic stability at the GH joint therefore requires healthy neuromuscular and musculoskeletal systems. These two

systems are functionally integrated through proprioceptive sensory receptors located within the GH joint's periarticular connective tissues.[116] As part of a reflex loop, these innervated connective tissues provide rapid and important information to the participating muscles. This feedback enhances the muscles' ability to control the arthrokinematics even at a subconscious level, as well as provide the needed dynamic stability. Challenging such a proprioceptive mechanism through functional exercise is a respected component of rehabilitation programs for persons with shoulder instability.[266]

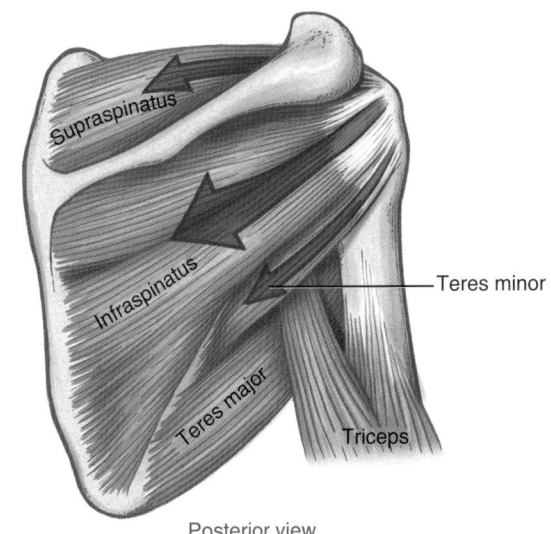

Posterior view

FIGURE 5.51 Posterior view of the right shoulder showing the activated supraspinatus, infraspinatus, and teres minor muscles. Note that the distal attachments of these muscles blend with the superior and posterior aspects of the glenohumeral joint. The teres major and parts of the long and lateral heads of the triceps brachii are also illustrated.

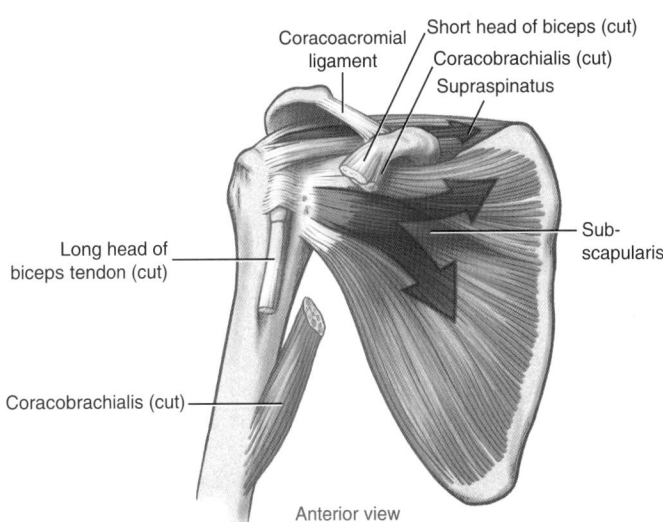

Anterior view

FIGURE 5.52 Anterior view of the right shoulder showing the subscapularis muscle blending into the anterior capsule of the glenohumeral joint before attaching to the lesser tubercle of the humerus. The subscapularis is shown with diverging arrows, reflecting two main fiber directions. The supraspinatus, coracobrachialis, tendon of the long head of the biceps, and coracoacromial ligament are also depicted.

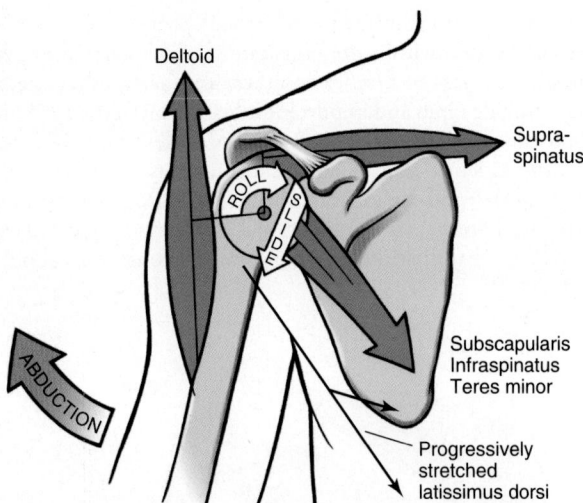

FIGURE 5.53 Anterior view of the right shoulder emphasizing the actions of the activated rotator cuff muscles during abduction of the GH joint. Note the internal moment arm used by both the deltoid and the supraspinatus. The latissimus dorsi is shown as a representative muscle that would generate an inferiorly directed passive tension on the humeral head when progressively stretched (elongated) during abduction.

Active Controllers of the Arthrokinematics at the Glenohumeral Joint

In the healthy shoulder, the rotator cuff muscles control much of the active arthrokinematics of the GH joint (Fig. 5.53). Contraction of the horizontally oriented supraspinatus produces a compression force directly into the glenoid fossa; this force stabilizes the humeral head firmly against the fossa during its superior roll into abduction.[273] During abduction, the muscle's contractile force rolls the humeral head superiorly while its semirigid structure serves as a musculotendinous "spacer" that restricts an excessive and counterproductive superior translation of the humeral head.[218,247,264] In addition, the remaining rotator cuff muscles (subscapularis, infraspinatus, and teres minor) have lines of force directed inferiorly on the humeral head during abduction (see Fig. 5.53).[82] The long head of the biceps, by crossing directly over the humeral head, also contributes in this fashion.[196] All the aforementioned inferior-directed forces on the humerus are necessary to help neutralize the contracting deltoid's strong superior translation effect on the humerus, especially at low abduction angles.[54,269] Indeed, contraction of the deltoid with a coexisting massive rotator cuff tear has been shown to cause excessive superior migration of the humeral head, measured by a corresponding reduction in size of the subacromial space.[124]

In addition to activation of the rotator cuff muscles, it is likely that forces produced by stretched antagonist (adductor) muscles throughout abduction also exert a useful inferior-directed force on the humeral head. As the arm is being raised overhead, these "antagonistic" muscle forces may be produced *passively* (as implied by the "progressively stretched" latissimus dorsi shown in Fig. 5.53) or *actively* through a low-level eccentric activation. Nevertheless, without the aforementioned set of inferior-directed myogenic forces, attempts at active abduction would likely allow the deltoid to pull the humeral head up against the coracoacromial arch, potentially blocking further abduction.

Finally, during abduction, the infraspinatus and teres minor muscles can also externally rotate the humerus to varying degrees to increase the clearance between the greater tubercle and the acromion (described earlier as the sixth kinematic principle of abduction). Realize that the overall effectiveness of the entire rotator cuff muscle group in controlling the arthrokinematics at the GH joint is based, in part, on optimal alignment of the scapula relative to the humerus.

> **Summary of the Functions of the Rotator Cuff Muscles in Controlling the Arthrokinematics of Abduction at the Glenohumeral Joint**
>
> **SUPRASPINATUS**
> - Drives the superior roll of the humeral head
> - Compresses the humeral head firmly against the glenoid fossa
> - Creates a semirigid spacer above the humeral head, restricting excessive superior translation of the humerus
>
> **INFRASPINATUS, TERES MINOR, AND SUBSCAPULARIS**
> - Exert a depression force on the humeral head
>
> **INFRASPINATUS AND TERES MINOR**
> - Externally rotate the humerus

Muscles That Adduct and Extend the Shoulder

The primary adductor and extensor muscles of the shoulder are the *posterior deltoid, latissimus dorsi, teres major, long head of the triceps brachii,* and *sternocostal head of the pectoralis major* (review Figs. 5.40, 5.42, 5.51, and 5.54, respectively). (The shoulder must be at least partially flexed to allow the line of force of the sternocostal fibers of the pectoralis major to be able to extend the shoulder back to the anatomic position.[234]) Of the muscles just listed, the latissimus dorsi, teres major, and pectoralis major have the largest moment arms for the combined motions of adduction and extension.[130] The *infraspinatus* (lower fibers) and *teres minor* muscles likely assist with these movements. As depicted in Fig. 5.55, the extensor and adductor muscles are capable of generating the largest torques of any muscle group of the shoulder.[97,227] Their high torque potential can be appreciated in tasks such as pulling the arm against resistance when climbing a rope or propelling through water, which requires forceful contractions of these potentially powerful muscles.

With the humerus held fixed, contraction of the latissimus dorsi can raise the pelvis upward. Persons with paraplegia often use this action during crutch- and brace-assisted ambulation as a substitute for weakened or paralyzed hip flexors.

Five of the seven adductor-extensor muscles have their primary proximal attachments on the inherently unstable scapula. It is therefore the responsibility of axial-scapular muscles to stabilize the scapula during active adduction and extension of the GH joint. Although the middle trapezius is well aligned to assist with this stabilization, the rhomboids and to a lesser extent levator scapulae are uniquely qualified based on their ability to combine the actions of downward rotation *and* retraction of the scapula[15] (Fig. 5.56). Based on bony attachments, the pectoralis minor (see Fig. 5.42B) and latissimus dorsi have lines of force to assist the rhomboids (and levator scapulae) with the downward rotation of the scapula. This action is most apparent when observed with the scapula already upwardly rotated and the shoulder abducted or flexed: positions that typically precede a vigorous shoulder adduction and extension effort, such as a propulsive swimming stroke or climbing up a rope.

As the shoulder is fully extending, the downwardly rotating scapula also anteriorly tilts.[70] This combined scapular motion, driven in part by contraction of the pectoralis minor, can functionally increase the extent of a backward reach.[15]

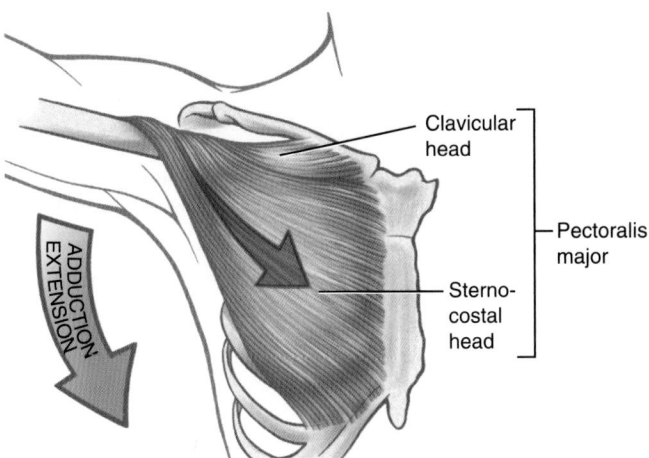

FIGURE 5.54 Anterior view of the right pectoralis major showing the adduction and extension function of the sternocostal head. The clavicular head of the pectoralis major is also shown.

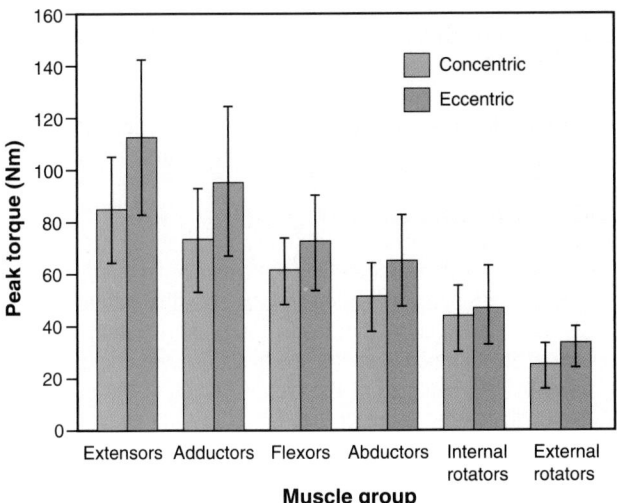

FIGURE 5.55 Graph shows a sample of peak torque data produced by the six shoulder muscle groups from a set of nonathletic, healthy men (N = 15, aged 22–35 years). The peak torques are shown in descending order. Data were collected during concentric and eccentric muscle activations using an isokinetic dynamometer set at an angular velocity of 60 degrees/sec. Means are expressed in newton-meters; brackets indicate standard deviation of the mean. (Data from Shklar A, Dvir Z: Isokinetic strength measurements in shoulder muscles, *J Biomech* 10:369, 1995.)

The entire rotator cuff group is active during shoulder adduction and extension.[15,129] Forces produced by these muscles assist with the action directly or stabilize the head of the humerus against the glenoid fossa. The subscapularis is particularly active during resisted extension, presumedly to counterbalance the strong posterior pull on the proximal humerus exerted by muscles such as the latissimus dorsi.[261]

Muscles That Internally and Externally Rotate the Shoulder

INTERNAL ROTATOR MUSCLES

The muscles that internally rotate the GH joint are the *subscapularis, pectoralis major, latissimus dorsi, teres major,* and *anterior*

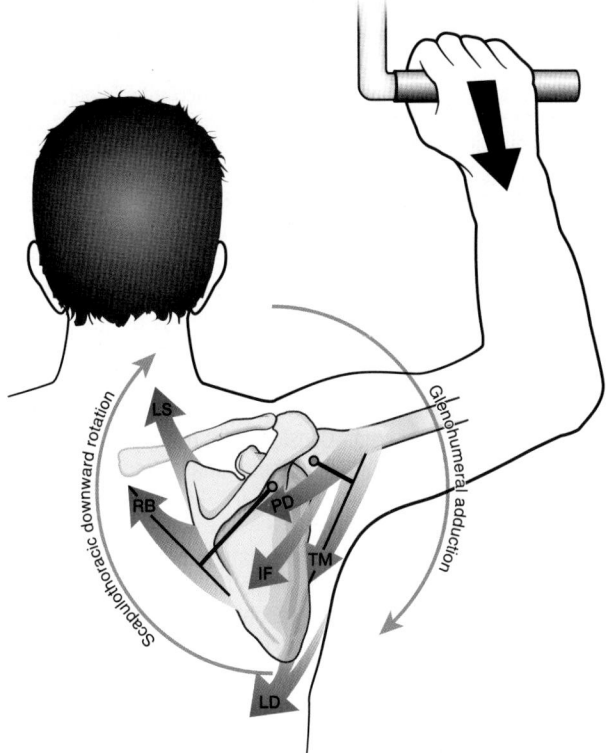

FIGURE 5.56 Posterior view of a shoulder showing the muscular interaction between scapulothoracic downward rotators and the glenohumeral adductors (and extensors). Two muscles are shown with moment arms: the teres major with its internal moment arm *(dark line)* extending from the glenohumeral joint, and rhomboids (combined major and minor) with its internal moment arm extending from the scapula's rotating axis of rotation. *IF,* infraspinatus and teres minor; *LD,* latissimus dorsi; *PD,* posterior deltoid; *RB,* rhomboids; *LS,* levator scapulae, *TM,* teres major. For clarity, the long head of the triceps is not shown.

deltoid. From a position of 30 degrees of abduction or flexion, the subscapularis has the greatest moment arm for internal rotation, whereas the anterior deltoid has, by far, the least.[2] Many of the internal rotators are also powerful extensors and adductors, such as those used during the propulsive phase of swimming.

The total muscle mass of the shoulder's internal rotators appreciably exceeds that of the external rotators. This fact is reflected by the larger maximal-effort torque produced by the internal rotators, during both eccentric and concentric activations (see Fig. 5.55).[227] On average, the internal rotators typically produce at least about 40% greater torque than the external rotators; however, this difference may be considerably greater based on the position of the shoulder during strength testing, type and speed of muscle activation, and specific sport participation.[20,122,165,173,236] One activity that naturally requires large internal rotation torque is high-speed throwing. Of particular interest in sports medicine is the large torque generated by these muscles in baseball pitchers just before the maximal external rotation (end of cocking) phase of overhead pitching. At this phase of a pitch, the internal rotator muscles must strongly decelerate a large external rotation torque that, in professional level athletes, peaks at approximately 70 to 90 Nm.[214] The opposing rotary torques create significant torsional shear on the shaft of the humerus. This

Shoulder Instability: A Final Look at This Important Clinical Issue

Maintaining stability at the glenohumeral (GH) joint requires a unique interaction among active and passive mechanisms around the shoulder. For several reasons, these mechanisms may fail, resulting in an unstable and potentially painful shoulder. The literature regarding the cause, diagnosis, classification, and treatment of shoulder instability lacks universal consensus.[18,92,93] The lack of agreement reflects the multiple causes of the instability, as well as its highly varied clinical expression. Although other schemes exist to classify shoulder instability,[93,232,268] this Special Focus concentrates on the three following types: posttraumatic, atraumatic, and acquired. Considerable overlap among these types of instability is common, further complicating the topic.

POSTTRAUMATIC INSTABILITY

Many cases of shoulder instability are attributed to a specific event involving a traumatic dislocation of the GH joint, most often in the anterior direction.[93,212] The pathomechanics of anterior dislocation often involve the motion or position of extreme external rotation in an abducted position. With the shoulder in this vulnerable position, the force of impact combined with strong muscle contraction can drive the humeral head off the anterior side of the glenoid fossa. This dislocation often injures the middle and inferior GH ligaments, anterior-inferior rim of the glenoid labrum, and potentially the tendons of the rotator cuff muscles.[212] Combined tears or lesions of the capsule or labrum that detach from the rim of the glenoid fossa are referred to as a *Bankart lesion*.[133]

Unfortunately, because of the associated injury to the labrum and capsular ligaments, posttraumatic shoulder instability often leads to repeated dislocations, each instance potentially causing additional damage to the joint, especially the labrum.[212,219,262] This likelihood is far greater in adolescents than in adults[98] due, in part, to differences in activity level and the natural increase in stiffness of periarticular connective tissues associated with aging.

Therapeutic measures to improve function and reduce the frequency of recurrent dislocations following the initial dislocation in younger persons typically include a brief period of immobilization and activity modification, followed by a multistaged physical rehabilitation program.[268] If this conservative approach fails to reduce the frequency or extent of the dislocations, surgery may be necessary. Opinions vary, however, on the need for or timing of surgery following a traumatic dislocation based on patient's age, activity level, degree of instability, associated trauma to the glenoid, and history of recurrent dislocations.[18,134] In certain cases, surgery may be the most appropriate treatment, especially in younger individuals wanting to return to sport.[104,126] Surgery typically involves a repair of the damaged tissues, often including techniques to tighten or plicate the anterior and inferior regions of the capsule.

ATRAUMATIC INSTABILITY

Persons diagnosed with atraumatic instability may display generalized ligamentous laxity throughout the body, often described as being congenital.[263] Even though the GH joint instability may not be attributed to an identifiable traumatic event, repeated microtrauma associated with ligamentous laxity may play a role in the pathogenesis.[133] The instability may be unidirectional or

multidirectional (i.e., in at least two directions), and bilateral. The cause of atraumatic instability may involve a combination of several factors, including but not limited to:

- Laxity or generalized weakness in periarticular and intramuscular connective tissues
- Bony dysplasia
- Reduced intra-articular pressure (reduced suction effect)
- Weakness, poor control, or increased fatigability of rotator cuff or scapular muscles
- Unusually large rotator cuff interval

Persons with atraumatic instability generally respond favorably to conservative therapy involving strengthening along with proprioceptive and motor control training exercises.[257,266] Those who do not adequately respond may be candidates for a surgical tightening of the GH joint by selectively cutting, folding, and suturing redundant regions of the anterior and inferior capsule.[219] At the time of surgery, persons with atraumatic instability have been shown to have a significant number of intra-articular lesions.[263] This finding suggests that excessive laxity—even with minimal or no history of actual dislocation—can precipitate articular damage.

ACQUIRED SHOULDER INSTABILITY

The pathomechanics of acquired shoulder instability are related to repeated cycles of overstretching the capsular ligaments within the GH joint. This condition is often associated with repetitive, high-velocity shoulder motions that involve extreme external rotation and abduction, common in sports like baseball, swimming, tennis, and volleyball.[268] Because of the biomechanics of the abducted and externally rotated shoulder (see Fig. 5.27), the anterior bands of the inferior and middle GH ligament become particularly vulnerable to plastic deformation. Once weakened by this process, the soft tissues are less able to hold the humeral head against the glenoid fossa. The tissue deformation can lead to increased joint laxity in multiple directions, possibly predisposing other stress-related pathologies such as *rotator cuff-related shoulder pain* (which includes subacromial impingement) and damage to the labrum and long head of the biceps. Acquired shoulder instability has also been associated with *internal impingement syndrome.* (The term "internal" refers to an impingement on the *inner or articular surface* of the rotator cuff and associated capsule, in contrast to the previously described "external" or subacromial impingement). Although not clearly understood, as the humerus moves into external rotation while approaching about 120 degrees of abduction, the greater tubercle may pinch the inner surface of the posterior-superior rotator cuff against the adjacent edge of the glenoid fossa to give rise to internal impingement.[28,107,119,217,268] This motion is inherent to many forms of overhead throwing and common reaching activities.

Surgical repair for acquired instability of the GH joint may be necessary depending on the extent of injury or impairment. The surgery may involve debridement of the rotator cuff, debridement or repair of the glenoid labrum, and anterior capsular plication.[208] Surgery is typically followed by an extensive postoperative rehabilitation program.[110,147,268]

SPECIAL FOCUS 5.9

Vulnerability of the Supraspinatus to Excessive Wear and Associated Pathology

Although all four rotator cuff muscles (RCM) are biomechanically vulnerable to overuse injuries and pain, the supraspinatus is especially at risk. The supraspinatus is a very active muscle, assisting the deltoid during abduction and also providing dynamic and, at times, static stability to the GH joint. The supraspinatus must produce relatively large forces, even during routine activities. Consider the demands on this muscle to hold a load by the hand at 90 degrees of abduction. At this point, the supraspinatus has an internal moment arm for abduction of about 2.5 cm (about 1 inch).[25] Supporting a load in the hand 50 cm (about 20 inches) distal to the GH joint creates a mechanical advantage of 1:20 (i.e., the ratio of internal moment arm of the supraspinatus to the external moment arm of the load). A 1:20 mechanical advantage implies that the supraspinatus must generate a force *20 times greater* than the weight of the load (see Chapter 1). Fortunately, the overlying deltoid muscle shares much of this demand. Nevertheless, the high forces imposed on the supraspinatus may, over time, cause excessive wear on the muscle's tendon near its insertion point (see MRI in Fig. 5.57). A preexisting reduced acromiohumeral distance may further exacerbate the stress on the tendon. Persons with a partially torn or inflamed supraspinatus tendon are often advised to hold objects close to the body in order to reduce the external moment arm of the load and thereby minimize the force demands on the musculotendinous unit.

Excessive deterioration of the supraspinatus tendon may be associated with stress-related degeneration of other RCM tendons. In addition to a more global tendinopathy, other pathologies may include adhesive capsulitis,[168] subacromial bursitis and pain, and osteoarthritis of AC joint (as indicated in Fig. 5.57). The underlying pathogenesis of these commonly related conditions is complex and not well understood, although advanced age, trauma, overuse, stress related to bony anomalies or poor neuromuscular control of GH and ST joints, and repeated impingement due to reduced acromiohumeral distance are often suspected as potential contributors.[e] Because tissues other than the RCM may also be involved in the genesis of this painful condition, the term *rotator cuff–related shoulder pain* has been recommended as the most encompassing diagnostic label, which may include RCM tendinopathy or tears, subacromial pain (impingement) and subacromial bursitis.[45,210] Regardless of involvement, the painful condition can disrupt the arthrokinematics and stability at the GH joint, thereby reducing the quality and strength of shoulder movement.

Persons with small or medium sized rotator cuff tears may benefit from physical therapy or primary surgical repair, however the later intervention may be more appropriate in younger and active persons.[174] Persons with irreparable or massive tears of their rotator cuff muscles often elect to receive a *reverse total shoulder arthroplasty* (RTSA) instead of an anatomic total shoulder arthroplasty.[30] The RTSA is termed "reverse" because the glenoid (scapular) prosthetic component is convex and the humeral component is concave. One functional goal of this design is to shift the axis of rotation medially and inferiorly relative to the scapula.[256] The design is intended to increase the tension (stretch) in the deltoid muscle as well as increase the muscle's abduction leverage. A desired functional outcome of the RTSA design is to allow the deltoid to better compensate for the reduced compression stabilization lost because of the deficient rotator cuff muscles. The improvement in RTSA design and surgical technique over time has led to favorable functional outcomes for persons with a wide range of significant rotator cuff tear pathology, including those with rheumatoid or osteoarthritis.[31,84,114]

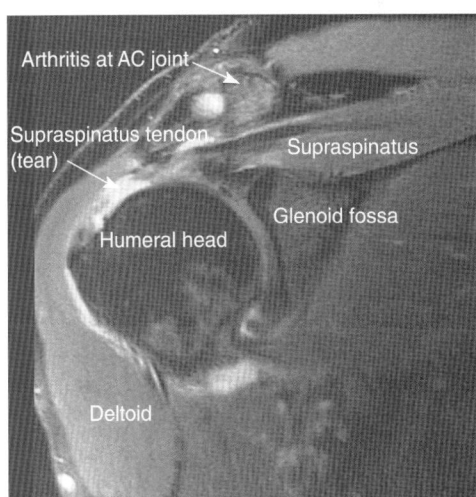

FIGURE 5.57 Frontal plane (T2 fat saturated) magnetic resonance image (MRI) showing a full-thickness supraspinatus tendon tear. Also note the degenerative osteoarthritis of the AC joint. (Courtesy Michael O'Brien, MD, Wisconsin Radiology Specialists, Milwaukee, WI.)

[e]13, 19, 124, 125, 143, 271,276

magnitude of shear is likely involved in the pathomechanics of "ball-thrower's fracture"—a relatively rare but serious injury involving a spontaneous spiral fracture of the middle and distal thirds of the humerus.[214] Similar biomechanical studies have focused on the late cocking phase of pitching in 12-year-old elite baseball pitchers. Although the torsional shear is much less because of the greatly reduced pitching velocity, the forces are likely related to the pathomechanics of proximal humeral epiphysiolysis ("Little League Shoulder") and to excessive retroversion of the humerus of the throwing limb.[213,243]

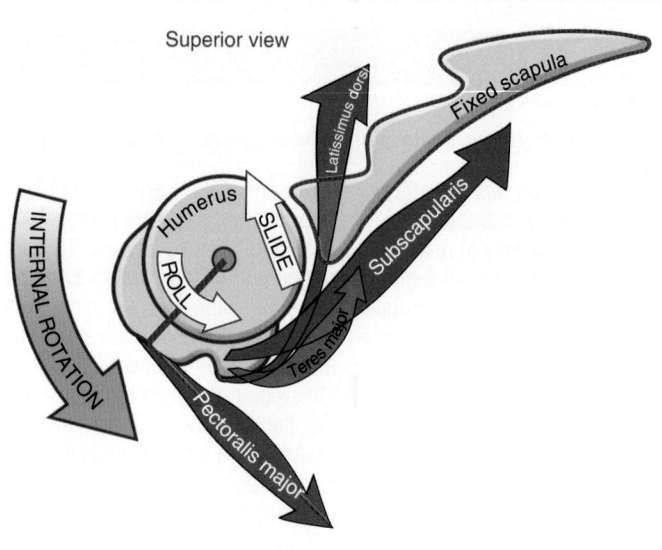

FIGURE 5.58 Superior view of the right shoulder showing the group action of the internal rotators around the glenohumeral joint's vertical axis of rotation. In this case the scapula is fixed and the humerus is free to rotate. The line of force of the pectoralis major is shown with its internal moment arm. Note the roll-and-slide arthrokinematics of the convex-on-concave motion. For clarity, the anterior deltoid is not shown.

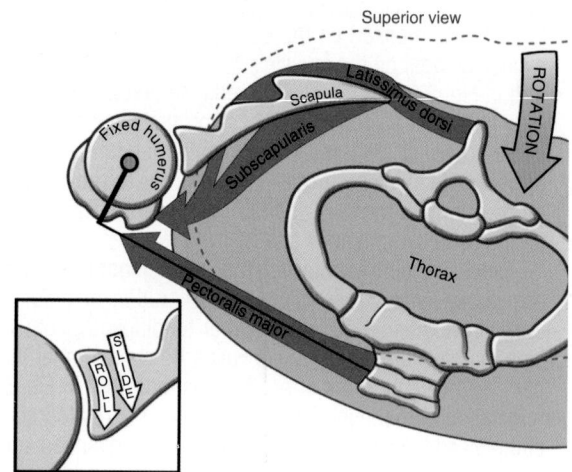

FIGURE 5.59 Superior view of the right shoulder showing actions of three internal rotators when the distal (humeral) segment is fixed and the scapula and trunk are free to rotate. The line of force of the pectoralis major is shown with its internal moment arm originating around the glenohumeral joint's vertical axis. Inset shows the roll-and-slide arthrokinematics during the concave-on-convex motion.

The muscles that internally rotate the GH joint are often described as rotators of the humerus relative to the scapula (Fig. 5.58). The arthrokinematics of this motion are based on the convex humeral head rotating on the fixed glenoid fossa. Consider, however, the muscle function and kinematics that occur when the humerus is held in a fixed position and the scapula is free to rotate. As depicted in Fig. 5.59, with sufficient muscle force, the scapula and trunk can rotate around a fixed humerus. Note that the arthrokinematics of the scapula-on-humerus rotation involve a concave glenoid fossa rolling and sliding in similar directions on the convex humeral head (see Fig. 5.59, inset).

EXTERNAL ROTATOR MUSCLES

The muscles that externally rotate the GH joint are the *infraspinatus, teres minor,* and *posterior deltoid* (see Figs. 5.40 and 5.51). From the anatomic position, the general horizontal lines of pull of the infraspinatus and teres minor are ideal for this action.

Unlike the internal rotator muscles of the shoulder, *all* the external rotators attach exclusively between the scapula and the humerus. Thus the ability of the external rotators to effectively transfer torque to the humerus requires that the scapula be firmly stabilized by the scapular retractor muscles to the axial skeleton[15] (Fig. 5.60). Consider, for example, the strong synergistic relationship between the middle-and-lower trapezius and the infraspinatus during resisted external rotation of the shoulder. With paralysis of the trapezius, a vigorous, resisted contraction in the infraspinatus (and other external rotators) causes the scapula to rotate unnaturally *toward the humerus,* creating excessive ST joint internal rotation. The muscular imbalance creates a scapular dyskinesis that is typically observed during resisted external rotation of the shoulder (Video 5.7).

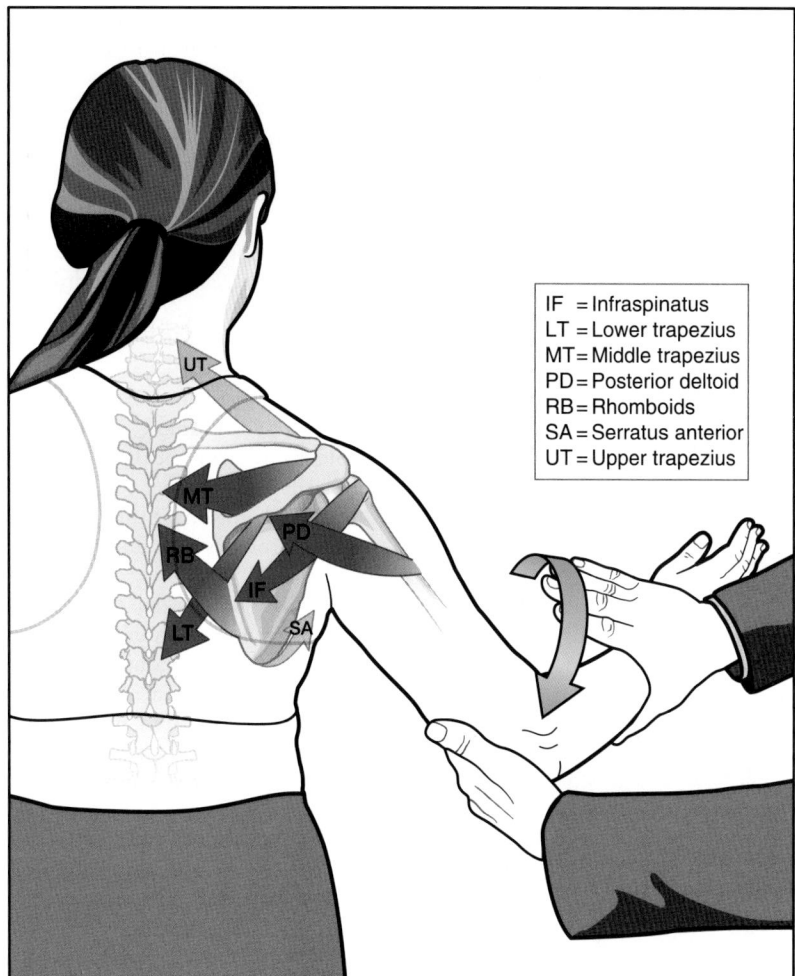

IF = Infraspinatus
LT = Lower trapezius
MT = Middle trapezius
PD = Posterior deltoid
RB = Rhomboids
SA = Serratus anterior
UT = Upper trapezius

FIGURE 5.60 Strong muscular interactions are shown between the primary scapulothoracic retractors and glenohumeral external rotators. The serratus anterior *(SA)* and upper trapezius *(UT)* are shown moderately active (in *light red*) helping to stabilize the scapula against undesired actions potentially caused by the dominating retractor muscles; for example, to counteract the strong downward rotation and depression forces exerted on the scapula by the rhomboids and lower trapezius, respectively. *IF,* infraspinatus (and teres minor); *LT,* lower trapezius; *MT,* middle trapezius; *PD,* posterior deltoid; *RB,* rhomboids

The external rotator muscles constitute a relatively small percentage of the total muscle mass at the shoulder. The external rotators therefore produce the lowest maximal-effort torque of any muscle group at the shoulder (see Fig. 5.55). Regardless of the muscles' relatively low maximal torque potentials, they are frequently used to generate high-velocity concentric contractions, such as during the cocking phase of winding up to pitch a baseball. Through eccentric activation, these same muscles must decelerate shoulder internal rotation at the release phase of pitching, which can reach a peak velocity of nearly 7000 degrees/sec.[59] These large force demands placed on the rapidly elongating and activated infraspinatus and teres minor may cause tears and chronic inflammation at the points of their distal attachment. Maintaining strength of the external rotators (especially relative to the more dominant strength of the internal rotators) may help minimize the risk of certain sporting-related injuries of the shoulder.[122,203]

SPECIAL FOCUS 5.10

A Closer Look at the Posterior Deltoid

The posterior deltoid is a shoulder extensor, adductor, and external rotator. In addition, this muscle is also the primary horizontal abductor at the shoulder. Vigorous contraction of the posterior deltoid during horizontal abduction requires that the scapula be firmly stabilized by the lower trapezius. Such a synergistic relationship becomes very evident by observing a person use a bow and arrow (Fig. 5.61). This muscular interaction forms a strong and nearly parallel link between the humerus and the vertebral column, with these landmarks serving as kinetic "proximal and distal attachments" of this muscular pair.

The posterior deltoid can be at least temporarily paralyzed from an overstretching of the axillary nerve. Persons with this paralysis frequently report difficulty in combining full shoulder extension and horizontal abduction, such as when placing the arm in the sleeve of a coat.

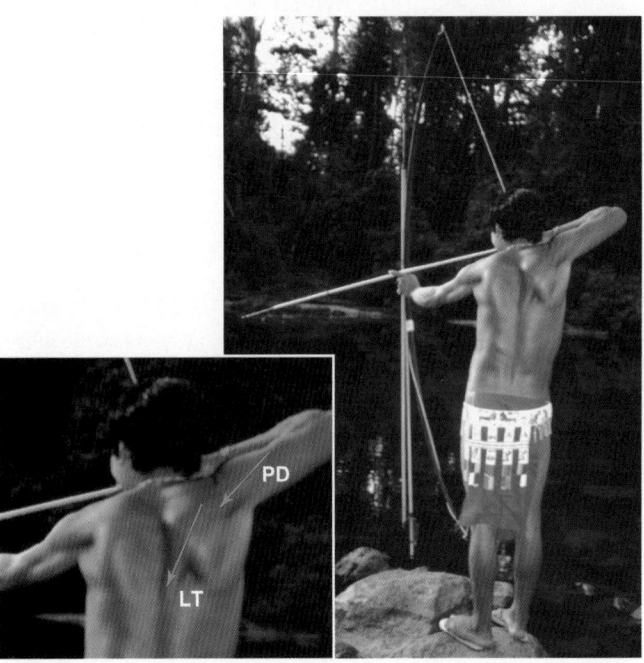

FIGURE 5.61 The hypertrophied right posterior deltoid and lower trapezius of an indigenous Tiriyo man engaged in bow fishing in the Amazon River region. Note the strong synergistic action between the right lower trapezius (*LT*) and right posterior deltoid (*PD*). The lower trapezius must anchor the scapula to the spine and provide a fixed proximal attachment for the strongly activated posterior deltoid. (Courtesy Plotkin MJ: *Tales of a shaman's apprentice,* New York, 1993, Viking-Penguin.)

SYNOPSIS

The four joints of the shoulder complex normally interact harmoniously to maximize the extent, stability, and ease of reach in the upper extremity. Each articulation contributes a unique element to these functions. Most proximally, the SC joint firmly attaches the shoulder to the axial skeleton. This joint is well stabilized by its interlocking saddle-shaped surfaces, combined with a capsule and articular disc. The SC joint serves as the basilar pivot point for virtually all movements of the shoulder.

The overall kinematics of the scapula are guided primarily by movement of the clavicle. The more specific path of the scapula, however, is governed by additional and equally important movements at the AC joint. This relatively flat and shallow AC joint is dependent on local capsular ligaments as well as the extrinsically located coracoclavicular ligament for its stability. Unlike the more stable SC joint, the AC joint dislocates relatively frequently after a strong medially and inferiorly directed force delivered to the shoulder.

The ST joint serves as an important mechanical platform for all active movements of the humerus. Consider full shoulder abduction, for example, which consists of nearly 60 degrees of scapular upward rotation coupled with varying amounts of posterior tilt and external rotation. Combined with the mechanically linked motions at the SC and AC joints, the well-positioned scapula provides a stable yet mobile base for the abducting humerus.

The GH joint is the most distal and mobile link within the shoulder complex. Mobility is enhanced by the naturally loose articular capsule, in conjunction with a relatively flat and small glenoid fossa. These same features that promote mobility at the GH joint often predispose it to instability, especially when associated with repetitive and vigorous motions near the end of the range of motion.

In addition to being prone to instability, the GH joints are frequently affected by degenerative pathologies. A common cause underlying many of these pathologies is excessive stress placed on periarticular connective tissues and the adjacent rotator cuff muscles. Stressed and damaged tissues often become inflamed and painful, as demonstrated in subacromial bursitis, rotator cuff tendonitis, and adhesive capsulitis.

Conservative treatment for many of the aforementioned degenerative or inflammatory conditions center around reducing the primary and secondary stresses on the joint, normalizing the arthrokinematics, restoring active and passive range of motion, improving strength, and reducing pain and inflammation.

At least 19 individual muscles power and control the wide range of movements available to the shoulder complex. Rather than working in isolation, these muscles interact synergistically to enhance their control over the multiple joints of the shoulder. Consider, for example, the muscular interactions required to abduct the shoulder in the plane of the scapula. Muscles such as the deltoid and rotator cuff require coactivation of at least the serratus anterior and trapezius to effectively stabilize the scapula and clavicle. Furthermore, these ST muscles can stabilize the scapula and clavicle only if their proximal skeletal attachments (cranium, ribs, and spine) are themselves well stabilized. Weakness anywhere along these links reduces the strength, ease, and control of active shoulder abduction. Factors that directly or indirectly disrupt these muscular-driven links include trauma, excessive stiffness of connective tissues, abnormal posture, joint instability, pain, peripheral nerve or spinal cord injuries, and diseases affecting the muscular or nervous system.

Appreciating how muscles naturally interact across the shoulder prepares the clinician to render an accurate diagnosis of the underlying pathomechanics of abnormal shoulder posture and movement. This knowledge is essential to the design of effective rehabilitation and treatment for a wide of shoulder impairments.

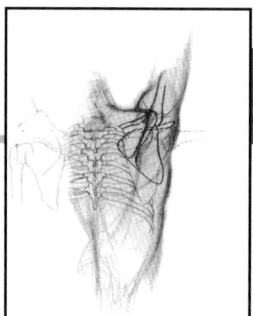

ADDITIONAL CLINICAL CONNECTIONS

CONTENTS

CLINICAL CONNECTION 5.1
Subacromial Pain Syndrome: A Summary of Possible Impingement-Based Pathomechanics

Subacromial pain syndrome is a common contributor to shoulder pain, often coexisting with inflammation and tears of the rotator cuff. A possible source of the pain is repeated and excessive impingement of the delicate tissues within the subacromial space during active shoulder movements. This impingement may be the result of an abnormally reduced volume within the subacromial space, often measured as a reduced acromiohumeral distance.[73,124,138] Fig. 5.62 shows an example of complete loss of the subacromial space as a person attempts active shoulder abduction. Tissues within the subacromial space likely to become inflamed and painful after repeated compression include the supraspinatus tendon, the tendon of the long head of the biceps, the superior capsule, and the subacromial bursa. Because of the functional importance of actively raising the arm overhead, pain during this action can cause significant functional limitations. The condition is particularly common in overhead-throwing athletes[128] and in workers that require prolonged or repeated shoulder abduction,[4,241] but it can also occur in relatively sedentary persons.

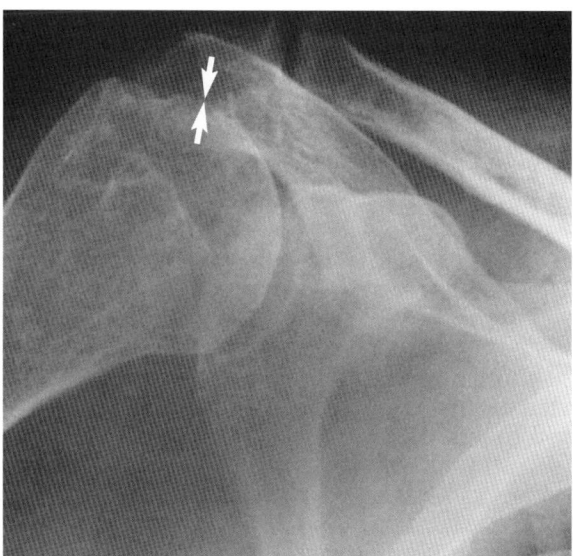

FIGURE 5.62 A radiograph of a person with subacromial impingement attempting abduction of the shoulder. The small arrows mark the impingement of the humeral head against the undersurface of the acromion. (Courtesy Gary L. Soderberg.)

For decades it was assumed that impingement of the supraspinatus tendon was central to the pathomechanics of subacromial pain, especially when the pain occurred at abduction angles that generally approached about 90 degrees. Although this assumption remains tenable, recent research questions its generalizability. For example, as abduction exceeds about 70 degrees, the bony attachment of the supraspinatus naturally shifts *medial* to the undersurface of the lateral acromion—outside the realm of the traditionally described location of "subacromial impingement."[73,136] Clearly, a more precise understanding of the pathomechanics of subacromial pain syndrome is needed, especially related to the dynamic anatomic and spatial relationships within the subacromial space during shoulder movement.[76,136,138]

As described earlier in this chapter, the height of the subacromial space in asymptomatic persons typically fluctuates between about 3 mm and almost 10 mm throughout abduction of the shoulder. Because of the many tissues occupying the relatively small subacromial space, the residing tissues likely experience some compression throughout at least part of the range of abduction. Such a natural and perhaps benign compression is likely for the supraspinatus tendon which, in the asymptomatic adult, has a thickness in the range of 4.9 to 6 mm.[103,170,224] For most persons, the bursa protects the tendons and capsule from excessive mechanical irritation. There is likely a threshold of cumulative compression that, once met, can cause pain in or near the subacromial tissues. This threshold may be partially related to the size of the subacromial space at any given point in the range of abduction, governed by kinesiologic and anatomic factors. One relevant kinesiologic factor involves abnormal arthrokinematics at the GH joint. As highlighted earlier, excessive superior migration of the humeral head during abduction can compress the contents within the subacromial space. The excessive superior migration of the humeral head may be caused by the inability of muscles, such as the rotator cuff, to coordinate the natural active arthrokinematics.

The pathomechanics associated with subacromial impingement has been studied from the perspectives of *both* humeral-on-scapular and scapular-on-humeral kinematics. Abnormal kinematics during either perspective can affect the volume of the subacromial space and therefore predispose painful impingement of the soft tissues. A considerable body of literature has specifically implicated abnormal ST kinematics (often labeled "scapular

Continued

ADDITIONAL CLINICAL CONNECTIONS

dyskinesis") as a contributing factor to subacromial impingement (or pain).[9,117,138,155,220] In the healthy pain-free shoulder, GH abduction conjointly involves significant ST upward rotation along with relatively subtle scapular adjustments such as posterior tilting and (in late abduction) external rotation. In contrast, several studies have shown that persons with painful subacromial impingement demonstrate at least one of the following kinematic signs during shoulder abduction: less than normal upward rotation, less posterior tilting, or less external rotation of the scapula.[75,139,152,156,239] These abnormal kinematics may contribute to subacromial impingement given that they can reduce the clearance between the humeral head and undersurface of the coracoacromial arch.[112,136,156,169] Interestingly, one study has demonstrated an *increase* in scapular upward rotation during active abduction in persons with experimentally induced subacromial pain.[260] These unexpected kinematics were considered a compensation strategy adapted to reduce the compression on the painful tissues. Whether abnormal scapular kinematics precede or follow a painful subacromial impingement is not always certain. Regardless of the specific pattern of scapular kinematics, the salient point is that even a small deviation in scapular kinematics likely has a disproportionately large effect on a volume as small (and crowded) as the subacromial space, especially in light of other concomitant factors such as swelling of the bursa or thickening of the supraspinatus tendon.

"Poor" or slumped resting posture of the shoulder or trunk has also been implicated as contributing factors to reducing the volume in the subacromial space.[24,102,118,144,155] Such posture, even in otherwise neurologically healthy persons, may be associated with a ST joint that is abnormally downwardly rotated and excessively protracted—positions typically associated with excessive anterior tilting and internal rotation of the scapula. Such a posture has indeed been correlated with a tight or overshortened pectoralis minor muscle.[23] By exerting an inferiorly directed tension on the coracoid process, tightness in this muscle could cause a scapular posture that positions the acromion closer to the subacromial tissues. In addition to a tight pectoralis minor, other factors predisposing abnormal posture or kinematics of the ST joint may include altered posture of the cervical and thoracic spine, including excessive thoracic kyphosis; increased activation of the upper trapezius, coupled with fatigue, reduced activation, or weakness of the serratus anterior, middle and lower trapezius, and rotator cuff group; and reduced coordination of the muscles that naturally sequence the kinematics between the scapula and humerus.[f]

Excessive subacromial impingement may be associated with pathologies directly related to the GH joint. These pathologies may include ligamentous instability, degeneration or tears of the tendons of the rotator cuff muscles and long head of the biceps,

adhesive capsulitis, excessive tightness in the posterior capsule (and associated excessive anterior migration of the humeral head toward a lower part of the coracoacromial arch), selected muscular tightness around the GH joint, and structurally induced changes in the volume of the subacromial space.[124,168,169,180,211] The last factor may result from osteophytes forming around the overlying AC joint, the presence of an abnormal hook-shaped acromion, or swelling and fragmentation of structures in and around the subacromial space.

The more popular factors purported to increase the risk for developing subacromial impingement are summarized in the following box.

> **Factors that May Increase the Risk for Developing Subacromial Impingement**
> - Abnormal kinematics at the GH joint
> - Scapular dyskinesis
> - "Slouched" trunk posture that affects the alignment of the ST joint, which may include excessive thoracic kyphosis
> - Fatigue, weakness, painful inhibition, poor control, or tightness of the muscles that control motions or postures at the GH and ST joints
> - Inflammation and swelling of tissues within and around the subacromial space
> - Degeneration or tears of the tendons of the rotator cuff muscles and long head of the biceps
> - Instability of the GH joint
> - Adhesions or stiffness within the inferior GH joint capsule
> - Excessive tightness in the posterior capsule of the GH joint (and associated anterior migration of the humeral head toward the lower margin of the coracoacromial arch)
> - Osteophytes forming around the AC joint
> - Abnormal shape of the acromion or coracoacromial arch

Nonsurgical treatment of subacromial pain due to suspected subacromial impingement typically include decreasing inflammation within the subacromial space; increasing control, strength or "balance" of the rotator cuff and axial-scapular muscles, improving kinesthetic awareness of movement and posture of the ST joint; attempting to restore the natural shoulder range of motion, tissue pliability, and arthrokinematics at the GH joint; providing education on the pathomechanics; and advice on pain management and activity modification. Exercise strategies aimed at addressing many of these objectives are based on an understanding of how an altered musculoskeletal system can adversely affect shoulder kinematics, ultimately reducing subacromial space and predisposing a person to subacromial impingement and potential pain (see the box on the following page).

[f]23,46,47,62,87,102,117,144,148,238

ADDITIONAL CLINICAL CONNECTIONS

CLINICAL CONNECTION 5.1
Subacromial Pain Syndrome: A Summary of Possible Impingement-Based Pathomechanics—cont'd

Studies and systematic reviews have demonstrated that treatments consisting of conventional physical therapy, including exercise and manual therapy, can be effective at reducing pain and improving function in some persons with suspected subacromial impingement pain.[66,85,200] Other studies have shown less clear outcomes, possibly attributable to poor research design.[226] In general, however, the effectiveness of exercise as a treatment approach will likely improve following a better understanding of how to match the type of exercise more precisely with the pathomechanics unique to the individual patient or client.

Proposed Mechanisms of How Alterations in the Musculoskeletal System Can Adversely Affect Shoulder Kinematics, and Ultimately Reduce the Subacromial Space

Altered Component of the Musculoskeletal System	Associated Adverse Kinematic Effect (reducing subacromial space)
Reduced activation of the serratus anterior, middle and lower trapezius	Reduced upward rotation, posterior tilt, and external rotation of the scapula
Excessive activation of the upper trapezius	May oppose posterior rotation of the clavicle;* through reciprocal inhibition, reduced activation of the lower trapezius
Reduced activation or degeneration/tears of the rotator cuff muscles	Excessive superior migration of the humeral head during abduction or flexion; reduced external rotation of the GH joint during abduction/flexion
Tightness of the posterior capsule of the GH joint and/or posterior rotator cuff muscles	Abnormal position of the humeral head relative to the glenoid fossa; excessive internal rotation bias of the scapula
Tightness of the pectoralis minor, coracobrachialis, or short head of the biceps brachii	Excessive internal rotation, anterior tilt, or downward rotation of the scapula
Excessive thoracic kyphosis	Excessive internal rotation or anterior tilt of the scapula; reduced upward rotation of the scapula

*Based on the line of force of the upper trapezius relative to the clavicle, which may be influenced by craniocervical posture

ADDITIONAL CLINICAL CONNECTIONS

Approximately 85% of the individual muscles of the shoulder attach directly to the scapula—a bone that in the adult weighs only about 160 g (just over ⅓ of a pound).[21] The miniscule inertial resistance of the scapula relative to the large, multidirectional forces produced by the muscles allows for even the smallest neuromuscular imbalance to cause abnormal positioning of the scapula, defined earlier as *scapular dyskinesis.* In essence, the relative bilateral orientation of the scapulae serves as a "window" into the neuromuscular environment within the shoulder. Depending on the severity and underlying cause, scapular dyskinesis can significantly disrupt the kinematics of the entire shoulder complex, thereby reducing the natural fluidity and comfort of movement.

The manner in which scapular dyskinesis affects shoulder kinematics can, at times, be hard to visualize. In certain cases, however, the abnormal kinematics can become clear with the aid of simple goniometric measurements, as explained in Fig. 5.63. To illustrate, first consider an analysis of normal scapulohumeral rhythm as an asymptomatic, male subject actively abducts his shoulder in the scapular plane (Fig. 5.63A). The picture shows the subject holding a position of 70 degrees of shoulder abduction, measured by a goniometer as the angle between a vertical reference line and the long axis of the humerus. The position depicted in Fig. 5.63A represents 1 of 17 static measurements made of *shoulder abduction,* between 10 and 170 degrees (see column of table and horizontal axis in the graph). At each 10-degree increment of shoulder abduction, the *scapulothoracic (ST) position* of upward rotation was recorded as the angle between a vertical reference line and the medial border of the scapula (see column of data and associated green data points in graph). These relatively simple measurements allow the amount of associated *glenohumeral (GH) joint abduction* to be roughly estimated as the *difference between shoulder abduction and the ST rotation position* (see blue data points in graph). Because the scapula is upwardly rotated 20 degrees at 70 degrees of shoulder abduction, the assumed angle of GH joint

abduction is about 50 degrees. Note that at 170 degrees of shoulder abduction, the scapula is upwardly rotated 54 degrees and the GH joint is assumed to be in 116 degrees of abduction: a kinematic pattern expected based on a normal scapulohumeral rhythm.

Fig. 5.63B shows the results of a similar analysis using a subject with marked scapular dyskinesis, which was associated with weakness of the right serratus anterior and complaints of subacromial pain with active abduction. The salient feature of the dyskinesis is that the scapula *downwardly* rotates (indicated by negative rotation values) through approximately the first half of shoulder abduction. Because the scapula is downwardly rotated 20 degrees at 70 degrees of shoulder abduction, the assumed angle of GH joint abduction angles is 90 degrees. In this situation, *the GH joint is in greater abduction than the shoulder.* Interestingly and inexplicably, the subject's scapula eventually began to upwardly rotate but only at shoulder abduction angles greater than 80 degrees. The subject was unable to actively abduct his shoulder beyond 150 degrees.

The excessively downwardly rotated position of the scapula during the first half of shoulder abduction can create several adverse conditions at the GH joint. One obvious factor is the likelihood of compressing the supraspinatus tendon within the subacromial space, especially at relatively low abduction angles.[137] Furthermore, the excessive GH joint abduction (caused by the excessive downward rotation of the scapula) would alter the natural lines of force of the rotator cuff muscles, thereby disrupting the arthrokinematics and associated dynamic stability of the joint. Also, the excessively downwardly rotated scapula would affect the length-tension relationships of the scapulohumeral muscles, possibly leading to weakness or muscular fatigue. Being able to visualize the altered kinematics of scapular dyskinesis can help clarify the associated pathokinesiology, an essential step in the diagnosis of movement impairment and in designing the most effective therapeutic intervention.

ADDITIONAL CLINICAL CONNECTIONS

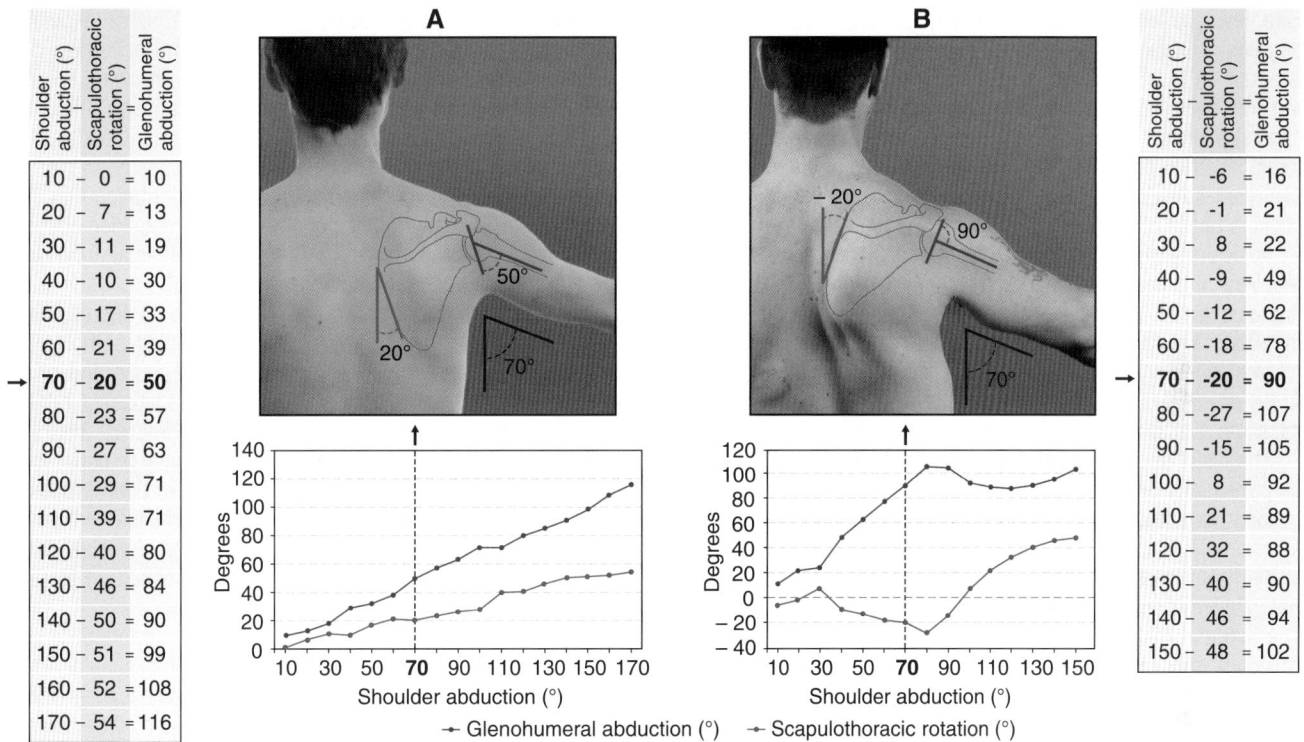

FIGURE 5.63 Goniometric measurements used to estimate glenohumeral joint abduction *(blue)* as the difference between shoulder abduction *(black;* plotted on the horizontal axis of the graphs) and the scapulothoracic rotation position *(green)*. A healthy male (A) and a male with scapular dyskinesis (B) are each shown holding their shoulder abducted to 70 degrees. Upward rotation of the scapula is indicated by positive angles; downward rotation by negative angles.

ADDITIONAL CLINICAL CONNECTIONS

CLINICAL CONNECTION 5.3
Excessive Humeral Retroversion with Reduced Internal Rotation of the Shoulder: Possible Clinical Implications

Elite level baseball pitchers generally exhibit about 40 to 45 degrees of humeral retroversion in the throwing arm.[192,266] This is about 10 to 15 degrees more than what is typically present in the non–throwing arm or what is expected in the adult. The excessive retroversion is believed to be a bony adaptation to cumulative torsional strain placed on the proximal humerus of the adolescent overhead-throwing athlete, specifically occurring during the late cocking phase of the throw.[94,249]

As depicted in Fig. 5.4 angle C, the normal 30 degrees of humeral retroversion is described as a fixed twist (or torsion) of the proximal humerus relative to the distal humerus. Because the torsion is evident throughout the entire shaft of the bone, it is equally valid to describe retroversion as an external rotation twist of the *distal humerus relative to the proximal humerus.* Either perspective is valid, each describing the same relative torsion along the long axis of the bone.

The distal perspective of describing humeral retroversion may be particularly useful in understanding some of the clinical implications purported to occur with excessive retroversion. Consider, for example, that a person with *45 degrees* of retroversion would likely display a resting arm posture of about 15 degrees of *external rotation* when the GH joint is in its neutral, anatomic position. The external rotation bias of the distal humerus (relative to the GH joint) may explain, in part, why elite level baseball pitchers typically demonstrate *greater* external rotation and less internal rotation in their throwing shoulder than in the non–throwing contralateral shoulder.[266] Note that with excessive retroversion, the *total* arc of internal and external rotation may not necessarily be different between the throwing and opposite shoulders. The critical difference is a 10 to 15-degree *shift* in the total arc of motion in the direction of external rotation. The greater external rotation of the limb allows an exaggerated "windup" of a pitch, which may improve performance by enabling increased pitching speed.[265]

Compared with the non–throwing arm, the reduced shoulder internal rotation often observed in the throwing arm of the elite level baseball pitcher has been referred to as *Glenohumeral Internal Rotation Deficit, or "GIRD."* Clinical interest in the pathomechanics of this condition is based primarily on the assumed increased risk of the throwing athlete with GIRD developing a wide range of painful shoulder or arm conditons.[166] Research has also shown an association between GIRD and increased thickness and stiffness of both the posterior (and posterior-inferior) capsule of the GH joint and external rotator muscles (infraspinatus, teres minor, and posterior deltoid).[83,171,198,211,249] The hypertrophy and stiffening of

these tissues might theoretically be attributed to large deceleration forces (reportedly 1–1.5 times body weight) occurring with internal rotation at every "release phase" of throwing.[166] The reduced end-range of internal rotation associated with GIRD may reduce the time that the posterior capsule and eccentrically active external rotator muscles have to decelerate and absorb the forces of the internally rotating humerus. The tissue adaptation may further limit internal rotation range of motion at the shoulder, possibly perpetuating the stress within the tissue, as well as altering optimal intra-articular paths of movement.

Throwing athletes with GIRD of at least 10 to 20 degrees have been shown to be at increased risk of developing pathology in the throwing shoulder.[33,94,225,266] Although direct cause-and-effect relationships are hard to show unequivocally, suspected related pathologies include subacromial (external) and internal impingement, tears of the labrum, and biceps and rotator cuff tendinopathy.[94,135,166,176,225] Further associations have been proposed between GIRD and injuries of the medial collateral ligament of the elbow in elite baseball players; however, evidence of a relationship between these is mixed[60,191,228,267] and varies based on starting pitching age.[115]

It is not always clear whether GIRD and its purported associated risk of injury is due to retroversion or to posterior shoulder stiffness, or both.[245] This is a relevant clinical question because limited internal rotation due to posterior shoulder stiffness may be responsive to physical therapy (muscular stiffness more so than capsular stiffness), in contrast to a limitation of internal rotation stemming exclusively from excessive humeral retroversion, which would not be responsive.[83] Recent research has also implicated an association between GIRD and scapular dyskinesis. Increased stiffness of the posterior capsule alone, for example, could cause excessive or prolonged *internal rotation* of the scapula while reaching overhead.[172] Recall that excessive or prolonged internal rotation of the scapula during shoulder abduction has been thought to increase the risk of subacromial impingement. Continued research is warranted to understand the biomechanical and biophysical relationships among humeral retroversion, GIRD, increased stiffness in the posterior capsular and/or external rotator muscles, scapular dyskinesis, and a host of possible stress-related injuries in the shoulder.[166] Greater knowledge may help with prevention, diagnosis, and treatment of the many stress-related injuries that have been associated with athletes engaged in overhead activities, as well as nonathletic but important movements.

REFERENCES

1. Abboud JA, Soslowsky LJ: Interplay of the static and dynamic restraints in glenohumeral instability, *Clin Orthop Relat Res* 400:48–57, 2002.

2. Ackland DC, Richardson M, Pandy MG: Axial rotation moment arms of the shoulder musculature after reverse total shoulder arthroplasty, *J Bone Joint Surg Am* 94(20):1886–1895, 2012.

3. Alexander S, Southgate DF, Bull AM, et al.: The role of negative intraarticular pressure and the long head of biceps tendon on passive stability of the glenohumeral joint, *J Shoulder Elbow Surg* 22(1):94–101, 2013.

4. Alexopoulos EC, Stathi IC, Charizani F: Prevalence of musculoskeletal disorders in dentists, *BMC Musculoskelet Disord* 5:16, 2004.

5. Aliaj K, Lawrence RL, Bo Foreman K, et al.: Kinematic coupling of the glenohumeral and scapulothoracic joints generates humeral axial rotation, *J Biomech* 136:111059, 2022.

6. Almajed YA, Hall AC, Gillingwater TH, et al.: Anatomical, functional and biomechanical review of the glenoid labrum, *J Anat* 00:1–11, 2021.

7. Almeida RF, Pereira ND, Ribeiro LP, et al.: Is the disabilities of the arm, shoulder and hand (Dash) questionnaire adequate to assess individuals with subacromial pain syndrome? Rasch model and international classification of functioning, disability and health, *Phys Ther* 101:1–11, 2021.

8. An KN, Browne AO, Korinek S, et al.: Three-dimensional kinematics of glenohumeral elevation, *J Orthop Res* 9(1):143–149, 1991.

9. Andres J, Painter PJ, McIlvain G, et al.: The effect of repeated shoulder motion on scapular dyskinesis in army ROTC cadets, *Mil Med* 185(5–6):e811–e817, 2020.

10. Assila N, Duprey S, Begon M: Glenohumeral joint and muscles functions during a lifting task, *J Biomech* 126:110641, 2021.

11. Bagg SD, Forrest WJ: A biomechanical analysis of scapular rotation during arm abduction in the scapular plane, *Am J Phys Med Rehabil* 67:238–245, 1988.

12. Bagg SD, Forrest WJ: Electromyographic study of the scapular rotators during arm abduction in the scapular plane, *Am J Phys Med* 65:111–124, 1986.

13. Barcia AM, Makovicka JL, Group MS, et al.: Scapular motion in the presence of rotator cuff tears: a systematic review, *J Shoulder Elbow Surg* 30(7):1679–1692, 2021.

14. Basmajian JV, Bazant FJ: Factors preventing downward dislocation of the adducted shoulder joint, *J Bone Joint Surg Am* 41:1182–1186, 1959.

15. Berckmans K, Castelein B, Borms D, et al.: Analysis of scapular kinematics and muscle activity by use of fine-wire electrodes during shoulder exercises, *Am J Sports Med* 48(5):1213–1219, 2020.

16. Berckmans KR, Castelein B, Borms D, et al.: Rehabilitation exercises for dysfunction of the scapula: exploration of muscle activity using fine-wire EMG, *Am J Sports Med* 49(10):2729–2736, 2021.

17. Bergmann G, Graichen F, Bender A, et al.: In vivo gleno-humeral joint loads during forward flexion and abduction, *J Biomech* 44(8):1543–1552, 2011.

18. Bishop JY, Hidden KA, Jones GL, et al.: Factors influencing surgeon's choice of procedure for anterior shoulder instability: a multicenter prospective cohort study, *Arthroscopy* 35(7):2014–2025, 2019.

19. Bodin J, Ha C, Petit Le MA, et al.: Risk factors for incidence of rotator cuff syndrome in a large working population, *Scand J Work Environ Health* 38(5):436–446, 2012.

20. Boettcher C, Halaki M, Holt K, et al.: Is the normal shoulder rotation strength ratio altered in elite swimmers? *Med Sci Sports Exerc* 52(3):680–684, 2020.

21. Borisov BK, Marei AN: Weight parameters of adult human skeleton, *Health Phys* 27(2):224–229, 1974.

22. Borstad JD, Ludewig PM: Comparison of three stretches for the pectoralis minor muscle, *J Shoulder Elbow Surg* 15(3):324–330, 2006.

23. Borstad JD, Ludewig PM: The effect of long versus short pectoralis minor resting length on scapular kinematics in healthy individuals, *J Orthop Sports Phys Ther* 35:227–238, 2005.

24. Borstad JD: Resting position variables at the shoulder: evidence to support a posture-impairment association, *Phys Ther* 86:549–557, 2006.

25. Bouaicha S, Ernstbrunner L, Jud L, et al.: The lever arm ratio of the rotator cuff to deltoid muscle explains and predicts pseudoparalysis of the shoulder: the shoulder abduction moment index, *Bone Joint Lett J* 100-b(12):1600–1608, 2018.

26. Bouaicha S, Slankamenac K, Moor BK, et al.: Cross-sectional area of the rotator cuff muscles in MRI - is there evidence for a biomechanical balanced shoulder? *PLoS One* 11(6):e0157946, 2016.

27. Braman JP, Engel SC, Laprade RF, et al.: In vivo assessment of scapulohumeral rhythm during unconstrained overhead reaching in asymptomatic subjects, *J Shoulder Elbow Surg* 18(6):960–967, 2009.

28. Braman JP, Zhao KD, Lawrence RL, et al.: Shoulder impingement revisited: evolution of diagnostic understanding in orthopedic surgery and physical therapy, *Med Biol Eng Comput* 52(3):211–219, 2014.

29. Brunnstrom S: Muscle testing around the shoulder girdle, *J Bone Joint Surg Am* 23:263–272, 1941.

30. Bullock GS, Garrigues GE, Ledbetter L, et al.: A systematic review of proposed rehabilitation guidelines following anatomic and reverse shoulder arthroplasty, *J Orthop Sports Phys Ther* 49(5):337–346, 2019.

31. Burden EG, Batten TJ, Smith CD, et al.: Reverse total shoulder arthroplasty, *Bone Joint Lett J* 103-b(5):813–821, 2021.

32. Burkart AC, Debski RE: Anatomy and function of the glenohumeral ligaments in anterior shoulder instability, *Clin Orthop Relat Res* 400:32–39, 2002.

33. Burkhart SS, Morgan CD, Kibler WB: The disabled throwing shoulder: spectrum of pathology. Part I: pathoanatomy and biomechanics, *Arthroscopy* 19:404–420, 2003.

34. Camargo PR, Neumann DA: Kinesiologic considerations for targeting activation of scapulothoracic muscles - Part 2: trapezius, *Braz J Phys Ther* 23(6):467–475, 2019.

35. Camargo PR, Phadke V, Braman JP, et al.: Three-dimensional shoulder kinematics after total claviculectomy: a biomechanical investigation of a single case, *Man Ther* 18(6):620–623, 2013.

36. Camci E, Duzgun I, Hayran M, et al.: Scapular kinematics during shoulder elevation performed with and without elastic resistance in men without shoulder pathologies, *J Orthop Sports Phys Ther* 43(10):735–743, 2013.

37. Chahla J, Aman ZS, Godin JA, et al.: Systematic review of the anatomic descriptions of the glenohumeral ligaments: a call for further quantitative studies, *Arthroscopy* 35(6):1917–1926.e2, 2019.

38. Chopp JN, Dickerson CR: Resolving the contributions of fatigue-induced migration and scapular reorientation on the subacromial space: an orthopaedic geometric simulation analysis, *Hum Mov Sci* 31(2):448–460, 2012.

39. Churchill RS, Brems JJ, Kotschi H: Glenoid size, inclination, and version: an anatomic study, *J Shoulder Elbow Surg* 10:327–332, 2001.

40. Coats-Thomas MS, Massimini DF, Warner JJP, et al.: In vivo evaluation of subacromial and internal impingement risk in asymptomatic individuals, *Am J Phys Med Rehabil* 97(9):659–665, 2018.

41. Cole A, Cox T: Treatment of glenohumeral subluxation: a review of the literature and considerations for pediatric population, *Am J Phys Med Rehabil* 98(8):706–714, 2019.

42. Colegate-Stone T, Allom R, Singh R, et al.: Classification of the morphology of the acromioclavicular joint using cadaveric and radiological analysis, *J Bone Joint Surg Br* 92(5):743–746, 2010.

43. Conway AM: Movements at the sternoclavicular and acromioclavicular joints, *Phys Ther* 41:421–432, 1961.

44. Cook JB, Krul KP: Challenges in treating acromioclavicular separations: current concepts, *J Am Acad Orthop Surg* 26(19):669–677, 2018.

45. Cook T, Lewis J: Rotator cuff-related shoulder pain: to inject or not to inject? *J Orthop Sports Phys Ther* 49(5):289–293, 2019.

46. Cools AM, Declercq GA, Cambier DC, et al.: Trapezius activity and intramuscular balance during isokinetic exercise in overhead athletes with impingement symptoms, *Scand J Med Sci Sports* 17(1):25–33, 2007.

47. Cools AM, Dewitte V, Lanszweert F, et al.: Rehabilitation of scapular muscle balance: which exercises to prescribe? *Am J Sports Med* 35(10):1744–1751, 2007.

48. Costic RS, Vangura Jr A, Fenwick JA, et al.: Viscoelastic behavior and structural properties of the coracoclavicular ligaments, *Scand J Med Sci Sports* 13:305–310, 2003.

49. De Rooij PP, Van Lieshout EMM, Schurink IJ, et al.: Current practice in the management of acromioclavicular joint dislocations; a national survey in The Netherlands, *Eur J Trauma Emerg Surg* 47(5):1417–1427, 2021.

50. Debski RE, Parsons IM, Woo SL, et al.: Effect of capsular injury on acromioclavicular joint mechanics, *J Bone Joint Surg* 83:1344–1351, 2001.

51. Debski RE, Sakone M, Woo SL, et al.: Contribution of the passive properties of the rotator cuff to glenohumeral stability during anterior-posterior loading, *J Shoulder Elbow Surg* 8:324–329, 1999.

52. Debski RE, Wong EK, Woo SL, et al.: An analytical approach to determine the in situ forces in the glenohumeral ligaments, *J Biomech Eng* 121:311–315, 1999.

53. DeFroda SF, Donnelly JC, Mulcahey MK, et al.: Shoulder instability in women compared with men: epidemiology, pathophysiology, and special considerations, *JBJS Rev* 7(9):e10, 2019.

54. DeFroda SF, Perry AK, Mehta N, et al.: Biomechanical role of the superior capsule in a rotator cuff sectioned and repaired state: a sequential sectioning study, *Am J Sports Med* 50(6):1541–1549, 2022.

55. Dekker TJ, Aman ZS, Peebles LA, et al.: Quantitative and qualitative analyses of the glenohumeral ligaments: an anatomic study, *Am J Sports Med* 48(8):1837–1845, 2020.

56. DePalma AF: *Degenerative changes in sternoclavicular and acromioclavicular joints in various decades*, Springfield, Ill, 1957, Charles C Thomas.

57. Dessaur WA, Magarey ME: Diagnostic accuracy of clinical tests for superior labral anterior posterior lesions: a systematic review, *J Orthop Sports Phys Ther* 38:341–352, 2008.

58. D'Hondt NE, Pool JJM, Kiers H, et al.: Validity of clinical measurement instruments assessing scapular function: insufficient evidence to recommend any instrument for assessing scapular posture, movement, and dysfunction-a systematic review, *J Orthop Sports Phys Ther* 50(11):632–641, 2020.

59. Dillman CJ, Fleisig GS, Andrews JR: Biomechanics of pitching with emphasis upon shoulder kinematics, *J Orthop Sports Phys Ther* 18:402–408, 1993.

60. Dines JS, Frank JB, Akerman M, et al.: Glenohumeral internal rotation deficits in baseball players with ulnar collateral ligament insufficiency, *Am J Sports Med* 37(3):566–570, 2009.

61. Dragoo JL, Braun HJ, Bartlinski SE, et al.: Acromioclavicular joint injuries in national collegiate athletic association football: data from the 2004-2005 through 2008-2009 national collegiate athletic association injury surveillance system, *Am J Sports Med* 40(9):2066–2071, 2012.

62. Ebaugh DD, Spinelli BA: Scapulothoracic motion and muscle activity during the raising and lowering phases of an overhead reaching task, *J Electromyogr Kinesiol* 20(2):199–205, 2010.

63. Ebaugh DD, McClure PW, Karduna AR: Effects of shoulder muscle fatigue caused by repetitive overhead activities on scapulothoracic and glenohumeral kinematics, *J Electromyogr Kinesiol* 16:224–235, 2006.

64. Edelson G: The development of humeral head retroversion, *J Shoulder Elbow Surg* 9(4):316–318, 2000.

65. Ekstrom RA, Donatelli RA, Soderberg GL: Surface electromyographic analysis of exercises for the trapezius and serratus anterior muscles, *J Orthop Sports Phys Ther* 33:247–258, 2003.

66. Eliason A, Harringe M, Engström B, et al.: Guided exercises with or without joint mobilization or no treatment in patients with subacromial pain syndrome: a clinical trial, *J Rehabil Med* 53(5):jrm00190, 2021.

67. Finley MA, Euiler E, Hiremath SV, et al.: Movement coordination during humeral elevation in individuals with newly acquired spinal cord injury, *J Appl Biomech* 1–6, 2020.

68. Friedenberg SM, Zimprich T, Harper CM: The natural history of long thoracic and spinal accessory neuropathies, *Muscle Nerve* 25:535–539, 2002.

69. Fukuda K, Craig EV, An KN, et al.: Biomechanical study of the ligamentous system of the acromioclavicular joint, *J Bone Joint Surg Am* 68:434–440, 1986.

70. Gava V, Rosa DP, Pereira ND, et al.: Ratio between 3D glenohumeral and scapulothoracic motions in individuals without shoulder pain, *J Electromyogr Kinesiol* 62:102623, 2022.

71. Gerber C, Blumenthal S, Curt A, et al.: Effect of selective experimental suprascapular nerve block on abduction and external rotation strength of the shoulder, *J Shoulder Elbow Surg* 16:815–820, 2007.

72. Giphart JE, Brunkhorst JP, Horn NH, et al.: Effect of plane of arm elevation on glenohumeral kinematics: a normative biplane fluoroscopy study, *J Bone Joint Surg Am* 95(3):238–245, 2013.

73. Giphart JE, van der Meijden OA, Millett PJ: The effects of arm elevation on the 3-dimensional acromiohumeral distance: a biplane fluoroscopy study with normative data, *J Shoulder Elbow Surg* 21(11):1593–1600, 2012.

74. Gohlke F: The pattern of the collagen fiber bundles of the capsule of the glenohumeral joint, *J Shoulder Elbow Surg* 3:111–128, 1994.

75. Goncalves DHM, de Oliveira AS, Freire LC, et al.: Three-dimensional kinematic analysis of upper limb movements between individuals with and without subacromial shoulder pain exploring the statistical parametric mapping, *J Biomech* 129:110806, 2021.

76. Gonçalves DHM, de Oliveira AS, Freire LC, et al.: Three-dimensional kinematic analysis of upper limb movements between individuals with and without subacromial shoulder pain exploring the statistical parametric mapping, *J Biomech* 129:110806, 2021.

77. Graichen H, Hinterwimmer S, von Eisenhart-Rothe R, et al.: Effect of abducting and adducting muscle activity on glenohumeral translation, scapular kinematics and subacromial space width in vivo, *J Biomech* 38:755–760, 2005.

78. Graichen H, Stammberger T, Bonél H, et al.: Three-dimensional analysis of shoulder girdle and supraspinatus motion patterns in patients with impingement syndrome, *J Orthop Res* 19:1192–1198, 2001.

79. Guney-Deniz H, Harput G, Toprak U, et al.: Relationship between middle trapezius muscle activation and acromiohumeral distance change during shoulder elevation with scapular retraction, *J Sport Rehab* 28(3):266–271, 2019.

80. Habechian FAP, Fornasari GG, Sacramento LS, et al.: Differences in scapular kinematics and scapulohumeral rhythm during elevation and lowering of the arm between typical children and healthy adults, *J Electromyogr Kinesiol* 24(1):78–83, 2014.

81. Hagiwara Y, Kanazawa K, Ando A, et al.: Effects of joint capsular release on range of motion in patients with frozen shoulder, *J Shoulder Elbow Surg* 29(9):1836–1842, 2020.

82. Halder AM, Zhao KD, Odriscoll SW, et al.: Dynamic contributions to superior shoulder stability, *J Orthop Res* 19:206–212, 2001.

83. Hall K, Borstad JD: Posterior shoulder tightness: to treat or not to treat? *J Orthop Sports Phys Ther* 48(3):133–136, 2018.

84. Hanisch K, Holte MB, Hvass I, et al.: Clinically relevant results of reverse total shoulder arthroplasty for patients younger than 65 years compared to the older patients, *Arthroplasty* 3(1):30, 2021.

85. Hanratty CE, McVeigh JG, Kerr DP, et al.: The effectiveness of physiotherapy exercises in subacromial impingement syndrome: a systematic review and meta-analysis [Review], *Semin Arthritis Rheum* 42(3):297–316, 2012.

86. Harris KD, Deyle GD, Gill NW, et al.: Manual physical therapy for injection-confirmed nonacute acromioclavicular joint pain, *J Orthop Sports Phys Ther* 42(2):66–80, 2012.

87. Harrison N, Garrett WZ, Timmons MK: Serratus anterior fatigue reduces scapular posterior tilt and external rotation during arm elevation, *J Sport Rehab* 30(8):1151–1157, 2021.

88. Harryman DT, Sidles JA, Clark JM, et al.: Translation of the humeral head on the glenoid with passive glenohumeral motion, *J Bone Joint Surg Am* 72:1334–1343, 1990.

89. Hashimoto T, Suzuki K, Nobuhara K: Dynamic analysis of intraarticular pressure in the glenohumeral joint, *J Shoulder Elbow Surg* 4(3):209–218, 1995.

90. Hatta T, Sano H, Zuo J, et al.: Localization of degenerative changes of the acromioclavicular joint: a cadaveric study, *Surg Radiol Anat* 35(2):89–94, 2013.

91. Hecker A, Aguirre J, Eichenberger U, et al.: Deltoid muscle contribution to shoulder flexion and abduction strength: an experimental approach, *J Shoulder Elbow Surg* 30(2):e60–e68, 2021.

92. Hegedus EJ, Michener LA, Seitz AL: Three key findings when diagnosing shoulder multidirectional instability: patient report of instability, hypermobility, and specific shoulder tests, *J Orthop Sports Phys Ther* 50(2):52–54, 2020.

93. Hettrich CM, Cronin KJ, Raynor MB, et al.: Epidemiology of the frequency, etiology, direction, and severity (feds) system for classifying glenohumeral instability, *J Shoulder Elbow Surg* 28(1):95–101, 2019.

94. Hibberd EE, Oyama S, Myers JB: Increase in humeral retrotorsion accounts for age-related increase in glenohumeral internal rotation deficit in youth and adolescent baseball players, *Am J Sports Med* 42(4):851–858, 2014.

95. Hik F, Ackland DC: The moment arms of the muscles spanning the glenohumeral joint: a systematic review, *J Anat* 234(1):1–15, 2019.

96. Hogan C, Corbett JA, Ashton S, et al.: Scapular dyskinesis is not an isolated risk factor for shoulder injury in athletes: a systematic review and meta-analysis, *Am J Sports Med* 49(10):2843–2853, 2021.

97. Holzbaur KR, Delp SL, Gold GE, et al.: Moment-generating capacity of upper limb muscles in healthy adults, *J Biomech* 40:2442–2449, 2007.

98. Hovelius L, Eriksson K, Fredin H, et al.: Recurrences after initial dislocation of the shoulder. Results of a prospective study of treatment, *J Bone Joint Surg Am* 65:343–349, 1983.

99. Howell SM, Galinat BJ: The glenoid-labral socket. A constrained articular surface, *Clin Orthop Relat Res* 122–125, 1989.

100. Howell SM, Imobersteg AM, Seger DH, et al.: Clarification of the role of the supraspinatus muscle in shoulder function, *J Bone Joint Surg Am* 68:398–404, 1986.

101. Hunt SA, Kwon YW, Zuckerman JD: The rotator interval: anatomy, pathology, and strategies for treatment, *J Am Acad Orthop Surg* 15:218–227, 2007.

102. Hunter DJ, Rivett DA, McKeirnan S, et al.: Relationship between shoulder impingement syndrome and thoracic posture, *Phys Ther* 100(4):677–686, 2020.

103. Hunter DJ, Rivett DA, McKiernan S, et al.: Acromiohumeral distance and supraspinatus tendon thickness in people with shoulder impingement syndrome compared to asymptomatic age and gender-matched participants: a case control study, *BMC Musculoskelet Disord* 22(1):1004, 2021.

104. Hurley ET, Manjunath AK, Bloom DA, et al.: Arthroscopic Bankart repair versus conservative management for first-time traumatic anterior shoulder instability: a systematic review and meta-analysis, *Arthroscopy* 36(9):2526–2532, 2020.

105. Inman VT, Saunders M, Abbott LC: Observations on the function of the shoulder joint, *J Bone Joint Surg Am* 26:1–32, 1944.

106. Inokuchi W, Sanderhoff OB, Søjbjerg JO, et al.: The relation between the position of the glenohumeral joint and the intraarticular pressure: an experimental study, *J Shoulder Elbow Surg* 6:144–149, 1997.

107. Ishikawa H, Kurokawa D, Muraki T, et al.: Increased external rotation related to the soft tissues is associated with pathologic internal impingement in high-school baseball players, *J Shoulder Elbow Surg* 31(9):1823–1830, 2022.

108. Johnson AJ, Godges JJ, Zimmerman GJ, et al.: The effect of anterior versus posterior glide joint mobilization on external rotation range of motion in patients with shoulder adhesive capsulitis, *J Orthop Sports Phys Ther* 37:88–99, 2007.

109. Johnson GR, Pandyan AD: The activity in the three regions of the trapezius under controlled loading conditions—an experimental and modelling study, *Clin Biomech* 20:155–161, 2005.

110. Johnson M: Rehabilitation following surgery for glenohumeral instability, *Sports Med Arthrosc Rev* 25(3):116–122, 2017.

111. Kaplan LD, Flanigan DC, Norwig J, et al.: Prevalence and variance of shoulder injuries in elite collegiate football players, *Am J Sports Med* 33(8):1142–1146, 2005.

112. Karduna AR, Kerner PJ, Lazarus MD: Contact forces in the subacromial space: effects of scapular orientation, *J Shoulder Elbow Surg* 14:393–399, 2005.

113. Kelley MJ, Kane TE, Leggin BG: Spinal accessory nerve palsy: associated signs and symptoms, *J Orthop Sports Phys Ther* 38(2):78–86, 2008.

114. Kennedy J, Klifto CS, Ledbetter L, et al.: Reverse total shoulder arthroplasty clinical and patient-reported outcomes and complications stratified by preoperative diagnosis: a systematic review, *J Shoulder Elbow Surg* 30(4):929–941, 2021.

115. Kennedy SM, Hannon JP, Conway JE, et al.: Effect of younger starting pitching age on humeral retrotorsion in baseball pitchers with an ulnar collateral ligament injury, *Am J Sports Med* 49(5):1160–1165, 2021.

116. Kholinne E, Kim D, Kwak JM, et al.: Topography of sensory receptors within the human glenohumeral joint capsule, *J Shoulder Elbow Surg* 30(4):779–786, 2021.

117. Kibler WB, Ludewig PM, McClure PW, et al.: Clinical implications of scapular dyskinesis in shoulder injury: the 2013 consensus statement from the 'Scapular Summit', *Br J Sports Med* 47(14):877–885, 2013.

118. Kibler WB, McMullen J: Scapular dyskinesis and its relation to shoulder pain, *J Am Acad Orthop Surg* 11:142–151, 2003.

119. Kibler WB, Sciascia A, Tokish JT, et al.: Disabled throwing shoulder 2021 update: part 1-anatomy and mechanics, *Arthroscopy* 38(5):1714–1726, 2022.

120. Kibler WB, Sciascia A, Wilkes T: Scapular dyskinesis and its relation to shoulder injury [Review], *J Am Acad Orthop Surg* 20(6):364–372, 2012.

121. Kibler WB, Sciascia AD, Uhl TL, et al.: Electromyographic analysis of specific exercises for scapular control in early phases of shoulder rehabilitation, *Am J Sports Med* 36:1789–1798, 2008.

122. Kim DK, Park G, Kuo LT, et al.: Isokinetic performance of shoulder external and internal rotators of professional volleyball athletes by different positions, *Sci Rep* 10(1):8706, 2020.

123. Kolz CW, Sulkar HJ, Aliaj K, et al.: Age-related differences in humerothoracic, scapulothoracic, and

glenohumeral kinematics during elevation and rotation motions, *J Biomech* 117:110266, 2021.

124. Kozono N, Okada T, Takeuchi N, et al.: In vivo dynamic acromiohumeral distance in shoulders with rotator cuff tears, *Clin Biomech* 60:95–99, 2018.

125. Kozono N, Takeuchi N, Okada T, et al.: Dynamic scapulohumeral rhythm: comparison between healthy shoulders and those with large or massive rotator cuff tear, *J* 28(3), 2020. 2309499020981779.

126. Kraeutler MJ, Belk JW, Carver TJ, et al.: Traumatic primary anterior glenohumeral joint dislocation in sports: a systematic review of operative versus nonoperative management, *Curr Sports Med Rep* 19(11):468–478, 2020.

127. Krahl VE: The torsion of the humerus; its localization, cause and duration in man, *Am J Anat* 80(3):275–319, 1947.

128. Krajnik S, Fogarty KJ, Yard EE, et al.: Shoulder injuries in US high school baseball and softball athletes, 2005-2008, *Pediatrics* 125(3):497–501, 2010.

129. Kronberg M, Nemeth G, Brostrom LA: Muscle activity and coordination in the normal shoulder. An electromyographic study, *Clin Orthop Relat Res* 257:76–85, 1990.

130. Kuechle DK, Newman SR, Itoi E, et al.: Shoulder muscle moment arms during horizontal flexion and elevation, *J Shoulder Elbow Surg* 6:429–439, 1997.

131. Kuhn JE, Huston LJ, Soslowsky LJ, et al.: External rotation of the glenohumeral joint: ligament restraints and muscle effects in the neutral and abducted positions, *J Shoulder Elbow Surg* 14:39S–48S, 2005.

132. Kurokawa D, Yamamoto N, Ishikawa H, et al.: Differences in humeral retroversion in dominant and nondominant sides of young baseball players, *J Shoulder Elbow Surg* 26(6):1083–1087, 2017.

133. Ladd LM, Crews M, Maertz NA: Glenohumeral joint instability: a review of anatomy, clinical presentation, and imaging, *Clin Sports Med* 40(4):585–599, 2021.

134. Lau BC, Hutyra CA, Gonzalez JM, et al.: Surgical treatment for recurrent shoulder instability: factors influencing surgeon decision making, *J Shoulder Elbow Surg* 30(3):e85–e102, 2021.

135. Laudner K, Meister K, Noel B, et al.: Anterior glenohumeral laxity is associated with posterior shoulder tightness among professional baseball pitchers, *Am J Sports Med* 40(5):1133–1137, 2012.

136. Lawrence RL, Braman JP, Ludewig PM: Shoulder kinematics impact subacromial proximities: a review of the literature, *Braz J Phys Ther* 24(3):219–230, 2020.

137. Lawrence RL, Braman JP, Ludewig PM: The impact of decreased scapulothoracic upward rotation on subacromial proximities, *J Orthop Sports Phys Ther* 49(3):180–191, 2019.

138. Lawrence RL, Braman JP, Keefe DF, et al.: The coupled kinematics of scapulothoracic upward rotation, *Phys Ther* 100(2):283–294, 2020.

139. Lawrence RL, Braman JP, LaPrade RF, et al.: Comparison of 3-dimensional shoulder complex kinematics in individuals with and without shoulder pain, part 1: sternoclavicular, acromioclavicular, and scapulothoracic joints, *J Orthop Sports Phys Ther* 44(9), 2014. 636–645–A8.

140. Lawrence RL, Braman JP, Staker JL, et al.: Comparison of 3-dimensional shoulder complex kinematics in individuals with and without shoulder pain, part 2: glenohumeral joint, *J Orthop Sports Phys Ther* 44(9):646–655B3, 2014.

141. Lawrence RL, Sessions WC, Jensen MC, et al.: The effect of glenohumeral plane of elevation on supraspinatus subacromial proximity, *J Biomech* 79:147–154, 2018.

142. Lawrence RL, Zauel R, Bey MJ: Measuring 3D in-vivo shoulder kinematics using biplanar videoradiography, *JoVE* 169(03):12, 2021.

143. Lee ECS, Roach NT, Clouthier AL, et al.: Three-dimensional scapular morphology is associated with rotator cuff tears and alters the abduction moment arm of the supraspinatus, *Clin Biomech* 78:105091, 2020.

144. Lewis JS, Wright C, Green A: Subacromial impingement syndrome: the effect of changing posture on

shoulder range of movement, *J Orthop Sports Phys Ther* 35:72–87, 2005.

145. Liu J, Hughes RE, Smutz WP, et al.: Roles of deltoid and rotator cuff muscles in shoulder elevation, *Clin Biomech* 12:32–38, 1997.

146. Lizaur A, Sanz-Reig J, Gonzalez-Parreno S: Long-term results of the surgical treatment of type III acromioclavicular dislocations: an update of a previous report, *J Bone Joint Surg Br* 93(8):1088–1092, 2011.

147. Lloyd G, Day J, Lu J, et al.: Postoperative rehabilitation of anterior glenohumeral joint instability surgery: a systematic review, *Sports Med Arthrosc Rev* 29(2):54–62, 2021.

148. Lopes AD, Timmons MK, Grover M, et al.: Visual scapular dyskinesis: kinematics and muscle activity alterations in patients with subacromial impingement syndrome, *Arch Phys Med Rehabil* 96(2):298–306, 2015.

149. Ludewig PM, Behrens SA, Meyer SM, et al.: Three-dimensional clavicular motion during arm elevation: reliability and descriptive data, *J Orthop Sports Phys Ther* 34:140–149, 2004.

150. Ludewig PM, Braman JP: Shoulder impingement: biomechanical considerations in rehabilitation, *Man Ther* 16(1):33–39, 2011.

151. Ludewig PM, Cook TM, Nawoczenski DA: Three-dimensional scapular orientation and muscle activity at selected positions of humeral elevation, *J Orthop Sports Phys Ther* 24:57–65, 1996.

152. Ludewig PM, Cook TM: Alterations in shoulder kinematics and associated muscle activity in people with symptoms of shoulder impingement, *Phys Ther* 80:276–291, 2000.

153. Ludewig PM, Hoff MS, Osowski EE, et al.: Relative balance of serratus anterior and upper trapezius muscle activity during push-up exercises, *Am J Sports Med* 32:484–493, 2004.

154. Ludewig PM, Phadke V, Braman JP, et al.: Motion of the shoulder complex during multiplanar humeral elevation, *J Bone Joint Surg Am* 91:378–389, 2009.

155. Ludewig PM, Reynolds JF: The association of scapular kinematics and glenohumeral joint pathologies, *J Orthop Sports Phys Ther* 39:90–104, 2009.

156. Lukasiewicz AC, McClure P, Michener L, et al.: Comparison of 3-dimensional scapular position and orientation between subjects with and without shoulder impingement, *J Orthop Sports Phys Ther* 29:574–583, 1999.

157. Lulic-Kuryllo T, Alenabi T, McDonald AC, et al.: Sub-regional activation of supraspinatus and infraspinatus muscles during activities of daily living is task dependent, *J Electromyogr Kinesiol* 54:102450, 2020.

158. Mall NA, Foley E, Chalmers PN, et al.: Degenerative joint disease of the acromioclavicular joint: a review [Review], *Am J Sports Med* 41(11):2684–2692, 2013.

159. Massimini DF, Boyer PJ, Papannagari R, et al.: In-vivo glenohumeral translation and ligament elongation during abduction and abduction with internal and external rotation, *J Orthop Surg Res* 7, 2012.

160. Matsuki K, Matsuki KO, Mu S, et al.: In vivo 3D analysis of clavicular kinematics during scapular plane abduction: comparison of dominant and non-dominant shoulders, *Gait Posture* 39(1):625–627, 2014.

161. Matsuki K, Matsuki KO, Yamaguchi S, et al.: Dynamic in vivo glenohumeral kinematics during scapular plane abduction in healthy shoulders, *J Orthop Sports Phys Ther* 42(2):96–104, 2012.

162. Matsumura N, Oki S, Fukasawa N, et al.: Glenohumeral translation during active external rotation with the shoulder abducted in cases with glenohumeral instability: a 4-dimensional computed tomography analysis, *J Shoulder Elbow Surg* 28(10):1903–1910, 2019.

163. McClure P, Balaicuis J, Heiland D, et al.: A randomized controlled comparison of stretching procedures for posterior shoulder tightness, *J Orthop Sports Phys Ther* 37:108–114, 2007.

164. McClure PW, Michener LA, Sennett B, et al.: Direct 3-dimensional measurement of scapular kinematics during dynamic movements in vivo, *J Shoulder Elbow Surg* 10:269–277, 2001.

165. McKay MJ, Baldwin JN, Ferreira P, et al.: Normative reference values for strength and flexibility of 1,000 children and adults, *Neurology* 88(1):36–43, 2017.

166. Medina G, Bartolozzi 3rd AR, Spencer JA, et al.: The thrower's shoulder, *JBJS Rev* 10(3), 2022.

167. Meehan K, Wassinger C, Roy JS, et al.: Seven key themes in physical therapy advice for patients living with subacromial shoulder pain: a scoping review, *J Orthop Sports Phys Ther* 50(6), 2020. 285-a12.

168. Michelin P, Delarue Y, Duparc F, et al.: Thickening of the inferior glenohumeral capsule: an ultrasound sign for shoulder capsular contracture, *Eur Radiol* 23(10):2802–2806, 2013.

169. Michener LA, McClure PW, Karduna AR: Anatomical and biomechanical mechanisms of subacromial impingement syndrome [Review], *Clin Biomech* 18:369–379, 2003.

170. Michener LA, Subasi Yesilyaprak SS, Seitz AL, et al.: Supraspinatus tendon and subacromial space parameters measured on ultrasonographic imaging in subacromial impingement syndrome, *Knee Surg Sports Traumatol Arthrosc* 23(2):363–369, 2015.

171. Mifune Y, Inui A, Nishimoto H, et al.: Assessment of posterior shoulder muscle stiffness related to posterior shoulder tightness in college baseball players using shear wave elastography, *J Shoulder Elbow Surg* 29(3):571–577, 2020.

172. Mihata T, McGarry MH, Akeda M, et al.: Posterior shoulder tightness can be a risk factor of scapular malposition: a cadaveric biomechanical study, *J Shoulder Elbow Surg* 29(1):175–184, 2020.

173. Mikesky AE, Edwards JE, Wigglesworth JK, et al.: Eccentric and concentric strength of the shoulder and arm musculature in collegiate baseball pitchers, *Am J Sports Med* 23:638–642, 1995.

174. Moosmayer S, Lund G, Seljom US, et al.: At a 10-year follow-up, tendon repair is superior to physiotherapy in the treatment of small and medium-sized rotator cuff tears, *J Bone Joint Surg Am* 101(12):1050–1060, 2019.

175. Morag Y, Jamadar DA, Miller B, et al.: The subscapularis: anatomy, injury, and imaging [Review], *Skelet Radiol* 40(3):255–269, 2011.

176. Morgan CD, Burkhart SS, Palmeri M, et al.: Type II SLAP lesions: three subtypes and their relationships to superior instability and rotator cuff tears, *Arthroscopy* 14(6):553–565, 1998.

177. Moseley HF: The clavicle: its anatomy and function, *Clin Orthop Relat Res* 58:17–27, 1968.

178. Kedadria A, Benabid Y, Remil O, et al.: A shoulder musculoskeletal model with three-dimensional complex muscle geometries, *Ann Biomed Eng* 51(5):1079–1093, 2023.

179. Mulla DM, Hodder JN, Maly MR, et al.: Glenohumeral stabilizing roles of the scapulohumeral muscles: implications of muscle geometry, *J Biomech* 100:109589, 2020.

180. Muraki T, Yamamoto N, Zhao KD, et al.: Effects of posterior capsule tightness on subacromial contact behavior during shoulder motions, *J Shoulder Elbow Surg* 21(9):1160–1167, 2012.

181. Murray IR, Goudie EB, Petrigliano FA, et al.: Functional anatomy and biomechanics of shoulder stability in the athlete [Review], *Clin Sports Med* 32(4):607–624, 2013.

182. Navarro-Ledesma S, Luque-Suarez A: Comparison of acromiohumeral distance in symptomatic and asymptomatic patient shoulders and those of healthy controls, *Clin Biomech* 53:101–106, 2018.

183. Neumann DA, Camargo PR: Kinesiologic considerations for targeting activation of scapulothoracic muscles - Part 1: serratus anterior, *Braz J Phys Ther* 23(6):459–466, 2019.

184. Neumann DA: The convex-concave rules of arthrokinematics: flawed or perhaps just misinterpreted? *J Orthop Sports Phys Ther* 42(2):53–55, 2012.

185. Nolte PC, Ruzbarsky JJ, Midtgaard KS, et al.: Quantitative and qualitative surgical anatomy of the acromioclavicular joint capsule and ligament: a cadaveric study, *Am J Sports Med* 49(5):1183–1191, 2021.

186. O'Brien SJ, Neves MC, Arnoczky SP, et al.: The anatomy and histology of the inferior glenohumeral ligament complex of the shoulder, *Am J Sports Med* 18:449–456, 1990.

187. O'Brien SJ, Schwartz RS, Warren RF, et al.: Capsular restraints to anterior-posterior motion of the abducted shoulder: a biomechanical study, *J Shoulder Elbow Surg* 4:298–308, 1995.

188. Oki S, Matsumura N, Iwamoto W, et al.: The function of the acromioclavicular and coracoclavicular ligaments in shoulder motion: a whole-cadaver study, *Am J Sports Med* 40(11):2617–2626, 2012.

189. Osias W, Matcuk Jr GR, Skalski MR, et al.: Scapulothoracic pathology: review of anatomy, pathophysiology, imaging findings, and an approach to management, *Skeletal Radiol* 47(2):161–171, 2018.

190. Ostermann RC, Moen TC, Siegert P, et al.: Acromioclavicular disk as a potential source of pain in AC joint injuries, *Am J Sports Med* 50(4):1039–1043, 2022.

191. Ostrander R, Escamilla RF, Hess R, et al.: Glenohumeral rotation deficits in high school, college, and professional baseball pitchers with and without a medial ulnar collateral ligament injury, *J Shoulder Elbow Surg* 28(3):423–429, 2019.

192. Oyama S, Hibberd EE, Myers JB: Changes in humeral torsion and shoulder rotation range of motion in high school baseball players over a 1-year period, *Clin Biomech* 28(3):268–272, 2013.

193. Pagnani MJ, Deng XH, Warren RF, et al.: Role of the long head of the biceps brachii in glenohumeral stability: a biomechanical study in cadaver, *J Shoulder Elbow Surg* 5:255–262, 1996.

194. Paletta Jr GA, Warner JJ, Warren RF, et al.: Shoulder kinematics with two-plane x-ray evaluation in patients with anterior instability or rotator cuff tearing, *J Shoulder Elbow Surg* 6:516–527, 1997.

195. Pallis M, Cameron KL, Svoboda SJ, et al.: Epidemiology of acromioclavicular joint injury in young athletes, *Am J Sports Med* 40(9):2072–2077, 2012.

196. Panico L, Roy T, Namdari S: Long Head of the biceps tendon ruptures: biomechanics, clinical ramifications, and management, *JBJS Rev* 9(10), 2021.

197. Paquet T, Van Den Broecke R, Casier S, et al.: Defining the shape of the scapulothoracic gliding surface, *Surg Radiol Anat* 41(11):1369–1375, 2019.

198. Paul RW, Sheridan B, Reuther KE, et al.: The contribution of posterior capsule hypertrophy to soft tissue glenohumeral internal rotation deficit in healthy pitchers, *Am J Sports Med* 50(2):341–346, 2022.

199. Phillips D, Kosek P, Karduna A: The contribution of the supraspinatus muscle at sub-maximal contractions, *J Biomech* 68:65–69, 2018.

200. Pieters L, Lewis J, Kuppens K, et al.: An update of systematic reviews examining the effectiveness of conservative physical therapy interventions for subacromial shoulder pain, *J Orthop Sports Phys Ther* 50(3):131–141, 2020.

201. Pikkarainen V, Kettunen J, Vastamaki M: The natural course of serratus palsy at 2 to 31 years, *Clin Orthop Relat Res* 471(5):1555–1563, 2013.

202. Plath JE, Aboalata M, Seppel G, et al.: Prevalence of and risk factors for dislocation arthropathy: radiological long-term outcome of arthroscopic Bankart repair in 100 shoulders at an average 13-year follow-up, *Am J Sports Med* 43(5):1084–1090, 2015.

203. Plummer HA, Plosser SM, Diaz PR, et al.: Effectiveness of a shoulder exercise program in division I collegiate baseball players during the fall season, *Int J Sports Phys Ther* 17(2):247–258, 2022.

204. Plummer HA, Sum JC, Pozzi F, et al.: Observational scapular dyskinesis: known-groups validity in patients with and without shoulder pain, *J Orthop Sports Phys Ther* 47(8):530–537, 2017.

205. Poppen NK, Walker PS: Forces at the glenohumeral joint in abduction, *Clin Orthop Relat Res*165–170, 1978.

206. Poppen NK, Walker PS: Normal and abnormal motion of the shoulder, *J Bone Joint Surg Am* 58:195–201, 1976.

207. Ranalletta M, Bongiovanni S, Suarez F, et al.: Do patients with traumatic recurrent anterior shoulder instability have generalized joint laxity? *Clin Orthop Relat Res* 470(4):957–960, 2012.

208. Reinold MM, Wilk KE, Hooks TR, et al.: Thermal-assisted capsular shrinkage of the glenohumeral joint in overhead athletes: a 15- to 47-month follow-up, *J Orthop Sports Phys Ther* 33:455–467, 2003.

209. Reis FP, de Camargo AM, Vitti M, et al.: Electromyographic study of the subclavius muscle, *Acta Anat* 105:284–290, 1979.

210. Requejo-Salinas N, Lewis J, Michener LA, et al.: International physical therapists consensus on clinical descriptors for diagnosing rotator cuff related shoulder pain: a Delphi study, *Braz J Phys Ther* 26(2):100395, 2022.

211. Rosa DP, Borstad JD, Ferreira JK, et al.: Comparison of specific and non-specific treatment approaches for individuals with posterior capsule tightness and shoulder impingement symptoms: a randomized controlled trial, *Braz J Phys Ther* 25(5):648–658, 2021.

212. Rutgers C, Verweij LPE, Priester-Vink S, et al.: Recurrence in traumatic anterior shoulder dislocations increases the prevalence of Hill-Sachs and Bankart lesions: a systematic review and meta-analysis. *Knee Surg Sports Traumatol Arthosc* 30(6):2130–2140, 2022.

213. Sabick MB, Kim YK, Torry MR, et al.: Biomechanics of the shoulder in youth baseball pitchers: implications for the development of proximal humeral epiphysiolysis and humeral retrotorsion, *Am J Sports Med* 33:1716–1722, 2005.

214. Sabick MB, Torry MR, Kim YK, et al.: Humeral torque in professional baseball pitchers, *Am J Sports Med* 32:892–898, 2004.

215. Sahara W, Sugamoto K, Murai M, et al.: Three-dimensional clavicular and acromioclavicular rotations during arm abduction using vertically open MRI, *J Orthop Res* 25:1243–1249, 2007.

216. Sahara W, Yamazaki T, Inui T, et al.: The glenohumeral micromotion and influence of the glenohumeral ligaments during axial rotation in varying abduction angle, *J Orthop Sci* 25(6):980–985, 2020.

217. Saini G, Lawrence RL, Staker JL, et al.: Supraspinatus-to-glenoid contact occurs during standardized overhead reaching motion, *Orthop J Sports Med* 9(10), 2021. 23259671211036908.

218. San Juan JG, Kosek P, Karduna AR: Humeral head translation after a suprascapular nerve block, *J Appl Biomech* 29(4):371–379, 2013.

219. Schrumpf MA, Maak TG, Delos D, et al.: The management of anterior glenohumeral instability with and without bone loss: AAOS exhibit selection, *J Bone Joint Surg Am* 96(2):e12, 2014.

220. Seitz AL, McClure PW, Lynch SS, et al.: Effects of scapular dyskinesis and scapular assistance test on subacromial space during static arm elevation, *J Shoulder Elbow Surg* 21(5):631–640, 2012.

221. Seitz AL, Michener LA: Ultrasonographic measures of subacromial space in patients with rotator cuff disease: a systematic review [Review], *J Clin Ultrasound* 39(3):146–154, 2011.

222. Sernandez H, Riehl J: Sternoclavicular joint dislocation: a systematic review and meta-analysis, *J Orthop Trauma* 33(7):e251–e255, 2019.

223. Seror P, Lenglet T, Nguyen C, et al.: Unilateral winged scapula: clinical and electrodiagnostic experience with 128 cases, with special attention to long thoracic nerve palsy, *Muscle Nerve* 57(6):913–920, 2018.

224. Sessions WC, Lawrence RL, Steubs JT, et al.: Thickness of the rotator cuff tendons at the articular margin: an anatomic cadaveric study, *Iowa Orthop J* 37:85–89, 2017.

225. Shanley E, Rauh MJ, Michener LA, et al.: Shoulder range of motion measures as risk factors for shoulder and elbow injuries in high school softball and baseball players, *Am J Sports Med* 39(9):1997–2006, 2011.

226. Shire AR, Staehr TAB, Overby JB, et al.: Specific or general exercise strategy for subacromial impingement syndrome-does it matter? a systematic literature review and meta analysis, *BMC Musculoskelet Disord* 18(1):158, 2017.

227. Shklar A, Dvir Z: Isokinetic strength measurements in shoulder muscles, *J Biomech* 10:369–373, 1995.

228. Smith DG, Swantek AJ, Gulledge CM, et al.: Relationship between glenohumeral internal rotation deficit and medial elbow torque in high school baseball pitchers, *Am J Sports Med* 47(12):2821–2826, 2019.

229. Soslowsky LJ, Flatow EL, LU B, et al.: Quantification of in situ contact areas at the glenohumeral joint: a biomechanical study, *J Orthop Res* 10:524–534, 1992.

230. Soslowsky LJ, Malicky DM, Blasier RB: Active and passive factors in inferior glenohumeral stabilization: a biomechanical model, *J Shoulder Elbow Surg* 6:371–379, 1997.

231. Spanhove V, Van Daele M, Van den Abeele A, et al.: Muscle activity and scapular kinematics in individuals with multidirectional shoulder instability: a systematic review, *Ann Phys Rehabil Med* 64(1):101457, 2021.

232. Staker JL, Braman JP, Ludewig PM: Kinematics and biomechanical validity of shoulder joint laxity tests as diagnostic criteria in multidirectional instability, *Braz J Phys Ther* 25(6):883–890, 2021.

233. Standring S: *Gray's anatomy: the anatomical basis of clinical practice*, ed 42, St Louis, 2021, Elsevier.

234. Steginik-Jansen CW, Buford Jr WL, Patterson RM, et al.: Computer simulation of pectoralis major muscle strain to guide exercise protocols for patients after breast cancer surgery, *J Orthop Sports Phys Ther* 41(6):417–426, 2011.

235. Steindler A: *Kinesiology of the human body: under normal and pathological conditions*, Springfield, Ill, 1955, Charles C Thomas.

236. Stickley CD, Hetzler RK, Freemyer BG, et al.: Isokinetic peak torque ratios and shoulder injury history in adolescent female volleyball athletes, *J Athl Train* 43(6):571–577, 2008.

237. Stokdijk M, Eilers PH, Nagels J, et al.: External rotation in the glenohumeral joint during elevation of the arm, *Clin Biomech* 18:296–302, 2003.

238. Struyf F, Cagnie B, Cools A, et al.: Scapulothoracic muscle activity and recruitment timing in patients with shoulder impingement symptoms and glenohumeral instability [Review], *J Electromyogr Kinesiol* 24(2):277–284, 2014.

239. Struyf F, Nijs J, Baeyens JP, et al.: Scapular positioning and movement in unimpaired shoulders, shoulder impingement syndrome, and glenohumeral instability [Review], *Scand J Med Sci Sports* 21(3):352–358, 2011.

240. Sugamoto K, Harada T, Machida A, et al.: Scapulohumeral rhythm: relationship between motion velocity and rhythm, *Clin Orthop Relat Res* 401:119–124, 2002.

241. Svendsen SW, Gelineck J, Mathiassen SE, et al.: Work above shoulder level and degenerative alterations of the rotator cuff tendons: a magnetic resonance imaging study, *Arthritis Rheum* 50:3314–3322, 2004.

242. Szucs KA, Borstad JD: Gender differences between muscle activation and onset timing of the four subdivisions of trapezius during humerothoracic elevation, *Hum Mov Sci* 32(6):1288–1298, 2013.

243. Takenaga T, Goto H, Tsuchiya A, et al.: Relationship between bilateral humeral retroversion angle and starting baseball age in skeletally mature baseball players-existence of watershed age, *J Shoulder Elbow Surg* 28(5):847–853, 2019.

244. Tamaoki MJ, Belloti JC, Lenza M, et al.: Surgical versus conservative interventions for treating acromioclavicular dislocation of the shoulder in adults, *Cochrane Database Syst Rev* 8:CD007429, 2010.

245. Tanaka K, Funasaki H, Murayama Y, et al.: Age-related differences in glenohumeral internal rotation deficit, humeral retrotorsion angle, and posterior shoulder tightness in baseball players, *J Shoulder Elbow Surg* 31(6):1184–1192, 2022.

246. Teece RM, Lunden JB, Lloyd AS, et al.: Three-dimensional acromioclavicular joint motions during elevation of the arm, *J Orthop Sports Phys Ther* 38:181–190, 2008.

247. Terrier A, Reist A, Vogel A, et al.: Effect of supraspinatus deficiency on humerus translation and glenohumeral contact force during abduction, *Clin Biomech* 22:645–651, 2007.

248. Teyhen DS, Christ TR, Ballas ER, et al.: Digital fluoroscopic video assessment of glenohumeral migration: static vs. dynamic conditions, *J Biomech* 43(7):1380–1385, 2010.

249. Thomas SJ, Swanik CB, Kaminski TW, et al.: Humeral retroversion and its association with posterior capsule thickness in collegiate baseball players, *J Shoulder Elbow Surg* 21(7):910–916, 2012.

250. Tran J, Switzer-McIntyre S, Agur AMR: Overview of innervation of shoulder and acromioclavicular joints, *Phys Med Rehabil Clin N Am* 32(4):667–674, 2021.

251. Urayama M, Itoi E, Sashi R, et al.: Capsular elongation in shoulders with recurrent anterior dislocation. Quantitative assessment with magnetic resonance arthrography, *Am J Sports Med* 31:64–67, 2003.

252. van der Helm FC, Pronk GM: Three-dimensional recording and description of motions of the shoulder mechanism, *J Biomech Eng* 117:27–40, 1995.

253. van Tongel A, MacDonald P, Leiter J, et al.: A cadaveric study of the structural anatomy of the sternoclavicular joint, *Clin Anat* 25(7):903–910, 2012.

254. Vangsness Jr CT, Jorgenson SS, Watson T, et al.: The origin of the long head of the biceps from the scapula and glenoid labrum. An anatomical study of 100 shoulders, *J Bone Joint Surg Br* 76:951–954, 1994.

255. Veeger HE, van der Helm FC: Shoulder function: the perfect compromise between mobility and stability, *J Biomech* 40:2119–2129, 2007.

256. Walker M, Brooks J, Willis M, et al.: How reverse shoulder arthroplasty works [Review], *Clin Orthop Relat Res* 469(9):2440–2451, 2011.

257. Warby SA, Ford JJ, Hahne AJ, et al.: Comparison of 2 exercise rehabilitation programs for multidirectional instability of the glenohumeral joint: a randomized controlled trial, *Am J Sports Med* 46(1):87–97, 2018.

258. Warner JJ, Deng XH, Warren RF, et al.: Static capsuloligamentous restraints to superior-inferior translation of the glenohumeral joint, *Am J Sports Med* 20:675–685, 1992.

259. Warth RJ, Spiegl UJ, Millett PJ: Scapulothoracic bursitis and snapping scapula syndrome: a critical review of current evidence, *Am J Sports Med* 43(1):236–245, 2015.

260. Wassinger CA, Sole G, Osborne H: Clinical measurement of scapular upward rotation in response to acute subacromial pain, *J Orthop Sports Phys Ther* 43(4):199–203, 2013.

261. Wattanaprakornkul D, Cathers I, Halaki M, et al.: The rotator cuff muscles have a direction specific recruitment pattern during shoulder flexion and extension exercises, *J Sci Med Sport* 14(5):376–382, 2011.

262. Wermers J, Schliemann B, Raschke MJ, et al.: The glenolabral articular disruption lesion is a biomechanical risk factor for recurrent shoulder instability, *Arthrosc Sports Med Rehabil* 3(6):e1803–e1810, 2021.

263. Werner AW, Lichtenberg S, Schmitz H, et al.: Arthroscopic findings in atraumatic shoulder instability, *Arthroscopy* 20:268–272, 2004.

264. Werner CM, Weishaupt D, Blumenthal S, et al.: Effect of experimental suprascapular nerve block on active glenohumeral translations in vivo, *J Orthop Res* 24:491–500, 2006.

265. Whiteley RJ, Ginn KA, Nicholson LL, et al.: Sports participation and humeral torsion, *J Orthop Sports Phys Ther* 39:256–263, 2009.

266. Wilk KE, Macrina LC, Arrigo C: Passive range of motion characteristics in the overhead baseball pitcher and their implications for rehabilitation, *Clin Orthop Relat Res* 470(6):1586–1594, 2012.

267. Wilk KE, Macrina LC, Fleisig GS, et al.: Deficits in glenohumeral passive range of motion increase risk of elbow injury in professional baseball pitchers: a prospective study, *Am J Sports Med* 42(9):2075–2081, 2014.

268. Wilk KE, Macrina LC: Nonoperative and postoperative rehabilitation for glenohumeral instability, *Clin Sports Med* 32(4):865–914, 2013.

269. Williamson PM, Hanna P, Momenzadeh K, et al.: Effect of rotator cuff muscle activation on glenohumeral kinematics: a cadaveric study, *J Biomech* 105:109798, 2020.

270. Wilson WR, Magnussen RA, Irribarra LA, et al.: Variability of the capsular anatomy in the rotator interval region of the shoulder, *J Shoulder Elbow Surg* 22(6):856–861, 2013.

271. Yamaguchi K, Ditsios K, Middleton WD, et al.: The demographic and morphological features of rotator cuff disease. A comparison of asymptomatic and symptomatic shoulders, *J Bone Joint Surg Am* 88:1699–1704, 2006.

272. Yamamoto N, Itoi E, Minagawa H, et al.: Why is the humeral retroversion of throwing athletes greater in dominant shoulders than in nondominant shoulders? *J Shoulder Elbow Surg* 15(5):571–575, 2006.

273. Yanagawa T, Goodwin CJ, Shelburne KB, et al.: Contributions of the individual muscles of the shoulder to glenohumeral joint stability during abduction, *J Biomech Eng* 130:210241–210249, 2008.

274. Yanai T, Fuss FK, Fukunaga T: In vivo measurements of subacromial impingement: substantial compression develops in abduction with large internal rotation, *Clin Biomech* 21:692–700, 2006.

275. Yang C, Goto A, Sahara W, et al.: In vivo three-dimensional evaluation of the functional length of glenohumeral ligaments, *Clin Biomech* 25(2):137–141, 2010.

276. Zdravkovic V, Alexander N, Wegener R, et al.: How do scapulothoracic kinematics during shoulder elevation differ between adults with and without rotator cuff arthropathy? *Clin Orthop Relat Res* 478(11):2640–2649, 2020.

STUDY QUESTIONS

1. How does the morphology (shape) of the sternoclavicular joint influence its arthrokinematics during elevation and depression, and during protraction and retraction?
2. Which periarticular connective tissues and muscles associated with the sternoclavicular joint become taut following full depression of the clavicle?
3. Describe how the osteokinematics at the sternoclavicular and acromioclavicular joints can combine to augment protraction of the scapulothoracic joint. Include axes of rotation and planes of motion in your answer.
4. Contrast the arthrokinematics at the glenohumeral joint during internal rotation from (A) the anatomic position and (B) a position of 90 degrees of abduction.
5. Injury to which spinal nerve roots would most likely severely weaken the movement of protraction of the scapulothoracic joint? Hɪɴᴛ: Refer to Appendix II, Part B.
6. With the arm well stabilized, describe the likely posture of the scapula following full activation of the teres major without activation of the rhomboid muscles.
7. Fig. 5.58 shows several internal rotator muscles of the glenohumeral joint. What role would these muscles have in directing the posterior slide of the humerus?
8. List all the muscles of the shoulder complex that are likely contracting during active shoulder abduction from the anatomic position. Consulting Appendix II, Part B, which pair of spinal nerve roots is most likely associated with the innervation of these active muscles?
9. With the aid of a skeletal model, image, or drawing, list muscles of the shoulder that, if either tight or weak, could favor an anteriorly tilted posture of the scapula.
10. In theory, how much active shoulder abduction is possible with a completely fused glenohumeral joint?
11. What motion simultaneously increases tension in all parts of the inferior glenohumeral ligament?
12. Describe the exact path of the long head of the biceps, from its distal to its proximal attachment. Where is the tendon vulnerable to entrapment and associated inflammation?
13. What active motion or motions are essentially impossible following an avulsion injury of the upper trunk of the brachial plexus?
14. How does the posture of the scapulothoracic joint affect the static stability of the glenohumeral joint?
15. Which movement combinations of the scapula would most likely reduce the volume within the subacromial space?
16. As described in this chapter, humeral retroversion is about 65 degrees at birth. How much retroversion is normally expected by the time a young person reaches his or her late teens?
17. Based on the line of force relative to the medial-lateral axis of rotation at the glenohumeral (GH) joint, compare the sagittal plane actions of the sternocostal fibers of the pectoralis major from the three starting positions: (A) near neutral anatomic position, (B) 30 degrees of extension beyond neutral position, and (C) 120 degrees of flexion.
18. Starting from the anatomic position, compare the likely relative tension (stretch) generated within the posterior capsule of the glenohumeral joint during (A) active and (B) passive external rotation of the shoulder.
19. Assume a teenager with cerebral palsy has trunk instability and significant thoracic kyphosis while sitting. Furthermore, while at rest, this "slumped" sitting posture is associated with a bilateral scapular posturing of 30 degrees of downward rotation, with significant anterior tilting and internal rotation. Cite kinesiologic factors associated with this overall posturing that may explain her inability to achieve enough active shoulder abduction to reach an elevated shelf in her closet.

Answers to the study questions can be found in the accompanying enhanced eBook version included with the print purchase of this textbook.

Additional Video Educational Content

- Fluoroscopic Observations of Selected Arthrokinematics of the Upper Extremity
- Fluoroscopic Comparison of the Arthrokinematics of Normal Shoulder versus Three Cases of Moderate to Severe Subacromial Impingement
- Isolated Paralysis of Right Trapezius Muscle: The physiotherapist performs a classic muscle test for each of the three parts of the trapezius muscle

- Isolated Paralysis of Right Trapezius Muscle: Reduced scapular retraction due to paralysis of middle trapezius

CLINICAL KINESIOLOGY APPLIED TO PERSONS WITH QUADRIPLEGIA (TETRAPLEGIA)
- Analysis of Coming to a Sitting Position (from the supine position) in a Person with C^6 Quadriplegia
- Analysis of Transferring from a Wheelchair to a Mat in a Person with C^6 Quadriplegia

- Analysis of Rolling (from the supine position) in a Person with C^6 Quadriplegia
- Functional Considerations of the Serratus Anterior Muscle in a Person with C^7 Quadriplegia
- Mechanics of a "Winging" Scapula in a Person with C^6 Quadriplegia
- Performance of a Sitting Push-Up by a Person with C^7 Quadriplegia

ALL VIDEOS in this chapter are available in the accompanying enhanced eBook version included with the print purchase of this textbook.

Elbow and Forearm

DONALD A. NEUMANN, PT, PhD, FAPTA

The elbow and forearm complex consists of three bones and four joints (Fig. 6.1). The *humero-ulnar* and *humeroradial joints* form the elbow. The motions of flexion and extension of the elbow provide a means to adjust the overall functional length of the upper limb. This mechanism is used for many important activities, such as feeding, reaching, throwing, and personal hygiene.

The radius and ulna articulate with each other within the forearm at the *proximal* and *distal radio-ulnar joints.* This pair of articulations allows the palm of the hand to be turned up (supinated) or down (pronated) without requiring motion of the shoulder. Supination and pronation can be performed in conjunction with, or independent from, elbow flexion and extension. The interaction between the elbow and forearm joints adds significantly to the versatility of

hand placement, thereby enhancing the overall function of the upper limb.

OSTEOLOGY

Mid-to-Distal Humerus

The anterior and posterior surfaces of the mid-to-distal humerus provide proximal attachments for the brachialis and the medial head of the triceps brachii (Figs. 6.2 and 6.3, respectively). The distal end of the shaft of the humerus terminates medially as the trochlea and the medial epicondyle, and laterally as the capitulum and lateral epicondyle. The *trochlea* resembles a rounded, empty spool of thread. The medial and lateral borders of the trochlea flare slightly to form *medial and lateral lips.* The medial lip is prominent and projects farther distally than the adjacent lateral lip. Midway between the medial and lateral lips is the *trochlear groove,* which, when one looks from posterior to anterior, spirals slightly toward the medial direction (Fig. 6.4). The *coronoid fossa* is located just proximal to the anterior aspect of the trochlea (see Fig. 6.2).

Four Articulations Within the Elbow and Forearm Complex

1. Humero-ulnar joint
2. Humeroradial joint
3. Proximal radio-ulnar joint
4. Distal radio-ulnar joint

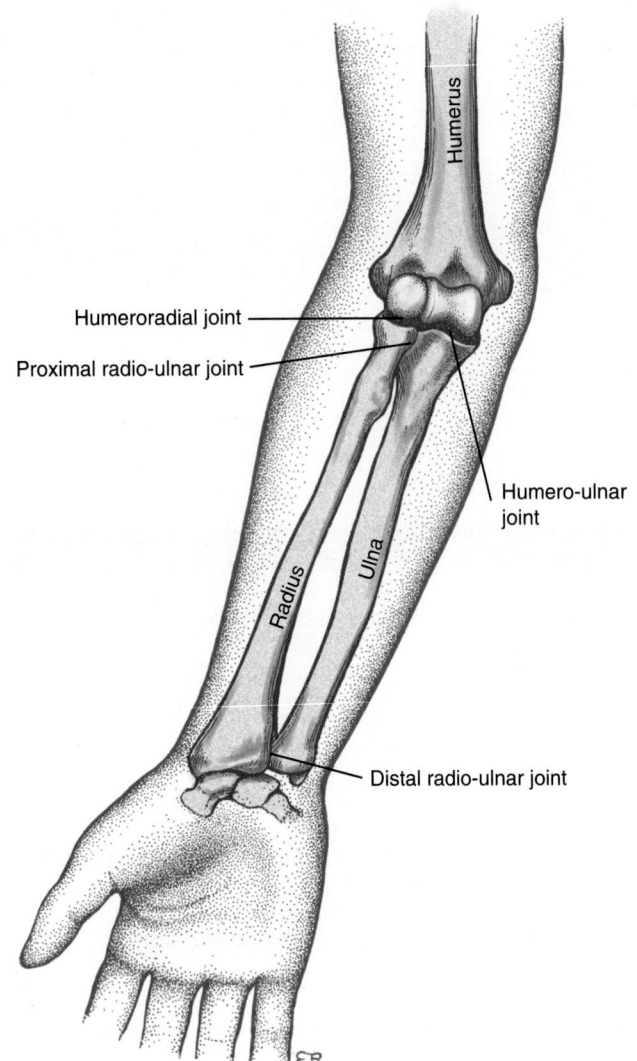

FIGURE 6.1 The articulations of the elbow and forearm complex.

Osteologic Features of the Mid-to-Distal Humerus

- Trochlea including groove and medial and lateral lips
- Coronoid fossa
- Capitulum
- Radial fossa
- Medial and lateral epicondyles
- Medial and lateral supracondylar ridges
- Olecranon fossa

Directly lateral to the trochlea is the rounded *capitulum.* The capitulum forms nearly one half of a sphere. A small *radial fossa* is located proximal to the anterior surface of the capitulum.

The *medial epicondyle* of the humerus projects medially from the trochlea (see Figs. 6.2 and 6.4). This prominent and easily palpable structure serves as the proximal attachment for the medial collateral ligament of the elbow as well as most forearm pronator and wrist flexor muscles.

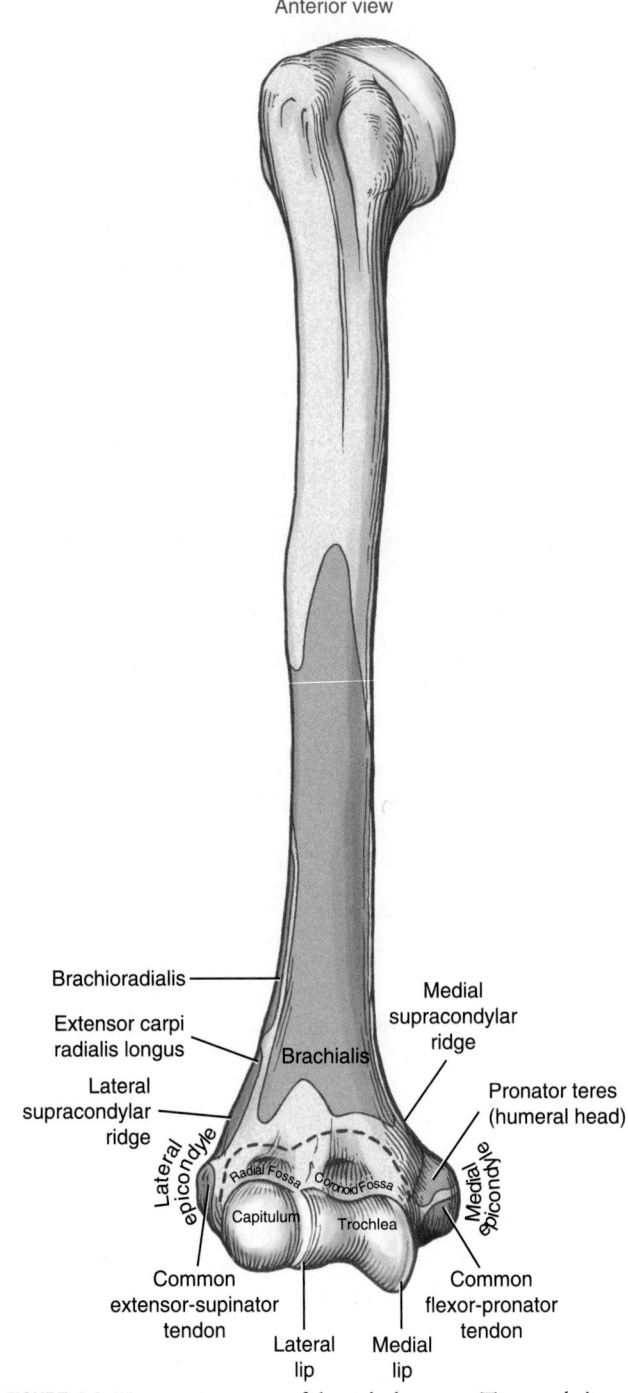

FIGURE 6.2 The anterior aspect of the right humerus. The muscles' proximal attachments are shown in red. The dashed lines show the capsular attachments of the elbow joint.

The *lateral epicondyle* of the humerus, less prominent than the medial epicondyle, serves as the proximal attachment for the lateral collateral ligament complex of the elbow as well as most forearm supinator and wrist extensor muscles. Immediately proximal to both epicondyles are the *medial* and *lateral supracondylar ridges,* which are relatively superficial and easily palpated.

On the posterior aspect of the humerus, just proximal to the trochlea, is the deep and broad *olecranon fossa.* Only a thin sheet of

Posterior view

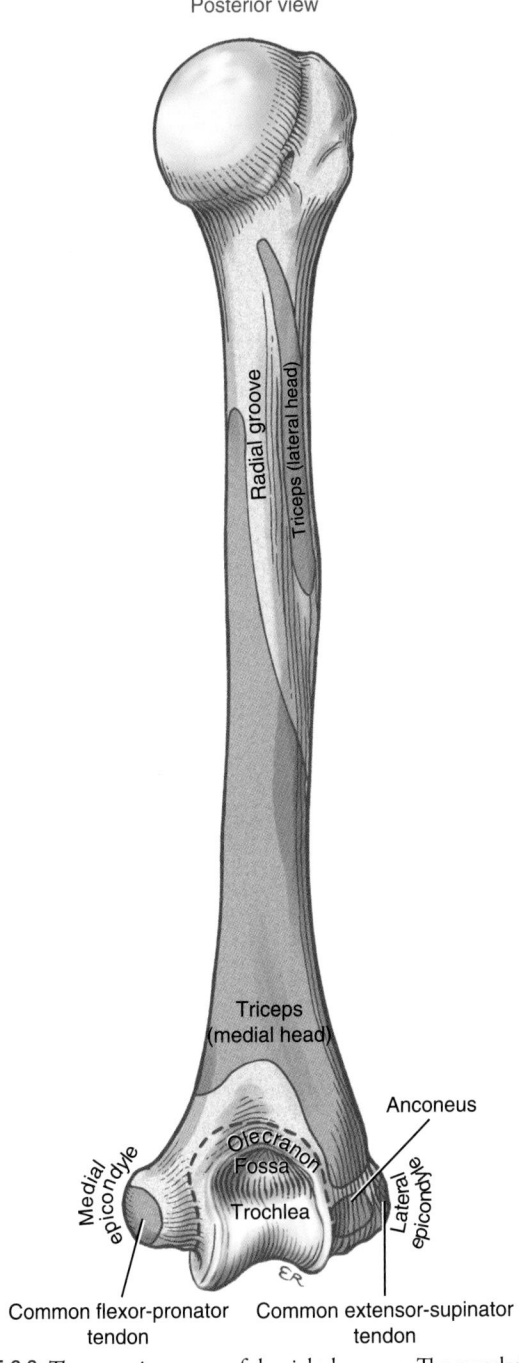

FIGURE 6.3 The posterior aspect of the right humerus. The muscles' proximal attachments are shown in red. The dashed lines show the capsular attachments around the elbow joint.

bone or membrane separates the olecranon fossa from the coronoid fossa.

Ulna

The ulna has a thick proximal end with distinct processes (Figs. 6.5 and 6.6). The *olecranon process* forms the large, blunt, proximal tip of the ulna, making up the "point" of the elbow (Fig. 6.7). The roughened posterior surface of the olecranon process accepts the

Right humerus: Inferior view

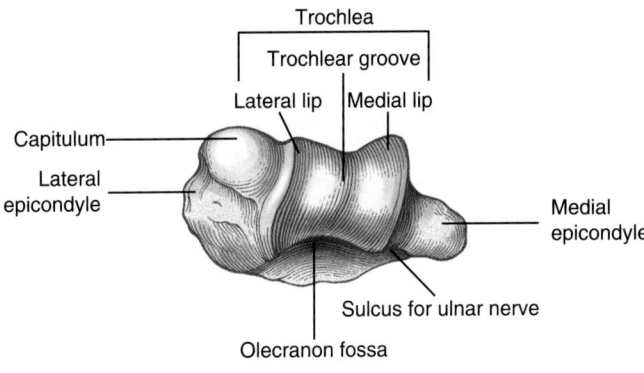

FIGURE 6.4 The distal end of the right humerus, inferior view.

insertion of the triceps brachii. The *coronoid process* projects sharply from the anterior body of the proximal ulna.

Osteologic Features of the Ulna

- Olecranon process
- Coronoid process
- Trochlear notch and longitudinal crest
- Radial notch
- Supinator crest
- Tuberosity of the ulna
- Ulnar head
- Styloid process
- Fovea

The *trochlear notch* of the ulna is the large jawlike process located between the anterior tips of the olecranon and coronoid processes. This concave notch articulates firmly with the reciprocally shaped trochlea of the humerus, forming the humero-ulnar joint. A thin raised *longitudinal crest* divides the trochlear notch down its midline.

The *radial notch* of the ulna is an articular depression just lateral to the inferior aspect of the trochlear notch (see Figs. 6.5 and 6.7). Extending distally and slightly dorsally from the radial notch is the *supinator crest*, marking the attachments for part of the lateral collateral ligament complex and the supinator muscle. The *tuberosity of the ulna* is a roughened impression just distal to the coronoid process, formed by the attachment of the brachialis muscle (see Fig. 6.5).

The *ulnar head* is located at the distal end of the ulna (Fig. 6.8). About three-quarters of the rounded ulnar head are covered with articular cartilage. The pointed *styloid process* (from the Greek root *stylos,* pillar) projects distally from the posterior-medial region of the extreme distal ulna. A small depression, known as the *fovea,* is located at the base of the styloid process. The fovea is normally filled by attachments of an articular disc and other ligaments.

Radius

In the fully supinated position, the radius lies approximately parallel and lateral to the ulna (see Figs. 6.5 and 6.6). The proximal end of the radius is small and therefore constitutes a relatively small structural component of the elbow. Its distal end, however, is enlarged, forming a major part of the wrist joint.

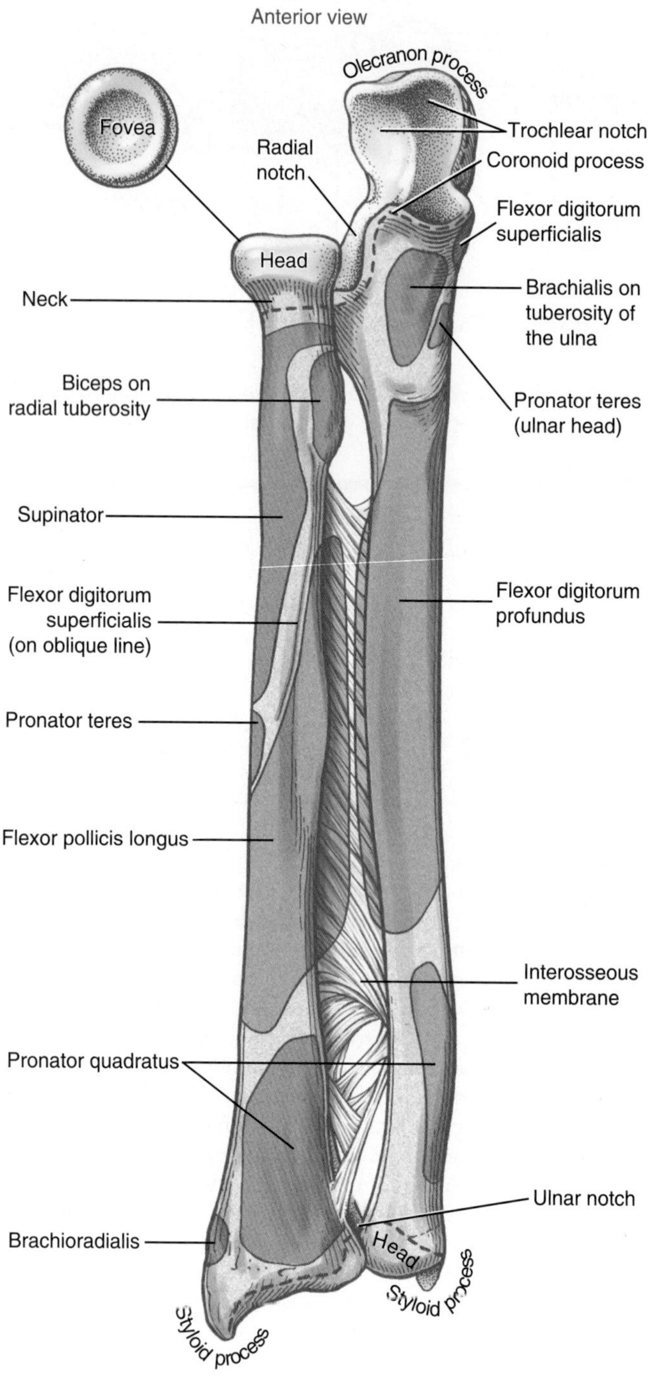

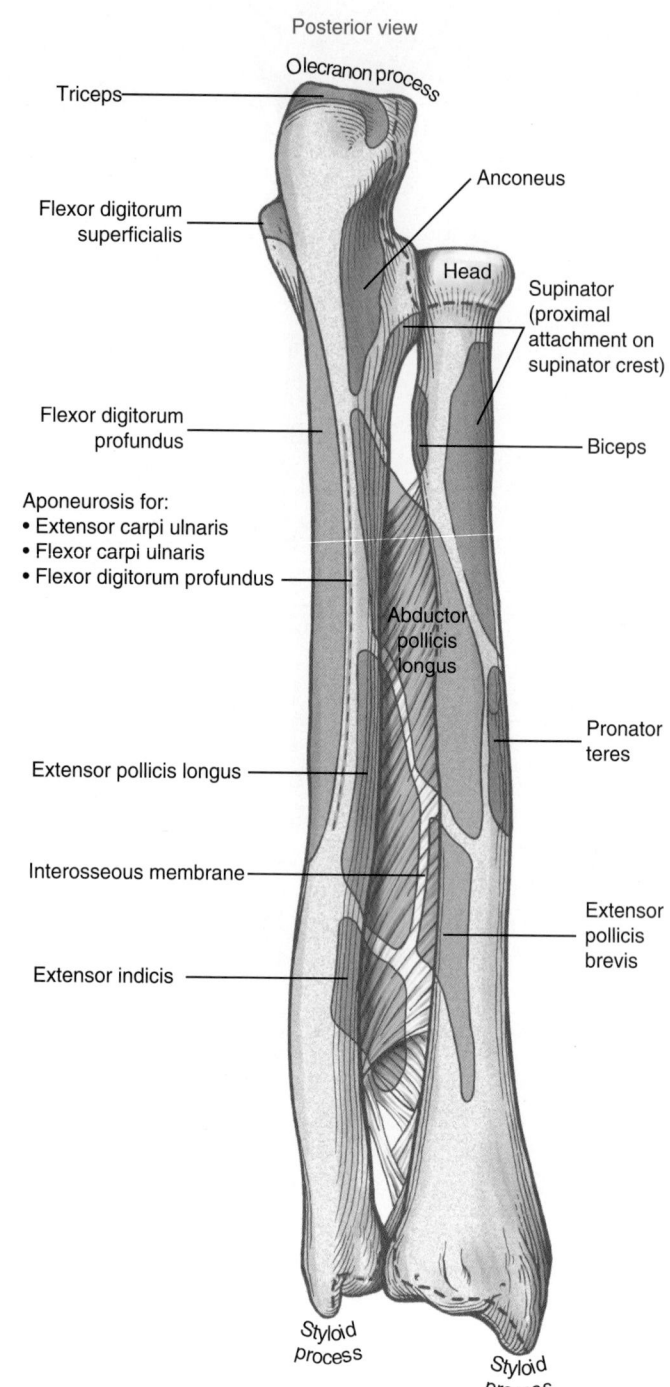

Anterior view

Fovea

Radial notch

Olecranon process

Trochlear notch

Coronoid process

Flexor digitorum superficialis

Brachialis on tuberosity of the ulna

Pronator teres (ulnar head)

Head

Neck

Biceps on radial tuberosity

Supinator

Flexor digitorum superficialis (on oblique line)

Pronator teres

Flexor pollicis longus

Flexor digitorum profundus

Pronator quadratus

Brachioradialis

Interosseous membrane

Ulnar notch

Head

Styloid process

Styloid process

FIGURE 6.5 The anterior aspect of the right radius and ulna. The muscles' proximal attachments are shown in red and distal attachments in gray. The dashed lines show the capsular attachments around the elbow and wrist and the proximal and distal radio-ulnar joints. The radial head is depicted from above to show the concavity of the fovea.

Posterior view

Triceps

Olecranon process

Anconeus

Flexor digitorum superficialis

Head

Supinator (proximal attachment on supinator crest)

Flexor digitorum profundus

Biceps

Aponeurosis for:
• Extensor carpi ulnaris
• Flexor carpi ulnaris
• Flexor digitorum profundus

Abductor pollicis longus

Pronator teres

Extensor pollicis longus

Interosseous membrane

Extensor indicis

Extensor pollicis brevis

Styloid process

Styloid process

FIGURE 6.6 The posterior aspect of the right radius and ulna. The muscles' proximal attachments are shown in red and distal attachments in gray. The dashed lines show the capsular attachments around the elbow and wrist and the proximal and distal radio-ulnar joints.

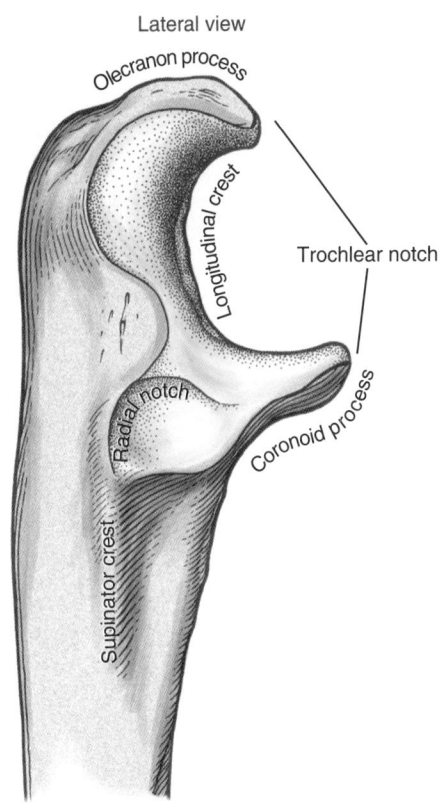

FIGURE 6.7 A lateral (radial) view of the right proximal ulna, with the radius removed. Note the jawlike shape of the trochlear notch.

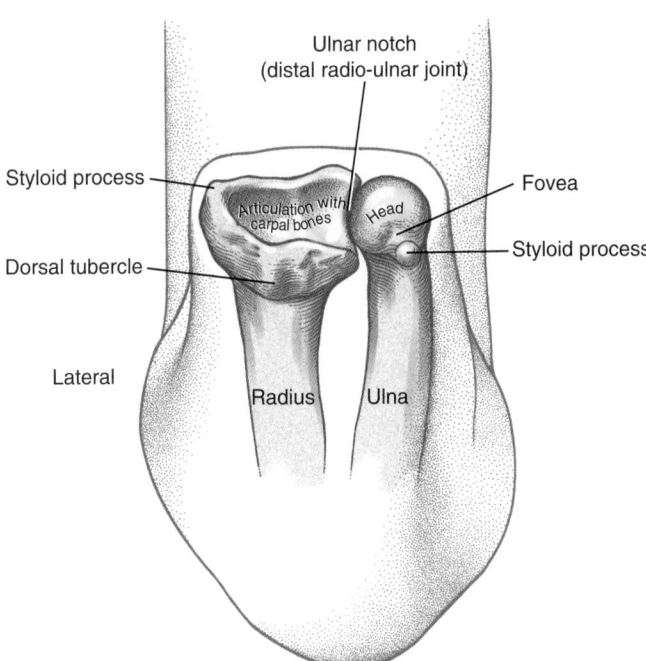

FIGURE 6.8 The distal end of the right radius and ulna with carpal bones removed. The forearm is in full supination. Note the prominent ulnar head and nearby styloid process of the ulna.

The *radial head* is a disclike structure located at the extreme proximal end of the radius. The rim of the radial head that articulates with the radial notch of the ulna is lined with a thin layer of articular cartilage, forming the proximal radio-ulnar joint. Immediately inferior to the radial head is the constricted *radial neck* (see Fig. 6.5).

The superior surface of the radial head consists of a shallow, cup-shaped depression known as the *fovea*. This cartilage-lined concavity articulates with the capitulum of the humerus, forming the humeroradial joint. The biceps brachii muscle attaches to the radius at the *radial (bicipital) tuberosity,* a roughened region located at the anterior-medial edge of the proximal radius.

Osteologic Features of the Radius
- Head
- Neck
- Fovea
- Radial (bicipital) tuberosity
- Ulnar notch
- Styloid process

The distal end of the radius articulates with carpal bones to form the radiocarpal joint at the wrist (see Fig. 6.8). The *ulnar notch* of the distal radius accepts the ulnar head at the distal radio-ulnar

joint. The prominent *styloid process* projects from the lateral surface of the distal radius, projecting farther distal than the ulnar styloid process.

ARTHROLOGY

Joints of the Elbow

GENERAL FEATURES OF THE HUMERO-ULNAR AND HUMERORADIAL JOINTS

The elbow consists of the humero-ulnar and humeroradial articulations (see Fig. 6.1). Although both joints contribute to the kinematics of flexion and extension, each has a different role in maintaining the overall three-dimensional stability of the elbow. The humero-ulnar joint provides much of its stability through the tight fit between the trochlea and trochlear notch. The less congruous humeroradial joint, in contrast, provides elbow stability through a buttressing of the radial head against the capitulum, in conjunction with its many capsuloligamentous connections.

Early anatomists classified the elbow as a *ginglymus* or *hinged joint* owing to its predominant uniplanar motion of flexion and extension. The term *modified hinge joint* is more appropriate because the ulna experiences a slight amount of axial rotation (i.e., rotation around its own longitudinal axis) and side-to-side motion as it flexes and extends.[91] Bioengineers must account for these relatively small "extra-sagittal" accessory motions to help improve the design of elbow joint prostheses. Premature loosening of an elbow prosthesis remains a leading surgical complication, especially in high demand patients.[35]

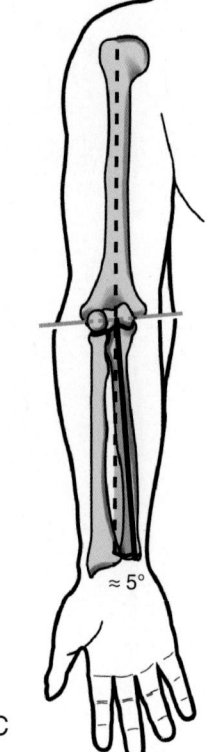

FIGURE 6.9 (A) The elbow's axis of rotation is shown extending slightly obliquely in a medial-lateral direction through the capitulum and the trochlea. An elbow with *normal cubitus valgus* is shown with an angle of about 15 degrees from the longitudinal axis of the humerus. (B) An example of *excessive cubitus valgus* deformity is shown with the forearm deviated laterally about 30 degrees. (C) An example of *cubitus varus* deformity is depicted with the forearm deviated medially about 5 degrees.

≈ 15°   ≈ 30°   ≈ 5°

A   B   C

Normal cubitus valgus   Excessive cubitus valgus   Cubitus varus

Normal "Valgus Angle" of the Elbow

Elbow flexion and extension occur around a near medial-lateral axis of rotation, passing through the vicinity of the lateral epicondyle, and ultimately through the convex members of the articulation (Fig. 6.9A). From medial to lateral, the axis courses slightly superiorly owing in part to the distal prolongation of the medial lip of the trochlea. This asymmetry in the trochlea causes the ulna to deviate laterally relative to the humerus. The natural frontal plane angle made by the extended elbow is referred to as *normal cubitus valgus*. (The term "carrying angle" is often used, reflecting the fact that the valgus angle tends to keep carried objects away from the side of the thigh during walking.) Paraskevas and co-workers reported an average cubitus valgus angle in healthy men and women of about 13 degrees, with a standard deviation close to 6 degrees.[82] Data on a healthy pediatric population revealed that the carrying angle naturally increases with age,[43] a point that may be relevant when evaluating bony alignment of the upper limb in children across a range of ages.

Occasionally the extended elbow may exhibit an *excessive cubitus valgus* that exceeds about 20 or 25 degrees (see Fig. 6.9B). In contrast, the forearm may less commonly show a *cubitus varus* (or "gunstock") deformity, where the forearm deviates toward the midline (see Fig. 6.9C). The terms *valgus* and *varus* are derived from the Latin *turned outward* (abducted) and *turned inward* (adducted), respectively.

A marked varus or valgus deformity may result from trauma, such as a severe fracture through the "growth plate" of the distal humerus in children. Excessive cubitus valgus may overstretch and damage the ulnar nerve as it crosses medial to the elbow.[25]

PERIARTICULAR CONNECTIVE TISSUE

The *articular capsule* of the elbow encloses the humero-ulnar joint, the humeroradial joint, and the proximal radio-ulnar joint (Fig. 6.10). The articular capsule surrounding these joints is thin and reinforced anteriorly by oblique and vertical bands of fibrous tissue. A *synovial membrane* lines the internal surface of the capsule (Fig. 6.11).

The articular capsule of the elbow is strengthened by collateral ligaments. These ligaments provide an important source of multiplanar stability to the elbow, most notably however within the frontal plane. Motions that increase tension in the ligaments are listed in Table 6.1. The *medial collateral ligament* (MCL) consists of anterior, posterior, and transverse fiber bundles (Fig. 6.12). The *anterior fibers* are the strongest and stiffest, providing the most significant resistance against a valgus (abduction) producing force to the elbow.[89] The anterior fibers arise from the anterior part of the medial epicondyle and insert on the medial part of the coronoid process of the ulna.[34] Careful dissection has identified nine separate components within the anterior set of fibers.[65] Because these fiber components span *both* sides of the axis of rotation, at least some are taut throughout the full range of motion: specifically, the anterior components are taut in extension, while the posterior components are taut in flexion.[52] When considered as a group, therefore, the

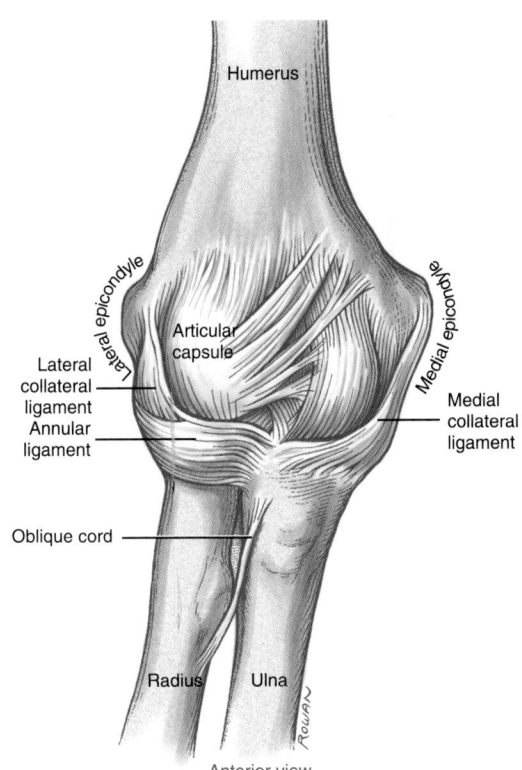

FIGURE 6.10 An anterior view of the right elbow showing the capsule and collateral ligaments.

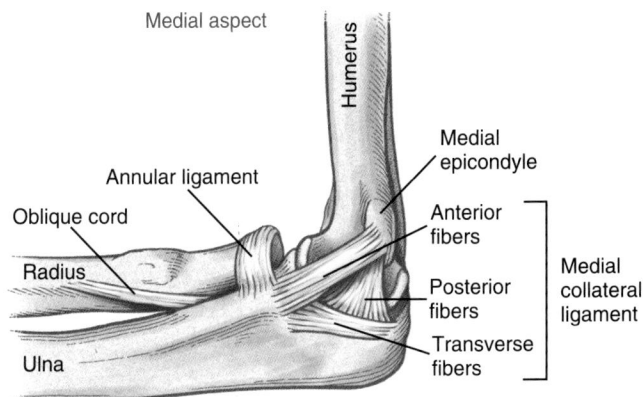

FIGURE 6.12 The fibers of the medial collateral ligament of the right elbow.

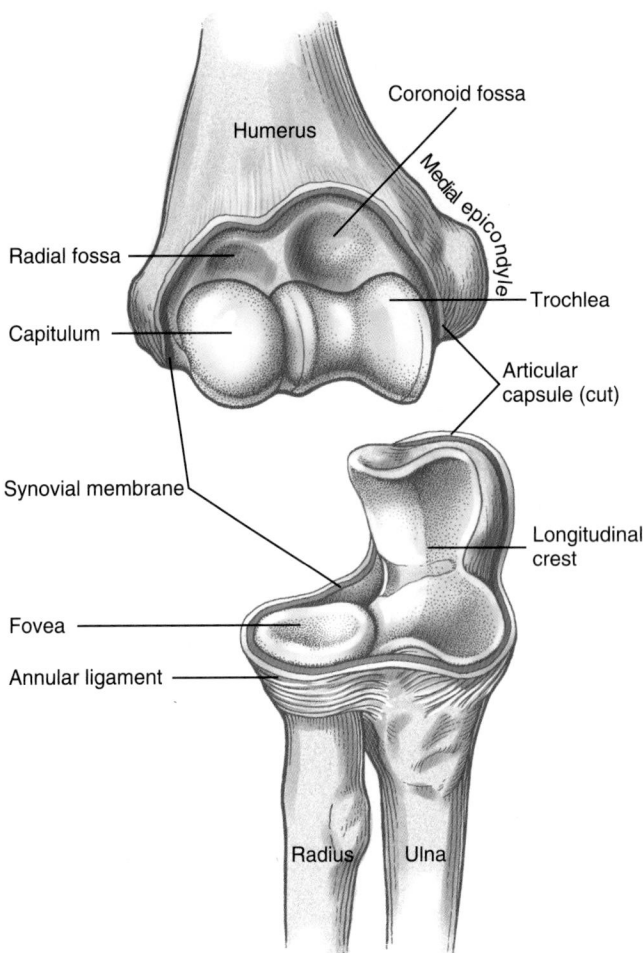

FIGURE 6.11 Anterior view of the right elbow disarticulated to expose the humero-ulnar and humeroradial joints. The margin of the proximal radio-ulnar joint is shown within the elbow's capsule. Note the small area on the trochlear notch lacking articular cartilage. The synovial membrane lining the internal side of the capsule is shown in blue.

anterior fibers of the MCL provide a global articular stability throughout the entire sagittal plane movement.

The *posterior fibers* of the MCL are less defined than the anterior fibers and are essentially fanlike thickenings of the posterior-medial capsule. As depicted in Fig. 6.12, the posterior fibers attach on the posterior part of the medial epicondyle and insert on the medial margin of the olecranon process. The posterior fibers resist a valgus-producing force, as well as become taut in the extremes of elbow flexion.[21,89] A third and poorly developed set of *transverse fibers* cross from the olecranon to the coronoid process of the ulna. Because these fibers originate and insert on the same bone, they provide only limited articular stability.

TABLE 6.1	**Primary Motions That Increase Tension in the Collateral Ligaments of the Elbow**
Ligament	**Motions That Increase Tension**
Medial collateral ligament (anterior fibers*)	Valgus
	Extension (anterior components) and flexion (posterior components)
Medial collateral ligament (posterior fibers)	Valgus
	Flexion
Radial collateral ligament	Varus
Lateral (ulnar) collateral ligament*	Varus
	External rotation of the proximal forearm relative to the humerus
	Flexion
Annular ligament	Distraction of the radius

*Primary valgus or varus stabilizers.

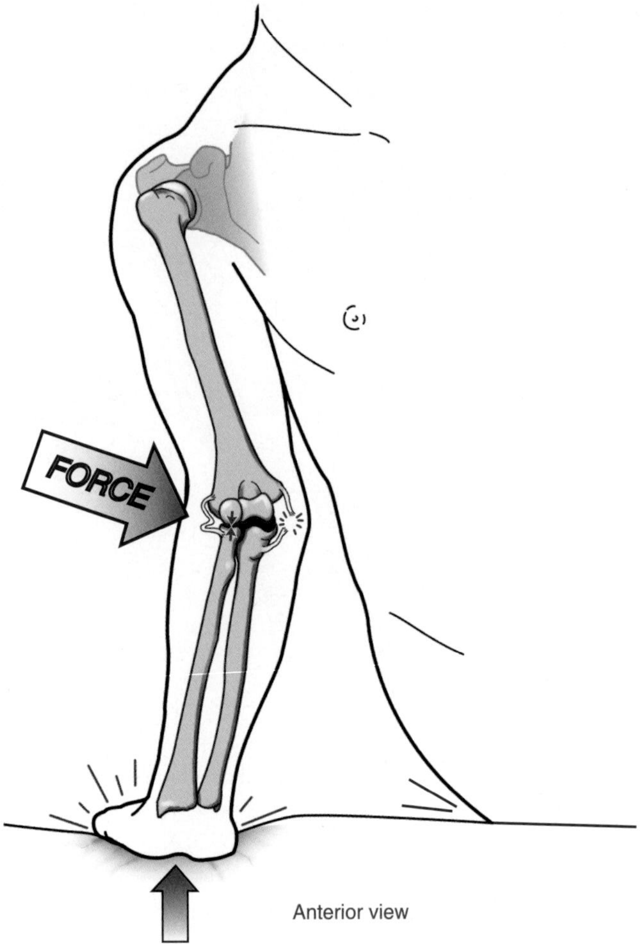

FIGURE 6.13 Attempts at catching oneself from a fall may create a severe valgus-producing force to the elbow, causing rupture of the medial collateral ligament and a potentially damaging compression force across the humeroradial joint, potentially fracturing the radial head.

Anterior view

In addition to the medial collateral ligaments, medially originating muscles including the flexor digitorum superficialis and the pronator-wrist flexor group can resist a significant component of a valgus-producing strain at the elbow.[20] For this reason, these muscles can be considered *dynamic medial stabilizers*, helping to partially unload and therefore protect the medial collateral ligament.

The MCL is susceptible to injury when the elbow is violently forced into excessive valgus, often from a fall onto an outstretched upper extremity (Fig. 6.13). The ligamentous injury may be associated with a compression fracture within the humeroradial joint or anywhere along the length of the radius—the forearm bone that accepts most of the compression force applied through the wrist. A severe valgus-producing force may also injure the ulnar nerve or muscles attaching to the medial epicondyle. Furthermore, this injury may be associated with excessive hyperextension of the elbow, injuring the anterior capsule.

The MCL is also susceptible to injury from non–weight-bearing, repetitive, and strenuous valgus-producing strains placed on the elbow. This injury is particularly common in all levels of baseball play, most notably in professional level pitchers.[38,108] Pain and valgus instability are typically evident during the late cocking and acceleration phase of throwing, when the valgus-producing torques at the elbow are at their greatest.[7,22] If ligamentous injury is significant, surgical reconstruction may be indicated, which typically involves repairing the anterior fibers by using an autologous tendon graft from the palmaris longus, gracilis, or plantaris—the so-called *Tommy John* surgery.[22,37,63] Most postoperative rehabilitation

facilities incorporate bracing with progressive range of motion, strengthening activities, and an interval throwing program.[55] Nonoperative treatment may be appropriate depending on the severity of injury and other factors such as age and desire to return to competitive sport.[53]

The *lateral collateral ligament complex* of the elbow is more variable in form than the medial collateral ligament (Fig. 6.14). The ligamentous complex originates on the lateral epicondyle and splits into two primary fiber bundles. One fiber bundle, traditionally known as the *radial collateral ligament,* fans out to merge primarily with the annular ligament, with some fibers also blending with the proximal attachments of the supinator and extensor carpi radialis brevis muscles. A second thicker fiber bundle, called the *lateral (ulnar) collateral ligament (LUCL),* attaches distally to the supinator crest on the lateral side of the ulna. The lateral location of both ligaments provides resistance against a varus-producing force at the elbow.

The relative posterior location of the LUCL renders most of its fibers taut at full flexion.[89] Furthermore, by attaching to the ulna, the LUCL functions along with the anterior fibers of the MCL as the primary frontal plane "guy wires" to the elbow. As a pair, the LUCL and anterior fibers of the MCL provide the primary soft tissue resistance against excessive varus and valgus movements, respectively, throughout most of the range of flexion and extension.

The relatively stout LUCL spans and structurally supports the radial head and proximal ulna (see Fig. 6.14). The orientation of the ligament limits excessive "external rotation" of the entire proximal forearm relative to the humerus. Proof of this function becomes

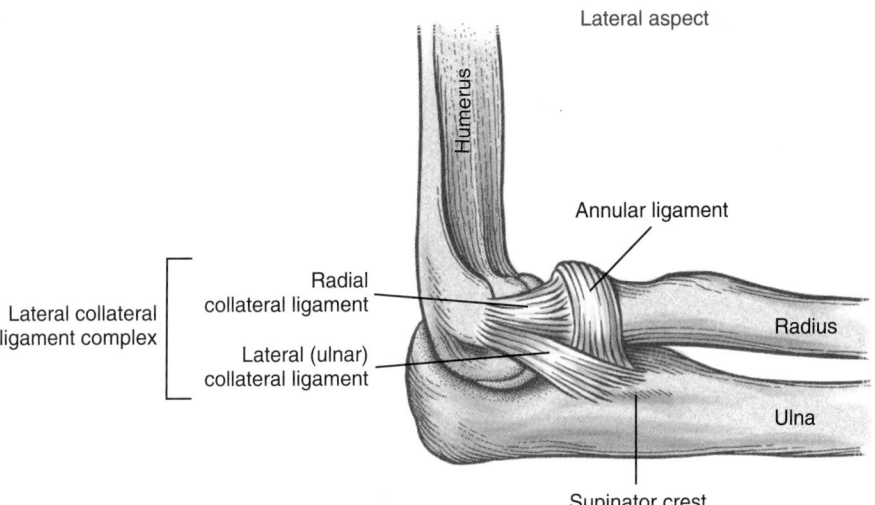

FIGURE 6.14 The components of the lateral collateral ligament complex of the right elbow.

SPECIAL FOCUS 6.1

Terrible Triad Injury of the Elbow

As described previously in relation to Fig. 6.13, falling onto an outstretched and often fully supinated forearm can result in injury to the MCL. In some cases, however, this type of fall can cause more extensive trauma, often described as the *terrible triad injury of the elbow.*[17,32] This serious and complex injury is classically defined as elbow joint dislocation (often with extensive ligamentous and soft tissue damage), fracture of the radial head, and fracture of the coronoid process. The extreme compression, often hyperextension, and valgus-producing force generated at ground contact can injure the MCL as well as fracture the bones. Often, in addition, at ground contact the distal humerus forcefully internally rotates relative to the fixed forearm. This produces a large posterior–lateral torsional (rotary) stress at the elbow, often completely tearing the LUCL and other adjacent soft tissues. The resulting posterior-lateral rotary instability of the elbow can be expressed clinically by manually placing an excessive external rotation (supination) stress to the entire proximal forearm (relative to a fixed humerus).[54,90] Depending on the severity of the injury, the rotary instability can involve both the humeroradial and the humero-ulnar joints. Because of the extensive trauma, treatment of this injury can pose a significant challenge to the surgeon and rehabilitation specialist.[24] In particularly severe cases, progress may be hindered by persistent instability, residuals of nerve damage, heterotopic ossification, and stiffness in the elbow. The goals of surgery typically include restoring bony and ligamentous integrity of the humero-ulnar and humeroradial joints. This restoration encourages earlier postsurgical movement, with aims of limiting long-term stiffness. Surgical treatment often involves the insertion of a prosthetic radial head, attempting to fortify the lateral column of the elbow.

apparent in some severe injuries that completely disrupt the LUCL. The radial head may dislocate from under the capitulum by twisting in a posterior and lateral direction, resulting in a posterior-lateral rotary instability of the entire elbow complex. The LUCL, therefore, is respected for its ability to provide both frontal and horizontal plane stability at the elbow.

As most joints do, the elbow joint has a measurable intracapsular pressure. This pressure, which is determined by the ratio of the volume of air to the volume of space, is lowest at about 80 degrees of flexion.[41] This joint position is often considered the "position of comfort" for persons with joint inflammation and swelling. Maintaining a swollen elbow in a flexed position may improve comfort but could predispose the person to an elbow flexion *contracture* (from the Latin root *contractura,* to draw together). This topic is explored further in Clinical Connection 6.1.

KINEMATICS

Functional Considerations of Flexion and Extension

Elbow flexion performs several important physiologic functions, such as pulling, lifting, feeding, and grooming.[79] The inability to actively bring the hand to the mouth for feeding, for example, significantly limits one's functional independence. Persons with a spinal cord injury above the C^5 nerve root, for example, may experience this profound functional impairment because of complete paralysis of elbow flexor muscles.

Elbow extension naturally occurs with activities such as throwing, pushing, and reaching. Loss of complete extension may be caused by marked stiffness in the elbow flexor muscles. The muscles become abnormally stiff after long periods of immobilization in a flexed and shortened position. Long-term flexion may be from prolonged casting for a fractured bone, or due to posttraumatic heterotopic ossification, osteophyte formation, elbow joint inflammation and effusion, muscle spasticity, paralysis of the triceps muscle, or scarring of the skin over the anterior elbow. In addition to the tightness in the flexor muscles, increased stiffness may occur in the anterior capsule and some anterior fibers of the medial collateral ligament.

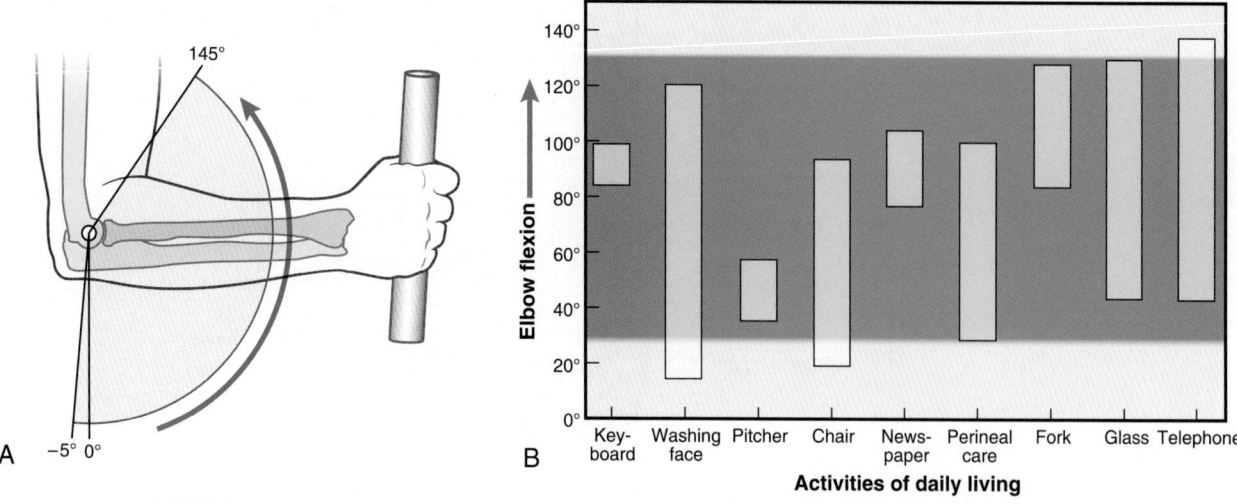

FIGURE 6.15 Range of motion at the elbow. (A) A healthy person showing an average range of elbow motion from 5 degrees beyond neutral extension through about 145 degrees of flexion. (B) The graph shows the range of motion at the elbow typically needed to perform the following activities: using a standard computer *keyboard, washing face,* pouring from a *pitcher,* rising from a *chair,* holding a *newspaper,* performing *perineal care,* bringing a *fork* to the mouth, bringing a *glass* to the mouth, and holding a *telephone.* The shaded area highlights the 100-degree "functional arc." (Data obtained from several sources; see text. Note: Data for perineal care represent the extremes of the maximal values used to perform the task.)

When measured by a goniometer, the maximal range of passive motion generally available to the elbow is from 5 degrees beyond neutral (0 degree) extension through about 145 degrees of flexion (Fig. 6.15A). As shown in Fig. 6.15B, many activities of daily living can be accomplished through a 100-degree "functional arc," from about 30 to 130 degrees of flexion.[61,69,88,91,104] Note the ample flexion needed to perform selected self-care and feeding activities. Understanding the kinematic demands naturally placed on the elbow helps clinicians set meaningful goals during physical rehabilitation programs.[33]

Arthrokinematics at the Humero-Ulnar Joint

The humero-ulnar joint is the articulation between the concave trochlear notch of the ulna and the convex trochlea of the humerus (Fig. 6.16). Hyaline cartilage covers about 300 degrees of articular surface on the trochlea, compared with only 180 degrees on the trochlear notch. The natural congruency and shape of this joint limits motion primarily to the sagittal plane. The sharp coronoid process of the ulna provides the primary source of bony resistance against a posterior translation of the ulna relative to the distal humerus, especially if the elbow is partially flexed.[51]

For the humero-ulnar joint to reach a fully extended position, sufficient extensibility is required in the dermis anterior to the elbow, flexor muscles, anterior capsule, and some anterior fibers of the medial collateral ligament (Fig. 6.17A). Full extension also requires that the prominent tip of the olecranon process become wedged into the olecranon fossa. Excessive ectopic (from the Greek root *ecto,* outside, + *topos,* place) bone formation around the olecranon fossa can therefore limit full extension. Normally, once in extension, the healthy humero-ulnar joint is stabilized primarily by articular congruency and by the increased tension in the stretched connective tissues.

During flexion at the humero-ulnar joint, the concave surface of the trochlear notch rolls and slides on the convex trochlea

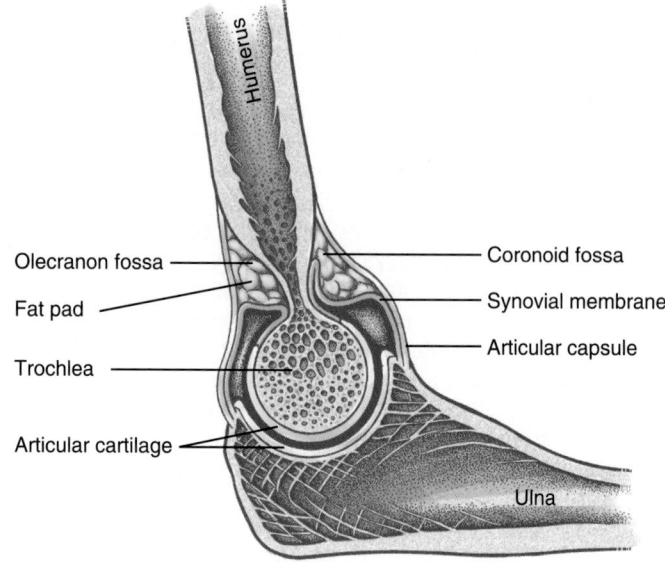

FIGURE 6.16 A sagittal section through the humero-ulnar joint showing the well-fitting joint surfaces between the trochlear notch and trochlea. The synovial membrane lining the internal side of the capsule is shown in blue.

(see Fig. 6.17B). Full elbow flexion requires elongation of the posterior capsule, extensor muscles, ulnar nerve, and certain portions of the collateral ligaments, especially the posterior fibers of the medial collateral ligament. Stretching of the ulnar nerve from prolonged or repetitive elbow flexion activities can lead to neuropathy.[15] A surgical treatment for this condition is to transfer the ulnar nerve anterior to the medial epicondyle, thereby reducing the tension in the nerve during flexion.

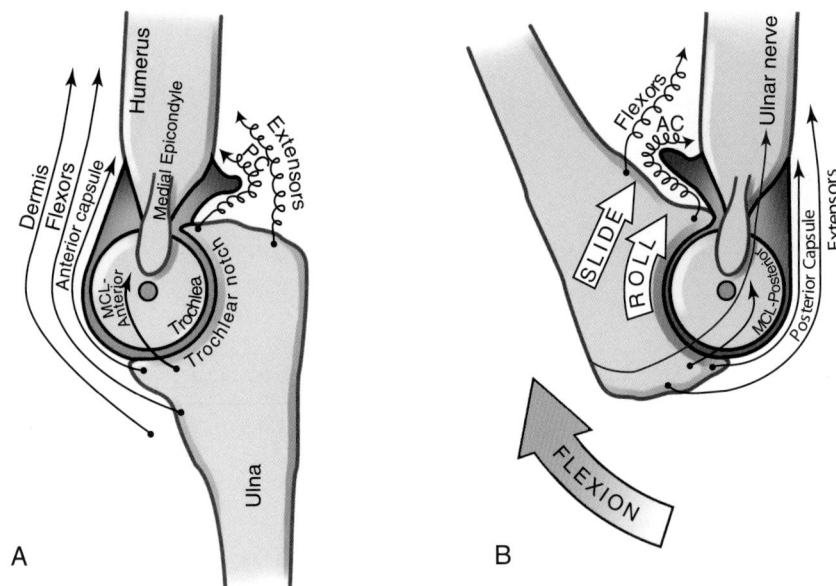

Resting in extension

FIGURE 6.17 (A) A sagittal section through the humero-ulnar joint. (A) The joint is resting in full extension. (B) The joint is passively flexed through full flexion. Note that in full flexion the coronoid process of the ulna fits into the coronoid fossa of the humerus. The medial-lateral axis of rotation is shown through the center of the trochlea. The stretched (taut) structures are shown as thin elongated arrows, and slackened structures are shown as wavy arrows. *AC,* Anterior capsule; *MCL-Anterior,* some anterior fibers of the medial collateral ligament; *MCL-Posterior,* posterior fibers of the medial collateral ligament; *PC,* posterior capsule.

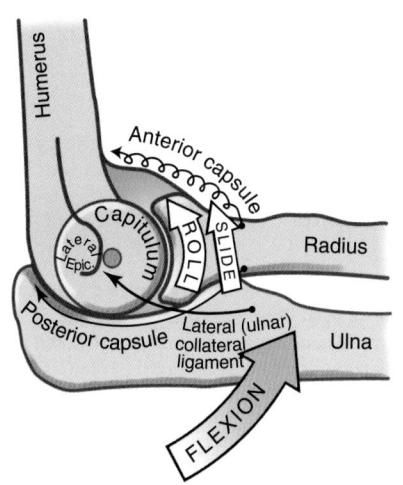

FIGURE 6.18 A sagittal section through the humeroradial joint during passive flexion. Note the medial-lateral axis of rotation in the center of the capitulum. The stretched (taut) structures are shown as thin elongated arrows, and slackened structures are shown as wavy arrows. Note the elongation of the lateral (ulnar) collateral ligament during flexion.

Arthrokinematics at the Humeroradial Joint

The humeroradial joint is an articulation between the cuplike fovea of the radial head and the reciprocally shaped rounded capitulum. The arthrokinematics of flexion and extension consist of the fovea of the radius rolling and sliding across the convexity of the capitulum (Fig. 6.18). During active flexion, the radial fovea is pulled firmly against the capitulum by contracting muscles.

Compared with the humero-ulnar joint, the humeroradial joint provides minimal anterior-posterior stability to the elbow. The humeroradial joint does, however, furnish significant lateral bracing to the elbow, providing about 50% of the resistance against a valgus-producing force.[70] The effectiveness of this resistance is based, in part, on the size and depth of the radial fovea and the compression forces produced by muscle activation.[94] Compression fracture, malunion, and/or surgical removal of the radial head may therefore predispose one to an excessive valgus deformity at the elbow.

Structure and Function of the Interosseous Membrane

The radius and ulna are bound together by the *interosseous membrane,* forming a fibrous, syndesmosis (Chapter 2). Most of the fibers of the interosseous membrane are referred to as the *central*

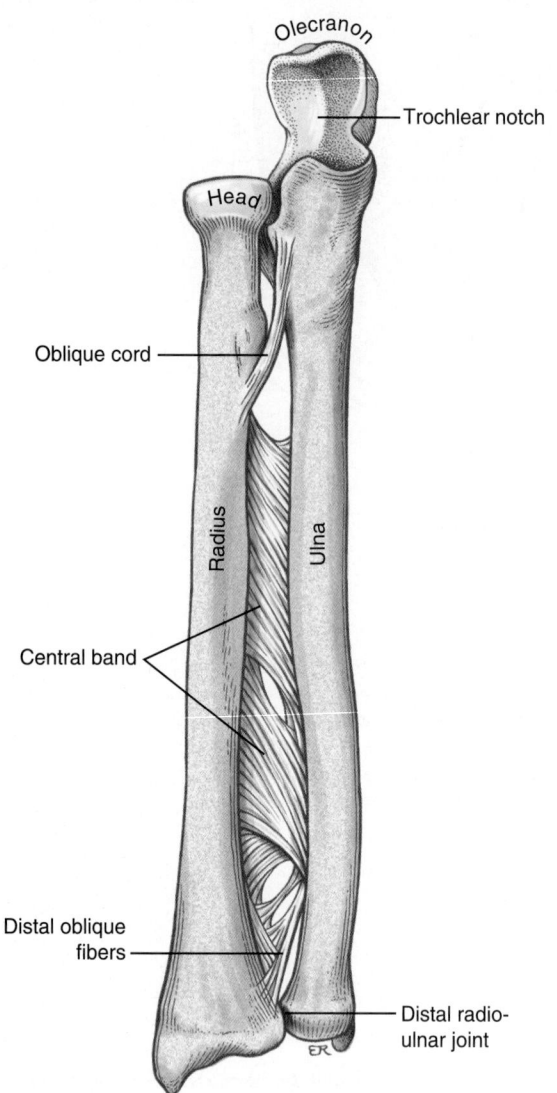

FIGURE 6.19 An anterior view of the right forearm, highlighting three components of the interosseous membrane. Note the more dominant central band.

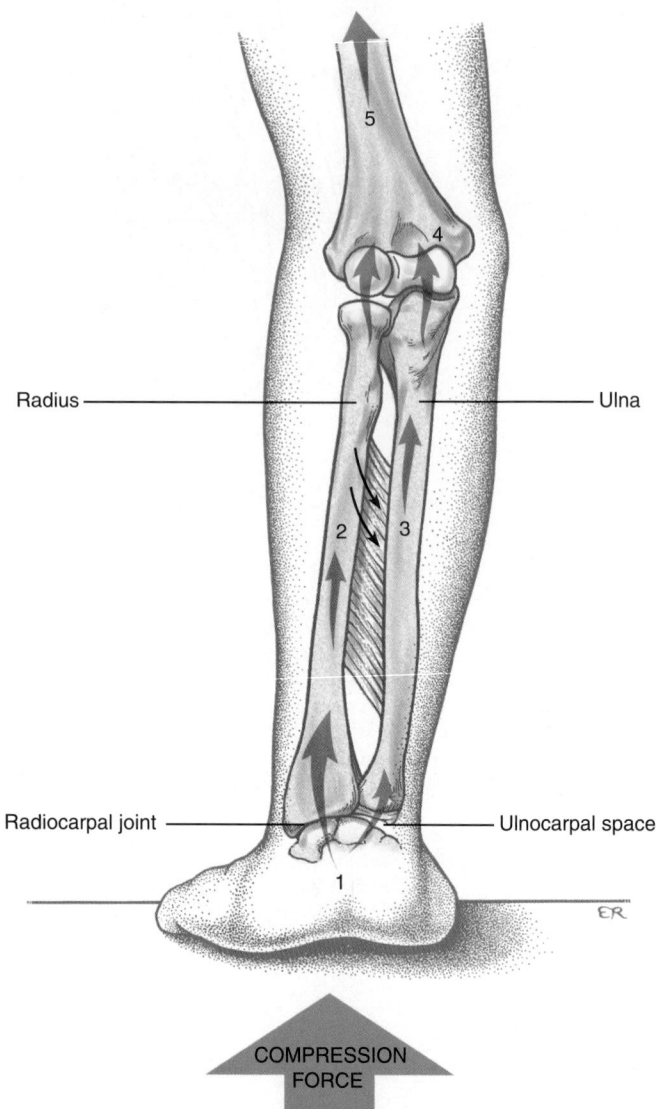

FIGURE 6.20 A *compression force* through the hand is transmitted primarily through the wrist *(1)* at the radiocarpal joint and to the radius *(2)*. This force pulls the central band of the interosseous membrane taut (shown by *two black arrows*), thereby transferring a significant part of the compression force to the ulna *(3)* and across the elbow at the humero-ulnar joint *(4)*. The compression forces that cross the elbow are finally directed toward the shoulder *(5)*. The stretched (taut) structures are shown as *thin elongated arrows*.

band (Fig. 6.19).[77] These prominent fibers are directed distal-medially from the radius, intersecting with the shaft of the ulna at about 20 degrees.[95] The central band has nearly twice the thickness of other fibers, with an ultimate tensile strength similar to that of the patellar tendon of the knee.[83]

In addition to the central band, several other smaller components of the interosseous membrane have been described.[77] Of these, two subsets are particularly noteworthy, both flowing generally perpendicular to the main central band (see Fig. 6.19). At the proximal forearm is a flattened *oblique cord,* which runs from the lateral side of the tuberosity of the ulna to just distal to the radial tuberosity. Functionally, the oblique cord helps limit distal migration of the radius relative to the ulna. Furthermore, based on fiber direction and attachments, the oblique cord, if tightened, may limit the extremes of forearm supination. Located at the extreme distal forearm are a small and poorly defined set of *distal oblique fibers,* which are only present in about 30% to 40% of membranes.[47,77] These fibers flow in an irregular fashion but are generally directed

distal-laterally from the distal one-sixth of the ulnar shaft, to the extreme distal radius at the margin of the distal radio-ulnar joint. These fibers are located directly deep to the pronator quadratus muscle. When present, the distal oblique fibers typically blend with connective tissues of the distal radio-ulnar joint, thereby adding some element of stability.

The primary functions of the *central band* of the interosseous membrane are to firmly bind the radius to the ulna, serve as an attachment site for extrinsic muscles of the hand, and provide a mechanism for transmitting force proximally through the upper limb. As illustrated in Fig. 6.20, about 80% of the compression force that crosses the wrist is directed through the radiocarpal joint. (This fact accounts, in part, for the relatively high likelihood of fracturing the radius from a fall on an outstretched hand.) The remaining 20% of the force crosses the medial side of the wrist, through the soft tissues located within the "ulnocarpal space."[81] Due to the fiber direction of the central band of the interosseous membrane, part of the proximal directed force through the radius is transferred across the membrane *to the ulna*. This mechanism allows a significant portion of the compression force that naturally acts on the radius to cross the elbow via the humero-ulnar joint. In this way, both the humero-ulnar and the humeroradial joints more equally "share" the compression forces that cross the elbow, thereby reducing each individual joint's long-term wear and tear.

Most elbow flexors, and essentially all primary supinator and pronator muscles, have their distal attachment on the radius. Consequently, during many functional activities, contraction of these muscles pulls the radius *proximally* against the capitulum of the humerus, especially when the elbow is at or near full extension. Biomechanical analysis indicates that the resulting compression force at the humeroradial joint reaches three to four times body weight during maximal-effort muscle contractions.[5] Based on the mechanism described in Fig. 6.20, the central band of the interosseous membrane helps shunt some of the muscular-produced compression forces *from the radius to the ulna*. In this way, the interosseous membrane helps protect the humeroradial joint from large myogenic compression forces. Tears within the interosseous membrane can result in a measurable proximal migration of the radius, caused either by contraction of regional muscles or by bearing weight through the wrist and forearm. Such undesired proximal migration of the radius can cause increased loading and, over time, excessive wear at the humeroradial joint.[78] In cases where the head of the radius has been severely fractured or surgically removed or replaced, the proximal migration is typically pronounced.[1] Over time, this proximal "drift" of the radius can place high stress not only on the humeroradial joint but also on certain bones within the wrist and the distal radio-ulnar joint, causing significant wrist pain and loss of function. (The pathomechanics associated with this topic are further explored in Chapter 7.) The potential multijoint pathomechanics resulting from the loss of structural integrity of the central band of the interosseous membrane reveal the important and global kinesiologic role of this structure—a role often underappreciated.

The predominant fiber direction of the central band of the interosseous membrane is *not* aligned to resist *distally applied* forces on the radius. For example, holding a heavy suitcase with the elbow extended causes a distracting force almost entirely through the radius (Fig. 6.21). The distal pull on the radius slackens, rather than tenses, most of the interosseous membrane, consequently placing larger demands on other tissues, such as the oblique cord and the annular ligament, to accept the load. Contraction of the brachioradialis or other muscles involved with grasp can assist with holding the radius and load firmly against the capitulum of the humerus. A deep aching in the forearm in persons who carry heavy loads (with elbow at the side and extended) may be from fatigue in these muscles. Supporting loads through the forearm at shoulder level, for example, like a waiter supporting a tray of food, directs the weight proximally through the radius, so that the interosseous membrane can assist with dispersing the load more evenly through the forearm.

Video 6.1 demonstrates the loading (tensing and slackening) of the interosseous membrane of a cadaver specimen.

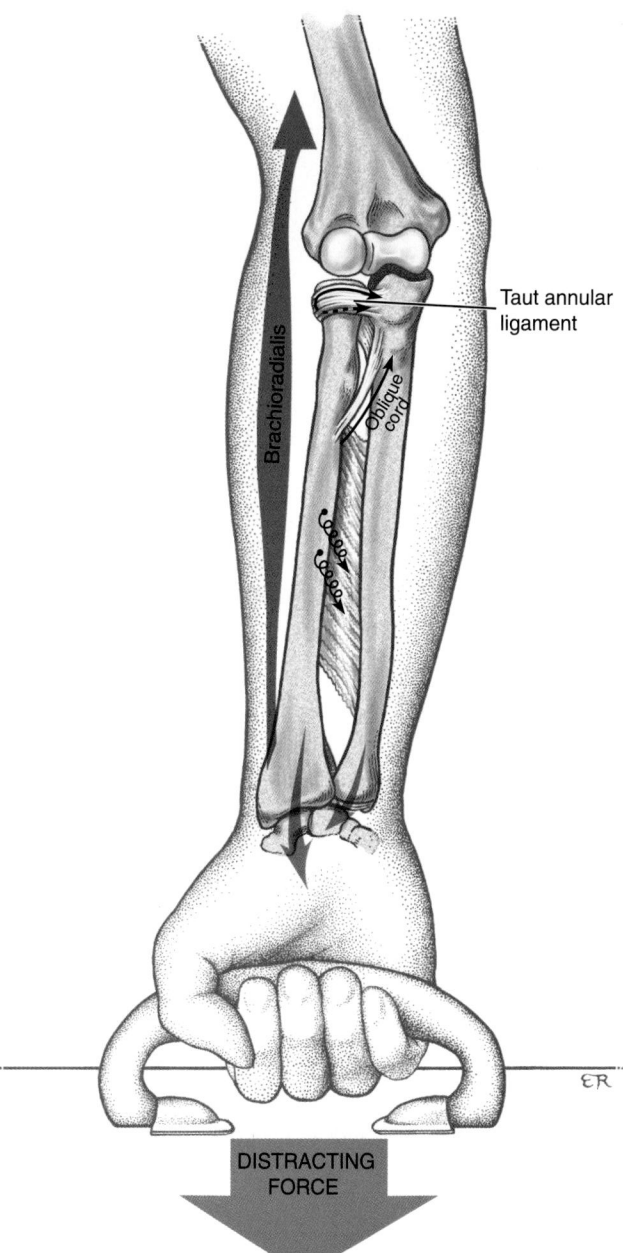

FIGURE 6.21 Holding a load, such as a suitcase, places a distal-directed *distracting force* predominantly through the radius. This distraction slackens most of the central band of the interosseous membrane (shown by *wavy arrows* over the membrane). Other structures, such as the oblique cord, the annular ligament, and the brachioradialis, must assist with the support of the load. The stretched (taut) structures are shown as *thin elongated arrows*.

Joints of the Forearm

GENERAL FEATURES OF THE PROXIMAL AND DISTAL RADIO-ULNAR JOINTS

The radius and ulna are bound together by the interosseous membrane and the proximal and distal radio-ulnar joints. This set of joints, situated at either end of the forearm, allows the forearm to rotate into pronation and supination. Forearm supination places the palm "up," or supine, and pronation places the palm "down," or prone. This forearm rotation occurs around an *axis of rotation* that extends from near the radial head through the ulnar head—an axis that intersects and connects both radio-ulnar joints (Fig. 6.22).[26] Pronation and supination provide a mechanism that allows independent rotation of the hand without an obligatory rotation of the ulna or humerus.

The kinematics of forearm rotation are more complicated than those implied by the simple "palm-up and palm-down" terminology. The palm does indeed rotate, but only because the hand and wrist connect firmly *to the radius* and not to the ulna. The space between the distal ulna and the medial side of the carpus allows the carpal bones to rotate freely, along with the radius, without interference from the distal ulna.

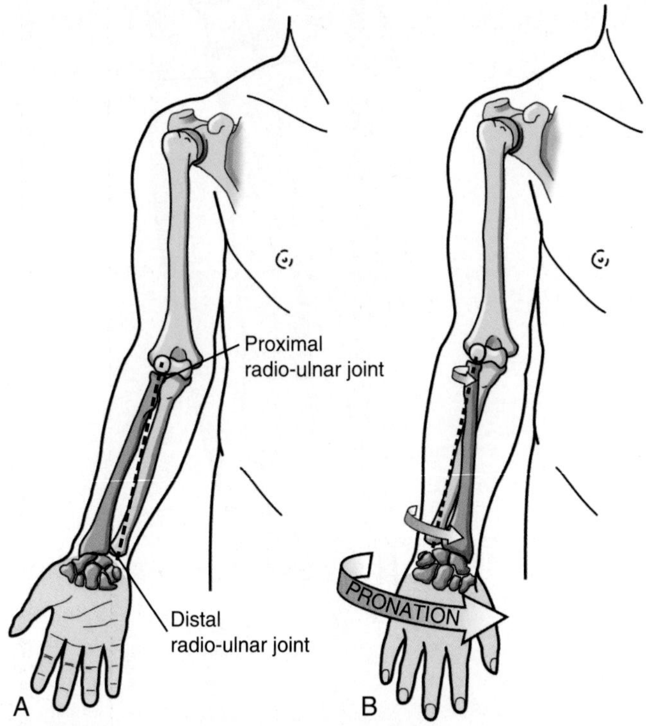

In the anatomic position the forearm is fully supinated when the ulna and radius lie nearly parallel to each other (see Fig. 6.22A). During pronation, the distal segment of the forearm complex (i.e., the radius and hand) rotates and crosses over an essentially fixed ulna (see Fig. 6.22B). The ulna, through its firm attachment to the humerus at the humero-ulnar joint, remains nearly stationary during an isolated pronation and supination movement. A stable humero-ulnar joint provides an essential rigid link on which the radius, wrist, and hand can pivot. Slight accessory movements occur at the humero-ulnar joint during pronation and supination; these motions being slight and not precisely defined in the literature. It certainly is possible for the ulna to rotate freely during pronation and supination, but only if the humerus is also freely rotating at the glenohumeral joint.

JOINT STRUCTURE AND PERIARTICULAR CONNECTIVE TISSUE

Proximal Radio-Ulnar Joint

The proximal radio-ulnar joint, the humero-ulnar joint, and the humeroradial joint all share one articular capsule. Within this capsule, the radial head is held against the proximal ulna by a fibro-osseous ring. This ring is formed by the radial notch of the ulna and the annular ligament (Fig. 6.23A). About 75% of the ring is formed by the annular ligament and 25% by the radial notch of the ulna.

The *annular* (from the Latin *annulus,* ring) *ligament* is a thick circular band of connective tissue attaching to the ulna on either side of the radial notch (see Fig. 6.23B). The ligament fits snugly around the radial head, holding the proximal radius against the ulna. The internal circumference of the annular ligament is lined with cartilage to reduce the friction against the radial head during

FIGURE 6.22 Anterior view of the right forearm. (A) In full supination the radius and ulna are parallel. (B) Moving into full pronation, the radius crosses over the ulna. The axis of rotation *(dashed line)* extends obliquely across the forearm from the radial head to the ulnar head. The radius and carpal bones (shown in *brown*) form the distal segment of the forearm complex. The humerus and ulna (shown in *yellow*) form the proximal segment of the forearm complex. Note that the thumb stays with the radius during pronation.

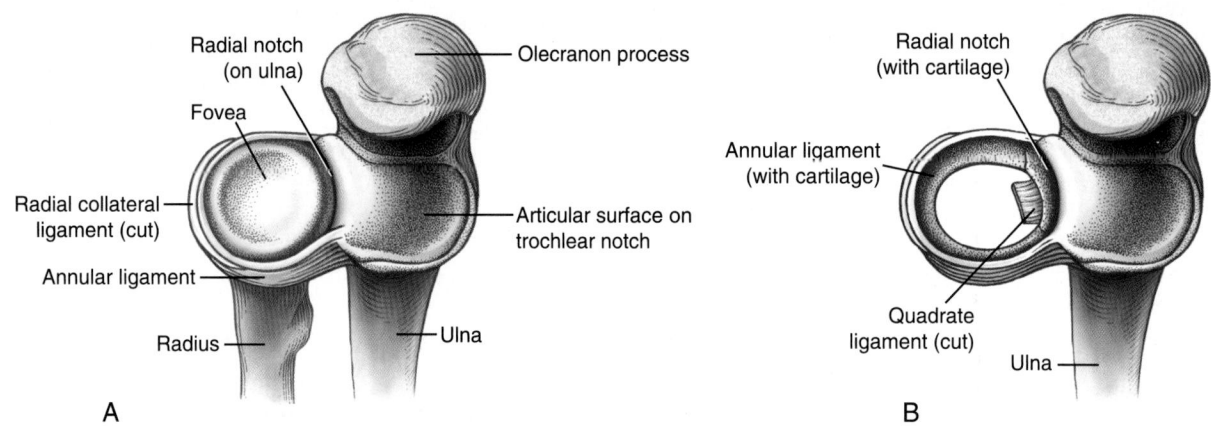

FIGURE 6.23 The right proximal radio-ulnar joint as viewed from above. (A) The radius is held against the radial notch of the ulna by the annular ligament. (B) The radius is removed, exposing the internal surface of the concave component of the proximal radio-ulnar joint. Note the cartilage lining the entire fibro-osseous ring. The quadrate ligament is cut near its attachment to the neck of the radius.

Dislocations of the Proximal Radio-Ulnar Joint

Because the hand attaches firmly to the radius through the wrist, a strenuous pull on the typically pronated hand can cause the radial head to slip distally through the annular ligament. This injury has been referred to by several names, including pulled elbow syndrome, nurse maid's elbow, or baby-sitter's elbow. Young children are particularly susceptible to this condition because of their ligamentous laxity, a nonossified radial head, relative reduced strength and slowed reflexes, and the increased likelihood of others forcefully pulling on their arms—such as a parent, guardian, or even a pet dog (Fig. 6.24). One of the best ways to prevent this dislocation is to explain to parents how a sharp pull on the child's hand can cause such a dislocation. The most common method for manually reducing this dislocation is through either a supination-and-flexion or a pronation maneuver applied to the child's forearm.[57]

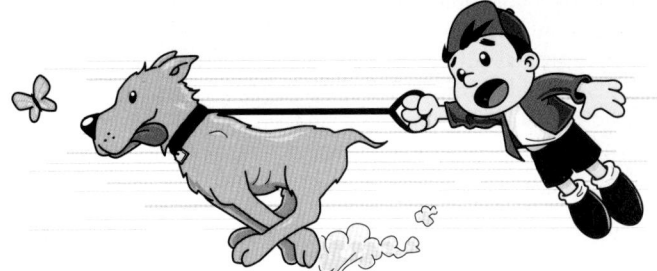

FIGURE 6.24 An example of a cause of "pulled-elbow syndrome" in a child. (Redrawn from Letts RM: Dislocations of the child's elbow. In Morrey BF, editor: *The elbow and its disorders,* ed 3, Philadelphia, 2000, Saunders. By permission of the Mayo Foundation for Medical Education and Research.)

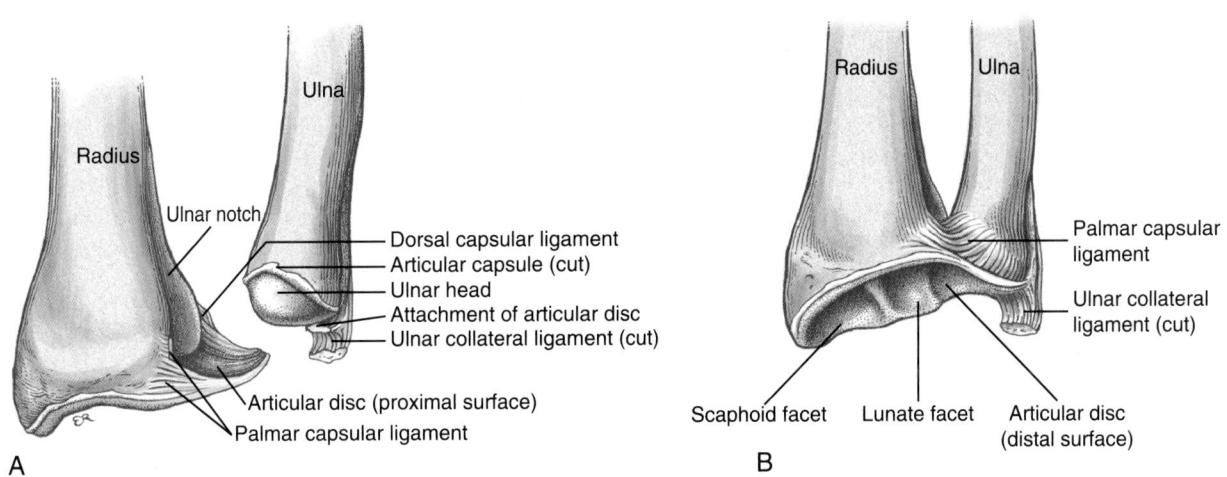

FIGURE 6.25 An anterior view of the right distal radio-ulnar joint. (A) The ulnar head has been pulled away from the concavity formed by the proximal surface of the articular disc and the ulnar notch of the radius. (B) The distal forearm has been tilted slightly to expose part of the distal surface of the articular disc and its connections with the more superficial layers of the palmar capsular ligament of the distal radio-ulnar joint. The scaphoid and lunate facets on the distal radius show impressions made by these carpal bones at the radiocarpal joint of the wrist.

pronation and supination. The external surface of the ligament receives attachments from the elbow capsule, the radial collateral ligament, and the supinator muscle.[16,96]

The *quadrate ligament* is thin and fibrous, arising just below the radial notch of the ulna and attaching distally to the medial surface of the neck of the radius (see Fig. 6.23B). The ligament stabilizes the proximal radio-ulnar joint, being stretched as the forearm approaches full rotation, most notably toward supination.[103]

Distal Radio-Ulnar Joint
The distal radio-ulnar joint consists of the convex head of the ulna positioned against the shallow concavity formed by the ulnar

notch on the radius and the proximal surface of an articular disc (Fig. 6.25). This important joint firmly connects the distal ends of the radius and ulna. The shallow and often irregularly shaped ulnar notch of the radius affords minimal osseous containment to the distal radio-ulnar joint. The majority of the stability of the joint is furnished through an elaborate set of connective tissues associated with the articular disc, plus activation of muscles.[97]

The articular disc at the distal radio-ulnar joint is also known as the *triangular fibrocartilage,* indicating its shape and predominant tissue type. As depicted in Fig. 6.25A, the lateral side of the disc attaches along the rim of the ulnar notch of the radius. The main body of the disc fans out horizontally into a triangular shape, with its apex attaching medially within the fovea and base of the styloid process of the ulna. The anterior and posterior edges of the disc are continuous with the relatively superficial *palmar (anterior)* and *dorsal (posterior) radio-ulnar joint capsular ligaments* (see Fig. 6.25). These well-defined ligaments share an attachment with the articular disc to the styloid process of the ulna; some deeper ligament fibers attach to the fovea.

The proximal surface of the disc, along with the attached capsular ligaments, holds the head of the ulna snugly against the ulnar notch of the radius during pronation and supination. This stabilizing mechanism guides the rotating distal end of the radius in a similarly secure manner as the annular ligament stabilizes and guides its proximal end.

The stability of the distal radio-ulnar joint is typically assessed clinically by applying dorsal- and palmar-directed forces to the distal radius relative to a well-fixed ulna.[19] Total translation of the radius as a result of this applied force is normally 5.5 mm (about ¼ inch) in healthy adults.[73] Translations exceeding this amount may be indicative of pathologic instability.

Introduction to the Triangular Fibrocartilage Complex

The articular disc at the distal radio-ulnar joint is part of a larger set of connective tissue known as the *triangular fibrocartilage complex*— typically abbreviated *TFCC*. The TFCC occupies most of the "ulnocarpal space" between the head of the ulna and the ulnar side of the wrist. Several adjacent and interconnected connective tissues are typically included with this complex, such as the capsular ligaments of the distal radio-ulnar joint and ulnar collateral ligament (see Fig. 6.25B).[105] The TFCC is the primary stabilizer of the distal radio-ulnar joint.[106] Significant attritional loss in the integrity of the TFCC is often associated with advanced rheumatoid arthritis. Weakness of the tissue can lead to marked multidirectional joint instability, often resulting in pain and difficulty in motions at the forearm and wrist.

Other structures that stabilize the distal radio-ulnar joint are the pronator quadratus, the tendon of the extensor carpi ulnaris, and the distal oblique fibers of the interosseous membrane.[4,67,76] The triangular fibrocartilage complex is anatomically and functionally associated with other structures of the wrist, and hence is discussed further in Chapter 7.

Stabilizers of the Distal Radio-Ulnar Joint

- Triangular fibrocartilage complex (TFCC)
- Pronator quadratus
- Tendon of the extensor carpi ulnaris
- Distal oblique fibers of the interosseous membrane

KINEMATICS

Functional Considerations of Pronation and Supination

Forearm supination occurs during many activities that involve bringing the palmar surface of the hand toward the face, such as when feeding, washing, and shaving. Forearm pronation, in contrast, is used to place the palmar surface of the hand down on an object, such as using a computer keyboard, grasping a coin, or pushing up from a chair.

The neutral or zero reference position of forearm rotation is the "thumb-up" position, midway between complete pronation and supination. On average, the forearm rotates through about 75 degrees of pronation and 85 degrees of supination (Fig. 6.26A). The literature indicates that many activities of daily living can be performed through a 100-degree "functional arc" of about 50 degrees of pronation to 50 degrees of supination.[104] This is apparent for most of the activities included in the graph in Fig. 6.26B.[69,88,91] To some extent, reduced pronation and

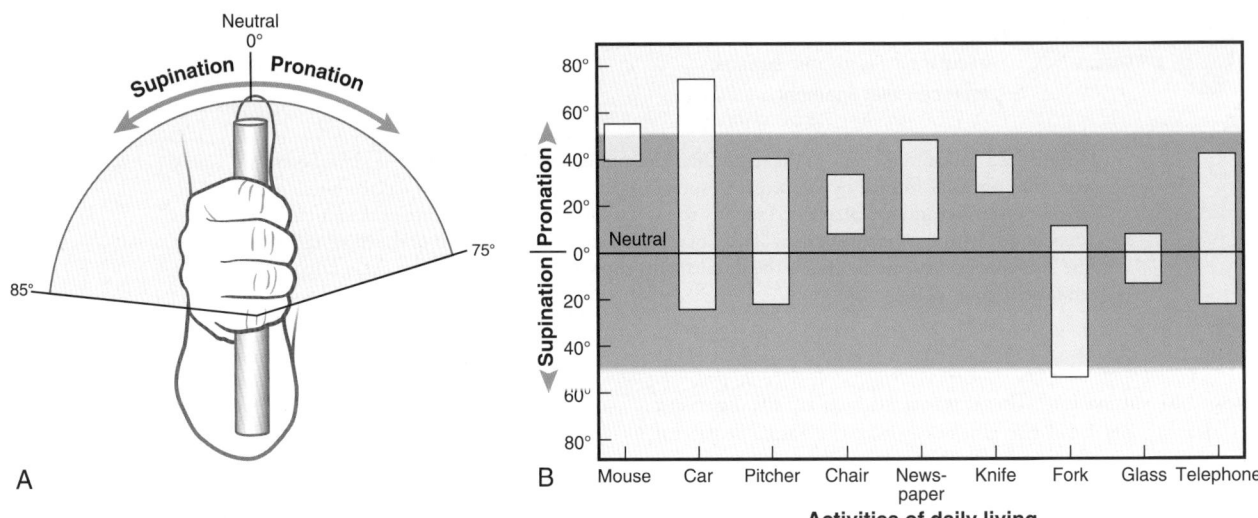

FIGURE 6.26 Range of motion at the forearm complex. (A) A healthy person generally allows 0 to 85 degrees of supination and 0 to 75 degrees of pronation. The 0-degree neutral position is shown with the thumb pointing straight up. (B) The graph shows the amount of forearm rotation usually required for healthy persons to perform the following activities: using a computer *mouse*, safely turning a steering wheel while driving a *car*, pouring from a *pitcher*, rising from a *chair*, reading a *newspaper*, cutting with a *knife*, bringing a *fork* to the mouth, bringing a *glass* to the mouth, and holding a *telephone*. The shaded area highlights the 100-degree "functional arc." (Data obtained from several sources; see text for more details.)

supination can be compensated through movements of the shoulder: internal rotation and abduction for pronation, and external rotation for supination.

Arthrokinematics at the Proximal and Distal Radio-Ulnar Joints

Pronation and supination require simultaneous movements at both the proximal and the distal radio-ulnar joints. As will be explained, pronation and supination also require movement at the adjacent humeroradial joint. A restriction at any one of these joints would restrict the overall movement of forearm rotation. Restrictions in passive range of motion can occur from tightness in muscle and/or connective tissues. Table 6.2 lists a sample of these tissues.

Supination

Supination at the *proximal radio-ulnar joint* occurs as a rotation of the radial head within the fibro-osseous ring formed by the annular ligament and radial notch of the ulna (Fig. 6.27, bottom box). The tight constraint of the radial head by the fibro-osseous ring prohibits standard roll-and-slide arthrokinematics.

Supination at the *distal radio-ulnar joint* occurs as the concave ulnar notch of the radius rolls and slides in similar directions on the head of the ulna (see Fig. 6.27, top box). During supination, the proximal surface of the articular disc slides (or "sweeps") firmly across the ulnar head. (The dynamic relationship between the disc and the ulna head can be appreciated by looking ahead at Fig. 6.47.) At the end range of supination, the palmar capsular

TABLE 6.2 Structures Most Capable of Restricting Full Supination and Pronation	
Restriction	**Structures**
Limit supination	Pronator teres, pronator quadratus, flexor carpi radialis, extrinsic finger flexors, articular disc and palmar capsular ligament at the distal radio-ulnar joint, interosseous membrane (central band), quadrate ligament, and oblique cord
Limit pronation	Biceps, supinator, radial wrist extensors, articular disc and dorsal capsular ligament at the distal radio-ulnar joint

ligament of the joint is stretched to its maximal length, creating a stiffness that naturally stabilizes the joint.[28,31] This stiffness provides increased stability at a position of reduced joint congruency. At the extremes of both supination and pronation, only about 10% of the surface of the ulnar notch of the radius is in direct contact with the ulnar head.[36] This is in sharp contrast with the more stable and congruent position of near neutral and slight supination,[42] where 60% of the articular surface is in contact, and the articular disc is pulled more directly over the center of the ulnar head.

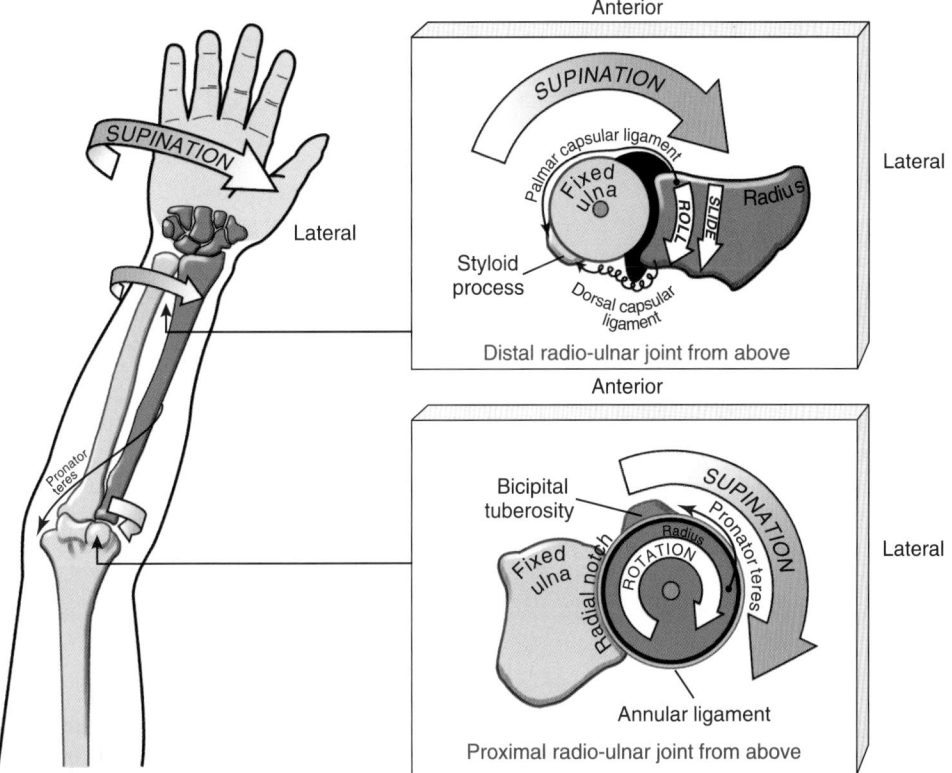

FIGURE 6.27 Illustration on the left shows the anterior aspect of a right forearm after completing full *supination*. During supination, the radius and carpal bones rotate around the fixed humerus and ulna. The inactive but stretched pronator teres is also shown. *Viewed as though looking down at your own right forearm,* the two insets depict a superior (cross-sectional) view of the arthrokinematics at the proximal and distal radio-ulnar joints. The articular disc at the distal radio-ulnar joint is not shown. The stretched (taut) structures are shown as thin elongated arrows, and slackened structures are shown as wavy arrows.

Pronation

The arthrokinematics of pronation at the proximal and distal radio-ulnar joints occur by mechanisms like those described for supination (Fig. 6.28). As depicted in the top inset of Fig. 6.28, full pronation elongates and thereby increases the tension in the dorsal capsular ligament at the distal radio-ulnar joint.[4,28,31,45] Full pronation slackens the palmar capsular ligament to about 70% of its original length.[93] Although not depicted in Fig. 6.28, the proximal surface of the articular disc slides across the ulnar head during pronation, thereby exposing much of its articular surface (see the asterisk in Fig. 6.28, top inset). This action allows the ulnar head to be readily palpated on the dorsal-ulnar side of the wrist.

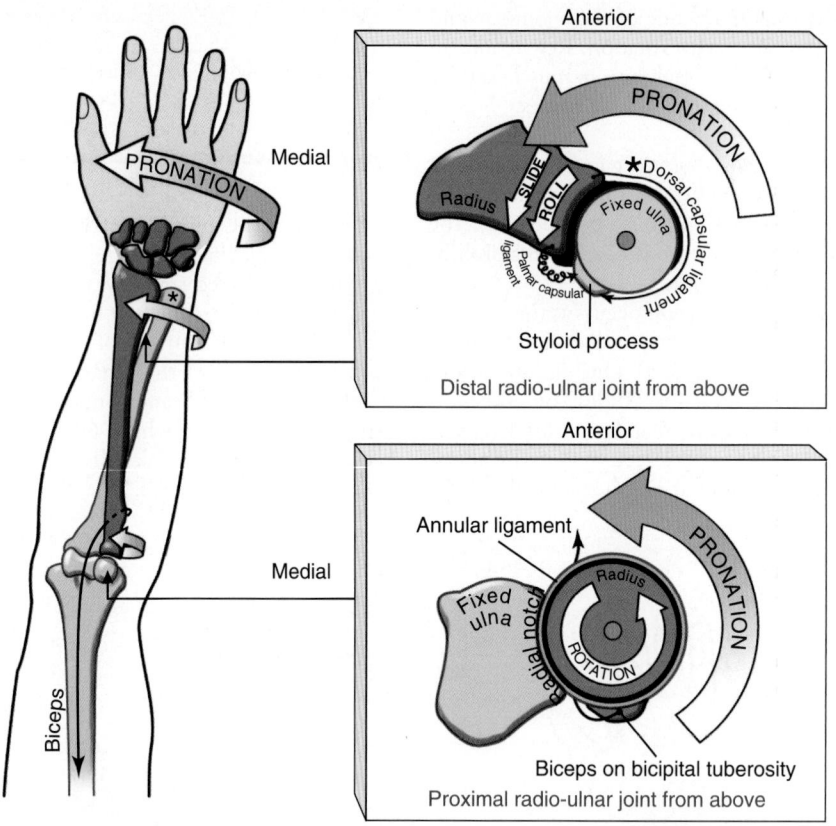

FIGURE 6.28 Illustration on the left shows the right forearm after completing full *pronation*. During pronation the radius and carpal bones rotate around the fixed humerus and ulna. The inactive but stretched biceps muscle is also shown. *Viewed as though looking down at your own right forearm,* the two insets show a superior (cross-sectional) view of the arthrokinematics at the proximal and distal radio-ulnar joints. The stretched (taut) structures are shown as thin elongated arrows, and slackened structures are shown as wavy arrows. The asterisks mark the exposed point on the anterior aspect of the ulnar head, which is apparent once the radius rotates fully around the ulna into complete pronation. The articular disc at the distal radio-ulnar joint is not shown.

SPECIAL FOCUS 6.3

Preventing Forearm Pronation Tightness

Splinting or rigid casting of parts of the upper extremity is often required following injury or surgery. The forearm is typically immobilized in some degree of pronation to optimize the use of the hand. The pronated bias during immobilization may explain, in some cases, why it is often more difficult for patients to regain full supination than pronation following the removal of their immobilization device. Pronation "tightness," or even permanent contracture, may be the result of adaptive shortening of several pronator muscles such as the pronator teres, pronator quadratus, flexor carpi radialis, and potentially the extrinsic finger flexors. In addition, full supination may be restricted by adaptive shortening and resultant stiffness in the quadrate ligament, oblique cord, palmar radio-ulnar joint capsular ligament, and interosseous membrane. Although not always practical or even possible, clinicians should nevertheless be aware of the possible therapeutic benefit of immobilizing a forearm in a partially *supinated* position, such that the muscles and connective tissues listed before are subjected to relative stretch while immobilized.

Near-Isometric Behavior of the Interosseous Membrane During Pronation and Supination

The axis of rotation for pronation and supination is oriented roughly parallel with most of the central band of the interosseous membrane, deviating by only about 10 to 12 degrees (compare Figs. 6.19 and 6.22A). This nearly parallel arrangement limits the change in length (or tension) of the membrane throughout pronation and supination.[67] (Recall from Chapter 1 that any force that acts *exactly parallel* to an axis of rotation produces no resistive torque.) The near-isometric behavior of much of the interosseous membrane is ideal because it provides a relatively constant level of stabilizing tension throughout movement. *Because the axis and the membrane are not precisely parallel, however, some change in length (and tension) must occur throughout the full range of forearm motion.* Research on this topic consistently shows that the tension in the central band of the interosseous membrane fluctuates only slightly throughout the full arc of movement, being least taut in full pronation and increasingly taut in supination.[30,48,62,67,107]

Humeroradial Joint: A "Shared" Joint between the Elbow and the Forearm

During pronation and supination, the proximal end of the radius rotates at both the *proximal radio-ulnar* and the *humeroradial joints.* Both joints have distinctive arthrokinematics during pronation and supination. The arthrokinematics at the proximal radio-ulnar joint were explained previously in Figs. 6.27 and 6.28. The arthrokinematics at the humeroradial joint involve a *spin* of the fovea of the radial head against the rounded capitulum of the humerus. Fig. 6.29 shows the arthrokinematics during active pronation under the muscular power of the pronator teres muscle. Contraction of this muscle—as well as others inserting on the radius—can generate significant compression force on the humeroradial joint, especially when the elbow

is near extension, a position that creates a lower angle-of-insertion of the muscle to the bone. This compression force is associated with a measurable proximal pull or migration of the radius, *most notably during pronation.*[68,86] Because the central band of the interosseous membrane is slightly less taut in pronation, it is less able to resist the proximal pull on the radius imparted by contraction of the pronator muscles. The natural proximal migration of the radius and associated increased joint compression of the humeroradial joint during active pronation has been referred to as the "screw home" mechanism of the elbow.[71]

Based on location, the humeroradial joint is mechanically linked to the kinematics of both the elbow and the forearm. *Any* motion performed at the elbow or forearm requires movement at this joint. A postmortem study of 32 cadavers (age at death ranging from 70–95 years) showed more frequent and severe degeneration across the humeroradial than the humero-ulnar joint.[2] The increased wear on the lateral compartment of the elbow can be explained in part by the frequent and complex arthrokinematics (spin and roll-and-slide), combined with varying amounts of muscular-produced compression force. Pain or limited motion at the humeroradial joint can significantly disrupt the functional mobility of the entire mid-to-distal upper extremity.

Pronation and Supination with the Radius and Hand Held Fixed

Up to this point in this chapter, the kinematics of pronation and supination have been described as a rotation of the *radius and hand* relative to a stationary, or fixed, humerus and ulna (see Figs. 6.27 and 6.28). The forearm rotation occurs when the upper limb is in a *non–weight-bearing position.* Pronation and supination are next described when the upper limb is in a weight-bearing position. In this case, the humerus and ulna rotate relative to a stationary, or fixed, radius and hand.

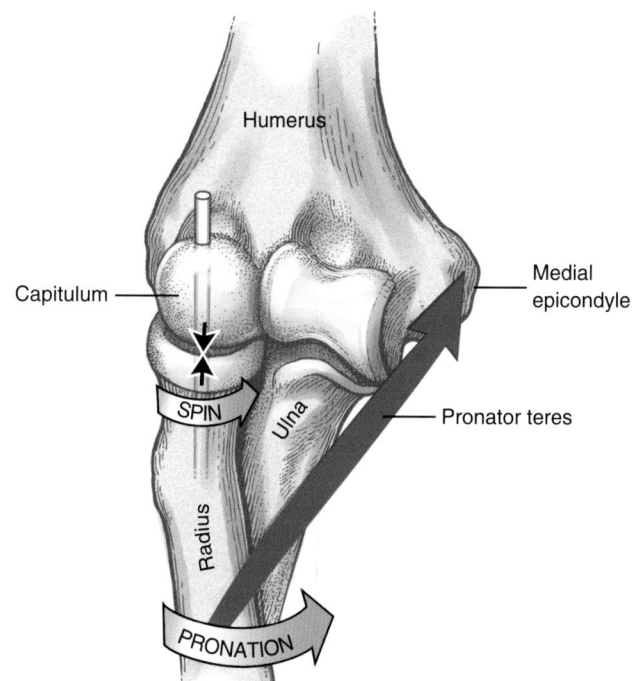

FIGURE 6.29 An anterior view of a right humeroradial joint during active pronation of the forearm. During pronation the fovea of the radial head spins against the capitulum. The spinning occurs around an axis that is nearly coincident with the axis of rotation through the proximal and distal radio-ulnar joints. The pronator teres muscle is shown active as it pronates the forearm and pulls the radius proximally against the capitulum. The opposing small arrows indicate an increased compression force at the humeroradial joint.

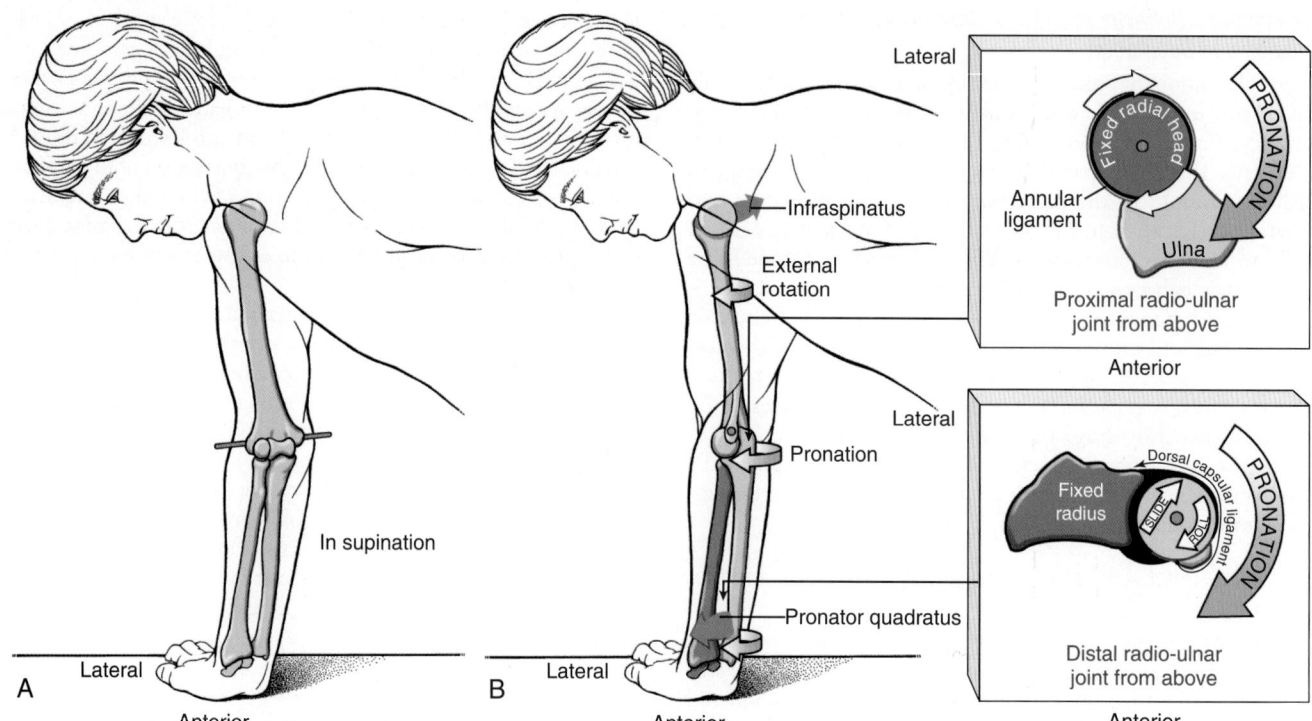

FIGURE 6.30 (A) A person is shown supporting his upper body weight through his right forearm, which is in full supination (i.e., the bones of the forearm are parallel). The radius is held fixed to the ground through the wrist; however, the humerus and ulna are free to rotate. (B) The humerus and ulna have rotated about 80 to 90 degrees externally from the initial position shown in (A). This rotation produces *pronation* at the forearm as the ulna rotates around the fixed radius. Note the activity depicted in the infraspinatus and pronator quadratus muscles. The two insets show a superior view of the arthrokinematics at the proximal and distal radio-ulnar joints. In the lower insert, stretched fibers of the dorsal capsular ligament (of the distal radio-ulnar joint) are shown as a *thin elongated arrow;* the articular disc is not shown.

Consider a person bearing weight through an upper extremity with elbow and wrist extended (Fig. 6.30A). The person's right glenohumeral joint is held partially internally rotated. The ulna and radius are positioned parallel in full supination. (The "rod" placed transversely through the epicondyles of the humerus helps with the orientation of this position.) With the radius and hand held firmly fixed with the ground, pronation of the forearm occurs by an *external rotation* of the humerus and ulna (see Fig. 6.30B). Because of the naturally tight structural fit of the humero-ulnar joint, rotation of the humerus is transferred, nearly degree for degree, to the rotating ulna. Moving back to the fully supinated position involves internal rotation of the humerus and ulna relative to the fixed radius and hand. It is important to note that these pronation and supination kinematics are essentially *an expression of active external and internal rotation of the glenohumeral joint, respectively.*

Fig. 6.30B depicts an interesting muscle "force-couple" used to pronate the forearm while in a weight-bearing position. The infraspinatus rotates the humerus relative to a fixed scapula, whereas the pronator quadratus rotates the ulna relative to a fixed radius. Both muscles, acting at either end of the upper extremity, produce forces that contribute to a pronation torque at the forearm. From a therapeutic perspective, an understanding of the muscular mechanics of pronation and supination from this weight-bearing perspective provides additional exercise strategies for strengthening or stretching muscles of the forearm and shoulder.

The far-right side of Fig. 6.30B illustrates the arthrokinematics at the radio-ulnar joints during pronation while the radius and hand are stationary. At the *proximal radio-ulnar joint* the annular ligament *and* radial notch of the ulna rotate around the fixed radial head (see Fig. 6.30B, top inset). Although not depicted, the capitulum of the humerus is spinning relative to the fovea of the fixed radius. At the *distal radio-ulnar joint* the head of the ulna rotates around the fixed ulnar notch of the radius (see Fig. 6.30B, bottom inset). Although not depicted in the previous illustration, the apex of the articular disc is pulled in the direction of the rotating styloid process of the ulna. Table 6.3 summarizes and compares the arthrokinematics at the radio-ulnar joints for both weight-bearing and non–weight-bearing conditions of the upper limb.

MUSCLE AND JOINT INTERACTION

Neuroanatomy Overview: Paths of the Musculocutaneous, Radial, Median, and Ulnar Nerves throughout the Elbow, Forearm, Wrist, and Hand

The musculocutaneous, radial, median, and ulnar nerves provide motor and sensory innervation to the muscles, ligaments, joint capsules, and skin of the elbow, forearm, wrist, and hand. The

TABLE 6.3 Arthrokinematics of Pronation and Supination

	Weight-Bearing (Radius and Hand Fixed)	Non–Weight-Bearing (Radius and Hand Free to Rotate)
Proximal radio-ulnar joint	Annular ligament *and* radial notch of the ulna rotate around a fixed radial head.	Radial head rotates within a ring formed by the annular ligament *and* the radial notch of the ulna.
Distal radio-ulnar joint	Convex ulnar head rolls and slides in opposite directions on the concave ulnar notch of the radius. The apex of the articular disc is pulled in the direction of the rotating styloid process of the ulna.	Concavity of the ulnar notch of the radius rolls and slides in similar directions on the convex ulna head. The lateral (radial) side of the articular disc is pulled in the direction of the rotating radius.

anatomic path of these nerves is described as a background for this chapter and the following two chapters on the wrist and the hand. The paths of these nerves, including the proximal-to-distal order in which they innervate muscles, are illustrated in Figs. II.1A–D found in Part A of Appendix II. These illustrations provide a useful visual accompaniment to the description of the following nerves.

The *musculocutaneous nerve,* formed from the C^5–C^7 spinal nerve roots, innervates the biceps brachii, coracobrachialis, and brachialis muscles (Fig. II.1A in Appendix II, Part A). As its name implies, the musculocutaneous nerve innervates muscle and then continues distally as a sensory nerve to the skin, supplying the lateral forearm and proximal wrist.

The *radial nerve,* formed from the C^5–T^1 spinal nerve roots, is a direct continuation of the posterior cord of the brachial plexus (see Fig. II.1B in Appendix II, Part A). This large nerve courses within the radial groove of the humerus to innervate the triceps and the anconeus. The radial nerve then emerges laterally at the distal humerus to innervate muscles that attach on or near the lateral epicondyle. Proximal to the elbow, the radial nerve innervates the brachioradialis (and a small lateral part of the brachialis) and the extensor carpi radialis longus. Distal to the elbow, the radial nerve consists of superficial and deep branches. The *superficial branch* is purely sensory, supplying the posterior-lateral aspects of the distal forearm, including the dorsal "web space" of the hand. The *deep branch* contains the remaining motor fibers of the radial nerve. This motor branch supplies the extensor carpi radialis brevis and the supinator muscle. After piercing through an intramuscular tunnel in the supinator muscle, the final section of the radial nerve courses toward the posterior side of the forearm. This terminal branch, often referred to as the *posterior interosseous nerve,* supplies the extensor carpi ulnaris and several muscles of the forearm, which function in extension of the digits.

The *median nerve,* formed from the C^6–T^1 spinal nerve roots, courses toward the elbow to innervate most muscles attaching on or near the medial epicondyle of the humerus. These muscles include the wrist flexors and forearm pronators (pronator teres, flexor carpi radialis, and palmaris longus) and the deeper located flexor digitorum superficialis (see Fig. II.1C in Appendix II, Part A). A deep branch of the median nerve, often referred to as the *anterior interosseous nerve,* innervates the deep muscles of the forearm: the lateral half of the flexor digitorum profundus, the flexor pollicis longus, and the pronator quadratus. The terminal part of the median nerve continues distally to cross the wrist through the carpal tunnel, under the cover of the transverse carpal

ligament. The nerve then innervates several of the intrinsic muscles of the thumb and the lateral fingers. The median nerve provides a rich source of sensation to the lateral palm, palmar surface of the thumb, and lateral two and one-half fingers (see Fig. II.1C in Appendix II, Part A, inset on median nerve sensory distribution).

The *ulnar nerve,* formed from the spinal nerve roots C^8–T^1, is formed by a direct branch of the medial cord of the brachial plexus (see Fig. II.1D in Appendix II, Part A). After passing posterior to the medial epicondyle, the ulnar nerve innervates the flexor carpi ulnaris and the medial half of the flexor digitorum profundus. The nerve then crosses the wrist external to the carpal tunnel and supplies motor innervation to many of the intrinsic muscles of the hand. The ulnar nerve supplies sensation to the skin on the ulnar side of the hand, including the medial side of the ring finger and entire small finger.

Innervation of Muscles and Joints of the Elbow and Forearm

Knowledge of the specific innervation to the muscle, skin, and joints is useful clinical information for treatment of persons who have sustained injury to the peripheral nerves or nerve roots. The informed clinician can anticipate not only the extent of the sensory and motor involvement after injury, but also the likely complications. Therapeutic activities, such as using splinting, performing selective strengthening and range-of-motion exercises, and providing patient education can often be initiated early after injury, provided there are no contraindications. This proactive approach minimizes the potential for permanent deformity and damage to insensitive skin and joints, thereby minimizing functional limitations.

INNERVATION OF MUSCLE

The *elbow flexors* have three different sources of peripheral nerve supply: the musculocutaneous nerve to the biceps brachii and brachialis, the radial nerve to the brachioradialis, and the median nerve to the pronator teres. In contrast, the *elbow extensors*—the triceps brachii and anconeus—have a single source of nerve supply through the radial nerve. Injury to this nerve can result in complete paralysis of the elbow extensors. Because three different nerves must be affected for all four elbow flexors to be paralyzed, important functions such as feeding and grooming are often at least partially preserved.

The muscles that *pronate the forearm* (pronator teres, pronator quadratus, and other secondary muscles that originate from the medial epicondyle) are innervated through the median nerve. *Supination of the forearm* is driven by the biceps brachii via the musculocutaneous nerve and the supinator muscle, plus secondary muscles that arise from the lateral epicondyle and dorsal forearm, via the radial nerve.

Table 6.4 summarizes the peripheral nerve and primary spinal nerve root innervation to the muscles of the elbow and forearm. This table was derived primarily from Appendix II, Part B, which lists the primary nerve roots that innervate the muscles of the upper extremity. Parts C–E of Appendix II include additional reference items to help guide the clinical assessment of the functional status of the C^5–T^1 spinal nerve roots and several major peripheral nerves of the upper limb.

SENSORY INNERVATION OF JOINTS

Humero-Ulnar and Humeroradial Joints

The humero-ulnar and humeroradial joints and the surrounding connective tissues receive their sensory innervation from the C^6–C^8 spinal nerve roots.[49] Fibers from these afferent nerve roots are carried primarily by the musculocutaneous and radial nerves and by the ulnar and median nerves.[96]

Proximal and Distal Radio-Ulnar Joints

The proximal radio-ulnar joint and surrounding elbow capsule receive sensory innervation from fibers within the median nerve that enter the C^6–C^7 spinal nerve roots.[96] The distal radio-ulnar joint receives most of its sensory innervation from fibers of the ulnar nerve that enter the C^8 nerve root.[49]

Function of the Elbow Muscles

Muscles that attach distally on the ulna flex or extend the elbow but possess no ability to pronate or supinate the forearm. In contrast, muscles that attach distally on the radius may, in theory, flex or extend the elbow, but also have a potential to pronate or supinate the forearm. This basic concept serves as the underlying theme through much of the remainder of this chapter.

Muscles acting primarily on the wrist also cross the elbow joint. For this reason, many of the wrist muscles have a potential to flex or extend the elbow. This potential is typically minimal and not discussed further. The proximal and distal attachments and nerve supply of the muscles of the elbow and forearm are listed in Appendix II, Part F. Also, as a reference, a list of cross-sectional areas of selected muscles of the elbow and forearm is found in Appendix II, Part G.

ELBOW FLEXORS

The biceps brachii, brachialis, brachioradialis, and pronator teres are primary elbow flexors. Each of these muscles produces a force that passes anterior to the medial-lateral axis of rotation at the elbow. Structural and related biomechanical variables of these muscles are included in Table 6.5 and will be referred to throughout this section.

TABLE 6.4 Primary Motor Innervation to the Muscles of the Elbow and Forearm

Muscle	Innervation*
Elbow Flexors	
Brachialis	Musculocutaneous nerve (C^5, C^6)
Biceps brachii	Musculocutaneous nerve (C^5, C^6)
Brachioradialis	Radial nerve (C^5, C^6)
Pronator teres	Median nerve (C^6, C^7)
Elbow Extensors	
Triceps brachii	Radial nerve (C^7, C^8)
Anconeus	Radial nerve (C^7, C^8)
Forearm Pronators	
Pronator quadratus	Median nerve (C^8, T^1)
Pronator teres	Median nerve (C^6, C^7)
Forearm Supinators	
Biceps brachii	Musculocutaneous nerve (C^5, C^6)
Supinator	Radial nerve (C^6)

*The primary spinal nerve root innervation of the muscles is in parentheses.

TABLE 6.5 Structural and Related Biomechanical Variables of the Primary Elbow Flexor Muscles*

Muscle	Work Capacity *Volume (cm³)*	Contraction Excursion *Length (cm)†*	Peak Force *Physiologic Cross-sectional Area (cm²)*	Leverage *Internal Moment Arm (cm)‡*
Biceps brachii (long head)	33.4	13.6	2.5	3.20
Biceps brachii (short head)	30.8	15.0	2.1	3.20
Brachialis	59.3	9.0	7.0	1.98
Brachioradialis	21.9	16.4	1.5	5.19
Pronator teres	18.7	5.6	3.4	2.01

Data from An KN, Hui FC, Morrey BF, et al: Muscles across the elbow joint: a biomechanical analysis, *J Biomech* 14:659, 1981.
*Structural properties are indicated by italics. The related biomechanical variables are indicated in boldface type.
†Muscle belly length measured at 70 degrees of flexion.
‡Internal moment arm measured with elbow flexed to 100 degrees and forearm fully supinated.

Individual Muscle Action of the Elbow Flexors

The *biceps brachii* attaches proximally on the scapula and distally on the radial tuberosity on the radius (Fig. 6.31). Secondary distal attachments include the deep fascia of the forearm through an aponeurotic sheet known as the *fibrous lacertus.*

The biceps produces its maximal electromyographic (EMG) activity when performing flexion and supination simultaneously, two primary actions of the muscle. These actions are very useful and important; for example, consider bringing a spoonful of soup to the mouth. The biceps exhibits relatively low levels of EMG activity when flexion is performed with the forearm deliberately held in pronation. This lack of muscle activation can be verified by self-palpation.

The *brachialis* lies deep to the biceps, originating on the anterior humerus and attaching distally on the extreme proximal ulna (Fig. 6.32). This muscle's sole function is to flex the elbow. As shown in Table 6.5, the brachialis has an average physiologic cross-section of 7 cm², the largest of any muscle crossing the elbow. For comparison, the long head of the biceps has a cross-sectional area of only 2.5 cm². Based on its large physiologic cross-section, the brachialis is expected to generate the greatest force of any muscle crossing the elbow.

The *brachioradialis* is the longest of all elbow muscles, attaching proximally on the lateral supracondylar ridge of the humerus and distally near the styloid process of the radius (see Fig. 6.31). Maximal shortening of the brachioradialis causes full elbow flexion and rotation of the forearm *to* the near neutral position. The dominant role of the brachioradialis as an elbow flexor has been well established.[11,14,39]

The brachioradialis muscle can be readily palpated on the anterior-lateral aspect of the forearm. Resisted elbow flexion, from a position of about 90 degrees of flexion and neutral forearm rotation, causes the muscle to stand out or "bowstring" sharply across

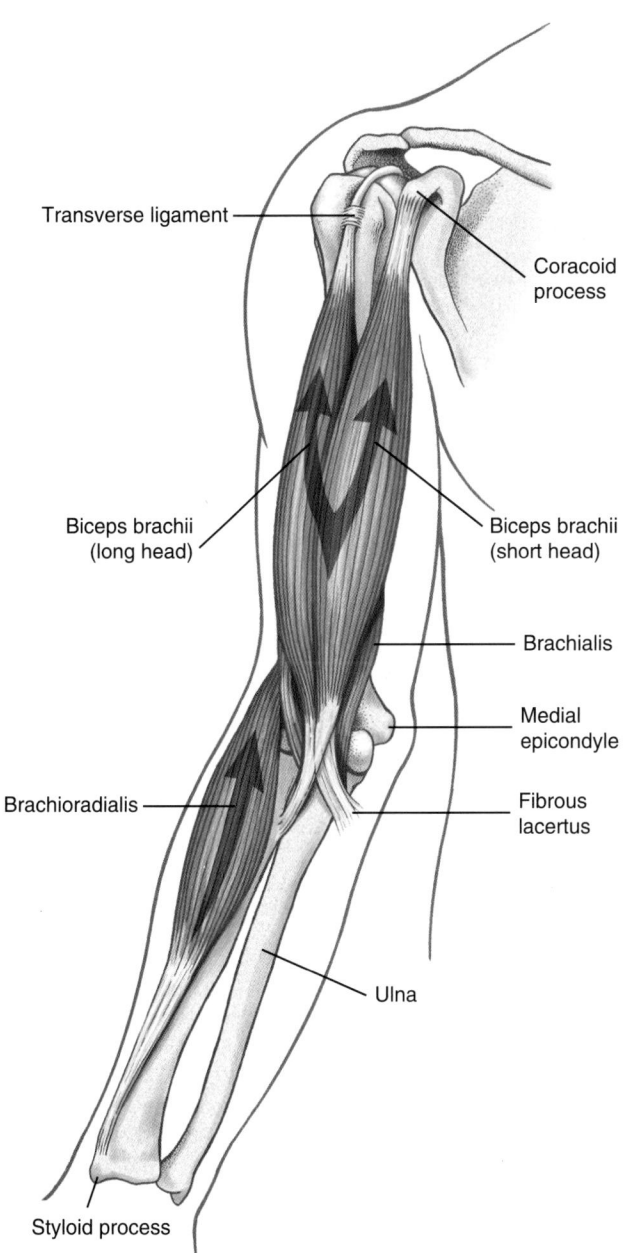

FIGURE 6.31 Anterior view of the right biceps brachii and brachioradialis muscles. The brachialis is deep to the biceps.

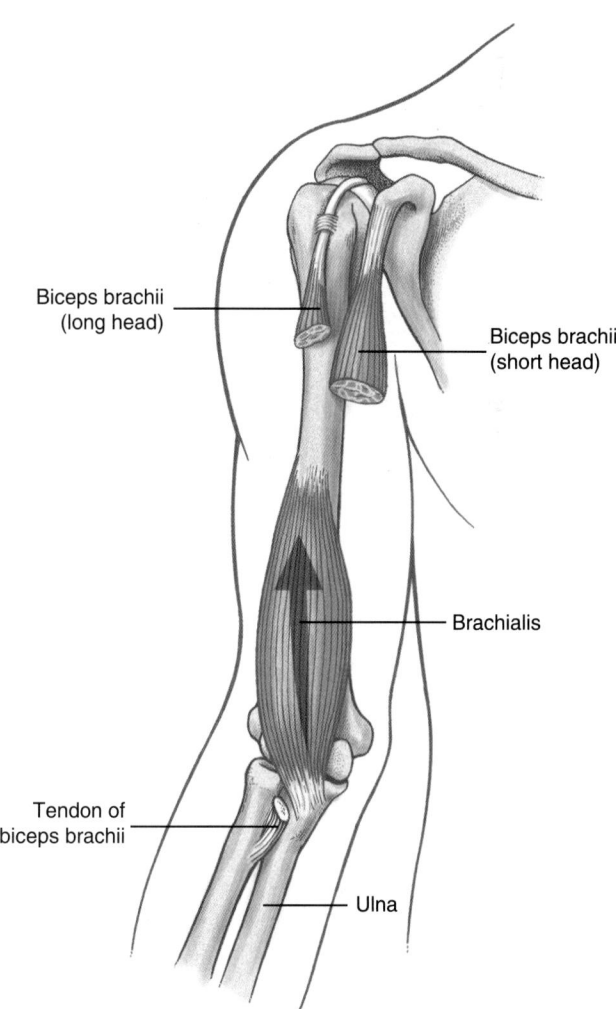

FIGURE 6.32 Anterior view of the right brachialis shown deep to the biceps muscle.

the elbow (Fig. 6.33). The bowstringing of this muscle increases its flexion moment arm to a length that exceeds that of the other flexors[3,87] (see Table 6.5).

The anatomy of the *pronator teres* is described under the section on pronator muscles (see Fig. 6.46). As a point of comparison, the pronator teres has a similar flexor moment arm as the brachialis, but only about 50% of its physiologic cross-sectional area (see Table 6.5).

Torque Generated by the Elbow Flexor Muscles

Fig. 6.34 shows the lines of force of three primary elbow flexors. Maximal-effort flexion torques of 725 kg-cm for men and 336 kg-cm for women have been reported for healthy middle-aged persons (Table 6.6).[8] Like most normative strength data, considerable variation exists within the literature.[56,64] The flexion torque data cited in Table 6.6 suggests that peak flexion torques are about 70% greater than peak extensor torques. In the knee, however, which is functionally analogous to the elbow in the lower extremity, the peak strength differential favors the extensor muscles, by an approximately similar magnitude. This difference likely reflects the greater relative functional demands typically placed on the flexors of the elbow compared with the flexors of the knee.

Elbow flexor torques produced with the forearm supinated are about 20% to 25% greater than those produced with the forearm fully pronated.[85] This difference is due primarily to the increased flexor moment arm of the biceps[72] and the brachioradialis when the forearm is in or approaches supination.

Most of the strength literature reports that maximal flexion torque at the elbow occurs near 85 to 95 degrees of flexion, although this may vary based on age, biologic sex, and methods of

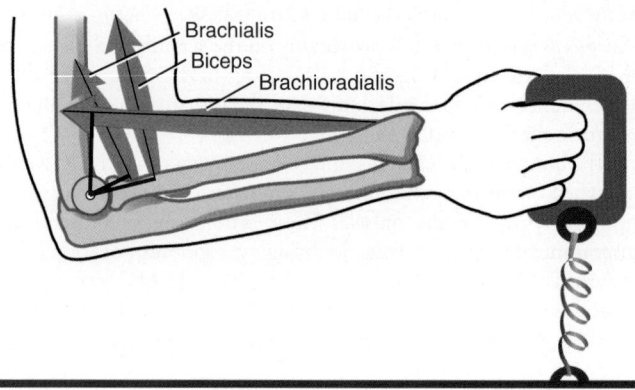

FIGURE 6.34 A lateral view showing the lines of force of three primary elbow flexors. The internal moment arm *(thick dark lines)* for each muscle is drawn to approximate scale. Note that the elbow has been flexed about 100 degrees, placing the biceps tendon at 90 degrees of insertion with the radius. See text for further details. The elbow's medial-lateral axis of rotation is shown piercing the capitulum.

TABLE 6.6 Average Maximal Isometric Internal Torques across the Elbow and Forearm

Movement	Torque (kg-cm)*	
	Males	**Females**
Flexion	725 (154)†	336 (80)
Extension	421 (109)	210 (61)
Pronation	73 (18)	36 (8)
Supination	91 (23)	44 (12)

Data from Askew LJ, An KN, Morrey BF, et al: Isometric elbow strength in normal individuals, *Clin Orthop Relat Res* 222:261, 1987.
*Conversions: 0.098 Nm/kg-cm.
†Standard deviations are in parentheses. Data are from 104 healthy subjects; average age male = 41 yr, average age female = 45.1 yr. The elbow is maintained in 90 degrees of flexion with neutral forearm rotation. Data are shown for dominant limb only.

SPECIAL FOCUS 6.4

Brachialis: The Workhorse of the Elbow Flexors

In addition to a large cross-sectional area, the brachialis muscle also has the largest volume of all elbow flexors (see Table 6.5). Muscle volume in general can be estimated by recording the volume of water displaced by the muscle or, perhaps more precisely, through MRI, CT, or ultrasound imaging. Large muscle volume suggests that the muscle has a large *work capacity*. For this reason, the brachialis has been called the "workhorse" of the elbow flexors.[11] This name is due in part to the muscle's large work capacity, but also to its active involvement in all types of elbow flexion activities, whether performed quickly or slowly or combined with pronation or supination. Because the brachialis attaches distally to the ulna, the motion of pronation or supination has no influence on its length, line of force, or internal moment arm.

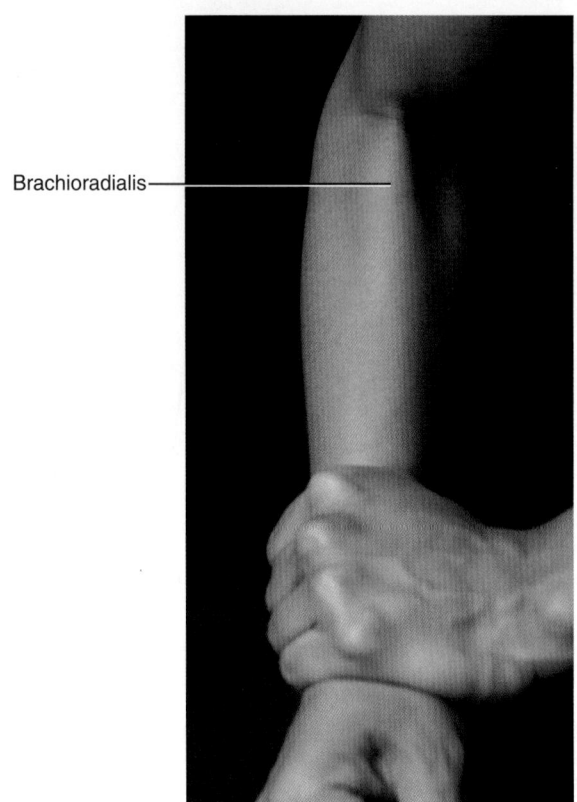

FIGURE 6.33 The right brachioradialis muscle is shown "bowstringing" over the elbow during a maximal-effort isometric activation.

Brachioradialis

testing.[40,84,102] Physiologic and biomechanical factors can help explain why the peak (isometric) flexion torque at the elbow tends to occur near 90 degrees of flexion. To explain, consider Fig. 6.35A, which shows a graph of the predicted relative torques produced by the three primary elbow flexor muscles across a full range of motion. The two primary factors responsible for the overall shape of the maximal torque-angle curve of the elbow flexors are (1) the muscle's maximal flexion *force* potential and (2) the internal *moment arm*

length. The data plotted in Fig. 6.35B predict that the maximal force of all muscles occurs at a muscle length that corresponds to about 80 degrees of flexion. The data plotted in Fig. 6.35C predict that the average maximal moment arm of all three muscles occurs at about 100 degrees of flexion. At about this joint angle, the insertion of the biceps tendon to the radius is near 90 degrees (see Fig. 6.34). This mechanical condition maximizes the internal moment arm of a muscle and thereby maximizes the conversion of a muscle force to

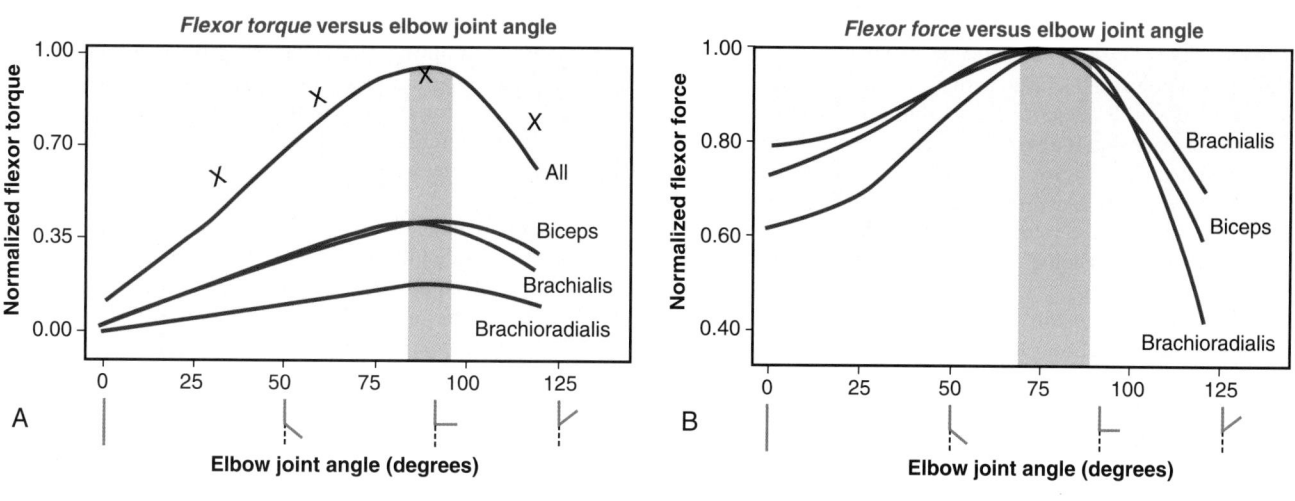

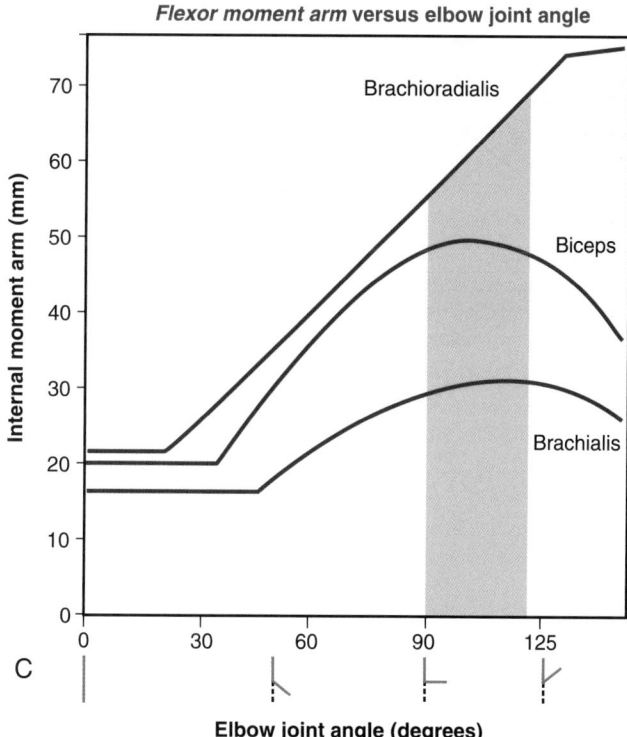

FIGURE 6.35 (A) Predicted maximal isometric *torque* versus joint angle curves for three primary elbow flexors based on a theoretical model that incorporates each muscle's architecture, length-tension relationship, and internal moment arm. (B) The length-tension relationships of the three muscles are shown as a normalized *flexor force* plotted against elbow joint angle. Note that muscle length decreases as joint angle increases. (C) The length of each muscle's *internal moment arm* is plotted against the elbow joint angle. The joint angle where each predicted variable is greatest is shaded in red. (Data for panels A and B from An KN, Kaufman KR, Chao EY: Physiological considerations of muscle force through the elbow joint, *J Biomech* 22:1249, 1989. Data for panel C from Amis AA, Dowson D, Wright V: Muscle strengths and musculoskeletal geometry of the upper limb, *Eng Med* 8:41, 1979.)

a joint torque. It is interesting that the data presented in Fig. 6.35B–C predict peak *torques* across generally similar joint angles. The natural ability to produce maximal elbow flexion torque at about 90 degrees of flexion functionally corresponds to the angle at which the greatest *external* torque (due to gravity) typically acts against the forearm, at least while standing or being in an upright sitting position. The relative "matching" of peak internal and external torques at similar elbow flexion angles is a factor used in the design of resistive exercise paradigms to strengthen the elbow flexor muscles. This concept was explored in Chapter 4.

Polyarticular Biceps Brachii: A Physiologic Advantage of Combining Elbow Flexion with Shoulder Extension

The biceps is a polyarticular muscle that produces force across multiple joints. As will be described, combining active elbow flexion with shoulder extension is a natural and effective way for producing biceps-generated elbow flexor torque. Consider the many examples of using this combination of movements, such as when sawing wood or pulling an object close to the body. The following hypothetical example proposes a physiologic mechanism that favors this natural movement combination.

For the sake of discussion, assume that at rest in the anatomic position the biceps is about 30 cm long (Fig. 6.36A). The biceps

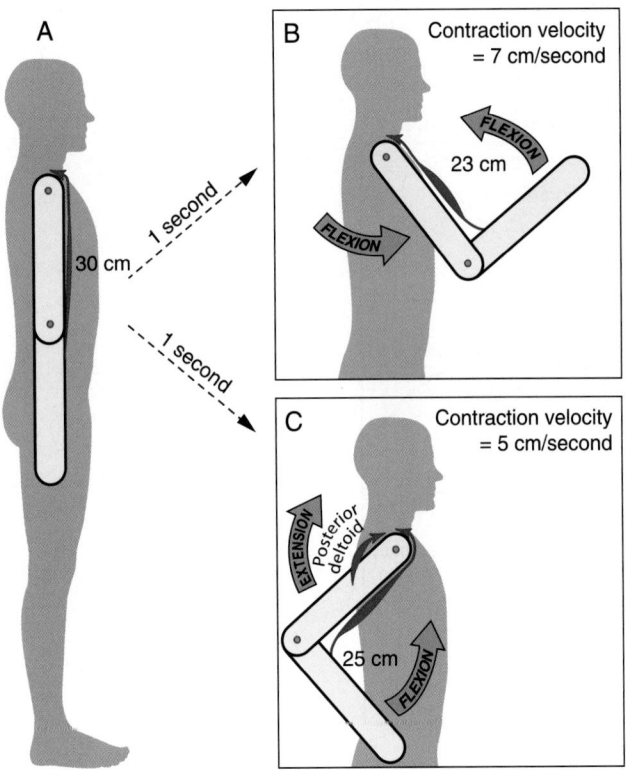

FIGURE 6.36 (A) This model shows a person with a 30-cm long biceps muscle. (B) After a 1-sec contraction, the biceps has contracted to a length of 23 cm, causing a simultaneous motion of 90 degrees of *elbow flexion* and 45 degrees of *shoulder flexion*. The biceps has shortened at a contraction velocity of 7 cm/sec. (C) The biceps *and* posterior deltoid are shown active in a typical pulling motion, which combines the simultaneous motions of 90 degrees of *elbow flexion* with 45 degrees of *shoulder extension*. The biceps is depicted as experiencing a net contraction to a length of 25 cm, over a 1-sec interval. Because of the simultaneous contraction of the posterior deltoid, the biceps shortened only 5 cm, at a contraction velocity of 5 cm/sec.

then shortens (contracts) to about 23 cm after an active motion that combines 90 degrees of elbow flexion with 45 degrees of shoulder flexion (see Fig. 6.36B). If the motion took 1 second to perform, the muscle experiences an average contraction velocity of 7 cm/sec. In contrast, consider a more natural and effective activation pattern involving both the biceps and the posterior deltoid to produce *elbow flexion* with *shoulder extension* (see Fig. 6.36C). During an activity such as pulling a heavy load up toward the side, for example, the activated biceps produces elbow flexion while at the same time it is *elongated across the extending shoulder*. By extending the shoulder, the contracting posterior deltoid, in effect, reduces the net shortening of the biceps. Based on the example in Fig. 6.36C, combining elbow flexion with shoulder extension reduces the average contraction velocity of the biceps to 5 cm/sec. This is 2 cm/sec slower than combining elbow flexion with shoulder flexion. As described in Chapter 3, the maximal force output of a muscle is greater when its contraction velocity is closer to zero, or near isometric.

The simple model described here illustrates one of many examples in which a one-joint muscle, such as the posterior deltoid, can enhance the force potential of another polyarticular muscle. In the example, the posterior deltoid serves as a powerful shoulder extensor for a vigorous pulling motion. In addition, the posterior deltoid assists in controlling the optimal contraction velocity and operational length of the biceps throughout the elbow flexion motion. The posterior deltoid, especially during high-power activities, is a very important synergist to the elbow flexors. Consider the consequences of performing the lift described in Fig. 6.36C with total paralysis of the posterior deltoid.

ELBOW EXTENSORS

Muscular Components

The primary elbow extensors are the *triceps brachii* and the *anconeus* (Figs. 6.37 and 6.38). The triceps converge to a common tendon attaching to the olecranon process of the ulna.

The triceps brachii has three heads: long, lateral, and medial. The *long head* has its proximal attachment on the infraglenoid tubercle of the scapula, thereby allowing the muscle to extend and adduct the shoulder. The long head has an extensive volume, exceeding all other muscles of the elbow (Table 6.7).

The *lateral* and *medial heads* of the triceps muscle have their proximal attachments on the humerus, on either side and along the radial groove. The medial head has an extensive proximal attachment on the posterior side of the humerus, occupying a location relatively similar to the brachialis on the bone's anterior side. Some of the more distal fibers of the medial head attach directly into the posterior capsule of the elbow. These fibers may be analogous to the articularis genu muscle at the knee, with a similar function in drawing the capsule taut during extension. Indeed, these muscle fibers at the elbow are often referred to as the *articularis cubiti*.

The *anconeus* is a small triangular muscle spanning the posterior side of the elbow. The muscle is located between the lateral epicondyle of the humerus and a strip of bone along the posterior aspect of the proximal ulna (see Fig. 6.37). Differing opinions can be found in the literature on the function of the anconeus in humans.[23] Compared with the triceps muscle, the anconeus has a relatively small cross-sectional area and a small moment arm for extension (see Table 6.7). Although the anconeus produces only about 15% of the total extension torque across the elbow,[109] its slow-twitch (type I) fiber type is ideal for providing relatively sustained, albeit low-level

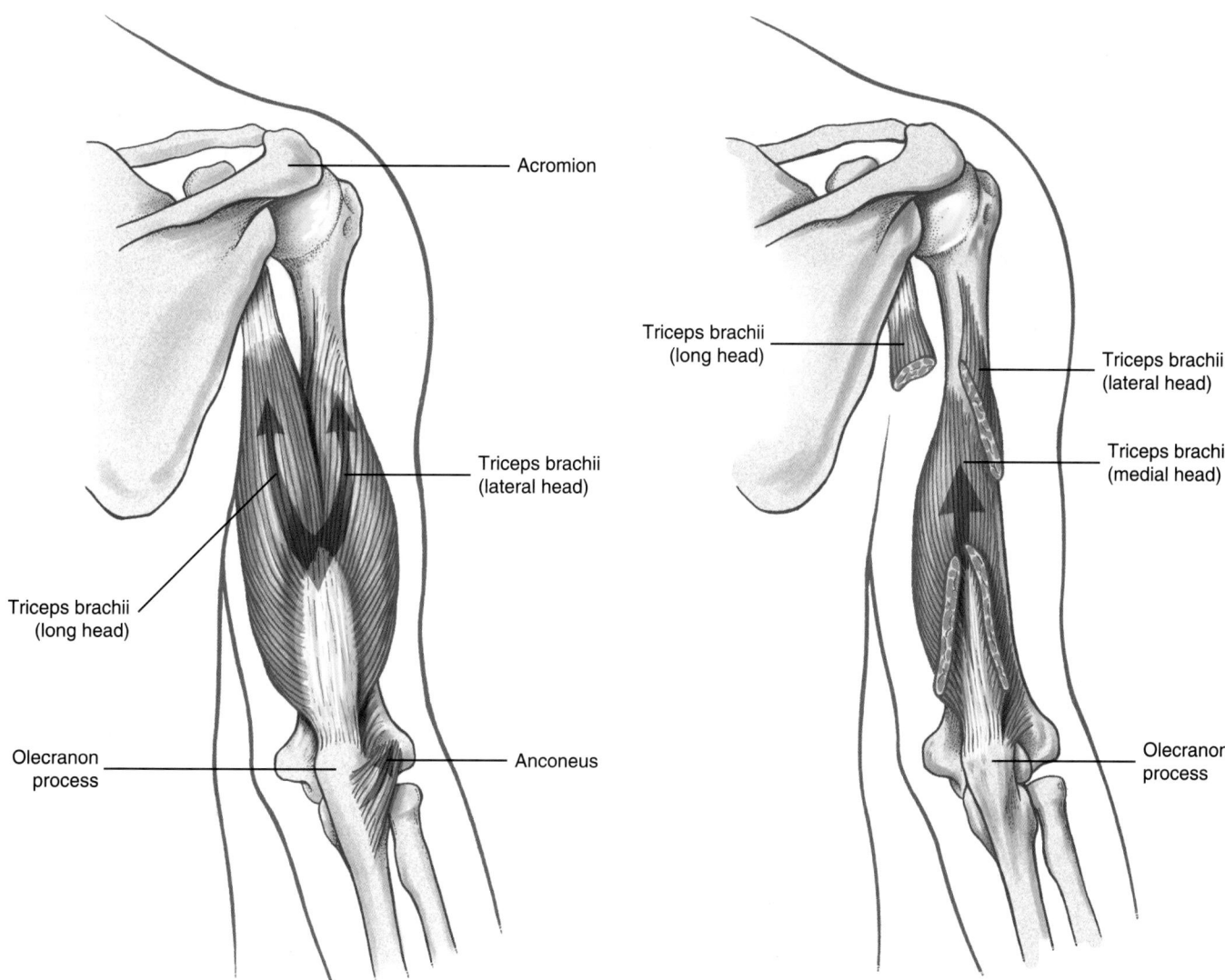

FIGURE 6.37 A posterior view shows the right triceps brachii and anconeus muscles. The medial head of the triceps is deep to the long and lateral heads and therefore not entirely visible.

FIGURE 6.38 A posterior view shows the right medial head of the triceps brachii. The long head and lateral head of the triceps are partially removed to expose the deeper medial head. The anconeus is not illustrated.

TABLE 6.7	**Structural and Related Biomechanical Variables of the Primary Elbow Extensor Muscles***			
	Work Capacity	**Contraction Excursion**	**Peak Force**	**Leverage**
Muscle	*Volume (cm³)*	*Length (cm)*†	*Physiologic Cross-sectional Area (cm²)*	*Internal Moment Arm (cm)*‡
Triceps brachii (long head)	66.6	10.2	6.7	1.87
Triceps brachii (medial head)	38.7	6.3	6.1	1.87
Triceps brachii (lateral head)	47.3	8.4	6.0	1.87
Anconeus	6.7	2.7	2.5	0.72

Data from An KN, Hui FC, Morrey BF, et al: Muscles across the elbow joint: a biomechanical analysis, *J Biomech* 14:659, 1981.
*Structural properties are indicated by italics. The related biomechanical variables are indicated in boldface type.
†Muscle belly length measured at 70 degrees of flexion.
‡Internal moment arm measured with elbow flexed to 100 degrees.

stability about the elbow. This function may help brace the humero-ulnar joint during active pronation and supination.[10,13]

The anconeus has a similar topographic orientation at the elbow as the oblique fibers of the vastus medialis have at the knee. This orientation is best appreciated by visually internally rotating the upper limb by 180 degrees, such that the olecranon faces anteriorly—a position more structurally and functionally analogous to the lower limb.

Electromyographic Analysis of Elbow Extension

Maximal-effort elbow extension generates high levels of EMG activity from all components of the elbow extensor group. During sub-maximal efforts of elbow extension, however, different parts of muscles are recruited only at certain levels of effort. The anconeus is usually the first muscle to initiate and maintain low levels of elbow extension force.[46,58,59,109] As extensor effort gradually increases, the medial head of the triceps is usually next in line to join the anconeus.[101] Because the medial head remains active throughout most levels of elbow extension, it may be considered the "workhorse" of the extensors, functioning as the extensor counterpart to the brachialis.[39]

Only after extensor demands at the elbow increase to moderate-to-high levels does the nervous system recruit the lateral head of the triceps, followed closely by the long head.[109] The long head functions as a "reserve" elbow extensor, equipped with a large volume suited for tasks that require high work performance.

Torque Generation by the Elbow Extensors

The elbow extensor muscles respond to many levels and types of functional demands. The muscles provide static stability to the elbow, similar to the way the quadriceps muscles are often used to stabilize the knee. Consider the common posture of bearing weight through the upper limb with elbows held partially flexed. The extensors stabilize the flexed elbow through isometric contraction or very low–velocity eccentric activation. In contrast, these same muscles are required to generate much larger and dynamic extensor torques through high-velocity concentric or eccentric activations. Consider activities such as throwing a ball, "breaking" a fall to the ground, or rapidly pushing open a door.

As with many explosive pushing activities, elbow extension is typically combined with some degree of shoulder flexion (Fig. 6.39). The shoulder flexion function of the anterior deltoid is an important synergistic component of the forward push. The anterior deltoid produces a shoulder flexion torque that drives the limb forward and neutralizes the shoulder extension potential of the long head of the triceps. From a physiologic perspective, combining

FIGURE 6.39 The triceps muscle is shown generating an extensor torque across the elbow to rapidly push open a door. Note that the elbow is extending as the anterior deltoid is flexing the shoulder. The anterior deltoid must oppose and exceed the shoulder extensor torque produced by the long head of the triceps. See text for further description. The internal moment arms are shown as bold lines originating at the joints' axes of rotation.

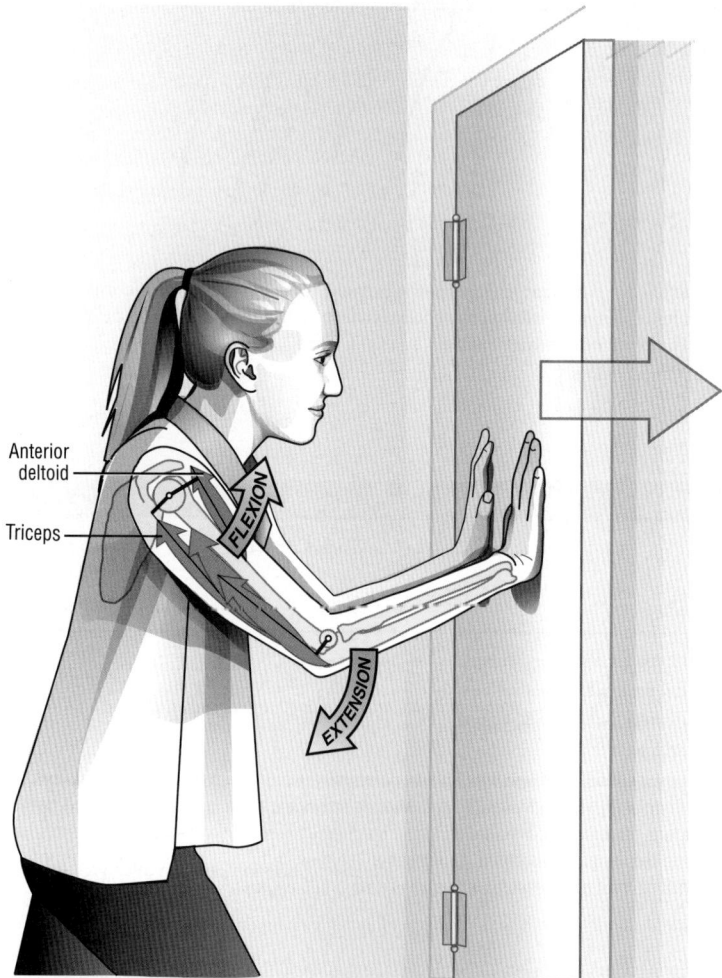

shoulder flexion with elbow extension minimizes the rate and amount of shortening required by the long head of the triceps to completely extend the elbow.

The elbow extensor muscles produce maximal-level torque when the elbow is flexed to about 80 to 90 degrees.[29,44,56,80,85] This joint position is similar to where the elbow flexor muscles, as a group, produce their maximum-flexion torque. Strong isometric coactivation of the elbow flexor and extensor muscles in a position near 90 degrees of flexion therefore produces a very stable fixed posture at the elbow. Such an isometric posture is often assumed naturally during activities that require a strong and rigid elbow, such as "arm wrestling" or using certain hand tools. Of interest, although both muscle groups produce peak, maximal-effort torques across similar joint angles, the largest internal moment arms for the two groups occur at very *different* joint angles: about 100 degrees of flexion for the elbow flexors (see Fig. 6.35C) and relatively close to full extension for the triceps (Fig. 6.40A).[98] The position of elbow extension increases the moment arm for the triceps because it places the thick olecranon process between the joint's axis of rotation and the line of force of the muscle's tendon (Fig. 6.40B–C). The fact that peak elbow extensor *torque* occurs at about 80 to 90 degrees of flexion instead of near extension suggests that muscle length may be more influential than moment arm (leverage) in determining where peak elbow extension torque naturally occurs in the range of motion.

SPECIAL FOCUS 6.5

Law of Parsimony

The hierarchic recruitment pattern described by the actions of the various members of the elbow extensors is certainly not the only strategy used by the nervous system to modulate the levels of extensor torque. As with most active movements, the pattern of muscle activation varies greatly from muscle to muscle and from person to person. It appears, however, that a general hierarchic recruitment pattern exists for the elbow extensors. This method of muscle group activation may be described as the *law of parsimony*. In the present context, the law of parsimony states that the nervous system tends to activate the fewest muscles or muscle fibers possible for the control of a given joint action. Recall that it is the responsibility of the small anconeus and medial head of the triceps to control activities that require lower-level extensor torque. Not until more dynamic or highly resisted extensor torque is needed does the nervous system select the larger, polyarticular, long head of the triceps. This hierarchic pattern of muscle recruitment makes practical sense from an energy perspective. Consider, for example, the inefficiency of having only the long head of the triceps, instead of the anconeus or medial head of the triceps, performing very low–level maintenance types of stabilization functions at the elbow. Additional muscular forces would be required from shoulder flexors, assuming gravitation forces are inadequate, to neutralize the undesired shoulder extension potential of the long head of the triceps. A simple task would require greater muscle activity than what is absolutely necessary. In general, as electromyographic evidence and general intuition suggest, tasks with low-level force demands are associated with relatively low "neural drive",[74] often involving dominant activation of the one-joint muscles.[46,100,109] As force demands increase, larger polyarticular muscles are recruited, along with the necessary neutralizer muscles.

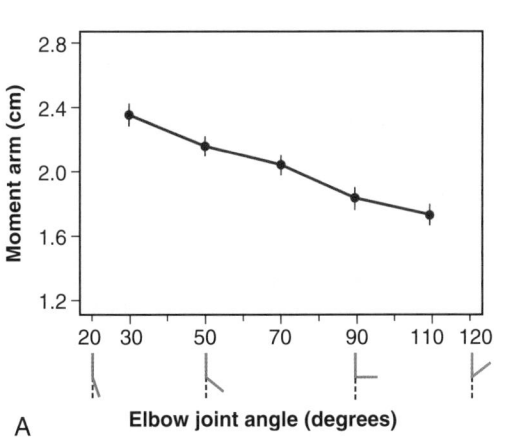

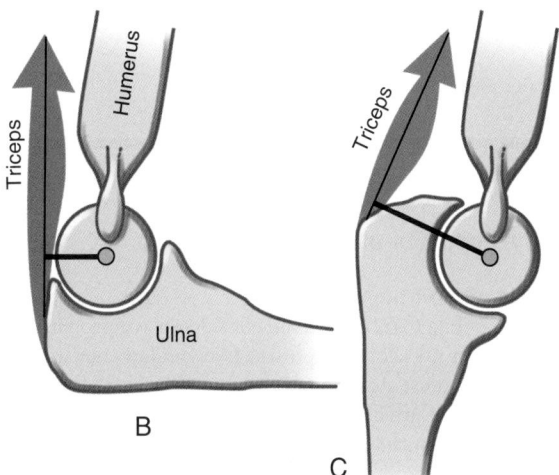

FIGURE 6.40 The extension moment arm of the triceps is plotted across multiple elbow joint angles (A). An anatomic model shows how the shape of the proximal ulna causes the moment arm to be less in 90 degrees of flexion (B) and more in near extension (C). The moment arm increases near extension because the olecranon process extends the distance between the axis of rotation and the perpendicular intersection with the line of force of the triceps. The moment arms are shown as thick black lines. See text for source of data.

Using Shoulder Muscles to Substitute for Triceps Paralysis

Cervical spine injury may result in C^6 tetraplegia (quadriplegia), with loss of motor and sensory function below the C^6 nerve root level. Symptoms may include total paralysis of the trunk and lower extremity muscles with partial paralysis of the upper extremity muscles. Because of the sparing of certain muscles innervated by C^6 and above, persons with this level of tetraplegia may still be able to perform many independent functional activities. Examples are moving to the sitting position from being supine, dressing, and transferring between a wheelchair and bed. Therapists who specialize in mobility training for persons with tetraplegia design movement strategies that allow an innervated muscle to substitute for part of the functional loss imposed by a paralyzed muscle.[75] This art of "muscle substitution" is an essential component to maximizing the movement efficiency in a person with paralysis.

Persons with C^6 tetraplegia have marked or total paralysis of their elbow extensors because these muscles receive most of their nerve root innervation below C^6. Loss of elbow extension reduces the ability to reach away from the body. In addition, activities such as sitting up in bed or transferring to and from a wheelchair become very difficult and labor intensive. A valuable method of muscle substitution uses innervated proximal shoulder muscles, such as the clavicular head of the pectoralis major and/or the anterior deltoid, to actively extend and lock the elbow (Fig. 6.41). This ability of a proximal muscle to extend the elbow requires that the hand be firmly fixed distally to some object. Under these circumstances, contraction of the shoulder musculature adducts and/or horizontally flexes the glenohumeral joint, pulling the humerus toward the midline. Controlling the stability of the elbow by using more proximal musculature is a very useful clinical concept. This concept also applies to the lower limb, as the hip extensors are able to extend the partially flexed knee even in the absence of the quadriceps muscle, as long as the foot is firmly fixed to the ground.

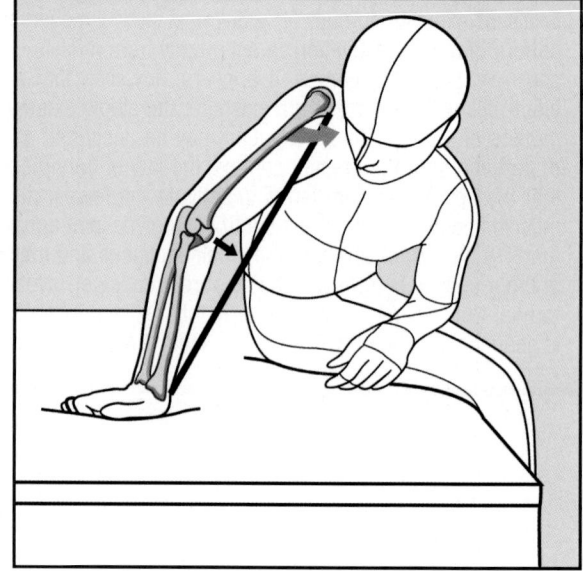

FIGURE 6.41 A depiction of a person with C^6 tetraplegia using the innervated clavicular portion of the pectoralis major and anterior deltoid *(red arrow)* to pull the humerus toward the midline. With the wrist and hand fixed to the bed, the muscles rotate the elbow into extension. Once locked into extension, the stable elbow allows the entire limb to accept weight without buckling at its middle link. The model in the illustration is assumed to have total paralysis of the triceps.

Function of the Supinator and Pronator Muscles

The lines of force of most pronator and supinator muscles of the forearm are shown in Fig. 6.42. To be even considered as a pronator or a supinator, a given muscle must possess two fundamental features. *First,* the muscle must attach on *both* sides of the axis of rotation—that is, a proximal attachment on the humerus or the ulna and a distal attachment on the radius or the hand. Muscles such as the brachialis or extensor pollicis brevis therefore cannot pronate or supinate the forearm, regardless of any other biomechanical variable. *Second,* the muscle must produce a force that acts with an *internal moment arm* about the axis of rotation for pronation and supination. The muscle's moment arm is greatest if its line of force is perpendicular to the axis of rotation. Although no pronator or supinator muscle (at least when considered in the anatomic position) has such an ideal line of force, the pronator quadratus comes close (see Fig. 6.42B).

Pronation and supination of the forearm are functionally associated with internal and external rotation at the shoulder. Shoulder internal rotation often occurs with pronation, whereas shoulder external rotation often occurs with supination. Combining these shoulder and forearm rotations allows the hand to rotate nearly 360 degrees in space, rather than only 170 to 180 degrees by pronation and supination alone.

When forearm muscle strength and range of motion are tested clinically, care must be taken to eliminate contributing motion or torque that has originated from the shoulder. To accomplish this, forearm pronation and supination are tested with the elbow held

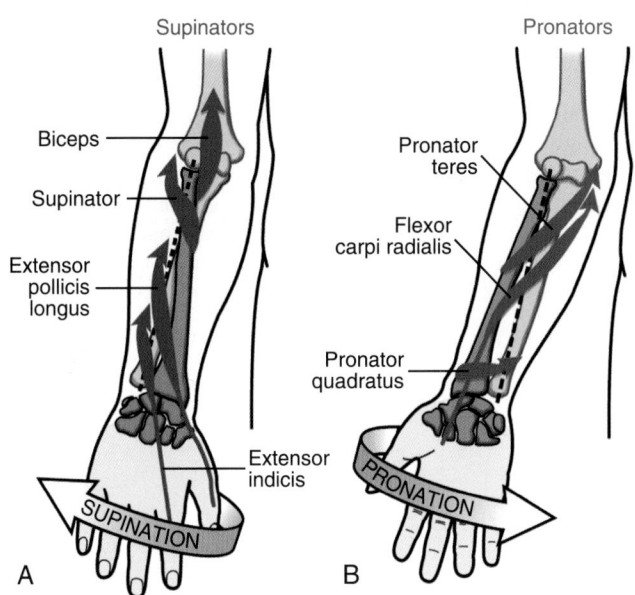

FIGURE 6.42 The line of force of supinators (A) and pronators (B) of the forearm. Note the degree to which all muscles intersect the forearm's axis of rotation *(dashed line)*.

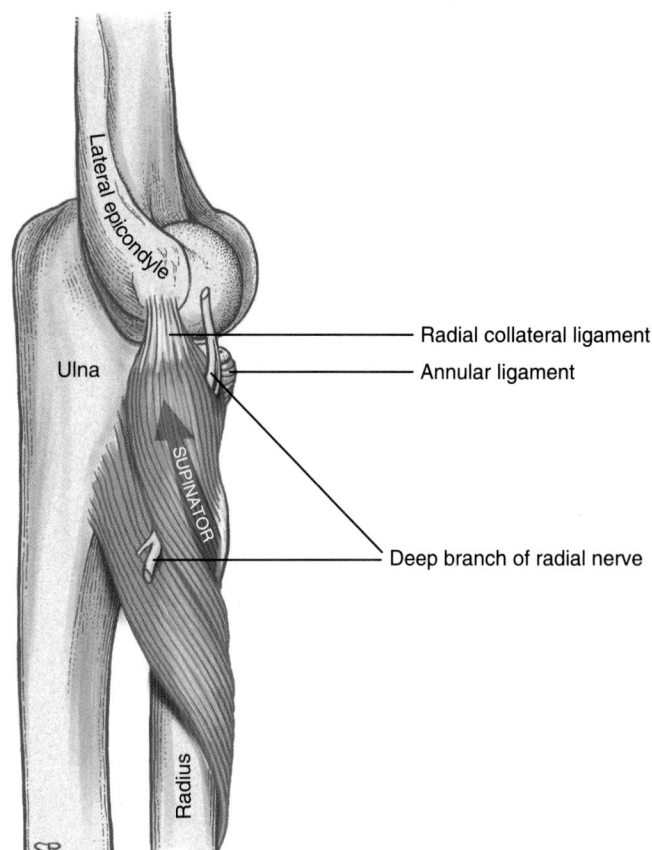

FIGURE 6.43 A lateral view of the right supinator muscle. The deep branch of the radial nerve is shown exiting between the superficial and deep fibers of the muscle. The radial nerve courses distally, as the posterior interosseous nerve, to innervate the finger and thumb extensors.

flexed to 90 degrees, with the medial epicondyle of the humerus pressed against the side of the body. In this position any undesired rotation at the shoulder is easily detected.

SUPINATOR MUSCLES

The primary supinator muscles are the *supinator* and *biceps brachii* (Fig. 6.42A). Secondary supinator muscles include the radial wrist extensors, which attach near the lateral epicondyle of the humerus, the extensor pollicis longus, and the extensor indicis. Although the moment arms of these secondary supinator muscles are small, they peak as the forearm moves closer to full supination. (Interestingly, with the forearm fully pronated, the extensor pollicis longus may actually possess a 1 mm moment arm to *pronate* the forearm.)[18]

The specific forearm function of the brachioradialis has long been debated, and some controversy persists. Consensus however is that the brachioradialis is a secondary supinator *and* a secondary pronator.[11,18,39,87] Regardless of the position of the forearm, muscle contraction rotates the forearm *toward* the neutral, thumb-up position. From a pronated position, therefore, the muscle supinates; from a supinated position, the muscle pronates. It is interesting that contraction of the brachioradialis rotates the forearm to a position between full supination and full pronation: the same position that also maximizes the muscle's moment arm as an elbow flexor.

PRIMARY SUPINATOR MUSCLES
- Supinator
- Biceps brachii

SECONDARY SUPINATOR MUSCLES
- Radial wrist extensors
- Extensor pollicis longus
- Extensor indicis
- Brachioradialis (from a pronated position)

Supinator versus Biceps Brachii

The *supinator muscle* has an extensive proximal muscle attachment (Fig. 6.43). A superficial set of fibers arises from the lateral epicondyle of the humerus and the radial collateral and annular ligaments. A deeper set of fibers arises from the ulna near and along the supinator crest. Both sets of muscle fibers attach distally along the proximal one-third of the radius. When pronated, the supinator muscle is wrapped around the radius, thereby maximizing its leverage to supinate the forearm.[18] The supinator has only minimal attachments to the humerus and passes too close to the medial-lateral axis of rotation at the elbow to produce significant flexion or extension torque.

The supinator muscle is a relentless forearm supinator, like the brachialis during elbow flexion. The supinator muscle generates significant EMG activity during forearm supination, regardless of the elbow angle or the speed or power of the action.[100] The biceps muscle, also a primary supinator, is normally recruited during higher power supination activities, especially those associated with elbow flexion.[27]

The nervous system usually recruits the supinator muscle for low-power tasks that require a supination motion only, while the biceps remains relatively inactive. (This is in accord with the law of parsimony described earlier in this chapter.) Only during moderate- or high-power supination motions does the biceps show significant EMG activity. Using the large polyarticular biceps to perform a simple, low-power supination task is not an efficient motor response.

Additional muscles, such as the triceps and posterior deltoid, would be required to neutralize any undesired biceps action at the shoulder and elbow. A simple movement then becomes increasingly more complicated and more energy-consuming than necessary.

The *biceps brachii* is a powerful supinator of the forearm. The biceps has about three times the physiologic cross-sectional area as the supinator muscle.[60] The dominant role of the biceps as a supinator can be verified by palpating the biceps during a series of rapid and forceful pronation-to-supination motions, especially with the elbow flexed to about 90 degrees. As the supinated forearm rotates toward pronation, the biceps tendon wraps around the proximal radius, and thus enhances its leverage to actively "unwrap" the radius back toward supination.[92]

The effectiveness of the biceps as a supinator is greatest when the elbow is flexed to about 90 degrees.[18] For this reason, the elbow is naturally held flexed to about 90 degrees during many high-powered supination tasks. At a 90-degree elbow angle, the tendon of the biceps approaches a 90-degree angle-of-insertion into the radius. This biomechanical situation allows essentially the *entire* magnitude of a maximal-effort biceps force to intersect

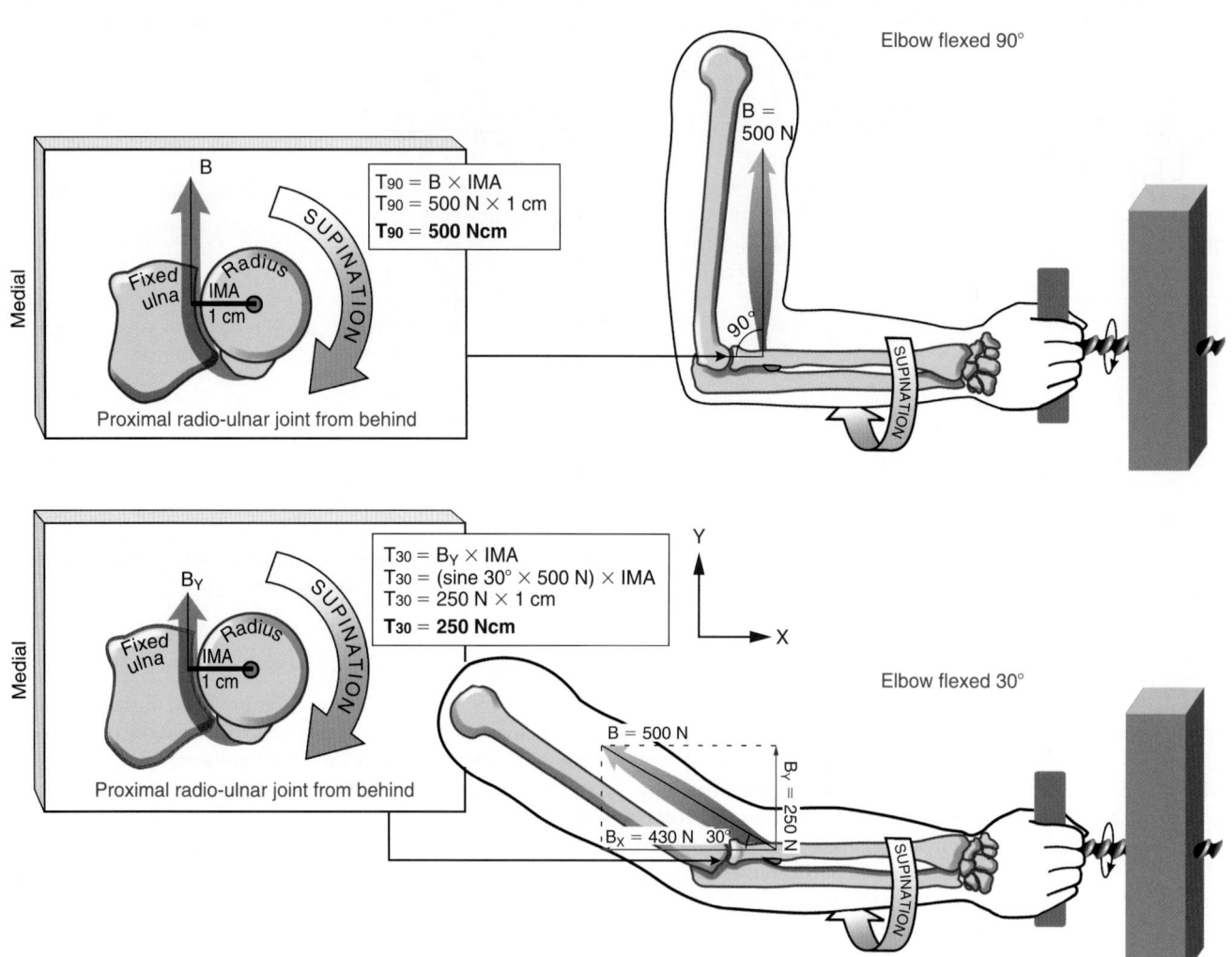

FIGURE 6.44 The difference in the mechanical ability of the biceps to produce a supination torque is estimated when the elbow is flexed 90 degrees and when the elbow is flexed 30 degrees. (Top) Lateral view shows the biceps attaching to the radius at a 90-degree angle. The muscle (B) is contracting to supinate the forearm with a maximal-effort force of 500 N. As shown from a superior view, 100% of the biceps force can be multiplied by the estimated 1-cm internal moment arm available for supination, producing 500 Ncm of torque (500 N × 1 cm). (Bottom) Lateral view shows that when the elbow is flexed to 30 degrees, the angle-of-insertion of the biceps to the radius is reduced to about 30 degrees. This change in angle reduces the force that the biceps can use to supinate (i.e., that generated perpendicular to the radius) to 250 N (B_Y). An even larger force component of the biceps, labeled B_X, is directed proximally through the radius in a direction nearly parallel with the forearm's axis of rotation. This force component has essentially no moment arm to supinate. The calculations show that the maximum supination torque with the elbow flexed 30 degrees is reduced to 250 Ncm (250 N × 1 cm) (sine 30 degrees = 0.5, and cosine 30 degrees = 0.86).

nearly perpendicular to the axis of rotation of the forearm. When the elbow is flexed to only 30 degrees, for example, the tendon of the biceps loses its right-angle intersection with the axis of rotation. As depicted by the calculations shown in Fig. 6.44, this change in angle reduces the mechanical supinator torque potential of the biceps by 50%. Clinically, this difference is important when evaluating the torque output from a strength-testing apparatus, designing resistive exercises, or providing advice about ergonomics.

When high-power supination torque is required to vigorously turn a screw, for example, the biceps is recruited by the nervous system to assist other muscles, such as the smaller supinator muscle and extensor pollicis longus. For reasons described previously, this task typically requires that the elbow be held flexed to about 90 degrees (Fig. 6.45). Maintaining this elbow posture during the task requires that the triceps muscle co-contract synchronously with the biceps muscle. The triceps muscle supplies an essential force during this activity because it prevents the biceps from flexing the elbow and shoulder during every supination effort. Unopposed biceps action would cause the screwdriver to be pulled away from the screw on every effort—hardly effective. By attaching to the ulna versus the radius, the triceps can neutralize the elbow flexion tendency of the biceps *without* interfering with the supination task. This muscular cooperation is an excellent example of how two muscles can function as synergists for one activity while at the same time remaining as direct antagonists.

SPECIAL FOCUS 6.7

Supination versus Pronation Torque Potential

According to data published by Askew et al, when averaged across sex, the supinator muscles produce about 23% greater isometric torque than the pronators.[8] Other values have been published from studies using different testing methods and sample demographics and anthropometrics but, in several comparable studies, the strength of the supinator muscles exceeds that of the pronator muscles.[9] This difference is partially explained by the fact that the supinator muscles possess about twice the physiologic cross-sectional area as the pronator muscles.[60] Many functional activities rely on the relative dominant strength of supination. Consider the activity of using a screwdriver to tighten a screw. When performed by the right hand, a clockwise tightening motion is driven by a contraction of several supinator muscles. The direction of the threads on a standard screw reflects the dominance in strength of the supinator muscles. Unfortunately for the left-hand–dominant person, a clockwise rotation of the left forearm must be performed by the *pronator muscles.* Left-handed persons often use the right hand for this activity, explaining why so many are somewhat ambidextrous.

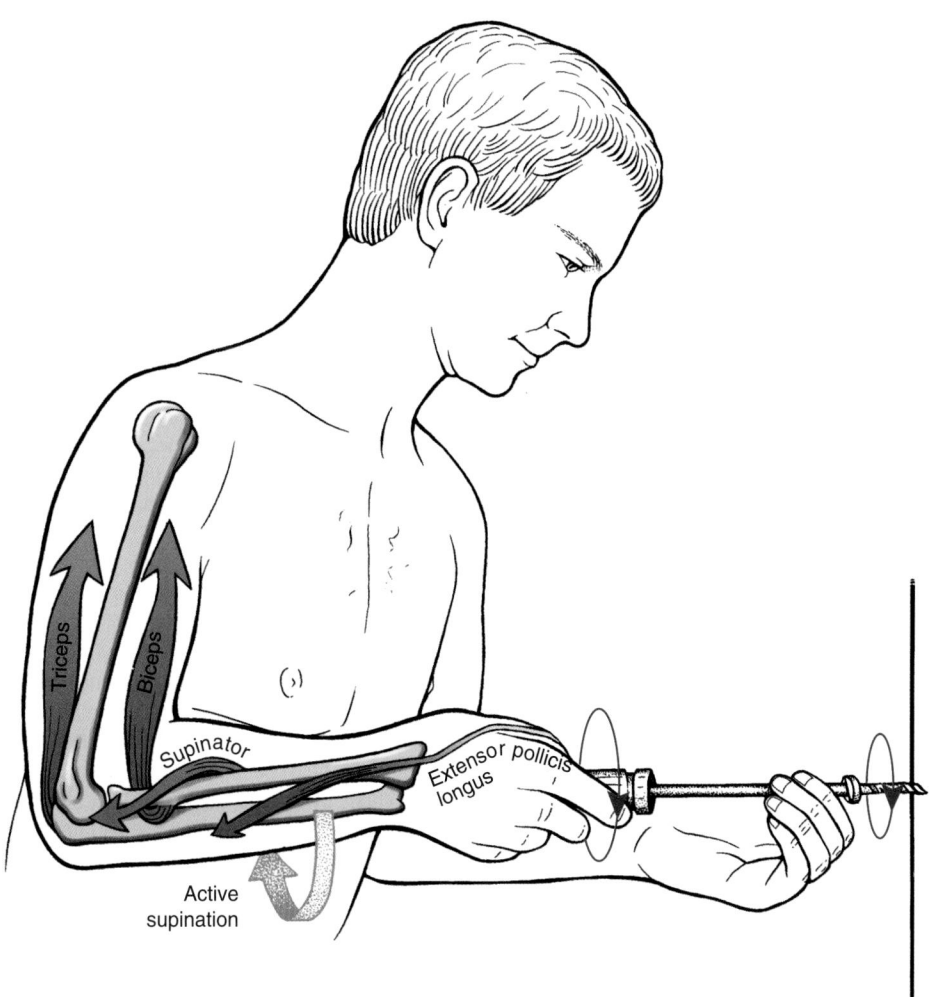

FIGURE 6.45 Vigorous contraction is shown of the biceps, supinator, and extensor pollicis longus to tighten a screw using a clockwise rotation with a screwdriver. The triceps muscle is activated isometrically to neutralize the strong elbow flexion tendency of the biceps. Note that coactivation of the triceps and biceps can help stabilize the glenohumeral joint.

PRONATOR MUSCLES

The primary muscles for pronation are the *pronator teres* and the *pronator quadratus* (Fig. 6.46).[18] The flexor carpi radialis and the palmaris longus are secondary pronators, both attaching to the medial epicondyle of the humerus (see Fig. 6.42B). In general, the pronation moment arms for all the aforementioned pronator muscles peak and remain relatively constant between about 40 degrees of supination and 40 degrees of pronation.[18] As described earlier, the brachioradialis is also a pronator, but only from a starting position of forearm supination.

> **PRIMARY PRONATOR MUSCLES**
> - Pronator teres
> - Pronator quadratus
>
> **SECONDARY PRONATOR MUSCLES**
> - Flexor carpi radialis
> - Palmaris longus
> - Brachioradialis (from a supinated position)

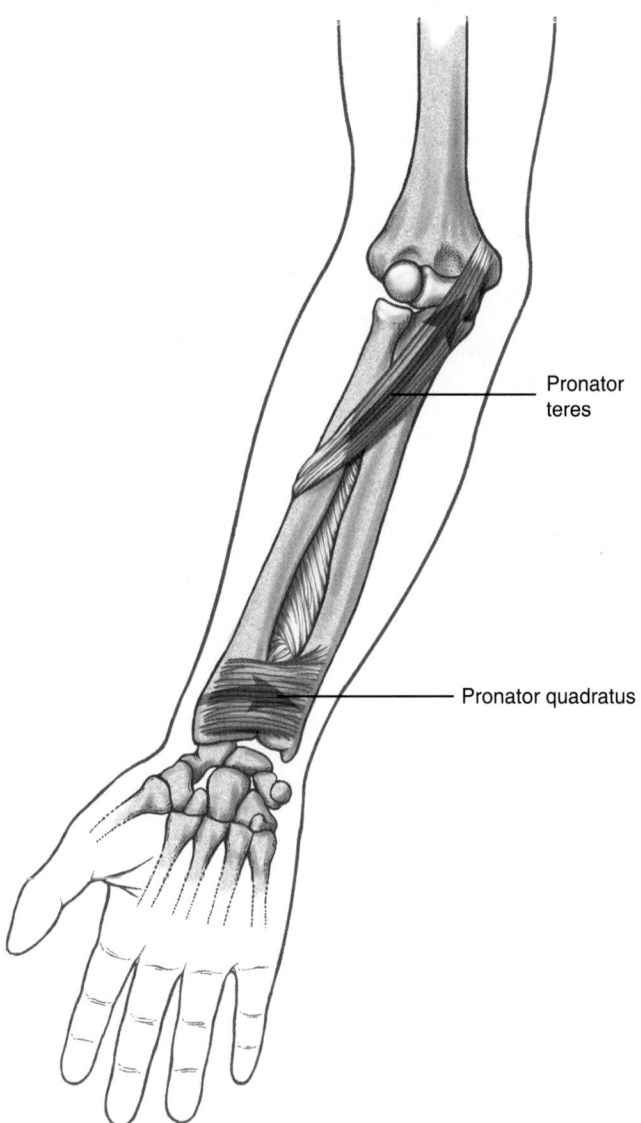

FIGURE 6.46 Anterior view of the right pronator teres and pronator quadratus.

In cases of a lacerated median nerve proximal to the elbow, the pronator teres and quadratus, and most secondary pronators, are typically paralyzed. Consequently, active, full range, pronation is essentially lost. The forearm tends to remain chronically supinated owing to the unopposed action of the innervated supinator and biceps muscles.

Pronator Teres versus Pronator Quadratus

The *pronator teres* has two heads: humeral and ulnar. The median nerve passes between these two heads and therefore is a site for possible nerve compression. The pronator teres functions as a primary forearm pronator, as well as an elbow flexor. This muscle produces its greatest EMG activity during higher-power pronation actions,[12] such as attempting to unscrew an overtightened screw with the right hand or just prior to the release phase of pitching a baseball. The triceps is an important synergist to the pronator teres, often required to neutralize the ability of the pronator teres to flex the elbow.

The *pronator quadratus* is located at the extreme distal end of the anterior forearm, deep to all the wrist flexors and extrinsic finger flexors. This flat, quadrilateral muscle attaches between the anterior surfaces of the distal one-fourth of the ulna and the radius. Overall, from proximal to distal, the pronator quadratus has a slight obliquity in fiber direction, similar to, but not quite as angled as, the pronator teres. Superficial and deep heads of this muscle are evident on cadaver dissection. In general, the pronator quadratus is the most active and consistently used pronator muscle, involved during all pronation movements, regardless of the power demands or the amount of associated elbow flexion.[12]

The pronator quadratus is well designed biomechanically as an effective torque producer and a stabilizer of the distal radio-ulnar joint. The pronator quadratus has a line of force oriented almost perpendicular to the forearm's axis of rotation (Fig. 6.47A). This design maximizes the potential of the muscle to produce torque. In addition to effectively producing a pronation torque, the muscle simultaneously compresses the ulnar notch of the radius directly against the ulnar head (see Fig. 6.47B). This compression force

SPECIAL FOCUS 6.8

A Return to the Law of Parsimony

Low-power activities that involve isolated pronation are generally initiated and controlled by the pronator quadratus. Throughout this chapter, a theme was developed between the function of a one-joint muscle and an associated polyarticular muscle. This hierarchic recruitment of the muscles followed the law of parsimony. At the *elbow,* low-power flexion or extension activities tend to be controlled or initiated by the brachialis, the anconeus, or the medial head of the triceps. Only when relatively high-power actions are required does the nervous system recruit the polyarticular biceps and long head of the triceps. At the *forearm,* low-power supination and pronation activities are controlled by the small supinator or the pronator quadratus; high-power actions require assistance from the biceps and pronator teres. Each time the typically expansive polyarticular muscles are recruited, however, additional muscles are needed to stabilize their undesired actions. Increasing the power of any action at the elbow and forearm creates a sharp disproportionate rise in overall muscle activity. Not only do the one-joint muscles increase their activity, but so do the polyarticular "reserve" muscles and a host of other neutralizer muscles.

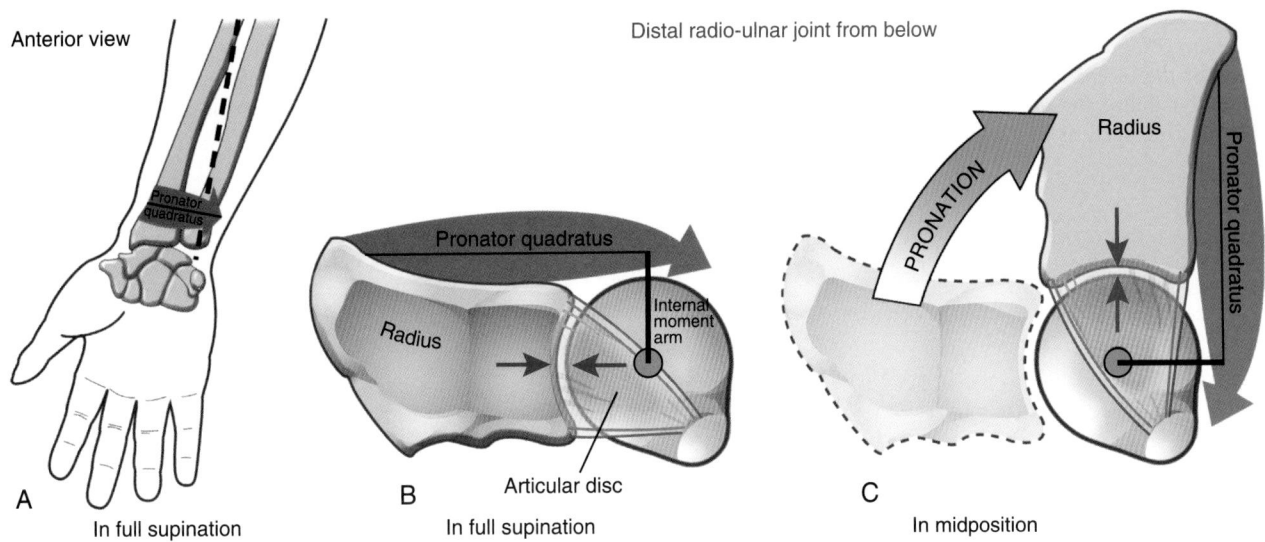

FIGURE 6.47 (A) Anterior view of the distal radio-ulnar joint shows the line of force of the pronator quadratus intersecting the forearm's axis of rotation *(dashed line)* at a near right angle. (B) The line of force of the pronator quadratus, with its internal moment arm, is shown with the carpal bones removed and forearm in full supination. The pronator quadratus produces a pronation torque, which is the product of the pronator muscle's force times the internal moment arm, *and* a compression force between the joint surfaces *(opposing arrows)*. (C) This dual function of the pronator quadratus is shown as the muscle pronates the forearm to the midposition. Also, the articular disc (of the TFCC) is shown as it follows the moving radius from supination (B) toward pronation (C).

stabilizes the distal radio-ulnar joint throughout the range of pronation (see Fig. 6.47C). This active force augments the passive force produced by the articular disc (within the triangular fibrocartilage complex). The force of the pronator quadratus also guides the joint through its natural arthrokinematics.

In the healthy joint, the compression force from the pronator quadratus and other muscles is absorbed by the joint without difficulty. In cases of severe rheumatoid arthritis, the articular cartilage, bone, and periarticular connective tissue lose their ability to adequately absorb joint forces. These myogenic compressive forces can become detrimental to joint stability. The same forces that help stabilize the joint in the healthy state may cause joint destruction in the diseased state.

SYNOPSIS

The shape of the proximal and distal ends of the radius and ulna provides insightful clues to the kinesiology of the regions. The large, C-shaped *proximal end of the ulna* provides a rigid, hinge-like stability to the humero-ulnar joint. The kinematics therefore are limited primarily to the sagittal plane. The rounded head of the *distal end of the ulna* articulates with the concave ulnar notch of the radius to form the distal radio-ulnar joint. Unlike the distal end of the radius, the distal ulna is *not* firmly articulated with the carpal bones. Any firm connection in this region would physically restrict pronation and supination.

The *proximal end of the radius* possesses a disclike head designed primarily to rotate against the capitulum and within the fibro-osseous ring of the proximal radio-ulnar joint. This rotation of the radius is the main kinematic component of pronation and supination. The ulna, in contrast, serves as a stable base for the rotating radius by virtue of its firm linkage to the humerus via the humero-ulnar joint. The relatively large *distal end of the radius* expands in both medial-lateral and anterior-posterior dimensions to accept the proximal row of carpal bones. This expanded surface area provides an excellent path for transmission of forces through the hand to the radius. Based on the prevailing fiber direction of the interosseous membrane, proximally directed forces acting on the radius are ultimately transmitted nearly equally across both medial and lateral compartments of the elbow.

Four major peripheral nerves cross the elbow: musculocutaneous, median, radial, and ulnar. Except for the musculocutaneous nerve, these nerves are injured with relative frequency, causing marked loss of sensory and muscle function distal to the site of trauma. Reduced muscular forces resulting from injury to any one of these nerves create a kinetic imbalance across the joints, which, if untreated, typically lead to deformity.

Essentially all muscles acting primarily on the elbow and forearm have their distal attachment on either the ulna or the radius. Those muscles that attach to the *ulna*—namely the brachialis and triceps—flex or extend the elbow but have no ability to pronate or supinate the forearm. The remaining muscles, in contrast, have their distal attachment on the *radius*. These muscles flex the elbow and, depending on their lines of force, also pronate or supinate the forearm. This anatomic arrangement allows the elbow to actively flex and extend while allowing the forearm to simultaneously pronate or supinate without any biomechanical interference among muscles. This design greatly enhances the ability of the upper extremity to interact with the surrounding environment, during activities that range from feeding, grooming, or preparing food to less refined actions such as thrusting the body upwards from a chair.

About half of the muscles studied in this chapter control multiple regions of the arm or forearm. For this reason, movements that appear quite simple and limited to just one region—such as the forearm, for example—are typically more complex and involve a larger than expected set of participating muscles. Reconsider the forceful biceps-driven supination action required to tighten a screw (previously highlighted in Fig. 6.45). During this task, triceps activation is also required to neutralize the strong (and unwanted) elbow flexion component of the biceps. The co-contraction of the long head of the biceps and triceps muscles must also kinetically balance and stabilize the glenohumeral joint. In addition, axial-scapular muscles, such as the trapezius, rhomboids, and serratus anterior, are needed to stabilize the scapula against the strong pull of the biceps and triceps muscles. Without this stabilization—be it from selective nerve injury, loss of motor control, pain, or simple disuse—the muscles of the elbow and forearm are less effective at performing their tasks.

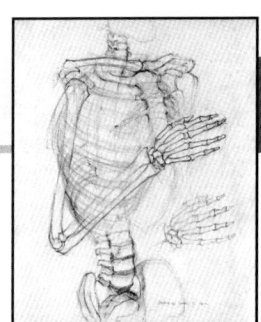

ADDITIONAL CLINICAL CONNECTIONS

CONTENTS

CLINICAL CONNECTION 6.1
Functional Implications of Reduced Elbow Extension

The term *contracture* is typically defined as a permanent tightening of muscular or nonmuscular tissues that restricts normal passive extension. One of the most disabling consequences of an elbow flexion contracture is reduced reaching capacity. As shown in Fig. 6.48, a fully extendable elbow (i.e., with a 0-degree contracture) demonstrates a 0-degree loss in area of forward reach. The area of forward reach diminishes only slightly (less than 6%) with a flexion contracture of less than 30 degrees. A flexion contracture that *exceeds* 30 degrees, however, results in a much greater loss of forward reach. As noted in the graph, a flexion contracture of 90 degrees reduces total reach by almost 50%. Minimizing a flexion contracture to less than 30 degrees can therefore have significant functional implications for patients.

The term joint *contracture* should be distinguished from the term joint *tightness,* which may not necessarily be permanent and

is often successfully treated using conservative therapy. Therapeutics may include reducing inflammation and swelling, positioning the joint in more extension (through using a continuous passive-motion device, serial casting, or static dynamic, or static progressive splinting), using "contract-relax" techniques to neurologically inhibit flexor muscles, suggesting activities or movements that encourage elbow extension, applying a long-duration low-load stretch to structures located on the anterior to the joint's medial-lateral axis of rotation, manually mobilizing the joint and relevant soft tissues, and strengthening muscles that produce elbow extension. If these conservative treatments fail to improve the range of extension then a surgical release may be considered, especially if function is significantly impaired and the condition is considered permanent. The most effective intervention for elbow flexion tightness or contracture is prevention.

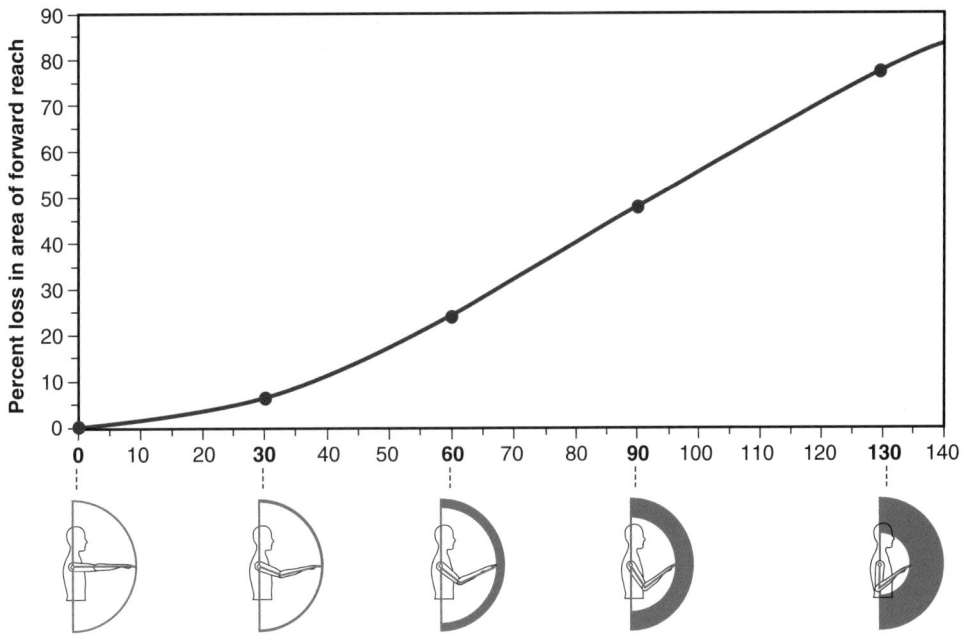

FIGURE 6.48 A graph showing the percent loss in area of forward reach of the arm, from the shoulder to finger, as a function of the severity of an elbow flexion contracture. Note the sharp increase in the reduction in reach as the flexion contracture exceeds 30 degrees. The figures across the bottom of the graph depict the progressive loss of reach, indicated by the increased semicircular area, as the flexion contracture becomes more severe.

Additional Clinical Connections

"Reverse Action" of the Elbow Flexor Muscles

During most typical activities of daily living, contraction of the elbow flexor muscles is performed to rotate the forearm toward the arm. Contraction of the same muscles, however, can rotate the arm *to* the forearm, provided that the distal aspect of the upper extremity is well fixed. A clinical example of the usefulness of such a "reverse contraction" of the elbow flexors is shown for a person with C[6] tetraplegia (Fig. 6.49). The person has complete paralysis of the trunk and lower extremity muscles but near-normal strength of the shoulder, elbow flexor, and wrist extensor muscles. With the distal aspect of the upper limb

well fixed with the assistance of the wrist extensor muscles and a strap, the elbow flexor muscles can generate sufficient force to rotate the *arm toward the forearm*. This maneuver allows the elbow flexor muscles to assist the person in moving up to a sitting position from supine. For this person, coming up to a sitting position is an essential step in preparing for other functional activities, such as dressing or transferring from the bed into a wheelchair.

As expected, the arthrokinematics at the humero-ulnar joint during this action involve a roll-and-slide in *opposite* directions.

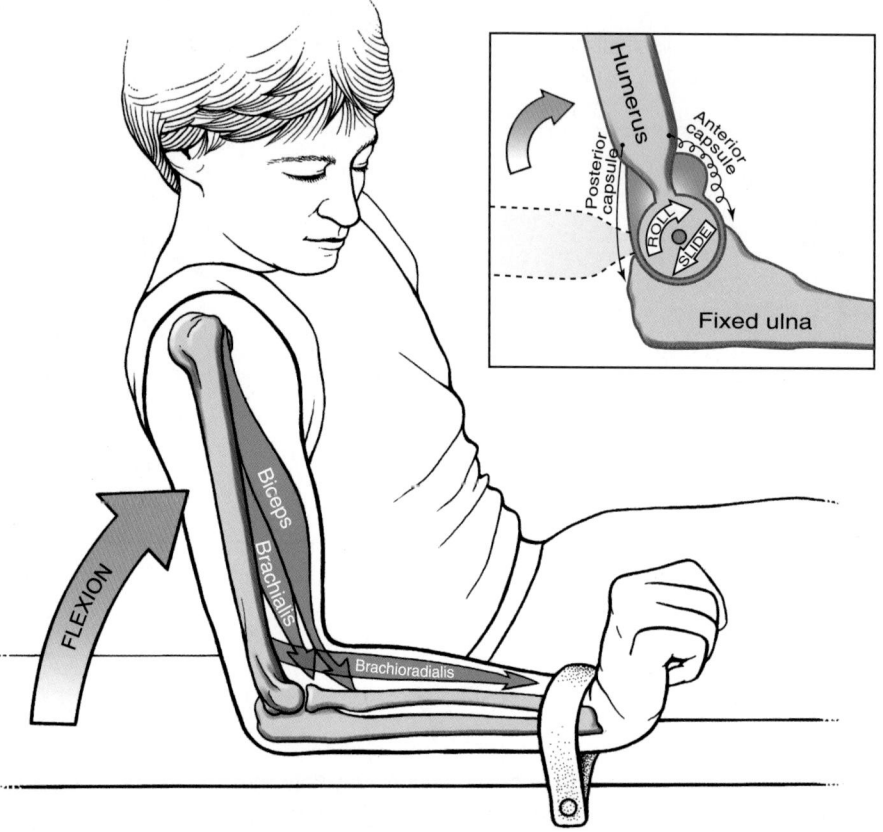

FIGURE 6.49 A person with midlevel tetraplegia using his elbow flexor muscles to flex the elbow and bring his trunk off the mat. Note that the distal forearm is securely stabilized. (Inset) The arthrokinematics at the humero-ulnar joint are shown during this movement. The anterior capsule is in a slackened position, and the posterior capsule is pulled relatively taut.

ADDITIONAL CLINICAL CONNECTIONS

CLINICAL CONNECTION 6.3

A Closer Look at the Distal Attachment of the Biceps Brachii

It has been generally assumed that the long and short heads of the biceps brachii share essentially identical distal attachments to the radius. Careful dissection of nonembalmed cadaveric material, however, has shown a slightly different anatomic picture.[50] Although both tendon bundles attach to the radial tuberosity, the attachment of the short head is slightly more *distal* and *closer to the apex* of the tuberosity than the long head (Fig. 6.50). Each distinct tendon bundle is separated by a thin areolar septum.

Analysis suggests that the different attachment sites of each of the tendon bundles have small but potentially relevant biomechanical implications. The tendon of the short head was found to have a greater internal moment arm for flexion based on its more distal attachment relative to the medial-lateral axis of rotation at the elbow. When equal muscle forces were experimentally passed through each tendon (with the elbow flexed to 90 degrees), the short head produced 15% greater elbow flexion torque than the

long head. Furthermore, because the tendon of the short head was found to attach closer to the raised apex of the radial tuberosity, it has a slightly greater moment arm for the production of forearm supination torque than the long head (when tested in neutral and pronated forearm positions). With equal forces passed through each tendon bundle, the short head produced an average of about 10% greater supination torque than the long head, depending on forearm position.

The relatively small difference in attachment sites (and hence differing biomechanics) between the two heads of the biceps is not likely important in ordinary clinical situations. However, the relatively small anatomic differences may be significant to the surgeon who is reattaching the tendon following a distal rupture of the biceps tendon. Respecting the precise anatomic detail may help optimize the functional results of the surgery.[92]

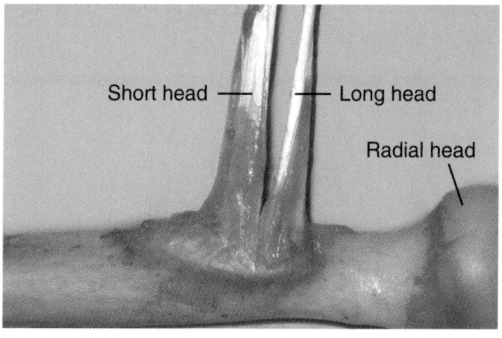

FIGURE 6.50 Photograph of a dissection of the two heads of the biceps brachii inserting into the radial tuberosity of a right radius. (Image from Jarrett CD, Weir DM, Stuffmann ES, et al: Anatomic and biomechanical analysis of the short and long head components of the distal biceps tendon, *J Shoulder Elbow Surg* 21[7]:942–948, 2012.)

ADDITIONAL CLINICAL CONNECTIONS

The radial nerve spirals obliquely around the posterior side of the humerus within the shallow radial groove of the humerus (see Fig. II.1B in Appendix II, Part A). Fractures or other trauma to the humerus in this region of the bone often injure the radial nerve. If the injury is severe enough, all radial nerve–innervated muscles distal to the site of injury may be paralyzed. The paralysis may be extensive, including the triceps, anconeus, brachioradialis, wrist extensor group, supinator, and all extrinsic extensor muscles to the digits. Loss of normal sensation typically includes the skin of the dorsal surface of the arm, most notably that covering the dorsal web space of the hand.

Because of the potential for regeneration of an injured peripheral nerve, the muscles may, in time, recover from the paralysis in an orderly proximal-to-distal fashion. Clues to whether the nerve has regenerated can be gained through electrophysiologic testing, in conjunction with palpation and manual testing of the strength of the affected musculature. One key muscle in this regard is the supinator muscle (see Fig. 6.43); reinnervation of this muscle would strongly suggest that the radial nerve has regenerated distally to within the proximal forearm. The deep lying supinator muscle, however, is difficult to palpate or isolate from other surrounding muscles.

In line with the law of parsimony, a clinical test exists that may help determine the relative activation of the supinator muscle in cases in which reinnervation is suspected. The "lap test," as it is sometimes called, requires the patient to support the forearm on the lap and *very slowly* supinate the forearm, free of any external resistance. Normally, with adequate practice, this very low–power supination can be performed without, or with very little, activation of the biceps. (You may want to practice this on yourself.) If the supinator muscle is innervated and functioning, the patient will usually be able to supinate *without* an accompanying contraction of the biceps. If, however, the supinator muscle is still paralyzed, even slow, low-power supination effort causes the biceps tendon to stand out sharply as it contracts to compensate for supinator muscle paralysis. Exaggerated biceps response to a very low–level supination task is a positive "lap test" result, suggesting marked weakness in the supinator muscle.

Although the diagnostic accuracy of the lap test is unknown, it does nevertheless show an example of applying kinesiologic and anatomic knowledge to clinical practice.

REFERENCES

1. Adams JE, Steinmann SP, Osterman AL: Management of injuries to the interosseous membrane [Review], *Hand Clin* 26(4):543–548, 2010.

2. Ahrens PM, Redfern DR, Forester AJ: Patterns of articular wear in the cadaveric elbow joint, *J Shoulder Elbow Surg* 10:52–56, 2001.

3. Akagi R, Iwanuma S, Hashizume S, et al.: In vivo measurements of moment arm lengths of three elbow flexors at rest and during isometric contractions, *J Appl Biomech* 28(1):63–69, 2012.

4. Altman E: The ulnar side of the wrist: clinically relevant anatomy and biomechanics, *J Hand Ther* 29(2):111–122, 2016.

5. Amis AA, Dowson D, Wright V: Elbow joint force predictions for some strenuous isometric actions, *J Biomech* 13:765–775, 1980.

6. An KN, Hui FC, Morrey BF, et al.: Muscles across the elbow joint: a biomechanical analysis, *J Biomech* 14:659–669, 1981.

7. Anz AW, Bushnell BD, Griffin LP, et al.: Correlation of torque and elbow injury in professional baseball pitchers, *Am J Sports Med* 38(7):1368–1374, 2010.

8. Askew LJ, An KN, Morrey BF, et al.: Isometric elbow strength in normal individuals, *Clin Orthop Relat Res* 222:261–266, 1987.

9. Axelsson P, Fredrikson P, Nilsson A, et al.: Forearm torque and lifting strength: normative data, *J Hand Surg Am* 43(7):677.e1–677.e17, 2018.

10. Basmajian JV, Griffin Jr WR: Function of anconeus muscle. An electromyographic study, *J Bone Joint Surg Am* 54(8):1712–1714, 1972.

11. Basmajian JV, Latif A: Integrated actions and functions of the chief flexors of the elbow: a detailed electromyographic analysis, *J Bone Joint Surg Am* 39:1106–1118, 1957.

12. Basmajian JV, Travill A: Electromyography of the pronator muscles of the forearm, *Anat Rec* 139:45–49, 1961.

13. Bergin MJ, Vicenzino B, Hodges PW: Functional differences between anatomical regions of the anconeus muscle in humans, *J Electromyogr Kinesiol* 23(6):1391–1397, 2013.

14. Boland MR, Spigelman T, Uhl TL: The function of brachioradialis, *J Hand Surg Am* 33(10):1853–1859, 2008.

15. Bordes Jr SJ, Jenkins S, Bang K, et al.: Ulnar nerve subluxation and dislocation: a review of the literature, *Neurosurg Rev* 44(2):793–798, 2021.

16. Bozkurt M, Acar HI, Apaydin N, et al.: The annular ligament: an anatomical study, *Am J Sports Med* 33:114–118, 2005.

17. Bozon O, Chrosciany S, Loisel M, et al.: Terrible triad injury of the elbow: a historical perspective, *Int Orthop* 46(10):2265–2272, 2022.

18. Bremer AK, Sennwald GR, Favre P, et al.: Moment arms of forearm rotators, *Clin Biomech* 21:683–691, 2006.

19. Brogan DM, Berger RA, Kakar S: Ulnar-sided wrist pain: a critical analysis review, *JBJS Rev* 7(5):e1, 2019.

20. Buffi JH, Werner K, Kepple T, et al.: Computing muscle, ligament, and osseous contributions to the elbow varus moment during baseball pitching, *Ann Biomed Eng* 43(2):404–415, 2015.

21. Buford Jr WL, Snijders JW, Patel VV, et al.: Specimen specific, 3D modeling of the elbow—prediction of strain in the medial collateral ligament, *Conf Proc IEEE Eng Med Biol Soc* 2012:3348–3351, 2012.

22. Cain Jr EL, Andrews JR, Dugas JR, et al.: Outcome of ulnar collateral ligament reconstruction of the elbow in 1281 athletes: results in 743 athletes with minimum 2-year follow-up, *Am J Sports Med* 38(12):2426–2434, 2010.

23. Capdarest-Arest N, Gonzalez JP, Turker T: Hypotheses for ongoing evolution of muscles of the upper extremity [Review], *Med Hypotheses* 82(4):452–456, 2014.

24. Chan K, MacDermid JC, Faber KJ, et al.: Can we treat select terrible triad injuries nonoperatively? *Clin Orthop Relat Res* 472(7):2092–2099, 2014.

25. Chang CW, Wang YC, Chu CH: Increased carrying angle is a risk factor for nontraumatic ulnar neuropathy at the elbow, *Clin Orthop Relat Res* 466:2190–2195, 2008.

26. Chin A, Lloyd D, Alderson J, et al.: A marker-based mean finite helical axis model to determine elbow rotation axes and kinematics in vivo, *J Appl Biomech* 26(3):305–315, 2010.

27. Cools AM, Borms D, Cottens S, et al.: Rehabilitation exercises for athletes with biceps disorders and slap lesions: a continuum of exercises with increasing loads on the biceps, *Am J Sports Med* 42(6):1315–1322, 2014.

28. Crowe MM, Martin JT, Grier AJ, et al.: In vivo mechanical function of the distal radial ulnar ligaments during rotation of the wrist, *J Hand Surg Am* 45(11):1012–1021, 2020.

29. Currier DP: Maximal isometric tension of the elbow extensors at varied positions. I. Assessment by cable tensiometer, *Phys Ther* 52:1043–1049, 1972.

30. DeFrate LE, Li G, Zayontz SJ, et al.: A minimally invasive method for the determination of force in the interosseous ligament, *Clin Biomech* 16:895–900, 2001.

31. DiTano O, Trumble TE, Tencer AF: Biomechanical function of the distal radioulnar and ulnocarpal wrist ligaments, *J Hand Surg Am* 28:622–627, 2003.

32. Dodds SD, Fishler TF: Terrible triad of the elbow, *Orthop Clin North Am* 44:47–58, 2013.

33. Dogan M, Kocak M, Onursal Kilinc O, et al.: Functional range of motion in the upper extremity and trunk joints: nine functional everyday tasks with inertial sensors, *Gait Posture* 70:141–147, 2019.

34. Dugas JR, Ostrander RV, Cain EL, et al.: Anatomy of the anterior bundle of the ulnar collateral ligament, *J Shoulder Elbow Surg* 16:657–660, 2007.

35. Egidy CC, Cross MB, Nam D, et al.: Total elbow arthroplasty: outcomes driving the evolution of implant design, *JBJS Rev* 7(5):e8, 2019.

36. Ekenstam F, Hagert CG: Anatomical studies on the geometry and stability of the distal radio ulnar joint, *Scand J Plast Reconstr Surg* 19:17–25, 1985.

37. Erickson BJ, Romeo AA: The ulnar collateral ligament injury: evaluation and treatment, *J Bone Joint Surg Am* 99(1):76–86, 2017.

38. Fleisig GS, Diffendaffer AZ, Ivey B, et al.: Changes in youth baseball pitching biomechanics: a 7-year longitudinal study, *Am J Sports Med* 46(1):44–51, 2018.

39. Funk DA, An KN, Morrey BF, et al.: Electromyographic analysis of muscles across the elbow joint, *J Orthop Res* 5:529–538, 1987.

40. Gallagher MA, Cuomo F, Polonsky L, et al.: Effects of age, testing speed, and arm dominance on isokinetic strength of the elbow, *J Shoulder Elbow Surg* 6:340–346, 1997.

41. Gallay SH, Richards RR, O'Driscoll SW: Intraarticular capacity and compliance of stiff and normal elbows, *Arthroscopy* 9:9–13, 1993.

42. Gammon B, Lalone E, Nishiwaki M, et al.: Arthrokinematics of the distal radioulnar joint measured using intercartilage distance in an in vitro model, *J Hand Surg Am* 43(3):283.e281–283.e289, 2018.

43. Golden DW, Jhee JT, Gilpin SP, et al.: Elbow range of motion and clinical carrying angle in a healthy pediatric population, *J Pediatr Orthop B* 16(2):144–149, 2007.

44. Guenzkofer F, Bubb H, Bengler K: Elbow torque ellipses: investigation of the mutual influences of rotation, flexion, and extension torques, *Work* 41(Suppl 7):2260–2267, 2012.

45. Hagert E, Hagert CG: Understanding stability of the distal radioulnar joint through an understanding of its anatomy [Review], *Hand Clin* 26(4):459–466, 2010.

46. Harwood B, Rice CL: Changes in motor unit recruitment thresholds of the human anconeus muscle during development preceding shortening elbow extensions, *J Neurophysiol* 107(10):2876–2884, 2012.

47. Hohenberger GM, Schwarz AM, Weiglein AH, et al.: Prevalence of the distal oblique bundle of the interosseous membrane of the forearm: an anatomical study, *J Hand Surg: European* 43(4):426–430, 2018.

48. Hotchkiss RN, An KN, Sowa DT, et al.: An anatomic and mechanical study of the interosseous membrane of the forearm: pathomechanics of proximal migration of the radius, *J Hand Surg Am* 14:256–261, 1989.

49. Inman VT, Saunders JB: Referred pain from skeletal structures, *J Nerv Ment Dis* 99:660–667, 1944.

50. Jarrett CD, Weir DM, Stuffmann ES, et al.: Anatomic and biomechanical analysis of the short and long head components of the distal biceps tendon, *J Shoulder Elbow Surg* 21(7):942–948, 2012.

51. Jeon IH, Sanchez-Sotelo J, Zhao K, et al.: The contribution of the coronoid and radial head to the stability of the elbow, *J Bone Joint Surg Br* 94(1):86–92, 2012.

52. Jordan D, Schimoler P, Kharlamov A, et al.: Correlation of force to deformation of the anterior bundle of the medial collateral ligament through consideration of band laxity, *J Orthop Res* 37(9):2027–2034, 2019.

53. Kadri OM, Okoroha KR, Patel RB, et al.: Nonoperative treatment of medial ulnar collateral ligament injuries in the throwing athlete: Indications, evaluation, and management, *JBJS Rev* 7(1):e6, 2019.

54. Kani KK, Chew FS: Terrible triad injuries of the elbow, *Emerg Radiol* 26(3):341–347, 2019.

55. Kemler BR, Rao S, Willier 3rd DP, et al.: Rehabilitation and return to sport criteria following ulnar collateral ligament reconstruction: a Systematic Review, *Am J Sports Med* 50(11):3112–3120, 2022.

56. Kotte SHP, Viveen J, Koenraadt KLM, et al.: Normative values of isometric elbow strength in healthy adults: a systematic review, *Shoulder Elbow* 10(3):207–215, 2018.

57. Krul M, van der Wouden JC, van Suijlekom-Smit LWA, et al.: Manipulative interventions for reducing pulled elbow in young children, *Cochrane Database Syst Rev* 1:CD007759, 2012.

58. Le Bozec S, Maton B, Cnockaert JC: The synergy of elbow extensor muscles during static work in man, *Eur J Appl Physiol Occup Physiol* 43:57–68, 1980.

59. Le Bozec S, Maton B: Differences between motor unit firing rate, twitch characteristics and fiber type composition in an agonistic muscle group in man, *Eur J Appl Physiol* 56:350–355, 1987.

60. Lehmkuhl LD, Smith LK: *Brunnstrom's clinical kinesiology*, ed 4, Philadelphia, 1983, FA Davis.

61. Magermans DJ, Chadwick EK, Veeger HE, et al.: Requirements for upper extremity motions during activities of daily living, *Clin Biomech* 20:591–599, 2005.

62. Malone PS, Cooley J, Morris J, et al.: The biomechanical and functional relationships of the proximal radioulnar joint, distal radioulnar joint, and interosseous ligament, *J Hand Surg: European* 40(5):485–493, 2015.

63. Marshall NE, Keller, Limpisvasti RO, et al.: Major league baseball pitching performance after Tommy John surgery and the effect of tear characteristics, technique, and graft type, *Am J Sports Med* 47(3):713–720, 2019.

64. McKay MJ, Baldwin JN, Ferreira P, et al.: Normative reference values for strength and flexibility of 1,000 children and adults, *Neurology* 88(1):36–43, 2017.

65. Miyake J, Moritomo H, Masatomi T, et al.: In vivo and 3-dimensional functional anatomy of the anterior bundle of the medial collateral ligament of the elbow, *J Shoulder Elbow Surg* 21(8):1006–1112, 2012.

66. Moritomo H, Noda K, Goto A, et al.: Interosseous membrane of the forearm: length change of ligaments during forearm rotation, *J Hand Surg Am* 34(4):685–691, 2009.

67. Moritomo H: The distal interosseous membrane: current concepts in wrist anatomy and biomechanics, *J Hand Surg Am* 37A:1501–1507, 2012.

68. Morrey BF, An KN, Stormont TJ: Force transmission through the radial head, *J Bone Joint Surg Am* 70:250–256, 1988.

69. Morrey BF, Askew LJ, Chao EY: A biomechanical study of normal functional elbow motion, *J Bone Joint Surg Am* 63:872–877, 1981.

70. Morrey BF, Tanaka S, An KN: Valgus stability of the elbow. A definition of primary and secondary constraints, *Clin Orthop Relat Res* 265(Apr):187–195, 1991.

71. Morrey BF: Radial head fracture. In Morrey BF, editor: *The elbow and its disorders*, ed 3, Philadelphia, 2000, Saunders.

72. Murray WM, Delp SL, Buchanan TS: Variation of muscle moment arms with elbow and forearm position, *J Biomech* 28:513–525, 1995.

73. Nagata H, Hosny S, Giddins GE: In-vivo measurement of distal radio-ulnar joint translation, *Hand Surg* 18(1):15–20, 2013.

74. Neumann DA, Soderberg GL, Cook TM: Electromyographic analysis of hip abductor musculature in healthy right-handed persons, *Phys Ther* 69:431–440, 1989.

75. Neumann DA: Use of diaphragm to assist rolling for the patient with quadriplegia, *Phys Ther* 59:39, 1979.

76. Nobauer-Huhmann IM, Pretterklieber M, Erhart J, et al.: Anatomy and variants of the triangular fibrocartilage complex and its MR appearance at 3 and 7T [Review], *Semin Musculoskelet Radiol* 16(2):93–103, 2012.

77. Noda K, Goto A, Murase T, et al.: Interosseous membrane of the forearm: an anatomical study of ligament attachment locations, *J Hand Surg Am* 34(3):415–422, 2009.

78. Ofuchi S, Takahashi K, Yamagata M, et al.: Pressure distribution in the humeroradial joint and force transmission to the capitulum during rotation of the forearm: effects of the Sauve-Kapandji procedure and incision of the interosseous membrane, *J Orthop Sci* 6:33–38, 2001.

79. Oosterwijk AM, Nieuwenhuis MK, van der Schans CP, et al.: Shoulder and elbow range of motion for the performance of activities of daily living: a systematic review, *Physiother Theory Pract* 34(7):505–528, 2018.

80. Osternig LR, Bates BT, James SL: Isokinetic and isometric torque force relationships, *Arch Phys Med Rehabil* 58(6):254–257, 1977.

81. Palmer AK, Werner FW: Biomechanics of the distal radioulnar joint, *Clin Orthop Relat Res* 187:26–35, 1984.

82. Paraskevas G, Papadopoulos A, Papaziogas B, et al.: Study of the carrying angle of the human elbow joint in full extension: a morphometric analysis, *Surg Radiol Anat* 26:19–23, 2004.

83. Pfaeffle HJ, Tomaino MM, Grewal R, et al.: Tensile properties of the interosseous membrane of the human forearm, *J Orthop Res* 14:842–845, 1996.

84. Pinter IJ, Bobbert MF, van Soest AJ, et al.: Isometric torque-angle relationships of the elbow flexors and extensors in the transverse plane, *J Electromyogr Kinesiol* 20(5):923–931, 2010.

85. Provins KA, Salter N: Maximum torque exerted about the elbow joint, *J Appl Physiol* 7:393–398, 1955.

86. Quigley RJ, Robicheaux GW, et al.: The proximal and distal position of the radius relative to the ulna through a full range of elbow flexion and forearm rotation, *J Hand Surg Eur Vol* 39(5):535–540, 2014.

87. Ramsay JW, Hunter BV, Gonzalez RV: Muscle moment arm and normalized moment contributions as reference data for musculoskeletal elbow and wrist joint models, *J Biomech* 42(4):463–473, 2009.

88. Rawal A, Chehata A, Horberry T, et al.: Defining the upper extremity range of motion for safe automobile driving, *Clin Biomech* 54:78–85, 2018.

89. Regan WD, Korinek SL, Morrey BF, et al.: Biomechanical study of ligaments around the elbow joint, *Clin Orthop Relat Res* 271:170–179, 1991.

90. Reichel LM, Milam GS, Sitton SE, et al.: Elbow lateral collateral ligament injuries, *J Hand Surg Am* 38(1):184–201, 2013.

91. Sardelli M, Tashjian RZ, MacWilliams BA: Functional elbow range of motion for contemporary tasks, *J Bone Joint Surg Am* 93(5):471–477, 2011.

92. Schmidt CC, Weir DM, Wong AS, et al.: The effect of biceps reattachment site, *J Shoulder Elbow Surg* 19(8):1157–1165, 2010.

93. Schuind F, An KN, Berglund L, et al.: The distal radioulnar ligaments: a biomechanical study, *J Hand Surg Am* 16:1106–1114, 1991.

94. Shukla DR, Fitzsimmons JS, An KN, et al.: Effect of radial head malunion on radiocapitellar stability, *J Shoulder Elbow Surg* 21(6):789–794, 2012.

95. Skahen 3rd JR, Palmer AK, Werner FW, et al.: The interosseous membrane of the forearm: anatomy and function, *J Hand Surg Am* 22:981–985, 1997.

96. Standring S: *Gray's anatomy: the anatomical basis of clinical practice*, ed 42, St Louis, 2021, Elsevier.

97. Stuart PR, Berger RA, Linscheid RL, et al.: The dorsopalmar stability of the distal radioulnar joint, *J Hand Surg Am* 25(4):689–699, 2000.

98. Sugisaki N, Wakahara T, Miyamoto N, et al.: Influence of muscle anatomical cross-sectional area on the moment arm length of the triceps brachii muscle at the elbow joint, *J Biomech* 43(14):2844–2847, 2010.

99. Topp KS, Boyd BS: Structure and biomechanics of peripheral nerves: nerve responses to physical stresses and implications for physical therapist practice, *Phys Ther* 86:92–109, 2006.

100. Travill A, Basmajian JV: Electromyography of the supinators of the forearm, *Anat Rec* 139:557–560, 1961.

101. Travill A: Electromyographic study of the extensor apparatus, *Anat Rec* 144:373–376, 1962.

102. Tsunoda N, O'Hagan F, Sale DG, et al.: Elbow flexion strength curves in untrained men and women and male bodybuilders, *Eur J Appl Physiol Occup Physiol* 66:235–239, 1993.

103. Tubbs RS, Shoja MM, Khaki AA, et al.: The morphology and function of the quadrate ligament, *Folia Morphol (Warsz)* 65(3):225–227, 2006.

104. Valone LC, Waites C, Tartarilla AB, et al.: Functional elbow range of motion in children and adolescents, *J Pediatr Orthop* 40(6):304–309, 2020.

105. van der Post AS, Jens S, Daams JG, et al.: The triangular fibrocartilage complex in the human wrist: a scoping review toward uniform and clinically relevant terminology, *Clin Anat* 35(5):626–648, 2022.

106. Ward LD, Ambrose CG, Masson MV, et al.: The role of the distal radioulnar ligaments, interosseous membrane, and joint capsule in distal radioulnar joint stability, *J Hand Surg Am* 25:341–351, 2000.

107. Watanabe H, Berger RA, Berglund LJ, et al.: Contribution of the interosseous membrane to distal radioulnar joint constraint, *J Hand Surg Am* 30:1164–1171, 2005.

108. Zaremski JL, Vincent KR, Vincent HK: Elbow ulnar collateral ligament: injury, treatment options, and recovery in overhead throwing athletes, *Curr Sports Med Rep* 18(9):338–345, 2019.

109. Zhang LQ, Nuber GW: Moment distribution among human elbow extensor muscles during isometric and submaximal extension, *J Biomech* 33(2):145–154, 2000.

STUDY QUESTIONS

1. List both muscular and nonmuscular tissues that can resist a distal pull (distraction) of the radius.
2. Describe how the different fibers of the medial collateral ligament of the elbow provide useful tension throughout the *entire* range of flexion and extension.
3. Describe the arthrokinematics at the humeroradial joint during a combined motion of elbow flexion and supination of the forearm.
4. Based on moment arm alone, which tissue shown in Fig. 6.17A could generate the greatest passive resistive torque opposing an elbow extension movement?
5. How many nerves innervate the primary muscles that flex the elbow (against gravity)?
6. Based on data provided in Table 6.7, which head of the triceps produces the greatest elbow extension torque?
7. Why was the extensor pollicis brevis *not* included in this chapter as a secondary supinator muscle of the forearm?
8. What is the kinesiologic role of the anterior deltoid during a "pushing" motion that combines elbow extension and shoulder flexion?
9. What muscle is the most direct antagonist to the brachialis muscle?
10. A patient has a 20-degree elbow flexion contracture that is assumed to originate from muscular tightness. As the clinician applies an extension stretch (torque) to the elbow near the end range of motion, the forearm passively "drifts" rather strongly toward supination. What clue does this observation provide as to which muscle or muscles are most tight (stiff)?
11. How would a radial nerve lesion in the axilla affect the task depicted in Fig. 6.45?
12. What position of the upper extremity maximally elongates the biceps brachii muscle?
13. Why would a surgeon be concerned about the integrity of the central band of the interosseous membrane before resecting a radial head or inserting a prosthetic radial head?
14. A patient has a median nerve injury at the midhumerus level. Would you expect any weakness in active flexion of the elbow? Over time, what deformity or "tightness pattern" is most likely to develop at the forearm?
15. Assume you want to maximally stretch (elongate) the brachialis muscle by passively extending the elbow. Would the effectiveness of the stretch be enhanced by combining full passive pronation or supination of the forearm to the elbow extension?
16. Describe a mechanism of injury at the elbow that could potentially injure the lateral (ulnar) collateral ligament (LUCL) from an excessive *valgus*-producing force applied to the elbow.
17. List some biomechanical benefits of the near-isometric behavior of the central band of interosseous membrane during pronation and supination.
18. In a weight-bearing position similar to that shown in Fig. 6.30 explain how, from a starting position of pronation, the latissimus dorsi could contribute to active *supination* of the forearm. Which tissues could restrict this active movement?
19. Assume a patent has complete severance of the median nerve, proximal to the elbow. Based on the innervation of the muscles of the elbow and forearm, you would expect at least near paralysis of active pronation. However, upon careful observation, you discover that the patient can actively pronate, although weakly, throughout full range of motion. How can you explain this ability?

Answers to the study questions are available in the accompanying enhanced eBook version included with the print purchase of this textbook.

Additional Video Educational Content

- Fluoroscopic Observations of Selected Arthrokinematics of the Upper Extremity
- Demonstration of Pronation and Supination of the Forearm with the Radius-and-Hand Held Fixed

CLINICAL KINESIOLOGY APPLIED TO PERSONS WITH QUADRIPLEGIA (TETRAPLEGIA)
- Analysis of Coming to a Sitting Position (from the supine position) in a Person with C^6 Quadriplegia

- Analysis of Transferring from a Wheelchair to a Mat in a Person with C^6 Quadriplegia
- Analysis of Rolling (from the supine position) in a Person with C^6 Quadriplegia
- Method for Actively Extending the Elbow with Weakened Triceps in a Person with Quadriplegia

ALL VIDEOS in this chapter are available in the accompanying enhanced eBook version included with the print purchase of this textbook.

Chapter

7

Wrist

DONALD A. NEUMANN, PT, PhD, FAPTA

CHAPTER AT A GLANCE

The wrist, or carpus, contains eight carpal bones that, as a group, act as a functional "spacer" between the forearm and hand. In addition to numerous small intercarpal joints, the wrist consists of two primary articulations: the radiocarpal and midcarpal joints (Fig. 7.1). The *radiocarpal joint* is located between the distal end of the radius and the proximal row of carpal bones. Just distal to this joint is the *midcarpal joint,* joining the proximal and distal rows of carpal bones. The two joints allow the wrist to flex and extend and to move from side to side in motions called radial and ulnar deviation. The nearby distal radio-ulnar joint was formally described in Chapter 6, primarily because of its functional role with pronation and supination of the forearm. The articular disc within the distal radio-ulnar joint will be revisited in this chapter because of its close anatomic relationship with the radiocarpal joint.

The position and stability of the wrist significantly affects the function of the hand. This is because many muscles that control the digits originate proximal to the hand, attaching to the forearm. A painful, unstable, or weak wrist often assumes a position that interferes with the optimal length in and passive tension within the extrinsic musculature, thereby reducing the effectiveness of grasp.

Several new terms are introduced here to describe the relative position and topography within the wrist and the hand. *Palmar* and *volar* are synonymous with *anterior; dorsal* is synonymous with *posterior.* These terms are used interchangeably throughout this chapter and the next chapter on the hand.

OSTEOLOGY

Distal Forearm

The dorsal surface of the distal radius has several grooves and raised areas that help guide or stabilize the tendons that course toward the wrist and hand (Fig. 7.2). Note, for example, the palpable *dorsal (Lister's) tubercle* that helps stabilize the position of the tendon of the extensor pollicis longus.

The palmar or volar surface of the distal radius is the location of the proximal attachments of the wrist capsule and the thick palmar radiocarpal ligaments (Fig. 7.3A). The *styloid process of the radius* projects distally from the lateral side of the radius. The *styloid process of the ulna,* sharper than its radial counterpart, extends distally from the posterior-medial corner of the distal ulna.

The *distal articular surface of the radius* is concave in both medial-lateral and anterior-posterior directions. Shallow concave facets are formed in the articular cartilage from indentations made by the scaphoid and lunate bones of the wrist (see Fig. 6.25B).

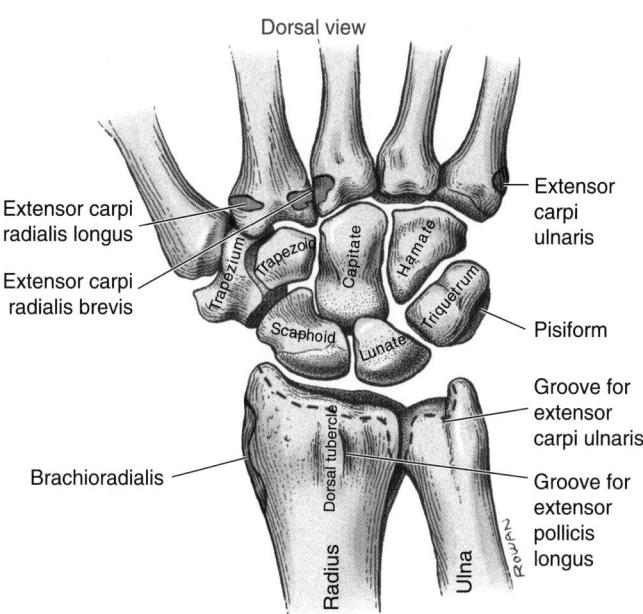

Dorsal view

FIGURE 7.2 The dorsal aspect of the bones of the right wrist. The muscles' distal attachments are shown in gray. The dashed lines show the proximal attachment of the dorsal capsule of the wrist.

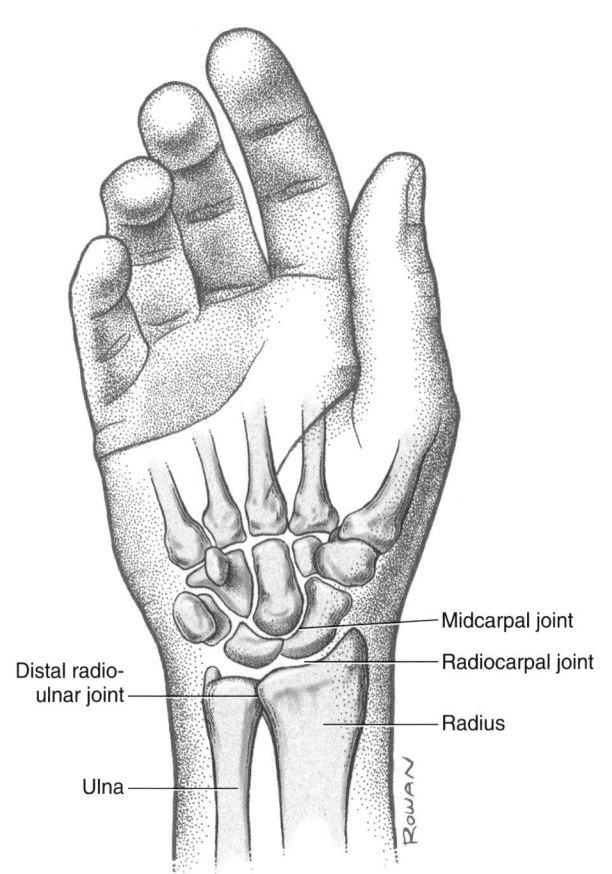

FIGURE 7.1 The bones and major articulations of the wrist.

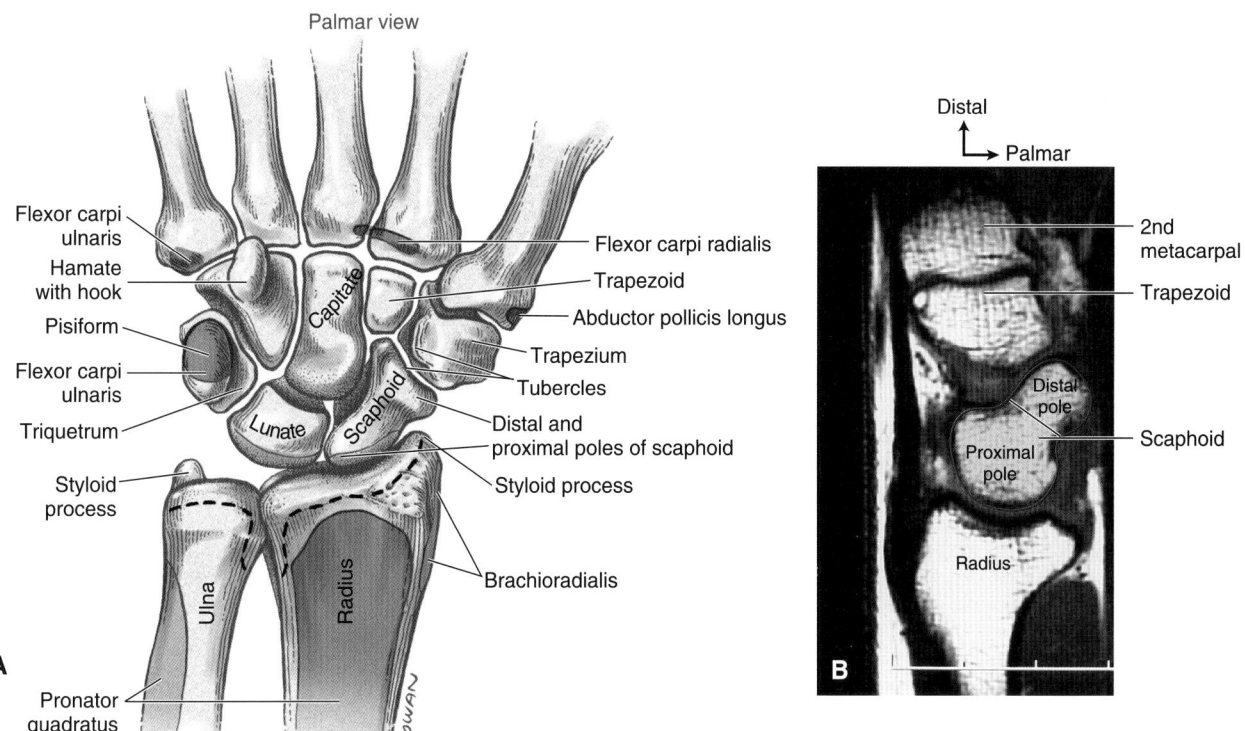

FIGURE 7.3 (A) The palmar aspect of the bones of the right wrist. The muscles' proximal attachments are shown in red and distal attachments in gray. The dashed lines show the proximal attachment of the palmar capsule of the wrist. (B) The full appreciation of the shape of the scaphoid is provided through a sagittal plane cross-section MR image. The thin black line marks the "waist" region of the bone, midway between the proximal and distal poles.

Osteologic Features of the Distal Forearm
- Dorsal tubercle of the radius
- Styloid process of the radius
- Styloid process of the ulna
- Distal articular surface of the radius

The distal end of the radius has two configurations of biomechanical importance. First, the distal end of the radius angles about 25 degrees toward the ulnar (medial) direction (Fig. 7.4A). This *ulnar tilt* allows the wrist and hand to rotate farther into ulnar deviation than into radial deviation. As a result of this tilt, radial deviation of the wrist is limited by bony impingement of the lateral side of the carpus against the styloid process of the radius. Second, the distal articular surface of the radius is angled about 10 degrees in the palmar direction (see Fig. 7.4B). This *palmar tilt* accounts, in part, for the slightly greater amounts of flexion than extension at the wrist.

Fractures of the distal end of the radius often affect the natural tilt of the distal radius. In the absence of proper orthopedic management, a permanent abnormal tilt of the distal radius can significantly alter the function of the radiocarpal and distal radio-ulnar joints. This topic is addressed in detail in Clinical Connection 7.3.

Carpal Bones

From a radial (lateral) to ulnar direction, the proximal row of carpal bones includes the scaphoid, lunate, triquetrum, and pisiform. The distal row includes the trapezium, trapezoid, capitate, and hamate (see Figs. 7.2 and 7.3).

The bones within the proximal row of the carpus are linked together in a relatively loose fashion. In contrast, the bones of the distal row of the carpus are rigidly joined by tight ligaments and irregular joint surfaces, thus providing a stable base for articulation with the metacarpal bones.

The following section presents a general anatomic description of each carpal bone. The ability to visualize each bone's relative position and shape is helpful in an understanding of the ligamentous anatomy and wrist kinematics.

SCAPHOID

The naming of the scaphoid is based on its vague resemblance to a boat (*scaphoid* from the Greek *skaphoeides,* like a boat). Most of the undersurface of the boat rides on the radius; the cargo area (or hull) of the "boat" is filled with part of the head of the capitate (see Fig. 7.3A). About 75% of the surface of the scaphoid is lined with articular cartilage, forming synovial joints with four other carpal bones and the radius. Because of its shape and unique position within the carpus, the scaphoid is functionally and anatomically associated with both the proximal and distal rows of carpal bones.

The scaphoid has two noteworthy *poles.* The gently rounded *proximal pole* articulates with the concave *scaphoid facet* of the radius (see Fig. 6.25B). The *distal pole* is slightly convex, articulating with the trapezium and trapezoid. The distal pole projects in a palmar direction about 30 degrees, which can be well appreciated from a sagittal plane slice provided by magnetic resonance (MR) imaging (see Fig. 7.3B). The distal pole possesses a blunt palmer *tubercle,* which is palpable at the base of the thenar musculature. Palpating this tubercle during wrist motion allows the clinician to assess the position and kinematics of this important bone.[92]

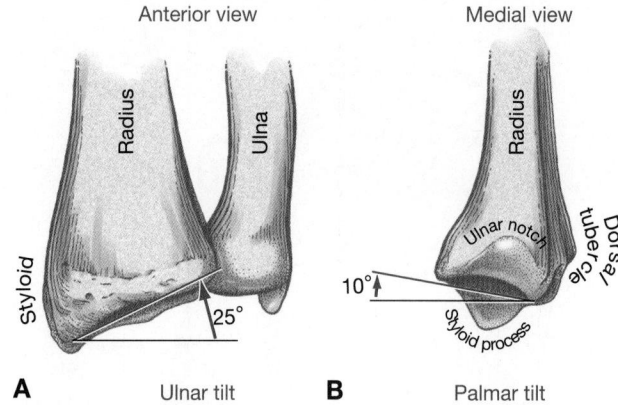

FIGURE 7.4 (A) Anterior view of the distal radius showing an *ulnar tilt* of about 25 degrees. (B) Medial view of the distal radius showing a *palmar tilt* of about 10 degrees.

Much of the medial surface of the scaphoid is deeply concave to accept the lateral half of the prominent head of the capitate bone (see Fig. 7.3A). Immediately proximal to this concavity is a facet for articulation with the lunate. This articulation, reinforced primarily by the scapholunate ligament, provides an important mechanical link within the proximal row of carpal bones.

LUNATE

The lunate (from the Latin *luna,* moon) is the central bone of the proximal row, wedged between the scaphoid and triquetrum. The lunate is the most inherently unstable of the carpal bones, in part because of its shape and lack of muscular attachments, but also because of its lack of strong ligamentous attachments to the rigidly held capitate bone.

Like the scaphoid, the lunate's proximal surface is convex, fitting into the concave facet on the radius (see Fig. 6.25B). The distal surface of the lunate is deeply concave, giving the bone its crescent moon–shaped appearance (see Fig. 7.3A). This articular surface most often accepts two convexities: the medial half of the head of the capitate and part of the apex of the hamate. The specific manner that the lunate contacts the hamate may affect carpal kinematics, possibly creating excessive stress within the ulnar side of the wrist.[1,100]

TRIQUETRUM

The triquetrum, or triangular bone, occupies the most ulnar position in the wrist, just medial and slightly distal to the lunate. It is palpable just distal to the ulnar styloid process, especially with the wrist radially deviated. The lateral surface of the triquetrum is long and flat for articulation with a similarly shaped surface on the hamate. An elliptical articular facet on the bone's palmar surface accepts the pisiform.

PISIFORM

The pisiform, meaning "shaped like a pea," articulates loosely with the palmar surface of the triquetrum. The bone is easily movable and palpable. The pisiform is embedded within the tendon of the flexor carpi ulnaris and therefore has the characteristics of a sesamoid bone. In addition, this bone serves as an attachment for the abductor digiti minimi muscle, transverse carpal ligament, and several other ligaments.

CAPITATE

The capitate is the largest of all carpal bones. This bone occupies a central location within the wrist, making articular contact with seven surrounding bones when considering the metacarpals (see Fig. 7.3A). The word *capitate* is derived from the Latin root meaning *head,* which describes the shape of the bone's prominent proximal surface. The large head articulates with the deep concavity provided by the scaphoid and lunate. The capitate is well stabilized between the hamate and trapezoid by short but strong ligaments.

The capitate's distal surface is rigidly joined to the base of the third and, to a lesser extent, the second and fourth metacarpal bones. This rigid articulation allows the capitate and the third metacarpal to function as a single column, providing significant longitudinal stability to the entire wrist and hand. The axis of rotation for all wrist motions passes through the capitate.

TRAPEZIUM

The trapezium is easily recognized by its distal saddle-shaped articular surface, which contributes to the first carpometacarpal joint. This critically important joint allows a wide range of motion of the thumb. The bone's proximal surface is slightly concave for its articulation with the distal pole of the scaphoid. Most of the trapezium's medial surface articulates with the trapezoid and the radial side of the base of the second metacarpal.

A slender and sharp *tubercle* projects from the palmar surface of the trapezium. This tubercle, along with the palmar tubercle of the scaphoid, provides attachment for the lateral side of the transverse carpal ligament (Fig. 7.5). Immediately medial to the palmar tubercle is a distinct groove for the tendon of the flexor carpi radialis.

TRAPEZOID

The trapezoid is a relatively small bone wedged tightly between the capitate and the trapezium. The trapezoid, like the trapezium, has a proximal surface that is slightly concave for articulation with the scaphoid. The bone makes a relatively firm articulation with the base of the second metacarpal bone.

HAMATE

The hamate is named after the large hooklike process that projects from its palmar surface. The hamate has the general shape of a pyramid. Its base, or distal surface, articulates with the bases of the fourth and fifth metacarpals. This articulation provides important functional mobility to the ulnar aspect of the hand, most noticeably when the hand is "cupped."

The apex of the hamate—its proximal surface—projects toward and most often contacts the lunate as it is wedged between the capitate laterally and triquetrum medially. The hook of the hamate (along with the pisiform) provides bony attachments for the medial side of the transverse carpal ligament (see Fig. 7.5).

Carpal Tunnel

As illustrated in Fig. 7.5, the palmar side of the carpal bones forms a concavity. Arching over this concavity is a thick fibrous band of connective tissue known as the *transverse carpal ligament.* This ligament is connected to four raised points on the palmar carpus, namely, the pisiform and the hook of the hamate on the ulnar side, and the tubercles of the scaphoid and the trapezium on the radial side. The transverse carpal ligament serves as an attachment site for many intrinsic muscles located within the hand and the palmaris longus, a wrist flexor muscle.

The transverse carpal ligament converts the palmar concavity made by the carpal bones into a *carpal tunnel.* The tunnel serves as a passageway for the median nerve and the tendons of extrinsic flexor muscles of the digits (Chapter 8). Furthermore, the transverse carpal ligament restrains the enclosed tendons from "bowstringing" anteriorly and out of the carpal tunnel, most notably during grasping actions performed with a partially flexed wrist.

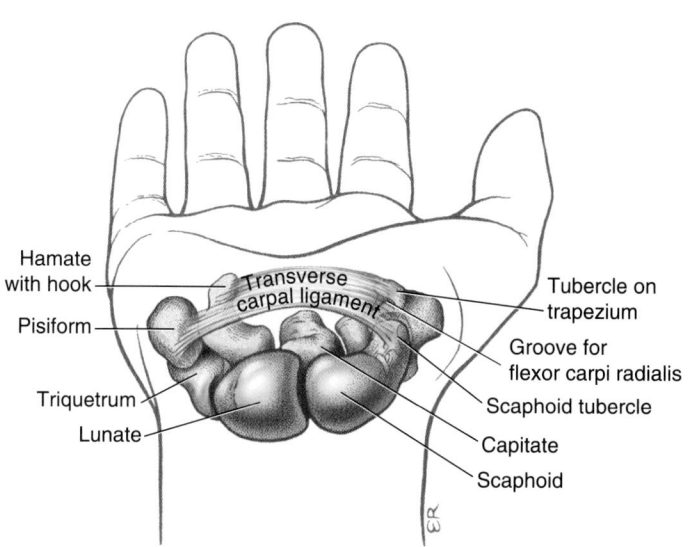

Hamate with hook
Pisiform
Triquetrum
Lunate
Transverse carpal ligament
Tubercle on trapezium
Groove for flexor carpi radialis
Scaphoid tubercle
Capitate
Scaphoid

FIGURE 7.5 A view through the carpal tunnel of the right wrist with all contents removed. The transverse carpal ligament is shown as the roof of the tunnel.

Scaphoid and Lunate: Vulnerability to Injury and Clinical Complications

It is likely that more has been written in the medical literature about the scaphoid and lunate than about all other carpal bones combined. Both bones are lodged between two rigid structures: the distal forearm and the distal row of carpal bones. Like a nut within a nutcracker, the scaphoid and lunate are vulnerable to compression-related injuries, with a relatively high probability of developing avascular necrosis.

THE SCAPHOID BONE AND ITS VULNERABILITY TO FRACTURE

The scaphoid is in the direct path of force transmission through the wrist. For this reason, the scaphoid is the most frequently fractured bone of the wrist. Actually, second only to fractures of the distal radius, the scaphoid is the most frequently fractured bone of the entire upper limb.[112] A common mechanism for fracturing this bone is to fall on a fully supinated forearm with the wrist extended and radially deviated. Persons with a fractured scaphoid typically show tenderness over the bone's palmar tubercle, as well as within the anatomic "snuffbox" of the wrist. Most fractures occur near or along the scaphoid's "waist," midway between the bone's two poles (see arrow in Fig. 7.6A). Because most blood vessels enter the scaphoid at and *distal* to its waist, fractures proximal to the waist may result in a delayed union or nonunion. If the fracture is untreated, the proximal pole may develop avascular necrosis and subsequent degenerative arthritis in the region. Fractures of the proximal pole often require surgery, followed by immobilization typically for at least 12 weeks or until there is evidence of radiographic union. Fractures of the distal pole typically do not require surgery, especially if nondisplaced, and generally require only 6 to 8 weeks of immobilization. Actual times of immobilization can vary greatly, based on the specific circumstances of the patient and the fracture.

Often a fractured scaphoid is associated with other injuries along the weight-bearing path of the wrist and hand. Associated injuries often involve fracture and/or dislocation of the lunate and fracture of the trapezium and distal radius.

KIENBÖCK'S DISEASE: AVASCULAR NECROSIS OF THE LUNATE

The condition of lunatomalacia (meaning literally "softening of the lunate") was first described by Kienböck in 1910.[90] *Kienböck's disease,* as it is called today, is described as a painful orthopedic disorder of uncertain origin, characterized by avascular necrosis of the lunate.[66,101] A history of trauma is frequently, but not universally, associated with the onset of the condition. Trauma may be linked to an isolated dislocation or fracture or to repetitive or near-constant lower-magnitude compression forces. It is not completely understood how the trauma, compression, and avascular necrosis are interrelated in the pathogenesis of the disease. What is clear, however, is that as avascular necrosis develops, the lunate often becomes fragmented and shortened, which may alter its relationship with the other adjoining carpal bones (see Fig. 7.6B). In severe cases the lunate may totally collapse, thereby altering the architecture, kinematics, and kinetics across the entire wrist. This consequence tends to occur more often in those involved in manual labor, such as pneumatic drill operators.

Treatment of Kienböck's disease may be conservative or radical, depending on the amount of functional limitation and pain, as well as the progression of the disease. In relatively mild forms of the disease—before the lunate fragments and becomes sclerotic—treatment may involve immobilization or unloading of the lunate, hand therapy to improve function and reduce pain, and modalities aimed to increase blood flow to the bone.[45,138] If the disease progresses, the length of the ulna, radius, or capitate bone may be surgically altered as a means to reduce the contact pressure on the lunate.[136] In more advanced cases, surgeries may include a partial or full excision of the lunate or a proximal row carpectomy.[134] Surgeries such as a capitate-hamate or capitate-third metacarpal arthrodesis (fusion) may also be considered to limit the proximal migration of the capitate against the fragmented lunate, with hopes of reducing a collapse of the carpus.[19,45]

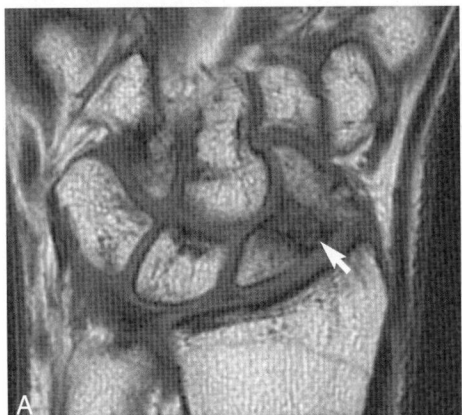
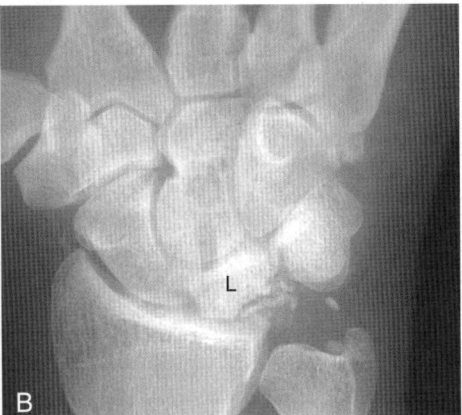

FIGURE 7.6 (A) A frontal (coronal) plane T1-weighted magnetic resonance image of the wrist of a patient showing a fracture of the scaphoid at the region of its waist *(arrow).* (B) An anterior-posterior view of a radiograph of the wrist of a patient with Kienböck's disease. Note that the lunate *(L)* is sclerotic, malformed, and fragmented. (From Helms CA: *Fundamentals of skeletal radiology,* ed 5, Philadelphia, 2020, Elsevier.)

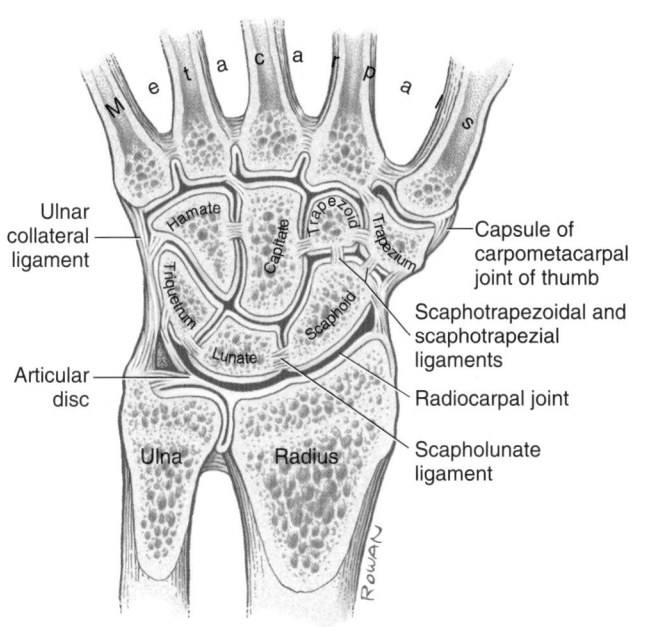

FIGURE 7.7 A frontal plane cross-section through the right wrist and distal forearm showing the shape of the bones and connective tissues.

ARTHROLOGY

Joint Structure and Ligaments of the Wrist

JOINT STRUCTURE

As illustrated in Fig. 7.1, the two primary articulations within the wrist are the *radiocarpal* and *midcarpal joints.* Many other *intercarpal joints* also exist between adjacent carpal bones (see Fig. 7.7).

Radiocarpal Joint

The *proximal components* of the radiocarpal joint are the concave surfaces of the radius and an adjacent articular disc (Figs. 7.7 and 7.8). As described in Chapter 6, this articular disc (often called the *triangular fibrocartilage*) is also an integral part of the distal radioulnar joint. The *distal components* of the radiocarpal joint are the convex proximal surfaces of the scaphoid and the lunate. The triquetrum is also considered part of the radiocarpal joint because at full ulnar deviation its medial surface contacts the articular disc.

The thick articular surface of the distal radius and the articular disc accept and disperse the forces that cross the wrist. Approximately 20% of the total compression force that crosses the radiocarpal joint passes through the articular disc to the ulna. The remaining 80% passes directly through the scaphoid and lunate to the radius.[87] The contact area at the radiocarpal joint tends to be greatest when the wrist is partially extended and slightly deviated in an ulnar direction.[65] This is also the wrist position at which maximal grip strength is obtained.

Midcarpal Joint

The midcarpal joint is the articulation between the proximal and distal rows of carpal bones (see Fig. 7.8). The capsule that surrounds the midcarpal joint is continuous with each of the many intercarpal joints.

The midcarpal joint can be divided descriptively into medial and lateral joint compartments. The larger and more prominent *medial*

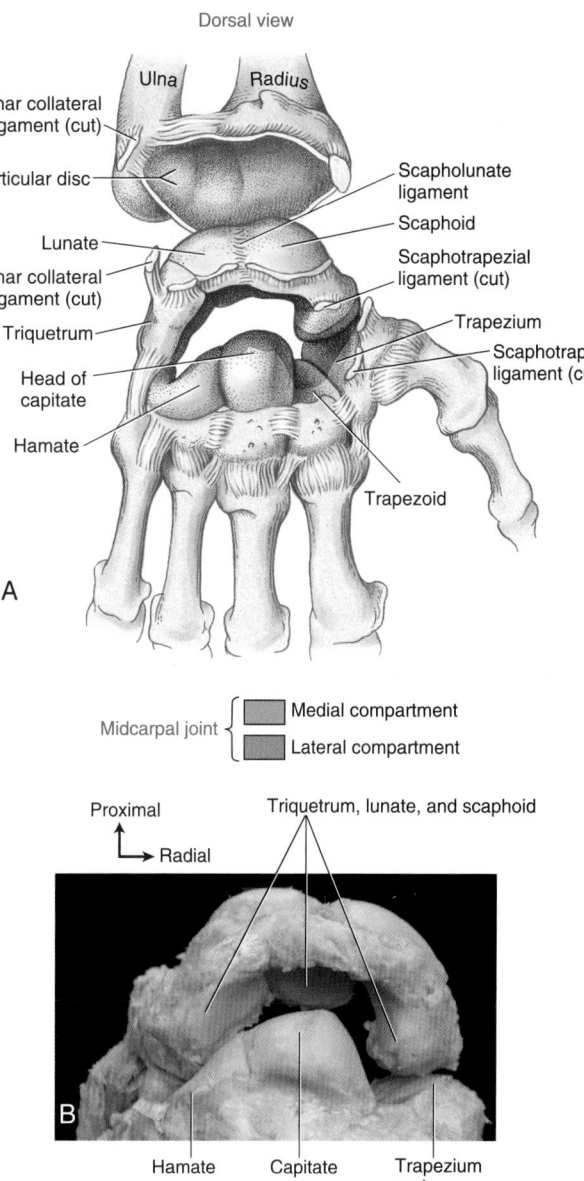

FIGURE 7.8 (A) Illustration of a dorsal view of a dissected right wrist showing several key structures associated with the radiocarpal and midcarpal joints. Red and gray colors highlight the medial and lateral compartments of the midcarpal joint, respectively. (B) Photograph of a dissected right wrist (as in image A), emphasizing the articular surfaces of the midcarpal joint. (Dissection prepared by Anthony Hornung, Rolandas Kesminas, and Donald A. Neumann, at Marquette University.)

compartment is formed by the convex head of the capitate and apex of the hamate, fitting into the concave recess formed by the distal surfaces of the scaphoid, lunate, and triquetrum (see Fig. 7.8). The head of the capitate fits into this concave recess much like a ball-and-socket joint.

The less conspicuous *lateral compartment* of the midcarpal joint is formed by the junction of the slightly convex distal pole of the scaphoid fitting against the contiguous and slightly concave proximal surfaces of the trapezium and the trapezoid (see Fig. 7.8). The lateral compartment lacks the pronounced ovoid shape of the medial compartment.

Intercarpal Joints

When including the pisotriquetral joint, 13 separate intercarpal articulations exist within the wrist, far too many to be formally described within this chapter (Fig. 7.7). Joint surfaces vary in shape between nearly flat to markedly convex or concave. As a whole, the many joints contribute to wrist motion through small gliding and rotary motions, occurring primarily between the bones within the proximal row of the carpus.[2] Compared with the large range of motion permitted at the radiocarpal and midcarpal joints, motion at the intercarpal joints is relatively small but nevertheless essential for normal wrist motion and natural posturing of the hand.

WRIST LIGAMENTS

The anatomy of wrist ligaments is typically studied through cadaver dissection, arthroscopy, and MR imaging. Many ligaments, however, are small and difficult to isolate from the surrounding tissues. The inconspicuous nature of some of the wrist ligaments should not, however, minimize their extreme kinesiologic importance. Wrist ligaments are essential to maintaining natural intercarpal alignment, as well as transferring and dissipating forces across the carpus. Muscle-produced forces transferred across ligaments provide important active control of the complex arthrokinematics of the wrist. Furthermore, when activated by stretch or mechanical disturbance, mechanoreceptors embedded within wrist ligaments contribute to wrist proprioception (position and motion awareness).[41,43] Sensory signals originating within a given stretched ligament travel to a specific set of muscles capable of reflexively protecting the wrist.[42] Wrist ligaments severely damaged through injury and disease may reduce the ability of the sensory receptors to communicate with the central nervous system. This loss of sensory information, when coupled with mechanical instability, can make a wrist vulnerable to further injury, deformity, and often degenerative arthritis.[29]

Wrist ligaments are classified as extrinsic or intrinsic (Box 7.1). Extrinsic ligaments have their proximal attachments on the radius or ulna and distal attachments within the wrist. As noted in Box 7.1, the triangular fibrocartilage complex (introduced previously in Chapter 6) includes structures associated with the wrist *and* the distal radio-ulnar joint. Intrinsic ligaments have both their proximal and distal attachments within the wrist.

The ligaments of the wrist are typically named according to the primary bones to which they attach. Despite this seemingly straightforward method of naming, some inconsistency exists in the literature on the naming of the ligaments. Additional resources should be consulted to appreciate alternative organization styles for classifying these ligaments, and for more extensive anatomic and functional descriptions.[14,29,33,120,123]

Extrinsic Ligaments

The extrinsic ligaments of the wrist are embedded within a fibrous capsule that surrounds both the wrist and the distal radio-ulnar joint. The *dorsal radiocarpal ligament* is thin and not easily distinguishable from the capsule itself. The ligament courses distally in an ulnar direction, attaching primarily between the distal radius and the dorsal surfaces of the lunate and triquetrum (Fig. 7.9). The dorsal radiocarpal ligament reinforces the dorsal side of the wrist and helps guide the natural arthrokinematics, especially of the bones of the proximal row.[115] The obliquely running fibers of this ligament limit an abnormal ulnar shift of the carpus.[94]

Although thin, the dorsal radiocarpal ligament is one of the richest sensory-innervated ligaments of the wrist, containing a

---

BOX 7.1   Extrinsic and Intrinsic Ligaments

EXTRINSIC LIGAMENTS OF THE WRIST

Dorsal radiocarpal
Radial collateral
Palmar radiocarpal
  - Radioscaphocapitate
  - Radiolunate (long and short)
Triangular fibrocartilage complex (TFCC)
  - Articular disc (triangular fibrocartilage)
  - Distal radio-ulnar joint capsular ligaments
  - Palmar ulnocarpal ligament
    - Ulnotriquetral
    - Ulnolunate
  - Ulnar collateral ligament
  - Fascial sheath that encloses the tendon of the extensor carpi ulnaris

INTRINSIC LIGAMENTS OF THE WRIST

Short (distal row)
  - Dorsal
  - Palmar
  - Interosseous
Intermediate
  - Lunotriquetral
  - Scapholunate
  - Scaphotrapezial and scaphotrapezoidal
Long
  - Palmar intercarpal ("inverted V")
    - Lateral leg (capitate to scaphoid)
    - Medial leg (capitate to triquetrum)
  - Dorsal intercarpal (trapezium-scaphoid-lunate-triquetrum)

---

relatively large number of mechanoceptors.[42] The dorsal radiocarpal ligament and associated radial nerve afferents therefore likely play an important role in wrist proprioception.

The *radial collateral ligament* consists of fibers embedded within the joint capsule that attach and cross the radial styloid process, scaphoid, and trapezium (Fig. 7.10).[128] The fibers blend with the lateral most fibers of palmar radiocarpal ligament.[83] The closely positioned tendons of the abductor pollicis longus and extensor pollicis brevis provide significant structural reinforcement to the relative thin fibers within the radial collateral ligament.

Deep and mostly separate from the palmar capsule of the wrist are several thick and strong ligaments known collectively as the *palmar radiocarpal ligament*. This ligament provides greater overall stability to the wrist than the thinner dorsal extrinsic ligament. Three dominant ligaments are typically described within this set: *radioscaphocapitate, long radiolunate,* and *short radiolunate* (see Fig. 7.10).[120,123] In general, each ligament arises from a roughened area on the distal palmar side of the radius, travels distally in an obliquely ulnar direction, and attaches to the palmar surfaces of several carpal bones. The short radiolunate ligament attaches distally to the lunate, whereas the more obliquely running long radiolunate ligament attaches not only to the lunate but also continues distally to blend with the lunotriquetral ligament.

As a whole, the palmar radiocarpal ligaments become maximally taut at full wrist extension, and thereby help limit impingement between the dorsal side of the radius and carpal bones. In addition, their oblique fiber direction assists the dorsal radiocarpal ligament in resisting abnormal ulnar shift of the carpus.

An example of the role that these ligaments play in guiding the arthrokinematics of the wrist will be provided later in this chapter.

Dorsal view

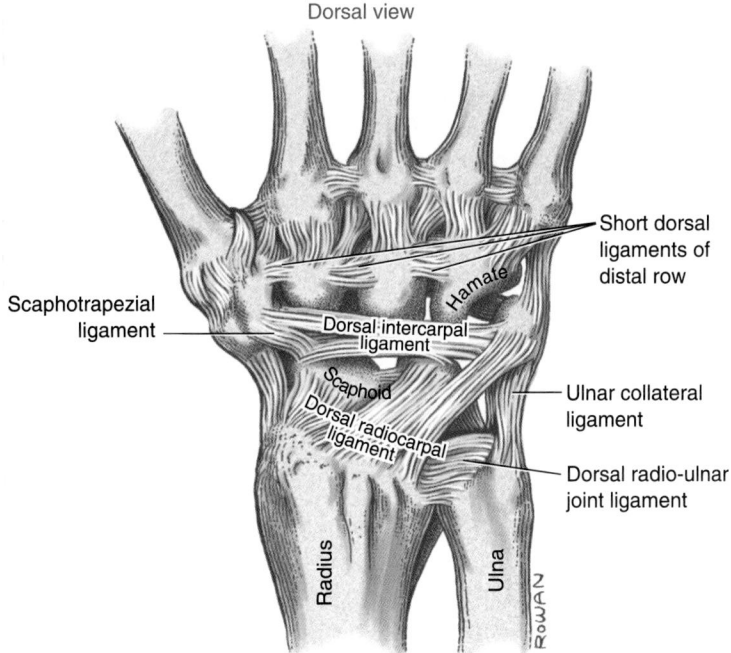

Short dorsal ligaments of distal row

Scaphotrapezial ligament

Dorsal intercarpal ligament

Hamate

Scaphoid

Dorsal radiocarpal ligament

Ulnar collateral ligament

Dorsal radio-ulnar joint ligament

Radius

Ulna

FIGURE 7.9 The primary dorsal ligaments of the right wrist.

Palmar view

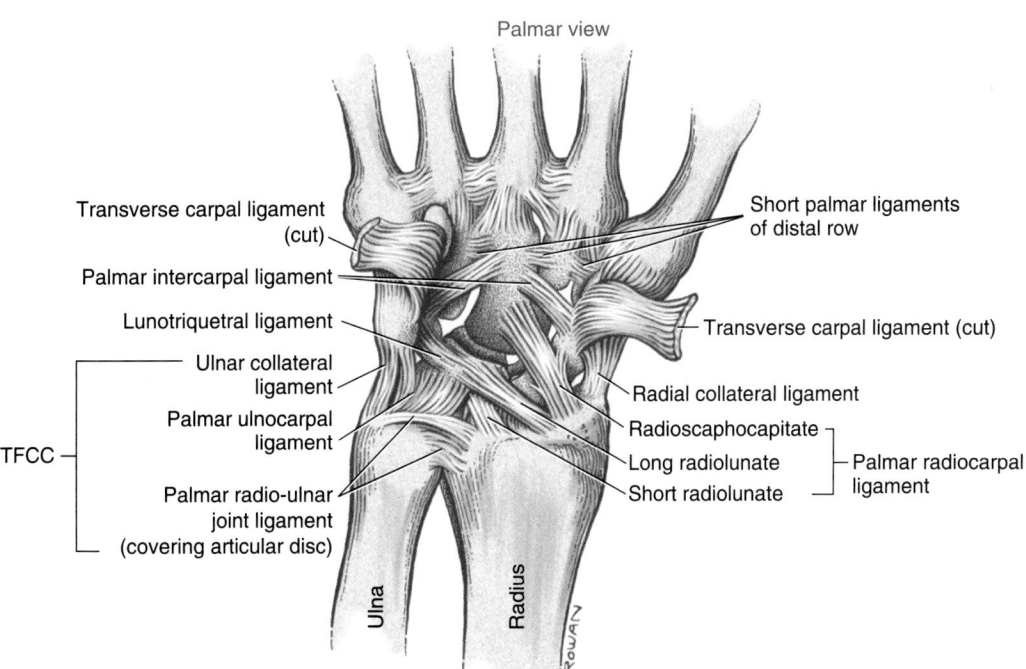

Transverse carpal ligament (cut)

Palmar intercarpal ligament

Lunotriquetral ligament

Ulnar collateral ligament

Palmar ulnocarpal ligament

TFCC

Palmar radio-ulnar joint ligament (covering articular disc)

Short palmar ligaments of distal row

Transverse carpal ligament (cut)

Radial collateral ligament

Radioscaphocapitate

Long radiolunate

Short radiolunate

Palmar radiocarpal ligament

Ulna

Radius

FIGURE 7.10 The primary palmar ligaments of the right wrist. The transverse carpal ligament has been cut and reflected to show the underlying ligaments. *TFCC,* triangular fibrocartilage complex.

Although the *ulnocarpal space* appears empty on a standard radiograph (Fig. 7.11A), it is filled with at least five interconnected tissues, known collectively as the *triangular fibrocartilage complex* (TFCC) (see Box 7.1). These constituents are depicted in Fig. 7.11B–C. The primary component of the TFCC is the *triangular fibrocartilage (TFC)*—the previously described *articular disc* located within both the distal radio-ulnar and the radiocarpal joints.

The primary global function of the TFCC is to securely bind the distal ends of the radius and ulna while simultaneously permitting the radius, with attached carpus, to freely rotate (pronate and supinate) around a fixed ulna. A summary of the more specific functions of the TFCC is included in Box 7.2. Anatomic details of the components of the TFCC are described in the following paragraphs. Be aware that many alternative names of the various components of the TFCC are common in the literature.[130]

The *triangular fibrocartilage* attaches directly or indirectly to all components of the TFCC and therefore forms the structural backbone of the entire complex (see Fig. 7.11B–C). The TFC is a biconcave articular disc, composed chiefly of fibrocartilage. The name "triangular" refers to the shape of the disc: its base attaches along the ulnar notch of the radius, and its apex into and near a depression (fovea) on the distal surface of the ulna (reviewed in Fig. 6.8). The sides of the "triangle" of the TFC (from base to apex) are strongly reinforced through connections to the *palmar* and *dorsal capsular ligaments* of the distal radio-ulnar joint.[4,36,] The disc's proximal surface accepts part of the head of the ulna at the distal radio-ulnar joint—the specific part depending on the exact pronation-supination position. The distal surface of the disc accepts the convex surfaces of part of the lunate and triquetrum at the radiocarpal joint (see Figs. 6.25 and 7.7). The central 80% to 85% of the TFC is avascular with poor or no healing potential.[70,124]

The *palmar ulnocarpal ligament* has two parts: ulnotriquetral and ulnolunate (see Fig. 7.11B–C).[14] This pair of ligaments has a common origin along part of the palmar radio-ulnar joint capsular ligament, continuing medially to the fovea of the ulna.[49,75] Both ligaments attach distally to the palmar aspects of the lunate and triquetrum. Because of the ulnocarpal ligaments shared proximal attachments with the palmar radio-ulnar joint capsular ligament, they help indirectly secure the position of the TFC.

The *ulnar collateral ligament* is a thickening of the medial capsule of the wrist, extending between the ulnar styloid process and the triquetrum[128] (see Fig. 7.10). Along with the flexor and extensor carpi ulnaris muscles, the often blended ulnotriquetral and ulnar collateral ligaments reinforce the ulnar side of the wrist. These ulnar ligaments must be sufficiently flexible, however, to allow the radius-and-hand to rotate freely, but securely, around the fixed ulna during forearm pronation and supination.

The *tendon* of the *extensor carpi ulnaris* courses through the sixth fibro-osseus compartment of the extensor retinaculum (see ahead

---

BOX 7.2 Specific Functions of the Triangular Fibrocartilage Complex

The triangular fibrocartilage complex (TFCC)
- Is the primary stabilizer of the distal radio-ulnar joint.
- Reinforces the ulnar side of the wrist.
- Forms part of the concavity of the radiocarpal joint.
- Helps transfer part of the compression forces that naturally cross the hand to the forearm. About 20% of the total compression force that crosses the wrist passes through the fibrocartilage disc component of the TFCC.

Refer to Box 7.1 for a list of the components of the TFCC.

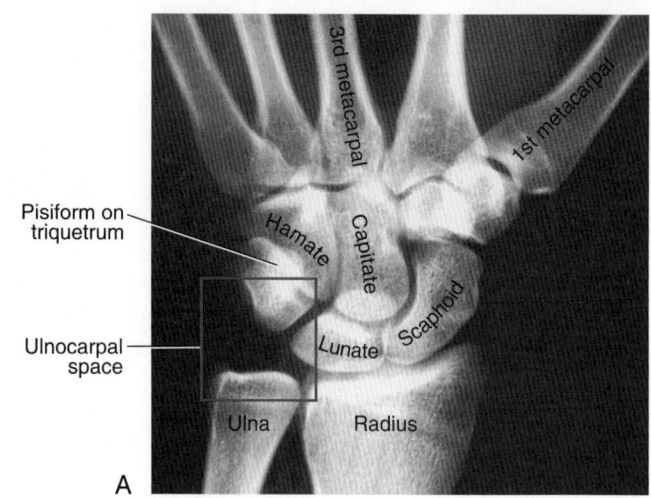

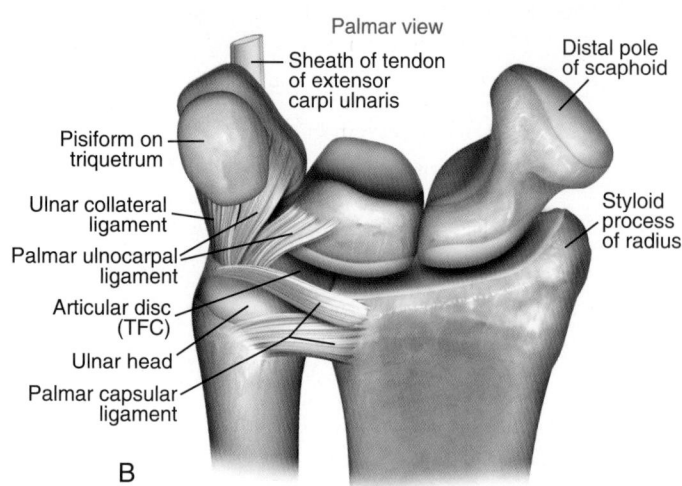

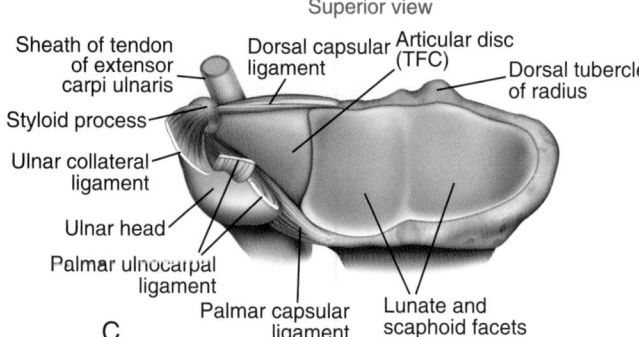

FIGURE 7.11 (A) Radiograph showing bones associated with the right wrist, including the "ulnocarpal space" (in red box). Panels B and C illustrate palmar and superior views of the wrist region, respectively, highlighting the triangular fibrocartilage complex (TFCC), which occupies much of the ulnocarpal space. The central feature of the TFCC is the triangular fibrocartilage *(TFC)*, often referred to simply as the articular disc.

Fig. 7.23). The floor of the compartment is adhered to the dorsal capsular ligament of the distal radio-ulnar joint. The floor of this fascial compartment and enclosed tendon thereby indirectly stabilizes the dorsal side of the triangular fibrocartilage.

A structurally intact TFCC is essential to normal function of the distal radio-ulnar joint and the wrist. As described in Chapter 6, degenerative changes within the TFCC can lead to pain and varying degrees of joint instability, often from an injury or secondary to advanced rheumatoid arthritis. In addition to pain and instability, symptoms of TFCC degeneration or inflammation may involve a weakened grip, crepitus, and reduced range of motion at the wrist and forearm. Injury to the more central part of the disc may not heal well and may benefit from arthroscopic intervention.[14]

Intrinsic Ligaments

Essentially every intercarpal junction is bound and strengthened by one or more intrinsic ligaments. Some of the ligaments are relatively thick and evident and others are small and not even formally named. Only the more defined and structurally relevant intrinsic ligaments will be described in this chapter.

The intrinsic ligaments of the wrist can be conveniently classified into three sets based on their relative length: short, intermediate, or long (see Box 7.1).[122] *Short ligaments* connect the bones of the distal row by their palmar, dorsal, or interosseous surfaces (see Figs. 7.9 and 7.10). The short ligaments firmly stabilize and unite the distal row of bones, permitting them to function effectively as a single mechanical unit.

Several intermediate ligaments exist within the wrist. The *lunotriquetral ligament* is an important stabilizer of the ulnar side of the lunate relative to the triquetrum. Although the ligament has multiple components, only the palmer fibers are shown in Fig. 7.10.[94] This ligament functions cooperatively with the very clinically relevant *scapholunate ligament*, the primary stabilizer of the scapholunate joint (see Figs. 7.7 and 7.8A). The scapholunate ligament has dorsal, palmar, and proximal fibers, by far, however, the dorsal fibers are the thickest and strongest.[9] The scapholunate ligament relies on its attachments to the mechanically stable scaphoid bone to secure the proper position of the inherently unstable lunate. The disproportionally high density of mechanoreceptors within the ligament adds to the functional importance of this structure.[42] The broader topic of the scapholunate ligament's important role in carpal stability will be described later in this chapter.

While the lunotriquetral and scapholunate ligaments provide an important element of stability *among* the proximal row of carpal bones, the *scaphotrapezial and scaphotrapezoidal ligaments* add significantly to the security to the junction *between* the two rows. These ligaments reinforce the articulation between the distal pole of the scaphoid with the trapezium and trapezoid (see Figs. 7.7 and 7.9).

Two relatively *long ligaments* are present within the wrist. First, the *palmar intercarpal ligament* attaches along palmar surfaces of the well-anchored capitate bone (see Fig. 7.10). From this stable origin, the ligament courses proximally as two discrete fiber groups, resembling the shape of an inverted V. The *lateral leg* of the inverted V attaches to the scaphoid, and the *medial leg* to the triquetrum. As depicted ahead in Fig. 7.17, these ligaments help guide certain arthrokinematics of the wrist.

The second of the two *long ligaments* is the thin *dorsal intercarpal ligament,* which provides transverse stability across the dorsum of the wrist (Fig. 7.9). The ligament attaches on the dorsal sides of the trapezium and scaphoid, then passes directly over (and frequently attaching to) the lunate as it courses ulnarly to attach to the dorsal side the triquetrum.[120,131] The ligament provides important structural reinforcement to the dorsal side of the scapholunate joint, lending an often much needed secondary stability to this articulation.[7,71,91] Similar to the dorsal radiocarpal and dorsal parts of the scapholunate ligaments, the dorsal intercarpal ligaments possess a disproportionally large number of radial nerve-associated mechanoreceptors, suggesting an important role in active coordination of wrist movement.[41,42]

Kinematics of Wrist Motion

OSTEOKINEMATICS

The osteokinematics of the wrist are formally defined for two degrees of freedom, each plane oriented at right angles to each other: flexion-extension in the sagittal plane and ulnar-radial deviation in the frontal plane (Fig. 7.12). Wrist circumduction—a full circular motion made by the wrist—is a combination of the aforementioned movements, not a distinct third degree of freedom.

The axis of rotation for the pure planar wrist movements passes through or near the head of the capitate (Fig. 7.13).[139] The axis runs in a near medial-lateral direction for flexion and extension and near anterior-posterior direction for radial and ulnar deviation. The firm articulation between the capitate and the base of the third metacarpal bone allows the rotation of the capitate to direct the osteokinematic path of the entire hand.

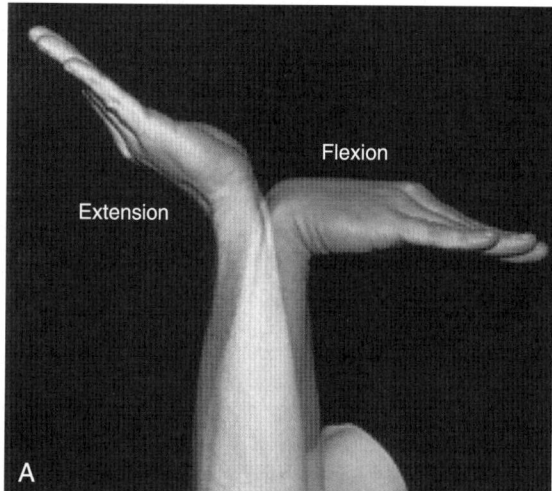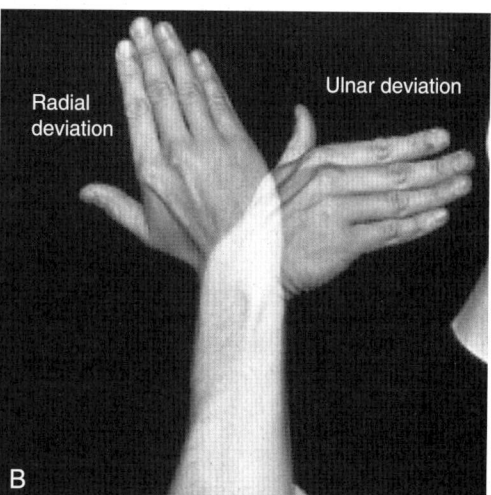

FIGURE 7.12 Osteokinematics of the wrist. (A) Flexion and extension. (B) Ulnar and radial deviation. Note that flexion exceeds extension and ulnar deviation exceeds radial deviation.

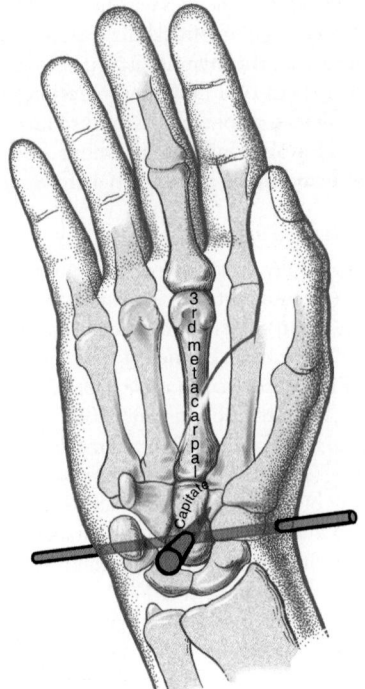

FIGURE 7.13 The medial-lateral *(green)* and anterior-posterior *(purple)* axes of rotation for wrist movement are shown piercing the head of the capitate bone.

The full range of motion of the wrist is typically measured by a standard goniometer or, equally well, through smartphone level or photography applications.[72,133] Typically, the wrist rotates about 130 to 160 degrees within the sagittal plane (see Fig. 7.12A). On average, the wrist flexes from 0 degrees to about 70 to 85 degrees and extends from 0 degrees to about 60 to 75 degrees.[104,109] The motion of flexion normally exceeds extension by about 10 to 15 degrees. End range extension is naturally limited by stiffness in the thick palmar radiocarpal ligaments. In some persons, a greater than average palmar tilt of the distal radius may also limit extension range (see Fig. 7.4B).

On average, the wrist rotates approximately 50 to 60 degrees in the frontal plane (see Fig. 7.12B).[104,139] The motion of radial and ulnar deviation is measured as the angle between the radius and the shaft of the third metacarpal. Ulnar deviation typically occurs from 0 degrees to about 35 to 40 degrees, while radial deviation typically occurs from 0 degrees to about 15 to 20 degrees. Primarily because of the ulnar tilt of the distal radius (see Fig. 7.4A), maximum ulnar deviation normally is double the maximum amount of radial deviation.

Ryu and colleagues measured the range of wrist motion needed to perform 24 common activities of 2 daily living (ADLs) in 40 healthy subjects.[104] The ADLs included personal care, hygiene, food preparation, writing, and using various tools or utensils. The researchers concluded that most of these ADLs could be comfortably performed using 40 degrees of flexion, 40 degrees of extension, 10 degrees of radial deviation, and 30 degrees of ulnar deviation. Three notable exceptions to this comfort range are: 1) pushing down with arms to help stand up from a seated position requires 60 degrees of wrist extension; 2) perineal care requires 54 degrees of wrist flexion; and 3) safely driving an automobile requires 38 degrees of ulnar deviation—essentially full range in most persons.[99,104]

Although wrist motions are typically described and often evaluated within the pure sagittal and frontal planes, the more functional

SPECIAL FOCUS 7.2

Passive Axial Rotation at the Wrist: How Much and Why?

In addition to flexion-extension and radial-ulnar deviation, the wrist allows a significant amount of passive axial rotation. This accessory motion (or joint "play") can be appreciated by firmly grasping your right clenched fist with your left hand. While securely holding your right hand from moving, strongly attempt to actively pronate and supinate the right forearm. The passive axial rotation at the right wrist is demonstrated by the rotation of the distal radius relative to the fixed base of the hand. Gupta and Moosawi reported an average of 34 degrees of total passive axial rotation in 20 asymptomatic wrists; the midcarpal joint permitted on average three times more passive axial rotation than the radiocarpal joint.[39]

The ultimate extent of axial rotation at the wrist is naturally limited by the shapes of the joints, especially the elliptic fit of the radiocarpal joint, and the tension in the obliquely oriented radiocarpal ligaments. Because the wrist's potential third degree of freedom is restricted, the hand ultimately must *follow* the pronating and supinating radius; and furthermore, the restriction allows the pronator and supinator muscles to effectively transfer their torques across the wrist to the working hand.

Accessory motions within the wrist—as in all synovial joints—enhance the overall function of the joint. For example, axial rotation at the wrist amplifies the total extent of functional pronation and supination of the hand relative to the forearm, as well as dampens the impact of reaching these end range movements. These functions are useful for activities such as wringing out clothes or turning doorknobs.

and natural path of motion involves a kinematic blend *among* planes: extension occurs with some radial deviation, and flexion with some ulnar deviation. The resulting path of motion follows an oblique path, similar to a *dart thrower's motion*.[21,74] This specific path varies depending on the task, but is usually angled out of the pure sagittal plane between about 25 and 50 degrees.[10,21,62,74] Such a movement is distinctively a human characteristic, likely associated with the human's unique skill in throwing objects. The full arc of a dart throwing motion is 35% to 40% greater than the full arc of a pure sagittal plane motion.[21,74] The kinematic coupling inherent to the functional dart thrower's motion is evident in many activities other than throwing, such as tying shoelaces, opening and closing a jar, drinking from a glass, casting a fishing pole, or combing hair. The dart throwing motion also reflects the dominant actions of many wrist muscles (to be described). For these reasons, the natural kinematics associated with the dart throwing motion should be considered during treatment and functional assessment of the wrist and hand.[10]

Decisions on the specific surgical management of a severely painful or unstable wrist is often dependent on factors such as the extent or type of pathology, or the anticipated physical demands required of the wrist after surgery. Some patients may require a *proximal row carpectomy,* allowing the capitate to articulate directly with the radius. In other cases, the wrist may require a partial or complete *arthrodesis* (surgical fusion). To minimize the functional impairment associated with a fusion, the wrist is often fused in an "average" static *position of function:* about 10 to 15 degrees of extension and 10 degrees of ulnar deviation.[105] Although permanently fusing a wrist (even partially) may seem like a radical option, the procedure may be the best treatment to achieve stability, relieve pain, and improve function. In some cases, a wrist arthrodesis may be a more practical surgical option than a *total wrist arthroplasty.* This is especially true in persons with a weakened bone stock from advanced rheumatoid arthritis or a history of bone infections, or for those who may be returning to a physically demanding occupation or lifestyle that may overstress the prosthesis.

The most common design of a total wrist arthroplasty replaces the degenerated distal radius and proximal row of carpal bones with metal-polyethylene implants. One obvious advantage of arthroplasty over wrist fusion is that it allows some movement of the hand. In general, the total wrist arthroplasty is considered a viable surgical option for treating a painful and arthritic wrist.[119] However, the total wrist arthroplasty has not reached the level of success of

arthroplasty of other joints in the body, such as the hip or knee.[46,77] One obstacle is the inherent mechanical complexity of the wrist; another is the small size of the replacement components, which concentrates high stress on the implanted material. Over time, high stress can contribute to premature loosening of the prosthesis.

The success rate of total wrist arthroplasty will likely continue to improve with continued advances in surgical technique, preoperative and postoperative management, knowledge of the natural biomechanics, and design of implants.[140]

ARTHROKINEMATICS

A wide range of methods have been used to study the detailed arthrokinematics of the wrist. Methods include linking cadaver material with electromechanical devices, planar radiography, biplanar cineradiography, dynamic 4D computed tomography, MRI, and computational modeling. Even with these sophisticated techniques, the resulting kinematic data do not always agree. Precise and repeatable descriptions of the kinematics are hampered by the sheer complexity and natural anatomic variation of the many moving articular interfaces.[56] Although much has been learned over the last several decades, the understanding of carpal kinematics continues to evolve.

Due to the structural complexity of the wrist, several conceptual models have evolved over the years to simplify the analysis and description of wrist kinematics.[97] This chapter describes the kinematics of the wrist assuming it is a double-joint system, with movement occurring simultaneously at both the *radiocarpal joint* and the *medial compartment of the midcarpal joint.* The exclusive focus on the medial compartment of the midcarpal joint is based on its structural prominence and proximity to the wrist's overall axis of rotation. The following discussion on arthrokinematics focuses on the dynamic relationship between these two joints.

Wrist Extension and Flexion

The essential kinematics of sagittal plane motion at the wrist can be appreciated by modeling the wrist as an articulated *central column,* formed by the linkages between the distal radius, lunate, capitate, and third metacarpal (Fig. 7.14).[97] Within this column, the *radiocarpal joint* is represented by the articulation between the radius and lunate, and the medial compartment of the *midcarpal joint* is represented by the articulation between the lunate and capitate. The carpometacarpal joint is a semirigid articulation formed between the capitate and the base of the third metacarpal.

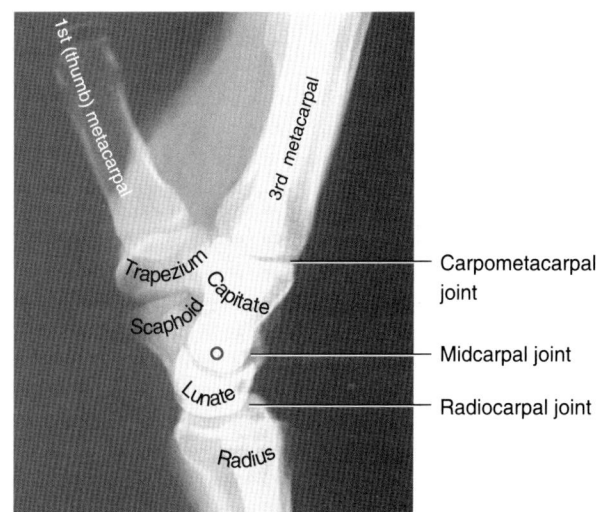

FIGURE 7.14 A lateral view of a radiograph of the central column of the wrist. The axis of rotation for flexion and extension is shown as a small circle at the base of the capitate. Observe the crescent shape of the lunate. For illustrative purposes, the lunate and capitate bones have been digitally enhanced.

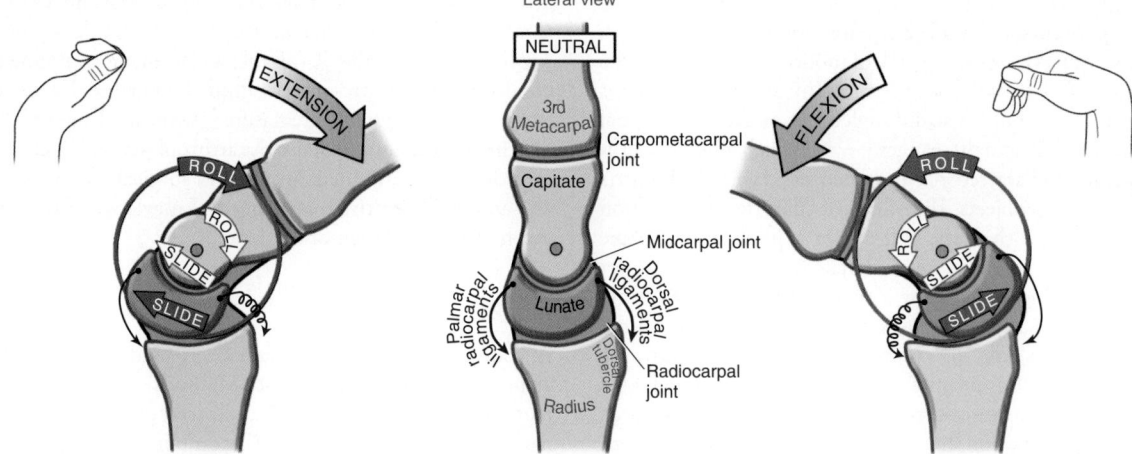

FIGURE 7.15 A model of the central column of the right wrist showing flexion and extension. The wrist in the center is shown at rest, in a neutral position. The roll-and-slide arthrokinematics are shown in the reddish color for the radiocarpal joint and in white for the midcarpal joint. During wrist extension *(left)*, the dorsal radiocarpal ligaments become slackened and the palmar radiocarpal ligaments become taut. The reverse arthrokinematics occur during wrist flexion *(right)*.

Dynamic Interaction within the Joints of the Central Column of the Wrist

The arthrokinematics of extension and flexion are based on synchronous convex-on-concave rotations at both the radiocarpal and the midcarpal joints. The arthrokinematics at the radiocarpal joint are highlighted by the reddish color in Fig. 7.15. *Extension* occurs as the convex surface of the lunate rolls dorsally on the radius and simultaneously slides in a palmar direction. The rolling motion directs the lunate's distal surface dorsally, toward the direction of extension. At the midcarpal joint, illustrated in white in Fig. 7.15, the head of the capitate rolls dorsally on the lunate and simultaneously slides in a palmar direction. Combining the arthrokinematics over both joints produces full wrist extension. This two-joint system has the advantage of yielding a significant total range of motion by requiring only moderate amounts of rotation at the individual joints. Mechanically, therefore, each joint moves within a relatively limited—and therefore more stable—arc of motion.

Full wrist extension elongates the palmar radiocarpal ligaments and all muscles that potentially flex the wrist. Tension within these stretched structures helps stabilize the wrist in its close-packed position of full extension.[67,96] Stability in full wrist extension is useful when weight is borne through the upper extremity during activities such as crawling on the hands and knees, using an assistive device for walking, and transferring one's own body from a wheelchair to a bed.

The arthrokinematics of wrist *flexion* are like those described for extension but occur in a reverse fashion (see Fig. 7.15).

Several studies have attempted to quantify the individual angular contributions of the radiocarpal and midcarpal joints to the total sagittal plane motion of the wrist.[8,24,62,73,121] Summarizing the detailed results of these studies is difficult given the large differences in research designs and methods of measurement. However, when considering the full range of motion, with few exceptions, most studies report synchronous and roughly equivalent—or at least significant—contributions from both joints.[60,62,85,97]

Using the simplified central column model to describe flexion and extension of the wrist offers an excellent conceptualization of a rather complex event. A limitation of the model, however, is that it does not account for *all* the carpal bones that participate in the motion. For example, the model ignores the kinematics of the

scaphoid bone at the radiocarpal joint. In brief, the arthrokinematics of the scaphoid on the radius are fundamentally like those of the lunate during flexion and extension, except for one feature. Based on different rotational axes, size, and curvature of the two bones, the scaphoid rolls on the radius at a different speed, magnitude, and path than the lunate.[8,11,96] This difference causes a linear and angular displacement between the scaphoid and lunate by the end of full motion. Normally, in the healthy wrist, the amount of displacement is minimized by the restraining action of ligaments, such as the scapholunate ligament (see Figs. 7.7 and 7.8A).

Ulnar and Radial Deviation of the Wrist
Dynamic Interaction Between the Radiocarpal and Midcarpal Joints

Like flexion and extension, ulnar and radial deviation occurs through synchronous convex-on-concave rotations at the radiocarpal joint and medial compartment of the midcarpal joint.[76] During *ulnar deviation,* the midcarpal and radiocarpal joints each contribute significant and, on average, roughly equivalent rotations to overall wrist motion (Fig. 7.16).[8,53,60] At the radiocarpal joint highlighted by the reddish color in Fig. 7.16, the scaphoid, lunate, and triquetrum roll in an ulnar direction and slide a significant distance radially. The extent of this radial slide is apparent by the final position of the lunate relative to the radius at full ulnar deviation. Ulnar deviation at the midcarpal joint occurs primarily from the capitate rolling in an ulnar direction and sliding slightly radially.

Radial deviation at the wrist occurs through similar arthrokinematics as described for ulnar deviation (see Fig. 7.16). The amount of radial deviation at the radiocarpal joint is limited because the radial side of the carpus impinges against the styloid process of the radius (refer to x-ray at top right of Fig. 7.16). Consequently, most of the radial deviation across the wrist occurs at the midcarpal joint.[8,53]

Additional Arthrokinematics Involving the Proximal Row of Carpal Bones

Careful observation of ulnar and radial deviation reveals more complicated arthrokinematics than described earlier. During the frontal plane movements, the proximal row of carpal bones "rocks" slightly into flexion and extension and, to a much lesser extent, "twists." The rocking motion is most noticeable in the scaphoid and, to a lesser

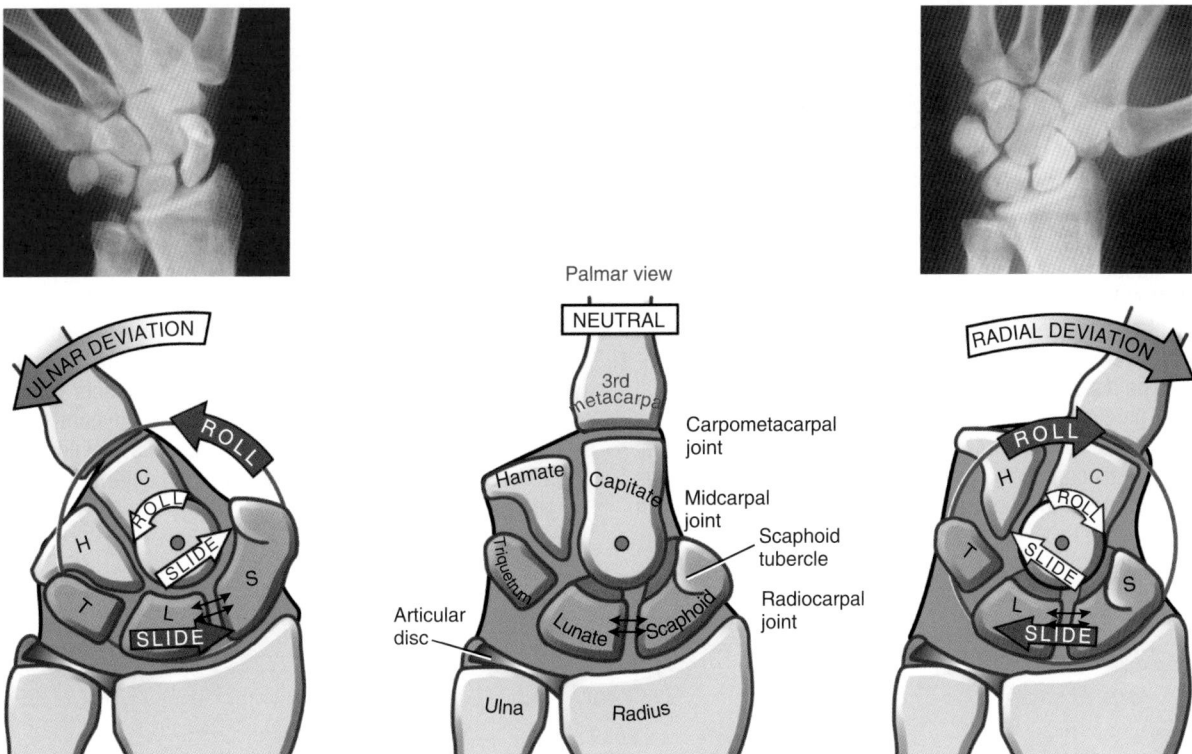

FIGURE 7.16 Radiographs and mechanical depiction of the arthrokinematics of ulnar and radial deviation for the right wrist. The roll-and-slide arthrokinematics are shown in reddish color for the radiocarpal joint and in white for the midcarpal joint. The scapholunate ligament is mechanically depicted in each drawing as two short arrows.

extent, the lunate. During radial deviation the proximal row *flexes* slightly; during ulnar deviation the proximal row *extends* slightly.[53,55] Note in Fig. 7.16, especially on the radiograph, the change in position of the scaphoid tubercle between the extremes of ulnar and radial deviation. According to Moojen and co-workers, at 20 degrees of ulnar deviation the scaphoid is rotated about 20 degrees into extension, relative to the radius.[73] The scaphoid appears to "stand up" or to lengthen with ulnar deviation, which projects its tubercle distally. At 20 degrees of radial deviation, the scaphoid flexes beyond neutral about 15 degrees, taking on a shortened stature with its tubercle having approached the radius. A functional shortening of the scaphoid may allow increased space for the carpus to more freely rotate towards end range of radial deviation (Video 7.1). The exact mechanism responsible for flexion and extension of bones within the proximal carpus during radial and ulnar deviation is not fully understood. Most likely, the mechanism is driven through a combination of forces produced by activated muscle, elongated and thus tensed ligaments, and compressions between adjacent bones. For such a complex mechanism to occur with only minimal carpal stress, adequate subconscious proprioceptive guidance is required through the many richly innervated structures.

The scaphoid's sagittal plane motion relative to the lunate during radial and ulnar deviation places natural stress within the scapholunate ligament (depicted as pairs of arrows in Fig. 7.16). In the normal wrist, this stress is typically well tolerated. In some cases, however, the repetitive and cyclic stress may weaken or rupture this or other ligaments, especially when combined with a preexisting injury or laxity. Rupture or weakness within this important ligament can significantly alter the arthrokinematics and transfer of

forces within the proximal row of carpal bones.[137] A mechanically unstable scapholunate articulation is typically associated with increased stress on other intercarpal joints, often leading to further carpal degenerative changes and pain.

Carpal Instability

Carpal instability describes a pathologic condition where any set of articulated carpal bones fails to remain normally aligned when challenged by a wide range of movements and loads. Carpal instability is typically associated with pain and a loss of function of the wrist and the hand. In its worst case, the increased carpal stress associated with the instability results in osteoarthritis.

The factor that typically initiates the events that lead to carpal instability is laxity or rupture of ligaments. The ultimate manifestation of the instability however depends on the severity and underlying cause for the ligaments' failure, combined with the overall health and responsiveness of the governing sensory-motor system.[42] The following examples (listed in the box below) introduce only two of many forms of carpal instability. A more detailed description of this extensive topic is beyond the scope of this textbook.

Two Common Forms of Carpal Instability
1. Rotational collapse of wrist: the "zigzag" deformity
   - Dorsal intercalated segment instability (DISI)
   - Volar intercalated segment instability (VISI)
2. Ulnar translocation of the carpus

SPECIAL FOCUS 7.3

Guiding Tensions within the "Double-V" System of Ligaments

The arthrokinematics of the wrist are ultimately driven by muscle but, to a large degree, are guided by intercarpal compression forces and by passive tension within ligaments. Fig. 7.17 illustrates one example of how a system of ligaments helps control the arthrokinematics of ulnar and radial deviation. In the neutral position, four ligaments appear as two inverted Vs, which have been referred to as the *double-V system of ligaments*.[122] The *distal inverted V* is formed by the medial and lateral legs of the palmar intercarpal ligament; the *proximal inverted V* is formed by the lunate attachments of the palmar ulnocarpal and palmar radiocarpal ligaments (see Fig. 7.10). All four legs of the ligamentous mechanism are under slight tension even in the neutral position. During ulnar deviation, passive tension increases diagonally across the wrist by the stretch placed in the lateral leg of the palmar intercarpal ligament and fibers of the palmar ulnocarpal ligament.[135] During *radial deviation,* tension is created in the opposite diagonal by a stretch in the medial leg of the palmar intercarpal ligament and fibers of the palmar radiocarpal ligament (in particular, the long radiolunate ligaments). A gradual increase in tension within these ligaments provides a source of control to the movement, as well as dynamic stability to the carpal bones. Tensions in stretched collateral ligaments of the wrist may assist the double-V system in determining the end range of radial and ulnar deviation.

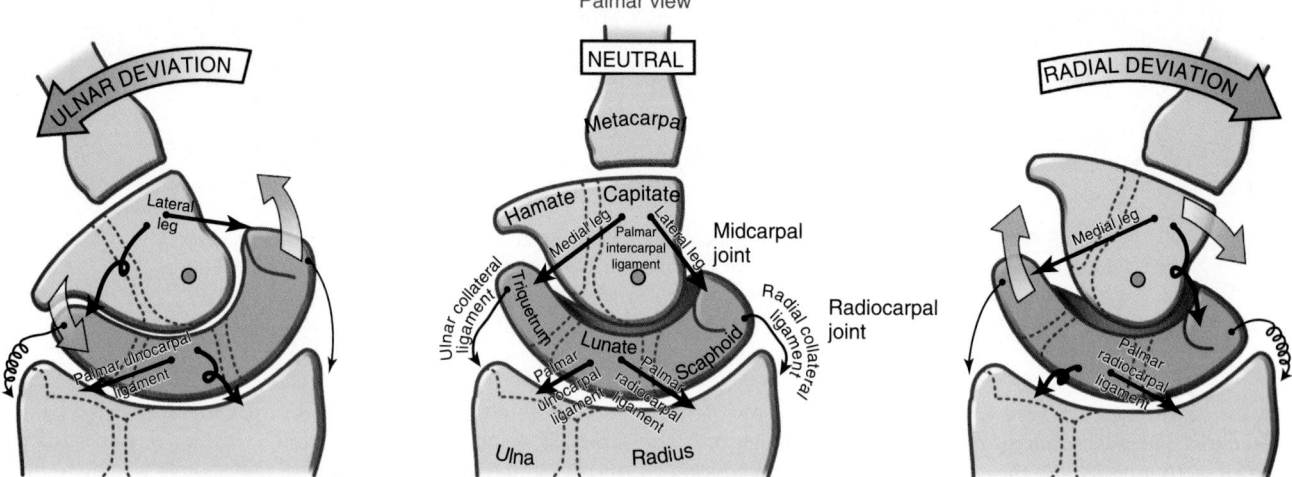

FIGURE 7.17 The tensing and slackening of the "double-V" system ligaments of the wrist are illustrated. The collateral ligaments are also shown. The bones have been blocked together for simplicity. Taut lines represent ligaments under increased tension.

ROTATIONAL COLLAPSE OF THE WRIST

Mechanically, the wrist consists of a mobile proximal row of carpal bones intercalated or interposed between two relatively rigid structures: the forearm (radius) and the distal row of carpal bones. Like cars of a freight train that are subject to derailment, the proximal row of carpal bones is susceptible to a rotational collapse in a "zigzag" fashion when compressed from both ends (Fig. 7.18). The compression forces that cross the wrist arise mainly from muscle activation and external contact. In most healthy persons, the wrist remains stable and well aligned when subjected to physiologic loads. Collapse and subsequent joint dislocation are prevented primarily by resistance from ligaments and muscles and by the position and articular shape of the adjoining carpal bones.[106] Although Fig. 7.18 depicts an oversimplification of the pathomechanics of most carpal instabilities, the figure nevertheless highlights an important underlying mechanical theme of the pathology.

The lunate is the most frequently dislocated carpal bone. Normally its stability is provided by ligaments and articular contact with adjacent bones of the proximal row, such as the scaphoid bone as depicted in Fig. 7.19A.[97] By virtue of its two poles, the scaphoid forms an important mechanical link between the lunate and the more stable, distal row of carpal bones. The continuity of this link typically requires that the scaphoid and adjoining ligaments be intact. Consider, as an example, a fall on an outstretched hand with a resulting fracture in the "waist" region of the scaphoid and tearing of the scapholunate ligament (see Fig. 7.19B). Disruption of the mechanical link between the two bones can result in *scapholunate dissociation* and subsequent malalignment of either or both bones.[91] As shown in Fig. 7.19B, the inherently less stable lunate may dislocate, or sublux, so its distal articular surface faces *dorsally.* This condition is referred to clinically as *dorsal intercalated segment instability* (DISI) (Fig. 7.20). The pathomechanics of DISI are often much more complicated or more varied than just described. For example, DISI can occur without scaphoid fracture but with tears of the scapholunate ligament along with other several secondary stabilizers of the scapholunate joint, such as the dorsal intercarpal, dorsal radiocarpal, or scaphotrapezial ligaments.[91,94]

For example, injury to the scapholunate and the scaphotrapezial ligaments may allow the scaphoid to excessively flex (rock forward) as the lunate progressively subluxes dorsally. In addition to the scapholunate malalignment, an excessive gap (or diastasis) typically forms between the scaphoid and lunate (as in Fig. 7.19B). Radiographic evidence of a gap of more than 3 mm is often used as a benchmark to suspect a clinically relevant scapholunate dissociation.[54] Active muscle contraction associated with grasp or bearing weight across the wrist with a DISI may force the capitate proximally between the scaphoid and lunate, thereby widening the preexisting gap.

Injury to other ligaments, such as the lunotriquetral ligament, may allow the lunate to dislocate such that its distal articular surface faces in a *volar* (palmar) orientation. This condition is referred to as *volar (palmar) intercalated segment instability* (VISI). Regardless of the type or direction of rotational collapse, the consequences can be painful and disabling. The abnormal arthrokinematics may create regions of high stress, possibly leading to more degeneration, chronic inflammation, and changes in the shapes of the bones. A painful and unstable wrist may fail to provide a stable platform for the hand. A collapsed wrist may also alter the length-tension relationship and moment arms of the muscles that cross the region. Surgery may be necessary to repair or augment a torn ligament.[59] A qualified hand therapist plays an important role in the management of both non-surgical and postsurgical rehabilitation.[28,52,116] Therapists need to understand the underlying pathomechanics to optimize the benefits of the medical intervention. Further discussions on the conservative treatment of scapholunate ligament injury can be found in Clinical Connection 7.3.

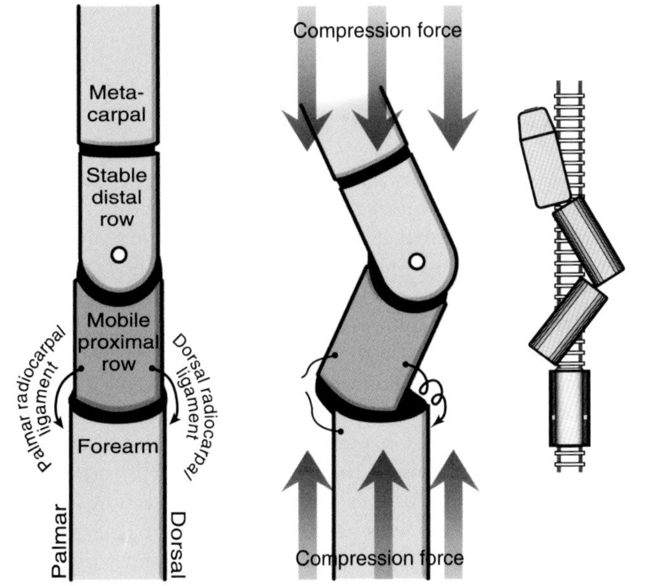

FIGURE 7.18 A highly diagrammatic depiction of a "zigzag" collapse of the central column of the wrist after a large compression force.

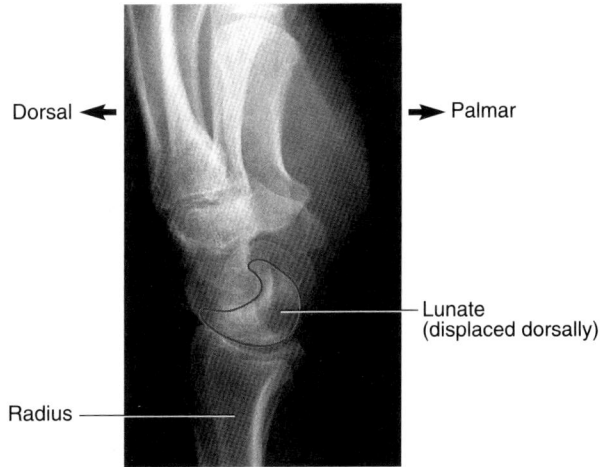

FIGURE 7.20 Lateral radiograph showing an abnormal *dorsal* position of the distal surface of the lunate, a condition referred to as *dorsal intercalated segment instability* (DISI). (Radiograph courtesy Jon Marion, CHT, OTR, and Thomas Hitchcock, MD, Marshfield Clinic, Marshfield, WI.)

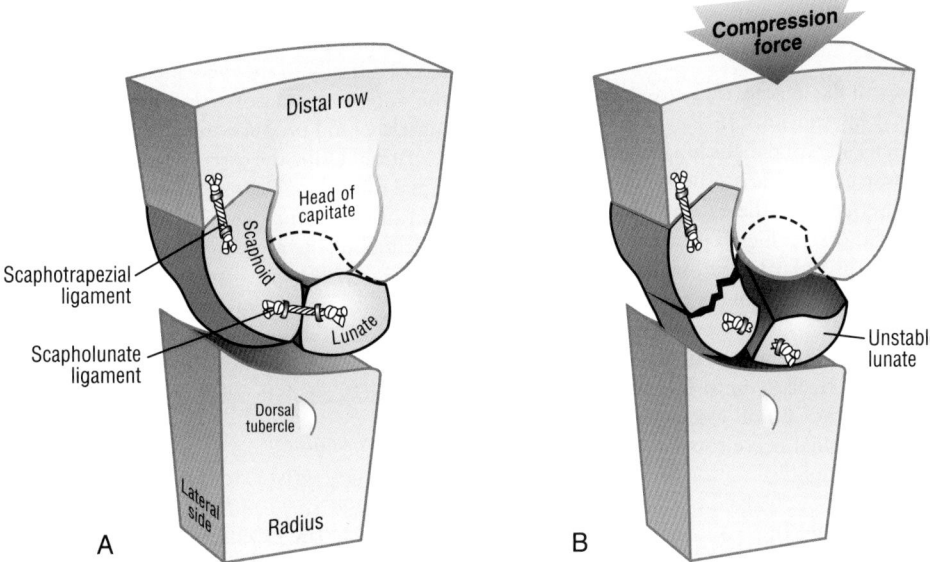

FIGURE 7.19 Highly mechanical model showing factors that maintain stability of the lunate. (A) Acting through ligaments, the scaphoid provides a mechanical linkage between the relatively mobile lunate and the rigid distal row of carpal bones. (B) Compression forces through the wrist from a fall may fracture the scaphoid and tear the scapholunate ligament. Loss of the mechanical link provided by the scaphoid often leads to lunate instability and/or dislocation. Note the excessive gap formed between the scaphoid and lunate bones.

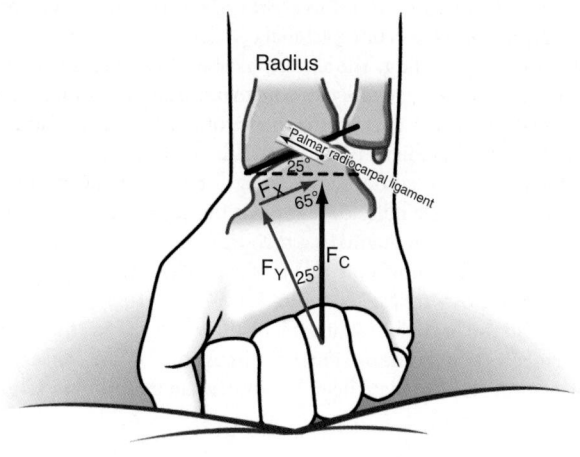

FIGURE 7.21 This illustration shows how the ulnar tilt of the distal radius can predispose to ulnar translocation of the carpus. Compression forces (F_C) that cross the wrist are resolved into (1) a force vector acting perpendicularly to the radiocarpal joint (F_Y) and (2) a force vector (F_X) running parallel to the radiocarpal joint. The F_Y force compresses and stabilizes the radiocarpal joint with a magnitude of about 90% of F_C (cosine 25° × F_C). The F_X force tends to translate the carpus in an ulnar direction, with a magnitude of 42% of F_C (sine 25° × F_C). Note that the fiber direction of the palmar radiocarpal ligament resists this natural ulnar translation of the carpus. The greater the ulnar tilt and/or compression force across the wrist, the greater the potential for the ulnar translation.

ULNAR TRANSLOCATION OF THE CARPUS

As pointed out earlier, the distal end of the radius is angled from side to side so that its articular surface is sloped in an ulnar about 25 degrees (see Fig. 7.4A). This *ulnar tilt* of the distal radius creates a natural tendency for the compressed carpus to slide (translate) in an ulnar direction. Fig. 7.21 shows that a wrist with an ulnar tilt of 25 degrees has an ulnar translation force of 42% of the total compression force that crosses the wrist. This translational force is naturally resisted by passive tension from various extrinsic ligaments, such as the obliquely oriented dorsal and palmar radiocarpal ligaments.[103,113] If these ligaments are weakened, the carpus may, over time, migrate in an ulnar direction. An excessive ulnar translocation can significantly alter the biomechanics of the wrist, potentially initiating a zigzag deformity that extends distally throughout the joints of the hand.

MUSCLE AND JOINT INTERACTION

Innervation of the Wrist Muscles and Joints

INNERVATION OF MUSCLE

The *radial nerve* innervates all the muscles that cross the dorsal side of the wrist (see Fig. II-1B in Appendix II, Part A). The primary wrist extensors are the extensor carpi radialis longus, extensor carpi radialis brevis, and extensor carpi ulnaris. The *median and ulnar nerves* innervate all muscles that cross the palmar side of the wrist, including the primary wrist flexors (see Figs. II-1C–D in Appendix II, Part A). The flexor carpi radialis and palmaris longus are innervated by the median nerve; the flexor carpi ulnaris is innervated by the ulnar nerve. As a reference, the primary spinal nerve roots that supply the muscles of the upper extremity are listed in Appendix II, Part B. In addition, Appendix II, Parts C to E include additional reference items to help guide the clinical assessment of the functional status of the C^5 to T^1 spinal nerve roots and several major peripheral nerves of the upper limb.

SENSORY INNERVATION OF THE JOINTS

The connective tissues associated with the radiocarpal and midcarpal joints receive sensory fibers predominantly from the C^6 and C^7 spinal nerve roots carried extensively in the radial nerve, but also in the median and lateral cutaneous nerve of the forearm.[30,38,42] The midcarpal joint is also innervated by sensory nerves traveling to the C^8 spinal nerve root via the deep branch of the ulnar nerve.

Function of the Muscles at the Wrist

The wrist is controlled by a primary and a secondary set of muscles. The muscles within the *primary set* attach distally within the carpus, or the adjacent proximal end of the metacarpals; these muscles act primarily on the wrist only. The muscles within the *secondary set* cross the carpus as they continue distally to attach to the digits. The secondary muscles therefore act on the wrist *and* the hand. This chapter focuses more on the muscles of the primary set. The anatomy and kinesiology of the muscles of the secondary set—such as the extensor pollicis longus and the flexor digitorum superficialis—are considered in detail in Chapter 8. The proximal and distal attachments and nerve supply of the muscles of the wrist are listed in Appendix II, Part F. Also, as a reference, cross-sectional areas of selected muscles of the wrist are listed in Appendix II, Part G.

As depicted in Fig. 7.13, the medial-lateral and anterior-posterior axes of rotation of the wrist intersect within the head of the capitate bone. Except for the palmaris longus, no muscle has a line of force that passes precisely *through* either axis of rotation. At least from the anatomic position, therefore, essentially all wrist muscles are equipped with moment arms to produce torques in both sagittal and frontal planes. The extensor carpi radialis longus, for example, passes dorsally to the medial-lateral axis of rotation and laterally to the anterior-posterior axis of rotation. Contraction of only this muscle would produce a combination of wrist extension *and* radial deviation. Using the extensor carpi radialis longus to produce a pure radial deviation motion, for example, would necessitate the activation of other muscles to neutralize the undesired wrist extension potential of the aforementioned muscle. Muscles of the wrist and hand rarely act in isolation when producing a meaningful movement. This theme of intermuscular cooperation will be further developed in this chapter and Chapter 8.

FUNCTION OF THE WRIST EXTENSORS

Muscular Anatomy

The primary wrist extensors are the *extensor carpi radialis longus,* the *extensor carpi radialis brevis,* and the *extensor carpi ulnaris* (Fig. 7.22). The extensor digitorum is also capable of generating significant wrist extension torque but is mainly involved with extension of the fingers. Other secondary wrist extensors are the extensor indicis, extensor digiti minimi, and extensor pollicis longus.

The proximal attachments of the primary wrist extensors are located on and near the lateral ("extensor-supinator") epicondyle of the humerus and dorsal border of the ulna (see Figs. 6.2 and 6.6).

Distally, the extensor carpi radialis longus and brevis attach side by side to the dorsal bases of the second and third metacarpals; the extensor carpi ulnaris attaches to the dorsal base of the fifth metacarpal.

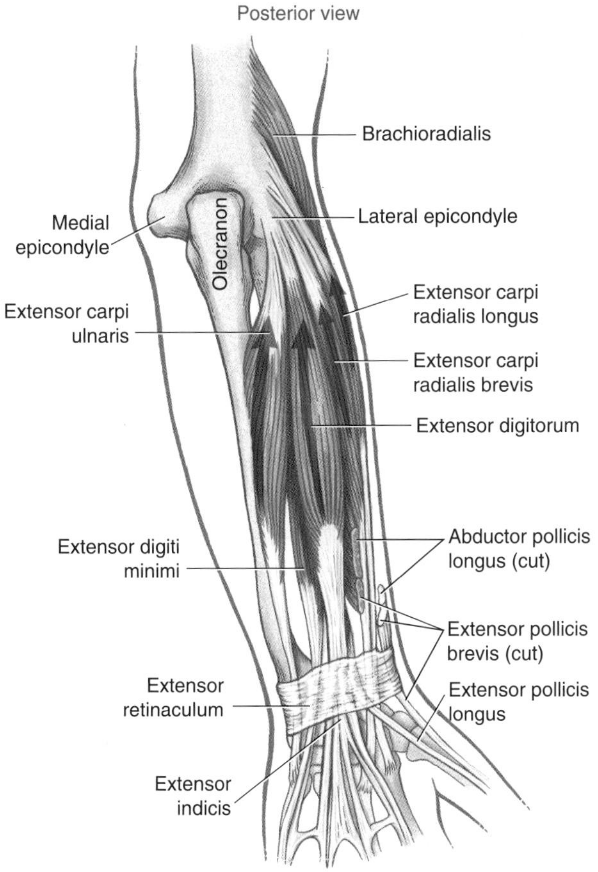

The tendons of the muscles that cross the dorsal and dorsal-radial side of the wrist are secured in place by the *extensor retinaculum* (Fig. 7.23). Ulnarly, the extensor retinaculum wraps around the styloid process of the ulna to attach palmar to the tendon of the flexor carpi ulnaris, pisiform bone, and pisometacarpal ligament. Radially, the retinaculum attaches to the region of the styloid process of the radius and the radial collateral ligament. The extensor retinaculum prevents the underlying tendons from "bowstringing" up and away from the radiocarpal joint during active movements of the wrist.

Between the extensor retinaculum and the underlying bones are six *fibro-osseus compartments* that house the tendons along with their synovial sheaths.[50] Clinicians frequently refer to these compartments by Roman numerals I to VI (see Fig. 7.23). Each compartment houses a specific set of tendons. Tenosynovitis frequently occurs within one or more of these compartments, often from repetitive or forceful activities that increase tension on the associated tendons. The tendons and surrounding synovial membranes within compartment I are particularly susceptible to inflammation, a condition called *de Quervain's tenosynovitis.* Activities that frequently cause this painful condition include repetitively pressing the trigger switch on a power tool, gripping tools while simultaneously supinating and pronating the forearm, or wringing out clothes. De Quervain's tenosynovitis is typically treated conservatively by using phonophoresis or iontophoresis, administering corticosteroid injections, applying ice, wearing a hand-wrist–based thumb splint, and modifying the activities that caused the inflammation.[68] If conservative therapy fails to reduce the inflammation, surgical release of the first compartment may be indicated.

FIGURE 7.22 A posterior view of the right forearm showing the primary wrist extensors: extensor carpi radialis longus, extensor carpi radialis brevis, and extensor carpi ulnaris. The extensor digitorum and other secondary wrist extensors are also evident.

Wrist Extensor Muscles
PRIMARY SET (ACT ON WRIST ONLY)
- Extensor carpi radialis longus
- Extensor carpi radialis brevis
- Extensor carpi ulnaris

SECONDARY SET (ACT ON WRIST AND HAND)
- Extensor digitorum
- Extensor indicis
- Extensor digiti minimi
- Extensor pollicis longus

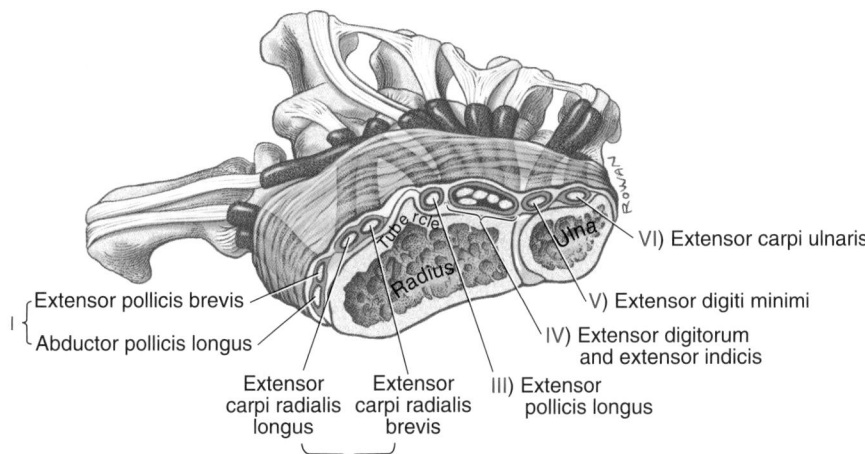

FIGURE 7.23 A dorsal oblique view shows a cross-section of the tendons of the extensor muscles of the wrist and digits passing through the extensor retinaculum of the wrist. All tendons that cross the dorsal aspect of the wrist travel within one of six fibro-osseus compartments embedded within the extensor retinaculum. Roman numerals indicate the specific fibro-osseus compartment, along with their associated set of tendons. Synovial linings are indicated in blue.

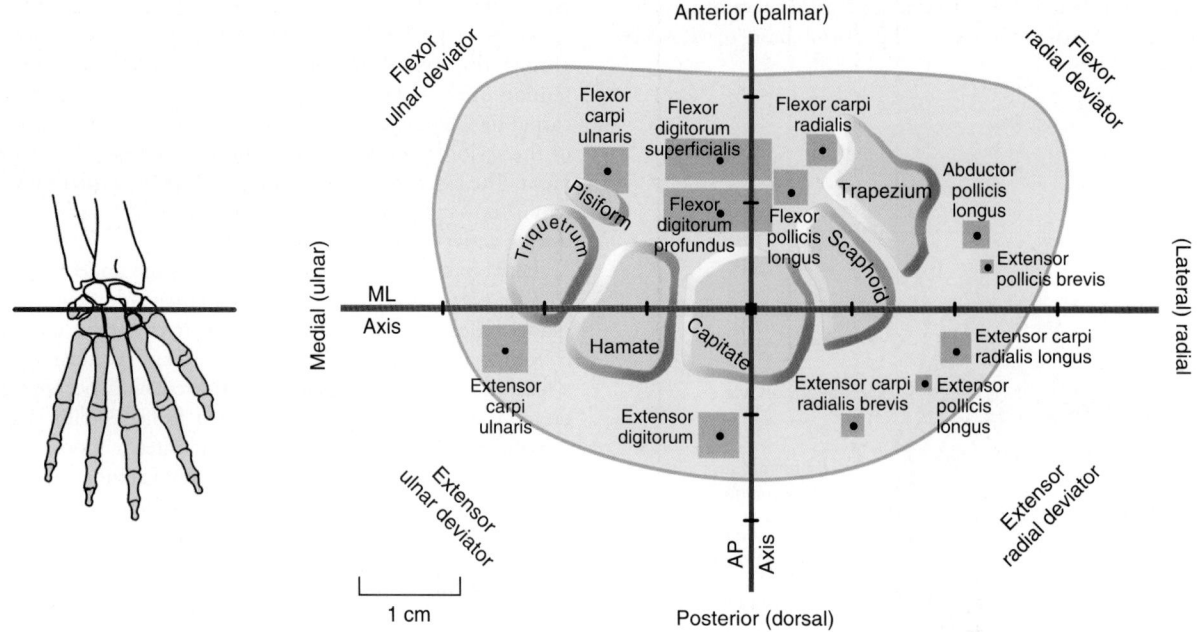

FIGURE 7.24 A cross-sectional view looking distally through the right carpal tunnel, similar to the perspective shown in Fig. 7.5. The plot depicts the *cross-sectional area, position,* and length of the *internal moment arms* for most muscles that cross the wrist at the level of the head of the capitate. The area within the red boxes on the grid is proportional to the cross-sectional area of the muscle's belly and therefore indicative of the relative maximal force production. The small black dot within each red box indicates the position of the muscle's tendon. The wrist's medial-lateral *(ML)* axis of rotation *(dark gray)* and anterior-posterior *(AP)* axis of rotation *(red)* intersect within the head of the capitate bone. Each muscle's moment arm for a particular action is equal to the perpendicular distance between the particular axis and the position of the muscle's tendon. The length of each moment arm (expressed in centimeters) is indicated by the major tick marks. Assume that the wrist is held in a neutral position.

Biomechanical Assessment of Wrist Muscles' Action and Torque Potential

Data are available on the relative position, cross-sectional area, and length of the internal moment arms of most muscles that cross the wrist.[13,63,98,126] By knowing the approximate location of the axes of rotation of the wrist, these data provide a useful method for estimating the action and relative torque potential of the wrist muscles (Fig. 7.24). Consider, for example, the extensor carpi ulnaris and the flexor carpi ulnaris. By noting the location of each tendon from the axis of rotation, it is evident that the extensor carpi ulnaris is an extensor and ulnar deviator and the flexor carpi ulnaris is a flexor and ulnar deviator. Because both muscles have similar cross-sectional areas, they likely produce comparable levels of maximal force. To estimate the relative *torque* production of the two muscles, however, each muscle's cross-sectional area must be multiplied by each muscle's specific moment arm length. The extensor carpi ulnaris therefore is considered a more potent ulnar deviator than an extensor; the flexor carpi ulnaris is considered both a potent flexor and a potent ulnar deviator.

The information portrayed in Fig. 7.24 will be referred to several times throughout this section to help explain the function of and interactions among muscles.

Wrist Extensor Activity While Making a Fist

The main function of the wrist extensors is to position and stabilize the wrist during activities involving active flexion of the digits. Of particular importance is the role of the wrist extensor muscles in making a fist or producing a strong grip. To demonstrate this, rapidly tighten and release the fist and note the strong synchronous

activity from the wrist extensors. The extrinsic finger flexor muscles, namely the flexor digitorum profundus and flexor digitorum superficialis, possess a significant internal moment arm as *wrist* flexors. The leverage of these muscles for wrist flexion is evident in Fig. 7.24. The wrist extensor muscles must counterbalance the significant *wrist flexion* torque produced by the finger flexor muscles (Fig. 7.25). As a strong, static grip is applied to an object, the wrist extensors typically hold the wrist in about 30 to 35 degrees of extension and about 5 to 15 degrees of ulnar deviation.[84] The extended position optimizes the length-tension relationship of the extrinsic finger flexors, thereby facilitating maximal grip strength (Fig. 7.26).[16]

The naturally large mechanical demand placed on the proximal attachments of the wrist extensors during grasp may cause degenerative pathology at the point of attachment to the lateral epicondyle.[40,69] Anatomic factors have implicated greater pathomechanical involvement in the extensor carpi radialis brevis compared with the other wrist extensors. The extensor carpi radialis brevis has a 14-fold *smaller* attachment area to the humerus compared with the extensor carpi radialis longus.[6] The smaller contact area could convert a large muscle force to a large and potentially damaging stress at the insertion site. Furthermore, the proximal tendon of the extensor carpi radialis brevis naturally contacts the lateral margin of the capitulum (of the distal humerus) during flexion and extension of the elbow. This sharp contact may abrade the undersurface of this muscle.[15]

As evident in Fig. 7.26, grip strength is significantly reduced when the wrist is flexed. A wrist held near the neutral position (4 degrees of flexion) is likely to experience a 33% reduction in maximum grip strength.[16] In healthy subjects, the decreased grip strength can be explained by a combination of factors. First, and likely foremost, the finger flexors cannot generate adequate force because they are functioning at an extremely shortened length respective to their length-tension curve. Second, the overstretched finger extensors, particularly the extensor digitorum, create a *passive* extensor torque at the fingers, which further reduces effective grip force. This combination

of physiologic and biomechanical events explains why a person with paralyzed or weakened wrist extensor muscles (from a radial nerve injury for example) has difficulty producing an effective grip, even though the finger flexor muscles are fully innervated.

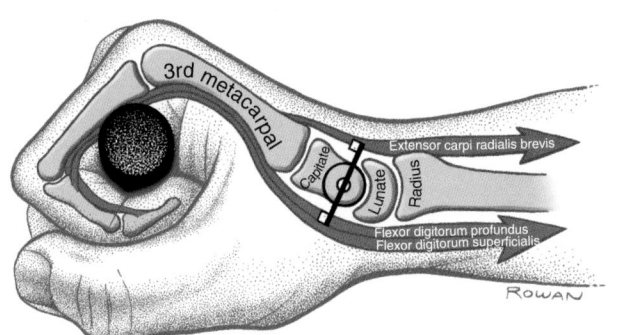

FIGURE 7.25 Muscle mechanics involved with the production of a strong grip. Contraction of the extrinsic finger flexors (flexor digitorum superficialis and profundus) flexes the fingers but also creates a simultaneous *wrist flexion* torque. Activation of the wrist extensors, such as the extensor carpi radialis brevis, is necessary to block the wrist flexion tendency caused by the activated finger flexor muscles. In this manner the wrist extensors maintain the optimal length of the finger flexors to effectively flex the fingers. The internal moment arms for the extensor carpi radialis brevis and extrinsic finger flexors are shown in dark bold lines. The small circle within the capitate marks the medial-lateral axis of rotation at the wrist.

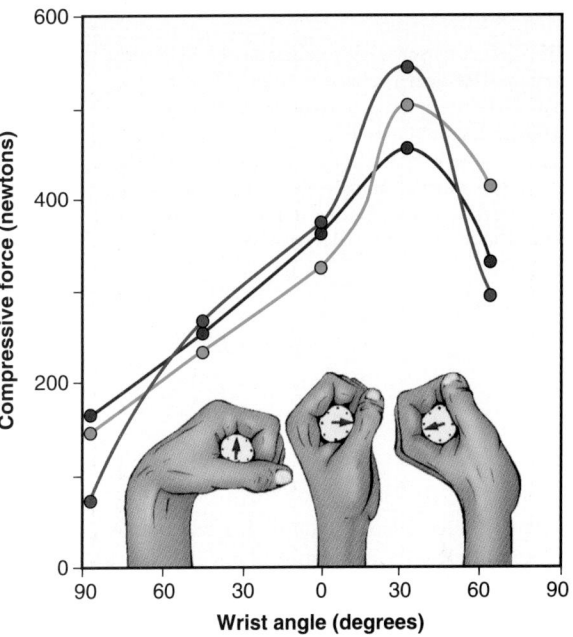

FIGURE 7.26 The compression forces produced by a maximal-effort grip are shown for three different wrist positions (for three subjects). Maximal grip force occurs at about 30 degrees of extension. (With permission from Inman VT, Ralston HJ, Todd F: *Human walking,* Baltimore, 1981, Williams & Wilkins.)

SPECIAL FOCUS 7.4

Overuse Syndrome of the Wrist Extensor Muscles: "Lateral Elbow Tendinopathy"

The most active wrist extensor muscle during a light grasp is the extensor carpi radialis brevis.[95] As the force of grip increases, the extensor carpi ulnaris and extensor carpi radialis longus also become active. Activities that require repetitive and forceful grasp, such as hammering or playing tennis, may overstress the proximal attachment of these muscles. This situation may lead to a painful and chronic condition referred to as *lateral elbow tendinopathy* or, more informally, "tennis elbow." The large force produced by the wrist extensor muscles to make a firm grasp is spread across a relatively small attachment site on the lateral epicondyle of the humerus, thereby creating large and potentially damaging stress at the point of attachment.

Because the risk of developing lateral elbow tendinopathy tends to be greatest in the workplace, the term "tennis elbow" is somewhat misleading.[40] Regardless of the name of the condition, symptoms universally include a painful and weakened grip, as well as pain with passive wrist flexion and forearm pronation, and point tenderness over the lateral epicondyle.[27]

There is a lack of consensus on the most effective treatment for this condition. Traditional conservative treatment with varying levels of success includes, but not limited to, splinting or counterforce bracing, icing often combined with nonsteroidal antiinflammatory

drugs, manual therapy (including cross-friction massage), stretching and strengthening of wrist extensor muscles (often using eccentrically activated muscle training), taping combined with exercise, dry needling, and other physical modalities such as low-intensity laser therapy, and iontophoresis.[a]

The pathophysiology of lateral elbow tendinopathy is not fully understood, evident by the plethora of terms used to describe the condition. The term *lateral epicondylitis* is still frequently encountered in the literature due to the original belief that the condition was primarily one of inflammation (hence the suffix -*itis*). Several lines of research have found, however, that the affected tendons do not show indicators of inflammation, but rather of degeneration with an incomplete reparative process, particularly in the tendon of the extensor carpi radialis brevis.[3,57,93] Histologic changes at the tendon include increased fibroblasts, vascular hyperplasia, and disorganized collagen fibrils—consistent with an "overuse tendinopathy."[6,61,102,127] It is possible that, in some cases, both inflammatory and degenerative processes persist throughout the course of the often self-limiting condition. Regardless of the actual pathologic process, the root of the problem is at least partially of biomechanical origin: a large stress is placed on the wrist extensor muscles to balance the strong wrist flexion potential of the extrinsic finger flexors.

[a]12,20,22,35,58,61,69,78,114,129

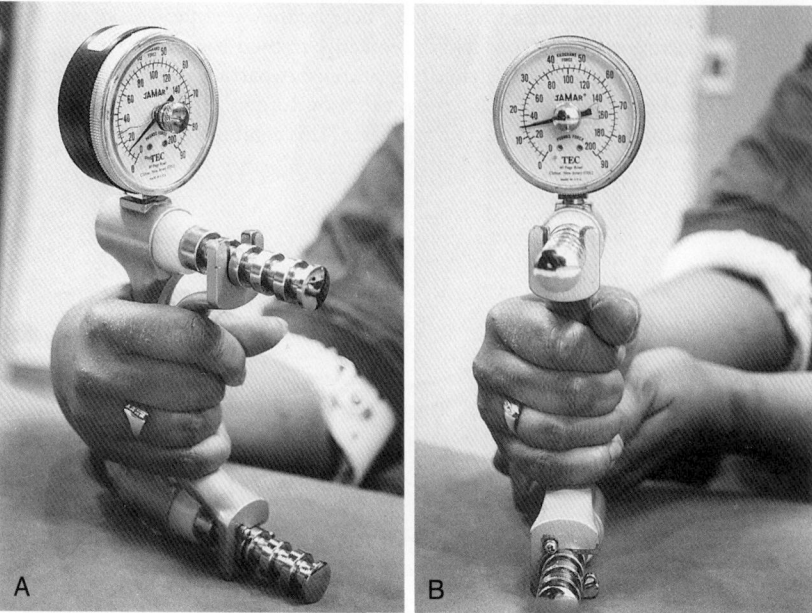

FIGURE 7.27 A person with paralysis of the right wrist extensor muscles (after a radial nerve injury) is performing a maximal-effort grip using a dynamometer. (A) Despite normally innervated finger flexor muscles, maximal grip strength measures only 10 pounds (about 4.5 kg). (B) The same person is shown manually stabilizing the weakened wrist to prevent it from flexing during the grip effort. Note that the grip force has nearly tripled.

Trying to produce a maximal-effort grip with paralyzed wrist extensors results in an abnormal posture of finger flexion *and* wrist flexion (Fig. 7.27A). Stabilizing the wrist in greater extension enables the finger flexor muscles to nearly triple their grip force (see Fig. 7.27B). Preventing the wrist from flexing maintains the extrinsic finger flexors at an elongated length more conducive to a higher force production.

Ordinarily the person depicted in Fig. 7.27 wears a splint that holds the wrist in 10 to 20 degrees of extension. If the radial nerve fails to reinnervate the wrist extensor muscles, a tendon from another muscle may be surgically rerouted to provide wrist extension torque. For example, the pronator teres muscle, innervated by the median nerve, is sutured to the tendon of the extensor carpi radialis brevis. Of the three primary wrist extensors, the extensor carpi radialis brevis is located most centrally at the wrist and has the greatest moment arm for wrist extension (see Fig. 7.24).

FUNCTION OF THE WRIST FLEXORS

Muscular Anatomy

The three primary wrist flexors are the *flexor carpi radialis,* the *flexor carpi ulnaris,* and the *palmaris longus* (Fig. 7.28). The palmaris longus is typically absent in about 15% of people, although this frequency may vary significantly according to ethnicity.[111,125] Even when present, the muscle often exhibits variation in shape and number of tendons. The tendon of this muscle is often used as a donor in tendon grafting surgery.

The tendons of the three primary wrist flexor muscles are easily identified on the anterior distal forearm, especially during strong isometric activation. The *palmar carpal ligament,* not easily identified by palpation, is located proximal to the transverse carpal ligament. This structure, analogous to the extensor retinaculum, stabilizes the tendons of the wrist flexors and prevents excessive bowstringing during flexion.

Other secondary muscles capable of flexing the wrist are the extrinsic flexors of the digits: the flexor digitorum profundus, flexor digitorum superficialis, and flexor pollicis longus. (The classification of these muscles as "secondary" wrist flexors should *not* imply they have a limited potential to perform this task. Actually, based on the muscles' cross-sectional areas and wrist flexor moment arms

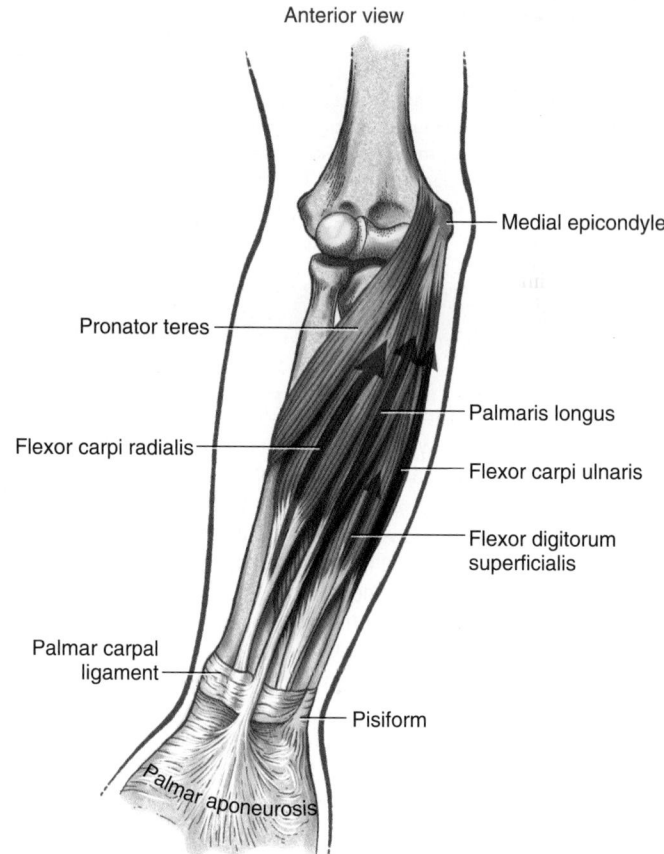

FIGURE 7.28 Anterior view of the right forearm showing the primary wrist flexor muscles: flexor carpi radialis, palmaris longus, and flexor carpi ulnaris. The flexor digitorum superficialis (a secondary wrist flexor) and pronator teres muscles are also shown.

(see Fig. 7.24), the wrist flexion torque potential of extrinsic flexors of the digits may *exceed* that of the primary wrist flexors.) With the wrist in a neutral position, the abductor pollicis longus and extensor pollicis brevis have a small moment arm for wrist flexion (see Fig. 7.24).

Wrist Flexor Muscles

PRIMARY SET (ACT ON WRIST ONLY)

- Flexor carpi radialis
- Flexor carpi ulnaris
- Palmaris longus

SECONDARY SET (ACT ON WRIST AND HAND)

- Flexor digitorum profundus
- Flexor digitorum superficialis
- Flexor pollicis longus
- Abductor pollicis longus
- Extensor pollicis brevis

TABLE 7.1 **Magnitude and Wrist Joint Position of Peak Isometric Torque Produced by Healthy Males**		
Wrist Muscle Group	**Mean Peak Torque (Nm)***	**Wrist Angle Coinciding with Peak Torque**
Flexors	12.2 (3.7)[†]	40 degrees of flexion
Extensors	7.1 (2.1)	From 30 degrees of flexion to 70 degrees of extension
Radial deviators	11.0 (2.0)	0 degrees (neutral)
Ulnar deviators	9.5 (2.2)	0 degrees (neutral)

*Conversions: 1.36 Nm/ft-lb.
[†]Standard deviations in parentheses.
Data from Delp SL, Grierson AE, Buchanan TS: Maximum isometric moments generated by the wrist muscles in flexion-extension and radial-ulnar deviation, *J Biomech* 29:1371, 1996.

The proximal attachments of the primary wrist flexors are located on and near the medial ("flexor-pronator") epicondyle of the humerus and dorsal border of the ulna (see Figs. 6.2 and 6.6). Technically, the tendon of the flexor carpi radialis does not cross the wrist *through* the carpal tunnel; rather, the tendon passes in a separate tunnel formed by a groove in the trapezium and fascia from the adjacent transverse carpal ligament (Fig. 7.29). The tendon of the flexor carpi radialis attaches distally to the palmar base of the second and sometimes the third metacarpal. The palmaris longus has a distal attachment primarily to the thick aponeurosis of the palm. The tendon of the flexor carpi ulnaris courses distally to attach to the pisiform bone and, in a plane superficial to the transverse carpal ligament, into the pisohamate and pisometacarpal ligaments and the base of the fifth metacarpal bone.

Functional Considerations

Based on moment arm and cross-sectional area (see Fig. 7.24), the flexor carpi ulnaris has the greatest wrist flexion torque potential of the three primary wrist flexor muscles. During active wrist flexion, the flexor carpi radialis and flexor carpi ulnaris act together as synergists while simultaneously opposing each other's radial and ulnar deviation ability.

An overly spastic or otherwise overactive flexor carpi ulnaris muscle frequently contributes to wrist flexion (and ulnar deviation) deformity in persons with cerebral palsy. A surgical tenotomy and

rerouting of the tendon of this muscle to the extensor side of the wrist is often performed to restore kinetic balance to the wrist. Research has shown, however, that even after a complete tenotomy of the flexor carpi ulnaris at the level of the pisiform bone, active force generated within this muscle is still capable of flexing the wrist.[23] Such a phenomenon can be explained by the presence of myofascial connections that naturally exist in the forearm between the muscle bellies of the flexor carpi ulnaris and other wrist flexor muscles, including the flexor digitorum profundus and superficialis. Such an intermuscular transfer of force is likely more common than what is typically believed, and likely occurs in other muscle groups that share similar proximal attachments.

As indicated in Table 7.1, maximal-effort strength testing has shown that the wrist flexor muscles are able to produce about 70% greater isometric torque than the wrist extensor muscles—12.2 Nm versus 7.1 Nm, respectively.[26] The greater total cross-sectional area of the wrist flexor muscles (including the extrinsic digital flexors) can account for much of this disparity.[47] Peak wrist flexion torque occurs between 30 and 40 degrees of flexion,[26,60] likely due to the sharp rise in overall wrist flexor moment arm as the wrist flexes.[37]

FUNCTION OF THE RADIAL AND ULNAR DEVIATORS

Muscles capable of producing *radial deviation* of the wrist are the extensor carpi radialis brevis and longus, extensor pollicis longus and brevis, flexor carpi radialis, abductor pollicis longus, and flexor pollicis longus (see in Fig. 7.24). In the neutral wrist position, the extensor carpi radialis longus and abductor pollicis longus possess the largest product of cross-sectional area and moment arm for radial deviation torque. The extensor pollicis brevis has the greatest moment arm of all radial deviators; however, because of a relatively small cross-sectional area, this muscle's torque production is relatively small. The abductor pollicis longus and extensor pollicis brevis provide important stability to the radial side of the wrist. As shown in Table 7.1, the radial deviator muscles generate about 15% greater isometric torque than the ulnar deviator muscles—11.0 Nm versus 9.5 Nm, respectively.

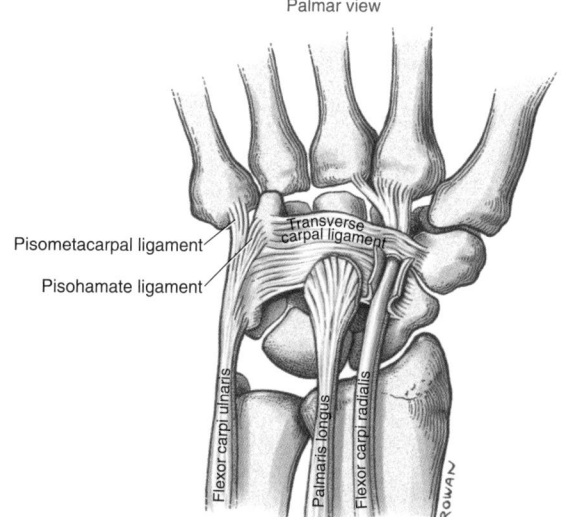

Palmar view

FIGURE 7.29 The palmar aspect of the right wrist showing the distal attachments of the primary wrist flexor muscles. Note that the tendon of the flexor carpi radialis courses through a sheath located within the superficial fibers of the transverse carpal ligament. Most of the distal attachment of the palmaris longus has been removed with the palmar aponeurosis.

Radial Deviators of the Wrist

- Extensor carpi radialis longus
- Extensor carpi radialis brevis
- Extensor pollicis longus
- Extensor pollicis brevis
- Flexor carpi radialis
- Abductor pollicis longus
- Flexor pollicis longus

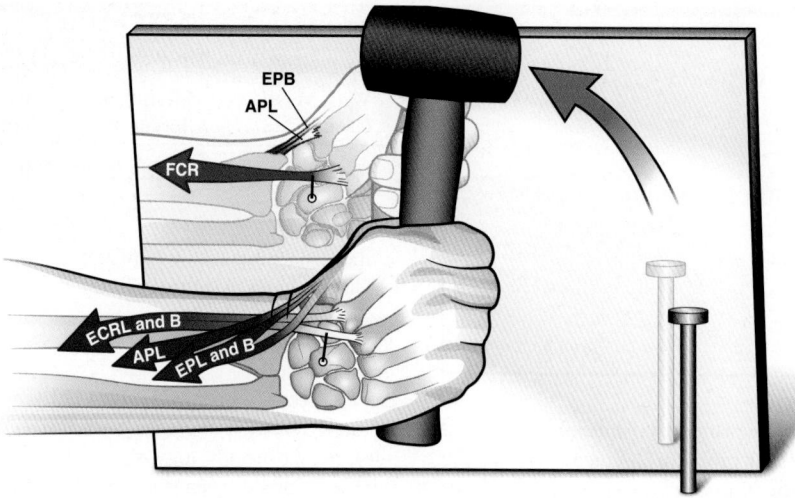

FIGURE 7.30 The muscles that perform radial deviation of the wrist are shown preparing to strike a nail with a hammer. The image in the background is a mirror reflection of the palmar surface of the wrist. The axis of rotation is through the capitate with the internal moment arms shown for the extensor carpi radialis brevis *(ECRB)* and the flexor carpi radialis *(FCR)* only. The flexor pollicis longus is not shown. *APL,* abductor pollicis longus; *ECRL and B,* extensor carpi radialis longus and brevis, respectively; *EPL and B,* extensor pollicis longus and brevis, respectively.

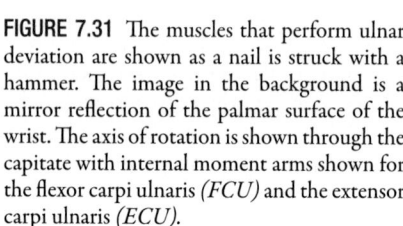

FIGURE 7.31 The muscles that perform ulnar deviation are shown as a nail is struck with a hammer. The image in the background is a mirror reflection of the palmar surface of the wrist. The axis of rotation is shown through the capitate with internal moment arms shown for the flexor carpi ulnaris *(FCU)* and the extensor carpi ulnaris *(ECU).*

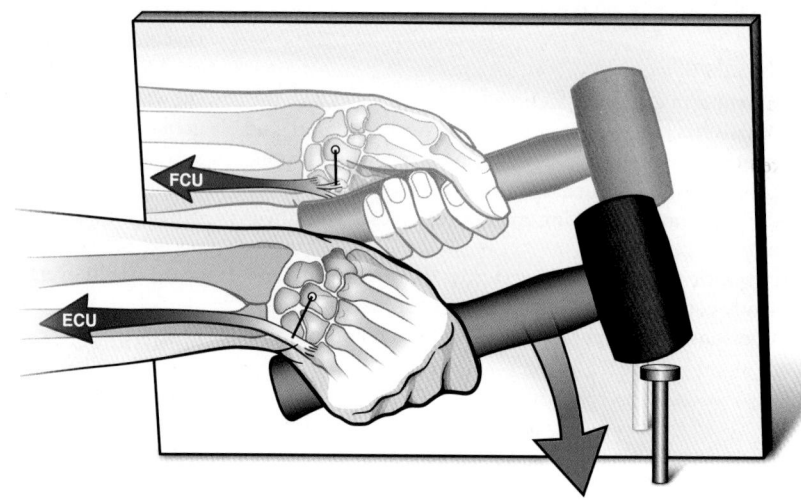

Active wrist extension is typically coupled with active radial deviation—a motion described earlier as the dart thrower's motion. This kinematic coupling can be observed as the radial deviator muscles contract to raise a hammer in preparation for striking a nail with the hammer (Fig. 7.30). Several activated muscles are depicted as passing lateral to the wrist's anterior-posterior axis of rotation. The action of the extensor carpi radialis longus and the flexor carpi radialis, shown with moment arms, illustrates a fine example of two muscles cooperating as synergists for one motion but as antagonists for another. The net effect of this muscular cooperation produces a radially deviated wrist, well stabilized in extension for optimal grasp of the hammer.

Muscles capable of *ulnar deviation* of the wrist are the extensor carpi ulnaris, flexor carpi ulnaris, flexor digitorum profundus and superficialis, and extensor digitorum (see Fig. 7.24). Because of moment arm length, however, the muscles most capable of this action, by far, are the extensor carpi ulnaris and flexor carpi ulnaris. Fig. 7.31 shows this strong pair of ulnar deviator muscles contracting to strike a nail with a hammer. The wrist is driven strongly into ulnar deviation as it flexes slightly. The overall posture of the wrist at nail strike remains biased toward extension however, a requirement for maintaining a firm grasp on the hammer.

Because of the strong functional association between the flexor and extensor carpi ulnaris during active ulnar deviation, injury to either muscle can incapacitate their combined effectiveness. For example, consider a painful tenosynovitis in the extensor carpi ulnaris tendon near its distal attachment. Attempts at active ulnar deviation with minimal to no activation in the painful extensor carpi ulnaris cause the action of the flexor carpi ulnaris to be unopposed. The resulting flexed posture of the wrist is thereby not suitable for maintaining an effective grasp.

Ulnar Deviators of the Wrist
- Extensor carpi ulnaris
- Flexor carpi ulnaris
- Flexor digitorum profundus and superficialis
- Extensor digitorum

SYNOPSIS

The wrist consists of two primary articulations: the radiocarpal and the midcarpal joints. The radiocarpal joint connects the distal end of the radius with bones of the proximal carpus; the midcarpal joint unites the proximal and distal rows of carpal bones. Rotations and translation among these joints produce movements in both frontal and sagittal planes, although most natural movements combine elements of both planes: the so-called "dart thrower's motion." This motion is used for many functions, including throwing, hammering, fly fishing, and grooming.

Forces produced by active muscle and subsequently stretched ligaments naturally guide the kinematics across the wrist. Following trauma, the ligaments of the wrist may lose their ability to maintain proper alignment between the bones. Ligamentous injury may also damage the imbedded sensory nerves, possibly reducing subconscious proprioceptive guidance to movement. The ensuing faulty arthrokinematics and increased stress on the joints often lead to further marked instability, pain, and potential deformity. Reduced or painful movements of the wrist can dramatically compromise the function of the hand and thus the entire upper limb.

In addition to providing optimal position of the hand, the wrist is also associated with two other important functions of the upper extremity: load acceptance and the kinematics of pronation and supination of the forearm. First, the wrist must be able to accept large compression forces that impact the distal end of the upper limb, similar to the way the ankle accepts forces during standing or walking. Compression forces that impact the wrist, however, occur not only from contact with the environment, such as pushing up from an armrest of a chair, but also from muscle forces produced to make a grasp. The naturally broadened shape of the distal radius helps reduce the contact pressure (i.e., force/area) against the carpal bones. The interosseous membrane and the relative flexible articulations within the proximal row of carpal bones further dissipate the compression forces that cross the wrist. Often, external forces may exceed the ability of these load dispersal mechanisms to protect the region, resulting in trauma such as fracture of the distal radius; tears in the interosseous membrane, triangular fibrocartilage complex (TFCC), scapholunate ligament; and fracture or dislocation of bones such as the scaphoid and lunate.

The natural design of the wrist is also strongly associated with the kinematics of pronation and supination of the forearm. Elements of this design are present on both sides of the wrist. Radially, the articular morphology of the radiocarpal joint partially restricts axial rotation between the carpus and the radius. By restricting this motion, the hand is obligated to follow the path of the pronating and supinating radius. As the wrist *limits* axial rotation on its radial side, it selectively *permits* this motion on its ulnar side. The large ulnocarpal space and associated soft tissues loosely bind the ulnar side of the carpus to the ulna. Acting as a semielastic tether, the TFCC allows the radius, with firmly attached carpus, to pronate and supinate freely about the distal end of the ulna. Without this freedom of motion on the ulnar side of the wrist, pronation and supination of the forearm would be significantly restricted.

Essentially all muscles that cross the wrist have multiple actions—either at the wrist itself or at the more distal digits. Consequently, relatively simple motions demand relatively complex muscular interactions. Consider, for example, that extending the wrist requires at least a pair of muscles to fine-tune the desired amount of radial deviation. Also consider the need for strong muscle activation from the wrist extensor muscles to stabilize the wrist during grasping. Without such proximal stability, the finger flexor muscles may be rendered essentially ineffective. Loss of proximal stability of the wrist can occur from several sources, including from injury or disease of the peripheral or central nervous center or from pain in the region of the lateral epicondyle, which is the proximal attachment site of the wrist extensor muscles, or in one of the six fibro-osseous compartments located on the dorsal side of the wrist. Understanding how these impairments affect the kinesiology of the wrist is a fundamental element of providing the most effective therapeutic intervention.

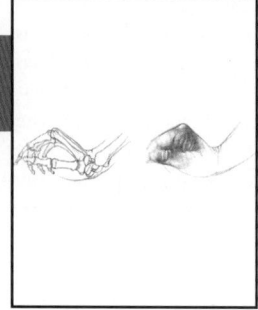

ADDITIONAL CLINICAL CONNECTIONS

CONTENTS

CLINICAL CONNECTION 7.1

Scapholunate Ligament: Potential Pathomechanics and Rehabilitation following Injury

Injury to the *scapholunate (SL) ligament* can initiate a cascading series of events that can lead to carpal instability and, in the worst-case scenario, to the structural collapse of the carpus.[88] Hand therapists play an essential role in the rehabilitation of persons following injury to this important ligament, both in nonoperative and postoperative care settings.[52] Certainly, this Clinical Connection could have featured other pathologies that affect the wrist. An injured SL ligament was chosen because of its relative frequency of involvement and, perhaps more importantly, because several tenets of wrist rehabilitation are based on anatomic, kinesiological, and pathomechanical concepts previously introduced in this chapter. This Clinical Connection is designed to reinforce and expand on these concepts, and to stimulate readers' interest in pursuing the advanced training required to specialize in this delivery of therapy.

FUNCTIONAL IMPORTANCE OF THE SCAPHOLUNATE LIGAMENT: A BRIEF OVERVIEW

The SL joint is a key, central articulation within the relatively loosely joined proximal row of carpal bones. As evident in Figs. 7.7 and 7.8, the distal aspect of the SL joint forms a deep socket to securely accept the large head of the capitate. During weight-bearing and movements driven by muscle contraction, the capitate (which is the base of the central column of the wrist and hand) is forced deeper into the SL socket. The structural security of the scapholunate joint is maintained primarily by the SL ligament. The joint is reinforced, however, by several secondary or indirect stabilizers—virtually any ligament that attaches to either the scaphoid or to the lunate—such as the scaphotrapezial and lunotriquetral ligaments (depicted in Figs. 7.9 and 7.10). These secondary ligaments, in conjunction with the dominant SL ligament, may be considered parts of a more global *scapholunate ligamentous complex*, helping to anchor the scaphoid and lunate to each other and to adjacent, stable carpal bones.

The SL ligament is strong, having the capacity to accept between 147 and 270 N (33 and 61 lbs) of tension before rupture.[79,88] This strength is necessary to statically support the SL joint under physiologic load, and also to dynamically support the joint as the scaphoid and lunate move in slightly different paths during wrist movements. Being well innervated with mechanoreceptors, a stretched SL ligament can reflexively activate appropriate muscles to help guide and compress the SL joint during its complex kinematics. Although the interaction between innervated ligaments and the neuromuscular system is not unique to the wrist, the topic has been particularly well described in this region.[33,42,43]

A POTENTIAL PATHOMECHANICAL SCENARIO AFTER INJURY TO THE SL LIGAMENT

Because the SL joint is in the direct path of compression across the wrist, the SL ligament is prone to injury from a fall onto an outstretched hand. A tear of the SL ligament can leave the SL joint mechanically unstable and painful. Depending on the extent of trauma to other carpal bones or ligaments, the SL joint may partially disassociate, forming a gap or a *diastasis.* Clinically, an SL disassociation can be observed on x-ray as one actively clenches the fist (Fig. 7.32). The SL gap shown in the x-ray is referred to as a *dynamic* disassociation because the gap occurs with active contraction of muscles that make a fist. The gap widens as the

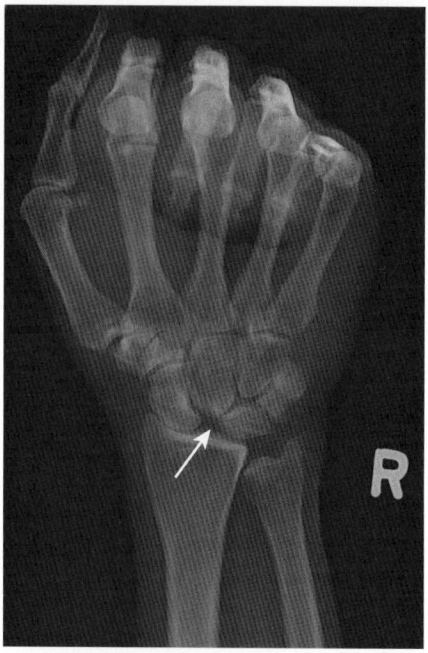

FIGURE 7.32 A posterior-anterior (PA) view of an x-ray showing a 4 mm gap within the unstable scapholunate joint (*arrow*) as a person makes a grip. (Radiograph Courtesy Ann Porretto-Loehrke, DPT, CHT, Hand to Shoulder Center, Appleton, WI.)

CLINICAL CONNECTION 7.1
Scapholunate Ligament: Potential Pathomechanics and Rehabilitation following Injury—cont'd

muscles pull the capitate (and third metacarpal) proximally into the weakened SL joint. A *static* SL dissociation may exist at rest or with a relaxed fist, typically indicating more severe or chronic injury with complete disruption of the SL ligament and attenuation of the secondary stabilizers.

Although difficult to appreciate on a planar x-ray, SL disassociation may also involve an abnormal torsion or twist of the scaphoid or the lunate. The combined gapping and torsion can, overtime, overstretch and weaken secondary SL joint stabilizers, even those that may not have been injured during the initial trauma. The compounding effect of ligamentous rupture and creep may lead to a gradual worsening of the SL disassociation.

The specific developing pathomechanics following a complete tear of the SL ligament are hard to predict, primarily because of the anatomic complexity of the wrist but also due to the unknown extent of injury or chronic stretch placed on the secondary SL stabilizers. The pathomechanics may be limited to only minimal SL dissociation, or it may progress to a substantial dissociation coupled with a generalized zigzag deformity of the proximal row, such as that described by the acronym *DISI* in Fig. 7.20. The ultimate clinical sequalae also depends on the amount of damage to the sensory nerve fibers and mechanoreceptors embedded within the injured ligaments. Reduced proprioceptive "guidance" likely results in more stressful arthrokinematics—aggravating an already precarious pathomechanical situation.[29]

If untreated or undiagnosed, the pathomechanics associated with SL dissociation can progress to severe and incapacitating osteoarthritis. A SL dissociation typically involves a separation and *radial* migration of the scaphoid against the adjacent styloid process of the radius. The ensuing abnormal bony contact can predispose degenerative osteoarthritis at the radial edge of the radioscaphoid junction. The degenerative process may then involve the capitate-lunate articulation (within the midcarpal joint), then eventually encompasses the entire radiocarpal joint. In later stages of this progression, the wrist may mechanically collapse, a pathologic situation referred to as *scapholunate advanced collapse,* or a "SLAC wrist."[18]

Medical and therapeutic intervention can often limit the progression of deformity, instability, and pain following a tear of the SL ligament. If the SL ligament is only partially or minimally torn, treatment may involve a conservative (nonoperative) approach. In more severe injuries, or in cases where a conservative approach

has been unsuccessful, surgery may be required. Surgical options depend on the extent of the injury and progression of the pathomechanics. Options range from repairing the injured ligament to more extensive surgery including augmenting secondary ligament stabilizers, or salvage procedures involving either a proximal row carpectomy or four-corner fusion, involving excision of the scaphoid and fusion of the capitate, hamate, lunate, and triquetrum.

SOME UNDERLYING PRINCIPLES BEHIND NONOPERATIVE REHABILITATION FOLLOWING INJURY TO THE SL LIGAMENT – A FOCUS ON THERAPEUTIC EXERCISE

The specifics of a nonoperative rehabilitation program following SL injury depends on several factors, including the extent and complexity of the injury, and the age, health, and activity level of the patient. Such information is determined as part of a thorough initial evaluation.[92] This section will briefly describe principles that support using exercise as a central part of the rehabilitation process. The following discussion assumes that the patient has only a partial tear of their SL ligament and has been appropriately advised by medical professionals to pursue a conservative, nonoperative, approach to their rehabilitation.

After allowing adequate time for ligament healing, a carefully prescribed, monitored, and dosed exercise program may be initiated with goals of improving wrist mobility and strength of the surrounding musculature. Besides the obvious benefits of strengthening muscles weakened through immobilization or guarding due to pain, improved strength aims to enhance neuromuscular control of the wrist. Better muscular control may allow the patient to dynamically self-stabilize a weakened or potentially unstable SL joint. Increased muscular stability may protect the joint against unnatural or extreme movements, thereby limiting excessive strain on the weakened SL ligament. In addition, patients are instructed in ways of performing daily activities without placing excessive load through the wrist.

Movements associated with wrist rehabilitation are often designed around the functional *dart thrower's movement (DTM).*[10,137] Like throwing a dart, the DTM is a coupled motion that combines wrist extension with radial deviation and wrist flexion with ulnar deviation. As described in this chapter, the oblique path of a functional DTM is naturally used during many common activities, such as combing hair, using a hammer, and casting a fishing rod. Depending on the specific task, the DTM is typically angled

Continued

ADDITIONAL CLINICAL CONNECTIONS

out of the pure sagittal plane by 25 to 50 degrees. Incorporating the DTM into active or passive exercise routines is believed to have advantages over pure planar motions, as it minimizes motion in the proximal row. Different lines of research have shown that, compared with pure sagittal and frontal plane motions, the DTM shifts a much greater proportion of wrist movement *from the radiocarpal to the midcarpal joint.*[21,74] In essence, the distal row of carpal bones rotates more-or-less as a fixed unit around the scaphoid. Reducing the kinematic demands on the proximal row of carpal bones likely reduces strain on the SL ligament. This allows the therapist to offer appropriately graded challenges to the musculature while minimizing the demands on the SL joint and ligament.[10,137] Although this premise is well considered and grounded on sound kinesiology, it is based primarily on the study of intact SL ligaments. More research is needed to determine the clinical efficacy and safety of this premise for persons with a structurally compromised SL ligament.

Therapeutic exercises are designed to strengthen and increase the neuromuscular control over muscles primarily responsible for the DTM, such as the extensor carpi radialis longus and abductor pollicis longus (radial-extensors) and the flexor carpi ulnaris (flexor-ulnar deviator). Not only are these muscles considered prime movers of a DTM, but tension in these muscles appears to "twist and close" the SL joint, thereby *reducing* the potential SL gapping. For this reason, the muscles previously listed are frequently referred to by clinicians as "SL friendly."[29,92] This contrasts with the extensor carpi ulnaris— often designated as a "SL unfriendly" muscle—based on its line of pull that has been shown by cadaver observation to twist the carpus in a way that *increases* SL gapping.[106–108]

Orthotics can be custom fabricated to encourage the DTM, thereby promoting effective and safe use of exercise during rehabilitation.[10,42] These devices help guide active wrist movements in a path consistent with a DTM, while simultaneously limiting the movement to the middle range of the motion. Additionally, this type of "dynamic" orthosis allows therapists to design actively engaging exercises that may improve the patient's proprioceptive awareness.[5,44] Ideally, this approach enhances the ability of certain muscles to subconsciously guide and stabilize the SL joint.[42,137] As a simple example, the patient can practice moving their affected wrist in a DTM that follows (or "mirrors") the movement performed by their unaffected wrist. This exercise can be repeated with and without visual guidance, and can, at least initially, be performed against gentle resistance. When deemed appropriate based on patient response and the integrity of the healed SL ligament, the range and scope of exercises may expand, and the patient may only need to rely on using a static orthosis while at rest.[10,137]

Exercises can continue to follow the DTM theme by having the patient hold or manipulate commercially available objects that offer oscillatory, plyometric or perturbation-type resistances.[137] The bottom line is to offer a wide range of appropriately dosed, conscious and subconscious challenges to movement, while maintaining the relative safety offered by the DTM.

In closing, it is important to bear in mind that although the DTM reduces the kinematic demands on the SL joint compared with pure planar motions, it does *not* eliminate it.[137] The reduction in SL joint and ligament motion depends on the task and angled path of the DTM, the specific arc used within the total available motion, and the level of demand placed on the muscles As a general guideline, most lines of research suggest that the greatest relative unloading of the SL ligament during active movement can be achieved by: (1) adhering to the oblique plane of the DTM, (2) reducing external resistance, and (3) avoiding the end or extreme ranges of motion. More research is needed to validate and expand the clinical utility of these guidelines.

ADDITIONAL CLINICAL CONNECTIONS

CLINICAL CONNECTION 7.2
"Ulnar Variance" at the Wrist: Associated Kinesiology and Clinical Implications

DEFINING "ULNAR VARIANCE"

The distal ends of the radius and the ulna approach the proximal side of the carpus at two locations: the radiocarpal joint and the ulnocarpal space. Excessive asymmetry in the length of either the radius or the ulna can place damaging stress on the soft tissues and bones of the wrist. Often, and especially when combined with excessive manual labor, increased carpal stress can cause chronic inflammation, pain, rupture or deformation of the ligaments, change in the shape of the bones and articular surfaces, reduced grip strength, and altered hemodynamics.

Variation in the length or position of the forearm bones can occur congenitally or can be acquired through trauma or disease. A method for quantifying the relative lengths of these bones at the wrist is referred to as *ulnar variance*.[86] This quantification is typically determined from a posterior-anterior (PA) radiograph, as shown in Fig. 7.33. An ulnar variance of zero, as indicated in the asymptomatic specimen illustrated in the figure, implies that the forearm bones extend distally the same length. *Positive ulnar variance* is the distance the ulnar head extends *distal* to the reference line; *negative ulnar variance* is the distance the ulnar head lies *proximal* to this line. Normative mean values for ulnar variance are generally reported to be between 0 and −1 mm, with a standard deviation of about 1.5 mm.[110]

A near neutral ulnar variance is expected in a healthy person when the variance is measured on a static radiograph. During certain active movements, however, ulnar variance fluctuates slightly. For example, as described in Chapter 6, contraction of the forearm pronator muscles pulls the radius slightly proximally. Although slight, this migration of the radius is evident at both the elbow and the wrist. As depicted in Fig. 6.29, the proximal migration of the radius during active *pronation* increases the compression force at the humeroradial joint. The natural, muscular-driven proximal translation of the radius creates a slight *positive* ulnar variance at the wrist (i.e., the ulnar head aligns more distally relative to the translated radius).[51] Muscle contraction involved with *making a grip* has also been shown to pull the radius proximally, increasing positive ulnar variance by 1 to 2 mm.[32] (Although the term *ulnar variance* implies displacement of the ulna, most often the variance is created by displacement of the *radius;* the stable humero-ulnar joint typically restricts migration of the ulna.)

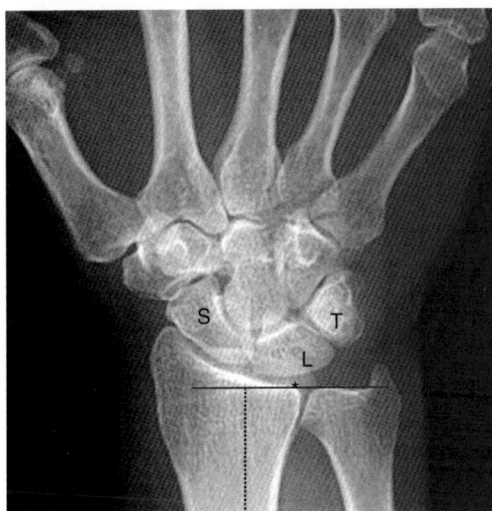

FIGURE 7.33 A posterior-anterior (PA) radiograph of an asymptomatic wrist, illustrating the measurement of ulnar variance. A dashed black line is drawn parallel with the long axis of the radius. Next, a red reference line is drawn perpendicular to the long axis of the radius at the level of the subchondral bone of the lunate facet of the radius (*indicated by the asterisk*). The distance between this reference line and the most distal portion of the ulnar head is the measure of ulnar variance. This image indicates an ulnar variance of zero—often referred to as "neutral" ulnar variance. *L,* Lunate; *S,* scaphoid; *T,* triquetrum. (Radiograph courtesy Jon Marion, OTR, CHT, and Thomas Hitchcock, MD, Marshfield Clinic, Marshfield, WI.)

The natural change in ulnar variance with forearm pronation and gripping activities is indeed small—on the order of 1 to 2 mm. The pliability of the triangular fibrocartilage complex (TFCC) and articular cartilage covering the adjacent bones typically accommodates this small movement without adverse physiologic consequence. Ulnar variance that significantly exceeds the natural 1 to 2 mm, however, can cause functional impairments at the wrist and distal radio-ulnar joint, which, over time, can be severe and disabling. The following sections highlight examples of such cases, including the relevant kinesiology and implications for medical treatment.

Continued

ADDITIONAL CLINICAL CONNECTIONS

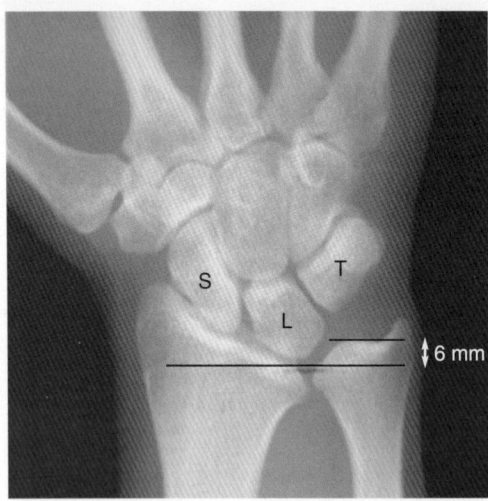

FIGURE 7.34 A posterior-anterior (PA) radiograph of a wrist with 6 mm of positive ulnar variance. Note the displaced distal radio-ulnar joint. *L,* lunate; *S,* scaphoid; *T,* triquetrum. (Radiograph courtesy Jon Marion, OTR, CHT, and Thomas Hitchcock, MD, Marshfield Clinic, Marshfield, WI.)

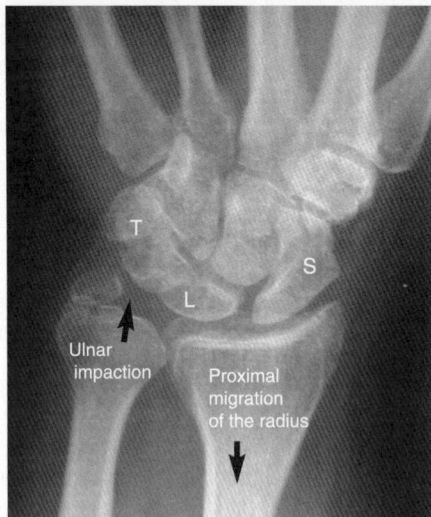

FIGURE 7.35 A posterior-anterior (PA) radiograph of the wrist of a patient diagnosed with "ulnar impaction syndrome." The patient has 5 mm of positive ulnar variance, secondary to a shortening (fracture) of the radius with subsequent proximal migration. Note the relative distal projection of the ulnar head into the ulnocarpal space. Also observe (1) the large osteophyte just distal to the ulnar head, (2) the loss of joint space between the lunate and the triquetrum, and (3) the scapholunate gap or diastasis (separation of bones without fracture), likely involving rupture of the scapholunate ligament. *L,* lunate; *S,* scaphoid; *T,* triquetrum. (Radiograph courtesy Ann Porretto-Loehrke, DPT, CHT, and John Bax, MD, PhD, Hand and Upper Extremity Center of Northeast Wisconsin, Appleton, WI.)

EXAMPLES OF CAUSE OF AND PATHOMECHANICS ASSOCIATED WITH EXCESSIVE ULNAR VARIANCE

POSITIVE ULNAR VARIANCE

Several factors can cause the ulna to extend farther distally than the radius. Fig. 7.34 shows an example of a patient who had dislocated her distal radio-ulnar joint and later developed 6 mm of positive ulnar variance. The patient experienced severe pain in the ulnocarpal space for 9 months, resulting in frequent loss of work. The patient ultimately required a surgical shortening of her ulna, thereby realigning the distal radio-ulnar joint.

Excessive positive ulnar variance is often associated with "ulnar impaction syndrome," characterized by distal encroachment of the ulna against the more central, avascular part of the triangular fibrocartilage (TFC), triquetrum, or lunate.[14] When severe, ulnar impaction may progress to inflammation and degeneration of the TFC. Fig. 7.35 illustrates a case of ulnar impaction syndrome in a physically active 54-year-old mill worker. The patient's pain was exacerbated by activities performed in ulnar deviation and by those that naturally increased his positive ulnar variance, such as weight-bearing through the upper extremity or making a strong

grip while pronating the forearm. This patient had fractured his radius while in his teens, resulting in a shortened radius with subsequent proximal migration. A shortened radius, either from a compression fracture or from surgical removal of the radial head, is a common precursor to ulnar impaction syndrome. In general, the likelihood of proximal migration of the radius is increased if the interosseous membrane is also torn. As described in Chapter 6, an important but subtle function of the interosseous membrane is to resist proximal migration of the radius.

NEGATIVE ULNAR VARIANCE

Fig. 7.36 shows a severe case of negative ulnar variance of the wrist secondary to a congenitally short ulna. The shortened ulna

ADDITIONAL CLINICAL CONNECTIONS

altered the natural congruence of the distal radio-ulnar joint, likely increasing intra-articular stress.[81] The increased stress placed on the joint, coupled with the patient's physically demanding occupation, eventually led to instability and degenerative arthritis, including rupture of most components of her TFCC. The chief complaint of this 42-year-old woman was unmanageable pain in the ulnar region of the wrist, instability (with "popping sounds"), and a significant loss of rotation of the forearm, especially supination.

Surgical intervention is often required in cases of severe pain and degeneration and loss of function in the distal radio-ulnar joint and ulnar side of the wrist. One such surgery to restore function primarily at the distal radio-ulnar joint is the *Sauvé-Kapandji* procedure.[34] The first step of the surgery is to fuse the unstable and painful distal radio-ulnar joint using a screw (Fig. 7.37). Next, a small 1-cm section of the ulna is removed at a point 1 to 2 cm proximal to the fused joint. This resulting space eventually forms a "pseudoarthrosis" (false joint), which serves as the "new" distal radio-ulnar joint. Pronation and supination now occur as the radius, carpal bones, and remaining distal ulna all rotate—as a fixed unit—about the more

proximal ulna. Efforts are usually taken to stabilize the remaining proximal "stump" of ulna, typically by using attachments of the pronator quadratus and extensor carpi ulnaris muscles. An intact interosseous membrane also provides stability to the proximal ulna.

A successful Sauvé-Kapandji operation typically restores at least functional, pain-free motion at the ulnar side of the wrist and distal forearm. Together with an intact TFCC, the short, distal (fused) segment of ulna acts as a stable base for the ulnar side of the wrist, which is especially useful during weight-bearing activities.

In addition to degeneration of the distal radio-ulnar joint and the TFCC, negative ulnar variance is often associated with *Kienböck's disease,* that is, fragmentation of the lunate (review Special Focus 7.1). As was also the case in the patient discussed in Fig. 7.36, the more distally projected radius jams against the lunate, perpetuating its fragmentation and avascular necrosis. Surgical treatment for Kienböck's disease may involve lengthening of the ulna, shortening of the radius, or, in very severe cases, partial or complete excision of the proximal row of carpal bones.[48,64] These procedures are all aimed at reducing the damaging stress on the lunate.

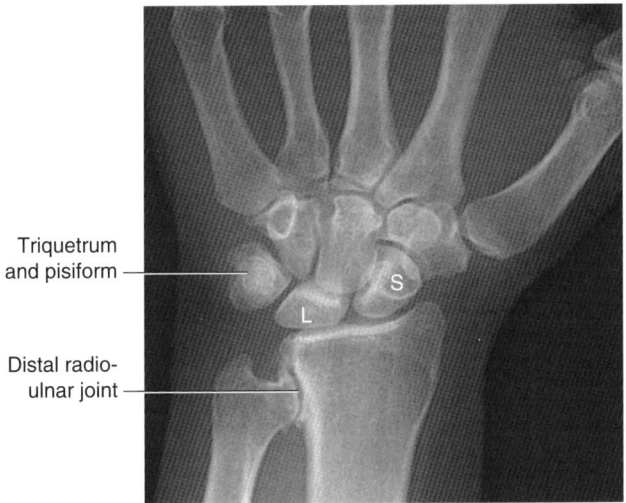

FIGURE 7.36 A posterior-anterior (PA) radiograph of a wrist with negative ulnar variance and associated degeneration of the distal radio-ulnar joint. *L,* lunate; *S,* scaphoid; *T,* triquetrum. (Radiograph courtesy Jon Marion, OTR, CHT, and Thomas Hitchcock, MD, Marshfield Clinic, Marshfield, WI.)

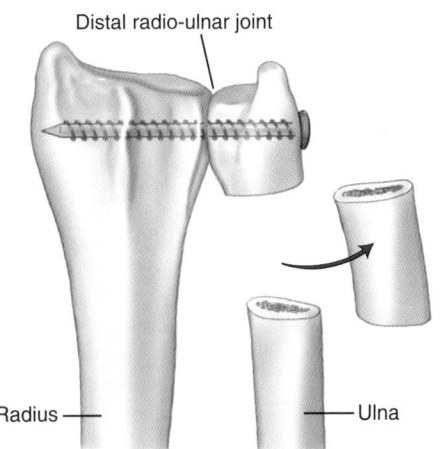

FIGURE 7.37 Sauvé-Kapandji procedure performed on the wrist. The distal radio-ulnar joint is fused, and a pseudoarthrosis is created in the ulna. (From Saunders R, Astifidis R, Burke SL, et al: *Hand and upper extremity rehabilitation: a practical guide,* ed 4, St Louis, 2015, Churchill Livingstone.)

Continued

ADDITIONAL CLINICAL CONNECTIONS

Fracture of the distal radius is one of the most common orthopedic injuries of the upper limb, often caused by a fall on an outstretched hand.[85] A fractured distal radius may be displaced or nondisplaced and may extend into the radiocarpal joint. The injury frequently involves other adjacent structures, such as a fracture of the scaphoid, an intra-articular fracture through the ulnar notch of the distal radio-ulnar joint, and a tear of the scapholunate ligament.[4,10]

Fig. 7.38 shows two orthogonal x-ray views of an extra-articular, displaced fractured radius in a 40-year-old female. Note that each view shows a different feature of the injury. The posterior-anterior (PA) view in Fig. 7.38A shows the transverse extent of the radial fracture *(arrow):* from about 2.5 cm proximal to the radial styloid process to near the ulnar notch. Note that on the PA view, the radius does not appear very displaced. The lateral view in Fig. 7.38B, however, shows that the distal radius is angulated (or displaced) *dorsally* about 25 degrees *(red line)* relative to the transverse plane of the image *(black line).* Because the distal radius normally exhibits about 10 degrees of *palmar* tilt (shown in the inset), the actual angulation caused by the fracture is closer to

35 degrees. It should be clear that at least two views of the x-ray are needed to assess the true severity and extent of the fracture; a third oblique view is often desired.

Most displaced fractures of the distal radius occur dorsally. If left untreated, the radius depicted in Fig. 7.38 would likely heal in this abnormal position, potentially altering the kinematics at the radiocarpal joint and, depending on the extent of the displacement, the distal radio-ulnar joint.[82,89] The resulting reduced natural congruency at these joints would create areas of high articular stress, serving as a potential precursor to degenerative arthritis. This potential would be even higher if the fracture were intra-articular, which occurs in about one in four wrist fractures in older women.[132] In addition, a fractured radius that remains significantly displaced or comminuted typically becomes functionally shortened, likely causing adverse consequences at the wrist. Biomechanically, these may include a *positive ulnar variance* with associated stress placed on the lunate and components within the distal radio-ulnar joint, including the triangular fibrocartilage (TFC). Physiologically, a permanently shortened radius may affect the length-tension relationship of muscles

Fractured distal radius

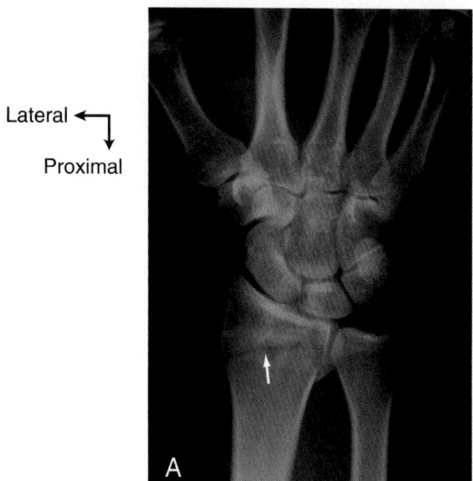

Lateral ←
Proximal ↓

A

Posterior-anterior (PA) view

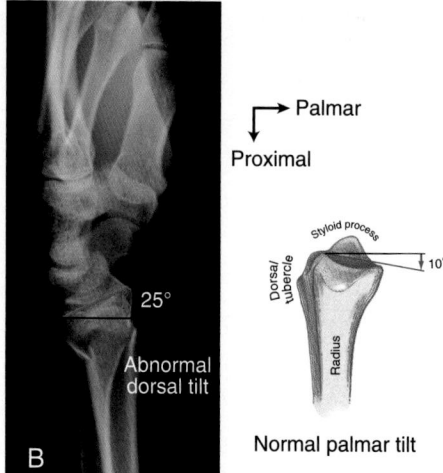

Palmar →
Proximal ↓

25°
Abnormal
dorsal tilt

B

Lateral view

Normal palmar tilt

FIGURE 7.38 Two views of a displaced, extra-articular fracture of the distal radius (Colles' fracture) in a 40-year-old female: (A) posterior-anterior view; (B) lateral view. Note in (B) that the distal fragment of the radius is abnormally displaced (angulated) *dorsally* about 25 degrees. The *inset* to the right shows the normal palmar tilt of the distal radius.

ADDITIONAL CLINICAL CONNECTIONS

that cross the wrist, such as the extrinsic digital flexor muscles. This situation may reduce grip strength. Kinematically, a significantly dorsally angulated distal radius may reduce the full range of functional flexion at the wrist, even if there is no soft tissue shortening. Interestingly, cadaver research simulating progressively increased dorsal angulation of the distal radius reported a progressive shift in the relative contribution of wrist flexion *to the radiocarpal* joint.[85] Possibility as a compensation, the greater kinematic demands placed on the radiocarpal (relative to the midcarpal) joint and proximal row of carpal bones may stress structures such as the vulnerable lunate and scapholunate ligament.[17] These pathomechanics may further contribute to the relatively high incidence of degenerative arthritis of the radiocarpal joint following a dorsal angulated fracture of the radius.

For reasons described earlier, attaining near normal alignment of the fractured distal radius is an important goal of orthopedic management. Distal radius fractures may be treated with immobilization through rigid casting or through surgery. Surgery often involves internal fixation using hardware or percutaneous external bony fixation. The specific choice of treatment depends on many factors, such as whether the fracture is significantly displaced or comminuted, the patient's age and activity level, and the presence of comorbidities such as osteoporosis.[25]

Regardless of the choice of orthopedic treatment, the goal is that the radius heals with optimal alignment. If the fracture is only slightly displaced and is stable, the treatment may involve simple casting following closed reduction. This treatment has the advantage of avoiding surgery, but, in some cases, may have the disadvantage of not *completely* immobilizing the fracture site. If the fracture site is not rigidly immobilized, excessive active movement or muscle activation, or weight-bearing (especially during the first few weeks) can cause the distal radius to "slip or settle" back to its precasted displacement. If this occurs or is suspected, the therapist may take a more conservative approach to the postfracture rehabilitation; however, if too conservative, the patient may develop tightness in the muscles and soft tissues around the wrist as well as those proximal and distal to the fractured region. Each patient's situation is unique and cannot be addressed in this chapter; specific guidelines on orthopedic and therapeutic management following distal radius fractures are available in other sources.[25,117,118]

Orthopedic surgery may be indicated when the distal radial fracture is markedly displaced or intra-articular, or in cases when it is not practical or prudent to immobilize with casting. Surgery has the inherent advantage of immediately and rigidly immobilizing the fracture site, thereby securing optimal position during healing. If medically appropriate, active range-of-motion exercise programs may be initiated sooner than with casting. Such an approach may limit immobilization-based muscle and soft tissue tightness throughout the upper limb.

REFERENCES

1. Abe S, Moritomo H, Oka K, et al.: Three-dimensional kinematics of the lunate, hamate, capitate and triquetrum with type 1 or 2 lunate morphology, *J Hand Surg: European* 43(4):380–386, 2018.
2. Akhbari B, Moore DC, Laidlaw DH, et al.: Predicting carpal bone kinematics using an expanded digital database of wrist carpal bone anatomy and kinematics, *J Orthop Res* 37(12):2661–2670, 2019.
3. Alfredson H, Ljung BO, Thorsen K, et al.: In vivo investigation of ECRB tendons with microdialysis technique—no signs of inflammation but high amounts of glutamate in tennis elbow, *Acta Orthop Scand* 71:475–479, 2000.
4. Altman E: The ulnar side of the wrist: clinically relevant anatomy and biomechanics. [review], *J Hand Ther* 29(2):111–122, 2016.
5. Anderson H, Hoy G: Orthotic intervention incorporating the dart-thrower's motion as part of conservative management guidelines for treatment of scapholunate injury, *J Hand Ther* 29(2):199–204, 2016.
6. Ando R, Arai T, Beppu M, et al.: Anatomical study of arthroscopic surgery for lateral epicondylitis, *Hand Surg* 13(2):85–91, 2008.
7. Athlani L, Pauchard N, Dautel G: Outcomes of scapholunate intercarpal ligamentoplasty for chronic scapholunate dissociation: a prospective study in 26 patients, *J Hand Surg: European* 43(7):700–707, 2018.
8. Bain GI, Clitherow HD, Millar S, et al.: The effect of lunate morphology on the 3-dimensional kinematics of the carpus, *J Hand Surg Am* 40(1), 2015. 81-9.e1.
9. Berger RA, Imeada T, Berglund L, et al.: Constraint and material properties of the subregions of the scapholunate interosseous ligament, *J Hand Surg Am* 24(5):953–962, 1999.
10. Bergner JL, Farrar JQ, Coronado RA: Dart thrower's motion and the injured scapholunate interosseous ligament: a scoping review of studies examining motion, orthoses, and rehabilitation, *J Hand Ther* 33(1):45–59, 2020.
11. Best GM, Mack ZE, Pichora DR, et al.: Differences in the rotation axes of the scapholunate joint during flexion-extension and radial-ulnar deviation motions, *J Hand Surg Am* 44(9):772–778, 2019.
12. Bisset LM, Collins NJ, Offord SS: Immediate effects of 2 types of braces on pain and grip strength in people with lateral epicondylalgia: a randomized controlled trial, *J Orthop Sports Phys Ther* 44(2):120–128, 2014.
13. Brand PW, Beach RB, Thompson DE: Relative tension and potential excursion of muscles in the forearm and hand, *J Hand Surg Am* 6:209–219, 1981.
14. Brogan DM, Berger RA, Kakar S: Ulnar-sided wrist pain: a critical analysis review, *JBJS Rev* 7(5):e1, 2019.
15. Bunata RE, Brown DS, Capelo R: Anatomic factors related to the cause of tennis elbow, *J Hand Surg Am* 89:1955–1963, 2007.
16. Burssens A, Schelpe N, Vanhaecke J, et al.: Influence of wrist position on maximum grip force in a post-operative orthosis, *Prosthet Orthot Int* 41(1):78–84, 2017.
17. Bushnell BD, Bynum DK: Malunion of the distal radius, *J Am Acad Orthop Surg* 15(1):27–40, 2007.
18. Campbell CC, Neustein TM, Daly CA, et al.: Surgical treatment of wrist arthritis in young patients, *JBJS Rev* 8(3):e0078, 2020.
19. Camus EJ, Van Overstraeten L, Schuind F: Lunate biomechanics: application to kienböck's disease and its treatment, *Hand Surg Rehabil* 40(2):117–125, 2021.
20. Chen Z, Baker NA: Effectiveness of eccentric strengthening in the treatment of lateral elbow tendinopathy: a systematic review with meta-analysis, *J Hand Ther* 34: 18–28, 2021.
21. Crisco JJ, Heard WM, Rich RR, et al.: The mechanical axes of the wrist are oriented obliquely to the anatomical axes, *J Bone Joint Surg Am* 93(2):169–177, 2011.
22. da Luz DC, de Borba Y, Ravanello EM, et al.: Iontophoresis in lateral epicondylitis: a randomized, double-blind clinical trial, *J Shoulder Elbow Surg* 28(9):1743–1749, 2019.

23. de Bruin M, Smeulders MJ, Kreulen M: Flexor carpi ulnaris tenotomy alone does not eliminate its contribution to wrist torque, *Clin Biomech* 26(7):725–728, 2011.
24. de Lange A, Kauer JM, Huiskes R: Kinematic behavior of the human wrist joint: a roentgen-stereophotogrammetric analysis, *J Orthop Res* 3:56–64, 1985.
25. DeGeorge Jr BR, Van Houten HK, Mwangi R, et al.: Outcomes and complications in the management of distal radial fractures in the elderly, *J Bone Joint Surg Am* 102(1):37–44, 2020.
26. Delp SL, Grierson AE, Buchanan TS: Maximum isometric moments generated by the wrist muscles in flexion-extension and radial-ulnar deviation, *J Biomech* 29:1371–1375, 1996.
27. Duncan J, Duncan R, Bansal S, et al.: Lateral epicondylitis: the condition and current management strategies, *Br J Hosp Med* 80(11):647–651, 2019.
28. Elnikety S, El-Husseiny M, Kamal T, et al.: Patient satisfaction with postoperative follow-up by a hand therapist, *Muscoskel Care* 10(1):39–42, 2012.
29. Esplugas M, Garcia-Elias M, Lluch A, et al.: Role of muscles in the stabilization of ligament-deficient wrists. [review], *J Hand Ther* 29(2):166–174, 2016.
30. Ferreres A, Suso S, Ordi J, et al.: Wrist denervation. Anatomical considerations, *J Hand Surg Br* 20:761–768, 1995.
31. Formica D, Charles SK, Zollo L, et al.: The passive stiffness of the wrist and forearm, *J Neurophysiol* 108(4):1158–1166, 2012.
32. Friedman SL, Palmer AK, Short WH, et al.: The change in ulnar variance with grip, *J Hand Surg Am* 18:713–716, 1993.
33. Garcia-Elias M, Puig de la Bellacasa I, Schouten C: Carpal ligaments: a functional classification, *Hand Clin* 33(3):511–520, 2017.
34. Giberson-Chen CC, Leland HA, Benavent KA, et al.: Functional outcomes after Sauvé-Kapandji arthrodesis, *J Hand Surg Am* 45(5):408–416, 2020.
35. Giray E, Karali-Bingul D, Akyuz G: The effectiveness of kinesiotaping, sham taping or exercises only in lateral epicondylitis treatment: a randomized controlled study, *Pm R* 11(7):681–693, 2019.
36. Gofton WT, Gordon KD, Dunning CE, et al.: Soft-tissue stabilizers of the distal radioulnar joint: an in vitro kinematic study, *J Hand Surg Am* 29:423–431, 2004.
37. Gonzalez RV, Buchanan TS, Delp SL: How muscle architecture and moment arms affect wrist flexion-extension moments, *J Biomech* 30(7):705–712, 1997.
38. Gray DJ, Gardner E: The innervation of the joints of the wrist and hand, *Anat Rec* 151:261–266, 1965.
39. Gupta A, Moosawi NA: How much can carpus rotate axially? An in vivo study, *Clin Biomech* 20:172–176, 2005.
40. Haahr JP, Andersen JH: Physical and psychosocial risk factors for lateral epicondylitis: a population based case-referent study, *Occup Environ Med* 60(5):322–329, 2003.
41. Hagert E, Garcia-Elias M, Forsgren S, et al.: Immunohistochemical analysis of wrist ligament innervation in relation to their structural composition, *J Hand Surg Am* 32(1):30–36, 2007.
42. Hagert E, Lluch A, Rein S: The role of proprioception and neuromuscular stability in carpal instabilities, *J Hand Surg Eur* 41(1):94–101, 2016.
43. Hagert E, Persson JKE, Werner M, et al.: Evidence of wrist proprioceptive reflexes elicited after stimulation of the scapholunate interosseous ligament, *J Hand Surg Am* 34:642–651, 2009.
44. Hagert E: Proprioception of the wrist joint: a review of current concepts and possible implications on the rehabilitation of the wrist [Review, 100 refs], *J Hand Ther* 23(1):2–16, 2010.
45. Hegazy G, Akar A, Abd-Elghany T, et al.: Treatment of Kienböck's disease with neutral ulnar variance by distal capitate shortening and arthrodesis to the base of the third metacarpal bone, *J Hand Surg Am* 44(6):518.e1–518.e9, 2019.

46. Holm-Glad T, Røkkum M, Röhrl SM, et al.: A randomized controlled trial comparing two modern total wrist arthroplasties:improved function with stable implants, but high complication rates in non-rheumatoid wrists at two years, *Bone Joint Lett J* 104-b(10):1132–1141, 2022.
47. Holzbaur KR, Delp SL, Gold GE, et al.: Moment-generating capacity of upper limb muscles in healthy adults, *J Biomech* 40:2442–2449, 2007.
48. Isa AD, McGregor ME, Padmore CE, et al.: Effect of radial lengthening on distal forearm loading following simulated in vitro radial shortening during simulated dynamic wrist motion, *J Hand Surg Am* 44(7):556–563.e5, 2019.
49. Ishii S, Palmer AK, Werner FW, et al.: An anatomic study of the ligamentous structure of the triangular fibrocartilage complex, *J Hand Surg Am* 23:977–985, 1998.
50. Iwamoto A, Morris RP, Andersen C, et al.: An anatomic and biomechanic study of the wrist extensor retinaculum septa and tendon compartments, *J Hand Surg Am* 31:896–903, 2006.
51. Jung JM, Baek GH, Kim JH, et al.: Changes in ulnar variance in relation to forearm rotation and grip, *J Bone Joint Surg Br* 83:1029–1033, 2001.
52. Kamal RN, Moore W, Kakar S: Team approach: management of scapholunate instability, *JBJS Rev* 7(2):e2, 2019.
53. Kaufmann R, Pfaeffle J, Blankenhorn B, et al.: Kinematics of the midcarpal and radiocarpal joints in radioulnar deviation: an in vitro study, *J Hand Surg Am* 30:937–942, 2005.
54. Kelly PM, Hopkins JG, Furey AJ, et al.: Dynamic CT scan of the normal scapholunate joint in a clenched fist and radial and ulnar deviation, *Hand* 13(6):666–670, 2018.
55. Kobayashi M, Berger RA, Nagy L, et al.: Normal kinematics of carpal bones: a three-dimensional analysis of carpal bone motion relative to the radius, *J Biomech* 30:787–793, 1997.
56. Kramer A, Allon R, Werner F, et al.: Distinct wrist patterns founded on measurements in plain radiographs, *J Wrist Surg* 7(5):366–374, 2018.
57. Kraushaar BS, Nirschl RP: Tendinosis of the elbow (tennis elbow). Clinical features and findings of histological, immunohistochemical, and electron microscopy studies, *J Bone Joint Surg Am* 81:259–278, 1999.
58. Kroslak M, Pirapakaran K, Murrell GAC: Counterforce bracing of lateral epicondylitis: a prospective, randomized, double-blinded, placebo-controlled clinical trial, *J Shoulder Elbow Surg* 28(2):288–295, 2019.
59. Kuo CE, Wolfe SW: Scapholunate instability: current concepts in diagnosis and management, *J Hand Surg Am* 33:998–1013, 2008.
60. La Delfa NJ, Potvin JR: A musculoskeletal model to estimate the relative changes in wrist strength due to interacting wrist and forearm postures, *Comput Methods Biomech Biomed Engin* 20(13):1403–1411, 2017.
61. Lenoir H, Mares O, Carlier Y: Management of lateral epicondylitis, *Orthop Traumatol Surg Res* 105(8s):S241–s246, 2019.
62. Leventhal EL, Moore DC, Akelman E, et al.: Carpal and forearm kinematics during a simulated hammering task, *J Hand Surg Am* 35(7):1097–1104, 2010.
63. Liber RL: *Skeletal muscle structure, function and plasticity: the physiologic basis of rehabilitation*, ed 3, Philadelphia, 2010, Lippincott Williams & Wilkins.
64. Lichtman DM, Lesley NE, Simmons SP: The classification and treatment of Kienböck's disease: the state of the art and a look at the future [Review], *J Hand Surg Eur Vol* 35(7):549–554, 2010.
65. Linscheid RL: Kinematic considerations of the wrist, *Clin Orthop Relat Res* 202:27–39, 1986.
66. Lutsky K, Beredjiklian PK: Kienböck disease [review], *J Hand Surg Am* 37(9):1942–1952, 2012.

67. Majima M, Horii E, Matsuki H, et al.: Load transmission through the wrist in the extended position, *J Hand Surg Am* 33:182–188, 2008.

68. McDermott JD, Ilyas AM, Nazarian LN, et al.: Ultrasound-guided injections for de Quervain's tenosynovitis, *Clin Orthop Relat Res* 470(7):1925–1931, 2012.

69. Meunier M: Lateral epicondylitis/extensor tendon injury, *Clin Sports Med* 39(3):657–660, 2020.

70. Mikić Z: The blood supply of the human distal radioulnar joint and the microvasculature of its articular disk, *Clin Orthop Relat Res* 275:19–28, 1992.

71. Mitsuyasu H, Patterson RM, Shah MA, et al.: The role of the dorsal intercarpal ligament in dynamic and static scapholunate instability, *J Hand Surg Am* 29:279–288, 2004.

72. Modest J, Clair B, DeMasi R, et al.: Self-Measured wrist range of motion by wrist-injured and wrist-healthy study participants using a built-in Iphone feature as compared with a universal goniometer, *J Hand Ther* 32(4):507–514, 2019.

73. Moojen TM, Snel JG, Ritt MJ, et al.: In vivo analysis of carpal kinematics and comparative review of the literature, *J Hand Surg Am* 28:81–87, 2003.

74. Moritomo H, Apergis EP, Garcia-Elias M, et al.: International federation of societies for surgery of the hand 2013 committee's report on wrist dart-throwing motion, *J Hand Surg Am* 39(7):1433–1439, 2014.

75. Moritomo H, Murase T, Arimitsu S, et al.: Change in the length of the ulnocarpal ligaments during radiocarpal motion: possible impact on triangular fibrocartilage complex foveal tears, *J Hand Surg Am* 33(8):1278–1286, 2008.

76. Moritomo H, Murase T, Goto A, et al.: Capitate-based kinematics of the midcarpal joint during wrist radioulnar deviation: an in vivo three-dimensional motion analysis, *J Hand Surg Am* 29:668–675, 2004.

77. Nair R: Total wrist arthroplasty [Review], *J Orthop Surg* 22(3):399–405, 2014.

78. Niedermeier SR, Crouser N, Speeckaert A, et al.: A survey of fellowship-trained upper extremity surgeons on treatment of lateral epicondylitis, *Hand* 14(5):597–601, 2019.

79. Nikolopoulos F, Apergis E, Kefalas V, et al.: Biomechanical properties of interosseous proximal carpal row ligaments, *J Orthop Res* 29(5):668–671, 2011.

80. Nikolopoulos FV, Apergis EP, Poulilios AD, et al.: Biomechanical properties of the scapholunate ligament and the importance of its portions in the capitate intrusion injury, *Clin Biomech* 26(8):819–823, 2011.

81. Nishiwaki M, Nakamura T, Nagura T, et al.: Ulnar-shortening effect on distal radioulnar joint pressure: a biomechanical study, *J Hand Surg Am* 33:198–205, 2008.

82. Nishiwaki M, Welsh M, Gammon B, et al.: Distal radioulnar joint kinematics in simulated dorsally angulated distal radius fractures, *J Hand Surg Am* 39(4):656–663, 2014.

83. Nozaki T, Wu W, Kaneko Y, et al.: High-resolution MRI of the ulnar and radial collateral ligaments of the wrist, *Acta Radiol* 58(12):1493–1499, 2017.

84. O'Driscoll SW, Horii E, Ness R, et al.: The relationship between wrist position, grasp size, and grip strength, *J Hand Surg Am* 17:169–177, 1992.

85. Padmore CE, Stoesser H, Nishiwaki M, et al.: The effect of dorsally angulated distal radius deformities on carpal kinematics: an in vitro biomechanical study, *J Hand Surg Am* 43(11):1036.e1–1036.e8, 2018.

86. Palmer AK, Glisson RR, Werner FW: Ulnar variance determination, *J Hand Surg Am* 7:376–379, 1982.

87. Palmer AK, Werner FW: Biomechanics of the distal radioulnar joint, *Clin Orthop Relat Res* 187:26–35, 1984.

88. Pang EQ, Douglass N, Behn A, et al.: Tensile and torsional structural properties of the native scapholunate ligament, *J Hand Surg Am* 43(9):864.e1–864.e7, 2018.

89. Park MJ, Cooney III WP, Hahn ME, et al.: The effects of dorsally angulated distal radius fractures on carpal kinematics, *J Hand Surg Am* 27:223–232, 2002.

90. Peltier LF: The classic. Concerning traumatic malacia of the lunate and its consequences: degeneration and compression fractures. Translation of 1910 article. Privatdozent Dr. Robert Kienbock, *Clin Orthop Relat Res* 150:4–8, 1980.

91. Perez AJ, Jethanandani RG, Vutescu ES, et al.: Role of ligament stabilizers of the proximal carpal row in preventing dorsal intercalated segment instability: a cadaveric study, *J Bone Joint Surg Am* 101(15):1388–1396, 2019.

92. Porretto-Loehrke A, Schuh C, Szekeres M: Clinical manual assessment of the wrist. [review], *J Hand Ther* 29(2):123–135, 2016.

93. Potter HG, Hannafin JA, Morwessel RM, et al.: Lateral epicondylitis: correlation of MR imaging, surgical, and histopathologic findings, *Radiology* 196:43–46, 1995.

94. Pulos N, Bozentka DJ: Carpal ligament anatomy and biomechanics, *Hand Clin* 31(3):381–387, 2015.

95. Radonjic D, Long C: Kinesiology of the wrist, *Am J Phys Med* 50:57–71, 1971.

96. Rainbow MJ, Kamal RN, Leventhal E, et al.: In vivo kinematics of the scaphoid, lunate, capitate, and third metacarpal in extreme wrist flexion and extension, *J Hand Surg Am* 38(2):278–288, 2013.

97. Rainbow MJ, Wolff AL, Crisco JJ, et al.: Functional kinematics of the wrist, *J Hand Surg Eur Vol* 41(1):7–21, 2016.

98. Ramsay JW, Hunter BV, Gonzalez RV: Muscle moment arm and normalized moment contributions as reference data for musculoskeletal elbow and wrist joint models, *J Biomech* 42(4):463–473, 2009.

99. Rawal A, Chehata A, Horberry T, et al.: Defining the upper extremity range of motion for safe automobile driving, *Clin Biomech* 54:78–85, 2018.

100. Rhee PC, Moran SL: The effect of lunate morphology in carpal disorders: review of the literature, *Curr Rheumatol Rev* 16(3):184–188, 2020.

101. Rioux-Forker D, Shin AY: Osteonecrosis of the lunate: kienböck disease, *J Am Acad Orthop Surg* 28(14):570–584, 2020.

102. Rose NE, Forman SK, Dellon AL: Denervation of the lateral humeral epicondyle for treatment of chronic lateral epicondylitis, *J Hand Surg Am* 38(2):344–349, 2013.

103. Rubensson C, Johansson T, Adolfsson L: Tensioning of the radioscaphocapitate and long radio-lunate ligaments for dynamic radiocarpal instability, *J Hand Surg: European* 43(4):369–374, 2018.

104. Ryu JY, Cooney III WP, Askew LJ, et al.: Functional ranges of motion of the wrist joint, *J Hand Surg Am* 16:409–419, 1991.

105. Safaee-Rad R, Shwedyk E, Quanbury AO, et al.: Normal functional range of motion of upper limb joints during performance of three feeding activities, *Arch Phys Med Rehabil* 71:505–509, 1990.

106. Salva-Coll G, Garcia-Elias M, Hagert E: Scapholunate instability: proprioception and neuromuscular control, *J Wrist Surg* 2(2):136–140, 2013.

107. Salva-Coll G, Garcia-Elias M, Leon-Lopez MT, et al.: Effects of forearm muscles on carpal stability, *J Hand Surg: European* 36(7):553–559, 2011.

108. Salva-Coll G, Garcia-Elias M, Lluch-Bergada A, et al.: Kinetic dysfunction of the wrist with chronic scapholunate dissociation. A cadaver study, *Clin Biomech* 77:105046, 2020.

109. Sarrafian SK, Melamed JL, Goshgarian GM: Study of wrist motion in flexion and extension, *Clin Orthop Relat Res* 126:153–159, 1977.

110. Schuind FA, Linscheid RL, An KN, et al.: A normal data base of posteroanterior roentgenographic measurements of the wrist, *J Bone Joint Surg Am* 74:1418–1429, 1992.

111. Sebastin SJ, Puhaindran ME, Lim AY, et al.: The prevalence of absence of the palmaris longus—a study in a Chinese population and a review of the literature, *J Hand Surg Br* 30:525–527, 2005.

112. Sendher R, Ladd AL: The scaphoid [Review], *Orthop Clin North Am* 44(1):107–120, 2013.

113. Shahabpour M, Van OL, Ceuterick P, et al.: Pathology of extrinsic ligaments: a pictorial essay [Review], *Semin Musculoskelet Radiol* 16(2):115–128, 2012.

114. Shakeri H, Soleimanifar M, Arab AM, et al.: The effects of Kinesiotape on the treatment of lateral epicondylitis, *J Hand Ther* 31(1):35–41, 2018.

115. Short WH, Werner FW, Green JK, et al.: The effect of sectioning the dorsal radiocarpal ligament and insertion of a pressure sensor into the radiocarpal joint on scaphoid and lunate kinematics, *J Hand Surg Am* 27:68–76, 2002.

116. Skirven TM, Osterman AL, Fedorczyk J, et al.: *Rehabilitation of the hand and upper extremity*, ed 7, St Louis, 2021, Elsevier, p 77. Chap 76.

117. Skirven TM, Osterman AL, Fedorczyk J: *Rehabilitation of the hand and upper extremity*, ed 6, St Louis, 2011, Elsevier, p 70. Chap 69.

118. Slutsky D, Osterman L: *Fractures and injuries of the distal radius and carpus*, ed 1, St Louis, 2008, Elsevier.

119. Srnec JJ, Wagner ER, Rizzo M: Total wrist arthroplasty, *JBJS Rev* 6(6):e9, 2018.

120. Standring S: *Gray's anatomy: the anatomical basis of clinical practice*, ed 42, St Louis, 2021, Elsevier.

121. Sun JS, Shih TT, Ko CM, et al.: In vivo kinematic study of normal wrist motion: an ultrafast computed tomographic study, *Clin Biomech* 15:212–216, 2000.

122. Taleisnik J: The ligaments of the wrist. In Taleisnik J, editor: *The wrist*, New York, 1985, Churchill Livingstone.

123. Taljanovic MS, Malan JJ, Sheppard JE: Normal anatomy of the extrinsic capsular wrist ligaments by 3-T MRI and high-resolution ultrasonography [Review], *Semin Musculoskelet Radiol* 16(2):104–114, 2012.

124. Thiru RG, Ferlic DC, Clayton ML, et al.: Arterial anatomy of the triangular fibrocartilage of the wrist and its surgical significance, *J Hand Surg Am* 11(2):258–263, 1986.

125. Thompson NW, Mockford BJ, Rasheed T, et al.: Functional absence of flexor digitorum superficialis to the little finger and absence of palmaris longus—is there a link? *J Hand Surg Br* 27:433–434, 2002.

126. Tolbert JR, Blair WF, Andrews JG, et al.: The kinetics of normal and prosthetic wrists, *J Biomech* 18:887–897, 1985.

127. Tosti R, Jennings J, Sewards JM: Lateral epicondylitis of the elbow [Review], *Am J Med* 126(4):357–366, 2013.

128. Türker T, Sheppard JE, Klauser AS, et al.: The radial and ulnar collateral ligaments of the wrist are true ligaments, *Diagn Interv Radiol* 25(6):473–479, 2019.

129. Uygur E, Aktaş B, Özkut A, et al.: Dry needling in lateral epicondylitis: a prospective controlled study, *Int Orthop* 41(11):2321–2325, 2017.

130. van der Post AS, Jens S, Daams JG, et al.: The triangular fibrocartilage complex in the human wrist: a scoping review toward uniform and clinically relevant terminology, *Clin Anat* 35(5):626–648, 2022.

131. Viegas SF, Yamaguchi S, Boyd NL, et al.: The dorsal ligaments of the wrist: anatomy, mechanical properties, and function, *J Hand Surg Am* 24:456–468, 1999.

132. Vogt M, Cauley JA, Tomaino MM, et al.: Distal radius fractures in older women: a 10-year follow-up study of descriptive characteristics and risk factors: the study of osteoporotic fractures, *J Am Geriatr Soc* 50(1):97–103, 2002.

133. Wagner ER, Conti Mica M, Shin AY: Smartphone photography utilized to measure wrist range of motion, *J Hand Surg: European* 43(2):187–192, 2018.

134. Wall LB, Stern PJ: Proximal row carpectomy [Review], *Hand Clin* 29(1):69–78, 2013.

135. Weaver L, Tencer AF, Trumble TE: Tensions in the palmar ligaments of the wrist. I. The normal wrist, *J Hand Surg Am* 19:464–474, 1994.

136. Werber KD, Schmelz R, Peimer CA, et al.: Biomechanical effect of isolated capitate shortening in Kienbock's disease: an anatomical study, *J Hand Surg Eur Vol* 38(5):500–507, 2013.

137. Wolff AL, Wolfe SW: Rehabilitation for scapholunate injury: application of scientific and clinical evidence to practice, *J Hand Ther* 29(2):146–153, 2016.

138. Wollstein R, Wollstein A, Rodgers J, et al.: A hand therapy protocol for the treatment of lunate overload or early Kienböck's disease, *J Hand Ther* 26(3):255–259, 2013.

139. Youm Y, McMurthy RY, Flatt AE, et al.: Kinematics of the wrist. I. An experimental study of radial-ulnar deviation and flexion-extension, *J Bone Joint Surg Am* 60:423–431, 1978.

140. Zijlker HJA, Ritt M, Beumer A: Fourth-Generation total wrist arthroplasty: a systematic review of clinical outcomes, *J Wrist Surg* 11(5):456–464, 2022.

STUDY QUESTIONS

1. How does the tendon of the flexor carpi radialis reach the base of the metacarpal bones without entering the carpal tunnel?
2. Cite factors that justify the greater range of ulnar deviation compared with radial deviation of the wrist.
3. Assume that trauma associated with a fractured distal radius created a permanent 25-degree *dorsal* tilt of the distal radius (review Fig. 7.4B). What are some probable functional impairments that may result from this malalignment?
4. Describe the arthrokinematic pattern for flexion and extension at the radiocarpal and medial compartment of the midcarpal joints.
5. Justify the importance of the capitate bone in osteokinematics of the entire wrist and hand.
6. The following questions are based on the data presented in Fig. 7.24.
   a. Which muscle would produce the greatest flexion torque at the wrist: the flexor carpi radialis or the flexor digitorum superficialis?
   b. Which muscle has the longest moment arm for ulnar deviation torque?
   c. Which muscle is the *most* direct antagonist to the flexor carpi ulnaris?
7. Define the kinematics of the "dart thrower's motion" at the wrist. Offer functional or therapeutic advantages of this motion compared with pure planar motions of the wrist.
8. Which two tendons of the thumb share the same fibrous tunnel within the extensor retinaculum of the wrist?
9. What is the role of the scaphoid in providing mechanical stability to the lunate?
10. How would you *maximally* stretch the extensor carpi radialis longus muscle?
11. Which extrinsic ligaments naturally resist ulnar translocation of the carpus?
12. A patient had severe trauma to the proximal radius and adjacent interosseous membrane that necessitated a partial resection of the radial head. Describe possible functional impairments or pathologies that might result from a subsequent 6- to 7-mm proximal migration of the radius.
13. Which carpal bones normally do *not* contact the capitate bone?
14. Compare the convex-concave joint relationships that exist within the medial and lateral compartments of the *midcarpal joint* of the wrist. Describe how these relationships affect the arthrokinematics of the joint during flexion and extension.
15. List all muscles that have a full or partial proximal attachment to the lateral epicondyle of the humerus. Which nerve innervates all these muscles?
16. Describe the muscular interaction between the flexor carpi ulnaris and flexor carpi radialis during active flexion of the wrist.
17. Contrast (a) the *position* of the wrist typically chosen to hold a hammer firmly and statically with (b) the *kinematics* at the wrist used during the preparatory and striking phases of striking a nail with a hammer.
18. Define wrist circumduction and offer reasons why this motion may be useful during a clinical evaluation.

Answers to the study questions can be found in the accompanying enhanced eBook version included with the print purchase of this textbook.

Additional Video Educational Content

- Fluoroscopic Observations of Selected Arthrokinematics of the Upper Extremity
- Overview of the Anatomy of the Carpal Bones in the Wrist of a Cadaver Specimen
- Overview of the Shapes of the Joints of the Right Wrist in a Cadaver Specimen

CLINICAL KINESIOLOGY APPLIED TO PERSONS WITH QUADRIPLEGIA (TETRAPLEGIA)
- Analysis of Transferring from a Wheelchair to a Mat in a Person with C^6 Quadriplegia

- Functional Considerations of the Wrist Extensor Muscles in a Person with C^6 Quadriplegia (includes "tenodesis action" at the wrist)

ALL VIDEOS in this chapter are available in the accompanying enhanced eBook version included with the print purchase of this textbook.

C h a p t e r

8

Hand

DONALD A. NEUMANN, PT, PhD, FAPTA

CHAPTER AT A GLANCE

Like our eyes, our hands function as an essential sensory organ for the perception of our surroundings (Fig. 8.1). The hand also allows for the physical manifestation of our most complex motor and emotional behaviors through gesture, touch, music, art, and writing.

Twenty-nine muscles drive the 19 bones and 19 articulations within the hand. Biomechanically, these structures interact with superb proficiency. The hand may be used in a very primitive fashion, as a hook or a club, or, more often, as a highly specialized instrument performing very complex manipulations requiring multiple levels of force and precision.

Because of the hand's enormous biomechanical complexity, its function involves a disproportionately large region of the cortex of the brain (Fig. 8.2). Accordingly, diseases or injuries affecting the hand often create a disproportionate loss of function. A hand totally incapacitated by rheumatoid arthritis, severe burn, or nerve or bone injury, for example, can dramatically reduce the function of the entire upper limb. This chapter describes the kinesiologic principles behind many of the musculoskeletal impairments of the hand frequently encountered in medical and rehabilitation

settings. These principles often serve as the basis for therapeutic intervention.

TERMINOLOGY

The wrist, or carpus, has eight carpal bones. The hand has five metacarpals, often referred to collectively as the "metacarpus." Each of the five digits contains a set of phalanges. The digits are designated numerically from 1 to 5, or as the thumb and the index, middle, ring, and small (little) fingers (Fig. 8.3A). A *ray* describes one metacarpal bone and its associated phalanges.

The articulations between the proximal end of the metacarpals and the distal row of carpal bones form the *carpometacarpal* (CMC) *joints* (see Fig. 8.3A). The articulations between the metacarpals and the proximal phalanges form the *metacarpophalangeal* (MCP) *joints.* Each finger has two *interphalangeal joints:* a proximal interphalangeal (PIP) and a distal interphalangeal (DIP) joint. The thumb has only two phalanges and therefore only one interphalangeal (IP) joint.

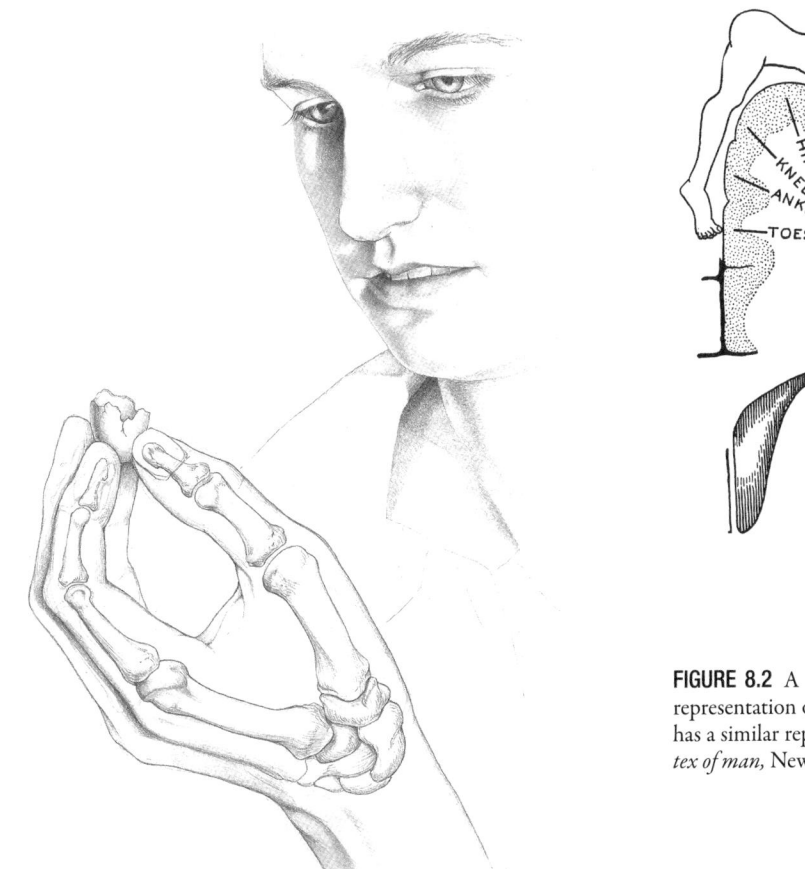

FIGURE 8.1 A very strong functional relationship exists between the hand and the eyes.

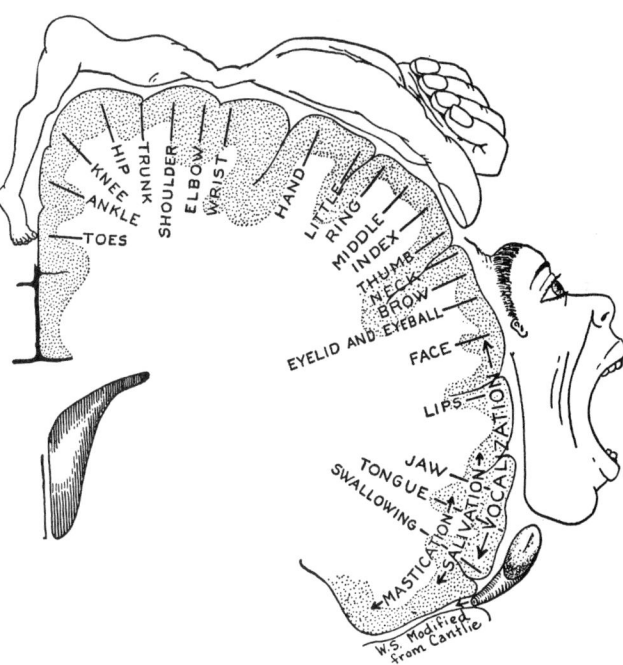

FIGURE 8.2 A motor homunculus of the brain showing the somatotopic representation of body parts. The sensory homunculus of the human brain has a similar representation. (From Penfield W, Rosnussen T: *Cerebral cortex of man,* New York, 1950, Macmillan, 1950.)

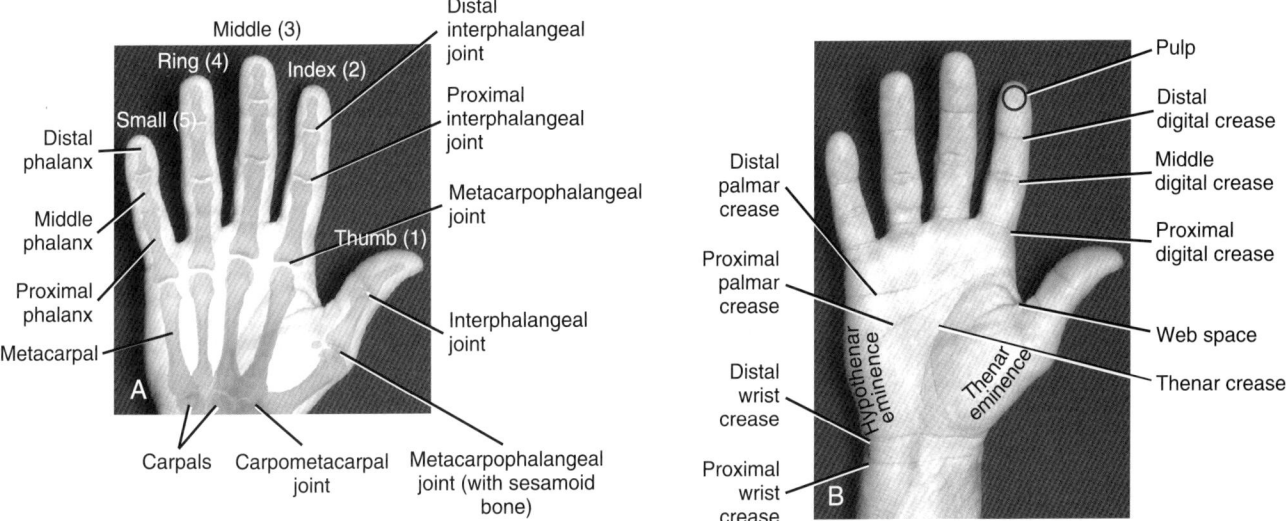

FIGURE 8.3 A palmar view of the basic anatomy of the hand. (A) Major bones and joints. (B) External landmarks.

Articulations Common to Each "Ray" of the Hand

- Carpometacarpal (CMC) joint
- Metacarpophalangeal (MCP) joint
- Interphalangeal (IP) joints
  - Thumb has one IP joint
  - Fingers have a proximal interphalangeal (PIP) joint and a distal interphalangeal (DIP) joint

Fig. 8.3B shows several features of the external anatomy of the hand. Note the *palmar creases,* or lines, that exist in the skin of the palm. They function as dermal "hinges," marking where the skin folds on itself during movement, and increase palmar skin adherence for enhancing the security of grasp. On the palmar (anterior) side of the wrist are the proximal and distal *wrist creases.* Of clinical interest is the fact that the distal wrist crease marks the location of the proximal margin of the underlying transverse carpal ligament. The *thenar crease* is formed by the folding of the dermis as the thumb is moved across the palm. The proximal *digital creases* are located distal to the actual joint line of the MCP joints. The distal and middle digital creases are superficial to the DIP and PIP joints, respectively. Clinicians use many of these creases as landmarks to help fabricate and apply hand orthoses (splints).

OSTEOLOGY

Metacarpals

The metacarpals, like the digits, are designated numerically as 1 through 5, beginning on the radial (lateral) side.

Each metacarpal has similar anatomic characteristics (Figs. 8.4 and 8.5). The first metacarpal (the thumb) is the shortest and stoutest; the second is usually the longest, and the length of the remaining three bones decreases from the radial to ulnar (medial) direction.

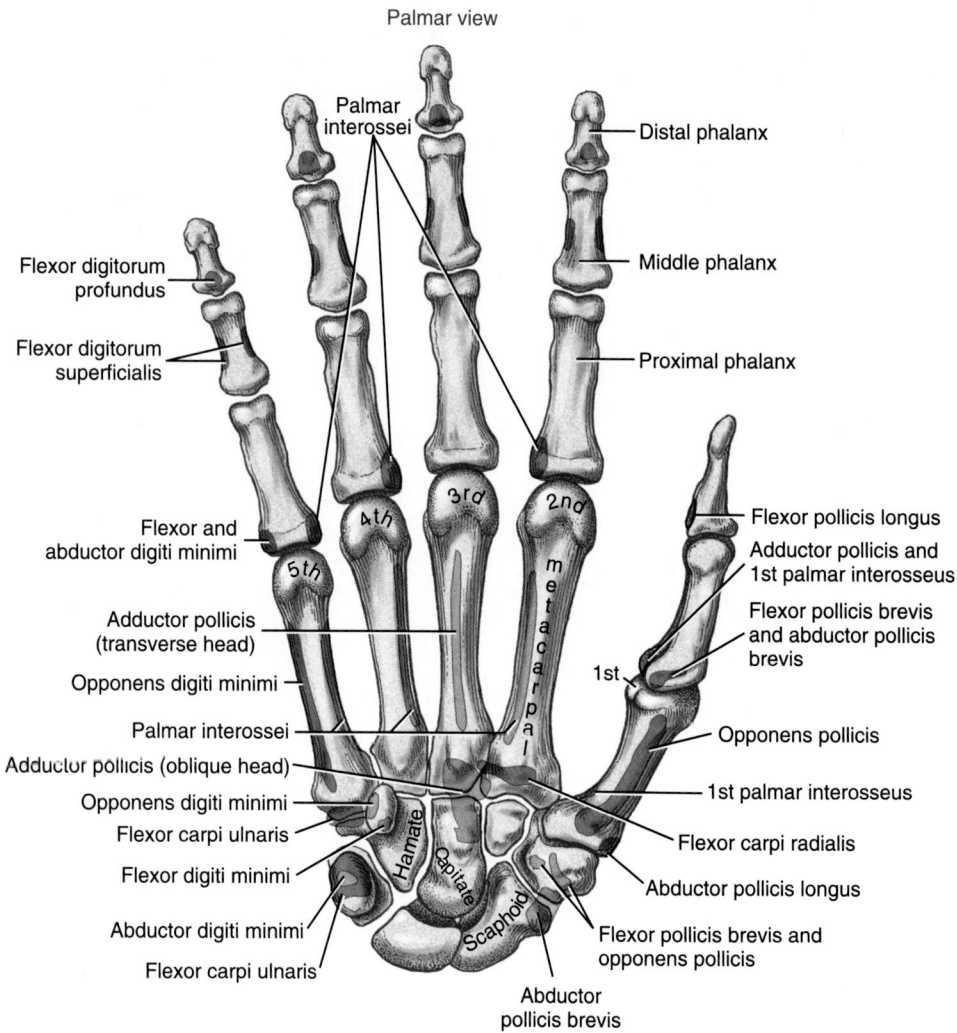

Palmar view

Palmar interossei

Distal phalanx

Middle phalanx

Proximal phalanx

Flexor digitorum profundus

Flexor digitorum superficialis

Flexor and abductor digiti minimi

Adductor pollicis (transverse head)

Opponens digiti minimi

Palmar interossei

Adductor pollicis (oblique head)

Opponens digiti minimi

Flexor carpi ulnaris

Flexor digiti minimi

Abductor digiti minimi

Flexor carpi ulnaris

Flexor pollicis longus

Adductor pollicis and 1st palmar interosseus

Flexor pollicis brevis and abductor pollicis brevis

Opponens pollicis

1st palmar interosseus

Flexor carpi radialis

Abductor pollicis longus

Flexor pollicis brevis and opponens pollicis

Abductor pollicis brevis

Hamate   Capitate   Scaphoid

FIGURE 8.4 A palmar view of the bones of the right wrist and hand. Proximal attachments of muscles are indicated in red and distal attachments in gray.

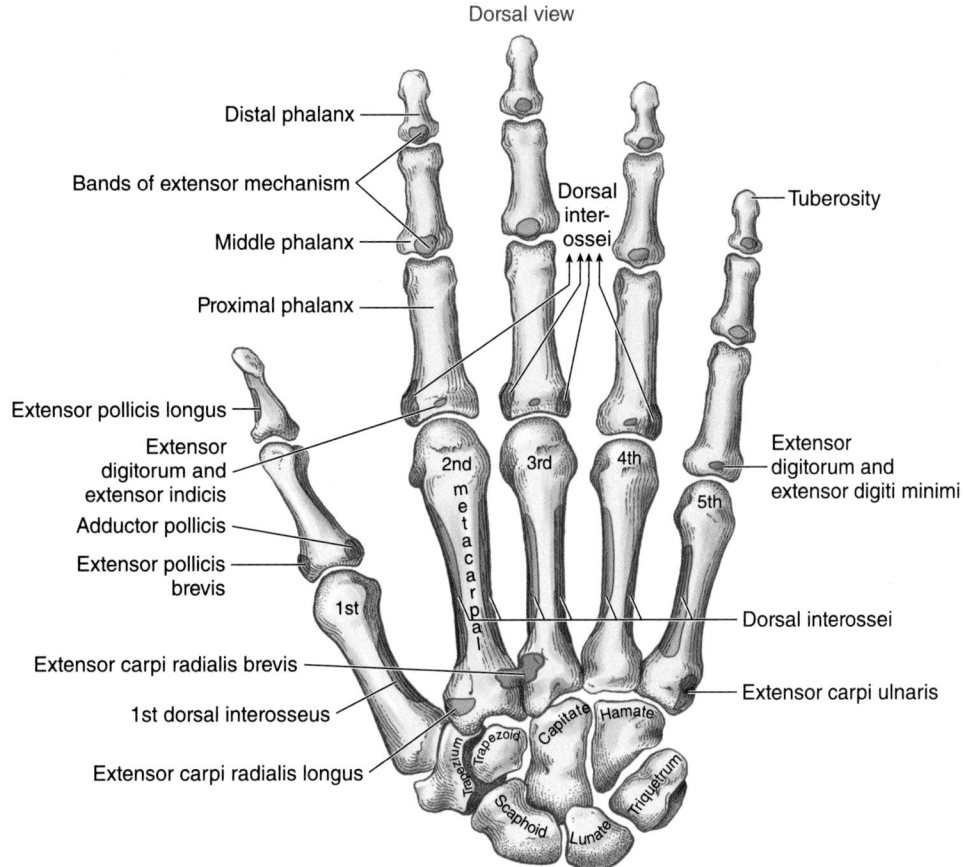

Dorsal view

Distal phalanx

Bands of extensor mechanism

Middle phalanx

Proximal phalanx

Dorsal interossei

Tuberosity

Extensor pollicis longus

Extensor digitorum and extensor indicis

Adductor pollicis

Extensor pollicis brevis

Extensor carpi radialis brevis

1st dorsal interosseus

Extensor carpi radialis longus

2nd metacarpal

3rd

4th

5th

1st

Extensor digitorum and extensor digiti minimi

Dorsal interossei

Extensor carpi ulnaris

Trapezium   Trapezoid   Capitate   Hamate

Scaphoid   Lunate   Triquetrum

FIGURE 8.5 A dorsal view of the bones of the right wrist and hand. Proximal attachments of muscles are indicated in red and distal attachments in gray.

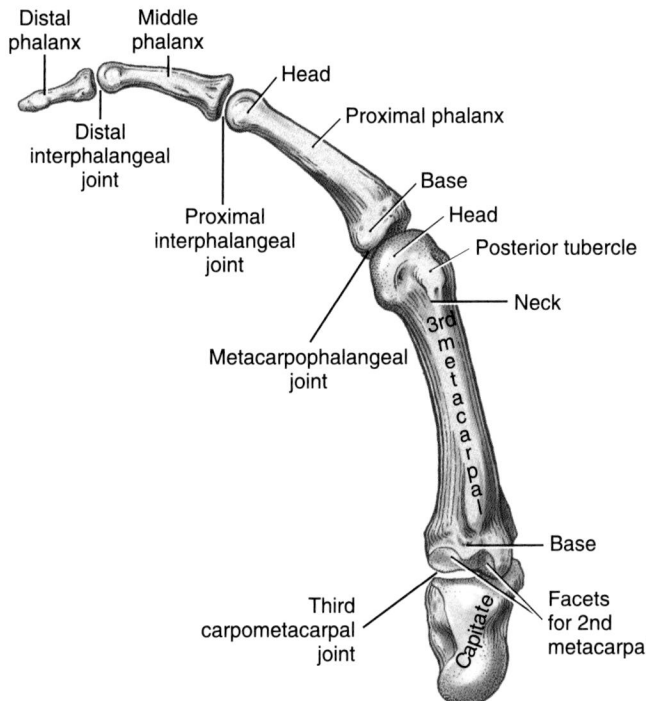

Distal phalanx   Middle phalanx

Head

Proximal phalanx

Distal interphalangeal joint

Distal

Base

Proximal interphalangeal joint

Head

Posterior tubercle

Metacarpophalangeal joint

Neck

3rd metacarpal

Base

Third carpometacarpal joint

Facets for 2nd metacarpal

Capitate

FIGURE 8.6 A lateral view of the bones of the third ray (metacarpal and associated phalanges), including the capitate bone of the wrist.

> **Osteologic Features of a Metacarpal**
> - Shaft
> - Base
> - Head
> - Neck
> - Posterior tubercles

Each metacarpal has an elongated *shaft* with articular surfaces at each end (Fig. 8.6). The palmar surface of the shaft is slightly concave longitudinally to accommodate many muscles and tendons in this region. Its proximal end, or *base*, articulates with one or more of the carpal bones. The bases of the second through the fifth metacarpals possess small facets for articulation with adjacent metacarpal bases.

The distal end of each metacarpal has a large convex *head*. The heads of the second through fifth metacarpals are evident as "knuckles" on the dorsal side of a clenched fist. Immediately proximal to the head is the metacarpal *neck*—a common site of fracture, especially of the fifth digit. A pair of *posterior tubercles* marks the attachment sites for the collateral ligaments of the MCP joints.

With the hand at rest in the anatomic position, the thumb's metacarpal is oriented in a different plane than the other digits. The second through the fifth metacarpals are aligned generally side by

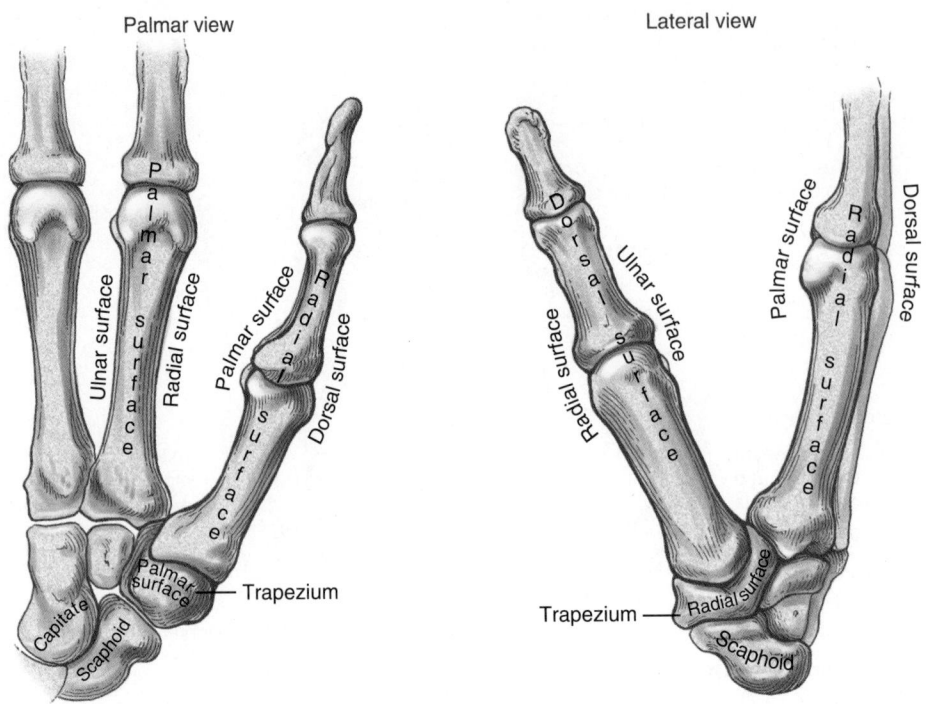

FIGURE 8.7 Palmar and lateral views of the hand showing the orientation of the bony surfaces of the right thumb. Note that the bones of the thumb are rotated approximately 90 degrees relative to the other bones of the wrist and the hand.

side, with their palmar surfaces facing anteriorly. The position of the thumb's metacarpal, however, is rotated almost 90 degrees medially (i.e., internally, relative to the other digits; see Fig. 8.3). Rotation places the very sensitive palmar surface of the thumb *toward* the midline of the hand. Optimum prehension requires that the thumb flexes in a plane that generally intersects, versus parallels, the plane of the flexing fingers. In addition, the thumb's metacarpal is positioned well anterior, or palmar, to the other metacarpals (see Fig. 7.14). This position of the first metacarpal and trapezium is strongly influenced by the palmar projection of the distal pole of the scaphoid.

The location of the first metacarpal allows the entire thumb to sweep freely across the palm toward the fingers. Virtually all prehensile motions, from grasping to pinching to precision handling, require the thumb to interact with the fingers. In the absence of a healthy and mobile thumb, the overall function of the hand is substantially reduced.

The medially rotated thumb requires unique terminology to describe its movement as well as its position. In the anatomic position, the dorsal surface of the bones of the thumb (i.e., the surface where the thumbnail resides) faces laterally (Fig. 8.7). The palmar surface therefore faces medially, the radial surface anteriorly, and the ulnar surface posteriorly. The terminology to describe the surfaces of the carpal bones and all other digital bones is standard: a palmar surface faces anteriorly, a radial surface faces laterally, and so forth.

Phalanges

The hand has 14 phalanges (from the Greek root *phalanx,* a line of soldiers). The phalanges within each finger are referred to as *proximal, middle,* and *distal* (see Fig. 8.3A). The thumb has only a proximal and a distal phalanx.

Osteologic Features of a Phalanx

- Base
- Shaft
- Head (proximal and middle phalanx only)
- Tuberosity (distal phalanx only)

Except for differences in sizes, all phalanges within a particular digit have similar morphology (see Fig. 8.5). The proximal and middle phalanges of each finger have a concave *base, a shaft,* and a convex *head.* As in the metacarpals, their palmar surfaces are slightly concave longitudinally. The distal phalanx of each digit has a concave base. At its distal end is a rounded *tuberosity* that anchors the fleshy pulp of soft tissue to the bony tip of each digit.

Arches of the Hand

Observe the natural concavity of the palmar surface of your relaxed hand. Control of this concavity allows the hand to securely hold and manipulate objects of many and varied shapes and sizes. This palmar concavity is supported by three integrated arch systems: two transverse and one longitudinal (Fig. 8.8). The *proximal transverse arch* is formed by the distal row of carpal bones. This is a static, rigid arch that forms the *carpal tunnel* (see Chapter 7). Like most arches in buildings and bridges, the arches of the hand are supported by a central *keystone* structure. The capitate bone is the keystone of the proximal transverse arch,

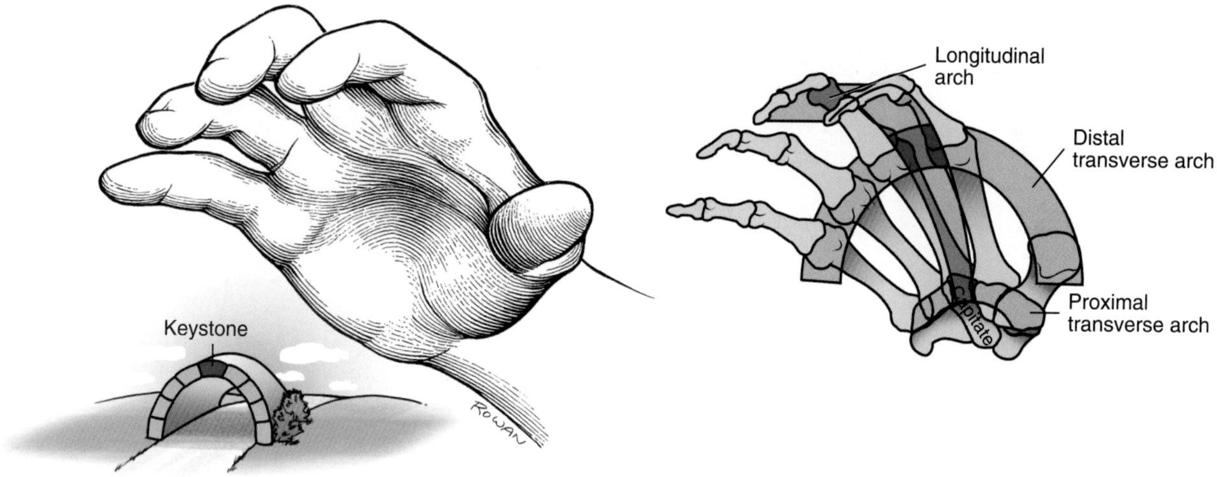

FIGURE 8.8 The natural concavity of the palm of the hand is supported by three integrated arch systems: one longitudinal and two transverse.

reinforced by multiple contacts with other bones, and strong intercarpal ligaments.

The *distal transverse arch* of the hand passes through the MCP joints. In contrast to the rigidity of the proximal arch, the sides of the distal arch are mobile. To appreciate this mobility, imagine transforming your hand from a completely flat surface to a cup-shaped surface that surrounds a baseball or a grapefruit. Transverse flexibility within the hand occurs as the peripheral metacarpals (first, fourth, and fifth) "fold" around the more stable central (second and third) metacarpals. The keystone of the distal transverse arch is formed by the MCP joints of these central metacarpals.

The *longitudinal arch* of the hand follows the general shape of the second and third rays. The proximal end of this arch is firmly linked to the carpus by the carpometacarpal (CMC) joints. These relatively rigid articulations provide an important element of longitudinal stability to the hand. The distal end of the arch is very mobile, which can be demonstrated by actively flexing and extending the fingers. The keystone of the longitudinal arch consists of the second and third MCP joints; note that these joints serve as keystones to *both* the longitudinal and the distal transverse arches.

As depicted in Fig. 8.8, all three arches of the hand are mechanically interlinked. Both transverse arches are joined by a "rigid tie-beam" provided by the second and third metacarpals. In the healthy hand, this mechanical linkage reinforces the entire arch system. In the hand with unstable or frail joints, however, a structural failure at any arch may weaken another. A classic example is the destruction of the MCP joints from severe or medically uncontrolled rheumatoid arthritis. This topic will be revisited at the end of this chapter.

ARTHROLOGY

Before progressing to the study of the structure and function of the joints, the terminology that describes the movement of the digits must be defined. The following descriptions assume that a particular movement starts from the anatomic position, with the elbow extended, forearm fully supinated, and wrist in a neutral position. Movement of the fingers is described in the standard fashion using the cardinal planes of the body: *flexion* and *extension* occur in the sagittal plane, and *abduction* and *adduction* occur in the frontal plane (Fig. 8.9A–D). The middle finger is the reference digit for naming abduction and adduction. The side-to-side movement of the middle finger is called *radial* and *ulnar deviation*.

Because the entire thumb is naturally rotated almost 90 degrees in relation to the fingers, the terminology used to describe thumb movement is different from that for the fingers (see Fig. 8.9E–I). *Flexion* is the movement of the palmar surface of the thumb in the frontal plane across the palm. *Extension* returns the thumb back toward its anatomic position. *Abduction* is the forward movement of the thumb away from the palm in a near sagittal plane. *Adduction* returns the thumb to the plane of the hand. (Although not used in this text, other terms frequently used to describe the movements of the thumb include *ulnar adduction* for flexion, *radial abduction* for extension, and *palmar abduction* for abduction.) *Opposition* is a special term describing a wide, sweeping arc of movement of the thumb across the palm, making direct contact with the tip of any of the fingers. As will be described, opposition of the thumb is a complex movement that is essential to the optimal function of the hand. *Reposition* is a movement from full opposition back to the anatomic position. This special terminology used to define the movement of the thumb serves as the basis for the naming of the muscles that act on the thumb (e.g., the opponens pollicis, extensor pollicis longus, and adductor pollicis).

Carpometacarpal Joints

The carpometacarpal (CMC) joints of the hand form the articulation between the distal row of carpal bones and the bases of the five metacarpal bones. These joints are positioned at the very proximal region of the hand.

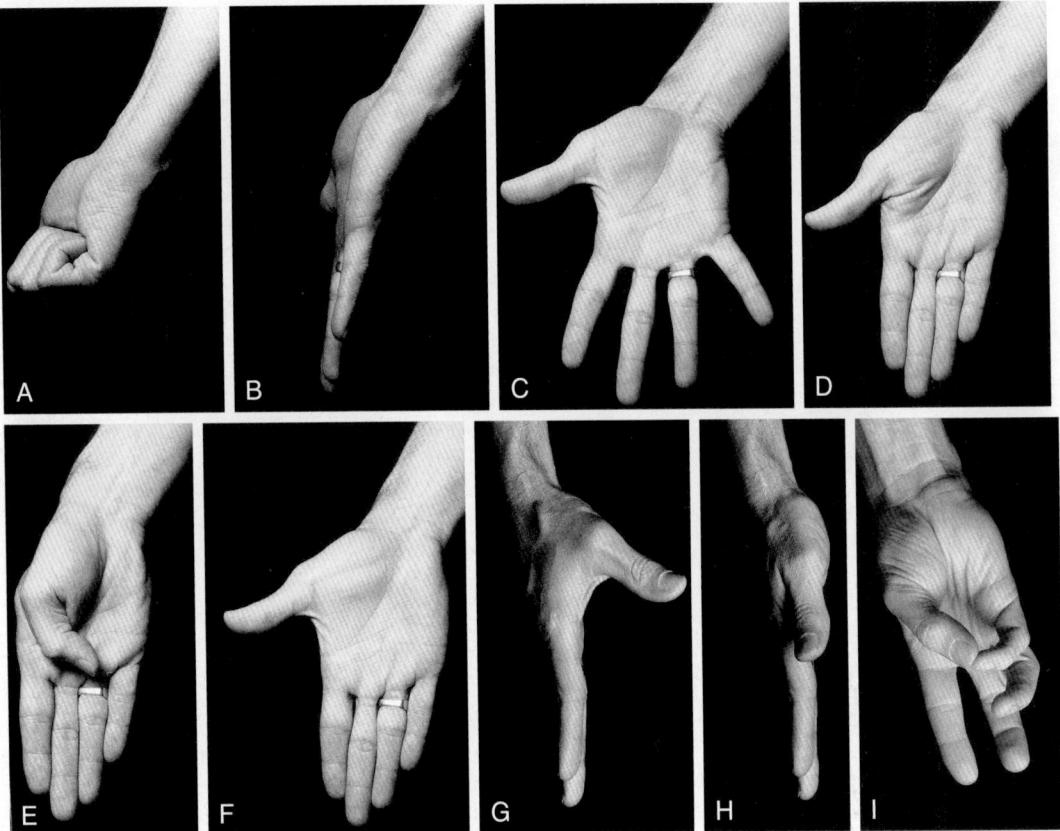

FIGURE 8.9 The system for naming the movements within the hand. (A–D) Finger motion. (E–I) Thumb motion. (A, Finger flexion; B, finger extension; C, finger abduction; D, finger adduction; E, thumb flexion; F, thumb extension; G, thumb abduction; H, thumb adduction; and I, thumb opposition.)

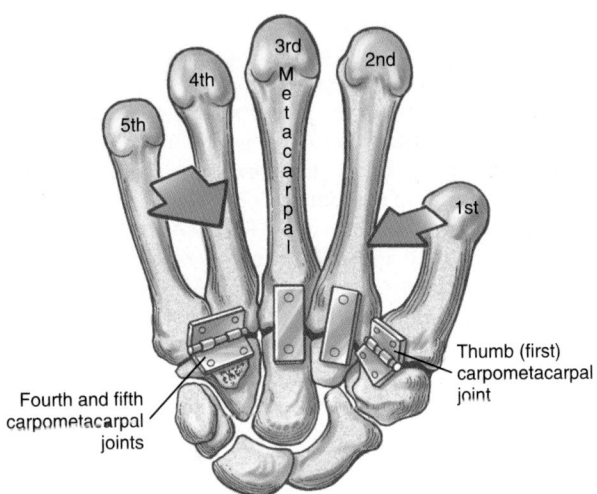

FIGURE 8.10 Palmar view of the right hand showing a highly mechanical depiction of the mobility across the five carpometacarpal joints. The peripheral joints—the first, fourth, and fifth—are much more mobile than the central two joints.

Fig. 8.10 shows a mechanical illustration of the relative mobility at the CMC joints. The second and third digits are rigidly joined to the distal carpus, forming a stable, fixed *central pillar* throughout the hand. In contrast, the more peripheral CMC joints form mobile radial and ulnar borders, which are capable of "folding" around the hand's central pillar. The function of the CMC joints allows the concavity of the palm to fit around many objects. This feature is one of the most impressive and unique functions of the human hand. Cylindrical objects, for example, can fit snugly into the palm, with the index and middle digits positioned to reinforce grasp. Without this ability, the dexterity of the hand is reduced to a primitive hinge like grasping motion.

SECOND THROUGH FIFTH CARPOMETACARPAL JOINTS

General Features and Ligamentous Support

The *second* CMC joint is formed through the articulation between the enlarged base of the second metacarpal and the distal surface of the trapezoid, and to a lesser extent the capitate and trapezium (see Figs. 8.4 and 8.5). The *third* CMC joint is formed primarily by the articulation between the base of the third metacarpal and the distal surface of the capitate. The *fourth* CMC joint consists of the articulation between the base of the fourth metacarpal and the distal surface of the hamate and to lesser extent the capitate. The *fifth* CMC joint consists of the articulation between the base of the fifth metacarpal and the distal surface of the hamate only. (The hamate accepts both fourth and fifth metacarpals, like the way the cuboid bone of the foot accepts both fourth and fifth metatarsals.) The bases of the second through fifth metacarpals have small facets for attachments to one another through *intermetacarpal joints*. These joints help stabilize the bases of the second through fifth metacarpals, thereby reinforcing the carpometacarpal joints.

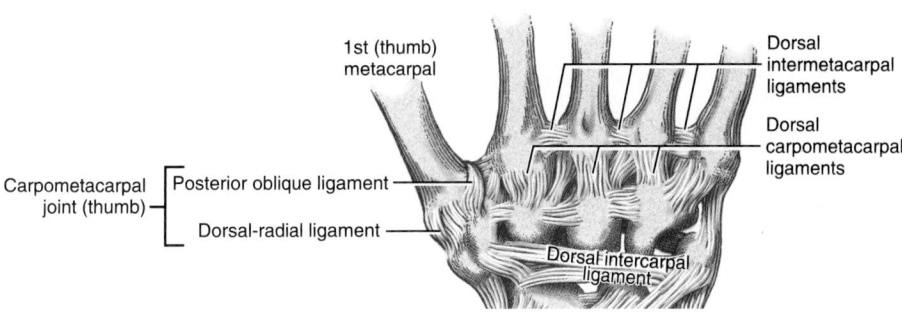

FIGURE 8.11 Dorsal side of the right hand showing the capsule and ligaments that stabilize the carpometacarpal joints.

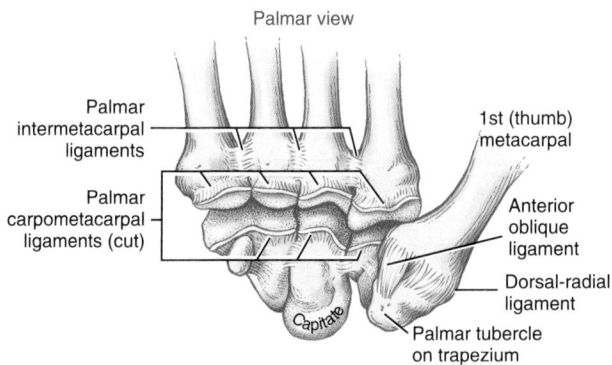

FIGURE 8.12 The palmar side of the right hand showing the articular surfaces of the second through the fifth carpometacarpal joints. The capsule and palmar carpometacarpal ligaments of digits 2 to 5 have been cut.

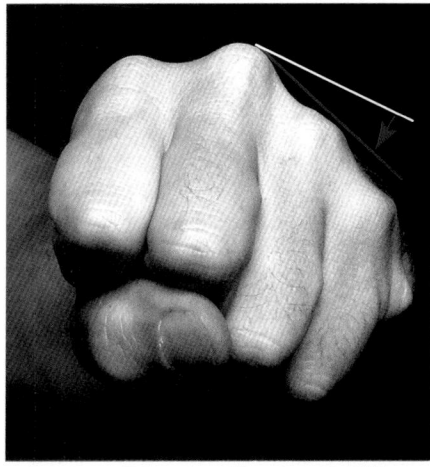

FIGURE 8.13 Mobility of the ulnar (fourth and fifth) carpometacarpal joints of the left hand. White line indicates the relaxed position of the distal metacarpals; red line indicates their position after the fist is clenched.

The CMC joints of the fingers are surrounded by articular capsules and strengthened by multiple dorsal and palmar carpometacarpal and intermetacarpal ligaments.[113] The dorsal ligaments are particularly well developed (Fig. 8.11).

Joint Structure and Kinematics

The CMC joints of the second and third digits are difficult to classify, varying between nearly planar to complex saddle articulations (Fig. 8.12).[142] Their jagged interlocking articular surfaces, coupled with strong ligaments, permit little movement. As mentioned earlier, stability at these joints forms the central pillar of the hand. The inherent stability of these radial-central metacarpals also provides a firm attachment for key muscles, including the extensor carpi radialis longus and brevis, and the adductor pollicis.

The slight and irregularly convex bases of the fourth and fifth metacarpals articulate with a slightly concave articular surface formed by the hamate. These two ulnar CMC joints allow the ulnar border of the hand to fold toward the center of the hand, thereby deepening the palmar concavity. This mobility—often referred to as a "cupping" motion—occurs primarily by flexion and medial rotation of the ulnar metacarpals toward the middle digit (Fig. 8.10).[20] Measurements of maximal passive mobility on cadaver hands have shown that, on average, the fourth CMC joint flexes and extends about 20 degrees and rotates medially about 27 degrees.[37] The fifth CMC joint (when tested with the fourth CMC joint firmly constrained) flexes and extends about 28 degrees and rotates medially about 22 degrees. The range of flexion and extension of the fifth CMC joint increases, however, to an average of 44 degrees when the closely positioned fourth CMC joint is unconstrained and free to move. This research demonstrates a strong kinematic linkage between the fourth and fifth CMC joints—a linkage that should be considered when evaluating and treating limitations of motion in this region of the hand.

The greater relative mobility allowed at the ulnar CMC joints is apparent by the movement of the fourth and fifth metacarpal heads while clenching a fist (Fig. 8.13). The increased mobility of the fourth and fifth CMC joints improves the effectiveness of grasp, as well as enhances the functional interaction with the opposable thumb.

CARPOMETACARPAL JOINT OF THE THUMB

The CMC joint of the thumb is located at the base of the first ray, between the metacarpal and the trapezium (see Fig. 8.7). This joint is by far the most complex of the CMC joints. The joint's unique saddle shape (see ahead Fig. 8.15) coupled with the natural "play" between the trapezium and adjacent carpal bones permit an essential array of thumb movements. The ultimate kinematic expression of the CMC joint is *opposition,* allowing the tip of the thumb to easily contact the tips of the other digits. Through this action, the thumb can securely encircle objects held within the palm. Opposition greatly enhances the dexterity of human prehension.

Capsule and Ligaments of the Thumb Carpometacarpal Joint

The capsule at the CMC joint of the thumb is naturally loose to accommodate a large and wide arc of motion. The capsule, however, is strengthened by several embedded ligaments. The many names used to describe these ligaments has led to confusion when studying their functional anatomy.[36,57,66,96,120] The number of named, distinct CMC joint ligaments reported in the literature ranges from just three

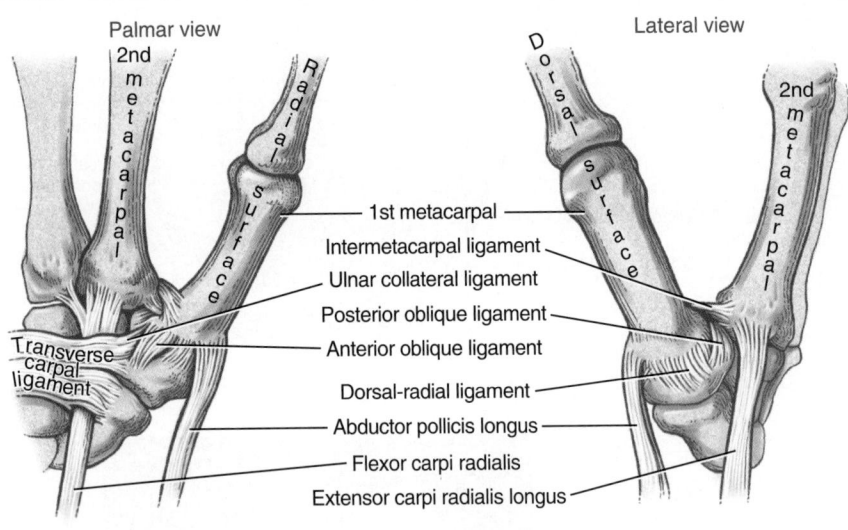

Palmar view

Lateral view

1st metacarpal
Intermetacarpal ligament
Ulnar collateral ligament
Posterior oblique ligament
Anterior oblique ligament
Dorsal-radial ligament
Abductor pollicis longus
Flexor carpi radialis
Extensor carpi radialis longus

FIGURE 8.14 Palmar and lateral views of the ligaments of the carpometacarpal joint of the right thumb.

TABLE 8.1 Ligaments of the Carpometacarpal Joint of the Thumb

Name	Proximal Attachment	Distal Attachment	Comments
Anterior (palmar) oblique*	Palmar tubercle on trapezium	Palmar base ("beak") of thumb metacarpal	Thin and weak; relatively slack during most movements; taut in full extension ("hitch hiker" position)
Ulnar collateral	Radial side of transverse carpal ligament	Palmar-ulnar base of thumb metacarpal	Taut in abduction and extension
Intermetacarpal	Dorsal-radial base of second metacarpal	Palmar-ulnar base of thumb metacarpal with ulnar collateral ligament	Taut in opposition, flexion, and abduction
Dorsal-radial†	Radial (lateral) surface of trapezium	Entire dorsal base of thumb metacarpal (fibers blend with tendon of abductor pollicis longus and posterior oblique ligament)	Densely populated with sensory fibers; taut in opposition, flexion, and combined flexion-and-adduction (e.g., key pinch); prime stabilizer of the CMC joint
Posterior oblique	Posterior-radial corner of trapezium	Palmar-ulnar base of thumb metacarpal	Taut in opposition, flexion, and abduction; prime stabilizer of the CMC joint

*Often described as having superficial and deep ("beak") fibers.
†Often referred to as the "dorsal ligamentous complex" when combined with the posterior oblique ligament.

to a bewildering sixteen.[36,86] This text describes five ligaments, each adding a unique element of stability to the CMC joint (Fig. 8.14). As a set, the ligaments help control the extent and direction of joint motion while helping to maintain joint alignment and stability. Table 8.1 summarizes the attachments of the ligaments of the CMC joint of the thumb and the motions that pull or wind them relatively taut.[a]

Although all the ligaments listed in Table 8.1 have an important role in maintaining joint stability, the *dorsal-radial* and *posterior oblique ligaments* excel in this ability (review Figs. 8.11, 8.12, and 8.14).[61,115,160] Based on their location relative to the surface of the thumb metacarpal, these ligaments have been referred to as the *"dorsal ligamentous complex."*[86,96] Originating off the radial (lateral) side of the trapezium, the dorsal ligamentous complex is pulled most taut when the CMC joint is either (1) fully opposed (which includes components of flexion and abduction), or (2) strongly flexed-and-adducted, such as during a "key pinch."[36,61,148] The tension produced within the dorsal ligamentous complex during these common and essential thumb positions helps maintain the natural alignment and stability of the CMC joint. Chronic and excessive overuse of the thumb in these positions can cause a stretch-induced weakness and

laxity within these ligaments.[52] This scenario is often observed in the thumbs of middle-to-later aged persons, especially those who have engaged in a hobby or occupation that has involved excessive use of their hands. Laxity within the dorsal ligamentous complex may contribute to the relatively common *dorsal-radial subluxation* of the thumb metacarpal (relative to the trapezium), forming a characteristic "hump" at the base of the thumb. If associated with severe osteoarthritis, the unstable CMC joint may come close to complete dislocation, as shown in e-Fig. 8.1.[131,144,160]

To achieve necessary physiologic stability at the CMC joint, the tension in the capsular ligaments must be supplemented by forces generated by activated muscle. In vivo research has established ample functional connections between sensory mechanoreceptors embedded within several ligaments, particularly the dorsal-radial ligament, and certain thumb muscles.[86,96,109] When the ligaments are stretched or otherwise perturbed by movement, the mechanoreceptors initiate a subconscious, stabilizing muscular response. Such a response is kinesiologically complex: muscles compress the saddle-shaped joint in just the precise and timely manner to ensure optimal mechanical stability.[2,108] As with many joints in the body, the stability and alignment of the CMC joint is dependent on an active interplay among the ligaments and the neuromuscular system.

[a]12,36,61,86,115,148,160

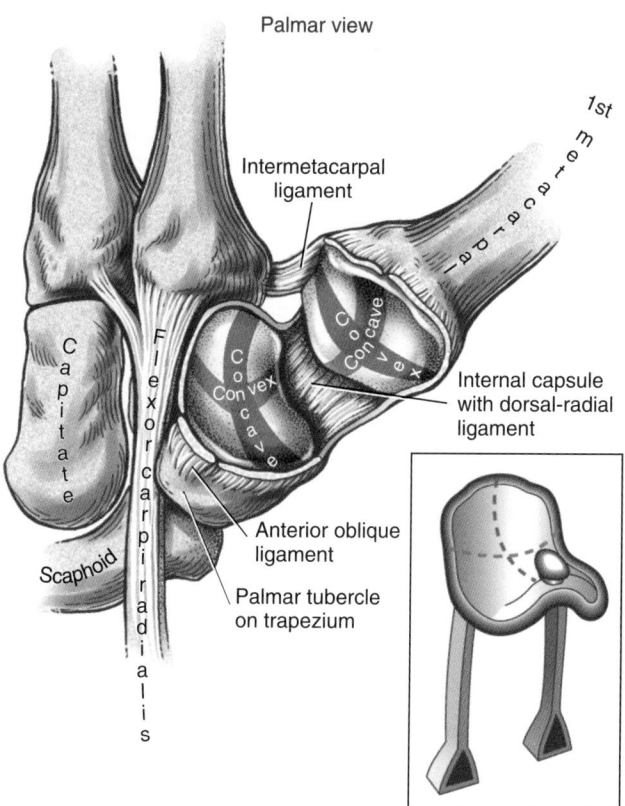

Palmar view

Intermetacarpal ligament

Internal capsule with dorsal-radial ligament

Anterior oblique ligament

Palmar tubercle on trapezium

FIGURE 8.15 The carpometacarpal joint of the right thumb is exposed to show its saddle-shaped appearance. The longitudinal diameters are shown in purple, and the transverse diameters in green.

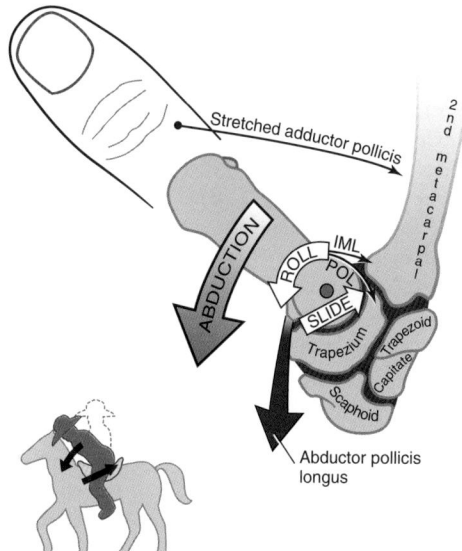

FIGURE 8.16 The arthrokinematics of abduction of the carpometacarpal joint of the thumb. Full abduction stretches the intermetacarpal ligament *(IML)*, the posterior oblique ligament *(POL)*, and the adductor pollicis muscle. The axis of rotation is depicted as a small circle at the base of the metacarpal. The abductor pollicis longus is shown actively rolling the articular surface of the thumb metacarpal in a palmar (anterior) direction. Note the analogy between the arthrokinematics of abduction and a "cowboy" falling forward on the horse's saddle: as the cowboy falls forward (toward abduction), a point on his chest "rolls" anteriorly, but a point on his rear end "slides" posteriorly.

Saddle Joint Structure

The CMC joint of the thumb is the classic saddle joint of the body (Fig. 8.15). The characteristic feature of a saddle joint is that each articular surface is convex in one dimension and concave in the other. The longitudinal diameter of the articular surface of the *trapezium* is generally concave from a palmar-to-dorsal direction. This surface is analogous to the front-to-rear contour of a horse's saddle. The transverse diameter on the articular surface of the trapezium is generally convex in a medial-to-lateral direction—a shape analogous to the side-to-side contour of a horse's saddle. The contour of the articular surface of the *thumb metacarpal* has the reciprocal shape of that described for the trapezium (see Fig. 8.15). The longitudinal diameter along the articular surface of the metacarpal is convex in a palmar-to-dorsal direction; its transverse diameter is concave in a medial-to-lateral direction.

Kinematics

The motions at the CMC joint occur primarily in two degrees of freedom. Abduction and adduction occur generally in the sagittal plane, and flexion and extension occur generally in the frontal plane. The axis of rotation for each plane of movement passes through the convex member of the articulation.[67,160]

Opposition and reposition of the thumb are mechanically derived from the two primary planes of motion at the CMC joint. The kinematics of these primary motions are discussed after the description of the two primary motions.

Abduction and Adduction at the Thumb Carpometacarpal Joint

In the position of adduction of the CMC joint, the thumb lies approximately within the plane of the hand. Maximum abduction, in contrast, positions the thumb metacarpal about 50 degrees anterior

to the plane of the palm.[163] Full abduction opens the web space of the thumb, forming a wide concave curvature useful for grasping large objects.

The arthrokinematics of abduction and adduction are based on the convex articular surface of the thumb metacarpal moving on the fixed concave (longitudinal) diameter of the trapezium (review Fig. 8.15). During *abduction,* the convex articular surface of the metacarpal rolls in a palmar (anterior) direction and slides dorsally on the concave surface of the trapezium (Fig. 8.16). Full abduction at the CMC joint elongates the adductor pollicis muscle and several ligaments (review Table 8.1). The arthrokinematics of *adduction* occur in the reverse order from those described for abduction.

Flexion and Extension at the Thumb Carpometacarpal Joint

Actively performing flexion and extension of the CMC joint of the thumb is associated with varying amounts of axial rotation of the metacarpal.[60] During flexion, the metacarpal rotates *medially* (i.e., toward the third digit); during extension, the metacarpal rotates *laterally* (i.e., away from the third digit). These "automatic" axial rotations are apparent by the change in orientation of the nail of the thumb between full extension and full flexion. This rotation is not considered a third degree of freedom because it cannot be executed independently of the other motions.

From the anatomic position, the CMC joint can be extended about 20 degrees. From full extension, the thumb metacarpal flexes across the palm about 40 degrees.[163]

The arthrokinematics of flexion and extension at the CMC joint are based on the concave articular surface of the metacarpal moving across the convex (transverse) diameter on the trapezium (review Fig. 8.15). During *flexion,* the concave surface of the metacarpal rolls and slides in an ulnar (medial) direction (Fig. 8.17A).[67] A shallow groove in the transverse diameter of the trapezium helps guide the slight medial rotation of the metacarpal. Full flexion elongates tissues such as the dorsal-radial ligament.

During *extension* of the CMC joint, the concave metacarpal rolls and slides in a lateral (radial) direction across the transverse diameter of the joint (see Fig. 8.17B). The groove on the articular surface of the trapezium guides the metacarpal into slight lateral rotation.[27] Full extension stretches ligaments situated on the ulnar side of the joint, such as the anterior oblique ligament. Table 8.2 summarizes the kinematics and articular geometry associated with flexion-extension and abduction-adduction at the CMC joint of the thumb.

Opposition of the Thumb Carpometacarpal Joint

The ability to precisely and firmly oppose the thumb to the tips of the other fingers is perhaps the definitive expression of the functional health of this digit—and arguably of the entire hand. It is often stated that the thumb is responsible for 40% to 50% of the overall function of the hand. The basis of this adage reflects the exceptional functionality of the opposable thumb and governing muscles.

The complex motion of opposition is a composite of the other primary motions already described for the CMC joint. For ease of discussion, Fig. 8.18A shows the full arc of opposition divided into two phases. In phase 1, the thumb metacarpal *abducts*. In phase 2, the abducted metacarpal *flexes and medially rotates* across the palm toward the small finger. Fig. 8.18B shows the detail of the kinematics of this complex movement. During *abduction,* the base of the thumb metacarpal follows a path in a palmar direction across the surface of the trapezium. Such a motion stretches certain ligaments across the CMC joint, such as those that comprise the dorsal ligamentous complex.[79] This stretch, in addition to activation of muscles such as the opponens pollicis, guides much of the kinematics of the flexion–medial rotation phase. The base of the flexing metacarpal rotates slightly medially, within a groove on the surface of the trapezium.[169] These muscular and ligamentous forces securely direct the path of the flexing and medially rotating metacarpal generally toward the medial articular

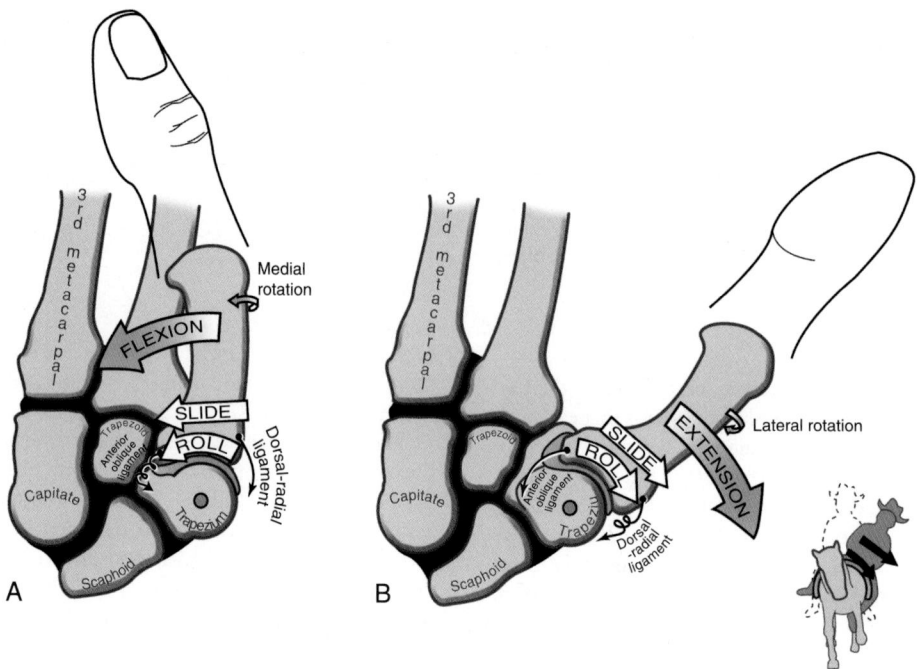

FIGURE 8.17 The arthrokinematics of flexion and extension at the carpometacarpal joint of the thumb. (A) Flexion is associated with a slight medial rotation, causing elongation in the dorsal-radial ligament. The anterior oblique ligament is slack. (B) Extension is associated with slight lateral rotation, causing elongation of the anterior oblique ligament. The axis of rotation is depicted as a small circle through the trapezium. Note the analogy between the arthrokinematics of extension and a "cowboy" falling sideways on the horse's saddle: as the cowboy falls sideways (toward extension), points on his chest and rear end both "roll and slide" in the same lateral direction.

TABLE 8.2 Factors Associated with Kinematics of the Primary Motions of the Carpometacarpal Joint of the Thumb*

Motion	Osteokinematics	Articular Geometry	Arthrokinematics
Abduction and adduction	Sagittal plane movement around a medial-lateral axis of rotation through the metacarpal	Convex (longitudinal) diameter of metacarpal moving on a concave surface of the trapezium	Abduction: palmar roll and dorsal slide Adduction: dorsal roll and palmar slide
Flexion and extension	Frontal plane movement around an anterior-posterior axis of rotation through the trapezium	Concave (transverse) diameter of the metacarpal moving on a convex surface of the trapezium	Flexion: medial roll and slide Extension: lateral roll and slide

*Opposition and reposition are not shown because they are derived from the two primary planes of motions (see text for further explanation).

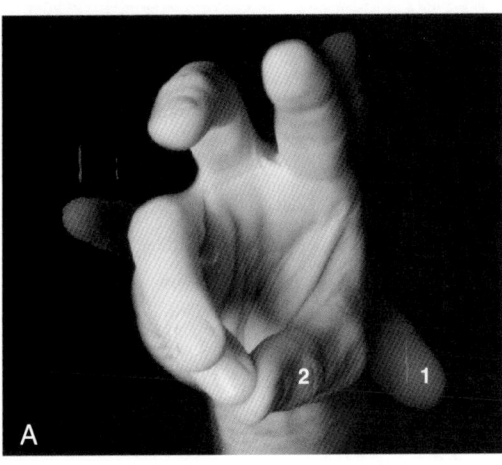
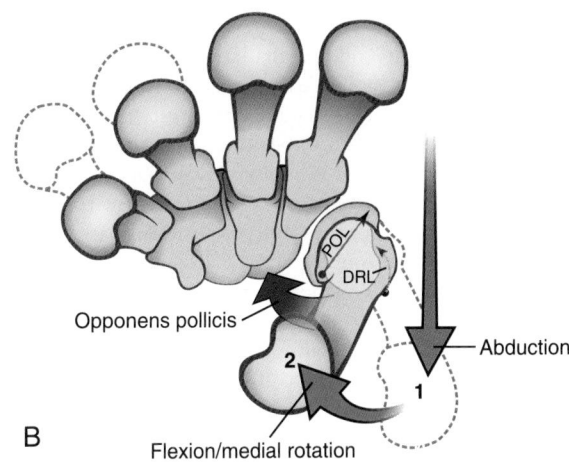

FIGURE 8.18 The arthrokinematics of opposition of the carpometacarpal joint of the thumb. (A) Two phases of opposition are shown: *(1)* abduction and *(2)* flexion with medial rotation. (B) The kinematics of the two phases of opposition: the posterior oblique ligament *(POL)* and dorsal-radial ligament *(DRL)*, constituting the dorsal ligamentous complex, are shown taut; the opponens pollicis is shown contracting *(red)*; the outline of the trapezium is indicated within the carpometacarpal joint.

SPECIAL FOCUS 8.1

Osteoarthritis of the Carpometacarpal Joint of the Thumb: A Common and Potentially Disabling Condition

Optimal function of the thumb CMC joint requires both mobility and stability. These seemingly contradictory functions are normally controlled by an interplay between tension in the capsular ligaments and activation of muscles. Because of the dominant role of muscles, relatively large forces are routinely generated across the joint. During a forceful key pinch, for example, a 12-fold greater compression force occurs within the thumb's CMC joint compared with the contact forces applied at the distal end of the thumb.[26] The magnitude of the joint "reaction" force, combined with the high frequency of its application, is theorized to be one of a set of factors accounting for the relatively frequent occurrence of osteoarthritis at this joint.[52,107,132] Radiologic evidence of osteoarthritis of the thumb CMC joint is indeed common: occurring in 13% of men in their fifth and sixth decades of life, 33% of postmenopausal women, and up to 90% of persons over the age of 80 years.[6,52,140]

The pathomechanics responsible for the frequent occurrence of osteoarthritis at the base of the thumb are not fully understood. Degeneration may develop secondary to acute injury or, perhaps more commonly, from cumulative relatively low-level trauma associated with an arduous occupation.[46,168] Predisposing factors other than mechanical overload may include systemic arthritis, obesity, ligamentous laxity, or high contact stress associated with subtle natural asymmetry of the articular surfaces.[52,56] Regardless of the specific cause, pain is typically the foremost symptom. A painful base of the thumb can reduce the functional potential of the entire hand, and therefore the entire upper extremity.

Articular degeneration associated with osteoarthritis of the CMC joint of the thumb tends to originate at the palmar articular surfaces.[31,137] Once advanced, the condition is typically associated with morphologic changes within the entire joint, osteophyte formation, weakened pinch, swelling, and dorsal-radial joint dislocation. Advanced stages may also involve degeneration of the

joints between the trapezium and the scaphoid, and the trapezium and the trapezoid: a condition often referred to as *basilar joint arthritis* of the thumb.

The prevalence of osteoarthritis of the CMC joint of the thumb occurs two to four times more often in women than in men.[56,110,132] This sex-related prevalence may be associated with hormonal-induced laxity in the joint's ligaments.[87,167] Also, because women, on average, have smaller CMC articular surfaces than men, perhaps the greater wear observed in females is, in part, from being subjected to larger articular contact pressure (i.e., force/area) when performing similar tasks as men.[59,132] Unscrewing a tight lid from a jar, for example, likely requires similar muscular (internal) torques, regardless of sex, but typically results in greater articular contact pressure in women.

Traditional conservative interventions for osteoarthritis of the thumb CMC joint include splinting; judicious and targeted exercise; mobilization techniques; implementation of physical modalities such as cold and heat; and utilization of nonsteroidal anti-inflammatory drugs (NSAIDs) and corticosteroid injections.[14,23,83,134,157] In addition, patients are instructed in ways to modify their activities to "protect" the base of the thumb from unnecessarily large forces and to preserve function in spite of the degenerative process.[106]

Surgical intervention may be required if conservative therapy is unsuccessful. Operative procedure followed by hand therapy may include arthroplasty with ligamentous reconstruction, partial or complete trapeziectomy with or without a biological joint "spacer," arthrodesis (fusion), prosthetic implant, or other interventions.[52,94,138,164] Although patients typically report improvement of function and reduced pain from a CMC prosthetic implant, the long-term success of this procedure remains hindered by the complex arthrokinematics coupled with the large forces that naturally occur at the CMC joint.[62,65]

surface of the trapezium. The last few degrees of opposition continue to stretch several ligaments, particularly the dorsal-radial ligament.[36,148,160] Forces from activated muscle and stretched ligaments are important in promoting maximal congruity and stability of the CMC joint once in full opposition. Accordingly, full opposition is considered the CMC joint's close-packed position.[142] Interestingly, the final rotation, or spin, of the thumb metacarpal as the joint approaches full opposition has been described as a "screw-home torque rotation"[79,160]—a mechanism similarly described for the knee when it is securely locked and rotated in full extension.

As noted by the change in orientation of the thumbnail in Fig. 8.18A, full opposition incorporates 45 to 60 degrees of medial rotation of the thumb.[24] Although the CMC joint of the thumb accounts for most of this rotation, lesser amounts occur in the form of accessory motions at the MCP and IP joints. Observations from cineradiography show that the trapezium also medially rotates slightly against the scaphoid and the trapezoid, thereby amplifying the final magnitude of the metacarpal rotation. The small and ring fingers contribute indirectly to opposition through a cupping motion at the fourth and fifth CMC joints. This motion allows the tip of the thumb to easily contact the tips of the small and ring fingers.

Reposition of the CMC joint returns the metacarpal from full opposition back to the anatomic position. This motion involves arthrokinematics of both adduction and extension–lateral rotation of the thumb metacarpal.

Metacarpophalangeal Joints

FINGERS

General Features and Ligaments

The metacarpophalangeal (MCP) joints of the fingers are relatively large, ovoid articulations formed between the convex heads of the metacarpals and the shallow concave proximal surfaces of the proximal phalanges (Fig. 8.19). Volitional motion at the MCP joint occurs predominantly in two planes: flexion and extension in the sagittal plane, and abduction and adduction in the frontal plane.

Mechanical stability at the MCP joint is critical to the overall biomechanics and architectural stability of the hand. As discussed earlier, the MCP joints serve as keystones that support the mobile arches of the hand. In the healthy hand, stability at the MCP joints is achieved by an elaborate set of interconnecting connective tissues. Embedded within the capsule of each MCP joint are a pair of radial and ulnar collateral ligaments and one palmar plate (Fig. 8.20). Each *collateral ligament* has its proximal attachment on and near the posterior tubercle of the metacarpal head. Crossing the MCP joint in an oblique palmar direction, the ligament forms two distinct parts. The more dorsal *cord part* of the ligament is thick and strong, attaching distally to the palmar region of the proximal end of the phalanx. The *accessory part* consists of thinner fan-shaped fibers, which attach distally along the edge of the palmar plate.[77]

Located palmar to each MCP joint are ligamentous-like structures called *palmar* (or *volar*) *plates* (see Fig. 8.20). The term *plate* describes a composition of dense, thick fibrocartilage. The distal end of each plate attaches firmly to the base of each proximal phalanx. The proximal, more elastic end attaches loosely to the metacarpal

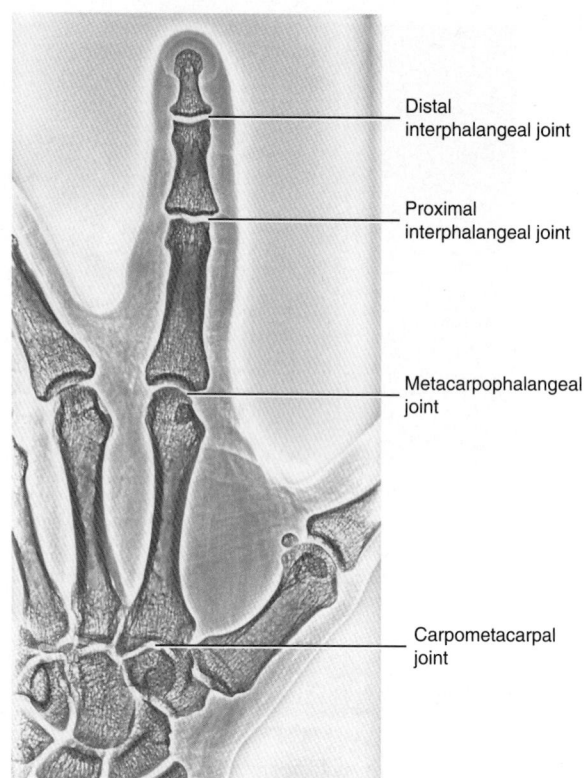

FIGURE 8.19 The joints of the index finger.

Distal interphalangeal joint

Proximal interphalangeal joint

Metacarpophalangeal joint

Carpometacarpal joint

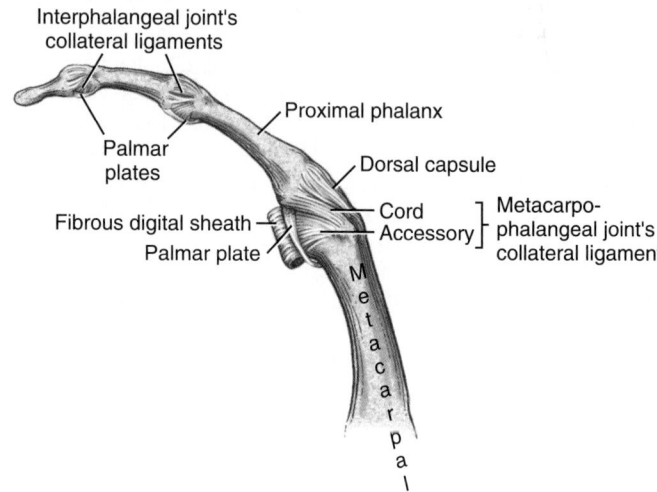

FIGURE 8.20 A lateral view of the two parts of the collateral ligament and associated connective tissues of the metacarpophalangeal, proximal interphalangeal, and distal interphalangeal joints of the finger.

Interphalangeal joint's collateral ligaments

Proximal phalanx

Palmar plates

Dorsal capsule

Fibrous digital sheath

Palmar plate

Cord

Accessory

Metacarpophalangeal joint's collateral ligament

Metacarpal

bone, just proximal to the head.[142] *Fibrous digital sheaths,* which form tunnels (typically referred to as "pulleys") for the extrinsic finger flexors, are anchored on the palmar (anterior) surface of the palmar plates. The primary function of the palmar plates is to strengthen the structure of the MCP joints and limit the extremes of extension.

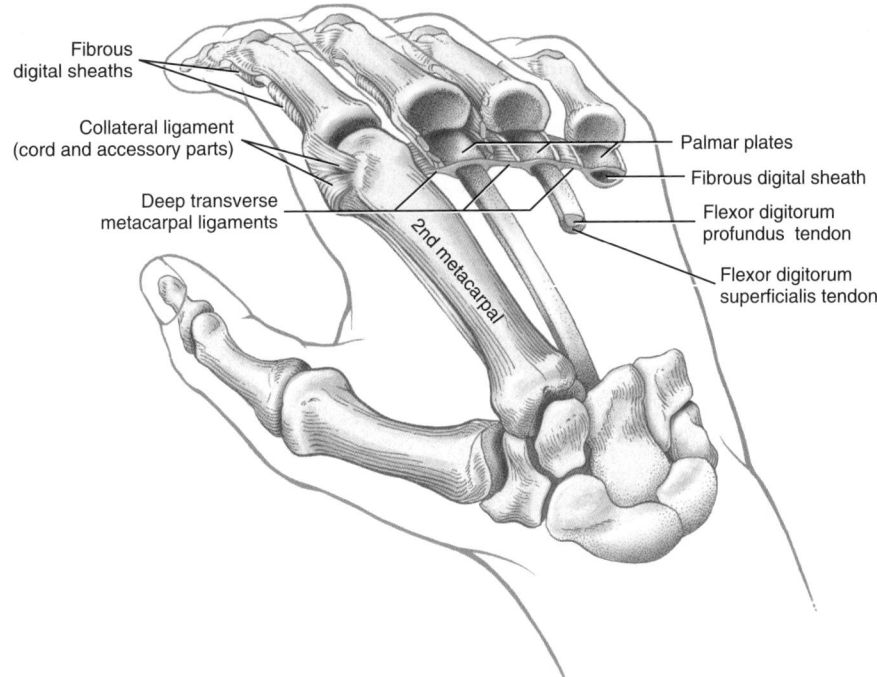

FIGURE 8.21 A dorsal view of the hand with an emphasis on the periarticular connective tissues at the metacarpophalangeal joints. Several metacarpal bones have been removed to expose various joint structures.

Fig. 8.21 illustrates several anatomic aspects of the MCP joints. The concave component of an MCP joint is formed by the articular surface of the proximal phalanx, the collateral ligaments (both cord and accessory parts), and the dorsal surface of the palmar plate. These tissues form a three-sided receptacle aptly suited to accept and stabilize the large metacarpal head. Attaching between the palmar plates of each MCP joint are three *deep transverse metacarpal ligaments*. The three ligaments merge into a wide, flat structure that interconnects and loosely binds the second through the fifth metacarpals.

Kinematics

Osteokinematics

In addition to the volitional motions expressed at the MCP joints, substantial accessory motions are possible, especially with the joint nearly extended. The joint can be distracted-compressed, translated in anterior-to-posterior and side-to-side directions, and axially rotated. The extent of passive axial rotation is particularly remarkable, allowing the fingers to better conform to the shapes of held objects, thereby increasing control of grasp (Fig. 8.22). The range of this passive axial rotation at the MCP joints is greatest at the ring and small fingers, with average rotations of about 30 to 40 degrees.[85]

The overall range of *flexion and extension* at the MCP joints increases gradually from the second to the fifth digit: the second (index) flexes to about 90 degrees, and the fifth to about 110 to 115 degrees.[9] The greater mobility allowed at the more ulnar MCP joints is like that expressed at the CMC joints. (The increased flexion at the more ulnar joints is apparent in the ergonomic design incorporated into many handles.) The MCP joints can be passively extended beyond the neutral (0-degree) position for a considerable range of 30 to 45 degrees. The joints can *abduct or adduct* (relative to the midline of the hand) between about 20 to 45 degrees, depending on the digit.[90]

The position of the wrist strongly influences the overall biplanar mobility of the MCP joints. This point becomes particularly

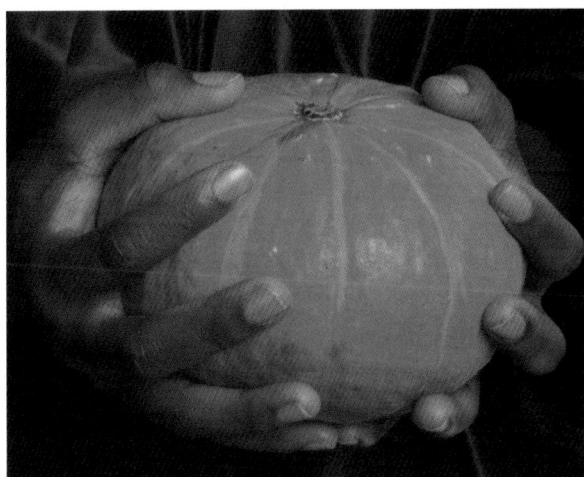

FIGURE 8.22 The accessory motions of axial rotation at the metacarpophalangeal joints are evident across several fingers during a grasp of a large, round object.

The Metacarpophalangeal Joints of the Fingers Permit Volitional Movements Primarily in Two Degrees of Freedom

- *Flexion* and *extension* occur in the sagittal plane around a medial-lateral axis of rotation.
- *Abduction* and *adduction* occur in the frontal plane around an anterior-posterior axis of rotation.

The axis of rotation for each movement passes through the head of the metacarpal.

---

relevant during a clinical evaluation. MCP joint mobility is least with the wrist fully extended.[90] Full wrist extension significantly stretches the extrinsic finger flexor muscles, producing a tension across the MCP joints that limits their overall extensibility.

Arthrokinematics

The head of each metacarpal has a slightly different shape but, in general, is rounded at the apex and nearly flat on the palmar surface (see Fig. 8.6). Articular cartilage covers the entire head and most of the palmar surface. The convex-concave relationship of the joint surfaces is readily apparent (Fig. 8.23).

The arthrokinematics at the MCP joint are based on the concave articular surface of the phalanx moving against the convex metacarpal head. Fig. 8.24A shows the arthrokinematics of active *flexion,* driven by one of the extrinsic flexor muscles: the flexor digitorum profundus. Flexion stretches and therefore increases the passive tension in the dorsal capsule and most of the thicker cord part of the collateral ligaments.[77] (As described in Special Focus 8.2 the accessory part of the

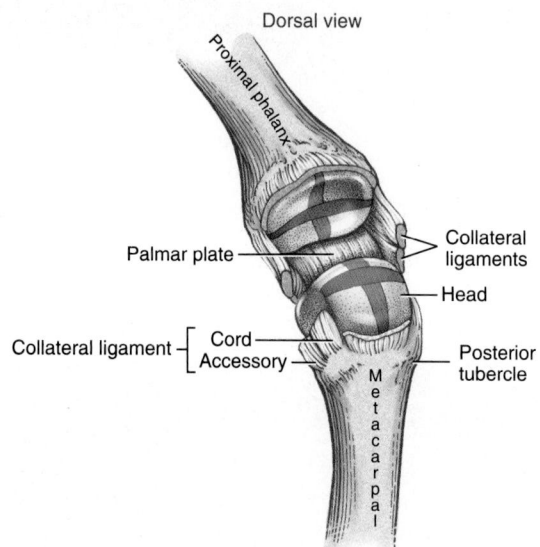

FIGURE 8.23 A dorsal view of the metacarpophalangeal joint opened to expose the shape of the articular surfaces. The longitudinal diameter of the joint is shown in green; the transverse diameter in purple.

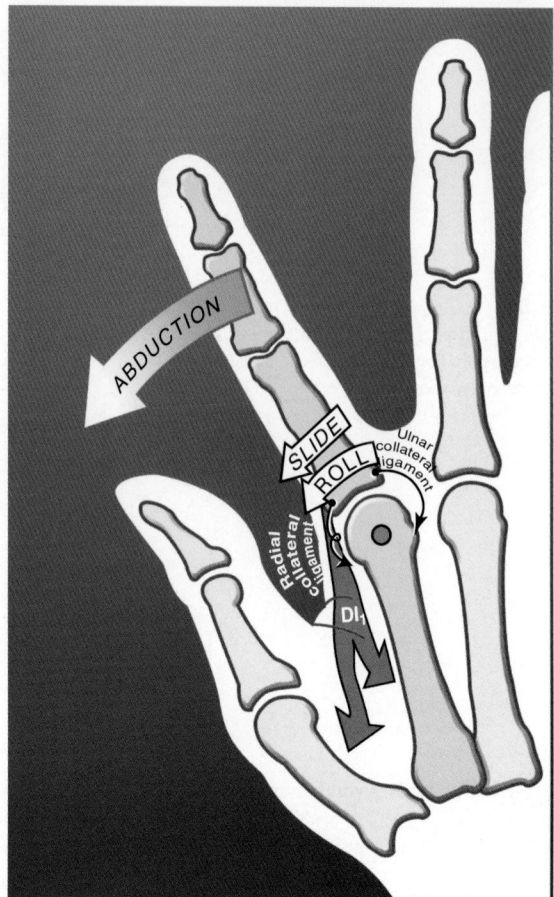

FIGURE 8.25 The arthrokinematics of active abduction at the metacarpophalangeal joint. Abduction is shown powered by the first dorsal interosseus muscle (DI_1). At full abduction, the ulnar collateral ligament is taut and the radial collateral ligament is slack. Note that the axis of rotation for this motion is in an anterior-posterior direction, through the head of the metacarpal.

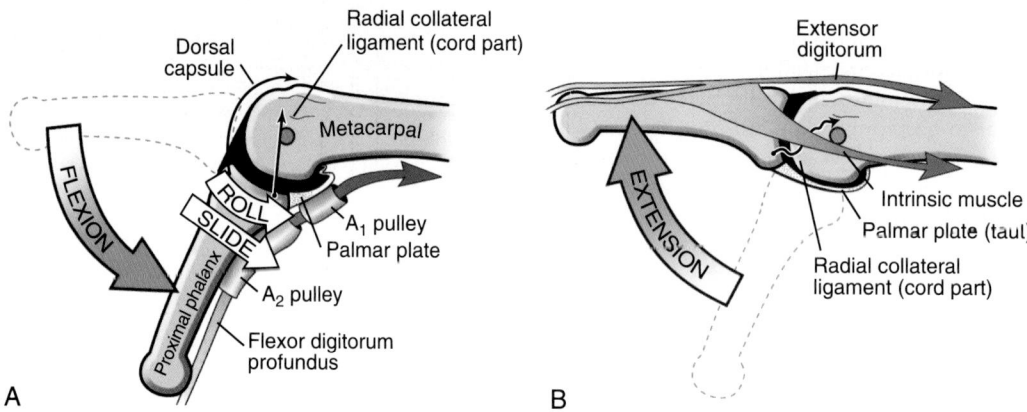

FIGURE 8.24 Lateral view of the arthrokinematics of active flexion and extension at the metacarpophalangeal (MCP) joint. (A) Flexion is shown during activation of the flexor digitorum profundus muscle. The tendon of this muscle is shown coursing through the A_1 and A_2 pulleys (specifically named pulleys within the fibrous digital sheaths). Flexion draws both the dorsal capsule and most of the cord part of the radial collateral ligament relatively taut. The arthrokinematics are shown as a roll and slide in similar directions. (B) Extension is shown controlled by coactivation of the extensor digitorum and one of the intrinsic muscles of the finger. The extended position draws the palmar plate taut while simultaneously creating relative slack in the cord part of the radial collateral ligament. Taut or stretched tissues are shown as thin elongated arrows; slack structures are shown as wavy arrows. The axis of rotation for this motion is in the medial-lateral direction, shown piercing the head of the metacarpal.

collateral ligaments remains nearly isometric in length throughout flexion and extension.) In the healthy state, the increased passive tension in elongated connective tissues helps guide the joint's natural arthrokinematics. For example, as depicted in Fig. 8.24A, the increased tension in the stretched dorsal capsule (depicted by the thin elongated arrow) prevents the joint from unnaturally "hinging" outward on its dorsal side. The tension helps maintain firm contact between the articular surfaces as the proximal phalanx slides and rolls in a palmar direction. The increased natural joint stability of the flexed MCP joints helps stabilize these joints during grasp.

Fig. 8.24B illustrates active *extension* of the MCP joint, driven through a coordinated coactivation of the extensor digitorum and one of the intrinsic muscles (to be further described later in this chapter). The arthrokinematics of extension are like those illustrated for flexion except that the roll and slide of the proximal phalanx occur in a dorsal direction. By 0 degrees of extension, the bulk of the cord part of the collateral ligaments has slackened while the palmar plate has elongated and unfolded to support the head of the metacarpal. The relative slackness created in most fibers of the collateral ligaments accounts, in part, for the increased passive mobility ("play") within the joint in the extended position. Active extension beyond the 0-degree position is typically limited by a combination of increased passive tension within the palmar plates coupled with activation of intrinsic muscles, such as the lumbricals.

The arthrokinematics of *abduction* and *adduction* of the MCP joints are similar to those described for flexion and extension. During abduction of the index MCP joint, for example, the proximal phalanx rolls and slides in a radial direction (Fig. 8.25). The first dorsal interosseus muscle not only directs the arthrokinematics of abduction but also stabilizes the joint radially as the radial collateral ligament progressively slackens.

The extent of active abduction and adduction at the MCP joints is significantly less when the motions are performed in full flexion compared with full extension. (This can be readily verified

SPECIAL FOCUS 8.2

Clinical Relevance of the Flexed Position of the Metacarpophalangeal Joints of the Fingers

It has long been recognized that the *flexed* MCP joint is more mechanically stable and exhibits less passive, accessory movement than an extended joint. Accordingly, flexion is considered the MCP joint's *close-packed position.*[142] As described in Chapter 1, the close-packed position of most joints is that unique position at which accessory movements (joint "play") are minimal and congruency within the joint is greatest. The close-packed, flexed position of the MCP joint is associated with increased tension primarily in the collateral ligaments. This tension adds stability to the base of the fingers during activities such as gripping, pinching, or using a key—activities that are typically performed in about 60 to 70 degrees of flexion.[64]

The increased stability associated with flexion of the MCP joint is in large part caused by the elongation and subsequent stretch placed on most of the *cord part* of the collateral ligaments. The stretch is caused by the eccentric or "out-of-round" cam shape of the metacarpal head. Because of this shape, flexion increases the distance between the proximal and distal attachments of these ligaments (Fig. 8.26). Because of different distal attachments, the relatively thin accessory part of the collateral ligaments remains at a near constant length (isometric) throughout flexion and extension, thereby exerting a more constant and lower level of stabilizing tension.[77]

After trauma or surgery, the hand may need to be immobilized by a cast or orthosis to promote healing and relieve pain. If the period of immobilization is prolonged, periarticular connective tissues positioned at a shortened (slackened) length will often remodel (i.e., adaptively shorten) in this position and subsequently generate greater resistance to elongation. In contrast, connective tissues immobilized in an elongated position are more likely to retain their normal stiffness. Consider, for example, a patient whose hand must be immobilized for 3 or 4 weeks after a fracture of the neck of the fourth or fifth metacarpal. A clinician will typically immobilize the hand with *the MCP joints flexed to about 60 to 70 degrees.* The flexed position of the MCP joints is designed to place

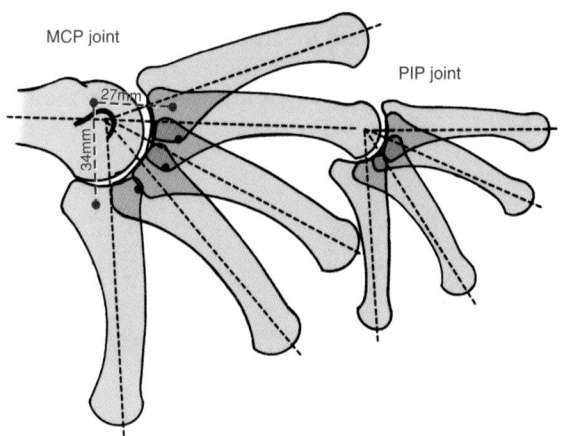

Lateral view

FIGURE 8.26 Because of the cam-shaped metacarpal head, flexion at the metacarpophalangeal *(MCP)* joint increases the distance between the attachment points of most of the cord part of the collateral ligaments (27 mm in extension and 34 mm in 90 degrees of flexion). This contrasts with the proximal interphalangeal *(PIP)* joint, where the distances between the proximal and distal attachments of the entire collateral ligaments remain essentially constant throughout flexion. (From Dubousset JF: The digital joints. In Tubiana R, editor: *The Hand,* Philadelphia, 1981, Saunders.)

a relative stretch on the cord parts of the collateral ligaments and thereby prevent their shortening. Preventing tightness within these fibers of the collateral ligaments reduces the likelihood of developing an "extension contracture" of the MCP joints.

In some cases, however, immobilizing the MCP joints in flexion may be inappropriate. For example, after surgical repair of the extensor tendon or dorsal capsule, or implantation of a total joint arthroplasty, the MCP joints must be immobilized in an extended (near 0-degree) position. This position reduces the strain on the healing tissues located on the dorsal aspect of the joint.

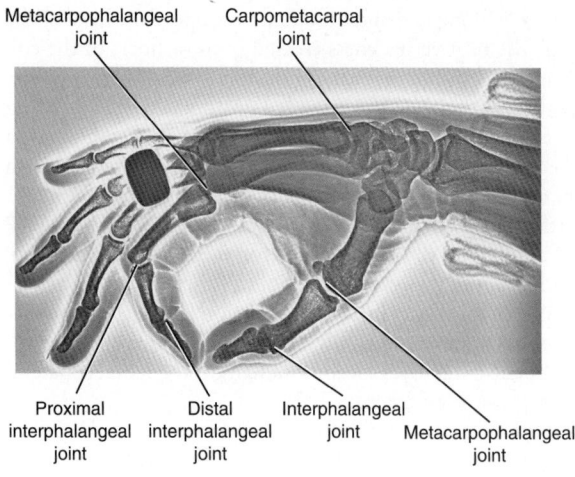

FIGURE 8.27 A side view of many of the joints of the wrist and hand. Note the sesamoid bone near the metacarpophalangeal joint of the thumb.

on your own hand.) Two factors can account for this difference. First, most of the cord parts of the collateral ligaments are taut near full flexion. Stored passive tension in these ligaments theoretically increases the compression force between the joint surfaces, thereby reducing available motion. Second, in the position of about 70 degrees of flexion, the articular surface of the proximal phalanges contacts the flattened palmar part of the metacarpal heads (see Fig. 8.24A). This relatively flat surface blocks the natural arthrokinematics required for maximal abduction and adduction range of motion.

THUMB

General Features and Ligaments

The MCP joint of the thumb consists of the articulation between the convex head of the first metacarpal and the concave proximal surface of the proximal phalanx of the thumb (Fig. 8.27). The basic structure and arthrokinematics of the MCP joint of the thumb are similar to those of the fingers. Marked differences exist, however, in osteokinematics. Active and passive motions at the MCP joint of the thumb are significantly less than those at the MCP joints of the fingers. For all practical purposes, the MCP joint of the thumb allows only one degree of freedom: flexion and extension within the frontal plane. Unlike the MCP joints of the fingers, extension of the thumb MCP joint is usually limited to just a few degrees (beyond the neutral, 0-degree position). The arthrokinematics of active flexion at the metacarpophalangeal joint of the thumb is illustrated in Fig. 8.28. From full extension, the proximal phalanx of the thumb can actively flex about 60 degrees across the palm toward the middle digit.[72]

Active abduction and adduction of the thumb MCP joint are very limited volitionally and therefore are considered accessory motions. This limitation can be observed by attempting to actively abduct or adduct the proximal phalanx while *firmly* stabilizing the thumb metacarpal. The structure of the collateral ligaments and the bony configuration of this joint are most likely responsible for restricting this motion—a restriction that lends natural longitudinal stability throughout the entire ray of the thumb.

Although the limited abduction and adduction at the MCP joint provide some natural stability to the thumb, the normally

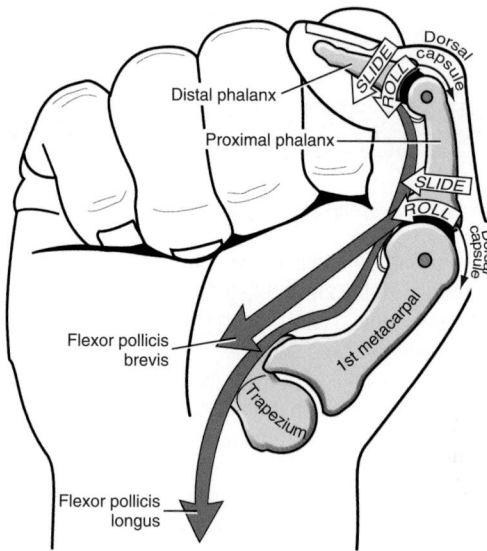

FIGURE 8.28 The arthrokinematics of active flexion are depicted for the metacarpophalangeal and interphalangeal joints of the thumb. Flexion is shown powered by the flexor pollicis longus and flexor pollicis brevis. The axis of rotation for flexion and extension at these joints is in the anterior-posterior direction, through the convex member of the joints. Taut or stretched tissues are shown as thin elongated arrows.

taut collateral ligaments at the joint are particularly vulnerable to injury from excessively large external torques. This is well exemplified by the relatively common "skier's injury" in which the handle and strap of the ski pole of a falling skier create a large (external) abduction torque at the MCP joint, damaging the joint's ulnar collateral ligament. The rupture point of this ligament has been experimentally shown to occur at about 45 degrees of abduction.[43]

Interphalangeal Joints

FINGERS

Distal to the MCP joints are the proximal and distal interphalangeal joints of the fingers (see Fig. 8.27). Each joint allows only one degree of freedom: flexion and extension.

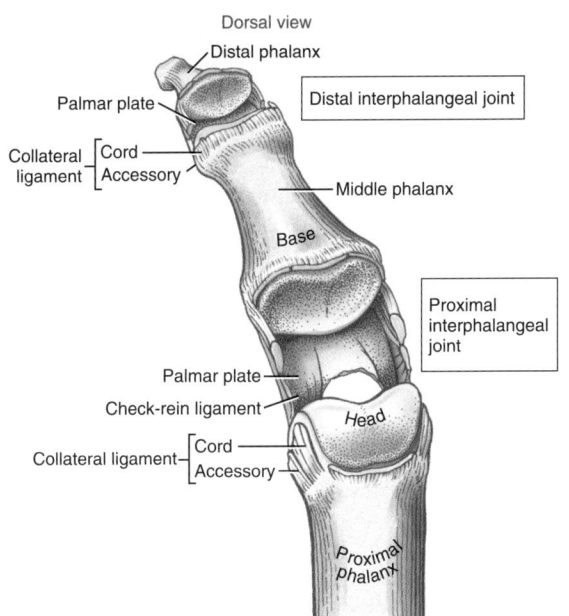

FIGURE 8.29 A dorsal view of the proximal interphalangeal and distal interphalangeal joints opened to expose the shape of the articular surfaces.

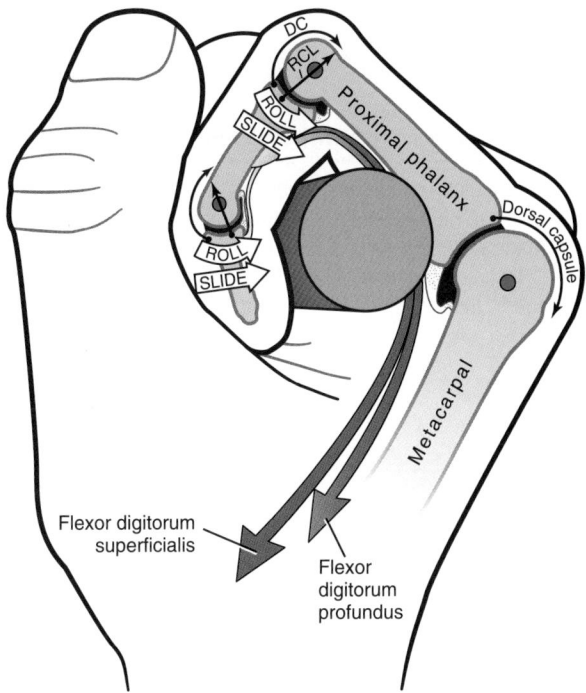

FIGURE 8.30 Illustration highlighting the active flexion arthrokinematics at the proximal and distal interphalangeal (PIP and DIP) joints of the index finger. At the PIP joint, the length of the dorsal capsule *(DC)* increases, while the length of the radial collateral ligament *(RCL)* remains nearly isometric (similar mechanics are shown at the DIP joint). The axis of rotation for each joint is in the medial-lateral direction. Relatively taut connective tissues are shown as thin elongated arrows.

General Features and Ligaments

The *proximal interphalangeal (PIP) joints* are formed by the articulation between the heads of the proximal phalanges and the bases of the middle phalanges. The articular surface of the joint appears as a tongue-in-groove articulation like that used in carpentry to join planks of wood (Fig. 8.29). The head of the proximal phalanx has two rounded condyles separated by a shallow central groove. The opposing surface of the middle phalanx has two shallow concave facets separated by a central ridge. The tongue-in-groove articulation helps guide the motion of flexion and extension as it restricts axial rotation.

Each PIP joint is surrounded by a capsule that is reinforced by radial and ulnar *collateral ligaments*.[142] The cord portion of the collateral ligament at the PIP joint significantly limits abduction and adduction motion. As with the MCP joint, the accessory part of the collateral ligament blends with and reinforces the *palmar plate* (see Fig. 8.29). The anatomic connections between the palmar plate and collateral ligaments form a secure seat for the head of the proximal phalanx. The palmar plate is the primary structure that limits hyperextension of the PIP joint.[123] In addition, the palmar surface of the plate serves as the attachment for the base of the *fibrous digital sheath*—the structure that houses the tendons of the extrinsic finger flexor muscles throughout the digits (see index and small fingers, Fig. 8.21).

The proximal-lateral regions of each palmar plate at the PIP joints thicken longitudinally, forming a fibrous tissue referred to as *check-rein ligaments* (see Fig. 8.29).[123] These tissues reinforce the proximal attachments of the palmar plate, as well as assist in limiting hyperextension of the joint. When enlarged, check-rein ligaments are often considered pathologic tissue and as such are often excised during surgical release of a flexion contracture at the PIP joint.

The *distal interphalangeal (DIP) joints* are formed through the articulation between the heads of the middle phalanges and the bases of the distal phalanges (see Fig. 8.29). The structures of the DIP joint and the surrounding connective tissue are like those of the PIP joint, except for the absence of the check-rein ligaments.

Kinematics

The PIP joints flex to about 100 to 120 degrees. The DIP joints allow less flexion, to about 70 to 90 degrees. As with the CMC and MCP joints of the fingers, flexion at the IP joints is generally *greater in the more ulnar digits*—a point that reflects the greater need for motion at these joints to perform many routine activities.[8] Minimal hyperextension is usually allowed at the PIP joints. The DIP joints, however, normally allow up to about 30 degrees of extension beyond the neutral (0-degree) position.

Similarities in joint structure cause similar arthrokinematics at the PIP and DIP joints. During active flexion at the PIP joint, for example, the concave base of the middle phalanx rolls and slides in a palmar direction by the pull of the extrinsic finger flexors (Fig. 8.30). During flexion, the passive tension created in the dorsal capsule helps guide and stabilize the roll-and-slide arthrokinematics.

In contrast to the MCP joints, passive tension throughout most fibers of the collateral ligaments at the IP joints remains *nearly constant* throughout the range of motion.[102] (This is implied in Fig. 8.30 by showing the tension within the relatively taut collateral ligaments coursing *through* the axes of rotation at the IP joints.) Perhaps the more spherical shape of the heads of the phalanges prevents a significant change in length in these collateral ligaments (see Fig. 8.26). The close-packed position of the PIP and DIP joints is full extension,[142] most likely because of the stretch placed on the palmar plates. During periods of immobilization of the hand, the PIP and DIP joints are often positioned in near extension. This position intentionally stretches the palmar plates, ideally to reduce the likelihood of developing a flexion contracture at these joints. Of the three joints of each finger, the PIP joint requires the greatest range of motion for performing most routine tasks.[8] Flexion contractures at these joints can therefore be particularly disruptive to hand function.

"Position of Function" of the Wrist and Hand

Some medical conditions, such as a traumatic head injury, stroke, or high-level tetraplegia (quadriplegia), can result in a permanent deformity of the wrist and hand. The deformity is caused by a combination of long-term paralysis, disuse, or abnormal tone in the muscles. Clinicians, therefore, often use orthoses that favor a position of the wrist and hand that maximally preserves functional potential. This position, often called the *position of function,* is shown in Fig. 8.31. This position provides an opened and cupped hand, with the wrist in position to maintain optimal length of the finger flexor muscles.

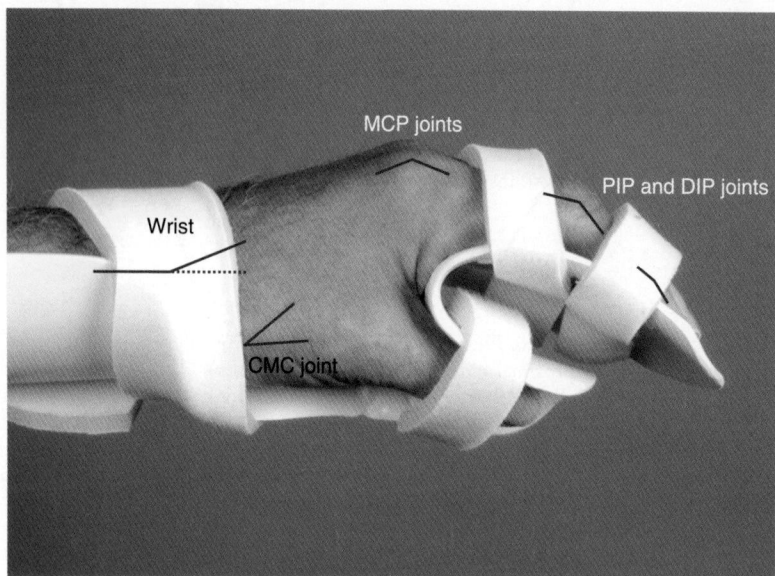

FIGURE 8.31 An orthotic device is used to support the wrist and hand in a "position of function." The person has flaccid paralysis from a stroke. The position of function incorporates the following: *wrist,* 20 to 30 degrees of extension with slight ulnar deviation; *fingers,* 35 to 45 degrees of metacarpophalangeal *(MCP)* joint flexion and 15 to 30 degrees of proximal interphalangeal *(PIP)* and distal interphalangeal *(DIP)* joint flexion; and *thumb,* 35 to 45 degrees of carpometacarpal *(CMC)* joint abduction. These positions may vary based on the patient's underlying physical or medical condition. (Courtesy Teri Bielefeld, PT, CHT: Zablocki VA Hospital, Milwaukee, WI.)

THUMB

The structure and function of the interphalangeal (IP) joint of the thumb are similar to those of the IP joints of the fingers. Motion is limited primarily to one degree of freedom, allowing active flexion to about 70 degrees (see Fig. 8.28).[72] The IP joint of the thumb can be passively extended beyond neutral to about 20 degrees. This motion is often employed to apply a force between the pad of the thumb and an object, such as pushing a thumbtack into a board.

MUSCLE AND JOINT INTERACTION

Innervation of Muscles, Skin, and Joints of the Hand

The complex and coordinated functions of the hand require a highly integrated interplay between the muscle and sensory systems. Consider, for example, the very precise and delicate movements of the digits performed by a concert violinist. One fact allowing for such precision is that a single axon traveling to an intrinsic muscle of the hand, such as the thumb, may innervate as few as 100 muscle fibers.[117] In this case, one axon would simultaneously activate *all* 100 muscle fibers. By contrast, a single axon traveling to the medial head of the gastrocnemius muscle—a muscle not involved with fine movements—may innervate about

2000 muscle fibers.[40] The smaller muscle fiber-to-axon ratio typical of most intrinsic muscles of the hand allows for a more precise gradation between levels of force, ultimately permitting finer control of movement.

Fine control over complex active movements of the digits also requires a constant stream of sensory information from different types of neuroreceptors from multiple regions of the hand, including skin, muscle, tendon, capsule, and ligaments.[166] How the nervous system interprets this information to guide and often predict complex and rapid movements is not fully understood despite years of research interest.[28] Consider the importance of this sensory information for allowing a person to quickly peel and eat a piece of fruit, with very little eye contact. This activity is controlled primarily through sensory input from the hands; much of the muscular activity is in *response* to this sensory information. Muscle activation devoid of sensory input typically results in a crude and uncoordinated movement. This is frequently observed in diseases that spare the motor system but affect primarily the sensory system, such as *tabes dorsalis,* a condition that affects the (sensory) afferent tracts within the spinal cord.

MUSCLE AND SKIN INNERVATION

Innervation to the muscles and the skin of the hand is illustrated in Fig. II.1B–D in Appendix II, Part A. The *radial nerve* innervates the extrinsic extensor muscles of the digits. These muscles, located on the dorsal aspect of the forearm, are the extensor digitorum, extensor digiti minimi, extensor indicis, extensor pollicis longus, extensor pollicis brevis, and abductor pollicis longus. The radial nerve is responsible for the sensation on the dorsal aspect of the wrist and hand, especially around the dorsal web space region and dorsal parts of the capsule of the CMC joint of the thumb.[57]

The *median nerve* innervates most of the extrinsic flexors of the digits. In the forearm the median nerve innervates the flexor digitorum superficialis. A branch of the median nerve (anterior interosseous nerve) then innervates the lateral half of the flexor digitorum profundus and the flexor pollicis longus.

Continuing distally, the median nerve enters the hand through the carpal tunnel, deep to the transverse carpal ligament. Once in the hand, the median nerve innervates the muscles that form the thenar eminence (flexor pollicis brevis, abductor pollicis brevis, and opponens pollicis) and the lateral two lumbricals. The median nerve is responsible for the sensation on the palmar-lateral aspect of the hand, including the tips and the palmar region of the lateral 3½ digits. Sensory fibers of the median nerve innervate the palmar aspects of the capsule of the CMC joint of the thumb.[57]

The *ulnar nerve* innervates the medial half of the flexor digitorum profundus. Distally the ulnar nerve crosses the wrist superficial to the carpal tunnel. In the hand, the deep motor branch of the ulnar nerve innervates the hypothenar muscles (flexor digiti minimi, abductor digiti minimi, opponens digiti minimi, and palmaris brevis) and the medial two lumbricals. The deep motor branch

continues laterally, deep in the hand, to innervate all palmar and dorsal interossei, and finally the adductor pollicis. The ulnar nerve is responsible for the sensation on the ulnar border of the hand, including most of the skin of the ulnar digits.

As a reference, the primary nerve roots that supply the muscles of the upper extremity are listed in Appendix II, Part B. In addition, Parts C–E of Appendix II include additional reference items to help guide the clinical assessment of the functional status of the C^5–T^1 nerve roots and several major peripheral nerves of the upper limb.

SENSORY INNERVATION TO THE JOINTS

For the most part, the *joints of the hand* receive sensation from sensory nerve fibers that supply the overlying dermatomes. (See dermatome chart in Appendix II, Part E.) These afferent nerve fibers merge with the following dorsal nerve roots at the spinal cord: C^6, carrying sensation from the thumb and index finger; C^7, carrying sensation from the middle finger; and C^8, carrying sensation from the ring and small fingers.[54,69,142]

Muscular Function of the Hand

Muscles that control the digits are classified as either *extrinsic* or *intrinsic* to the hand (Table 8.3). Extrinsic muscles have their proximal attachments in the forearm or, in some cases, as far proximal as the epicondyles of the humerus. Intrinsic muscles, in contrast, have both their proximal and their distal attachments within the hand. As a summary and reference, the detailed bony attachments and nerve supply of the muscles of the hand are included in Appendix II, Part F. In addition, a list of cross-sectional areas of selected muscles of the hand are listed in Appendix II, Part G.

Most active movements of the hand, such as opening and closing the fingers, require precise cooperation between the

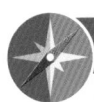

SPECIAL FOCUS 8.4

The "Protective" Role of Normal Sensation

Normal sensation to the hand is essential for its protection against mechanical and thermal injury. Persons with peripheral neuropathy, spinal cord trauma, or peripheral nerve injury, for example, often lose varying levels of sensation in their extremities, making them very vulnerable to injury. Persons afflicted with the relatively rare condition of Hansen's disease (formerly called "leprosy"[161]) may have totally insensitive digits, as well as dermatologic lesions. Over time—and especially without medical care—persons with severe or uncontrolled Hansen's disease may experience a partial or complete loss of their digits. This phenomenon is only indirectly related to the infecting bacteria; the more direct cause stems from the unnecessarily large, and often damaging, contact forces applied to the insensitive digits. With normal sensation, persons typically apply a relatively low amount of force to their hands while performing most routine activities—usually just the minimum needed to adequately perform a given task. In Hansen's disease, however, a greater than normal force is often applied to compensate for the diminished sensation. Although the increased force may be slight for any given application, multiple applications over an extended period can damage skin and other connective tissue. Regardless of the pathology that causes the loss of sensation, clinicians must educate their patients about their increased vulnerability to injury and suggest methods for protecting the region.[104]

TABLE 8.3 Extrinsic and Intrinsic Muscles to the Hand	
Extrinsic Muscles	
Flexors of the digits	Flexor digitorum superficialis Flexor digitorum profundus Flexor pollicis longus
Extensors of the fingers	Extensor digitorum Extensor indicis Extensor digiti minimi
Extensors of the thumb	Extensor pollicis longus Extensor pollicis brevis Abductor pollicis longus
Intrinsic Muscles	
Thenar eminence	Abductor pollicis brevis Flexor pollicis brevis Opponens pollicis
Hypothenar eminence	Abductor digiti minimi Flexor digiti minimi Opponens digiti minimi Palmaris brevis
Other	Adductor pollicis (two heads) Lumbricals (four) Interossei (four palmar and four dorsal)

extrinsic and the intrinsic muscles of the hand and the muscles of the wrist. This important topic is addressed in detail later in this chapter.

EXTRINSIC FLEXORS OF THE DIGITS

Anatomy and Joint Action of the Extrinsic Flexors of the Digits

The extrinsic flexor muscles of the digits are the flexor digitorum superficialis, flexor digitorum profundus, and flexor pollicis longus (Figs. 8.32 and 8.33). These muscles have extensive proximal attachments from the medial epicondyle of the humerus and forearm.

The muscle belly of the *flexor digitorum superficialis* is in the anterior forearm, just deep to the three wrist flexors and the pronator teres muscle (see Fig. 8.32). Its four tendons cross the wrist and enter the palmar aspect of the hand. At the level of the proximal phalanx, each tendon splits to allow passage of the tendon of the flexor digitorum profundus (Fig. 8.34, middle and index fingers). The two split parts of each tendon cross the PIP joint before attaching to the sides of the palmar aspect of the middle phalanx.

The primary action of the flexor digitorum superficialis is to flex the PIP joints. This muscle, however, flexes *all* the joints it crosses. In general, except for the small finger, each tendon can be controlled relatively independently of the other. This independence of function is especially evident at the index finger.

The muscle belly of the *flexor digitorum profundus* is in the deepest muscular plane of the forearm, deep to the flexor digitorum superficialis muscle (see Fig. 8.33). Each of the four tendons of flexor digitorum profundus passes through the split tendon of the flexor digitorum superficialis. Each profundus tendon then continues distally to attach to the palmar side of the base of the distal phalanx. The flexor digitorum profundus is the sole flexor of the DIP joint, but, like the superficialis, can assist in flexing every joint it crosses.

The flexor digitorum profundus to the index finger can often be controlled relatively independently of the other profundus tendons. The remaining three tendons, however, are interconnected through various muscular fasciculi, which usually prohibit isolated DIP joint flexion of a single finger.

The *flexor pollicis longus* resides in the deepest muscular plane of the forearm, just lateral to the flexor digitorum profundus (see Fig. 8.33). This muscle crosses the wrist and attaches distally to the palmar side of the base of the distal phalanx of the thumb. The flexor pollicis longus is the sole flexor at the IP joint of the thumb, and it also exerts a substantial flexion torque at the MCP and CMC joints of the thumb. If not opposed, the flexor pollicis longus also flexes and radially deviates the wrist.

All three extrinsic digital flexor muscles are often active in unison, especially when a firm grip of the entire hand is required. The actions of these muscles curl the digits into flexion while also assisting with opposition of the first, fourth, and fifth digits' CMC joints. This action is most evident when a fist is alternately tightly clenched and released. Although subtle, these opposition actions assist certain intrinsic muscles in raising the borders of the hand, thereby improving the effectiveness and security of grasp.

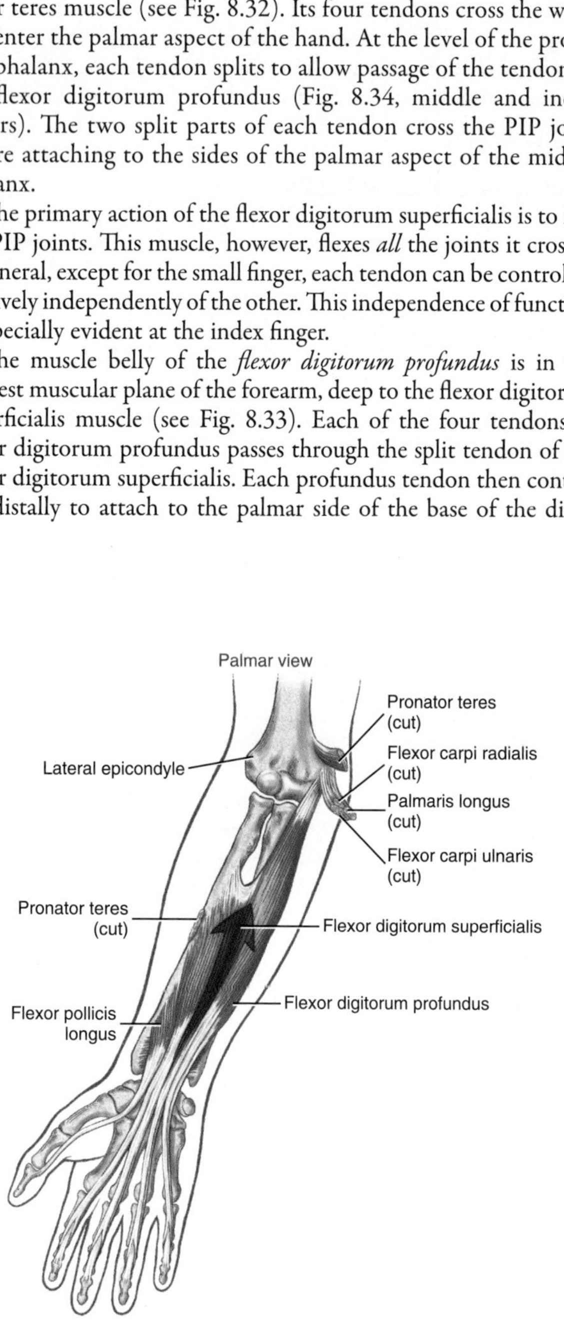

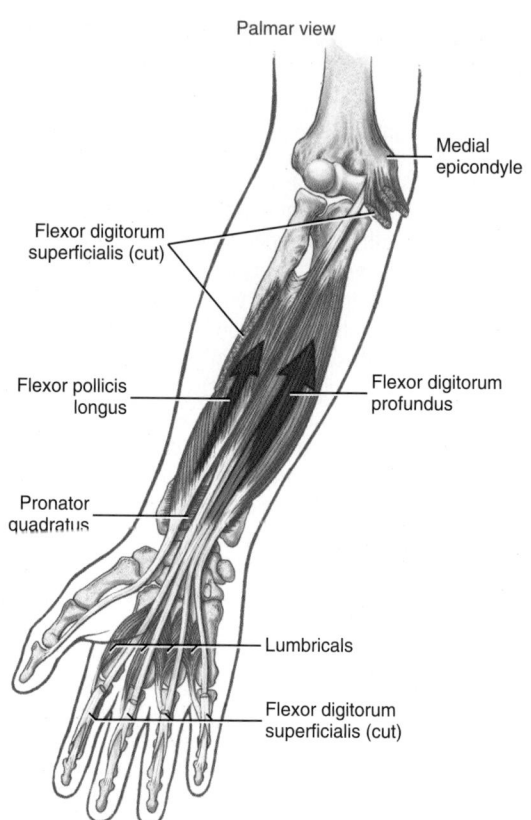

FIGURE 8.32 An anterior view of the right forearm highlighting the action of the flexor digitorum superficialis muscle. Note the cut proximal ends of the wrist flexors and pronator teres muscles.

FIGURE 8.33 An anterior view of the right forearm highlighting the action of the flexor digitorum profundus and the flexor pollicis longus muscles. The lumbrical muscles are shown attaching to the tendons of the flexor digitorum profundus. Note the cut proximal and distal ends of the flexor digitorum superficialis.

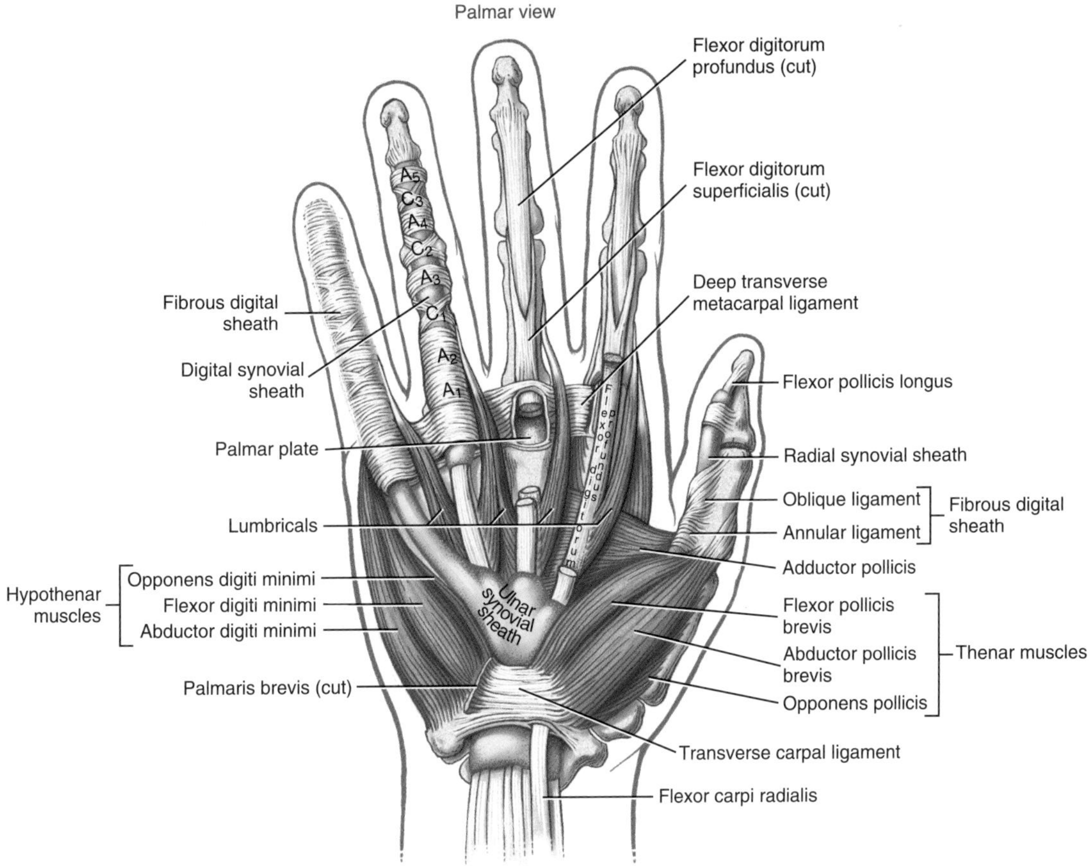

Palmar view

FIGURE 8.34 A palmar view illustrates several important structures of the right hand. Note the *small finger* showing the fibrous digital sheath and ulnar synovial sheath *(blue)* encasing the extrinsic flexor tendons. The *ring finger* has the fibrous digital sheath removed, thereby highlighting the digital synovial sheath *(blue)* and the annular (A_1 to A_5) and cruciate (C_1 to C_3) pulleys. The *middle finger* shows the synovial sheath and pulleys removed to expose the distal attachments of the flexor digitorum superficialis and profundus. The *index finger* has a portion of the flexor digitorum superficialis tendon removed, thereby exposing the deeper tendon of the flexor digitorum profundus and attached lumbrical. The *thumb* highlights the oblique and annular pulleys, along with the radial synovial sheath *(blue)* surrounding the tendon of the flexor pollicis longus.

An extensive synovial membrane surrounds the nine extrinsic digital flexor tendons as they pass through the carpal tunnel: An *ulnar synovial sheath* encloses the flexor digitorum superficialis and profundus, and a smaller *radial synovial sheath* encloses the flexor pollicis longus (see ahead Fig. 8.35). These synovial sheaths surround most of the length of the flexor tendons as they course throughout the hand (shown in blue in select digits in Fig. 8.34).[142] The synovial-ensheathed tendons travel within protective fibro-osseous tunnels known as *fibrous digital sheaths* (see Fig. 8.34, small finger). Throughout the length of each digit, the fibrous digital sheaths are anchored to the phalanges and the palmar plates (see Fig. 8.21, index finger). Embedded within each fibrous sheath are discrete bands of tissue called *flexor pulleys* (see Fig. 8.34, A_1 to A_5, C_1 to C_3 in ring finger).

The fibrous digital sheaths and associated flexor pulleys provide a structural passageway for the flexor tendons and their surrounding synovial sheaths. The synovial sheaths are physiologically and biomechanically important, as they provide nutrition and lubrication to their enclosed tendons. The synovial fluid secreted from the inner walls of the synovial sheath reduces the friction between adjacent flexor tendons and between the tendons and the fibrous sheath. After surgical repair of a flexor tendon injury, adhesions may develop within the fibrous sheath, typically between the sheath's proximal margin and the attachment of the flexor digitorum superficialis to the middle phalanx. Following surgery, a trained hand therapist is needed to closely monitor an exercise program designed to facilitate the careful gliding of the repaired tendon.[76,126,152]

The tendons of the flexor digitorum superficalis and profundus and surrounding synovial membranes within the hand may become chronically inflamed, often from repetitive overuse. In certain cases, the associated swelling narrows the space within the flexor digital sheath and thereby restricts the free gliding of the tendons. This often painful and inflammatory condition is commonly referred to as "trigger finger," or more formally *stenosing flexor tenosynovitis*. The inflamed region of the tendon may develop a nodule that occasionally becomes wedged within the stenosed region of the sheath (usually involving the A_1 pulley), thereby blocking movement of the digit. The involved finger may become temporarily stuck in a certain position, however upon muscular contraction the tendon may suddenly slip through the constriction and rapidly flex or extend with an audible snap (hence the term "trigger finger"). Conservative management of this condition may include the use of NSAIDS, cortisone injection, activity modification, and orthotic intervention.[103] If these approaches are unsuccessful, a surgical release of the constricted region of the sheath may be considered.

SPECIAL FOCUS 8.5

Structural and Functional Basis for "Carpal Tunnel Syndrome"

The nine extrinsic flexor tendons of the digits and the median nerve pass through the carpal tunnel (Fig. 8.35). These tendons are surrounded by moist synovial sheaths and other connective tissues, designed to reduce friction between the structures. The median nerve may be compressed and mechanically stressed as it passes through this crowded and relatively unyielding tunnel. Over time this stress can cause *carpal tunnel syndrome* (CTS), a problem cited as the most frequent compression neuropathy of the upper extremity.[30] CTS is characterized by pain and paresthesia in the sensory distribution of the median nerve, often interfering with sleep. Weakness and atrophy can occur in the muscles of the thenar eminence. When severe, CTS can significantly interfere with the ease and comfort of performing routine activities.

Diagnosing CTS is often difficult due to the myriad of conditions that may have similar or overlapping symptoms.[30,32] Furthermore, the cause of CTS is not completely understood and is likely multifactorial. Two potentially interrelated mechanisms may be involved with its pathogenesis. First, an overcrowding of the tendons or their protective sheaths can increase carpal tunnel pressure, thereby compressing the median nerve. This may occur, for example, from the presence of an abnormally small tunnel, systemic water retention, or inflammation and subsequent swelling of the tendons or synovial membranes. Second, extreme or repetitive wrist movements may place excessive stress on the median nerve within the carpal tunnel. This may be associated with repetitive use of the wrist and hand in certain work-related professions.[21] Occupations

that involve the use of vibration tools, excessive bending of the wrist, or repetitive or forceful grips have been associated with increased incidence of CTS.[121,128,154] These potentially stressful activities may place direct stress on the median nerve itself, or cause inflammation and swelling of tissues that surround it.

Conservative treatments may be effective at reducing symptoms of CTS.[41] These may include using a nighttime wrist orthosis, selected biophysical agents (such as superficial heat or short-wave diathermy), a combined orthotic and stretching program, manual therapy, and education to teach ways to limit stress on the wrist, such as finding alternate ways of using a keyboard or mouse. Other conservative treatments exist with varying levels of research support.[41] If conservative treatment is ineffective, surgical decompression of the carpal tunnel may be performed, often with favorable results.[135,136]

In closing, research continues to evaluate wrist and hand movements or postures that may cause excessive stress to the structures within the carpal tunnel. An in vivo study using ultrasonic images of healthy wrists has shown that the *dart thrower's motion* (discussed in Chapter 7) is associated with *minimal* displacement or deformation of the median nerve or changes in the width of the carpal arch.[88] This oblique wrist motion, recognized for minimizing stress on the often-vulnerable scapholunate ligament, may also be considered relatively "safe" for minimizing stress on the median nerve within the carpal tunnel.

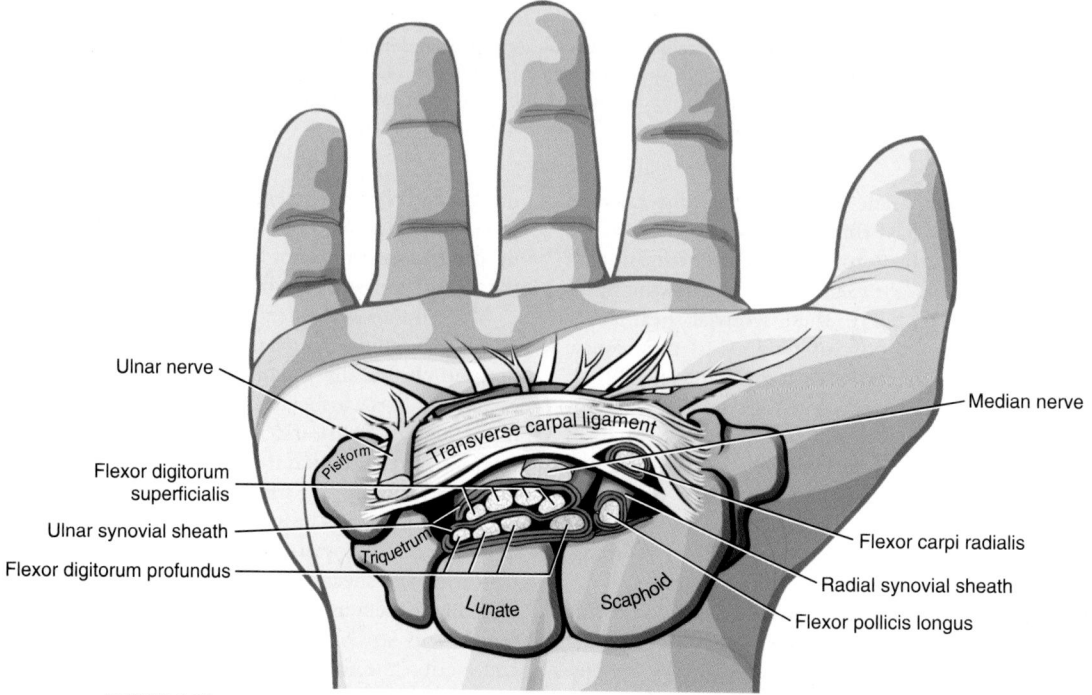

FIGURE 8.35 A transverse view through the entrance of the carpal tunnel of the right wrist. The ulnar synovial sheath *(blue)* surrounds the tendons of the flexors digitorum superficialis and profundus. The radial synovial sheath surrounds the tendon of the flexor pollicis longus. Note the position of the median and ulnar nerves relative to the transverse carpal ligament.

Anatomy and Function of the Flexor Pulleys

Fig. 8.34 shows the flexor pulleys that are embedded within the fibrous digital sheath. Five *annular pulleys* have been described for each finger, designated as A_1 to A_5. The major pulleys (A_2 and A_4) attach to the shafts of the proximal and middle phalanges. The minor pulleys (A_1, A_3, and A_5) attach directly to the palmar plate at each of the three joints within a finger. Three less distinct *cruciate pulleys* (C_1 to C_3) exist. These secondary pulleys are made of thin, flexible fibers that crisscross over the tendons at regions where the digital sheaths bend during flexion. The *annular and oblique ligaments* of the thumb function as pulleys for the passage of the tendon of the flexor pollicis longus (see Fig. 8.34).

Flexor pulleys, the palmar aponeurosis, and skin all share a similar function of holding the underlying tendons at a relatively close distance to the joints. Without the restraint provided by these tissues, the force of a strong contraction of the extrinsic finger flexors causes the tendon to pull away from the joint's axis of rotation, a phenomenon referred to as "bowstringing" of the tendon. The flexor pulleys have a particularly important role in naturally preventing bowstringing of the tendons.[129] The pulleys may be overstretched or torn, however, secondary to trauma, overuse, or disease. (Of interest, overstretching and subsequent bowstringing of the flexor tendons have been observed in 26% of elite rock climbers, most often in the ring and middle fingers.[156]) A severing or overstretching of the major A_2 or A_4 pulley significantly alters the moment arms of the flexor tendons, thereby altering the biomechanics of finger flexion—a point further discussed in Clinical Connection 8.2.

Role of Proximal Stabilizer Muscles during Active Finger Flexion

The extrinsic digital flexors are mechanically capable of flexing multiple joints, from the DIP joint to, at least theoretically for the flexor digitorum superficialis, the elbow. For these muscles to isolate their flexion potential across a single joint, other muscles must contract synergistically along with the extrinsic digital flexors. Consider the flexor digitorum superficialis performing isolated PIP joint flexion (Fig. 8.36). At the onset of contraction, the extensor digitorum must act as a proximal stabilizer to prevent the flexor digitorum superficialis from flexing the MCP joint and the wrist. Because the flexor moment arm length of the flexor digitorum superficialis progressively *increases* at the more proximal joints, a relatively small force applied to a distal joint is amplified to a greater torque at the more proximal joints.[49,50] Fig. 8.36 shows that a 20-N (4.5-lb) force within the superficialis tendon produces a 15-Ncm torque at the PIP joint, a 20-Ncm torque at the MCP joint, and a 25-Ncm torque at the midcarpal joint of the wrist. The greater the force produced by the flexor digitorum superficialis, the greater the force demands placed on the proximal stabilizers. The proximal stabilizers include the extensor digitorum and, when needed, the wrist extensors. The amount of muscle force and coordination required for a simple action of PIP joint flexion is actually more than it first appears. Paralysis or weakness of proximal stabilizers can significantly disrupt the effectiveness of more distal muscle function.

Passive Finger Flexion via "Tenodesis Action" of the Extrinsic Digital Flexors

The extrinsic flexors of the digits—namely, the flexor digitorum profundus and superficialis and the flexor pollicis longus—cross anterior to the wrist. The position of the wrist therefore significantly

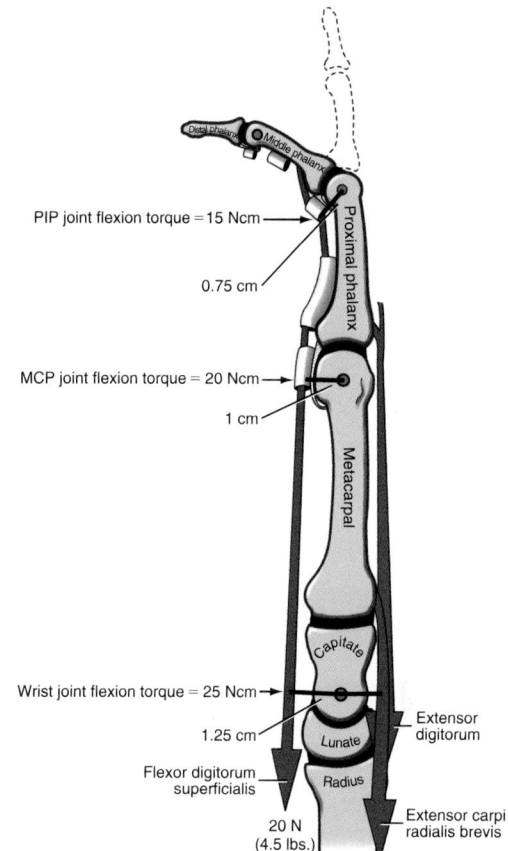

PIP joint flexion torque = 15 Ncm

0.75 cm

MCP joint flexion torque = 20 Ncm

1 cm

Wrist joint flexion torque = 25 Ncm

1.25 cm

Flexor digitorum superficialis

Extensor digitorum

Extensor carpi radialis brevis

20 N (4.5 lbs.)

FIGURE 8.36 The muscle activation required to produce the simple motion of proximal interphalangeal joint flexion. A 20-N (4.5-lb) force produced by the flexor digitorum superficialis creates a flexion torque across every joint it crosses. Because of the progressively larger moment arms in the more proximal joints, the flexor torques progressively increase in a proximal direction from 15 to 25 Ncm. To isolate only flexion at the proximal interphalangeal joint, the extensor digitorum and the extensor carpi radialis brevis must resist the flexion effect of the flexor digitorum superficialis across the wrist and metacarpophalangeal joints.

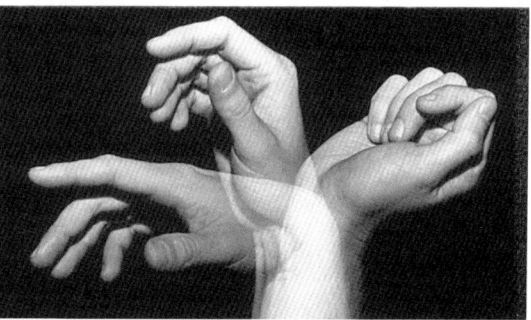

FIGURE 8.37 "Tenodesis action" of the finger flexors in a healthy person. As the wrist is extended, the thumb and fingers automatically flex because of the stretch placed on the extrinsic digital flexors. The flexion occurs passively, without effort from the subject.

alters the length and subsequent passive tension in these muscles. One implication of this arrangement can be appreciated by actively extending the wrist and observing the *passive flexion* of the fingers and thumb (Fig. 8.37). The digits automatically flex (with wrist extension) because of the increased passive tension in the stretched digital flexor muscles. The stretching of a polyarticular muscle across one joint, which generates a passive movement at other joints, is referred to as a *tenodesis action* of a muscle.

The amount of passive flexion of the fingers caused by the aforementioned tenodesis action is surprisingly large; in healthy subjects, on average, completely extending the wrist from full flexion automatically flexes the DIP joint about 20 degrees, the PIP joint about 50 degrees, and the MCP joint about 35 degrees.[146] Fig. 8.37 also demonstrates that in the position of full wrist flexion, the fingers, most notably the index, passively extend because of a similar tenodesis action of the stretched extrinsic digital extensor muscles. Essentially all polyarticular muscles in the body demonstrate some degree of tenodesis action.

EXTRINSIC EXTENSORS OF THE FINGERS

Muscular Anatomy

The extrinsic extensors of the fingers are the extensor digitorum, the extensor indicis, and the extensor digiti minimi (see Fig. 7.22). The extensor digitorum and the extensor digiti minimi originate from a common tendon off the lateral epicondyle of the humerus. The extensor indicis has its proximal attachment on the dorsal surface of the ulna and adjacent regions of the interosseous membrane. The *extensor digitorum,* in terms of cross-sectional area, is the predominant finger extensor.[95] In addition to functioning as a finger extensor, the extensor digitorum has an excellent moment arm as a wrist extensor (see Fig. 7.24).

SPECIAL FOCUS 8.6

The Usefulness of Tenodesis Action in Some Persons with Tetraplegia

The natural tenodesis action of the extrinsic digital flexor muscles has important clinical implications. One example involves a person with C[6] tetraplegia who has near or complete paralysis of the digital flexors and extensors, but well-innervated wrist extensors. People with this level of spinal cord injury often employ a tenodesis action for many functions, such as holding a cup of water. To open the hand to grasp the cup, the person allows gravity to first flex the wrist. This, in turn, stretches the partially paralyzed extensors of the fingers and thumb (see "taut" muscles in Fig. 8.38A).

In Fig. 8.38B, *active contraction of a wrist extensor muscle* (shown in red) slackens the extensor digitorum but also, more importantly, stretches the paralyzed finger and thumb flexor muscles, such as the flexor digitorum profundus and flexor pollicis longus. The stretch in these flexor muscles creates enough passive tension to effectively flex the digits and grasp the cup. The amount of passive tension in the digital flexors is controlled indirectly by the degree of active wrist extension.

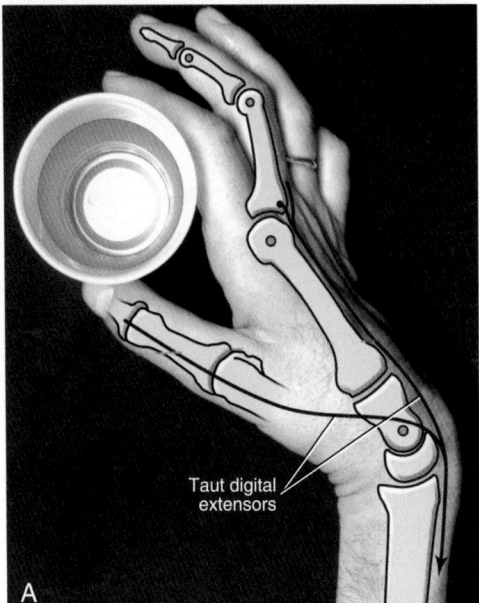

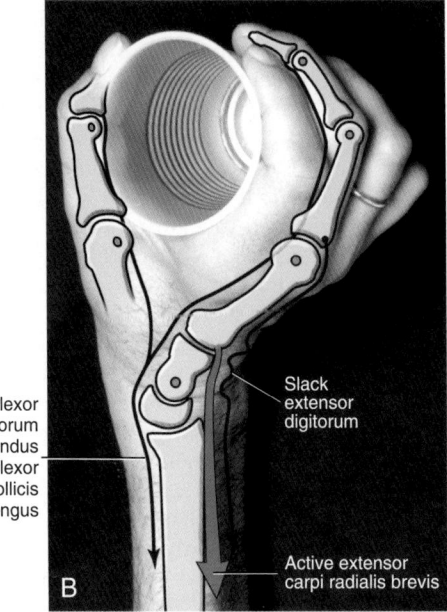

Taut flexor digitorum profundus and flexor pollicis longus

Slack extensor digitorum

Taut digital extensors

Active extensor carpi radialis brevis

FIGURE 8.38 A person with C[6] level tetraplegia using "tenodesis action" to grasp a cup of water. (A) Gravity-induced wrist flexion causes the hand to open. (B) Active wrist extension by contraction of the innervated extensor carpi radialis brevis (shown in *red*) creates enough passive tension in the paralyzed digital flexors to hold the cup of water.

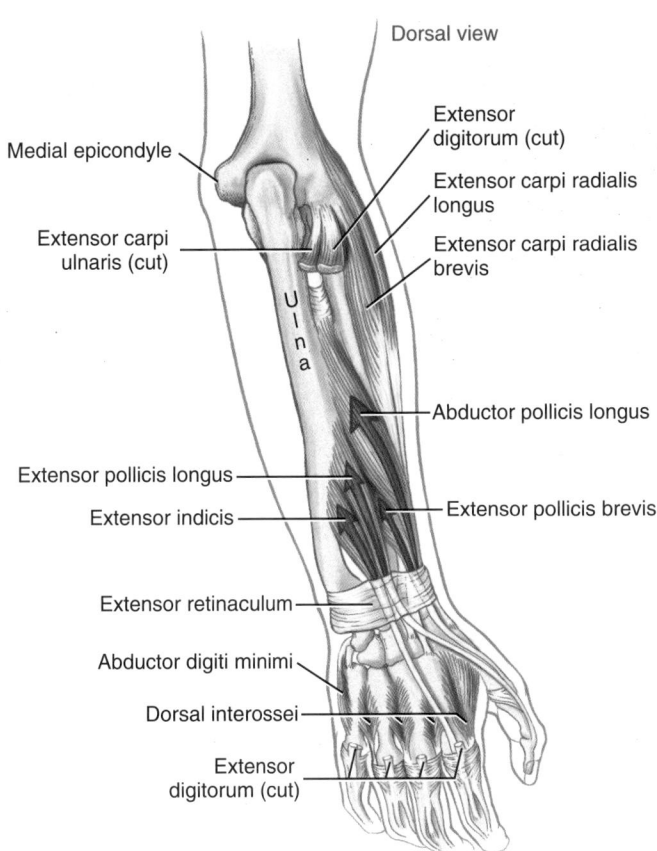

Dorsal view

Medial epicondyle

Extensor carpi ulnaris (cut)

Ulna

Extensor digitorum (cut)

Extensor carpi radialis longus

Extensor carpi radialis brevis

Abductor pollicis longus

Extensor pollicis longus

Extensor indicis

Extensor pollicis brevis

Extensor retinaculum

Abductor digiti minimi

Dorsal interossei

Extensor digitorum (cut)

FIGURE 8.39 A dorsal view of the right upper extremity highlighting the digital extensors: the extensor indicis, extensor pollicis longus, extensor pollicis brevis, and abductor pollicis longus. Note the cut proximal ends of the extensor carpi ulnaris and the extensor digitorum.

Dissecting the extensor digitorum and extensor minimi exposes the deeper *extensor indicis* and the extrinsic extensor muscles of the thumb (Fig. 8.39). The extensor indicis muscle has only one tendon, which serves the index finger. The *extensor digiti minimi* is a small fusiform muscle often interconnected with the extensor digitorum. As depicted in Fig. 8.40, the extensor digiti minimi often has two tendons.

Tendons of the extensor digitorum, extensor indicis, and extensor digiti minimi cross the wrist in synovial-lined compartments located within the extensor retinaculum (see Fig. 7.23). Distal to the extensor retinaculum, the tendons course toward the fingers, dorsal to the metacarpals (see Fig. 8.40). The tendons of the extensor digitorum are interconnected by several *juncturae tendinae*. These thin strips of connective tissue stabilize the angle of approach of the tendons to the base of the MCP joints and may limit independent movement of the individual tendons.

The anatomic organization of the extensor tendons of the fingers is very different from that of the finger flexors. The flexor tendons travel in well-defined digital sheaths toward single bony attachments. In contrast, distal to the wrist, the extensor tendons lack a defined digital sheath or pulley system. The extensor tendons eventually become integrated into a fibrous expansion of connective tissues, located along the length of the dorsum of each finger (see Fig. 8.40). The complex set of connective tissue is called the *extensor mechanism,* although other terms have been used over the years, including the *extensor expansion, dorsal aponeurosis, extensor apparatus,* and *extensor assembly.*[25,33,141] The extensor mechanism serves as a primary distal attachment for the extensor digitorum, indicis, and digiti minimi and for most of the intrinsic muscles acting on the fingers. The following section describes the anatomy of the extensor mechanism. A similar but less organized extensor mechanism exists for the thumb.

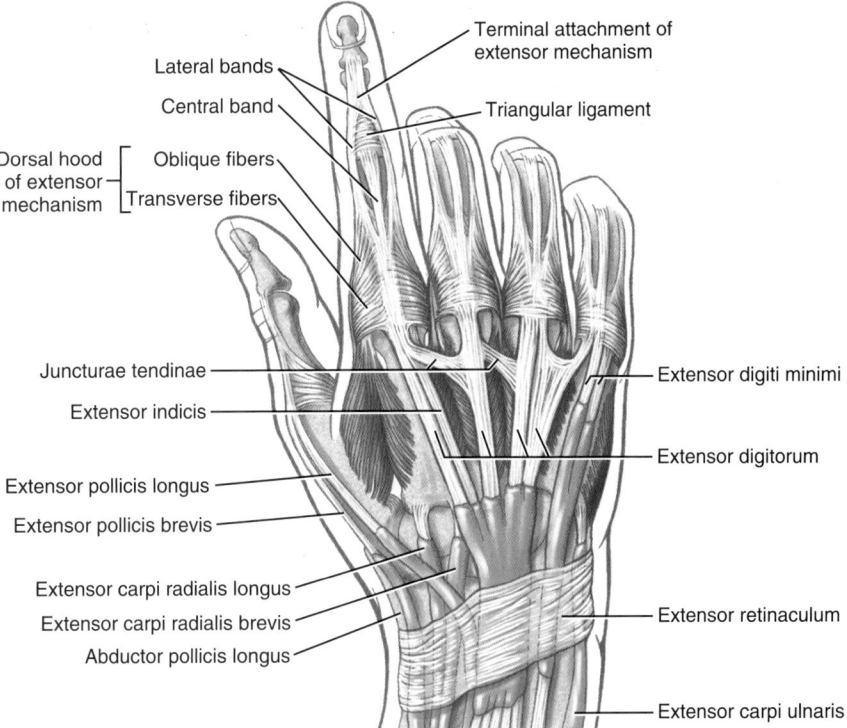

Lateral bands

Terminal attachment of extensor mechanism

Central band

Triangular ligament

Dorsal hood of extensor mechanism

Oblique fibers

Transverse fibers

Juncturae tendinae

Extensor indicis

Extensor digiti minimi

Extensor digitorum

Extensor pollicis longus

Extensor pollicis brevis

Extensor carpi radialis longus

Extensor carpi radialis brevis

Abductor pollicis longus

Extensor retinaculum

Extensor carpi ulnaris

FIGURE 8.40 A dorsal view of the muscles, tendons, and extensor mechanism of the right hand. The synovial sheaths (in *blue*) and the extensor retinaculum are also depicted. The dorsal interosseus muscles and abductor digiti minimi muscles are also evident on the dorsal aspect of the hand.

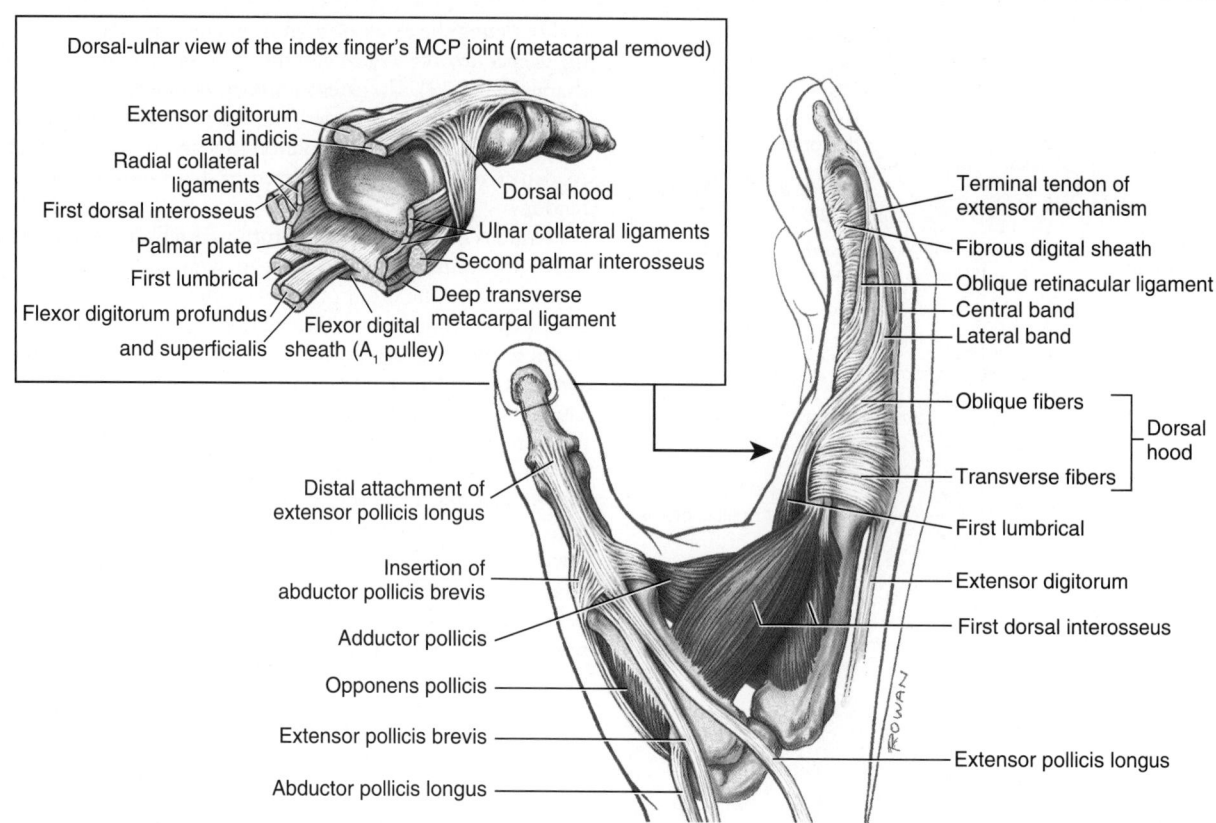

Dorsal-ulnar view of the index finger's MCP joint (metacarpal removed)

Extensor digitorum
and indicis
Radial collateral
ligaments
First dorsal interosseus
Palmar plate
First lumbrical
Flexor digitorum profundus
and superficialis
Flexor digital
sheath (A₁ pulley)
Dorsal hood
Ulnar collateral ligaments
Second palmar interosseus
Deep transverse
metacarpal ligament

Terminal tendon of
extensor mechanism
Fibrous digital sheath
Oblique retinacular ligament
Central band
Lateral band
Oblique fibers
Dorsal hood
Transverse fibers
First lumbrical
Extensor digitorum
First dorsal interosseus

Distal attachment of
extensor pollicis longus
Insertion of
abductor pollicis brevis
Adductor pollicis
Opponens pollicis
Extensor pollicis brevis
Abductor pollicis longus
Extensor pollicis longus

FIGURE 8.41 A lateral view of the muscles, tendons, and extensor mechanism of the right hand. The illustration in the box highlights the anatomy associated with the metacarpophalangeal joint of the index finger.

TABLE 8.4   Anatomy and Primary Function of the Components of the Extensor Mechanism

Component	Pertinent Anatomy	Primary Function
Central band	Direct continuation of the tendon of the extensor digitorum; attaches to the dorsal side of the base of the middle phalanx	Serves as the "backbone" of the extensor mechanism Transmits extensor force from the extensor digitorum across the PIP joint
Lateral bands	Formed from divisions off the central band; pair of bands fuse as a single attachment to the dorsal side of the distal phalanx; the lateral bands are loosely interconnected dorsally by the triangular ligament	Transmit extensor force from the extensor digitorum, lumbricals, and interossei across the PIP and DIP joints
Dorsal hood (transverse and oblique fibers)	*Transverse fibers:* Connect the extensor tendon with the palmar plate at the MCP joint	Stabilize the extensor digitorum tendon over the dorsal aspect of the MCP joint Form a sling around the proximal end of the proximal phalanx, thereby assisting the extensor digitorum in extending the MCP joint
	Oblique fibers: Course distally and dorsally to fuse with the lateral bands	Transfer force from lumbricals and interossei to the lateral bands of the extensor mechanism, thereby assisting with extension of the PIP and DIP joints
Oblique retinacular ligament	Slender, oblique-running fibers connecting the fibrous digital sheaths to the lateral bands of the extensor mechanism	Helps coordinate movement between the PIP and DIP joints of the fingers

DIP, distal interphalangeal; *MCP,* metacarpophalangeal; *PIP,* proximal interphalangeal.

Extensor Mechanism of the Fingers

A small slip of the tendon of the extensor digitorum attaches to the base of the dorsal side of the proximal phalanx. The remaining tendon flattens into a *central band,* forming the "backbone" of the extensor mechanism to each finger (see Figs. 8.40 and 8.41). The central band courses distally to attach to the dorsal base of the middle phalanx. Before crossing the PIP joint, two *lateral bands* diverge from the central band. More distally, the lateral bands fuse into a single terminal tendon that attaches to the dorsal base of the distal phalanx. Note in Fig. 8.40 that the lateral bands are loosely interconnected dorsally by a thin *triangular ligament.* The attachment of the central and lateral bands into the phalanges allows the extensor digitorum to transfer extensor force distally throughout the entire finger.

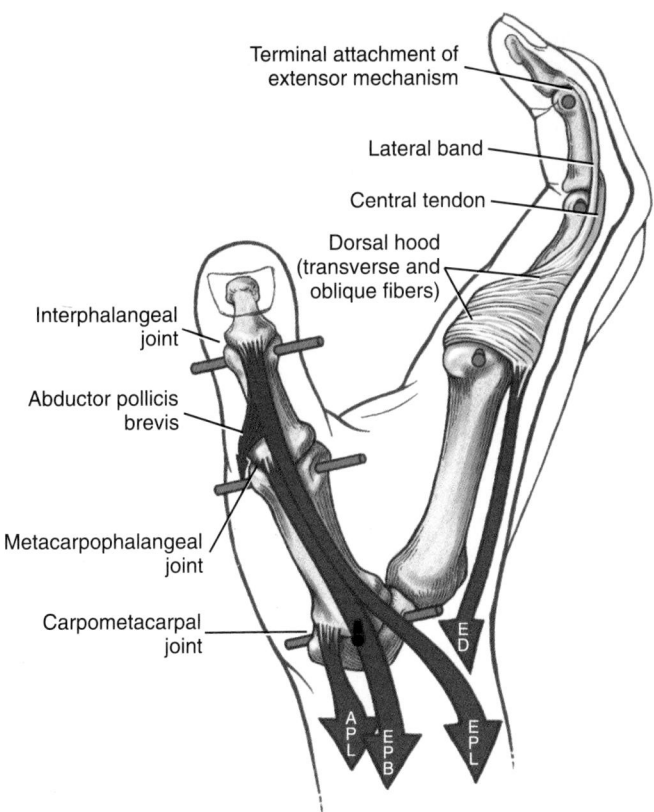

Terminal attachment of
extensor mechanism

Lateral band

Central tendon

Dorsal hood
(transverse and
oblique fibers)

Interphalangeal
joint

Abductor pollicis
brevis

Metacarpophalangeal
joint

Carpometacarpal
joint

FIGURE 8.42 The function of the extrinsic extensor muscles of the hand is demonstrated. Each muscle's action is determined by the orientation of the line of force relative to the axes of rotation at each joint. (The axes of rotation for all flexion and extension movements are depicted in green. The axis of rotation for abduction and adduction movements at the base of the thumb is indicated in purple.) Isolated contraction of the extensor digitorum *(ED)* hyperextends the metacarpophalangeal joints. The extensor pollicis longus *(EPL)*, the extensor pollicis brevis *(EPB)*, and the abductor pollicis longus *(APL)* are all primary thumb extensors. Attachments of the abductor pollicis brevis are shown blending into the distal tendon of the extensor pollicis longus.

Each extensor mechanism of a given finger has a bilateral pair of *oblique retinacular ligaments*.[153] Fig. 8.41 shows the oblique retinacular ligament on the radial side of the index finger. The slender fibers arise proximally from the fibrous digital sheath, just proximal to the PIP joint, and course obliquely and distally to insert into the lateral bands. The ligaments help coordinate movement between the PIP and DIP joints of the fingers, a point to be discussed later in this chapter.

The most prominent feature of the proximal end of the extensor mechanism is the *dorsal hood*, located immediately dorsal to the MCP joint (see Figs. 8.40 and 8.41). This thin, almost translucent sheet of connective tissue is triangular in shape (with its base being proximal), possessing both transverse and oblique fibers. The *transverse fibers* run on either side of and nearly perpendicular to the tendon of the extensor digitorum. The fibers course in a palmar direction (often referred to as "sagittal" bands) and attach loosely to the palmar plate and deep transverse metacarpal ligament.[142] Although loosely anchored palmarly, the transverse fibers still exert a restraining tension that centralizes the extensor digitiorum tendon over the dorsal side of the MCP joint.[80] The transverse fibers also form a functional "sling" around the base of the proximal phalanx (Fig. 8.42). This sling assists the extensor digitorum muscle in extending the MCP joint. The *oblique fibers* of the dorsal hood

course more distally and dorsally to eventually fuse with the lateral bands (see Fig. 8.41).

As a general rule, the intrinsic muscles of the fingers (specifically the lumbricals and interossei) attach into the extensor mechanism via the oblique fibers and, to a lesser extent, the transverse fibers of the dorsal hood. Fig. 8.41 shows this arrangement for the first dorsal interosseus and lumbrical of the index finger. Via these important connections, the intrinsic muscles assist the extensor digitorum with extension of the PIP and DIP joints.

The anatomic and functional components of the extensor mechanism are summarized in Table 8.4. The overall kinesiologic relevance of the extensor mechanism will be made clear later in the chapter.

Action of the Extrinsic Finger Extensors

Isolated contraction of the extensor digitorum produces hyperextension of the MCP joints. Only in the presence of activated intrinsic muscles of the fingers can the extensor digitorum fully extend the PIP and DIP joints. This important point will be reinforced later in this chapter.

EXTRINSIC EXTENSORS OF THE THUMB

Anatomic Considerations

The extrinsic extensors of the thumb are the *extensor pollicis longus, extensor pollicis brevis,* and *abductor pollicis longus* (see Figs. 8.39 and 8.41). These radial innervated muscles have their proximal attachments on the dorsal region of the forearm. The tendons of these muscles compose the "anatomic snuffbox" located on the radial side of the wrist. The tendons of the abductor pollicis longus and the extensor pollicis brevis together pass through the first dorsal compartment within the extensor retinaculum of the wrist (see Fig. 7.23). Distal to the extensor retinaculum, the tendon of the abductor pollicis longus inserts primarily into the radial-dorsal surface of the base of the thumb metacarpal. Additional distal attachments of this muscle attach into the trapezium and blend with fibers of the intrinsic thenar muscles.[133,145] The extensor pollicis brevis attaches distally to the dorsal base of the proximal phalanx of the thumb. The tendon of the extensor pollicis longus crosses the wrist in the third compartment in a groove just medial to the dorsal tubercle of the radius (see Fig. 7.23). The extensor pollicis longus attaches distally to the dorsal base of the distal phalanx of the thumb. Fibers from both extrinsic extensor tendons contribute to the central tendon of the extensor mechanism of the thumb.

Functional Considerations

The multiple actions of the extensor pollicis longus, extensor pollicis brevis, and abductor pollicis longus can be understood by noting their line of force relative to the axes of rotation at the joints they cross (see Fig. 8.42). The *extensor pollicis longus* extends the IP, MCP, and CMC joints of the thumb. The muscle passes to the dorsal side of the medial-lateral axis of the CMC joint and is therefore also capable of adducting this joint. The extensor pollicis longus is unique in its ability to perform all actions that reposition the opposed thumb back to the anatomic position: extension (with slight lateral rotation) and adduction of the first metacarpal.

Fig. 8.42 also illustrates that the *extensor pollicis brevis* is an extensor of the MCP and CMC joints of the thumb; the *abductor pollicis longus* extends only at the CMC joint. At least in theory, the long abductor muscle can also abduct the CMC joint, based on its line of force passing just anterior (palmar) to the joint's medial-lateral axis of rotation. The combined extension-abduction action of the abductor pollicis longus reflects its attachment on the radial-dorsal corner of the base of the thumb metacarpal. The actions of all the muscles that cross the joints of the thumb are summarized in Box 8.1.

The extensor pollicis longus and the abductor pollicis longus are potent radial deviators at the wrist (see Fig. 7.24). During extension of the thumb, therefore, an ulnar deviator muscle must be activated to stabilize the wrist against unwanted radial deviation. This activation is apparent by palpating the raised tendon of the flexor carpi ulnaris, located just proximal to the pisiform, during rapid, vigorous, and full extension of the thumb.

INTRINSIC MUSCLES OF THE HAND

The hand contains 20 intrinsic muscles. Despite their relatively small size, these muscles are essential to the fine control and alignment of the digits. Topographically, the intrinsic muscles are divided into four sets, as follows:

1. Muscles of the thenar eminence
   - Abductor pollicis brevis
   - Flexor pollicis brevis
   - Opponens pollicis
2. Muscles of the hypothenar eminence
   - Flexor digiti minimi
   - Abductor digiti minimi
   - Opponens digiti minimi
   - Palmaris brevis
3. Adductor pollicis
4. Lumbricals and interossei

Muscles of the Thenar Eminence
Anatomic Considerations
The *abductor pollicis brevis, flexor pollicis brevis, and opponens pollicis* make up the bulk of the thenar eminence (see Fig. 8.34). The flexor pollicis brevis is often described as having two heads: a *superficial head,* which comprises most of the muscle, and a *deep head,* which may be small, poorly defined, or absent.[142] This chapter considers only

---

BOX 8.1   Actions of Muscles That Cross the Joints of the Thumb

CARPOMETACARPAL JOINT

FLEXION	**EXTENSION**
Adductor pollicis	Extensor pollicis brevis
Flexor pollicis brevis	Extensor pollicis longus
Flexor pollicis longus	Abductor pollicis longus
Opponens pollicis	
Abductor pollicis brevis*	

ABDUCTION	**ADDUCTION**
Abductor pollicis brevis	Adductor pollicis
Abductor pollicis longus	Extensor pollicis longus
Flexor pollicis brevis*	First dorsal interosseus*
Opponens pollicis*	

OPPOSITION	**REPOSITION**
Opponens pollicis	Extensor pollicis longus
Flexor pollicis brevis	
Abductor pollicis brevis	
Flexor pollicis longus	
Abductor pollicis longus	

METACARPOPHALANGEAL JOINT†

FLEXION	**EXTENSION**
Adductor pollicis	Extensor pollicis longus
Flexor pollicis brevis	Extensor pollicis brevis
Flexor pollicis longus	
Abductor pollicis brevis*	

INTERPHALANGEAL JOINT

FLEXION	**EXTENSION**
Flexor pollicis longus	Extensor pollicis longus
	Abductor pollicis brevis and adductor pollicis (due to attachment into extensor mechanism of thumb)‡

*Secondary action.
†Only one degree of freedom is considered for the metacarpophalangeal joint.
‡Slight volitional extension may be noted in cases of radial nerve injury.

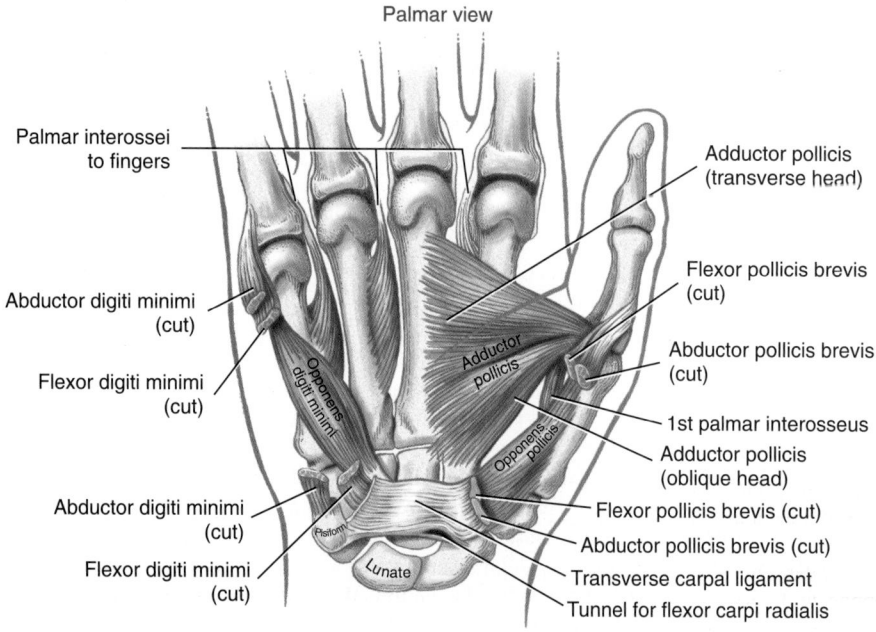

Palmar view

Palmar interossei to fingers

Abductor digiti minimi (cut)

Flexor digiti minimi (cut)

Abductor digiti minimi (cut)

Flexor digiti minimi (cut)

Opponens digiti minimi

Pisiform

Lunate

Adductor pollicis (transverse head)

Flexor pollicis brevis (cut)

Abductor pollicis brevis (cut)

1st palmar interosseus

Adductor pollicis (oblique head)

Opponens pollicis

Adductor pollicis

Flexor pollicis brevis (cut)

Abductor pollicis brevis (cut)

Transverse carpal ligament

Tunnel for flexor carpi radialis

FIGURE 8.43 A palmar view of the deep muscles of the right hand. The abductor and flexor muscles of the thenar and hypothenar eminences have been cut away to expose the underlying opponens pollicis and opponens digiti minimi.

the superficial head when discussing the flexor pollicis brevis. Deep to the abductor pollicis brevis is the opponens pollicis (Fig. 8.43). All three thenar muscles have their proximal attachments on the transverse carpal ligament and adjacent carpal bones. Both the short abductor and flexor muscles have their distal attachments on the radial side of the base of the proximal phalanx. In addition, the abductor pollicis brevis attaches partially to the radial side of the extensor mechanism of the thumb. The deeper opponens pollicis attaches distally to the entire radial border of the thumb metacarpal.

Functional Considerations

By attaching into the transverse carpal ligament, the palmaris longus helps stabilize the common proximal attachment of all three muscles of the thenar eminence. Once stabilized, the thenar muscle can securely position the thumb in varying amounts of opposition, usually to facilitate grasping. As discussed earlier, opposition combines elements of CMC joint abduction, flexion, and medial rotation. Each muscle within the thenar eminence is a prime mover for at least one component of opposition, and an assistant for several others (see Box 8.1).[78,139]

The actions of the thenar muscles across the CMC joint become apparent when each muscle's line of force relative to a particular axis of rotation is viewed (Fig. 8.44). Note that the opponens pollicis has a line of force to *medially rotate* the thumb toward the fingers. Because the opponens pollicis attaches distally to the metacarpal (and therefore proximal to the MCP joint), its entire contractile force is dedicated to controlling the CMC joint.

Implications of Median Nerve Injury

A severance of the median nerve paralyzes all three muscles of the thenar eminence: namely the opponens pollicis, flexor

pollicis brevis, and abductor pollicis brevis. Consequently, opposition of the thumb is essentially disabled. The thenar eminence region becomes flat because of muscle atrophy. The functional loss of opposition, in conjunction with the anesthesia of the tips of the thumb and radial fingers, greatly reduces precision grip and other manipulative functions of the hand.

In addition to the important medial rotation function of the opponens pollicis, all three muscles of the thenar eminence independently perform the combined actions of *flexion and abduction* of the CMC joint. These kinematics are essential to lifting the thumb up and over the palm during opposition. Fig. 8.45 compares these and other combined actions of the muscles that cross the CMC joint of the thumb. As noted by the location of the black dots, almost all the muscles have a combined action as a *flexor-abductor*, a *flexor-adductor*, an *extensor-adductor*, or an *extensor-abductor*. As indicated, the median nerve is the only source of innervation of the *flexion-abduction quadrant* of muscles. Although abduction of the thumb is still possible primarily because of the radial nerve–innervated abductor pollicis longus,[15] this action is usually overruled by the stronger remaining adduction torque potential of the ulnar nerve–innervated adductor pollicis muscle (see ADPo and ADPt). For this reason, persons with a median nerve injury are susceptible to an adduction contracture of the CMC joint of the thumb. As described earlier, an adduction bias

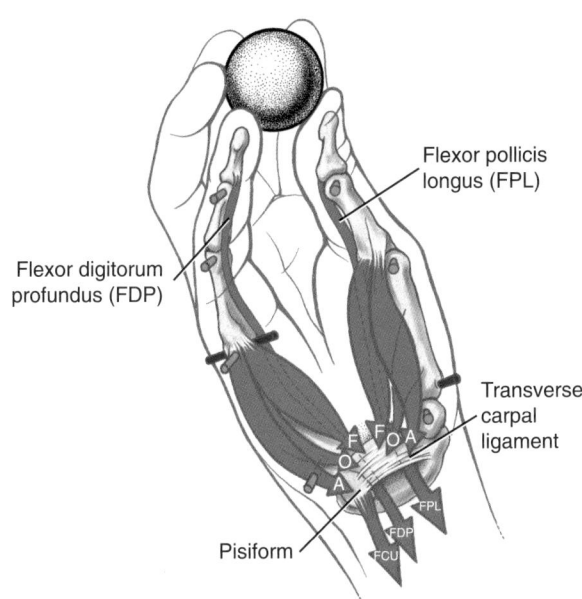

FIGURE 8.44 The actions of the thenar and hypothenar muscles are depicted during opposition of the thumb and small finger. (The axes of rotation for all flexion and extension movements are depicted in green. The axes of rotation for abduction and adduction movements at the metacarpophalangeal joint of the small finger and the carpometacarpal joint of the thumb are indicated in purple.) Other active muscles include the flexor pollicis longus and flexor digitorum profundus of the small finger. The flexor carpi ulnaris *(FCU)* stabilizes the pisiform bone for the abductor digiti minimi. *A,* abductor pollicis brevis and abductor digiti minimi; *F,* flexor pollicis brevis and flexor digiti minimi; *O,* opponens pollicis and opponens digiti minimi.

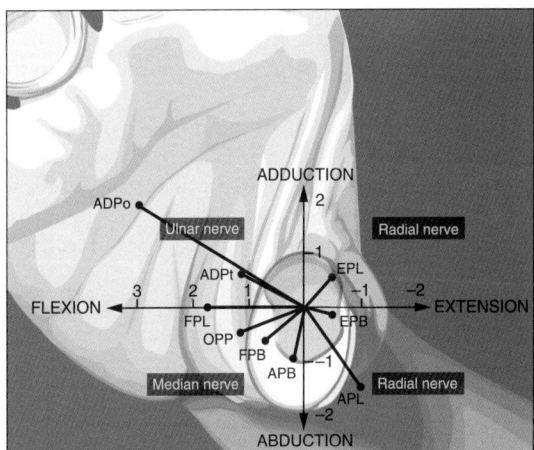

FIGURE 8.45 An illustration that associates the potential torque (strength) and combined actions of the muscles that cross the carpometacarpal *(CMC)* joint of the right thumb. The trapezium is outlined in light yellow at the base of the thumb. The black dots represent the location of each muscle relative to the two (primary) degrees of freedom of movement at the CMC joint: flexion-extension and adduction-abduction. Except for the flexor pollicis longus *(FPL),* each muscle is classified as a flexor-abductor, a flexor-adductor, an extensor-adductor, or an extensor-abductor. Furthermore, the length of each line associated with each muscle is proportional to the maximum torque potential of the muscle, which considers *both* the muscle's moment arm and the cross-sectional area. The units used on the axes indicate torque in Nm. Observe that the muscles that fall within each of the four quadrants share the same source of innervation. *ADPo,* adductor pollicis, oblique head; *ADPt,* adductor pollicis, transverse head; *APB,* abductor pollicis brevis; *APL,* abductor pollicis longus; *EPB,* extensor pollicis brevis; *EPL,* extensor pollicis longus; *FPB,* flexor pollicis brevis; *FPL,* flexor pollicis longus; *OPP,* opponens pollicis. (The diagram is based on data originally plotted by Smutz WP, Kongsayreepong A, Hughes RE, et al: Mechanical advantage of the thumb muscles, *J Biomech* 31:565–570, 1998. From Neumann DA, Bielefeld TB: The carpometacarpal joint of the thumb: stability, deformity, and therapeutic intervention, *J Orthop Sports Phys Ther* 33:386, 2003.)

to the thumb is certainly counterproductive to the natural kinematics of opposition.

Muscles of the Hypothenar Eminence
Anatomic Considerations

The muscles of the hypothenar eminence consist of the *flexor digiti minimi, abductor digiti minimi, opponens digiti minimi,* and *palmaris brevis* (see Figs. 8.34 and 8.43). The abductor digiti minimi is the most superficial and medial of these muscles, occupying the extreme ulnar border of the hand. The relatively small flexor digiti minimi is located just lateral to, and often blended with, the abductor. Deep to these muscles is the opponens digiti minimi, the largest of the hypothenar muscles. The palmaris brevis is a thin and relatively insignificant muscle about the thickness of a postage stamp. It attaches between the transverse carpal ligament and an area of skin just distal to the pisiform bone (see Fig. 8.34). The palmaris brevis raises the height of the hypothenar eminence, typically to assist with a deepening of the concavity of the palm.

The overall anatomic plan of the hypothenar muscles is like that of the muscles of the thenar eminence.[124] Both the flexor digiti minimi and the opponens digiti minimi have their proximal attachments on the transverse carpal ligament and the hook of the hamate. The abductor digiti minimi has extensive proximal attachments from the pisohamate ligament, pisiform bone, and flexor carpi ulnaris tendon. During resisted or rapid abduction of the small finger, the flexor carpi ulnaris contracts to stabilize the attachment for the abductor digiti minimi. This effect can be verified by palpating the tendon of the flexor carpi ulnaris just proximal to the pisiform bone.

The abductor and flexor digiti minimi both have their distal attachments on the ulnar border of the base of the proximal phalanx of the small finger. Some fibers from the abductor also blend with the ulnar side of the extensor mechanism. The opponens digiti minimi has its distal attachment along the ulnar border of the fifth metacarpal, proximal to the MCP joint.

Functional Considerations

A common function of the hypothenar muscles is to raise and "cup" the ulnar border of the hand. This action deepens the distal transverse arch and enhances digital contact with held objects (see Fig. 8.44). When necessary, the abductor digiti minimi can spread the small finger for greater control of grasp. The opponens digiti minimi rotates, or opposes, the fifth metacarpal toward the middle digit. Contraction of the long finger flexors of the small finger, such as the flexor digitorum profundus, also contributes to raising the ulnar border of the hand. The actions of all the muscles that cross the joints of the small finger are listed in Box 8.2.

Injury to the ulnar nerve can completely paralyze the hypothenar muscles. The hypothenar eminence becomes flat because of muscle atrophy. The action of raising and cupping the ulnar border of the hand is significantly reduced. Anesthesia over the entire small finger can contribute to a loss of dexterity.

Adductor Pollicis Muscle

The *adductor pollicis* is a two-headed muscle lying deep in the web space of the thumb, palmar to the second and third metacarpals (see Fig. 8.43). The muscle has its proximal attachments on the most stable skeletal region of the hand. The thicker *oblique head* arises from the capitate bone, bases of the second and third metacarpals, and other adjacent connective tissues.[142] The thinner, triangular *transverse head* attaches on the palmar surface of the third

---

> **BOX 8.2   Actions of Muscles That Cross the Joints of the Small Finger**
>
> **CARPOMETACARPAL JOINT**
>
> | **FLEXION AND OPPOSITION** | **EXTENSION** |
> | --- | --- |
> | Flexor digiti minimi | Extensor digitorum |
> | Opponens digiti minimi | Extensor digiti minimi |
> | Flexor digitorum superficialis and profundus | |
> | Palmaris brevis | |
>
> **METACARPOPHALANGEAL JOINT**
>
> | **FLEXION** | **EXTENSION** |
> | --- | --- |
> | Flexor digiti minimi | Extensor digitorum |
> | Abductor digiti minimi* | Extensor digiti minimi |
> | Lumbrical | |
> | Palmar interosseus | |
> | Flexor digitorum superficialis and profundus | |
>
> | **ABDUCTION** | **ADDUCTION** |
> | --- | --- |
> | Abductor digiti minimi | Palmar interosseus |
>
> **PROXIMAL INTERPHALANGEAL JOINT**
>
> | **FLEXION** | **EXTENSION** |
> | --- | --- |
> | Flexor digitorum superficialis and profundus | Extensor digitorum |
> | | Extensor digiti minimi |
> | | Lumbrical |
> | | Palmar interosseus |
>
> **DISTAL INTERPHALANGEAL JOINT**
>
> | **FLEXION** | **EXTENSION** |
> | --- | --- |
> | Flexor digitorum profundus | Extensor digitorum |
> | | Extensor digiti minimi |
> | | Lumbrical |
> | | Palmar interosseus |

*Secondary action.

---

metacarpal bone. Both heads join for a common distal attachment on the ulnar side of the base of the proximal phalanx of the thumb; the tendon frequently sends fibers into the extensor mechanism of the thumb.

The adductor pollicis is a dominant muscle at the CMC joint, producing the greatest combination of flexion and adduction torque.[17] This important source of torque is applied to many activities, such as pinching an object between the thumb and index finger or closing a pair of scissors (Fig. 8.46). The transverse head of the adductor pollicis uses a very long moment arm to generate both *flexion* (Fig. 8.46A) and *adduction* (Fig. 8.46B) torque at the base of the thumb. Although the transverse fibers have the greater leverage at the CMC joint, the thicker oblique head generates the greater flexion and adduction torque (compare ADPo and ADPt in Fig. 8.45).[97,139]

Lumbricals and Interosseus Muscles

The *lumbricals* (from the Latin root *lumbricus,* earthworm) are four slender muscles that originate from the tendons of the flexor digitorum profundus (see Figs. 8.33 and 8.34). More specifically, the lumbricals associated with the index and middle fingers arise from the radial sides of their respective profundus tendons. Although variable, the lumbricals associated with the ring and small fingers are often bipennate, arising from the radial sides of their respective

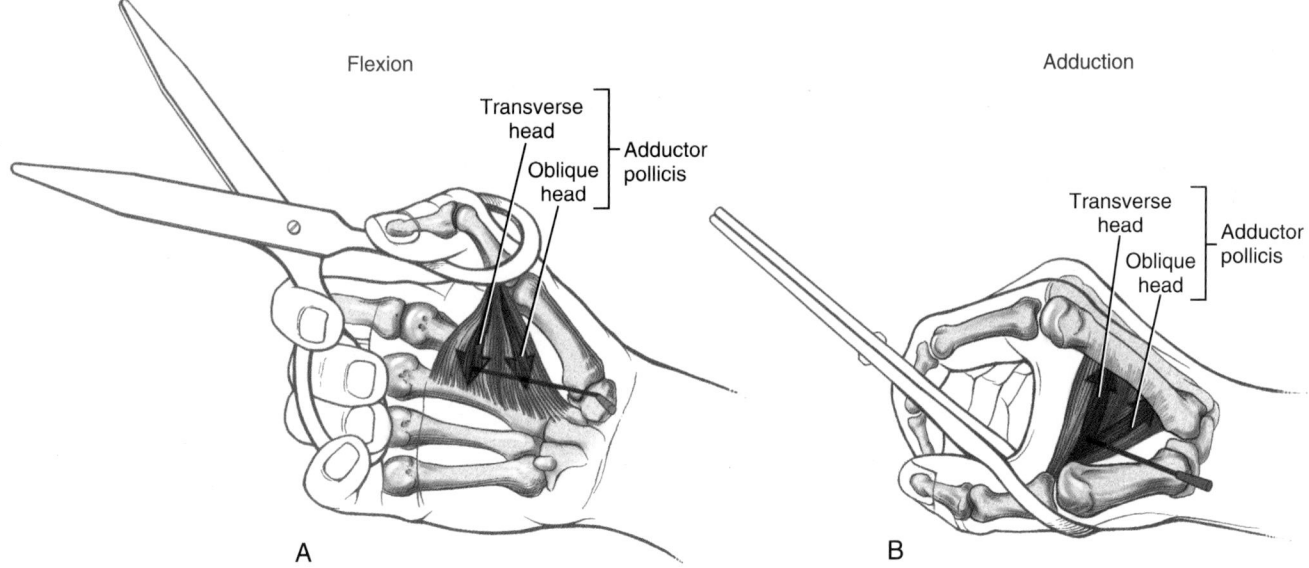

Flexion

Transverse
head

Oblique
head

} Adductor
pollicis

Adduction

Transverse
head

Oblique
head

} Adductor
pollicis

A

B

FIGURE 8.46 The biplanar action of the adductor pollicis muscle is illustrated using a pair of scissors for flexion (A) and adduction (B) at the thumb's carpometacarpal joint. In both (A) and (B) the transverse head of the adductor pollicis produces a significant torque because of its long moment arm about an anterior-posterior axis (*green,* part A) and medial-lateral axis (*purple,* part B). Both heads of the adductor pollicis are also strong flexors of the thumb's metacarpophalangeal joint.

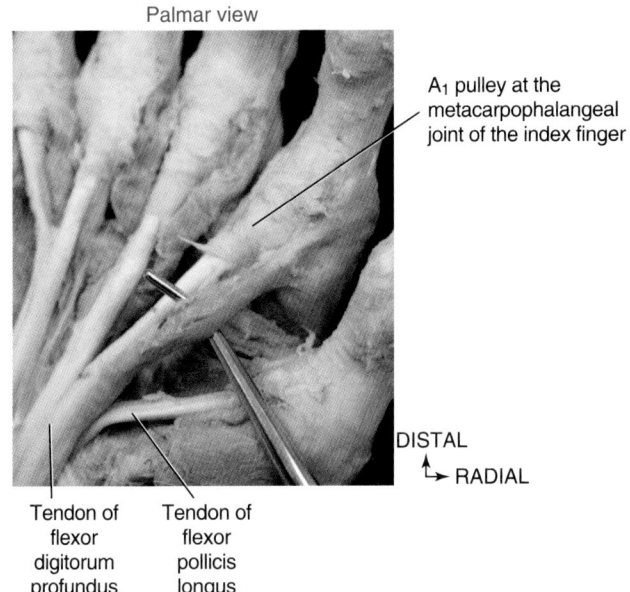

Palmar view

A₁ pulley at the
metacarpophalangeal
joint of the index finger

DISTAL

RADIAL

Tendon of
flexor
digitorum
profundus

Tendon of
flexor
pollicis
longus

FIGURE 8.47 A palmar view of the right hand of an embalmed cadaver, highlighting the first lumbrical muscle. The probe is lifting the muscle belly of the first lumbrical from the underlying adductor pollicis muscle. The proximal attachment of the first lumbrical is shown arising from the tendon of the flexor digitorum profundus. The distal attachment of the first lumbrical can be seen blending with the oblique fibers of the dorsal hood of the extensor mechanism of the index finger.

profundus tendons as well as the ulnar sides of the adjacent tendons. Like the flexor digitorum profundus, the lumbricals have a dual source of innervation: the two lateral lumbricals by the median nerve, and the two medial lumbricals by the ulnar nerve.

All four lumbricals show marked variation in both size and attachments.[122] From their tendinous proximal attachments, the lumbricals course *palmar* to the deep transverse metacarpal ligament and then *radial* to the MCP joints (see Fig. 8.41, first lumbrical). Distally, a typical lumbrical attaches to the adjacent lateral band of the extensor mechanism, most often via the oblique fibers of the dorsal hood (see close-up view of first lumbrical in Fig. 8.47). This distal attachment enables the lumbricals to exert a proximal pull throughout the extensor mechanism.

The overall role of the lumbricals in hand function has been studied and debated for many years.[25,93,99,127,150] What is known for certain is that their contraction produces flexion at the MCP joints and extension at the PIP and DIP joints.[162] This seemingly paradoxical action is possible because the lumbricals pass *palmar* to the MCP joints but *dorsal* to the PIP and DIP joints (Fig. 8.48). By also passing on the *radial* side of the MCP joint, the lumbrical assists with radial deviation of this joint (abduction or adduction depending on the finger), although this action is slight compared with the interossei muscles.

Of all the intrinsic muscles of the hand, the lumbricals have the greatest muscle fiber length as a proportion of their total muscle length, but the smallest cross-sectional area.[16,97] This anatomic design suggests that these muscles can generate small amounts of force over a relatively long distance. Although a low force potential in a muscle generally suggests a limited role in controlling movement, this is not always the case. Muscles have other important kinesiologic functions besides producing force. The first lumbrical, for example, possesses a very rich source of muscle spindles—sensory organs that closely monitor changes in the length of the muscle. The average spindle density of the first lumbrical is approximately three

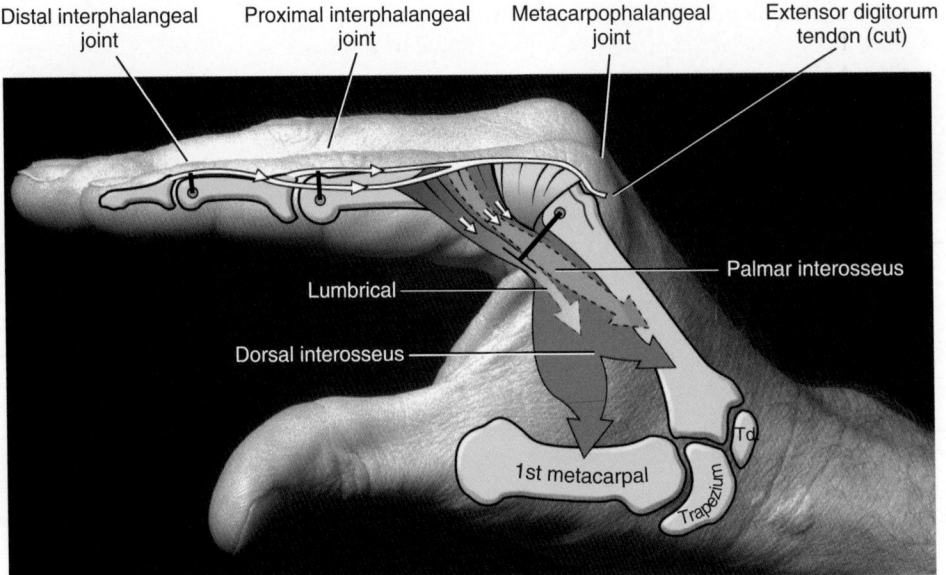

Distal interphalangeal joint
Proximal interphalangeal joint
Metacarpophalangeal joint
Extensor digitorum tendon (cut)

Palmar interosseus
Lumbrical
Dorsal interosseus

1st metacarpal
Td
Trapezium

FIGURE 8.48 The combined actions of the lumbricals and interossei are shown as flexors at the metacarpophalangeal joint and extensors at the interphalangeal joints. The lumbrical is shown with the greatest moment arm for flexion at the metacarpophalangeal joint. The medial-lateral axis of rotation at each joint is shown as a small circle. Moment arms are depicted as thick black lines, originating at each axis of rotation. *Td,* trapezoid bone.

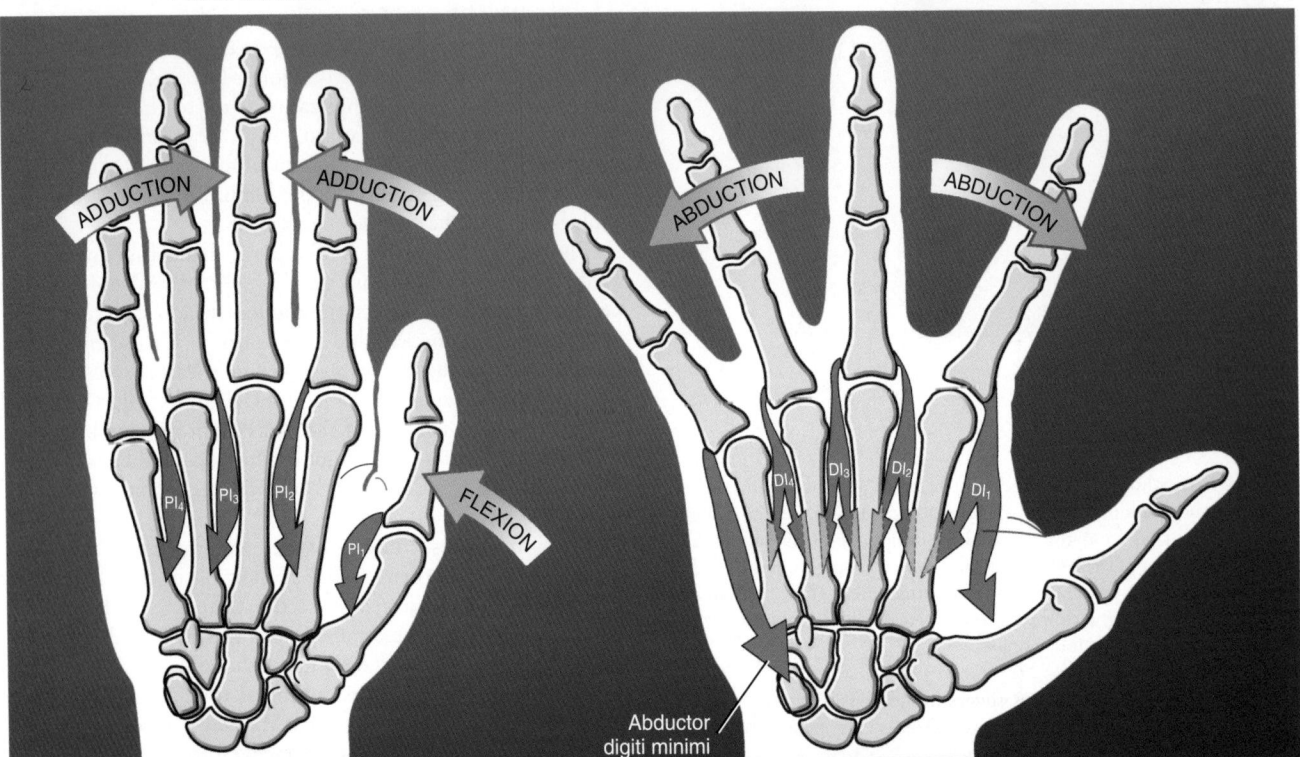

Palmar interossei
Dorsal interossei

ADDUCTION
ADDUCTION
ABDUCTION
ABDUCTION

PI₄ PI₃ PI₂ PI₁
FLEXION

DI₄ DI₃ DI₂ DI₁

Abductor digiti minimi

FIGURE 8.49 A palmar view of the frontal plane action of the palmar interossei (PI_1 to PI_4) and dorsal interossei (DI_1 to DI_4) at the metacarpophalangeal joints of the hand. The abductor digiti minimi is shown abducting the small finger.

times greater than that of the interosseus muscles within the hand and eight times greater than that of the biceps brachii muscle.[125] This large density of muscle spindles in the lumbricals suggests a role in providing sensory feedback during complex movements.[127,159] By also attaching to the tendons of the flexor digitorum profundus, perhaps the lumbricals are in position to help coordinate the interactions between the intrinsic and extrinsic muscles.

The *interosseus muscles* are named according to their general location between the metacarpal bones (see Figs. 8.4 and 8.5). As with the lumbricals, variations in attachments and morphology are more the rule than the exception.[38,142] In general, the interossei act at the MCP joints to spread the digits apart (abduction) or bring them together (adduction).

The four *palmar interossei* of the hand are slender, typically single-headed muscles that occupy the palmar region of the interosseous spaces. The three palmar interossei to the fingers have their proximal attachments on the palmar surfaces and sides of the second, fourth, and fifth metacarpals (see Fig. 8.43). The muscles' distal attachments vary but typically include the oblique fibers of the dorsal hood, and the sides of the bases of the proximal phalanges.[38] These muscles *adduct* the second, fourth, and fifth MCP joints toward the midline of the hand (Fig. 8.49). The palmar interosseus muscle to the thumb is typically small and often poorly defined.[111] This deep muscle has its distal attachment on the ulnar side of the proximal phalanx of the thumb, and often attaches to a sesamoid bone at the MCP joint.[142] Although controversy exists in the anatomic literature, the first palmar interosseus may be a small part of the oblique head of the adductor pollicis.[10] Regardless of its origin, this small muscle is positioned to help flex the MCP joint of the thumb, bringing the first metacarpal toward the midline of the hand.

The four *dorsal interossei* fill the dorsal sides of the interosseous spaces (see Fig. 8.39). In contrast to the palmar interossei, the dorsal muscles have a bipennate shape. Although variations are common, the general rule is that the dorsal interossei have distal attachments to the oblique fibers of the dorsal hood, as well as to the sides of the bases of the proximal phalanges.[68,98] Some distal attachments may blend with more palmar aspects of the transverse fibers of the dorsal hood and the palmar plate.[38] The first dorsal interosseus (formerly *abductor indicis*) is the largest and most accessible for clinical inspection.[68] With the index finger well stabilized, the first dorsal interosseus can assist the adductor pollicis in *adducting* the thumb at the CMC joint. (This can be visualized by reversing the direction of the arrow of the first dorsal interosseus to the thumb in Fig. 8.48.)

As a set, the dorsal interossei *abduct* the MCP joints of the index, middle, and ring fingers away from an imaginary reference line through the middle digit (see Fig. 8.49). Abduction of the fifth MCP joint is performed by the abductor digiti minimi of the hypothenar group.

In addition to abducting and adducting the fingers, the interossei and abductor digiti minimi provide an important source of dynamic stability to the MCP joints. When the two hands shown in Fig. 8.49 are visually superimposed, it is apparent that each MCP joint of the fingers is equipped with a pair of abducting and adducting muscles. The pairs act as dynamic collateral ligaments, providing strength to the MCP joints. Acting in pairs, this interosseus musculature also controls the extent of axial rotation permitted at the MCP joints.

To varying degrees, both palmar and dorsal interossei have a line of force that passes *palmar* to the MCP joints, especially when the MCP joints are flexed. The interossei, via their attachments into the extensor mechanism, pass *dorsal* to the IP joints of the fingers (see index finger in Fig. 8.48). Like the lumbricals, therefore, contraction of the interossei flexes the MCP joints and extends the IP joints. Compared with the lumbricals, the interossei produce greater flexion torques at the MCP joints. Even though the lumbricals have the larger moment arm for this action, the overwhelmingly larger cross-sectional area of the interossei empowers them with the greater flexion torque potential. In contrast to the lumbricals, the interossei produce relatively larger forces but over a shorter contraction distance (Table 8.5).[70]

TABLE 8.5   **Selected Anatomic and Functional Comparisons between the Lumbrical and Interosseus Muscles**

	Lumbricals	Dorsal Interossei	Palmar Interossei
Innervation	Lateral: Median nerve Medial: Ulnar nerve	Ulnar nerve	Ulnar nerve
Primary distal attachments	Oblique fibers of the dorsal hood, and ultimately to the adjacent lateral band of the extensor mechanism	Oblique fibers of the dorsal hood (and ultimately to the adjacent lateral band), and to the side of the base of the proximal phalanx	Oblique fibers of the dorsal hood (and ultimately to the adjacent lateral band), and to the side of the base of the proximal phalanx
Contractile characteristics	Generate relatively small force over a relatively long distance	Generate relatively large force over a relatively short distance	Nondistinct
Primary actions	MCP joint flexion and PIP and DIP joint extension	*Abduction* of fingers; MCP joint flexion and PIP and DIP joint extension	*Adduction* of fingers; MCP joint flexion and PIP and DIP joint extension
Comments	Relatively large endowment of muscle spindles, suggesting an important source of sensory feedback to help guide movement	Distal attachments typically include bone and extensor mechanism Usually bipennate, with proximal attachments arising by two heads	Distal attachments typically include bone and extensor mechanism; usually single-headed muscles First palmar interosseus (to the thumb) may assist with flexion of MCP joint

DIP, distal interphalangeal; *MCP*, metacarpophalangeal; *PIP*, proximal interphalangeal.

Interaction of the Extrinsic and Intrinsic Muscles of the Fingers

As described in Fig. 8.48, simultaneous contraction of the intrinsic muscles of the fingers (lumbricals and interossei) produces a combined MCP joint flexion and IP joint extension. This position of the hand is referred to as the *intrinsic-plus position*. In contrast, simultaneous contraction of the extrinsic muscles of the fingers (extensor digitorum, flexor digitorum superficialis, and flexor digitorum profundus) produces MCP joint hyperextension and IP joint flexion: the *extrinsic-plus position*. The two opposite positions of the fingers are presented in Fig. 8.50. A very important kinesiologic principle of the hand is that many functional or complex digital movements require a synergistic *blending* of these two opposite actions. This point is reinforced in the next sections.

The interaction between the extrinsic and intrinsic muscles of the hand can produce many combinations of movements used to perform a seemingly infinite number of functions.[73] The following analysis, however, addresses the muscular interaction within a typical finger during two fundamental functions: *opening* and *closing of the hand*. The precise muscular interactions used to perform these actions are not completely understood, despite years of research and study based on anatomy, biomechanics, electromyography, and computer-simulated modeling.[b]

Part of the obstacle in understanding the muscular interactions is that similar movements can be performed by different combinations of muscles, both within and between persons. Precise muscular interaction also depends on the speed or power of an activity, the skill of the performer, the weight and shape of the manipulated object, and the natural variability of human movement. Of interest, much of what is absolutely known has been learned by carefully observing the pathomechanic impairments of the hand that resulted from a disruption of the neuromusculoskeletal system.

OPENING THE HAND: FINGER EXTENSION

Primary Muscular Activity

Opening the hand is often performed in preparation for grasp. The greatest resistance to extension of the fingers across the MCP and IP joints is usually not from gravity but from the viscoelastic resistance generated by the stretching of the extrinsic finger flexors. The passive "recoil" force generated within these muscles is largely responsible for the partially flexed posture of a relaxed hand.

The primary extensors of the fingers are the *extensor digitorum* and the *intrinsic muscles,* specifically the lumbricals and interossei. In general, the lumbricals show a greater and more consistent level of electromyographic (EMG) activity than the interossei during finger extension.[99]

Fig. 8.51A shows the extensor digitorum exerting a force on the extensor mechanism, pulling the MCP joint toward extension. The intrinsic muscles furnish both direct and indirect effects on the mechanics of extension of the IP joints (see Fig. 8.51B,C). The *direct effect* is provided by the proximal pull placed on the extensor mechanism; the *indirect effect* is provided by the production of a flexion torque at the MCP joint.[158] The opposing flexion torque prevents the extensor digitorum from hyperextending the MCP joint—an action that prematurely dissipates most of its contractile force. *Only with the MCP joint blocked from being hyperextended can the extensor digitorum effectively tense the extensor mechanism sufficiently to completely extend the IP joints.*

[b]16,25,48,75,82,92,99,100,112,158

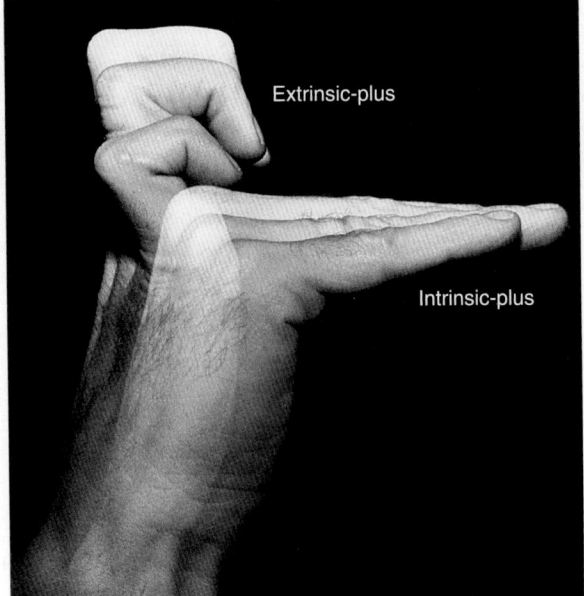

FIGURE 8.50 The extrinsic-plus and intrinsic-plus positions of the healthy hand.

The extensor digitorum and intrinsic muscles of the fingers cooperate synergistically to extend the finger. Paradoxically, it is the *opposing* actions of the extensor digitorum and the intrinsic muscles across the MCP joint that allow them to synergistically extend the IP joints. This relationship can be observed in a person with an injury of the ulnar nerve (Fig. 8.52A). With paralysis of the intrinsic muscles of the medial two fingers, activation of the extensor digitorum causes a characteristic "clawing" of the digits: the MCP joints hyperextend and the IP joints remain partially flexed.[158] This is often called the "intrinsic-minus" posture because of the lack of intrinsic-innervated muscles. (This posture is fundamentally similar to the "extrinsic-plus" posture depicted in Fig. 8.50.) Without the MCP joint flexion torque normally provided by the intrinsic muscles, the extensor digitorum functions *only* to hyperextend the MCP joints. This posture stretches the extrinsic finger flexors, thereby adding further resistance against extension of the IP joints. As shown in Fig. 8.52B, with manual application of a flexion torque across the MCP joint (i.e., a force normally furnished by the intrinsic muscles), contraction of the extensor digitorum is able to fully extend the IP joints. Blocking the MCP joint from hyperextending also slackens the extrinsic flexor tendons, thereby minimizing much of the passive resistance to extension of the IP joints. Preventing the MCP joints from hyperextending is one form of therapeutic intervention after paralysis of the intrinsic muscles of the fingers. Therapists may fabricate an orthosis that limits extension of the MCP joints; surgeons may devise a block against hyperextension by rerouting a tendon from a stronger, innervated muscle to the flexor side of the involved MCP joints.

Function of Wrist Flexors during Finger Extension

Activation of the wrist flexor muscles normally accompanies active finger extension, especially when performed rapidly. Although this activity is depicted only in the flexor carpi radialis in Fig. 8.51, other wrist flexors are also active. The wrist flexors offset the large extension potential of the extensor digitorum at the wrist. The wrist flexes slightly during rapid and complete finger extension. (Compare Fig. 8.51A with Fig. 8.51C.) Wrist flexion helps maintain optimal length of the extensor digitorum during active finger extension.

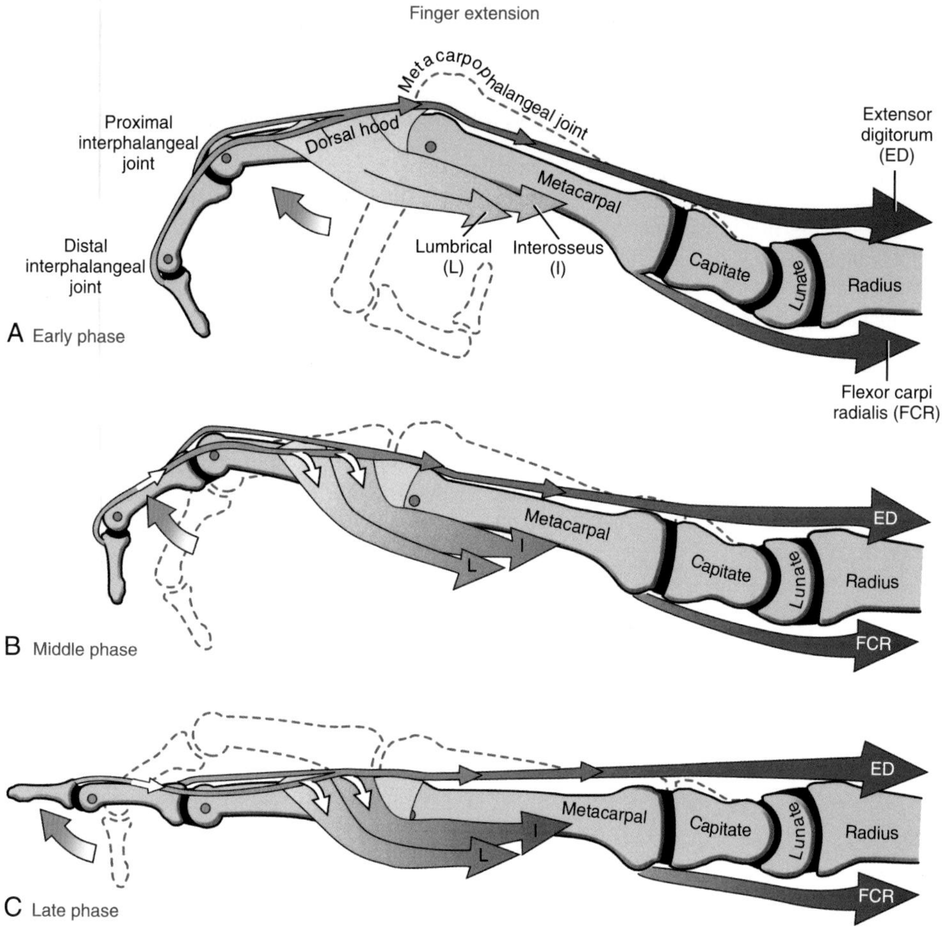

Finger extension

Proximal
interphalangeal
joint

Metacarpophalangeal joint

Dorsal hood

Metacarpal

Capitate

Lunate

Radius

Extensor
digitorum
(ED)

Distal
interphalangeal
joint

Lumbrical
(L)

Interosseus
(I)

A Early phase

Flexor carpi
radialis (FCR)

Metacarpal

Capitate

Lunate

Radius

ED

L

I

FCR

B Middle phase

Metacarpal

Capitate

Lunate

Radius

ED

L

I

FCR

C Late phase

FIGURE 8.51 A lateral view depicting the intrinsic and extrinsic muscular interactions at one finger during *full extension*. The dashed outlines depict starting positions. (A) Early phase: The extensor digitorum is shown primarily extending the metacarpophalangeal joint. (B) Middle phase: The intrinsic muscles (lumbricals and interossei) assist the extensor digitorum with extension of the proximal and distal interphalangeal joints. The intrinsic muscles also produce an opposing flexion torque at the metacarpophalangeal joint that prevents the extensor digitorum from hyperextending the metacarpophalangeal joint. (C) Late phase: Muscle activation continues through full finger extension. Note the activation in the flexor carpi radialis to slightly flex the wrist. Observe the proximal migration of the dorsal hood between flexion and full extension. (The intensity of the red indicates the relative intensity of the muscle activity.)

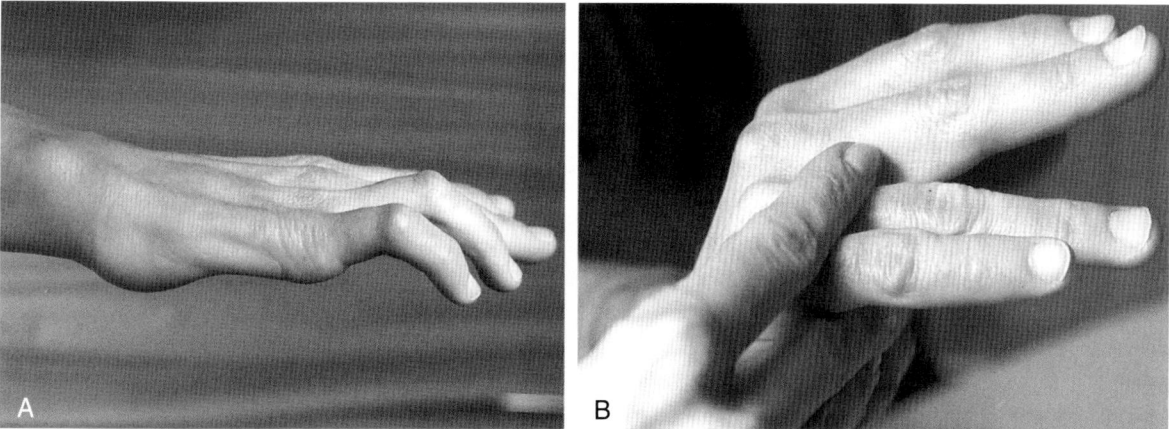

FIGURE 8.52 Attempts to extend the fingers with an ulnar nerve lesion with paralysis of most intrinsic muscles of the fingers. (A) The medial fingers show a "clawing" of the fingers: hyperextended metacarpophalangeal joints with interphalangeal joints partially flexed. Note the atrophy in the hypothenar eminence and interosseous spaces. (B) By manually holding the metacarpophalangeal joints into flexion, the extensor digitorum, innervated by the radial nerve, can fully extend the interphalangeal joints.

SPECIAL FOCUS 8.7

Oblique Retinacular Ligaments: Transfer of Passive Extension Force from the Proximal Interphalangeal Joint to the Distal Interphalangeal Joint

As depicted in Fig. 8.41, the oblique retinacular ligaments course from the palmar side of the PIP joint to the dorsal side of the distal interphalangeal (DIP) joint. Although controversy exists regarding their relative importance, their oblique direction across the PIP and DIP joints allows them to coordinate extension between these two joints.[58] The extensor digitorum and intrinsic muscles extend the PIP joint through the extensor mechanism; such an action stretches the oblique retinacular ligament (Fig. 8.53, steps 1 to 3). The passive force in the stretched oblique ligament is transferred distally, helping to *extend* the DIP joint (see Fig. 8.53, step 4). The oblique retinacular ligament is sometimes called the "link ligament," suggesting its probable role in helping to synchronize extension at both joints.

The oblique retinacular ligament may become tight because of arthritis, connective tissue disease, or trauma. Tightness in these ligaments may be associated with *Dupuytren's contracture,* a condition involving a progressive thickening and shortening of the palmar and digital fascia of the hand.[101] The condition often results in a flexed posture of the fingers, especially on the ulnar side of the hand. The oblique retinacular ligament may also be involved, resulting in an exaggerated flexion contracture at the PIP joint. Attempts at passively extending a PIP joint with a tight oblique retinacular ligament often causes the DIP joint to passively extend.

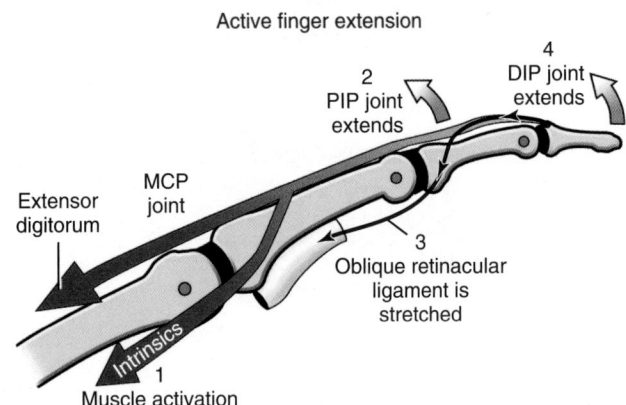

FIGURE 8.53 The transfer of passive force in the stretched oblique retinacular ligament during active extension of the finger. The numbered sequence *(1–4)* indicates the chronologic order of events.

CLOSING THE HAND: FINGER FLEXION

Primary Muscle Action

The muscles used to close the hand depend in part on the specific joints that need to be flexed, and on the force and velocity demands of the action. Flexing the fingers against resistance or at relatively high speed requires activation of the *flexor digitorum profundus, flexor digitorum superficialis,* and, to a lesser extent, the *interosseus* muscles (Fig. 8.54A). Forces produced by the flexor digitorum profundus and superficialis flex all three joints of the fingers; the flexing finger pulls the extensor mechanism distally by several millimeters.

Although typically inactive while the hand is closing, the *lumbricals* may still passively assist with this action. Recall that the lumbricals attach between the flexor digitorum profundus and the extensor mechanism. During active finger flexion, the lumbricals are stretched in a proximal direction because of the contracting flexor digitorum profundus and at the same time are stretched in a distal direction owing to the distal migration of the extensor mechanism (see Fig. 8.54B, bidirectional arrow in lumbrical). Between full extension and full active flexion, a lumbrical must stretch an extraordinary distance.[127] The stretch generates a *passive flexion torque* across the MCP joint. Although small, this passive torque may supplement the *active flexion torque* produced by the interossei and, primarily, the extrinsic flexor musculature.[91]

Injury to the ulnar nerve can cause paralysis of most of the intrinsic muscles that act on the fingers. Maximal-effort grip strength has been shown to be reduced by 38% in healthy persons who were subjected to a temporary ulnar nerve block at the level of the wrist.[84] In addition, marked paralysis of the intrinsic muscles alters the timing or sequencing of flexion across the various finger joints.[74] Normally, the PIP and DIP joints flex first, followed closely in time by flexion at the MCP joints. With paralyzed intrinsic muscles, especially if overstretched by chronic hyperextension of the MCP joints, the initiation of flexion at the MCP joints is significantly delayed. Consequently, the fingers "roll" into flexion from a distal to proximal perspective, losing the characteristic wide sweeping flexion motion apparent in normally innervated hands.[7] The resulting asynchronous flexion can interfere with the quality of grasp. The distal-to-proximal roll-up flexion pattern can push some objects out of the grasping hand.

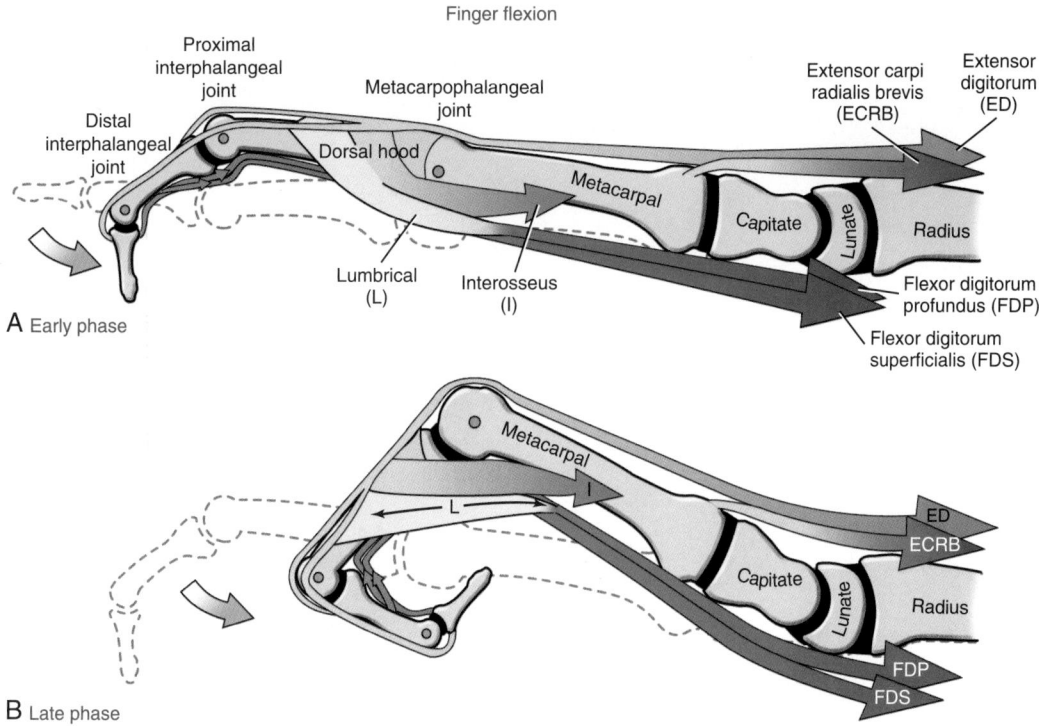

FIGURE 8.54 A side view depicting the intrinsic and extrinsic muscular interaction at one finger during a relatively "high-powered" finger *flexion*. The dashed line outlines depict the starting positions. (A) Early phase: The flexor digitorum profundus, flexor digitorum superficialis, and interosseus muscles actively flex the joints of the finger. The lumbrical is shown as being essentially inactive. (B) Late phase: Muscle activation continues essentially unchanged through full flexion. The lumbrical remains essentially inactive but is stretched across both ends. The extensor carpi radialis brevis is shown extending the wrist slightly. The extensor digitorum helps decelerate flexion of the metacarpophalangeal joint. Note the distal migration of the dorsal hood between the early and late phases of flexion. (The intensity of the red indicates the relative intensity of muscle activity.)

The extensor digitorum shows consistent EMG activity while the hand is closing.[100] This activity reflects the muscle's role as an extension brake at the MCP joint. This important stabilization function allows the long finger flexors to shift their action distally to the PIP and DIP joints. Without coactivation of the extensor digitorum, the long finger flexors exhaust most of their flexion potential over the MCP joints, reducing their potential for more refined actions at the more distal joints.

Function of Wrist Extensors during Finger Flexion
Making a strong fist requires strong synergistic activation from the wrist extensor muscles (see Fig. 8.54, extensor carpi radialis brevis). Wrist extensor activity can be verified by palpating the dorsum of the forearm while a fist is made. As explained in Chapter 7, the primary function of the wrist extensors, including the extensor digitorum, is to neutralize the strong wrist flexion tendency of the activated extrinsic finger flexor muscles (review Fig. 7.25). While the fingers are actively flexing, wrist extension also helps maintain more optimal length of the extrinsic finger flexors. If the wrist extensors are paralyzed, attempts at making a fist result in a posture of wrist flexion *and* finger flexion. When combined with the increased passive tension in the overstretched extensor digitorum, the overshortened, activated finger flexors are typically incapable of producing an effective grip (see Fig. 7.27).

THE WIDE FUNCTIONAL VERSATILITY OF THE HAND

Although 23 unique "grasps" have been defined and quantified,[71] the actual number of different functional expressions of the human hand is virtually limitless. To begin to appreciate the scope of this topic, it may be useful to consider three broad categories of hand function: *support, manipulation, and prehension.* As a *support,* the hand can act in a nonspecific manner to brace or stabilize an object, often freeing the other hand for a more specific task. The hand may also be used as a simple platform to transfer or accept forces, such as when supporting the head when tired or to assist in standing from a seated position.

Functions of the Hand
- Support
- Manipulation
  - Repetitive and blunt
  - Continuous and fluid
- Prehension used during grip and pinch
  - Power grip
  - Precision grip
  - Power (key) pinch
  - Precision pinch
  - Hook grip

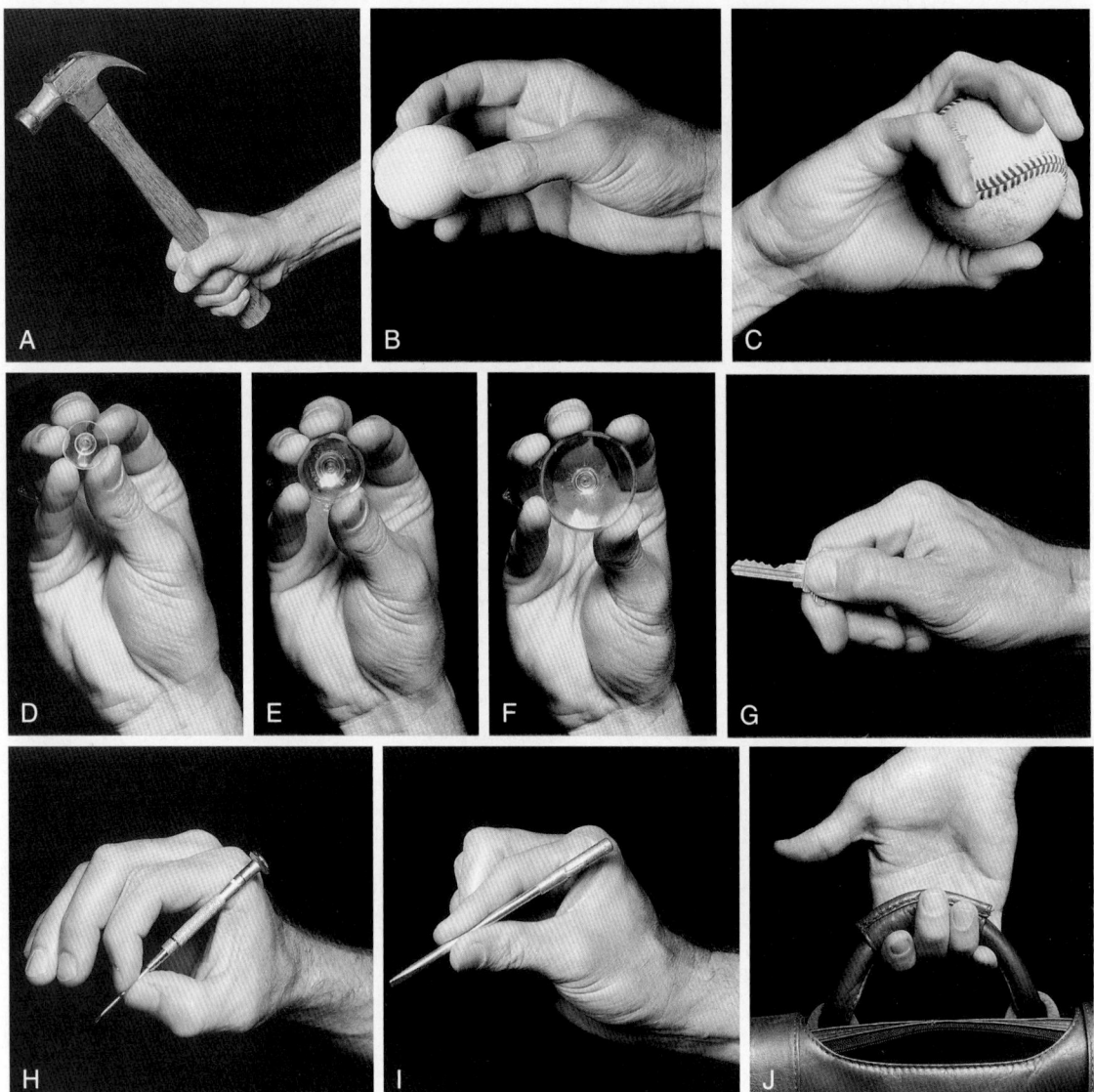

FIGURE 8.55 A healthy hand is shown performing common types of prehension functions. (A) Power grip. (B) Precision grip to hold an egg. (C) Precision grip to throw a baseball. (D–F) Modifications of the precision grip by altering the concavity of the distal transverse arch. (G) Power key pinch. (H) Tip-to-tip prehension pinch. (I) Pad-to-pad prehension pinch. (J) Hook grip.

Perhaps the most varied function of the hand is its ability to *manipulate* objects. In a very general sense, the hand manipulates objects in two fundamental ways: digital motions may be *repetitive* and *blunt*, such as texting, typing, or scratching, or, in contrast, *continuous* and *fluid*, in which the rate and intensity of motion is controlled, such as when writing or sewing. And, of course, many, if not most, types of digital manipulations combine both ways of movement.

Prehension describes the ability of the fingers and thumb to grasp or to seize, often for holding, securing, and picking up objects. Several different terms have evolved over the years to describe the many forms of prehension.[89,116,143] Many forms of prehension can be described as a *grip* (or grasp), in which all digits are used, or as a *pinch,* in which primarily the thumb and index finger are used. Each form can be further classified based on the need for *power* (loosely defined as high force with less regard to

the exactness of the task) or *precision* (i.e., high level of exactness with low force). The specific classifications of prehension subsequently described are not intended to include *all* possible ways that the hand can be used. These definitions are nevertheless useful to establish a common reference for clinical communication and research.

Basically, most types of prehension activities fall into one of the following five types:

1. The *power grip* is used when stability and large forces are needed, without the need for precision. The shape of held objects tends to be spherical or cylindrical. Using a hammer is a good example of a power grip (Fig. 8.55A). This activity requires strong forces from the finger flexors, especially from the fourth and fifth digits; intrinsic muscles of the fingers, especially the interossei; and the thumb adductor and flexor muscles. Wrist extensors are needed to stabilize the wrist.

2. The *precision grip* is used when control and/or delicate action is needed during prehension, often involving a spheroidal shape (see Fig. 8.55B,C). The thumb is usually held partially abducted, and the fingers partially flexed. The precision grip uses the thumb and one or more of the digits to improve grip security or, if needed, to add variable amounts of force. Clinically, the term *three-point pinch* (or three-jaw chuck) specifically describes when the index and middle fingers meet the thumb. The precision grip can be modified to fit objects of varied sizes by altering the contour of the distal transverse arch of the hand (see Fig. 8.55D–F).

3. The *power (key) pinch* (also referred to as lateral pinch) is used when large forces are needed to stabilize an object between the thumb and the lateral border of the index finger (see Fig. 8.55G). The power pinch is an extremely useful form of prehension, combining the force of the adductor pollicis and first dorsal interosseus with the dexterity and sensory acuity of the thumb and index finger.

4. The *precision pinch* is used to provide fine control to objects held between the thumb and index finger, without the need for high power. This type of pinch has many forms, such as the *tip-to-tip* or *pad-to-pad* method of holding an object (see panels H and I, respectively, of Fig. 8.55). The tip-to-tip pinch is used especially for tiny objects when skill and precision are required. The pad-to-pad pinch provides greater surface area for contact with larger objects, thereby increasing prehensile security.

5. The *hook grip* is a form of prehension that does not involve the thumb. A hook grip is formed by the partially flexed PIP and DIP joints of the fingers, held in position primarily by the flexor digitorum profundus.[48] This grip is often used in a static manner for prolonged periods of time, such as holding a luggage strap (see Fig. 8.55J).

JOINT DEFORMITIES TYPICALLY CAUSED BY RHEUMATOID ARTHRITIS

One of the more destructive aspects of advanced rheumatoid arthritis is chronic synovitis. Over time, synovitis can reduce the tensile strength of the periarticular connective tissues. Adequate tensile strength in these tissues is critical to withstanding the nearly constant volley of forces that arise from external contact with the environment and, more significantly, muscle activation. Even an action as relatively light as naturally striking a computer keyboard can generate more than 11 N (about 2.5 lb) of force across the MCP joint of the finger.[22] Without adequate restraint provided by healthy periarticular connective tissues, these forces and others that are typically much higher can eventually weaken or even destroy the mechanical integrity of the joint. When the connective tissues are weakened by a combination of disease and repetitive microtrauma, the joint structure can become misaligned, painful, unstable, and frequently deformed permanently. Knowledge of the pathomechanics of hand deformities associated with rheumatoid arthritis is a prerequisite for effective treatment. This holds true because so many traditional treatments for hand deformity address the mechanical cause of the problem.

Zigzag Deformity of the Thumb

Advanced rheumatoid arthritis often results in a zigzag deformity of the thumb. As defined in Chapter 7, a *zigzag deformity* results from the collapse of multiple interconnected joints in alternating directions. Although several combinations of deformity have been described, one relatively common deformity involves CMC joint flexion and adduction, MCP joint hyperextension, and IP joint flexion (Fig. 8.56).[11,114] In this example the collapse of the thumb starts with instability at the CMC joint. Ligaments that normally reinforce the joint, such as the anterior oblique and dorsal-radial ligaments, can become weak and completely or partially rupture because of the disease process. Subsequently the base of the thumb metacarpal dislocates off the radial or dorsal-radial edge of the trapezium (see arrow at base of first metacarpal in Fig. 8.56). Once this dislocation occurs, the adductor and short flexor muscles, which are often in spasm, hold the thumb metacarpal rigidly against the palm. In time, rheumatoid disease may cause the muscles to become fibrotic and permanently shortened, maintaining the deformity at the CMC joint. In efforts to extend the rigid thumb out of the palm, a compensatory hyperextension deformity at the MCP joint often occurs. A weakened and overstretched palmar plate at this joint offers little resistance to the extension forces produced by the extensor pollicis longus and brevis or contact forces produced during pinch. Eventual bowstringing of these tendons across the MCP joint increases their extension moment arms, thereby further contributing to the hyperextension deformity. The IP joint tends to remain flexed because of the passive tension in the stretched flexor pollicis longus.

Clinical interventions for a zigzag deformity of the thumb depend on the specific mechanics of the collapse and the severity of the underlying rheumatoid disease. Nonsurgical intervention includes orthotic intervention to encourage more normal joint

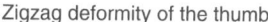

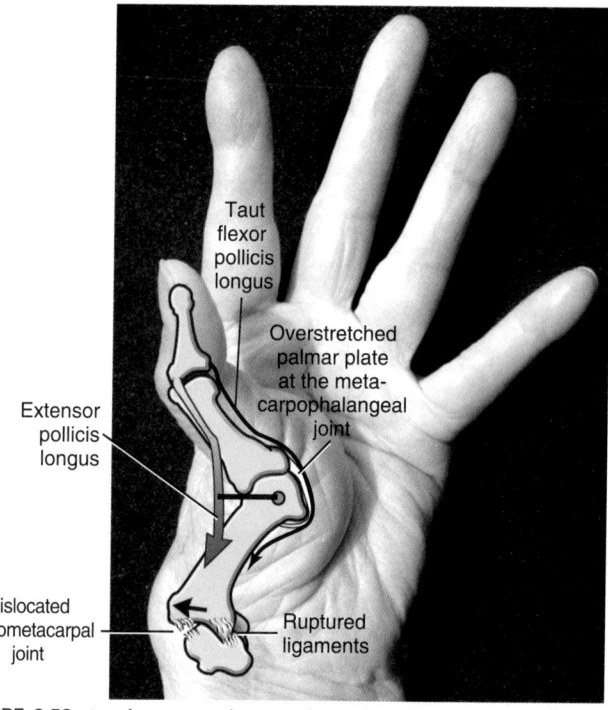

FIGURE 8.56 A palmar view showing the pathomechanics of a common zigzag deformity of the thumb caused by advanced, chronic rheumatoid arthritis. The base of the thumb metacarpal dislocates at the carpometacarpal joint *(arrow)*, initiating a series of events that lead to hyperextension at the metacarpophalangeal joint. The interphalangeal joint remains partially flexed because of the passive tension in the stretched flexor pollicis longus.

alignment, medications to reduce chronic inflammation, and patient education of ways to compensate for lost function and to minimize everyday stress on the joint.[14,83,118,119,149] Surgery may be considered if more conservative intervention fails to slow the progression of the deformity.

Destruction of the Metacarpophalangeal Joints of the Finger

Advanced rheumatoid arthritis is often associated with deformities at the MCP joint of the fingers. The two most common deformities are *palmar dislocation* and *ulnar drift* (Fig. 8.57). Although these two deformities typically occur together, they are discussed separately in the following sections.

PALMAR DISLOCATION OF THE METACARPOPHALANGEAL JOINT

When the fingers flex during grip, the tendons of the flexor digitorum superficialis and profundus are naturally deflected in a palmar direction across the MCP joint (Fig. 8.58A). This natural bend generates a bowstringing force in the palmar direction. As indicated in Fig. 8.58A, the bowstringing force is transferred through much of the MCP joint's periarticular connective tissue: from flexor A₁ pulley, palmar plate, collateral ligaments, and, finally, to posterior tubercle of the metacarpal head. The greater the degree of flexion at the MCP joint, the greater the

magnitude of the bowstringing force. In the healthy hand, this force is safely dissipated throughout the natural elasticity and strength of the tissues.

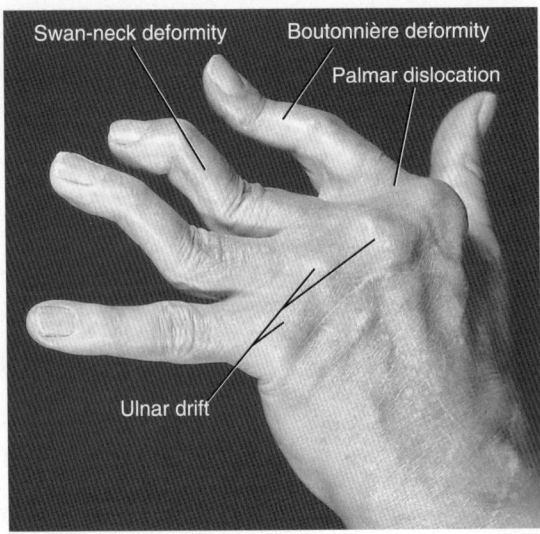

FIGURE 8.57 A hand showing the common deformities caused by severe rheumatoid arthritis. Particularly evident are the following: *palmar dislocation* of the metacarpophalangeal joint; *ulnar drift; swan-neck deformity;* and *boutonnière deformity.* See text for further details. (Courtesy Teri Bielefeld, PT, CHT: Zablocki VA Hospital, Milwaukee, WI.)

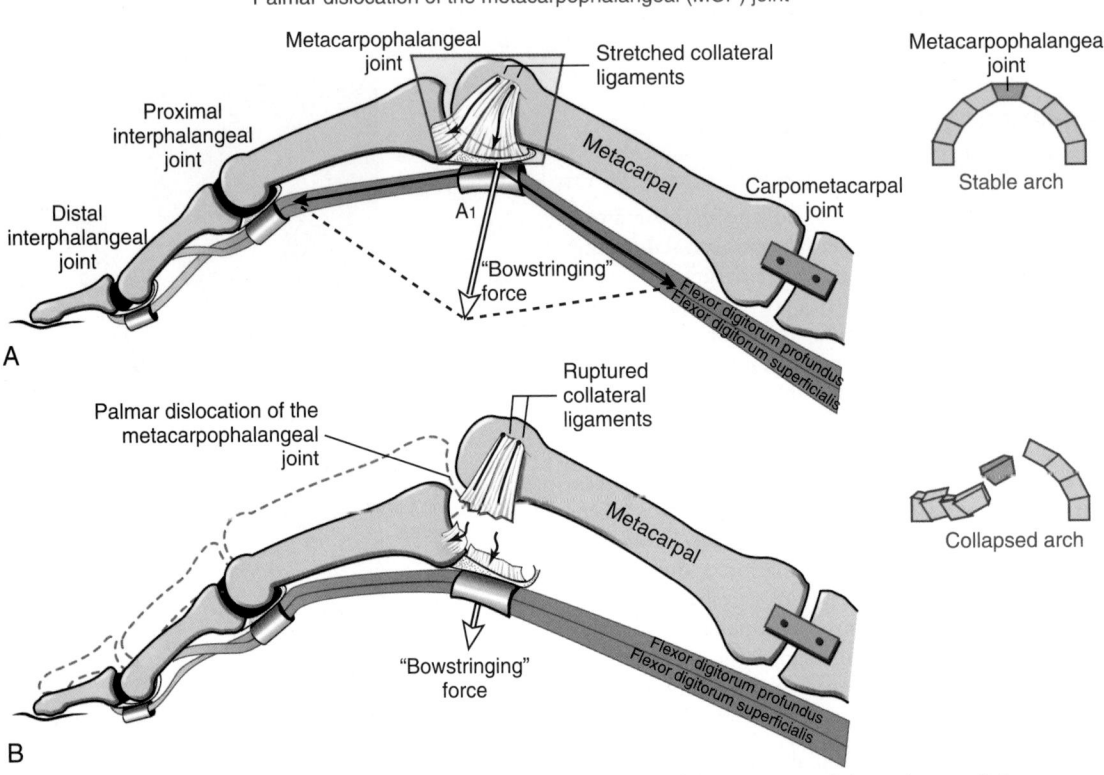

FIGURE 8.58 Pathomechanics of progressive palmar dislocation of the metacarpophalangeal joint of the finger. (A) The bend in the activated flexor tendons across the metacarpophalangeal joint produces a palmar-directed, bowstringing force against the joint. In the healthy hand, the passive tension in the stretched collateral ligaments adequately resists the palmar pull on the joint structures. (B) In a finger with advanced rheumatoid arthritis, the bowstringing force can rupture the weakened collateral ligaments. As a result, the proximal phalanx may eventually dislocate in a palmar direction.

In the hand with severe rheumatoid arthritis, the collateral ligaments may rupture because of the constant bowstringing force. In time, the proximal phalanx may translate excessively in a palmar direction, resulting in a completely dislocated MCP joint (see Fig. 8.58B). Palmar dislocation may collapse both the longitudinal and the transverse arches of the hand, causing it to appear relatively flat.

Patient education on ways to "protect" the MCP joint from further palmar dislocation is an important part of treatment.[13] Patients are instructed on how to perform functional activities that place limited demands on their finger flexor muscles.

ULNAR DRIFT

Ulnar "drift" deformity at the MCP joint consists of an excessive ulnar deviation and ulnar translation (slide) of the proximal phalanx. This deformity is common in advanced stages of rheumatoid arthritis and often occurs in conjunction with a palmar dislocation of the MCP joint (as indicated in Fig. 8.57).

To fully understand the pathomechanics of ulnar drift, it is important to realize that all hands—healthy or otherwise—are constantly subjected to factors that favor an ulnar-deviated posture of the fingers.[13,44,147] These factors include the force of gravity, an asymmetric slope of the metacarpal heads, and the prevailing ulnar (medial) line of pull of the extrinsic flexor tendons as they pass the MCP joints. But perhaps the most influential factor stems from the relentless, ulnar-directed forces applied against the proximal phalanges of the radial fingers. These forces are produced by contact from handheld objects and large "pinching" forces generated by the flexor muscles of the thumb. Fig. 8.59A shows these ulnar-directed forces pushing the index finger in an ulnar direction. The subsequent ulnar deviation of the MCP joint increases the ulnar deflection—or bend—in the extensor digitorum (ED) tendon as its crosses the dorsal side of the joint. The deflection creates a potentially destabilizing bowstringing force on the tendon. In the healthy hand, however, the transverse fibers of the dorsal hood and radial collateral ligament maintain the extensor tendon *over* the axis of rotation, thereby protecting the joint from drifting further into ulnar deviation.

The previous description reinforces the important role that healthy connective tissue plays in maintaining the stability of a joint. Often, in severe cases of rheumatoid arthritis, the transverse fibers of the dorsal hood rupture or overstretch, allowing the tendon of the extensor digitorum to slip toward the *ulnar* side of the joint's axis of rotation (see Fig. 8.59B). In this position, the force produced by the extensor digitorum acts with a moment arm that amplifies the ulnar-deviated posture. This situation initiates a self-perpetuating process: the greater the ulnar deviation, the greater the associated moment arm, and the greater the deforming ulnar deviation torque. In time, a weakened and overstretched radial collateral ligament may also rupture, allowing the proximal phalanx to rotate and slide in an ulnar direction, leading to complete joint dislocation. Persons with severe ulnar drift that affects multiple fingers are typically most concerned about appearance and the reduced function—especially related to pinch and power grip.[42]

Pathomechanics associated with ulnar drift at the metacarpophalangeal joint

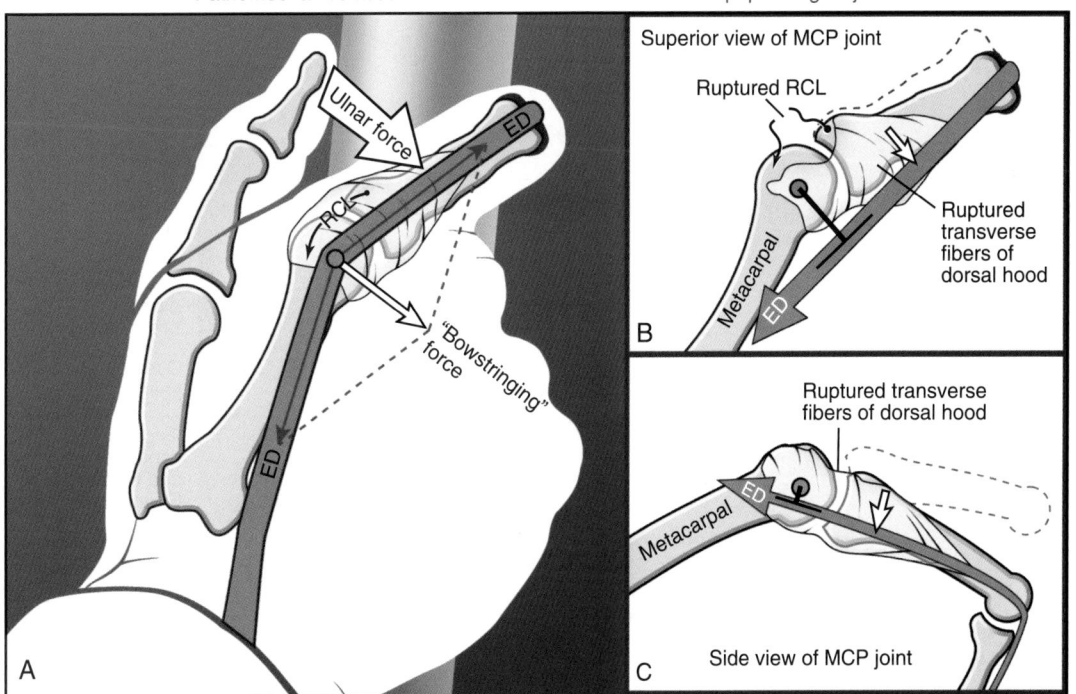

FIGURE 8.59 Pathomechanics associated with ulnar drift at the metacarpophalangeal *(MCP)* joint of the index finger. (A) Ulnar-directed forces generated primarily by the thumb produce a natural bowstringing force on the deflected tendon of the extensor digitorum *(ED)*. The radial collateral ligament *(RCL)* is shown being naturally stretched. (B) Superior view. In rheumatoid arthritis, rupture of the transverse fibers of the dorsal hood can allow the extensor tendon to migrate in an ulnar direction. (C) Side view. Once unstable, the extensor digitorum tendon may also displace *palmar* to the MCP joint. In this case the displaced tendon creates a flexion torque at the MCP joint—often favoring a palmar dislocation of the joint, in addition to the ulnar drift. The axis of rotation at each MCP joint is shown as a circle at the center of the metacarpal head. (In parts B and C, the moment arms are depicted as *thick black lines* originating at the axis of rotation.)

The pathomechanics of ulnar drift often involve a secondary destabilizing process at the MCP joints. In addition to ulnar migration, the tendon of the extensor digitorum may also slip in a palmar direction into the natural "gullies" between the prominent metacarpal heads. This abnormal palmar position reduces the moment arm of the extensor digitorum for extending the MCP joint. As depicted in a side view in Fig. 8.59C, the extensor tendon may displace *palmar* to the medial-lateral axis of rotation. In this case the displaced tendon creates a flexion torque; any active attempt at extending the fingers will result in a paradoxical *flexion* at the MCP joint. These abnormal mechanics favor the palmar dislocation deformity previously described.

Treatment for ulnar drift typically includes normalizing the alignment of the joint and, when possible, minimizing the underlying mechanics that are responsible for the instability or deformity. Common nonsurgical treatment includes using orthotics and specialized assistive devices, and advising patients on how to minimize the deforming forces across the MCP joint.[13,105,149] Consider the strong ulnar deviation (external) torque placed on the MCP joints of the right hand when the lid of a jar is loosened or a pitcher of water is held. This torque may, over time, predispose or accentuate ulnar drift. In general, patients are advised to avoid most heavy gripping and forceful key pinch activities, especially during the acute inflammation or painful stage of rheumatoid arthritis.

Surgical intervention for excessive ulnar drift may include transferring the extensor digitorum tendon to the *radial* side of the MCP joint's anterior-posterior axis of rotation. In more severe cases the damaged MCP joint may be replaced with a total joint arthroplasty.[42] This usually provides relief of pain and restores some function, although the patient typically will not regain full range of motion. This surgery is often performed in conjunction with reconstruction of the joint's periarticular connective tissues. A fusion or arthroplasty of the wrist may also be indicated because the mechanics associated with a misaligned wrist can create potentially deforming forces on the MCP joint. Regardless of the specific surgery, proper postsurgical treatment is critical for successful rehabilitation. This treatment is typically provided by certified hand therapists who have specialized in hand rehabilitation.[119]

Zigzag Deformities of the Fingers

Two classic zigzag deformities of the finger can occur: swan-neck deformity and boutonnière deformity (see Fig. 8.57). The pathomechanics behind these deformities are often centered at the PIP joint and are typically, but not exclusively, associated with advanced rheumatoid arthritis. As noted in the previous photograph, these zigzag deformities often occur in conjunction with ulnar drift and palmar dislocation of the MCP joints.

SWAN-NECK DEFORMITY

Swan-neck deformity is characterized by hyperextension of the PIP joint with flexion at the DIP joint (see Fig. 8.57, middle finger). The intrinsic muscles within the fingers affected by rheumatoid arthritis

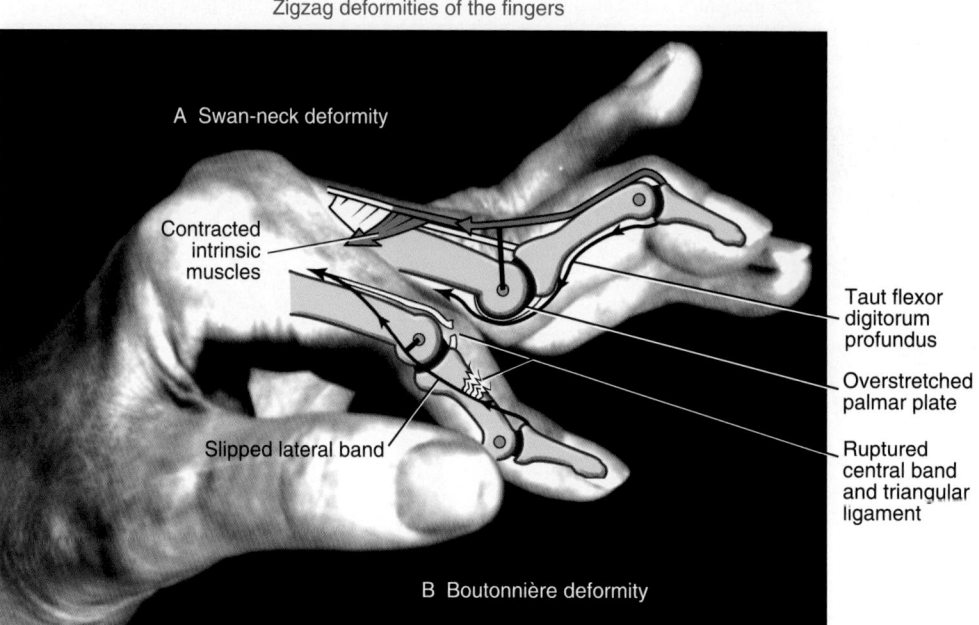

FIGURE 8.60 Two common zigzag deformities of the finger with severe rheumatoid arthritis. (A) The middle finger shows the pathomechanics of the *swan-neck deformity*. The contracted intrinsic muscle—such as a lumbrical or a second dorsal interosseus muscle (in red)—is creating an extension torque on the proximal interphalangeal (PIP) joint. Over time, the weakened palmar plate becomes overstretched, allowing the PIP joint to deform into severe hyperextension. The moment arm used by the extensor mechanism is shown as a black line originating at the axis of rotation at the PIP joint. The distal interphalangeal (DIP) joint remains partially flexed because of the increased passive tension in the stretched flexor digitorum profundus tendon. (B) The index finger depicts the pathomechanics of the *boutonnière deformity*. The central band and triangular ligament have ruptured, causing the lateral bands to slip in a *palmar* direction relative to the PIP joint; thus the joint loses its only means of extension. The moment arm used by the slipped lateral bands is shown as a short black line originating at the axis of rotation at the PIP joint. The DIP joint remains hyperextended because of increased passive tension in the taut lateral bands.

may become fibrotic and contracted. With weakened palmar plates at the PIP joint, the tension within the intrinsic muscles may eventually collapse the PIP joints into hyperextension (Fig. 8.60A). The hyperextended position of the PIP joint causes the lateral bands of the extensor mechanism to bowstring *dorsally,* away from the joint's axis of rotation. Bowstringing increases the moment arm for the intrinsic muscles to extend the PIP joint, thereby accentuating the hyperextension deformity. The DIP joint tends to remain flexed because of the stretch placed on the tendon of the flexor digitorum profundus across the PIP joint.

Although swan-neck deformity is typically associated with rheumatoid arthritis, it also can develop from trauma to the palmar plate at the PIP joint, or from spasticity or chronic hypertonus of the intrinsic muscles of the fingers, such as in persons with cerebral palsy. Regardless of cause, treatment typically involves orthotic intervention to block hyperextension of the PIP joint, or surgery to repair the palmar plate or to implant a total joint arthroplasty.[39,47,130]

BOUTONNIÈRE DEFORMITY

The *boutonnière deformity* is described as flexion of the PIP joint and hyperextension of the DIP joint (see Fig. 8.57, index finger). (The term *boutonnière*—a French word meaning buttonhole—describes the appearance of the head of the proximal phalanx as it slips through the "buttonhole" created by the displaced lateral bands.) The interphalangeal joints collapse essentially in a reciprocal pattern to that described for the swan-neck deformity. The primary cause of the boutonnière deformity typically involves a rupture or attenuation of the central band of the extensor mechanism along with the triangular ligament that interconnects the lateral bands (review normal anatomy in Fig. 8.40).[53] The weakness of these structures is often the result of chronic synovitis involving the PIP joint but may also occur from direct trauma. Rupture of the triangular ligament allows the lateral bands to slip toward the palmar side of the axis of rotation at the PIP joint (see Fig. 8.60B). Consequently, forces transferred across the slipped lateral bands (either from active

---

 SPECIAL FOCUS 8.8

Instability of the Metacarpophalangeal Joint: Additional Pathomechanics Associated with Instability of the Wrist

From a proximal to distal perspective, the wrist-and-hand unit consists of six major articulations. Such a long, continuous series of links is inherently mechanically unstable. Often, instability at a more proximal joint predisposes instability at a more distal joint: the so-called "zigzag" deformity. One classic zigzag deformity associated with the wrist and hand involves *ulnar drift of the metacarpophalangeal (MCP) joints and excessive radial deviation of the wrist.*

As a background to this discussion, recall that the potentially deforming ulnar-directed "bowstringing" force across the dorsum of the MCP joints is naturally minimized by the central alignment of the tendons of the extensor digitorum. This is illustrated in Fig. 8.61A. Instability of the wrist, however, can change the alignment between the extensor tendons and the MCP joints. As a possible

sequela of either chronic inflammation or trauma, the entire carpus may shift (or translocate) in an ulnar direction (Fig. 8.61B).[5] (These pathomechanics were described in Chapter 7.) The ulnar shift increases the moment arms of the radial deviator muscles of the wrist. Over time, therefore, the carpus and metacarpals may assume a more *radially rotated* position.[13] As depicted in Fig. 8.61C, the radially positioned metacarpals accentuate the ulnar bowstringing torque across the MCP joints. If the extensor mechanism cannot stabilize the tendons of the extensor digitorum, the tendons migrate in an ulnar direction, gaining moment arm length (as shown on the index finger), which fuels the MCP joint's ulnar drift pathomechanics. Surgeons and therapists need to consider these pathomechanics as part of the assessment and treatment for ulnar drift.

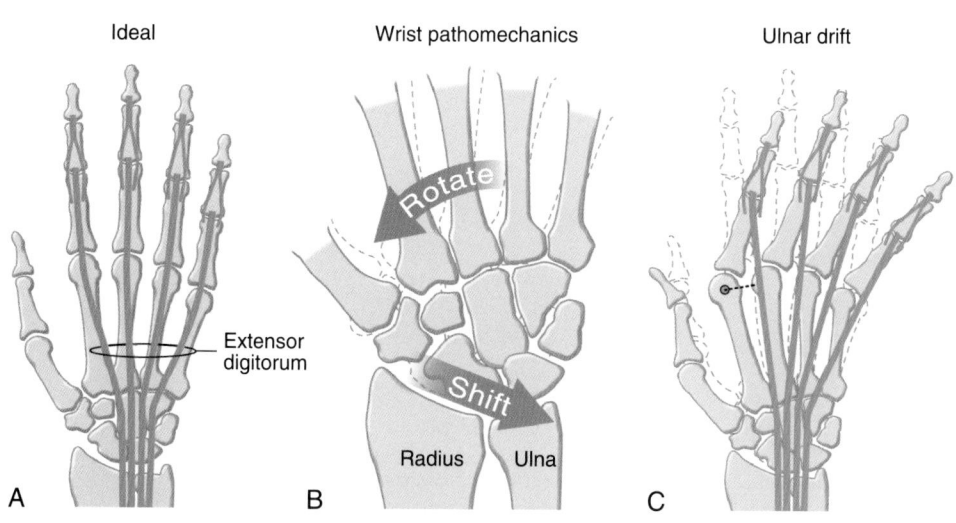

FIGURE 8.61 (A) In the ideal or normal wrist, the tendons of the extensor digitorum are centrally maintained over or close to the dorsal side of the metacarpophalangeal (MCP) joints. (B) Because of the natural *ulnar tilt* of the distal radius, compressive forces that cross a weakened wrist can eventually shift the carpus in an ulnar direction. The altered mechanics often cause the distal wrist and metacarpals to rotate in a radial direction. (C) Pathomechanics of the wrist ultimately leading to excessive ulnar drift of the MCP joints. The axis of rotation and increased moment arm for ulnar deviation are depicted for the index finger. (Figure from Bielefeld TB, Neumann DA: The unstable metacarpophalangeal joint in rheumatoid arthritis: anatomy, pathomechanics, and physical rehabilitation considerations, *J Orthop Sports Phys Ther* 35:502, 2005.)

or from passive sources) cause *flexion* at the PIP joint instead of normal extension. Essentially, the PIP joint loses all muscular sources of extension, which can be functionally significant given the relatively large range of motion normally required at this joint.[8]

As depicted in Fig. 8.60, the DIP joint in the boutonnière deformity remains hyperextended because of the increased tension in the stretched lateral bands. The inability to flex the DIP joint interferes with the ease of picking up small objects, such as a coin from a table.

Early boutonnière deformity may be treated conservatively by splinting the PIP joint in extension or by using corticosteroid injections.[130,155] Surgery may be required to repair the central band and/or realign the lateral bands dorsal to the PIP joint.[39,47,165]

SYNOPSIS

The kinesiology of the hand is as fascinating as it is complex. On careful observation, it becomes clear that all 19 bones and 19 joints are morphologically different, and therefore each possesses a unique function.

The joints of the hand are organized into three sets of articulations: CMC, MCP, and IP. The *CMC* joints form the functional transition between the wrist and the hand. Located most proximally within the hand, these joints are fundamentally responsible for adjusting the curvature of the palm, from flat to deeply cup-shaped. The more peripheral CMC joints of the hand are particularly important in this regard because they allow the thumb to approach the tips of the other digits and they raise the ulnar border of the hand. In collaboration with the more stable second and third CMC joints, the peripheral joints allow the hand to securely hold a near-infinite number of irregularly curved shapes. Very specialized muscles, such as the opponens pollicis and opponens digiti minimi, are dedicated solely to controlling the first and fifth CMC joints. Trauma or disease involving these joints can deprive the hand of many postures that are unique to human prehension.

The relatively large *MCP* joints are stabilized by an elaborate set of periarticular connective tissues—a necessity, considering that each joint must support the weight of an entire set of phalanges. In addition, the MCP joints are subjected to particularly high loads as they function as the keystones for both the longitudinal and the distal transverse arches of the hand. Specialized tissues such as palmar plates and thickened collateral ligaments are required to stabilize these articulations while simultaneously permitting a relatively wide arc of movement. Trauma and disease, such as advanced or chronic rheumatoid arthritis, can lead to instability of the MCP joints, which can disrupt the mechanical integrity of the entire hand.

Although the MCP joint of the thumb is limited primarily to flexion and extension, the MCP joints of the fingers move in two degrees of freedom. The combined motions of abduction and extension of the fingers, for example, maximize the breadth of the hand, which is especially useful for holding broad objects of varying curvatures. The fit of the object within the hand is further enhanced by the mobility profile expressed across all CMC joints, and by the passive, axial rotation permitted by the MCP joints.

The *IP joints* of the hand are located most distally within the upper extremity and therefore are most frequently in physical contact with surrounding objects. The distal pads of the digits, therefore, are soft to dampen contact forces; the distal digits also contain a very high density of sensory receptors, maximizing tactile sensitivity. Ironically, although the IP joints are most intimately involved with manipulation and grasp, they possess the most elementary kinematics of the digits. The IP joints flex and extend only; the other potential planes of motion are blocked by the bony fit of the joint and by periarticular connective tissues. The functional potential of the IP joints therefore is highly dependent on the more complex kinematics permitted in the more proximal joints of the hand.

Flexion range of motion is nevertheless extensive at the IP joints—from 70 degrees at the IP joint of the thumb to 120 degrees at the more ulnar located proximal interphalangeal joints of the fingers. Such motion is needed to fully close the fist, hold a handbag, or otherwise maximize digital contact with objects. Full extension at these joints is equally important to open the hand in preparation for grasp.

Located most distally, the IP joints are vulnerable to direct trauma, such as a lacerated tendon or a fracture within the joint. Such injuries can significantly reduce the functional mobility of the IP joints. Also, spastic paralysis from injury to the central nervous system can reduce the control over movement of the IP joints. Regardless of the cause, reduced control or loss of mobility of the IP joints can significantly minimize the functional potential of the hand.

The 29 muscles of the hand have been classified into extrinsic and intrinsic groups, primarily to facilitate anatomic organization. The muscular kinesiology, however, is based more on the functional interaction and synergy *between* the two groups. It is rare that an isolated contraction of single extrinsic or intrinsic muscle produces a meaningful movement. A simple example supporting this premise is related to the kinesiology of extending the finger. One could assume that a muscle bearing the name *extensor digitorum* would independently perform this action. This is not the case; isolated contraction of the extensor digitorum only hyperextends the MCP joints, causing the proximal and distal IP joints to collapse into

flexion. As described earlier in this chapter, simultaneous extension of all three joints of the fingers requires a coordinated interplay among the extensor digitorum *and* the intrinsic muscles, such as the lumbricals and interossei. More complex and rapid movements of the digits demand an even greater functional interdependence between the intrinsic and extrinsic muscles.

Valuable insights into the normal kinesiology of the hand can be discovered by carefully studying the pathomechanics after trauma, disease, or muscle paralysis. Typically the pathomechanics—and often the resulting deformity—reflect the *loss* of a critical force once supplied by muscle or connective tissue. Restoring kinetic balance to the region is often a major component underlying surgical and therapeutic intervention for impairments of the hand. The hand surgeon, for example, may route the tendon of the extensor digitorum more radially over the MCP joints to overcompensate for an exaggerated "ulnar drift" posture; the therapist, for example, may devise an orthotic device that prevents unwanted hyperextension of the MCP joints after paralysis of interosseus and lumbrical muscles—in essence, replacing the force otherwise produced by these now paralyzed muscles.

In closing, it is important to consider that the intent of most movements routinely performed throughout the upper limb relates indirectly or directly to optimizing prehension. Disease or injury that incapacitates the hand, therefore, significantly reduces the demands placed on the entire limb. This becomes apparent in a person with a severe hand injury who invariably develops observable disuse muscle atrophy and restriction of movement as far proximally as the shoulder. This strong functional association between the hand and the entire upper limb should be considered during all clinical assessments of the upper limb.

ADDITIONAL CLINICAL CONNECTIONS

CONTENTS

CLINICAL CONNECTION 8.1

"Tendon Transfer" Surgery to Restore Kinetic Balance and Function to the Partially Denervated Hand: A Look at Some Underlying Kinesiology

The median, ulnar, and radial nerves are all vulnerable to injury as they course throughout the upper limb. The nerves may be severely compressed or stretched, lacerated by fractured bone, or penetrated by foreign objects, including glass, knives, and bullets. These same nerves may also be involved in neuropathies. Injury or pathology involving these peripheral nerves can cause varying degrees of muscular paralysis, loss of sensation, and trophic changes in the skin.

The resulting impairments of a peripheral nerve injury or neuropathy can have devastating functional effects on the involved region of the body. Especially with peripheral nerve injuries, certain muscular actions of the wrist and hand may be completely lost. Furthermore, the skin in the associated region becomes vulnerable to injury because of the loss of sensation. Selective muscular paralysis results in a kinetic imbalance across the joint or joints, thereby increasing the likelihood of deformity. Consider, for example, a complete laceration of the median nerve at the level of the wrist. Paralysis of the muscles of the thenar eminence can disable the important movement of opposition of the thumb. Without therapeutic intervention, the thumb metacarpal may also develop an adduction and lateral rotation contracture because of the unopposed pull of (1) the ulnar nerve–innervated adductor pollicis and (2) the radial nerve–innervated extensor pollicis longus. Such a deformity is the antithesis of the position of opposition.

Injury to the major nerves of the upper limb often results in a predictable pattern of muscle paralysis, sensory loss, and potential deformity. (Neuroanatomic illustrations such as that contained in Appendix II, Part C can serve as useful guides for anticipating which muscles may be paralyzed after a nerve injury.) Regeneration of an injured nerve with return of motor and sensory function is physiologically possible; however, the extent of neuronal growth depends on several factors, including the continuity of the connective tissue sheath (endoneurial tube) that surrounds the individual axons. Crush and traction injuries that leave the endoneurial tube intact but destroy the axon have a better prognosis for regeneration. After a complete laceration of the axon and endoneurial tube, surgical repair of the nerve is a necessary prerequisite for regeneration. In ideal circumstances, a peripheral nerve can regenerate at a rate of about 1 mm/day (or about 1 inch/month). During this time, therapists often assume an important therapeutic role, including educating the patient about the medical condition (including the risk of injuring insensitive skin), providing the patient

with selected strengthening and stretching exercises, training the patient to compensate for persistent muscular weakness, and providing the patient with orthotic interventions to reduce deformity and assist or compensate for lost active motion.

In cases in which paralysis after nerve injury appears permanent, surgeons may perform a *"tendon transfer."* This surgical procedure reroutes the tendon of an innervated muscle in such a manner that all or parts of the lost actions of the paralyzed muscle are restored. A tendon transfer surgery is particularly indicated when paralysis significantly diminishes the performance of an important function—such as the loss of opposition of the thumb. A tendon transfer to restore opposition of the thumb is referred to as an *opponensplasty.* Although many types of opponensplasty techniques have been described, one common method involves surgically redirecting the tendon of the flexor digitorum superficialis (of the ring finger) to the thumb (Fig. 8.62A).[34] The natural split in the superficialis tendon is expanded and then the split tendon is sutured to both sides of the MCP joint of the thumb, at the point of attachment of the abductor pollicis brevis. To mimic the line of force of the paralyzed thenar muscles, the transferred tendon is secured by a connective tissue pulley to the distal attachment of the flexor carpi ulnaris muscle. The restoration of abduction and medial rotation of the thumb is essential to the success of the operation (see Fig. 8.62B). Therapists must devise creative methods to train patients to use the transferred musculotendinous unit to accomplish its new action. Training is greatly enhanced if the patient has at least partial sensation in the involved digits and if the transferred muscle is a natural synergist to the paralyzed one.

Several types of tendon transfer surgeries have been devised following injury or pathology of the nerves within the distal upper extremity.[17,151] The specific choice of surgery depends on the location and extent of nerve damage, the loss of function, the amount of residual sensation, and the passive range of motion of the involved joints. Equally important is the availability of a suitable musculotendinous unit for surgical transfer. Of particular interest to the surgeon is the transferred muscle's maximum *torque* potential. Because torque is the product of the muscle's force production and its internal moment arm, both variables need to be considered.

The relative force potential of a muscle that is considered for tendon transfer surgery can be estimated by its cross-sectional area. These data are published in the literature.[16,63,95] During

ADDITIONAL CLINICAL CONNECTIONS

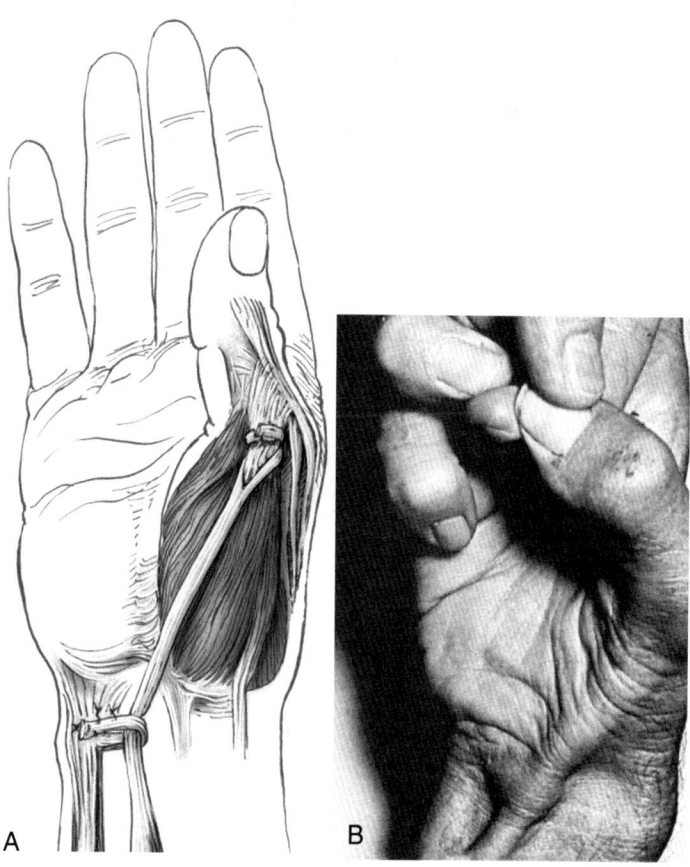

FIGURE 8.62 (A) After an injury to the median nerve at the wrist, this relatively common type of opponensplasty intends to restore at least partial opposition of the thumb. The tendon of the flexor digitorum superficialis of the ring finger has been surgically rerouted to the MCP joint of the thumb. (B) Photograph showing the results of opponensplasty. Observe the medial rotation and abduction of the thumb. The tendon of the flexor digitorum superficialis is evident under the skin. (From Hentz VR, Chase RA: *Hand surgery: a clinical atlas,* Philadelphia, 2001, Saunders.)

A

B

surgery, it is difficult to make a direct measurement of a transferred muscle's *moment arm* about a joint, for a given action. This variable of leverage, however, is very important. To optimize the functional results of the tendon transfer, it is often desirable that the surgeon closely match the transferred muscle's moment arm with that of the paralyzed one. As introduced in Chapter 1, two identical muscles with different moment arms will produce different kinetics and kinematics across a joint. For example, if a surgeon positions a muscle's tendon *too close* to the joint's axis of rotation, the reduced moment arm would minimize the muscle's torque potential; the operation, therefore, may fail to

match the muscle's strength to its functional demand. Alternatively, positioning the muscle's tendon *too far* from the joint's axis (i.e., creating an abnormally large moment arm) would create a situation in which a given amount of muscle shortening would produce a limited—and perhaps ineffective—amount of joint rotation.

Given the importance of knowing the transferred muscle's potential moment arm for an action, the late Dr. Paul Brand—a preeminent hand surgeon—devised a method to estimate this variable at the time of operation.[17] The power of this technique lies in its elegant simplicity: the geometric principle of a *radian*. As

Continued

Additional Clinical Connections

depicted by Fig. 8.63A, one radian (θ) is defined as the angle at the center of a circle that has an arc (s) equal to its radius (r): 1 radian equals 57.3 degrees. The concept of a radian can be extended to a rope rotating around a pulley, as shown in Fig. 8.63B. When the pulley is rotated 57.3 degrees, the rope that runs off the pulley (s) is equal to the radius of the pulley (r). (This concept can be expressed mathematically as s = θ times r.) Brand used the rope-and-pulley system as a model for a tendon and anatomic joint system, respectively; the radius of the pulley (r) is analogous to the internal moment arm of the muscle, and the rope (s) is analogous to the excursion of its tendon. At the time of surgery, Brand estimated the internal moment arm of both the transferred tendon and the tendon of the paralyzed muscle by simply measuring the excursion of the tendon as the joint was passively rotated approximately 57 degrees (see Fig. 8.63C). *After 57 degrees of joint rotation, the resulting tendon excursion (labeled s) is approximately equal to the internal moment arm available to the muscle.* Brand sutured the transferred tendon in place when the moment arm approximated

that of the tendon of the paralyzed muscle (or that established by normative data[17]). In cases in which the moment arm of the transferred muscle was not acceptable, Brand attempted to reconcile the problem by redirecting the line of pull of the tendon or by selecting another one for use in the transfer.

Brand's use of the radian to estimate a muscle's internal moment arm assumes that the curvatures of the joint surfaces are perfect spheres. Because the surfaces of most joints of the hand are only approximately spherical, these estimates contain some error. Nevertheless, the error is likely small and clinically insignificant, especially when comparing moment arm lengths of the same joint within a given patient. Using the concept of a radian to mathematically relate the excursion of a tendon to its moment arm is employed relatively often in biomechanical research.[1,19,45] The technique, commonly referred to as the "tendon-excursion method," has been used with cadaver specimens to measure the natural change in moment arm length throughout the range of motion for most muscles of the hand.[50,81,82,139]

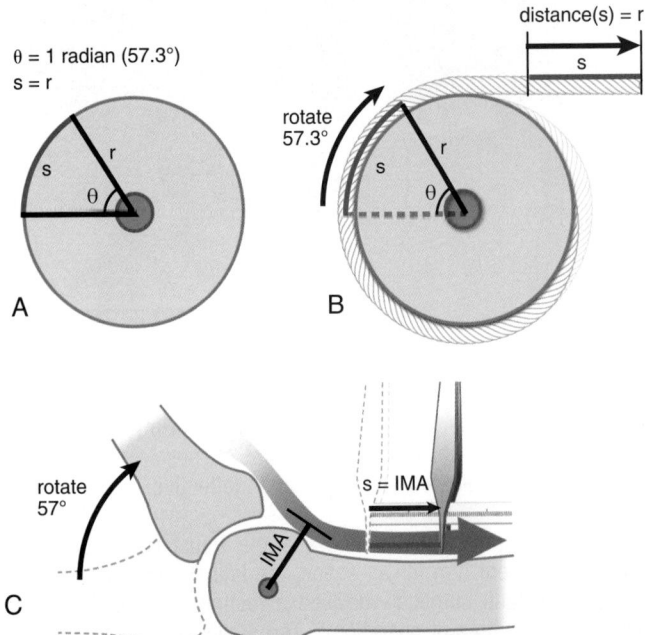

FIGURE 8.63 (A) One radian (θ) equals 57.3 degrees. The arc of the circle *(s)* formed by a radian is equal to its radius *(r)*. (This relationship can be stated mathematically: s = θ × r.) (B) The concept of the radian extended to a rope and rotating pulley. The radius of the pulley *(r)* equals s when θ = 1 radian (57.3 degrees). (C) The concept of the radian applied to an anatomic joint, such as the MCP joint. The tendon excursion *(s)* resulting from approximately 57 degrees of joint rotation is the approximate length of the internal moment arm *(IMA)*.

ADDITIONAL CLINICAL CONNECTIONS

CLINICAL CONNECTION 8.2
Biomechanical Consequences of Damaged Flexor Pulleys of the Hand

An important function of the flexor pulleys of the hand is to maintain a relatively constant moment arm length of the extrinsic flexor tendons as they cross the joints of the fingers. If the pulleys are overstretched, lacerated, or torn, the force of the contracting muscle causes the tendon to bowstring away from the joint. Bowstringing of a tendon significantly increases its moment arm and, in turn, increases the mechanical advantage of the muscle at the joint. As described in Chapter 1, increasing a muscle's mechanical advantage has two effects on joint mechanics: (1) amplification of the torque produced per level of muscle force and (2) reduction of the angular rotation of the joint per linear distance of muscle contraction. The negative clinical implication of a torn, cut, or overstretched flexor pulley primarily involves the second factor. To illustrate this effect on grasping, assume that with intact A_2, A_3, and A_4 pulleys, the moment arm of the flexor digitorum profundus tendon is about 0.75 cm at the PIP joint (Fig. 8.62A).[50] Based on the geometric principle of a *radian,* a muscle that shortens a length equal to its own moment arm at a joint will produce 1 radian (57 degrees) of joint rotation.[17] Accordingly, with intact pulleys, 1.5 cm of contraction of the flexor

digitorum profundus with a 0.75-cm moment arm would theoretically produce 114 degrees (2 radians) of PIP joint flexion. This biomechanical situation is desirable because it allows a relatively small muscle contraction to produce a relatively large rotation at the joint. A finger with cut A_2 and A_3 pulleys, as shown in Fig. 8.62B, could theoretically *double* the length of the moment arm of the flexor digitorum profundus across the PIP joint. Consequently, a muscle contraction of 1.5 cm would, in theory, produce only about 57 degrees of joint rotation (i.e., one radian)—*about half the motion produced with intact pulleys.* Assuming that the near maximal shortening range of the flexor digitorum profundus is 2 cm, a finger with a ruptured pulley will not be able to flex fully, regardless of effort.[3] Although all five annular pulleys are biomechanically important, surgeons traditionally have placed a higher priority on repairing or preserving the "major" A_2 and A_4 pulleys. Practically however, other factors must be considered, such as the structural integrity and health of the remaining or adjacent pulleys, specific goals of the surgery, and morphology of the embedded tendons.[29]

FIGURE 8.62 Pathomechanics of torn flexor pulleys. (A) With intact pulleys, the moment arm of the flexor digitorum profundus (FDP) across the proximal interphalangeal *(PIP)* joint is about 0.75 cm. Theoretically, a 1.5-cm contraction of this muscle would cause about 114 degrees (or about 2 radians) of flexion at the PIP joint. (B) A rupture of the A_2 and A_3 pulleys may increase the flexor moment arm of the FDP to 1.5 cm. A 1.5-cm contraction of the FDP would now produce only about 57 degrees of flexion of the PIP joints.

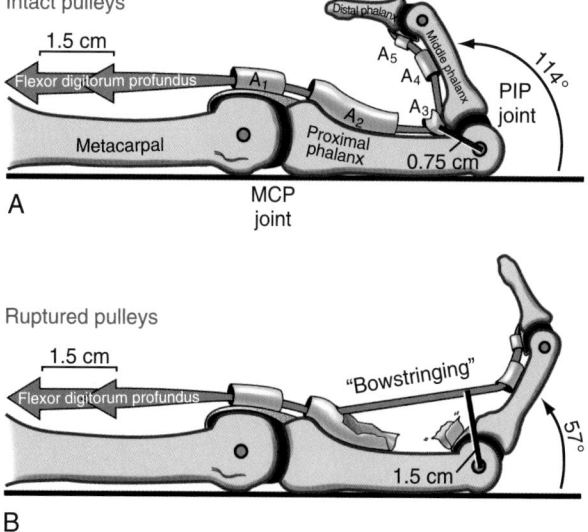

Additional Clinical Connections

CLINICAL CONNECTION 8.3

Muscular Biomechanics of a "Key Pinch": Highlighting the Demands Placed on the First Dorsal Interosseus Muscle

Pinching an object between the thumb and lateral side of the index finger is an important prehensile function, typically referred to as a "key pinch." An effective key pinch places especially large force demands on the first dorsal interosseus (FDI) muscle. (This demand can be appreciated by palpating its prominent belly during the pinch, about 2.5 cm proximal to the lateral side of the metacarpophalangeal joint of the index finger.) The FDI must generate a strong enough *abduction* force at the MCP joint of the index finger to counteract the very potent *flexion* force produced by the many muscles of the thumb. The effect of these opposing muscular forces generates a pinch force between the index finger and thumb (indicated as F_T versus F_I in Fig. 8.65). Flexion, the strongest of all thumb movements,[78] is driven primarily by the adductor pollicis, the flexor pollicis longus, and muscles within the thenar eminence. As indicated in the figure, the *internal* moment arm used by the FDI to stabilize the MCP joint of the index finger is about 1 cm. Furthermore, the pinch force generated by the thumb (F_T) against the MCP joint of the index finger acts with an *external* moment arm of about 5 cm (compare IMA and EMA in Fig. 8.65). This fivefold difference in leverage across the MCP joint requires that the FDI must produce a force about five times the pinching force applied to the distal thumb. Because many functional activities demand a pinch force that exceeds 45 N (10 lb), the FDI must therefore be able to produce an abduction force of about 225 N (50 lb, i.e., five times more than the pinch force experienced at the tips of the digits). To determine whether this is physiologically possible, first consider that as a rough estimate, skeletal muscle produces a maximum force of about 30 N/cm^2 (43.5 lb/in^2). An average-sized FDI (with a cross-sectional area of about 3.8 cm^2)[35] would therefore be expected to produce about 114 N (26 lbs) of force—only about half of the required force estimated earlier. Even based on this rough estimate, it is still likely that a maximal-effort key pinch requires greater abduction torque than what the FDI is physiologically capable of producing to stabilize the index finger. The torque deficit may be met by the second dorsal interosseus, and possibly with the assistance of the radial-positioned lumbricals of the index and middle fingers.

With an ulnar nerve lesion, the adductor pollicis muscle—the dominant pinching muscle of the thumb—and all interosseus muscles may be paralyzed. Paralysis of these muscles typically decreases key pinch by almost 80%.[84] The region around the dorsal web space becomes hollow due to atrophy in the previously mentioned muscles (Fig. 8.66). A person with an ulnar nerve lesion often relies on the flexor pollicis longus (a median nerve–innervated muscle) to partially compensate for the loss of key pinch. This compensation is evident by the increased flexion at the interphalangeal (IP) joint of the thumb—known as *Froment's sign.* Pinch remains weak, however, primarily because of the inability of the paralyzed FDI to counteract the flexor force of the flexor pollicis longus.

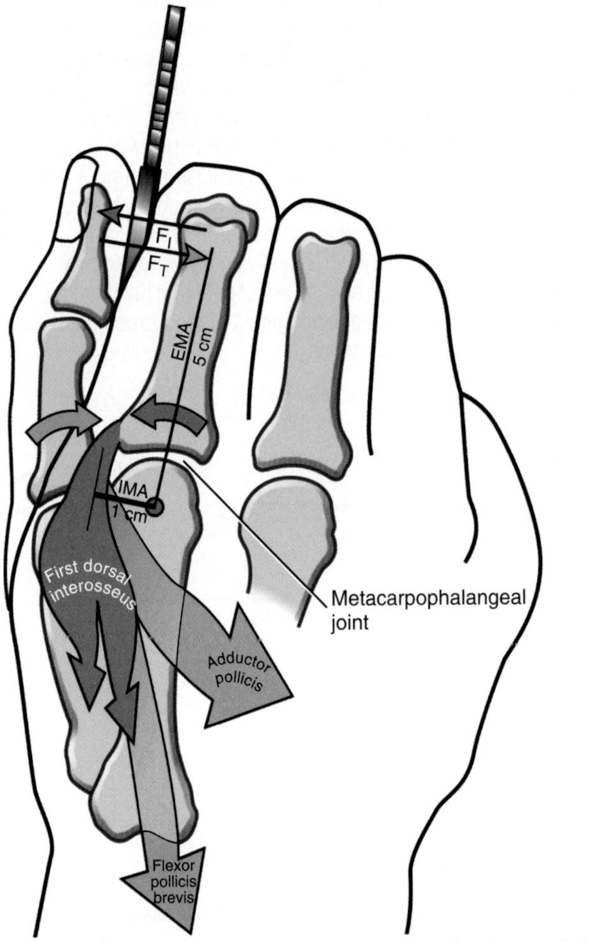

FIGURE 8.65 A dorsal view of the muscle mechanics of a "key pinch." Illustrated in lighter red, the adductor pollicis and flexor pollicis brevis are shown producing a pinch force through the thumb *(F_T)*. In dark red, the first dorsal interosseus is shown opposing the thumb's flexor force by producing a force through the index finger *(F_I)*. The external moment arm *(EMA)* at the metacarpophalangeal joint is 5 cm; the internal moment arm *(IMA)* at the metacarpophalangeal joint is 1 cm.

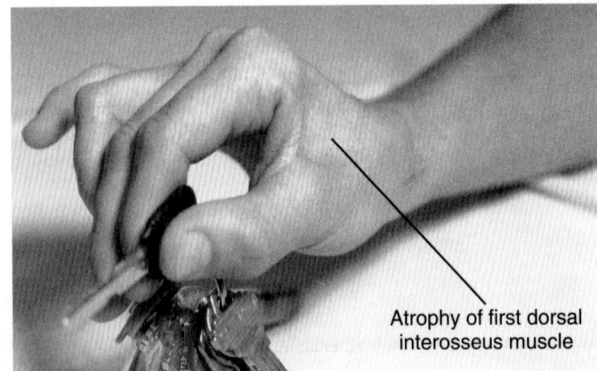

FIGURE 8.66 A person with an ulnar nerve lesion attempting to perform a key pinch. The flexion at the interphalangeal joint of the thumb is an attempt to compensate for the paralysis of the adductor pollicis muscle.

REFERENCES

1. Ackland DC, Merritt JS, Pandy MG: Moment arms of the human neck muscles in flexion, bending and rotation, *J Biomech* 44(3):475–486, 2011.
2. Adams JE, O'Brien V, Magnusson E, et al.: Radiographic analysis of simulated first dorsal interosseous and opponens pollicis loading upon thumb CMC joint subluxation: a cadaver study, *Hand (N Y)* 13(1):40–44, 2018.
3. An KN, Ueba Y, Chao EY, et al.: Tendon excursion and moment arm of index finger muscles, *J Biomech* 16:419–425, 1983.
4. Armbruster EJ, Tan V: Carpometacarpal joint disease: addressing the metacarpophalangeal joint deformity, *Hand Clin* 24:295–299, 2008.
5. Arimitsu S, Murase T, Hashimoto J, et al.: A three-dimensional quantitative analysis of carpal deformity in rheumatoid wrists, *J Bone Joint Surg Br* 89:490–494, 2007.
6. Armstrong AL, Hunter JB, Davis TR: The prevalence of degenerative arthritis of the base of the thumb in post-menopausal women, *J Hand Surg Br* 19(3):340–341, 1994.
7. Arnet U, Muzykewicz DA, Friden J, et al.: Intrinsic hand muscle function, part 1: creating a functional grasp, *J Hand Surg Am* 38(11):2093–2099, 2013.
8. Bain GI, Polites N, Higgs BG, et al.: The functional range of motion of the finger joints, *J Hand Surg Eur* 40(4):406–411, 2015.
9. Batmanabane M, Malathi S: Movements at the carpometacarpal and metacarpophalangeal joints of the hand and their effect on the dimensions of the articular ends of the metacarpal bones, *Anat Rec* 213:102–110, 1985.
10. Bello-Hellegouarch G, Aziz MA, Ferrero EM, et al.: "Pollical palmar interosseous muscle" (musculus adductor pollicis accessorius): attachments, innervation, variations, phylogeny, and implications for human evolution and medicine [Review], *J Morphol* 274(3):275–293, 2013.
11. Belt E, Kaarela K, Lehtinen J, et al.: When does subluxation of the first carpometacarpal joint cause swan-neck deformity of the thumb in rheumatoid arthritis: a 20-year follow-up study, *Clin Rheumatol* 17:135–138, 1998.
12. Bettinger PC, Linscheid RL, Berger RA, et al.: An anatomic study of the stabilizing ligaments of the trapezium and trapeziometacarpal joint, *J Hand Surg Am* 24:786–798, 1999.
13. Bielefeld T, Neumann DA: The unstable metacarpophalangeal joint in rheumatoid arthritis: anatomy, pathomechanics, and physical rehabilitation considerations, *J Orthop Sports Phys Ther* 35:502–520, 2005.
14. Bielefeld T, Neumann DA: Therapist's management of the thumb carpometacarpal joint with osteoarthritis. In Skirven TM, et al.: *Rehabilitation of the hand and upper extremity*, ed 6, St Louis, 2011, Elsevier.
15. Boatright JR, Kiebzak GM: The effects of low median nerve block on thumb abduction strength, *J Hand Surg Am* 22:849–852, 1997.
16. Brand PW, Beach RB, Thompson DE: Relative tension and potential excursion of muscles in the forearm and hand, *J Hand Surg Am* 6:209–219, 1981.
17. Brand PW, Hollister A: *Clinical biomechanics of the hand*, ed 2, St Louis, 1993, Mosby Year-Book.
18. Brand PW: The reconstruction of the hand in leprosy, *Clin Orthop Relat Res* 396:4–11, 2002.
19. Bremer AK, Sennwald GR, Favre P, et al.: Moment arms of forearm rotators, *Clin Biomech* 21:683–691, 2006.
20. Buffi JH, Crisco JJ, Murray WM: A method for defining carpometacarpal joint kinematics from three-dimensional rotations of the metacarpal bones captured in vivo using computed tomography, *J Biomech* 46(12):2104–2108, 2013.
21. Burt S, Deddens JA, Crombie K, et al.: A prospective study of carpal tunnel syndrome: workplace and individual risk factors, *Occup Environ Med* 70(8):568–574, 2013.
22. Butz KD, Merrell G, Nauman EA: A biomechanical analysis of finger joint forces and stresses developed during common daily activities, *Comput Methods Biomech Biomed Engin* 15(2):131–140, 2012.
23. Cantero-Téllez R, Villafañe JH, Valdes K, et al.: Effect of immobilization of metacarpophalangeal joint in thumb carpometacarpal osteoarthritis on pain and function. A quasi-experimental trial, *J Hand Ther* 31(1):68–73, 2018.
24. Cheema TA, Cheema NI, Tayyab R, et al.: Measurement of rotation of the first metacarpal during opposition using computed tomography, *J Hand Surg Am* 31:76–79, 2006.
25. Close JR, Kidd CC: The functions of the muscles of the thumb, the index, and long fingers. Synchronous recording of motions and action potentials of muscles, *J Bone Joint Surg Am* 51:1601–1620, 1969.
26. Cooney WP, Chao EY: Biomechanical analysis of static forces in the thumb during hand function, *J Bone Joint Surg Am* 59(1):27–36, 1977.
27. Cooney III WP, Lucca MJ, Chao EY, et al.: The kinesiology of the thumb trapeziometacarpal joint, *J Bone Joint Surg Am* 63:1371–1381, 1981.
28. Cordo PJ, Horn JL, Kunster D, et al.: Contributions of skin and muscle afferent input to movement sense in the human hand, *J Neurophysiol* 105(4):1879–1888, 2011.
29. Cox HG, Hill JB, Colon AF, et al.: The impact of dividing the flexor tendon pulleys on tendon excursion and work of flexion in a cadaveric model, *J Hand Surg Am* 46(12):1064–1070, 2021.
30. Dabbagh A, MacDermid JC, Yong J, et al.: Diagnosing carpal tunnel syndrome: diagnostic test accuracy of scales, questionnaires, and hand symptom diagrams-a systematic review, *J Orthop Sports Phys Ther* 50(11):622–631, 2020.
31. D'Agostino P, Dourthe B, Kerkhof F, et al.: In vivo biomechanical behavior of the trapeziometacarpal joint in healthy and osteoarthritic subjects, *Clin Biomech* 49:119–127, 2017.
32. Dengler J, Stephens JD, Bamberger HB, et al.: Mimickers of carpal tunnel syndrome, *JBJS Rev* 8(2):e0087, 2020.
33. Dogadov A, Alamir M, Serviere C, et al.: The biomechanical model of the long finger extensor mechanism and its parametric identification, *J Biomech* 58:232–236, 2017.
34. Duymaz A, Karabekmez FE, Zhao C, et al.: Tendon transfer for the restoration of thumb opposition: the effects of friction and pulley location, *Plast Reconstr Surg* 132(3):604–609, 2013.
35. Dvir Z: Biomechanics of muscle. In Dvir Z, editor: *Clinical biomechanics*, Philadelphia, 2000, Churchill Livingstone.
36. Edmunds JO: Current concepts of the anatomy of the thumb trapeziometacarpal joint [Review], *J Hand Surg Am* 36(1):170–182, 2011.
37. El Shennawy M, Nakamura K, Patterson RM, et al.: Three-dimensional kinematic analysis of the second through fifth carpometacarpal joints, *J Hand Surg Am* 26:1030–1035, 2001.
38. Eladoumikdachi F, Valkov PL, Thomas J, et al.: Anatomy of the intrinsic hand muscles revisited: part I. Interossei, *Plast Reconstr Surg* 110:1211–1224, 2002.
39. Elzinga K, Chung KC: Managing swan neck and boutonniere deformities, *Clin Plast Surg* 46(3):329–337, 2019.
40. Enoka RM: *Neuromechanics of human movement*, ed 5, Champaign, Ill, 2015, Human Kinetics.
41. Erickson M, Lawrence M, Jansen CWS, et al.: Hand pain and sensory deficits: carpal tunnel syndrome, *J Orthop Sports Phys Ther* 49(5):Cpg1–cpg85, 2019.
42. Estermann L, Marks M, Herren DB, et al.: Determinants of long-term satisfaction after silicone MCP arthroplasty in patients with inflammatory diseases, *Hand Surg Rehabil* 39(6):545–549, 2020.
43. Firoozbakhsh K, Yi IS, Moneim MS, et al.: A study of ulnar collateral ligament of the thumb metacarpophalangeal joint, *Clin Orthop Relat Res* 403:240–247, 2002.
44. Flatt AE: Ulnar drift, *J Hand Ther* 9:282–292, 1996.
45. Fletcher JR, MacIntosh BR: Estimates of Achilles tendon moment arm length at different ankle joint angles: effect of passive moment, *J Appl Biomech* 1–22, 2018.
46. Fontana L, Neel S, Claise JM, et al.: Osteoarthritis of the thumb carpometacarpal joint in women and occupational risk factors: a case-control study, *J Hand Surg Am* 32:459–465, 2007.
47. Fox PM, Chang J: Treating the proximal interphalangeal joint in swan neck and boutonniere deformities, *Hand Clin* 34(2):167–176, 2018.
48. Fox PM, Oliver JD, Nguyen V, et al.: Electromyographic analysis of grip, *Orthopedics* 42(6):e555–e558, 2019.
49. Francis-Pester FW, Thomas R, Sforzin D, et al.: The moment arms and leverage of the human finger muscles, *J Biomech* 116:110180, 2021.
50. Franko OI, Winters TM, Tirrell TF, et al.: Moment arms of the human digital flexors, *J Biomech* 44(10):1987–1990, 2011.
51. Goodman HJ, Choueka J: Biomechanics of the flexor tendons, *Hand Clin* 21:129–149, 2005.
52. Gottschalk MB, Patel NN, Boden AL, et al.: Treatment of basilar thumb arthritis: a critical analysis review, *JBJS Rev* 6(7):e4, 2018.
53. Grau L, Baydoun H, Chen K, et al.: Biomechanics of the acute boutonniere deformity, *J Hand Surg Am* 43(1):80.e1–80.e6, 2018.
54. Gray DJ, Gardner E: The innervation of the joints of the wrist and hand, *Anat Rec* 151:261–266, 1965.
55. Gupta S, Michelsen-Jost H: Anatomy and function of the thenar muscles [Review], *Hand Clin* 28(1):1–7, 2012.
56. Haara MM, Heliovaara M, Kroger H, et al.: Osteoarthritis in the carpometacarpal joint of the thumb. Prevalence and associations with disability and mortality, *J Bone Joint Surg Am* 86-A(7):1452–1457, 2004.
57. Hagert E, Lee J, Ladd AL: Innervation patterns of thumb trapeziometacarpal joint ligaments, *J Hand Surg Am* 37(4):706–714, 2012.
58. Hahn P, Krimmer H, Hradetzky A, et al.: Quantitative analysis of the linkage between the interphalangeal joints of the index finger. An in vivo study, *J Hand Surg Br* 20:696–699, 1995.
59. Halilaj E, Moore DC, Laidlaw DH, et al.: The morphology of the thumb carpometacarpal joint does not differ between men and women, but changes with aging and early osteoarthritis, *J Biomech* 47(11):2709–2714, 2014.
60. Halilaj E, Rainbow MJ, Got C, et al.: In vivo kinematics of the thumb carpometacarpal joint during three isometric functional tasks, *Clin Orthop Relat Res* 472(4):1114–1122, 2014.
61. Halilaj E, Rainbow MJ, Moore DC, et al.: In vivo recruitment patterns in the anterior oblique and dorsoradial ligaments of the first carpometacarpal joint, *J Biomech* 48(10):1893–1898, 2015.
62. Hentz VR: Surgical treatment of trapeziometacarpal joint arthritis: a historical perspective [Review], *Clin Orthop Relat Res* 472(4):1184–1189, 2014.
63. Holzbaur KR, Murray WM, Gold GE, et al.: Upper limb muscle volumes in adult subjects, *J Biomech* 40:742–749, 2007.
64. Hume MC, Gellman H, McKellop H, et al.: Functional range of motion of the joints of the hand, *J Hand Surg Am* 15:240–243, 1990.
65. Igoe D, Middleton C, Hammert W: Evolution of basal joint arthroplasty and technology in hand surgery [Review], *J Hand Ther* 27(2):115–120, 2014.
66. Imaeda T, An KN, Cooney III WP, et al.: Anatomy of trapeziometacarpal ligaments, *J Hand Surg Am* 18:226–231, 1993.
67. Imaeda T, Niebur G, Cooney III WP, et al.: Kinematics of the normal trapeziometacarpal joint, *J Orthop Res* 12:197–204, 1994.

68. Infantolino BW, Challis JH: Architectural properties of the first dorsal interosseous muscle, *J Anat* 216(4):463–469, 2010.

69. Inman VT, Saunders JB: Referred pain from skeletal structures, *J Nerv Ment Dis* 99:660–667, 1944.

70. Jacobson MD, Raab R, Fazeli BM, et al.: Architectural design of the human intrinsic hand muscles, *J Hand Surg Am* 17:804–809, 1992.

71. Jarque-Bou NJ, Vergara M, Sancho-Bru JL, et al.: A calibrated database of kinematics and EMG of the forearm and hand during activities of daily living, *Sci Data* 6(1):270, 2019.

72. Jenkins M, Bamberger HB, Black L, et al.: Thumb joint flexion. What is normal? *J Hand Surg Br* 23:796–797, 1998.

73. Kamakura N: *Postures and movement patterns of the human hand*, Boca Raton, 2022, BrownWalker Press.

74. Kamata Y, Nakamura T, Tada M, et al.: How the lumbrical muscle contributes to placing the fingertip in space: a three-dimensional cadaveric study to assess fingertip trajectory and metacarpophalangeal joint balancing, *J Hand Surg: European* 41(4):386–391, 2016.

75. Kamper DG, George HT, Rymer WZ: Extrinsic flexor muscles generate concurrent flexion of all three finger joints, *J Biomech* 35:1581–1589, 2002.

76. Kannas S, Jeardeau TA, Bishop AT: Rehabilitation following Zone II flexor tendon repairs, *Tech Hand Up Extrem Surg* 19(1):2–10, 2015.

77. Kataoka T, Moritomo H, Miyake J, et al.: Changes in shape and length of the collateral and accessory collateral ligaments of the metacarpophalangeal joint during flexion, *J Bone Joint Surg Am* 93(14):1318–1325, 2011.

78. Kaufman KR, An KN, Litchy WJ, et al.: In-vivo function of the thumb muscles, *Clin Biomech* 14:141–150, 1999.

79. Kawanishi Y, Oka K, Tanaka H, et al.: In vivo 3-dimensional kinematics of thumb carpometacarpal joint during thumb opposition, *J Hand Surg Am* 43(2):182.e1–182.e7, 2018.

80. Kichouh M, Vanhoenacker F, Jager T, et al.: Functional anatomy of the dorsal hood of the hand: correlation of ultrasound and MR findings with cadaveric dissection, *Eur Radiol* 19(8):1849–1856, 2009.

81. Kociolek AM, Keir PJ: Modelling tendon excursions and moment arms of the finger flexors: anatomic fidelity versus function, *J Biomech* 44(10):1967–1973, 2011.

82. Koh S, Buford Jr WL, Andersen CR, et al.: Intrinsic muscle contribution to the metacarpophalangeal joint flexion moment of the middle, ring, and small fingers, *J Hand Surg Am* 31:1111–1117, 2006.

83. Kolasinski SL, Neogi T, Hochberg MC, et al.: 2019 American College of Rheumatology/Arthritis Foundation guideline for the management of osteoarthritis of the hand, hip, and knee, *Arthritis Rheumatol* 72(2):220–233, 2020.

84. Kozin SH, Porter S, Clark P, et al.: The contribution of the intrinsic muscles to grip and pinch strength, *J Hand Surg Am* 24:64–72, 1999.

85. Krishnan J, Chipchase L: Passive axial rotation of the metacarpophalangeal joint, *J Hand Surg Br* 22:270–273, 1997.

86. Ladd AL, Lee J, Hagert E: Macroscopic and microscopic analysis of the thumb carpometacarpal ligaments: a cadaveric study of ligament anatomy and histology, *J Bone Joint Surg Am* 94(16):1468–1477, 2012.

87. Ladd AL, Weiss AP, Crisco JJ, et al.: The thumb carpometacarpal joint: anatomy, hormones, and biomechanics, *Instr Course Lect* 62:165–179, 2013.

88. Lakshminarayanan K, Shah R, Li ZM: Morphological and positional changes of the carpal arch and median nerve associated with wrist deviations, *Clin Biomech* 71:133–138, 2020.

89. Landsmeer JF: Power grip and precision handling, *Ann Rheum Dis* 21:164–170, 1962.

90. Latz D, Koukos C, Boeckers P, et al.: Influence of wrist position on the metacarpophalangeal joint motion of the index through small finger, *Hand* 14(2):259–263, 2019.

91. Leijnse JN, Kalker JJ: A two-dimensional kinematic model of the lumbrical in the human finger, *J Biomech* 28:237–249, 1995.

92. Leijnse JN, Spoor CW, Shatford R: The minimum number of muscles to control a chain of joints with and without tenodeses, arthrodeses, or braces—application to the human finger, *J Biomech* 38:2028–2036, 2005.

93. Leijnse JN: Why the lumbrical muscle should not be bigger—a force model of the lumbrical in the unloaded human finger, *J Biomech* 30:1107–1114, 1997.

94. Lerebours A, Marin F, Bouvier S, et al.: Trends in trapeziometacarpal implant design: a systematic survey based on patents and administrative databases, *J Hand Surg Am* 45(3):223–238, 2020.

95. Liber RL: *Skeletal muscle structure, function and plasticity: the physiologic basis of rehabilitation*, ed 3, Philadelphia, 2009, Lippincott Williams & Wilkins.

96. Lin JD, Karl JW, Strauch RJ: Trapeziometacarpal joint stability: the evolving importance of the dorsal ligaments [Review], *Clin Orthop Relat Res* 472(4):1138–1145, 2014.

97. Linscheid RL, An KN, Gross RM: Quantitative analysis of the intrinsic muscles of the hand, *Clin Anat* 4:265–284, 1991.

98. Liss FE: The interosseous muscles: the foundation of hand function [Review], *Hand Clin* 28(1):9–12, 2012.

99. Long C, Brown TD: Electromyographic kinesiology of the hand: muscles moving the long finger, *J Bone Joint Surg Am* 46:1683–1706, 1964.

100. Long C: Intrinsic-extrinsic muscle control of the fingers. Electromyographic studies, *J Bone Joint Surg Am* 50:973–984, 1968.

101. Loos B, Puschkin V, Horch RE: 50 years experience with Dupuytren's contracture in the Erlangen University Hospital—a retrospective analysis of 2919 operated hands from 1956 to 2006, *BMC Musculoskelet Disord* 8:60, 2007.

102. Loubert PV, Masterson TJ, Schroeder MS, et al.: Proximity of collateral ligament origin to the axis of rotation of the proximal interphalangeal joint of the finger, *J Orthop Sports Phys Ther* 37:179–185, 2007.

103. Lunsford D, Valdes K, Hengy S: Conservative management of trigger finger: a systematic review, *J Hand Ther* 32(2):212–221, 2019.

104. MacMoran JW, Brand PW: Bone loss in limbs with decreased or absent sensation: ten year follow-up of the hands in leprosy, *Skeletal Radiol* 16:452–459, 1987.

105. Masiero S, Boniolo A, Wassermann L, et al.: Effects of an educational-behavioral joint protection program on people with moderate to severe rheumatoid arthritis: a randomized controlled trial, *Clin Rheumatol* 26:2043–2050, 2007.

106. Melvin JL: Therapist's management of osteoarthritis in the hand. In Skriven TM, Osterman AL, Fedorczyk J, et al.: *Rehabilitation of the hand and upper extremity*, ed 6, St Louis, 2011, Elsevier.

107. Miyamura S, Oka K, Sakai T, et al.: Cartilage wear patterns in severe osteoarthritis of the trapeziometacarpal joint: a quantitative analysis, *Osteoarthritis Cartilage* 27(8):1152–1162, 2019.

108. Mobargha N, Esplugas M, Garcia-Elias M, et al.: The effect of individual isometric muscle loading on the alignment of the base of the thumb metacarpal: a cadaveric study, *J Hand Surg Eur Vol* 41(4):374–379, 2016.

109. Mobargha N, Rein S, Hagert E: Ligamento-muscular reflex patterns following stimulation of a thumb carpometacarpal ligament: an electromyographic study, *J Hand Surg Am* 44(3):248.e1–248.e9, 2019.

110. Moriatis Wolf J, Turkiewicz A, Atroshi I, et al.: Prevalence of doctor-diagnosed thumb carpometacarpal joint osteoarthritis: an analysis of Swedish health Care, *Arthritis Care Res* 66(6):961–965, 2014.

111. Morrison PE, Hill RV: And then there were four: anatomical observations on the pollical palmar interosseous muscle in humans, *Clin Anat* 24(8):978–983, 2011.

112. Murai S, Tanaka T, Aoki M: Combinatorial roles of extrinsic and intrinsic muscles in extension strength of the distal interphalangeal joint, *J Orthop Res* 30(6):893–896, 2012.

113. Nakamura K, Patterson RM, Viegas SF: The ligament and skeletal anatomy of the second through fifth carpometacarpal joints and adjacent structures, *J Hand Surg Am* 26:1016–1029, 2001.

114. Nalebuff EA: Diagnosis, classification and management of rheumatoid thumb deformities, *Bull Hosp Jt Dis* 29:119–137, 1968.

115. Nanno M, Kodera N, Tomori Y, et al.: Three-dimensional dynamic motion analysis of the first carpometacarpal ligaments, *J Ortho Surg* 25(1):1–6, 2017.

116. Napier JR: The prehensile movements of the human hand, *J Bone Joint Surg Br* 38:902–913, 1956.

117. Neto HS, Filho JM, Passini Jr R, et al.: Number and size of motor units in thenar muscles, *Clin Anat* 17:308–311, 2004.

118. Neumann DA, Bielefeld TB: The carpometacarpal joint of the thumb: stability, deformity, and therapeutic intervention, *J Orthop Sports Phys Ther* 33:386–399, 2003.

119. O'Shaughnessy MA, Kannas S, Ernste F, et al.: Team approach: role of medical and surgical management in rheumatoid arthritis of the hand and wrist, *JBJS Rev* 7(8):e10, 2019.

120. Pagalidis T, Kuczynski K, Lamb DW: Ligamentous stability of the base of the thumb, *Hand* 13:29–36, 1981.

121. Palmer KT: Carpal tunnel syndrome: the role of occupational factors [Review], *Best Pract Res Clin Rheumatol* 25(1):15–29, 2011.

122. Palti R, Vigler M: Anatomy and function of lumbrical muscles [Review], *Hand Clin* 28(1):13–17, 2012.

123. Pang EQ, Yao J: Anatomy and biomechanics of the finger proximal interphalangeal joint, *Hand Clin* 34(2):121–126, 2018.

124. Pasquella JA, Levine P: Anatomy and function of the hypothenar muscles [Review], *Hand Clin* 28(1):19–25, 2012.

125. Peck D, Buxton DF, Nitz A: A comparison of spindle concentrations in large and small muscles acting in parallel combinations, *J Morphol* 180:243–252, 1984.

126. Pettengill K, et al.: Postoperative management of flexor tendon injuries. In Skriven TM, Osterman AL, Fedorczyk J, et al.: *Rehabilitation of the hand and upper extremity*, ed 6, St Louis, 2011, Elsevier.

127. Ranney D, Wells R: Lumbrical muscle function as revealed by a new and physiological approach, *Anat Rec* 222:110–114, 1988.

128. Rempel DM, Keir PJ, Bach JM: Effect of wrist posture on carpal tunnel pressure while typing, *J Orthop Res* 26:1269–1273, 2008.

129. Roloff I, Schöffl VR, Vigouroux L, et al.: Biomechanical model for the determination of the forces acting on the finger pulley system, *J Biomech* 39:915–923, 2006.

130. Rosenthal EA, Elhassan BT: The extensor tendons: evaluation and surgical management. In Skriven TM, et al.: *Rehabilitation of the hand and upper extremity*, ed 6, St Louis, 2011, Elsevier.

131. Rust PA, Ek ETH, Tham SKY: Assessment of normal trapeziometacarpal joint alignment, *J Hand Surg: European* 42(6):605–609, 2017.

132. Schneider MTY, Zhang J, Crisco JJ, et al.: Trapeziometacarpal joint contact varies between men and women during three isometric functional tasks, *Med Eng Phys* 50:43–49, 2017.

133. Schulz CU, Anetzberger H, Pfahler M, et al.: The relation between primary osteoarthritis of the trapeziometacarpal joint and supernumerary slips of the abductor pollicis longus tendon, *J Hand Surg Br* 27:238–241, 2002.

134. Scott A: Is a joint-specific home exercise program effective for patients with first carpometacarpal joint osteoarthritis? A critical review, *Hand Ther* 23(3):83–94, 2018.

135. Shi Q, Bobos P, Lalone EA, et al.: Comparison of the short-term and long-term effects of surgery and nonsurgical intervention in treating carpal tunnel syndrome: a systematic review and meta-analysis, *Hand (N Y)* 15(1):13–22, 2020.
136. Shi Q, MacDermid JC: Is surgical intervention more effective than non-surgical treatment for carpal tunnel syndrome? A systematic review [Review], *J Orthop Surg* 6:17, 2011.
137. Shih JG, Mainprize JG, Binhammer PA: Comparison of computed tomography articular surface geometry of male versus female thumb carpometacarpal joints, *Hand* 13(1):33–39, 2018.
138. Siegel P, Jackson D, Baugh C: Practice patterns following carpometacarpal (CMC) arthroplasty, *J Hand Ther* 35(1):67–73, 2022.
139. Smutz WP, Kongsayreepong A, Hughes RE, et al.: Mechanical advantage of the thumb muscles, *J Biomech* 31:565–570, 1998.
140. Sodha S, Ring D, Zurakowski D, et al.: Prevalence of osteoarthrosis of the trapeziometacarpal joint, *J Bone Joint Surg Am* 87(12):2614–2618, 2005.
141. Stack HG: Muscle function in the fingers, *J Bone Joint Surg Br* 44:899–902, 1962.
142. Standring S: *Gray's anatomy: the anatomical basis of clinical practice*, ed 42, St Louis, 2021, Elsevier.
143. Stival F, Michieletto S, Cognolato M, et al.: A quantitative taxonomy of human hand grasps, *J NeuroEng Rehabil* 16(1):28, 2019.
144. Strauch RJ, Rosenwasser MP, Behrman MJ: A biomechanical assessment of ligaments preventing dorsoradial subluxation of the trapeziometacarpal joint, *J Hand Surg Am* 24(1):198–199, 1999.
145. Strong CL, Perry J: Function of the extensor pollicis longus and intrinsic muscle of the thumb, *J Am Phys Ther Assoc* 46:939–945, 1966.
146. Su FC, Chou YL, Yang CS, et al.: Movement of finger joints induced by synergistic wrist motion, *Clin Biomech* 20:491–497, 2005.
147. Taguchi M, Zhao C, Zobitz ME, et al.: Effect of finger ulnar deviation on gliding resistance of the flexor digitorum profundus tendon within the A₁ and A₂ pulley complex, *J Hand Surg Am* 31:113–117, 2006.
148. Tan J, Xu J, Xie RG, et al.: In vivo length and changes of ligaments stabilizing the thumb carpometacarpal joint, *J Hand Surg Am* 36(3):420–427, 2011.
149. Terrino AL, et al.: The rheumatoid thumb. In Skriven TM, Osterman AL, Fedorczyk J, et al.: *Rehabilitation of the hand and upper extremity*, ed 6, St Louis, 2011, Elsevier.
150. Thomas DH, Long C: Biomechanical considerations of lumbricalis behavior in the human finger, *J Biomech* 1:107–115, 1968.
151. Tordjman D, d'Utruy A, Bauer B, et al.: Tendon transfer surgery for radial nerve palsy, *Hand Surg Rehabil* 41s:s90–s97, 2022.
152. Trumble TE, Vedder NB, Seiler 3rd JG, et al.: Zone-II flexor tendon repair: a randomized prospective trial of active place-and-hold therapy compared with passive motion therapy, *J Bone Joint Surg Am* 92(6):1381–1389, 2010.
153. Ueba H, Moradi N, Erne HC, et al.: An anatomic and biomechanical study of the oblique retinacular ligament and its role in finger extension, *J Hand Surg Am* 36(12):1959–1964, 2011.
154. Ugbolue UC, Hsu WH, Goitz RJ, et al.: Tendon and nerve displacement at the wrist during finger movements, *Clin Biomech* 20:50–56, 2005.
155. Valdes K, Boyd JD, Povlak SB, et al.: Efficacy of orthotic devices for increased active proximal interphalangeal extension joint range of Motion: a systematic review, *J Hand Ther* 32(2):184–193, 2019.
156. Vigouroux L, Quaine F, Paclet F, et al.: Middle and ring fingers are more exposed to pulley rupture than index and little during sport-climbing: a biomechanical explanation, *Clin Biomech* 23:562–570, 2008.
157. Villafane JH, Cleland JA, Fernandez-de-las-Penas C: The effectiveness of a manual therapy and exercise protocol in patients with thumb carpometacarpal osteoarthritis: a randomized controlled trial, *J Orthop Sports Phys Ther* 43(4):204–213, 2013.
158. Wachter NJ, Mentzel M, Krischak GD, et al.: Predictive value of metacarpophalangeal stabilization tests for simulated ulnar nerve lesion measured by a sensor glove, *J Hand Ther* 32(1):64–70, 2019.
159. Wang K, McGlinn EP, Chung KC: A biomechanical and evolutionary perspective on the function of the lumbrical muscle, *J Hand Surg Am* 39(1):149–155, 2014.
160. Wang KK, Zhang X, McCombe D, et al.: Quantitative analysis of in-vivo thumb carpometacarpal joint kinematics using four-dimensional computed tomography, *J Hand Surg Eur Vol* 43(10):1088–1097, 2018.
161. Wariyar B: Hansen's disease (leprosy), *Nebr Med J* 81:147–148, 1996.
162. Wells RP, Ranney DA: Lumbrical length changes in finger movement: a new method of study in fresh cadaver hands, *J Hand Surg Am* 11:574–577, 1986.
163. White J, Coppola L, Skomurski A, et al.: Influence of age and gender on normative passive range of motion values of the carpometacarpal joint of the thumb, *J Hand Ther* 31(3):390–397, 2018.
164. Wilkens SC, Meghpara MM, Ring D, et al.: Trapeziometacarpal arthrosis, *JBJS Rev* 7(1):e8, 2019.
165. Williams K, Terrono AL: Treatment of boutonnière finger deformity in rheumatoid arthritis, *J Hand Surg Am* 36(8):1388–1393, 2011.
166. Windhorst U: Muscle proprioceptive feedback and spinal networks [Review, 411 refs], *Brain Res Bull* 73(4–6):155–202, 2007.
167. Wolf JM, Scher DL, Etchill EW, et al.: Relationship of relaxin hormone and thumb carpometacarpal joint arthritis, *Clin Orthop Relat Res* 472(4):1130–1137, 2014.
168. Wolf JM, Turkiewicz A, Atroshi I, et al.: Occupational load as a risk factor for clinically relevant base of thumb osteoarthritis, *Occup Environ Med* 77(3):168–171, 2020.
169. Zancolli EA, Ziadenberg C, Zancolli Jr E: Biomechanics of the trapeziometacarpal joint, *Clin Orthop Relat Res* 220:14–26, 1987.

STUDY QUESTIONS

1. Compare the relative mobility permitted at the proximal and distal transverse arches of the hand.
2. List regions within the hand where you would most expect muscle atrophy after a longstanding (a) ulnar neuropathy and (b) median neuropathy.
3. The adductor pollicis is a forceful muscle requiring stable proximal bony attachments. After reviewing the muscle's proximal attachments, state whether this requirement has been met.
4. Which movements at the carpometacarpal joint of the thumb constitute opposition? Which muscles are most responsible for performing these individual movements?
5. Describe the path of the lumbrical muscle of the index finger, from its proximal to its distal attachment. Explain how this muscle can flex the metacarpophalangeal joint and simultaneously extend the interphalangeal joints.
6. Fig. 8.42 shows the lines of force of the extensor pollicis longus, extensor pollicis brevis, and abductor pollicis longus at the carpometacarpal joint. Of the three muscles, which (a) is capable of adduction, (b) is capable of abduction, and (c) has neither potential? Finally, which of these muscles can extend the carpometacarpal joint?
7. What is the role of the lumbricals and interossei in opening the hand (i.e., extending the fingers)?
8. Contrast the underlying pathomechanics in the swan-neck and boutonnière deformities.
9. Which of the three intrinsic muscles illustrated in Fig. 8.48 has the greatest moment arm for flexion of the metacarpophalangeal joint of the index finger?
10. Clinicians frequently immobilize the hand of a person with a fractured metacarpal in a position of flexion of the metacarpophalangeal joint and near extension of the interphalangeal joints. What is the reason for doing this? Which muscle could eventually become tight (contracted) from this prolonged position?
11. A person with a damaged ulnar nerve at the level of the pisiform bone typically shows marked weakness of adduction of the carpometacarpal joint of the thumb. Why would this occur? Which muscle could substitute for some of the loss of adduction at this joint?
12. How does the saddle-shaped joint structure of the carpometacarpal joint of the thumb influence the arthrokinematics of flexion and extension and abduction and adduction?
13. Rank the passive mobility of the carpometacarpal joints of the hand from least to most. What is the functional significance of this mobility pattern?
14. A patient shows marked weakness in the active movements of abduction and adduction of the fingers and in making a "key pinch." In addition, the patient shows atrophy of the muscles of the hypothenar eminence and decreased sensation over the ulnar border of the hand and distal forearm. Based on information displayed in Appendix II, Parts B through E, which spinal nerve roots are most likely associated with these impairments?

STUDY QUESTIONS—cont'd

15. Assume a person has a completely lacerated flexor digitorum profundus (FDP) tendon of the ring finger at the level of the A_4 pulley. Furthermore, the person reports that attempts at making a fist result in extension rather than flexion of the distal interphalangeal joint of the ring finger. (This observation is often referred to by clinicians as "paradoxical extension.") Please offer a possible kinesiologic explanation for this phenomenon.

16. Describe the position of the fingers in someone diagnosed with "intrinsic muscle contracture." Which position of the fingers would stretch the tightened muscles?

17. Assume you are evaluating the passive range of motion (ROM) of the PIP joint of your patient's index finger. Your measurements show a ROM from 110 degrees of flexion to 30 degrees short of neutral extension (i.e., 0 degrees). How could you distinguish if the 30-degree loss of extension is due to tightness in an extrinsic finger flexor muscle or tightness in the palmar plate at the PIP joint?

Answers to the study questions are available in the accompanying enhanced eBook version included with the print purchase of this textbook.

Additional Video Educational Content

- Fluoroscopic Observations of Selected Arthrokinematics of the Upper Extremity
- Kinesiology of Flexing and Extending the Finger (using a cadaveric finger model)
- Prototype of a Large Mechanical Finger

CLINICAL KINESIOLOGY APPLIED TO PERSONS WITH QUADRIPLEGIA (TETRAPLEGIA)
- Analysis of Transferring from a Wheelchair to a Mat in a Person with C^6 Quadriplegia

- Functional Considerations of the Wrist Extensor Muscles in a Person with C^6 Quadriplegia (includes "tenodesis action" at the wrist)

ALL VIDEOS in this chapter are available in the accompanying enhanced eBook version included with the print purchase of this textbook.

APPENDIX

II

Reference Materials for Muscle Attachments and Innervations, Muscle Cross-Sectional Areas, and Dermatomes of the Upper Extremity

Part A: Paths of the Peripheral Nerves throughout the Elbow, Wrist, and Hand

The following figures illustrate the path and general proximal-to-distal order of muscle innervation. The location of some muscles is altered slightly for illustration purposes. The primary nerve roots that form each nerve are shown in parentheses.

Musculocutaneous nerve (C⁵⁻⁷)

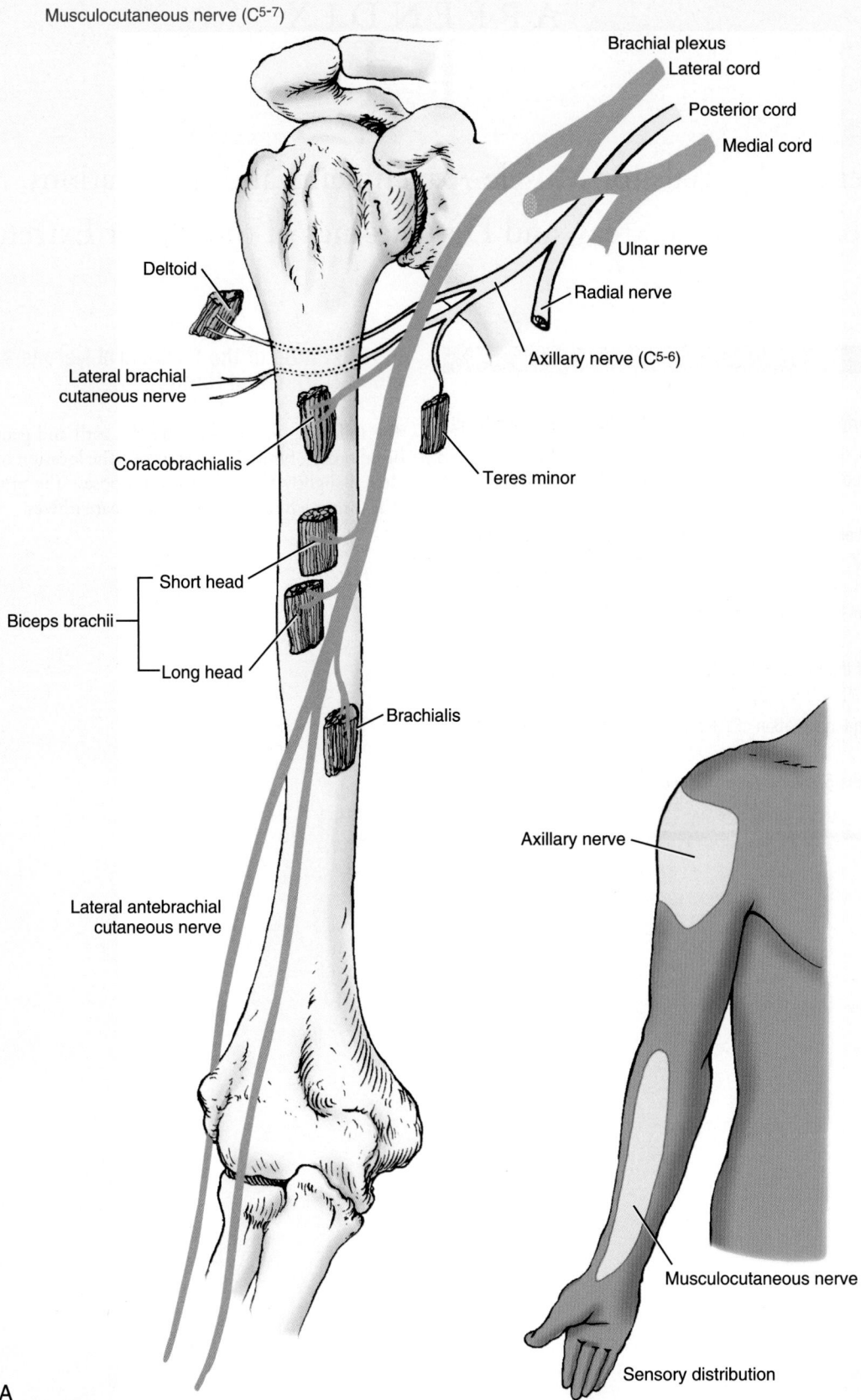

Brachial plexus
Lateral cord
Posterior cord
Medial cord

Ulnar nerve

Radial nerve

Axillary nerve (C⁵⁻⁶)

Deltoid

Lateral brachial
cutaneous nerve

Coracobrachialis

Teres minor

Biceps brachii — Short head

Long head

Brachialis

Lateral antebrachial
cutaneous nerve

Axillary nerve

Musculocutaneous nerve

Sensory distribution

A

FIGURE II.1A   The path of the musculocutaneous nerve is shown as it innervates the coracobrachialis, biceps brachii, and brachialis muscles. The sensory distribution of this nerve is shown as the lighter region along the lateral forearm. The motor and sensory components of the axillary nerve are also shown.

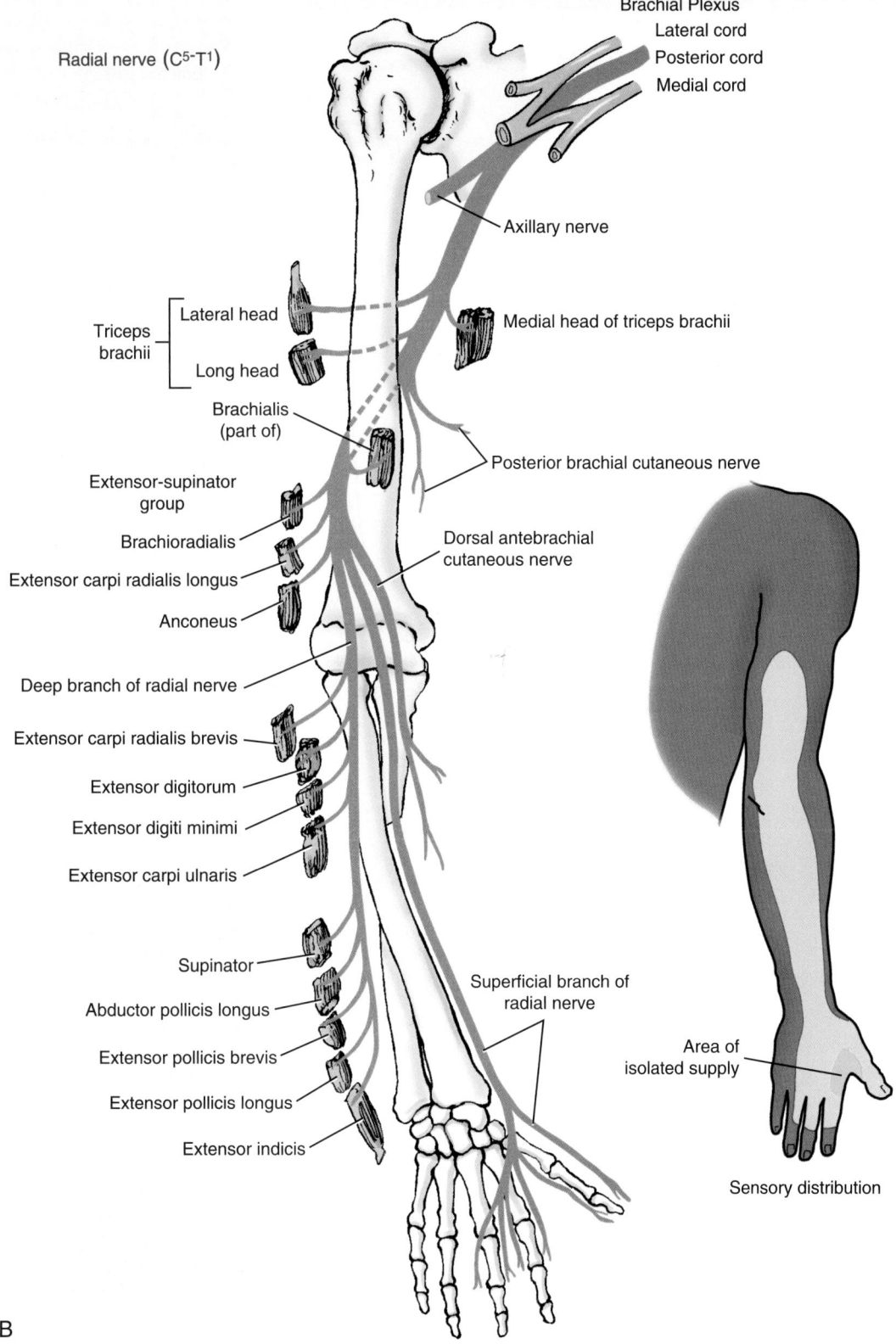

Radial nerve (C⁵-T¹)

Brachial Plexus
Lateral cord
Posterior cord
Medial cord

Axillary nerve

Triceps brachii
Lateral head
Long head

Medial head of triceps brachii

Brachialis (part of)

Posterior brachial cutaneous nerve

Extensor-supinator group

Brachioradialis

Extensor carpi radialis longus

Anconeus

Dorsal antebrachial cutaneous nerve

Deep branch of radial nerve

Extensor carpi radialis brevis

Extensor digitorum

Extensor digiti minimi

Extensor carpi ulnaris

Supinator

Abductor pollicis longus

Extensor pollicis brevis

Extensor pollicis longus

Extensor indicis

Superficial branch of radial nerve

Area of isolated supply

Sensory distribution

B

FIGURE II.1B   The path of the radial nerve is shown as it innervates most of the extensors of the arm, fore-arm, wrist, and digits. See text for more detail on the proximal-to-distal order of muscle innervation. The general sensory distribution of this nerve is shown as the lighter region along the dorsal aspect of the upper extremity. The dorsal "web space" of the hand is innervated solely by sensory branches of the radial nerve (depicted in green). This area of "isolated" nerve supply makes it a preferred location for testing the sensory function of this nerve.

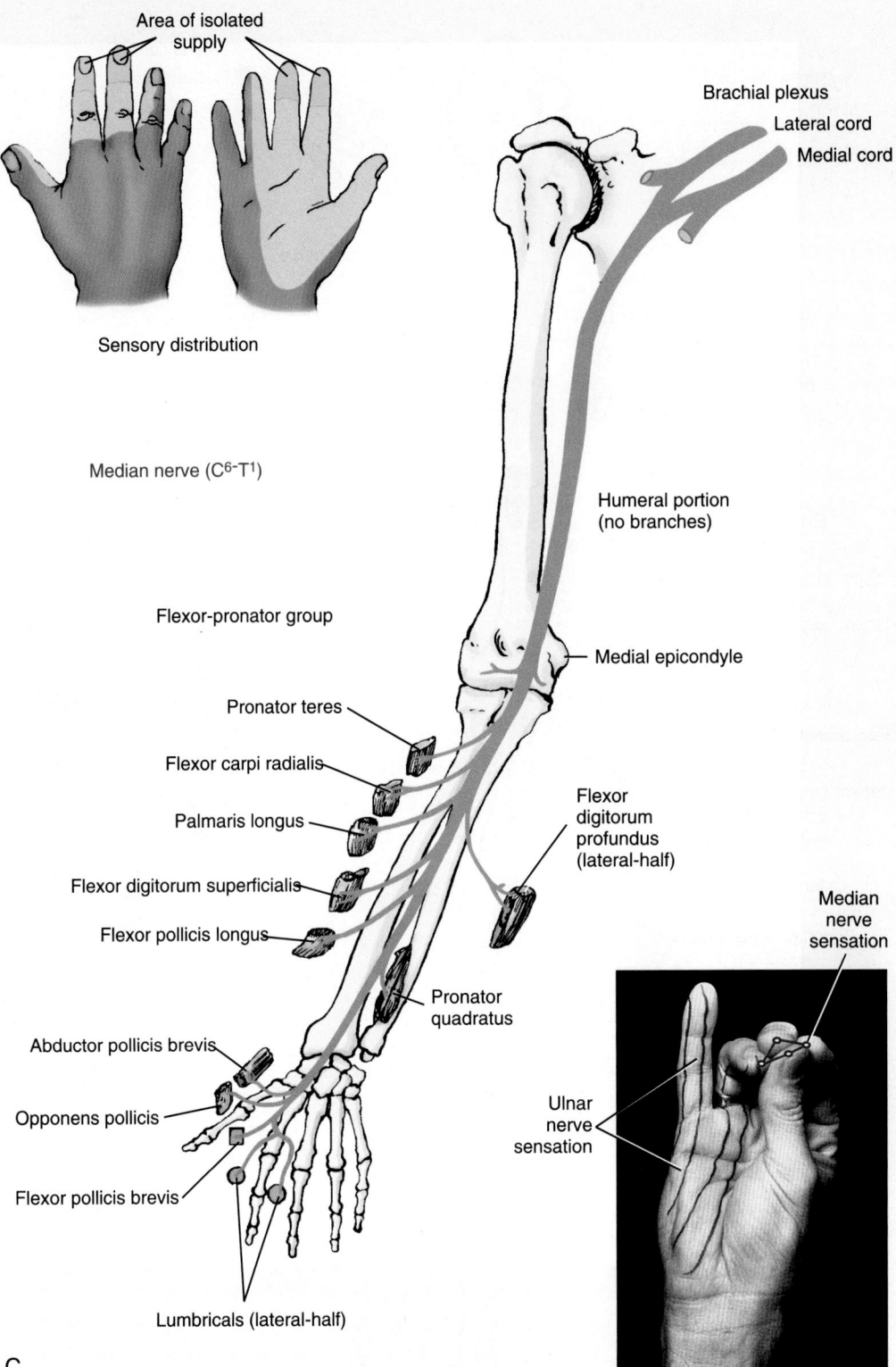

Area of isolated supply

Sensory distribution

Median nerve (C⁶-T¹)

Flexor-pronator group

Pronator teres

Flexor carpi radialis

Palmaris longus

Flexor digitorum superficialis

Flexor pollicis longus

Abductor pollicis brevis

Opponens pollicis

Flexor pollicis brevis

Lumbricals (lateral-half)

Brachial plexus
Lateral cord
Medial cord

Humeral portion (no branches)

Medial epicondyle

Flexor digitorum profundus (lateral-half)

Pronator quadratus

Median nerve sensation

Ulnar nerve sensation

C

FIGURE II.1C   The path of the median nerve is shown supplying the pronators, wrist flexors, long (extrinsic) flexors of the digits (except the flexor digitorum profundus to the ring and small finger), most intrinsic muscles to the thumb, and two lateral lumbricals. The general sensory distribution of this nerve is shown as the lighter region within the hand. The area of skin that receives isolated median nerve sensation is indicated (in green) along the distal end of the index and middle fingers. *Inset,* the median nerve supplies the sensation of the skin that naturally makes contact in a pinching motion between the thumb and fingers. (Photograph by Donald A. Neumann.)

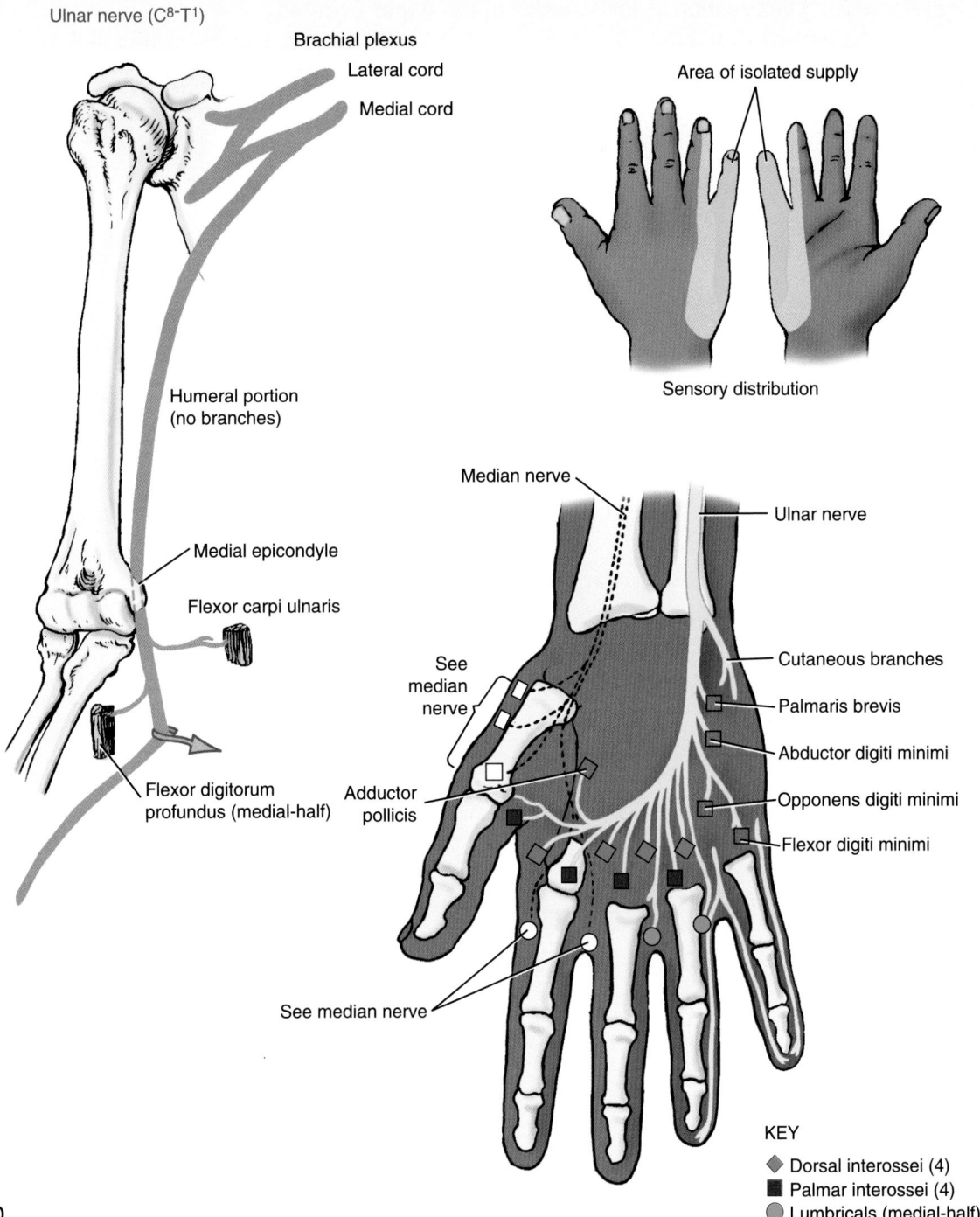

Ulnar nerve (C⁸-T¹)

Brachial plexus

Lateral cord

Medial cord

Area of isolated supply

Sensory distribution

Humeral portion
(no branches)

Median nerve

Ulnar nerve

Medial epicondyle

Flexor carpi ulnaris

See
median
nerve

Cutaneous branches

Palmaris brevis

Abductor digiti minimi

Opponens digiti minimi

Flexor digiti minimi

Adductor
pollicis

Flexor digitorum
profundus (medial-half)

See median nerve

KEY

◆ Dorsal interossei (4)
■ Palmar interossei (4)
● Lumbricals (medial-half)

D

FIGURE II.1D   The path of the ulnar nerve is shown supplying most of the intrinsic muscles of the hand, including the two medial lumbricals. The general sensory distribution of this nerve covers the skin on the ulnar side of the hand, including the medial side of the ring finger and entire small finger. The area of skin that receives isolated ulnar nerve sensation is depicted in green, which includes the entire small finger and the extreme ulnar side of the hand. (A to D modified from de Groot JH: *Correlative neuroanatomy,* ed 21, Norwalk, 1991, Appleton & Lange.)

Part B: Spinal Nerve Root Innervation of the Muscles of the Upper Extremity

Muscle					Nerve Root				
	C¹	C²	C³	C⁴	C⁵	C⁶	C⁷	C⁸	T¹
Serratus anterior					X	X	X	*X*	
Rhomboids, major and minor				*X*	X				
Subclavius					X	X			
Supraspinatus					X	X			
Infraspinatus					X	X			
Subscapularis					X	X	*X*		
Latissimus dorsi						X	X	X	
Teres major					*X*	X	*X*		
Pectoralis major (clavicular)					X	X			
Pectoralis major (sternocostal)						*X*	*X*	X	X
Pectoralis minor							*X*	X	*X*
Teres minor					X	X			
Deltoid					X	X			
Coracobrachialis					*X*	X	X		
Biceps					X	X			
Brachialis					X	X			
Triceps						*X*	X	X	*X*
Anconeus							X	X	
Brachioradialis					X	X			
Extensor carpi radialis longus and brevis					*X*	X	X	*X*	
Supinator					*X*	X			
Extensor digitorum						*X*	X	X	
Extensor digiti minimi						*X*	X	X	
Extensor carpi ulnaris						*X*	X	X	
Abductor pollicis longus						*X*	X	X	
Extensor pollicis brevis						*X*	X	X	
Extensor pollicis longus						*X*	X	X	
Extensor indicis						*X*	X	X	
Pronator teres						X	X		
Flexor carpi radialis						X	X	*X*	
Palmaris longus							X	X	*X*
Flexor digit. superficialis							*X*	X	X
Flexor digit. profundus I and II							*X*	X	X
Flexor pollicis longus							*X*	X	X
Pronator quadratus							*X*	X	X
Abductor pollicis brevis							*X*	*X*	*X*
Opponens pollicis							*X*	*X*	*X*
Flexor pollicis brevis							*X*	*X*	*X*
Lumbricals I and II							*X*	X	X
Flexor carpi ulnaris							*X*	X	*X*
Flexor digit. profundus III and IV								X	X
Palmaris brevis								X	X
Abductor digiti minimi								X	X
Opponens digiti minimi								X	X
Flexor digiti minimi								X	X
Palmar interossei								X	X
Dorsal interossei								X	X
Lumbricals III and IV								X	X
Adductor pollicis								X	X

Data compiled primarily from Kendall FP, McCreary EK, Provance PG, et al: *Muscles: testing and function with posture and pain,* ed 5, Philadelphia, 2005, Lippincott Williams & Wilkins; Standring S: *Gray's anatomy: the anatomical basis of clinical practice,* ed 42, St Louis, 2021, Elsevier; and unpublished clinical observations of persons with spinal cord injury.
X, minor-to-moderate distribution; **X**, major distribution.

Part C: Five Major Nerves and Their Motor Innervation Pattern throughout the Upper Extremity

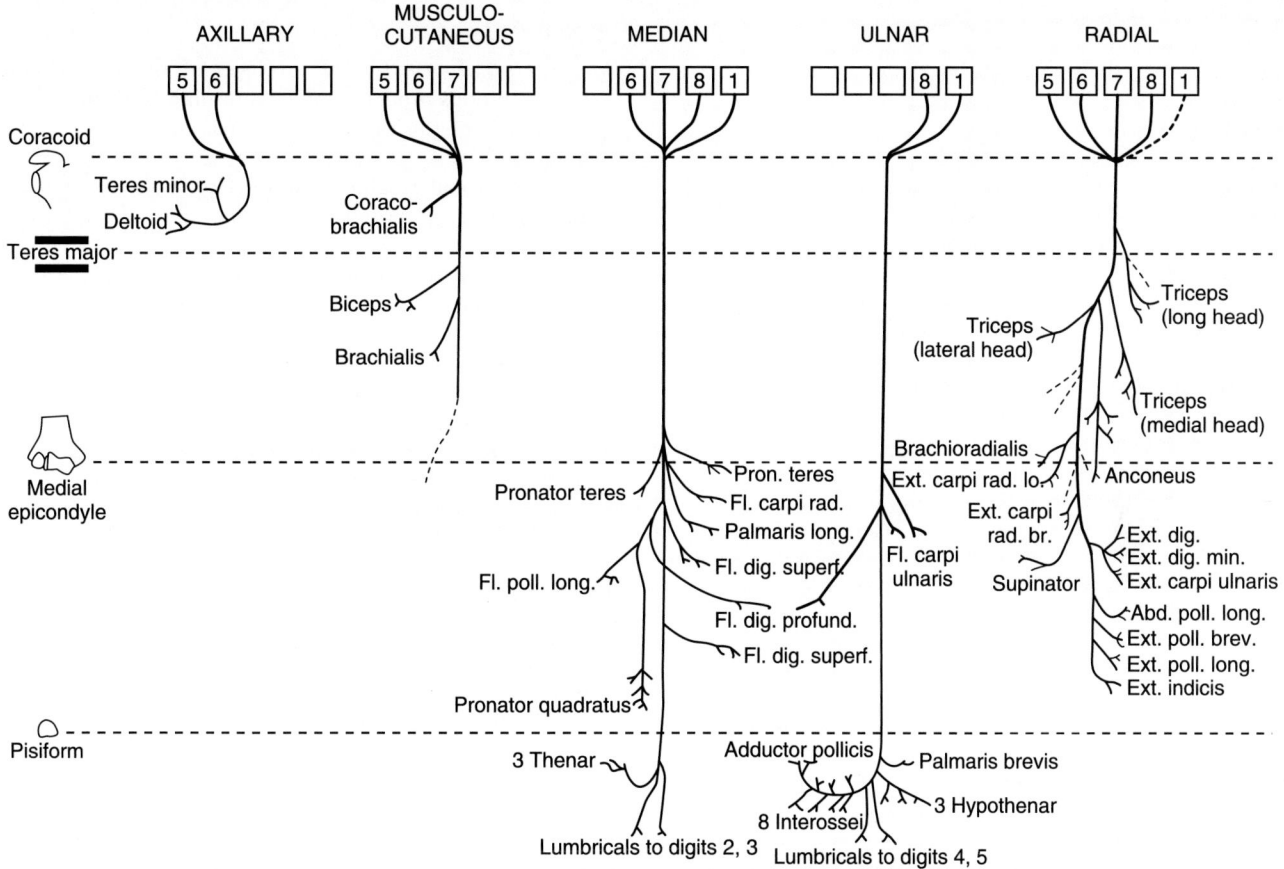

FIGURE II.2   Motor innervations of the upper extremity. (From Swanson AB, de Groot Swanson G: Principles and methods of impairment evaluation in the hand and upper extremity. In American Medical Association: *Guides to the evaluation of permanent impairment,* ed 4, Chicago, 1993, AMA.)

Part D: Key Muscles for Testing the Function of Spinal Nerve Roots (C^5 to T^1)

The table shows the key muscles typically used to test the function of individual nerve roots of the brachial plexus (C^5–T^1). Reduced strength in a key muscle may indicate an injury to or a pathologic process within the associated nerve root.

Key Muscles	Nerve Root	Sample Test Movements
Biceps brachii	C^5	Elbow flexion with forearm supinated
Middle deltoid	C^5	Shoulder abduction
Extensor carpi radialis longus	C^6	Wrist extension with radial deviation
Triceps brachii	C^7	Elbow extension
Extensor digitorum	C^7	Finger extension (metacarpophalangeal joint only)
Flexor digitorum profundus	C^8	Flexion of middle finger (distal interphalangeal joint)
Abductor digiti minimi	T^1	Abduction of little finger (metacarpophalangeal joint)

Part E: Dermatomes of the Upper Extremity

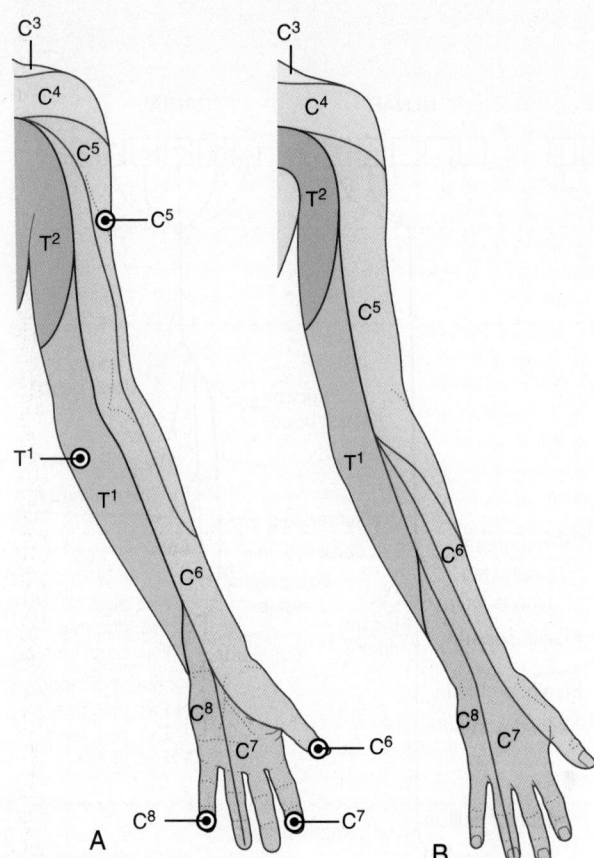

FIGURE II.3 Dermatomes of the upper limb. (A) Anterior view of the left side. (B) Posterior (dorsal) view of the right side. Bold dots indicate regions often used clinically to test each dermatome. Variations are common. *C⁷*, Seventh cervical nerve root; *T¹*, first thoracic nerve root; and so on. (Modified from Drake R, Vogl W, Mitchell A: *Gray's anatomy for students,* ed 3, Philadelphia, 2014, Churchill Livingstone.)

Part F: Attachments and Innervation of the Muscles of the Upper Extremity

SHOULDER MUSCULATURE

CORACOBRACHIALIS

Proximal attachment: apex of the coracoid process by a common tendon with the short head of the biceps
Distal attachment: medial aspect of middle shaft of the humerus
Innervation: musculocutaneous nerve

DELTOID

Proximal attachments:
Anterior part: anterior surface of the lateral end of the clavicle
Middle part: superior surface of the lateral edge of the acromion
Posterior part: posterior border of the spine of the scapula
Distal attachment: deltoid tuberosity of the humerus
Innervation: axillary nerve

INFRASPINATUS

Proximal attachment: infraspinous fossa
Distal attachment: middle facet of the greater tubercle of the humerus; part of the capsule of the glenohumeral joint
Innervation: suprascapular nerve

LATISSIMUS DORSI

Proximal attachments: posterior layer of the thoracolumbar fascia, spinous processes, and supraspinous ligaments of the lower half of the thoracic vertebrae and all lumbar vertebrae; median sacral crest; posterior crest of the ilium; lower four ribs; small area near the inferior angle of the scapula; and muscular interdigitations from the obliquus external abdominis
Distal attachment: floor of the intertubercular groove of the humerus
Innervation: thoracodorsal (middle subscapular) nerve

LEVATOR SCAPULA

Proximal attachments: transverse processes of C1 and C2 and posterior tubercles of transverse processes of C3 and C4
Distal attachment: medial border of the scapula between the superior angle and root of the spine
Innervation: ventral rami of spinal nerves (C³–C⁴) and the dorsal scapular nerve

PECTORALIS MAJOR

Proximal attachments:
Clavicular head: anterior margin of the medial half of the clavicle
Sternocostal head: lateral margin of the manubrium and body of the sternum and cartilages of the first six or seven ribs; costal fibers blend with muscular slips from obliquus external abdominis
Distal attachment: crest of the greater tubercle of the humerus
Innervation: lateral and medial pectoral nerves

PECTORALIS MINOR

Proximal attachments: external surfaces of the third through fifth ribs
Distal attachment: medial border of the coracoid process
Innervation: medial pectoral nerve

RHOMBOID MAJOR AND MINOR

Proximal attachments: ligamentous nuchae and spinous processes of C7 to T5
Distal attachment: medial border of scapula, from the root of the spine to the inferior angle
Innervation: dorsal scapular nerve

SERRATUS ANTERIOR

Proximal attachments: external surface of the lateral region of the first to ninth ribs
Distal attachment: entire medial border of the scapula, with a concentration of fibers near the inferior angle
Innervation: long thoracic nerve

SUBCLAVIUS

Proximal attachment: at the extreme anterior end of the first rib
Distal attachment: inferior middle one-third of the clavicle
Innervation: subclavian nerve

SUBSCAPULARIS
Proximal attachment: subscapular fossa
Distal attachment: lesser tubercle of the humerus; part of the capsule of the glenohumeral joint
Innervation: upper and lower subscapular nerves

SUPRASPINATUS
Proximal attachment: supraspinous fossa
Distal attachment: upper facet of the greater tubercle of the humerus; part of the capsule of the glenohumeral joint
Innervation: suprascapular nerve

TERES MAJOR
Proximal attachment: inferior angle of the scapula
Distal attachment: crest of the lesser tubercle of the humerus
Innervation: lower subscapular nerve

TERES MINOR
Proximal attachment: posterior surface of the lateral border of the scapula
Distal attachment: lower facet of the greater tubercle of the humerus; part of the capsule of the glenohumeral joint
Innervation: axillary nerve

TRAPEZIUS
Proximal attachments:
Upper part: medial aspect of superior nuchal line and external occipital protuberance, upper and middle parts of cervical ligamentum nuchae
Middle part: lower part of cervical ligamentum nuchae, spinous processes and supraspinous ligaments of T1- T6
Lower part: spinous processes and supraspinous ligaments of T7-T12
Distal attachments:
Upper part: posterior-superior edge of the lateral one-third of the clavicle
Middle part: medial margin of the acromion and upper lip of the spine of the scapula
Lower part: medial end of the spine of the scapula, just lateral to the root
Innervation: primarily by the spinal accessory nerve (cranial nerve XI); secondary innervation directly from ventral rami of C^2–C^4

ELBOW AND FOREARM MUSCULATURE
ANCONEUS
Proximal attachment: posterior side of the lateral epicondyle of the humerus
Distal attachment: between the olecranon process and proximal surface of the posterior side of the ulna
Innervation: radial nerve

BICEPS BRACHII
Proximal attachments:
Long head: supraglenoid tubercle of the scapula
Short head: apex of the coracoid process of the scapula
Distal attachments: bicipital tuberosity of the radius; also to deep connective tissue within the forearm via the fibrous lacertus
Innervation: musculocutaneous nerve

BRACHIALIS
Proximal attachment: distal aspect of the anterior surface of the humerus

Distal attachments: coronoid process and tuberosity on the proximal ulna
Innervation: musculocutaneous nerve (small contribution from the radial nerve)

BRACHIORADIALIS
Proximal attachment: upper two-thirds of the lateral supracondylar ridge of the humerus
Distal attachment: lateral side of the distal radius, just proximal to the styloid process
Innervation: radial nerve

PRONATOR TERES
Proximal attachments:
Humeral head: medial epicondyle
Ulnar head: medial to the tuberosity of the ulna
Distal attachment: lateral surface of the middle radius
Innervation: median nerve

PRONATOR QUADRATUS
Proximal attachment: anterior surface of the distal ulna
Distal attachment: anterior surface of the distal radius
Innervation: median nerve

SUPINATOR
Proximal attachments: lateral epicondyle of the humerus, radial collateral and annular ligaments, and supinator crest of the ulna
Distal attachment: lateral surface of the proximal radius
Innervation: radial nerve

TRICEPS BRACHII
Proximal attachments:
Long head: infraglenoid tubercle of the scapula
Lateral head: posterior humerus, superior and lateral to the radial groove
Medial head: posterior humerus, inferior and medial to the radial groove
Distal attachment: olecranon process of the ulna
Innervation: radial nerve

WRIST MUSCULATURE
EXTENSOR CARPI RADIALIS BREVIS
Proximal attachment: common extensor-supinator tendon attaching to the lateral epicondyle of the humerus, and radial collateral ligament
Distal attachment: dorsal-radial base of third metacarpal and dorsal-ulnar base of second metacarpal
Innervation: radial nerve

EXTENSOR CARPI RADIALIS LONGUS
Proximal attachments: common extensor-supinator tendon attaching to the lateral epicondyle of the humerus and the distal part of the lateral supracondylar ridge of the humerus
Distal attachment: radial-posterior surface of the base of the second metacarpal
Innervation: radial nerve

EXTENSOR CARPI ULNARIS
Proximal attachments: common extensor-supinator tendon attaching to the lateral epicondyle of the humerus and the posterior border of the middle one-third of the ulna

Distal attachment: posterior-ulnar surface of the base of the fifth metacarpal
Innervation: radial nerve

FLEXOR CARPI RADIALIS

Proximal attachment: common flexor-pronator tendon attaching to the medial epicondyle of the humerus
Distal attachments: palmar surface of the base of the second metacarpal and a small slip to the base of the third metacarpal
Innervation: median nerve

FLEXOR CARPI ULNARIS

Proximal attachments:
Humeral head: common flexor-pronator tendon attaching to the medial epicondyle of the humerus
Ulnar head: posterior border of the middle one-third of the ulna
Distal attachments: pisiform bone, pisohamate and pisometacarpal ligaments, and palmar base of the fifth metacarpal bone
Innervation: ulnar nerve

PALMARIS LONGUS

Proximal attachment: common flexor-pronator tendon attaching to the medial epicondyle of the humerus
Distal attachment: central part of the transverse carpal ligament and palmar aponeurosis of the hand
Innervation: median nerve

EXTRINSIC HAND MUSCULATURE
ABDUCTOR POLLICIS LONGUS

Proximal attachments: posterior surface of the middle part of the radius and ulna, and adjacent interosseous membrane
Distal attachments: radial-dorsal surface of the base of the thumb metacarpal; occasional secondary attachments to the trapezium and thenar muscles
Innervation: radial nerve

EXTENSOR DIGITORUM

Proximal attachment: common extensor-supinator tendon attaching to the lateral epicondyle of the humerus
Distal attachments: by four tendons, each to the base of the extensor mechanism and to the dorsal base of the proximal phalanx of the fingers
Innervation: radial nerve

EXTENSOR DIGITI MINIMI

Proximal attachment: ulnar side of the belly of the extensor digitorum
Distal attachments: tendon usually divides, joining the ulnar side of the tendon of the extensor digitorum
Innervation: radial nerve

EXTENSOR INDICIS

Proximal attachments: posterior surface of the middle to distal part of the ulna and adjacent interosseous membrane
Distal attachment: tendon blends with the ulnar side of the index tendon of the extensor digitorum
Innervation: radial nerve

EXTENSOR POLLICIS BREVIS

Proximal attachments: posterior surface of the middle to distal parts of the radius and adjacent interosseous membrane
Distal attachment: dorsal base of the proximal phalanx and extensor mechanism of the thumb
Innervation: radial nerve

EXTENSOR POLLICIS LONGUS

Proximal attachments: posterior surface of the middle part of the ulna and adjacent interosseous membrane
Distal attachment: dorsal base of the distal phalanx and extensor mechanism of the thumb
Innervation: radial nerve

FLEXOR DIGITORUM PROFUNDUS

Proximal attachments: proximal three-fourths of the anterior and medial sides of the ulna and adjacent interosseous membrane
Distal attachments: by four tendons, each to the palmar base of the distal phalanges of the fingers
Innervation:
Medial half: ulnar nerve
Lateral half: median nerve

FLEXOR DIGITORUM SUPERFICIALIS

Proximal attachments:
Humeroulnar head: common flexor-pronator tendon attaching to the medial epicondyle of the humerus and the medial side of the coronoid process of the ulna
Radial head: oblique line just distal and lateral to the bicipital tuberosity
Distal attachments: by four tendons, each to the sides of the palmar aspect of the middle phalanges of the fingers
Innervation: median nerve

FLEXOR POLLICIS LONGUS

Proximal attachments: middle part of the anterior surface of the radius and adjacent interosseous membrane
Distal attachment: palmar base of the distal phalanx of the thumb
Innervation: median nerve

INTRINSIC HAND MUSCULATURE
ABDUCTOR DIGITI MINIMI

Proximal attachments: pisohamate ligament, pisiform bone, and tendon of the flexor carpi ulnaris
Distal attachments: ulnar side of the base of the proximal phalanx of the little finger; also attaches into the extensor mechanism of the little finger
Innervation: ulnar nerve

ABDUCTOR POLLICIS BREVIS

Proximal attachments: transverse carpal ligament, palmar tubercles of the trapezium and scaphoid bones
Distal attachments: radial side of the base of the proximal phalanx of the thumb; also attaches into the extensor mechanism of the thumb
Innervation: median nerve

ADDUCTOR POLLICIS

Proximal attachments:

Oblique head: capitate bone, base of the second and third metacarpals, adjacent capsular ligaments of the carpometacarpal joints, and sheath of the tendon of the flexor carpi radialis

Transverse head: palmar surface of the third metacarpal

Distal attachments: both heads attach on the ulnar side of the base of the proximal phalanx of the thumb and to the medial sesamoid bone at the metacarpophalangeal joint; also attaches into the extensor mechanism of the thumb

Innervation: ulnar nerve

DORSAL INTEROSSEI

Proximal attachments:

First: adjacent sides of the first (thumb) and second metacarpals

Second: adjacent sides of the second and third metacarpals

Third: adjacent sides of the third and fourth metacarpals

Fourth: adjacent sides of the fourth and fifth metacarpals

Distal attachments:

First: radial sides of the oblique fibers of the dorsal hood and base of the proximal phalanx of the index finger

Second: radial sides of the oblique fibers of the dorsal hood and base of the proximal phalanx of the middle finger

Third: ulnar sides of the oblique fibers of the dorsal hood and base of the proximal phalanx of the middle finger

Fourth: ulnar sides of the oblique fibers of the dorsal hood and base of the proximal phalanx of the ring finger

Innervation: ulnar nerve

FLEXOR DIGITI MINIMI

Proximal attachments: transverse carpal ligament and hook of the hamate

Distal attachment: ulnar side of the base of the proximal phalanx of the little finger

Innervation: ulnar nerve

FLEXOR POLLICIS BREVIS

Proximal attachments: transverse carpal ligament and palmar tubercle of the trapezium

Distal attachments: radial side of the base of the proximal phalanx of the thumb; also to the lateral sesamoid bone at the metacarpophalangeal joint

Innervation: median nerve

LUMBRICALS

Proximal attachments:

Medial two: adjacent sides of the flexor digitorum profundus tendons of the little, ring, and middle fingers

Lateral two: lateral sides of the flexor digitorum profundus tendons of the middle and index fingers

Distal attachment: lateral margin of the extensor mechanism via the oblique fibers of the dorsal hood

Innervation:

Medial two: ulnar nerve

Lateral two: median nerve

OPPONENS DIGITI MINIMI

Proximal attachments: transverse carpal ligament and hook of the hamate

Distal attachment: ulnar surface of the shaft of the fifth metacarpal

Innervation: ulnar nerve

OPPONENS POLLICIS

Proximal attachments: transverse carpal ligament and palmar tubercle of the trapezium

Distal attachment: radial surface of the shaft of the thumb metacarpal

Innervation: median nerve

PALMARIS BREVIS

Proximal attachments: transverse carpal ligament and palmar fascia just distal and lateral to the pisiform bone

Distal attachment: skin on the ulnar border of the hand

Innervation: ulnar nerve

PALMAR INTEROSSEI

Proximal attachments:

First: ulnar side of the thumb metacarpal

Second: ulnar side of the second metacarpal

Third: radial side of the fourth metacarpal

Fourth: radial side of the fifth metacarpal

Distal attachments:

First: ulnar side of the proximal phalanx of the thumb, blending with the adductor pollicis; also attaches to the medial sesamoid bone at the metacarpophalangeal joint

Second: ulnar sides of the oblique fibers of the dorsal hood and base of the proximal phalanx of the index finger

Third: radial sides of the oblique fibers of the dorsal hood and base of the proximal phalanx of the ring finger

Fourth: radial sides of the oblique fibers of the dorsal hood and base of the proximal phalanx of the small finger

Innervation: ulnar nerve

Part G: Physiologic Cross-Sectional Areas of Selected Muscles of the Upper Extremity

Physiologic Cross-Sectional Areas (PCSAs) of a Sample of Adult Human Upper Extremity Muscles*

Muscle	PCSA (cm^2) (mean ± SD)	Muscle	PCSA (cm^2) (mean ± SD)
Shoulder Musculature		Extensor pollicis brevis	0.5 ± 0.3[2]
Supraspinatus	6.7 ± 0.6[5]	Extensor pollicis longus	1.0 ± 0.1[3]
Infraspinatus	10.7 ± 1.0[5]	Extensor indicis	0.6 ± 0.1[3]
Subscapularis	15.5 ± 1.4[5]	Flexor digitorum superficialis I	2.5 ± 1.6[1]
Teres minor	3.2 ± 0.3[5]	Flexor digitorum superficialis II	1.7 ± 0.6[1]
Coracobrachialis	2.0[4]	Flexor digitorum superficialis III	1.2 ± 0.7[1]
Elbow and Forearm Musculature		Flexor digitorum superficialis IV	0.7 ± 0.4[1]
Biceps (long head)	2.5 ± 0.2[1]	Flexor digitorum profundus I	1.8 ± 0.2[3]
Biceps (short head)	2.1 ± 0.5[1]	Flexor digitorum profundus II	2.2 ± 0.2[3]
Brachialis	7.0 ± 1.9[1]	Flexor digitorum profundus III	1.7 ± 0.2[3]
Triceps (medial head)	6.1 ± 2.3[1]	Flexor digitorum profundus IV	2.2 ± 0.3[3]
Triceps (lateral head)	6.0 ± 1.2[1]	Flexor pollicis longus	2.1 ± 0.2[3]
Triceps (long head)	6.7 ± 2.0[1]	**Intrinsic Hand Musculature**	
Anconeus	2.5 ± 1.2[1]	Abductor pollicis brevis	0.7 ± 0.3[2]
Brachioradialis	1.5 ± 0.5[1]	Opponens pollicis	1.0 ± 0.4[2]
Pronator teres	3.4 ± 1.5[1]	Flexor pollicis brevis	0.7 ± 0.2[2]
Supinator	3.4 ± 1.0[1]	Lumbrical I	0.1 ± 0.0[2]
Pronator quadratus	2.1 ± 0.3[3]	Lumbrical II	0.1 ± 0.0[2]
Wrist Musculature		Lumbrical III	0.1 ± 0.0[2]
Extensor carpi radialis brevis	2.9 ± 1.4[1]	Lumbrical IV	0.1 ± 0.0[2]
Extensor carpi radialis longus	2.4 ± 1.0[1]	Abductor digiti minimi	0.9 ± 0.5[2]
Extensor carpi ulnaris	3.4 ± 1.3[1]	Opponens digiti minimi	1.1 ± 0.4[2]
Flexor carpi radialis	2.0 ± 0.6[1]	Flexor digiti minimi	0.5 ± 0.4[2]
Flexor carpi ulnaris	3.2 ± 0.0[1]	Palmar interosseus II	0.8 ± 0.3[2]
Palmaris longus	0.9 ± 0.6[1]	Palmar interosseus III	0.7 ± 0.3[2]
Extrinsic Hand Musculature		Palmar interosseus IV	0.6 ± 0.2[2]
Extensor digitorum I	0.5 ± 0.1[3]	Dorsal interosseus I	1.5 ± 0.4[2]
Extensor digitorum II	1.0 ± 0.2[3]	Dorsal interosseus II	1.3 ± 0.8[2]
Extensor digitorum III	0.9 ± 0.1[3]	Dorsal interosseus III	1.0 ± 0.5[2]
Extensor digitorum IV	0.4 ± 0.1[3]	Dorsal interosseus IV	0.9 ± 0.4[2]
Extensor digiti minimi	0.6 ± 0.1[3]	Adductor pollicis	1.9 ± 0.4[2]
Abductor pollicis longus	1.9 ± 0.6[2]		

*Muscles are listed in a general proximal-to-distal order. Data are from five sources (see superscripts).
Data compiled with the assistance of Jonathon Senefeld.

References

1. An KN, Hui FC, Morrey BF, et al.: Muscles across the elbow joint: a biomechanical analysis, *J Biomech* 14:659–669, 1981.
2. Jacobson MD, Raab R, Fazeli BM, et al.: Architectural design of the human intrinsic hand muscles, *J Hand Surg [Am]* 17:804–809, 1992.
3. Lieber RL, Jacobson MD, Fazeli BM, et al.: Architecture of selected muscles of the arm and forearm: anatomy and implications for tendon transfer, *J Hand Surg [Am]* 17:787–798, 1992.
4. Veeger HE, Yu B, An KN, et al.: Parameters for modeling the upper extremity, *J Biomech* 30:647–652, 1997.
5. Ward SR, Hentzen ER, Smallwood LH, et al.: Rotator cuff muscle architecture: implications for glenohumeral stability, *Clin Orthop Relat Res* 448:157–163, 2006.

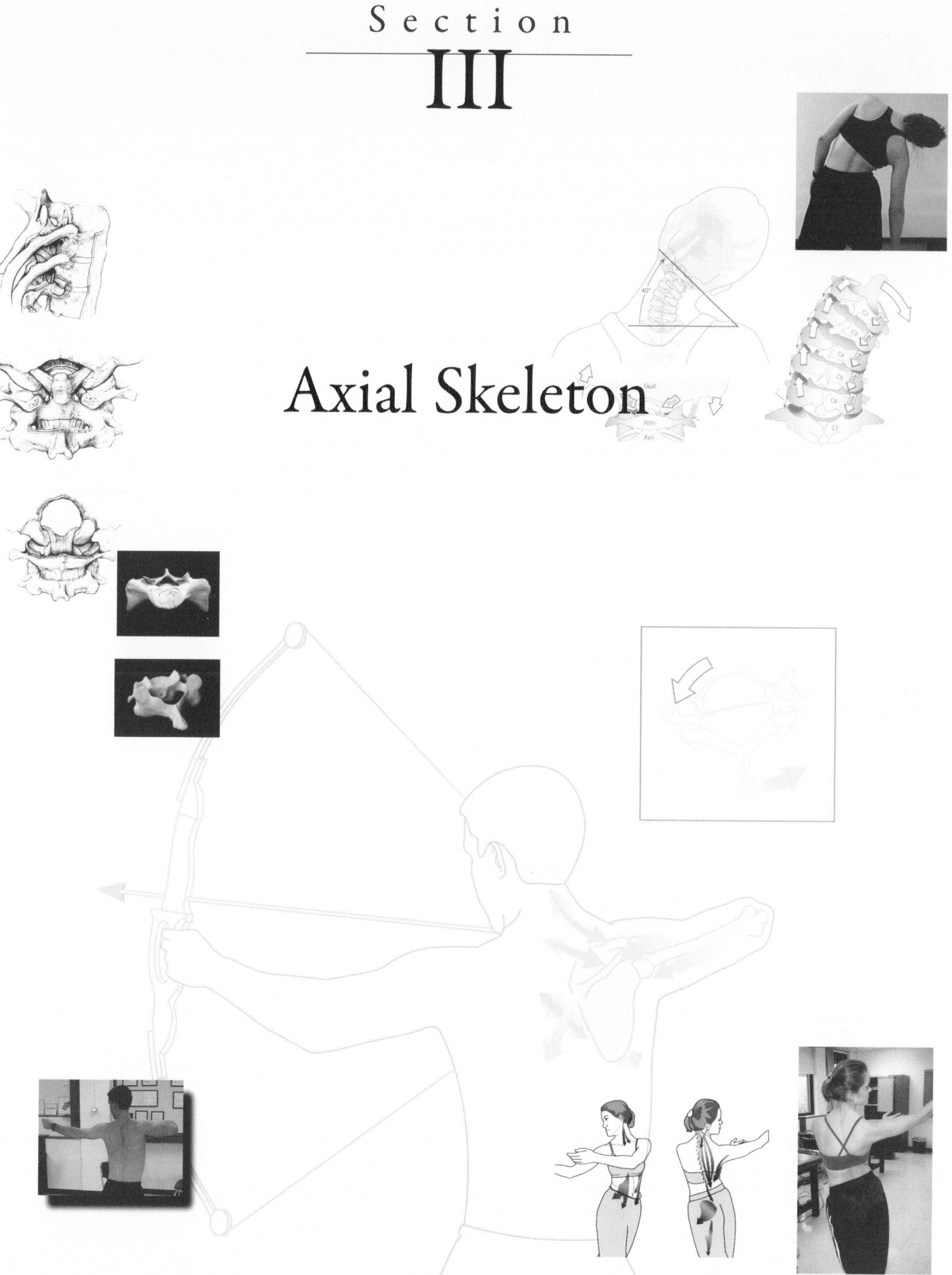

Axial Skeleton

Section III

Axial Skeleton

Section III focuses on the kinesiology of the axial skeleton: the cranium, vertebrae, sternum, and ribs. The section is divided into three chapters, each describing a different kinesiologic aspect of the axial skeleton. Chapter 9 presents osteology and arthrology, and Chapter 10 presents muscle and joint interactions. Chapter 11 describes two special topics related to the axial skeleton: the kinesiology of mastication (chewing) and ventilation.

Section III presents several overlapping functions that involve the axial skeleton. These functions include (1) provision of axial stability plus overall mobility to the body; (2) optimal placement of the senses of vision, hearing, and smell; (3) protection to the spinal cord, brain, and internal organs; and (4) control of bodily activities such as the mechanics of ventilation, mastication, childbirth, coughing, and defecation. Musculoskeletal impairments within the axial skeleton can cause limitation in any of these four functions.

EDUCATIONAL eCONTENT

Chapters 9-11 contain several videos that are designed to enhance the understanding of the kinesiology presented within Section III. Material includes videos of fluoroscopy of cervical and TMJ arthrokinematics, special teaching models, visual EMG-based display of activated muscles during exercises involving the trunk and upper extremity, examples of persons displaying abnormal kinesiology, and more.

Certain videos relate specifically to the text material. Other material, referred to as *additional video educational content* are not indicated in the text but are listed at the very end of each chapter.

How to view? The videos and e-figures are available in the accompanying enhanced eBook version included with the print purchase of this textbook. Visit Elsevier eBooks+ (eBooks.Health.Elsevier.com) to access this content.

ADDITIONAL CLINICAL CONNECTIONS

Additional Clinical Connections are included at the end of each chapter. This feature is intended to highlight or expand on a particular clinical concept associated with the kinesiology covered in the chapter.

STUDY QUESTIONS

Study Questions are also included at the end of each chapter. These questions are designed to challenge the reader to review or reinforce some of the main concepts contained within the chapter. The process of answering these questions is an effective way for students to prepare for examinations. The answers to the questions are available in the accompanying enhanced eBook version included with the print purchase of this textbook.

Chapter
9

Axial Skeleton: Osteology and Arthrology

DONALD A. NEUMANN, PT, PhD, FAPTA

GUY G. SIMONEAU, PT, PhD, FAPTA

As a whole, the skeleton is comprised of axial and appendicular components. The *appendicular skeleton* consists of the bones of the extremities, including the clavicle, scapula, and pelvis; the *axial skeleton,* in contrast, consists of the cranium, vertebral column (spine), ribs, and sternum (Fig. 9.1). As indicated in Fig. 9.1, the axial and appendicular skeletons articulate superiorly at the sternoclavicular joints and inferiorly at the sacroiliac joints.

The osteology and associated arthrology presented in this chapter focus primarily on the axial skeleton. This focus includes the craniocervical region, vertebral column, and sacroiliac joints, describing how these articulations provide stability, movement, and load transfer throughout the axial skeleton. Muscles play a large role in this function and are the primary focus of Chapter 10.

Disease, trauma, overuse, and normal aging can cause a host of neuromuscular and musculoskeletal conditions involving the axial skeleton. Disorders of the vertebral column are often associated with neurologic impairment, primarily because of the close anatomic relationship between neural tissue (spinal cord and nerve roots) and connective tissue (vertebrae and associated ligaments, intervertebral discs, and synovial joints). A herniated disc, for example, can increase pressure on the adjacent neural tissues, resulting in local inflammation and weakness, sensory disturbances, and reduced reflexes throughout the lower limb. Furthermore, certain movements and habitual postures of the vertebral column may increase the likelihood of connective tissues impinging on neural tissues, such as a spinal nerve root. An understanding of the detailed osteology and arthrology of the axial skeleton is crucial to an appreciation of the associated pathomechanics, as well as the rationale for many clinical examinations and interventions.

Table 9.1 summarizes the terminology used to describe the relative location or region within the axial skeleton.

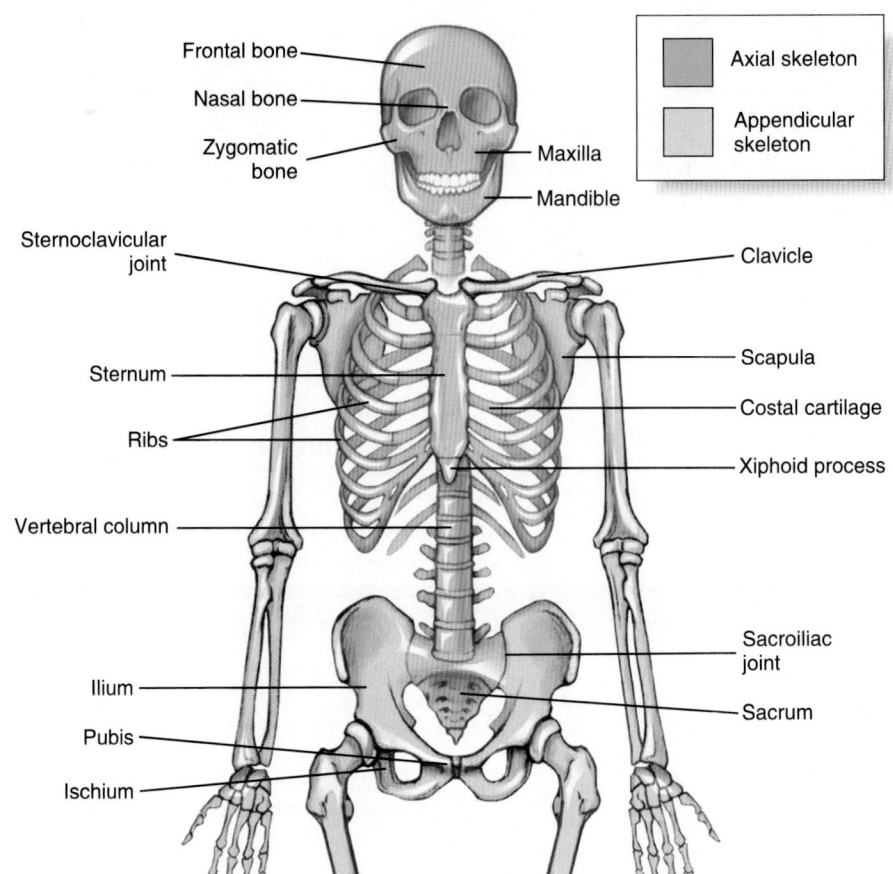

FIG. 9.1 Human skeleton. The axial skeleton is highlighted in blue. (From Thibodeau GA, Patton KT: *Structure and function of the body,* ed 14, St Louis, 2011, Elsevier.)

TABLE 9.1 Terminology Describing Relative Location or Region within the Axial Skeleton*		
Term	**Synonym**	**Definition**
Posterior	Dorsal	Back of the body
Anterior	Ventral	Front of the body
Medial	None	Midline of the body
Lateral	None	Away from the midline of the body
Superior	Cranial	Head or top of the body
Inferior	Caudal (the "tail")	Tail, or the bottom of the body

*The definitions assume a person is in the anatomic position.

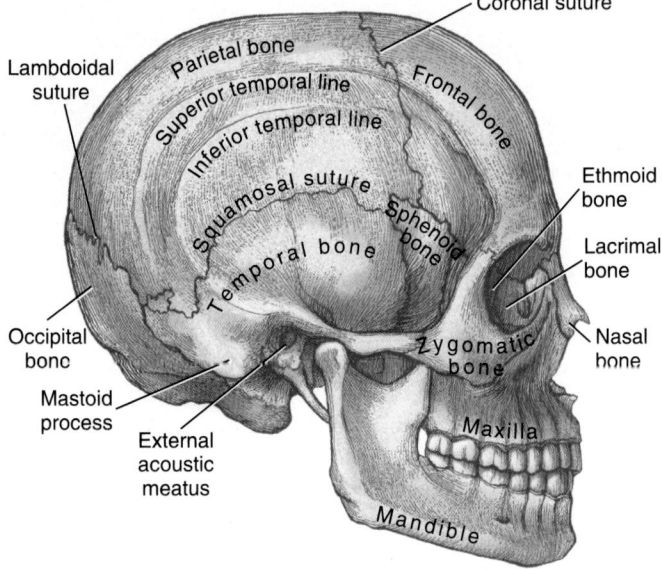

FIG. 9.2 Lateral view of the skull.

OSTEOLOGY

Components within the Axial Skeleton

CRANIUM

The cranium encases and protects the brain and several essential sensory organs (eyes, ears, nose, and vestibular system). Of the many individual bones of the cranium, only the temporal and occipital bones are relevant to the material covered in Chapters 9 and 10.

Temporal and Occipital Bones

Each of the two *temporal* bones forms part of the lateral external surface of the skull, immediately surrounding and including the external acoustic meatus (Fig. 9.2). The *mastoid process,* easily palpable, is

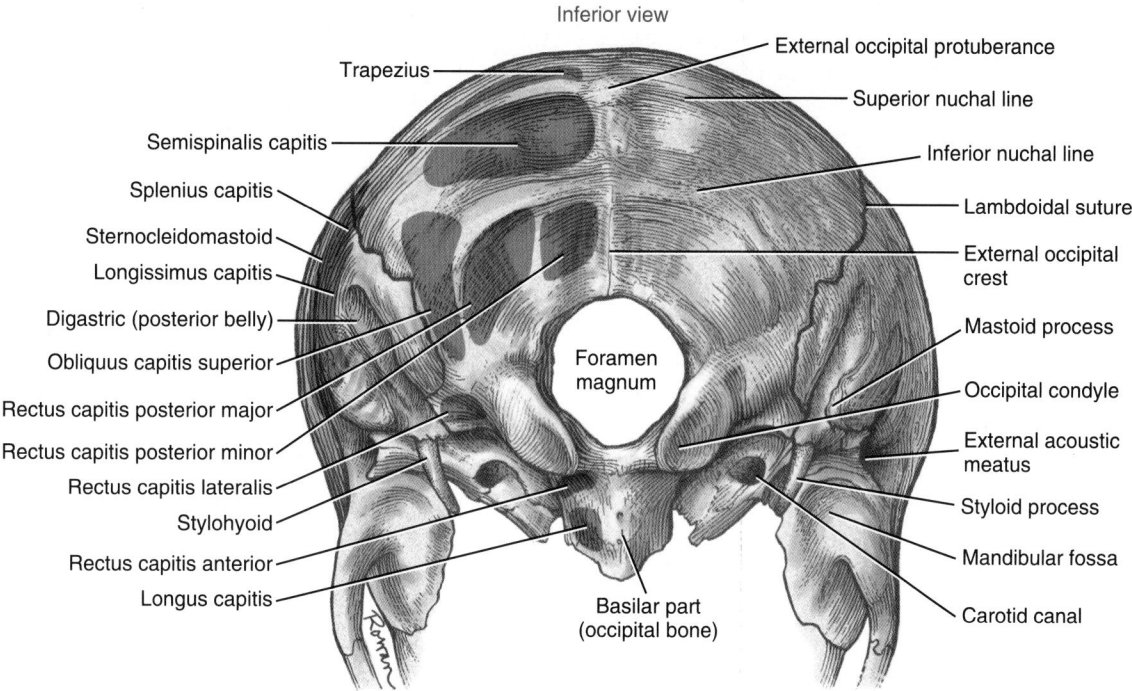

Inferior view

Trapezius — External occipital protuberance

Semispinalis capitis — Superior nuchal line

Splenius capitis — Inferior nuchal line

Sternocleidomastoid — Lambdoidal suture

Longissimus capitis — External occipital crest

Digastric (posterior belly) — Mastoid process

Obliquus capitis superior — Occipital condyle

Rectus capitis posterior major — External acoustic meatus

Rectus capitis posterior minor — Styloid process

Rectus capitis lateralis — Mandibular fossa

Stylohyoid — Carotid canal

Rectus capitis anterior — Basilar part (occipital bone)

Longus capitis

Foramen magnum

FIG. 9.3 Inferior view of the occipital and temporal bones. The lambdoidal sutures separate the occipital bone medially from the temporal bones laterally. Distal muscle attachments are indicated in gray, and proximal attachments are indicated in red.

just posterior to the ear. This prominent process serves as an attachment for many muscles, such as the sternocleidomastoid.

The *occipital bone* forms much of the posterior base of the skull (Fig. 9.3). The *external occipital protuberance* is a palpable midline point, serving as the most cranial attachment for the ligamentum nuchae and the medial part of the upper trapezius muscle. The *superior nuchal line* extends laterally from the external occipital protuberance to the base of the mastoid process. This thin but distinct line marks the attachments of several extensor muscles of the head and neck, such as the trapezius and splenius capitis muscles. The *inferior nuchal line* marks the anterior edge of the attachment of the semispinalis capitis muscle.

Relevant Osteologic Features

TEMPORAL BONE
- Mastoid process

OCCIPITAL BONE
- External occipital protuberance
- Superior nuchal line
- Inferior nuchal line
- Foramen magnum
- Occipital condyles
- Basilar part

The *foramen magnum* is a large circular hole located at the base of the occipital bone, serving as the passageway for the spinal cord. A pair of prominent *occipital condyles* projects from the anterior-lateral margins of the foramen magnum, forming the convex component of the atlanto-occipital joint. The *basilar part* of the occipital bone lies just anterior to the anterior rim of the foramen magnum.

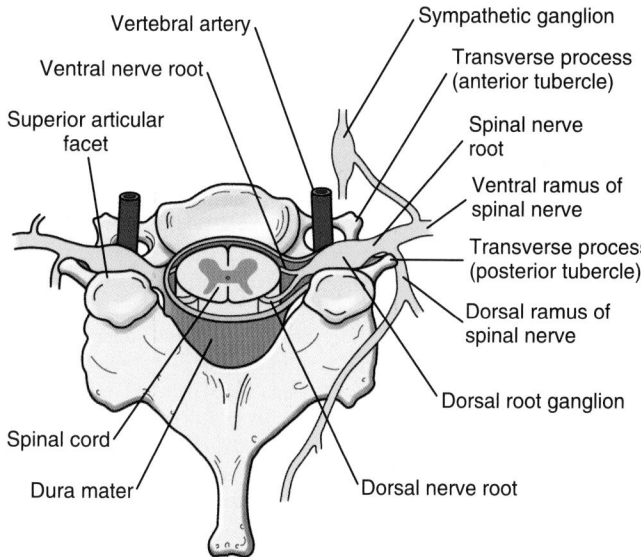

Vertebral artery — Sympathetic ganglion

Ventral nerve root — Transverse process (anterior tubercle)

Superior articular facet — Spinal nerve root

Ventral ramus of spinal nerve

Transverse process (posterior tubercle)

Dorsal ramus of spinal nerve

Dorsal root ganglion

Spinal cord — Dorsal nerve root

Dura mater

FIG. 9.4 A cross-section of a spinal cord is shown. Note the relationship among the neural tissues, components of the cervical vertebra, and the vertebral artery. (Modified with permission from Magee DL: *Orthopedic physical assessment,* ed 3, Philadelphia, 1997, Saunders.)

VERTEBRAE: BUILDING BLOCKS OF THE SPINE

In addition to providing vertical stability throughout the trunk and neck, the vertebral column protects the spinal cord, ventral and dorsal nerve roots, and exiting spinal nerve roots (Fig. 9.4). The relationship between the spinal cord and exiting nerve roots throughout the entire vertebral column is schematically shown in Fig. III.1 in Appendix III, Part A.

The midthoracic vertebrae demonstrate many of the essential anatomic and functional characteristics of any given vertebra (Fig. 9.5). As a general orientation, a vertebra can be subdivided into three sections. Anteriorly is the large vertebral *body*—the primary weight-bearing component of a vertebra. Posteriorly are the transverse and spinous processes, laminae, and articular processes, collectively referred to as *posterior elements.* The *pedicles,* the third section, act as bridges that connect the body with the posterior elements. Thick and strong, the pedicles transfer forward the muscle forces applied to posterior elements for dispersion across the vertebral body and intervertebral discs. Table 9.2 provides greater detail on the structure and function of the components of a typical midthoracic vertebra.

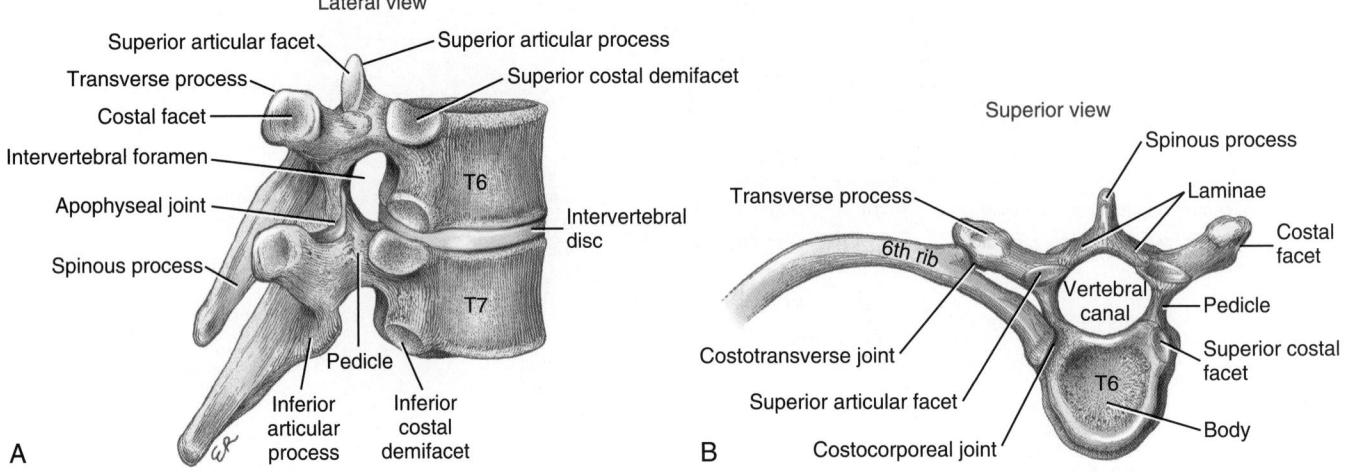

FIG. 9.5 The essential characteristics of a vertebra. (A) Lateral view of the sixth and seventh vertebrae (T6 and T7). (B) Superior view of the sixth vertebra with right rib.

TABLE 9.2 **Major Parts of a Midthoracic Vertebra**

Part	Description	Primary Function
Body	Large cylindrical mass of trabecular bone lined by a thin cortex of bone. The trabecular core is lightweight while still offering excellent resistance against compression	Primary weight-bearing structure of each vertebra
Intervertebral disc	Thick ring of specialized fibrocartilage located between vertebral bodies below C2	Shock absorber and spacer throughout the vertebral column
Interbody joint	A cartilaginous joint formed between the superior and inferior surfaces of an intervertebral disc and adjacent vertebral bodies	Primary bond between vertebrae
Pedicle	Short, thick dorsal projection of bone from the middle to superior part of the vertebral body	Connects the vertebral body to the posterior elements of a vertebra
Lamina	Thin vertical plate of bone connecting the base of the spinous process to each transverse process (The term *laminae* refers to both right lamina and left lamina)	Protects the posterior aspect of the spinal cord
Vertebral canal	Central canal located just posterior to the vertebral body; the canal is surrounded by the pedicles and laminae	Houses and protects the spinal cord and meninges
Intervertebral foramen	Lateral opening between adjacent vertebrae	Passageway for spinal nerve roots exiting the vertebral canal
Transverse process	Horizontal projection of bone from the junction of a lamina and a pedicle	Attachments for muscles, ligaments, and ribs
Costal facets (on body)	Rounded impressions formed on the lateral sides of the thoracic vertebral bodies; most thoracic vertebral bodies have partial superior and inferior facets (called *demifacets*)	Attachment sites for the heads of ribs (costocorporeal joints)
Costal facets (on transverse process)	Oval facets located at the anterior tips of most thoracic transverse processes	Attachment sites for the articular tubercle of ribs (costotransverse joints)
Spinous process	Dorsal midline projection of bone from the laminae	Midline attachments for muscles and ligaments
Superior and inferior articular processes, including articular facets and apophyseal joints	Paired articular processes arising from the junction of a lamina and a pedicle; each process has smooth cartilage-lined articular facets; as a general rule, superior articular facets face posteriorly and inferior articular facets face anteriorly	Superior and inferior articular facets form paired apophyseal joints; these synovial joints guide the direction and magnitude of intervertebral movement

RIBS

Twelve pairs of ribs enclose the thoracic cavity, forming a protective cage for the cardiopulmonary organs. The posterior end of a typical rib has a *head,* a *neck,* and an *articular tubercle* (Fig. 9.6). The head and tubercle articulate with a thoracic vertebra, forming two synovial *costovertebral joints:* costocorporeal and costotransverse, respectively (Fig. 9.5B). These joints anchor the posterior end of a rib to its corresponding vertebra. A typical *costocorporeal joint* connects the head of a rib to a pair of *costal demifacets* that span two adjacent vertebrae and the intervening intervertebral disc. A *costotransverse joint* connects the articular tubercle of a rib with a costal facet on the transverse process of a corresponding vertebra.

The anterior end of a rib consists of flattened hyaline cartilage. Ribs 1 through 10 attach either directly or indirectly to the sternum, thereby completing the thoracic rib cage anteriorly. The cartilage of ribs 1 to 7 attaches directly to the lateral border of the sternum via seven sternocostal joints (Fig. 9.7). The cartilage of ribs 8 to 10 attaches to the sternum by fusing to the cartilage of the immediately superior rib. Ribs 11 and 12 are referred to as "free floating" because they do not attach anteriorly to the sternum.

STERNUM

The sternum is slightly convex and rough anteriorly, and slightly concave and smooth posteriorly. The bone has three parts: the manubrium (Latin, meaning "handle"), the body, and the xiphoid process (from the Greek, "sword") (Fig. 9.7). Developmentally, the *manubrium* fuses with the body of the sternum at the *manubriosternal joint,* a cartilaginous (synarthrodial) articulation that often ossifies later in life. Just lateral to the *jugular notch* of the manubrium are the *clavicular facets* of the *sternoclavicular joints.* Immediately inferior to the sternoclavicular joint is a *costal facet* that accepts the head of the first rib at the first *sternocostal joint.*

Osteologic Features of the Sternum

- Manubrium
- Jugular notch
- Clavicular facets for sternoclavicular joints
- Body
- Costal facets for sternocostal joints
- Xiphoid process

Intrasternal Joints

- Manubriosternal joint
- Xiphisternal joint

The lateral edge of the body of the sternum is marked by a series of *costal facets* that accept the cartilages of ribs 2 to 7. The

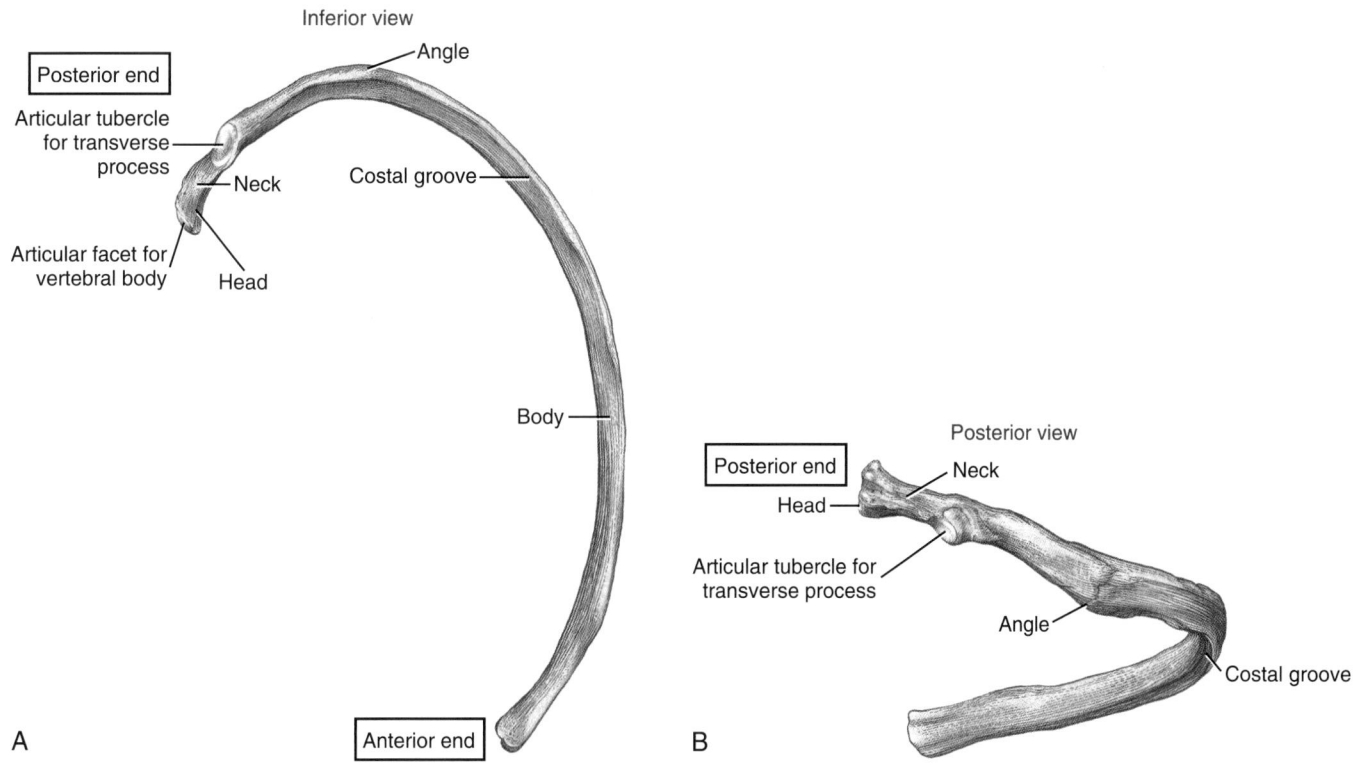

FIG. 9.6 A typical right rib. (A) Inferior view. (B) Posterior view.

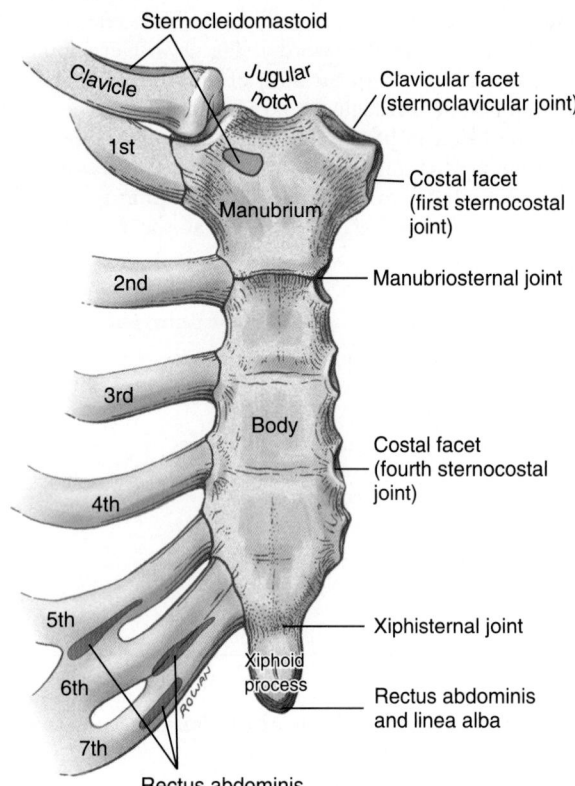

FIG. 9.7 Anterior view of the sternum, part of the right clavicle, and the first seven ribs. The following articulations are seen: (1) intrasternal joints (manubriosternal and xiphisternal), (2) sternocostal joints, and (3) sternoclavicular joints. The attachment of the sternocleidomastoid muscle is indicated in red. The attachments of the rectus abdominis and linea alba are shown in gray.

arthrology of the sternocostal joints is discussed in greater detail in Chapter 11, within the context of ventilation. The *xiphoid process* is attached to the inferior end of the body of the sternum by the *xiphisternal joint.* Like the manubriosternal joint, the xiphisternal joint is connected primarily by fibrocartilage. The xiphisternal joint is commonly ossified by the time of adulthood.[275]

Vertebral Column as a Whole

The *vertebral (spinal) column* usually consists of 33 vertebral bony *segments* divided into five regions. Normally there are 7 *cervical,* 12 *thoracic,* 5 *lumbar,* 5 *sacral,* and 4 *coccygeal segments.* The sacral and coccygeal vertebrae are usually fused in the adult, forming individual sacral and coccygeal bones. Individual vertebrae are abbreviated alphanumerically; for example, C2 for the second cervical, T6 for the sixth thoracic, and L1 for the first lumbar. Each region of the vertebral column (e.g., cervical and lumbar) has a distinct morphology that reflects its specific function and movement potential. Vertebrae located at the cervicothoracic, thoracolumbar, and lumbosacral junctions often share characteristics that reflect the transition between major regions of the vertebral column. It is not uncommon, for example, for the transverse processes of C7 to have thoracic-like facets to accept a rib or for L5 to be "sacralized" (i.e., fused with the base of the sacrum).

NORMAL CURVATURES WITHIN THE VERTEBRAL COLUMN

The human vertebral column consists of a series of reciprocal curvatures within the sagittal plane (Fig. 9.8A). These natural curvatures contribute to what is often perceived as "ideal" spinal posture. The curvatures also define the anatomic (or neutral) position of the different regions of the spine. In the anatomic position, the cervical and lumbar regions are naturally convex anteriorly and concave posteriorly, exhibiting an alignment called *lordosis,* meaning to "bend backward." The degree of lordosis is usually less in the cervical region than in the lumbar region. A recent study, for example, reported that about 25% of a group of more than 1000 asymptomatic individuals had a straight or slightly kyphotic cervical spine.[143,323] The thoracic and sacrococcygeal regions, in contrast, exhibit a natural *kyphosis.* Kyphosis describes a curve that is concave anteriorly and convex posteriorly. The anterior concavity provides space for the organs within the thoracic and pelvic cavities.

The natural curvatures within most of the vertebral column are not fixed but are dynamic and change shape during movements and adjustment of posture. Further extension of the vertebral column accentuates the cervical and lumbar lordosis but reduces the thoracic kyphosis (Fig. 9.8B). In contrast, flexion of the vertebral column decreases, or flattens, the cervical and lumbar lordosis but accentuates the thoracic kyphosis (Fig. 9.8C). In contrast, the sacrococcygeal curvature is fixed.

The vertebral column of the fetus is mostly kyphotic throughout its length with the development of a more obvious lordosis in the cervical and lumbar spines after birth. Some evidence via magnetic resonance (MR) images suggests the presence of a slight lordotic curvature forming in the lumbar region during fetal development.[45] Ultimately, though, the full extent of lordosis in both the cervical and the lumbar spine develops in association with motor maturation and the assumption of a more upright posture. In the cervical spine, extensor muscles pull on the head and neck as the prone-lying infant begins to lift their heads to observe and explore their surrounding environment. More caudally, the developing hip flexor muscles pull inferiorly on the front of the pelvis as the infant developmentally prepares for walking. This muscular pull rotates (or tilts) the pelvis anteriorly relative to the hips, thereby positioning the lumbar spine into a relative lordosis. Once the child stands, the natural lordosis of the lumbar spine directs the body's line of gravity through or near the first lumbar vertebra (L1) and the base of the sacrum. The natural lordosis of the lumbar spine is a biomechanically favorable adaptation in humans, minimizing the local muscular effort required to maintain erect posture.[307]

The sagittal plane curvatures within the vertebral column also provide strength and resilience to the axial skeleton. A reciprocally curved vertebral column acts like a pliable but stable arch. Near vertical compression forces between vertebrae are partially shared by tension in stretched connective tissues and muscles located along the convex side of each curve. As is true with long bones such as the femur, the vertebral column's strength and stability are derived more so from its ability to "give" slightly under a load rather than its ability to support large compression forces statically.

A potentially negative consequence of the natural spinal curvatures is the presence of shear forces at regions of transition *between* curves. For example, shear forces can cause premature loosening of surgical spinal fusions, especially those performed in

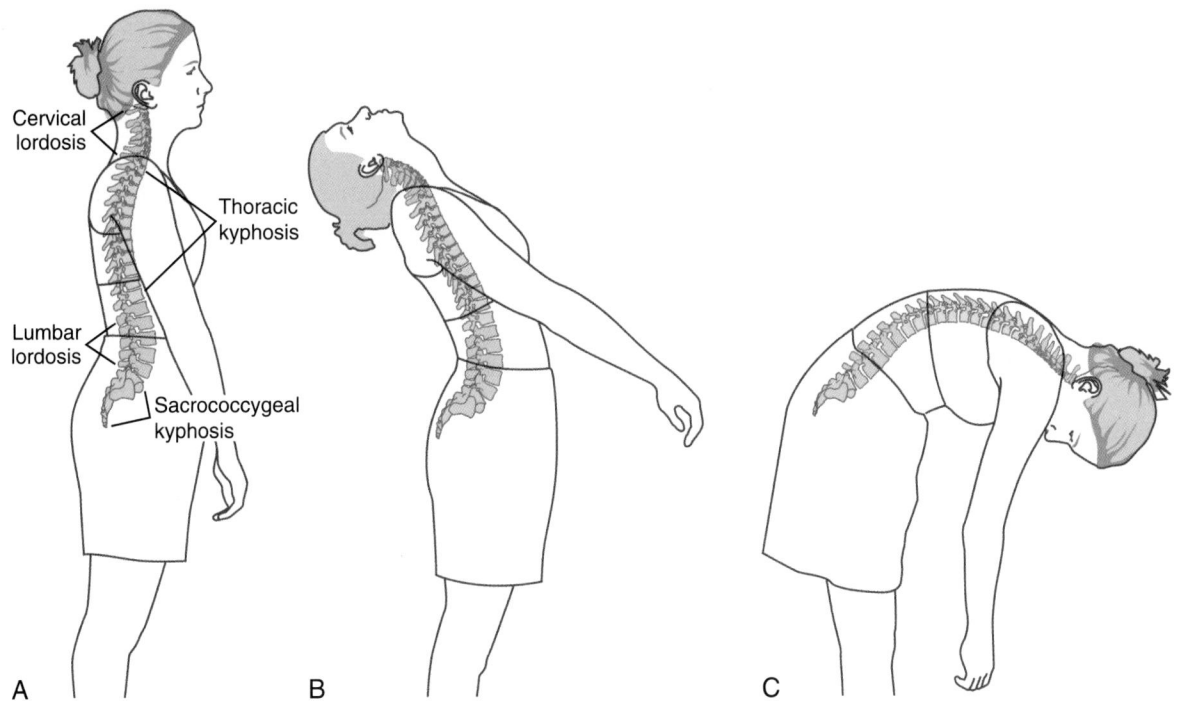

FIG. 9.8 A side view shows the normal sagittal plane curvatures of the vertebral column. (A) The anatomic (neutral) position while one is standing. (B) Full extension of the vertebral column increases the cervical and lumbar lordosis but reduces (straightens) the thoracic kyphosis. (C) Flexion of the vertebral column decreases the cervical and lumbar lordosis but increases the thoracic kyphosis.

the cervicothoracic and thoracolumbar regions. Also, under certain pathologic conditions within the lumbosacral region, the lower lumbar vertebrae may slide excessively anterior relative to the sacrum—a potentially serious condition referred to as anterior spondylolisthesis.

LINE OF GRAVITY PASSING THROUGH THE BODY

Although highly variable, the line of gravity acting on a standing person with typical posture passes near the mastoid process of the temporal bone, anterior to the second sacral vertebra, just posterior to the hip joints, and anterior to the knee and ankle (Fig. 9.9). In the vertebral column, the line of gravity typically falls just to the *concave* side of the apex of each region's curvature. Ideal posture therefore allows the line of gravity to produce modest sagittal plane torques that can help maintain the optimal shape of each curvature. Furthermore, ideal posture allows the force of gravity to produce torques in alternating flexion and extension directions throughout the major regions of the vertebral column. Alternating and partially offsetting torques minimize the *net* external torque acting across the vertebral column as a whole. This mechanical situation minimizes the overall neutralizing torques required of the muscles and ligaments.

The model depicted in Fig. 9.9 is more ideal than real because each person's posture is unique and transient. Factors that alter the spatial relationship between the line of gravity and the spinal curvatures include fat deposition, age, biologic sex, phenotype, bone maturity, the specific shapes of the regional spinal curvatures, posturing of the head and the limbs, muscle strength and endurance, and connective tissue extensibility.[198] The actual orientation of the line of gravity relative to the axial skeleton has distinctive biomechanical consequences on the spine. For example, gravitation force passing posterior to the lumbar region produces a constant extension torque on the low back, facilitating an increase in natural lordosis. Conversely, gravity passing anterior to the lumbar region

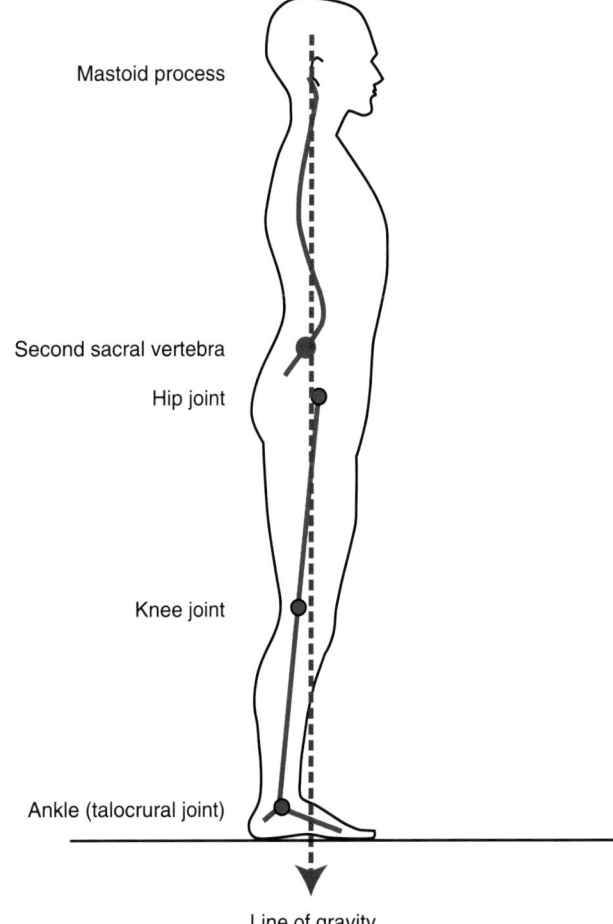

FIG. 9.9 A sagittal plane model illustrating the line of gravity as it passes through the body of a person standing with ideal posture. (Modified from Neumann DA: Arthrokinesiologic considerations for the aged adult. In Guccione AA, editor: *Geriatric physical therapy,* ed 2, Chicago, 2000, Mosby.)

produces a constant flexion torque. In both cases the external torque created by gravity (and its associated external moment arm) must be neutralized by torques produced actively by muscle and passively by connective tissues. In extreme postures, these torque demands and therefore compressive forces may be high; if persistent, they may lead to muscular overuse and fatigue, undesirable postural compensations, as well as progressive structural changes, potentially leading to painful conditions.

Anatomic factors can also influence the unique shape of the spinal curves throughout the vertebral column; these include wedged-shaped intervertebral discs or vertebral bodies, spatial orientation of apophyseal joints (often referred to as "facet" joints), histologic composition of ligaments, and the degree of natural muscle stiffness. The intervertebral discs in the cervical and lower lumbar regions are slightly thicker anteriorly, for example, thereby favoring an anterior convexity in these regions.

The normal sagittal plane alignment of the vertebral column may be altered by many factors: disease, such as in ankylosing spondylosis, poliomyelitis, or muscular dystrophy; trauma, such as severe fracture or spinal cord injury; or changes related to advanced age or reduced activity, such as osteoporosis or muscle weakness. Often, relatively minor forms of abnormal or deviated postures occur in otherwise healthy persons. These deviations may be subtle at first, starting as mechanical responses to postural deviations in other regions of the body. As illustrated in Fig. 9.10, excessive lumbar lordosis may develop as compensation for excessive thoracic kyphosis and vice versa. The goal of this type of postural compensation may be to help maintain a near horizontal line of vision and/or to offset the excessive torque demands created by an exaggerated curvature in just one part of the spine. The "swayback" posture shown in Fig. 9.10C, for example, illustrates a combined exaggerated lumbar lordosis and thoracic kyphosis. Often, other unexplainable postures exist such as the "rounded back" appearance in Fig. 9.10E. This posture shows a combined excessive thoracic kyphosis with reduced lumbar lordosis. Regardless of the cause or location of the postural deviation, the associated abnormal curvatures alter the spatial relation between the line of gravity and each spinal region. When severe, abnormal vertebral curvatures can increase stress on muscles, ligaments, bones, intervertebral discs, apophyseal joints, and exiting spinal nerve roots. Abnormal curves also change the volume of body cavities. An exaggerated

thoracic kyphosis, for example, can significantly reduce the space for the lungs to expand during deep breathing.

LIGAMENTOUS SUPPORT OF THE VERTEBRAL COLUMN

The vertebral column is supported by an extensive set of ligaments. Spinal ligaments limit motion, help maintain natural spinal curvatures, and, by stabilizing the spine, protect the delicate spinal cord and spinal nerve roots. These ligaments, described in the following paragraphs and illustrated in Fig. 9.11, all possess slightly different strengths and functions depending on their locations within the vertebral column. The basic structure and functions of each ligament are summarized in Table 9.3.

The *ligamentum flavum* originates on the anterior surface of one lamina and inserts on the posterior surface of the lamina below. Consisting of a series of paired ligaments, the ligamenta flava (plural) extend throughout the vertebral column, situated immediately posterior to the spinal cord. The ligamenta flava and adjacent laminae form the posterior wall of the vertebral canal.

Ligamentum flavum literally means "yellow ligament," reflecting its high content of light-yellow elastic connective tissue. Histologically, the ligamentum flavum consists of about 80% elastin and 20% collagen.[318] The tissue's highly elastic nature is ideal for exerting a relatively constant, although modest, resistance throughout a wide range of flexion. Such resistance may absorb or "soften" some of the intervertebral compression force generated at the near end range of spinal flexion. Measurements have shown that between the anatomic (neutral) position and full flexion, the ligamentum flavum experiences an approximately 35% increase in strain (elongation) (Fig. 9.12).[193] Extreme and forceful flexion beyond this length can ultimately lead to its rupture and, in addition, possibly causing damaging compressive forces on the anterior side of the intervertebral disc. The ligamenta flava are thickest in the lumbar region,[275] where the magnitude of intervertebral flexion is the largest of any region within the vertebral column.

The highly elastic nature of the ligamentum flavum is interesting from both a functional and a structural perspective. In addition to providing gradual resistance to the full range of flexion, its inherent elasticity also exerts a small but constant compression force between vertebrae, even in the anatomic position.[28] The elasticity may prevent the ligament from buckling inward during full extension. A forceful buckling, or in-folding, might otherwise pinch and, in certain scenarios, injure the adjacent spinal cord.[173]

The *interspinous ligaments* fill much of the space between adjacent spinous processes. The deeper, more elastin-rich fibers blend with the ligamenta flava; the more superficial fibers contain more collagen, and blend with the supraspinous ligaments. The fiber direction and organization of the interspinous ligaments vary from region to region.[122] The interspinous ligaments in the lumbar region, for example, fan in an oblique posterior-cranial direction (Fig. 9.11A). Fibers in this region are drawn taut only at the more extremes of flexion.

As evident by their name, the *supraspinous ligaments* attach between the tips of the spinous processes. As with the interspinous ligaments, these ligaments resist separation of adjacent spinous processes, thereby resisting flexion. The ability to resist flexion is greatest in regions of the vertebral column where these structures are more robust and contain a greater proportion of collagen. Throughout the lumbar region, for example, the ligaments are not extensively developed; they are either sparse (especially between L4 and L5) or partially replaced by strands of thoracolumbar

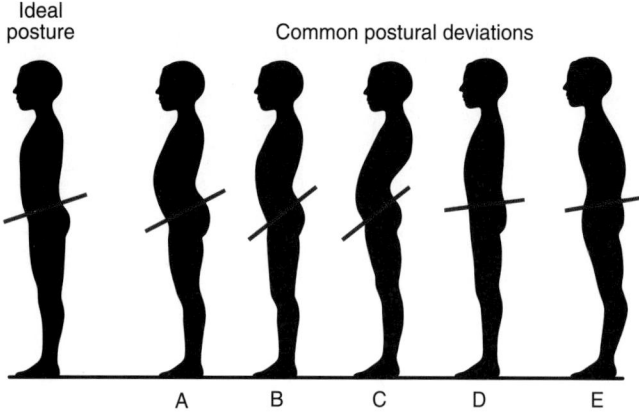

Ideal posture   Common postural deviations

A   B   C   D   E

FIG. 9.10 A drawing showing common postural deviations of the vertebral column and pelvis within the sagittal plane. All subjects in the figure are considered typical, from a neuromuscular perspective. The red line at each iliac crest indicates the varying degree of pelvic tilt (or lumbar lordosis). (Modified from McMorris RO: Faulty postures, *Pediatr Clin North Am* 8:217, 1961.)

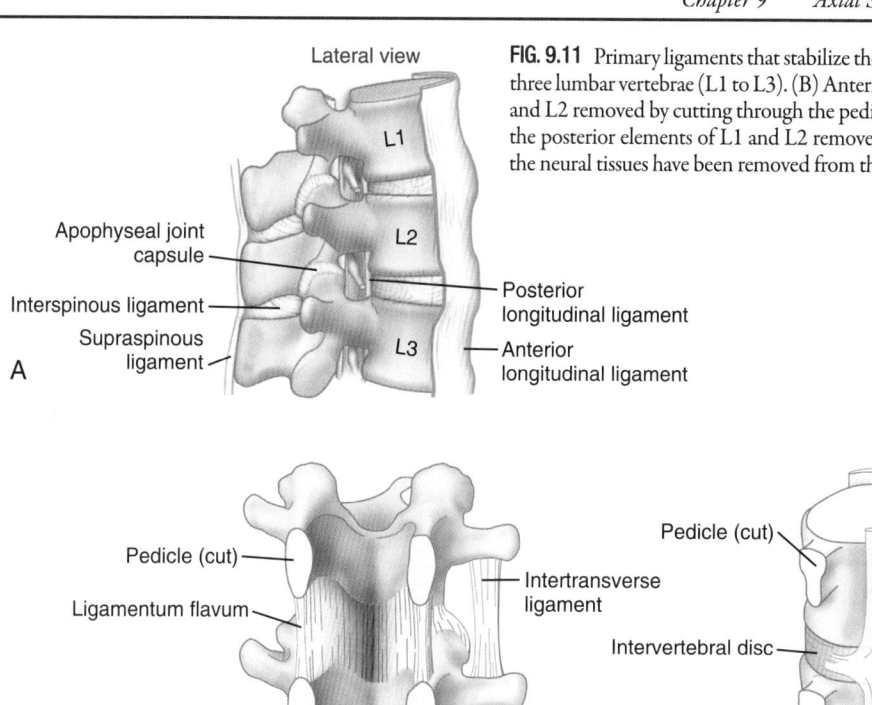

Lateral view

Apophyseal joint capsule

Interspinous ligament

Supraspinous ligament

A

FIG. 9.11 Primary ligaments that stabilize the vertebral column. (A) Lateral overview of the first three lumbar vertebrae (L1 to L3). (B) Anterior view of L1 to L3 vertebrae with the bodies of L1 and L2 removed by cutting through the pedicles. (C) Posterior view of L1 to L3 vertebrae with the posterior elements of L1 and L2 removed by cutting through the pedicles. In (B) and (C), the neural tissues have been removed from the vertebral canal.

L1

L2

L3

Posterior longitudinal ligament

Anterior longitudinal ligament

Pedicle (cut)

Ligamentum flavum

Posterior longitudinal ligament

Intervertebral disc

Anterior longitudinal ligament

B

Intertransverse ligament

Apophyseal joint capsule

Anterior view

Anterior longitudinal ligament

Pedicle (cut)

Intervertebral disc

Posterior longitudinal ligament

Vertebral canal

Ligamentum flavum

C

Posterior view

TABLE 9.3 Major Ligaments of the Vertebral Column

Name	Attachments	Function	Comment
Ligamentum flavum	Between the anterior surface of one lamina and the posterior surface of the lamina below	Limits and "softens" end range intervertebral flexion	Contains a high percentage of elastin; lies immediately posterior to the spinal cord; thickest in the lumbar region
Supraspinous and interspinous ligaments	Between the adjacent spinous processes from C7 to the sacrum	Limit flexion	Ligamentum nuchae is the cervical and cranial extension of the supraspinous ligaments, providing a midline structure for muscle attachments, and support to the head
Intertransverse ligaments	Between adjacent transverse processes	Limits contralateral lateral flexion and forward flexion	Few fibers exist in the cervical region; in the thoracic region, the ligaments are intertwined with local muscle; in the lumbar region, the ligaments are thin and membranous
Anterior longitudinal ligament	Between the basilar part of the occipital bone and the entire length of the anterior surfaces of all vertebral bodies, including the sacrum	Limits extension or excessive lordosis in the cervical and lumbar regions; reinforces the anterior sides of the intervertebral discs	Best developed in the lumbar spine; about twice the tensile strength as that of the posterior longitudinal ligament
Posterior longitudinal ligament	Throughout the length of the posterior surfaces of all vertebral bodies, between the axis (C2) and the sacrum	Limits flexion; reinforces the posterior sides of the intervertebral discs	Lies within the vertebral canal, just anterior to the spinal cord
Capsules of the apophyseal joints	Margin of each apophyseal joint	Strengthen the apophyseal joints	Loose in the near-neutral (anatomic) position but become increasingly taut at the extremes of all other positions

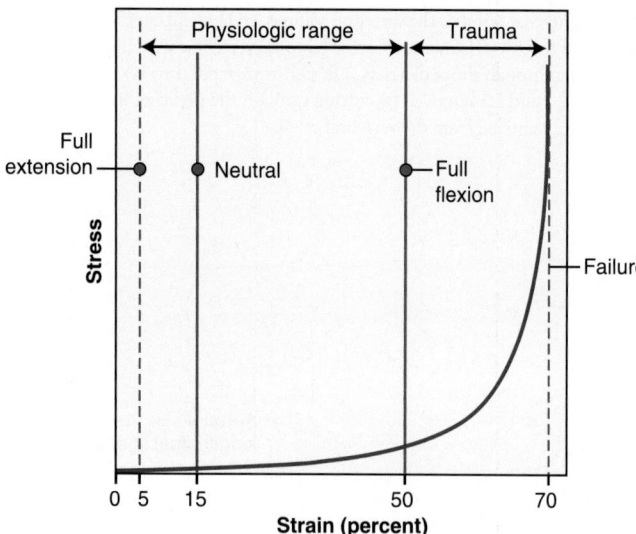

FIG. 9.12 The stress-strain relationship of the ligamentum flavum is shown between full extension and the point of tissue failure beyond full normal-range flexion. Note that the ligament fails at a point 70% beyond its fully slackened length. (See text for source of data.)

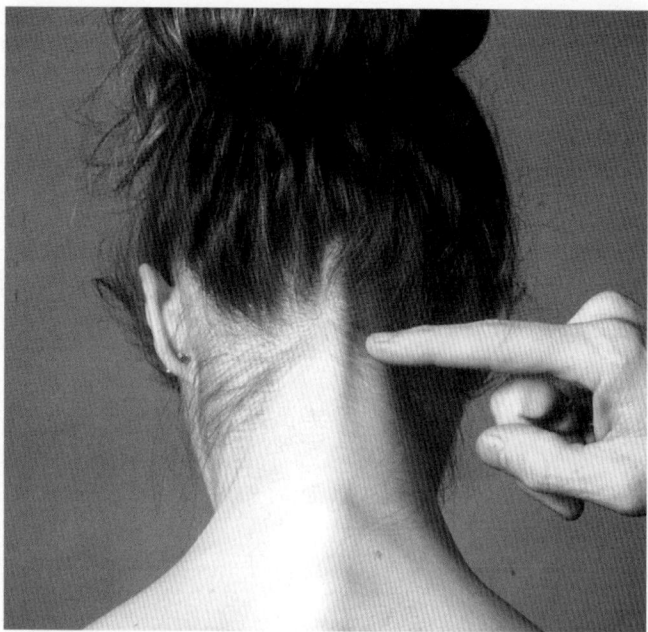

FIG. 9.13 A prominent ligamentum nuchae in a thin healthy woman.

fascia (described ahead) or small musculotendinous fibers.[28] Not surprisingly, therefore, the supraspinous ligaments within the lumbar region are typically the first structures to rupture in extreme flexion.[2]

In the cervical region the supraspinous ligaments are very well developed and extend cranially as the *ligamentum nuchae.* This tough bilaminar strip of fibroelastic tissue attaches between the cervical spinous processes and external occipital protuberance. The ligamentum nuchae does not function as a ligament in the pure sense (i.e., by stabilizing one bone to another), rather it provides a shared midline attachment site for many muscles, such as the trapezius and splenius capitis and cervicis.[275] Passive tension in a stretched ligamentum nuchae likely adds useful support to a partially flexed head and neck. A prominent ligamentum nuchae accounts for some of the difficulty often encountered in palpating the spinous process in the middle to upper cervical region (Fig. 9.13).

The *intertransverse ligaments* are poorly defined, thin, and membranous structures that extend between adjacent transverse processes.[275] These tissues become only slightly taut in contralateral lateral flexion and, to a lesser degree, forward flexion.[313]

The *anterior longitudinal ligament* is a long, strong, straplike structure attaching to the basilar part of the occipital bone and the entire length of the anterior surfaces of all vertebral bodies, including the sacrum. The deeper fibers blend with and reinforce the anterior portions of the intervertebral discs. The anterior longitudinal ligament becomes taut in extension and slack in flexion.[313] In the cervical and lumbar regions, tension in the anterior longitudinal ligament helps limit the degree of natural lordosis. This ligament is narrow at its cranial end but widens as it courses caudally.

The *posterior longitudinal ligament* is a continuous band of connective tissue that attaches to the posterior surfaces of the vertebral bodies, between the axis (C2) and the sacrum. The posterior longitudinal ligament is located within the vertebral canal, immediately anterior to the spinal cord (see Fig. 9.11A). (It is important to note that the posterior and anterior longitudinal ligaments are named according to their relationship to the

vertebral body, not the spinal cord.) Throughout its length, the deeper fibers of the posterior longitudinal ligament blend with and reinforce the posterior side of the intervertebral discs. Cranially, the posterior longitudinal ligament is a broad structure, narrowing as it descends toward the lumbar region. The slender lumbar portion limits its ability to restrain a posterior bulging (or herniated) disc. As with most ligaments of the vertebral column, the posterior longitudinal ligament becomes increasingly taut with flexion.[114]

Capsular ligaments of the apophyseal joints attach along the entire rim of the facet surfaces (see Fig. 9.11A). As will be described in an upcoming section on arthrology, apophyseal joints help interconnect and stabilize the intervertebral junctions. Equally important are the apophyseal joints' unique role in guiding the dominant direction of movement direction of a particular intervertebral junction. The capsular ligaments that surround the apophyseal joints contain a blend of elastin and collagen fibers that render them strong enough to maintain the physical integrity of the apophyseal joint, yet pliable enough to allow the intervertebral translations inherent to spinal kinematics.[130] The apophyseal joint capsules are reinforced by adjacent muscles (multifidus) and ligamenta flava, most notably in the lumbar region.

The capsular ligaments are relatively loose (lax) in the anatomic (neutral) position, but at least some fibers become increasingly taut as the joint approaches the extremes of all its movements.[94] Passive tension is naturally greatest in motions that create the largest relative movement between joint surfaces, such as full flexion in the cervical region.[8] The kinematics are highly specific to the particular region of the vertebral column and will be revisited in subsequent sections of this chapter.

In closing, knowledge of a spinal ligament's location relative to the axis of rotation within a given intervertebral junction provides important insight into its primary functions. As will be further described in an upcoming section, the axis of rotation for intervertebral movement is near or through the region of the *vertebral body.* When sagittal plane movement is considered, for example, any ligament located posterior to the vertebral body is stretched (and thereby pulled taut) during flexion. Conversely, any ligament located anterior to the vertebral body is stretched during extension. As noted by reviewing Fig. 9.11A, *all ligaments except the anterior longitudinal ligament would become taut in flexion.*[133,313] Appreciating how movement and posture stretch spinal ligaments is fundamental to understanding the mechanisms by which ligaments limit motions and are potentially injured, as well as how ligaments indirectly protect the spinal cord and nerve roots. This is a very clinically relevant issue because at some critical length or force, a chronically overstretched and weakened ligament will either remain in a permanent state of relative elongation (or creep) or reach its ultimate failure point. A ruptured or lax ligament is typically not capable of adequately stabilizing its associated intervertebral junction. Ensuing spinal instability may result. *Spinal instability*—a term used extensively in the medical, research, and rehabilitation literature—has been formally defined as the loss of natural intervertebral stiffness that can lead to abnormal and increased intervertebral motion.[128,232,261] To experimentally study and quantify spinal instability, the concept of a kinematic neutral zone has been used. The *neutral zone,* typically defined through cadaver or animal research, is the range (or "zone") of intervertebral movement that generates minimal passive resistance from the surrounding connective tissues.[261,313] The neutral zone typically increases with injury or laxity of the connective tissues. Consequently, the responsibility for controlling spinal motion shifts from passive restraints offered through the connective tissues to active restraints offered through the muscular system. If marked or chronic, spinal instability in live humans is believed to cause further injury to local ligaments, as well as injury to apophyseal joints, intervertebral discs, and, perhaps more importantly, the delicate neural elements. Spinal instability may be associated with painful movements of the trunk, or indirectly, the extremities. As will be described in Chapter 10, depending on the nature of the instability, treatment may involve exercises or activities aimed at improving the ability of the neuromuscular system to better control motion and potentially increase the natural stiffness within a given spinal region.[240] However, if the condition is severe, treatment for spinal instability may require surgical intervention, such as a surgical fusion.

Regional Osteologic Features of the Vertebral Column

The adage that "function follows structure" is very applicable to the study of the vertebral column. Although all vertebrae have a common morphologic theme, each also has a specific shape that reflects its unique function. The following section, along with Table 9.4, highlights specific osteologic features of each region of the vertebral column.

CERVICAL REGION

The cervical vertebrae are the smallest and most mobile vertebrae. The high extent of mobility is designed to maximize the movement of the head and special senses like vision and hearing. Perhaps the most unique anatomic feature of the cervical vertebrae is the presence of *transverse foramina* located within the transverse processes (Fig. 9.14). The important vertebral artery ascends through this foramen, coursing toward the foramen magnum to transport blood to the brain and spinal cord. In the neck, the vertebral artery is located immediately anterior to the exiting spinal nerve roots (see Fig. 9.4).

The third through the sixth cervical vertebrae show nearly identical features and are therefore considered typical of this region. The upper two cervical vertebrae, the atlas (C1) and the axis (C2), and

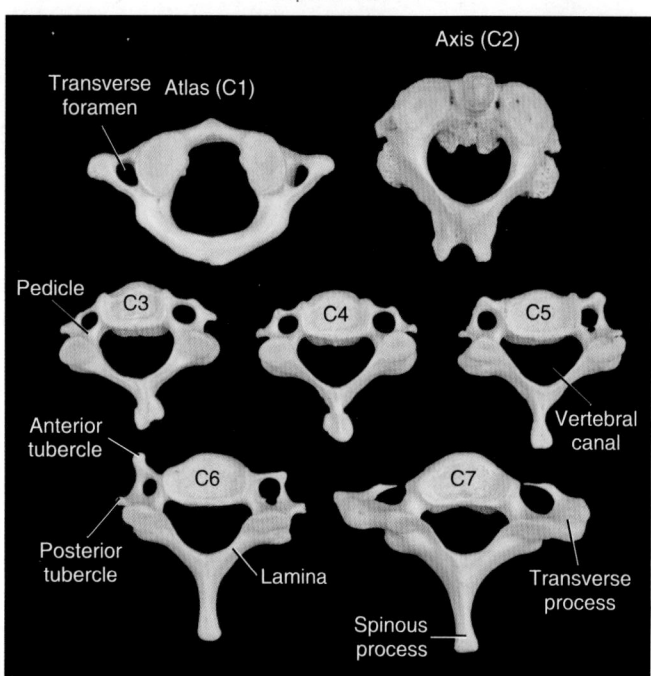

FIG. 9.14 A superior view of all seven cervical vertebrae from the same specimen.

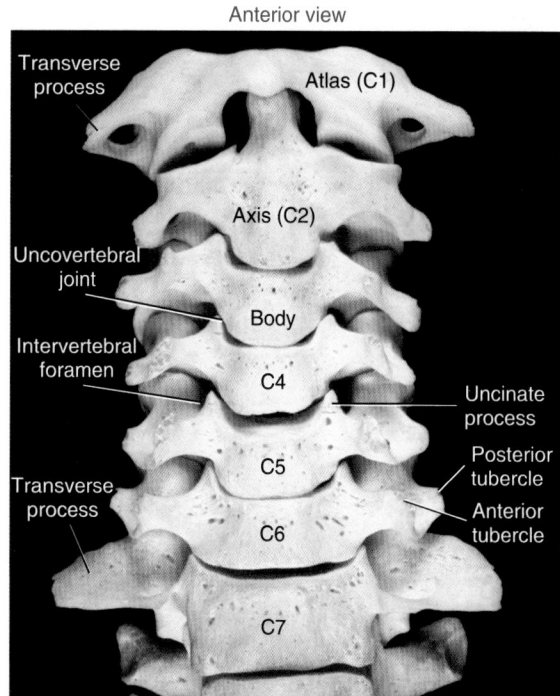

FIG. 9.15 An anterior view of the cervical vertebral column.

the seventh cervical vertebra (C7) are atypical for reasons described in a subsequent section.

Typical Cervical Vertebrae (C3 to C6)

C3 to C6 have small rectangular *bodies* made of a relatively dense and strong cortical shell. The bodies are wider from side to side than from front to back (Figs. 9.14 and 9.15). The superior and inferior

TABLE 9.4 Osteologic Features of the Vertebral Column

	Body	Superior Articular Facets	Inferior Articular Facets	Spinous Processes	Vertebral Canal	Transverse Processes	Comments
Atlas (C1)	None	Concave, face generally superior	Flat to slightly concave, face generally inferior	None, replaced by a small posterior tubercle	Triangular, largest of cervical region	Largest of cervical region	Two large lateral masses, joined by anterior and posterior arches
Axis (C2)	Tall with a vertical projecting dens	Flat to slightly convex, face generally superior	Flat, face anterior and inferior	Bifid, thick and broad	Large and triangular	Small and rounded	Large superior articular processes that support the atlas and cranium
C3–C6	Wider than deep; have uncinate processes	Flat, face posterior and superior	As above	Typically bifid	Large and triangular	End as anterior and posterior tubercles	Considered typical cervical vertebrae
C7	Wider than deep	As above	Transition to typical thoracic vertebrae	Large and prominent, easily palpable	Triangular	Thick and prominent, may have a large anterior tubercle forming an "extra rib"	Often called "vertebral prominens" because of large spinous process
T2–T9	Equal width and depth as costal demifacets for attachment of the heads of ribs 2–9	Flat, face mostly posterior	Flat, face mostly anterior	Long and pointed, slant inferiorly	Round, smaller than cervical	Project horizontally and slightly posterior, have costal facets for tubercles of ribs	Considered typical thoracic vertebrae
T1 and T10–T12	T1 has a full costal facet for rib 1 and a partial demifacet for rib 2 T10–T12 each has a full costal facet	As above	As above	As above	As above	T10–T12 may lack costal facets	Considered "atypical" thoracic vertebrae primarily because of manner of rib attachment
L1–L5	Wider than deep L5 is slightly wedged (i.e., higher height anteriorly than posteriorly)	Slightly concave, face medial to posterior-medial	L1–L4 slightly convex, face lateral to anterior-lateral L5: flat, faces anterior and slightly lateral	Stout and rectangular	Triangular, contains cauda equina	Slender, project laterally	Superior articular processes have mammillary bodies
Sacrum	Fused Body of first sacral vertebra most evident	Flat, face posterior and slightly medial	None	None, replaced by multiple spinous tubercles	As above	None, replaced by multiple transverse tubercles	
Coccyx	Fusion of four rudimentary vertebrae	Rudimentary	Rudimentary	Rudimentary	Ends at the first coccyx	Rudimentary	

Cervical Osteophytes Causing Neurologic Symptoms in the Upper Extremity: One Possible Consequence of a Degenerated Intervertebral Disc

Fully hydrated and normal intervertebral discs naturally act as "spacers" between individual vertebrae. One possible benefit of the spacing is to partially unload the nearby *uncovertebral joints.* Lacking substantial articular cartilage, the relatively small uncovertebral joints are not designed to tolerate compression and shear forces, especially if these forces are repetitive or large. Fig. 9.16 illustrates how a healthy, hydrated, and full disc located between C3 and C4 creates a protective gap between the adjacent C3–C4 uncovertebral joint. Fig. 9.16 also shows how a degenerated, dehydrated, and thinned disc between C4 and C5 increases the contact force at the C4–C5 uncovertebral joint. Over time, the increased force can stimulate growth of an osteophyte ("bone spur"). The osteophyte is shown compressing the C^5 spinal nerve root, which may cause radiating (radicular) pain, muscle weakness, or altered sensations throughout that nerve's peripheral distribution, typically down the lateral aspect of the arm. In an indirect way, healthy intervertebral discs protect not only the surrounding bone, but also the nerve roots.

Anterior view

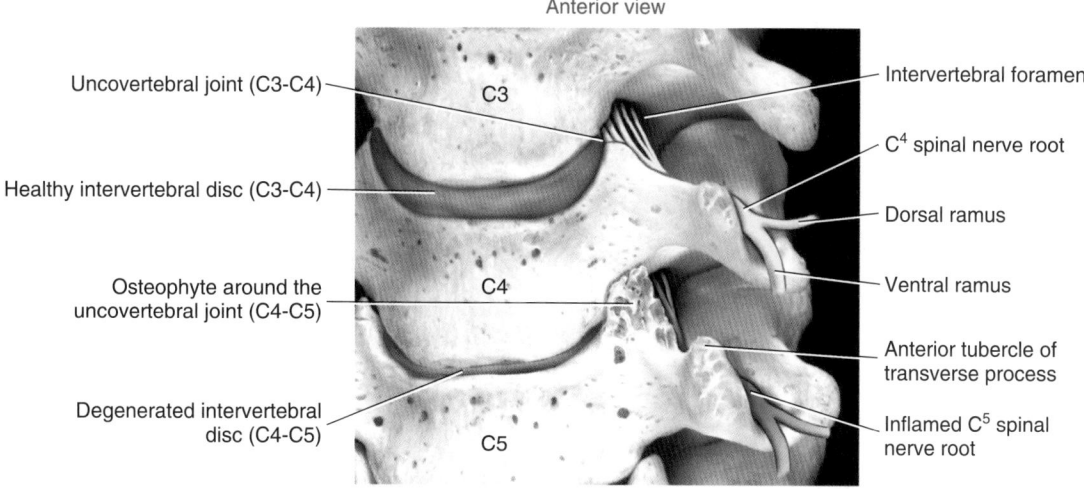

FIG. 9.16 A digitally enhanced image comparing the relative loading of the uncovertebral joints based on the health of the adjacent intervertebral discs. The osteophyte formed at the C4–C5 uncovertebral joint is shown to compress and inflame the exiting C^5 spinal nerve root.

surfaces of the bodies are not as flat as those of most other vertebrae but are curved or notched. The superior surfaces are concave side to side, with raised lateral hooks called *uncinate processes* (*uncus* means "hook"). The inferior surfaces, in contrast, are concave anterior-posterior, with elongated anterior and posterior margins. When articulated, small *uncovertebral joints* form between the uncinate process and a recess on the lateral-inferior edge of the superior adjoining vertebral body. As noted in Fig. 9.15, the uncovertebral joints form part of the medial wall of the intervertebral foramen. These joints (also called "Joints of Luschka"[111]) typically exist bilaterally from C2–C3 to C6–C7 intervertebral junctions. Whether these joints are truly synovial is uncertain.[195] Furthermore, the biomechanical role of the uncovertebral joints is unclear, although they likely have both structural and kinematic functions. The uncinate processes may help centralize the position of the adjacent intervertebral disc, especially during motion.[109,290] Furthermore, the uncovertebral joints may be associated with the mechanical "coupling" that naturally occurs between axial rotation and lateral flexion throughout much of the cervical region (described ahead).[195,251] Clinically these joints become important when the uncinate processes are unnaturally large or angulated, or when osteophytes form around their margins, thereby reducing the size of the adjacent intervertebral foramen. In either case, the uncinate processes or associated osteophytes may impinge on and irritate exiting cervical spinal nerve roots, thereby causing neurologic symptoms in the ipsilateral upper extremity.

The *pedicles* of C3 to C6 are short and curved posterior-lateral (see Fig. 9.14). Very thin *laminae* extend posterior-medially from each pedicle (Fig. 9.17). The triangular *vertebral canal* is large in the cervical region to accommodate the thickening of the spinal cord associated with the formation of the cervical plexus and brachial plexus.

Within the C3 to C6 region, consecutive superior and inferior articular processes form a continuous articular "pillar," interrupted by apophyseal joints (Fig. 9.18). The articular facets within each apophyseal joint are smooth and flat, with joint surfaces oriented midway between the frontal and horizontal planes. The *superior articular facets* face posterior and superior, whereas the *inferior articular facets* face anterior and inferior.

The *spinous processes* of C3 to C6 are short, with some processes being bifid (i.e., having two distinct processes) (see Fig. 9.14, C3).[171] The *transverse processes* are short lateral extensions that terminate as variably shaped *anterior* and *posterior tubercles.* These tubercles are unique to C3–C6, serving as attachment sites for muscles such as the scalenus anterior, levator scapulae, and splenius cervicis.

Posterior-lateral view

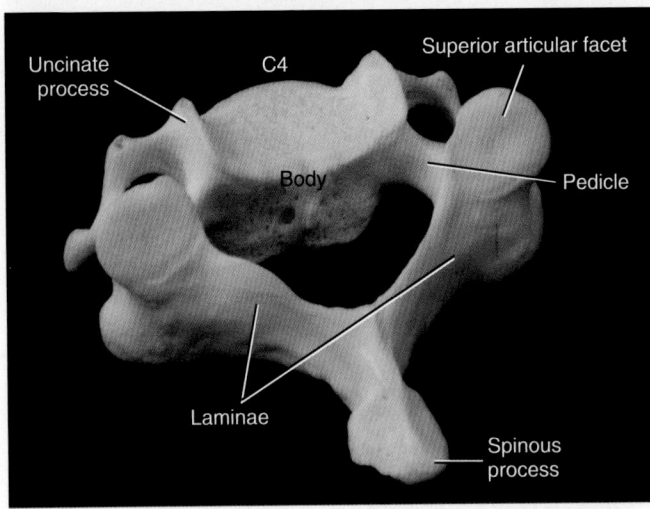

FIG. 9.17 A posterior-lateral view of the fourth cervical vertebra.

Lateral view

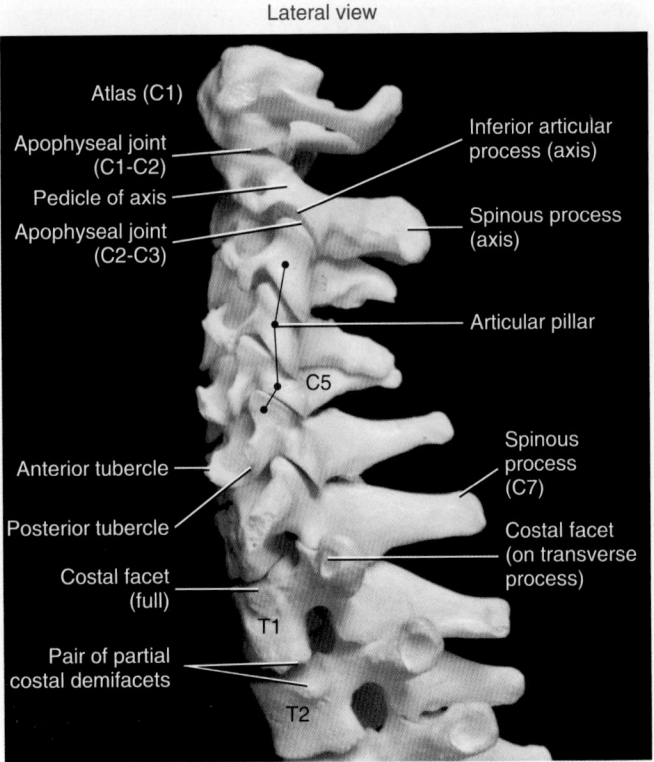

FIG. 9.18 A lateral view of the cervical vertebral column.

Superior view

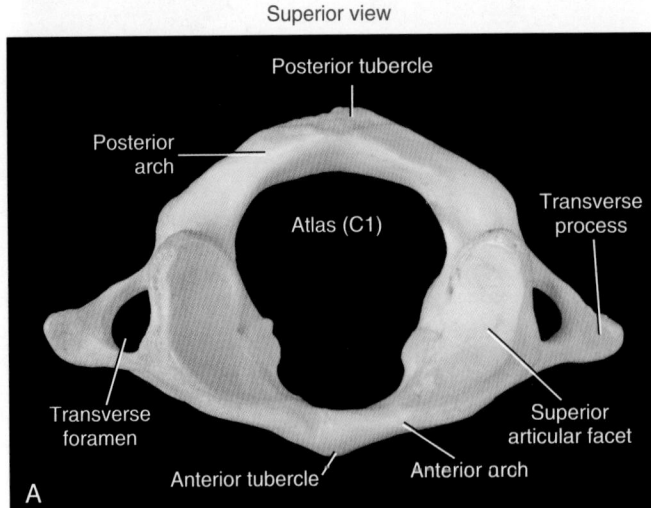

Anterior view

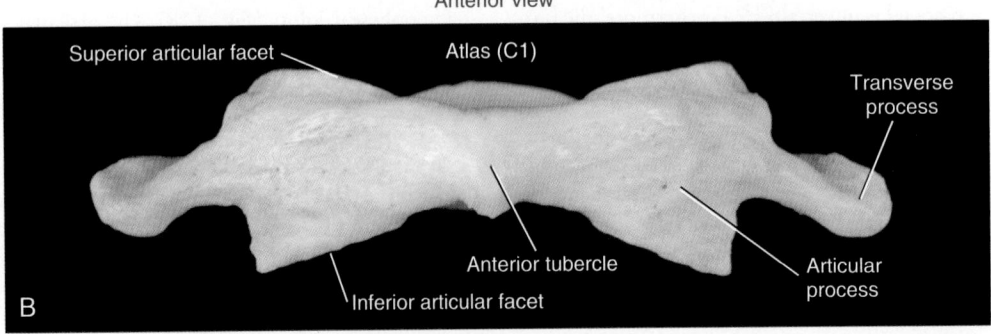

FIG. 9.19 The atlas. (A) Superior view. (B) Anterior view.

Anterior view

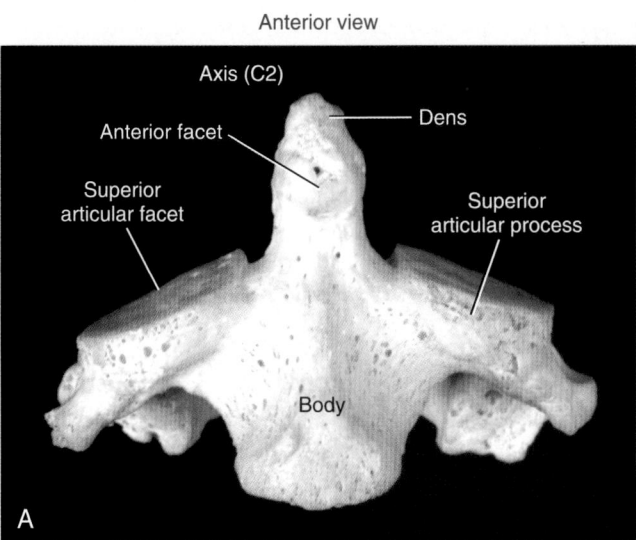

FIG. 9.20 The axis. (A) Anterior view. (B) Superior view.

Superior view

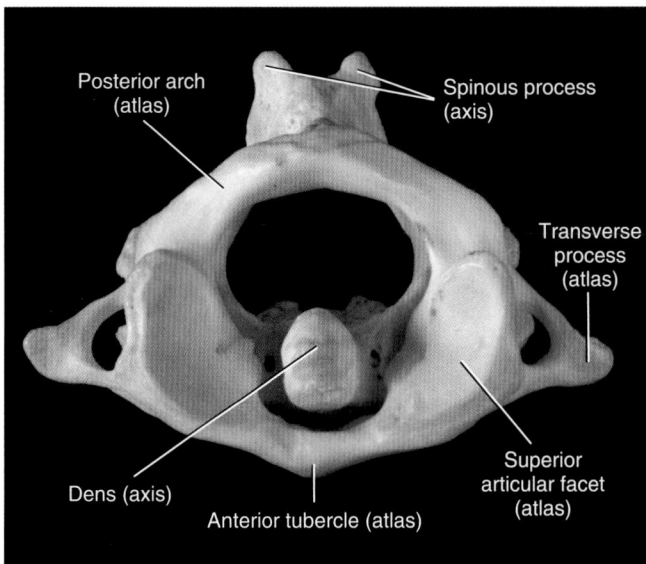

FIG. 9.21 A superior view of the median atlanto-axial articulation.

Atypical Cervical Vertebrae (C1, C2, and C7)
Atlas (C1)
As indicated by the name, the primary function of the atlas is to support the head. Possessing no body, pedicle, lamina, or spinous process, the atlas is essentially two large lateral masses joined by anterior and posterior arches (Fig. 9.19A). The short *anterior arch* has an *anterior tubercle* for attachment of the anterior longitudinal ligament. The much larger *posterior arch* forms nearly half the circumference of the entire atlantal ring. A small *posterior tubercle* marks the midline of the posterior arch. The lateral masses support the prominent superior articular processes, which in turn support the cranium.

The large and concave *superior articular facets* of the atlas generally face cranially, in a position to accept the large, convex occipital condyles. The *inferior articular facets* are generally flat to slightly concave. These facet surfaces generally face inferiorly, with their lateral edges sloped downward, approximately 20 degrees from the horizontal plane (Fig. 9.19B). The atlas has large, palpable *transverse processes,* usually the most prominent of the cervical vertebrae. These transverse processes serve as attachment points for several small but important muscles that control fine movements of the cranium.

Axis (C2)
The axis has a large, tall *body* that serves as a base for the upwardly projecting *dens (odontoid process)* (Fig. 9.20). Part of the elongated body is formed from remnants of the body of the atlas and the intervening disc. The dens provides a rigid vertical axis of rotation for the atlas and head (Fig. 9.21). Projecting laterally from the body is a pair of superior articular processes (Fig. 9.20A). These large processes have slightly convex *superior articular facets* that are oriented about 20 degrees from the horizontal plane, matching the slope of the inferior articular facets of the atlas. Projecting from the prominent superior articular processes of the axis are a pair of stout *pedicles* and a pair of very short *transverse processes* (Fig. 9.20B). A pair of inferior articular processes projects inferiorly from the pedicles, with *inferior articular facets* facing anteriorly and inferiorly (Fig. 9.18). The *spinous process* of the axis is bifid and broad. The palpable spinous process serves as an attachment for many muscles, such as the semispinalis cervicis.

"Vertebra Prominens" (C7)
C7 is the largest of all cervical vertebrae, having many characteristics of thoracic vertebrae. C7 can have large *transverse processes,* as illustrated in Fig. 9.15. A hypertrophic anterior tubercle on the transverse process may sprout an extra cervical rib, which may impinge on the brachial plexus. This vertebra also has a large *spinous process,* characteristic of other thoracic vertebrae (Fig. 9.18).[171] Anatomists often refer to C7 as the "vertebra prominens," reflecting its typically large and readily palpable spinous process.

THORACIC REGION

Typical Thoracic Vertebrae (T2 to T9)

The second through the ninth thoracic vertebrae usually demonstrate similar features (see T6 and T7 in Fig. 9.5). *Pedicles* are directed posteriorly from the body, making the vertebral canal narrower than in the cervical region. The large *transverse processes* project posterior-laterally, each containing a *costal facet* that articulates with the tubercle of the corresponding rib (at the *costotransverse joint*). Short, thick *laminae* form a broad base for the downward-slanting *spinous processes.*

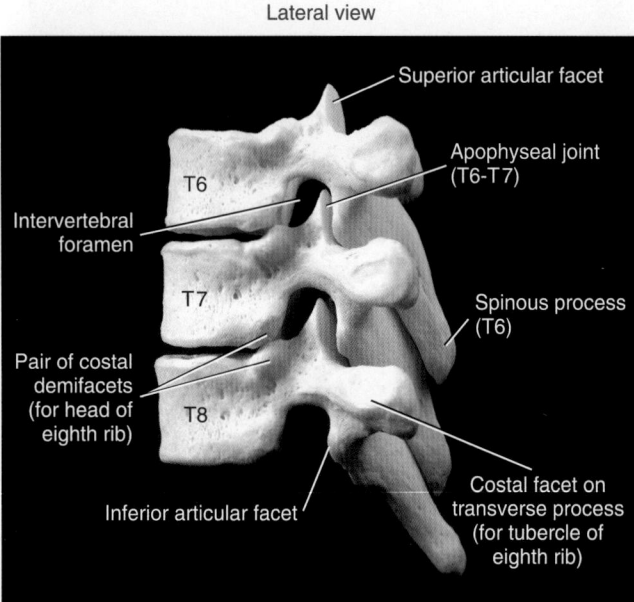

Lateral view

FIG. 9.22 A lateral view of the sixth through eighth thoracic vertebrae.

The superior and inferior articular facets in the thoracic region are oriented vertically with a slight forward pitch (Fig. 9.22). The *superior articular facets* face generally posterior; the *inferior articular facets* face generally anterior. Once articulated, the superior and inferior facets form apophyseal joints, which are aligned relatively close to the frontal plane.

Each of the heads of ribs 2 through 9 typically articulates with a pair of *costal demifacets* that span one thoracic intervertebral junction (see pair of costal demifacets for the eighth rib in Fig. 9.22). As described earlier, these articulations are called *costocorporeal joints.* A thoracic (intercostal) spinal nerve exits through a corresponding thoracic *intervertebral foramen,* located just anterior to the apophyseal joints.

Atypical Thoracic Vertebrae (T1 and T10 to T12)

The first and usually last three thoracic vertebrae are considered atypical mainly because of the particular manner of rib attachment. T1 has a *full costal facet* superiorly that accepts the entire head of the first rib and a *demifacet* inferiorly that accepts part of the head of the second rib (see Fig. 9.18). The spinous process of T1 is especially elongated and often as prominent as the spinous process of C7. Although variable, the bodies of T10 through T12 may have a single, *full costal facet* for articulation with the heads of the 10th, 11th, and 12th ribs, respectively. T11 and to T12 usually lack costotransverse joints.

LUMBAR REGION

Lumbar vertebrae have massive wide *bodies,* suitable for supporting the entire superimposed weight of the head, trunk, and arms (Fig. 9.23). The total mass of the five lumbar vertebrae is approximately twice that of all seven cervical vertebrae.

For the most part, the lumbar vertebrae possess similar characteristics. *Laminae* and *pedicles* are short and thick, forming the posterior and lateral walls of the nearly triangular *vertebral canal. Transverse processes* project almost laterally; those associated with

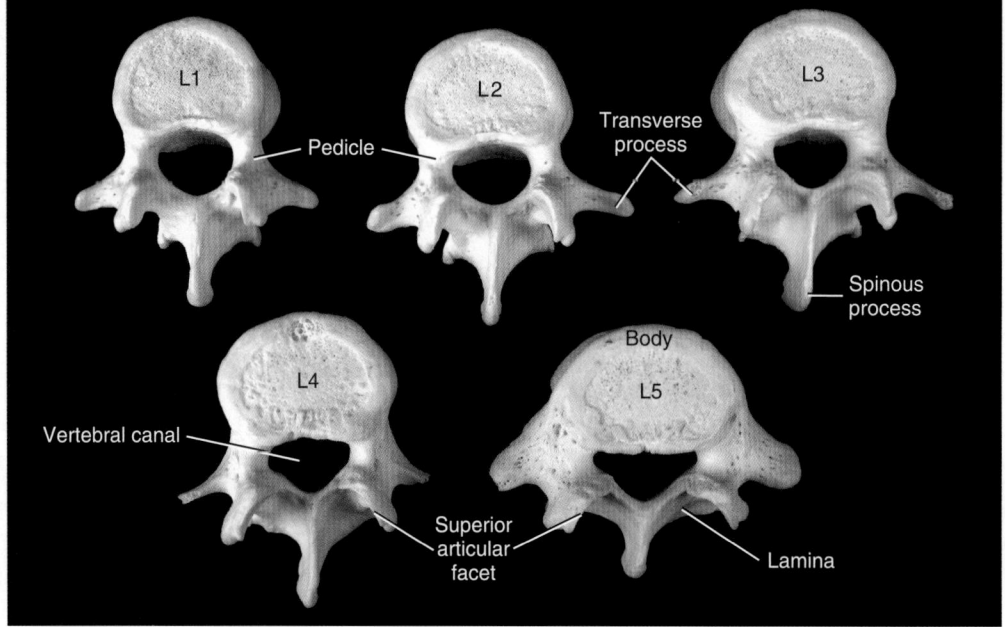

Superior view

FIG. 9.23 A superior view of the five lumbar vertebrae.

Lateral view

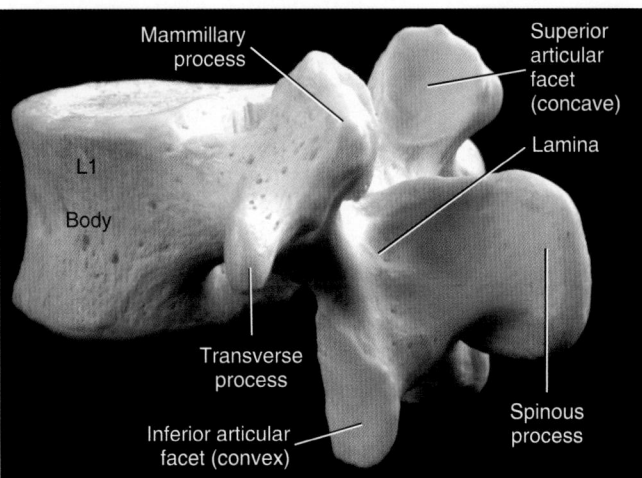

FIG. 9.24 A lateral and slightly posterior view of the first lumbar vertebra.

L1 to L4 are thin and tapered; however, the transverse processes of L5 are short, thick, and strong. *Spinous processes* are broad and rectangular, projecting horizontally from the junction of each lamina (Fig. 9.24). This shape is strikingly different from the pointed, sloped spinous processes of the thoracic region. Short *mammillary processes* project from the posterior surfaces of each superior articular process. These structures serve as attachment sites for the multifidus muscle.

The articular facets of the lumbar vertebrae are oriented nearly vertically. The *superior articular facets* are moderately concave, facing medial to posterior-medial. As depicted in Fig. 9.23, the superior facet surfaces in the upper lumbar region tend to be oriented closest with the sagittal plane, and the superior facet surfaces in the middle to lower lumbar region are oriented approximately midway between the sagittal and frontal planes. The *inferior articular facets* are reciprocally matched to the shape and orientation of the superior articular facets. In general, the inferior articular facets are slightly convex, facing generally lateral to anterior-lateral (Fig. 9.24).

The inferior articular facets of L5 articulate with the superior articular facets of the sacrum. The resulting *L5–S1 apophyseal joints* are typically oriented much closer to the frontal plane than the other lumbar articulations. The L5–S1 apophyseal joints provide an important source of anterior-posterior stability to the lumbosacral junction.

SACRUM

The sacrum is a triangular bone with its base facing superiorly and apex inferiorly (Fig. 9.26). An important function of the sacrum is to transmit the weight of the vertebral column to the pelvis. In childhood, each of five separate sacral vertebrae is joined by a cartilaginous membrane. By adulthood, however, the sacrum has fused into a single bone, which still retains some anatomic features of generic vertebrae.

The anterior (pelvic) surface of the sacrum is smooth and concave, forming part of the posterior wall of the pelvic cavity. Four paired *ventral (pelvic) sacral foramina* transmit the ventral rami of spinal nerve roots that form much of the sacral plexus. The dorsal surface of the sacrum is convex and rough because of the

SPECIAL FOCUS 9.2

Developmental Anomalies of the Lumbar Apophyseal Joints

At birth, the articular surfaces of the apophyseal joints within the lumbar spine are oriented very close to the frontal plane, similar to most thoracic apophyseal joints. Between birth and about 11 or 12 years of age, however, the orientation within all but the lower lumbar apophyseal joints gradually transforms to their final adult position biased slightly closer to the sagittal plane (Fig. 9.25).[28,241] The slow structural transformation is governed by different rates of ossification within the articular processes. Bogduk describes the possibility that this transformation may be influenced by the developing upright posture of the child and the demands placed on certain muscles, such as the lumbar multifidus.[28] Although the apophyseal joints continue to grow throughout adolescence, their spatial orientation is essentially established before the teenage years.

Natural variations in the development of the lumbar apophyseal joints in childhood can create structural asymmetries that persist into adulthood—a condition often referred to as "facet joint tropism."[313] Although variations can be extreme, most are relatively minor, such as a slight bilateral asymmetry between the right and left articular surfaces of the joints. (An example of this asymmetry is evident by comparing the superior articular facets of the lumbar vertebrae illustrated in Fig. 9.23.) Slight bilateral asymmetries exist in about 20% to 30% of all adult lumbar vertebrae, although they are likely inconsequential.[28] In more extreme cases, however, the bilateral asymmetry could create uneven stress throughout the intervertebral junctions.[54] Although evidence is mixed, the increased stress could potentially predispose a person to premature degeneration in the apophyseal joints.[78]

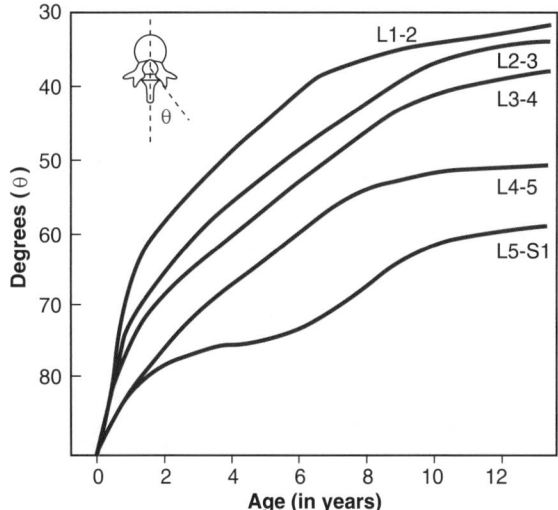

FIG. 9.25 Graph showing the orientation of the articular surfaces of the lumbar apophyseal joints as a function of age. (Based on Lutz G, Die Entwicklung der Kleinen Wirbelgelenke: *Z Orth* 104:19–28, 1967. In Bogduk N: *Clinical and radiological anatomy of the lumbar spine,* ed 5, St Louis, 2012, Churchill Livingstone.)

Anterior view

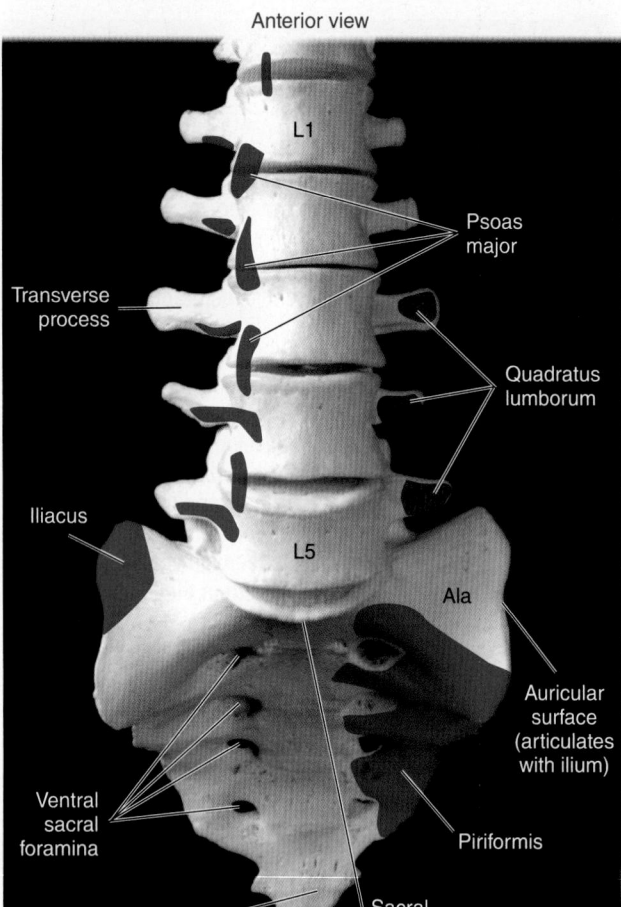

Psoas major

Transverse process

Quadratus lumborum

Iliacus

L5

Ala

Auricular surface (articulates with ilium)

Ventral sacral foramina

Piriformis

Coccyx

Sacral promontory

FIG. 9.26 An anterior view of the lumbosacral region. Attachments of the piriformis, iliacus, and psoas major are indicated in red. Attachments of the quadratus lumborum are indicated in gray.

Posterior-lateral view

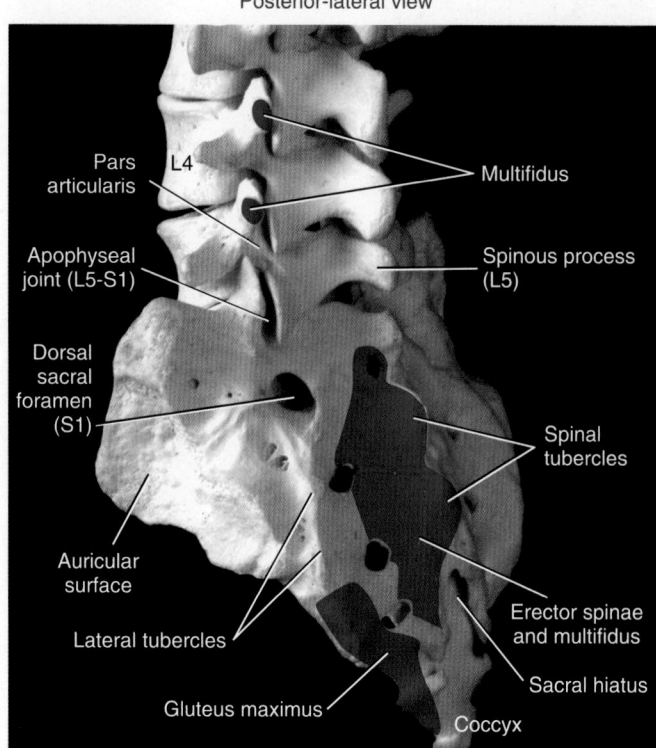

Pars articularis

L4

Multifidus

Apophyseal joint (L5-S1)

Spinous process (L5)

Dorsal sacral foramen (S1)

Spinal tubercles

Auricular surface

Erector spinae and multifidus

Lateral tubercles

Sacral hiatus

Gluteus maximus

Coccyx

FIG. 9.27 A posterior-lateral view of the lumbosacral region. Attachments of the multifidus, erector spinae, and gluteus maximus are indicated in red.

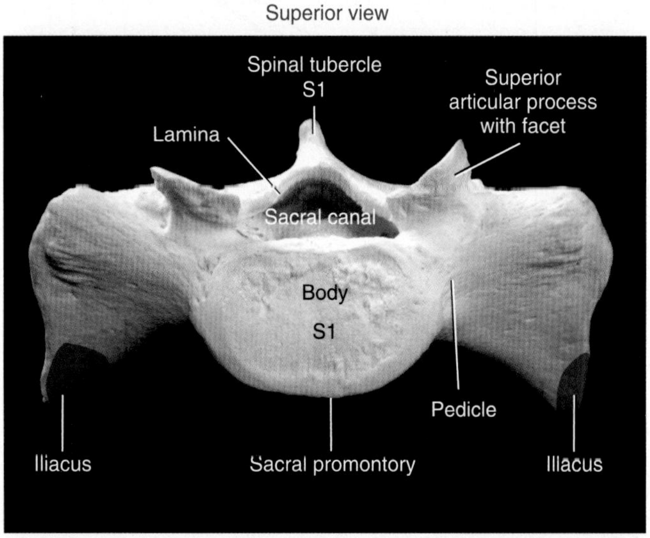

attachments of muscle and ligaments (Fig. 9.27). Several *spinal and lateral tubercles* mark the remnants of fused spinous and transverse processes, respectively. Four paired *dorsal sacral foramina* transmit the dorsal rami of sacral spinal nerve roots.

The superior surface of the sacrum shows a clear representation of the *body* of the first sacral vertebra (Fig. 9.28). The sharp anterior edge of the body of S1 is called the *sacral promontory*. The triangular *sacral canal* houses and protects the cauda equina. *Pedicles* are very thick, extending laterally as the *ala* (pair of wings) of the sacrum. Stout superior articular processes have *superior articular facets* that face generally posterior-medially. These facets articulate with the inferior facets of L5 to form L5–S1 apophyseal joints (Fig. 9.27). The large *auricular surfaces* articulate with the ilia, forming the sacroiliac joint. The sacrum narrows caudally to form its *apex,* a point of articulation with the coccyx.

COCCYX

The coccyx is a small triangular bone consisting of four fused vertebrae (Fig. 9.27). The base of the coccyx joins the apex of the sacrum at the *sacrococcygeal joint.* The joint has a fibrocartilaginous disc and is held together by several small ligaments. The sacrococcygeal joint usually fuses late in life. In youths, small *intercoccygeal joints* persist; however, these typically are fused in adults.[275]

Superior view

Spinal tubercle S1

Superior articular process with facet

Lamina

Sacral canal

Body S1

Pedicle

Iliacus

Sacral promontory

Iliacus

FIG. 9.28 A superior view of the sacrum. Attachments of the iliacus muscles are indicated in red.

At birth, the spinal cord and vertebral column are nearly the same length. Thereafter, however, the vertebral column grows at a slightly faster rate than the spinal cord. Consequently, in the adult, the caudal end of the spinal cord terminates generally adjacent to the L1 vertebra. The lumbosacral spinal nerve roots therefore must travel a great distance caudally before reaching their corresponding intervertebral foramina (see Fig. III.1 in Appendix III, Part A). As a group, the elongated nerves resemble a horse's tail, hence the term *cauda equina.*

The cauda equina is a set of peripheral nerves that are bathed in cerebrospinal fluid and located within the lumbosacral vertebral canal. Severe fracture or trauma in the lumbosacral region may damage the cauda equina but spare the spinal cord. Damage to the cauda equina, a component of the peripheral nervous system, may result in muscle paralysis and atrophy, altered sensation, and reduced reflexes. In contrast, spasticity with exaggerated reflexes typically occurs with damage to the spinal cord—a component of the central nervous system. If severed, therefore, the nerves of the cauda equina possess at least the physiologic potential for regeneration.

ARTHROLOGY

Typical Intervertebral Junction

The typical intervertebral junction has three functional components: (1) the transverse and spinous processes, (2) the apophyseal joints, and (3) an interbody joint (Fig. 9.29). The *transverse and spinous processes* provide mechanical outriggers, or levers, that increase the mechanical leverage of muscles and ligaments. *Apophyseal joints* are primarily responsible for guiding intervertebral motion, much as railroad tracks guide the direction of a train.[29] As will be emphasized, the geometry, height, and spatial orientation of the articular facets within the apophyseal joints greatly influence the prevailing direction as well as extent of intervertebral motion. *Interbody joints* connect an intervertebral disc with a pair of vertebral bodies. An essential function of the interbody joints is to absorb and distribute loads across the vertebral column. Normally, at least in the lumbar region, the interbody joint accepts most of the weight that is borne through the intervertebral junction. As indicated in Fig. 9.29, flexion of the spine shifts an even greater proportion of the superimposed body weight forward to the interbody joint. In addition, the interbody joints provide the greatest source of adhesion between vertebrae,[114] serve as the approximate axes of rotation, and function as deformable intervertebral spacers. As spacers, the intervertebral discs constitute about 25% of the total height of the vertebral column. The functional importance of the space created by a healthy intervertebral disc cannot be overstated. The greater the relative intervertebral space, the greater the ability of one vertebral body to "rock" forward and backward on another, for example. Without any disc space, the nearly flat bone-on-bone interface between two consecutive bodies would block rotation in the sagittal

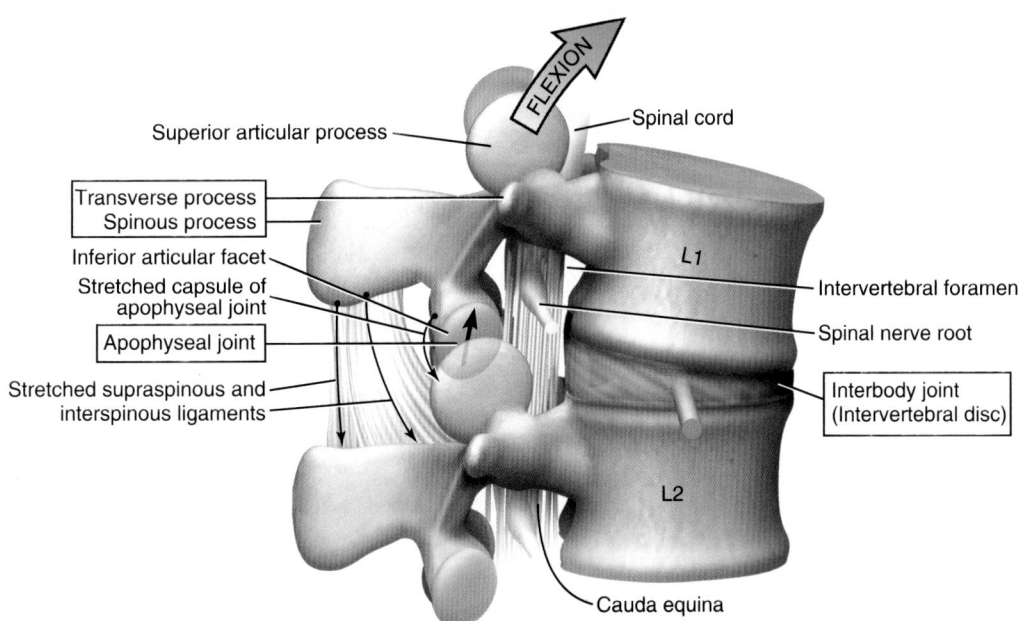

FIG. 9.29 A model highlights the three functional components of a typical intervertebral junction: transverse and spinous processes, apophyseal joints, and interbody joint, including the intervertebral disc. The L1–L2 junction is shown flexing, guided by the sliding between the articular facet surfaces of the apophyseal joints *(black, thicker arrow)*. The medial-lateral axis of rotation is shown through the interbody joint. The interspinous and supraspinous ligaments are shown stretched. Note the compression of the front of the intervertebral disc. Also note that the spinal cord terminates near the L1 vertebra and then forms the cauda equina.

and frontal planes—allowing only tipping or translation. Finally, the space created by the intervertebral discs provides adequate passage for the exiting spinal nerve roots.

Functional impairments involving the apophyseal or the interbody joints can result from trauma, excessive use and cumulative stress, osteoarthritis or other disease processes, advanced age, or combinations thereof. Regardless of cause, impairments involving these joints can lead to abnormal and painful kinematics, distorted posture, remodeling of local bone, and mechanical impingement of neural tissues. Appreciating the spatial and physical relationships between the neurology, osteology, and arthrology of a typical intervertebral junction may help understand and evaluate the many approaches used to treat spinal-related pain and dysfunction.

TERMINOLOGY DESCRIBING MOVEMENT

With a few important exceptions, movement within any given intervertebral junction is relatively small. When added across the entire vertebral column, however, these small movements can yield considerable angular rotation. The *osteokinematics* across the entire axial skeleton (which includes the vertebral column and cranium) are described as rotations within the three cardinal planes. Each plane, or degree of freedom, is associated with one axis of rotation, directed through or near the interbody joint (Fig. 9.30).[257,313] By convention, movement throughout the vertebral column, including the head on the cervical spine, is described in a cranial-to-caudal fashion, with the direction of movement referenced by a point on the *anterior* side of the more cranial (superior) vertebral segment.

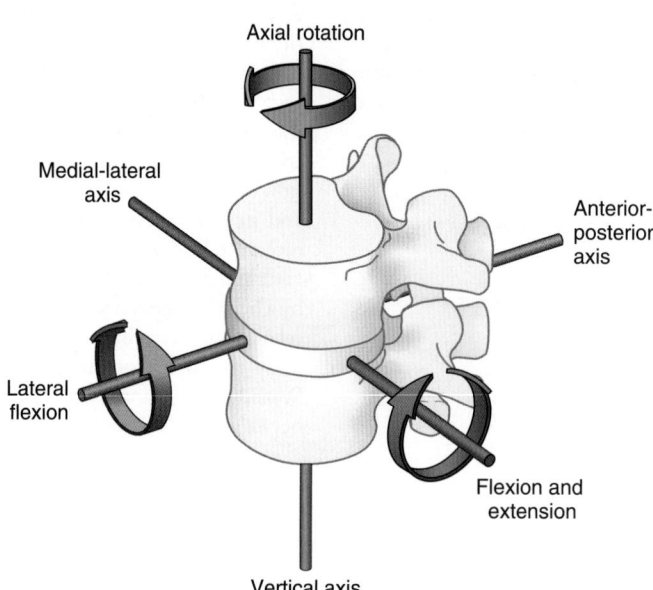

Terminology Describing the Osteokinematics of the Axial Skeleton

Common Terminology	Plane of Movement	Axis of Rotation	Other Terminology
Flexion and extension	Sagittal	Medial-lateral	Forward and backward bending
Lateral flexion to the right or left	Frontal	Anterior-posterior	Side bending to the right or left
Axial rotation to the right or left*	Horizontal	Vertical	Rotation, torsion

*Axial rotation of the spine is defined by the direction of movement of a point on the *anterior side* of the vertebral body.

FIG. 9.30 Terminology describing the osteokinematics of the vertebral column; illustrated for a typical lumbar intervertebral junction.

TABLE 9.5 Terminology Describing the Arthrokinematics at the Apophyseal Joints

Terminology	Definition	Functional Example
Approximation of joint surfaces	An articular facet surface tends to move closer to its partner facet; joint approximation is usually caused by a *compression* force	Axial rotation between L1 and L2 typically causes an approximation (compression) of the contralateral apophyseal joint
Separation (gapping) between joint surfaces	An articular facet surface tends to move away from its partner facet; joint separation is usually caused by a *distraction* force	Therapeutic traction as a way to decompress or separate the apophyseal joints
Sliding (gliding) between joint surfaces	An articular facet translates in a linear or curvilinear direction relative to another articular facet; sliding between joint surfaces is caused by a force directed tangential to the joint surfaces	Flexion-extension of the middle to lower cervical spine

During C4–C5 axial rotation to the left, for example, a point on the anterior body of C4 rotates to the left, although the spinous process rotates to the right.

Arthrokinematics of intervertebral motion describe the relative movement *between* articular facet surfaces within the apophyseal joints. Most facet surfaces are flat or nearly flat, and terms such as *approximation, separation* (or *gapping*), and *sliding* adequately describe the arthrokinematics (Table 9.5).

STRUCTURE AND FUNCTION OF THE APOPHYSEAL JOINTS

The vertebral column contains 24 pairs of apophyseal joints. Each apophyseal joint is formed between opposing articular facet surfaces (Fig. 9.31).* Mechanically classified as *plane joints,* apophyseal joints are lined with articular cartilage and enclosed by a synovial-lined, well-innervated capsule.[42,130] Sensory stimuli arising from the capsule and local, deep muscles help guide intervertebral movement as well as protect the joints from excessive stress. Although exceptions and natural variations are common, the articular surfaces of most apophyseal joints are essentially flat. Slightly curved joint surfaces are present primarily in the upper cervical and throughout the lumbar regions.

The word *apophysis* means "outgrowth," emphasizing the protruding nature of the articular processes. Acting as mechanical barricades, the articular processes permit certain movements but block others. In general, the near–vertically oriented apophyseal joints within the lower thoracic, lumbar, and lumbosacral regions block excessive anterior translation of one vertebra on another. Functionally this is important because excessive anterior translation significantly compromises the volume of the vertebral canal—the space occupied by the spinal cord or passing spinal nerve roots.

---

*This textbook uses the formal term *apophyseal* when referring to these joints, which is an abbreviated form of the term *zygapophyseal.* It should be recognized however that the more commonly used clinical term for apophyseal joint is simply "facet joint."

The orientation of the plane of the facet surfaces within each joint strongly influences the kinematics at different regions across the vertebral column. Generally, *horizontal facet surfaces favor axial rotation,* whereas *vertical facet surfaces* (in either sagittal or frontal planes) *block axial rotation.* Most apophyseal joint surfaces, however, are oriented somewhere between the horizontal and vertical.[130] Fig. 9.32 shows the typical joint orientation for superior articular facets in the cervical, thoracic, and lumbar regions. The plane of the facet surfaces explains, in part, why axial rotation is far greater in the cervical region than in the lumbar region. Additional factors that influence the predominant motion at each spinal region include the sizes of the intervertebral discs (relative to the associated vertebral bodies), the overall shape of the vertebrae, local muscle actions, and attachments made by ribs or ligaments.

STRUCTURE AND FUNCTION OF THE INTERBODY JOINTS

The spinal column has 23 interbody joints, extending from C2–C3 to L5–S1. Each interbody joint contains an intervertebral disc, vertebral endplates, and adjacent vertebral bodies. Anatomically, this joint is classified as a cartilaginous *synarthrosis* (see Chapter 2).

Structural Considerations of the Lumbar Intervertebral Discs

Most of what is known about the structure and function of intervertebral discs is based on research performed in the lumbar region. The research focus reflects the region's high frequency of disc degeneration, especially in the lower vertebral segments.

A lumbar intervertebral disc consists of a central nucleus pulposus surrounded by an annulus fibrosus (Fig. 9.33). The *nucleus pulposus* is a pulplike gel, normally located in the middle to posterior part of the disc. In youth, the nucleus pulposus within the lumbar discs consists of 70% to 90% water.[275] The hydrated nucleus allows the

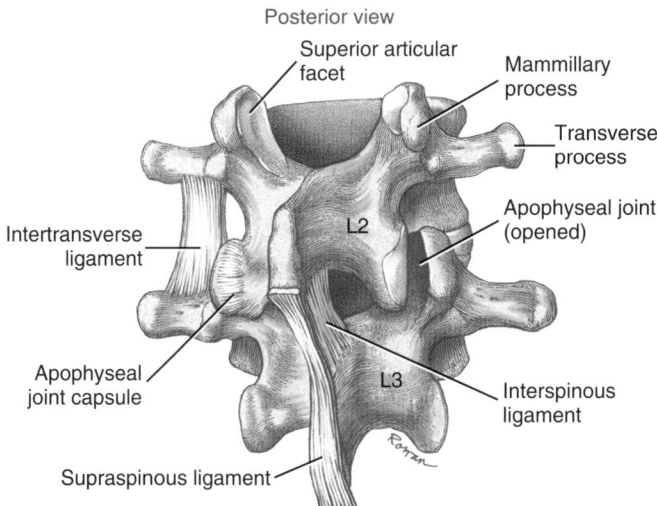

FIG. 9.31 A posterior view of the second and third lumbar vertebrae. The capsule and associated ligaments of the right apophyseal joint are removed to show the vertical alignment of the joint surfaces. The top vertebra is rotated to the *right* to maximally expose the articular surfaces of the right apophyseal joint. Note the gapping within the right apophyseal joint.

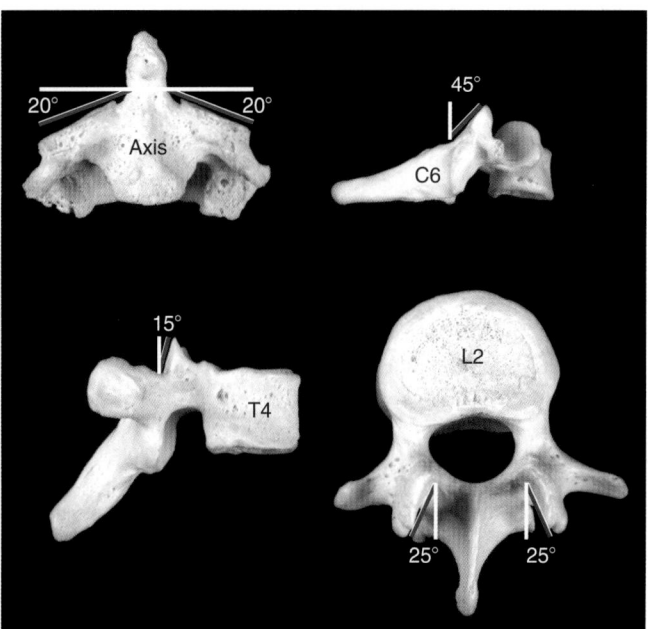

FIG. 9.32 Spatial orientations are displayed for a typical set of superior articular facet surfaces (of apophyseal joints) from cervical, thoracic, and lumbar vertebrae. The red line indicates the plane of the superior articular facet, measured against a vertical or horizontal reference line.

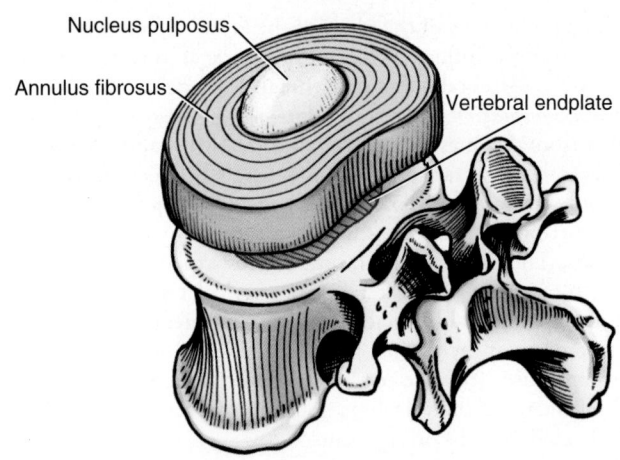

Nucleus pulposus

Annulus fibrosus

Vertebral endplate

FIG. 9.33 The intervertebral disc is shown lifted away from the underlying vertebral endplate. (Modified from Kapandji IA: *The physiology of joints,* ed 3, New York, 1974, Churchill Livingstone.)

SPECIAL FOCUS 9.4

Intra-articular Structures Located within Apophyseal Joints

Small and inconsistently formed accessory structures (inclusions) may exist around the margins of apophyseal joints, most frequently described in the upper cervical and the lumbar regions. In the lumbar spine, Bogduk describes two primary types of accessory structures: subcapsular fat pads and fibro-adipose meniscoids.[28] *Subcapsular fat pads* fill small crevices formed between the capsule and the underlying synovial membrane, typically at the superior and inferior margins of the joint. The subcapsular fat pads may extend outside the joint through very small crevices in the capsule. When fully formed, larger extracapsular fat pads within the lumbar region fill part of the space between the lamina and the overlying multifidus muscle.

Fibro-adipose meniscoids are another set of connective tissue found at the periphery of apophyseal joints. These structures range from thickenings or "pleats" of connective tissue variously placed along the internal surface of the joint capsule, to folds of synovium that encapsulate small fat pads, collagen fibers, and blood vessels. The larger fibro-adipose meniscoids can extend several millimeters into the apophyseal joint.[28]

The specific function of intra-articular inclusions within apophyseal joints is not universally accepted. Some authors have described them as deformable spacers that help dissipate compression forces within the joint.[183] Others have speculated that the structures are designed to partially cover the articular cartilage that becomes exposed at the extremes of motion.[28] This transient coverage may protect and lubricate the exposed surfaces until the joint is returned to its natural anatomic position. Although opinions vary, the intra-articular inclusions may have important clinical relevance. The larger fibro-adipose meniscoids in cervical regions may become impinged as the apophyseal joints forcefully hyperextend, such as during a cervical whiplash injury. Because these tissues are well innervated, they may be a nociceptive source of pain.[95] Meniscoids may proliferate to a point that they "lock" an apophyseal joint by physically restricting the natural arthrokinematics.[208]

disc to function as a modified hydraulic shock absorption system, capable of continuously dissipating and transferring loads across consecutive vertebrae. The nucleus pulposus is thickened into a gel-like consistency by relatively large branching proteoglycans. Each proteoglycan is an aggregate of many water-binding glycosaminoglycans linked to core proteins (see Chapter 2).[3,85] Dispersed throughout the hydrated proteoglycan mixture are thin type II collagen fibers, elastin fibers, and other proteins. The collagen forms an infrastructure that helps support the proteoglycan network. Very small numbers of chondrocytes and fibrocytes are interspersed throughout the nucleus, ultimately responsible for the synthesis and regulation of the proteins and proteoglycans. In the very young, the nucleus pulposus contains a few chondrocytes that are remnants of the primitive notochord.[275]

The *annulus fibrosus* in the lumbar discs consists primarily of 10 to 20 concentric layers, or rings, of collagen fibers.[28] Like dough surrounding jelly in a doughnut, the collagen rings encase and physically entrap the liquid-based central nucleus. The annulus fibrosus contains material and cells similar to what is found in the nucleus pulposus, differing mainly in proportion. In the annulus, collagen makes up about 50% to 60% of the dry weight, compared with only 15% to 20% in the nucleus pulposus. Abundant elastin and fibrillin proteins are interspersed in parallel to the rings of collagen, bestowing an element of circumferential elasticity to the annulus fibrosus.[322]

The outermost or peripheral layers of the annulus fibrosus consist primarily of type I and type II collagen.[41] This arrangement provides circumferential strength and flexibility to the disc, as well as a way to bond the annulus to the anterior and posterior longitudinal ligaments and to the adjacent rim of the vertebral bodies and endplates. (The outer layers of the annulus fibrosus contain the disc's only sensory nerves; see innervation of the disc, Chapter 10.) The deeper, internal layers of the annulus contain less type I collagen and more water—gradually transforming into tissue with characteristics similar to those of the centrally located nucleus pulposus.

Normally, compression forces acting on the disc increase the hydrostatic pressure within the water-logged nucleus pulposus. This rise in and containment of hydrostatic pressure ultimately absorb and evenly distribute loads across the entire intervertebral junction. Fully hydrated and pressurized discs protect not only the interbody joints, but also, indirectly, the apophyseal joints. A dehydrated and thinned disc increases the compressive loads and affects the kinematics on the associated apophyseal joints.[161] Degenerative disc disease, therefore, is believed to be a natural precursor to arthritis (or arthrosis) of the apophyseal joints.[17,130,161]

The intervertebral discs are important mechanical stabilizers of the spine. This stabilizing function is primarily a result of the structural configuration of the collagen fibers within the annulus fibrosus.[204] As shown in Fig. 9.34, most fibers are oriented in a rather precise geometric pattern. In the lumbar region, collagen rings are oriented, on average, about 65 degrees from the vertical, with fibers of adjacent layers traveling in opposite directions.[28,130] This structural arrangement offers resistance against intervertebral distraction (vertical separation), shear (sliding), and torsion (twisting) while still allowing essential osteokinematics. If the embedded collagen fibers ran nearly vertically, the disc would most effectively resist distraction forces, but not sliding or torsion. In contrast, if all fibers ran nearly parallel to the top of the vertebral body, the disc would most effectively resist shear and torsion, but not distraction. The 65-degree angle likely represents a geometric compromise that permits tensile forces to be applied primarily against the most

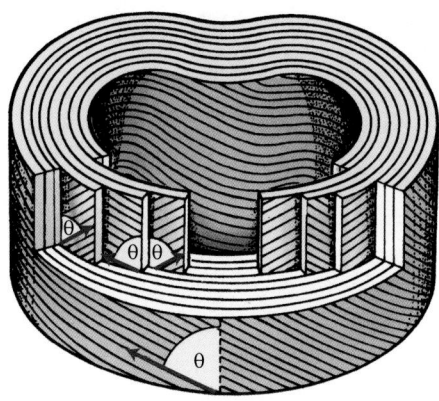

FIG. 9.34 The detailed organization of the annulus fibrosus shown with the nucleus pulposus removed. Collagen fibers are arranged in multiple concentric layers, with fibers in every other layer running in identical directions. The orientation of each collagen fiber (depicted as θ) is about 65 degrees from the vertical. (Modified from Bogduk N: *Clinical and radiological anatomy of the lumbar spine,* ed 5, New York, 2012, Churchill Livingstone.)

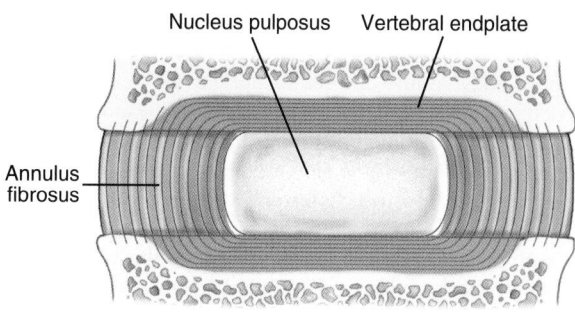

FIG. 9.35 A vertical slice through the interbody joint shows the relative position of the vertebral endplates. (Modified from Bogduk N: *Clinical and radiological anatomy of the lumbar spine,* ed 5, New York, 2012, Churchill Livingstone.)

natural movements of the lumbar spine. Distraction forces are an inherent component of flexion, extension, and lateral flexion, occurring as one vertebral body tips slightly and thus separates from its neighbor. Shear and torsion forces are produced during virtually all horizontal plane movements of the vertebral column. The presence of torsional forces is especially pertinent because of the orientation of the annular fibers. Because the collagen rings are oriented only 25 degrees *from the horizontal plane,* about 90% of the torsional force applied to the disc (i.e., cosine of 25°) will potentially stretch the annular fibers. Also, because of the alternating layering of the annulus, only the collagen fibers oriented in the direction of the slide or twist become taut; fibers in every other layer slacken. These factors may explain, at least in part, why activities that involve repetitive and forceful axial rotation of the trunk are potential risk factors for causing back injury.[51,66]

Not all annular rings in the lumbar disc completely encircle the nucleus, as implied in Fig. 9.34.[28] Some rings are incomplete and fuse with adjacent rings, particularly in the posterior-lateral quadrant of the disc. The literature also reports incomplete annular rings in the cervical discs.[184] When a cervical disc is viewed from above, the annulus has a near-crescent shape, thick along the anterior rim and progressively tapering to a very thin layer at the disc's lateral margins. Little or no annular fibers exist at the region of the uncovertebral joints. A small fissure (or cleft) typically extends horizontally inward from each uncovertebral joint, coursing to the deeper regions of the disc.[184] Although the function of the fissures is uncertain, they likely function with the uncovertebral joints by increasing the freedom of movement within the cervical region.

Vertebral Endplates

The *vertebral endplates* in the adult are relatively thin cartilaginous caps of connective tissue that cover most of the superior and inferior surfaces of the vertebral bodies (Fig. 9.33). At birth, the endplates are thick, accounting for about 50% of the height of each intervertebral space. During childhood, the endplates function as growth plates for the vertebrae; in the adult, the endplates recede and occupy only about 5% of the height of each intervertebral space.[245]

The surface of the vertebral endplate that faces the disc is composed primarily of fibrocartilage, which binds directly and strongly to the collagen within the annulus fibrosus (Fig. 9.35). This fibrocartilaginous bond forms the primary adhesion between consecutive vertebrae. In contrast, the surface of the endplate that faces the vertebral body is composed primarily of calcified cartilage that is weakly affixed to the bone. This endplate-bone interface is often described as the "weak link" within the interbody joint, often the first component of the interbody joint to fracture under high or repetitive compressive loading.[190,238] A perforated or fractured endplate can allow the proteoglycan gel to leak from the nucleus pulposus, causing structural disruption of the disc.[98,233]

Only the outer, more peripheral rings of the annulus fibrosus normally contain blood vessels. For this reason, most of the disc has an inherently limited healing capacity. Essential nutrients, such as glucose and oxygen, must diffuse a great distance to reach the deeper cells that sustain the disc's low but essential metabolism. The source of these nutrients is carried in blood vessels located in the more superficial annulus and, more substantially, blood stored in the adjacent vertebral bodies.[98] Most of these nutrients must diffuse across the vertebral endplate and through the disc's extracellular matrix, eventually reaching the cells residing deep in the disc.[237] These cells must receive nourishment to manufacture essential extracellular proteoglycans. Aged discs, for example, typically show reduced permeability and increased calcification of the vertebral endplates, which, in turn, reduce the flow of nutrients and oxygen into the disc.[30,64,245] This age-related process can inhibit cellular metabolism and synthesis of proteoglycans. Less proteoglycan content reduces the ability of the nucleus to attract and retain water, thereby limiting its ability to effectively absorb and transfer loads.[15,320]

Reduced diffusion of nutrients across the vertebral endplates and subsequent poor nutrition of the nucleus pulposus are not limited to just the aging population. Even in the young, excessive or abnormal mechanical loading and subsequent degeneration of the vertebral endplates reduce the ability of nutrients to flow deep into the nucleus. Research on chronically and abnormally loaded vertebral endplates harvested during surgery for the correction of advanced scoliosis in individuals aged 11 to 17 years showed widespread altered diffusion and poor nutrition of the disc's nuclear material.[239] This is an important consideration, because optimal function of vertebral endplates is essential to the health and subsequent shock absorption function of the intervertebral disc throughout one's lifetime.

Intervertebral Disc as a Hydrostatic Pressure Distributor

The vertebral column is the primary support structure for the trunk and upper body. While one stands upright for example, approximately 80% of the load supported by two adjoining lumbar vertebrae is carried through the interbody joint; the remaining 20% is carried by posterior elements, such as apophyseal joints and laminae. As will be described later in this chapter and in Chapter 10, the relative sharing of load across the intervertebral junction is strongly influenced both by the region and by the position of the spinal column.

The intervertebral discs are uniquely designed shock absorbers that protect the vertebral bone from potentially damaging loading that may arise from body weight and activation of muscle. The collagen-based annulus fibrosus can share a significant part of the intervertebral load based purely on its structural bulk.[14] However, a more elaborate and dynamic load-sharing system is required to protect the vertebrae against larger, sustained, and repetitive loading. This system is based on a biomechanical interaction between the water-based nucleus pulposus and the annular rings. Compressive loads push the endplates inward and toward the nucleus pulposus. Being filled mostly with water and therefore essentially incompressible, the young and healthy nucleus responds by slowly deforming radially and outwardly against the annulus fibrosus (Fig. 9.36A). Radial deformation is resisted by the tension created within the stretched rings of collagen and elastin of the annulus fibrosus (Fig. 9.36B). Pressure within the entire disc is thus uniformly elevated and transmitted evenly to the adjacent vertebra (Fig. 9.36C). When the compressive force is removed from the endplates, the stretched elastin and collagen fibers return to their original preloaded length, ready for another compressive force. This mechanism allows sustained compressive forces to be shared by multiple structures, thereby preventing "spot loading" (i.e., highly concentrated forces acting on a small surface area of a tissue). Because it has viscoelastic properties, the intervertebral disc can resist a fast or strongly applied compression more than a slow or light compression.[140] The disc therefore can be flexible at lower loads and more rigid at higher loads.

In Vivo Pressure Measurements from the Nucleus Pulposus

In vivo human studies have measured the pressure within the nucleus pulposus in the lumbar region during different activities.[7,194,315] Data generally agree that the pressure is relatively low at rest in the supine position but increases significantly during activities that combine forward bending of the trunk and the need for vigorous trunk muscle contraction. When high, the intradiscal pressure can produce transient changes in the shape of the intervertebral disc, even in healthy specimens. Sustained flexion in the lumbar spine, for example, can reduce the height of the disc slightly as water is slowly forced outward. Sustained and full lumbar *extension,* in contrast, reduces the pressure in the disc; this allows water to be reabsorbed into the disc, thus reinflating it to its natural level.

Analysis of in vivo pressure data within the disc during movement and varying body position has a long history, and has established some of the early concepts on possible mechanisms for lumbar disc injury.[160] Data produced by two well cited studies are compared in Fig. 9.37.[192,315] Although somewhat dated, both studies reinforce three general points: (1) disc pressures are large when one holds a load in front of the body, especially when bending forward; (2) lifting a load with the knees flexed places less pressure on the lumbar disc than does lifting a load with the knees straight (the latter method typically generating more demands on the back muscles); and (3) sitting in a forward-slouched position produces greater disc pressure than sitting

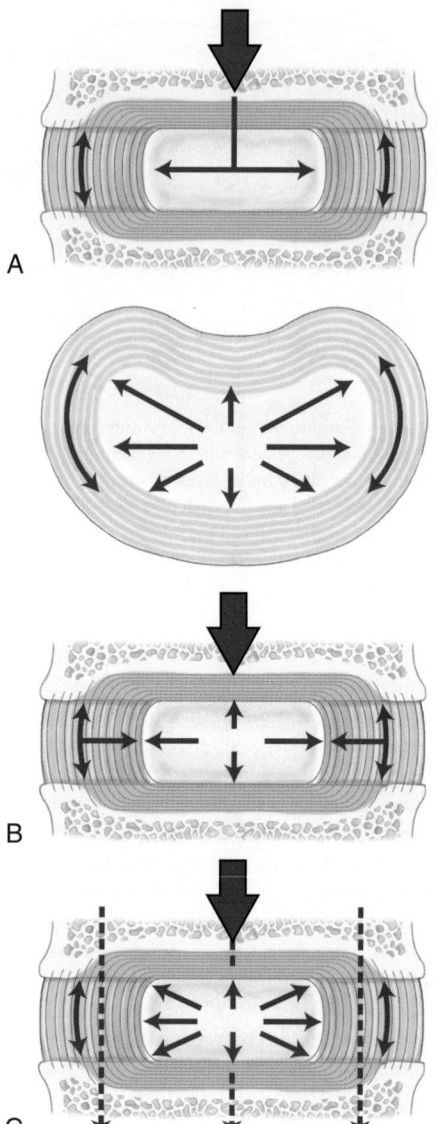

FIG. 9.36 The mechanism of force transmission through an intervertebral disc. (A) Compression force from body weight and muscle contraction *(straight arrows)* raises the hydrostatic pressure in the nucleus pulposus. In turn, the increased pressure elevates the tension in the annular fibrosus *(curved arrows)*. (B) The increased tension in the annulus inhibits radial expansion of the nucleus. The rising nuclear pressure is also exerted upward and downward against the vertebral endplates. (C) The pressure within the disc is evenly redistributed to several tissues as it is transmitted across the endplates to the adjacent vertebra. (Modified from Bogduk N: *Clinical and radiological anatomy of the lumbar spine,* ed 5, New York, 2012, Churchill Livingstone.)

erect. These points serve as a theoretical basis for many education and prevention programs aimed at protecting the intervertebral discs and low back region in general from potentially excessive damaging stress.[63]

Diurnal Fluctuations in the Water Content within the Intervertebral Discs

When a healthy spine is unloaded, such as during bed rest, the pressure within the nucleus pulposus is relatively low.[192] This relatively low pressure, combined with the hydrophilic nature of the nucleus pulposus, attracts water into the disc. As a result, the disc swells

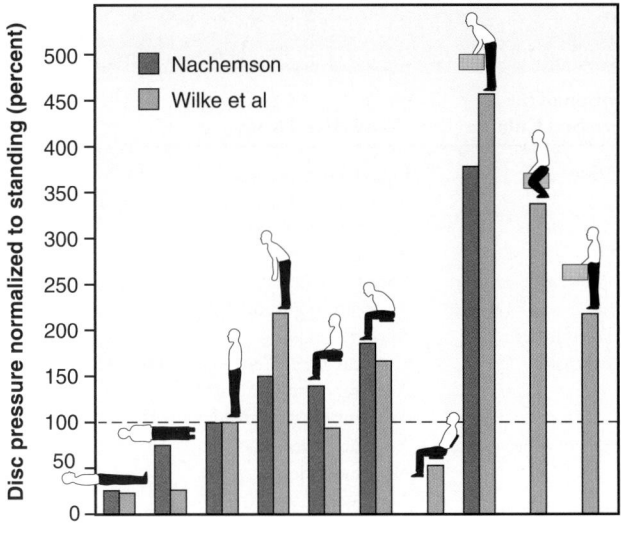

FIG. 9.37 A comparison between data from two intradiscal pressure studies. Each study measured in vivo pressures from a lumbar nucleus pulposus in a 70-kg subject during common postures and activities. The pressures are normalized to standing. (Modified from Wilke H-J, Neef P, Caimi M, et al: New in vivo measurements of pressures in the intervertebral disc in daily life, *Spine* 24:755, 1999.)

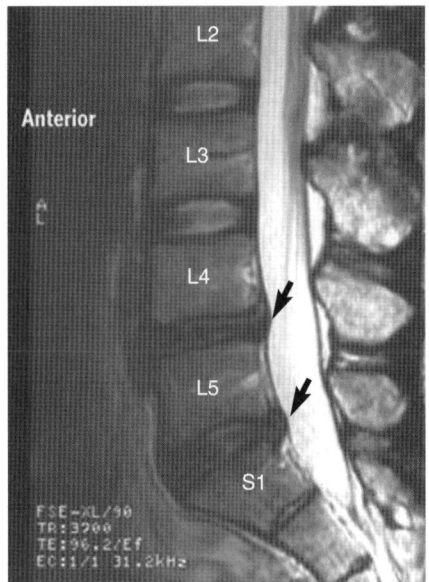

FIG. 9.38 A midsagittal T2-weighted MRI scan of a 35-year-old man with a history of recurrent low back pain that is provoked by prolonged or repeated lumbar flexion. Evidence of disc degeneration is indicated by a diminished (darker) signal intensity in the nuclear regions of L4–L5 and L5–S1. Modest posterior displacement or "bulging" of the disc is also noticeable at the L4–L5 and L5–S1 junctions *(arrows)*. (Image courtesy Paul F. Beattie PT, PhD, FAPTA.)

A relatively dehydrated nucleus pulposus exerts less hydrostatic pressure when compressed.[28] Once relatively depressurized, the disc may bulge outward when compressed, like a "flat tire." The older, degenerated intervertebral disc is subsequently less able to uniformly cushion the vertebral body and endplates against compressive loads.[203] As a consequence, disc degeneration increases with age and affects most persons, to varying extent, who are at least 35 or 40 years old.[102,228,234,296] A diagnosis of *disc degeneration* is most effectively made using MR imaging, typically based on a diminished signal intensity of the T2-weighted image (indicative of reduced water content), loss of distinction between the border of the annulus fibrosus and the nucleus pulposus, disc (nuclear) bulging, and loss of disc space.[102,227] The MR image scan in Fig. 9.38 shows diminished signal intensity between L4–L5 and L5–S1 along with slight bulging of the disc. Furthermore, a degenerated disc may display circumferential, radial, and peripheral fissures (clefts) within the annulus.[102] According to Adams, these fissures can often be observed even in young adolescent persons.[3] Excessive degeneration may also be associated with complete depressurization of the nucleus in conjunction with delamination of the annular fibers and microfractures of the vertebral endplates.[64,102] In some cases, the internal disruption of the annular fibers may lead to a herniation (prolapse) of the nucleus pulposus (typically posteriorly toward or into the spinal canal). Remarkably, a significant percentage of persons with observable signs of disc degeneration on MR image remain asymptomatic, *without* experiencing continued mechanical deterioration or loss of function.[132] The important topic of disc degeneration, including disc herniation, is described in more detail later in this chapter.

slightly overnight when one is sleeping, increasing its relative hydration volume by about 10%.[15] When one is awake and upright, however, weight bearing produces compression forces across the vertebral endplates that push water out of the disc.[131] The natural cycle of swelling and contraction of the disc produces on average a 1% diurnal variation in overall body height.[291] This daily variation has a strong inverse relationship to age. Karakida and colleagues used MR imaging to measure the variation in water content in the discs of a group of working persons between the ages of 23 and 56 years old, with no medical history of low back pain.[137] Remarkably, significant diurnal variation in water content was found only in the discs of persons *younger than* 35 years of age. These findings are consistent with the fact that the water-retaining capacity of intervertebral discs naturally declines with increasing age.[3] The relative dehydration is caused by the parallel, age-related decline in the discs' proteoglycan content.[64,228,292]

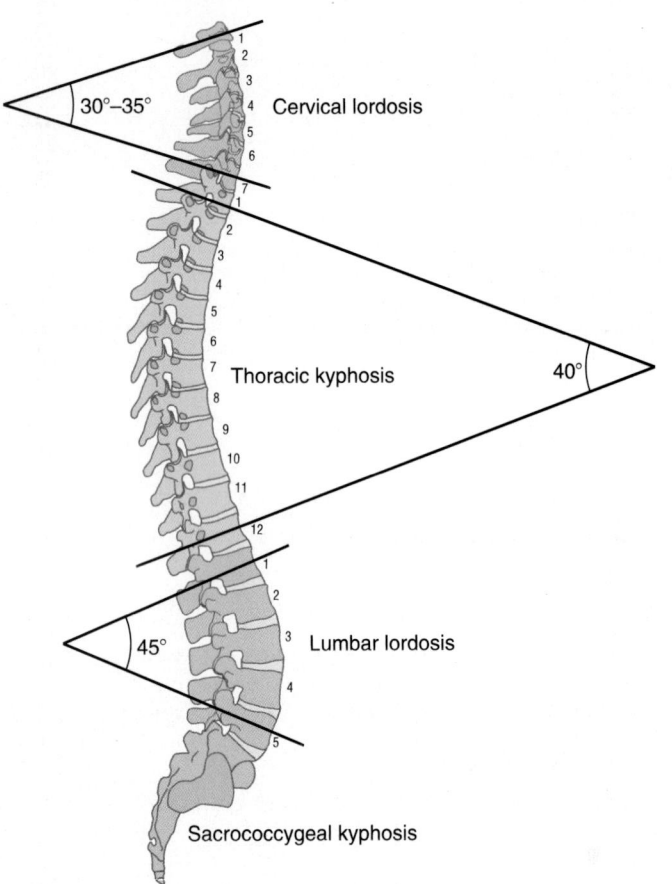

FIG. 9.39 A sample of normal sagittal plane curvatures across regions of the vertebral column. The curvatures define the anatomic position for each region, often referred to as "ideal" posture while standing.

REGIONAL ANATOMY AND KINEMATICS ACROSS THE VERTEBRAL COLUMN

This section describes the anatomy and kinematics throughout the various regions of the vertebral column. For each region, a maximum expected range of motion will be cited, assuming a starting, anatomic position (Fig. 9.39).[107,147,175] The reported range of motion in the literature is highly variable, reflecting differences in test position (sitting versus standing, for example), subjects' sex, age, and body type.[12,71,323] Data also vary for active and passive movements and whether radiologic or nonradiologic devices were used to measure the motion.[214] Methods typically include the use of goniometers (manual, electrical, or fiberoptic), flexible rulers, or inclinometers or more sophisticated tools that employ three-dimensional MR imaging, incremental biplanar and single plane radiography, videofluoroscopy, ultrasonography, and computerized analysis using electromechanical, potentiometric, optical, or electromagnetic tracking systems. The connective tissues within the vertebral column play a major role in limiting and therefore defining the normal limits of motion across regions; selected examples are provided in Table 9.6.[135] In cases of disease, trauma, or extended periods of immobilization, these connective tissues may become abnormally stiff or lax, thus interfering with normal kinematics. Understanding the structures' normal function is a prerequisite for the design of treatments aimed to restore normal intervertebral kinematics.

TABLE 9.6 Selected Examples of Connective Tissues That May Limit Motions of the Vertebral Column

Motion of the Vertebral Column	Connective Tissues
Flexion	Ligamentum nuchae Interspinous and supraspinous ligaments Ligamentum flavum Apophyseal joints* Posterior annulus fibrosus Posterior longitudinal ligament
Beyond neutral extension	Apophyseal joints Cervical viscera (esophagus and trachea) Anterior annulus fibrosus Anterior longitudinal ligament
Axial rotation	Annulus fibrosus Apophyseal joints Alar ligaments
Lateral flexion	Intertransverse ligaments Contralateral annulus fibrosus Apophyseal joints

*Depending on the movement, resistance generated by apophyseal joints may be caused by excessive approximation within the joint, increased tension within the capsule, or a combination of factors.

Introduction to Spinal Coupling

Movement performed within any given plane throughout the vertebral column is usually associated with an automatic, and often clinically imperceptible, movement in another plane. This kinematic phenomenon is called *spinal coupling*. Although spinal coupling can involve both rotation and translation, more clinical attention is paid to the rotational kinematics.

The mechanical explanations for the cause of most purported spinal coupling patterns are varied and typically unclear. Explanations may include muscle action, articular facet alignment within apophyseal joints, pre-existing posture, attachment of ribs, stiffness of connective tissues, and geometry of the physiologic curve itself.[48,70,99,155,269] The last explanation, rooted more in mechanics than biology, may be demonstrated by using a flexible rod as a model of the spine. Bend the rod about 30 to 40 degrees in one plane to mimic the natural lordosis or kyphosis of a particular region. While maintaining this curve, "laterally flex" the rod and note a slight automatic axial rotation. The biplanar bend placed on a flexible rod apparently creates unequal strains that are dissipated as torsion. This demonstration does not explain all coupling patterns observed clinically throughout the vertebral column, however.

Although some manual therapists incorporate spinal coupling into their assessment and treatment of spinal dysfunction, little consensus exists as to which coupling pattern is considered normal for a specific region.[48,155,269] One important exception is the relatively consistent coupling pattern that is naturally expressed between lateral flexion and ipsilateral axial rotation in the middle and lower cervical spine.[48,99,126,251] The specifics of this coupling pattern are described in detail in the section on kinematics of the craniocervical region.

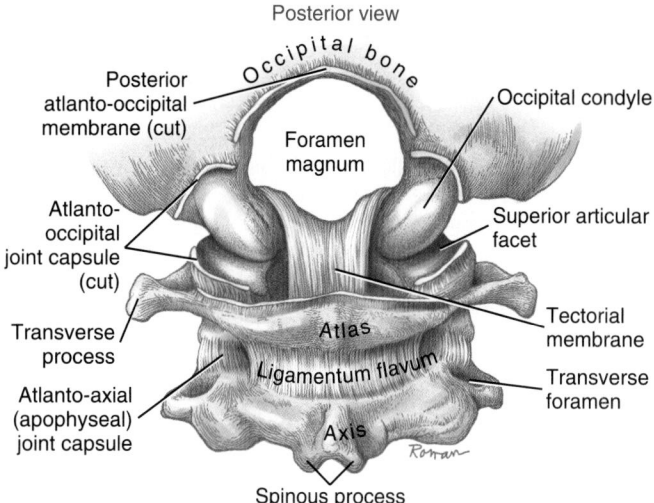

FIG. 9.40 A posterior view of exposed atlanto-occipital joints. The cranium is rotated forward to expose the articular surfaces of the joints. Note the tectorial membrane as it crosses between the atlas and the cranium.

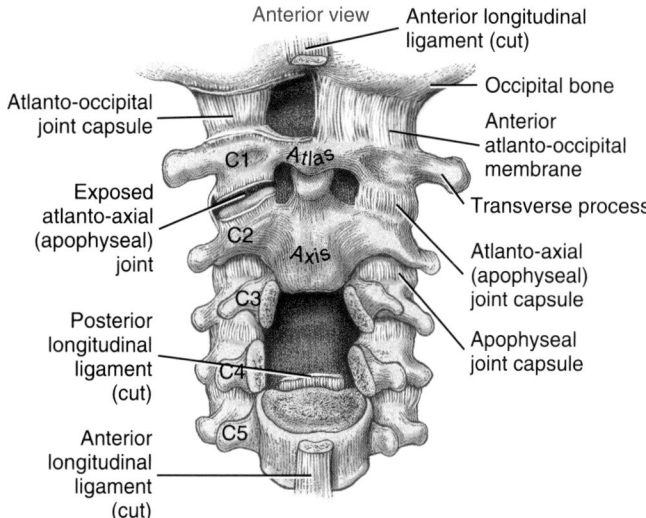

FIG. 9.41 An anterior view illustrates the connective tissues associated with the atlanto-occipital joint and the atlanto-axial joint complex. The right side of the atlanto-occipital membrane is removed to show the capsule of the atlanto-occipital joint. The capsule of the right atlanto-axial (apophyseal) joint is also removed to expose its articular surfaces. The spinal cord and the bodies of C3 and C4 are removed to show the orientation of the posterior longitudinal ligament.

The motions of lateral flexion and axial rotation have been shown to be coupled in various manners in the thoracic and lumbar regions, although not consistently reported across multiple studies.[100,155,156,215,269] The inconsistency may reflect the natural variability of the phenomenon in these regions, as well as different testing methodologies or conditions, dissimilar subject populations, or, more likely, a combination of these factors.

Craniocervical Region

The terms "craniocervical region" and "neck" are used interchangeably. Both terms refer to the combined set of three articulations: *atlanto-occipital joint, atlanto-axial joint complex,* and *intracervical apophyseal joints* (C2 to C7). The overall organization used to present the regional anatomy and kinematics of the craniocervical region is outlined in Box 9.1. The upcoming section begins with an overview of the anatomy followed by a discussion of kinematics, organized by plane of movement.

ANATOMY OF JOINTS

Atlanto-Occipital Joint

The atlanto-occipital joints provide independent movement of the cranium relative to the atlas (C1). The joints are formed by the protruding convex condyles of the occipital bone fitting into the reciprocally concave superior articular facets of the atlas (Fig. 9.40). The congruent convex-concave relationship provides inherent structural stability to the articulation.

Anteriorly, the capsule of each atlanto-occipital joint blends with the *anterior atlanto-occipital membrane* (Fig. 9.41). Posteriorly, the capsule is covered by a thin, broad *posterior atlanto-occipital membrane* (Fig. 9.42). As depicted on the right side of Fig. 9.42, the vertebral artery pierces the posterior atlanto-occipital membrane to enter the foramen magnum. This crucial artery supplies blood to the brain.

FIG. 9.42 A posterior view illustrates the connective tissues associated with the atlanto-occipital joint and atlanto-axial joint complex. The left side of the posterior atlanto-occipital membrane and the underlying capsule of the atlanto-occipital joint are removed. The laminae and spinous processes of C2 and C3, the spinal cord, and the posterior longitudinal ligament and tectorial membrane are also removed to expose the posterior sides of the vertebral bodies and the dens.

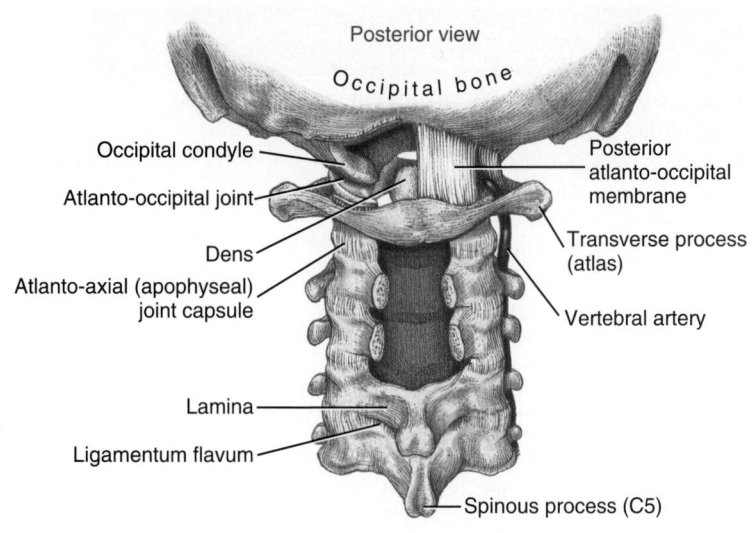

FIG. 9.43 A superior view of the dens and its structural relationship to the median atlanto-axial joint. The spinal cord and the alar ligaments have been removed and the tectorial membrane is cut. Synovial membranes are in blue.

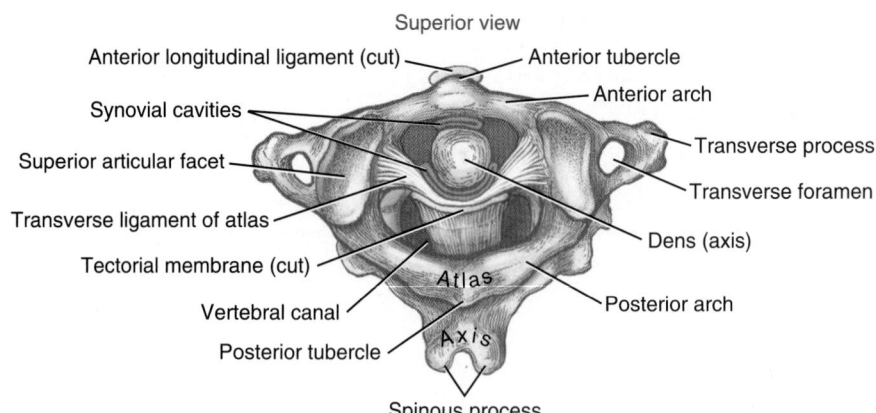

The concave-convex structure of the atlanto-occipital joints permits angular rotation primarily in two degrees of freedom.[284] The primary motions are flexion and extension. Lateral flexion is slight. Axial rotation is significantly limited and will not be considered as a third degree of freedom.

Atlanto-Axial Joint Complex

The atlanto-axial joint complex has two articular components: a median joint and a pair of laterally positioned apophyseal joints. The median joint is formed by the dens of the axis (C2) projecting through an osseous-ligamentous ring created by the anterior arch of the atlas and the transverse ligament (Fig. 9.43). Because the dens serves as a vertical axis for horizontal plane rotation of the atlas, the atlanto-axial joint is often described as a pivot joint.

The *median joint* within the atlanto-axial joint complex has two synovial cavities. The smaller, anterior cavity is formed between the anterior side of the dens and the posterior border of the anterior arch of the atlas (Fig. 9.43). An anterior facet on the anterior side of the dens marks this articulation (see Fig. 9.20A). The much larger posterior cavity separates the posterior side of the dens and a cartilage-lined section of the *transverse ligament of the atlas*. This strong, 2-cm long ligament is essential to the horizontal plane stability of the atlanto-axial articulation.[39] Without its restraint, the atlas (and articulated cranium) can slip anteriorly relative to the axis, possibly resulting in compression or injury to the spinal cord.

The two *apophyseal joints* of the atlanto-axial joint are formed by the articulation of the inferior articular facets of the atlas with the superior facets of the axis (see exposed right joint in Fig. 9.41). The surfaces of these apophyseal joints are generally flat and oriented close to the horizontal plane, a design that maximizes the freedom of axial rotation.

The atlanto-axial joint complex allows two degrees of freedom. Roughly 50% of the total horizontal plane rotation within the craniocervical region occurs at the atlanto-axial joint complex. The second degree of freedom at this joint complex is flexion-extension. Lateral flexion is relatively limited and will not be considered as a third degree of freedom.

Tectorial Membrane and the Alar Ligaments

A review of the anatomy of the atlanto-axial joint complex must include a brief description of the tectorial membrane and the alar ligaments, connective tissues that help connect the cranium to the upper cervical spine. As discussed, the transverse ligament of the atlas makes firm contact with the posterior side of the dens (Fig. 9.43). Just posterior to the transverse ligament is a broad, firm sheet of connective tissue called the *tectorial membrane* (Figs. 9.40 and 9.43). As a continuation of the posterior longitudinal ligament, the tectorial membrane ascends intracranially to attach to the basilar part of the occipital bone, just anterior to the rim of the foramen magnum. En route to this cranial attachment, the edges of the tectorial membrane blend with part of the capsule

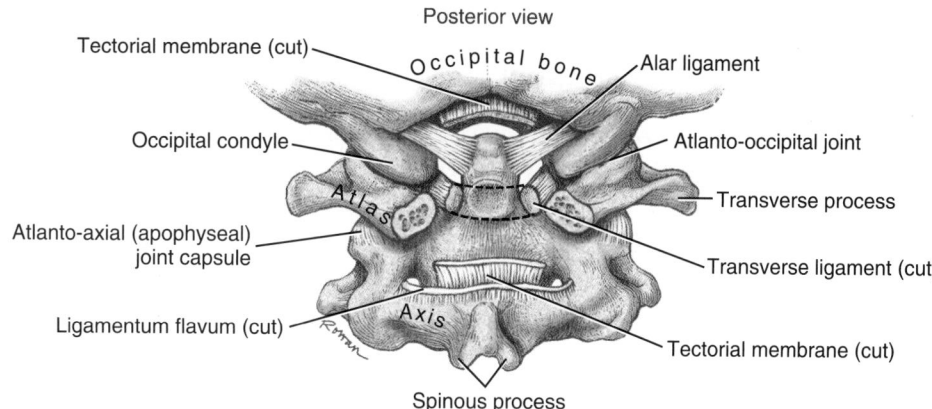

FIG. 9.44 A posterior view of the atlanto-axial joint complex. The posterior arch of the atlas, tectorial membrane, and transverse ligament of the atlas are cut to expose the posterior side of the dens and the alar ligaments. The dashed lines indicate the removed segment of the transverse ligament of the atlas.

TABLE 9.7 Approximate Range of Motion for the Three Planes of Movement for the Joints of the Craniocervical Region*

Joint or Region	Flexion and Extension (Sagittal Plane, Degrees)	Axial Rotation (Horizontal Plane, Degrees)	Lateral Flexion (Frontal Plane, Degrees)
Atlanto-occipital joint	Flexion: 5 Extension: 10 Total: 15	Negligible	About 5
Atlanto-axial joint complex	Flexion: 5 Extension: 5 Total: 10	35–40	Negligible
Intracervical region (C2–C7)	Flexion: 35–40 Extension: 55–65 Total: 90–105	30–35	30–35
Total across craniocervical region	Flexion: 45–50 Extension: 70–80 Total: 115–130	65–75	35–40

*The horizontal and frontal plane motions are to one side only. Data in table are approximate and compiled from multiple sources.

of the adjacent atlanto-occipital joints. There is limited published information on the function of the tectorial membrane. Based on attachments, however, the ligament likely provides generalized multidirectional stability to the craniocervical junction.

The *alar ligaments* are tough fibrous cords each approximately 1 cm in length.[275] As shown in Fig. 9.44, each ligament passes laterally and slightly superiorly from the posterior-lateral region of the upper dens to medial side of the occipital condyle.[211] Clinically referred to as "check ligaments," the alar ligaments are recognized for their ability to resist, or check, *axial rotation* of the head-and-atlas relative to the dens.[115,212,217] The pair of ligaments is relatively loose in the anatomic position but becomes increasingly taut during axial rotation; the ligament located contralateral to the side of the rotation exhibits slightly greater resistance to the movement.[52,69,250] In addition to limiting axial rotation, the alar ligaments also restrict the extremes of all other potential motions at the atlanto-occipital joint.[284]

Direct trauma to the craniocervical region or indirect trauma in the form of whiplash injury has the potential to injure the alar ligaments. But the ability to diagnose an injury to the alar ligaments accurately through special clinical tests is questionable. Accurate diagnosis through imaging is also challenging.[284]

Intracervical Apophyseal Joints (C2 to C7)
The facet surfaces within apophyseal joints of C2 to C7 are orientated like shingles on a 45-degree sloped roof, approximately halfway between the frontal and horizontal planes (see Fig. 9.18, C2–C3 articulation). This orientation enhances the freedom of movement in all three planes, a hallmark of cervical arthrology.

SAGITTAL PLANE KINEMATICS

The craniocervical region is the most mobile region within the entire vertebral column. Highly specialized joints facilitate precise positioning of the head, often associated with vision, hearing, smell, and equilibrium. The individual joints within the craniocervical region normally interact in a highly coordinated manner. Table 9.7 lists typical ranges of motion contributed by each area of the craniocervical region.[a] Because of the large range and variability in the data presented in the literature, the actual values listed in this table are more useful for appreciating the *relative* kinematics among joints, and less as a strict objective guide for evaluating movement in individual patients.

[a] 24, 29, 70, 209, 214, 225, 260, 280

Osteokinematics of Flexion and Extension

About 115 to 130 degrees of combined flexion and extension occur across the entire craniocervical region. From the anatomic position of about 30 to 35 degrees of extension (resting lordosis), the craniocervical region *extends* approximately an additional 70 to 80 degrees and *flexes* 45 to 50 degrees (Figs. 9.45 and 9.46). Although highly variable, most research data indicate that extension typically exceeds flexion throughout the craniocervical region, generally by a ratio of 1.5 to 1.

In addition to muscles, connective tissues limit the extremes of craniocervical motion. For example, the ligamentum nuchae and interspinous ligaments provide significant restraint to the extremes of flexion, whereas the approximation of the apophyseal joints limits the extremes of extension. Flexion is also limited by compression forces from the anterior margin of the annulus fibrosus, whereas extension is limited by the compression forces from the posterior margin of the annulus fibrosus. Additional tissues that limit or restrict sagittal plane motion across the craniocervical region are listed in Table 9.6.

About 20% of the total sagittal plane motion at the craniocervical region occurs at the atlanto-occipital joint and atlanto-axial joint complex, and the remainder occurs at the apophyseal joints of C2 to C7. The axis of rotation for flexion and extension is directed in a medial-lateral direction through each of the three joint regions: near the occipital condyles at the atlanto-occipital joint, the dens at the atlanto-axial joint complex, and the bodies or adjacent interbody joints of C2 to C7.[40,68]

The volume of the cervical vertebral canal is greatest in full flexion and least in full extension.[120] For this reason, a person with stenosis (narrowing) of the vertebral canal may be more vulnerable to spinal cord injury during full, end range extension activities. Repeated episodes of hyperextension-related injuries may lead to cervical myelopathy (from the Greek root *myelo,* denoting spinal cord, and *pathos,* suffering) and related neurologic deficits.

Arthrokinematics of Flexion and Extension
Atlanto-Occipital Joint

Like the rockers on a rocking chair, the convex occipital condyles *roll* backward in extension and forward in flexion within the concave superior articular facets of the atlas. Based on traditional convex-on-concave arthrokinematics, the condyles are expected to simultaneously *slide* slightly in the direction opposite to the roll (Fig. 9.45A and Fig. 9.46A). Tension in articular capsules, associated atlanto-occipital membranes, and alar ligaments limits the extent of the arthrokinematics.

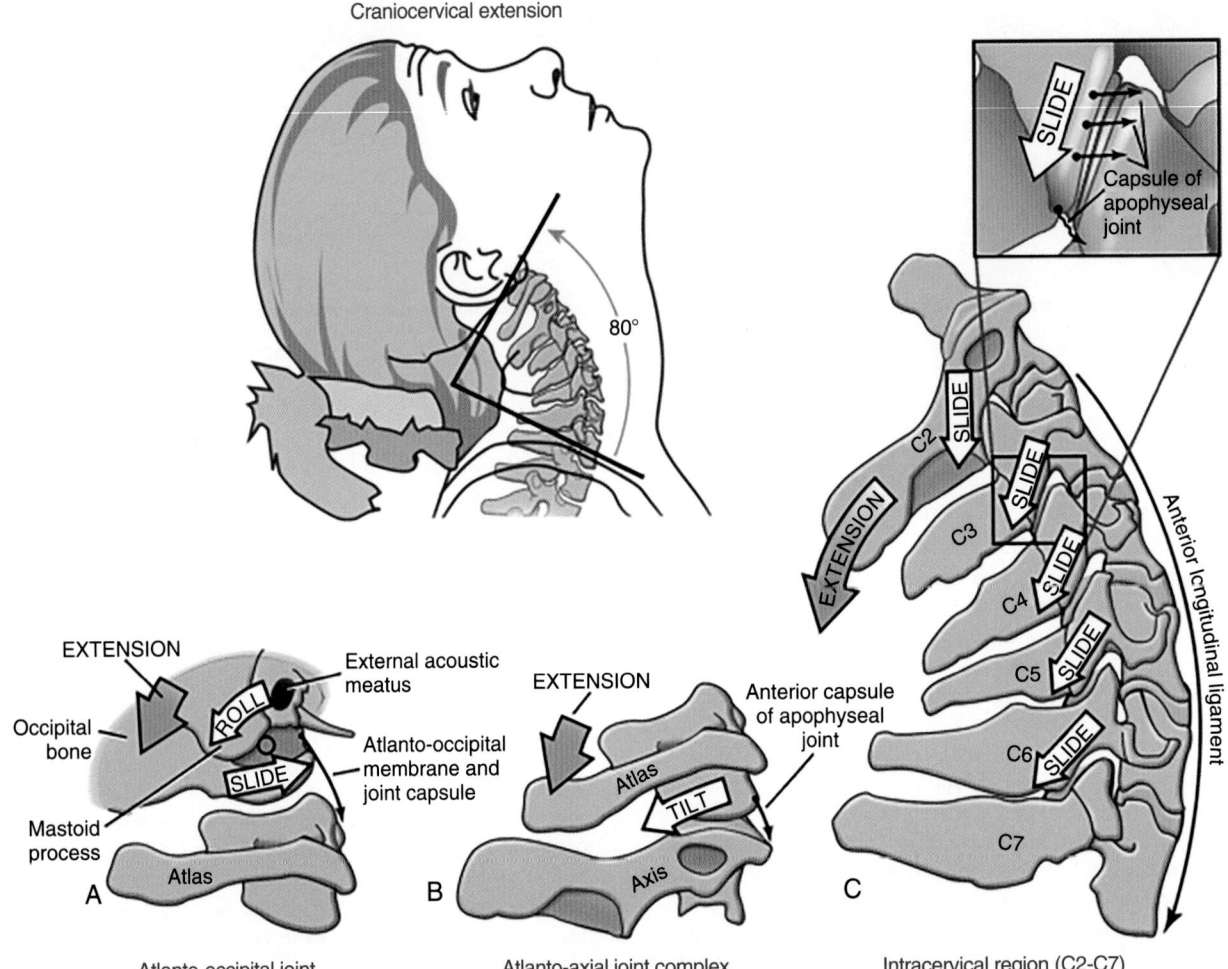

FIG. 9.45 Kinematics of craniocervical extension. (A) Atlanto-occipital joint. (B) Atlanto-axial joint complex. (C) Intracervical region (C2 to C7). Elongated, taut tissues are indicated by thin black arrows; slackened tissue is indicated by a wavy black arrow.

Atlanto-Axial Joint Complex

Although the primary motion at the atlanto-axial joint complex is axial rotation, the joint structure allows roughly 10 degrees of total flexion and extension. Acting as a spacer between the cranium and axis, the ring-shaped atlas tilts forward during flexion and backward during extension (Figs. 9.45B and 9.46B). The extent of the tilting is limited, in part, by contact between the transverse ligament of the atlas and dens (at full flexion) and between the anterior arch of the atlas and dens (at full extension).

Intracervical Articulations (C2 to C7)

Flexion and extension throughout the C2 to C7 vertebrae occur through an arc that follows the oblique plane set by the articular facets of the apophyseal joints. During *extension* the inferior articular facets of the superior vertebrae slide *inferiorly* and *posteriorly*, relative to the superior articular facets of the inferior vertebrae (see Fig. 9.45C). These movements produce approximately 55 to 65 degrees of extension, stretching primarily the anterior and lateral capsule of the apophyseal joints (see inset Fig. 9.45C). At full extension, the combined inferior and posterior sliding arthrokinematics concentrates the loading on the inferior part of the apophyseal joints.[129]

In general, the anatomic or slightly extended position of the cervical region increases the area of contact within the apophyseal joints. For this reason, this position may be considered the apophyseal joints' *close-packed position.* In fact, the anatomic or slightly extended position may be considered the close-packed position for *all* apophyseal joints across the vertebral column; moderate flexion is considered the joints' loose- or open-packed position. (As described for most synovial joints in the body, the close-packed position is a unique position that increases the area of joint contact *and* increases the tension in the surrounding capsular ligaments. Because at least some fibers of the capsular ligaments of apophyseal joints become increasingly taut on either side of the anatomic or slightly extended position, these joints are an exception to this general rule.)

The arthrokinematics of *flexion* throughout the intracervical region occur in a reverse fashion to that described for extension. The inferior articular facets of the superior vertebrae slide *superiorly* and *anteriorly*, relative to the superior articular facets of the inferior vertebrae. As depicted in Fig. 9.46C, the sliding between the articular facets produces approximately 35 to 40 degrees of flexion. Flexion stretches all the components of the capsule of the apophyseal joints[8] and reduces the area of joint contact.

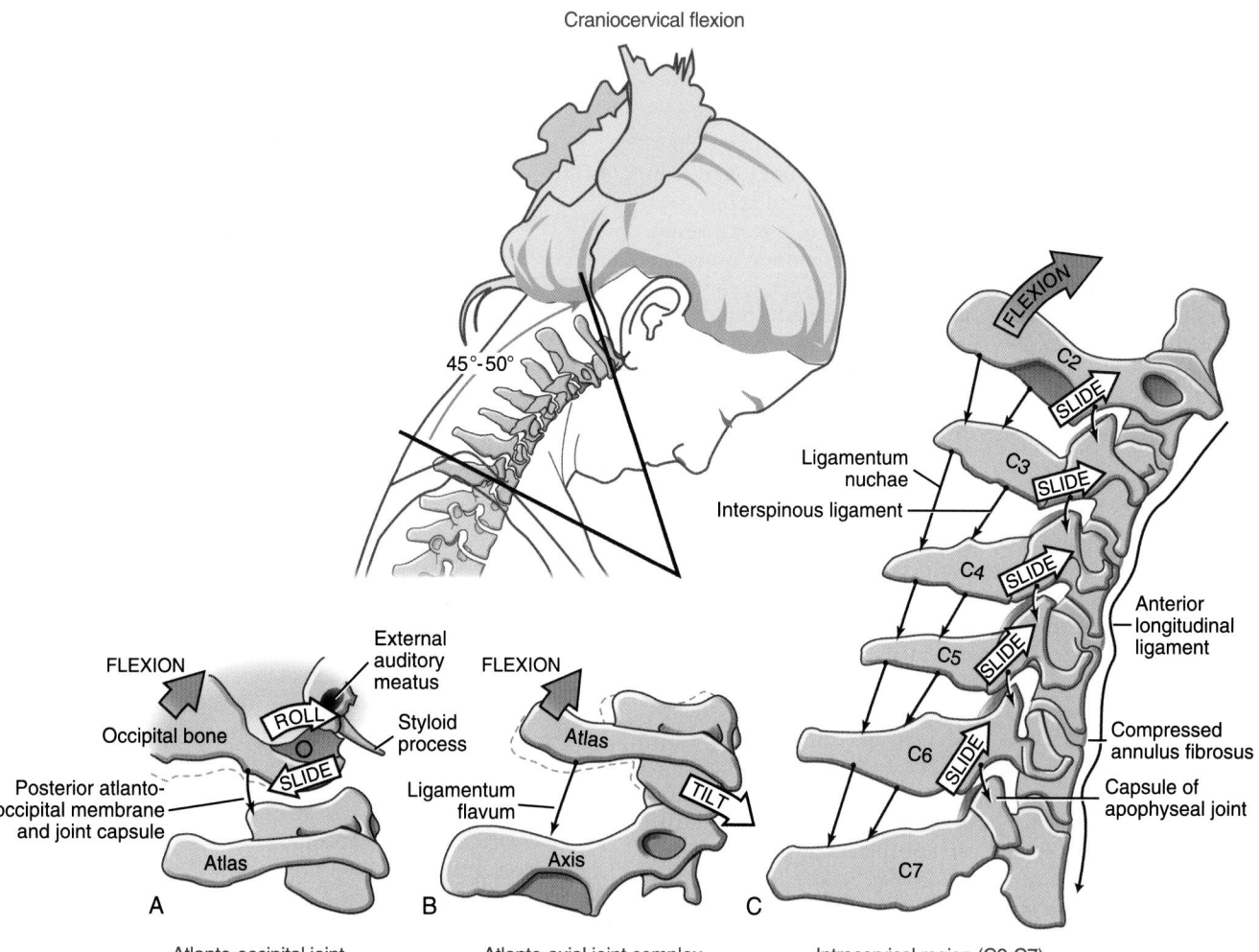

FIG. 9.46 Kinematics of craniocervical flexion. (A) Atlanto-occipital joint. (B) Atlanto-axial joint complex. (C) Intracervical region (C2 to C7). Note in (C) that flexion slackens the anterior longitudinal ligament and increases the space between the adjacent laminae and spinous processes. Elongated, taut tissues are indicated by thin black arrows; relatively slackened tissue is indicated by a wavy black arrow.

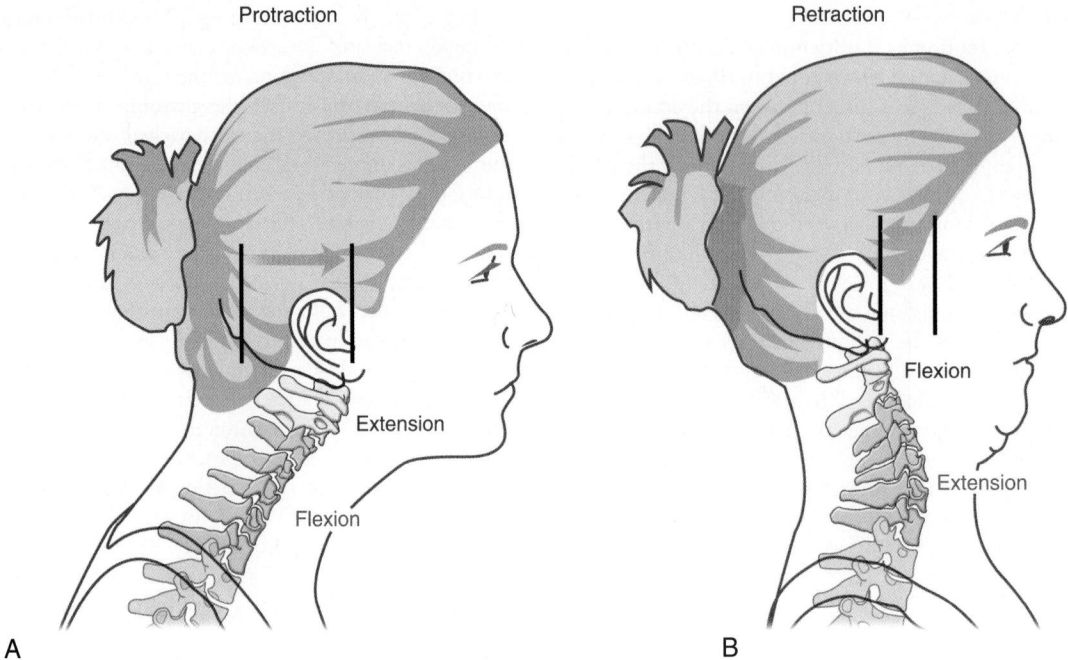

Protraction   Retraction

FIG. 9.47 Protraction and retraction of the cranium. (A) During protraction of the cranium, the lower-to-mid cervical spine flexes as the upper craniocervical region extends. (B) During retraction of the cranium, in contrast, the lower-to-mid cervical spine extends as the upper craniocervical region flexes. Note the change in distance between the C1 and C2 spinous processes during the two movements.

Overall, about 90 to 105 degrees of cervical flexion and extension occur because of the sliding within the cervical apophyseal joint surfaces. This extensive range of motion is in part a result of the relatively long and unobstructed arc of motion provided by the oblique plane of the facet surfaces. On average, about 15 degrees of total sagittal plane motion occur at each intervertebral junction between C2–C3 and C7–T1. The largest sagittal plane angular displacement tends to occur at the C4–C5 or C5–C6 levels,[235,267] possibly accounting for the relatively high incidence of spondylosis and hyperflexion-related fractures at these levels.[226]

Osteokinematics of Protraction and Retraction

In addition to flexion and extension in the craniocervical region, the head can also translate forward (protraction) and backward (retraction) within the sagittal plane.[210] As indicated in Fig. 9.47, from the natural resting position, full range of protraction typically exceeds full range of retraction by about 80% (6.23 cm versus 3.34 cm in the normal adult, respectively).[70] The natural resting position is usually about 35% *forward* from the fully retracted position.

Typically, *protraction* of the head flexes the lower-to-mid cervical spine and simultaneously extends the upper craniocervical region (Fig. 9.47A). *Retraction* of the head, in contrast, extends or straightens the lower-to-mid cervical spine and simultaneously flexes the upper craniocervical region (Fig. 9.47B). In both movements, *the lower-to-mid cervical spine follows the translation of the head.* Protraction and retraction of the head are physiologically normal and useful motions, often associated with enhancing vision. Prolonged periods of protraction, however, may lead to a chronic forward head posture, causing increased strain on the craniocervical extensor muscles.

HORIZONTAL PLANE KINEMATICS

Osteokinematics of Axial Rotation

Axial rotation of the head and neck is a very important function, intimately related to vision and hearing, and ultimately personal safety. For example, a functional kinematic study by Cobian and colleagues has shown that backing up a car or looking for traffic before crossing a road typically requires 42% to 48% of one's maximal axial rotation.[46]

The full range of craniocervical rotation is about 65 to 75 degrees to each side, but this varies considerably with age.[46,214,285] For example, healthy children between the ages of 3.5 and 5 years have on average 100 degrees of passive rotation to each side.[207] Fig. 9.48 shows a young adult with about 80 degrees of active rotation to one side, for a total bilateral range of about 160 degrees. With an additional 160 to 170 degrees of total horizontal plane movement of the eyes, the bilateral visual field approaches 330 degrees, with little or no movement of the trunk.

Although values vary considerably based on type of study, up to roughly half of the axial rotation of the craniocervical region occurs at the atlanto-axial joint complex, with the remaining throughout C2 to C7.[251,325,326] Rotation at the atlanto-occipital joint is restricted to just a few degrees because of the deep-seated placement of the occipital condyles within the superior articular facets of the atlas.

Arthrokinematics of Axial Rotation
Atlanto-Axial Joint Complex
The atlanto-axial joint complex is designed for maximal rotation within the horizontal plane. The design is most evident in the structure of the axis, with its vertical dens and near horizontal superior articular facets (see Fig. 9.32). The ring-shaped atlas and attached transverse ligament "twist" about the dens, producing about 35 to 40 degrees of axial rotation in each direction (Fig. 9.48A). The

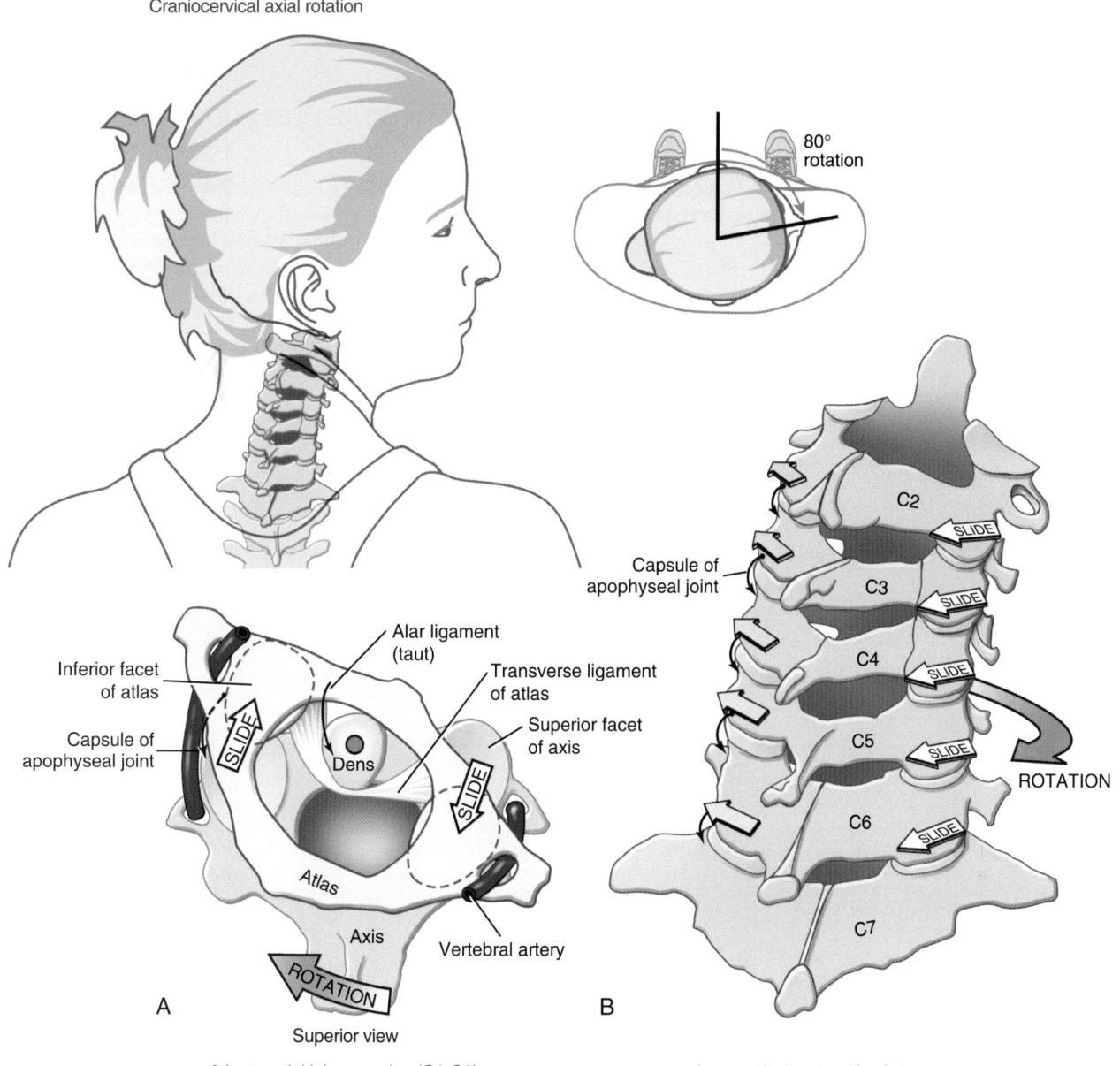

FIG. 9.48 Kinematics of craniocervical axial rotation. (A) Atlanto-axial joint complex. (B) Intracervical region (C2 to C7).

generally flat inferior articular facets of the atlas slide in a curved path across the broad "shoulders" of the superior articular facets of the axis. Because of the limited axial rotation permitted at the atlanto-occipital joint, the cranium follows the rotation of the atlas nearly degree for degree. The axis of rotation for the head-and-atlas is provided by the vertically projected dens.

The extremes of axial rotation are limited primarily by contralaterally located alar ligaments, ligamentous tension in the apophyseal joints, and the many muscles that cross the craniocervical region (see Chapter 10). Although full rotation stretches both vertebral arteries (Fig. 9.48A), in most people this action does not typically impede blood flow.[148]

Intracervical Articulations (C2 too C7)

Rotation throughout C2 to C7 is guided primarily by the spatial orientation of the facet surfaces within the apophyseal joints. The facet surfaces are oriented about 45 degrees between the horizontal and frontal planes (see Fig. 9.32).[226] The inferior facets of the superior vertebrae slide *posteriorly* and *slightly inferiorly* on the same side as the rotation, and *anteriorly* and *slightly superiorly* on the side opposite the rotation (Fig. 9.48B). These arthrokinematics result in approximately 30 to 35 degrees of axial rotation to each side over the C2 to C7 region, nearly equal to that permitted at the atlanto-axial joint complex. Rotation is greatest in the more cranial vertebral segments.

FRONTAL PLANE KINEMATICS

Osteokinematics of Lateral Flexion

Approximately 35 to 40 degrees of lateral flexion are available to each side throughout the craniocervical region (Fig. 9.49).[46] The extremes of this movement can be demonstrated by attempting to touch the ear to the tip of the shoulder. Most of this movement occurs at the C2 to C7 region; however, about 5 degrees in each direction may occur at the atlanto-occipital joint. Lateral flexion at the atlanto-axial joint complex is negligible.

Arthrokinematics of Lateral Flexion

Atlanto-Occipital Joint

A small amount of side-to-side *rolling* of the occipital condyles occurs over the superior articular facets of the atlas. Based on the convex-on-concave relationship of the joints, the occipital condyles are expected to *slide* slightly in a direction opposite to the roll (Fig. 9.49A).

Intracervical Articulations (C2 to C7)

The arthrokinematics of lateral flexion at the C2 to C7 vertebral segments are illustrated in Fig. 9.49B. The inferior articular facets of the superior vertebrae on the same side as the lateral flexion slide

inferiorly and *slightly posteriorly,* and the inferior articular facets on the side opposite the lateral flexion slide *superiorly* and *slightly anteriorly.*

SPINAL COUPLING BETWEEN LATERAL FLEXION AND AXIAL ROTATION

The approximate 45-degree inclination of the articular facets of C2 to C7 promotes a mechanical *spinal coupling* between movements in the frontal and horizontal planes. Because the plane of the inferior articular facet of an upper vertebra follows the plane of the superior articular facet of a lower vertebra, a component of lateral flexion and axial rotation occur simultaneously. For this reason, lateral flexion and axial rotation in the *middle and lower* cervical region are mechanically coupled in an *ipsilateral fashion;* for example, lateral flexion to the right occurs with slight axial rotation to the right, and vice versa.[126,251] Although it is speculation, the uncovertebral joints, located exclusively in the mid and lower regions of the cervical spine, may facilitate this coupled horizontal and frontal plane motion.[195,251]

The ipsilateral spinal coupling just described for the middle to lower craniocervical region is the most accepted and least

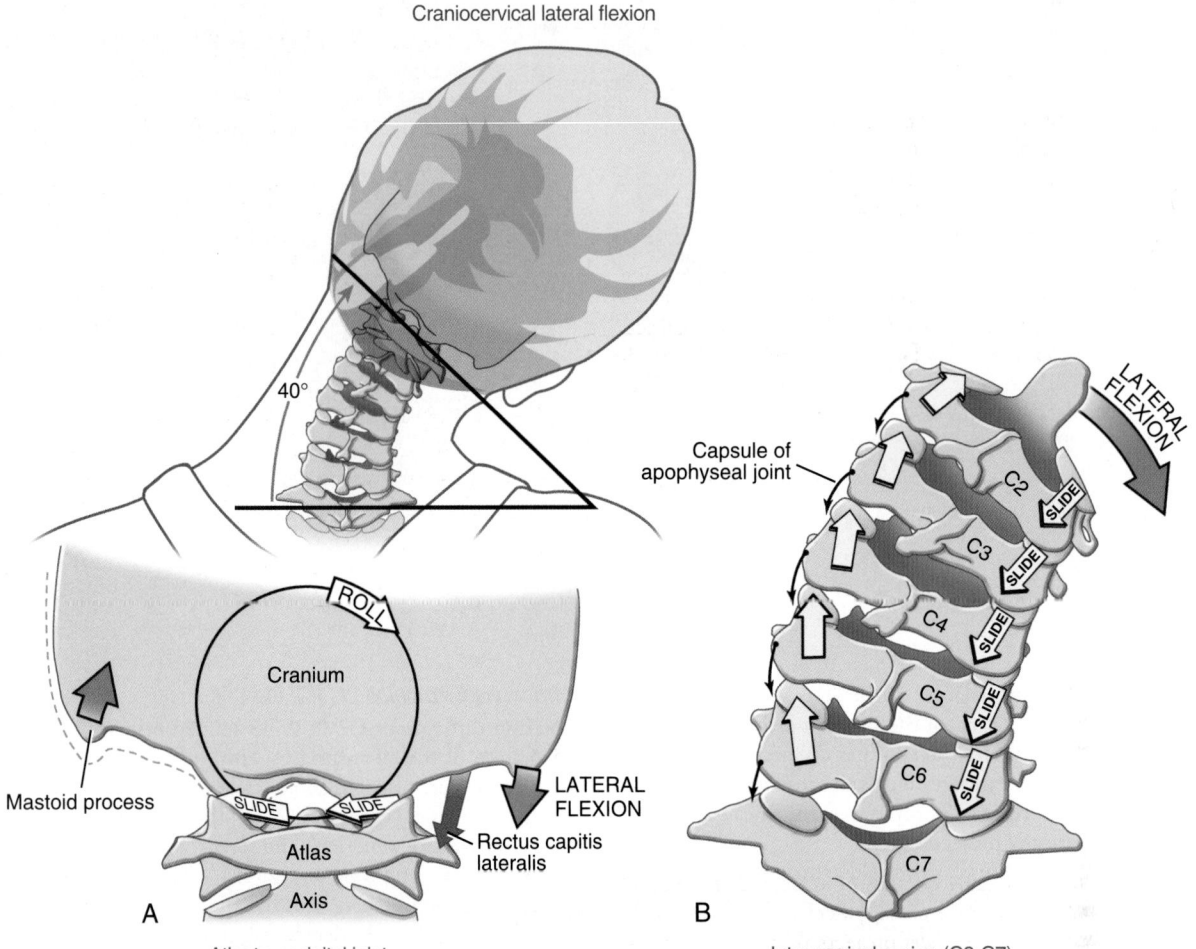

Craniocervical lateral flexion

FIG. 9.49 Kinematics of craniocervical lateral flexion. (A) Atlanto-occipital joint. The rectus capitis lateralis is shown laterally flexing the joint. (B) Intracervical region (C2 to C7). Note the ipsilateral coupling pattern between axial rotation and lateral flexion (see text for further details). Elongated, taut tissues are indicated by thin black arrows.

SPECIAL FOCUS 9.5

Cervical Motion and Its Effect on the Diameter of the Intervertebral Foramina

Movement in the cervical region significantly affects the size of the intervertebral foramina. The difference in size can be large, especially during motions of flexion and extension.[145] This issue has important clinical implications because of the location of the exiting spinal nerve roots. MR imaging has shown that from the anatomic position, 40 degrees of cervical flexion *increases* the opening of the individual cervical intervertebral foramen by 31%; cervical extension of 30 degrees, in contrast, *decreases* the opening by 20%.[191] The mechanical association between flexion and increased area in the C3–C4 intervertebral foramen can be appreciated by comparing the anatomic position (Fig. 9.50A) to an extreme flexed cervical spine position, shown in Fig. 9.50B. During flexion, an upward and forward slide of the inferior articular facet of C3 significantly widens the C3–C4 intervertebral foramen. Full flexion, therefore, allows greater room for passage of a spinal nerve root.

In addition to sagittal plane motion, the area of the intervertebral foramina also varies in size during lateral flexion and axial rotation. Lateral flexion increases the area of the contralateral intervertebral foramina, while narrowing the foramina on the ipsilateral side—obvious consequences of the arthrokinematics of this motion. Axial rotation also increases the area within the contralateral intervertebral foramina by as much as 20% after 40 degrees of craniocervical rotation.

The mechanics described thus far in this Special Focus have clinical relevance in cases of a stenosed (narrowed)

intervertebral foramen, secondary to either an osteophyte or a swelling of the connective tissue sheath surrounding the spinal nerve root. If the compression inflames the spinal nerve root, it may precipitate *radicular* ("shooting") *pain* down a person's arm usually in a path along the corresponding cervical dermatome. Compression against the spinal nerve root can also result in *radiculopathy,* altered or blocked transmission of motor or sensory nerve impulses, leading to ipsilateral weakness and paresthesia of the corresponding cervical myotome and dermatome, respectively. These neurologic responses may be initiated or exacerbated by craniocervical motion. Consider, for example, a person with a severely stenosed intervertebral foramen on the right. A motion likely to compress the exiting nerve root would be full extension, especially if combined with the coupled motions of right lateral flexion and right axial rotation. This combination of movements may occur, for example, when shaving under the chin on the left side.

Mechanical or manual traction of the cervical region is often used in efforts to decompress a spinal nerve root that is compressed by a stenosed intervertebral foramen.[88] Careful positioning of the cervical region in conjunction with the traction can in theory widen the intervertebral foramen. This may be accomplished by positioning the neck in some flexion, sometimes combined with some lateral flexion and, potentially, axial rotation *away from* the side of the suspected pathology.

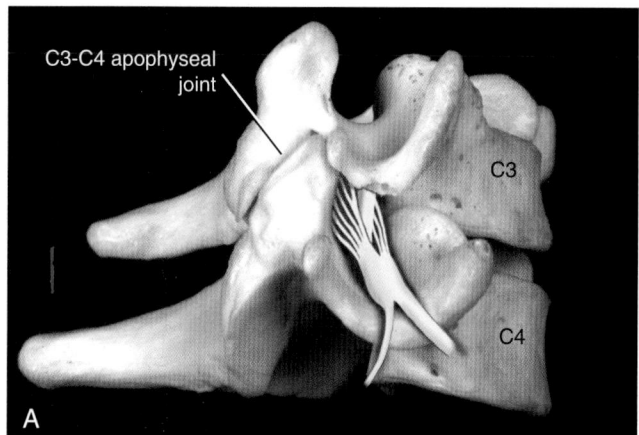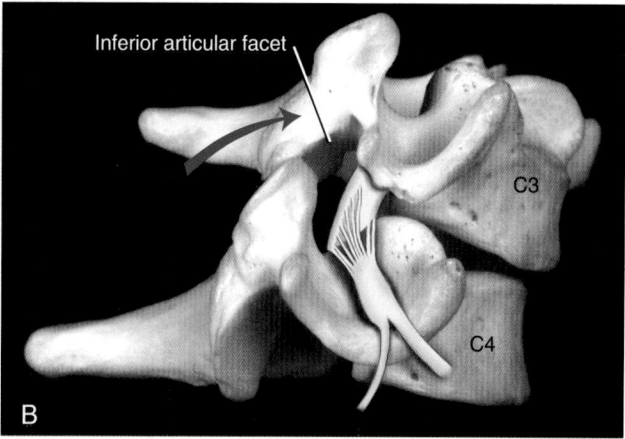

FIG. 9.50 Illustration designed to show how full flexion between C3 and C4 affects the size of the intervertebral foramen. (A) In the anatomic position the facet surfaces within the apophyseal joint are in full contact. (B) Maximum flexion is associated with an upward and forward movement of the inferior articular facet of C3. This "opening" of the apophyseal joint significantly increases the size of the intervertebral foramen, thereby providing greater room for passage of the C^4 spinal nerve root. Note the reduced contact area within the flexed apophyseal joint.

controversial coupling pattern of the entire vertebral column.[47] On casual visual observation, however, this coupling pattern is not so apparent. Most persons appear to laterally flex the craniocervical region *without* an obligatory axial rotation of the face (or chin) to the side of the lateral flexion, or vice versa. The lack of a perceptible ipsilateral coupling is achieved by independent actions of either the atlanto-axial or the atlanto-occipital joints. Consider, for example, lateral flexion of C2 to C7 to the right. During this active motion, the atlanto-axial joint typically demonstrates a *contralateral* spinal coupling pattern by slightly rotating the atlas-and-cranium to the left, which conceals the fact that the C2 to C7 region actually rotated to the right.[126,127] This compensatory action of the atlanto-axial joint minimizes the overall rotation of the head, which helps the eyes fixate on an anteriorly located stationary object during lateral flexion of the neck.

For reasons similar to those discussed in the previous paragraph, a compensatory *contralateral* coupling pattern usually also exists at the atlanto-occipital joints. This coupling may reduce part of the undesired lateral flexion of the head during axial rotation of the neck, allowing, for example, a near horizontal plane of vision when rotating to look over your shoulder while driving.[126,127,251] The contralateral coupling patterns expressed at both atlanto-axial and atlanto-occipital joints are controlled subconsciously by the actions of specialized muscles (addressed further in Chapter 10). Tension in the alar ligament may also play a role in guiding this contralateral coupling pattern in the axial–atlanto-occipital complex.[251] Consider, for example, axial rotation of the upper craniocervical region to the right. Selective tension in the *left* alar ligament may pull the left occipital condyle inferiorly, causing slight left lateral flexion of the atlanto-occipital joint.

Thoracic Region

The thorax consists of a relatively rigid rib cage, formed by the ribs, thoracic vertebrae, and sternum. The rigidity of the region provides (1) a stable base for muscles to control the craniocervical region, (2) a protective area for the intrathoracic organs, and (3) a mechanical bellows for breathing (see Chapter 11).

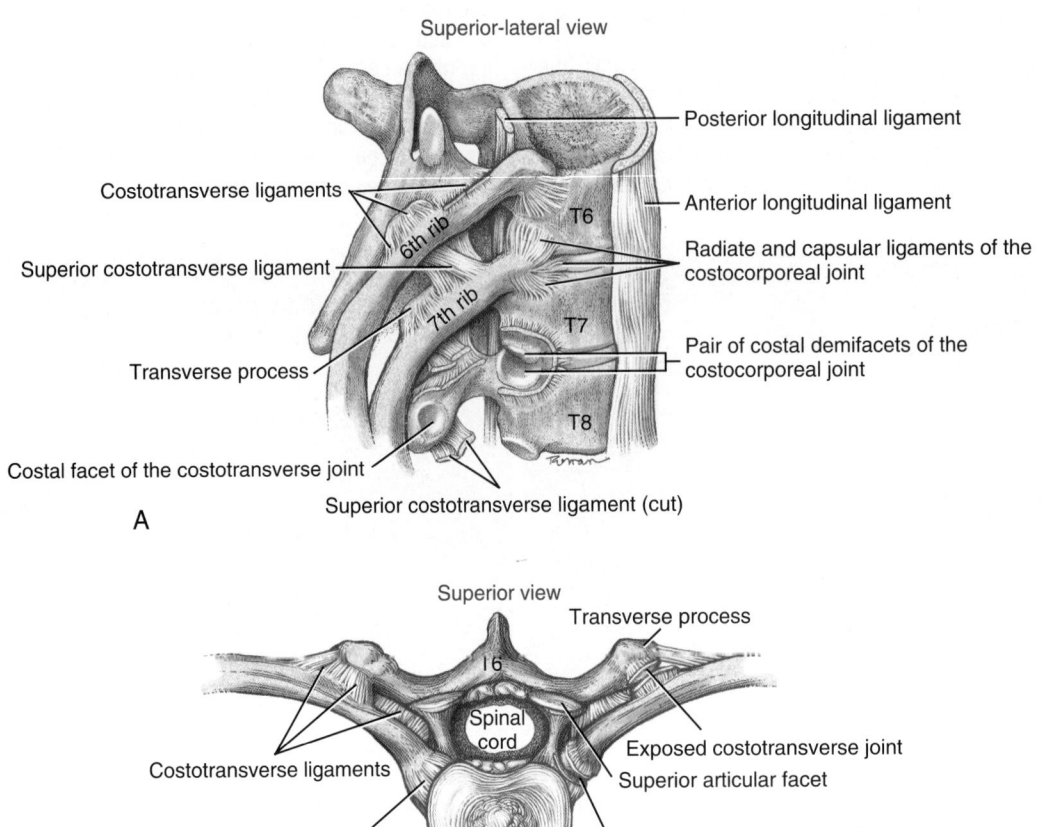

Superior-lateral view

Posterior longitudinal ligament

Costotransverse ligaments

Superior costotransverse ligament

Anterior longitudinal ligament

6th rib   T6

Radiate and capsular ligaments of the costocorporeal joint

7th rib   T7

Transverse process

Pair of costal demifacets of the costocorporeal joint

T8

Costal facet of the costotransverse joint

Superior costotransverse ligament (cut)

A

Superior view

Transverse process

I6

Spinal cord

Exposed costotransverse joint

Superior articular facet

Costotransverse ligaments

Exposed costocorporeal joint

Capsular and radiate ligaments

Annulus fibrosus

B

Nucleus pulposus

FIG. 9.51 The costotransverse and costocorporeal joints of the midthoracic region. (A) Superior-lateral view highlights the structure and connective tissues of the costotransverse and costocorporeal joints associated with the sixth through the eighth thoracic vertebrae. The eighth rib is removed to expose the costal facets of the associated costocorporeal and costotransverse joints. (B) Superior view shows the capsule of the left costocorporeal and costotransverse joints cut to expose joint surfaces. Note the spatial relationships among the nucleus pulposus, annulus fibrosus, and spinal cord.

ANATOMY OF THORACIC ARTICULAR STRUCTURES

The thoracic spine has 24 apophyseal joints, 12 on each side. Each joint possesses articular facets that face generally in the frontal plane, with a mild forward slope that averages about 15 to 25 degrees from the vertical (see example of T4 in Fig. 9.32).[177,218] The movement potential of these apophyseal joints is limited by the relative immobility of the adjacent costovertebral (costocorporeal and costotransverse) joints.[32] Indirectly, this pair of joints mechanically links most of the thoracic vertebrae anteriorly to the fixed sternum.

Most *costocorporeal joints* connect the head of a rib with a pair of costal demifacets on thoracic vertebral bodies and with the adjacent margin of an intervening intervertebral disc (Fig. 9.51). The articular surfaces of the costocorporeal joints are slightly ovoid,[275] held together primarily by *capsular* and *radiate ligaments.*

Costotransverse joints connect the articular tubercle of most ribs to the costal facet on the transverse process of the corresponding thoracic vertebrae. An articular capsule surrounds this synovial joint. The extensive (nearly 2-cm long) *costotransverse ligament* firmly anchors the neck of a rib to the entire length of a corresponding transverse process (Fig. 9.51). In addition, each costotransverse joint is stabilized by a *superior costotransverse ligament.* This strong ligament attaches between the superior margin of the neck of one rib and the inferior margin of the transverse process of the vertebra located above (Fig. 9.51A). Ribs 11 and 12 usually lack costotransverse joints.

Because the ribs attach to the thoracic vertebrae, the kinematics of the thorax and the costocorporeal and costotransverse joints are mechanically interrelated, although in vivo research on this topic has not been extensively published. This text focuses on the kinematics of the costocorporeal and costotransverse joints as they relate primarily to ventilation, which will be described in Chapter 11.

Key Anatomic Aspects of the Costocorporeal and Costotransverse Joints

EACH COSTOCORPOREAL JOINT
- Usually connects the head of a rib with a pair of costal demifacets and the adjacent margin of an intervening intervertebral disc
- Is stabilized by radiate and capsular ligaments

EACH COSTOTRANSVERSE JOINT
- Usually connects the articular tubercle of a rib with the costal facet on the transverse process of a corresponding thoracic vertebra
- Is stabilized by the costotransverse and the superior costotransverse ligaments

---

With the exception of the sacroiliac joints, the thoracic region as a whole is normally the most mechanically stable portion of the vertebral column. Much of this inherent stability is afforded through attachments between the thoracic vertebrae and the rib cage.[158] The constituents of the rib cage include the costocorporeal and costotransverse joints, ribs, sternocostal joints, and the sternum. In vitro cadaver testing has shown that the rib cage (including the sternum) provides between 36% and 78% of the total passive resistance to full

TABLE 9.8 Approximate Range of Motion for the Three Planes of Movement for the Thoracic Region*

Flexion and Extension (Sagittal Plane, Degrees)	Axial Rotation (Horizontal Plane, Degrees)	Lateral Flexion (Frontal Plane, Degrees)
Flexion: 30–40 Extension: 15–20 Total: 45–60	25–35	25–30

*The horizontal and frontal plane motions are to one side only.

thoracic motion.[32,309] Although the cadaver studies provide important data, they do not account for additional factors that exist in the living, such as volitionally increasing intra-abdominal pressure (via a Valsalva maneuver) and activating intercostal and other trunk muscles. Nevertheless, it is clear that the presence of an intact and stable rib cage protects the thoracic spine, including the spinal cord. During a fall, for example, the impact to the thoracic spine is partially absorbed and dissipated by the rib cage and the associated muscles and connective tissues. Evidence for this can be found by the relatively high frequency of fractures of the sternum that occur in combination with thoracic spine injuries.[32,309]

KINEMATICS

When an adult is standing, the thoracic region typically exhibits about 35 to 45 degrees of natural kyphosis (refer to Fig. 9.39).[215] From the anatomic position, motion occurs in all three planes. Although the range of motion at each thoracic intervertebral junction is relatively small, cumulative motion is considerable when expressed over the entire thoracic spine (Table 9.8).[71,90,175,215,314]

The direction and extent of thoracic movement within any given plane are influenced by several factors, including the resting posture of the region, specific orientation of the apophyseal joints, splinting action of the rib cage, and relative heights of the intervertebral discs. Compared with the cervical and lumbar regions, the thoracic region has by far the smallest disc-to-vertebral body height ratio. The relatively thin discs naturally limit the extent to which one vertebral body can rotate (or rock) on another before being blocked by bony compression, at least in the sagittal and frontal planes. Although this factor limits thoracic mobility slightly, it provides another element of overall stability to the region.

Kinematics of Flexion and Extension

Approximately 30 to 40 degrees of flexion and 15 to 20 degrees of extension are typically available throughout the thoracic region. These kinematics are shown in context with flexion and extension over the entire thoracolumbar region in Figs. 9.52 and 9.53, respectively. The extremes of *flexion* are limited by tension in connective tissues located posterior to the vertebral bodies, such as the capsule of the apophyseal joints and supraspinous and posterior longitudinal ligaments. The extremes of *extension,* on the other hand, are limited by tension in the anterior longitudinal ligament and by potential impingement between laminae or between adjacent downward-sloping spinous processes, especially in the upper and middle thoracic vertebrae. The magnitude of thoracic flexion and extension tends to be greater in the extreme caudal regions, in great part because of the "free-floating" most caudal ribs and the shift to a more sagittal plane orientation of the apophyseal joints.

The arthrokinematics at the apophyseal joints in the thoracic spine are generally similar to those described for the C2 to C7 region. Subtle differences are related primarily to different shapes of the vertebrae, presence or absence of rib attachments, and different spatial orientations of the articular facets of apophyseal joints. *Flexion* between T5 and T6, for example, occurs by a superior and slightly anterior sliding of the inferior facet surfaces of T5 on the superior facet surfaces of T6 (Fig. 9.52A). The moderately forward-sloped articular surfaces of the apophyseal joints naturally facilitate flexion throughout the region. *Extension* occurs by a reverse process (Fig. 9.53A).

Kinematics of Axial Rotation

Approximately 25 to 35 degrees of horizontal plane (axial) rotation occur to each side throughout the thoracic region. This motion is depicted in conjunction with axial rotation across the entire thoracolumbar region in Fig. 9.54. Rotation between T6 and T7, for example, occurs as the near–frontal plane–aligned inferior articular facets of T6 slide for a short distance against the similarly aligned superior articular facets of T7 (see Fig. 9.54A). Although this isolated rotation is indeed small and virtually imperceptible, the overall osteokinematics are, however, easily observable when added across the entire thoracic region. The freedom of this axial rotation declines in the lower thoracic spine.[90,314] In this region, the apophyseal joints are slightly more vertically oriented as they shift to a more sagittal plane orientation.

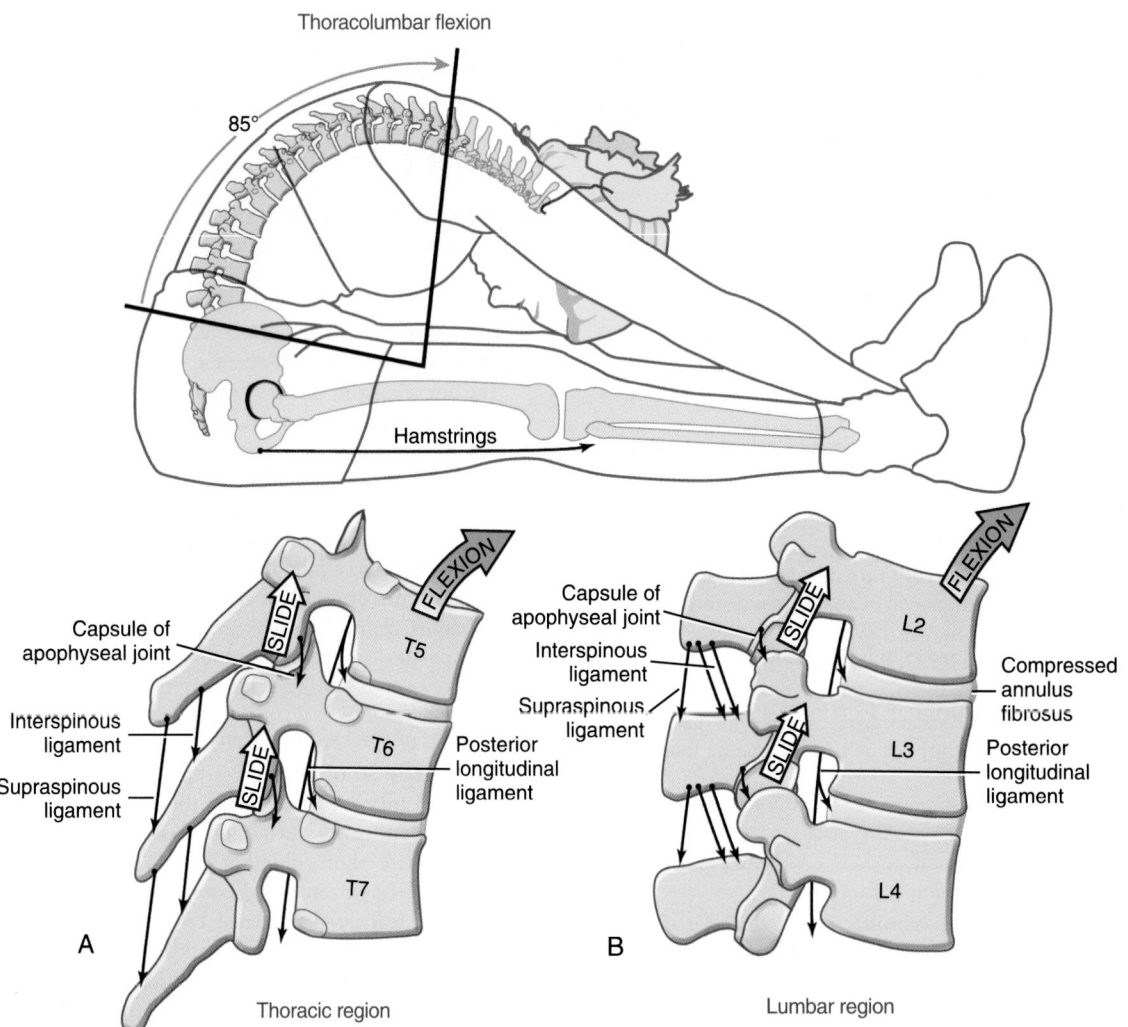

FIG. 9.52 The kinematics of thoracolumbar flexion are shown through an 85-degree arc: in this subject, the sum of 35 degrees of thoracic flexion and 50 degrees of lumbar flexion. (A) Kinematics at the thoracic region. (B) Kinematics at the lumbar region. Elongated, taut tissues are indicated by thin black arrows.

Kinematics of Lateral Flexion

The predominant frontal plane orientation of the thoracic facet surfaces suggests a relative freedom of lateral flexion. This potential freedom of movement is never fully expressed, however, because of the stabilization provided by the attachments to the ribs. Lateral flexion in the thoracic region is illustrated in context with lateral flexion over the entire thoracolumbar region in Fig. 9.55. Approximately 25 to 30 degrees of lateral flexion occur to each side in the thoracic region. As depicted in Fig. 9.55A, lateral flexion of T6 on T7 occurs as the inferior facet surface of T6 slides superiorly on the side contralateral to the lateral flexion and inferiorly on the side ipsilateral to the lateral flexion. Note that the ribs drop slightly on the side of the lateral flexion and rise slightly on the side opposite the lateral flexion.[158]

Lumbar Region

ANATOMY OF THE ARTICULAR STRUCTURES

L1–L4 Region

The facet surfaces of most lumbar apophyseal joints are oriented nearly vertically, with a moderate-to-strong sagittal plane bias (Fig. 9.56). The orientation of the superior articular facets of L2, for example, is on average about 25 degrees from the sagittal plane (see Fig. 9.32). This orientation favors sagittal plane motion at the expense of rotation in the horizontal plane.[215]

L5–S1 Junction

Like any typical intervertebral junction, the L5–S1 junction has an interbody joint anteriorly and a pair of apophyseal joints posteriorly. The facet surfaces of the L5–S1 apophyseal joints are usually oriented in a more frontal plane than those of other lumbar regions (see Fig. 9.56).

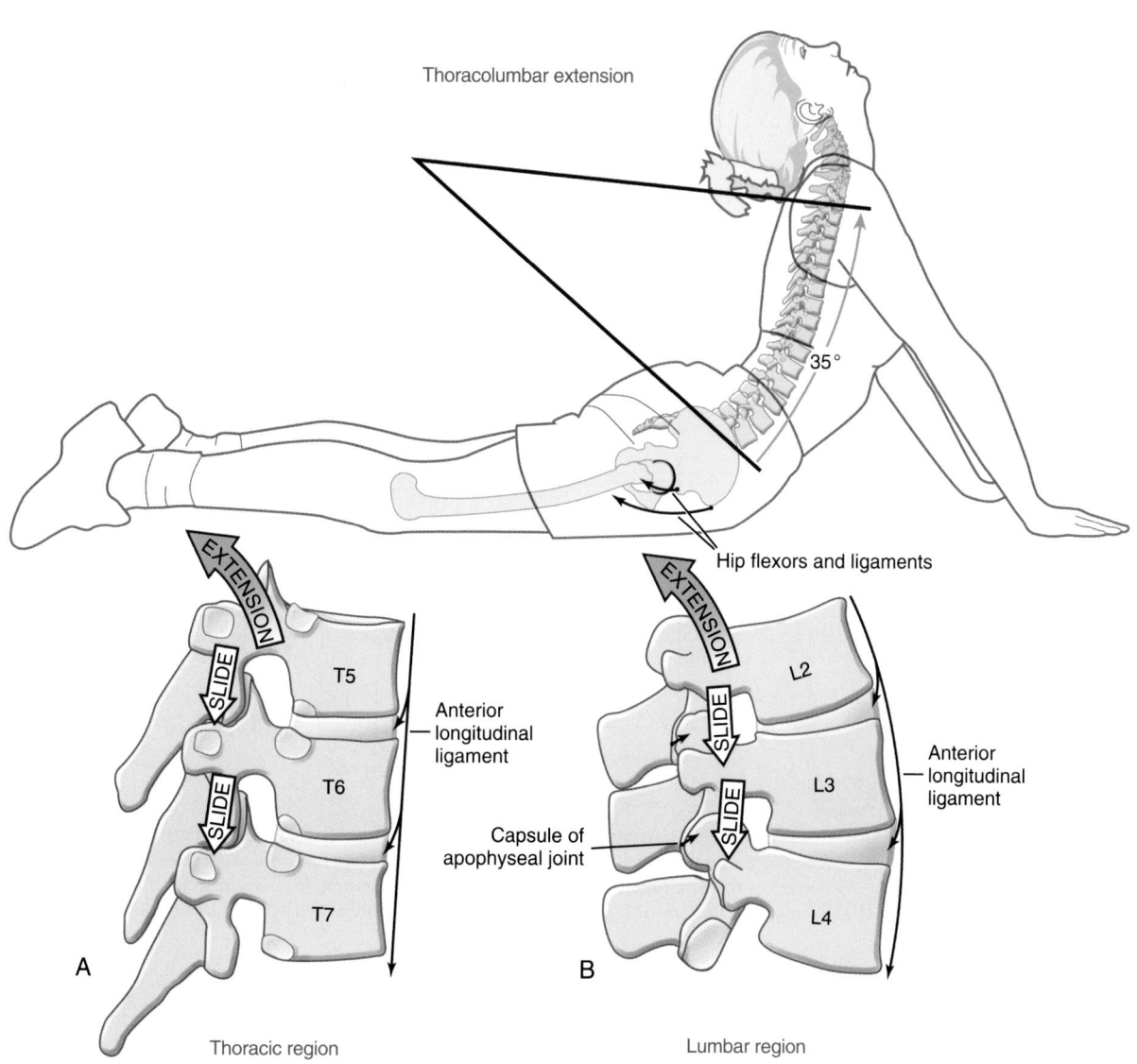

FIG. 9.53 The kinematics of thoracolumbar extension are shown through an arc of about 35 degrees: the sum of 20 degrees of thoracic extension and 15 degrees of lumbar extension. (A) Kinematics at the thoracic region. (B) Kinematics at the lumbar region. Elongated, taut tissues are indicated by thin black arrows.

Thoracolumbar axial rotation

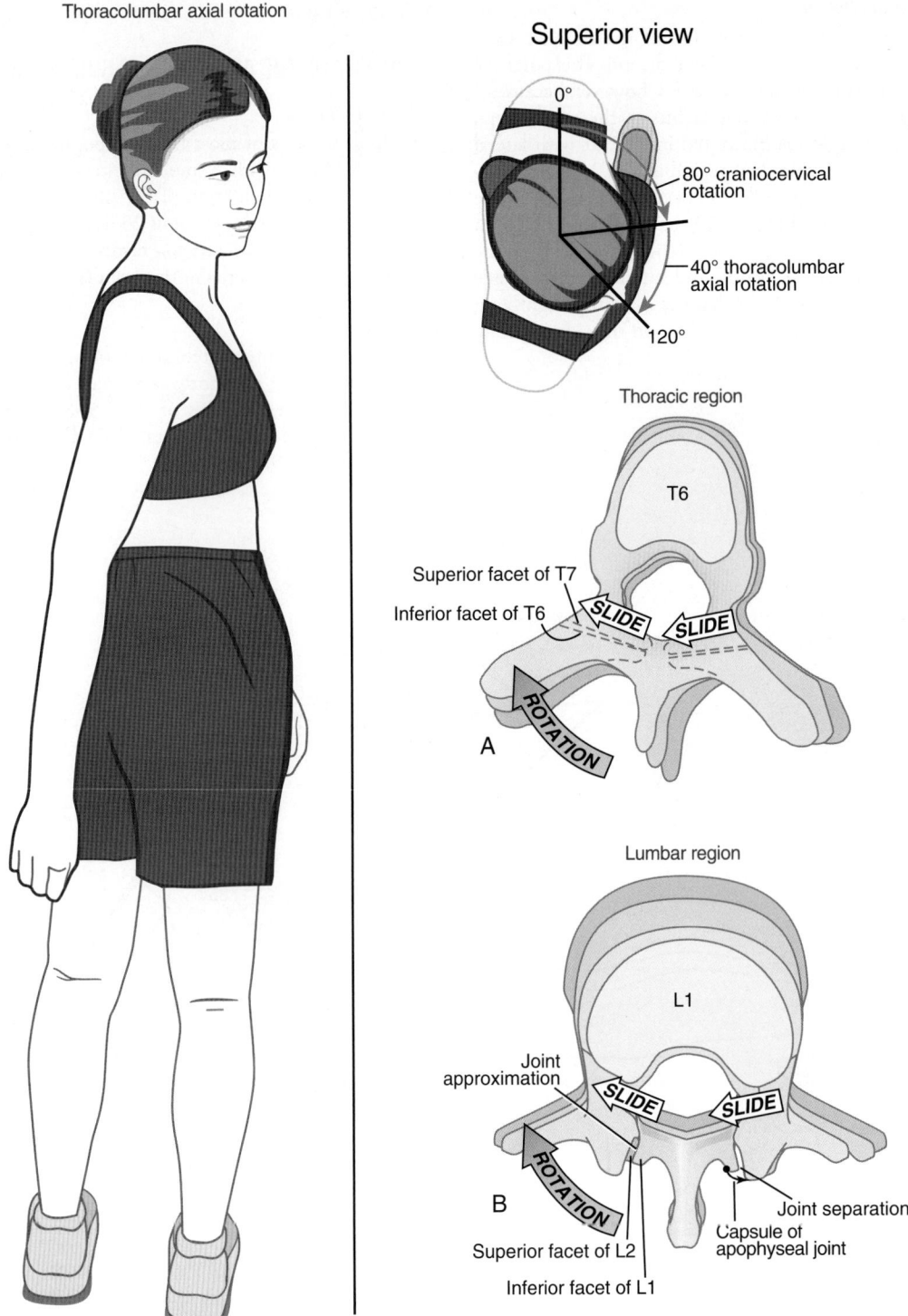

FIG. 9.54 The kinematics of thoracolumbar axial rotation is depicted as the subject rotates her face 120 degrees to the right. The thoracolumbar axial rotation is shown through an approximate 40-degree arc: the sum of about 35 degrees of thoracic rotation and 5 degrees of lumbar rotation. (A) Kinematics at the thoracic region. (B) Kinematics at the lumbar region. Elongated, taut tissue is indicated by thin black arrow.

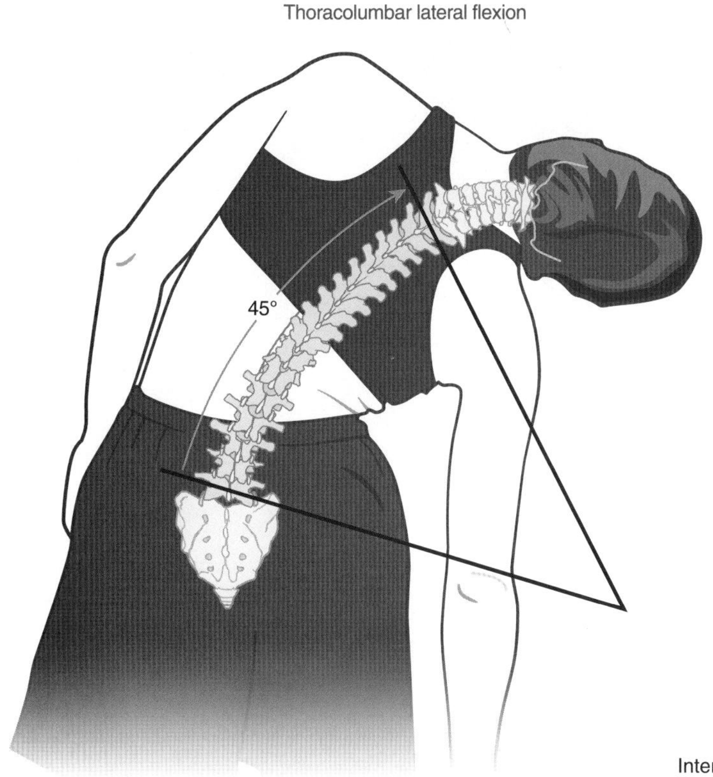

Thoracolumbar lateral flexion

45°

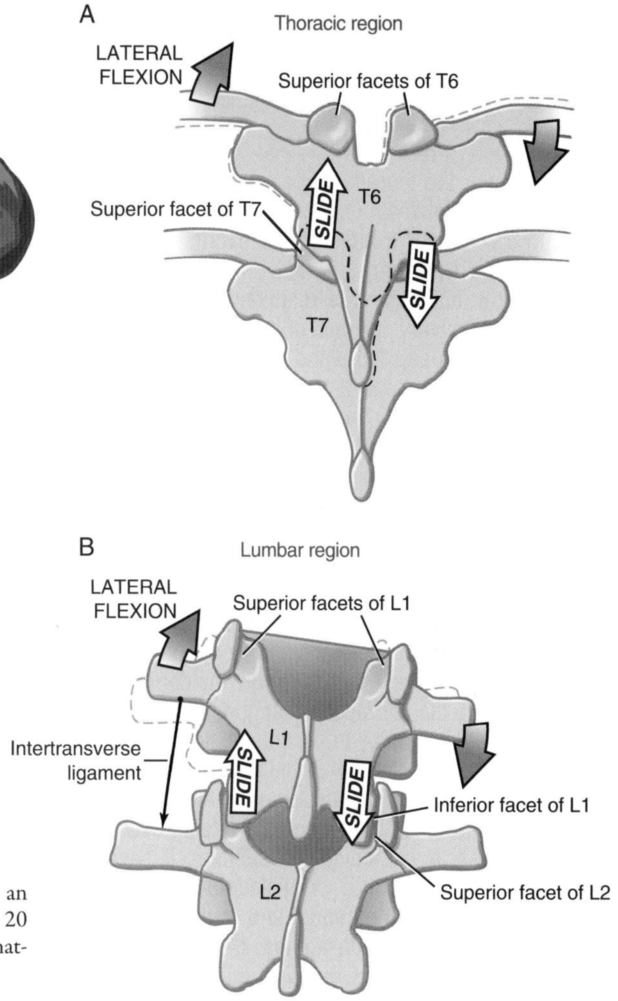

A   Thoracic region

LATERAL FLEXION   Superior facets of T6

Superior facet of T7   T6   SLIDE   SLIDE

T7

B   Lumbar region

LATERAL FLEXION   Superior facets of L1

Intertransverse ligament   L1   SLIDE   SLIDE

Inferior facet of L1

Superior facet of L2

L2

FIG. 9.55 The kinematics of thoracolumbar lateral flexion are shown through an approximate 45-degree arc: the sum of 25 degrees of thoracic lateral flexion and 20 degrees of lumbar lateral flexion. (A) Kinematics at the thoracic region. (B) Kinematics at the lumbar region. Elongated, taut tissue is indicated by a thin black arrow.

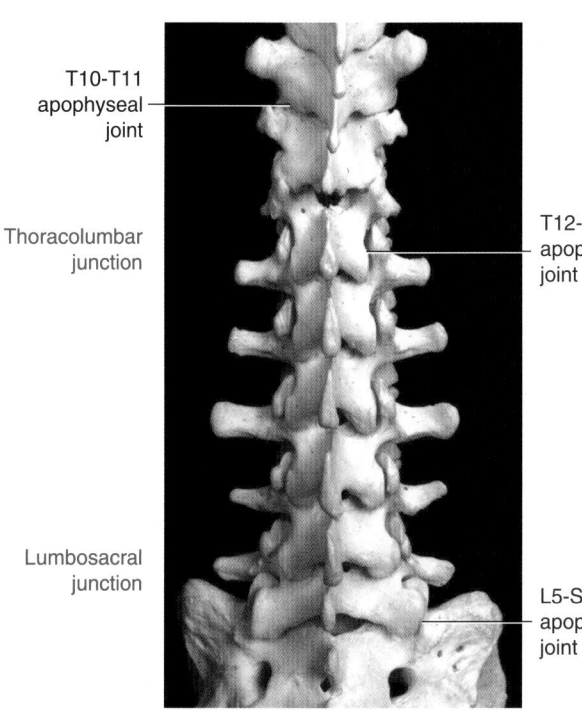

T10-T11 apophyseal joint

Thoracolumbar junction

Lumbosacral junction

T12-L1 apophyseal joint

L5-S1 apophyseal joint

FIG. 9.56 A posterior view of the thoracolumbar and lumbosacral junctions. Note the transition in the orientation of the facet surfaces within the apophyseal joints at the two junctions. Also note that the bony specimen demonstrates a frontal plane bias at both L4–L5 and L5–S1 apophyseal joints. This variation is not uncommon.

Some Clinical Implications Regarding the Thoracolumbar Junction

At or near the thoracolumbar junction, the facet surfaces of the apophyseal joints change their orientation rather abruptly, from near frontal to near sagittal planes.[130,177] The point of this transition is T12-L1 for the specimen shown in Fig. 9.56, although it is relatively common for the transition point to vary by one or two junctions. This relative sharp frontal-to-sagittal plane transition in apophyseal joint orientation may create a sagittal plane hypermobility and mechanical instability in this region.[185] This is evident in Fig. 9.57 as a young boy with cerebral palsy attempts to support himself up on his knees. The lack of control and weakness of his trunk muscles allows the thoracolumbar junction to collapse into the plane of least bony resistance—in this case, into marked thoracolumbar hyperextension. This collapse creates a severe hyperlordosis in the region.

As a second clinical example, the aforementioned sharp frontal-to-sagittal plane transition in apophyseal joints may partially explain the relatively high incidence of traumatic paraplegia at the thoracolumbar junction. In certain high-impact accidents involving trunk flexion, the thorax, held relatively rigid by the rib cage, is free to violently flex as a unit over the upper lumbar region. A large flexion torque delivered to the thorax may concentrate an excessive hyperflexion stress at the point of transition. If severe enough, the stress may fracture or dislocate the bony elements and possibly injure the caudal end of the spinal cord or the cranial end of the cauda equina. Surgical fixation devices implanted to immobilize an unstable thoracolumbar junction are particularly susceptible to stress failure, compared with devices implanted in other regions of the vertebral column.

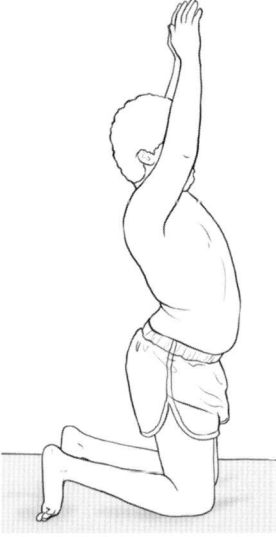

FIG. 9.57 Illustration of a young boy with cerebral palsy with weak and poor control of his trunk muscles. Note the excessive hyperextension in the region of the thoracolumbar junction. (Courtesy Lois Bly, PT, MA.)

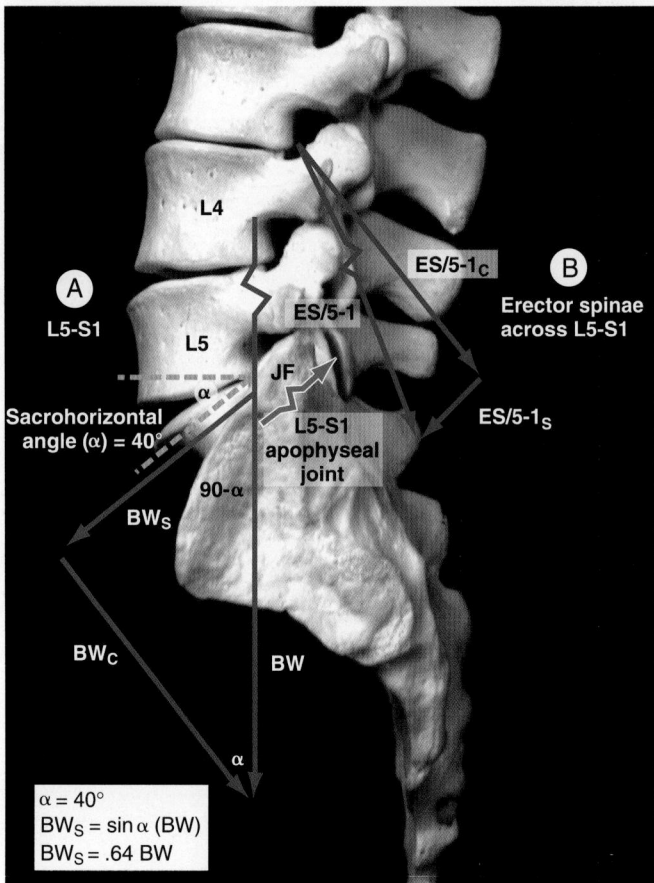

FIG. 9.58 Lateral view shows the biomechanics responsible for the shear forces at the interbody joints of L5–S1. (A) The sacrohorizontal angle (α) at L5–S1 is the angle between the horizontal plane and the superior surface of the sacrum. BW (body weight) is the weight of the body located above the sacrum. BW_C is the force of body weight directed perpendicular to the superior surface of the sacrum. BW_S is the shear force of body weight directed parallel to the superior surface of the sacrum. The joint force *(JF)* at the L5–S1 apophyseal joint is shown as a short blue arrow. (B) The force vector of the active erector spinae is shown as it crosses L5–S1 (ES/5–1). $ES/5\text{-}1_C$ is the force of the muscle directed perpendicular to the superior surface of the sacrum. $ES/5\text{-}1_S$ is the shear force of the muscle directed parallel to the superior surface of the sacrum.

The base (top) of the sacrum is naturally inclined anteriorly and inferiorly, forming an approximate 40-degree *sacrohorizontal angle* when standing (Fig. 9.58A).[61] Given this angle, the force from body weight (BW) creates an *anterior* shear force (BW_S) acting parallel to the superior surface of the sacrum, and a compressive force (BW_C) acting perpendicular to the superior surface of the sacrum. The magnitude of the anterior shear force is equal to the product of BW times the sine of the sacrohorizontal angle. A typical sacrohorizontal angle of 40 degrees produces an anterior shear force at the L5–S1 junction equal to 64% of the superimposed BW. Increasing the degree of lumbar lordosis enlarges the sacrohorizontal angle, which in effect amplifies the anterior shear at the L5–S1 junction. If the sacrohorizontal angle were increased to 55 degrees, for example, the anterior shear force would increase to 82% of the superimposed BW. While standing or sitting, the magnitude of lumbar lordosis (and corresponding sacrohorizontal angle) can be increased by anterior tilting the pelvis (see ahead Fig. 9.63A). (Tilting the pelvis is defined as a short-arc sagittal plane rotation of the pelvis relative to both femoral heads. The direction of the tilt is indicated by the direction of rotation of the iliac crests.)

SPECIAL FOCUS 9.7

Anterior Spondylolisthesis at L5–S1

*A*nterior *spondylolisthesis* is a general term that describes an anterior slipping or displacement of one vertebra relative to another. This condition most often occurs at the L5–S1 junction, as illustrated in Fig. 9.59, but may occur in other regions of the lumbar spine, notably L4–L5.[11] The term *spondylolisthesis* is derived from the Greek *spondylo,* meaning vertebra, and *listhesis,* meaning to slip. This condition may be acquired after excessive stress or pathology, or it may be congenital. Rarely does one vertebra slide forward more than about 25% to 30% the width of the underlying vertebra.[196] In more severe anterior spondylolisthesis, the slippage may be associated with a bilateral fracture (or deficit) through the *pars articularis,* a section of a lumbar vertebra midway between the superior and inferior articular processes (see Fig. 9.27). The acquired form of anterior spondylolisthesis at L5–S1 may be progressive and in part likely caused by repetitive physical activities that involve full and forceful extension of the region. Severe anterior spondylolisthesis may compress the cauda equina, as this bundle of nerves passes by the L5–S1 junction.

As described in Fig. 9.58A, an increased lumbar lordosis increases the normal sacrohorizontal angle, thereby magnifying the anterior shear force between L5 and S1. Exercises or other actions that create a forceful and full extension of the lower lumbar spine should therefore be avoided, or at least minimized, for persons with anterior spondylolisthesis, especially if the condition is unstable or progressive.[297] As shown in Fig. 9.58B, the force vector of the erector spinae muscle that crosses L5–S1 (ES/5–1) creates an anterior shear force (ES/5–1$_S$) parallel to the superior body of the sacrum. The direction of this shear is a function of the orientation of the adjacent erector spinae fibers and the 40-degree sacrohorizontal angle. In theory, a greater muscular force increases the anterior shear at the L5–S1 junction, especially if the muscle activation exaggerates the lordosis.

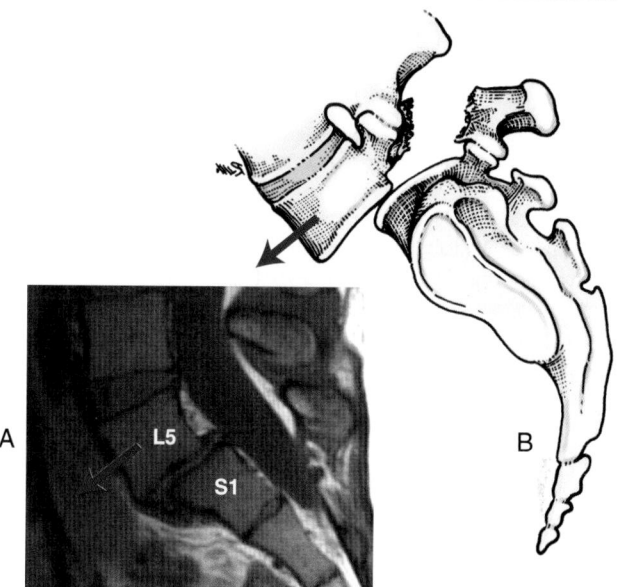

FIG. 9.59 (A) T1-weighted MR image showing an anterior spondylolisthesis of L5 on S1, with an enlarged central canal. (B) Drawing showing severe anterior spondylolisthesis of L5 on S1 after a fracture of the pars articularis. (A from Krishnan A, Silbergleit R: Imaging in spinal stenosis, *Seminars in spine surgery* 19:3, 2007. pp. 126-142; B modified from Canale ST, Beaty JH: *Campbell's operative orthopedics,* ed 11, St Louis, 2008, Mosby.)

Several structures resist the natural anterior shearing force produced at the L5–S1 junction. These include the intervening intervertebral disc, the capsule of the apophyseal joints, the wide and strong anterior longitudinal ligament, and the iliolumbar ligaments. The *iliolumbar ligament* arises from the inferior aspect of the transverse processes of L4 and L5 and adjacent fibers of the quadratus lumborum muscle.[303] The ligament attaches inferiorly to the ilium, just anterior to the sacroiliac joint, and to the upper-lateral aspect of the sacrum (see ahead Fig. 9.70). Bilaterally, the iliolumbar ligaments provide a firm anchor between the naturally stout transverse processes of L5 and the underlying ilium and sacrum.[28,91,319]

In addition to the aforementioned connective tissues, the wide, sturdy articular facets of the L5–S1 apophyseal joints provide bony stabilization to the L5–S1 junction. The near–frontal plane inclination of the facet surfaces is ideal for resisting the anterior shear at this region. This resistance creates a compression force within the L5–S1 apophyseal joints (see blue force vector in Fig. 9.58A, labeled JF). Without adequate stabilization and structural integrity, L5 can slip forward relative to the sacrum.[97] This abnormal, potentially serious condition is known as *anterior spondylolisthesis.*

KINEMATICS

Typically, lumbar lordosis is greater when standing than when sitting.[124] While standing, the typical adult lumbar spine exhibits about 40 to 50 degrees of lordosis, although even wider ranges have been reported based on different measurement systems and studied populations.[12,28,147,246] Across adult age groups, females tend to exhibit greater lumbar lordosis than males.[12] From an anatomically neutral (lordotic) position, the lumbar spine can move in three degrees of freedom. Data on the range of lumbar motion are highly variable across studies and populations; typical values are listed in Table 9.9.[b] The following sections focus on the kinematics of each plane of motion within the lumbar region.

Sagittal Plane Kinematics: Flexion and Extension

On average, about 45 to 55 degrees of flexion and 15 to 25 degrees of extension are available in the adult lumbar spine. The total 60- to 80-degree arc of sagittal plane motion is substantial, considering it occurs across only five intervertebral junctions. This predominance of

[b] 12, 46, 100, 146, 175, 202, 222, 288, 305, 325

TABLE 9.9 Approximate Range of Motion for the Three Planes of Movement for the Lumbar Region*

Flexion and Extension (Sagittal Plane, Degrees)	Axial Rotation (Horizontal Plane, Degrees)	Lateral Flexion (Frontal Plane, Degrees)
Flexion: 45–55 Extension: 15–25 Total: 60–80	5–10	20

*The horizontal and frontal plane motions are to one side only.

BOX 9.2 Order of the Subtopics Involving the Sagittal Plane Kinematics at the Lumbar Region

Flexion of the lumbar spine
Extension of the lumbar spine
Lumbopelvic rhythm during trunk flexion and extension
- Variations of lumbopelvic rhythms during *trunk flexion* from a standing position: a kinematic analysis
- Lumbopelvic rhythm during *trunk extension* from a forward bent position: a muscular analysis

Effect of pelvic tilting on the kinematics of the lumbar spine
- Kinesiologic correlations between anterior pelvic tilt and increased lumbar lordosis
- Kinesiologic correlations between posterior pelvic tilt and decreased lumbar lordosis

sagittal plane motion is largely a result of the prevailing sagittal plane orientation of the facet surfaces of the lumbar apophyseal joints.

Many important and common activities of daily living involve a flexion and extension "folding" of the midsection of the body. Consider, for example, bending forward to pick up on object from the floor, donning socks, putting on pants, ascending steep steps, or getting out of an automobile; also consider a young child transitioning between crawling and sitting. All these activities involve a kinematic interaction among the middle and upper trunk and lumbar spine, and between the pelvis and femurs (hips). As described later in this chapter, this kinematic interaction takes place as far cranially as the craniocervical region.

The following section of the chapter focuses on several subtopics within the broad topic of sagittal plane kinematics of the lumbar spine. Box 9.2 lists the order of these subtopics.

Flexion of the Lumbar Region

Fig. 9.52B shows the kinematics of flexion of the lumbar region in context with flexion of the trunk and hips. Pelvic-on-femoral (hip) flexion increases the passive tension in the stretched muscles, such as the hamstrings. With the lower end of the vertebral column fixed by the sacroiliac joints, continued flexion of the middle and upper lumbar region reverses the natural lordosis in the low back.

Typical kinematic patterns of lumbar flexion from a standing position have been well studied. Throughout a 24-hour period, asymptomatic adults across a wide age range perform an average of 4400 sagittal plane motions of at least 5 degrees in the lumbar spine.[247] Most of these motions are in the direction of flexion. Furthermore, full lumbar flexion from upright standing tends to occur more within the middle and lower lumbar segments—particularly within the region with the greatest lordosis while standing.[150,324] The variability of the relative intervertebral contribution to total lumbar motion has been shown to increase in the presence of low back pain.[181]

Lumbar flexion kinematics are often described based on movement at the apophyseal joints. During flexion between L3 and L4, for example, the inferior articular facets of L3 slide superiorly and anteriorly, roughly 5 mm relative to the superior facets of L4.[279] When considering the summation of these active kinematics across the entire lumbar region, compression forces generated between vertebrae shift *away* from the apophyseal joints (which normally support less than 20% of the total spinal load in erect standing) and *toward* the discs and vertebral bodies.[2,94] The compressed anterior aspects of the discs and stretched posterior ligaments support more of the total load as the trunk is progressively flexed. In extreme flexion, the fully stretched articular capsules of the apophyseal joints restrain further forward migration of the superior vertebra. The capsular ligaments of the apophyseal joints are strong, capable of supporting up to 1000 N (225 lb) of tension before failure.[55]

The extreme flexed position of the lumbar spine significantly reduces the contact area within the apophyseal joints. Paradoxically, although a fully flexed lumbar spine significantly reduces the total load on a given apophyseal joint, it is possible that the *contact pressure* (force per unit area) increases because of the reduced surface area to distribute the load. The absolute increase in contact pressure may or may not be excessive, however, depending on the total magnitude of the forces that are acting on the flexed joint. The presence of strong trunk muscle activation in a flexed position can generate very high contact pressures. Exceedingly high pressure can damage the flexed apophyseal joints, especially if sustained over a prolonged period or if the articular surfaces are abnormally shaped.

The amount of flexion across the lumbar spine affects the size of the intervertebral foramina and vertebral canal, and the potential for deforming the nucleus pulposus.[94,163] Relative to the anatomic position, flexion *increases* the cross-sectional area of the lumbar intervertebral foramina and vertebral canal by 11% to 12%.[125] Lumbar flexion, therefore, may potentially be used therapeutically to temporarily reduce impingement of the cauda equina within a stenosed vertebral canal or a compressed nerve root within an obstructed intervertebral foramen.[254] In certain circumstances, however, this potential therapeutic advantage may be associated with a potential therapeutic disadvantage. For example, excessive or prolonged flexion of the lumbar region generates increased compression force on the anterior portion of the disc, ultimately deforming the gel-like nucleus pulposus in a *posterior* direction.[4,26,82,86,94] In the healthy spine, the magnitude of the posterior deformation is small and usually of no consequence. Significant migration of the disc material can be naturally resisted by increased tension in the stretched posterior side of the annulus fibrosus. A disc with a weak, cracked, or distended posterior annulus may, however, experience a posterior migration (or oozing) of the nucleus pulposus. In some cases, the nuclear material may impinge against the spinal cord or nerve roots (Fig. 9.60). This potentially painful impairment is frequently referred to as a *herniated* or *prolapsed disc*, or more formally a *herniated nucleus pulposus*. Persons with a herniated disc may experience severe pain and altered sensation, muscle weakness, and reduced reflexes in the lower extremity, consistent with the specific motor and sensory distribution of the impinged nerve root.

Extension of the Lumbar Region

Extension of the lumbar region is essentially the reverse kinematics of flexion, and it increases the natural lordosis (see Fig. 9.53). When lumbar extension is combined with full hip extension, the increased passive tension in the stretched flexor muscles and capsular ligaments of the hip limits pelvic-on-femoral extension, thereby promoting further lordosis in the lumbar spine.

In contrast to flexion, extension between L3 and L4, for example, occurs as the inferior articular facets of L3 slide inferiorly and slightly posteriorly relative to the superior facets of L4. From a flexed position, moving into the anatomic or slightly extended position increases the contact area within the apophyseal joints, at a time when these joints are typically accepting a greater percentage of body weight.[257,264]

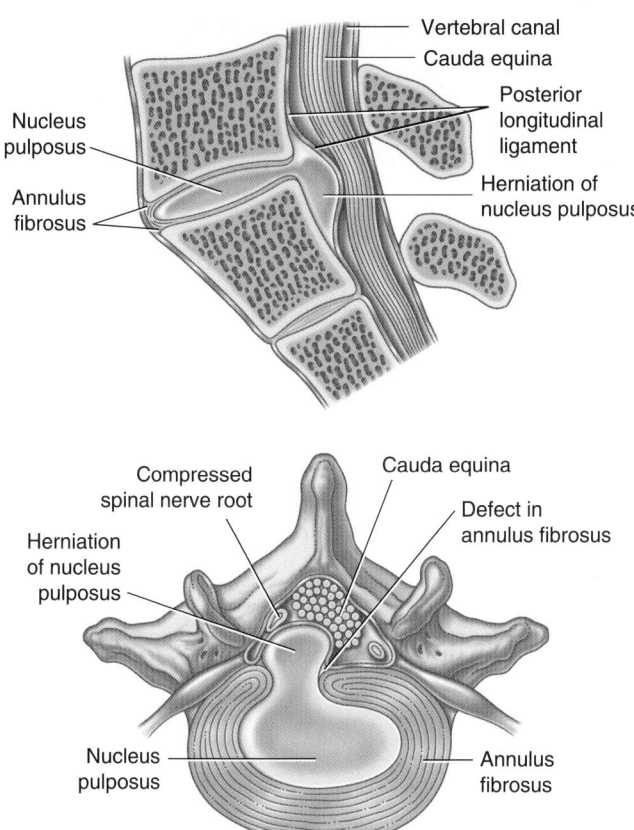

FIG. 9.60 Two views of a full herniated nucleus pulposus in the lumbar region. (From Standring S: *Gray's anatomy,* ed 41, New York, 2015, Churchill Livingstone.)

This situation may limit the contact pressure within the joints. This protective scenario does not apply, however, to the physiologic *extremes* of lumbar extension. In full lumbar extension, the tips of the inferior articular facets (of a top vertebra) slide inferiorly beyond the joint surface of the superior articular facets of the vertebra below.[94] Contact pressures can therefore rise significantly in the hyperextended lumbar spine as the relatively "sharp" tips of the inferior articular facet contact the adjacent lamina region. For this reason, a chronic posture of lumbar *hyperlordosis* can place large and potentially damaging stress on the apophyseal joints and adjacent regions. Furthermore, hyperextension of the lumbar spine can compress the interspinous ligaments, possibly creating a source of low back pain.[114]

As with flexion, extension of the lumbar spine affects the size of the intervertebral foramina and vertebral canal, and the potential for altering the shape of the nucleus pulposus.[4,86] Relative to the anatomic position, full lumbar extension *reduces* the diameters of the intervertebral foramina and vertebral canal by 15% and 11%, respectively.[125] Because of this, a person with a stenosed intervertebral foramen or vertebral canal may be advised to limit activities that involve full, end range extension, especially if they cause weakness or altered sensations in the extremities. Full extension, however, also tends to "push" the nucleus pulposus in an *anterior* direction,[26,81,94,289] thereby potentially resisting posterior migration or deformation of the nucleus.[4,21] Full sustained lumbar extension has been shown to reduce pressure within the disc[192,258] and in some cases to reduce the contact pressure between the displaced nuclear material and the

neural tissues. Evidence of the latter is assumed to occur based on "centralization" of symptoms, meaning that the pain or altered sensation (perceived in the lower extremities presumably because of nerve root impingement) migrates *toward* the low back.[311] Centralization therefore suggests reduced contact pressure between the displaced nuclear material and a nerve root. Although not certain, the reduced symptoms after sustained full extension may occur because either the nuclear material is pushed forward and away from the neural tissues, or because the neural tissues are pulled posteriorly and away from the nuclear material, or a combination of both, or other reasons not yet understood. Full extension of the lumbar region (as well as the hip joints) may also partially unload, or slacken, local and adjacent neural tissues, thereby reducing the intensity of neurogenic pain. Emphasizing lumbar extension exercises and postures as a way to reduce radiating pain and radiculopathy from a posterior herniated nucleus pulposus was popularized by Robin McKenzie, and such exercises are well-known as "McKenzie exercises" (or more recently as Mechanical Diagnosis and Therapy).[152,252] Therapeutic approaches that emphasize sustained active and passive extension have been shown to offer varying degrees of relief of symptoms and improvement of function in persons with a known posterior or posterior-lateral disc herniation and associated radiculopathy.[35,43,92] This specific therapeutic approach, however, would not be appropriate for everyone with a painful herniated disc and associated radiculopathy.[172] For example, consider a person with an acute and fully herniated and sequestered disc at the L5/S1 level compressing against the S^1 nerve root in the vertebral canal. Because full extension of the lumbar spine reduces the size of the vertebral canal slightly, this motion may further compress an inflamed and swollen S^1 nerve root, thereby increasing radiating pain down the leg.

Lumbopelvic Rhythm during Trunk Flexion and Extension

In conjunction with the hip joints, the lumbar spine provides the central flexion and extension pivot point for the human body as a whole. Consider, in this respect, activities such as fully flexing and extending the trunk from a standing position. The kinematic relationship between the lumbar spine and hip joints during such sagittal plane movements has been referred to as *lumbopelvic rhythm.* (A loose analogy of this concept exists for the shoulder and was described as *scapulohumeral rhythm* in Chapter 5.) Paying attention to the lumbopelvic rhythm and relative activation patterns of the extensor muscles can provide clues for detecting abnormal muscle and joint interactions and associated movement dysfunctions within the region.[106,164,216,295] These clues may provide valuable insight into effective treatment of the underlying pathomechanics.

Variations of Lumbopelvic Rhythms during Trunk Flexion from a Standing Position: A Kinematic Analysis. Consider the common action of bending forward toward the ground while keeping the knees nearly straight. Although highly variable, a healthy adult may perform this motion by combining about 45 degrees of lumbar flexion with a nearly simultaneous 60 degrees of hip (pelvic-on-femoral) flexion (Fig. 9.61A).[76,142,282] (It may be worth noting that these values correspond to about 50% of the total hip flexion typically allowed, but about 90% of the total lumbar flexion typically allowed.) Typically, lumbar flexion occurs more during the first 25% of the bend, while hip flexion occurs slightly more during the last 25% of the bend.[58,142,282] Although other generally similar kinematic strategies are common, those that deviate significantly from this typical lumbopelvic rhythm may help distinguish pathology or impairments affecting the lower spine from those affecting the hip joints.[142,249,265]

Variations of lumbopelvic rhythms during trunk flexion: A kinematic analysis

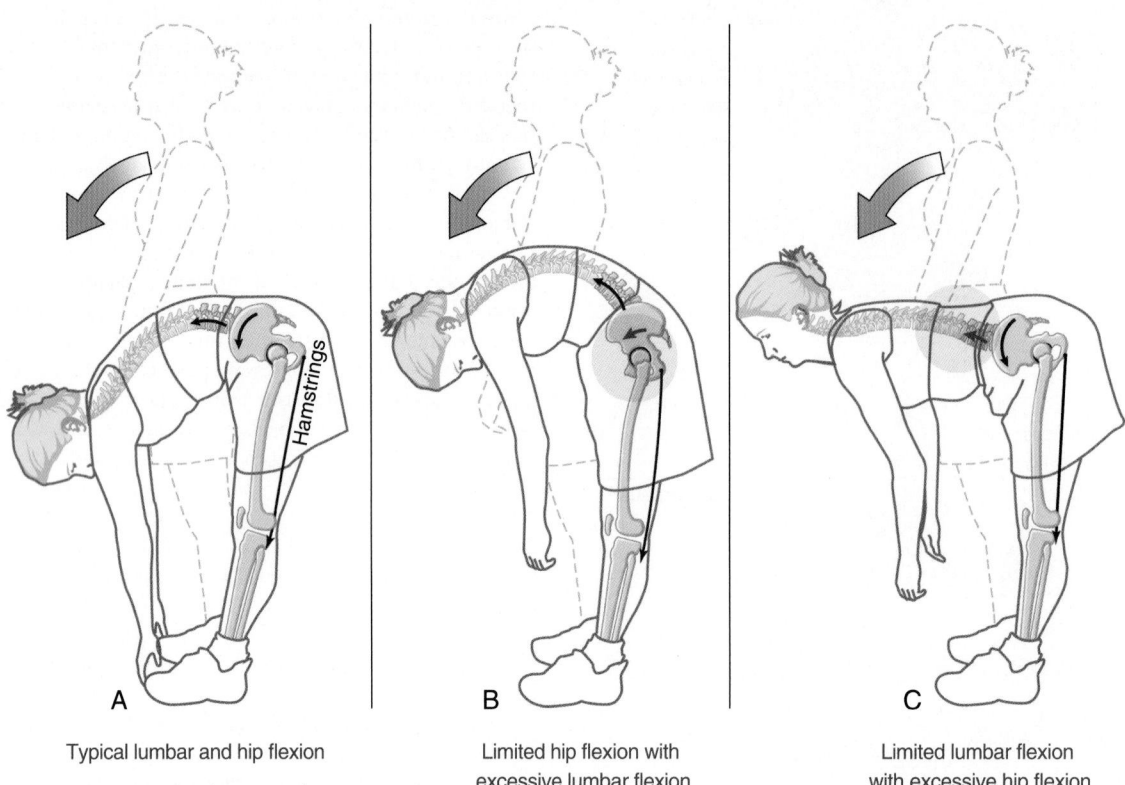

Typical lumbar and hip flexion

Limited hip flexion with
excessive lumbar flexion

Limited lumbar flexion
with excessive hip flexion

FIG. 9.61 Three different lumbopelvic rhythms used to flex the trunk forward toward the floor with knees held straight. (A) A typical kinematic strategy used to flex the trunk from a standing position, incorporating a near simultaneous 45 degrees of flexion of the lumbar spine and 60 degrees of hip (pelvic-on-femoral) flexion. (B) With limited flexion in the hips (for example, from tight hamstrings), greater flexion is required of the lumbar and lower thoracic spines. (C) With limited lumbar mobility, greater flexion is required of the hip joints. In (B) and (C), the red shaded circles and red arrows indicate regions of restricted mobility.

Fig. 9.61B–C shows lumbopelvic rhythms associated with marked restriction in mobility at the hip joints (B) or lumbar region (C). In both parts B and C, the amount of overall trunk flexion is reduced. If greater flexion is required, the hip joints or lumbar region may mutually compensate for the other's limited mobility. This situation may increase the stress on the compensating region. As depicted in Fig. 9.61B, with *limited hip flexion* from, for example, restricted hamstring extensibility or hip arthritis, bending the trunk toward the ground requires greater flexion in the lumbar and lower thoracic spinal regions. Eventually, exaggerated flexion may overstretch and subsequently weaken the posterior connective tissues within the region (including the thoracolumbar fascia), thereby reducing the ability of these tissues to limit further flexion. A chronic posture of increased flexion of the lumbar spine places a disproportionally larger compressive load on the intervertebral discs, theoretically increasing their likelihood for degeneration.

Fig. 9.61C demonstrates a kinematic scenario where *flexion of the lumbar spine is limited,* which may be associated with low back pathology or perhaps a chosen strategy related to culture or work demands. Regardless, reaching toward the ground requires disproportionally greater flexion of the hip joints, thereby creating greater demands on the hip extensor muscles. Consequently, the hip joints are subjected to greater compression loads. In persons with healthy hips, this relatively low-level increase in compression force is usually well tolerated. In a person with a pre-existing hip condition (such as osteoarthritis), however, the increased compression force may be painful and possibly accelerate a degenerative process.

Lumbopelvic Rhythm during Trunk Extension from a Forward Bent Position: A Muscular Analysis. A typical lumbopelvic

rhythm used to extend the trunk from a forward bent position is depicted in a series of consecutive phases for a healthy person in Fig. 9.62A–C. Although lumbar extension and hip extension occur nearly simultaneously throughout the movement, typically the early phase is associated with enhanced activation of the hip extensor muscles (Fig. 9.62A).[142] Significant activation of the lumbar extensor muscles is typically delayed slightly until the middle phase (Fig. 9.62B).[142,199] The short delay in lumbar extension places greater extension torque demands on the powerful hip extensor muscles (such as the hamstrings and gluteus maximus) at the time when the external flexion torque on the lumbar region is greatest (see external moment arm depicted as a dark black line in Fig. 9.62A). This may be a beneficial strategy to naturally protect the low back muscles and underlying joints from large forces. In this scenario, the demand on the lumbar extensor muscles increases only after the trunk has been sufficiently raised and the external moment arm, relative to body weight, has been minimized (Fig. 9.62B). Persons with low back pain or existing degenerative conditions of the low back may purposely further delay strong activation of the lumbar extensor muscles until the trunk is closer to vertical. Once standing fully upright, hip and back muscles are typically relatively inactive as long as the force vector resulting from body weight falls either through or posterior to the hip joints (Fig. 9.62C).

Effect of Pelvic Tilting on the Kinematics of the Lumbar Spine
Flexion and extension of the lumbar spine typically occur by one of two fundamentally different movement strategies. The first strategy is often used to maximally displace the upper trunk and upper extremities relative to the thighs, such as when lifting or reaching. This

Lumbopelvic rhythm during trunk extension: A muscular analysis

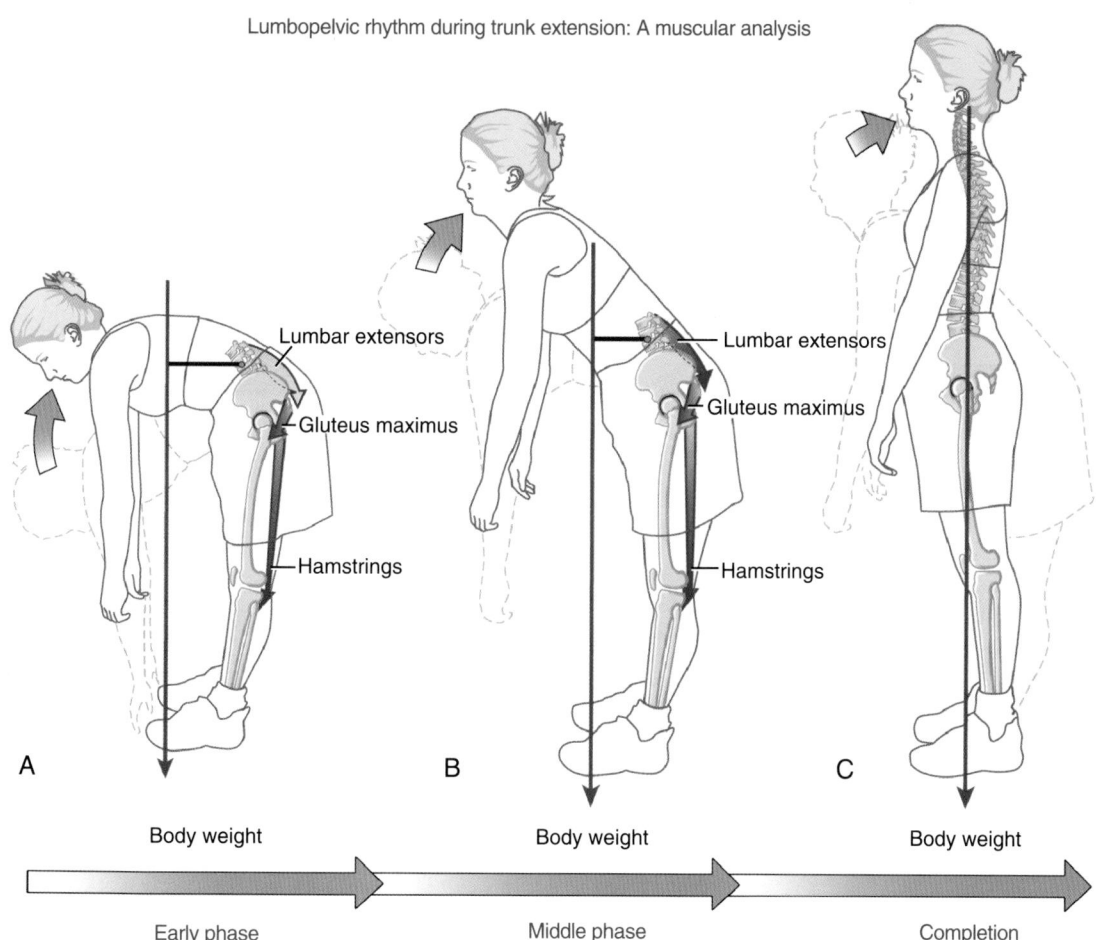

FIG. 9.62 A typical lumbopelvic rhythm is shown as a healthy person extends their trunk from a forward bent position. The motion is conveniently divided into three consecutive phases (A–C). In each phase the axis of rotation for trunk extension is arbitrarily placed through the body of L3. (A) In the *early phase,* trunk extension occurs to a greater extent through extension of the hips (pelvis on femurs), under relatively strong activation of hip extensor muscles (gluteus maximus and hamstrings). (B) In the *middle phase,* trunk extension occurs through a shared activation of the hip and lumbar extensors. (C) At the *completion* of the event, muscle activity typically ceases once the line of force from body weight falls posterior to the hips. The external moment arm used by body weight is depicted as a solid black line. The greater intensity of red indicates relatively greater intensity of muscle activation.

strategy, depicted in Figs. 9.61A and 9.62, combines near-maximal flexion and extension of the lumbar spine with a wide arc of pelvic-on-femoral (hip) and trunk motion. A second and more subtle movement strategy, which is the focus of this current discussion, involves a relatively *short-arc* forward or backward tilt (or rotation) *of the pelvis,* with the trunk remaining nearly stationary. As depicted ahead in Fig. 9.63A–D, an anterior pelvic tilt accentuates lumbar lordosis, whereas a posterior pelvic tilt reduces lumbar lordosis.[112] Because the pelvis is located at the very base of the trunk, its posture can have important kinesiologic and clinical consequences. The amount of pelvic tilt directly influences the amount of lumbar lordosis and, especially while sitting, the alignment of the superimposed vertebral column and craniocervical region. Furthermore, the extremes of the postures depicted in Fig. 9.63A–D can significantly alter the diameter of the lumbar vertebral canal and intervertebral foramina and create a pressure gradient that may deform or push the nucleus pulposus slightly—in a direction *away from* the compressed side of the disc.

The axis of rotation for pelvic tilting is in a medial-lateral direction through both hip joints. This mechanical association strongly links the (pelvic-on-femoral) movement of the hip joints with that

of the lumbar spine. This relationship is discussed further in the next section and again in Chapter 12.

Kinesiologic Correlations between Anterior Pelvic Tilt and Increased Lumbar Lordosis. Active anterior pelvic tilt can be achieved by simultaneous contraction of the hip flexor and back extensor muscles (Fig. 9.63A). Strengthening and increasing the postural control or awareness of these muscles can favor a more lordotic posture of the lumbar spine.[254] Depending on the circumstances, increasing the lumbar lordosis may be therapeutically desirable. Typically, however, a chronic posture of excessive or exaggerated lumbar lordosis is functionally undesirable. This could be caused by marked muscle weakness, such as weakness of the hip extensor and abdominal muscles in a child with severe muscular dystrophy. The pathomechanics of exaggerated anterior pelvic tilt and associated exaggerated lumbar lordosis may also involve a hip flexion contracture with increased passive tension (tightness) in the hip flexor muscles (Fig. 9.64). As described earlier in this chapter, possible negative consequences of exaggerated lordosis include increased compression within the lumbar apophyseal joints or increased contact pressure between posterior elements of lumbar vertebrae.

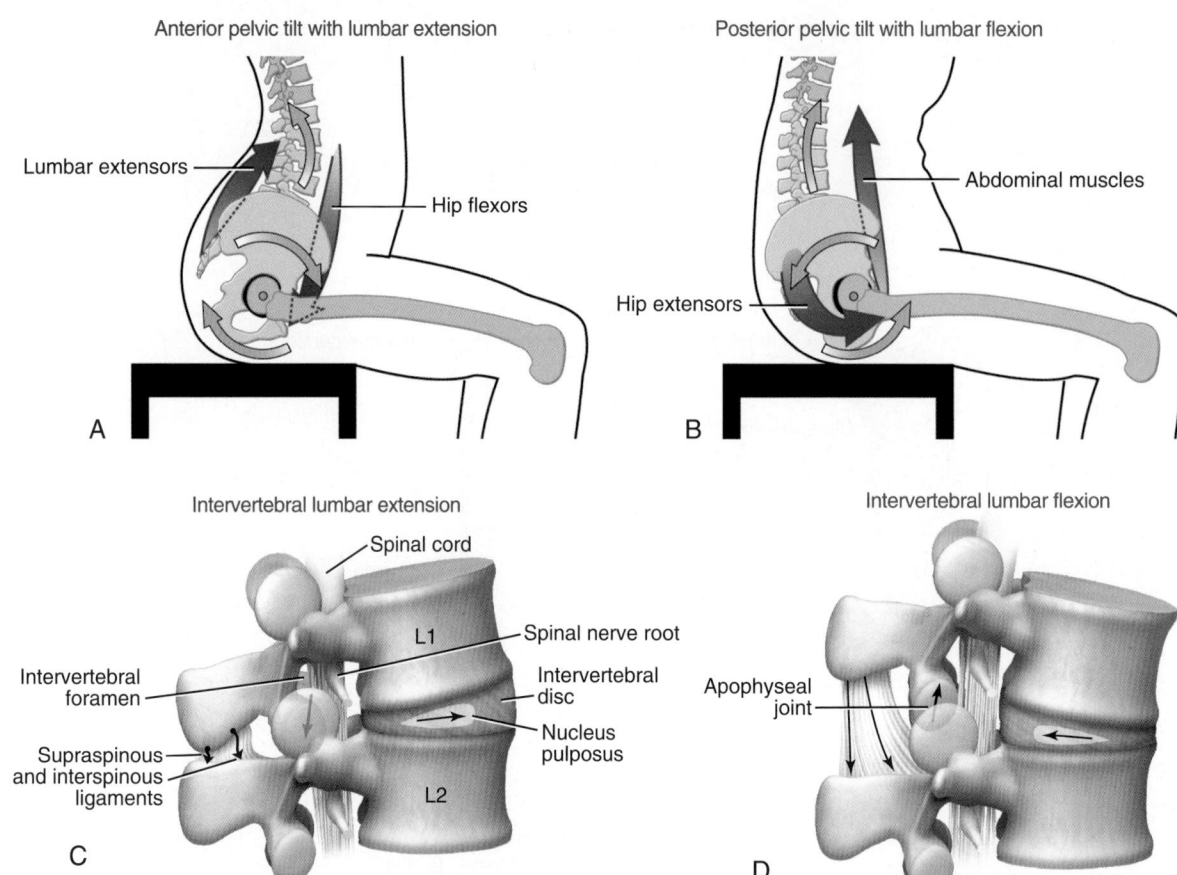

FIG. 9.63 Anterior and posterior tilting of the pelvis and its effect on the kinematics of the lumbar spine. (A and C) *Anterior pelvic tilt* extends the lumbar spine and increases the lordosis. This action tends to shift the nucleus pulposus anteriorly and reduces the diameter of the intervertebral foramen. (B and D) *Posterior pelvic tilt* flexes the lumbar spine and decreases the lordosis. This action tends to shift the nucleus pulposus posteriorly and increases the diameter of the intervertebral foramen. Muscle activity is shown in red.

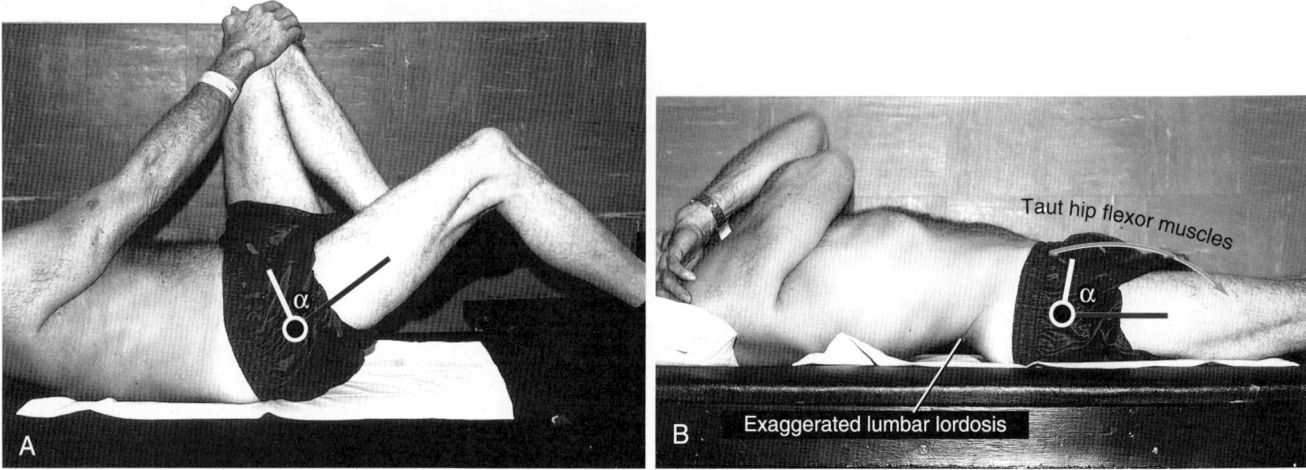

FIG. 9.64 The relationship between taut hip flexor muscles, excessive anterior pelvic tilt, and exaggerated lumbar lordosis in a person with marked right hip osteoarthritis. The medial-lateral axis of rotation of the hip is shown as an open white circle. (A) A right hip flexion contracture is shown by the angle (α) formed between the femur *(red line)* and a white line representing the iliac crest of the pelvis. The left normal hip is held flexed to keep the pelvis as posteriorly tilted as possible. (B) With both legs allowed to lie against the mat, tension created in the taut and shortened right hip flexors tilts the pelvis anteriorly, exaggerating the lumbar lordosis. The increased lordosis is evident by the hollow in the low back region. The hip flexion contracture is still present but is masked by the anteriorly tilted position of the pelvis. (Photograph from the archives of the late Mary Pat Murray, PT, PhD, FAPTA, Marquette University.)

SPECIAL FOCUS 9.8

More about the Herniated Nucleus Pulposus

The formal name for a herniated or prolapsed disc is a *herniated nucleus pulposus.* Herniations typically involve a posterior-lateral or posterior migration of the nucleus pulposus toward the very sensitive neural tissues (i.e., the spinal cord, cauda equina, ventral or dorsal nerve roots, or exiting spinal nerve roots). In vivo research strongly suggests that the herniated material is not just the nucleus but also fragments of dislodged vertebral endplates.[238] The term herniated *nucleus pulposus* (or disc) therefore may not be totally correct. However, because the term is so well embedded in the literature it will be used throughout this chapter.

Not all herniated discs are as remarkable as that illustrated in Fig. 9.60. In relatively mild cases the displaced nucleus migrates posteriorly but remains well within the confines of the annulus fibrosus. More moderate cases, however, may progress to a point at which the nuclear material, although still remaining within the posterior annulus, *bulges* or *protrudes* beyond the circumference of the posterior rim of the vertebral body. In more severe cases, this nuclear material completely herniates through the annular wall (or posterior longitudinal ligament) and *extrudes* into the epidural space (depicted in Fig. 9.60). In some cases, the extruded material may become lodged in the epidural space—frequently referred to as *sequestration* of the herniated disc. Extruded or sequestered herniations may have a better prognosis than a protruded or bulging disc.[64] Once displaced into the spinal canal, the herniated nucleus attracts macrophages that can assist with resorption of the displaced material.[132] Even a small amount of resorption can significantly reduce the mechanical pressure placed on the neural tissues. This mechanism may partially explain why, in some persons, pain associated with a herniated disc may resolve over time without surgical intervention.

Disc-related pain may result from the degenerated disc itself or from consequences of a herniated nucleus pulposus. Pain associated with a degenerated disc may be from damage to the innervated periphery of the posterior annulus fibrosus, posterior longitudinal ligament, or vertebral endplates. Perhaps more serious, however, is the pain and radiculopathy caused by the herniated disc compressing the neural tissues within the spinal canal (as seen in Fig. 9.60). In both scenarios, pain increases when the local tissues are swollen and inflamed.[168] If compressed, the inflamed nerves within the spinal canal or intervertebral foramina typically produce pain and altered sensations that are topographically associated with the dermatomes in the lower extremities. The symptoms are often referred to as "sciatica" because of the strong likelihood that the herniated disc affects nerve roots that ultimately form the sciatic nerve (L^4–S^3). Although pain may be a large component of a herniated nucleus pulposus, it is not a universal consequence of the pathlogy.[31]

Posterior disc herniation in the lumbar region typically involves two often interrelated mechanisms. The first involves a large, sudden compression or shear force delivered against an otherwise relatively healthy lumbar spine. This mechanism of injury may be associated with a single traumatic event, such as extremely strenuous coughing or vomiting[223] or the lifting or carrying of large loads.[246] A second and much more common mechanism involves a series of lower-magnitude forces delivered against the lumbar spine over the course of several years, often involving *preexisting disc degeneration.*[64,78,306,308] A degenerated disc may possess radial clefts (or fissures) that serve as a path of least resistance for the posterior-directed flow of the nuclear material.

Repetitive or chronic flexion of the lumbar spine likely increases the vulnerability of a posterior or posterior-lateral disc herniation. Flexion stretches and thins the posterior side of the annulus while the nuclear gel is forced posteriorly, often under high hydrostatic pressure. These pressures increase during strenuous lifting or bending activities that require strong activation of trunk muscles.[192,258] With sufficiently high hydrostatic pressure, the nuclear gel can create or find a pre-existing fissure in the posterior annulus.

Lumbar flexion combined with a twisting motion (i.e., axial rotation combined with lateral flexion) further increases the vulnerability of a posterior or posterior-lateral disc herniation.[66,238] When the spine is rotated, only half the posterior fibers of the annulus are taut, reducing its resistance to the migrating nuclear gel. Computer modeling and cadaveric research have also shown that combined axial rotation and lateral flexion concentrate large circumferential tensions in the annular fibers located within the posterior-lateral quadrant of the disc.[258,289] Over time, this region is more prone to develop fissures or cracks, thereby providing less resistance to the forces from the nuclear material.

It has been argued that a severely degenerated (and dehydrated) disc seldom experiences the classic herniated nucleus pulposus.[34] Apparently, a dehydrated nucleus is too dry and not under sufficient hydrostatic pressure to flow through the annulus. Although exceptions certainly exist, the classic herniated nucleus pulposus tends to occur more frequently in persons younger than age 40 years, at a time when the nucleus is still able to retain a relatively large volume of water. Furthermore, the chance of experiencing pain from a bulging disc may, in some persons, be greater in the morning, when the nucleus is pressurized by its relatively high diurnal water content.[13,170]

MECHANICAL OR STRUCTURAL FACTORS THAT MAY FAVOR A HERNIATED NUCLEUS PULPOSUS IN THE LUMBAR SPINE
1. Pre-existing disc degeneration with radial fissures, cracks, or tears in the posterior annulus that allow a path for the flow of nuclear material
2. Sufficiently hydrated nucleus capable of exerting high intradiscal pressure
3. Inability of the posterior annulus to resist pressure from a potentially migrating or deforming nucleus
4. Sustained or repetitive loading applied over a flexed and rotated (twisted) spine

Furthermore, exaggerated lumbar lordosis is associated with an increased anterior shear force across the lower lumbar spine and lumbosacral junction, which in some persons favors the development of an anterior spondylolisthesis.

Kinesiologic Correlations between Posterior Pelvic Tilt and Decreased Lumbar Lordosis. Active posterior pelvic tilt is produced by contraction of the hip extensor and abdominal muscles (see Fig. 9.63B). Strengthening and increasing the patient's conscious control over these muscles theoretically favor a reduced lumbar lordosis. This concept was the trademark of the once popular "Williams flexion exercises," a therapeutic approach that stressed stretching the hip flexor and low back extensor muscles while strengthening the abdominal and hip extensor muscles.[317] In principle, these exercises were considered most appropriate for persons with low back pain caused by excessive lumbar lordosis.

Horizontal Plane Kinematics: Axial Rotation

Only about 5 to 10 degrees of horizontal plane rotation occur to each side throughout the lumbar region.[89,221,287] Clinical measurements often exceed this amount, likely because of extraneous motion at the hip joint (pelvis rotating on the femur) and the lower thoracic region. The kinematics of lumbar axial rotation are shown in context with the rotation of the entire thoracolumbar region in Fig. 9.54B. Axial rotation between L1 and L2 to the right, for example, occurs as the left inferior articular facet of L1 approximates or compresses against the left superior articular facet of L2. Simultaneously, the right inferior articular facet of L1 separates (distracts or gaps) slightly from the right superior articular facet of L2.

The limited amount of axial rotation usually permitted within the lumbar region is remarkable. For example, some studies report measuring only about 1 or 2 degrees of unilateral axial rotation across the L3-4 intervertebral junction.[89,276,325] The relatively strong sagittal plane orientation of the lumbar apophyseal joints physically restricts axial rotation throughout the region. As indicated in Fig. 9.54B, the apophyseal joints located contralateral to the side of the rotation compress (or approximate), thereby blocking further movement.[25] Much of the actual rotation is accompanied by compression of the articular cartilage within the contralateral apophyseal joint. (Recall that the direction of rotation of any part of the axial skeleton is based on a point on the *anterior* side of the region, not the spinous process.) Axial rotation is also limited by tension created in the stretched annulus fibrosus as well as stretched capsules of the apophyseal joints on the side of the rotation (Fig. 9.54B).[149,313] In theory, an axial rotation of 3 degrees at any lumbar intervertebral junction would damage the articular facet surfaces and tear the collagen fibers in the annulus fibrosus.[28] Most normal physiologic movements likely remain safely under this potentially damaging limit.

The natural bony resistance to axial rotation in the lumbar region provides vertical stability throughout the lower end of the vertebral column. The well-developed lumbar multifidus and relatively rigid sacroiliac joints reinforce this stability.

Frontal Plane Kinematics: Lateral Flexion

About 20 degrees of lateral flexion occur to each side in the lumbar region. Except for differences in orientation and structure of the apophyseal joints, the arthrokinematics of lateral flexion are nearly the same in the lumbar region as in the thoracic region. Ligaments on the side opposite the lateral flexion limit the motion (see Fig. 9.55B). In addition, lateral flexion to the right, for example, significantly compresses the right side of the disc, also limiting motion. Normally, with lateral flexion, the nucleus pulposus deforms slightly *away* from the direction of the movement, or, stated differently, toward the convex side of the bend.[83,313]

Sitting Posture and Its Effect on Alignment within the Lumbar and Craniocervical Regions

Although the pelvis is technically part of the lower extremity, while sitting it functions in a postural sense as the "lowest" vertebra. Consequently, the sagittal plane posture of the pelvis (relative to the femoral heads) while sitting can have a significant influence on the spinal alignment throughout the entire vertebral column. The topic of sitting posture and pelvic position, therefore, has important therapeutic implications on the treatment and prevention of problems throughout the axial skeleton.[38,63] The following discussion highlights the effects of *sagittal plane* posturing of the pelvis, specifically as it affects the lumbar and craniocervical regions.

Consider the classic contrast made between "poor" and "ideal" sitting postures (Fig. 9.65). In the poor or slouched posture depicted in Fig. 9.65A, the pelvis is posteriorly tilted with a relatively flexed (flattened) lumbar spine. Eventually this posture may lead to adaptive shortening in connective tissues and muscles, ultimately perpetuating the undesirable posture.

A slouched sitting posture increases the external moment arm between the line of force of the upper body and lumbar vertebrae (see red line in Fig. 9.65A). This situation places greater demands on tissues that normally resist flexion of the lower trunk, including the intervertebral discs. As explained earlier in this chapter, in vivo pressure measurements typically demonstrate larger pressures within the lumbar discs in slouched sitting compared with erect sitting.[315] Even in healthy persons, the increased pressures from the slouched sitting position can deform the nucleus pulposus posteriorly slightly, especially in the L4–L5 and L5–S1 regions.[4] A habitually slouched sitting posture may, in time, result in *creep* in certain spinal connective tissues.[36] Creep and associated weakness of the posterior annulus fibrosus, for example, would reduce the tissues' ability to block a posteriorly protruding nucleus pulposus. This biomechanical scenario may be related to the pathogenesis of a subset of cases of nonspecific low back pain. The position of the pelvis and lumbar spine during sitting influences the posture of the axial skeleton as far cranially as the craniocervical region.[179] On average, the flat posture of the low back is associated with a more protracted position of the craniocervical region (i.e., a "forward head" posture) (see Fig. 9.65A).[27] Sitting with the lumbar spine flexed tips the thoracic and lower cervical regions forward slightly, toward flexion. To maintain a horizontal visual gaze—such as that typically required to view a computer monitor—the *upper* craniocervical region must compensate by extending slightly. Over time, this posture may result in adaptive shortening in the small posterior suboccipital muscles (see Chapter 10) and posterior ligaments and membranes associated with the atlanto-axial and atlanto-occipital joints. There is generally consistent but mixed level of evidence in the literature that forward head posturing is associated with neck pain, reduced range of motion, and headache.[9,74,136] The evidence for this association is generally stronger in adults and older adults, but lacking or weak in adolescents.[174,236,242]

As depicted in Fig. 9.65B, a more ideal sitting posture that includes the natural lordosis (and increased anterior pelvic tilt) extends the lumbar spine. The change in posture at the base (caudal aspect) of the spine has an optimizing influence on the adjacent more cranial segments. The more upright and extended thoracic spine facilitates a more retracted (extended) base of the cervical spine, yielding a more desirable "chin-in" position. Because the base of the cervical spine is more extended, the upper craniocervical region tends to flex slightly to a more neutral posture.

The ideal sitting posture depicted in Fig. 9.65B is difficult for many persons to maintain, especially for several hours at a time. Fatigue often develops in the lumbar extensor muscles. A prolonged, slouched

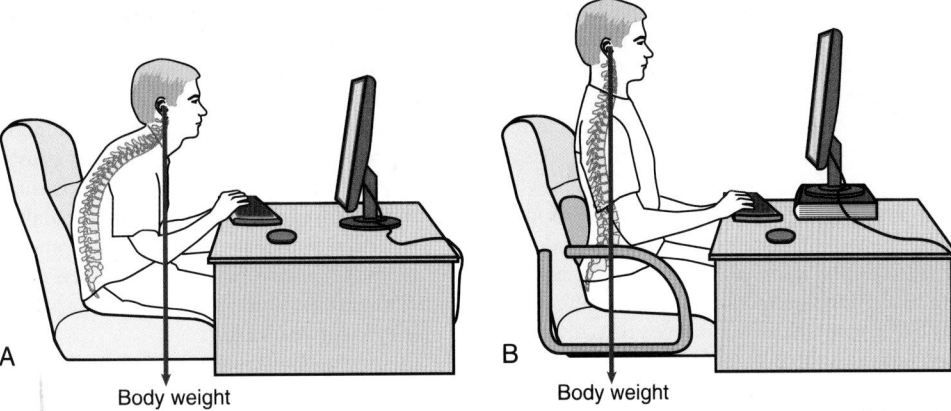

FIG. 9.65 Sitting posture and its effects on the alignment of the lumbar and craniocervical regions. (A) With a slouched posture, the lumbar spine flexes, which reduces its normal lordosis. The head, therefore, assumes a forward (protracted) posture. (B) With ideal sitting posture, the lumbar spine assumes a more normal lordosis, which facilitates a more desirable "chin-in" (retracted) position of the head. In some cases, adjusting the height of the monitor may favor a more ideal sitting posture. The line of gravity resulting from body weight is shown in red.

SPECIAL FOCUS 9.9

Using Knowledge of Kinesiology to Help Guide Some Therapeutic Interventions for Treating Chronic Low Back Pain: A Selected Example

Low back pain with disability is extremely common throughout the world.[96] Key factors believed to contribute to this condition include various comorbidities coupled with biophysical, social, psychologic, and genetic factors.[110] There are many nonsurgical, conservative approaches for treating persons with chronic low back pain, far beyond the scope of this chapter to elucidate.[c] Overarching goals behind many of these conservative treatments are to improve function and quality of life and to reduce pain, ideally with an emphasis on nonpharmacologic interventions. Broadly speaking, physical therapy interventions with varying levels of evidence fall within three areas: patient education, exercise, and manual therapy. These interventions are often guided by classification systems that help clinicians match subgroups of patients (based on their clinical presentation) with interventions that have the highest likelihood of success.[93,116] *Patient education* focuses on the importance of staying active and other aspects of rehabilitation, such as pacing strategies, graded exposures, and adapting activities based on individual characteristics. Facilitating a general understanding of the neuroscience of pain, as well as encouraging active pursuits in activities such as yoga,

stretching, Pilates, aerobic exercises, and other activities of interest to the patient are also key components. Specific therapeutic *exercise* includes those that aim to increase muscle strength and endurance, as well as improve trunk mobility and movement control. These exercises may target activation of specific trunk muscles (Chapter 10) or be a more global approach incorporating aerobic, aquatic, general fitness, or multimodal activities. *Manual therapy* includes joint mobilization, soft tissue mobilization, and neural mobilization techniques, and may be provided in conjunction with other interventions such as dry needling.

Many of the therapeutic approaches mentioned earlier require a sound understanding of the mechanical and functional interactions among the bones, joints (and closely associated nerve roots), and muscles within the lumbopelvic region. This assertion is the basis for much of the material presented thus far in this chapter and throughout Chapter 10. To highlight just one such mechanical interaction, consider the marked and usually contrasting biomechanical effects that are associated with flexion and extension of the lumbar intervertebral junctions (Table 9.10). The contrasting biomechanics may potentially contribute important clues as far as the source of pain or mechanical dysfunction, and potentially guide effective treatment.

[c] 44, 93, 110, 113, 118, 159, 213, 220, 244, 252

TABLE 9.10 Some Contrasting Kinesiologic Effects of Lumbar Flexion and Extension

Structure	Effect of Flexion	Effect of Extension
Nucleus pulposus	Deformed or pushed posteriorly	Deformed or pushed anteriorly
Annulus fibrosus	Posterior side stretched	Anterior side stretched
Apophyseal joint	Capsule stretched Minimizes articular contact area Articular loading decreased	Capsule slackened (neutral extension only) Maximizes articular contact area (neutral extension only) Articular loading increased
Intervertebral foramina	Widened	Narrowed
Vertebral canal	Volume increases slightly	Volume decreases slightly
Posterior longitudinal ligament	Increased tension (elongated)	Decreased tension (slackened)
Ligamentum flavum	Increased tension (elongated)	Decreased tension (slackened)
Interspinous ligament	Increased tension (elongated)	Decreased tension (slackened)
Supraspinous ligament	Increased tension (elongated)	Decreased tension (slackened)
Anterior longitudinal ligament	Decreased tension (slackened)	Increased tension (elongated)
Spinal cord (cauda equina)	Increased tension (elongated)	Decreased tension (slackened)

sitting posture may thus be an unavoidable occupational hazard for some persons. In addition to the possible negative effects of a chronically flexed lumbar region, the slouched sitting posture may increase the muscular stress at the base of the cervical spine. The forward-head posture increases the external flexion torque on the cervical column as a whole, necessitating greater force production from the extensor muscles and local connective tissues. Sitting posture may be improved by a combination of efforts, such as improving awareness of one's alignment; strengthening and stretching appropriate muscles; adjusting the position of the visual display terminal;[154] wearing eyeglasses if needed; and improving or altering the ergonomic design of the chair including adequate lumbar support. Realize, however, that advice or efforts to adjust a person's sitting posture should be highly individualized. Because each person's head posture and overall body anthropometrics are so unique, one cannot assume that a single "ideal" posture is biomechanically best suited for all persons.

SUMMARY OF THE KINEMATICS WITHIN THE VERTEBRAL COLUMN

With the visual aid of Fig. 9.66, the following points summarize several kinematic themes of the vertebral column.

1. The *cervical spine* permits relatively large amounts of motion in all three planes. Most notable is the high degree of axial rotation permitted at the atlanto-axial joint. Ample range of motion is necessary to maximize the movement of the head—the site of many important functions, including hearing, sight, smell, and equilibrium.

2. The *thoracic spine* permits a relatively constant amount of lateral flexion. This kinematic feature reflects the general frontal plane orientation of the apophyseal joints combined with the stabilizing effect of the ribs. The thoracic spine supports and protects the thorax and its enclosed organs. As described in Chapter 11, an important function of the thorax is to provide a mechanical bellows for ventilation.

3. The *thoracolumbar spine*, from a cranial-to-caudal direction, permits increasing amounts of flexion and extension at the expense of axial rotation. This feature reflects, among other things, the progressive transformation of the orientation of the apophyseal joints, from the horizontal and frontal planes in the cervical-thoracic junction to the near sagittal plane in the lumbar region. The prevailing near sagittal plane and vertical orientation of the lumbar region naturally favor flexion and extension but restrict axial rotation.

4. The *lumbar spine*, in combination with flexion and extension of the hips, forms the primary pivot point for sagittal plane motion of the entire trunk.

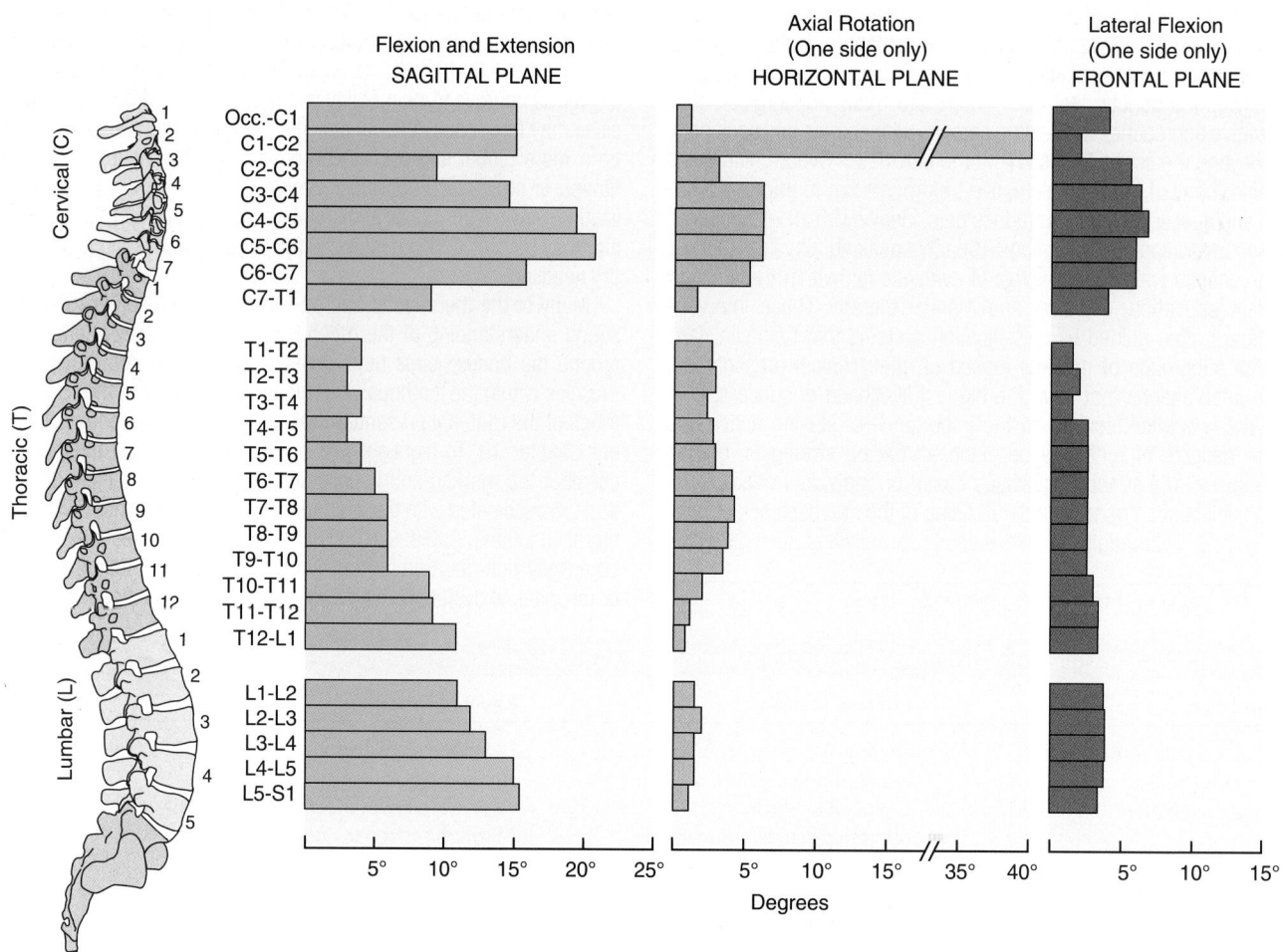

FIG. 9.66 A graph summarizing the overall maximal range of motion (in degrees) allowed across three planes, throughout the cervical, thoracic, and lumbar regions. Data represent a compilation of several sources indicated in the text. (Figure styled after White AA, Panjabi MM: Kinematics of the spine. In White AA, Panjabi MM, editors: *Clinical biomechanics of the spine*, Philadelphia, 1990, Lippincott.)

SACROILIAC JOINTS

The sacroiliac joints consist of the junction between the sides of the sacrum and the opposing surface of each ilium (Fig. 9.1). The wedging of the sacrum between the ilia provides effective transfer of potentially large forces between the vertebral column, the lower extremities, and ultimately the ground. As highlighted in Fig. 9.1, the sacroiliac joints mark the transition between the caudal end of the axial skeleton and the appendicular skeleton of the lower limbs. The analogous articulations at the *cranial* end of the axial skeleton are the sternoclavicular joints of the shoulder complex. Both the sternoclavicular and the sacroiliac joints possess unique structural characteristics that satisfy their distinctive functions. The saddle-shaped sternoclavicular joint is designed primarily for extensive triplanar mobility, a definite necessity for providing wide placement of the upper limbs in space. In contrast, the large, tight-fitting sacroiliac joint is designed primarily for stability and effective load transfer.

Although difficult to accurately diagnose, sacroiliac joints are believed to be the source of pain in about 15% to 30% of persons with chronic low back pain.[206] Sacroiliac joint pain may be secondary to injury to the joint or the surrounding periarticular connective tissues. Injury may be the result of obvious trauma, such as falling directly onto the region or unexpectedly stepping into a hole or off a steep step. Trauma to the region may be associated with difficult childbirth. In both males and females, injury to the sacroiliac joints may be related to repetitive unilateral or unidirectional torsions applied to the pelvis and low back, such as during figure skating or in other sports that demand frequent kicking or high-velocity throwing. Finally, the sacroiliac joint may be injured from excessive stress caused by postural or structural abnormalities. Examples include pelvic asymmetry resulting from misaligned ilia, excessive lumbar lordosis, scoliosis, or unequal leg lengths. Finite element modeling estimates that a leg length asymmetry of only 1 cm would result in a fivefold increase in the compression load across the sacroiliac joint while performing active trunk movements.[141] Of

clinical interest, the aforementioned modeling study predicted that the sacroiliac joint on the side of the *longer* limb would experience the greater increase in load.

Often, the mechanism of injury or pathology underlying a painful sacroiliac joint is not readily apparent, regardless of a careful joint- and region-specific evaluation.[259,283] If pain persists that cannot be attributed to pathology involving the sacroiliac joint, a thorough medical evaluation is needed to rule out other conditions, such as a herniated disc or inflamed lumbar or lumbosacral apophyseal joint, or even more serious pathology.

Much remains to be learned about the clinical evaluation and management of a painful sacroiliac joint. The best diagnostic evidence for determining whether the sacroiliac joint is the actual source of back pain is to assess the reduction in pain following controlled injections of an anesthetic into the joint.[266,283] In general, however, the literature reports only fair to limited diagnostic accuracy of most other clinical and medical imaging tests.[104,153,180,243,266] Adding to the joint's clinical ambiguity is the lack of a consistent terminology for describing biomechanics. For all these reasons, the clinical importance of this joint may be either understated or exaggerated.

Anatomic Considerations

The structural demands placed on the sacroiliac joints are best considered in context of the entire *pelvic ring*. The components of the pelvic ring are the sacrum, the pair of sacroiliac joints, the three bones of each hemipelvis (ilium, pubis, and ischium), and the pubic symphysis joint (Fig. 9.67). The pelvic ring transfers body weight bidirectionally between the trunk and femurs. The strength of the pelvic ring depends primarily on the tight fit of the sacrum wedged between the two halves of the pelvis. The sacrum, anchored by the two sacroiliac joints, is the keystone of the pelvic ring. The pubic symphysis joint, joining the right and left pubic bones anteriorly, adds an additional element of structural stability to the pelvic ring.

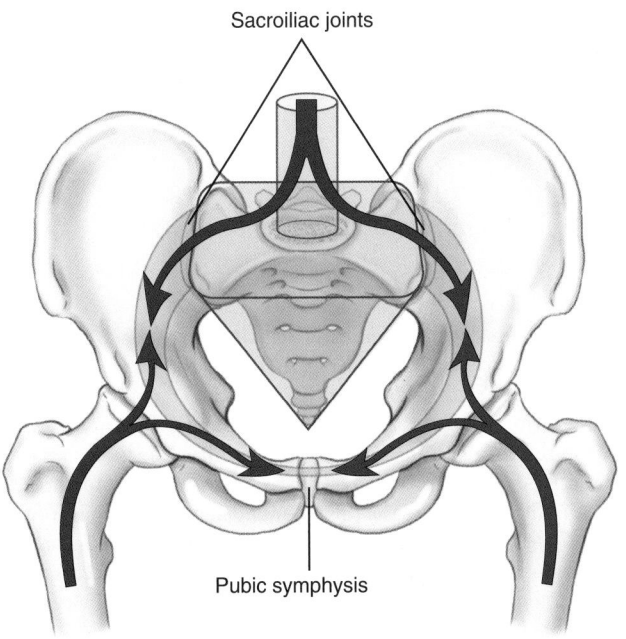

FIG. 9.67 The components of the pelvic ring. The arrows show the direction of body weight force as it is transferred between the pelvic ring, trunk, and femurs. The keystone of the pelvic ring is the sacrum, which is wedged between the two ilia and secured bilaterally by the sacroiliac joints. (Redrawn after Kapandji IA: *The physiology of joints,* vol 3, New York, 1974, Churchill Livingstone.)

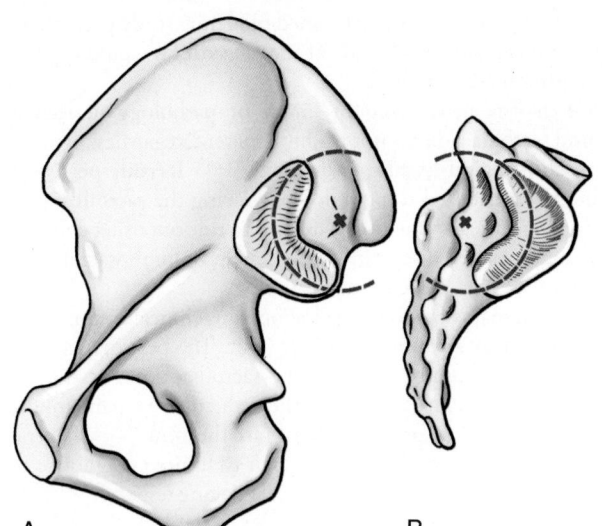

FIG. 9.68 The exposed articular surfaces of the right sacroiliac joint are shown. (A) Iliac surface. (B) Sacral surface. (Modified from Kapandji IA: *The physiology of joints,* vol 3, New York, 1974, Churchill Livingstone.)

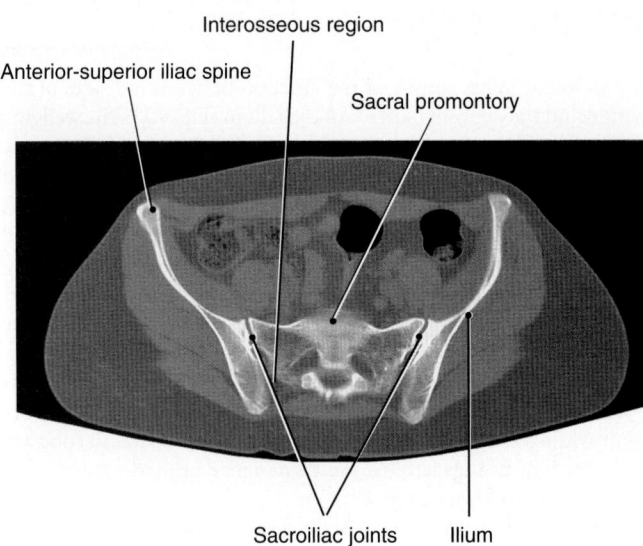

FIG. 9.69 A horizontal cross-sectional computed tomographic scan at the level of the sacroiliac joints. Note the irregular articular surfaces. (From Kelley LL, Petersen CM: *Sectional anatomy for imaging professionals,* ed 3, St Louis, 2012, Mosby.)

JOINT STRUCTURE

The sacroiliac joint is located just anterior to the readily palpable posterior-superior iliac spine of the ilium. Structurally, the joint consists of a relatively rigid articulation between the *auricular surface* (from Latin *auricle,* meaning little ear) of the sacrum and the matching *auricular surface* of the ilium. The articular surfaces of the joint have a semicircular, boomerang shape, with the open angle of the boomerang facing posteriorly (Fig. 9.68).

The evolving structure of the sacroiliac joint throughout the lifespan has contributed to discrepancies in the literature on the joint's anatomic classification.[229] In childhood the sacroiliac joint has all the characteristics of a diarthrodial joint, being relatively mobile and possessing a synovial membrane and articular cartilage. Between puberty and adulthood, however, the sacroiliac joint gradually transforms from a diarthrodial (synovial) joint to a modified synarthrodial joint.[206,275] Most notably, the articular surfaces change from smooth to rough. A mature sacroiliac joint possesses numerous, reciprocally contoured elevations and depressions, etched within the subchondral bone and articular cartilage (Fig. 9.69). These roughened areas increase the coefficient of friction within the joint, enhancing the resistance against vertical shear between the joint surfaces. While aging throughout adulthood, the joint capsule becomes increasingly fibrotic, less pliable, and less mobile. Degenerative-like changes of the sacroiliac joint have been identified through CT scans in more than 85% of asymptomatic (pain-free) adults greater than 60 years of age.[75] By the eighth decade of life, about 10% of the population have completely ossified or fused sacroiliac joints—far more often in men than in women.[60,263] The stiffer and less mobile aged joint, coupled with decreased bone density, may partially explain the increased risk of sacral fractures in the elderly. Anthropologists routinely use the structural condition of the sacroiliac joint as a method to determine the approximate age of a specimen.

The rather dramatic changes in the articular structure of the sacroiliac joints between birth and older age are in some ways like those of joints that develop osteoarthrosis. Degenerative-like changes occur more often on the iliac side of the joint, possibly due to its naturally thinner layer of articular cartilage.[283] It is likely that these typically asymptomatic changes are not pathologic, in the strict sense of the word, but rather a structural remodeling to accommodate to the increased loading associated with physical maturation. As with all joints, however, the sacroiliac joint may become inflamed at any age, often associated with ankylosing spondylitis.

LIGAMENTS

The sacroiliac joint is reinforced by an extensive and thick set of ligaments.[229] These ligaments include the anterior sacroiliac, interosseous, and posterior sacroiliac ligaments.[73,303] Although the iliolumbar, sacrotuberous, and sacrospinous ligaments do not directly cross the joint, they nevertheless provide significant articular stability.[103,231]

Ligaments That Stabilize the Sacroiliac Joint

- Anterior sacroiliac
- Interosseous
- Short and long posterior sacroiliac
- Iliolumbar
- Sacrotuberous and sacrospinous

The *anterior sacroiliac ligament* is a thickening of the anterior and inferior regions of the capsule (Fig. 9.70).[229] The *interosseous ligament* has been partially exposed in Fig. 9.70 by removing part of the left side of the sacrum and other local ligaments. The interosseous ligament, the strongest ligament of the sacroiliac joint, consists of a set of very dense and short fibers that tightly fills most of the gap that naturally exists along the posterior and superior margins of the joint.[73,303] (This gap, evident in Fig. 9.69, has been referred to as the "interosseous region" of the sacroiliac joint.[248]) The interosseous ligament rigidly binds the sacrum with the ilium, forming a syndesmosis (Chapter 2).

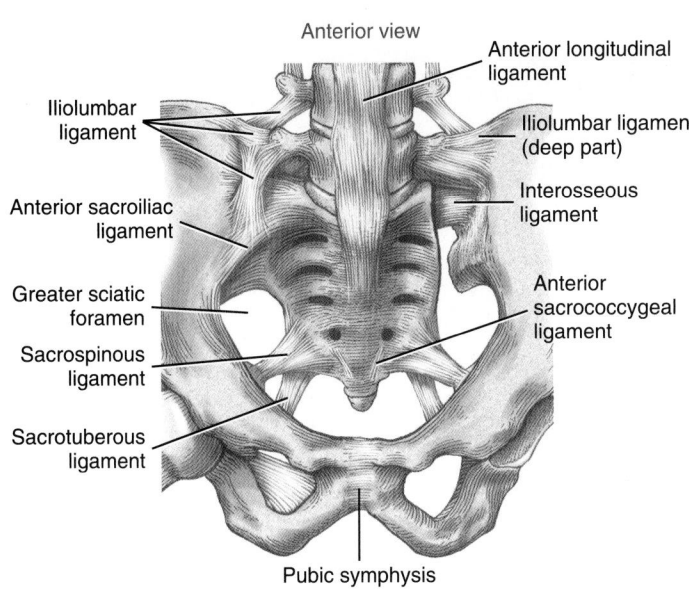

FIG. 9.70 An anterior view of the lumbosacral region and pelvis shows the major ligaments in the region, especially those of the sacroiliac joint. On the specimen's left side, part of the sacrum, superficial parts of the iliolumbar ligament, and the anterior sacroiliac ligament are removed to expose the auricular surface of the ilium and deeper interosseous ligament.

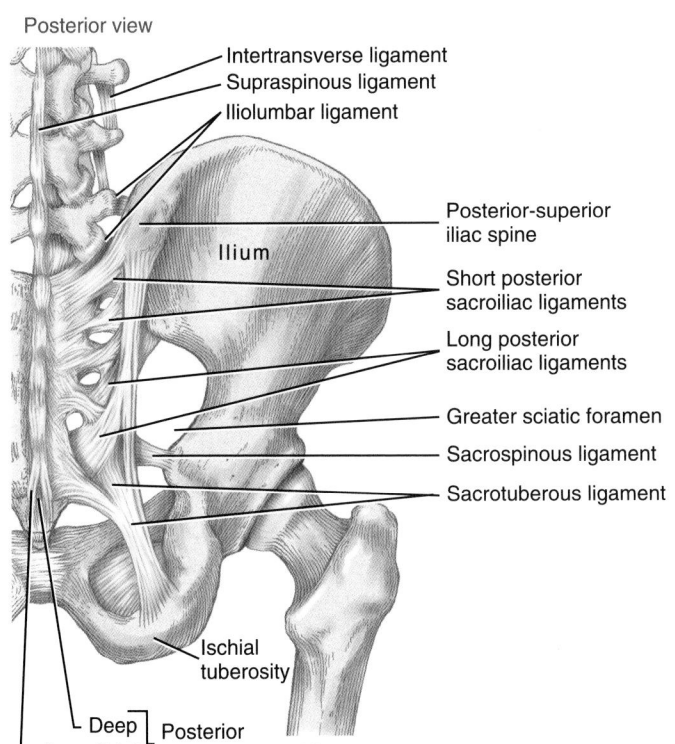

FIG. 9.71 A posterior view of the right lumbosacral region and pelvis shows the major ligaments that reinforce the sacroiliac joint.

Short and long *posterior sacroiliac ligaments* cross the posterior side of the sacroiliac joint (Fig. 9.71). The extensive but relatively thin set of *short posterior sacroiliac ligaments* originates along the posterior-lateral side of the sacrum. The ligaments run superiorly and laterally to insert on the ilium, near the iliac tuberosity and the posterior-superior iliac spine. Many of these fibers blend with the deeper interosseous ligament. Fibers of the well-developed *long posterior sacroiliac ligament* originate in the regions of the third and fourth sacral segments and then course toward an attachment on the posterior-superior iliac spine of the ilium.

The *iliolumbar ligament,* described earlier as a stabilizer of the lumbosacral joint, blends with and reinforces the anterior sacroiliac ligament (Fig. 9.70). The *sacrotuberous ligament* is large, arising from the posterior-superior iliac spine, lateral sacrum, and coccyx, attaching distally to the ischial tuberosity (Fig. 9.71). The distal attachment blends with the tendon of the biceps femoris (lateral hamstring) muscle. The *sacrospinous ligament* is located deep to the sacrotuberous ligament, arising from the lateral margin of the caudal end of the sacrum and coccyx, attaching distally to the ischial spine.

Superior view

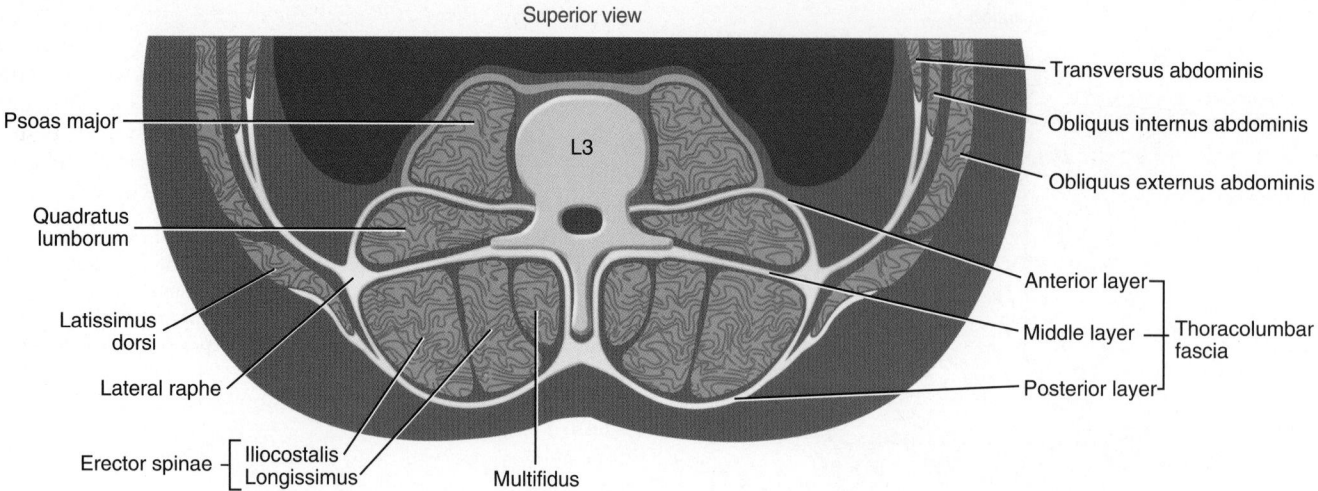

FIG. 9.72 A superior view of a horizontal cross-sectional drawing through the low back at the level of the third lumbar vertebra. The anterior, middle, and posterior layers of the thoracolumbar fascia are shown surrounding various muscle groups.

INNERVATION

Sensory nerve fibers have been identified within the periarticular connective tissues of the sacroiliac joints.[178,299,303] Many of these sensory nerve fibers have tested positive for substance P and calcitonin gene–related polypeptides.[281] The presence of these peptides strongly suggests a role in the transmission of pain. Anatomic reviews on the joint's innervation consistently include the dorsal rami of the L[5]–S[4] spinal nerve roots, and less often the ventral rami of L[4]–S[2].[229,303] Persons with a painful sacroiliac joint often report symptoms in the ipsilateral lower lumbar and medial buttock area, near the posterior-superior iliac spine and adjacent the long and short posterior sacroiliac joint ligaments.[303]

THORACOLUMBAR FASCIA

The thoracolumbar fascia plays an important functional role in the mechanical stability of the low back, including the sacroiliac joint.[301,316] This fascia is most extensive in the lumbar region, where it is organized into anterior, middle, and posterior layers. Three layers of the thoracolumbar fascia partially surround and compartmentalize the posterior muscles of the lower back, as illustrated in Fig. 9.72.

The *anterior and middle layers* of the thoracolumbar fascia are named according to their position relative to the quadratus lumborum muscle. Both layers are anchored medially to the transverse processes of the lumbar vertebrae and inferiorly to the iliac crests. The *posterior layer* of the thoracolumbar fascia covers the posterior surface of the erector spinae and multifidus and, more superficially, the latissimus dorsi muscle. This layer of the thoracolumbar fascia attaches to the spinous processes of all lumbar vertebrae and the sacrum, and to the ilium near the posterior-superior iliac spines. These attachments provide mechanical stability to the sacroiliac joint. Stability is enhanced by attachments of the gluteus maximus and latissimus dorsi.

The posterior and middle layers of the thoracolumbar fascia fuse at their lateral margins, forming a *lateral raphe*. This tissue blends with fascia of the transversus abdominis and, to a lesser extent, with the obliquus internus abdominis (internal oblique) muscle. The

functional significance of these muscular attachments is addressed in greater detail in Chapter 10.

Kinematics

Relatively small and poorly defined three-dimensional rotational and translational movements have been described at the sacroiliac joint. Although difficult to measure, the magnitude of these movements in the adult has been reported to be from 1 to 4 degrees for rotation, and from 1 to 2 mm for translation.[72,144,206,278,303]

Although no terminology completely describes the complex rotational and translational movements at the sacroiliac joint, two terms, nevertheless, are typically used for this purpose: *nutation* and *counternutation*. These terms describe movements limited to the near sagittal plane, around a near medial-lateral axis of rotation that traverses the interosseous ligament[73] (Fig. 9.73). *Nutation* (meaning to nod forward) is defined as the relative *anterior tilt* of the base (top) of the sacrum relative to the ilium. *Counternutation* is a reverse motion defined as the relative *posterior tilt* of the base of the sacrum relative to the ilium. (Note the term *relative* used in the previous definitions.) As depicted in Fig. 9.73, nutation and counternutation can occur by sacral-on-iliac rotation (as previously defined), by iliac-on-sacral rotation, or by both motions performed simultaneously.

Terms Describing Motion at the Sacroiliac Joint

- *Nutation* occurs by anterior sacral-on-iliac rotation, posterior iliac-on-sacral rotation, or both motions performed simultaneously.
- *Counternutation* occurs by posterior sacral-on-iliac rotation, anterior iliac-on-sacral rotation, or both motions performed simultaneously.

FUNCTIONAL CONSIDERATIONS

The sacroiliac joints perform two main functions: (1) a stress relief mechanism within the pelvic ring and (2) a stable means for load transfer between the axial skeleton and lower limbs.

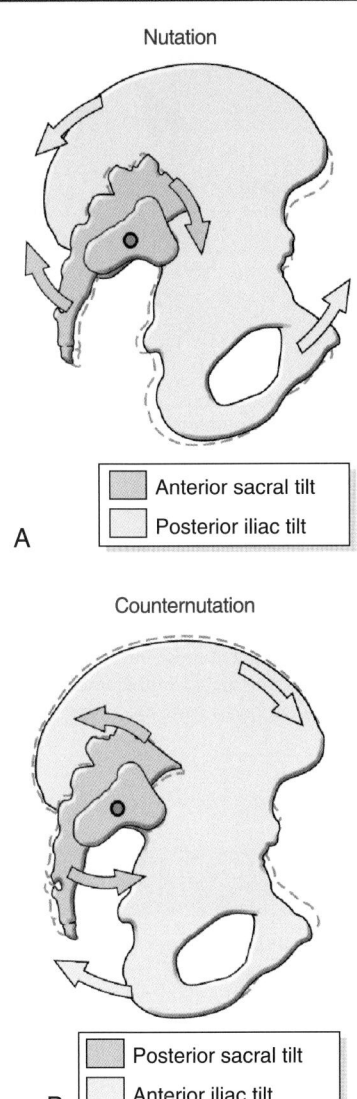

Nutation

Anterior sacral tilt
Posterior iliac tilt

A

Counternutation

Posterior sacral tilt
Anterior iliac tilt

B

FIG. 9.73 The kinematics at the sacroiliac joints. (A) Nutation. (B) Counternutation. (See text for definitions.) Sacral rotations are indicated by the darker shade of tan, iliac rotations are indicated by the lighter shade of tan. The axis of rotation for sagittal plane movement is indicated by the small green circle.

Stress Relief

The movements at the sacroiliac joints, although slight, permit an important element of stress relief within the entire pelvic ring. This stress relief is especially important during walking and running and, in women, during childbirth.

During walking, the reciprocal flexion and extension pattern of the lower limbs causes each side of the pelvis to rotate slightly out of phase with the other. For example, at normal speed of walking, the heel of the advancing lower limb strikes the ground as the toes of the opposite limb are still in contact with the ground. Finite element analysis of the sacrum during gait predicts that the sacroiliac joint on the stance side nutates as the sacroiliac joint on the swing side counternutates.[286] These sacroiliac torsions are likely amplified with increased walking speed. Although relatively slight, these reciprocal movements at each sacroiliac joint during walking help dissipate stress that would otherwise occur in the pelvic ring if it were a solid and continuous structure.[302] The pubic symphysis joint has a similar role in relieving stress throughout the pelvic ring.

Movement of the sacroiliac joints increases during labor and delivery.[37] A significant increase in joint laxity occurs during the last trimester of pregnancy and is especially notable in women during their second pregnancy compared with their first. Increased nutation during childbirth rotates the lower part of the sacrum posteriorly, thereby increasing the size of the pelvic outlet and favoring the passage of the infant. The articular surfaces of the sacroiliac joints are smoother in women, presenting less resistance to these slight physiologic motions.

Sacroiliac joint pain is not uncommon in women during pregnancy and may persist after delivery as a poorly defined condition termed *pelvic girdle pain syndrome*.[300,303] In addition to the pain, women with this painful syndrome tend to have trouble performing an active straight leg raise—a clinical test believed to specifically challenge the load transfer mechanics through the pelvic ring.[19,268] The combination of weight gain and altered center of mass, increased lumbar lordosis, increased torque demand in lumbar region while walking, and hormone-induced laxity of ligaments may biomechanically overstress the sacroiliac joints.[101] Pregnant women with asymmetric sacroiliac joint laxity have been shown to be statistically more likely to develop moderate to severe pelvic girdle pain compared with pregnant women who have symmetric laxity.[56] However, the specific pathogenesis of *chronic* postpartum pelvic pain is not well understood. Some studies suggest that the chronic pain may be associated with fatigue and reduced control of selective lumbopelvic muscles, potentially contributing to the instability and increased stress on the sacroiliac joints.[19,44,62] Continued research is needed to firmly establish an effective, multidisciplined approach of treatment for this condition.[87,119]

Stability During Load Transfer: Mechanics of Generating a Nutation Torque at the Sacroiliac Joints

The plane of the articular surfaces of the sacroiliac joint is largely vertical. This orientation renders the joint vulnerable to vertical slipping, especially when subjected to large forces. In most persons, nutation at the sacroiliac joints *increases* the compression and shear forces between joint surfaces, thereby increasing articular stability.[19,303] For this reason, the close-packed position of the sacroiliac joint is considered full nutation. *Forces that create a nutation torque are therefore considered the primary stabilizing forces at the sacroiliac joint.* This stabilizing torque is created by gravity, stretched ligaments, and muscle activation. When unloaded, such as when lying down, the sacroiliac joints naturally return to a less stable, or counternutated, position.

Nutation Torque Increases the Stability at the Sacroiliac Joints

This torque is produced by three forces:
- Gravity
- Passive tension from stretched ligaments
- Muscle activation

Stabilizing Effect of Gravity

The downward force of gravity resulting from body weight passes through the lumbar vertebrae, usually just anterior to an imaginary line connecting the midpoints of the two sacroiliac joints. At the same time, the femoral heads produce an upward-directed compression force through the acetabula. Each of these two forces acts with a separate moment arm to create a *nutation torque* about the sacroiliac joints (Fig. 9.74A). The torque resulting from body weight rotates the *sacrum* anteriorly relative to the ilium, whereas the

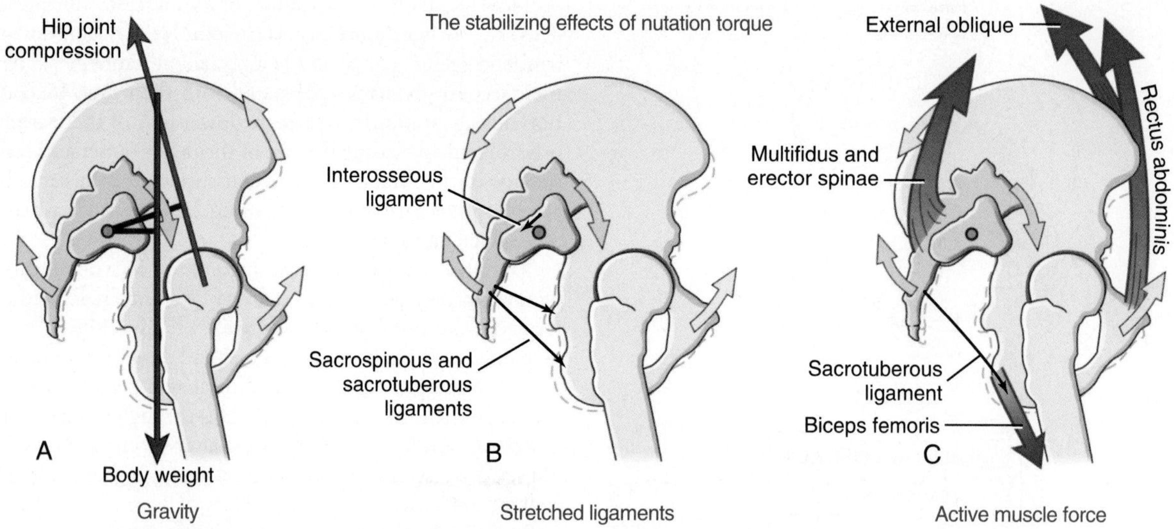

FIG. 9.74 Nutation torque increases the stability at the sacroiliac joints. (A) Two forces resulting primarily from gravity from body weight *(red downward-directed arrow)* and hip joint compression *(brown upward-directed arrow)* generate a nutation torque at the sacroiliac joints. Each force has a moment arm *(black line)* that acts from the axis of rotation *(green circle at joint)*. (B) The nutation torque stretches the interosseous, sacrospinous, and sacrotuberous ligaments, ultimately compressing and stabilizing the sacroiliac joints. (C) Muscle contraction *(red)* creates an active nutation torque across the sacroiliac joints. Note the biceps femoris transmitting tension through the sacrotuberous ligament.

torque resulting from hip compression force rotates the *ilium* posteriorly relative to the sacrum. This nutation torque "locks" the joints by increasing the friction between the rough and reciprocally contoured articular surfaces.[303,304] This locking mechanism relies primarily on gravity and congruity of the joint surfaces rather than on tension within extra-articular structures such as ligaments and muscles. (This locking mechanism has been described as *"form closure"* by Vleeming et al, in contrast to "force closure" described below.[302])

Stabilizing Effect of Ligaments and Muscles

As described previously, the first line of stability of the sacroiliac joints is created through a nutation torque created through the actions of gravity and weight bearing through the pelvis. The resulting stability is adequate for activities that involve relatively low, static loading between the pelvis and the vertebral column, such as sitting and standing. For larger and more repetitive and dynamic loading, however, the stability at the sacroiliac joints relies on an interaction of forces produced by ligaments and muscles to produce a firmly nutated position (i.e., through *"force* closure"). As described in Fig. 9.74B, nutation torque stretches several connective tissues at the sacroiliac joint, notably the sacrotuberous, sacrospinous, and interosseous ligaments.[73] Increased tension in these ligaments further compresses the surfaces of the sacroiliac joints, thereby adding to their transarticular stability.[28] In stark contrast is the long posterior sacroiliac joint ligament, which is slackened by nutation and tensed by counternutation.[73]

In addition to ligaments, several trunk, hip, and lumbopelvic muscles reinforce and stabilize the sacroiliac joints (Box 9.3). Such myogenic stability is likely necessary during activities such as jogging or lifting. The stabilizing action of many of these muscles is based on their attachments to the thoracolumbar fascia and to the sacrospinous and sacrotuberous ligaments.[271,302,303] Contractile forces from muscles listed in Box 9.3 can stabilize the sacroiliac joints by (1) generating active compression forces against the articular

---

> **BOX 9.3   Muscles That Help Reinforce and Stabilize the Sacroiliac Joint**
>
> Erector spinae and lumbar multifidus
> Diaphragm and pelvic floor muscles
> Abdominal muscles
> - Rectus abdominis
> - Obliquus abdominis internus and externus
> - Transversus abdominis
>
> Hip extensor muscles (such as biceps femoris and gluteus maximus)
> Latissimus dorsi
> Iliacus and piriformis

---

surfaces, (2) increasing the magnitude of nutation torque and subsequently engaging an active locking mechanism, (3) pulling or tensing connective tissues that directly or indirectly reinforce the joints, and (4) employing any combination of these effects. As one example, consider the muscular interaction depicted in Fig. 9.74C. Contraction of the multifidus and erector spinae muscles rotates the sacrum anteriorly, whereas contraction of the rectus abdominis, external oblique, and biceps femoris (one of the hamstring muscles) rotates the ilium posteriorly, two elements that produce nutation torque. (Activation of many of these same muscles, along with the gluteus maximus, would naturally occur during relative strenuous activities, such as lifting or pulling.) Through direct attachments, the biceps femoris (and gluteus maximus) increases the tension within the sacrotuberous ligament. The muscular interaction explains, in part, why strengthening and improving the control of many of the muscles listed in Box 9.3 is recommended for treatment of an unstable sacroiliac joint.[16,294,302,303] Furthermore, increased strength or control of muscles such as the latissimus dorsi and gluteus maximus, erector spinae, internal oblique, and transversus abdominis muscles provides stability to the sacroiliac joints via their connections into the thoracolumbar fascia. Coactivation of the diaphragm and pelvic floor muscles (as part of a Valsalva maneuver) has been postulated as a means to increase the stiffness of the lumbopelvic region and sacroiliac joint.[303] Furthermore, the more horizontally disposed muscles, such as the internal oblique and especially the transversus abdominis, may also provide joint stability directly by compressing the ilia inward toward the sacrum. The logic and purported benefits of wearing a pelvic belt as a form of treatment for sacroiliac joint pain or instability are based, in large part, on the same stabilizing mechanics normally provided by many of the aforementioned muscles.[57,182,303]

Finally, the iliacus (part of the iliopsoas) and piriformis muscles, by attaching directly into the capsule or margins of the sacroiliac joints (review Fig. 9.26), also provide a secondary source of stability to the sacroiliac articulation.[270] Without adequate stabilization provided by the muscles listed in Box 9.3, the sacroiliac joints may be more vulnerable to malalignment or hypermobility—two factors that can potentially stress the joint and contribute to a painful condition.

SYNOPSIS

The bony components of the axial skeleton include the cranium, vertebral column, sternum, and ribs. Of these four components, the vertebral column is most aptly designed to accept the loads produced by body weight and activated muscle. The absorption and distribution of these loads are a prime function of the intervertebral discs. The strength and compliance of the vertebral column is governed by ligaments and muscles, acting in conjunction with the normal, reciprocally shaped curvatures of the spine.

Each vertebra within a given vertebral region has a unique shape. Consider, for example, the contrasting shapes between the axis (C2) and L4; their very different morphology contrasts the different functional demands imposed on the two ends of the vertebral column. The axis, with its vertically projecting dens, is a central pivot point for the wide range of axial rotation allowed by the head and neck. The body of L4, in contrast, is designed to support large, superimposed loads.

The typical intervertebral junction has three important elements: transverse and spinal processes for attachments of muscles and ligaments, interbody joints for intervertebral adhesion and shock absorption, and finally the apophyseal joints for guiding the relative kinematics of each region. This third element is particularly important in understanding the kinematics throughout the axial skeleton. Remarkably, much of the characteristic motion allowed within each region of the vertebral column is dictated by the spatial orientation of apophyseal joints. Consider, most cranially, the geometric disposition of the apophyseal joints within the cervical region. The articular surfaces are oriented nearly horizontally at the atlanto-axial joint and at nearly 45 degrees between the horizontal and frontal planes throughout the remainder of the cervical region. This specific geometry bestows the craniocervical region with the greatest potential for three-dimensional movement of any region in the vertebral column—a necessity considering the location of the sources of many special senses within the head.

Although the 12 pairs of apophyseal joints within the thoracic region are oriented close to the frontal plane, the expected freedom of lateral flexion is limited because of the splinting action of the ribs. Relative rigidity within the thoracic cage is a requirement for the mechanics of ventilation and for protection of the heart and lungs.

The near sagittal plane orientation of middle and upper apophyseal joints within the lumbar region allows ample flexion and extension of the lower end of the vertebral column while simultaneously resisting horizontal plane rotation. The combined sagittal plane motion provided by the lumbar spine and the pelvis (relative to the hip joints) provides an important flexion and extension hinging point for the entire body. The "lumbopelvic rhythm" expressed in this region amplifies the reach of the upper extremities and hands, important for bending down to pick objects off the floor or reaching upward to a high shelf.

The relative frontal plane bias of the apophyseal joints of the L5–S1 junction provides important restraint to potentially damaging anterior shear force created between the caudal end of the lumbar spine and the base of the sacrum. This forward shear increases with increased lumbar lordosis, often performed in conjunction with an excessive anterior tilt of the pelvis relative to the femoral heads.

The most caudal articulations of the axial skeleton are the sacroiliac joints. These joints provide a relatively rigid junction for the transmission of large forces between the end of the axial spine and the lower extremities. These relatively large joints are naturally well stabilized, although they must permit small movements that help open the birth canal and dissipate stress within the pelvic ring while walking and running.

When optimally aligned and supported by healthy connective tissues and muscles, the vertebral column and craniocervical region provide mobility and vertical stability to the body as a whole. The important role of muscle in providing vertical stability to the axial skeleton is a recurring theme throughout Chapter 10. An abnormally aligned axial skeleton can exaggerate the deforming potential of gravity and active muscles, which can cause excessive and often damaging stress to bone, discs, ligaments, and the neural tissues. The rationale for many treatments for impairments of the axial skeleton is based on optimizing ideal posture throughout the body.

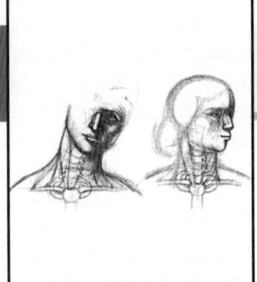

ADDITIONAL CLINICAL CONNECTIONS

CONTENTS

Clinical Connection 9.1: Degenerative Disc Disease: Interactions between Mechanical and Biologic Factors, 390

Clinical Connection 9.2: Scoliosis and Hyperkyphosis: Classic Examples of Structural Deformity Involving the Thoracic Spine, 392

CLINICAL CONNECTION 9.1

Degenerative Disc Disease: Interactions between Mechanical and Biologic Factors

Depending on severity, disc degeneration may be associated with other conditions of the spine, such as annular tears, partial or complete nuclear prolapse, disc narrowing, and the presence of vertebral osteophytes. Many of these conditions are directly or indirectly associated with the reduced ability of the disc to adequately absorb forces.

As described in this chapter, the load absorption quality of the intervertebral discs is based on biomechanical interactions among the annulus fibrosus, a hydrated nucleus pulposus, and the vertebral endplates. The ability of the disc to optimally absorb and redistribute loads may start to decline at a relatively (and surprisingly) young age. Consequently, early signs of disc degeneration may begin as early as the second decade and affects most persons to varying degrees by their third and fourth decades of life.[102,188] Although the data vary considerably, studies report that 30% to 70% of all adults have at least some detectable signs of disc degeneration on MR imaging;[274,308] however, most persons are essentially asymptomatic and report little or no loss of function. Disc degeneration, at least in its modest form, can therefore be considered a natural part of the aging process. The development of more severe disc degeneration associated with marked pain and loss of function is *not,* however, a normal part of aging. Disc degeneration associated with marked pain, and its associated functional limitations, should more appropriately be called *degenerative disc disease (DDD).*

DDD is a major medical and economic problem, accounting for up to 90% of all adult spinal surgeries in the United States.[5] Researchers strive to understand and improve the treatment for persons with DDD; however, its epidemiology and etiology are complicated and multifactorial. Epidemiologic research is hampered by unclear operational definitions of the disease, in addition to the fact that so many adults with significant disc degeneration remain asymptomatic.[3,102] Furthermore, it is difficult to distinguish which elements of disc degeneration occur naturally with aging (and associated wear and tear) and which are strictly pathologic.

Much of the research on the pathogenesis of DDD focuses on the interaction between mechanical and biologic factors.[10,64,123,228,238] *Mechanical factors* are the most intuitive and easiest to understand. There is little doubt that excessive loading of a disc over a prolonged time frame can contribute to its degeneration.[64,272] Ensuing mechanical instability of the intervertebral junction (which may involve the apophyseal joints) can create higher stress and

biochemical changes within the disc, thereby continuing the cycle of stress-induced degeneration.[64,168,327]

The fact that mechanical overload may initiate the process of disc degeneration in some persons and not others is a mystery. Other risk factors besides mechanical overload are obviously involved. The strongest risk factor for DDD is related to genetic inheritance.[18,219] Secondary risk factors include advanced age, poor disc nutrition (which may implicate smoking), occupation, anthropometrics (i.e., body size and proportion), and long-term exposure to total body vibration.[18,105,187,205,298] Except for genetics, several of the aforementioned factors may need to be present together to significantly increase the risk for developing DDD.

Although excessive forces delivered to a partially dehydrated disc may help explain the *initiation* of DDD, it cannot explain the large intersubject variations in pain and inflammation or rate of disease progression. Evidence suggests that the severity and progression of disc disease is strongly associated with the body's *biologic response* to the degenerative process.[3,64,123,228] Following tears of the annulus fibrosus, for example, vascularized granulation tissue invades the injured region (a phenomenon referred to as *neovascularization*), apparently as a normal component of inflammatory healing. Afferent neurons transmitting pain (nociceptors) also invade the vascularized granulation tissue, even in areas where nerves and blood vessels normally do not exist.[50,134] In addition, mast cells, macrophages, enzymes, and a host of *cytokines* (proteins and peptides that mediate and regulate specific cellular functions, such as tissue growth and inflammation) have been found within the granulation tissue.[224,262] Through a complicated and only partially understood process, the cytokines indirectly stimulate growth and sensitivity of the nociceptors, as well as increase the inflammation in the region.[1,117,228,321] In some persons this inflammatory response may prolong and amplify the pain. This process may also promote the release of more proinflammatory cytokines, which stimulate additional nociceptors in the annulus as well as the adjacent spinal canal and nerve sheaths surrounding the spinal nerve roots.[28] As a result, pain that originated as a torn annulus may also be expressed clinically as radiating pain down the course of the associated dermatome of the lower extremity. This process may help explain why a relatively nonstressful movement of the back in a person with degenerated discs may produce a heightened pain response, involving both the back and the lower extremity.

Degenerative Disc Disease: Interactions between Mechanical and Biologic Factors—cont'd

The chondrocytes and fibroblasts located within the intervertebral discs are able to detect minute physical characteristics of the surrounding physical environment, such as the magnitude and duration of tension and compressive forces, osmotic pressure, and nuclear hydrostatic pressure.[84] Through a complex and not well understood process known as *mechanotransduction,* cells within the disc (or any tissue) are able to respond to mechanical stimuli by altering their cellular metabolism, gene expression, and protein synthesis; ideally for the purposes of adapting to the mechanical environment.[64,84,117] Excessive compression on the disc, for example, has been experimentally shown to produce cell-mediated responses that include excessive release of proteinases, cytokines, interleukins, and nitric oxide.[228] These substances can alter the biosynthesis and distribution of the extracellular matrix, including proteoglycans and collagen.[6,123] In a degenerating disc, however, this process can produce a structurally and functionally inferior matrix, which is less able to absorb or distribute loads. Left unregulated, this process may accelerate the degenerative process. If normally regulated, however, this process may remodel the structure of the disc, allowing it to better tolerate varying loads throughout one's lifetime. Fig. 9.75 summarizes one possible set of mechanical and biologic interactions that may be involved in the development of DDD.

To improve the understanding of the multifactorial processes underlying DDD, Adams and Roughley proposed the following definition: "The process of disc degeneration is an aberrant, cell mediated response to progressive structural failure."[3] This definition succinctly incorporates the interactions between mechanical and biologic factors and serves as a model for clinical research. Beattie and colleagues, for example, have raised the hypothesis that controlled loading and unloading of the spine through therapeutic efforts, such as traction, graded muscle contractions, joint manipulations, and repeated movements, may improve the hydration of a moderately degenerated disc.[20,22] Perhaps greater hydration can improve the mechanical properties and biochemical environment within the damaged disc, thereby reducing the cycle of inflammation and further degeneration. Such a hypothesis requires integrated research among clinical and research scientists who study the pathogenesis and treatment of DDD. Ultimately, understanding more about this interaction will hopefully lead to improved patient care.

**Mechanical and Biologic Interactions
that May Be Associated with Degenerative Disc Disease**

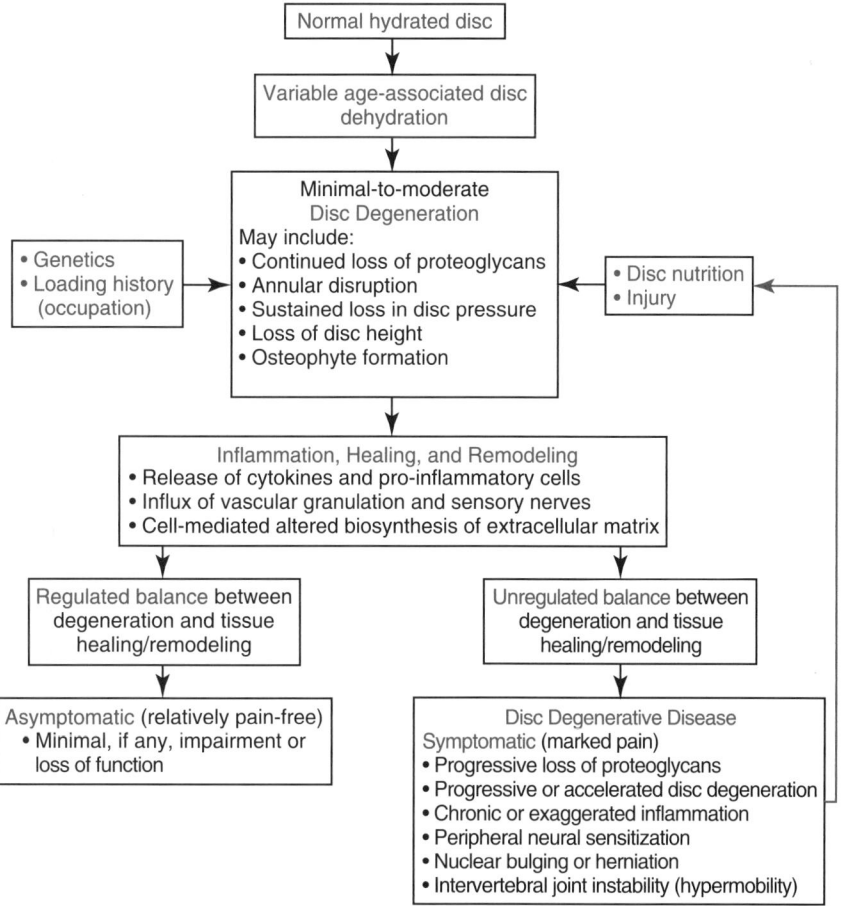

FIG. 9.75 A series of mechanical and biologic interactions that may be associated with degenerative disc disease. The red arrow indicates possible feedback loops that may perpetuate the disease process. See text for further details.

ADDITIONAL CLINICAL CONNECTIONS

CLINICAL CONNECTION 9.2
Scoliosis and Hyperkyphosis: Classic Examples of Structural Deformity Involving the Thoracic Spine

Maintaining the spine in normal alignment throughout life requires that extrinsic forces, governed by gravity and physical contact, are balanced by intrinsic forces, governed by muscles and osseous-ligamentous structures. When this delicate balance fails, varying amounts of deformity typically ensues. Herniated discs and nerve root impingements are relatively uncommon in the thoracic spine. This may be a result of, in part, the relatively low intervertebral mobility and high stability provided by the rib cage. Postural abnormalities, deformity, or malalignment, however, may occur relatively frequently in the thoracic region. The thoracic spine, constituting about half the entire length of the vertebral column, is particularly vulnerable to the effects of asymmetric or exaggerated forces created by gravity, muscle, or connective tissue. Scoliosis and hyperkyphosis are classic examples of significant deformity involving the thoracic spine and are thus featured in this two-part Additional Clinical Connection.

PART I: SCOLIOSIS

Scoliosis (from the Greek word meaning curvature) is a deformity of the vertebral column characterized by abnormal curvatures *in all three planes*—most notably, however, in the frontal and horizontal planes (Fig. 9.76A). The deformity most often involves the thoracic spine; however, other closely mechanically linked regions such as the lumbar spine, pelvis, and hips may be involved.[138] Scoliosis is typically defined as either functional or structural. *Functional scoliosis* can be corrected by a volitional shift in posture, whereas *structural scoliosis* is a fixed deformity that cannot be corrected fully by an active shift in posture.

Approximately 80% of all cases of structural scoliosis are termed *idiopathic,* meaning the condition has no apparent biologic or mechanical cause.[293] For unknown reasons, progressive idiopathic scoliosis affects adolescent females four times as often as males, especially those experiencing a rapid growth spurt.[166,176] Overall, approximately 2% to 3% of the adolescent population aged 10 to 16 years exhibits a lateral (frontal plane) curvature that exceeds 10 degrees.[166]

Although the underlying cause of adolescent idiopathic scoliosis is not known, several theories have been developed to help explain its pathogenesis. Some of these theories include: uneven growth or abnormal histologic structure of connective tissues (such as the vertebral endplates, intertransverse ligaments, and annulus fibrosus); asymmetry in paraspinal muscle activation; uncontrolled thoracic coupling between frontal and horizontal plane movements, asymmetry in intrapleural pressure distribution, and asymmetry in spinal loading leading to abnormal growth and remodeling of the vertebral bodies or intervertebral discs.[156,255,256,277,293] Also, because adolescent idiopathic scoliosis seems to occur only in humans, some theories have focused on biomechanical interactions between gravity and the upright posture.[253]

Approximately 20% of cases of structural scoliosis are caused by neuromuscular or muscular pathology, trauma, or congenital abnormalities.[79] Examples of pathology include poliomyelitis, muscular dystrophy, spinal cord injury, and cerebral palsy. In these cases, scoliosis is typically initiated by an asymmetry of muscular forces acting on the vertebral column.

Typically, scoliosis is described by the location, direction, and number of fixed frontal plane curvatures (lateral bends) within the vertebral column. The most common pattern of scoliosis consists of a single lateral curve with an apex in the T7–T9 region.[49] Other patterns may involve a secondary or compensatory curve, most often in the thoracolumbar or lumbar regions. The direction of the primary lateral curve is defined by the *side of the convexity* of the lateral deformity. The magnitude of the lateral curvature is typically measured on a radiograph by drawing the *Cobb angle* (Fig. 9.77). Because the thoracic vertebrae are most often involved with scoliosis, asymmetry of the rib cage is common. The ribs on the side of the thoracic concavity are pulled together, and the ribs on the side of the convexity are spread apart. The degree of torsion, or horizontal plane deformity, can be measured on an anterior-posterior radiograph by noting the rotated position of the vertebral pedicles.

The deformity in structural scoliosis typically has a fixed *contralateral* spinal coupling pattern involving lateral flexion and axial rotation.[293] The spinous processes of the involved vertebrae are rotated in the horizontal plane, typically toward the side of the concavity of the fixed thoracic curvature. The ribs therefore are forced to follow the horizontal plane rotation of the thoracic vertebrae. This explains why the *rib hump* is typically on the convex side of the frontal plane curvature (Fig. 9.76A). The exact mechanism responsible for the typically fixed contralateral coupling pattern is not understood.

Several factors are considered when deciding on the method of treating adolescent idiopathic scoliosis, including the magnitude of the frontal plane curve, the degree of progression, the cosmetic appearance of the deformity, and, particularly important, whether the child is in a growth spurt. In general, the larger the frontal plane curve and the younger the skeletal maturation of the child, the greater the likelihood of significant progression of the deformity.

ADDITIONAL CLINICAL CONNECTIONS

Scoliosis and Hyperkyphosis: Classic Examples of Structural Deformity Involving the Thoracic Spine—cont'd

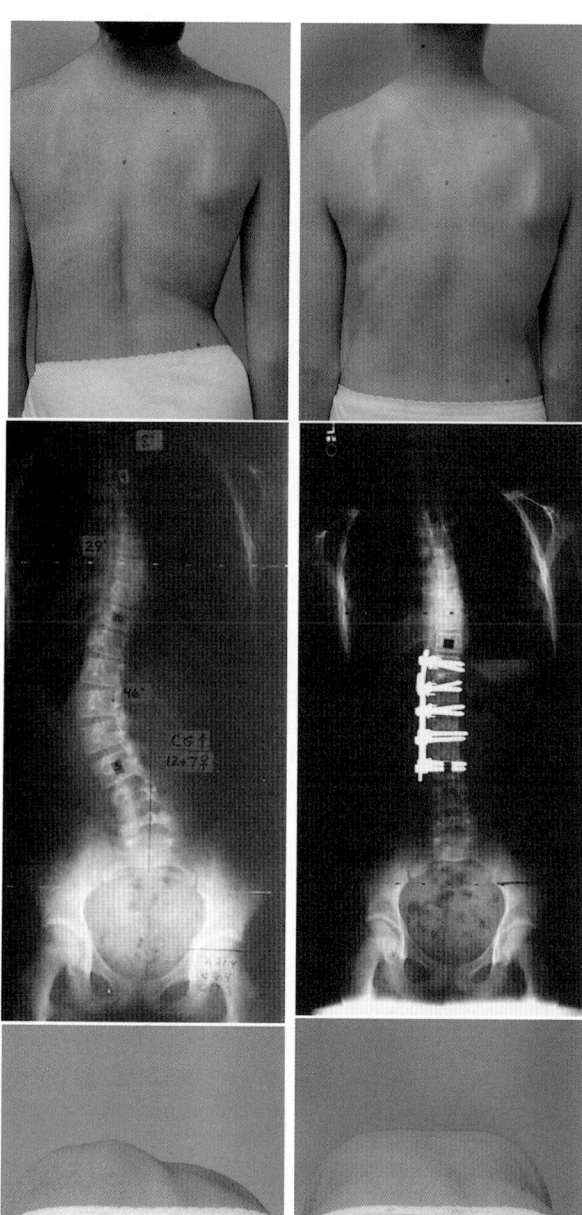

Pre-operative

Postoperative

A

B

FIG. 9.76 Illustration of a 12-year-old, skeletally immature girl with structural scoliosis. (A) Preoperative photographs and radiograph show the primary frontal plane curve in the thoracolumbar region. The lateral bend is 46 degrees, with its convexity (apex) to the girl's left side. The bottom photograph shows the girl bent forward at the waist, displaying the horizontal plane component of scoliosis, or "rib hump," on the subject's left side. (B) Postoperative photographs and radiograph of the same girl after an anterior spinal fusion and placement of instrumentation. Note the correction of the rib hump in the accompanying bottom photograph. (From Lenke LG: *CD Horizon Legacy Spinal System anterior dual-rod surgical technique manual,* Memphis, TN, 2002, Medtronic Sofamor Danek.)

Continued

ADDITIONAL CLINICAL CONNECTIONS

CLINICAL CONNECTION 9.2
Scoliosis and Hyperkyphosis: Classic Examples of Structural Deformity Involving the Thoracic Spine—cont'd

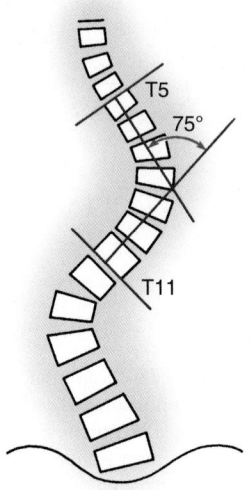

FIG. 9.77 A *Cobb angle* measures the degree of lateral bend in a spinal curvature associated with scoliosis. In this example the thoracic spine shows a Cobb angle of 75 degrees, with the apex of the curve at the T8–T9 junction. The Cobb angle is measured from a radiograph showing an anterior-posterior view. (From Canale ST, Beaty JH: *Campbell's operative orthopaedics,* ed 12, Philadelphia, 2012, Mosby.)

Depending on the severity and progression of the deformity, treatment options may include careful observation for progression of scoliosis, physical therapy, bracing, and surgery. (Fig. 9.76B shows the clinical and radiographic views of a young girl after anterior spinal fusion and placement of instrumentation.) Several studies indicate that bracing and surgery can control or partially correct the curves in adolescent idiopathic scoliosis.[d] The objective of bracing is usually to prevent a small curve from progressing to a large one. The immediate objective of surgery is to stabilize the curve and provide partial correction. The long-term objective of surgery is to prevent future pain and disability, although the certainty and degree of these complications are not known.[312] Surgery is extensive and is not without an inherent risk to the child. Although the strength of the evidence is mixed, several studies have reported modest therapeutic benefits of using scoliosis-specific exercises, often in conjunction with bracing, to limit the progression of a relatively mild frontal plane curvature (typically those with a Cobb angle of less than

[d] 59, 65, 80, 166, 167, 197, 201, 273, 310, 312

25 degrees).[77,151,162,189,197] Published clinical guidelines suggest that the exercises should be administered regularly and progressively by specifically trained therapists, and that the exercises incorporate postural "self-correction" and task-oriented activities, tailored to each patient's unique curve pattern.[197]

A very general guideline is used by some physicians to help decide between bracing and surgery options. Children with a thoracic Cobb angle of about 40 degrees or less are stronger candidates for bracing; those with a Cobb angle greater than about 45 to 50 degrees, however, are stronger candidates for surgery. Children with a Cobb angle between 40 and 50 degrees are in a "gray area" as to which is the more effective treatment. It is important to realize that the aforementioned guidelines are very general and vary based on other factors, such as the child's skeletal maturity, degree of curve progression, cosmetic appearance, and presence of multiple curves. The presence of a significantly reduced thoracic kyphosis (or actual lordosis) warrants stronger consideration for surgery, based on the likely ineffectiveness of bracing and the potential compromise in pulmonary function.[67,166]

PART II: HYPERKYPHOSIS OF THE THORACIC REGION
On average, about 40 to 45 degrees of natural kyphosis exist when one is standing at ease. In some persons, however, *excessive thoracic kyphosis* (formally termed *hyperkyphosis*) may develop and cause functional limitations. Hyperkyphosis may occur due to trauma, abnormal growth and development of vertebrae, severe degenerative disc disease, or marked osteoporosis and subsequent vertebral fractures—typically associated with advanced aging.[186] A modest increase in thoracic kyphosis and associated loss in body height is a normal aspect of reaching advanced age and is usually not debilitating.

The two most common conditions associated with progressive thoracic kyphosis are Scheuermann's kyphosis and osteoporosis. *Scheuermann's kyphosis,* or "juvenile kyphosis," is the most common cause of thoracic hyperkyphosis in adolescence. Although the cause of the condition is unknown, it is characterized primarily by the abnormal growth rate of different parts of the vertebrae, resulting in excessive anterior wedging of the thoracic and upper lumbar vertebral bodies. This condition appears to have a significant genetic predisposition, with a reported incidence of 1% to 8% of the general population.[169] The developing hyperkyphosis is rigid and cannot be volitionally reversed. Bracing may be effective in reducing the progression of the deformity in modest cases; surgery, however, may be warranted in severe cases that do not respond to conservative treatment.[165]

ADDITIONAL CLINICAL CONNECTIONS

Osteoporosis of the spine and associated compression fractures may lead to the genesis and ultimate progression of thoracic hyperkyphosis often seen in elderly women.[139] Osteoporosis is a chronic metabolic bone disease that affects primarily postmenopausal women; this condition is not a normal part of aging. Multiple vertebral fractures resulting from osteoporosis may lead to reduced height of the anterior sides of vertebral bodies, thereby promoting the progression of excessive thoracic kyphosis. One such scenario is demonstrated by analyzing the postures depicted in Fig. 9.78A–C, each modeled after actual radiographs of live subjects. In the ideal spinal posture, the line of force from body weight falls slightly to the concave side of the apex of the normal cervical and thoracic curvatures (see Fig. 9.78A). Gravity therefore can act with an external moment arm that favors normal thoracic and cervical curvatures. The ideal posture shown in Fig. 9.78A creates a small cervical extension torque and a small thoracic flexion torque. In the thoracic spine, the tendency to collapse further into kyphosis is normally resisted, in part, by compression forces between the

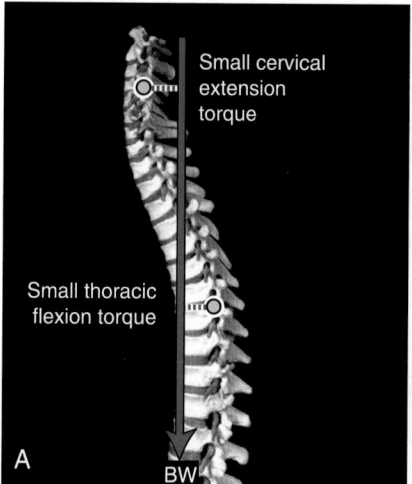

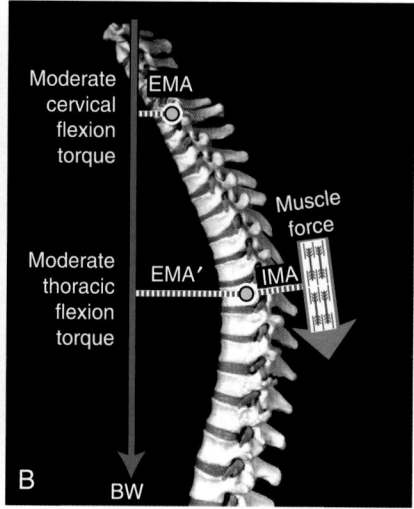

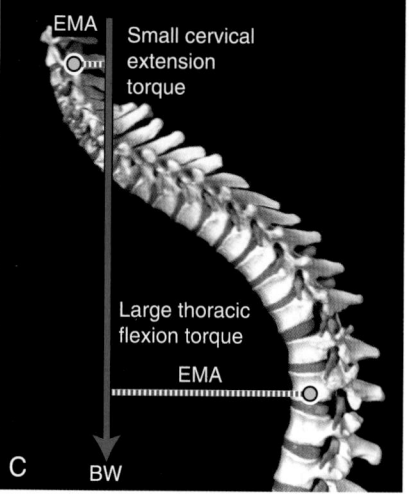

FIG. 9.78 Lateral views show the biomechanical relationships between the line of gravity from body weight (BW) and varying degrees of thoracic kyphosis. In each of the three models, the axes of rotation are depicted as the near midpoint of the thoracic and cervical regions *(green circles).* (A) In a person with ideal standing posture and normal thoracic kyphosis, body weight creates a small cervical extension torque and a small thoracic flexion torque. The external moment arms used by body weight are shown as dashed red lines. (B) In a person with moderate thoracic hyperkyphosis, body weight creates a moderate cervical and thoracic flexion torque *(EMA'*, external moment arm at midthoracic spine; *EMA*, external moment arm at midcervical spine; *IMA*, internal moment arm for trunk extensor muscle force). (C) In a person with severe thoracic hyperkyphosis, body weight causes a small cervical extension torque and a large thoracic flexion torque. Skeletal models are based on lateral radiographs of actual standing persons.

Continued

ADDITIONAL CLINICAL CONNECTIONS

anterior sides of the interbody joints. Vertebrae weakened from osteoporosis may be unable to resist the anterior compression forces.[230] Over time, the compression forces may produce excessive anterior wedging of the vertebral bodies, thereby accentuating the slow collapse into hyperkyphosis.

Furthermore, if significant disc degeneration and dehydration of the nucleus are present, the hyperkyphotic posture may further compress the anterior side of the discs.[227] At this point, a pathologic deforming process has been well initiated (see Fig. 9.78B). The increased flexed posture shifts the line of force resulting from body weight farther anteriorly, thus increasing the length of the external moment arm (EMA') and the magnitude of the flexed kyphotic posture. As a result, both thoracic and cervical spine regions may be subjected to a moderate flexion torque (see Fig. 9.78B). Increased extensor muscle and posterior ligamentous tension is needed to hold the trunk, neck, and head upright. The increased force passing through the interbody joints can create compression fractures in the vertebral bodies along with the formation of osteophytes. At this point, the vicious cycle is well established.

The magnitude of the compression force exerted between vertebrae of a hyperkyphotic thoracic spine can be surprisingly large. The amount of compression force associated with the posture depicted in Fig. 9.78B can be estimated by assuming a condition of static equilibrium within the sagittal plane: the product of body weight (BW) force and the external moment arm (EMA') equals the product of the muscle force times the internal moment arm (IMA). Assuming that the EMA' is about twice the length of the IMA, rotary equilibrium in the sagittal plane requires a muscle force of twice the body weight. Assume that a 180-lb person (1 lb = 4.448 N) has about 60% of body weight (108 lb) located above the midthoracic region. An extensor muscle force of approximately 216 lb (2 × 108 lb) is needed to hold the flexed posture. When considering superimposed body weight, a total of about 324 lb of compression force

(216 lb of muscle force plus 108 lb of body weight) is exerted on a midthoracic interbody joint. Applying this same biomechanical solution to the ideal posture shown in Fig. 9.78A yields a 50% *reduction* in total interbody joint compression force. This reduction is based on the ideal posture having an external moment arm approximately half the length of the IMA. Although this simple mathematic model is not absolutely accurate and does not consider dynamic aspects of movement, it emphasizes how posture can have a profound effect on the forces produced across an interbody joint.[108]

The thoracic posture shown in Fig. 9.78B may progress, in extreme cases, to that shown in Fig. 9.78C. As shown, the line of force from body weight has produced a small upper cervical extension torque and a large thoracic flexion torque. Note that despite the large thoracic kyphosis, the person can extend her upper craniocervical region enough to maintain a horizontal visual gaze. The main point of Fig. 9.78C, however, is to appreciate the biomechanical effect that a large external flexion torque can have on the progression of severe thoracic hyperkyphosis. Such severe hyperkyphosis has been shown to negatively affect one's quality of life, reduce inspiratory and vital capacity of the lungs, as well as increase the risk of falling because of a reduced sense of balance.[53,139] The hyperkyphosis may even further progress with a continued history of multiple compression fractures, untreated osteoporosis, progressive degenerative disc disease, and weakening of the trunk extensor muscles.[186] Muscle weakness may be the result of reduced activity as well as an altered length-tension relationship within the overstretched trunk extensor muscles.[33,200]

Treatment of excessive thoracic kyphosis depends strongly on the severity of the deformity, age, and health of the person. Options may include pharmacologic agents to reduce osteoporosis, surgery, and physical therapy—including exercise, postural education, taping, bracing, and balance training if applicable.[33,139]

REFERENCES

1. Abe Y, Akeda K, An HS, et al.: Proinflammatory cytokines stimulate the expression of nerve growth factor by human intervertebral disc cells, *Spine* 32:635–642, 2007.
2. Adams MA, Hutton WC, Stott JR: The resistance to flexion of the lumbar intervertebral joint, *Spine* 5:245–253, 1980.
3. Adams MA, Roughley PJ: What is intervertebral disc degeneration, and what causes it? *Spine* 31:2151–2161, 2006.
4. Alexander LA, Hancock E, Agouris I, et al.: The response of the nucleus pulposus of the lumbar intervertebral discs to functionally loaded positions, *Spine* 32:1508–1512, 2007.
5. An HS, Anderson PA, Haughton VM, et al.: Introduction: disc degeneration: summary, *Spine* 29:2677–2678, 2004.
6. An HS, Masuda K: Relevance of in vitro and in vivo models for intervertebral disc degeneration, *J Bone Joint Surg Am* 88(Suppl 2):88–94, 2006.
7. Andersson GB, Ortengren R, Nachemson A: Intradiskal pressure, intra-abdominal pressure and myoelectric back muscle activity related to posture and loading, *Clin Orthop Relat Res* 129:156–164, 1977.
8. Anderst WJ, Donaldson III WF, Lee JY, et al.: In vivo cervical facet joint capsule deformation during flexion-extension, *Spine* 39(8):E514–E520, 2014.
9. Andias R, Silva AG: A systematic review with meta-analysis on functional changes associated with neck pain in adolescents, *Muscoskel Care* 17(1):23–36, 2019.
10. Ansaripour H, Ferguson SJ, Flohr M: In vitro biomechanics of the cervical spine: a systematic review, *J Biomech Eng* 144(10), 2022.
11. Aono K, Kobayashi T, Jimbo S, et al.: Radiographic analysis of newly developed degenerative spondylolisthesis in a mean twelve-year prospective study, *Spine* 35(8):887–891, 2010.
12. Arshad R, Pan F, Reitmaier S, et al.: Effect of age and sex on lumbar lordosis and the range of motion. A systematic review and meta-Analysis, *J Biomech* 82:1–19, 2019.
13. Awad JN, Moskovich R: Lumbar disc herniations: surgical versus nonsurgical treatment, *Clin Orthop Relat Res* 443:183–197, 2006.
14. Ayturk UM, Garcia JJ, Puttlitz CM: The micromechanical role of the annulus fibrosus components under physiological loading of the lumbar spine, *J Biomech Eng* 132(6):061007, 2010.
15. Baldoni M, Gu W: Effect of fixed charge density on water content of ivd during bed rest: a numerical analysis, *Med Eng Phys* 70:72–77, 2019.
16. Barker PJ, Hapuarachchi KS, Ross JA, et al.: Anatomy and biomechanics of gluteus maximus and the thoracolumbar fascia at the sacroiliac joint, *Clin Anat* 27(2):234–240, 2014.
17. Bashkuev M, Reitmaier S, Schmidt H: Relationship between intervertebral disc and facet joint degeneration: a probabilistic finite element model study, *J Biomech* 102:109518, 2020.
18. Battie MC, Videman T: Lumbar disc degeneration: epidemiology and genetics, *J Bone Joint Surg Am* 88(Suppl 2):3–9, 2006.
19. Beales DJ, O'Sullivan PB, Briffa NK: The effects of manual pelvic compression on trunk motor control during an active straight leg raise in chronic pelvic girdle pain subjects, *Man Ther* 15(2):190–199, 2010.
20. Beattie PF: Current understanding of lumbar intervertebral disc degeneration: a review with emphasis upon etiology, pathophysiology, and lumbar magnetic resonance imaging findings, *J Orthop Sports Phys Ther* 38:329–340, 2008.
21. Beattie PF, Brooks WM, Rothstein JM, et al.: Effect of lordosis on the position of the nucleus pulposus in supine subjects. A study using magnetic resonance imaging, *Spine* 19:2096–2102, 1994.
22. Beattie PF, Butts R, Donley JW, et al.: The within-session change in low back pain intensity following spinal manipulative therapy is related to differences in diffusion of water in the intervertebral discs of the upper lumbar spine and L5-S1, *J Orthop Sports Phys Ther* 44(1):19–29, 2014.
23. Bell JA, Stigant M: Development of a fibre optic goniometer system to measure lumbar and hip movement to detect activities and their lumbar postures, *J Med Eng Technol* 31:361–366, 2007.
24. Bergman GJ, Knoester B, Assink N, et al.: Variation in the cervical range of motion over time measured by the "flock of birds" electromagnetic tracking system, *Spine* 30:650–654, 2005.
25. Bermel EA, Barocas VH, Ellingson AM: The role of the facet capsular ligament in providing spinal stability, *Comput Methods Biomech Biomed Engin* 21(13):712–721, 2018.
26. Berry DB, Hernandez A, Onodera K, et al.: Lumbar spine angles and intervertebral disc characteristics with end-range positions in three planes of motion in healthy people using upright MRI, *J Biomech* 89:95–104, 2019.
27. Black KM, McClure P, Polansky M: The influence of different sitting positions on cervical and lumbar posture, *Spine* 21:65–70, 1996.
28. Bogduk N: *Clinical and radiological anatomy of the lumbar spine*, ed 5, New York, 2012, Churchill Livingstone.
29. Bogduk N, Mercer S: Biomechanics of the cervical spine. I: normal kinematics, *Clin Biomech (Bristol, Avon)* 15:633–648, 2000.
30. Boos N, Weissbach S, Rohrbach H, et al.: Classification of age-related changes in lumbar intervertebral discs: 2002 Volvo Award in basic science, *Spine* 27:2631–2644, 2002.
31. Borenstein DG, O'Mara Jr JW, Boden SD, et al.: The value of magnetic resonance imaging of the lumbar spine to predict low-back pain in asymptomatic subjects: a seven-year follow-up study, *J Bone Joint Surg Am* 83:1306–1311, 2001.
32. Brasiliense LB, Lazaro BC, Reyes PM, et al.: Biomechanical contribution of the rib cage to thoracic stability, *Spine* 36(26):E1686–E1693, 2011.
33. Briggs AM, van Dieën JH, Wrigley TV, et al.: Thoracic kyphosis affects spinal loads and trunk muscle force, *Phys Ther* 87:595–607, 2007.
34. Brisby H: Pathology and possible mechanisms of nervous system response to disc degeneration, *J Bone Joint Surg Am* 88(Suppl 2):68–71, 2006.
35. Browder DA, Childs JD, Cleland JA, et al.: Effectiveness of an extension-oriented treatment approach in a subgroup of subjects with low back pain: a randomized clinical trial, *Phys Ther* 87:1608–1618, 2007.
36. Busscher I, van Dieen JH, van der Veen AJ, et al.: The effects of creep and recovery on the in vitro biomechanical characteristics of human multi-level thoracolumbar spinal segments, *Clin Biomech (Bristol, Avon)* 26(5):438–444, 2011.
37. Calguneri M, Bird HA, Wright V: Changes in joint laxity occurring during pregnancy, *Ann Rheum Dis* 41:126–128, 1982.
38. Castanharo R, Duarte M, McGill S: Corrective sitting strategies: an examination of muscle activity and spine loading, *J Electromyogr Kinesiol* 24(1):114–119, 2014.
39. Cattrysse E, Barbero M, Kool P, et al.: 3D morphometry of the transverse and alar ligaments in the occipito-atlanto-axial complex: an in vitro analysis, *Clin Anat* 20:892–898, 2007.
40. Chancey VC, Ottaviano D, Myers BS, et al.: A kinematic and anthropometric study of the upper cervical spine and the occipital condyles, *J Biomech* 40:1953–1959, 2007.
41. Chelberg MK, Banks GM, Geiger DF, et al.: Identification of heterogeneous cell populations in normal human intervertebral disc, *J Anat* 186:43–53, 1995.
42. Chen C, Lu Y, Kallakuri S, et al.: Distribution of A-delta and C-fiber receptors in the cervical facet joint capsule and their response to stretch, *J Bone Joint Surg Am* 88:1807–1816, 2006.
43. Choi G, Raiturker PP, Kim MJ, et al.: The effect of early isolated lumbar extension exercise program for patients with herniated disc undergoing lumbar discectomy, *Neurosurgery* 57:764–772, 2005.
44. Cholewicki J, Breen A, Popovich Jr JM, et al.: Can biomechanics research lead to more effective treatment of low back pain? A point-counterpoint debate, *J Orthop Sports Phys Ther* 49(6):425–436, 2019.
45. Choufani E, Jouve JL, Pomero V, et al.: Lumbosacral lordosis in fetal spine: genetic or mechanic parameter, *Eur Spine J* 18(9):1342–1348, 2009.
46. Cobian DG, Daehn NS, Anderson PA, et al.: Active cervical and lumbar range of motion during performance of activities of daily living in healthy young adults, *Spine* 38(20):1754–1763, 2013.
47. Cook C, Hegedus E, Showalter C, et al.: Coupling behavior of the cervical spine: a systematic review of the literature, *J Manip Physiol Ther* 29:570–575, 2006.
48. Cook C, Showalter C: A survey on the importance of lumbar coupling biomechanics in physiotherapy practice, *Man Ther* 9:164–172, 2004.
49. Coonrad RW, Murrell GA, Motley G, et al.: A logical coronal pattern classification of 2,000 consecutive idiopathic scoliosis cases based on the scoliosis research society-defined apical vertebra, *Spine* 23:1380–1391, 1998.
50. Coppes MH, Marani E, Thomeer RT, et al.: Innervation of "painful" lumbar discs, *Spine* 22:2342–2349, 1997.
51. Craig BN, Congleton JJ, Beier E, et al.: Occupational risk factors and back injury, *Int J Occup Saf Ergon* 19(3):335–345, 2013.
52. Crisco III JJ, Panjabi MM, Dvorak J: A model of the alar ligaments of the upper cervical spine in axial rotation, *J Biomech* 24:607–614, 1991.
53. Culham EG, Jimenez HA, King CE: Thoracic kyphosis, rib mobility, and lung volumes in normal women and women with osteoporosis, *Spine* 19:1250–1255, 1994.
54. Cyron BM, Hutton WC: Articular tropism and stability of the lumbar spine, *Spine* 5:168–172, 1980.
55. Cyron BM, Hutton WC: The tensile strength of the capsular ligaments of the apophyseal joints, *J Anat* 132(Pt 1):145–150, 1981.
56. Damen L, Buyruk HM, Guler-Uysal F, et al.: Pelvic pain during pregnancy is associated with asymmetric laxity of the sacroiliac joints, *Acta Obstet Gynecol Scand* 80(11):1019–1024, 2001.
57. Damen L, Spoor CW, Snijders CJ, et al.: Does a pelvic belt influence sacroiliac joint laxity? *Clin Biomech (Bristol, Avon)* 17(7):495–498, 2002.
58. Damm P, Reitmaier S, Hahn S, et al.: In vivo hip and lumbar spine implant loads during activities in forward bent postures, *J Biomech* 102:109517, 2020.
59. Danielsson AJ, Hasserius R, Ohlin A, et al.: A prospective study of brace treatment versus observation alone in adolescent idiopathic scoliosis: a follow-up mean of 16 years after maturity, *Spine* 32:2198–2207, 2007.
60. Dar G, Peleg S, Masharawi Y, et al.: Sacroiliac joint bridging: demographical and anatomical aspects, *Spine* 30:E429–E432, 2005.
61. De Carvalho DE, Soave D, Ross K, et al.: Lumbar spine and pelvic posture between standing and sitting: a radiologic investigation including reliability and repeatability of the lumbar lordosis measure, *J Manip Physiol Ther* 33(1):48–55, 2010.
62. Deering RE, Senefeld J, Pashibin T, et al.: Fatigability of the lumbopelvic stabilizing muscles in women 8 and 26 weeks postpartum, *J Womens Health Phys Therap* 42(3):128–138, 2018.
63. Del Pozo-Cruz B, Adsuar JC, Parraca J, et al.: A web-based intervention to improve and prevent low back pain among office workers: a randomized controlled trial. [Reprint in *Arch Prev Riesgos Labor* 16(3):138, 2013; PMID: 23930271], *J Orthop Sports Phys Ther* 42(10):831–841, 2012.
64. Desmoulin GT, Pradhan V, Milner TE: Mechanical aspects of intervertebral disc injury and implications on biomechanics, *Spine* 45(8):E457–E464, 2020.

65. Dolan LA, Weinstein SL: Surgical rates after observation and bracing for adolescent idiopathic scoliosis: an evidence-based review, *Spine* 32:S91–S100, 2007.

66. Drake JD, Aultman CD, McGill SM, et al.: The influence of static axial torque in combined loading on intervertebral joint failure mechanics using a porcine model, *Clin Biomech (Bristol, Avon)* 20(10):1038–1045, 2005.

67. Dreimann M, Hoffmann M, Kossow K, et al.: Scoliosis and chest cage deformity measures predicting impairments in pulmonary function: a cross-sectional study of 492 patients with scoliosis to improve the early identification of patients at risk, *Spine* 39(24):2024–2033, 2014.

68. Dvorak J, Panjabi MM, Novotny JE, et al.: In vivo flexion/extension of the normal cervical spine, *J Orthop Res* 9:828–834, 1991.

69. Dvorak J, Schneider E, Saldinger P, et al.: Biomechanics of the craniocervical region: the alar and transverse ligaments, *J Orthop Res* 6:452–461, 1988.

70. Edmondston SJ, Henne SE, Loh W, et al.: Influence of cranio-cervical posture on three-dimensional motion of the cervical spine, *Man Ther* 10:44–51, 2005.

71. Edmondston SJ, Waller R, Vallin P, et al.: Thoracic spine extension mobility in young adults: influence of subject position and spinal curvature, *J Orthop Sports Phys Ther* 41(4):266–273, 2011.

72. Egund N, Olsson TH, Schmid H, et al.: Movements in the sacroiliac joints demonstrated with roentgen stereophotogrammetry, *Acta Radiol Diagn (Stockh)* 19:833–846, 1978.

73. Eichensehr PH, Sybert DR, Cotton JR: A finite element analysis of sacroiliac joint ligaments in response to different loading conditions, *Spine* 36(22):E1446–E1452, 2011.

74. Elizagaray-Garcia I, Beltran-Alacreu H, Angulo-Díaz S, et al.: Chronic primary headache subjects have greater forward head posture than asymptomatic and episodic primary headache sufferers: systematic review and meta-analysis, *Pain Med* 21(10):2465–2480, 2020.

75. Eno JJ, Boone CR, Bellino MJ, et al.: The prevalence of sacroiliac joint degeneration in asymptomatic adults, *J Bone Joint Surg Am* 97(11):932–936, 2015.

76. Esola MA, McClure PW, Fitzgerald GK, et al.: Analysis of lumbar spine and hip motion during forward bending in subjects with and without a history of low back pain, *Spine* 21:71–78, 1996.

77. Fan Y, Ren Q, To MKT, et al.: Effectiveness of scoliosis-specific exercises for alleviating adolescent idiopathic scoliosis: a systematic review, *BMC Musculoskelet Disord* 21(1):495, 2020.

78. Farfan HF, Huberdeau RM, Dubow HI: Lumbar intervertebral disc degeneration: the influence of geometrical features on the pattern of disc degeneration—a post mortem study, *J Bone Joint Surg Am* 54:492–510, 1972.

79. Farley FA, Li Y, Jong N, et al.: Congenital scoliosis SRS-22 outcomes in children treated with observation, surgery, and VEPTR, *Spine* 39(22):1868, 2014.

80. Farshad M, Kutschke L, Laux CJ, et al.: Extreme long-term outcome of operatively versus conservatively treated patients with adolescent idiopathic scoliosis, *Eur Spine J* 29(8):2084–2090, 2020.

81. Fazey PJ, Song S, Mønsås S, et al.: An MRI investigation of intervertebral disc deformation in response to torsion, *Clin Biomech (Bristol, Avon)* 21:538–542, 2006.

82. Fazey PJ, Song S, Price RI, et al.: Nucleus pulposus deformation in response to rotation at L1-2 and L4-5, *Clin Biomech (Bristol, Avon)* 28(5):586–589, 2013.

83. Fazey PJ, Takasaki H, Singer KP: Nucleus pulposus deformation in response to lumbar spine lateral flexion: an in vivo MRI investigation, *Eur Spine J* 19(7):1115–1120, 2010.

84. Fearing BV, Hernandez PA, Setton LA, et al.: Mechanotransduction and cell biomechanics of the intervertebral disc, *JOR Spine* 1(3), 2018.

85. Feng H, Danfelter M, Strømqvist B, et al.: Extracellular matrix in disc degeneration, *J Bone Joint Surg Am* 88(Suppl 2):25–29, 2006.

86. Fennell AJ, Jones AP, Hukins DW: Migration of the nucleus pulposus within the intervertebral disc during flexion and extension of the spine, *Spine* 21:2753–2757, 1996.

87. Filipec M, Matijevic R: Expert advice about therapeutic exercise during pregnancy reduces the symptoms of sacroiliac dysfunction, *J Perinat Med* 48(6):559–565, 2020.

88. Fritz JM, Thackeray A, Brennan GP, et al.: Exercise only, exercise with mechanical traction, or exercise with over-door traction for patients with cervical radiculopathy, with or without consideration of status on a previously described subgrouping rule: a randomized clinical trial, *J Orthop Sports Phys Ther* 44(2):45–57, 2014.

89. Fujii R, Sakaura H, Mukai Y, et al.: Kinematics of the lumbar spine in trunk rotation: in vivo three-dimensional analysis using magnetic resonance imaging, *Eur Spine J* 16(11):1867–1874, 2007.

90. Fujimori T, Iwasaki M, Nagamoto Y, et al.: Kinematics of the thoracic spine in trunk rotation: in vivo 3-dimensional analysis, *Spine* 37(21):E1318–E1328, 2012.

91. Fujiwara A, Tamai K, Yoshida H, et al.: Anatomy of the iliolumbar ligament, *Clin Orthop Relat Res* 380:167–172, 2000.

92. Garcia AN, Costa LC, da Silva TM, et al.: Effectiveness of back school versus McKenzie exercises in patients with chronic nonspecific low back pain: a randomized controlled trial, *Phys Ther* 93(6):729–747, 2013.

93. George SZ, Fritz JM, Silfies SP, et al.: Interventions for the management of acute and chronic low back pain: Revision 2021, *J Orthop Sports Phys Ther* 51(11):CPG1–CPG60, 2021.

94. Ghezelbash F, Schmidt H, Shirazi-Adl A, et al.: Internal load-sharing in the human passive lumbar spine: review of in vitro and finite element model studies, *J Biomech* 102:109441, 2020.

95. Giles LG, Taylor JR: Human zygapophyseal joint capsule and synovial fold innervation, *Br J Rheumatol* 26:93–98, 1987.

96. Global regional: , and national incidence, prevalence, and years lived with disability for 310 diseases and injuries, 1990-2015: a systematic analysis for the global burden of disease study 2015, *Lancet* 388(10053):1545–1602, 2016.

97. Grobler LJ, Robertson PA, Novotny JE, et al.: Etiology of spondylolisthesis. Assessment of the role played by lumbar facet joint morphology, *Spine* 18:80–91, 1993.

98. Grunhagen T, Wilde G, Soukane DM, et al.: Nutrient supply and intervertebral disc metabolism, *J Bone Joint Surg Am* 88(Suppl 2):30–35, 2006.

99. Guo R, Zhou C, Wang C, et al.: In vivo primary and coupled segmental motions of the healthy female head-neck complex during dynamic head axial rotation, *J Biomech* 123:110513, 2021.

100. Ha TH, Saber-Sheikh K, Moore AP, et al.: Measurement of lumbar spine range of movement and coupled motion using inertial sensors—a protocol validity study, *Man Ther* 18(1):87–91, 2013.

101. Haddox AG, Hausselle J, Azoug A: Changes in segmental mass and inertia during pregnancy: a musculoskeletal model of the pregnant woman, *Gait Posture* 76:389–395, 2020.

102. Haefeli M, Kalberer F, Saegesser D, et al.: The course of macroscopic degeneration in the human lumbar intervertebral disc, *Spine* 31:1522–1531, 2006.

103. Hammer N, Höch A, Klima S, et al.: Effects of cutting the sacrospinous and sacrotuberous ligaments, *Clin Anat* 32(2):231–237, 2019.

104. Hancock MJ, Maher CG, Latimer J, et al.: Systematic review of tests to identify the disc, SIJ or facet joint as the source of low back pain, *Eur Spine J* 16(10):1539–1550, 2007.

105. Hangai M, Kaneoka K, Kuno S, et al.: Factors associated with lumbar intervertebral disc degeneration in the elderly, *Spine J* 8:732–740, 2008.

106. Harris-Hayes M, Sahrmann SA, Van Dillen LR: Relationship between the hip and low back pain in athletes who participate in rotation-related sports [Review, 66 refs], *J Sport Rehabil* 18(1):60–75, 2009.

107. Harrison DD, Janik TJ, Troyanovich SJ, et al.: Comparisons of lordotic cervical spine curvatures to a theoretical ideal model of the static sagittal cervical spine, *Spine* 21:667–675, 1996.

108. Harrison DE, Colloca CJ, Harrison DD, et al.: Anterior thoracic posture increases thoracolumbar disc loading, *Eur Spine J* 14:234–242, 2005.

109. Hartman J: Anatomy and clinical significance of the uncinate process and uncovertebral joint: a comprehensive review [Review], *Clin Anat* 27(3):431–440, 2014.

110. Hartvigsen J, Hancock MJ, Kongsted A, et al.: What low back pain is and why we need to pay attention, *Lancet* 391(10137):2356–2367, 2018.

111. Hayashi K, Yabuki T: Origin of the uncus and of Luschka's joint in the cervical spine, *J Bone Joint Surg Am* 67:788–791, 1985.

112. Hayden AM, Hayes AM, Brechbuhler JL, et al.: The effect of pelvic motion on spinopelvic parameters, *Spine J* 18(1):173–178, 2018.

113. Henry SM, Fritz JM, Trombley AR, et al.: Reliability of a treatment-based classification system for subgrouping people with low back pain, *J Orthop Sports Phys Ther* 42(9):797–805, 2012.

114. Heuer F, Schmidt H, Klezl Z, et al.: Stepwise reduction of functional spinal structures increase range of motion and change lordosis angle, *J Biomech* 40:271–280, 2007.

115. Hidalgo-García C, Lorente AI, Lucha-López O, et al.: The effect of alar ligament transection on the rotation stress test: a cadaveric Study, *Clin Biomech (Bristol, Avon)* 80:105185, 2020.

116. Hill JC, Whitehurst DG, Lewis M, et al.: Comparison of stratified primary care management for low back pain with current best practice (Start Back): a randomised controlled trial, *Lancet* 378(9802):1560–1571, 2011.

117. Hiyama A, Sakai D, Mochida J: Cell signaling pathways related to pain receptors in the degenerated disk, *Global Spine J* 3(3):165–174, 2013.

118. Hodges PW: Hybrid approach to treatment tailoring for low back pain: a proposed model of care, *J Orthop Sports Phys Ther* 49(6):453–463, 2019.

119. Hodges PW, Cholewicki J, Popovich Jr JM, et al.: Building a collaborative model of sacroiliac joint dysfunction and pelvic girdle pain to understand the diverse perspectives of experts, *PM&R* 11(Suppl 1):S11–S23, 2019.

120. Holmes A, Han ZH, Dang GT, et al.: Changes in cervical canal spinal volume during in vitro flexion-extension, *Spine* 21:1313–1319, 1996.

121. Howarth SJ, Gallagher KM, Callaghan JP: Postural influence on the neutral zone of the porcine cervical spine under anterior-posterior shear load, *Med Eng Phys* 35(7):910–918, 2013.

122. Hukins DW, Kirby MC, Sikoryn TA, et al.: Comparison of structure, mechanical properties, and functions of lumbar spinal ligaments, *Spine* 15:787–795, 1990.

123. Iatridis JC, MaClean JJ, Roughley PJ, et al.: Effects of mechanical loading on intervertebral disc metabolism in vivo, *J Bone Joint Surg Am* 88(Suppl 2):41–46, 2006.

124. Ike H, Dorr LD, Trasolini N, et al.: Spine-Pelvis-Hip relationship in the functioning of a total hip replacement, *J Bone Joint Surg Am* 100(18):1606–1615, 2018.

125. Inufusa A, An HS, Lim TH, et al.: Anatomic changes of the spinal canal and intervertebral foramen associated with flexion-extension movement, *Spine* 21:2412–2420, 1996.

126. Ishii T, Mukai Y, Hosono N, et al.: Kinematics of the cervical spine in lateral bending: in vivo three-dimensional analysis, *Spine* 31:155–160, 2006.

127. Ishii T, Mukai Y, Hosono N, et al.: Kinematics of the subaxial cervical spine in rotation: in vivo three-dimensional analysis, *Spine* 29:2826–2831, 2004.

128. Izzo R, Guarnieri G, Guglielmi G, et al.: Biomechanics of the spine. Part I: spinal stability [Review], *Eur J Radiol* 82(1):118–126, 2013.

129. Jaumard NV, Bauman JA, Weisshaar CL, et al.: Contact pressure in the facet joint during sagittal bending of the cadaveric cervical spine, *J Biomech Eng* 133(7):071004, 2011.

130. Jaumard NV, Welch WC, Winkelstein BA: Spinal facet joint biomechanics and mechanotransduction in normal, injury and degenerative conditions [Review], *J Biomech Eng* 133(7):071010, 2011.

131. Jenkins JP, Hickey DS, Zhu XP, et al.: MR imaging of the intervertebral disc: a quantitative study, *Br J Radiol* 58:705–709, 1985.

132. Jensen MC, Brant-Zawadzki MN, Obuchowski N, et al.: Magnetic resonance imaging of the lumbar spine in people without back pain, *N Engl J Med* 331:69–73, 1994.

133. John JD, Saravana Kumar G, Yoganandan N: Cervical spine morphology and ligament property variations: a finite element study of their influence on sagittal bending characteristics, *J Biomech* 85:18–26, 2019.

134. Johnson WE, Evans H, Menage J, et al.: Immunohistochemical detection of Schwann cells in innervated and vascularized human intervertebral discs, *Spine* 26:2550–2557, 2001.

135. Jonas R, Demmelmaier R, Wilke HJ: Influences of functional structures on the kinematic behavior of the cervical spine, *Spine J* 20(12):2014–2024, 2020.

136. Kalmanson OA, Khayatzadeh S, Germanwala A, et al.: Anatomic considerations in headaches associated with cervical sagittal imbalance: a cadaveric biomechanical study, *J Clin Neurosci* 65:140–144, 2019.

137. Karakida O, Ueda H, Ueda M, et al.: Diurnal T2 value changes in the lumbar intervertebral discs, *Clin Radiol* 58:389–392, 2003.

138. Karam M, Bizdikian AJ, Khalil N, et al.: Alterations of 3D acetabular and lower limb parameters in adolescent idiopathic scoliosis, *Eur Spine J* 29(8):2010–2017, 2020.

139. Katzman WB, Wanek L, Shepherd JA, et al.: Age-related hyperkyphosis: its causes, consequences, and management [Review, 63 refs], *J Orthop Sports Phys Ther* 40(6):352–360, 2010.

140. Keller TS, Spengler DM, Hansson TH: Mechanical behavior of the human lumbar spine. I: creep analysis during static compressive loading, *J Orthop Res* 5:467–478, 1987.

141. Kiapour A, Abdelgawad AA, Goel VK, et al.: Relationship between limb length discrepancy and load distribution across the sacroiliac joint—a finite element study, *J Orthop Res* 30(10):1577–1580, 2012.

142. Kim MH, Yi CH, Kwon OY, et al.: Comparison of lumbopelvic rhythm and flexion-relaxation response between 2 different low back pain subtypes, *Spine* 38(15):1260–1267, 2013.

143. Kim SW, Kim TH, Bok DH, et al.: Analysis of cervical spine alignment in currently asymptomatic individuals: prevalence of kyphotic posture and its relationship with other spinopelvic parameters, *Spine J* 18(5):797–810, 2018.

144. Kissling RO, Jacob HA: The mobility of the sacroiliac joint in healthy subjects, *Bull Hosp Jt Dis* 54:158–164, 1996.

145. Kitagawa T, Fujiwara A, Kobayashi N, et al.: Morphologic changes in the cervical neural foramen due to flexion and extension: in vivo imaging study, *Spine* 29:2821–2825, 2004.

146. Kondratek M, Krauss J, Stiller C, et al.: Normative values for active lumbar range of motion in children, *Pediatr Phys Ther* 19:236–244, 2007.

147. Korovessis PG, Stamatakis MV, Baikousis AG: Reciprocal angulation of vertebral bodies in the sagittal plane in an asymptomatic Greek population, *Spine* 23:700–704, 1998.

148. Kranenburg HAR, Tyer R, Schmitt M, et al.: Effects of head and neck positions on blood flow in the vertebral, internal carotid, and intracranial arteries: a systematic review, *J Orthop Sports Phys Ther* 49(10):688–697, 2019.

149. Krismer M, Haid C, Rabl W: The contribution of anulus fibers to torque resistance, *Spine* 21:2551–2557, 1996.

150. Kuai S, Guan X, Zhou W, et al.: Continuous lumbar spine rhythms during level walking, stair climbing and trunk flexion in people with and without lumbar disc herniation, *Gait Posture* 63:296–301, 2018.

151. Kuznia AL, Hernandez AK, Lee LU: Adolescent idiopathic scoliosis: common questions and answers, *Am Fam Physician* 101(1):19–23, 2020.

152. Lam OT, Strenger DM, Chan-Fee M, et al.: Effectiveness of the Mckenzie method of mechanical diagnosis and therapy for treating low back pain: literature review with meta-analysis, *J Orthop Sports Phys Ther* 48(6):476–490, 2018.

153. Laslett M, Aprill CN, McDonald B, et al.: Diagnosis of sacroiliac joint pain: validity of individual provocation tests and composites of tests, *Man Ther* 10:207–218, 2005.

154. Lee TH, Liu TY: Postural and muscular responses while viewing different heights of screen, *Int J Occup Saf Ergon* 19(2):251–258, 2013.

155. Legaspi O, Edmond SL: Does the evidence support the existence of lumbar spine coupled motion? A critical review of the literature, *J Orthop Sports Phys Ther* 37:169–178, 2007.

156. Liebsch C, Graf N, Wilke HJ: The effect of follower load on the intersegmental coupled motion characteristics of the human thoracic spine: an in vitro study using entire rib cage specimens, *J Biomech* 78:36–44, 2018.

157. Liebsch C, Graf N, Wilke HJ: In vitro analysis of kinematics and elastostatics of the human rib cage during thoracic spinal movement for the validation of numerical models, *J Biomech* 94:147–157, 2019.

158. Liebsch C, Graf N, Appelt K, et al.: The rib cage stabilizes the human thoracic spine: an in vitro study using stepwise reduction of rib cage structures, *PLoS One* 12(6):e0178733, 2017.

159. Liew BXW, Ford JJ, Scutari M, et al.: How does individualised physiotherapy work for people with low back pain? A bayesian network analysis using randomised controlled trial data, *PLoS One* 16(10):e0258515, 2021.

160. Li JQ, Kwong WH, Chan YL, et al.: Comparison of in vivo intradiscal pressure between sitting and standing in human lumbar spine: a systematic review and meta-analysis, *Life (Basel)* 12(3), 2022.

161. Li W, Wang S, Xia Q, et al.: Lumbar facet joint motion in patients with degenerative disc disease at affected and adjacent levels: an in vivo biomechanical study, *Spine* 36(10):E629–E637, 2011.

162. Liu D, Yang Y, Yu X, et al.: Effects of specific exercise therapy on adolescent patients with idiopathic scoliosis: a prospective controlled cohort Study, *Spine (Phila Pa 1976)* 45(15):1039–1046, 2020.

163. Liu T, El-Rich M: Effects of nucleus pulposus location on spinal loads and joint centers of rotation and reaction during forward flexion: a combined finite element and musculoskeletal study, *J Biomech* 104:109740, 2020.

164. Liu T, Khalaf K, Adeeb S, et al.: Effects of lumbopelvic rhythm on trunk muscle forces and disc loads during forward flexion: a combined musculoskeletal and finite element simulation study, *J Biomech* 82:116–123, 2019.

165. Lonner BS, Newton P, Betz R, et al.: Operative management of Scheuermann's kyphosis in 78 patients: radiographic outcomes, complications, and technique, *Spine* 32:2644–2652, 2007.

166. Lonstein JE: Scoliosis: surgical versus nonsurgical treatment, *Clin Orthop Relat Res* 443:248–259, 2006.

167. Lonstein JE, Winter RB: The Milwaukee brace for the treatment of adolescent idiopathic scoliosis. A review of one thousand and twenty patients, *J Bone Joint Surg Am* 76:1207–1221, 1994.

168. Lotz JC, Ulrich JA: Innervation, inflammation, and hypermobility may characterize pathologic disc degeneration: review of animal model data, *J Bone Joint Surg Am* 88(Suppl 2):76–82, 2006.

169. Lowe TG, Line BG: Evidence based medicine: analysis of Scheuermann kyphosis, *Spine* 32:S115–S119, 2007.

170. Lu YM, Hutton WC, Gharpuray VM: Do bending, twisting, and diurnal fluid changes in the disc affect the propensity to prolapse? A viscoelastic finite element model, *Spine* 21:2570–2579, 1996.

171. Ludwisiak K, Podgorski M, Biernacka K, et al.: Variation in the morphology of spinous processes in the cervical spine - an objective and parametric assessment based on ct study, *PLoS One [Electronic Resource]* 14(6):e0218885, 2019.

172. Machado LA, de Souza MS, Ferreira PH, et al.: The McKenzie method for low back pain: a systematic review of the literature with a meta-analysis approach, *Spine* 31:E254–E262, 2006.

173. Maeda T, Ueta T, Mori E, et al.: Soft-tissue damage and segmental instability in adult patients with cervical spinal cord injury without major bone injury, *Spine* 37(25):E1560–E1566, 2012.

174. Mahmoud NF, Hassan KA, Abdelmajeed SF, et al.: The relationship between forward head and neck pain: a systematic review and meta-analysis, *Curr Rev Musculoskelet Med* 12(4):562–577, 2019.

175. Mannion AF, Knecht K, Balaban G, et al.: A new skin-surface device for measuring the curvature and global and segmental ranges of motion of the spine: reliability of measurements and comparison with data reviewed from the literature, *Eur Spine J* 13:122–136, 2004.

176. Marks M, Petcharaporn M, Betz RR, et al.: Outcomes of surgical treatment in male versus female adolescent idiopathic scoliosis patients, *Spine* 32:544–549, 2007.

177. Masharawi Y, Rothschild B, Dar G, et al.: Facet orientation in the thoracolumbar spine: three-dimensional anatomic and biomechanical analysis, *Spine* 29:1755–1763, 2004.

178. McGrath MC, Zhang M: Lateral branches of dorsal sacral nerve plexus and the long posterior sacroiliac ligament, *Surg Radiol Anat* 27:327–330, 2005.

179. McLean L: The effect of postural correction on muscle activation amplitudes recorded from the cervicobrachial region, *J Electromyogr Kinesiol* 15:527–535, 2005.

180. Mekhail N, Saweris Y, Sue Mehanny D, et al.: Diagnosis of sacroiliac joint pain: predictive value of three diagnostic clinical tests, *Pain Pract* 21(2):204–214, 2021.

181. Mellor FE, Thomas PW, Thompson P, et al.: Proportional lumbar spine inter-vertebral motion patterns: a comparison of patients with chronic, non-specific low back pain and healthy controls, *Eur Spine J* 23(10):2059–2067, 2014.

182. Mens JM, Damen L, Snijders CJ, et al.: The mechanical effect of a pelvic belt in patients with pregnancy-related pelvic pain, *Clin Biomech (Bristol, Avon)* 21(2):122–127, 2006.

183. Mercer S, Bogduk N: Intra-articular inclusions of the cervical synovial joints, *Br J Rheumatol* 32:705–710, 1993.

184. Mercer S, Bogduk N: The ligaments and annulus fibrosus of human adult cervical intervertebral discs, *Spine* 24:619–626, 1999.

185. Miele VJ, Panjabi MM, Benzel EC: Anatomy and biomechanics of the spinal column and cord, *Handb Clin Neurol* 109:31–43, 2012.

186. Mika A, Unnithan VB, Mika P: Differences in thoracic kyphosis and in back muscle strength in women with bone loss due to osteoporosis, *Spine* 30:241–246, 2005.

187. Mikkonen P, Leino-Arjas P, Remes J, et al.: Is smoking a risk factor for low back pain in adolescents? A prospective cohort study, *Spine* 33:527–532, 2008.

188. Miller JA, Schmatz C, Schultz AB: Lumbar disc degeneration: correlation with age, sex, and spine level in 600 autopsy specimens, *Spine* 13:173–178, 1988.

189. Monticone M, Ambrosini E, Cazzaniga D, et al.: Active self-correction and task-oriented exercises reduce spinal deformity and improve quality of life in subjects with mild adolescent idiopathic scoliosis. results of a randomised controlled trial, *Eur Spine J* 23(6):1204–1214, 2014.

190. Moore RJ: The vertebral endplate: disc degeneration, disc regeneration, *Eur Spine J* 15(Suppl 3):S333–S337, 2006.

191. Muhle C, Resnick D, Ahn JM, et al.: In vivo changes in the neuroforaminal size at flexion-extension and axial rotation of the cervical spine in healthy persons examined using kinematic magnetic resonance imaging, *Spine* 26:E287–E293, 2001.

192. Nachemson A: Lumbar intradiscal pressure. Experimental studies on post-mortem material, *Acta Orthop Scand Suppl* 43:1–104, 1960.

193. Nachemson A: Some mechanical properties of the third lumbar interlaminar ligament (ligamentum flavum), *J Biomech* 1:211–220, 1968.

194. Nachemson A: The load on lumbar disks in different positions of the body, *Clin Orthop Relat Res* 45:107–122, 1966.

195. Nagamoto Y, Ishii T, Iwasaki M, et al.: Three-dimensional motion of the uncovertebral joint during head rotation, *J Neurosurg Spine* 17(4):327–333, 2012.

196. Nava-Bringas TI, Romero-Fierro LO, Trani-Chagoya YP, et al.: Stabilization exercises versus flexion exercises in degenerative spondylolisthesis: a randomized controlled trial, *Phys Ther* 101(8), 2021.

197. Negrini S, Donzelli S, Aulisa AG, et al.: 2016 SOSORT guidelines: orthopaedic and rehabilitation treatment of idiopathic scoliosis during growth, *Scoliosis Spinal Disord* 13:3, 2018.

198. Negrini A, Vanossi M, Donzelli S, et al.: Spinal coronal and sagittal balance in 584 healthy individuals during growth: normal plumb line values and their correlation with radiographic measurements, *Phys Ther* 99(12):1712–1718, 2019.

199. Nelson JM, Walmsley RP, Stevenson JM: Relative lumbar and pelvic motion during loaded spinal flexion/extension, *Spine* 20:199–204, 1995.

200. Neumann DA, Soderberg GL, Cook TM: Electromyographic analysis of hip abductor musculature in healthy right-handed persons, *Phys Ther* 69:431–440, 1989.

201. Newman JM, Shah NV, Diebo BG, et al.: The top 100 classic papers on adolescent idiopathic scoliosis in the past 25 years: a Bibliometric Analysis of the Orthopaedic Literature, *Spine Deform* 8(1):5–16, 2020.

202. Ng JK, Kippers V, Richardson CA, et al.: Range of motion and lordosis of the lumbar spine: reliability of measurement and normative values, *Spine* 26:53–60, 2001.

203. Niosi CA, Oxland TR: Degenerative mechanics of the lumbar spine, *Spine J* 4:202S–208S, 2004.

204. O'Connell GD, Sen S, Elliott DM: Human annulus fibrosus material properties from biaxial testing and constitutive modeling are altered with degeneration, *Biomech Model Mechanobiol* 11:493–503, 2012.

205. Oda H, Matsuzaki H, Tokuhashi Y, et al.: Degeneration of intervertebral discs due to smoking: experimental assessment in a rat-smoking model, *J Orthop Sci* 9:135–141, 2004.

206. Odeh K, Wu W, Taylor B, et al.: In-Vitro 3d Analysis of sacroiliac joint kinematics: primary and coupled motions, *Spine* 46(8):E467–E473, 2021.

207. Ohman AM, Beckung ER: A pilot study on changes in passive range of motion in the cervical spine, for children aged 0-5 years, *Physiother Theory Pract* 29(6):457–460, 2013.

208. Olson KA: *Manual physical therapy of the spine,* ed 3, St Louis, 2021, Elsevier.

209. Ordway NR, Seymour R, Donelson RG, et al.: Cervical sagittal range-of-motion analysis using three methods. Cervical range-of-motion device, 3D space, and radiography, *Spine* 22:501–508, 1997.

210. Ordway NR, Seymour RJ, Donelson RG, et al.: Cervical flexion, extension, protrusion, and retraction. A radiographic segmental analysis, *Spine* 24:240–247, 1999.

211. Osmotherly PG, Rivett DA, Mercer SR: Revisiting the clinical anatomy of the alar ligaments, *Eur Spine J* 22(1):60–64, 2013.

212. Osmotherly PG, Rivett D, Rowe LJ: Toward understanding normal craniocervical rotation occurring during the rotation stress test for the alar ligaments, *Phys Ther* 93(7):986–992, 2013.

213. Owen PJ, Miller CT, Mundell NL, et al.: Which specific modes of exercise training are most effective for treating low back pain? Network meta-analysis, *Br J Sports Med* 54(21):1279–1287, 2020.

214. Pan F, Arshad R, Zander T, et al.: The effect of age and sex on the cervical range of motion - a systematic review and meta-analysis, *J Biomech* 75:13–27, 2018.

215. Pan F, Firouzabadi A, Reitmaier S, et al.: The shape and mobility of the thoracic spine in asymptomatic adults - a systematic review of in vivo studies, *J Biomech* 78:21–35, 2018.

216. Pan F, Firouzabadi A, Zander T, et al.: Sex-dependent differences in lumbo-pelvic coordination for different lifting tasks: a study on asymptomatic adults, *J Biomech* 102:109505, 2020.

217. Panjabi M, Dvorak J, Crisco III JJ, et al.: Effects of alar ligament transection on upper cervical spine rotation, *J Orthop Res* 9:584–593, 1991.

218. Panjabi MM, Oxland T, Takata K, et al.: Articular facets of the human spine. Quantitative three-dimensional anatomy, *Spine* 18:1298–1310, 1993.

219. Patel AA, Spiker WR, Daubs M, et al.: Evidence for an inherited predisposition to lumbar disc disease, *J Bone Joint Surg Am* 93(3):225–229, 2011.

220. N92 Peacock M, Douglas S, Nair P: Neural mobilization in low back and radicular pain: a systematic review, *J Man Manip Ther* 1–9, 2022.

221. Pearcy M, Portek I, Shepherd J: The effect of low-back pain on lumbar spinal movements measured by three-dimensional x-ray analysis, *Spine* 10:150–153, 1985.

222. Pearcy MJ, Tibrewal SB: Axial rotation and lateral bending in the normal lumbar spine measured by three-dimensional radiography, *Spine* 9:582–587, 1984.

223. Pecha MD: Herniated nucleus pulposus as a result of emesis in a 20-yr-old man, *Am J Phys Med Rehabil* 83:327–330, 2004.

224. Peng B, Hao J, Hou S, et al.: Possible pathogenesis of painful intervertebral disc degeneration, *Spine* 31:560–566, 2006.

225. Penning L: Normal movements of the cervical spine, *AJR Am J Roentgenol* 130:317–326, 1978.

226. Pesenti S, Lafage R, Lafage V, et al.: Cervical facet orientation varies with age in children: an MRI study, *J Bone Joint Surg Am* 100(9):e57, 2018.

227. Pfirrmann CW, Metzdorf A, Elfering A, et al.: Effect of aging and degeneration on disc volume and shape: a quantitative study in asymptomatic volunteers, *J Orthop Res* 24:1086–1094, 2006.

228. Podichetty VK: The aging spine: the role of inflammatory mediators in intervertebral disc degeneration, *Cell Mol Biol* 53:4–18, 2007.

229. Poilliot AJ, Zwirner J, Doyle T, et al.: A Systematic review of the normal sacroiliac joint anatomy and adjacent tissues for pain physicians, *Pain Physician* 22(4):E247–e274, 2019.

230. Pollintine P, Dolan P, Tobias JH, et al.: Intervertebral disc degeneration can lead to "stress-shielding" of the anterior vertebral body: a cause of osteoporotic vertebral fracture? *Spine* 29:774–782, 2004.

231. Pool-Goudzwaard A, Hoek vD, Mulder P, et al.: The iliolumbar ligament: its influence on stability of the sacroiliac joint, *Clin Biomech (Bristol, Avon)* 18:99–105, 2003.

232. Pope MH, Panjabi M: Biomechanical definitions of spinal instability, *Spine* 10(3):255–256, 1985.

233. Przybyla A, Pollintine P, Bedzinski R, et al.: Outer annulus tears have less effect than endplate fracture on stress distributions inside intervertebral discs: relevance to disc degeneration, *Clin Biomech (Bristol, Avon)* 21:1013–1019, 2006.

234. Pye SR, Reid DM, Smith R, et al.: Radiographic features of lumbar disc degeneration and self-reported back pain, *J Rheumatol* 31:753–758, 2004.

235. Qu N, Graven-Nielsen T, Lindstrom R, et al.: Recurrent neck pain patients exhibit altered joint motion pattern during cervical flexion and extension movements, *Clin Biomech* 71:125–132, 2020.

236. Quek J, Pua YH, Clark RA, et al.: Effects of thoracic kyphosis and forward head posture on cervical range of motion in older adults, *Man Ther* 18(1):65–71, 2013.

237. Rajasekaran S, Babu JN, Arun R, et al.: ISSLS prize winner: a study of diffusion in human lumbar discs: a serial magnetic resonance imaging study documenting the influence of the endplate on diffusion in normal and degenerate discs, *Spine* 29:2654–2667, 2004.

238. Rajasekaran S, Bajaj N, Tubaki V, et al.: ISSLS Prize winner: the anatomy of failure in lumbar disc herniation: an in vivo, multimodal, prospective study of 181 subjects, *Spine* 38(17):1491–1500, 2013.

239. Rajasekaran S, Vidyadhara S, Subbiah M, et al.: ISSLS prize winner: a study of effects of in vivo mechanical forces on human lumbar discs with scoliotic disc as a biological model: results from serial postcontrast diffusion studies, histopathology and biochemical analysis of twenty-one human lumbar scoliotic discs, *Spine* 35(21):1930–1943, 2010.

240. Reeves NP, Cholewicki J, van Dieën JH, et al.: Are stability and instability relevant concepts for back pain? *J Orthop Sports Phys Ther* 49(6):415–424, 2019.

241. Reichmann S: The postnatal development of form and orientation of the lumbar intervertebral joint surfaces, *Z Anat Entwicklungsgesch* 133:102–123, 1971.

242. Richards KV, Beales DJ, Smith AL, et al.: Is neck posture subgroup in late adolescence a risk factor for persistent neck pain in young adults? A Prospective Study, *Phys Ther* 101(3), 2021.

243. Riddle DL, Freburger JK: Evaluation of the presence of sacroiliac joint region dysfunction using a combination of tests: a multicenter intertester reliability study, *Phys Ther* 82:772–781, 2002.

244. Riley SP, Swanson BT, Cleland JA: The why, where, and how clinical reasoning model for the evaluation and treatment of patients with low back pain, *Braz J Phys Ther* 25(4):407–414, 2021.

245. Roberts S, Evans H, Trivedi J, et al.: Histology and pathology of the human intervertebral disc, *J Bone Joint Surg Am* 88(Suppl 2):10–14, 2006.

246. Rodriguez-Soto AE, Jaworski R, Jensen A, et al.: Effect of load carriage on lumbar spine kinematics, *Spine* 38(13):E783–E791, 2013.

247. Rohlmann A, Consmüller T, Dreischarf M, et al.: Measurement of the number of lumbar spinal movements in the sagittal plane in a 24-hour period, *Eur Spine J* 23(11):2375–2384, 2014.

248. Rosatelli AL, Agur AM, Chhaya S: Anatomy of the interosseous region of the sacroiliac joint, *J Orthop Sports Phys Ther* 36:200–208, 2006.

249. Sahrmann SA: *Diagnosis and treatment of movement impairment syndromes,* St Louis, 2002, Mosby.

250. Saldinger P, Dvorak J, Rahn BA, et al.: Histology of the alar and transverse ligaments, *Spine* 15:257–261, 1990.

251. Salem W, Lenders C, Mathieu J, et al.: In vivo three-dimensional kinematics of the cervical spine during maximal axial rotation, *Man Ther* 18(4):339–344, 2013.

252. Sanchis-Sánchez E, Lluch-Girbés E, Guillart-Castells P, et al.: Effectiveness of mechanical diagnosis and therapy in patients with non-specific chronic low back pain: a literature review with meta-analysis, *Braz J Phys Ther* 25(2):117–134, 2021.

253. Sarwark JF, Castelein RM, Maqsood A, et al.: The biomechanics of induction in adolescent idiopathic scoliosis: theoretical factors, *J Bone Joint Surg Am* 101(6):e22, 2019.

254. Scannell JP, McGill SM: Lumbar posture—should it, and can it, be modified? A study of passive tissue stiffness and lumbar position during activities of daily living, *Phys Ther* 83:907–917, 2003.

255. Schlager B, Krump F, Boettinger J, et al.: Characteristic morphological patterns within adolescent idiopathic scoliosis may be explained by mechanical loading, *Eur Spine J* 27(9):2184–2191, 2018.

256. Schlager B, Niemeyer F, Galbusera F, et al.: Asymmetrical intrapleural pressure distribution: a cause for scoliosis? A computational analysis, *Eur J Appl Physiol* 118(7):1315–1329, 2018.

257. Schmidt H, Heuer F, Claes L, et al.: The relation between the instantaneous center of rotation and facet joint forces—a finite element analysis, *Clin Biomech (Bristol, Avon)* 23:270–278, 2008.

258. Schmidt H, Kettler A, Heuer F, et al.: Intradiscal pressure, shear strain, and fiber strain in the intervertebral disc under combined loading, *Spine* 32:748–755, 2007.

259. Schneider BJ, Rosati R, Zheng P, et al.: Challenges in diagnosing sacroiliac joint pain: a narrative review, *PM&R* 11(Suppl 1):S40–S45, 2019.

260. Seacrist T, Saffioti J, Balasubramanian S, et al.: Passive cervical spine flexion: the effect of age and gender, *Clin Biomech (Bristol, Avon)* 27(4):326–333, 2012.

261. Sengupta DKM, Fan HP: The basis of mechanical instability in degenerative disc disease: a cadaveric study of abnormal motion versus load distribution, *Spine* 39(13):1032–1043, 2014.

262. Setton LA, Chen J: Mechanobiology of the intervertebral disc and relevance to disc degeneration, *J Bone Joint Surg Am* 88(Suppl 2):52–57, 2006.

263. Shibata Y, Shirai Y, Miyamoto M: The aging process in the sacroiliac joint: helical computed tomography analysis, *J Orthop Sci* 7:12–18, 2002.

264. Shirazi-Adl A, Drouin G: Load-bearing role of facets in a lumbar segment under sagittal plane loadings, *J Biomech* 20:601–613, 1987.

265. Shojaei I, Salt EG, Bazrgari B: A prospective study of lumbo-pelvic coordination in patients with non-chronic low back pain, *J Biomech* 102:109306, 2020.

266. Simopoulos TT, Manchikanti L, Singh V, et al.: A systematic evaluation of prevalence and diagnostic accuracy of sacroiliac joint interventions [Review], *Pain Physician* 15(3):E305–E344, 2012.

267. Simpson AK, Biswas D, Emerson JW, et al.: Quantifying the effects of age, gender, degeneration, and adjacent level degeneration on cervical spine range of motion using multivariate analyses, *Spine* 33:183–186, 2008.

268. Sjodahl J, Gutke A, Ghaffari G, et al.: Response of the muscles in the pelvic floor and the lower lateral abdominal wall during the active straight leg raise in women with and without pelvic girdle pain: an experimental study, *Clin Biomech* 35:49–55, 2016.

269. Sizer Jr PS, Brismee JM, Cook C: Coupling behavior of the thoracic spine: a systematic review of the literature, *J Manip Physiol Ther* 30:390–399, 2007.

270. Snijders CJ, Hermans PF, Kleinrensink GJ: Functional aspects of cross-legged sitting with special attention to piriformis muscles and sacroiliac joints, *Clin Biomech (Bristol, Avon)* 21:116–121, 2006.

271. Snijders CJ, Ribbers MT, de Bakker HV, et al.: EMG recordings of abdominal and back muscles in various standing postures: validation of a biomechanical model on sacroiliac joint stability, *J Electromyogr Kinesiol* 8:205–214, 1998.

272. Sorensen IG, Jacobsen P, Gyntelberg F, et al.: Occupational and other predictors of herniated lumbar disc disease—a 33-year follow-up in the Copenhagen male study, *Spine* 36(19):1541–1546, 2011.

273. Sponseller PD: Bracing for adolescent idiopathic scoliosis in practice today, *J Pediatr Orthop* 31(1:Suppl 69), 2011.

274. Stadnik TW, Lee RR, Coen HL, et al.: Annular tears and disk herniation: prevalence and contrast enhancement on MR images in the absence of low back pain or sciatica, *Radiology* 206:49–55, 1998.

275. Standring S: *Gray's anatomy: the anatomical basis of clinical practice*, ed 42, St Louis, 2021, Elsevier.

276. Steffen T, Rubin RK, Baramki HG, et al.: A new technique for measuring lumbar segmental motion in vivo. Method, accuracy, and preliminary results, *Spine* 22:156–166, 1997.

277. Stokes IA, Gardner-Morse M: Muscle activation strategies and symmetry of spinal loading in the lumbar spine with scoliosis, *Spine* 29:2103–2107, 2004.

278. Sturesson B, Selvik G, Uden A: Movements of the sacroiliac joints. A roentgen stereophotogrammetric analysis, *Spine* 14:162–165, 1989.

279. Svedmark P, Tullberg T, Noz ME, et al.: Three-dimensional movements of the lumbar spine facet joints and segmental movements: in vivo examinations of normal subjects with a new non-invasive method, *Eur Spine J* 21(4):599–605, 2012.

280. Swinkels RA, Swinkels-Meewisse IE: Normal values for cervical range of motion, *Spine* 39(5):362–367, 2014.

281. Szadek KM, Hoogland PV, Zuurmond WW, et al.: Possible nociceptive structures in the sacroiliac joint cartilage: an immunohistochemical study, *Clin Anat* 23(2):192–198, 2010.

282. Tafazzol A, Arjmand N, Shirazi-Adl A, et al.: Lumbopelvic rhythm during forward and backward sagittal trunk rotations: combined in vivo measurement with inertial tracking device and biomechanical modeling, *Clin Biomech (Bristol, Avon)* 29(1):7–13, 2014.

283. Thawrani DP, Agabegi SS, Asghar F: Diagnosing sacroiliac joint pain, *J Am Acad Orthop Surg* 27(3):85–93, 2019.

284. Tisherman R, Hartman R, Hariharan K, et al.: Biomechanical contribution of the alar ligaments to upper cervical stability, *J Biomech* 99:109508, 2020.

285. Tousignant M, Smeesters C, Breton AM, et al.: Criterion validity study of the cervical range of motion (CROM) device for rotational range of motion on healthy adults, *J Orthop Sports Phys Ther* 36:242–248, 2006.

286. Toyohara R, Kurosawa D, Hammer N, et al.: Finite element analysis of load transition on sacroiliac joint during bipedal walking, *Sci Rep* 10(1):13683, 2020.

287. Troke M, Moore AP, Maillardet FJ, et al.: A normative database of lumbar spine ranges of motion, *Man Ther* 10:198–206, 2005.

288. Trudelle-Jackson E, Fleisher LA, Borman N, et al.: Lumbar spine flexion and extension extremes of motion in women of different age and racial groups: the WIN Study, *Spine* 35(16):1539–1544, 2010.

289. Tsantrizos A, Ito K, Aebi M, et al.: Internal strains in healthy and degenerated lumbar intervertebral discs, *Spine* 30:2129–2137, 2005.

290. Tubbs RS, Rompala OJ, Verma K, et al.: Analysis of the uncinate processes of the cervical spine: an anatomical study, *J Neurosurg Spine* 16(4):402–407, 2012.

291. Tyrrell AR, Reilly T, Troup JD: Circadian variation in stature and the effects of spinal loading, *Spine* 10:161–164, 1985.

292. Urban JP, McMullin JF: Swelling pressure of the lumbar intervertebral discs: influence of age, spinal level, composition, and degeneration, *Spine* 13:179–187, 1988.

293. Van der Plaats A, Veldhuizen AG, Verkerke GJ: Numerical simulation of asymmetrically altered growth as initiation mechanism of scoliosis, *Ann Biomed Eng* 35:1206–1215, 2007.

294. van Wingerden JP, Vleeming A, Buyruk HM, et al.: Stabilization of the sacroiliac joint in vivo: verification of muscular contribution to force closure of the pelvis, *Eur Spine J* 13:199–205, 2004.

295. van Wingerden JP, Vleeming A, Ronchetti I: Differences in standing and forward bending in women with chronic low back or pelvic girdle pain: indications for physical compensation strategies, *Spine* 33(11):E334–E341, 2008.

296. Vernon-Roberts B, Moore RJ, Fraser RD: The natural history of age-related disc degeneration: the pathology and sequelae of tears, *Spine* 32:2797–2804, 2007.

297. Vibert BT, Sliva CD, Herkowitz HN: Treatment of instability and spondylolisthesis: surgical versus nonsurgical treatment, *Clin Orthop Relat Res* 443:222–227, 2006.

298. Videman T, Levalahti E, Battie MC: The effects of anthropometrics, lifting strength, and physical activities in disc degeneration, *Spine* 32:1406–1413, 2007.

299. Vilensky JA, O'Connor BL, Fortin JD, et al.: Histologic analysis of neural elements in the human sacroiliac joint, *Spine* 27:1202–1207, 2002.

300. Vleeming A, Albert HB, Ostgaard HC, et al.: European guidelines for the diagnosis and treatment of pelvic girdle pain Review, 155 refs, *Eur Spine J* 17(6):794–819, 2008.

301. Vleeming A, Pool-Goudzwaard AL, Stoeckart R, et al.: The posterior layer of the thoracolumbar fascia. Its function in load transfer from spine to legs, *Spine* 20:753–758, 1995.

302. Vleeming A, Schuenke M: Form and force closure of the sacroiliac joints, *PM&R* 11(Suppl 1):S24–s31, 2019.

303. Vleeming A, Schuenke MD, Masi AT, et al.: The sacroiliac joint: an overview of its anatomy, function and potential clinical implications [Review], *J Anat* 221(6):537–567, 2012.

304. Vleeming A, Volkers AC, Snijders CJ, et al.: Relation between form and function in the sacroiliac joint. Part II: biomechanical aspects, *Spine* 15:133–136, 1990.

305. Waddell G, Somerville D, Henderson I, et al.: Objective clinical evaluation of physical impairment in chronic low back pain (see comment), *Spine* 17:617–628, 1992.

306. N91 Wade K, Berger-Roscher N, Saggese T, et al.: How annulus defects can act as initiation sites for herniation, *Eur Spine J* 31(6):1487–1500, 2022.

307. Wagner H, Liebetrau A, Schinowski D, et al.: Spinal lordosis optimizes the requirements for a stable erect posture, *Theor Biol Med Model* 9(13), 2012.

308. Waris E, Eskelin M, Hermunen H, et al.: Disc degeneration in low back pain: a 17-year follow-up study using magnetic resonance imaging, *Spine* 32:681–684, 2007.

309. Watkins R, 4th, Watkins 3rd R, Williams L, et al.: Stability provided by the sternum and rib cage in the thoracic spine, *Spine* 30:1283–1286, 2005.

310. Weinstein SL, Dolan LA, Wright JG, et al.: Effects of bracing in adolescents with idiopathic scoliosis, *N Engl J Med* 369(16):1512–1521, 2013.

311. Werneke MW, Hart DL, Cutrone G, et al.: Association between directional preference and centralization in patients with low back pain, *J Orthop Sports Phys Ther* 41(1):22–31, 2011.

312. Westrick ER, Ward WT: Adolescent idiopathic scoliosis: 5-year to 20-year evidence-based surgical results, *J Pediatr Orthop* 31(1:Suppl 8), 2011.

313. Widmer J, Fornaciari P, Senteler M, et al.: Kinematics of the spine under healthy and degenerative conditions: a systematic review, *Ann Biomed Eng* 47(7):1491–1522, 2019.

314. Wilke HJ, Herkommer A, Werner K, et al.: In vitro analysis of the segmental flexibility of the thoracic spine, *PLoS One* 12(5):e0177823, 2017.

315. Wilke HJ, Neef P, Caimi M, et al.: New in vivo measurements of pressures in the intervertebral disc in daily life, *Spine* 24:755–762, 1999.

316. Willard FH, Vleeming A, Schuenke MD, et al.: The thoracolumbar fascia: anatomy, function and clinical considerations [Review], *J Anat* 221(6):507–536, 2012.

317. Williams PC: Examination and conservative treatment for disk lesions of the lower spine, *Clin Orthop Relat Res* 5:28–40, 1955.

318. Yahia LH, Garzon S, Strykowski H, et al.: Ultrastructure of the human interspinous ligament and ligamentum flavum. A preliminary study, *Spine* 15:262–268, 1990.

319. Yamamoto I, Panjabi MM, Oxland TR, et al.: The role of the iliolumbar ligament in the lumbosacral junction, *Spine* 15:1138–1141, 1990.

320. Yang B, O'Connell GD: Intervertebral disc swelling maintains strain homeostasis throughout the annulus fibrosus: a finite element analysis of healthy and degenerated discs, *Acta Biomater* 100:61–74, 2019.

321. Yang G, Marras WS, Best TM: The biochemical response to biomechanical tissue loading on the low back during physical work exposure, *Clin Biomech (Bristol, Avon)* 26(5):431–437, 2011.

322. Yu J, Fairbank JC, Roberts S, et al.: The elastic fiber network of the anulus fibrosus of the normal and scoliotic human intervertebral disc, *Spine* 30:1815–1820, 2005.

323. Yukawa Y, Kato F, Suda K, et al.: Age-related changes in osseous anatomy, alignment, and range of motion of the cervical spine. Part I: radiographic data from over 1,200 asymptomatic subjects, *Eur Spine J* 21(8):1492–1498, 2012.

324. Zander T, Bashkuev M, Schmidt H: Are there characteristic motion patterns in the lumbar spine during flexion? *J Biomech* 70:77–81, 2018.

325. Zhang C, Mannen EM, Sis HL, et al.: Moment-Rotation behavior of intervertebral joints in flexion-extension, lateral bending, and axial rotation at all levels of the human spine: a structured review and meta-regression analysis, *J Biomech* 100:109579, 2020.

326. Zhang QH, Teo EC, Ng HW, et al.: Finite element analysis of moment-rotation relationships for human cervical spine, *J Biomech* 39:189–193, 2006.

327. Zhao F, Pollintine P, Hole BD, et al.: Discogenic origins of spinal instability, *Spine* 30:2621–2630, 2005.

STUDY QUESTIONS

1. Describe the osteokinematics at the craniocervical region during cranial protraction (from a fully retracted position). Which tissues, if normal, would become relatively slackened in a position of full protraction?

2. How could the natural elasticity of the ligamentum flavum protect the interbody joint against excessive and potentially damaging compression forces?

3. Based on moment arm length alone, which connective tissue most effectively limits flexion torque within the thoracolumbar region?

4. Are the intertransverse ligaments between L3 and L4 positioned to limit sagittal plane rotation? If so, which motion?

5. Describe the arthrokinematics at the apophyseal joints between L2 and L3 during full axial rotation to the right.

6. From an anterior to posterior direction, list, in order, the connective tissues that exist at the atlanto-axial joint. Start anteriorly with the anterior arch of the atlas, and finish posteriorly at the tips of the spinous processes. Be sure to include the dens and transverse ligament of the atlas in your answer.

7. Define nutation and counternutation at the sacroiliac joint.

8. Which ligament of the sacroiliac joint is slackened by the motion of nutation? Why?

9. Persons with a history of a posterior herniated disc are usually advised against lifting a large load held in front the body, especially with a flexed lumbar spine. How would you justify this advice?

10. Describe the articulations between the sixth rib and the midthoracic spine.

11. Explain how a severely degenerated disc can lead to osteophyte formation in the midcervical spine.

12. Assume the subject depicted in Fig. 9.10C has increased lumbar lordosis caused primarily by tightened (shortened) hip flexor muscles. Describe the possible negative kinesiologic or biomechanical consequences that may result within the lumbar and lumbosacral regions.

13. Describe the mechanical role of the annulus fibrosis in distributing compression forces across the interbody joint.

14. With the visual aid of Fig. III-1 (in Appendix III, Part A), explain why a severe posterior herniated disc between the bodies of L4 and L5 can compress the L^4 spinal nerve root, but possibly L^5 and all sacral nerve roots as well.

15. Describe the general transition in spatial orientation of the articular surfaces of the apophyseal joints, starting with the atlanto-axial joint and finishing with the lumbosacral junction. Explain how this transition influences the predominant kinematics across the various regions. Include in your answer the kinematics associated with the most often expressed spinal coupling pattern within the mid and lower craniocervical region.

16. Describe arthrokinematics at the apophyseal joints between C4 and C5 during full extension.

17. Assume the active motion of full craniocervical rotation to the left. Explain the most likely change in size (area) of the left C5-C6 intervertebral foramen.

Answers to the study questions are available in the accompanying enhanced eBook version included with the print purchase of this textbook.

Additional Video Educational Content

A Fluoroscopic Observation of Flexion and Extension of the Craniocervical Region in an Adult Male.

All videos in this chapter are included in the accompanying enhanced eBook version included with the print purchase of this textbook.

Chapter

10

Axial Skeleton: Muscle and Joint Interactions

DONALD A. NEUMANN, PT, PhD, FAPTA

GUY G. SIMONEAU, PT, PhD, FAPTA

The osteology and arthrology of the axial skeleton are presented in Chapter 9. Chapter 10 now focuses on the many muscle and joint interactions occurring within the axial skeleton. The muscles control posture and stabilize the axial skeleton, protect the spinal cord and internal organs, generate intrathoracic and intra-abdominal pressures for many physiologic functions, produce torques required for movement of the body as a whole, and, lastly, furnish fine mobility to the head and neck for optimal placement of the eyes, ears, nose, and organs of equilibrium. It is striking that many of the muscles within the axial skeleton actively participate in several of these functions simultaneously.

The anatomic structure of the muscles within the axial skeleton varies considerably in length, shape, fiber direction, cross-sectional area, and leverage across the underlying joints. Such variability reflects the broad range of functional demands placed on the musculature, from manually lifting and transporting heavy objects to

producing subtle motions of the head for accenting a lively conversation.

Muscles within the axial skeleton cross multiple regions of the body. The trapezius muscle, for example, attaches to the clavicle and the scapula within the appendicular skeleton and to the vertebral column and the cranium within the axial skeleton. These extensive attachments have clinical relevance, as protective guarding of the upper trapezius due to an underlying painful condition can affect the quality of motion throughout both the upper extremity and craniocervical region.

The primary aim of this chapter is to elucidate the structure and function of the muscles within the axial skeleton. This information is essential when considering the clinical examination and management of possible impairments associated with posture, tissue extensibility, muscle strength or endurance, and movement in people with neck or back pain.

Muscles associated with ventilation and mastication (chewing) are presented in Chapter 11.

INNERVATION OF THE MUSCLES AND JOINTS WITHIN THE TRUNK AND CRANIOCERVICAL REGIONS

An understanding of the organization of the innervation of the craniocervical and trunk muscles begins with an appreciation of the formation of a typical *spinal nerve root* (Fig. 10.1). Each spinal nerve root is formed by the union of ventral and dorsal *nerve roots:* the *ventral nerve roots* contain primarily "outgoing" (efferent) axons

that supply motor commands to muscles and other effector organs associated with the autonomic nervous system. The *dorsal nerve roots* contain primarily "incoming" (afferent) dendrites, with the cell body of the neuron located in an adjacent *dorsal root ganglion.* Sensory neurons transmit information to the spinal cord from the muscles, joints, skin, and other organs associated with the autonomic nervous system.

Near or within the intervertebral foramen, the ventral and dorsal nerve roots join to form a *spinal nerve root.* (Spinal nerve roots are often described as "mixed," emphasizing that they contain varying combinations of *both* sensory and motor fibers.) The spinal nerve root thickens due to the merging of the motor and sensory neurons and the presence of the dorsal root ganglion.

The vertebral column contains 31 pairs of spinal nerve roots: 8 cervical, 12 thoracic, 5 lumbar, 5 sacral, and 1 coccygeal. The abbreviations *C, T, L,* and *S* with the appropriate superscript number designate each spinal nerve root—for example, C^5 and T^6. The cervical region has seven vertebrae but eight cervical nerve roots. The suboccipital nerve (C^1) leaves the spinal cord between the occipital bone and the atlas (C1). Similarly, the rest of the cervical nerve roots, down to C^7, exit the spinal cord just superior or cranial to their respective vertebral bodies. The C^8 spinal nerve root exits the spinal cord between the seventh cervical vertebra and the first thoracic vertebra. Spinal nerve roots T^1 and below exit the spinal cord just inferior or caudal to their respective vertebral bodies.

Once a spinal nerve root exits its intervertebral foramen, it immediately divides into a *ventral and dorsal ramus* (the Latin word *ramus* means "branch") (Fig. 10.1). Depending on location, the ventral ramus forms nerves that innervate, in general, the muscles, joints, and skin of the *anterior-lateral trunk and neck, and the extremities.* The dorsal ramus, in contrast, forms nerves that innervate, in general, the muscles, joints, and skin of the *posterior trunk and neck.* This anatomic organization is depicted generically by the illustration in Fig. 10.2.

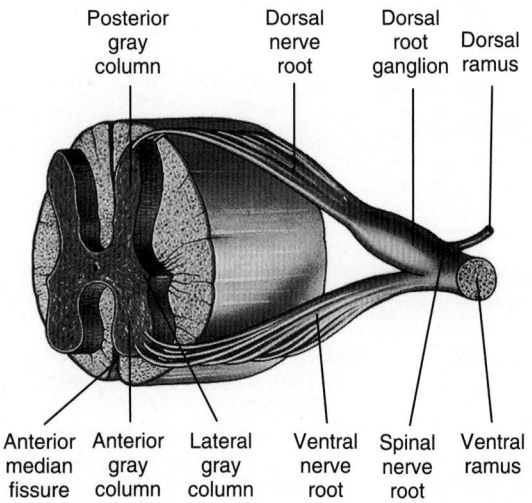

FIGURE 10.1 A cross-section of the spinal cord and a typical spinal nerve root are illustrated. Multiple *ventral and dorsal nerve roots,* flowing from and to the gray matter of the spinal cord, respectively, fuse into a single *spinal nerve root.* The enlarged dorsal root ganglion contains the cell bodies of the afferent (sensory) neurons. The spinal nerve root immediately divides into a relatively small dorsal ramus and a much larger ventral ramus. (Modified from Standring S: *Gray's anatomy: the anatomical basis of clinical practice,* ed 41, St Louis, 2016, Elsevier.)

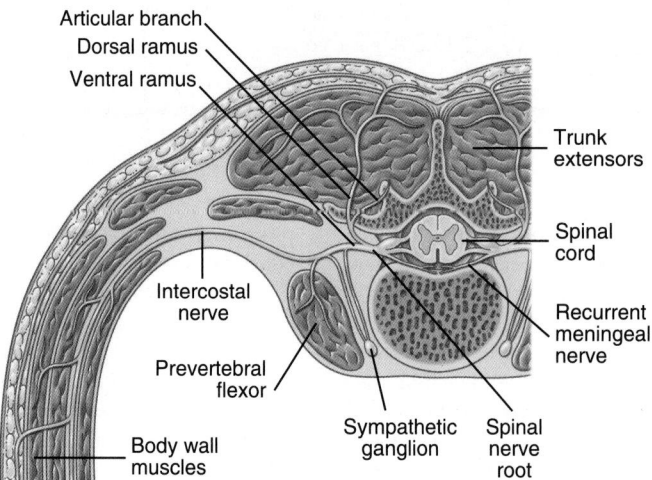

FIGURE 10.2 A cross-sectional view of an unspecified region of the thoracic trunk, highlighting a typical spinal nerve root and the path of its ventral and dorsal rami. The ventral ramus is shown forming an intercostal nerve, which innervates muscles in the anterior-lateral trunk, such as the intercostal and abdominal muscles. The dorsal ramus is shown innervating trunk extensor muscles, such as the erector spinae and multifidus. Although not depicted, the ventral and dorsal rami also contain sensory fibers that innervate ligaments and other connective tissues. (Modified from Standring S: *Gray's anatomy: the anatomical basis of clinical practice,* ed 41, St Louis, 2016, Elsevier.)

Ventral Ramus Innervation

Throughout the vertebral column, each ventral ramus of a spinal nerve root either forms a plexus or continues as an individual named nerve.

PLEXUS

A plexus is an intermingling of ventral rami that form peripheral nerves, such as the radial, phrenic, or sciatic nerve. The four major plexuses are formed by the following ventral rami: cervical (C^1–C^4), brachial (C^5–T^1), lumbar (T^{12}–L^4) and sacral (L^4–S^4).* Most of the nerves that flow from the brachial, lumbar, and sacral plexuses innervate structures associated with the limbs, or, more precisely, the appendicular skeleton. Most nerves that flow from the cervical plexus, however, innervate structures associated with the axial skeleton.

INDIVIDUAL NAMED NERVES

Many of the ventral rami within the trunk and craniocervical regions do not contribute to the formation of a plexus; rather, they remain as individual named nerves. Each of these nerves typically innervates only a part or a segment of a muscle or connective tissue. This is why, for example, many muscles that extend across a large part of the axial skeleton possess *multiple* levels of segmental innervation. The two most recognized sets of individual segmental nerves derived from the ventral rami are the intercostal (thoracic) and the recurrent meningeal nerves (see Fig. 10.2).

Intercostal Nerves (T^1 to T^{12})

Each of the 12 ventral rami of the thoracic spinal nerve roots forms an *intercostal nerve,* innervating an intercostal dermatome and the set of intercostal muscles that share the same intercostal space. (Refer to the dermatome chart in Appendix III, Part B, Fig. III.2.) Most of the T^1 ventral ramus forms the lower trunk of the brachial plexus, with a smaller branch forming the first intercostal nerve. The ventral rami of T^7–T^{12} also innervate the muscles of the anterior-lateral trunk (i.e., the "abdominal" muscles). The T^{12} ventral ramus forms the last intercostal (subcostal) nerve, frequently sending a branch that joins the L^1 ventral ramus of the lumbar plexus.

Recurrent Meningeal Nerves

A single recurrent meningeal (sinuvertebral) nerve branches off the extreme proximal aspect of each ventral ramus. After its bifurcation, the recurrent meningeal nerve courses back into the intervertebral foramen (hence the name "recurrent" [Fig. 10.2]). As a set, these often very small nerves provide sensory and sympathetic nerve supply to the meninges that surround the spinal cord, and to connective tissues associated with the interbody joints.[22] Most notably, the recurrent meningeal nerve supplies sensation to the posterior longitudinal ligament and adjacent areas of the superficial part of the annulus fibrosus. Sensory nerves innervating the anterior longitudinal ligament reach the spinal cord via small branches from nearby ventral rami and adjacent sympathetic connections.

Dorsal Ramus Innervation

A dorsal ramus branches from every spinal nerve root, innervating structures in the posterior trunk usually in a highly segmental fashion. With the exception of the C^1 and C^2 dorsal rami, which are discussed separately, all dorsal rami are smaller than their ventral rami counterparts (see Fig. 10.2). In general, dorsal rami course a relatively short distance posteriorly (dorsally) before innervating selected adjacent muscles and connective tissues on the back of the trunk (Box 10.1).

The dorsal ramus of C^1 ("suboccipital" nerve) is primarily a motor nerve, innervating the suboccipital muscles. The dorsal ramus of C^2 is the largest of the cervical dorsal rami, innervating local muscles as well as contributing to the formation of the greater occipital nerve (C^2 and C^3)—a sensory nerve to the posterior and superior scalp region.

> **BOX 10.1   Structures Innervated by Dorsal Rami of Spinal Nerve Roots (C^1–S^5)**
>
> **MUSCLES**
> - Deep layer of muscles of the posterior trunk
> - Muscles of the posterior craniocervical region
>
> **SKIN**
> - Dermatome (sensory) distribution across the posterior trunk, on either side of the vertebral column
>
> **JOINTS**
> - Ligaments attaching to the posterior side of the vertebrae
> - Capsule of the apophyseal joints
> - Dorsal ligaments of the sacroiliac joints

TRUNK AND CRANIOCERVICAL REGIONS

The muscles of the axial skeleton are organized into two broad and partially overlapping areas: the *trunk* and the *craniocervical region.* The muscles within each area are further organized into sets, based more specifically on their location.

The muscles within each area of the body are presented in two sections, the first covering anatomy and individual muscle actions, and the second covering examples of the functional interactions among related muscles. Throughout this chapter, the reader is encouraged to consult Chapter 9 for a review of the pertinent osteology related to the attachments of muscles. Part C of Appendix III should be consulted for a summary of more detailed muscular anatomy and innervation of the muscles of the axial skeleton.

Before beginning the description of the muscles of the trunk, a few fundamental topics will be reviewed, some of which are specifically related to the kinesiology of the axial skeleton.

Production of Internal Torque

By convention, the "strength" of a muscle action within the axial skeleton is expressed as an *internal torque,* defined for the sagittal, frontal, and horizontal planes. Within each plane, the torque potential is equal to the product of (1) the muscle force generated parallel

---

*The small coccygeal plexus is formed by the ventral ramus of S^5 and the solitary ventral coccygeal nerve root. The plexus exits the sacral hiatus and supplies sensation to the sacrotuberous ligament and adjacent skin.

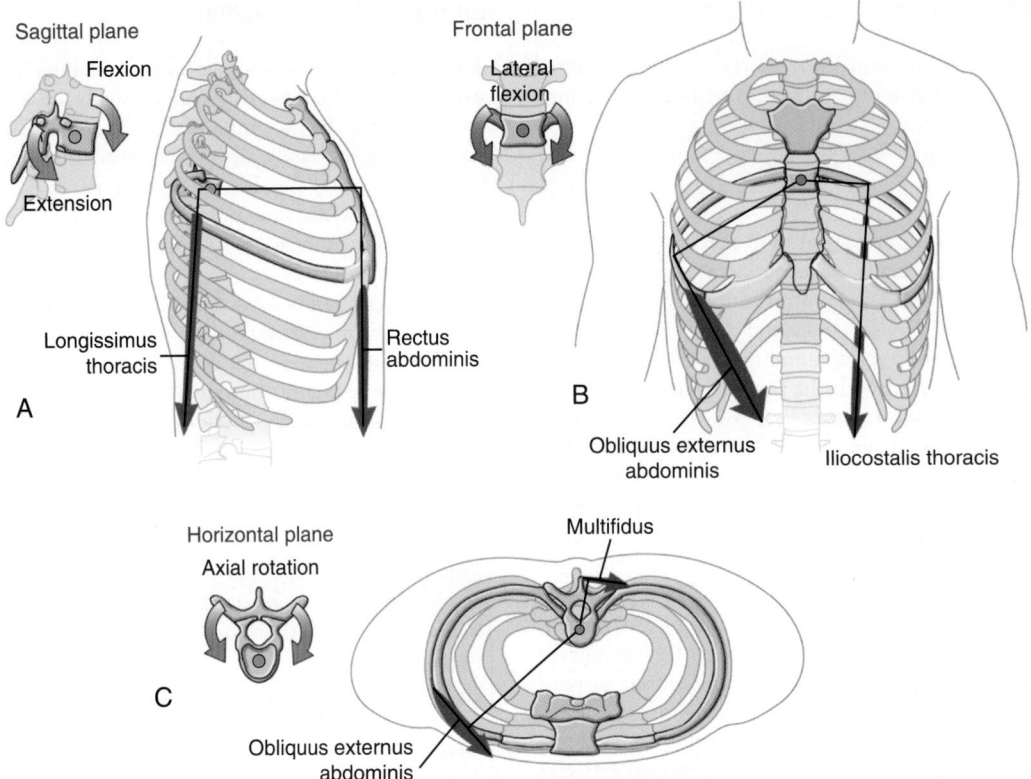

FIGURE 10.3 Selected muscles of the trunk are shown producing an internal torque within each of the three cardinal planes. The torque is equal to the product of the muscle force *(red arrows)* within a given plane and its internal moment arm *(black lines from each axis of rotation)*. The body of T6 is chosen as the representative axis of rotation *(small open circle)*. In each case the strength of a muscle action is determined by the distance and spatial orientation of the muscle's line of force relative to the axis of rotation.

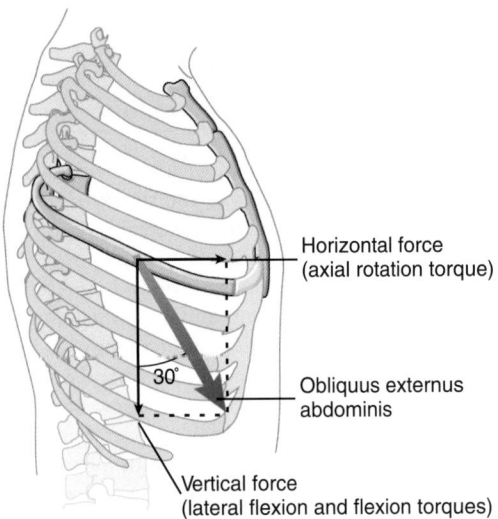

FIGURE 10.4 The line of force of the obliquus externus abdominis muscle is shown directed in the sagittal plane, with a spatial orientation about 30 degrees from the vertical. The resultant muscle force vector *(red)* is trigonometrically partitioned into a vertical force to produce lateral flexion and flexion torques, and a horizontal force to produce axial rotation torque.

to a given plane, and (2) the length of the internal moment arm available to the muscle (Fig. 10.3).

The spatial orientation of a muscle's line of force determines its effectiveness for producing a torque for a particular action.

Consider, for example, the obliquus externus abdominis muscle producing a force across the lateral thorax, with a line of force oriented about 30 degrees from the vertical (Fig. 10.4). The muscle's resultant force vector can be trigonometrically partitioned into unequal vertical and horizontal force components. The vertical force component—about 86% of the muscle's maximal force—is available for producing lateral flexion or flexion torques. The horizontal force component—about 50% of the muscle's maximal force—is available for producing an axial rotation torque. (This estimation is based on the cosine and sine values of 30 degrees, respectively.) For any muscle of the axial skeleton to contribute *all* its force potential toward axial rotation, its overall line of force must be directed solely in the horizontal plane. For a muscle to contribute *all* its force potential toward either lateral flexion or flexion-extension, its overall line of force must be directed vertically. (Realize, though, that a vertically oriented muscle cannot produce any axial rotation because it lacks the moment arm required to produce a torque in the horizontal plane. As described in Chapter 1, a muscle force is *incapable* of producing a torque within a given plane if it either *parallels* or *pierces* the associated axis of rotation.)

The lines of force of muscles that control movement of the axial skeleton have a spatial orientation that varies over a wide spectrum, from nearly vertical to nearly horizontal. This fact is important with regard to a muscle's or muscle group's torque potential for a given action. For example, because more of the total muscle mass of the trunk is biased vertically than horizontally, maximal efforts usually produce greater frontal and sagittal plane torques than horizontal plane torques.

Special Considerations for the Study of Muscle Actions within the Axial Skeleton

To understand the actions of muscles located within the axial skeleton, it is necessary to first consider the muscle during both unilateral and bilateral activations. *Bilateral contraction* usually produces pure flexion or extension of the axial skeleton. Any potential for lateral flexion or axial rotation is neutralized by opposing forces in contralateral muscles. *Unilateral contraction,* in contrast, tends to produce flexion or extension of the axial skeleton, with some combination of lateral flexion and contralateral or ipsilateral axial rotation. (The term *lateral flexion* of the axial skeleton implies "ipsilateral" lateral flexion and therefore is not so specified throughout this chapter.)

The action of a muscle within the axial skeleton depends, in part, on the relative extent of fixation, or stabilization, of the body segments to which the muscle attaches. As an example, consider the effect of a bilateral contraction of a member of the erector spinae group—a muscle that attaches to both the thorax and the pelvis. With the pelvis stabilized, the muscle can extend the thorax; with the thorax stabilized, the muscle can anteriorly rotate (tilt) the pelvis. (Both of these motions occur in the sagittal plane.) If the thorax and pelvis are both free to move, the muscle can simultaneously extend the thorax *and* anteriorly tilt the pelvis. Unless otherwise stated, however, this chapter assumes that the superior (cranial) end of a muscle is less constrained and therefore freer to move than its inferior or caudal counterpart.

Depending on body position, gravity may assist or resist movements of the axial skeleton. Slowly flexing the head from the anatomic (standing) position, for example, is normally controlled by *eccentric* activation of the neck *extensor* muscles. Gravity, in this case, is the prime "flexor" of the head, whereas the extensor muscles control the speed and extent of the action. Rapidly flexing the head, however, requires a burst of concentric activation from the neck flexor muscles, because the desired speed of the motion may be greater than that produced by action of gravity alone. Unless otherwise stated, it is assumed that the action of a muscle is performed via a concentric contraction, rotating a body segment against gravity or against some other form of external resistance.

Muscles of the Trunk: Anatomy and Their Individual Actions

The following section focuses primarily on the relationships between the anatomy and the individual actions of the muscles of the trunk. Musculature is divided into three sets: (1) muscles of the *posterior trunk,* (2) muscles of the *anterior-lateral trunk,* and (3) *additional muscles* (Table 10.1).

TABLE 10.1 Anatomic Organization of the Muscles of the Axial Skeleton*

Anatomic Region	Set	Muscles
Muscles of the trunk	Set 1: Muscles of the posterior trunk ("back" muscles)	**Superficial Layer** Trapezius, latissimus dorsi, rhomboids, levator scapula, serratus anterior **Intermediate Layer**[†] Serratus posterior superior Serratus posterior inferior **Deep Layer** Three groups: Erector spinae group (spinalis, longissimus, iliocostalis) Transversospinal group (semispinalis muscles, multifidus, rotators) Short segmental group (interspinalis muscles, intertransversarius muscles)
	Set 2: Muscles of the anterior-lateral trunk ("abdominal" muscles)	Rectus abdominis Obliquus internus abdominis Obliquus externus abdominis Transversus abdominis
	Set 3: Additional muscles	Iliopsoas Quadratus lumborum
Muscles of the craniocervical region	Set 1: Muscles of the anterior-lateral craniocervical region	Sternocleidomastoid Scalenus anterior Scalenus medius Scalenus posterior Longus colli Longus capitis Rectus capitis anterior Rectus capitis lateralis
	Set 2: Muscles of the posterior craniocervical region	**Superficial Group** Splenius cervicis Splenius capitis **Deep Group ("Suboccipital" Muscles)** Rectus capitis posterior major Rectus capitis posterior minor Obliquus capitis superior Obliquus capitis inferior

*A muscle is classified as belonging to the "trunk" or "craniocervical region" based on the location of most of its attachments.
[†]These muscles are discussed in Chapter 11.

SET 1: MUSCLES OF THE POSTERIOR TRUNK ("BACK" MUSCLES)

The muscles of the posterior trunk are organized into three layers: superficial, intermediate, and deep (see Table 10.1).

Muscles in the Superficial and Intermediate Layers of the Back

The muscles in the *superficial layer* of the back are presented in the study of the shoulder (see Chapter 5). They include the trapezius, latissimus dorsi, rhomboids, levator scapula, and serratus anterior. The trapezius and latissimus dorsi are most superficial, followed by the deeper rhomboids and levator scapula. The serratus anterior muscle is located more laterally on the thorax.

Bilateral contraction of most of the muscles of the superficial layer extends the adjacent region of the axial skeleton. Unilateral contraction, however, laterally flexes and, in most cases, axially rotates the region. The right middle trapezius, for example, assists with right lateral flexion and left axial rotation of the upper thoracic region.

The muscles included in the *intermediate layer* of the back are the serratus posterior superior and the serratus posterior inferior. They are located just deep to the rhomboids and latissimus dorsi. The serratus posterior superior and inferior are thin muscles that contribute little to the movement or stability of the trunk. Their function is more likely related to the mechanics of ventilation, and therefore they are described in Chapter 11.

Muscles within the superficial and intermediate layers of the back may be classified as being "foreign" to the region because, from an embryologic perspective, they were originally associated with the front "limb buds" and only later in their development migrated dorsally to their final position on the back. Although muscles such as the levator scapula, rhomboids, and serratus anterior are located within the back, technically they belong with upper limb muscles. The superficial and intermediate layer of back muscles are therefore innervated by ventral rami of spinal nerves (i.e., the brachial plexus or intercostal nerves).

Muscles in the Deep Layer of the Back

Muscles in the deep layer of the back are the (1) erector spinae group, (2) transversospinal group, and (3) short segmental group (Table 10.2). The anatomic organization of the erector spinae and transversospinal groups is illustrated in Fig. 10.6.

In general, from superficial to deep, the fibers of the muscles in the deep layer become progressively shorter and more angulated. A muscle within the more superficial erector spinae group may extend virtually the entire length of the vertebral column. In contrast, each muscle within the deeper, short segmental group crosses only one intervertebral junction.

Although there are a few exceptions, muscles in the deep layer of the back are innervated segmentally through the dorsal rami of adjacent spinal nerves.[193] A particularly long muscle within the erector spinae group, for example, is innervated by multiple dorsal rami throughout the spinal cord. A shorter muscle, such as the rotator longus, for example, is innervated by a single dorsal ramus.

Embryologically, and unlike the muscles in the extremities and anterior-lateral trunk, the muscles in the deep layer of the back have retained their original location dorsal to the neuraxis. For this reason, these muscles may be classified as being "native" to the back. As a general rule, most of the deep muscles of the back are innervated by dorsal rami of adjacent spinal nerves.

SPECIAL FOCUS 10.1

Muscles of the Superficial Layer of the Back: An Example of Muscles "Sharing" Actions between the Axial and Appendicular Skeletons

Chapter 5 describes the actions of the muscles of the superficial layer of the back, based on their ability to rotate the appendicular skeleton (i.e., humerus, scapula, or clavicle) toward a fixed axial skeleton (i.e., head, sternum, vertebral column, or ribs). The same muscles, however, are equally capable of performing the "reverse" action (i.e., rotating segments of the axial skeleton toward the fixed appendicular skeleton). This muscular action is demonstrated by highlighting the functions of the trapezius during use of a bow and arrow. As indicated in Fig. 10.5, several muscles produce a force needed to stabilize the position of the scapula and abducted arm. Forces produced in the upper and middle trapezius simultaneously rotate the cervical and upper thoracic spine to the left, indicated by the bidirectional arrows. This "contralateral" axial rotation effect is shown for C6 in the inset within Fig. 10.5. As the muscle pulls the spinous process of C6 to the *right,* the anterior side of the vertebra is rotated to the *left.* The right trapezius (and rhomboids) stabilizes the scapula against the pull of the posterior deltoid, long head of the triceps, and serratus anterior. The shared actions of these muscles demonstrate the inherent efficiency of the musculoskeletal system. In this example, a few muscles accomplish multiple actions across both the axial and the appendicular skeletons.

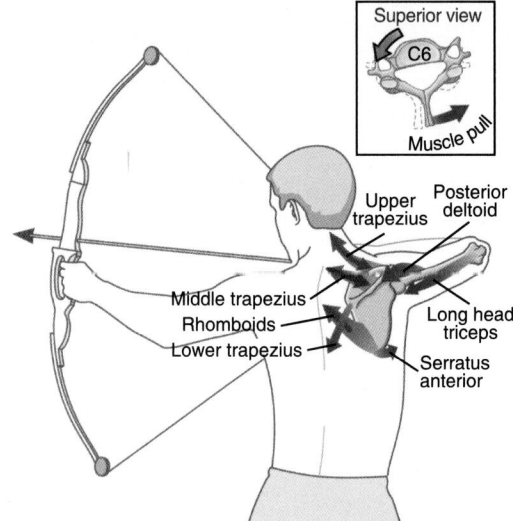

FIGURE 10.5 The actions of several muscles of the right shoulder and upper trunk are shown as an archer uses a bow and arrow. The upper trapezius and middle trapezius demonstrate the dual action of (1) rotating the cervical and upper thoracic spine *to the left* (see inset) and (2) stabilizing the position of the right scapula relative to the thorax. The bidirectional arrows indicate the muscles simultaneously rotating the spinous process toward the scapula and stabilizing the scapula against the pull of the long head of the triceps, posterior deltoid, and serratus anterior.

TABLE 10.2 **Muscles in the Deep Layer of the Back**			
Group (and Relative Depth)	**Individual Muscles**	**General Fiber Direction**	**Comments**
Erector spinae (superficial)	Iliocostalis lumborum	Cranial and lateral	Most effective leverage for lateral flexion
	Iliocostalis thoracis	Vertical	
	Iliocostalis cervicis	Cranial and medial	
	Longissimus thoracis	Vertical	Most developed of erector spinae group
	Longissimus cervicis	Cranial and medial	
	Longissimus capitis	Cranial and lateral	
	Spinalis thoracis	Vertical	Poorly defined, the spinalis capitis usually fuses with the semispinalis capitis
	Spinalis cervicis	Vertical	
	Spinalis capitis	Vertical	
Transversospinal (intermediate)	Semispinalis		
	Semispinalis thoracis	Cranial and medial	Cross six to eight intervertebral junctions; fibers travel cranial-medially, except for the large superficial part of the semispinalis capitis, which courses vertically
	Semispinalis cervicis	Cranial and medial	
	Semispinalis capitis	Overall near vertical	
	Multifidus	Cranial and medial	Fibers cross two to four intervertebral junctions
	Rotatores		
	Rotator brevis	Horizontal	Rotator brevis crosses just one intervertebral junction; rotator longus crosses two
	Rotator longus	Cranial and medial	Rotatores are most developed in thoracic region
Short segmental (deep)	Interspinalis	Vertical	Both muscles cross one intervertebral junction and are most developed in the cervical region
	Intertransversarius	Vertical	Interspinalis muscles are mixed with the interspinous ligaments

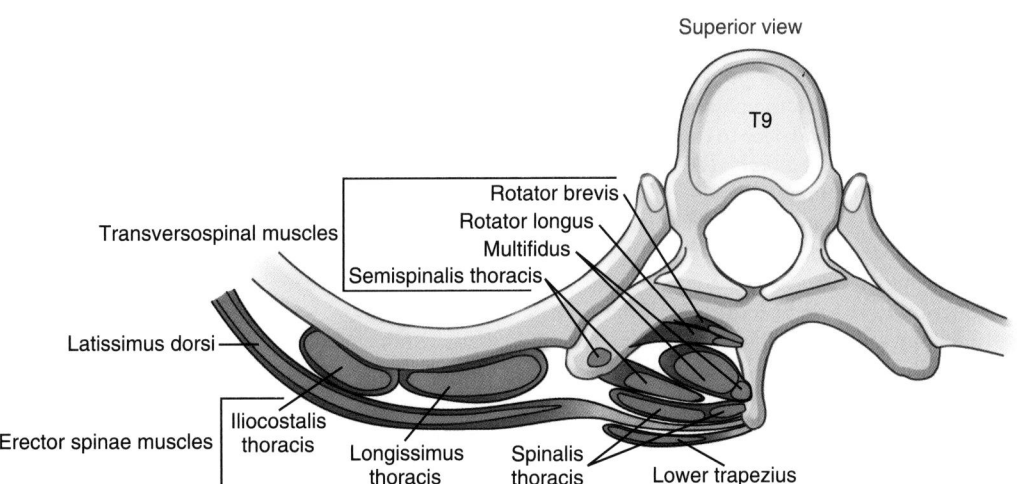

FIGURE 10.6 Cross-sectional view through T9 highlighting the topographic organization of the erector spinae and the transversospinal group of muscles. The short segmental group of muscles is not shown.

Posterior view

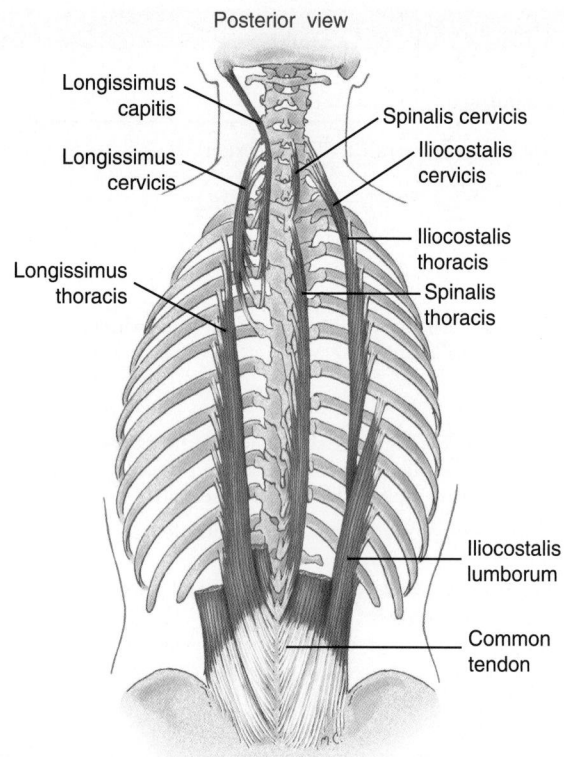

FIGURE 10.7 The muscles of the erector spinae group. For clarity, the left iliocostalis, left spinalis, and right longissimus muscles are cut just superior to the common tendon. (Modified from Luttgens K, Hamilton N: *Kinesiology: scientific basis of human motion,* ed 9, Madison, WI, 1997, Brown & Benchmark.)

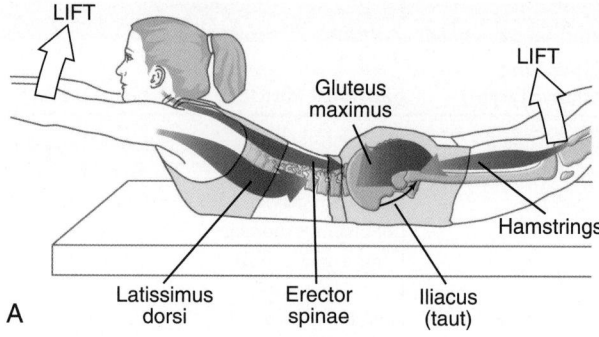

A

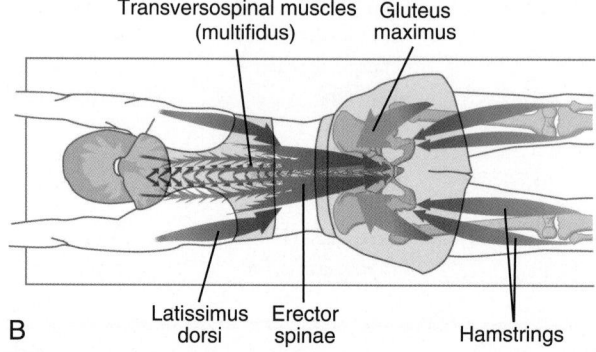

B

FIGURE 10.8 Muscle activation patterns of a healthy person during extension of the trunk and head. The upper and lower extremities are also being lifted away from the supporting surface. (A) Side view. (B) Top view. Note in (A) that the stretched iliacus muscle contributes to the anterior-tilted position of the pelvis.

Erector Spinae Group

The erector spinae are an extensive and poorly defined group of muscles that run on both sides of the vertebral column, roughly within one hand's width from the spinous processes (Fig. 10.7). Most of the muscles are located deep to the posterior layer of the thoracolumbar fascia (see Chapter 9) and deep to the muscles in the intermediate and superficial layers of the back. The erector spinae consist of the *spinalis, longissimus,* and *iliocostalis* muscles. Each muscle is further subdivided topographically into three regions, producing a total of nine named muscles (see Table 10.2).

The bulk of the erector spinae muscles have a common attachment on a broad and thick *common tendon,* located in the region of the sacrum (see Fig. 10.7). This common tendon anchors the erector spinae to many locations (Box 10.2). From this firm caudal origin arise three poorly organized vertical columns of muscle: the spinalis, longissimus, and iliocostalis. The general muscle attachments are described in the following sections; more specific attachments can be found in Appendix III, Part C.

Spinalis Muscles. Spinalis muscles include the *spinalis thoracis, spinalis cervicis,* and *spinalis capitis.* In general, this small and often indistinct (or missing) column of muscle arises from the upper part of the common tendon. The muscle ascends by attaching to adjacent spinous processes of most thoracic vertebrae or, in the cervical region, the ligamentum nuchae. The spinalis capitis, if present, often blends with the medial part of the semispinalis capitis.[193]

Longissimus Muscles. The longissimus muscles include the longissimus thoracis, longissimus cervicis, and longissimus capitis. As a set, these muscles form the largest and most developed column of the erector spinae group. The fibers of the *longissimus thoracic*

BOX 10.2 **Attachments Made by the Common Tendon of the Erector Spinae**

- Spinal tubercles of the sacrum
- Spinous processes and supraspinous ligaments in the lower thoracic and entire lumbar region
- Iliac crest and tuberosity
- Sacrotuberous and sacroiliac ligaments
- Gluteus maximus
- Multifidus

muscles fan cranially from the common tendon, attaching primarily to the posterior end of most ribs. In the neck, the *longissimus cervicis* angles slightly medially before attaching to the posterior tubercle of the transverse processes of the cervical vertebrae (see Fig. 10.7). The *longissimus capitis,* in contrast, courses slightly laterally and attaches to the posterior margin of the mastoid process of the temporal bone. The slightly more oblique angulation of the superior portion of the longissimus capitis and cervicis suggests that these muscles assist with *ipsilateral* axial rotation of the craniocervical region. Using a piece of string to mimic the muscles' line of pull on an articulated skeleton model is a useful way to visualize these muscular actions.

Iliocostalis Muscles. The iliocostalis muscles include the iliocostalis lumborum, iliocostalis thoracis, and iliocostalis cervicis. This group occupies the most lateral column of the erector spinae. The *iliocostalis lumborum* arises from the common tendon and courses upward and slightly outward to attach lateral to the angle of the

Posterior view

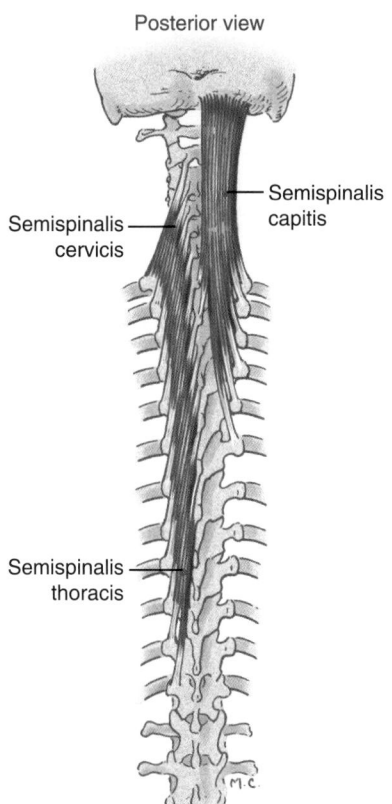

FIGURE 10.9 A posterior view shows the more superficial semispinalis muscles within the transversospinal group. For clarity, only the left semispinalis cervicis, left semispinalis thoracis, and right semispinalis capitis are included. (Modified from Luttgens K, Hamilton N: *Kinesiology: scientific basis of human motion,* ed 9, Madison, WI, 1997, Brown & Benchmark.)

lower ribs. The *iliocostalis thoracis* continues vertically to attach just lateral to the angle of the middle and upper ribs. From this point, the *iliocostalis cervicis* continues cranially and slightly medially to attach to posterior tubercles of the transverse processes of the mid-cervical vertebrae, along with the longissimus cervicis.

Summary. The erector spinae muscles cross a considerable distance throughout the axial skeleton (Fig. 10.7). This anatomic feature suggests a design more suited for control of gross movements across a large part of axial skeleton (such as extending the trunk while rising from a low chair) rather than finer movements at selected intervertebral junctions. *Bilateral contraction* of the erector spinae as a group extends the trunk, neck, or head (Fig. 10.8). The muscles' relatively large cross-sectional areas enable them to generate large extension torque across the axial spine, suitable for lifting or carrying heavy objects.

By attaching to the sacrum and to the pelvis, the erector spinae can anteriorly tilt the pelvis, thereby accentuating the lumbar lordosis. (Pelvic tilt describes a sagittal plane rotation of the pelvis around the hip joints. The direction of the tilt is indicated by the rotation direction of the iliac crests.) As depicted in Fig. 10.8A, the anterior pelvic tilt is accentuated by the increased tension in stretched hip flexor muscles, such as the iliacus.

Contracting unilaterally, the more laterally positioned iliocostalis muscles are the most effective lateral flexors of the erector spinae group. The cranial or cervical components of the longissimus and iliocostalis muscles assist with ipsilateral axial rotation, especially when the head and neck are first fully contralaterally rotated. The iliocostalis lumborum assists slightly with ipsilateral axial rotation.

Posterior view

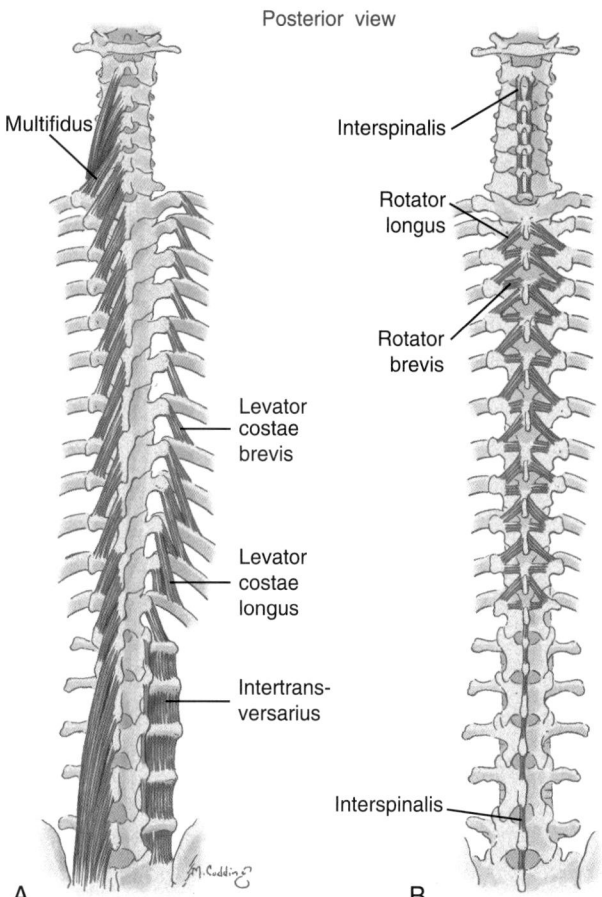

A   B

FIGURE 10.10 A posterior view shows the deeper muscles within the transversospinal group: multifidus on entire left side of (A); rotatores bilaterally in (B). The muscles within the short segmental group (intertransversarius and interspinalis) are depicted in (A) and (B), respectively. Note that intertransversarius muscles are shown for the right side of the lumbar region only. The levatores costarum muscles are involved with ventilation and are discussed in Chapter 11. (Modified from Luttgens K, Hamilton N: *Kinesiology: scientific basis of human motion,* ed 9, Madison, WI, 1997, Brown & Benchmark.)

Transversospinal Muscles

Located immediately deep to the erector spinae muscles is the transversospinal muscle group: the *semispinalis, multifidus,* and *rotatores* (Figs. 10.9 and 10.10). Semispinalis muscles are located superficially; the multifidus, intermediately; and the rotatores, deeply.

The name *transversospinal* refers to the general attachments of most of the muscles (i.e., from the transverse processes of one vertebra to the spinous processes of a more superiorly located vertebra). With a few exceptions, these attachments align most muscle fibers in a cranial-and-medial direction. Many of the muscles within the transversospinal group are morphologically similar, varying primarily in *length* and in the *number* of intervertebral junctions that each muscle crosses (see ahead Fig. 10.11). Although somewhat oversimplified, this concept can greatly assist in learning the overall anatomy and actions of these muscles.

Semispinalis Muscles. The semispinalis muscles consist of the semispinalis thoracis, semispinalis cervicis, and semispinalis capitis (Fig. 10.9). In general, each muscle, or main set of fibers within each muscle, crosses six to eight intervertebral junctions. The *semispinalis thoracis* consists of many thin muscle fasciculi,

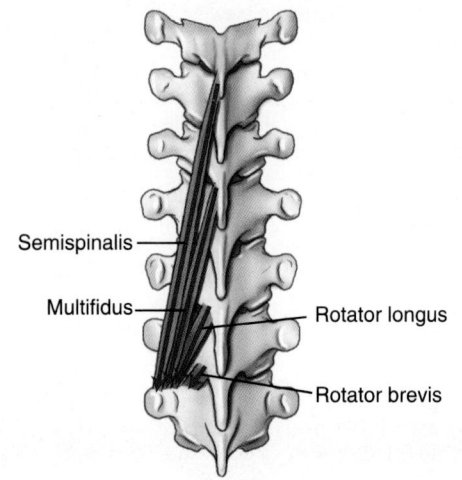

Semispinalis

Multifidus

Rotator longus

Rotator brevis

Muscle group	Relative length and depth	Average number of crossed intervertebral junctions
Semispinalis	Long; superficial	6-8
Multifidus	Intermediate	2-4
Rotatores	Short; deep	1-2

FIGURE 10.11 Simplified depiction of the spatial orientation of muscles within the left transversospinal muscle group. Additional information is listed in tabular format. (Note that the muscles illustrated normally exist bilaterally, throughout the entire cranial-caudal aspect of the vertebral column; their unilateral location in the figure is simplified for the sake of clarity.)

interconnected by long tendons. Muscle fibers attach from transverse processes of T6 to T10 to spinous processes of C6 to T4. The *semispinalis cervicis,* much thicker and more developed than the semispinalis thoracis, attaches from upper thoracic transverse processes to spinous processes of C2 to C5. Muscle fibers that attach to the prominent spinous process of the axis (C2) are particularly well developed, serving as important stabilizers for the suboccipital muscles (described ahead).

The *semispinalis capitis* lies deep to the splenius and trapezius muscles. The muscle arises from the tips of transverse processes of C7 to T7. The deeper part of the muscle consists of fasciculi that course cranially and slightly medially to attach to posterior surfaces of articular processes of midcervical vertebrae. The more superficial and thicker part of the muscle continues cranially, attaching to a relatively large region on the occipital bone, filling much of the area between the superior and inferior nuchal lines (see Fig. 9.3). (Note that the muscle's deeper cervical attachments are not evident in Fig. 10.9.)

The semispinalis cervicis and capitis are the largest muscles that cross the posterior side of the neck.[23] Their large size, favorable moment arm length, and strong overall vertical fiber direction empower them to produce 35% to 40% of the total extension torque of the craniocervical region.[2,201,214] Right and left semispinalis capitis muscles are readily palpable as thick and round cords on either side of the midline of the upper neck, especially evident in infants and in thin, muscular adults (Fig. 10.12).

Multifidus. The multifidus muscle group is situated just deep to the semispinalis muscles. The multiple fasciculi that comprise the multifidus share a similar fiber direction and length, extending between the posterior sacrum and the axis (C2). In general, the multifidus originates from the transverse process of one vertebra and insert on the spinous process of a vertebra located two to four intervertebral junctions above (see Fig. 10.10A).

The fibers of the multifidus are thickest and most developed in the lumbosacral region (see multiple attachments listed in Box 10.3). The overlapping fibers fill much of the concave space formed between the spinous and transverse processes. The fibers within the muscles are short with relatively large cross-sectional

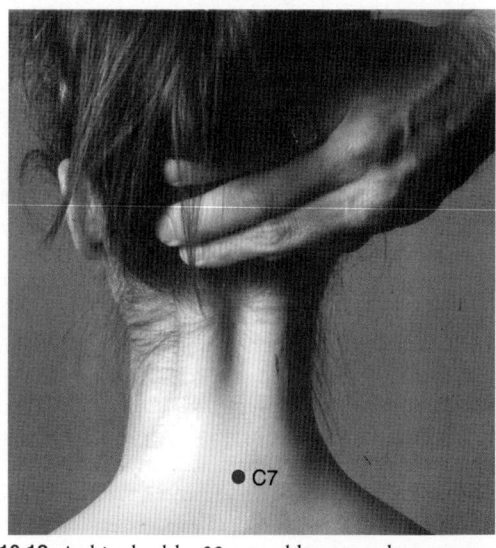

● C7

FIGURE 10.12 A thin, healthy 22-year-old woman demonstrates the contours of the activated right and left semispinalis capitis muscles. Manual resistance is applied against a strong extension effort of the head. The *dot* indicates the spinous process of the C7 vertebra.

areas—an architectural design that provides excellent stability to the base of the spine.[222]

Rotatores. The rotatores are the deepest of the transversospinal group of muscles. The rotatores consist of several individual sets of muscle fibers, most developed in the thoracic region (see Fig. 10.10B).[193] Each fiber group attaches between the transverse process of one vertebra and the lamina and base of the spinous process of a vertebra located one or two intervertebral junctions above. By definition, the *rotator brevis* spans one intervertebral junction, and the *rotator longus* spans two intervertebral junctions.

Summary. On average, the transversospinal muscles cross fewer intervertebral junctions than the erector spinae group. This feature suggests that, in general, the transversospinal muscles favor a design for producing relatively fine controlled movements and stabilizing forces across the axial skeleton.

Contracting bilaterally, the transversospinal muscles extend the axial skeleton (see Fig. 10.8B). Increased extension torque exaggerates the cervical and lumbar lordosis and decreases the thoracic kyphosis. The size and thickness of the transversospinal muscles are greatest at either end of the axial skeleton. *Cranially,* the semispinalis cervicis and capitis are very well-developed extensors of the craniocervical region; *caudally,* the multifidus are very well-developed extensors of the lower lumbar region, accounting for two-thirds of the muscular-based stability in this region.[230]

Contracting unilaterally, the transversospinal muscles laterally flex the spine; however, their leverage for this action is limited because of their proximity to the vertebral column. (One notable exception is the semispinalis capitis, which has favorable leverage for lateral flexion of the cranium and, thus indirectly, of the entire craniocervical region.) The more obliquely oriented transversospinal muscles assist with *contralateral* axial rotation. From a relatively fixed transverse process, contraction of an isolated region of the left multifidus or left rotator longus, for example, can rotate a superiorly located spinous process toward the left and, as a result, rotate the anterior side of the vertebra to the right. Compared with all the trunk muscles, however, the transversospinal muscles are secondary axial rotators. The leverage for this rotation is relatively poor because of the muscle's overall proximity to the vertebral column. (Compare the multifidus with the obliquus abdominis externus, for example, in Fig. 10.3C). Furthermore, the prevailing lines of force of most transversospinal muscle fibers is directed more vertically than horizontally, thereby providing a greater force potential for extension than for axial rotation.

Short Segmental Group of Muscles

The short segmental group of muscles consists of the *interspinalis* and the *intertransversarius muscles* (see Fig. 10.10). (The plural "interspinales and intertransversarii" is often used to describe all the members within the entire set of these muscles.) They lie deep to the transversospinal group of muscles. The name "short segmental" refers to the extremely short length and highly segmented organization of the muscles. Each individual interspinalis or intertransversarius muscle crosses just one intervertebral junction. These muscles are most developed in the cervical region, where fine control of the head and neck is so critical.[193]

Each pair of interspinalis muscles is located on both sides of, and often blends with, the corresponding interspinous ligament. The interspinales have a relatively favorable leverage and optimal fiber direction for producing extension torque. The magnitude of this

torque, however, is relatively small considering the muscles' small size and therefore low force potential.

Each right and left pair of intertransversarius muscles is located between adjacent transverse processes. The anatomy of the intertransversarii as a group is more complex than that of the interspinales. In the cervical region, for example, each intertransversarius muscle is divided into small anterior and posterior muscles, between which pass the ventral rami of spinal nerves.

Unilateral contraction of the intertransversarii as a group laterally flexes the vertebral column. Although the magnitude of the lateral flexion torque is relatively small compared with that of other muscle groups, it still likely provides an important source of intervertebral stability.

Summary. The highly segmented nature of the interspinalis and intertransversarius muscles is ideal for fine motor control of the axial skeleton. Because these unisegmental muscles possess a relatively high density of muscle spindles, they likely provide the nervous system (and therefore other muscles) a rich source of sensory feedback, especially in the craniocervical region.

SET 2: MUSCLES OF THE ANTERIOR-LATERAL TRUNK ("ABDOMINAL" MUSCLES)

The muscles of the anterior-lateral trunk include the rectus abdominis, obliquus externus abdominis, obliquus internus abdominis, and transversus abdominis (Fig. 10.13). As a group, these muscles are often collectively referred to as the "abdominal" muscles. The rectus abdominis is a long, straplike muscle located on both sides of the midline of the body. The obliquus externus abdominis, obliquus internus abdominis, and transversus abdominis—the lateral abdominals—are wide and flat, layered superficial to deep, across the anterior-lateral aspects of the abdomen.

The abdominal muscles have several important physiologic functions, including supporting and protecting abdominal viscera and increasing intrathoracic and intra-abdominal pressures. As will be further described in Chapter 11, increasing the pressures in these cavities assists with functions such as forced expiration of air from the lungs, coughing, vocalization, defecation, and childbirth. This chapter focuses more on the kinesiologic functions of the abdominal muscles as they move and stabilize the trunk. Another important role of the abdominal muscles is to provide a stable pelvic attachment site for hip muscles, which is described in Chapter 12.

Formation of the Rectus Sheaths and Linea Alba

The obliquus externus abdominis, obliquus internus abdominis, and transversus abdominis muscles from the right and left sides of the body fuse at the midline of the abdomen through a blending of connective tissues. Each muscle contributes a thin bilaminar sheet of connective tissue that ultimately forms the *anterior and posterior rectus sheaths*. As depicted in Fig. 10.14, the anterior rectus sheath is formed from connective tissues from the obliquus externus abdominis and the obliquus internus abdominis muscles. The posterior rectus sheath is formed from connective tissues from the obliquus internus abdominis and transversus abdominis. Both sheaths surround the vertically oriented rectus abdominis muscle and continue medially to fuse with matching connective tissues from the other side of the abdomen. The connective tissues thicken and crisscross as they traverse the midline, forming the *linea alba* (the Latin word *linea* means "line," and *albus,* "white"). The linea alba runs longitudinally between the xiphoid process and pubic symphysis and pubic crest.

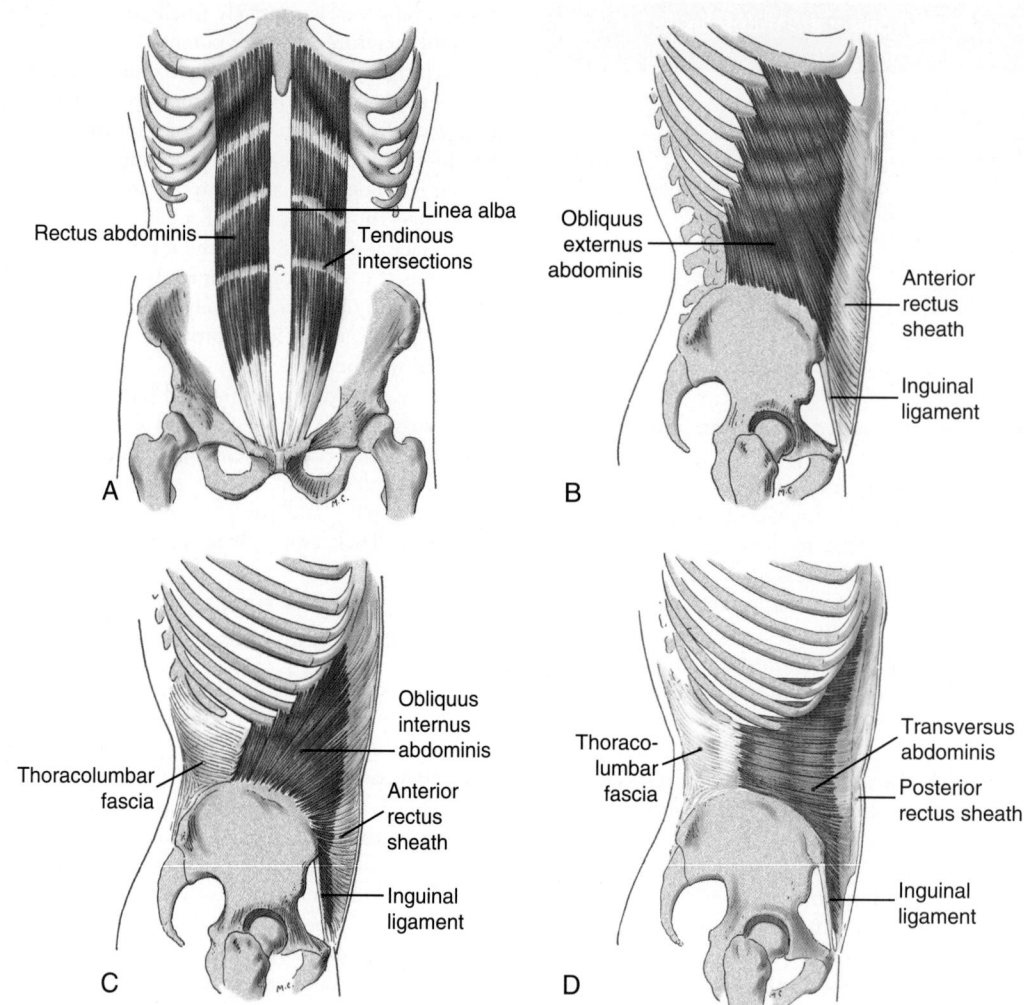

FIGURE 10.13 The abdominal muscles of the anterior-lateral trunk. (A) Rectus abdominis with the anterior rectus sheath removed. (B) Obliquus externus abdominis. (C) Obliquus internus abdominis, deep to the obliquus externus abdominis. (D) Transversus abdominis, deep to other abdominal muscles. (Modified from Luttgens K, Hamilton N: *Kinesiology: scientific basis of human motion,* ed 9, Madison, WI, 1997, Brown & Benchmark.)

The crisscross arrangement of the fibers within the linea alba adds strength to the abdominal wall, much like the laminated structure of plywood. The linea alba also mechanically links the right and left lateral abdominal muscles, providing an effective way to transfer muscular force across the midline of the body.

Anatomy of the Abdominal Muscles

The *rectus abdominis* muscle consists of right and left halves, separated by the linea alba (Fig. 10.13A). Each half of the muscle runs vertically, widening as it ascends within an open sleeve formed between the anterior and posterior rectus sheaths. In pregnant women, the distance between right and left sides of the muscle (interrectus distance) often increases because of the abdominal distension that occurs during the second and third trimesters of pregnancy—a condition referred to as diastasis rectus abdominis.[45]

Of all the abdominal muscles, the rectus abdominis has the longest fascicle length but smallest physiologic cross-sectional area.[27] The straplike muscle is intersected and reinforced by three transverse or oblique fibrous bands, known as *tendinous intersections*. These bands blend with the anterior rectus sheath.*

The rectus abdominis attaches superiorly on the xiphoid process and cartilages of the fifth through seventh ribs. Caudally, the muscle arises from the region on and surrounding the crest of the pubis, often partially blending with the proximal attachment of the adductor longus. As a result of their common attachments, excessive force transmitted through these muscles may strain the connective tissue attachments to bone, potentially leading to a myriad of painful conditions generally referred to as "groin-related pain in athletes" (previously referred to as athletic pubalgia or sports hernia).[164,225]

---

* The specific function of the tendinous intersections is unknown. Although speculation, the connective tissue may partition the muscle into smaller segments, thereby reducing the relative amount of shortening required of the individual muscle fibers to actively flex the trunk. Another possibility is that the tendinous intersections are connective tissue septa that roughly define several of the myotomes of the muscle.

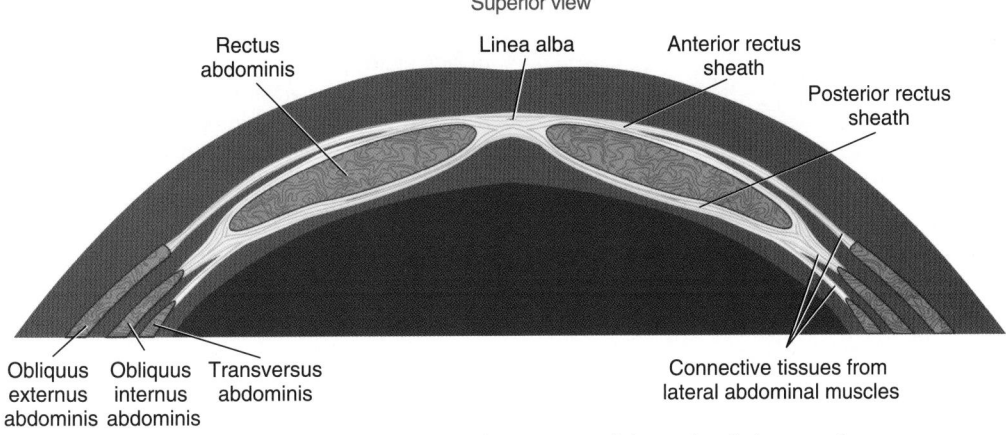

Superior view

Rectus abdominis Linea alba Anterior rectus sheath Posterior rectus sheath

Obliquus externus abdominis Obliquus internus abdominis Transversus abdominis Connective tissues from lateral abdominal muscles

FIGURE 10.14 Horizontal cross-sectional view of the anterior abdominal wall shown at the approximate level of the third lumbar vertebra.

TABLE 10.3 Attachments and Individual Actions of the Lateral Abdominal Muscles

Muscle	Lateral Attachments	Medial Attachments	Actions on the Trunk
Obliquus externus abdominis	Lateral side of ribs 5–12	Iliac crest, linea alba, and contralateral rectus sheaths	*Bilaterally:* flexion of the trunk and posterior tilt of the pelvis *Unilaterally:* lateral flexion and contralateral rotation of the trunk
Obliquus internus abdominis	Iliac crest, inguinal ligament, and thoracolumbar fascia	Ribs 9 to 11 (or 12), linea alba, and contralateral rectus sheaths	*Bilaterally:* as above, plus increases tension in the thoracolumbar fascia *Unilaterally:* lateral flexion and ipsilateral rotation of the trunk
Transversus abdominis	Iliac crest, thoracolumbar fascia, inner surface of the cartilages of ribs 6–12, and the inguinal ligament	Linea alba and contralateral rectus sheaths	*Bilaterally:* stabilization of attachment sites for other abdominal muscles; compression of the abdominal cavity; increases tension in the thoracolumbar fascia

The anatomic organization of the obliquus externus abdominis, obliquus internus abdominis, and transversus abdominis muscles is different from that of the rectus abdominis. As a group, the more laterally placed muscles originate laterally or posterior-laterally on the trunk and run in a different direction toward the midline, eventually blending with the linea alba and contralateral rectus sheaths (Table 10.3).

The *obliquus externus abdominis* (informally referred to as the "external oblique") is the most superficial of the lateral abdominal muscles. The external oblique muscle travels in an inferior-and-medial direction, similar to the direction of the hands placed diagonally in front pockets of pants (Fig. 10.13B). The *obliquus internus abdominis* (or informally the "internal oblique") is located immediately deep to the external oblique muscle, forming the second layer of the lateral abdominals. The internal oblique muscle possesses the largest physiologic cross-sectional area of all the abdominal muscles, and therefore presumably can generate the largest isometric force.[27] Fibers attaching on the iliac crest blend to varying degrees with the adjacent thoracolumbar fascia. From this lateral attachment point, the fibers course in a cranial-and-medial direction toward the linea alba and lower ribs. As evident in Fig. 10.13C, the inferior attachments of the internal oblique muscle extend to the inguinal ligament. The average fiber direction of the internal oblique muscle is nearly perpendicular to the average fiber direction of the overlying external oblique muscle.

The *transversus abdominis* is the deepest of the abdominal muscles (Fig. 10.13D). The muscle is also known anatomically as the "corset muscle," reflecting its role in compressing the abdomen as well as stabilizing the lower back through attachments into the thoracolumbar fascia.[193,232] Of all the abdominal muscles, the transversus abdominis has the most extensive and consistent attachments into the thoracolumbar fascia,[204] followed closely by the internal oblique muscle.

Actions of the Abdominal Muscles

Bilateral action of the rectus abdominis and oblique abdominal muscles reduces the distance between the xiphoid process and the pubic symphysis.[218] Depending on which body segment is more stable, bilateral contraction of these abdominal muscles flexes the thorax and upper lumbar spine, posteriorly tilts the pelvis, or both. Fig. 10.15 depicts a diagonally performed sit-up maneuver that places a relatively large demand on the oblique abdominal muscles.[218] During a standard sagittal plane sit-up, however, the opposing axial rotation and lateral flexion tendencies of the various abdominal muscles are neutralized by opposing right and left muscles.

As described in Chapter 9, the axes of rotation for all motions of the vertebral column are located in the region of the interbody joints. The relative posterior placement of the axes relative to the trunk equips the abdominal muscles, most notably the rectus abdominis, with very favorable leverage for generating trunk flexion

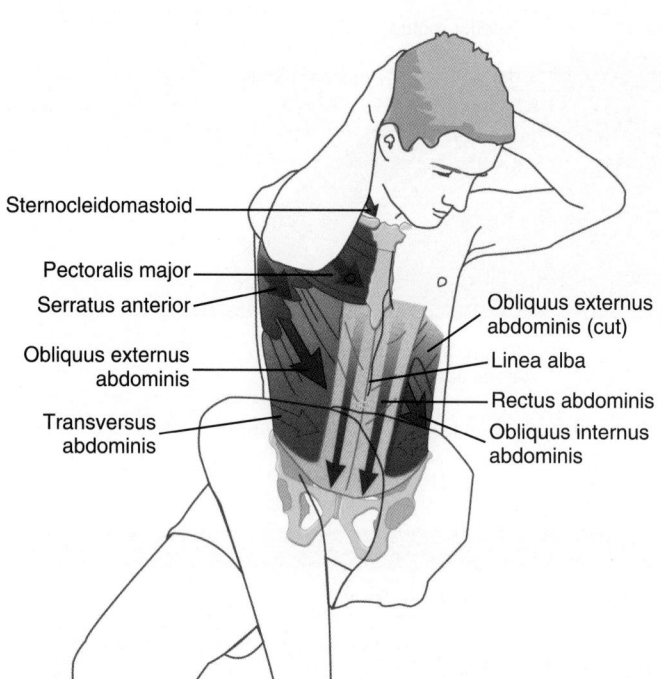

FIGURE 10.15 Typical muscle activation pattern of a healthy person performing a diagonal sit-up maneuver that incorporates trunk flexion and axial rotation to the left. During this action, the right external oblique muscle acts synergistically with the left internal oblique muscle. Note the simultaneous bilateral activation of the rectus abdominis and the deeper transversus abdominis.

torque (Fig. 10.16). Note in Fig. 10.16 that, with the exception of the psoas major, all muscles have a moment arm to produce torques in *both* sagittal and frontal planes.

Contracting unilaterally, the abdominal muscles laterally flex the trunk. The external and internal obliques are particularly effective in this action owing to their relatively favorable leverage (i.e., long moment arms) (Fig. 10.16) and, as a pair, relatively large cross-sectional area. The combined cross-sectional area of the external and internal obliques at the level of the L4–L5 junction is almost twice that of the rectus abdominis muscle.[141]

Lateral flexion of the trunk often involves activation of both trunk flexor and extensor muscles. For example, lateral flexion against resistance to the right demands a contraction from the right external and internal obliques, right erector spinae, and right transversospinal muscles. Coactivation amplifies the total frontal torque while simultaneously stabilizing the trunk within the sagittal plane.[12]

By far, the internal and external oblique muscles are the most effective axial rotators of the trunk.[7,12,97] The external oblique muscle is a contralateral rotator, and the internal oblique muscle is an ipsilateral rotator. The strong axial rotation potential of these muscles reflects their relatively large cross-sectional area and favorable leverage (see Fig. 10.3C for long moment arm length of the obliquus externus abdominis). During active axial rotation in a particular direction, the external oblique muscle on one side functions synergistically with the internal oblique on the other side.[211] This functional synergy produces a diagonal line of force that crosses the midline through the muscles' mutual attachment into the linea alba (see highlighted muscles in Fig. 10.15). Contraction of the two muscles therefore reduces the distance between one shoulder and the contralateral iliac crest.

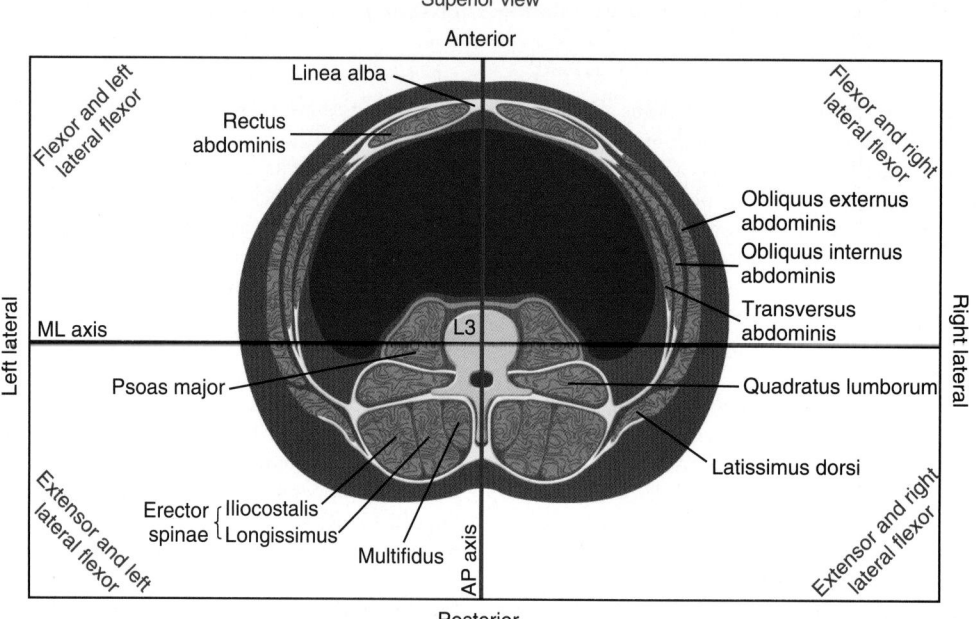

FIGURE 10.16 Horizontal cross-sectional view through several muscles of the trunk at the approximate level of the third lumbar vertebra *(L3).* The potential of muscles to produce a torque in both sagittal and frontal planes is shown. The anterior-posterior *(AP)* axis of rotation *(red)* and medial-lateral *(ML)* axis of rotation *(black)* intersect in the center of the third lumbar vertebra. Muscles located anterior and posterior to the medial-lateral axis have the potential to flex and extend the trunk, respectively; muscles located right and left to the anterior-posterior axis have the potential to laterally flex the trunk to right and left, respectively.

Several electromyographic (EMG) studies using intramuscular (fine-wire) electrodes demonstrate some degree of bilateral activation of the *transversus abdominis* during axial rotation.[43,109,211] Furthermore, it has been shown that during axial rotation the middle and lower fibers of the transversus abdominis coactivate at slightly different times than the upper fibers.[211] Although the exact role of the transversus abdominis during axial rotation is uncertain, the muscle appears to function more as a *stabilizer* for the oblique abdominal muscles than a torque generator of axial rotation. Bilateral activation of the transversus abdominis can stabilize the ribs, linea alba, and thoracolumbar fascia—areas that serve as attachments for the internal or external oblique muscles.

In general, the torque demands placed on the axial rotators of the trunk vary considerably based on the nature of an activity and the position of the body.[12] Torque demands are relatively large during high-power axial rotations, such as sprinting, wrestling, and throwing a discus or javelin. The demands may be very low, however, during activities that involve slow, relatively unresisted twisting of the trunk while in an upright position, such as during walking over level surfaces. Axial rotation performed primarily within the horizontal plane places little to no gravity-induced external torque on the rotator muscles. The muscles' primary resistance, in this case, is caused by the inertia of the trunk and the passive tension created by stretching of various connective tissues and antagonist muscles.

SPECIAL FOCUS 10.2

Role of Trunk Extensors as "Rotational Synergists" to the Oblique Abdominal Muscles

The external and internal oblique muscles are the primary axial rotators of the trunk. Secondary axial rotators include the ipsilateral latissimus dorsi, the more oblique components of the ipsilateral iliocostalis lumborum, and the contralateral transversospinal muscles. These secondary axial rotators are also effective extensors of the trunk. During a strong axial rotation movement, these extensor muscles are able to offset or neutralize *the potent trunk flexion potential of the oblique abdominal muscles*. Without this neutralizing action, a strenuous action of axial rotation would automatically be combined with flexion of the trunk. The aforementioned extensor muscles resist the flexion tendency of the oblique abdominal muscles but also contribute to the axial rotation torque.

The multiple and relatively thick fibers of the multifidus provide a particularly important element of extension stability to the lumbar region during axial rotation. Pain and inflammation involving the apophyseal joints or discs in the lumbar region may be associated with weakness, atrophy, fatty infiltration, reflexive inhibition, or "guarding" of these muscles.[79,90] Without adequate activation and force production from the multifidus during axial rotation, the partially unopposed oblique muscles may, in theory, create a subtle and possibly undesirable flexion bias to the base of the spine.

Comparing Trunk Flexor versus Trunk Extensor Peak Torque

In the healthy adult, the magnitude of a maximal-effort trunk flexion torque is typically *less than* the maximal-effort trunk extension torque. Although data vary based on age, sex, history of back pain, and angular velocity of the testing device, the *flexor-to-extensor*

torque ratios determined isometrically for the trunk and craniocervical regions are between 0.45 and 0.77.[56,107,149,157,214] Although the trunk flexor muscles normally possess greater overall leverage for sagittal plane torque (see Fig. 10.16), the trunk extensor muscles possess greater cross-sectional area and, perhaps equally important, greater overall vertical orientation of muscle fibers.[56,141] The typically greater torque potential of the trunk extensor muscles reflects the muscles' predominant role in counteracting gravity, either for maintaining upright posture or for carrying loads in front of the body.

SET 3: ADDITIONAL MUSCLES (ILIOPSOAS AND QUADRATUS LUMBORUM)

Although the iliopsoas and quadratus lumborum are not anatomically considered muscles of the trunk, they are strongly associated with the kinesiology of the region.[167]

Iliopsoas

The iliopsoas is a large muscle consisting of two parts: the iliacus and the psoas major (see Fig. 12.25). As are most hip flexors, the iliopsoas is innervated by the femoral nerve, a large branch from the lumbar plexus. The iliacus has a proximal attachment on the iliac fossa and lateral sacrum, just anterior and superior to the sacroiliac joint. The psoas major attaches proximally to the transverse processes of T12 to L5, including the intervertebral discs. The two muscles fuse distal and deep to the inguinal ligament to form one or more tendons that attach to the lesser trochanter and adjacent regions of the femur.

The iliopsoas is a long muscle, exerting a potent kinetic influence across the trunk, lumbar spine, lumbosacral junction, and pelvofemoral (hip) joints. Crossing anterior to the hip, the muscle is a dominant flexor, drawing the femur toward the pelvis or the pelvis toward the femur. In the latter movement, the iliopsoas can anteriorly tilt the pelvis, a motion that increases the lordosis of the lumbar region assuming the trunk remains relatively stationary (review in Fig. 9.63A). With muscular assistance from the abdominal muscles, a strong bilateral contraction of the iliopsoas can also rotate the pelvis *and* superimposed trunk over fixed femurs. Based on this ability, the iliopsoas is as much a respected trunk flexor as a hip flexor. This discussion resumes later in this chapter and again in Chapter 12.

Actions of the Iliopsoas

ILIACUS
- Predominant hip flexor, both femur-on-pelvis and pelvis-on-femur

PSOAS MAJOR
- Predominant hip flexor, both femur-on-pelvis and pelvis-on-femur
- Lateral flexor of the lumbar region
- Flexor of the lower lumbar spine relative to the sacrum
- Vertical stabilizer of the lumbar spine

Function of the Psoas Major at the Lumbosacral Region

In the anatomic position, the psoas major demonstrates leverage for lateral flexion of the lumbar spine (see Fig. 10.16).[126] Little—if any—leverage exists for axial rotation. As expected, therefore, the muscle is highly active during resisted lateral flexion of the trunk.[168]

The flexor and extensor capacity of the psoas major differs throughout the lumbosacral region. Across the L5–S1 junction, the

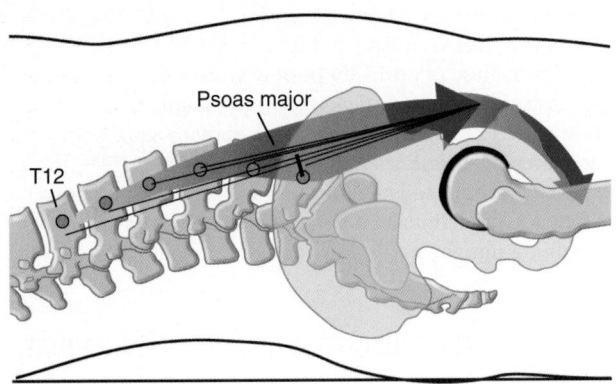

FIGURE 10.17 A lateral view of the psoas major highlights its multiple lines of force relative to the medial-lateral axes of rotation within the T12–L5 and L5–S1 segments. Note that the lines of force pass near or through the axes, with the exception of L5–S1. The flexion moment arm of the psoas major at L5–S1 is shown as the *short black line.*

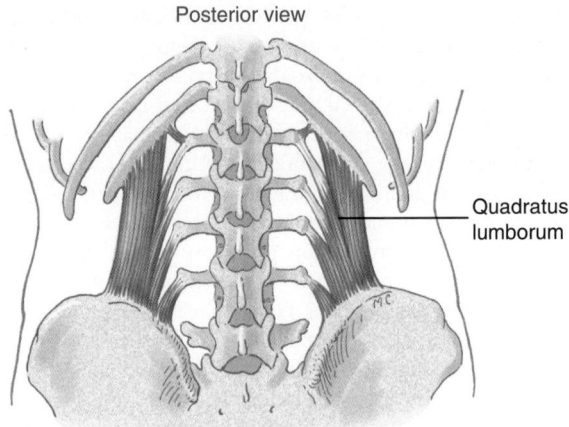

FIGURE 10.18 A posterior view of the quadratus lumborum muscles. (Modified from Luttgens K, Hamilton N: *Kinesiology: scientific basis of human motion,* ed 9, Madison, WI, 1997, Brown & Benchmark.)

psoas major has an approximate 2-cm moment arm for flexion (Fig. 10.17).[142] The psoas major is therefore an effective flexor of the lower end of the lumbar spine relative to the sacrum. Progressing cranially toward L1, however, the line of force of the psoas major gradually shifts slightly *posterior,* falling either through or just posterior to the multiple medial-lateral axes of rotation (see cross-section at L3 in Fig. 10.16). The muscle's location reduces or eliminates its flexor or extensor capacity. The psoas major therefore is neither a dominant flexor nor an extensor of the lumbar region but rather an important vertical stabilizer of the region.[78,168,178,185] (The term "vertical stabilizer" describes a muscular function of stabilizing a region of the axial skeleton in a near-vertical, or longitudinal, orientation while maintaining its natural physiologic curve.) Because of the lack of effective net leverage throughout the lumbar region, the psoas major (as a whole) likely has only a moderate role in directly influencing the degree of lumbar lordosis, at least while standing upright with a neutral posture.[185] The iliopsoas, however (as all hip flexor muscles), has the potential to indirectly increase the lordotic posture of the lumbar spine by tilting the pelvis anteriorly across the hip joints.

Quadratus Lumborum

Anatomically, the quadratus lumborum is considered a muscle of the posterior abdominal wall. The muscle attaches inferiorly to the iliolumbar ligament and iliac crest and superiorly to the twelfth rib and the tips of the stout transverse processes of L1 to L4 (Fig. 10.18). The relative thickness of the muscle and its relative location to the lumbar bodies are evident by viewing Fig. 10.16. The quadratus lumborum is innervated by the ventral rami of spinal nerves T[12] and L[1]-L[3].

Contracting *bilaterally,* the quadratus lumborum is an extensor of the lumbar region.[199] Contracting *unilaterally,* the quadratus lumborum laterally flexes the lumbar region.[78,199] The axial rotation potential of the quadratus lumborum, however, is likely extremely minimal at least when the spine is in a neutral anatomic position.

Clinically, the quadratus lumborum is often called a "hip hiker" when its role in walking is being described, especially for persons with paraplegia at or below the L[1] neurologic level. By elevating (hiking) one side of the pelvis, the quadratus lumborum may assist with raising the lower limb to clear the foot from the ground during the swing phase of brace-assisted ambulation.

The psoas major and the quadratus lumborum run nearly vertically on both sides of the lumbar vertebrae (see Fig. 10.16). A strong bilateral contraction of these muscles may provide useful vertical

stability to the lumbar spine, including the L5–S1 junction, although the potential physiologic effectiveness of the quadratus lumborum in this manner has been questioned.[172]

> **Actions of the Quadratus Lumborum**
> **ACTING BILATERALLY**
> - Extension of the lumbar region
> - Vertical stabilization of the lumbar spine, including the lumbosacral junction
>
> **ACTING UNILATERALLY**
> - Lateral flexion of the lumbar region
> - Elevation of one side of the pelvis ("hip hiking")

Muscles of the Trunk: Functional Interactions among Muscles

Thus far in this chapter, the discussion on the muscles of the trunk has focused primarily on their anatomy and, for the most part, individual actions (Table 10.4). The upcoming discussion pays more attention to the functional interactions *among* the muscles or muscle groups. Two themes are explored: (1) muscular-based stability of the trunk and (2) muscular kinesiology of performing a standard sit-up movement.

MUSCULAR-BASED STABILITY OF THE TRUNK

The central nervous system uses muscle as its primary means for actively stabilizing the inherently mechanically, unstable axial skeleton, including the trunk.[40] This process is executed through planned intention, or use of more subconscious feedback and feedforward mechanims.[177] Although gravity, ligaments, fascia, and discs all provide an important source of this stability, only muscles can adjust both the magnitude and the timing of their forces. The fundamental role of trunk muscles as dynamic stabilizers of the region becomes readily apparent when these muscles are either partially or fully paralyzed or lack virtually all motor control. Such a profound motor deficit may be present in persons with severe spinal cord injury, muscular dystrophy, or cerebral palsy. In these relatively extreme cases, the absence of muscular support can, over time, cause the spinal column to literally collapse under the weight of the trunk. This postural collapse can lead to severe deformities, interfering with ventilation or

TABLE 10.4 Actions of Most Muscles of the Trunk*				
Muscle	**Flexion**	**Extension**	**Lateral Flexion**	**Axial Rotation**[†]
Trapezius	—	XX	XX	XX (CL)
Spinalis muscles (as a group)	—	XX	X	—
Longissimus thoracis	—	XXX	XX	—
Longissimus cervicis	—	XXX	XX	XX (IL)
Longissimus capitis	—	XXX	XX	XX (IL)
Iliocostalis lumborum	—	XXX	XXX	X (IL)
Iliocostalis thoracis	—	XXX	XXX	—
Iliocostalis cervicis	—	XXX	XXX	XX (IL)
Semispinalis thoracis	—	XXX	X	X (CL)
Semispinalis cervicis	—	XXX	X	X (CL)
Semispinalis capitis	—	XXX	XX	X (CL); cervical spine only
Multifidus	—	XXX	X	XX (CL)
Rotatores	—	XX	X	XX (CL)
Interspinalis muscles	—	XX	—	—
Intertransversarius muscles	—	X	XX	—
Rectus abdominis	XXX	—	XX	—
Obliquus externus abdominis	XXX	—	XXX	XXX (CL)
Obliquus internus abdominis	XXX	—	XXX	XXX (IL)
Transversus abdominis[‡]	—	—	—	—
Psoas major	X	X	XX	—
Quadratus lumborum	—	XX	XX	—

*Unless otherwise stated, the actions describe movement of the muscle's superior or lateral aspect relative to its fixed inferior or medial aspect. The actions are assumed to occur from *the anatomic position*, against an external resistance. A muscle's relative torque or strength potential for a given action is assigned X (minimal), XX (moderate), or XXX (maximum), based on moment arm (leverage), cross-sectional area, and fiber direction — indicates no effective or conclusive action.

[†]*CL*, contralateral rotation; *IL*, ipsilateral rotation.

[‡]Acts primarily to increase intra-abdominal pressure and, via attachments to the thoracolumbar fascia, to stabilize the lumbar region. Also stabilizes the attachment sites for the other lateral abdominal muscles.

with sitting upright. In contrast to these extreme motor deficits, persons with an apparently intact neuromuscular system may still lack the necessary muscle strength and/or motor control to adequately stabilize their trunk. Such functional spinal instability may be related to neural inhibition, physical inactivity, atrophy and other histologic changes in muscle, the neurologic processing of pain, or pre-existing degenerative changes in the spine.[42,177] Although often subtle and difficult to clinically validate, lack of muscular control of the trunk may theoretically result in undesired intervertebral micromotion throughout the axial spine that, over time, could place cumulative and excessive stress on the vertebral column and neural elements. This clinical scenario is typically less outwardly severe than the extreme cases cited earlier but nevertheless may have the potential to cause spinal-related pain, at least in a certain subset of the population.

In general terms, muscular-based stability of the trunk is often referred to as "core stability," although this term is often overused clinically and not well defined. Nevertheless, such muscular stability infers a near-static posture of the trunk even under the influence of destabilizing external forces. Consider, for example, the wave of muscular activation experienced throughout the trunk when one attempts to stand or sit upright in an accelerating bus or train. Normally, trunk muscles can subconsciously stabilize the position of the trunk relative to the surrounding environment and, equally important, to stabilize the individual spinal segments within the axial skeleton. Ideally, a stable "core" provided by the muscles of the trunk provides structural integrity to the region, optimizes postural alignment, and limits excessive, and potentially stressful, micromotions between intervertebral junctions. Finally, stability of the trunk also establishes a firm base for muscles to move and adequately control the limbs. This control is especially important for control of the knee while landing from a jump.[31]

This chapter partitions the muscular stabilizers of the trunk into two anatomic groups, based on their attachments. *Intrinsic muscular stabilizers* include the relatively short, deep, and segmented muscles that attach primarily *within* the region of the vertebral column. *Extrinsic muscular stabilizers,* in contrast, include relatively long muscles that attach, either partially or totally, to structures *outside* the region of the vertebral column, such as the cranium, pelvis, ribs, and lower extremities.

Intrinsic Muscular Stabilizers of the Trunk

- Transversospinal group
  - Semispinalis muscles
  - Multifidus
  - Rotatores
- Short segmental group
  - Interspinalis muscles
  - Intertransversarius muscles

Extrinsic Muscular Stabilizers of the Trunk

- Muscles of the anterior-lateral trunk ("abdominals")
  - Rectus abdominis
  - Obliquus externus abdominis
  - Obliquus internus abdominis
  - Transversus abdominis
- Erector spinae
- Quadratus lumborum
- Psoas major
- Hip muscles that connect the lumbopelvic regions with the lower extremity

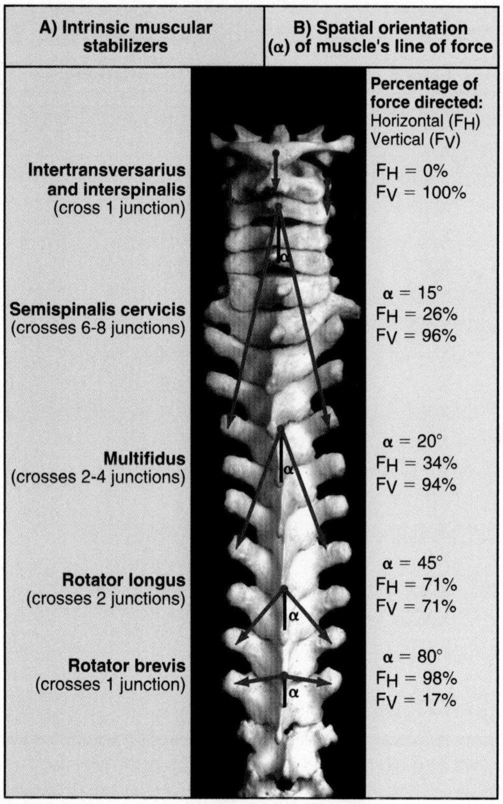

A) Intrinsic muscular stabilizers	B) Spatial orientation (α) of muscle's line of force
	Percentage of force directed: Horizontal (F_H) Vertical (F_V)
Intertransversarius and interspinalis (cross 1 junction)	F_H = 0% F_V = 100%
Semispinalis cervicis (crosses 6-8 junctions)	α = 15° F_H = 26% F_V = 96%
Multifidus (crosses 2-4 junctions)	α = 20° F_H = 34% F_V = 94%
Rotator longus (crosses 2 junctions)	α = 45° F_H = 71% F_V = 71%
Rotator brevis (crosses 1 junction)	α = 80° F_H = 98% F_V = 17%

FIGURE 10.19 Diagrammatic representation of the spatial orientation of the lines of force of the intrinsic muscular stabilizers. (A) The lines of force of muscles are shown within the frontal plane. (B) The spatial orientation of the line of force of each muscle is indicated by the angle (α) formed relative to the vertical position. The percentage of muscle force directed vertically is equal to the cosine of α; the percentage of muscle force directed horizontally is equal to the sine of α. Assuming adequate leverage, the vertically directed muscle forces produce extension and lateral flexion, and the more horizontally directed muscle forces produce axial rotation. Note that the muscles illustrated exist throughout the entire vertebral column; their location in the figure is simplified for the sake of clarity.

Intrinsic Muscular Stabilizers of the Trunk

The intrinsic muscular stabilizers of the trunk include the *transversospinal* and *short segmental* groups of muscles. These deep and relatively short muscles are depicted in a highly diagrammatic fashion in Fig. 10.19A. In general, these muscles stabilize the spine by precisely controlling alignment and stiffness among a relatively few intervertebral junctions at a time.[177] The relative high density of muscle spindles residing in many of these segmental muscles enhances their fine-tuning ability.[155]

As indicated in Fig. 10.19B, the spatial orientation of each muscle's line of force (depicted by α) produces a unique stabilization effect on the vertebral column. Vertically running interspinalis and intertransversarius muscles produce 100% of their force in the vertical direction (F_V). In contrast, the near horizontally oriented rotator brevis muscle produces close to 100% of its force in the horizontal direction (F_H). All of the remaining muscles produce forces that are directed diagonally at some angle between 0 and 90 degrees. The muscles act as an array of bilaterally matched guy wires, specifically aligned to compress as well as control the shear between intervertebral junctions. In addition to effectively securing both vertical and horizontal stability, collectively these muscles exert extension, lateral flexion, and axial rotation torques across the entire vertebral column.

Without such fine muscle control, the multisegmented vertebral column becomes very vulnerable to exaggerated spinal curvature, excessive interspinal mobility, and, in some cases, may lead to painful structural instability.

Extrinsic Muscular Stabilizers of the Trunk

The primary extrinsic muscular stabilizers of the trunk include the abdominal muscles, erector spinae, quadratus lumborum, psoas major, and the hip muscles (by connecting the lumbopelvic region with the lower extremities). (See box on previous page.) These relatively long and often thick muscles stabilize the trunk by creating a strong and semirigid link between the cranium, vertebral column, pelvis, and lower extremities. Because many of these muscles cross a broad region of the body or trunk, they likely provide relatively coarse control over intersegmental mobility and stability. In addition, because many of these muscles possess a sizable cross-sectional area and leverage, they are, as a group, also important torque generators for the trunk and adjacent hip joints.

External forces applied against the upper trunk (and upper limbs) can produce substantial destabilizing leverage against the more caudal or inferior regions of the axial skeleton. The stabilization function of the extrinsic muscles is therefore particularly important in the lower trunk, including the lumbopelvic region. Although difficult to show a consistent causal relationship, muscular instability at the base of the spine may lead to postural malalignment throughout the entire vertebral column, as well as potentially lead to excessive wear of the lumbar apophyseal, interbody, and sacroiliac joints.

To further illustrate the potential role of the extrinsic stabilizers, Fig. 10.20 shows a person activating their external muscular stabilizers in response to an impending external perturbation. Note the concentration of muscular activity in the lower region of the trunk. Activation of the psoas major, quadratus lumborum, erector spinae, and abdominal muscles have the potential to provide substantial stability to the lumbopelvic region, in all three planes. Strong activation of abdominal muscles also helps to increase intra-abdominal pressure—a mechanism believed to exert a stabilizing effect throughout the lumbar region.[58,198] The horizontally oriented transversus abdominis, in particular, creates a circumferential splinting effect across the entire low back region, including the sacroiliac joints.[220]

Activation of the abdominal muscles also helps stabilize the pelvis against the pull of extensor muscles such as the erector spinae and quadratus lumborum. With the pelvis and caudal end of the spine well stabilized, forces that have an effect on the trunk are effectively transferred across the sacroiliac joints, through the hips, and ultimately through the lower extremities. Exercises designed to increase the muscular stability of the low back and lower trunk regions ideally should include creative activities that challenge both the trunk and the hip muscles, in all three planes of motion.

In closing, although the external and internal muscular stabilizers have been presented separately, there is a large overlap and redundancy in their functions. This may be appreciated by mentally superimposing the muscular arrows depicted in both Figs. 10.19 and 10.20. In ideal health, all muscles of the trunk contribute to the stabilization of the trunk, in both static and dynamic conditions.[26,113,162,202,217] The specific strategy used by any single muscle differs, however, based on factors such as its depth, cross-sectional area, fiber type, morphology, spatial orientation, and skeletal or connective tissue attachments.

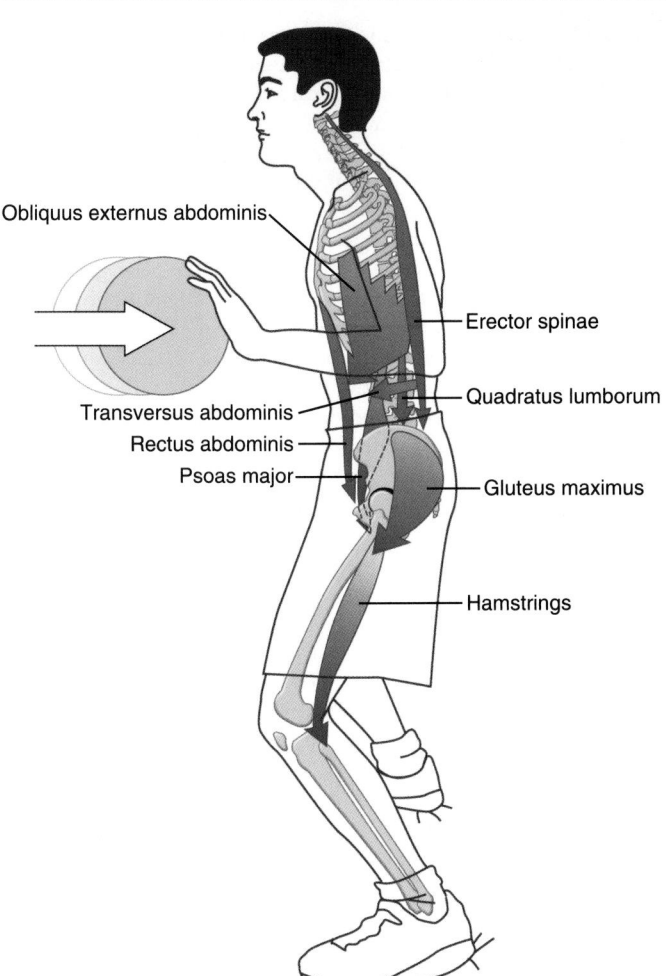

FIGURE 10.20 A typical activation pattern for a sample of external muscular stabilizers.

In the figure, the following labels appear:
- Obliquus externus abdominis
- Erector spinae
- Quadratus lumborum
- Transversus abdominis
- Rectus abdominis
- Psoas major
- Gluteus maximus
- Hamstrings

PERFORMING A STANDARD SIT-UP MOVEMENT

Most whole-body functional activities require concurrent activation of both the trunk and hip muscles. Consider, for example, the combined movements of the trunk and hips while one lifts a child, swings a baseball bat or golf club, reaches toward the floor, or shovels snow or dirt. To introduce this important synergistic relationship, the following discussion focuses on the muscular actions of performing a standard full *sit-up* movement.

In addition to being a very important functional activity, components of the full sit-up maneuver are often performed to challenge and strengthen the abdominal muscles. The common goal of resistive exercise is to increase the strength and control of these muscles, often to improve overall stability of the trunk. In a very broad sense, the strategies used to strengthen abdominal muscles usually fall into one of four categories (Fig. 10.21). In column 1 of Fig. 10.21, the abdominal muscles contract to produce a near isometric force to maintain a relative *constant distance* between the xiphoid process and the anterior pelvis. In columns 2 to 4, the abdominal muscles contract to *reduce* the distance between the xiphoid process and the anterior pelvis. (By acting eccentrically, the same muscles could also be challenged to slowly resist an *increase* in distance between these two regions of the body.)

#1 Isometric activity	#2 Rotating the trunk toward the stationary pelvis	#3 Rotating the trunk and pelvis toward the stationary legs	#4 Rotating the pelvis (and/or legs) toward the stationary trunk
Pictured example: 1. While in quadruped position, maintain rigid trunk and pelvis. Progress to raising arm and contralateral leg while balancing knee on an unstable surface, like an inflatable ball. **Other examples:** 2. Maintain upright trunk while seated on a relatively unstable surface. 3. Hold trunk rigid in a prone "plank" position with elbows extended and hands placed under shoulders. Progress to side plank position, varying the amount of ground contact made by the supporting limbs.	**Pictured example:** 1. Partial sit-ups ("crunches") with or without a foot stool. **Other examples:** 2. As above, but incorporate diagonal or rotational movements of the trunk. Add external resistance or perform exercise on a slightly reclined surface. 3. Lateral trunk curls ("crunches"), adding resistance as needed.	**Pictured example:** 1. Traditional full sit-up **Other examples:** 2. As above, but apply external resistance, or vary external moment arm by changing the position of the arms. 3. Perform traditional sit-up as pictured, but from a slightly reclined or unstable surface. 4. Perform traditional sit-up as pictured, but add diagonal or rotational movements of the trunk and pelvis.	**Pictured example:** 1. While holding the suspended trunk vertical, perform slow and deliberate bilateral or unilateral hip flexion motions. Progress to adding posterior pelvic tilt motions. **Other examples:** 2. As above but incorporate diagonal or rotational movements of the legs. 3. Unilateral or bilateral straight-leg raises from supine; adjust resistance by bending the knee and thereby changing the "length" of the lower extremities.

FIGURE 10.21 Four strategies typically used to perform abdominal strengthening exercises. Pictured examples are illustrated across the bottom row.

A full sit-up performed in a bent-knee position can be conveniently divided into two overlapping phases, based on the primary pivot point assumed for the motion. The "trunk flexion" phase involves primarily a modest amount of flexion of the thoracolumbar region, terminating when both scapulae are raised off the mat (Fig. 10.22A). The "hip flexion" phase involves continued flexion of the thoracolumbar region combined with marked pelvic-on-femoral (hip) flexion, yielding an additional 70 to 90 degrees of flexion of the trunk (see Fig. 10.22B).

As depicted in Fig. 10.22A, the *trunk flexion phase* is driven primarily by contraction of the abdominal muscles, most notably the rectus abdominis.[28,59,162] Contraction of these muscles flexes the trunk about a medial-lateral axis of rotation estimated near the thoracolumbar junction. The flexion of the trunk is typically accompanied by a posterior (tilt) rotation of the pelvis, thereby flattening the lumbar spine. During this phase, the EMG level of the hip flexor muscles is relatively low, regardless of the position of the hips and knees.[8,59] Partially flexing the hips before performing the exercise releases the passive tension in the hip flexor muscles (notably the dominant iliopsoas) while simultaneously increasing the passive tension in the gluteus maximus. These combined effects may assist the abdominal muscles in first producing and then maintaining a posteriorly tilted pelvis.

Finally, as illustrated in Fig. 10.22A, the latissimus dorsi, by passing anterior to the upper thoracic spine, may assist in flexing this region of the thorax.[218] Additionally, the sternal head of the pectoralis major may assist in advancing the upper extremities toward the pelvis.

During the *hip flexion phase* of the sit-up, the pelvis-and-trunk rotate as a single unit toward the relatively fixed femurs, dominated by strong contraction of the hip flexor muscles.[59] Although any hip flexor muscle can assist with this action, Fig. 10.22B shows the iliacus and rectus femoris as the active participants. Relative levels of EMG signal intensity from the iliacus, sartorius, and rectus femoris are significantly greater when the legs are actively held fixed to the supporting surface.[8] The heels of the shoes are shown in Fig. 10.22B being pulled into the supporting surface to fixate the

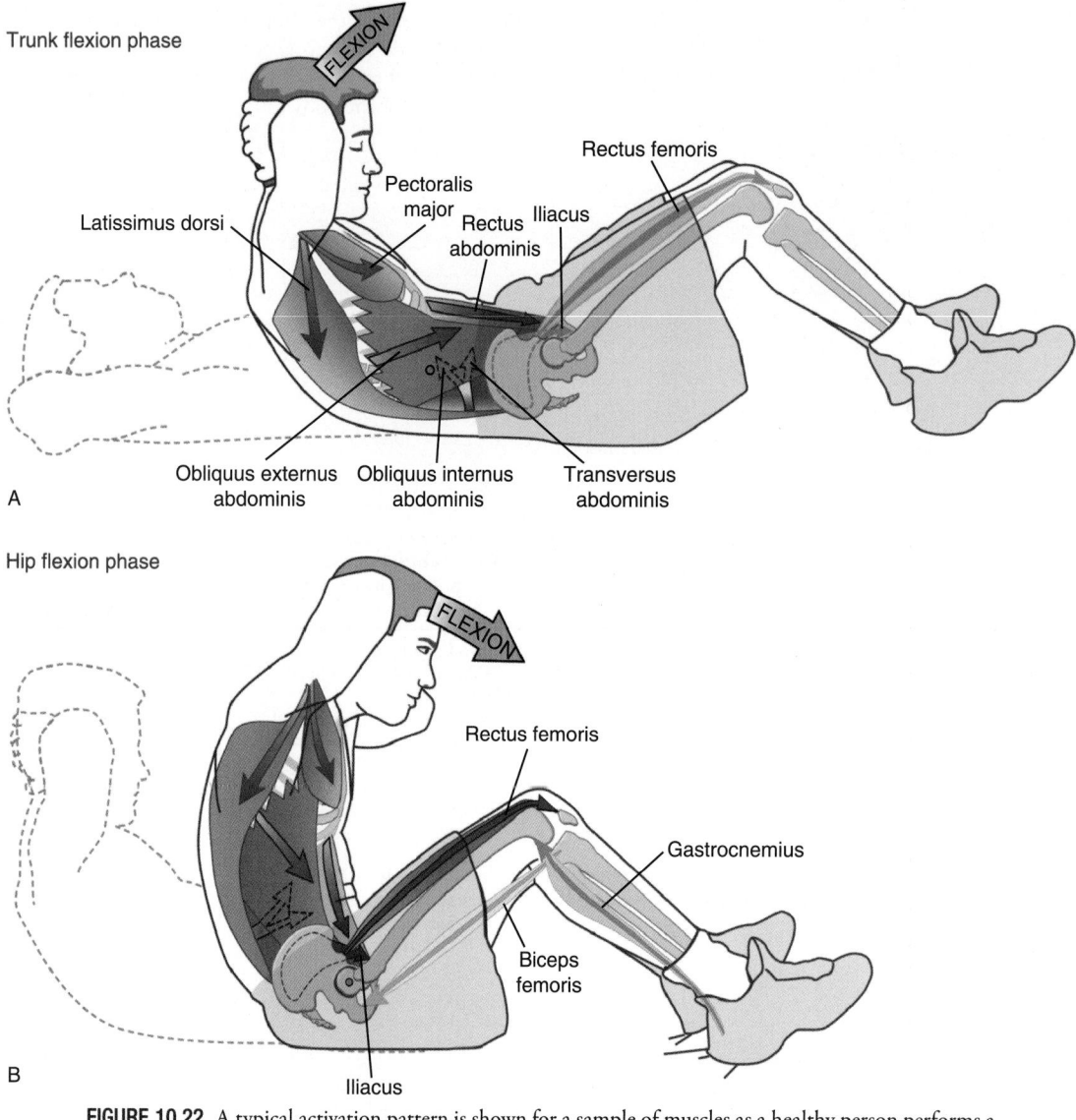

FIGURE 10.22 A typical activation pattern is shown for a sample of muscles as a healthy person performs a standard full *sit-up*. The intensity of the red color is related to the assumed intensity of the muscle activation. The full sit-up is divided into two phases: the trunk flexion phase, followed by the hip flexion phase. (A) The *trunk flexion phase* of the sit-up involves strong activation of the abdominal muscles, especially the rectus abdominis. (B) The *hip flexion phase* of the sit-up involves continued activation of the abdominal muscles but, more important, also the hip flexor muscles. Note in (B) the large pelvic-on-femoral contribution to the sit-up maneuver. The axes of rotation for movements performed in (A) and (B) are depicted by a *small circle*.

lower extremities relative to the pelvis and trunk. This stabilizing action produces relatively modest activation of the biceps femoris—a representative hamstring muscle, and moderate activation of the gastrocnemius.[154] Interestingly, activation of any of the bi-articular hamstring muscles must be of the eccentric type, given that the pelvis is simultaneously rotating in the direction of hip flexion.

The axis of rotation during the hip flexion phase of the full sit-up ultimately shifts toward the hip joints. Depending on the movement strategy, the abdominal muscles may continue to contract to create additional thoracolumbar flexion or remain nearly isometrically active through the completion of the sit-up. Their activation, however, does not contribute to hip (pelvic-on-femoral) flexion; rather, these muscles hold the flexed thoracolumbar region firmly in place while the pelvis is anteriorly rotating.

Persons with weakness of their abdominal muscles typically display a characteristic posture when attempting to perform a full sit-up. The hip flexor muscles tend to dominate the activity, often causing an exaggerated lumbar lordosis by excessively anterior tilting the pelvis, especially evident at the initiation of the maneuver.

Muscles of the Craniocervical Region: Anatomy and Their Individual Actions

The following sections describe the anatomy and individual actions of the muscles that act exclusively within the craniocervical region. Musculature is divided into two sets: (1) muscles of the *anterior-lateral* craniocervical region and (2) muscles of the *posterior* craniocervical region (listed in Table 10.1).

Fig. 10.23 serves as an introduction to the potential actions of many muscles in the craniocervical region. The illustration depicts selected muscles as flexors or extensors, or right or left lateral flexors, depending on their attachment relative to the axes of rotation through the atlanto-occipital joints. Although Fig. 10.23 indicates

SPECIAL FOCUS 10.3

Comparing the Abdominal "Curl-up" Exercise with the Standard Full Sit-up

The early, trunk flexion phase of the full sit-up (depicted in Fig. 10.22A) is similar in many respects to the popular, and often recommended, "curl-up" or "crunch" exercise, often defined as ending when both scapulae are raised off the mat, for strengthening the abdominal muscles. Both the curl-up and the full sit-up can place significant and challenging demands on the abdominal muscles as a whole. Notably, however, the curl-up produces significant activation from the rectus abdominis.[77,162] Furthermore, compared with a full (bent-knee) sit-up, the curl-up exercise (as depicted in Fig. 10.22A) places only marginal demands on the hip flexor muscles—typically not the muscles targeted for strengthening. Perhaps the most clinically significant difference in the two exercises is the fact that the curl-up exercise involves only modest flexion of the lumbar spine, likely less than about 5 degrees.[77] This is typically less than the degree of lumbar flexion that accompanies a *full* (bent-knee) sit-up. The flexion of the lumbar spine during the full sit-up can create greater pressure on the discs (see Chapter 9). For select subgroups, such as those who encounter significant pain with lumbar flexion or those with lumbar disc herniation, the curl-up exercise may therefore be more appropriate than the full sit-up. This precaution appears prudent, especially considering that the curl-up exercise still places significant demands on the abdominal muscles.[77]

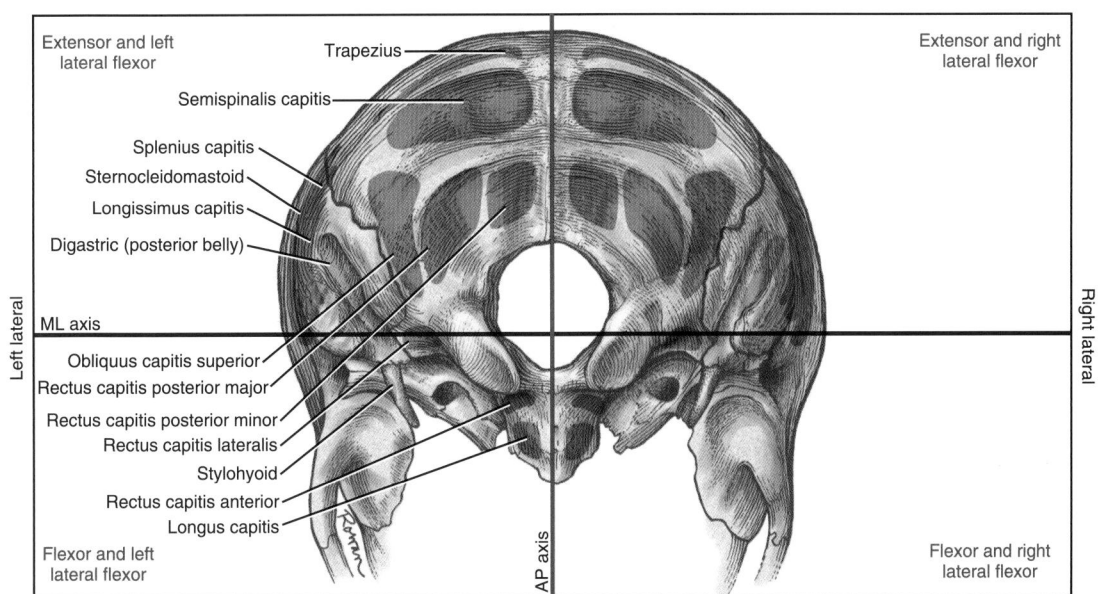

FIGURE 10.23 The potential action of muscles that attach to the inferior surface of the occipital and temporal bones is highlighted. The actions of the muscles across the atlanto-occipital joint are based on their location relative to the medial-lateral *(ML) (black)* and anterior-posterior *(AP) (red)* axis of rotation at the level of the occipital condyles. Note that the actions of most muscles fit into one of four quadrants. (Distal muscle attachments are indicated in *gray*, and proximal attachments are indicated in *red*.)

the muscle actions at the atlanto-occipital joint only, the relative position of the muscles provides a useful guide for an understanding of the actions at other joints within the craniocervical region. This figure is referenced throughout the upcoming sections.

SET 1: MUSCLES OF THE ANTERIOR-LATERAL CRANIOCERVICAL REGION

The muscles of the anterior-lateral craniocervical region are listed in Box 10.4. With the exception of the sternocleidomastoid, which is innervated primarily by the spinal accessory nerve (cranial nerve XI), the muscles in this region are innervated by small unnamed nerves that branch from the ventral rami of the cervical plexus.

Moment arm data for many of the muscles of the craniocervical region are listed as a resource in Appendix III, Part D, Fig. III.3.

Sternocleidomastoid

The sternocleidomastoid is typically a prominent muscle located superficially on the anterior aspect of the neck. Inferiorly the muscle attaches by two heads: medial (sternal) and lateral (clavicular) (Fig. 10.24). From this attachment, the muscle ascends obliquely

> **BOX 10.4 Muscles of the Anterior-Lateral Craniocervical Region**
>
> - Sternocleidomastoid
> - Scalenes
>   - Scalenus anterior
>   - Scalenus medius
>   - Scalenus posterior
> - Longus colli
> - Longus capitis
> - Rectus capitis anterior
> - Rectus capitis lateralis

across the neck to attach to the cranium, specifically between the mastoid process of the temporal bone and the lateral half of the superior nuchal line.

Acting unilaterally, the sternocleidomastoid is a dominant lateral flexor and contralateral axial rotator of the craniocervical region.[2] Contracting bilaterally, a pair of sternocleidomastoid muscles can flex *or* extend the craniocervical region depending on the specific area. Evident from a lateral view of a neutral cervical spine, the line of force of the right sternocleidomastoid is directed across the neck in an oblique fashion (Fig. 10.24, inset). Below approximately C3, the sternocleidomastoid crosses well *anterior* to the medial-lateral axes of rotation; above C3, however, the sternocleidomastoid crosses just *posterior* to the medial-lateral axes of rotation.[214] Acting together, the sternocleidomastoid muscles provide a strong *flexion* torque to the mid-to-lower cervical spine and a minimal *extension* torque to the upper cervical spine, including the atlanto-axial and atlanto-occipital joints. It is worth noting that this combined sagittal plane action favors a forward (protracted) head posture (review Chapter 9 and Fig. 9.47A)

Computer modeling indicates that the sagittal plane torque potential of the different regions of the sternocleidomastoid is strongly affected by the initial position of the craniocervical region.[214] Primarily because of moment arm length, the flexed position of the mid-to-lower cervical spine, for example, nearly doubles the muscle's flexion torque potential in this region. This becomes especially relevant in persons with an established marked forward head posture. Because this posture involves excessive flexion at the mid-to-lower cervical region, it may perpetuate the biomechanics that strongly favor a forward head posture.

Scalenes

The scalene muscles attach between the tubercles of the transverse processes of the middle to lower cervical vertebrae and the first two ribs (Fig. 10.25). (As a side note, the Latin or Greek root of the word *scalene* refers to a triangle with three unequal sides.) The specific attachments of these muscles are listed in Appendix III, Part C. The brachial plexus courses between the scalenus anterior and scalenus medius. Hypertrophy, spasm, or excessive stiffness of these muscles may compress the brachial plexus and cause motor and sensory disturbances in the upper extremity.

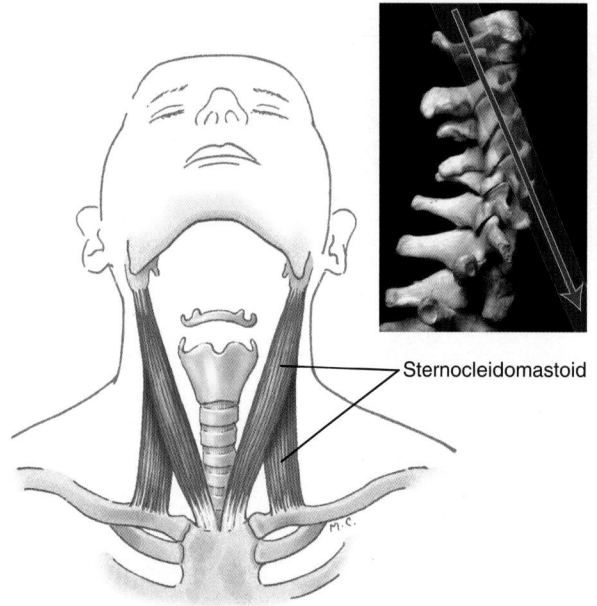

FIGURE 10.24 An anterior view of the sternocleidomastoid muscles. The inset shows a lateral view of the oblique orientation of the sternocleidomastoid muscle *(arrow)* as it crosses the craniocervical region. (Modified from Luttgens K, Hamilton N: *Kinesiology: scientific basis of human motion,* ed 9, Madison, WI, 1997, Brown & Benchmark; Photograph of inset by Donald A. Neumann.)

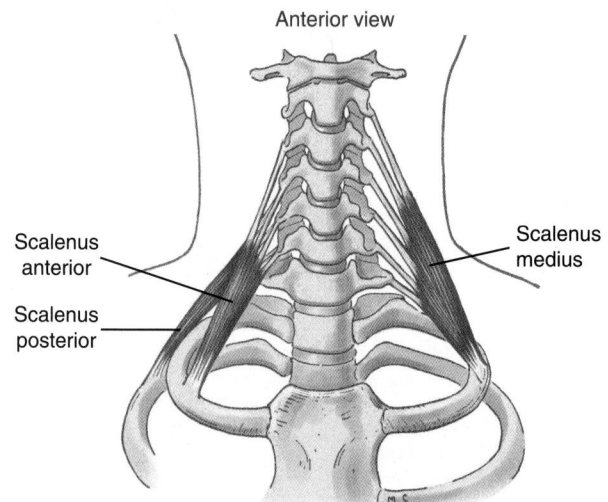

FIGURE 10.25 An anterior view of the right scalenus posterior and scalenus anterior, and the left scalenus medius. (Modified from Luttgens K, Hamilton N: *Kinesiology: scientific basis of human motion,* ed 9, Madison, WI, 1997, Brown & Benchmark.)

The function of the scalene muscles depends on which skeletal attachments are most fixed. With the cervical spine well stabilized, the scalene muscles raise the ribs to assist with inspiration during breathing. Alternatively, with the first two ribs well stabilized, contraction of the scalene muscles moves the cervical spine.

Contracting unilaterally, the scalene muscles laterally flex the cervical spine.[2,28] The scalenus anterior, arising from the anterior-lateral region of the first rib, has the greatest moment arm of all the scalenes for this action, second only to the cranial fibers of the sternocleidomastoid.[2] The horizontal plane (axial rotation) action of the scalenes is not really clear. Based on the limited publications on this topic, when analyzed from the anatomic position, the muscles have only a slight and short-range *ipsilateral* rotation function.[2,34] This limited axial rotation potential is because the scalenes' averaged line of force nearly pierces the vertical axis of rotation. The muscles' full axial rotation potential, however, is likely realized only when the craniocervical region is well outside the anatomic position. The axial rotation actions of the scalenes are therefore dependent on the overall posture of the region and, even more importantly, on the starting position from which the muscles contract. It appears that an important function of the scalene muscles is their ability to *return* the craniocervical region to a near-neutral position from a previously contralaterally or ipsilaterally rotated position. This more global and perhaps primary function may be overlooked when the neutral (anatomic) position is used as a starting point to analyze the muscles' action. This may be true for many muscles throughout the axial spine (and the body). In the axial spine, for example, the rectus abdominis and quadratus lumborum may have minimal axial rotation ability from the anatomic position but perhaps a greater ability to rotate the body *back* to the anatomic position from a pre-rotated position.

Contracting bilaterally, the scalenus anterior muscles have a limited moment arm to flex the cervical spine.[2] The muscles' bilateral activity is most likely related to ventilation (as described previously) and providing stability to the cervical region. The cervical attachments of all three scalene muscles split into several individual fasciculi (Fig. 10.25). Like a system of guy wires that stabilize a large antenna, the scalene muscles provide excellent bilateral and vertical stability to the middle and lower cervical spine. Fine control of the upper craniocervical region is more the responsibility of the shorter, more specialized muscles, such as the rectus capitis anterior and the suboccipital muscles (discussed ahead).

Longus Colli and Longus Capitis

The longus colli and longus capitis are located deep to the cervical viscera (trachea and esophagus), on both sides of the cervical column (Fig. 10.26). The muscles' deep location limits their moment arm lengths for producing sagittal or frontal plane torques.[201] These muscles function primarily as a *dynamic anterior longitudinal ligament,* providing an active element of vertical stability to the region.[62,116]

The *longus colli* consists of multiple fascicles that closely adhere to the anterior surfaces of the upper three thoracic and all cervical vertebrae. This segmented muscle ascends the cervical region through multiple attachments between the vertebral bodies, anterior tubercles of transverse processes, and anterior arch of the atlas. The longus colli is the only muscle that attaches in its entirety to the anterior surface of the vertebral column. Compared with the scalene and sternocleidomastoid muscles, the longus colli is a relatively thin muscle. The more anterior fibers of the longus colli flex the cervical region, reducing cervical lordosis. The more lateral

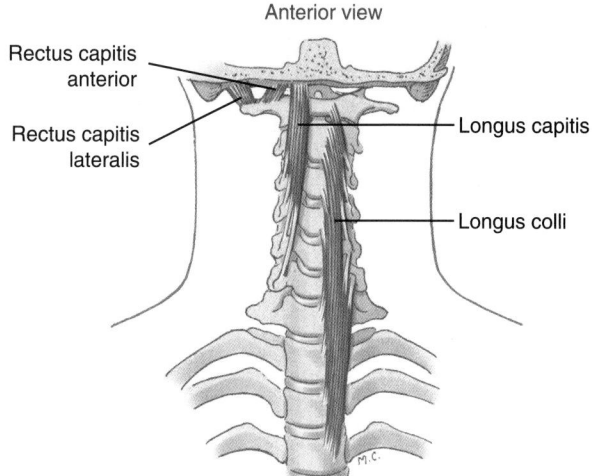

FIGURE 10.26 An anterior view of the deep muscles in the neck. The following muscles are shown: right longus capitis, right rectus capitis anterior, right rectus capitis lateralis, and left longus colli. (Modified from Luttgens K, Hamilton N: *Kinesiology: scientific basis of human motion,* ed 9, Madison, WI, 1997, Brown & Benchmark.)

fibers act in conjunction with the scalene muscles to vertically stabilize the region.

The *longus capitis* arises from the anterior tubercles of the transverse processes of the mid-to-lower cervical vertebrae and inserts into the basilar part of the occipital bone (see Fig. 10.23). The primary action of the longus capitis is to flex and stabilize the upper craniocervical region. Lateral flexion is a secondary action.

Rectus Capitis Anterior and Rectus Capitis Lateralis

The rectus capitis anterior and rectus capitis lateralis are two short, deep muscles that arise from the elongated transverse processes of the atlas (C1) and insert on the inferior surface of the occipital bone (Fig. 10.26). The rectus capitis anterior, the smaller of the recti, attaches immediately anterior to the occipital condyle; the rectus capitis lateralis attaches laterally to the occipital condyle (see Fig. 10.23).

The actions of the rectus capitis anterior and lateralis muscles are limited to the atlanto-occipital joint; each muscle controls one of the joint's two degrees of freedom (see Chapter 9). The rectus capitis anterior is a flexor, and the rectus capitis lateralis is a lateral flexor.

SET 2: MUSCLES OF THE POSTERIOR CRANIOCERVICAL REGION

The muscles of the posterior craniocervical region are listed in Box 10.5. They are innervated by dorsi rami of cervical spinal nerves.

BOX 10.5   Muscles of the Posterior Craniocervical Region

- Splenius muscles
  - Splenius cervicis
  - Splenius capitis
- Suboccipital muscles
  - Rectus capitis posterior major
  - Rectus capitis posterior minor
  - Obliquus capitis superior
  - Obliquus capitis inferior

Posterior view

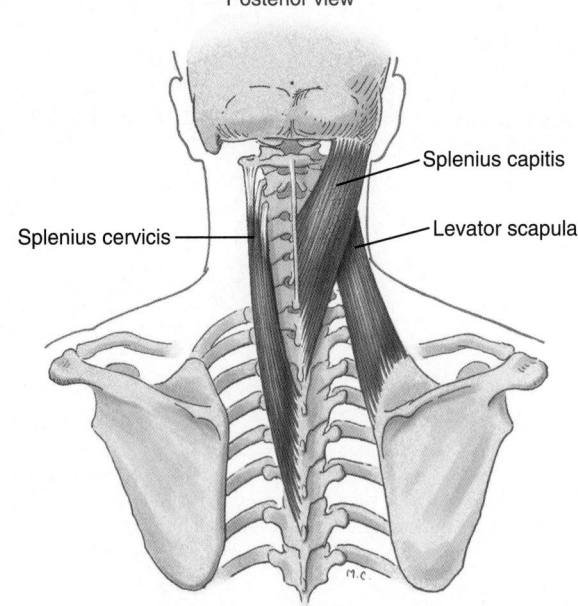

FIGURE 10.27 A posterior view of the left splenius cervicis, right splenius capitis, and right levator scapula. Although not visible, the cervical attachments of the levator scapula are similar to the cervical attachments of the splenius cervicis. (Modified from Luttgens K, Hamilton N: *Kinesiology: scientific basis of human motion,* ed 9, Madison, WI, 1997, Brown & Benchmark.)

Splenius Cervicis and Capitis

The splenius cervicis and capitis muscles are a long and thin pair of muscles, named by their resemblance to a bandage (from the Greek *splenion,* "bandage") (Fig. 10.27). As a pair, the splenius muscles arise from the inferior half of the ligamentum nuchae and spinous processes of C7 to T6, just deep to the trapezius muscles. The *splenius capitis* attaches to the occipital bone, just inferior to the sternocleidomastoid (see Fig. 10.23). The *splenius cervicis* attaches to the posterior tubercles of the transverse processes of C1 to C3. Much of this cervical attachment is shared by the attachments of the levator scapula muscle.

Contracting unilaterally, the splenius muscles perform lateral flexion and ipsilateral axial rotation of the head and cervical spine. Based on a larger cross-sectional area and a more oblique fiber direction, the splenius capitis is, by far, the more dominant axial rotator.[2,23] Contracting bilaterally, the splenius muscles possess excellent leverage to extend the upper craniocervical region.[201]

Suboccipital Muscles

The suboccipital muscles consist of four paired muscles located very deep in the posterior neck, immediately superficial to the atlanto-occipital and atlanto-axial joints (Fig. 10.28). These relatively short but thick muscles attach among the atlas, axis, and occipital bone. (Their specific muscular attachments are listed in Appendix III, Part C.)

The suboccipital muscles are not easily palpable. They lie deep to the upper trapezius, splenius group, and semispinalis capitis muscles (see Fig. 10.23). In conjunction with the rectus capitis anterior and lateralis, the suboccipital muscles provide precise control over the atlanto-occipital and atlanto-axial joints. Each muscle has a distinctive set of bony attachments and line of force. Consequently, as indicated in Fig. 10.29, each suboccipital muscle (plus each short rectus muscle) has a unique level of control and dominance over the joints of the upper craniocervical region.[2,23] This level of control is essential for optimal positioning of the many special senses associated with the head. The

Posterior view

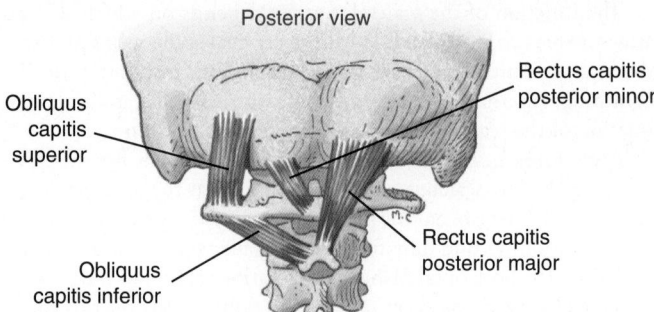

FIGURE 10.28 A posterior view of the suboccipital muscles. The left obliquus capitis superior, left obliquus capitis inferior, left rectus capitis posterior minor, and right rectus capitis posterior major are shown. (Modified from Luttgens K, Hamilton N: *Kinesiology: scientific basis of human motion,* ed 9, Madison, WI, 1997, Brown & Benchmark.)

relatively large density of muscle spindles within these muscles also suggests an important role in providing neural feedback regarding the position and rate of head movement, thus indirectly contributing to balance, equilibrium, and eye-head coordination.[53,170]

In closing, dissection study has shown that the medial and deeply situated rectus capitis posterior minor muscles share fascial attachments with the immediately adjacent (and deep) posterior atlanto-occipital membrane (see Fig. 9.42).[216] Because this membrane also attaches to the spinal dura mater, a contracting muscle could pull the dura posteriorly slightly. Functionally, the posterior pull on the dura mater during full extension may be a natural protective mechanism that limits an inward bulging of the dura against the spinal cord. Research interests into these fascial connections has been prompted, in part, by the possibility that excessive tension in the suboccipital muscles may be associated with the pathogenesis of cervicogenic headaches.

Muscles of the Craniocervical Region: Functional Interactions among Muscles That Cross the Craniocervical Region

Nearly 30 pairs of muscles cross the craniocervical region. These include the muscles that act exclusively within the craniocervical region (see Fig. 10.29 and Table 10.5), plus those classified as muscles of the posterior trunk that cross the craniocervical region (e.g., trapezius and longissimus capitis).

This section highlights the functional interactions among the muscles that cross the craniocervical regions during two activities: (1) stabilizing the craniocervical region and (2) producing the movements of the head and neck that optimize the function of visual, auditory, and olfactory systems. Although many other functional interactions exist for these muscles, the two activities provide a format for describing key kinesiologic principles involved in this important region of the body.

STABILIZING THE CRANIOCERVICAL REGION

The muscles that cross the craniocervical region comprise much of the bulk of the neck, especially in the regions lateral and posterior to the cervical vertebrae. When strongly activated, this mass of muscle serves to protect the cervical viscera and blood vessels, intervertebral discs, apophyseal joints, and neural tissues.

Athletes involved in contact sports may benefit from resistive or so-called "stabilization" exercises to hypertrophy this musculature. Hypertrophy alone, however, may not necessarily prevent neck

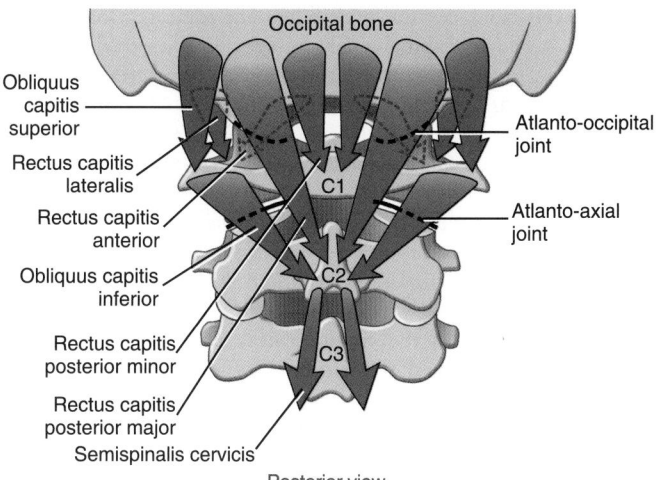

Occipital bone

Obliquus capitis superior

Rectus capitis lateralis

Rectus capitis anterior

Obliquus capitis inferior

Rectus capitis posterior minor

Rectus capitis posterior major

Semispinalis cervicis

Atlanto-occipital joint

Atlanto-axial joint

C1

C2

C3

Posterior view

MUSCLES	ATLANTO-OCCIPITAL JOINT			ATLANTO-AXIAL JOINT		
	FLEXION	EXTENSION	LATERAL FLEXION	FLEXION	EXTENSION	AXIAL ROTATION*
Rectus capitis anterior	XX	–	X	–	–	–
Rectus capitis lateralis	–	–	XX	–	–	–
Rectus capitis posterior major	–	XXX	XX	–	XXX	XX(IL)
Rectus capitis posterior minor	–	XX	X	–	–	–
Obliquus capitis inferior	–	–	–	–	XX	XXX(IL)
Obliquus capitis superior	–	XXX	XXX	–	–	–

*IL = ipsilateral rotation

FIGURE 10.29 A posterior view depicts the lines of force of muscles relative to the underlying atlanto-occipital and atlanto-axial joints. Each of these joints allows two primary degrees of freedom. Note that the attachment of the semispinalis cervicis muscle provides a stable base for the rectus capitis posterior major and the obliquus capitis inferior, two of the larger and more dominant suboccipital muscles. The chart summarizes the actions of the muscles at the atlanto-occipital and atlanto-axial joints. A muscle's relative torque or strength potential for a given action is assigned one of three scores: X, minimal; XX, moderate; and XXX, maximum. The *dash* indicates no effective torque production.

 S P E C I A L F O C U S 1 0 . 4

Specialized Muscles That Control the Atlanto-axial and Atlanto-occipital Joints: An Example of Fine-Tuning of Cervical Spinal Coupling

The highly specialized muscles listed in Fig. 10.29 exert fine control over the movements of the upper craniocervical region. One benefit of this control is related to the *spinal coupling pattern* typically expressed within the cervical region. As described in Chapter 9, an ipsilateral spinal coupling pattern exists in the mid-and-lower cervical region between the motions of axial rotation and lateral flexion. Axial rotation, resulting primarily from the orientation of the facet surfaces within the apophyseal joints, is mechanically associated with slight ipsilateral lateral flexion, and vice versa. The expression of this coupling pattern can be obscured, however, by the action of the specialized muscles that control the atlanto-occipital and atlanto-axial joints. Consider, for example, right axial rotation of the craniocervical region. For a level horizontal visual gaze to be maintained throughout axial rotation, the left rectus capitis lateralis, for example, produces a slight left lateral flexion torque to the head. This muscular action offsets the tendency of the head to laterally flex to the right with the rest of the cervical region during the right axial rotation.[75] Similarly, right lateral flexion of the mid-to-lower cervical region (which is coupled with slight right axial rotation) may be accompanied by a slight offsetting left axial rotation torque applied to the head by the obliquus capitis inferior muscle. In both examples, the muscular actions allow the head and eyes to fix on an object more precisely visually.

TABLE 10.5 Actions of Selected Muscles Located within the Craniocervical Region*

Muscle	Flexion	Extension	Lateral Flexion	Axial Rotation†
Sternocleidomastoid	XXX	X‡	XXX	XXX (CL)
Scalenus anterior	X	—	XXX	X (IL)
Scalenus medius	—	—	XX	X (IL)
Scalenus posterior	—	—	XX	X (IL)
Longus colli	XX	—	X	—
Longus capitis	XX	—	X	—
Splenius capitis	—	XXX	XX	XXX (IL)
Splenius cervicis	—	XXX	XX	XX (IL)

*The actions are assumed to occur *from the anatomic (neutral) position,* against an external resistance. A muscle's relative torque or strength potential for a given action is scored as X (minimal), XX (moderate), or XXX (maximum) based on moment arm (leverage), cross-sectional area, and fiber direction—indicates no effective or conclusive action.
†*CL,* contralateral rotation; *IL,* ipsilateral rotation.
‡Upper parts of sternocleidomastoid extend the upper cervical region, atlanto-axial joint, and atlanto-occipital joint.

injury. Data on the biomechanics of whiplash injury, for example, suggest that the time required to react to an impending injury and generate a substantial stabilizing force may exceed the time of the whiplash event.[50] For this reason, athletes need to anticipate a potentially harmful situation and activate the neck musculature *before* impact.[105] It may be possible that appropriately timed activation of craniocervical muscles may stiffen the neck and thereby limit the transfer of acceleration-related whiplash energy between the head and brain, potentially reducing the risk of sport-related concussion.[105,200]

In addition to stabilizing and protecting the neck, forces produced by muscles provide the primary source of vertical stability to the craniocervical region. The "critical load" of the cervical spine (i.e., maximum compressive load that the neck, unsupported by muscle, can sustain before buckling) is between 10.5 and 40 N (between 2.4 and 9 lb). Remarkably, this may be less than the actual weight of the head.[165,169] A coordinated interaction of craniocervical muscles generates forces that are, on average, directed nearly *through* the instantaneous axis of rotation at each intervertebral junction. By passing through or close to these multiple axes, the forces compress the vertebral segments together, thereby stabilizing them without buckling. The magnitude of these compression forces generated across the craniocervical region is quite high—nearly three times the weight of the head during the low-level muscle activation required to balance the head during upright standing, and up to 23 times the weight of the head (or 1.7 times body weight) during maximal-effort muscle activation.[146,169]

Much of the muscular stabilization of the craniocervical region is accomplished by the relatively short, segmented muscles, such as the relatively thick cervical multifidus. The rotatores, longus colli and capitis, and interspinalis muscles provide additional stabilization. The relatively short fibers and multiple bony attachments of these muscles as a whole exert a fine, coordinated control of the stability in the region. This stability is augmented by other longer and typically much thicker muscles, including the scalenes, sternocleidomastoid, levator scapula, semispinalis capitis and cervicis, and trapezius. When needed, these muscles form an extensive and strong guy-wire system that ensures vertical stability, most notably in frontal and sagittal planes. Fig. 10.30A highlights a sample of muscles that act as guy wires to maintain ideal anterior-posterior alignment throughout the craniocervical region. Ideally, the co-contraction of flexor and extensor muscles counterbalances, and as a consequence vertically stabilizes, the region. Note that the muscles depicted in Fig. 10.30A are anchored inferiorly to several different structures: the sternum, clavicle, ribs, scapula, and vertebral column. These bony structures themselves must be stabilized by other muscles, such as the lower trapezius and subclavius, to secure the scapula and clavicle, respectively.

PRODUCING EXTENSIVE AND WELL-COORDINATED MOVEMENTS OF THE HEAD AND NECK: OPTIMIZING THE PLACEMENT OF THE EYES, EARS, AND NOSE

The craniocervical region allows the greatest triplanar mobility of any region of the axial skeleton. Ample movement is essential for optimal spatial orientation of the eyes, ears, and nose. Although all planes of motion are equally important in this regard, the following section highlights movement within the horizontal plane.

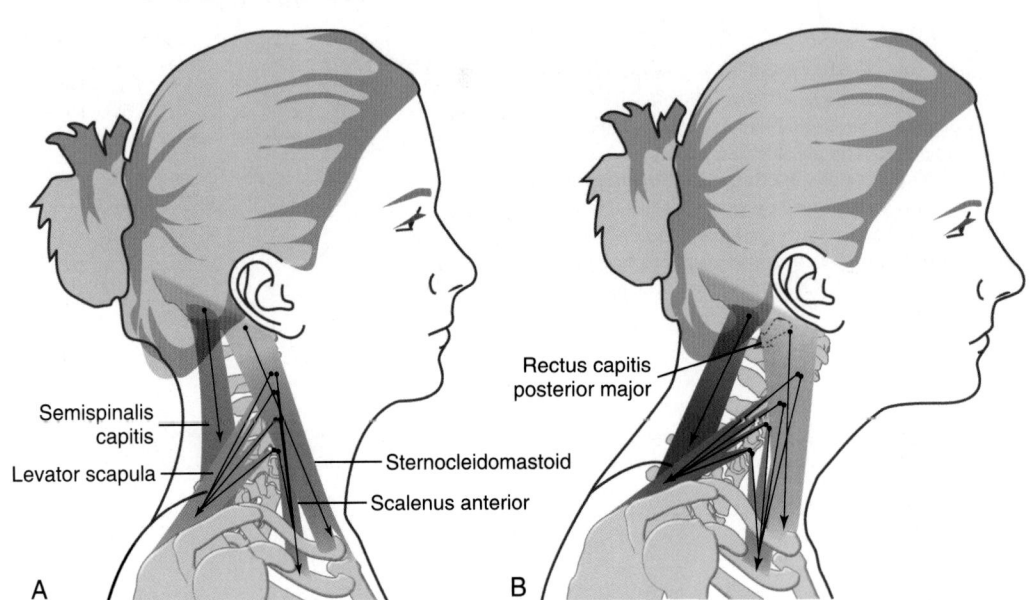

FIGURE 10.30 (A) Four muscles are acting as guy wires to maintain ideal posture within the craniocervical region. (B) Mechanics associated with a chronic forward head posture as discussed in Special Focus 10.5. The protracted position of the craniocervical region places greater stress on the levator scapula and semispinalis capitis muscles. The rectus capitis posterior major—one of the suboccipital muscles—is shown actively extending the upper craniocervical region. The highly active and stressed muscles are depicted in *brighter red*.

SPECIAL FOCUS 10.5

Muscular Imbalance Associated with Chronic Forward Head Posture

The ideal posture shown in Fig. 10.30A depicts an optimally balanced craniocervical "guy-wire" system. Excessive muscular tension in any of the muscles, however, can alter the vertical stability of the region. One such alteration is a chronic forward (protracted) head posture (see Fig. 10.30B).[36] Habitual forward head posture may be associated with several, often interrelated pathomechanical scenarios. Consider the three following possibilities. First, an excessive or violent hyperextension movement of the craniocervical region can strain muscles such as the sternocleidomastoid, longus colli, and scalenus anterior. As a result, chronic spasm or protective guarding in the strained muscles can bias a flexed position of the lower-to-mid cervical region, thereby initiating the mechanics of a protracted (or forward head) posture (review Chapter 9). A clinical sign often associated with forward head posturing is a realignment of the sternocleidomastoid within the sagittal plane. The cranial end of the muscle, normally aligned posterior to the sternoclavicular joint, shifts anteriorly with the head to a position directly above the sternoclavicular joint (compare Fig. 10.30A with Fig. 10.30B).

A second pathomechanical scenario that may cause or predispose forward head posturing relates to neural inhibition, pain, weakness, or fatigability of the deeper craniocervical flexor muscles, specifically the longus colli and capitis.[48] Why these particular muscles are more susceptible to relative deactivation is not entirely clear. Nevertheless, and perhaps as a compensation, the more superficial sternocleidomastoid or scalenus anterior may become the dominant kinetic influence in the region.[110] The biomechanics and neuromuscular control of the deep and superficial craniocervical flexor muscles is complex and not fully understood, and has been a topic of physical therapy research for neck pain and associated headache or temporomandibular joint pain.[15,29,60,61] Some therapeutic approaches to this impairment focus on exercises that increase the activation of the longus colli and capitis while minimizing the activation of the dominant sternocleidomastoid.[30,48,62,206] One such exercise is performed using EMG biofeedback and asking the supine-lying person to perform a craniocervical flexion (nodding) movement (an action of the longus capitis) while simultaneously flattening the cervical lordosis against a pressure gauge (an action of the longus colli). A successful movement is achieved if the action can be performed (and verified by the pressure gauge) with minimal activation of the sternocleidomastoid. Greater relative activation of the longus colli and capitis during head and neck movements is believed to provide better intrinsic vertical stability without a strong forward translation effect on the craniocervical region—a hallmark of dominant bilateral sternocleidomastoid activation.

Finally, a chronic forward head posture may be related to ergonomics. One such scenario involves purposely protracting the entire craniocervical region to improve visual contact with objects positioned in front of the body, such as when viewing a computer screen, mobile phone, or television.[131] A forward head position, if used for an extended period, may alter the functional resting length of the craniocervical muscles, possibly transforming the forward posture into a person's "natural" posture.

It is likely that the pathomechanics of forward head posturing is often the result of a combination of the scenarios described earlier rather than any one particular cause. Regardless of the predisposing factors, a chronic forward head posture stresses extensor muscles, such as the levator scapula and semispinalis capitis (see Fig. 10.30B).[144] Suboccipital muscles, such as the rectus capitis posterior major (or minor), may become overloaded and fatigued as a result of its prolonged extension activity required to "level" the head and eyes (review Fig. 9.47A).[111] Over time, increased muscular stress throughout the entire craniocervical region can lead to localized and painful muscle spasms, or "trigger points," common in the levator scapula and suboccipital muscles. This condition may be associated with headaches, reduced neck mobility, and radiating pain into the scalp and temporomandibular joints.[9,57,111,161] This association between posture and pain tends to be stronger in the adult and older adult population but generally lacking for adolescents.[136,175,179] In either group, however, an overall definitive causal relationship between chronic forward head posture and pain has not been well established. Common interventions for forward head posturing often focus on ways of restoring optimal craniocervical posture, which may include improved postural awareness, selective muscle activation and stretching, ergonomic workplace redesign,[238] and specific manual therapy techniques.

SPECIAL FOCUS 10.6

Whiplash Injury: Wide-Ranging Clinical Implications

The soft tissues of the cervical spine are particularly vulnerable to injury from a whiplash event, often associated with an automobile accident. In some cases, the injury can result in a myriad of severe and long-lasting symptoms, typically involving neck pain, dizziness, headache, and complaints of reduced neck mobility. A wider range of clinical findings are often included within the broad term *whiplash-associated disorder,* including muscle weakness, disturbed nociceptive processing, nerve root or brachial plexus injury, altered cervical posturing, concussion-related symptoms, cognitive changes, cutaneous hypersensitivity on the neck and upper limb, stress-related anxiety, and more.[74,115,124,176,231] Treatment for such a complex and intermixing of clinical findings likely benefits from the expertise of multiple health professionals.[231]

Whiplash associated with cervical hyperextension generally creates greater strain on soft tissues than does whiplash associated with cervical hyperflexion.[196] Hyperextension occurs over a relatively large range of motion and therefore can severely strain the craniocervical flexor muscles, cervical viscera, and other anteriorly located connective tissues, as well as excessively compress the apophyseal joints, discs, and posterior elements of the cervical spine (Fig. 10.31A).[101] In contrast, the maximum extent of flexion is partially blocked by the chin striking the chest (see Fig. 10.31B). Ideally, head restraints placed within automobiles help limit the extent of hyperextension and reduce injury from a collision.[101]

Hyperextension injuries tend to occur more often from rear-end impact automobile collisions. Careful measurements of human replicas and cadaver material show that immediately on contact the craniocervical region sharply *retracts,* followed by a more prolonged hyperextension.[123,166] The brief retraction phase, due to the person's trunk being rapidly pushed forward by the back of the car seat, is usually completed *before* the cranium hits the head restraint. The *anterior longitudinal ligament* within the mid-and-lower cervical spine is particularly vulnerable to injury during this unprotected phase of the whiplash event.[101]

The *alar ligaments* are vulnerable to injury during the prolonged hyperextension phase of a rear-end collision, especially when the

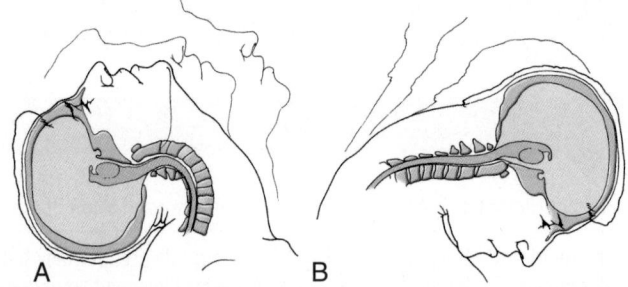

FIGURE 10.31 During whiplash injuries, cervical hyperextension (A) typically exceeds cervical flexion (B). As a result, the anterior structures of the cervical region are more vulnerable to strain injury. (From Porterfield JA, DeRosa C: *Mechanical neck pain: perspectives in functional anatomy,* Philadelphia, 1995, Saunders.)

head is rotated at the time of the collision.[195] Rotation of the head stretches the alar ligaments, which places them closer to their point of mechanical failure.

In addition, research has shown that the severe hyperextension associated with whiplash places excessive strain on flexor muscles, in particular the deeper *longus colli and longus capitis.*[144] In one study, a 56% strain (elongation) was measured in the longus colli—a level that can cause tissue damage. Often a person with a hyperextension injury shows a correlating pattern of marked tenderness with possible protective spasm in the region of the longus colli. Spasm in the longus colli would theoretically decrease the lordosis in the cervical spine. Persons with a strained and painful longus colli may have difficulty shrugging their shoulders—an action produced primarily by the upper trapezius. When the longus colli and other flexors are too painful to strongly contract, the upper trapezius muscle loses some of its stable cervical attachment and therefore becomes less effective as an active elevator of the shoulder girdle. This clinical scenario is an excellent example of the interdependence of muscle function, in which one muscle's action depends on the stabilization force of another.

Fig. 10.32 illustrates a total body movement that exhibits a sample of the muscular interactions used to maximize the extent of right axial rotation of the craniocervical region. Note that full axial rotation of the craniocervical region provides the eyes with much more than 180 degrees of visual scanning. As depicted, rotation to the right is driven by simultaneous activation of the left sternocleidomastoid and left trapezius (see Fig. 10.32A); right splenius capitis and cervicis; right upper erector spinae, such as the longissimus capitis; and left transversospinal muscles, such as the multifidus (see Fig. 10.32B). Although not depicted, several suboccipital muscles (namely the right rectus capitis posterior major and right obliquus capitis inferior) are actively controlling atlanto-axial joint rotation.

Activation of the muscles listed provides the required rotational power and control to the head and neck, as well as simultaneously stabilizing the craniocervical region in both the frontal and the sagittal planes. For example, the extension potential provided by the splenius capitis and cervicis, trapezius, and upper erector spinae is balanced by the flexion potential of the sternocleidomastoid.

Furthermore, the left lateral flexion potential of the left sternocleidomastoid and left trapezius is balanced by the right lateral flexion potential of the right splenius capitis and cervicis.

Full axial rotation of the craniocervical region requires muscular interactions that extend into the trunk and lower extremities. Consider, for example, the activation of the right and left oblique abdominal muscles as well as the transversus abdominis (see Fig. 10.32A). These muscles provide much of the torque needed to rotate and transfer forces dynamically throughout the entire body—ultimately from the lower extremities to the craniocervical region. Furthermore, as suggested by Fig. 10.32B, the erector spinae and transversospinal muscles are active throughout the posterior trunk to offset the potent trunk flexion tendency of the oblique abdominal muscles. The latissimus dorsi is an ipsilateral rotator of the trunk assuming the glenohumeral joint is well stabilized by other muscles.[12] The left gluteus maximus is shown actively rotating the pelvis and attached lumbosacral region to the right, relative to the fixed left femur. Furthermore, the right adductor longus muscle is also shown

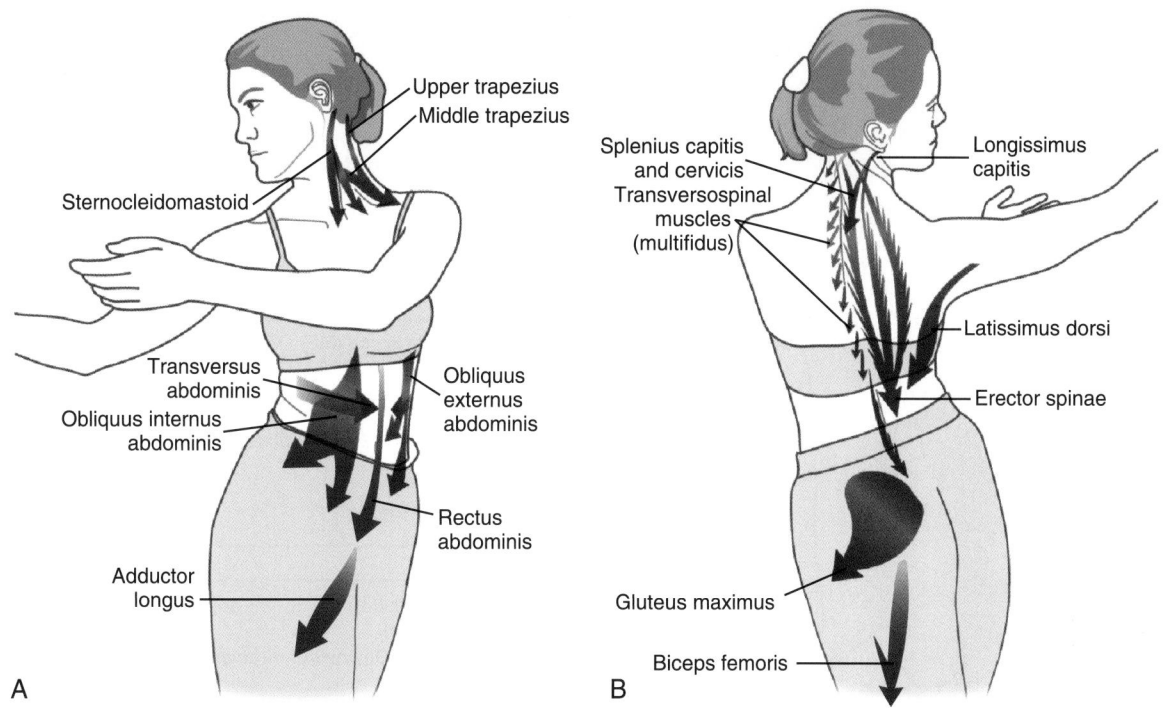

FIGURE 10.32 A typical activation pattern of selected muscles of the craniocervical region, trunk, and hip as a healthy person rotates the entire body to the right within the horizontal plane. (A) Anterior view. (B) Posterior view.

assisting the horizontal plane rotation of the pelvis relative to the fixed right femur. Note the near continuous line of force shared between the rectus abdominis and adductor longus. This kinetic interaction shows a nice example of muscles from different regions working synergistically to transfer forces between the trunk, through the pelvis, and to the lower limb.

SELECTED BIOMECHANICAL ISSUES OF LIFTING: A FOCUS ON REDUCING BACK INJURY

Lifting heavy objects can generate large compression, tension, and shear forces throughout the body, most notably across the low back region. At some critical point, forces acting on the low back may exceed the structural tolerance of the local muscles, ligaments, or apophyseal and interbody joints. The ensuing injury may be at macroscopic or microscopic levels, causing a release of inflammatory cytokines that may result in acute or potentially chronic low back pain.[51,236] Lifting is a major risk factor associated with the development of low back pain, especially secondary to the frequent and repetitive lifting of relatively large loads required in many occupations.[38,39,41,114,173]

Furthermore, inadequate strength and poor lifting mechanics may predispose workers to low back pain: an estimated 30% of the workforce in the United States regularly handles materials in a potentially harmful manner, including tasks related to lifting.[151]

This topic of the biomechanics of lifting describes (1) *why* the low back experiences high forces that may make this region biomechanically vulnerable to lifting-related injury and (2) *how* the forces in the low back may be minimized with the intent of reducing the chance of injury. Although this chapter focuses on the mechanics of lifting as a risk factor for developing low back pain, it does not discuss the many other possible factors that may be associated with this condition, such as age, sex, history of injury, underlying medical conditions, or lifting frequency. The causes and prevention of low back pain related to lifting is complex, multifactorial, and not well understood.

Muscular Mechanics Associated with Extension of the Low Back While Lifting

Studies have shown that compared with upright standing, bending fully forward at the waist typically doubles or triples the forces placed on the lumbar spine.[46] The majority of these forces are caused by activation of extensor muscles of the posterior trunk. Lifting or lowering objects to and from the floor can place even larger demands on the trunk extensor muscles. By necessity, these muscle forces are transferred either directly or indirectly to the joints and connective tissues (tendons, ligaments, fascia, and discs) within the low back. These forces generated while lifting clearly appear to be associated with back injury.[152] The following sections therefore focus on the role of the muscles during lifting, and how forces produced by muscles may be modified to reduce the stress on the structures in the low back region.

ESTIMATING THE MAGNITUDE OF FORCE IMPOSED ON THE LOW BACK DURING LIFTING

Considerable research has been undertaken to quantify the relative demands placed on the various structures in the low back during lifting or performance of other strenuous activities.[a] This research helps clinicians and governmental agencies develop safety guidelines and limits for lifting, especially in the workplace.[47,99,134,138] Of particular interest with regard to lifting injury are the variables of peak active force (or torque) produced by muscles; tension developed within stretched ligaments and muscles; and compression and shear forces developed against the intervertebral discs and apophyseal joints. Although direct in vivo measurements of these variables have been reported, they are typically estimated indirectly through a laboratory-based inverse dynamics approach, often in conjunction with computer-based models.[11,39,129,150,221] A simple but less accurate method of estimating

---

[a]3,39,46,67,68,72,174,221,229,235

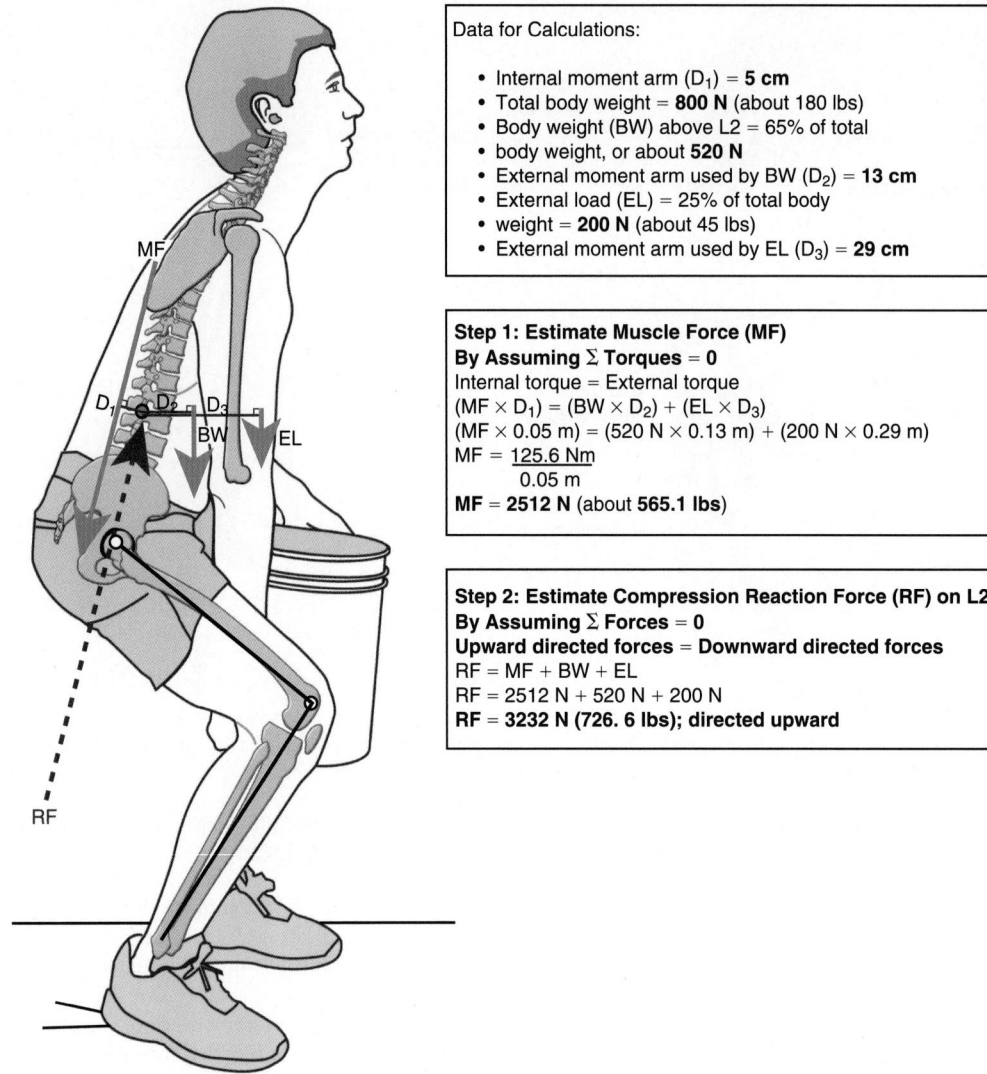

Data for Calculations:

- Internal moment arm (D₁) = **5 cm**
- Total body weight = **800 N** (about 180 lbs)
- Body weight (BW) above L2 = 65% of total
- body weight, or about **520 N**
- External moment arm used by BW (D₂) = **13 cm**
- External load (EL) = 25% of total body
- weight = **200 N** (about 45 lbs)
- External moment arm used by EL (D₃) = **29 cm**

Step 1: Estimate Muscle Force (MF)
By Assuming Σ Torques = 0
Internal torque = External torque
$(MF \times D_1) = (BW \times D_2) + (EL \times D_3)$
$(MF \times 0.05\ m) = (520\ N \times 0.13\ m) + (200\ N \times 0.29\ m)$
MF = 125.6 Nm / 0.05 m
MF = 2512 N (about 565.1 lbs)

Step 2: Estimate Compression Reaction Force (RF) on L2
By Assuming Σ Forces = 0
Upward directed forces = Downward directed forces
RF = MF + BW + EL
RF = 2512 N + 520 N + 200 N
RF = 3232 N (726. 6 lbs); directed upward

FIGURE 10.33 The steps used to estimate the approximate compressive reaction force *(RF)* on the L2 vertebra while a load is lifted. The biomechanics are limited to the sagittal plane, around an axis of rotation arbitrarily set at L2 *(green circle)*. The mathematic solutions assume a condition of static equilibrium. All abbreviations are defined in the boxes. (To simplify the mathematics, the calculations assume that all forces are acting in a vertical direction. This assumption introduces modest error in the results. All moment arm directions are designated as positive.)

forces imposed on the low back uses calculations based on the assumption of static equilibrium, as explained ahead.

The following section presents steps used in making a static-based estimation of the compression force on the L2 vertebra while a load is lifted in the sagittal plane. Although this example provides a limited amount of information on a rather complex biomechanical event, it does yield valuable insight into the relationship between the force produced by the muscle and the compression force imposed on a representative structure within the low back.

Fig. 10.33 (top box) shows the data required to make an approximate estimate of the compression force placed on the L2 vertebra during lifting. The individual in the figure is depicted midway through a vertical lift of a moderately heavy load, weighing 25% of body weight. The axis of rotation for the sagittal plane motion is oriented in the medial-lateral direction, arbitrarily set at L2 (see Fig. 10.33, open circle). Estimating the compression force is a two-step process; each step assumes a condition of static, rotary and linear equilibrium.

Step 1 solves for extensor muscle force by assuming that the sum of the internal and external torques within the sagittal plane is equal to zero (Σ Torques = 0). Note that two external torques are described: one resulting from the external load (EL) and one resulting from the individual's body weight (BW) located above L2. The extensor muscle force (MF) is defined as the MF generated on the posterior (extensor) side of the axis of rotation. If the back extensor muscles are assumed to have an average internal moment arm of 5 cm, the extensor muscles must produce at least 2512 N (565.1 lb) of force to lift the load.

Step 2 estimates the compressive reaction force (RF) imposed on the L2 vertebra during lifting. (This *reaction force* implies that the L2 vertebra must "push" back against the downward acting forces.) A rough estimate of this force can be made by assuming static linear equilibrium. (For the sake of simplicity, the calculations assume that MF acts totally in the vertical direction and is therefore parallel with BW and the EL forces.) The RF vector (see Fig. 10.33) is also assumed to be equal in magnitude but opposite in direction to the sum of MF, BW, and EL.

The solution to this example suggests that a compression force of approximately 3232 N (greater than 725 lb) is exerted on L2 when an external load weighing 200 N (about 45 lb) is lifted with the trunk in a relatively erect position and the weight held near the body. To put this magnitude of force into practical perspective, consider the following two points. First, the National Institute of Occupational Safety and Health (NIOSH) has set guidelines to protect workers from excessive loads on the lumbar region caused by lifting and handling materials. NIOSH has recommended an upper safe limit of 3400 N (764 lb) of compression force on the L5–S1 junction.[72,223,224] Second, the maximal load-carrying capacity of the lumbar spine is estimated to be 6400 N (1439 lb),[102] almost twice the maximal safe force recommended by NIOSH. The limit of 6400 N of force applies to a 40-year-old man; this limit decreases by 1000 N each subsequent decade. These force values are very general guidelines that typically would not apply to all persons in all lifting situations.[71,191]

The static model described before likely underestimates the actual compressive force on the L2 vertebra by as much as 20%.[212] Two factors can explain much of this underestimation. First, the model accounts for muscle force produced by the back extensors only. Other muscles, especially those with near vertical fiber orientation such as the rectus abdominis and the psoas major, certainly add to the muscular-based compression on the lumbar spine. Second, the model assumes *static* equilibrium, thereby ignoring the additional forces needed to accelerate the body and load upward. A *rapid* lift requires greater muscle force and imposes greater compression and shear on the joints and connective tissues in the low back. For this reason, it is usually recommended that a person lift loads slowly and smoothly, a condition not always practical in all settings.

WAYS TO REDUCE THE FORCE DEMANDS ON THE BACK MUSCLES DURING LIFTING

The calculations performed in Step 2 of Fig. 10.33 show that muscle force (MF) is, by far, the most influential variable for determining the magnitude of the compressive (reaction) force on the lumbar spine. Proportional reductions in muscle force, therefore, can very effectively reduce the overall compression force on the structures in the low back.

An important factor responsible for the large forces in the low back muscles during lifting is the disparity in the length of the associated internal and external moment arms. The internal moment arm (D_1) depicted in Fig. 10.33 is assumed to be 5 cm. The extensor muscles are therefore at a sizable mechanical *disadvantage* and must produce a force many times larger than the weight of the load being lifted. As previously demonstrated, lifting an external load weighing 25% of one's body weight produces a compression force on L2 of four times one's body weight!

Therapeutic and educational programs are often designed to reduce the likelihood of back injury by minimizing the need for very large extensor muscle forces during lifting. In theory, this can be accomplished in four ways. *First,* as previously stated, reducing the acceleration which a load is lifted proportionately decreases the amount of back extensor muscle force required for the task.

Second, reduce the weight of the external load. Although this point is obvious, it is not always possible.

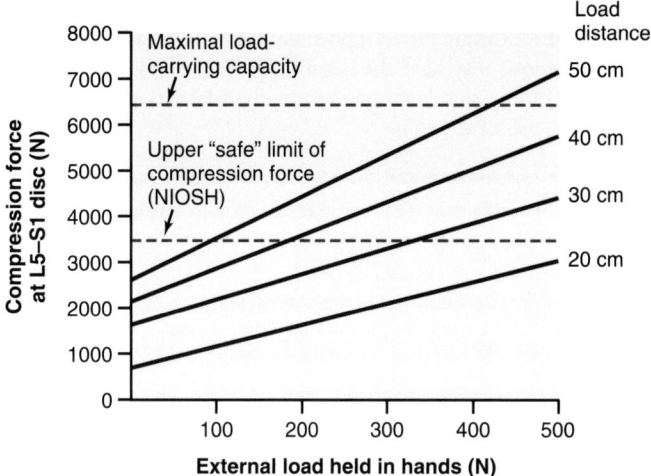

FIGURE 10.34 Graph shows the predicted compression force at the L5–S1 disc as a function of load size and the distance the loads are held in front of the body (1 lb = 4.448 N). The two red horizontal lines indicate (1) the maximal load-carrying capacity of the lumbar region before structural failure and (2) the upper safe limits of compression force on the lumbar spine as determined by the National Institute of Occupational Safety and Health. (Plot modified from Chaffin DB, Andersson GBJ: *Occupational biomechanics,* ed 2, New York, 1991, John Wiley & Sons.)

Third, reduce the length of the external moment arm of the external load. This is likely the most effective and practical method of decreasing compressive reaction forces on the low back.[46] As demonstrated in Fig. 10.33, ideally a load should be lifted from between the knees, thereby minimizing the distance between the load and the lumbar region. Based on the calculations, this ideal method of lifting produced a compression force on the lumbar region that remained close to the upper limits of safety proposed by NIOSH. Lifting the same load with a *longer* external moment arm may create very large and potentially harmful compression forces on the low back. Fig. 10.34 shows a plot of predicted compression (reaction) forces on the L5–S1 disc as a function of both load size and distance between the load and the front of the chest.[32] Although perhaps an extreme and unrealistic example, the plot predicts that holding an external load weighing 200 N (45 lb) 50 cm in front of the body creates about 4500 N of compression force, greatly exceeding the upper safe limit of 3400 N.

In everyday life, lifting an object from between the knees or in a similar manner is not always practical. Consider the act of sliding a patient toward the head of a hospital bed. The inability to reduce the distance between the patient's center of mass (located anterior to S2) and the lifter can compromise the safety of the lifter.

Fourth, increase the *internal* moment arm available to the low back extensor muscles. A larger internal moment arm for extension allows a given extension torque to be generated with less muscle force. As stated, less muscle force typically equates to less force on the vertebral elements. Accentuated lumbar lordosis has been reported to increase the internal moment arm available to the lumbar erector spinae by 6% to 15% compared with a neutral posture.[13,209] Lifting with an accentuated lumbar lordosis, however, is not always possible or desirable. Lifting a very heavy load off the floor, for example, typically requires a flexed lumbar spine, which would decrease the extensor muscles' moment arm by 3% to 7% compared with a neutral posture.[13,108] (Biomechanically, this situation would require proportionally greater muscle force per given extensor torque.) Even if possible, maintaining an exaggerated lumbar lordosis may have the negative consequences of generating excessive compression loads on the apophyseal joints and other posterior elements of the spine.

Four Ways to Reduce the Amount of Force Required of the Back Extensor Muscles during Lifting

- Reduce the acceleration of lifting
- Reduce the magnitude of the external load
- Reduce the length of the external moment arm
- Increase the length of the internal moment arm

ROLE OF INCREASING INTRA-ABDOMINAL PRESSURE DURING LIFTING

Activities that involve lifting, especially relatively heavy loads, are typically associated with the production of a *Valsalva maneuver*. The Valsalva maneuver describes the action of voluntarily increasing intra-abdominal pressure by vigorous contraction of the abdominal muscles against a closed glottis. The Valsalva maneuver creates a rigid column of high pressure within the abdomen that pushes upward against the diaphragm muscle, anteriorly against the deeper abdominal muscles (transversus abdominis and internal oblique), posteriorly against the lumbar spine and posterior abdominal wall, and downward against the pelvic floor muscles (levator ani and coccygeus). As described by Bartelink many years ago,[18] this rigid pneumatic column acts as an inflated "intra-abdominal balloon," which creates a modest *extension* torque on the lumbar spine, thereby reducing the demands on the lumbar extensor muscles and ultimately lowering the muscular-based compression forces on the lumbar spine.

Research supports the idea that generating a Valsalva maneuver while lifting does indeed partially unload the lumbar intervertebral junctions as well as increase the muscular stiffness and stability of the lumbar region.[14,89,199] The degree to which the Valsalva maneuver unloads the lumbar spine, however, is not fully understood or resolved. There are several potentially offsetting biomechanical factors at play. Although the Valsalva maneuver reduces the force demands on the lumbar extensor muscles (and therefore the lumbar spine) while lifting, the strong concurrent activation of the abdominal muscles that is needed to increase intra-abdominal pressure *increases* the compression force on the lumbar spine. Because all abdominal muscles (except perhaps the transversus abdominis) are dominant and direct flexors of the trunk and lumbar spine, their strong activation requires additional counterbalancing forces from the extensor muscles. The resulting increased activation of virtually *all* trunk muscles (flexors and extensors) may offset some of the unloading effect achieved by the increased abdominal pressure. This is especially the case for the more vertically-oriented muscles, which contribute a greater percentage of the compression forces across the lumbar spine. Nevertheless, it is generally agreed that producing a Valsalva maneuver while lifting is mechanically beneficial, as it achieves a *net* reduction in lumbar compression force—although the exact amount of reduction and related muscular biomechanics are not fully elucidated.[198]

In addition to increasing intra-abdominal pressure, a strong contraction of the abdominal muscles while lifting also provides a bracing effect around the lumbopelvic region, which is helpful in resisting unwanted torsions created by the asymmetric lifting of external loads.[43,44] Furthermore, forces produced by the transversus abdominis may be particularly effective in stabilizing the lumbopelvic region for at least two reasons. First, the transversus abdominis has extensive horizontally-oriented attachments into the thoracolumbar fascia.[220] Forces produced by this muscle activation therefore generate a circumferential corset effect around the entire low back region. Second, by acting primarily in the transverse direction, the transversus abdominis can increase intra-abdominal pressure *without* creating a concurrent flexion torque or an increase in vertical compression force on the lumbar spine.[14] The more transverse fibers of the internal oblique muscles are able to assist the transversus abdominis with these aforementioned functions.

In closing, one should not overlook the role of the diaphragm muscle in generating muscular stability in the low back or lumbopelvic regions.[91,120] During inhalation, contraction of the diaphragm muscle pulls the dome of this muscle inferiorly—deeper into the abdomen, which increases intra-abdominal pressure and generates a local pneumatic stiffness in the lumbopelvic region. To be fully effective, this muscular effort requires simultaneous activation of the abdominal and pelvic floor muscles. This multi-muscular effort reinforces the low back not only for lifting but also for activities involving external resistance applied to the limbs.[76,122] Research suggests that some persons with low back pain do not adequately engage their diaphragm muscle during lifting or resisted trunk movements, perhaps leaving the low back vulnerable to injury.[76,121] Whether the reduced activation or control of the diaphragm muscle directly or indirectly causes low back pain, or is simply the consequence of muscular guarding due to back pain, is not known. The vital role of the diaphragm muscle in ventilation will be described in Chapter 11.

ADDITIONAL SOURCES OF EXTENSION TORQUE USED FOR LIFTING

The maximal force-generating capacity of the low back extensor muscles in a typical young adult is estimated to be approximately 4000 N (900 lb).[22] If an average internal moment arm of 5 cm is assumed, this muscle group is then expected to produce about *200 Nm* of trunk extension torque (i.e., 4000 N × 0.05 m). What is perplexing, however, is the fact that maximal-effort lifting likely requires extensor torques that may greatly *exceed* 200 Nm. For example, the person depicted lifting the load in Fig. 10.33 would have exceeded the theoretical 200-Nm strength limit if the external load were increased to about 80% of the lifter's body weight. Although this is a considerable weight, it is not unusual for a person to successfully lift much greater loads, such as those regularly encountered by heavy labor workers and by competitive "power lifters." In attempts to explain this apparent discrepancy, two secondary sources of extension torque are proposed: (1) passive tension generated from stretching the posterior ligamentous system and (2) muscular-generated tension transferred through the thoracolumbar fascia.

Passive Tension Generation from Stretching the Posterior Ligamentous System

When stretched, healthy ligaments and fascia exhibit some degree of natural elasticity. This feature allows connective tissue to temporarily store a portion of the force that initially causes the elongation. Bending forward in preparation for lifting progressively elongates several connective tissues in the lumbar region, and presumably the passive tension developed in these tissues can assist with an extension torque.[13,52] These connective tissues, collectively known as the *posterior ligamentous system,* include the posterior longitudinal ligament, ligamentum flavum, apophyseal joint capsule, interspinous ligament, and the thoracolumbar fascia.

In theory, about 72 Nm of total passive extensor torque are produced by maximally stretching the posterior ligamentous system (Table 10.6).[22] Adding this passive torque to the hypothetical 200 Nm of active torque yields a total of 272 Nm of extension torque available for lifting. A fully engaged (stretched) posterior ligamentous system can therefore generate about 25% of the total extension torque for lifting. Note, however, that this 25% passive torque reserve is available only after the lumbar spine is maximally flexed, which is rare during lifting. Even competitive power lifters, who appear to lift with a fully rounded low back, avoid the extremes of flexion.[37] Many researchers generally believe that maximum or near-maximum flexion of the lumbar spine should be avoided during heavy and repetitive lifting.[22,140] Although it has not been unequivocally shown to reduce lifting-related injuries in all situations,[186] it is nevertheless usually suggested that the lumbar region be held in a near-neutral (mid-range) position when lifting.[117,143] The neutral position may favor near-maximal surface contact area within the apophyseal joints, which may help reduce articular contact pressure. Furthermore, maintaining the neutral position during lifting may limit flexion-induced creep in the posterior ligamentous tissues as well as align the local extensor muscles to be most effective at resisting anterior shear.[143]

Although maintaining a neutral lumbar spine while lifting may have some purported benefits in reducing local stress-related injuries, it engages only a small portion of the total passive torque reserve available to assist with extension. Most of the extension torque must therefore be generated by active muscle contraction. It is important, therefore, that the extensor muscles be strong enough to meet the potentially large demands placed on the low back by heavy lifting. Adequate strength in the lumbar multifidus is particularly critical in this regard.[78,222] Without adequate strength in these muscles, the lumbar spine may be pulled into excessive flexion by the external torque imposed by the large load, creating a posture potentially unsafe for some individuals involved with repetitive lifting.

Muscular-Generated Tension Transferred through the Thoracolumbar Fascia

The thoracolumbar fascia is thickest and most extensively developed in the lumbar region.[232] As noted in Fig. 9.72, the fascia is arranged in anterior, middle, and posterior layers. Much of the tissue attaches to the lumbar spine, sacrum, and pelvis in a position well *posterior* to the axis of rotation at the lumbar region. Theoretically, therefore, passive tension within stretched thoracolumbar fascia can produce an extension torque in the lumbar region and thus augment the torque created by the low back musculature.[139]

As alluded to earlier, for the thoracolumbar fascia to generate useful tension, it must be first stretched and rendered taut. This can occur in two ways. First, the fascia is stretched simply when one bends forward and flexes the lumbar spine in preparation for lifting. Second, and more significant, the fascia is stretched by active contraction of muscles that attach directly into the middle and posterior layer of the thoracolumbar fascia, namely the transversus abdominis, internal oblique, and latissimus dorsi.[58] The prevailing horizontal fiber direction of most of the thoracolumbar fascia, however, limits the amount of extension torque that can be produced at the lumbar spine. Theoretically, maximal activation of the three aforementioned muscles can pull on the thoracolumbar fascia with a force that could produce up to 10 Nm of extension torque across the lower lumbar spine.[70] Although this magnitude of lumbar extensor torque is relatively small (compared with a theoretical maximum of 200 Nm produced volitionally), it nevertheless furnishes additional stabilization to the region.

The gluteus maximus and latissimus dorsi indirectly contribute to a low back extension torque through their extensive attachments to the thoracolumbar fascia.[220] Both are active during lifting but for different reasons. The gluteus maximus controls the hips while stabilizing the sacroiliac joints. The latissimus dorsi helps transfer the external load being lifted from the arms to the trunk. In addition to attaching into the posterior layer of the thoracolumbar fascia, the latissimus dorsi attaches into the posterior aspect of the pelvis, sacrum, and spine. Based on these attachments and their relative moment arms for producing lumbar extension (see Fig. 10.16), the latissimus dorsi has all the attributes of a respected extensor of the low back. The oblique fiber direction of the muscle as it ascends the

TABLE 10.6 Maximal Passive Extensor Torque Produced by Stretched Connective Tissues in the Lumbar Region

Connective Tissue	Average Maximum Tension (N)*	Extensor Moment Arm (m)†	Maximal Passive Extensor Torque (Nm)‡
Posterior longitudinal ligament	90	0.02	1.8
Ligamentum flava	244	0.03	7.3
Capsule of apophyseal joints	680	0.04	27.2
Interspinous ligament	107	0.05	5.4
Posterior layer of thoracolumbar fascia, including supraspinous ligaments and the aponeurosis covering the erector spinae muscles	500	0.06	30.0
TOTAL			71.7

*Average maximum tension is the tension (force) within each stretched tissue at the point of rupture.
†Extensor moment arm is the perpendicular distance between the attachment sites of the ligaments and the medial-lateral axis of rotation within a representative lumbar vertebra.
‡Maximal passive extensor torque is estimated by the product of maximum tension (force) and extensor muscle moment arm.
Data from Bogduk N: *Clinical and radiological anatomy of the lumbar spine,* ed 5, New York, 2012, Churchill Livingstone.

trunk can also provide torsional stability to the axial skeleton, especially when bilaterally active.[218] This stability may be especially useful when large loads are handled in an asymmetric fashion.

Summary of Factors That Likely Contribute to Safe Lifting

The lifting technique used in Fig. 10.33 illustrates two fundamental features that likely contribute to the safe lifting technique: (1) the lumbar spine is held in a neutral lordotic position and (2) the load is lifted from between the knees. The rationales for these and other factors considered to contribute to safe lifting are listed in Table 10.7. Other, more general considerations include (1) knowing one's physical limits, (2) thinking the lift through before the event, and (3) within practical and health limits, remaining in optimal physical and cardiovascular condition.

TABLE 10.7 Factors Considered to Contribute to Safe Lifting Techniques

Consideration	Rationale	Comment
A lifted load should be as light and infrequently as practical and held as close to the body as possible.	Minimizes the total volume of external torque load, thereby minimizing the force demands on the back muscles.	Lifting an external load from between the knees is an effective way to reduce the load's external moment arm, although not always practical to implement.
Lift with the lumbar spine as close as possible to its neutral (lordotic) position (i.e., avoid *extremes* of flexion and extension).	Vigorous contraction of the back extensor muscles with the lumbar spine *maximally flexed* may potentially overload the intervertebral discs. In contrast, vigorous contraction of the back extensor muscles with the lumbar spine *maximally extended* may potentially overload the apophyseal joints.	Lifting with limited flexion or extension in the lumbar spine may be acceptable for some persons, depending on the health and experience of the lifter. Varying amounts of flexion or extension each have biomechanical advantages. • Lifting with the lumbar spine in *minimal-to-moderate flexion* increases the passive tension generated by the posterior ligamentous system, possibly reducing the force demands on extensor muscles. • Lifting with the lumbar spine *near complete extension* may augment the moment arm for some of the extensor muscles while the apophyseal joints remain in or near their close-packed position.
When lifting, activate the hip and knee extensor muscles to minimize the force demands on the low back muscles.	Large forces produced by low back extensor muscles can injure discs, vertebral endplates, apophyseal joints or the muscles themselves.	A person with hip or knee arthritis may be unable to effectively use the muscles in the legs to assist the back muscles.
Minimize the vertical and horizontal distance that a load must be lifted throughout a given work period.	Minimizing the cumulative distance the load is moved reduces the total work caused by repetitive lifting, thereby reducing fatigue; minimizing the distance the load is moved reduces the extremes of movement in the low back region.	Using handles or an adjustable-height platform may be helpful.
Minimize the weight of loads lifted in an asymmetric manner.	Asymmetric loads (for example, unilateral loads held out and away from the body) may concentrate large forces on a relatively small number of muscles or connective tissues.	Lifting asymmetric loads may also destabilize one's balance.
Avoid twisting when lifting.	Torsional forces applied to vertebrae can predispose the person to intervertebral disc injury.	A properly designed work environment can reduce the need for twisting during lifting.
Lift as slowly and smoothly as conditions allow.	A slow and smooth lift (i.e., with minimal acceleration) minimizes the peak force generated in muscles and connective tissues.	
Lift with a moderately wide and slightly staggered base of support provided by the legs.	A relatively wide base of support affords greater overall stability of the body, thereby reducing the chance of a fall or slip.	
Use the assistance of a mechanical device or additional people to lift something.	Using assistance in lifting can reduce the demand on the back of the primary lifter.	Using a mechanical hoist (Hoyer lift) or a "two-person" transfer may be prudent in many settings.

SPECIAL FOCUS 10.7

Two Contrasting Lifting Techniques: The Stoop versus the Squat Lift

The stoop lift and the squat lift represent one biomechanical extreme within a broad continuum of possible lifting strategies (Fig. 10.35)[125] Understanding some of the biomechanic and physiologic differences between these rather extreme methods of lifting may provide insight into the advantages or disadvantages of other, more common lifting techniques.

The *stoop lift* is performed primarily by extending the hips and lumbar region while the knees remain slightly flexed (see Fig. 10.35A). This lifting strategy is associated with greater flexion of the low back, especially at the initiation of the lift. By necessity, the stoop lift creates a long external moment arm between the trunk (and load) and the low back. The greater external torque requires greater extension forces from the low back and trunk extensor muscles. In combination with a markedly flexed lumbar spine, the stoop lift has the potential to create large compression and shear forces on the discs.

The *squat lift,* in contrast, typically begins with near maximally flexed knees (see Fig. 10.35B). The knees and hips extend during the lift, powered by the quadriceps and hip extensor muscles. Depending on the physical characteristics of the load and the initial depth of the squat, the lumbar region may remain extended, in a neutral position, or partially flexed throughout the lift. Perhaps the greatest advantage of the squat lift is that it can allow the load to be raised from between the knees. This placement of the lifted load can significantly reduce the external moment arm of the load and trunk and, as a consequence, diminish the extensor torque demands on the muscles of the back.

The squat lift is most often advocated by health or ergonomic professionals as the safer of the two techniques in terms of producing less stress on the low back and therefore preventing back injuries.[1,16,19] Little direct proof, however, can be found to support this strongly held popular belief.[1,13,46,213,219] Nevertheless, the often-promoted advantage of the squat lift technique needs to be considered in terms of potential tradeoffs. Although the squat lift may reduce the demands on the extensor muscles and other tissues in the low back, it usually creates greater demands on the knees.[190] The high amount of initial knee flexion associated with the full squat places high force demands on the quadriceps muscles to extend the knees. The forces impose very large pressures across the tibiofemoral and patellofemoral joints. Healthy persons may tolerate high pressures at these joints without negative consequences; however, someone with painful or arthritic knees may not. The adage that lifting with the legs "spares the back and spoils the knees" does, therefore, have some validity.

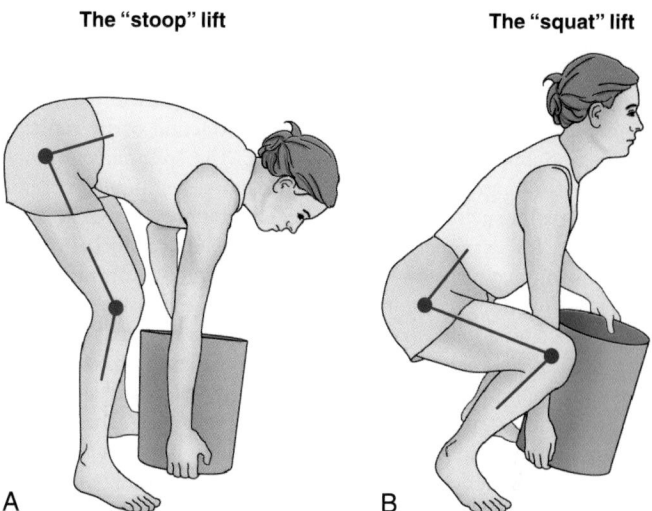

FIGURE 10.35 Two contrasting styles of lifting. (A) The initiation of the stoop lift. (B) The initiation of the squat lift. The axes of rotation at the hip and knee joints are represented as *red circles.*

Another factor to consider when comparing the benefits of the squat lift over the stoop lift is the *total work* required to lift the load. The mechanical work performed during lifting is equal to the weight of the body and the load multiplied by the vertical displacement of the body and the load. The stoop lift is 23% to 34% more metabolically "efficient" than the squat lift in terms of work performed per level of oxygen consumption.[226] The squat lift requires greater work because a greater proportion of the total body mass must be moved through space.

Rather than performing a squat lift or a stoop lift, many people choose an individualized or freestyle lifting technique. A freestyle technique allows the lifter to combine some of the benefits of the squat lift with the more metabolically efficient stoop lift. Workers have reported a higher self-perceived maximal safe limit when allowed to lift with a freestyle technique rather than with a set technique.[125]

In closing, although the specific lifting technique may be an important consideration for safe lifting, other equally important variables exist. These include the lifter's physical strength, health, experience, comfort, or personal preference for a lifting technique; history of previous injury; ergonomic design of the workplace; stability of the load being lifted; or work productivity incentives.[16,80,156,227]

SYNOPSIS

The muscles of the trunk and craniocervical regions have a wide range of often interrelated functions. These range from moving and stabilizing the body to assisting with or optimizing activities such as vision and equilibrium, ventilation, chewing and swallowing, defecation, and childbirth. This chapter focuses primarily on movement and stabilization.

Ultimately, muscles that control movement of the trunk and craniocervical regions do so either by contracting or by resisting elongation by a more dominating force. The specificity of such control can be greatly enhanced by the muscles' unique anatomic characteristics, such as shape, size, fiber orientation, and innervation. Consider, for example, the very short and vertical rectus capitis lateralis muscle in the upper craniocervical region. Contraction of this muscle is designed to make small and precise adjustments to the atlanto-occipital joint, perhaps to help track an object as it crosses the visual field. Such an action is primarily reflexive in nature and linked to neural centers that help coordinate vision and associated righting and postural reactions of the head and neck. The nervous system likely provides ample neural connections between the rectus capitis lateralis and a host of other structures, including other craniocervical muscles, apophyseal joints, and the vestibular-and-ocular apparatus. Injury to the small and deep muscles of the craniocervical region may potentially disrupt this stream of neurologic signaling. In cases of reduced or distorted craniocervical proprioception, movements may become slightly uncoordinated and subsequently place higher than normal stress on the local joints. This stress may prolong or exaggerate symptoms after an injury, as is often the case with trauma associated with whiplash or concussion.

In contrast to small muscles, such as the rectus capitis lateralis, consider the much larger internal oblique that courses obliquely across the middle and lower abdomen. This muscle extends between the linea alba anteriorly and the thoracolumbar fascia posteriorly. During a 100-meter sprint, for example, this muscle is repetitively strongly activated as it accelerates and decelerates rotation of the trunk. The highly segmental innervation of this muscle may allow a more sequential activation across the whole muscle, perhaps facilitating a "wave" of contractile force that is transmitted throughout the abdomen and low back. During the strong activation of the abdominal muscles during sprinting, the diaphragm muscle must contract and descend against a very high intra-abdominal pressure. This topic is further explored in the next chapter.

In addition to generating forces required for movement, the muscles of the trunk and craniocervical regions also have the primary responsibility of stabilizing the spine. This stability must occur in three dimensions, across multiple segments, and for an infinite number of both anticipated and unexpected environmental situations. Consider, for example, the need to stabilize the trunk before landing from a jump or while attempting to stand upright on a rocking boat. One primary benefit of this stabilization is to protect the joints, discs, and ligaments within the axial skeleton and, perhaps more important, the delicate spinal cord and exiting spinal nerve roots.

Muscular stabilization can be provided simply through large muscle bulk. This is particularly evident at the craniocervical and lumbosacral regions, where the cross-sectional areas of the paravertebral muscles are the largest. At the lumbosacral region, for example, the vertebral column is closely surrounded by thick, oblique to vertically oriented muscles, such as the psoas major, multifidus, and lower erector spinae.

Other, more complex methods of muscular stability exist across the axial spine, much of which may be "preprogrammed" within the nervous system. For example, certain trunk muscles subconsciously contract slightly before active movements of the upper limbs, especially when performed rapidly. This preparatory activity helps stabilize the trunk against unwanted reactive movements that may, over time, damage the spine. Furthermore, during lower extremity movements, the activation of trunk muscles is essential to stabilize and fixate the proximal attachments of several muscles that cross the hips and knees. The importance of this muscular stabilization is often evident in persons with weakened abdominal muscles secondary to pathology, such as a child with muscular dystrophy. In this case a strong contraction of the hip flexor muscles, for example, produces an excessive and undesired anterior tilting of the pelvis relative to the hip joints. This position of the pelvis, in turn, creates an exaggerated lordosis of the lumbar spine. Over time, this abnormal posture may increase the stress on the apophyseal joints and increase anterior shearing across the lumbosacral junction.

In closing, persons with injury and disease involving the axial skeleton often demonstrate a complicated set of musculoskeletal clinical findings, typically affecting their ability to move freely and comfortably and potentially affecting the amount of stress placed on their vertebral and neural tissues. The complexity and often uncertainty of the underlying pathomechanics in these conditions partially accounts for the many different therapeutic and rehabilitation options used to treat the associated disorders, especially those that involve chronic pain. The degree of uncertainty can be minimized only by continued and focused clinical and laboratory research in this area.

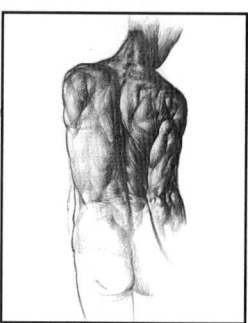

ADDITIONAL CLINICAL CONNECTIONS

CLINICAL CONNECTION 10.1

A Closer Look at the Spinal Stabilizing Functions of Selected Abdominal Muscles and the Lumbar Multifidus

The following discussion highlights examples of spinal stabilization performed by selected *abdominal muscles* and the lumbar *multifidus*. These muscles are featured primarily because of the large body of research that has focused on their ability (or lack thereof) to stabilize the lumbopelvic region (which includes the lumbar spine, lumbosacral junction, and sacroiliac joints).[44,202,210] The topic has attracted significant attention primarily because of the high incidence of instability and stress-related degeneration in this region.

ABDOMINAL MUSCLES

Much of what is known about the kinesiology of the muscular stabilizers of the lumbopelvic region is based on ultrasound imaging, or on electromyographic (EMG) technology, using surface or fine-wire (needle) electrodes.[25,130,147,211,228] One methodology used in

the EMG research involves the recording of the order in which various trunk muscles respond to expected or unexpected whole-body perturbations. As an example, Fig. 10.36A shows the onset of the EMG responses of a selected set of abdominal muscles as a healthy, pain-free person rapidly flexes the arm after a visual stimulus.[210] The top EMG signal (depicted in red) is from the anterior deltoid and the remaining EMG signals are from the *external oblique,* the middle and lower regions of the *internal oblique,* and the upper, middle, and lower regions of the *transversus abdominis.* All muscles recorded from this one subject responded at slightly different times (indicated by vertical arrows) relative to the initiation of the deltoid's EMG signal (red dashed line). Fig. 10.36B shows the overall relative onset data based on 11 healthy subjects.

As previously reported, the lower and middle fibers of the transversus abdominis and internal oblique muscles consistently

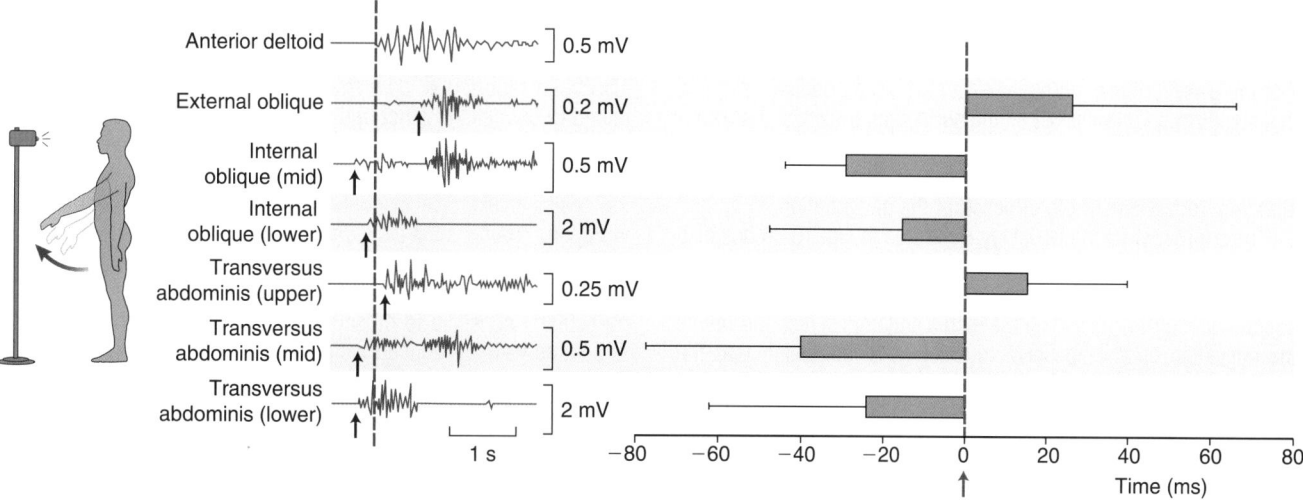

FIGURE 10.36 (A) The electromyographic (EMG) responses are shown from selected abdominal muscles as a healthy person rapidly flexes their arm after a visual stimulus. The different onset times of EMG signals from the abdominal muscles *(vertical dark arrows)* are compared with the onset of the EMG signal from the anterior deltoid *(red),* a shoulder flexor muscle. (B) The means *(purple bars)* and standard deviations of the muscle onset times are shown, averaged across 110 trials, for all 11 healthy subjects. (Data redrawn from Urquhart DM, Hodges PW, Story IH: Postural activity of the abdominal muscles varies between regions of these muscles and between body positions, *Gait Posture* 22:295, 2005.)

activate *before* the activation of the deltoid muscle.[211] This anticipatory response is believed to be a subconscious, feedforward mechanism employed by the nervous system to minimize reactive countermovements of the trunk.[210] Although subtle and difficult to prove, this anticipatory muscular response may help protect the lumbopelvic region from potentially damaging shear forces.

It is interesting that multiple regions of the transversus abdominis and internal oblique activate at different times in response to the rapidly elevated arm. It is as though the different regions within these muscles respond as distinct anatomic entities. Although separated by only a very short time, the sequential muscular responses provide insight into the complex stabilizing functions of these muscles. Consider, in this regard, the following proposed functions for each of the three regions of the transversus abdominis.[181,192,210] Contraction of the *upper fibers* of the transversus abdominis may help stabilize the rib cage and linea alba. The *lower fibers* are believed to compress and thereby help stabilize the sacroiliac joints.[92] Contraction of the *middle fibers* of the transversus abdominis transfers tension directly to the lumbar spinous processes and sacrum by connections into the thoracolumbar fascia (see Chapter 9). This action is part of the "corset" effect described earlier in this chapter for this muscle.

Furthermore, bilateral contraction of the *middle fibers* of the transversus abdominis is particularly effective (along with other abdominal muscles) at compressing the abdominal cavity and thereby increasing intra-abdominal pressure. Evidence exists that the rise in intra-abdominal pressure not only exerts a modest extension torque on the lumbar spine but also stabilizes the region.[44,89,92] For the most effective stabilization, the cylinderlike abdominal cavity must also be simultaneously compressed from both its cranial and its caudal ends. This is normally accomplished by concurrent activation and descent of the diaphragm muscle—the roof of the abdominal cavity—and activation and ascent of the pelvic floor muscles—the ultimate floor of the abdominal cavity.[91,122] Interestingly, EMG research on healthy subjects suggests that the transversus abdominis has a particularly dedicated role in this stabilization process. Of all the abdominal muscles, the transversus abdominis most consistently responds to postural perturbations intended to destabilize the body's center of mass while standing, regardless of the direction of the perturbation.[44]

The experimental methodology illustrated in Fig. 10.36 has also been used to study the sequential activation of the abdominal muscles in response to rapidly flexing the lower limb.[93] Consistently, the abdominal muscles (including the rectus abdominis) respond *before* the activation of the hip flexor muscles. It is interesting that the transversus abdominis and internal oblique are consistently the first of the trunk muscles to respond, on average 50 to 100 msec before the hip flexor muscles. This activation pattern of the abdominal muscles, as a group, reflects their need to stabilize the lower trunk during the leg movement, as well as to fixate the lumbopelvic region against the pull of the contracting hip flexor muscles. The transversus abdominis and the oblique abdominal muscles also respond before rapid activation of selected hip *abductor* and *extensor* muscles.[93] These abdominal muscles appear "dedicated" to stabilizing the lower trunk, regardless of the direction of the forces produced by the contracting hip musculature.

Hodges and colleagues used a similar experimental protocol to study the sequential muscle activation in persons with chronic low back pain.[94,148] Remarkably, this research showed a consistent, short delay in the onset of EMG signals from the transversus abdominis—the activation of this muscle occurring most often *after* the activation of the prime movers of the rapid limb motion. Whether a short delay in abdominal muscle activation can create sufficient reactive stress in the lumbopelvic region to ultimately cause low back pain is not known, although it is an intriguing question. Cadaveric studies have indeed shown that axial rotation of as little as 2 to 3 degrees per intervertebral lumbar junction can potentially injure the apophyseal and interbody joints (see Chapter 9). A single "unprotected" stress event may not be significant; however, multiple events that accumulate over many years may predispose the region to injury.

LUMBAR MULTIFIDUS

Research has shown that like the transversus abdominis and internal oblique, the *lumbar multifidus* consistently activates relatively early as healthy persons respond to various perturbations imposed against the body.[24,118] The multifidus is believed to be a very capable stabilizer of the lumbar spine.[180,222,230] The muscle's regional strength is augmented by its relatively large size; they account for about one-third of the total cross-sectional area of all deep paraspinal muscles at the L4 level.[22,135] In addition to their thickness, the fibers within the multifidus also have a highly segmented organization. These features favor precise and authoritative control over intersegmental lumbar stability.[21,119,222,230]

The multifidus in persons with low back pain disorders typically show increased fat infiltration plus persistent atrophy and neuromuscular inhibition.[42,64,79,197,237] Increased local proinflammatory macrophages and cytokines may mediate some of these changes in multifidus composition.[103] These findings are noteworthy, considering the muscles' proposed importance in stabilizing the lumbar region. The amount of atrophy in the lumbar multifidus is striking; a 30% reduction in cross-sectional area has been reported,[87] in some cases within days of the onset of the painful symptoms.[88]

Marked and persisting atrophy of the lumbar multifidus has also been reported in *pain-free* healthy subjects who were subjected to 8 weeks of strict bed rest.[17,21] Of particular interest was the response of a subgroup of the subjects who, while remaining on strict bed rest, were allowed to exercise twice daily (performing resistive exercise in conjunction with receiving whole-body vibration). These subjects demonstrated statistically less multifidus atrophy, and the atrophy did not persist as long as in the inactive, control group. It appears that the lumbar multifidus is particularly sensitive to musculoskeletal pathology in the lumbar region, as well as reduced weight bearing through the axial skeleton. Regardless of the underlying mechanism, it is reasonable to assume that marked and prolonged atrophy of these muscles reduces the mechanical stability of the lumbar spine, potentially leaving it vulnerable to stress-related injury. Furthermore, although limited to animal research, it appears that increased thickness in the connective tissues within muscle spindles of the multifidus are associated with pathology of the lumbar intervertebral discs.[104] Although speculation, similar changes in the structure of the muscle spindle within the multifidus of persons with low back pain could partially explain reduced spinal proprioception in this population. These findings support continued research in how to design exercises that best increase the strength, control, and stabilization of the lumbar multifidus in persons with low back pain.[66,79,86,90,234]

ADDITIONAL CLINICAL CONNECTIONS

A significant percentage of the stress-related musculoskeletal pathology of the trunk occurs at the lumbopelvic region. This region includes the lumbar spine, lumbosacral junction, and the sacroiliac joints. Although an evolving and imprecise clinical term, *lumbopelvic instability* typically describes a painful, usually nonspecific condition, that is assumed to be associated with poor control, reduced stiffness, and hypermobility at one or more of the articulated segments within the region.[177] The amount of hypermobility may be slight and often difficult to determine when assessing for structural instability.[4] This condition, nevertheless, is thought to have the potential to generate damaging stress on spinal-related structures, including the interbody joint and disc, apophyseal and sacroiliac joints, spinal ligaments, and neural tissues. The clinical picture of this condition is often complicated by the uncertainty regarding whether lumbopelvic instability is the *cause* or the *effect* of other impairments in the low back, such as degenerative disc disease.[20]

Weakness, fatigue, reflex inhibition, and/or the inability of trunk muscles to specifically control the timing or magnitude of forces have long been suspected as a potential cause, or at least an associated factor, in the pathogenesis of lumbopelvic instability and associated low back pain. For this reason, exercise is often considered an essential component of treatment for this condition, especially when the exercises are chosen for the appropriate subgroups of patients who are likely to respond in a favorable manner.[63,85,96,163] It is beyond the scope of this chapter to describe the details and effectiveness of the many types of exercises designed to reduce pain by improving lumbopelvic stability; a sample of this extensive literature can be found in other sources.[b] As a summary, the following discussion briefly describes five clinical themes that relate to the design of exercises that intend to reduce pain associated with lumbopelvic instability. These clinical themes will undoubtedly evolve as research continues in this important area.

1. Train persons in exercises aimed to *selectively activate deeper stabilizers* of the trunk, most notably the lumbar multifidus, transversus abdominis, and internal oblique. Activation of these muscles appears important for establishing a baseline stability and stiffness of the lumbopelvic region, especially in advance of unexpected or sudden movements of the trunk or extremities.[40,95,177,182,202] The literature suggests that some persons with low back pain have difficulty selectively and appropriately activating these muscles, especially while maintaining a neutral position of the lumbar spine.[84] As a part of the initial treatment, clinicians often attempt to instruct persons to "draw in" (or hollow) the abdomen, an action assumed to be performed almost exclusively by bilateral contraction of the transversus abdominis and internal oblique.[81,84,128] Teaching individuals to engage in activities that selectively activate these deeper muscles may need to be reinforced or confirmed by using real-time ultrasound imaging.[82,130,205] Such confirmation may be inconclusive through simple clinical palpation or observation. Once it is assumed that an individual has learned to selectively activate these muscles, the next critical step is to maintain the activation while challenging the muscles during functional or recreational activities—a concept often referred to as "core awareness."

2. Design exercises that simultaneously challenge a *wide range* of *muscles* of the trunk. The biomechanical complexity required to effectively stabilize the trunk during whole-body activities demands the *interaction* of several muscles, rather than isolated activation of any single muscle. Optimal stability of the trunk requires coordinated actions of *both* the intrinsic and the extrinsic muscular stabilizers.[55,83,162] Lumbopelvic stability, in general, requires activation from deeper segmental muscles, such as the multifidus and the transversus abdominis but also requires synergistic activation from more superficial muscles, such as the quadratus lumborum, erector spinae, psoas major, rectus abdominis, and oblique abdominals. By attaching into thoracolumbar fascia, activation of the gluteus maximus and latissimus dorsi have also been shown to increase lumbopelvic stability, at least over the short term.[202] Coactivation of the diaphragm muscle assists with this stability by way of helping to increase intra-abdominal pressure. Ample data exist in the literature that can assist the clinician in designing exercises that vary the demands on a wide range of muscles. Many of the exercises are relatively simple to teach to patients or clients and require little to no equipment, yet they place relatively demanding and simultaneous challenges on several important trunk muscles. The relative exercise demands placed on many of these muscles have been well studied using EMG by Okubo and colleagues.[162] As an example, consider the classic, supine *"bridge"* exercise where the trunk and both hips are held extended and the knees are flexed to 90 degrees. Holding this position while alternating bouts of unilateral knee extension produces EMG levels from the erector spinae and multifidus of about 35% and 50% of that produced by a maximum voluntary isometric contraction (MVIC), respectively.[162] As a second example, consider a derivative of the common *prone "plank"* exercise, where the trunk and hips are held suspended straight in extension while only the

[b]5,69,79,85,137,153,163,182,202,215

Continued

ADDITIONAL CLINICAL CONNECTIONS

toes and forearms are contacting the ground. Holding this position while alternating lifts of the upper limb and contralateral lower limb places demands on the transversus abdominis, rectus abdominis, and external oblique of 30%, 35%, and 80% MVIC, respectively.[162] Interestingly, the demands placed against the right and left sides of many of the muscles studied while performing the modified plank and bridge exercises can be selectively and significantly increased based on the particular side of the moved limbs. The most dramatic example of this bilateral asymmetry of muscle action was shown by the transversus abdominis. Specifically, performing the prone plank exercise while lifting the *left arm* with the *right leg* produced an average EMG level from the *left* transversus abdominis that was four times greater than that produced by the right side of this muscle during the same exercise. The strong ipsilateral coupling between the side of the raised arm and side of dominant muscle activation during the performance of the prone plank exercise may be yet another strategy to challenge the transversus abdominis muscle, in addition to the common "drawing in" (or hollowing) maneuver so often recommended.

3. Design exercises that intend to optimize lumbopelvic stability while discouraging "offending" lumbopelvic movements or alignments that stress the musculoskeletal system to the point of producing or sustaining overly painful symptoms.[85,98,184] In short, the clinician helps the patient exchange the offending movements (or postures) for those that are assumed less stressful to the local tissues and therefore provoke less pain or discomfort.[100,137]

Prescribing exercises that appropriately alter a patients' conscious control of their movements can be challenging, especially if the patient's tissues have structurally accommodated to an offending movement. In practice, the clinician must extensively assess the unique alignment, movement, and associated symptom profile of their patients; then prescribe exercises that incorporate alternative movements and alignments that may *avoid* or *modify* stressful and excessively symptomatic responses. The most appropriate movement pattern is determined by noting the patient's immediate symptomatic response to their preferred (and often potentially stressful) movement pattern; or by consulting a body of knowledge that has classified specific lumbopelvic-and-hip movement patterns according to their likelihood of stressing

musculoskeletal tissues.[85] Once the most kinesiologically optimal movement is adopted (for example, performing an appropriate and relatively comfortable lumbopelvic rhythm while flexing the trunk toward the floor—see Chapter 9), exercises are given to help incorporate the "new" movement skills into normal daily activities.

Movement patterns believed to provoke microtrauma to tissues within the lumbopelvic and hip regions have been formally classified into several *movement system impairment syndromes.*[85,184] These classifications are designed to help guide the treatment. Recognizing a given impairment syndrome followed by teaching specific exercises that most likely reestablish a patient's motor control requires keen clinical observations of movement, often supplemented with advanced training.[85]

4. Design resistive exercises that favor an increase not only in muscle strength and control but also *endurance.* During most routine activities, only modest levels of muscle force are required to establish a baseline stability of the lumbopelvic region.[143] Although this level of muscular effort may be relatively low, it typically must be sustained over several hours. In theory, reduced muscular endurance would reduce the lumbopelvic region's ability to sustain a relatively rigid or stiff posture over time, especially when engaging in more rigorous activities.

Studies showing a direct cause-and-effect relationship between reduced lumbopelvic muscular endurance and low back injury are lacking in the research literature. However, some evidence lends partial support to this general premise. As reported by Lopes et al, reduced trunk endurance as measured by the prone plank test, coupled with reduced "posterior chain" flexibility and previous history of musculoskeletal pain, predicted overuse injury in the low back and lower extremities in a subset of 545 Naval cadets.[133]

5. Provide exercises that challenge *postural control, equilibrium, and positional awareness of the body as a whole.*[54] Some persons with chronic low back pain have shown reduced proprioception (position sense) of the lumbopelvic region and reduced standing balance, compared with healthy controls.[69,145] Whether these deficits are related to each other and to the cause of low back pain is unknown. Some authors assert that the deficits may be related to delayed muscle reaction times coupled with impaired neuromuscular feedback.[59]

ADDITIONAL CLINICAL CONNECTIONS

CLINICAL CONNECTION 10.3
Torticollis and Sleeping Position: Is There a Link?

Torticollis (from the Latin *tortus,* twisted, + *collum,* neck) typically describes a pathologic condition of chronic, unilateral shortening of the sternocleidomastoid muscle. The condition, generally identified in the young child or infant, is most often congenital but may also be acquired after birth because of positioning of the child's head. Regardless of onset, a child or infant with torticollis typically has an asymmetric craniocervical posture that reflects the primary actions of the tightened muscle. The child illustrated in Fig. 10.37 has a tight left sternocleidomastoid (see arrow), with a corresponding posture of slight left lateral flexion combined with right axial rotation of the craniocervical region.

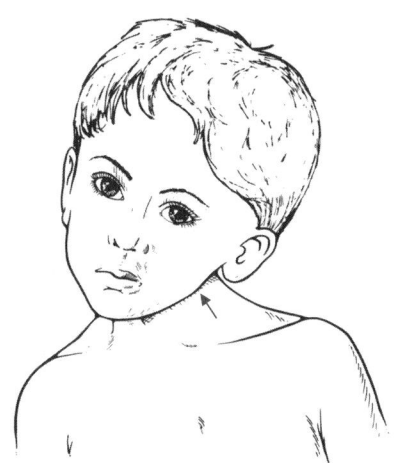

FIGURE 10.37 Torticollis affecting the left sternocleidomastoid of a young boy *(arrow).* Note the posture of slight left lateral flexion combined with right axial rotation of his craniocervical region. (From Herring JA: *Tachdjian's pediatric orthopaedics,* ed 3, Philadelphia, 2002, Saunders.)

The reported incidence of torticollis varies considerably because of different methods for detecting the condition as well as inconsistent definitions of the condition. Estimates of the incidence of congenital torticollis range from 0.4% to 3.9% to as high as 16% of births.[34,49,194]

Although torticollis most often involves muscle, it may be associated with non-muscular systems. The far more common congenital, muscular-based torticollis usually is associated with excessive fibrous tissue (with a proliferation of type III collagen) and varying amounts of adipocyte hyperplasia within the sternocleidomastoid.[33,49,132] Although the exact cause of this condition is unknown, it is frequently associated with a difficult childbirth, breech delivery, or intrauterine malpositioning or crowding.[34,127,187] The more potentially serious, non–muscular-based torticollis may involve pathology associated with the nervous system (including vision) or the skeletal system (typically associated with cervical dysplasia). Several thorough reviews of the clinical expressions, causes, and treatments of torticollis exist in the literature.[187,207]

Approximately one-third of infants with torticollis also develop *plagiocephaly.*[49] This condition is an abnormal molding and subsequent distortion in the shape of a young infant's naturally soft cranium.[127] The distorted shape is typically caused by the infant's head resting in a single prolonged position against another surface. Some authors believe that an infant with an *existing* torticollis may develop a secondary plagiocephaly (involving the posterior-lateral cranium) before or shortly after birth because of the prolonged and concentrated contact against the infant's rotated cranium. Alternately, other authors assert that an infant born *free of* torticollis may eventually develop plagiocephaly with a secondary torticollis simply because of a favored rotated position of the head while the infant sleeps in a supine position.[6] Once developed, the positional plagiocephaly strongly reinforces the established asymmetric (rotated) head position adapted for sleeping. The constant rotated position of the head produces a chronically shortened contralateral sternocleidomastoid, which eventually develops into a contracture and the classic expression of torticollis. Many infants who develop torticollis after plagiocephaly do not have fibrotic changes in the tightened sternocleidomastoid muscle; the deformity develops purely because of muscle tightness caused by the abnormal craniocervical positioning.[49,233] This clinical expression of torticollis in the infant is often referred to as positional or postural torticollis.

The notion that plagiocephaly can, in some cases, lead to a positional torticollis was reinforced by a series of events that occurred in the 1990s. Within this decade, the American Academy of Pediatrics published recommendations that healthy infants be placed in a supine position for sleeping to reduce the incidence of sudden infant death syndrome (SIDS).[233] The "*back*-to-sleep" recommendation had a dramatic effect on the sleeping pattern of many infants in the United States. The incidence of infants positioned prone for sleep decreased by 66% from 1992 to 1996.[10,208]

Continued

ADDITIONAL CLINICAL CONNECTIONS

Although a direct cause-and-effect relationship cannot be unequivocally stated, the rate of SIDS declined approximately 38% to 50% during this same time period.[49,183] The remarkable and simultaneous decline in the incidence of SIDS strongly reinforced the fundamental premise of the "Back-to-Sleep" campaign (which has been updated, expanded, and later renamed the "Safe-to-Sleep" campaign[203]). Evidence strongly suggests that the increased frequency of supine-only sleeping has also led to an increase in the incidence of positional plagiocephaly, most notably affecting the posterior-lateral cranium.[106] Furthermore, additional data show that the dramatic increase in positional plagiocephaly has led to a parallel increase in positional torticollis.[171]

Without a doubt, the huge and life-saving success of the Back-to-Sleep campaign of the 1990s far outweighs the potential negative consequence caused by the increased incidence of plagiocephaly and secondary torticollis. Efforts are ongoing to minimize the incidence of these two potentially related conditions. Clinicians often advise parents or guardians to alternate the head position of the supine-positioned infant.[73,112] Clinicians also advocate that parents or guardians set aside short periods of supervised and interactive "prone-play" (or "tummy time") with the infant several times during daytime awake hours, while still strictly adhering to the Back-to-Sleep principle.[35,112] Encouraging more prone-lying while infants are awake will very likely reduce the likelihood of developing plagiocephaly (and secondary torticollis), and may also facilitate the infant's natural neuromuscular development.[112] Some authors feel that excessive time spent in the supine position may cause delays in achieving certain milestones of motor development, although the long-term consequence of these delays, if any, is not clear.[158,160,188,189]

Regardless of the exact cause of torticollis, medical intervention is typically conservative and includes physical therapy.[65] Early intervention is key to successful conservative therapy.[187] Therapy most often involves educating the parent or caregiver on the condition, stretching the affected muscle while strengthening its contralateral pair, and encouraging activities that facilitate normal motor development, such as rolling or maintaining control of the head.[159] Parents or guardians of a child with torticollis are instructed on how to stretch the tight muscle and how to position and handle the child to promote elongation (stretch) of the involved muscle (e.g., encouraging activities that place the chin of the child *toward* the affected muscle). Although relatively rare, in more severe cases of contracture, the muscle may be injected with botulinum toxin (Botox) or be surgically released.[127,207]

REFERENCES

1. Abdoli-Eramaki M, Agababova M, Janabi J, et al.: Evaluation and comparison of lift styles for an ideal lift among individuals with different levels of training, *Applied Ergonomics* 78:120–126, 2019.

2. Ackland DC, Merritt JS, Pandy MG: Moment arms of the human neck muscles in flexion, bending and rotation, *J Biomech* 44(3):475–486, 2011.

3. Adams MA, Dolan P: A technique for quantifying the bending moment acting on the lumbar spine in vivo, *J Biomech* 24:117–126, 1991.

4. Alqarni AM, Schneiders AG, Hendrick PA: Clinical tests to diagnose lumbar segmental instability: a systematic review [Review], *J Orthop Sports Phys Ther* 41:130–140, 2011.

5. Amaral DDV, Miyamoto GC, Franco KFM, et al.: Examination of a subgroup of patients with chronic low back pain likely to benefit more from Pilates-based exercises compared to an educational booklet, *J Orthop Sports Phys Ther* 50(4):189–197, 2020.

6. American Academy of Pediatrics Task Force on Infant Positioning and SIDS: Positioning and sudden infant death syndrome (SIDS): update, *Pediatrics* 98:1216–1218, 1996.

7. Andersson EA, Grundstrom H, Thorstensson A: Diverging intramuscular activity patterns in back and abdominal muscles during trunk rotation, *Spine* 27:E152–E160, 2002.

8. Andersson EA, Nilsson J, Ma Z, et al.: Abdominal and hip flexor muscle activation during various training exercises, *Eur J Appl Physiol Occup Physiol* 75:115–123, 1997.

9. Andias R, Silva AG: A systematic review with meta-analysis on functional changes associated with neck pain in adolescents, *Muscoskel Care* 17(1):23–36, 2019.

10. Argenta LC, David LR, Wilson JA, et al.: An increase in infant cranial deformity with supine sleeping position, *J Craniofac Surg* 7:5–11, 1996.

11. Arjmand N, Plamondon A, Shirazi-Adl A, et al.: Predictive equations for lumbar spine in load-dependent asymmetric one- and two-handed lifting activities, *Clin Biomech* 27(6):537–544, 2012.

12. Arjmand N, Shirazi-Adl A, Parnianpour M: Trunk biomechanics during maximum isometric axial torque exertions in upright standing, *Clin Biomech* 23:969–978, 2008.

13. Arjmand N, Shirazi-Adl A: Biomechanics of changes in lumbar posture in static lifting, *Spine* 30:2637–2648, 2005.

14. Arjmand N, Shirazi-Adl A: Role of intra-abdominal pressure in the unloading and stabilization of the human spine during static lifting tasks, *Eur Spine J* 15:1265–1275, 2006.

15. Armijo-Olivo S, Silvestre R, Fuentes J, et al.: Electromyographic activity of the cervical flexor muscles in patients with temporomandibular disorders while performing the craniocervical flexion test: a cross-sectional study, *Phys Ther* 91(8):1184–1197, 2011.

16. Armstrong DP, Fischer SL: Understanding individual differences in lifting mechanics: do some people adopt motor control strategies that minimize biomechanical exposure, *Hum Mov Sci* 74:102689, 2020.

17. Barr KP, Griggs M, Cadby T: Lumbar stabilization: a review of core concepts and current literature, Part 2, *Am J Phys Med Rehabil* 86:72–80, 2007.

18. Bartelink DL: The role of abdominal pressure in relieving the pressure on the lumbar intervertebral discs, *J Bone Joint Surg Br* 39:718–725, 1957.

19. Bazrgari B, Shirazi-Adl A, Arjmand N: Analysis of squat and stoop dynamic liftings: muscle forces and internal spinal loads, *Eur Spine J* 16:687–699, 2007.

20. Beattie PF: Current understanding of lumbar intervertebral disc degeneration: a review with emphasis upon etiology, pathophysiology, and lumbar magnetic resonance imaging findings, *J Orthop Sports Phys Ther* 38:329–340, 2008.

21. Belavý DL, Hides JA, Wilson SJ, et al.: Resistive simulated weightbearing exercise with whole body vibration reduces lumbar spine deconditioning in bedrest, *Spine* 33:E121–E131, 2008.

22. Bogduk N: *Clinical and radiological anatomy of the lumbar spine*, ed 5, New York, 2012, Churchill Livingstone.

23. Borst J, Forbes PA, Happee R, et al.: Muscle parameters for musculoskeletal modelling of the human neck, *Clin Biomech* 26(4):343–351, 2011.

24. Briggs AM, Greig AM, Bennell KL, et al.: Paraspinal muscle control in people with osteoporotic vertebral fracture, *Eur Spine J* 16:1137–1144, 2007.

25. Brown SH, McGill SM: A comparison of ultrasound and electromyography measures of force and activation to examine the mechanics of abdominal wall contraction, *Clin Biomech* 25(2):115–123, 2010.

26. Brown SH, Vera-Garcia FJ, McGill SM: Effects of abdominal muscle coactivation on the externally preloaded trunk: variations in motor control and its effect on spine stability, *Spine* 31:E387–E393, 2006.

27. Brown SH, Ward SR, Cook MS, et al.: Architectural analysis of human abdominal wall muscles: implications for mechanical function, *Spine* 36(5):355–362, 2011.

28. Buford JA, Yoder SM, Heiss DG, et al.: Actions of the scalene muscles for rotation of the cervical spine in macaque and human, *J Orthop Sports Phys Ther* 32:488–496, 2002.

29. Cagnie B, Dickx N, Peeters I, et al.: The use of functional MRI to evaluate cervical flexor activity during different cervical flexion exercises, *J Appl Physiol* 104(1):230–235, 2008.

30. Cagnie B, Dolphens M, Peeters I, et al.: Use of muscle functional magnetic resonance imaging to compare cervical flexor activity between patients with whiplash-associated disorders and people who are healthy, *Phys Ther* 90(8):1157–1164, 2010.

31. Cannon J, Cambridge EDJ, McGill SM: Increased core stability is associated with reduced knee valgus during single-leg landing tasks: investigating lumbar spine and hip joint rotational stiffness, *J Biomech* 116:110240, 2021.

32. Chaffin DB, Andersson GBJ: *Occupational biomechanics*, ed 2, New York, 1991, John Wiley and Sons.

33. Chen HX, Tang SP, Gao FT, et al.: Fibrosis, adipogenesis, and muscle atrophy in congenital muscular torticollis, *Medicine (Baltim)* 93(23):e138, 2014.

34. Chen MM, Chang HC, Hsieh CF, et al.: Predictive model for congenital muscular torticollis: analysis of 1021 infants with sonography, *Arch Phys Med Rehabil* 86:2199–2203, 2005.

35. Cheng JC, Wong MW, Tang SP, et al.: Clinical determinants of the outcome of manual stretching in the treatment of congenital muscular torticollis in infants. A prospective study of eight hundred and twenty-one cases, *J Bone Joint Surg Am* 83:679–687, 2001.

36. Cho J, Lee E, Lee S: Upper thoracic spine mobilization and mobility exercise versus upper cervical spine mobilization and stabilization exercise in individuals with forward head posture: a randomized clinical trial, *BMC Musculoskelet Disord* 18(1):525, 2017.

37. Cholewicki J, McGill SM: Lumbar posterior ligament involvement during extremely heavy lifts estimated from fluoroscopic measurements, *J Biomech* 25:17–28, 1992.

38. Coenen P, Gouttebarge V, van der Burght AS, et al.: The effect of lifting during work on low back pain: a health impact assessment based on a meta-analysis, *Occup Environ Med* 71(12):871–877, 2014.

39. Coenen P, Kingma I, Boot CR, et al.: Cumulative low back load at work as a risk factor of low back pain: a prospective cohort study, *J Occup Rehabil* 23(1):11–18, 2013.

40. Cort JA, Dickey JP, Potvin JR: Trunk muscle contributions to L4-5 joint rotational stiffness following sudden trunk lateral bend perturbations, *J Electromyogr Kinesiol* 23(6):1334–1342, 2013.

41. Craig BN, Congleton JJ, Beier E, et al.: Occupational risk factors and back injury, *Int J Occup Saf Ergon* 9(3):335–345, 2013.

42. Crawford RJ, Fortin M, Weber KA, et al.: Are magnetic resonance imaging technologies crucial to our understanding of spinal conditions? *J Orthop Sports Phys Ther* 49(5):320–329, 2019.

43. Cresswell AG, Grundstrom H, Thorstensson A: Observations on intra-abdominal pressure and patterns of abdominal intra-muscular activity in man, *Acta Physiol Scand* 144:409–418, 1992.

44. Crommert ME, Ekblom MM, Thorstensson A: Activation of transversus abdominis varies with postural demand in standing, *Gait Posture* 33(3):473–477, 2011.

45. Crommert ME, Flink I, Gustavsson C: Predictors of disability attributed to symptoms of increased interrecti distance in women after childbirth: an observational study, *Phys Ther* 101(6):1–6, 2021.

46. Damm P, Reitmaier S, Hahn S, et al.: In vivo hip and lumbar spine implant loads during activities in forward bent postures, *J Biomech* 102:109517, 2020.

47. Dawson AP, McLennan SN, Schiller SD, et al.: Interventions to prevent back pain and back injury in nurses: a systematic review, *Occup Environ Med* 64:642–650, 2007.

48. de Araujo FX, Ferreira GE, Scholl Schell M, et al.: Measurement properties of the craniocervical flexion test: a systematic review, *Phys Ther* 100(7):1094–1117, 2020.

49. de Chalain TM, Park S: Torticollis associated with positional plagiocephaly: a growing epidemic, *J Craniofac Surg* 16:411–418, 2005.

50. Deng YC, Goldsmith W: Response of a human head/neck/upper-torso replica to dynamic loading—I. Physical model, *J Biomech* 20:471–486, 1987.

51. Desmoulin GT, Pradhan V, Milner TE: Mechanical aspects of intervertebral disc injury and implications on biomechanics, *Spine* 45(8):E457–E464, 2020.

52. Dolan P, Mannion AF, Adams MA: Passive tissues help the back muscles to generate extensor moments during lifting, *J Biomech* 27:1077–1085, 1994.

53. Dugailly PM, Sobczak S, Moiseev F, et al.: Musculoskeletal modeling of the suboccipital spine: kinematics analysis, muscle lengths, and muscle moment arms during axial rotation and flexion extension, *Spine* 36(6):E413–E422, 2011.

54. Ebenbichler GR, Oddsson LI, Kollmitzer J, et al.: Sensory-motor control of the lower back: implications for rehabilitation, *Med Sci Sports Exerc* 33:1889–1898, 2001.

55. Ekstrom RA, Osborn RW, Hauer PL: Surface electromyographic analysis of the low back muscles during rehabilitation exercises, *J Orthop Sports Phys Ther* 38:736–745, 2008.

56. El Ouaaid Z, Shirazi-Adl A, Plamondon A, et al.: Trunk strength, muscle activity and spinal loads in maximum isometric flexion and extension exertions: a combined in vivo-computational study, *J Biomech* 46(13):2228–2235, 2013.

57. Elizagaray-Garcia I, Beltran-Alacreu H, Angulo-Díaz S, et al.: Chronic primary headache subjects have greater forward head posture than asymptomatic and episodic primary headache sufferers: systematic review and meta-analysis, *Pain Med* 21(10):2465–2480, 2020.

58. El-Monajjed K, Driscoll M: A finite element analysis of the intra-abdominal pressure and paraspinal muscle compartment pressure interaction through the thoracolumbar fascia, *Comput Methods Biomech Biomed Engin* 23(10):585–596, 2020.

59. Escamilla RF, Babb E, DeWitt R, et al.: Electromyographic analysis of traditional and nontraditional abdominal exercises: implications for rehabilitation and training, *Phys Ther* 86:656–671, 2006.

60. Falla D, Jull G, Dall'Alba P, et al.: An electromyographic analysis of the deep cervical flexor muscles in performance of craniocervical flexion, *Phys Ther* 83(10):899–906, 2003.

61. Falla D, Jull G, Hodges P, et al.: An endurance-strength training regime is effective in reducing

myoelectric manifestations of cervical flexor muscle fatigue in females with chronic neck pain, *Clin Neurophysiol* 117(4):828–837, 2006.

62. Falla D, Jull G, Russell T, et al.: Effect of neck exercise on sitting posture in patients with chronic neck pain, *Phys Ther* 87:408–417, 2007.

63. Ferreira PH, Ferreira ML, Maher CG, et al.: Specific stabilisation exercise for spinal and pelvic pain: a systematic review, *Aust J Physiother* 52:79–88, 2006.

64. Fortin M, Macedo LG: Multifidus and paraspinal muscle group cross-sectional areas of patients with low back pain and control patients: a systematic review with a focus on blinding [Review], *Phys Ther* 93(7):873–888, 2013.

65. Fradette J, Gagnon I, Kennedy E, et al.: Clinical decision making regarding intervention needs of infants with torticollis, *Pediatr Phys Ther* 23(3):249–256, 2011.

66. Freeman MD, Woodham MA, Woodham AW: The role of the lumbar multifidus in chronic low back pain: a review [Review, 25 refs], *Pharm Manag PM R* 22(2):142–146, 2010.

67. Gagnon D, Plamondon A, Lariviere C: A Comparison of lumbar spine and muscle loading between male and female workers during box transfers, *J Biomech* 81:76–85, 2018.

68. Gallagher S, Marras WS: Tolerance of the lumbar spine to shear: a review and recommended exposure limits [Review], *Clin Biomech* 27(10):973–978, 2012.

69. Gatti R, Faccendini S, Tettamanti A, et al.: Efficacy of trunk balance exercises for individuals with chronic low back pain: a randomized clinical trial, *J Orthop Sports Phys Ther* 41(8):542–552, 2011.

70. Gatton ML, Pearcy MJ, Pettet GJ, et al.: A three-dimensional mathematical model of the thoracolumbar fascia and an estimate of its biomechanical effect, *J Biomech* 43(14):2792–2797, 2010.

71. Ghezelbash F, Shirazi-Adl A, El Ouaaid Z, et al.: Subject-specific regression equations to estimate lower spinal loads during symmetric and asymmetric static lifting, *J Biomech* 102:109550, 2020.

72. Ghezelbash F, Shirazi-Adl A, Plamondon A, et al.: Comparison of different lifting analysis tools in estimating lower spinal loads - evaluation of NIOSH criterion, *J Biomech* 112:110024, 2020.

73. Graham Jr JM: Tummy time is important, *Clin Pediatr (Phila)* 45:119–121, 2006.

74. Greening J, Anantharaman K, Young R, et al.: Evidence for increased magnetic resonance imaging signal intensity and morphological changes in the brachial plexus and median nerves of patients with chronic arm and neck pain following whiplash injury, *J Orthop Sports Phys Ther* 48(7):523–532, 2018.

75. Guo R, Zhou C, Wang C, et al.: In vivo primary and coupled segmental motions of the healthy female head-neck complex during dynamic head axial rotation, *J Biomech* 123:110513, 2021.

76. Hagins M, Lamberg EM: Individuals with low back pain breathe differently than healthy individuals during a lifting task, *J Orthop Sports Phys Ther* 41(3):141–148, 2011.

77. Halpern AA, Bleck EE: Sit-up exercises: an electromyographic study, *Clin Orthop Relat Res* 145:172–178, 1979.

78. Hansen L, de Zee M, Rasmussen J, et al.: Anatomy and biomechanics of the back muscles in the lumbar spine with reference to biomechanical modeling, *Spine* 31:1888–1899, 2006.

79. Hebert JJ, Koppenhaver SL, Magel JS, et al.: The relationship of transversus abdominis and lumbar multifidus activation and prognostic factors for clinical success with a stabilization exercise program: a cross-sectional study, *Arch Phys Med Rehabil* 91(1):78–85, 2010.

80. Heidari E, Arjmand N, Kahrizi S: Comparisons of lumbar spine loads and kinematics in healthy and nonspecific low back pain individuals during unstable lifting activities, *J Biomech* 144:111344, 2022.

81. Henry SM, Teyhen DS: Ultrasound imaging as a feedback tool in the rehabilitation of trunk muscle

dysfunction for people with low back pain, *J Orthop Sports Phys Ther* 37:627–634, 2007.

82. Herbert WJ, Heiss DG, Basso DM: Influence of feedback schedule in motor performance and learning of a lumbar multifidus muscle task using rehabilitative ultrasound imaging: a randomized clinical trial, *Phys Ther* 88:261–269, 2008.

83. Hesse B, Frober R, Fischer MS, et al.: Functional differentiation of the human lumbar periphvertebral musculature revisited by means of muscle fibre type composition, *Ann Anat* 195(6):570–580, 2013.

84. Hides J, Wilson S, Stanton W, et al.: An MRI investigation into the function of the transversus abdominis muscle during "drawing-in" of the abdominal wall, *Spine* 31:E175–E178, 2006.

85. Hides JA, Donelson R, Lee D, et al.: Convergence and divergence of exercise-based approaches that incorporate motor control for the management of low back pain, *J Orthop Sports Phys Ther* 49(6):437–452, 2019.

86. Hides JA, Stanton WR, McMahon S, et al.: Effect of stabilization training on multifidus muscle cross-sectional area among young elite cricketers with low back pain, *J Orthop Sports Phys Ther* 38:101–108, 2008.

87. Hides JA, Stokes MJ, Saide M, et al.: Evidence of lumbar multifidus muscle wasting ipsilateral to symptoms in patients with acute/subacute low back pain, *Spine* 19:165–172, 1994.

88. Hodges P, Holm AK, Hansson T, et al.: Rapid atrophy of the lumbar multifidus follows experimental disc or nerve root injury, *Spine* 31:2926–2933, 2006.

89. Hodges P, Kaigle HA, Holm S, et al.: Intervertebral stiffness of the spine is increased by evoked contraction of transversus abdominis and the diaphragm: in vivo porcine studies, *Spine* 28:2594–2601, 2003.

90. Hodges PW, Danneels L: Changes in structure and function of the back muscles in low back pain: different time points, observations, and mechanisms, *J Orthop Sports Phys Ther* 49(6):464–476, 2019.

91. Hodges PW, Butler JE, McKenzie DK, et al.: Contraction of the human diaphragm during rapid postural adjustments, *J Physiol (Lond)* 505(Pt 2):539–548, 1997.

92. Hodges PW, Cresswell AG, Daggfeldt K, et al.: In vivo measurement of the effect of intra-abdominal pressure on the human spine, *J Biomech* 34:347–353, 2001.

93. Hodges PW, Richardson CA: Contraction of the abdominal muscles associated with movement of the lower limb, *Phys Ther* 77:132–142, 1997.

94. Hodges PW, Richardson CA: Feedforward contraction of transversus abdominis is not influenced by the direction of arm movement, *Exp Brain Res* 114:362–370, 1997.

95. Hodges PW, Richardson CA: Inefficient muscular stabilization of the lumbar spine associated with low back pain. A motor control evaluation of transversus abdominis, *Spine* 21:2640–2650, 1996.

96. Hodges PW: Hybrid approach to treatment tailoring for low back pain: a proposed model of care, *J Orthop Sports Phys Ther* 49(6):453–463, 2019.

97. Hoek van Dijke GA, Snijders CJ, Stoeckart R, et al.: A biomechanical model on muscle forces in the transfer of spinal load to the pelvis and legs, *J Biomech* 32:927–933, 1999.

98. Hoffman SL, Harris-Hayes M, Van Dillen LR: Differences in activity limitation between 2 low back pain subgroups based on the movement system impairment model, *Pm R* 2(12):1113–1118, 2010.

99. Hoogendoorn WE, Bongers PM, de Vet HC, et al.: Flexion and rotation of the trunk and lifting at work are risk factors for low back pain: results of a prospective cohort study, *Spine* 25:3087–3092, 2000.

100. Hooker QL, Lanier VM, Roles K, et al.: Motor skill training versus strength and flexibility exercise in people with chronic low back pain: Preplanned analysis of effects on kinematics during a functional activity, *Clin Biomech* 92:105570, 2022.

101. Ivancic PC: Facet joint and disc kinematics during simulated rear crashes with active injury prevention systems, *Spine* 36(18):E1215–E1224, 2011.

102. Jager M, Luttmann A: The load on the lumbar spine during asymmetrical bi-manual materials handling, *Ergonomics* 35:783–805, 1992.

103. James G, Chen X, Diwan A, et al.: Fat Infiltration in the multifidus muscle is related to inflammatory cytokine expression in the muscle and epidural adipose tissue in individuals undergoing surgery for intervertebral disc herniation, *Eur Spine J* 30(4):837–845, 2021.

104. James G, Stecco C, Blomster L, et al.: Muscle spindles of the multifidus muscle undergo structural change after intervertebral disc degeneration, *Eur Spine J* 31(7):1879–1888, 2022.

105. Jin X, Feng Z, Mika V, et al.: The role of neck muscle activities on the risk of mild traumatic brain injury in American football, *J Biomech Eng* 139(10), 2017.

106. Jones MW: The other side of "back to sleep, *Neonatal Netw* 22:49–53, 2003.

107. Jordan A, Mehlsen J, Bülow PM, et al.: Maximal isometric strength of the cervical musculature in 100 healthy volunteers, *Spine* 24:1343–1348, 1999.

108. Jorgensen MJ, Marras WS, Gupta P, et al.: Effect of torso flexion on the lumbar torso extensor muscle sagittal plane moment arms, *Spine* 3:363–369, 2003.

109. Juker D, McGill S, Kropf P, et al.: Quantitative intramuscular myoelectric activity of lumbar portions of psoas and the abdominal wall during a wide variety of tasks, *Med Sci Sports Exerc* 30:301–310, 1998.

110. Jull G, Falla D: Does increased superficial neck flexor activity in the craniocervical flexion test reflect reduced deep flexor activity in people with neck pain? *Man Ther* 25:43–47, 2016.

111. Kalmanson OA, Khayatzadeh S, Germanwala A, et al.: Anatomic considerations in headaches associated with cervical sagittal imbalance: a cadaveric biomechanical study, *J Clin Neurosci* 65:140–144, 2019.

112. Kaplan SL, Coulter C, Sargent B: Physical therapy management of congenital muscular torticollis: a 2018 evidence-based clinical practice guideline from the APTA Academy of Pediatric Physical Therapy, *Pediatr Phys Ther* 30(4):240–290, 2018.

113. Kavcic N, Grenier S, McGill SM: Determining the stabilizing role of individual torso muscles during rehabilitation exercises, *Spine* 29:1254–1265, 2004.

114. Kemp PA, Burnham BR, Copley GB, et al.: Injuries to air force personnel associated with lifting, handling, and carrying objects, *Am J Prev Med* 38(Suppl. 1):S148–S155, 2010.

115. Kennedy E, Quinn D, Chapple C, et al.: Can the neck contribute to persistent symptoms post concussion? A prospective descriptive case series, *J Orthop Sports Phys Ther* 49(11):845–854, 2019.

116. Kettler A, Hartwig E, Schultheiss M, et al.: Mechanically simulated muscle forces strongly stabilize intact and injured upper cervical spine specimens, *J Biomech* 35:339–346, 2002.

117. Khoddam-Khorasani P, Arjmand N, Shirazi-Adl A: Effect of changes in the lumbar posture in lifting on trunk muscle and spinal loads: a combined in vivo, musculoskeletal, and finite element model study, *J Biomech* 104:109728, 2020.

118. Kiefer A, Shirazi-Adl A, Parnianpour M: Synergy of the human spine in neutral postures, *Eur Spine J* 7:471–479, 1998.

119. Kjaer P, Bendix T, Sorensen JS, et al.: Are MRI-defined fat infiltrations in the multifidus muscles associated with low back pain? *BMC Med* 5:2, 2007.

120. Kocjan J, Adamek M, Gzik-Zroska B, et al.: Network of breathing. multifunctional role of the diaphragm: a review, *Adv Respir Med* 85(4):224–232, 2017.

121. Kolar P, Sulc J, Kyncl M, et al.: Postural function of the diaphragm in persons with and without chronic low back pain, *J Orthop Sports Phys Ther* 42(4):352–362, 2012.

122. Kolar P, Sulc J, Kyncl M, et al.: Stabilizing function of the diaphragm: dynamic MRI and synchronized spirometric assessment, *J Appl Physiol* 109:1064–1071, 2010.

123. Krakenes J, Kaale BR: Magnetic resonance imaging assessment of craniovertebral ligaments and membranes after whiplash trauma, *Spine* 31:2820–2826, 2006.

124. Kristjansson E, Gislason MK: Women with late whiplash syndrome have greatly reduced load-bearing of the cervical spine. In-vivo biomechanical, cross-sectional, lateral radiographic study, *Eur J Phys Rehabil Med* 54(1):22–33, 2018.

125. Kuijer PP, van Oostrom SH, Duijzer K, et al.: Maximum acceptable weight of lift reflects peak lumbosacral extension moments in a functional capacity evaluation test using free style, stoop and squat lifting, *Ergonomics* 55(3):343–349, 2012.

126. Kumar S: Moment arms of spinal musculature determined from CT scans, *Clin Biomech* 3:137–144, 1988.

127. Kuo AA, Tritasavit S, Graham Jr JM: Congenital muscular torticollis and positional plagiocephaly, *Pediatr Rev* 35(2):79–87, 2014.

128. Lariviere C, Boucher JA, Mecheri H, et al.: Maintaining lumbar spine stability: a study of the specific and combined effects of abdominal activation and lumbosacral orthosis on lumbar intrinsic stiffness, *J Orthop Sports Phys Ther* 49(4):262–271, 2019.

129. Larsen FG, Svenningsen FP, Andersen MS, et al.: Estimation of spinal loading during manual materials handling using inertial motion capture, *Ann Biomed Eng* 48(2):805–821, 2020.

130. Lee DH, Hong SK, Lee YS, et al.: Is abdominal hollowing exercise using real-time ultrasound imaging feedback helpful for selective strengthening of the transversus abdominis muscle?: a prospective, randomized, parallel-group, comparative study, *Medicine (Baltim)* 97(27):e11369, 2018.

131. Lee TH, Liu TY: Postural and muscular responses while viewing different heights of screen, *Int J Occup Saf Ergon* 19(2):251–258, 2013.

132. Li D, Wang K, Zhang W, et al.: Expression of Bax/Bcl-2, Tgf-B1, and Type III collagen fiber in congenital muscular torticollis, *Med Sci Monit* 24:7869–7874, 2018.

133. Lopes TJA, Simic M, Chia L, et al.: Trunk Endurance, Posterior chain flexibility, and previous history of musculoskeletal pain predict overuse low back and lower extremity injury: a prospective cohort study of 545 navy cadets, *J Sci Med Sport* 24(6):555–560, 2021.

134. Lu ML, Waters TR, Krieg E, et al.: Efficacy of the revised NIOSH lifting equation to predict risk of low-back pain associated with manual lifting: a one-year prospective study, *Hum Factors* 56(1):73–85, 2014.

135. Macintosh JE, Bogduk N: The biomechanics of the lumbar multifidus, *Clin Biomech* 1:205–213, 1986.

136. Mahmoud NF, Hassan KA, Abdelmajeed SF, et al.: The relationship between forward head posture and neck pain: a systematic review and meta-analysis, *Curr Rev Musculoskelet Med* 12(4):562–577, 2019.

137. Marich AV, Lanier VM, Salsich GB, et al.: Immediate effects of a single session of motor skill training on the lumbar movement pattern during a functional activity in people with low back pain: a repeated-measures study, *Phys Ther* 98(7):605–615, 2018.

138. Martimo KP, Verbeek J, Karppinen J, et al.: Manual material handling advice and assistive devices for preventing and treating back pain in workers, *Cochrane Database Syst Rev* 3:CD005958, 2007.

139. Mawston G, Holder L, O'Sullivan P, et al.: Flexed lumbar spine postures are associated with greater strength and efficiency than lordotic postures during a maximal lift in pain-free individuals, *Gait Posture* 86:245–250, 2021.

140. McGill SM, Hughson RL, Parks K: Changes in lumbar lordosis modify the role of the extensor muscles, *Clin Biomech* 15:777–780, 2000.

141. McGill SM, Patt N, Norman RW: Measurement of the trunk musculature of active males using CT scan radiography: implications for force and moment generating capacity about the L4/L5 joint, *J Biomech* 21:329–341, 1988.

142. McGill SM, Santaguida L, Stevens J: Measurement of the trunk musculature from T5 to L5 using MRI scans of 15 young males corrected for muscle fibre orientation, *Clin Biomech* 8:171–178, 1993.

143. McGill SM: Biomechanics of the thoracolumbar spine. In Dvir Z, editor: *Clinical biomechanics*, Philadelphia, 2000, Churchill Livingstone.

144. McLean L: The effect of postural correction on muscle activation amplitudes recorded from the cervicobrachial region, *J Electromyogr Kinesiol* 15:527–535, 2005.

145. Mok NW, Brauer SG, Hodges PW: Changes in lumbar movement in people with low back pain are related to compromised balance, *Spine* 36(1):E45–E52, 2011.

146. Moroney SP, Schultz AB, Miller JA: Analysis and measurement of neck loads, *J Orthop Res* 6:713–720, 1988.

147. Morris SL, Lay B, Allison GT: Transversus abdominis is part of a global not local muscle synergy during arm movement, *Hum Mov Sci* 32:1176–1185, 2013.

148. Moseley GL, Hodges PW, Gandevia SC: External perturbation of the trunk in standing humans differentially activates components of the medial back muscles, *J Physiol* 547:581–587, 2003.

149. Mueller J, Mueller S, Stoll J, et al.: Trunk extensor and flexor strength capacity in healthy young elite athletes aged 11-15 years, *J Strength Cond Res* 28(5):1328–1334, 2014.

150. Muller A, Pontonnier C, Robert-Lachaine X, et al.: Motion-Based prediction of external forces and moments and back loading during manual material handling tasks, *Appl Ergon* 82:102935, 2020.

151. National Institute for Occupational Safety and Health (NIOSH): *The national occupational exposure survey, report No. 89-103*, Cincinnati, 1989, NIOSH.

152. National Research C, Institute of Medicine Panel: On musculoskeletal D, and the W. In *Musculoskeletal disorders and the workplace: low back and upper extremities*, National Academies Press (US), 2001.

153. Nava-Bringas TI, Romero-Fierro LO, Trani-Chagoya YP, et al.: Stabilization exercises versus flexion exercises in degenerative spondylolisthesis: a randomized controlled trial, *Phys Ther* 101(8), 2021.

154. Neumann DA, Malloy P: *Unpublished EMG observations*, Marquette University, 2016.

155. Nitz AJ, Peck D: Comparison of muscle spindle concentrations in large and small human epaxial muscles acting in parallel combinations, *Am Surg* 52:273–277, 1986.

156. Nolan D, O'Sullivan K, Newton C, et al.: Are there differences in lifting technique between those with and without low back pain? A systematic review, *Scand J Pain* 20(2):215–227, 2020.

157. Nordin M, Kahanovitz N, Verderame R, et al.: Normal trunk muscle strength and endurance in women and the effect of exercises and electrical stimulation. Part 1: normal endurance and trunk muscle strength in 101 women, *Spine* 12:105–111, 1987.

158. Ohman A, Beckung E: Children who had congenital torticollis as infants are not at higher risk for a delay in motor development at preschool age, *Pharm Manag PM R* 5(10):850–855, 2013.

159. Ohman A, Nilsson S, Beckung E: Stretching treatment for infants with congenital muscular torticollis: physiotherapist or parents? A randomized pilot study, *Pharm Manag PM R* 2(12):1073–1079, 2010.

160. Ohman A, Nilsson S, Lagerkvist AL, et al.: Are infants with torticollis at risk of a delay in early motor milestones compared with a control group of healthy infants? *Dev Med Child Neurol* 51(7):545–550, 2009.

161. Okeson JP: *Management of temporomandibular disorders and occlusion*, ed 8, St Louis, 2020, Elsevier.

162. Okubo Y, Kaneoka K, Imai A, et al.: Electromyographic analysis of transversus abdominis and lumbar multifidus using wire electrodes during lumbar stabilization exercises, *J Orthop Sports Phys Ther* 40(11):743–750, 2010.

163. Owen PJ, Miller CT, Mundell NL, et al.: Which specific modes of exercise training are most effective for treating low back pain? Network meta-Analysis, *Br J Sports Med* 54(21):1279–1287, 2020.

164. Palisch A, Zoga AC, Meyers WC: Imaging of athletic pubalgia and core muscle injuries: clinical and therapeutic correlations [Review], *Clin Sports Med* 32(3):427–447, 2013.

165. Panjabi MM, Cholewicki J, Nibu K, et al.: Critical load of the human cervical spine: an in vitro experimental study, *Clin Biomech* 13:11–17, 1998.

166. Panjabi MM, Ivancic PC, Maak TG, et al.: Multiplanar cervical spine injury due to head-turned rear impact, *Spine* 31:420–429, 2006.

167. Park RJ, Tsao H, Cresswell AG, et al.: Anticipatory postural activity of the deep trunk muscles differs between anatomical regions based on their mechanical advantage, *Neuroscience* 261:161–172, 2014.

168. Park RJ, Tsao H, Cresswell AG, et al.: Differential activity of regions of the psoas major and quadratus lumborum during submaximal isometric trunk efforts, *J Orthop Res* 30(2):311–318, 2012.

169. Patwardhan AG, Havey RM, Ghanayem AJ, et al.: Load-carrying capacity of the human cervical spine in compression is increased under a follower load, *Spine* 25:1548–1554, 2000.

170. Peck D, Buxton DF, Nitz A: A comparison of spindle concentrations in large and small muscles acting in parallel combinations, *J Morphol* 180(3):243–252, 1984.

171. Persing J, James H, Swanson J, et al.: Prevention and management of positional skull deformities in infants. American academy of pediatrics committee on practice and ambulatory medicine, section on plastic surgery and section on neurological surgery, *Pediatrics* 112:199–202, 2003.

172. Phillips S, Mercer S, Bogduk N: Anatomy and biomechanics of quadratus lumborum, *Proc Inst Mech Eng H* 222(2):151–159, 2008.

173. Punnett L, Pruss-Utun A, Nelson DI, et al.: Estimating the global burden of low back pain attributable to combined occupational exposures, *Am J Ind Med* 48(6):459–469, 2005.

174. Punt M, Nematimoez M, van Dieën JH, et al.: Real-time feedback to reduce low-back load in lifting and lowering, *J Biomech* 102:109513, 2020.

175. Quek J, Pua YH, Clark RA, et al.: Effects of thoracic kyphosis and forward head posture on cervical range of motion in older adults, *Man Ther* 18(1):65–71, 2013.

176. Rebbeck T, Evans K, Elliott JM: Concussion in combination with whiplash-associated disorder may be missed in primary care: key recommendations for assessment and management, *J Orthop Sports Phys Ther* 49(11):819–828, 2019.

177. Reeves NP, Cholewicki J, van Dieën JH, et al.: Are stability and instability relevant concepts for back pain? *J Orthop Sports Phys Ther* 49(6):415–424, 2019.

178. Regev GJ, Kim CW, Tomiya A, et al.: Psoas muscle architectural design, in vivo sarcomere length range, and passive tensile properties support its role as a lumbar spine stabilizer, *Spine* 36(26):E1666–E1674, 2011.

179. Richards KV, Beales DJ, Smith AL, et al.: Is neck posture subgroup in late adolescence a risk factor for persistent neck pain in young adults? A prospective study, *Phys Ther* 101(3), 2021.

180. Richardson C, Hodges PW, Hides JA: *Therapeutic exercise for lumbopelvic stabilization*, ed 2, St Louis, 2004, Churchill Livingstone.

181. Richardson CA, Snijders CJ, Hides JA, et al.: The relation between the transversus abdominis muscles, sacroiliac joint mechanics, and low back pain, *Spine* 27:399–405, 2002.

182. Rowley KM, Smith JA, Kulig K: Reduced trunk coupling in persons with recurrent low back pain is associated with greater deep-to-superficial trunk muscle activation ratios during the balance-dexterity task, *J Orthop Sports Phys Ther* 49(12):887–898, 2019.

183. Safe to Sleep-Public Education Program https://safetosleep.nichd.nih.gov/safesleepbasics/about

184. Sahrmann SA: *Diagnosis and treatment of movement impairment syndromes*, St Louis, 2013, Elsevier Health Sciences/Mosby.

185. Santaguida PL, McGill SM: The psoas major muscle: a three-dimensional geometric study, *J Biomech* 28:339–345, 1995.

186. Saraceni N, Kent P, Ng L, et al.: To Flex or Not to Flex? Is there a relationship between lumbar spine flexion during lifting and low back pain? A systematic review with meta-analysis, *J Orthop Sports Phys Ther* 50(3):121–130, 2020.

187. Sargent B, Kaplan SL, Coulter C, et al.: Congenital muscular torticollis: Bridging the gap between research and clinical practice, *Pediatrics* 144(2), 2019.

188. Schertz M, Zuk L, Green D: Long-term neurodevelopmental follow-up of children with congenital muscular torticollis, *J Child Neurol* 28(10):1215–1221, 2013.

189. Schertz M, Zuk L, Zin S, et al.: Motor and cognitive development at one-year follow-up in infants with torticollis, *Early Hum Dev* 84:9–14, 2008.

190. Schipplein OD, Trafimow JH, Andersson GB, et al.: Relationship between moments at the L5/S1 level, hip and knee joint when lifting, *J Biomech* 23:907–912, 1990.

191. Skals S, Blafoss R, Andersen LL, et al.: Manual material handling in the supermarket sector. part 2: knee, spine and shoulder joint reaction forces, *Appl Ergon* 92:103345, 2021.

192. Snijders CJ, Ribbers MT, de Bakker HV, et al.: EMG recordings of abdominal and back muscles in various standing postures: validation of a biomechanical model on sacroiliac joint stability, *J Electromyogr Kinesiol* 8:205–214, 1998.

193. Standring S: *Gray's anatomy: the anatomical basis of clinical practice*, ed 42, St Louis, 2021, Elsevier.

194. Stellwagen LM, Hubbard ET, Chambers C, et al.: Torticollis, facial asymmetry and plagiocephaly in normal newborns, *Arch Dis Child* 93:827–831, 2008.

195. Stemper BD, Pintar FA, Rao RD: The influence of morphology on cervical injury characteristics [Review], *Spine* 36(Suppl. 25), 2011.

196. Stemper BD, Yoganandan N, Pintar FA, et al.: Anterior longitudinal ligament injuries in whiplash may lead to cervical instability, *Med Eng Phys* 28:515–524, 2006.

197. Stevens S, Agten A, Timmermans A, et al.: Unilateral changes of the multifidus in persons with lumbar disc herniation: a systematic review and meta-analysis, *Spine J* 20(10):1573–1585, 2020.

198. Stokes IA, Gardner-Morse MG, Henry SM: Abdominal muscle activation increases lumbar spinal stability: analysis of contributions of different muscle groups, *Clin Biomech* 26(8):797–803, 2011.

199. Stokes IA, Gardner-Morse MG, Henry SM: Intra-abdominal pressure and abdominal wall muscular function: spinal unloading mechanism, *Clin Biomech* 25(9):859–866, 2010.

200. Streifer M, Brown AM, Porfido T, et al.: The potential role of the cervical spine in sports-related concussion: clinical perspectives and considerations for risk reduction, *J Orthop Sports Phys Ther* 49(3):202–208, 2019.

201. Suderman BL, Vasavada AN: Neck Muscle moment arms obtained in-vivo from MRI: effect of curved and straight modeled paths, *Ann Biomed Eng* 45(8):2009–2024, 2017.

202. Sung W, Hicks GE, Ebaugh D, et al.: Individuals with and without low back pain use different motor control strategies to achieve spinal stiffness during the prone instability test, *J Orthop Sports Phys Ther* 49(12):899–907, 2019.

203. Task Force on Sudden Infant Death Syndrome, Moon RY: SIDS and other sleep-related infant deaths: expansion of recommendations for a safe infant sleeping environment], *Pediatrics* 128(5):1030–1039, 2011.

204. Tesh KM, Dunn JS, Evans JH: The abdominal muscles and vertebral stability, *Spine* 12:501–508, 1987.

205. Teyhen DS, Gill NW, Whittaker JL, et al.: Rehabilitative ultrasound imaging of the abdominal muscles, *J Orthop Sports Phys Ther* 37:450–466, 2007.

206. Thoomes-de GM, Schmitt MS: The effect of training the deep cervical flexors on neck pain, neck mobility, and dizziness in a patient with chronic nonspecific neck pain after prolonged bed rest: a case report, *J Orthop Sports Phys Ther* 42(10):853–860, 2012.

207. Tomczak KK, Rosman NP: Torticollis [review], *J Child Neurol* 28(3):365–378, 2013.

208. Turk AE, McCarthy JG, Thorne CH, et al.: The "back to sleep campaign" and deformational plagiocephaly: is there cause for concern? *J Craniofac Surg* 7:12–18, 1996.

209. Tveit P, Daggfeldt K, Hetland S, et al.: Erector spinae lever arm length variations with changes in spinal curvature, *Spine* 19:199–204, 1994.

210. Urquhart DM, Hodges PW, Story IH: Postural activity of the abdominal muscles varies between regions of these muscles and between body positions, *Gait Posture* 22:295–301, 2005.

211. Urquhart DM, Hodges PW: Differential activity of regions of transversus abdominis during trunk rotation, *Eur Spine J* 14:393–400, 2005.

212. van Dieen JH, Faber GS, Loos RC, et al.: Validity of estimates of spinal compression forces obtained from worksite measurements, *Ergonomics* 53(6):792–800, 2010.

213. van Dieen JH, Hoozemans MJ, Toussaint HM: Stoop or squat: a review of biomechanical studies on lifting technique, *Clin Biomech* 14:685–696, 1999.

214. Vasavada AN, Li S, Delp SL: Influence of muscle morphometry and moment arms on the moment-generating capacity of human neck muscles, *Spine* 23:412–422, 1998.

215. Vasseljen O, Unsgaard-Tondel M, Westad C, et al.: Effect of core stability exercises on feed-forward activation of deep abdominal muscles in chronic low back pain: a randomized controlled trial, *Spine* 37(13):1101–1108, 2012.

216. Venne G, Rasquinha BJ, Kunz M, et al.: Rectus capitis posterior minor: histological and biomechanical links to the spinal dura mater, *Spine* 42(8):E466–e473, 2017.

217. Vera-Garcia FJ, Elvira JL, Brown SH, et al.: Effects of abdominal stabilization maneuvers on the control of spine motion and stability against sudden trunk perturbations, *J Electromyogr Kinesiol* 17:556–567, 2007.

218. Vera-Garcia FJ, Moreside JM, McGill SM: Abdominal muscle activation changes if the purpose is to control pelvis motion or thorax motion, *J Electromyogr Kinesiol* 21(6):893–903, 2011.

219. Villumsen M, Samani A, Jørgensen MB, et al.: Are forward bending of the trunk and low back pain associated among Danish blue-collar workers? A cross-sectional field study based on objective measures, *Ergonomics* 58(2):246–258, 2015.

220. Vleeming A, Mooney V, Stoeckart R: *Movement stability and lumbopelvic pain integration of research and therapy*, St Louis, 2007, Churchill Livingstone.

221. Wang S, Park WM, Kim YH, et al.: In vivo loads in the lumbar L3-4 disc during a weight lifting extension, *Clin Biomech* 29(2):155–160, 2014.

222. Ward SR, Kim CW, Eng CM, et al.: Architectural analysis and intraoperative measurements demonstrate the unique design of the multifidus muscle for lumbar spine stability, *J Bone Joint Surg Am* 91:176–185, 2009.

223. Waters TR, Putz-Anderson V, Garg A, et al.: *Applications manual for the revised NIOSH lifting equation (Pub. No. 94-110)*, Cincinnati, OH, 1994, U.S. Department of Health and Human Services, National Institute for Occupational Safety and Health.

224. Waters TR, Putz-Anderson V, Garg A, et al.: Revised NIOSH equation for the design and evaluation of manual lifting tasks, *Ergonomics* 36:749–776, 1993.

225. Weir A, Brukner P, Delahunt E, et al.: Doha agreement meeting on terminology and definitions in groin pain in athletes, *Br J Sports Med* 49(12):768–774, 2015.

226. Welbergen E, Kemper HC, Knibbe JJ, et al.: Efficiency and effectiveness of stoop and squat lifting at different frequencies, *Ergonomics* 34:613–624, 1991.

227. Weston EB, Aurand AM, Dufour JS, et al.: One versus two-handed lifting and lowering: lumbar spine loads and recommended one-handed limits protecting the lower back, *Ergonomics* 63(4):505–521, 2020.

228. Whittaker JL, Warner MB, Stokes M: Comparison of the sonographic features of the abdominal wall muscles and connective tissues in individuals with and without lumbopelvic pain, *J Orthop Sports Phys Ther* 43:11–19, 2013.

229. Wilke HJ, Rohlmann A, Neller S, et al.: ISSLS prize winner: a novel approach to determine trunk muscle forces during flexion and extension—a comparison of data from an in vitro experiment and in vivo measurements, *Spine* 28:2585–2593, 2003.

230. Wilke HJ, Wolf S, Claes LE, et al.: Stability increase of the lumbar spine with different muscle groups. A biomechanical in vitro study, *Spine* 20:192–198, 1995.

231. Willaert W, Leysen L, Lenoir D, et al.: Combining stress management with pain neuroscience education and exercise therapy in people with whiplash-associated disorders: a clinical perspective, *Phys Ther* 101(7), 2021.

232. Willard FH, Vleeming A, Schuenke MD, et al.: The thoracolumbar fascia: anatomy, function and clinical considerations [Review], *J Anat* 221(6):507–536, 2012.

233. Willinger M, Hoffman HJ, Wu KT, et al.: Factors associated with the transition to nonprone sleep positions of infants in the United States: the National Infant Sleep Position Study, *JAMA* 280:329–335, 1998.

234. Winder B, Keri PA, Weberg DE, et al.: Postural cueing increases multifidus activation during stabilization exercise in participants with chronic and recurrent low back pain: an electromyographic study, *J Electromyogr Kinesiol* 46:28–34, 2019.

235. Wurzelbacher SJ, Lampl MP, Bertke SJ, et al.: The effectiveness of ergonomic interventions in material handling operations, *Appl Ergon* 87:103139, 2020.

236. Yang G, Marras WS, Best TM: The biochemical response to biomechanical tissue loading on the low back during physical work exposure, *Clin Biomech* 26(5):431–437, 2011.

237. Yanik B, Keyik B, Conkbayir I: Fatty degeneration of multifidus muscle in patients with chronic low back pain and in asymptomatic volunteers: quantification with chemical shift magnetic resonance imaging, *Skeletal Radiol* 42(6):771–778, 2013.

238. Yim J, Park J, Lohman E, et al.: Comparison of cervical muscle activity and spinal curvatures in the sitting position with 3 different sloping seats, *Med* 99(28):e21178, 2020.

STUDY QUESTIONS

1. Describe the most likely craniocervical posture resulting from (a) unilateral and (b) bilateral spasm (or shortening) in the sternocleidomastoid muscle(s).
2. Why are the superficial and intermediate muscles of the posterior back classified as "foreign" to the region? Describe how the specific innervation of these muscles is associated with this classification.
3. List structures that receive sensory innervation from the recurrent meningeal nerve. What nerves provide sensory innervation to the capsule of the apophyseal joints?
4. Justify why an isolated strong contraction of the semispinalis thoracis would likely produce *contralateral* axial rotation, whereas a strong isolated contraction of the longissimus cervicis or capitis would likely produce *ipsilateral* axial rotation. Use Figs. 10.7 and 10.9 as a reference for answering this question.
5. Assume a person has a complete spinal cord injury at the level of T8. Based on your knowledge of muscle innervation, predict which muscles of the trunk would be unaffected and which would be partially or completely paralyzed. Consider only the abdominal muscles, multifidus, and erector spinae in your response.
6. List three muscles that attach to *anterior* tubercles and three that attach to *posterior* tubercles of transverse processes of cervical vertebrae. What important structure passes between these muscle attachments?
7. As a group, the trunk extensor muscles produce greater maximal-effort torque than the trunk flexor muscles (abdominals). Cite two factors that can account for this difference in strength.
8. Which of the major trunk muscles would experience the most significant stretch (elongation) after a motion of full trunk extension, right lateral flexion, and right axial rotation?
9. Based on Fig. 10.16, which muscle has the greatest moment arm for (a) flexion and (b) lateral flexion at L3?
10. Describe how an overshortened (contracted) iliacus muscle can cause an increased lumbar lordosis while a person is standing. What effect could this posture have on the stress at the lumbosacral junction?
11. At the level of the third lumbar vertebra, which connective tissues form the anterior rectus sheath (of the abdominal wall)?
12. What is the primary difference between a dorsal ramus of a spinal nerve root and a dorsal nerve root?
13. Describe the similarities and differences in the structure of the multifidus and the semispinales muscles.
14. As indicated in Fig. 10.29, why is the axial rotation function of the rectus capitis posterior major muscle limited to the atlanto-axial joint only?
15. With the aid of a plastic skeleton model or other visual resource, describe the rotational (horizontal plane) action of the right scalenus anterior muscle from (A) the anatomic position, (B) a position of full rotation to the right, (C) a position of full rotation to the left.
16. As described in the chapter, the Valsalva maneuver is often used to increase pneumatic-based stability within the lumbopelvic region when lifting or performing other activities. List three muscle groups within the axial skeleton that are directly involved with this activity, and describe the common mechanical principle by which they, acting in concert, increase stability within the region.
17. Which muscle is a direct antagonist to the left external oblique muscle?

Answers to the Study Questions are available in the accompanying enhanced eBook version included with the print purchase of this textbook.

Additional Video Educational Content

Videos of a healthy male exercising with surface EMG-driven light bulbs attached to the skin over various muscles of the upper extremity and trunk. Exercises are designed primarily to coactivate certain muscles of the upper extremity and trunk. Exercises include the use of TRX© Suspension Training, Body Blade©, Battle Rope©, and a medicine ball.

Videos

1. Row, posterior muscles with TRX
2. Push-up, anterior muscles with TRX
3. Using two small Body Blades
4. Using one large Body Blade
5. Using Battle Rope
6. Throwing and catching a medicine ball

All videos for this chapter are available in the accompanying enhanced eBook version included with the print purchase of this textbook.

Chapter

11

Kinesiology of Mastication and Ventilation

DONALD A. NEUMANN, PT, PhD, FAPTA

CHAPTER AT A GLANCE

PART 1: MASTICATION

Mastication is the process of chewing, tearing, and grinding food with the teeth. This mechanical process, the first step in digestion, involves an interaction among the central nervous system and the muscles of mastication—the teeth, the tongue, and the pair of temporomandibular joints (TMJs). The joints form the pivot point between the lower jaw (mandible) and the base of the cranium. The TMJ is one of the most important and continuously used joints in the body, not only during mastication but also during swallowing and speaking. Pain associated with reduced function of the TMJ can therefore have a significant effect on one's overall health and well-being. Effective clinical intervention for painful dysfunctions

of this often-complicated area requires a sound understanding of the kinesiology of the TMJ and surrounding craniocervical region. The first part of this chapter focuses on the kinesiology of the TMJs during mastication.

OSTEOLOGY AND TEETH

Regional Surface Anatomy

Fig. 11.1 highlights some of the surface anatomy associated with the TMJ. The *mandibular condyle* fits within the mandibular fossa of the temporal bone. The condyle can be palpated just anterior to the *external auditory meatus* (i.e., the opening into the ear). The cranial

451

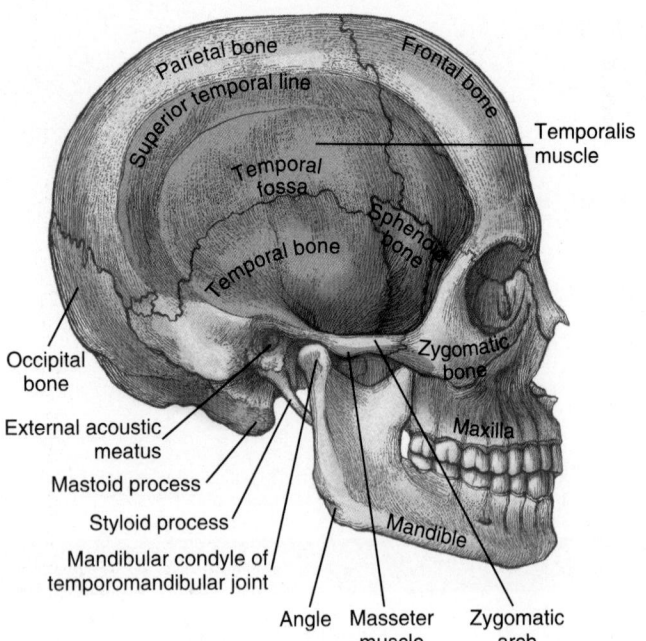

FIGURE 11.1 Lateral view of the skull with emphasis on bony landmarks associated with the temporomandibular joint. The proximal attachments of the temporalis and masseter muscles are indicated in red.

attachment of the temporalis muscle fills a broad, slightly concave region of the skull known as the *temporal fossa.* The temporal, parietal, frontal, sphenoid, and zygomatic bones all contribute to the temporal fossa.

Additional surface anatomy associated with the TMJ includes the *mastoid process* of the temporal bone, the *angle of the mandible,* and the *zygomatic arch.* The zygomatic arch is formed by the union of the zygomatic process of the temporal bone and the temporal process of the zygomatic bone.

Individual Bones

The mandible, maxilla, temporal, zygomatic, sphenoid, and hyoid bones are all related to the structure or function of the TMJ (Fig. 11.1).

MANDIBLE

The mandible is the largest and most mobile of the facial bones, suspended from the cranium by the muscles, ligaments, and capsule of the TMJ. Muscles of mastication attach either directly or indirectly to the mandible. Muscle contraction positions the teeth embedded within the mandible firmly against the teeth embedded within the fixed maxilla.

Relevant Osteologic Features of the Mandible

- Body
- Ramus
- Angle
- Coronoid process
- Condyle
- Notch
- Neck
- Pterygoid fossa

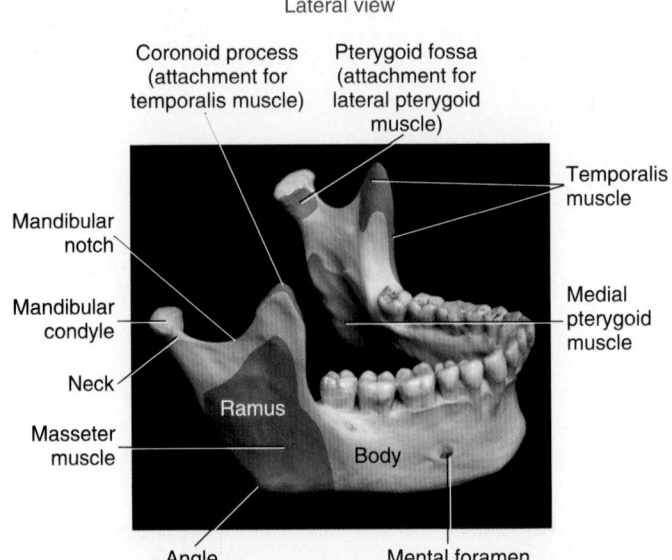

FIGURE 11.2 Lateral view of the mandible. Distal attachments of muscles are shown.

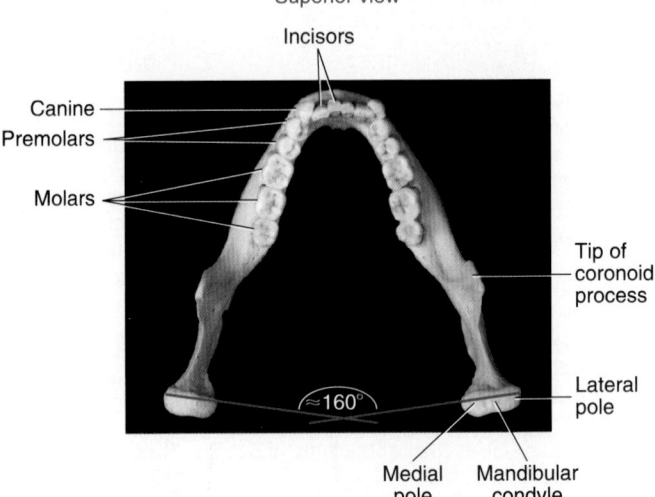

FIGURE 11.3 The mandible as viewed from above. The names of the permanent teeth are indicated. The long (side-to-side) axis through each mandibular condyle intersects at an approximately 160-degree angle.

The two main parts of the mandible are the body and the two rami (Fig. 11.2). The *body,* the horizontal portion of the bone, accepts the lower 16 adult teeth (Fig. 11.3). The *rami* of the mandible project vertically from the posterior aspect of the body (see Fig. 11.2). Each ramus has an external and an internal surface and four borders. The posterior and inferior borders of the ramus join at the readily palpable *angle* of the mandible. The masseter and medial pterygoid muscles—two powerful muscles of mastication—share similar attachments in the region of the angle of the mandible.

At the superior end of the ramus are the coronoid process, mandibular condyle, and mandibular notch. The *coronoid process* is a triangular projection of thin bone that extends upward from the anterior border of the ramus. This process is the primary inferior attachment of the temporalis muscle. The mandibular *condyle* extends upward from the posterior border of the ramus. The condyle forms the convex bony component of the TMJ. Extending between the coronoid process and mandibular condyle is the mandibular

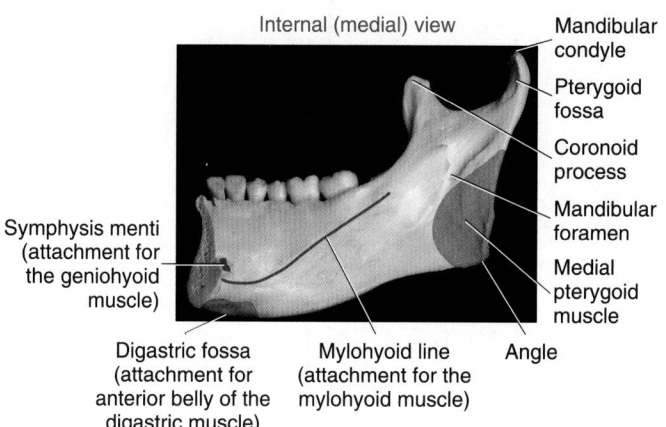

Internal (medial) view

Mandibular condyle
Pterygoid fossa
Coronoid process
Mandibular foramen
Medial pterygoid muscle
Angle
Mylohyoid line (attachment for the mylohyoid muscle)
Digastric fossa (attachment for anterior belly of the digastric muscle)
Symphysis menti (attachment for the geniohyoid muscle)

FIGURE 11.4 Internal view of the right side of the mandible. The bone is bisected in the near sagittal plane. The attachments of the mylohyoid and geniohyoid muscles are indicated in red; the attachments of the anterior belly of the digastric and medial pterygoid muscles are indicated in gray. Note the one missing third molar ("wisdom tooth").

notch. The mandibular *neck* is a slightly constricted region located immediately below the condyle. The lateral pterygoid muscle attaches to the anterior-medial surface of the mandibular neck, within a depression called the *pterygoid fossa* (Figs. 11.2 and 11.4).

MAXILLA

The right and left maxillae fuse to form a single maxilla, or upper jaw. The maxilla is fixed within the skull through rigid articulations to adjacent bones (see Fig. 11.1). The maxilla extends superiorly, forming the floor of the nasal cavity and the orbit of the eyes. The lower horizontal portions of the maxilla accept the upper teeth.

TEMPORAL BONE

Two temporal bones exist—one on each side of the cranium. The *mandibular fossa* forms the bony concavity of the TMJ, highlighted in a side view in the lower part of Fig. 11.5. The highest point of the fossa is the *dome,* often very thin and membranous (see main illustration in Fig. 11.5). The fossa is bound anteriorly by the *articular eminence* and posteriorly by the *postglenoid tubercle* and the tympanic part of the temporal bone. On full opening of the mouth, the condyles of the mandible slide anteriorly and inferiorly across the pair of sloped articular eminences.

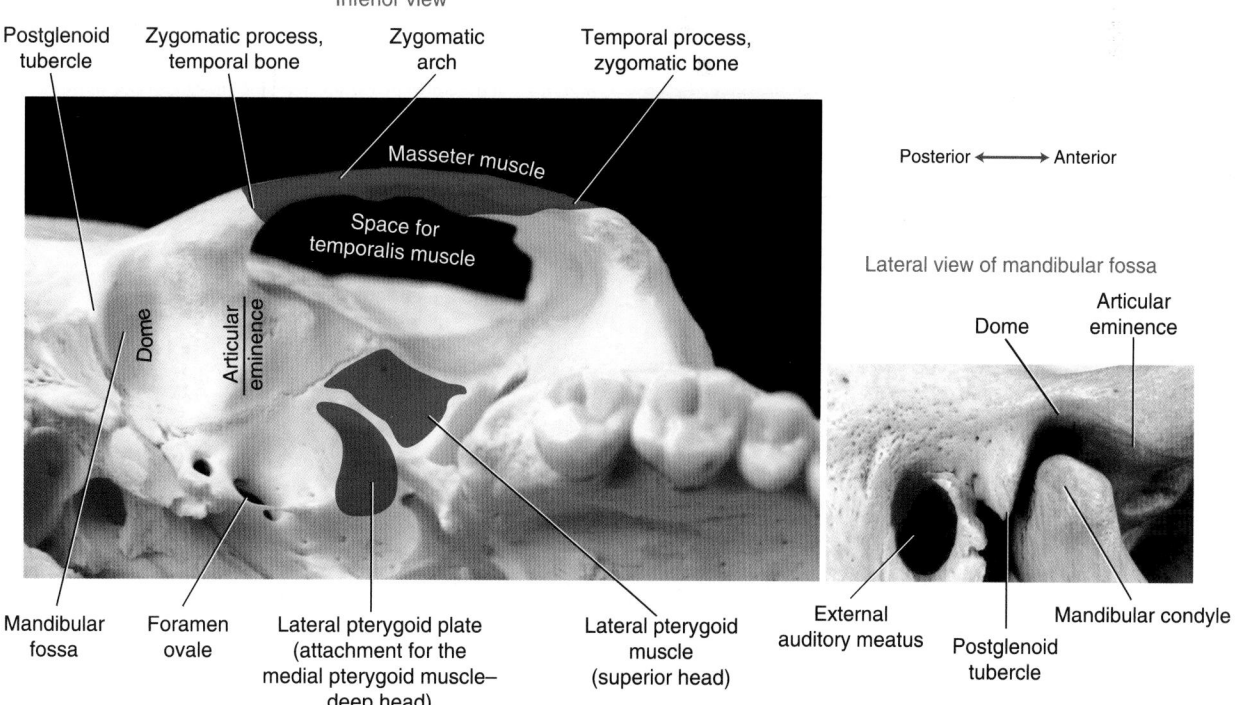

Inferior view

Postglenoid tubercle
Zygomatic process, temporal bone
Zygomatic arch
Temporal process, zygomatic bone
Masseter muscle
Space for temporalis muscle
Dome
Articular eminence
Mandibular fossa
Foramen ovale
Lateral pterygoid plate (attachment for the medial pterygoid muscle–deep head)
Lateral pterygoid muscle (superior head)

Posterior ←——→ Anterior

Lateral view of mandibular fossa

Dome
Articular eminence
External auditory meatus
Postglenoid tubercle
Mandibular condyle

FIGURE 11.5 Main photograph: Inferior view of the skull highlighting the right mandibular fossa, lateral pterygoid plate, and zygomatic arch. The proximal attachments of the masseter, medial pterygoid (deep head), and lateral pterygoid (superior head) muscles are shown in red. Small photograph at right shows a close-up, lateral perspective of the mandibular fossa and adjacent bony features.

Relevant Osteologic Features of the Temporal Bone

- Mandibular fossa
- Dome
- Articular eminence
- Postglenoid tubercle
- Styloid process
- Zygomatic process

The *styloid process* is a long slender extension of bone that protrudes from the inferior aspect of the temporal bone (see Fig. 11.1). The pointed process serves as an attachment for the stylomandibular ligament (to be discussed further) and three small muscles (styloglossus, stylohyoid, and stylopharyngeus). The *zygomatic process* of the temporal bone forms the posterior half of the zygomatic arch (see main illustration in Fig. 11.5).

ZYGOMATIC BONE

The right and left zygomatic bones constitute a major part of the cheeks and the lateral orbits of the eyes (see Fig. 11.1). The *temporal process* of the zygomatic bone contributes to the anterior half of the zygomatic arch (see Fig. 11.5). A large part of the masseter muscle attaches to the zygomatic bone and the adjacent zygomatic arch.

SPHENOID BONE

Although the sphenoid bone does not contribute to the structure of the TMJ, it does provide proximal attachments for the medial and lateral pterygoid muscles. When articulated within the cranium, the sphenoid bone lies transversely across the base of the skull. The relevant osteologic features of the sphenoid bone are its *greater wing, medial pterygoid plate,* and *lateral pterygoid plate* (Fig. 11.6). With a section of the zygomatic arch removed, the lateral surfaces of the greater wing and lateral pterygoid plate are revealed (Fig. 11.7).

Relevant Osteologic Features of the Sphenoid Bone

- Greater wing
- Medial pterygoid plate
- Lateral pterygoid plate

HYOID BONE

The hyoid is a U-shaped bone that can be palpated at the base of the throat, just anterior to the body of the third cervical vertebra (Fig. 11.8). The *body* of the hyoid is convex anteriorly. The bilateral *greater horns* form its slightly curved sides. The hyoid is suspended primarily by a bilateral pair of stylohyoid ligaments. Several muscles involved with moving of the tongue, swallowing, and speaking attach to the hyoid bone (see Fig. 11.21).

Teeth

The maxilla and mandible each contain 16 permanent teeth (see Fig. 11.3 for names of lower teeth). The structure of each tooth reflects its function in mastication (Table 11.1).

Each tooth has two basic parts: crown and root (Fig. 11.9). Normally the *crown* is covered with enamel and is located above the gingiva (gum). The *root* of each tooth is embedded in relatively thick

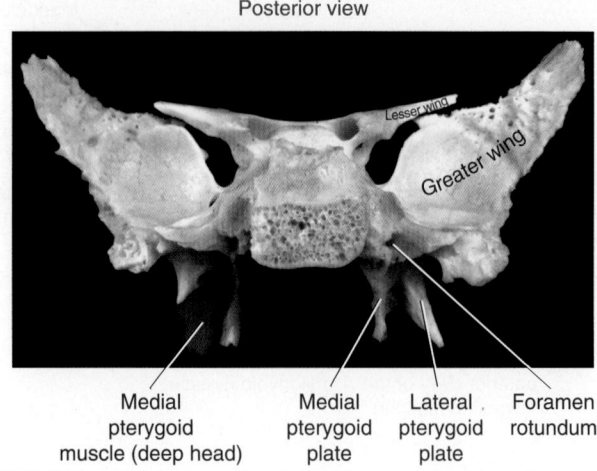

FIGURE 11.6 Posterior view of a sphenoid bone removed from the cranium. The proximal attachment of the medial pterygoid muscle (deep head) is indicated in red.

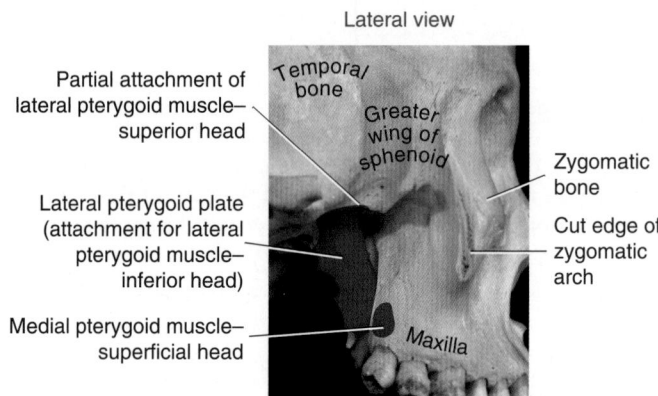

FIGURE 11.7 Lateral view of the right side of the cranium with a section of the zygomatic arch removed. The greater wing and lateral side of the lateral pterygoid plate are visible. Note the attachments in red for the pterygoid muscles.

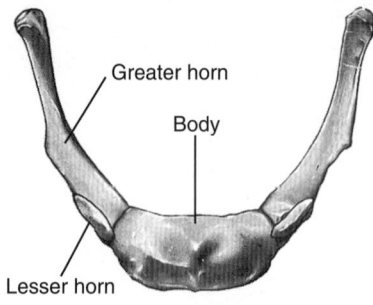

FIGURE 11.8 Superior view of the hyoid bone, located at the base of the throat. (From Standring S: *Gray's anatomy: the anatomical basis of clinical practice,* ed 39, St Louis, 2005, Elsevier.)

alveolar bone. The *periodontal ligaments* help attach the roots of the teeth within their sockets.

Cusps are conical elevations that arise on the surface of a tooth. *Maximal intercuspation* describes the position of the mandible when the cusps of the opposing teeth are in maximal contact. The

TABLE 11.1 Permanent Teeth

Names	Functions	Numbers	Structural Characteristics
Incisors	Cut food	Maxillary, 4 Mandibular, 4	Sharp edges
Canines	Tear food	Maxillary, 2 Mandibular, 2	Longest permanent teeth; crown has a single cusp
Premolars	Crush food	Maxillary, 4 Mandibular, 4	Crown has two cusps (bicuspid); lower second premolars may have three cusps
Molars	Grind food into small particles for swallowing	Maxillary, 6 Mandibular, 6	Crown has four or five cusps

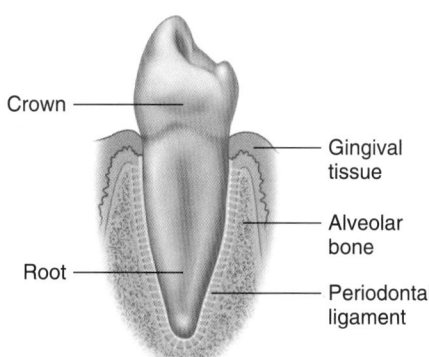

FIGURE 11.9 The tooth and its periodontal supportive structures. The width of the periodontal ligaments is greatly exaggerated for illustrative purposes. (From Okeson JP: *Management of temporomandibular disorders and occlusion,* ed 8, St Louis, 2013, Mosby.)

term is used interchangeably with *centric occlusion. Central relation* describes the relative resting position of the articular surfaces within the TMJ. The relaxed *postural position* of the mandible allows a slight "freeway space" (interocclusal clearance) between the upper and lower teeth. Normally the teeth make contact (occlude) only during chewing and swallowing.

ARTHROLOGY OF THE TEMPOROMANDIBULAR JOINT

The temporomandibular joint (TMJ) is a loosely fitting articulation formed between the mandibular condyle and the mandibular fossa (see Figs. 11.1 and 11.5, illustration on the right). It is a synovial joint that permits a wide range of rotation as well as translation. An *articular disc* cushions the potentially large and repetitive forces inherent to mastication. The disc separates the joint into two synovial joint cavities (Fig. 11.10). The *inferior joint cavity* is between the inferior aspect of the disc and the mandibular condyle. The larger *superior joint cavity* is between the superior surface of the disc and the segment of bone formed by the mandibular fossa and the articular eminence.

Osseous Structure

MANDIBULAR CONDYLE

The prominent condyle of the mandible is flattened from front to back, with its medial-lateral length twice as long as its

anterior-posterior length (see Fig. 11.3). The condyle is generally convex, possessing short projections known as *medial* and *lateral poles.* The medial pole is typically more prominent than the lateral. While the mouth is opening and closing, the outside edge of the lateral pole can be palpated as a point under the skin just anterior to the external auditory meatus.

The articular surface of the mandibular condyle is lined with a thin but dense layer of *fibrocartilage.*[135] This tissue absorbs forces associated with mastication better than hyaline cartilage, and it has a superior reparative process.[121] Both of these functions are important given the extraordinary demands placed on the TMJ.

MANDIBULAR FOSSA

The mandibular fossa of the temporal bone is divided into two surfaces: articular and nonarticular. The *articular surface* of the fossa is formed by the articular eminence, occupying the sloped anterior wall of the fossa (see Figs. 11.5 and 11.10). The articular eminence functions as a load-bearing surface and therefore consists of thick compact bone, lined with fibrocartilage. Full opening of the mouth requires that each condyle slides forward across the articular eminence. Excessive shear and compression at this interface may eventually cause fragmentation of the fibrocartilage, a common indicator of early degenerative arthritis at the TMJ.[107]

The slope of the articular eminence is, on average, 55 degrees from the horizontal plane.[55] The steepness of the slope partially determines the kinematic path of the condyle during opening and closing of the mouth.

The *nonarticular surface* of the mandibular fossa consists of a very thin layer of bone and fibrocartilage that occupies much of the superior (dome) and posterior walls of the fossa (see Fig. 11.5). According to Okeson,[108] this thin region is not an adequate load-bearing surface. A large upward force applied to the chin can fracture this region of the fossa, possibly even sending bone fragments into the cranium.

Articular Disc

The articular disc within the TMJ consists primarily of dense fibrocartilage which, except for its periphery, lacks a blood supply and sensory innervation. The histology of this tissue is generally like that of other load-bearing intra-articular discs of the body, such as the disc within the distal radio-ulnar joint and the meniscus of the knee. The disc within the TMJ is flexible but firm owing to its high collagen content. The entire periphery of the disc attaches to the surrounding capsule of the joint.

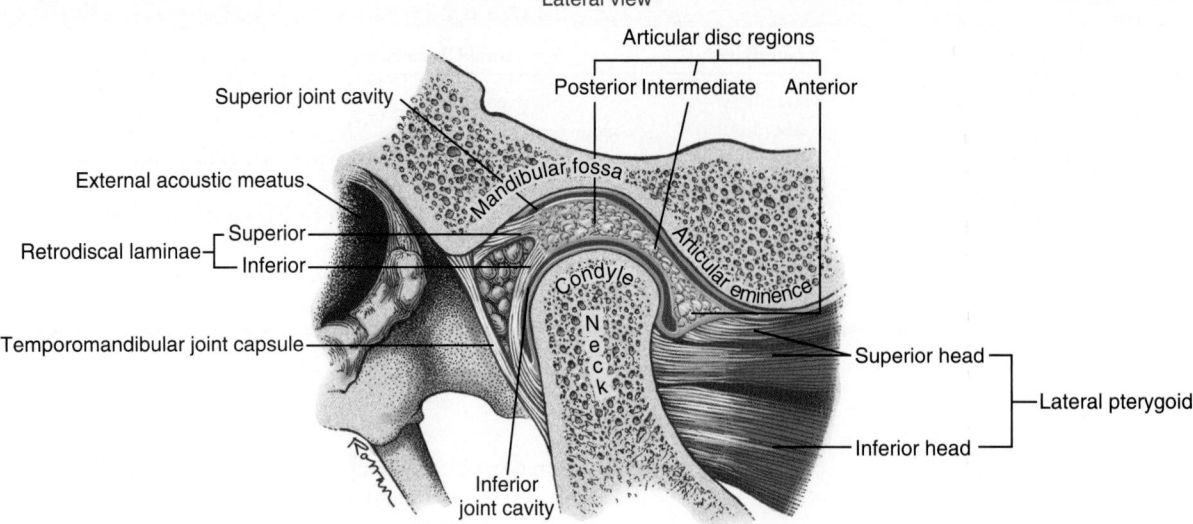

FIGURE 11.10 A lateral view of a sagittal plane cross-section through a normal right temporomandibular joint. The mandible is in a position of maximal intercuspation, with the disc in its ideal position relative to the condyle and the temporal bone.

The disc is divided into three regions: posterior, intermediate, and anterior (see Fig. 11.10). The shape of each region allows the disc to accommodate to the varying contours of the condyle and the fossa. The *posterior region* of the disc is convex superiorly and concave inferiorly. The concavity accepts most of the condyle, much like a ball-and-socket joint. The extreme posterior region attaches to the loosely organized *retrodiscal laminae,* containing collagen and elastin fibers. Connections made by the laminae anchor the disc posteriorly to bone. A meshwork of fat, blood vessels, and sensory nerves fills the space between the superior and inferior laminae.

The *posterior region* of the articular disc attaches to the following:
- Collagen-rich *inferior retrodiscal lamina,* which in turn attaches to the periphery of the superior neck of the mandible along with the capsule of the TMJ
- Elastin-rich *superior retrodiscal lamina,* which in turn attaches to the tympanic plate of the temporal bone just posterior to the mandibular fossa

---

The *intermediate region* of the disc is concave inferiorly and generally flat superiorly. The *anterior region* is nearly flat inferiorly and slightly concave superiorly to accommodate the convexity of the articular eminence. The anterior region of the disc attaches to several tissues.

The *anterior region* of the articular disc attaches to the following:
- Periphery of the superior neck of the mandible, along with the anterior capsule of the TMJ
- Tendon of the superior head of the lateral pterygoid muscle
- Temporal bone just anterior to the articular eminence

The thickness of the disc varies between its anterior and posterior regions. The thinnest intermediate region is only 1 mm thick.[59] The

anterior and posterior regions, however, are about two to three times thicker. The disc is constricted at its intermediate region.[108] The constriction, flanked by the adjacent thicker anterior and posterior regions, forms a dimple on the disc's inferior surface. In maximal intercuspation, the dimpled intermediate region of the disc should fit between the anterior-superior edge of the condyle and the articular eminence of the fossa. The properly positioned disc affords maximal protection to the mandibular condyle as it slides forward across the articular eminence during the later phase of opening the mouth widely.

The articular disc maximizes the congruency within the TMJ to reduce contact pressure. The disc also adds stability to the joint and helps guide the condyle of the mandible during movement. In the healthy TMJ, the disc slides with the translating condyle. Movement is governed by intra-articular contact pressure, by muscle forces, and by collateral ligaments that attach the periphery of the disc to the condyle.

Capsular and Ligamentous Structures

FIBROUS CAPSULE

The TMJ and disc are surrounded by a loose *fibrous capsule.* The internal surfaces of the capsule are lined with a synovial membrane. Superiorly the capsule attaches to the rim of the mandibular fossa of the temporal bone, as far anterior as the articular eminence. Inferiorly the capsule attaches to the periphery of the articular disc and to the superior neck of the mandible. Anteriorly the capsule and part of the anterior edge of disc attach to the tendon of the superior head of the lateral pterygoid muscle (see Fig. 11.10).

The capsule of the TMJ provides significant support to the articulation. Medially and laterally the capsule is relatively firm, providing stability to the joint during lateral movements such as those produced during chewing. Anteriorly and posteriorly, however, the capsule is relatively lax, allowing the condyle and disc to translate forward when the mouth is opened.

LATERAL LIGAMENT

The primary ligament reinforcing the TMJ is the *lateral (temporomandibular) ligament* (Fig. 11.11A). The lateral ligament has been described as a combination of horizontal and oblique fibers (see Fig. 11.11B).[108] The more superficial *oblique fibers* course in an anterior-superior direction, from the posterior neck of the mandible to the lateral margins of the articular eminence and zygomatic arch. The deeper *horizontal fibers* share similar temporal attachments. They course horizontally and posteriorly to attach into the lateral pole of the mandibular condyle.

The primary function of the lateral ligament is to stabilize the lateral side of the capsule. Tears or excessive elongation of the lateral ligament may cause the disc to migrate medially by an unopposed pull of the superior head of the lateral pterygoid muscle. As described in the discussion of arthrokinematics, the oblique fibers of the lateral ligament help guide the movement of the condyle during opening of the mouth.

ACCESSORY LIGAMENTS

The *stylomandibular* and *sphenomandibular ligaments* are accessory ligaments of the TMJ. Both are located medial to the joint capsule (Fig. 11.12). The ligaments help suspend the mandible from the cranium and likely have only a limited dynamic role in mastication.

> **Supporting Connective Tissues within the Temporomandibular Joint**
> - Articular disc
> - Fibrous capsule
> - Lateral temporomandibular joint ligament
> - Sphenomandibular ligament
> - Stylomandibular ligament

Osteokinematics

The primary osteokinematics of the mandible are most often described as protrusion and retrusion, lateral excursion, and depression and elevation (Figs. 11.13 to 11.15). Varying degrees of combined mandibular translation and rotation occur during all primary movements. These combined kinematics optimize the mechanical process of mastication, and are routinely measured clinically as an indicator of TMJ function.[145] A thorough description of these kinematics can be found in a textbook by Okeson.[108]

PROTRUSION AND RETRUSION

Protrusion of the mandible occurs as it translates *anteriorly* without significant rotation (see Fig. 11.13A). *Retrusion* of the mandible occurs in the reverse direction (see Fig. 11.13B). As will be described ahead, protrusion and retrusion are fundamental components of full opening and closing of the mouth, respectively.

LATERAL EXCURSION

Lateral excursion of the mandible occurs primarily as a side-to-side translation (see Fig. 11.14A). The direction (right or left) of active lateral excursion can be described as either contralateral or ipsilateral to the side of the primary muscle action. In the adult, an average of 11 mm (almost ½ inch) of maximal unilateral excursion is considered normal.[132] Lateral excursion of the mandible is usually combined with relatively slight rotational movements. Normally, the specific path of movement is guided through an interplay of several factors, including contact made between upper and lower teeth (occlusion), action of the muscles, shape of the mandibular fossa and mandibular condyle, and position of the articular disc. For purposes of evaluating dental occlusion, dentists frequently refer to the side of the lateral excursion movement as the "working" side of the mandible.

DEPRESSION AND ELEVATION

Depression of the mandible causes the mouth to *open,* an action that is naturally combined with some protrusion (see Fig. 11.15A).[25] Maximal opening of the mouth typically occurs during actions such as yawning and singing. In the adult, the mouth can be opened an average of 45 to 50 mm as measured between the incisal edges of the upper and lower front teeth.[58,132] The interincisal opening is typically large enough to fit three adult "knuckles" (proximal interphalangeal joints). Typical mastication, however, requires an average

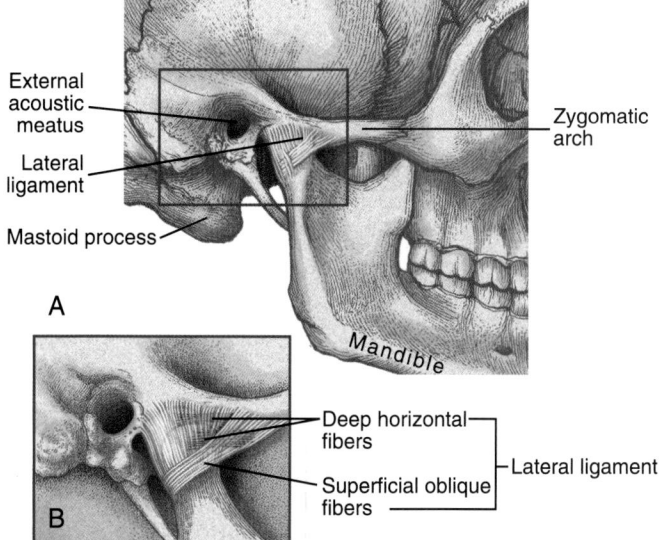

FIGURE 11.11 (A) The lateral ligament of the temporomandibular joint. (B) The lateral ligament's main fibers: oblique and horizontal.

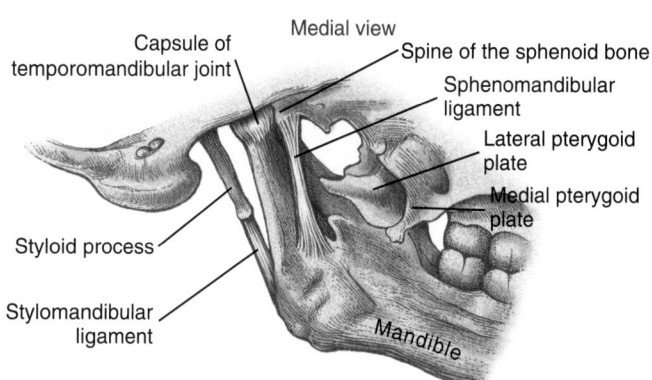

FIGURE 11.12 A medial view of the temporomandibular joint capsule shows the stylomandibular and sphenomandibular ligaments.

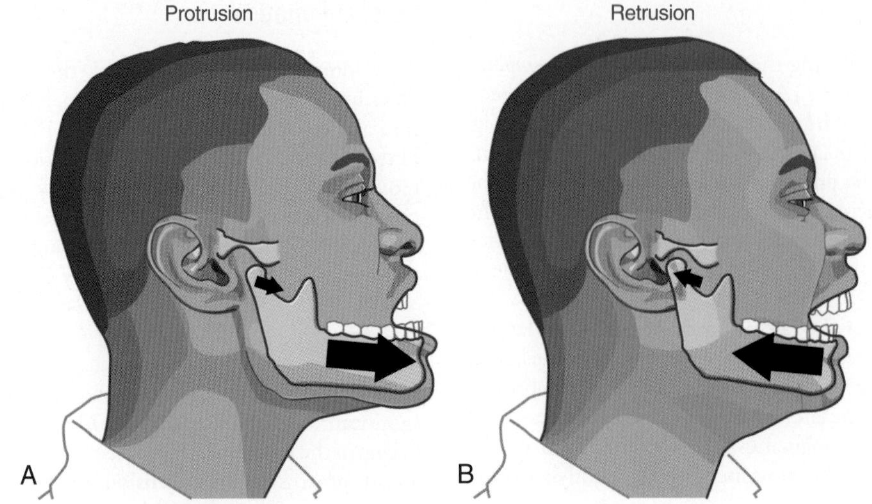

Protrusion

Retrusion

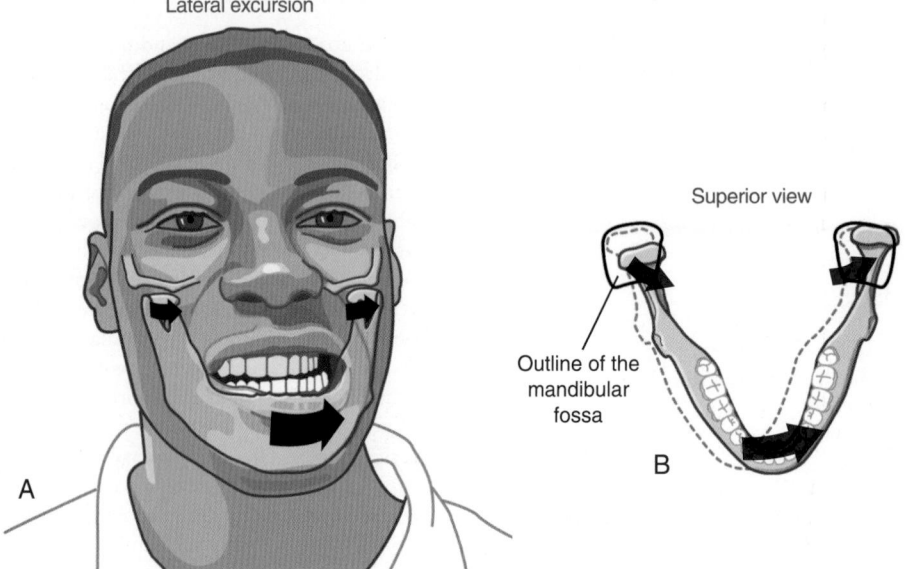

FIGURE 11.13 Protrusion (A) and retrusion (B) of the mandible.

Lateral excursion

Superior view

Outline of the
mandibular
fossa

FIGURE 11.14 Lateral excursion of the mandible (A) shown combined with horizontal plane rotation (B).

Depression

Elevation

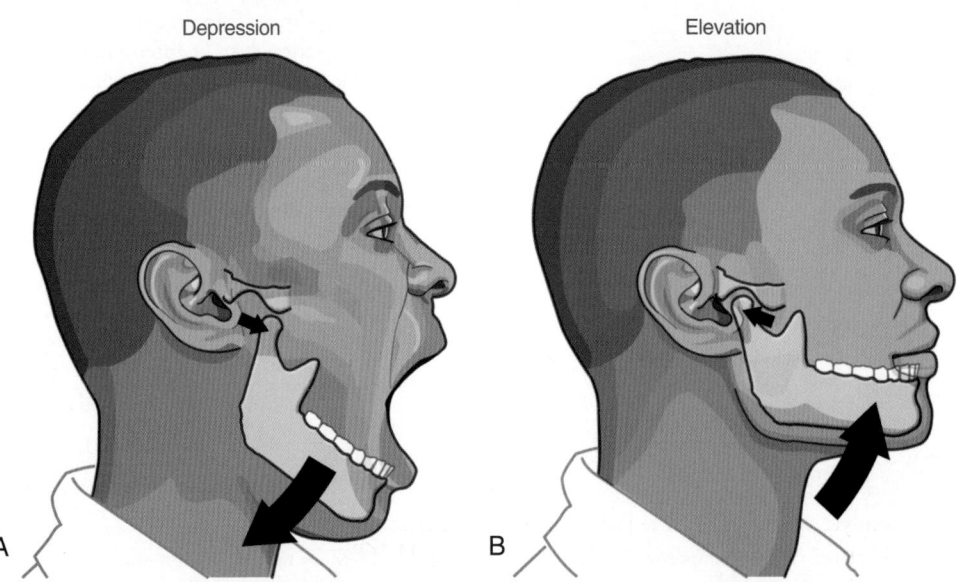

FIGURE 11.15 Depression (A) and elevation (B) of the mandible.

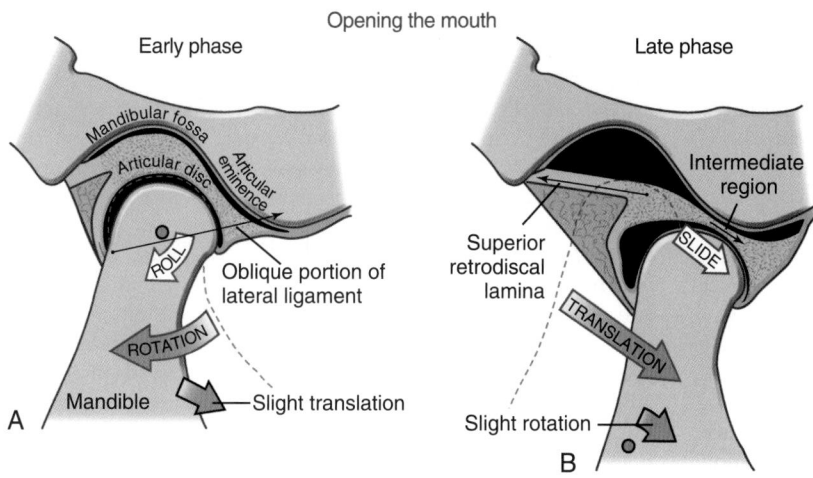

Opening the mouth

Early phase

Late phase

FIGURE 11.16 Arthrokinematics of opening the mouth, illustrated for the right temporomandibular joint only: early phase (A) and late phase (B).

maximal opening of 18 mm—about 38% of maximum (sufficient to accept one adult knuckle). Being unable to fit two knuckles (i.e., about 40 mm) between the edges of the upper and lower incisors is usually considered abnormal in the average sized adult.[128]

From a fully opened position, *elevation* of the mandible *closes* the mouth, an action that is combined with some retrusion (see Fig. 11.15B).[25] During this process, the teeth within the elevating mandible strongly oppose the teeth within the fixed maxilla, typically used to crush food during mastication.

Arthrokinematics

Movement of the mandible typically involves bilateral action of the TMJs. Abnormal function in one joint naturally interferes with the function of the other. Similar to the osteokinematics, the arthrokinematics of the TMJ normally involve a combination of rotation and translation. In general, during *rotational movement* the mandibular condyle rotates relative to the inferior surface of the disc, and during *translational movement* the mandibular condyle *and* disc slide essentially together.[108] The disc usually moves in the direction of the translating condyle.

PROTRUSION AND RETRUSION

During protrusion and retrusion the mandibular condyle and disc translate anteriorly and posteriorly, respectively, relative to the fossa (see Fig. 11.13). Maximum condylar translation of about 1.25 cm (about ½ inch) has been measured in each direction in healthy adults.[16] The condyle and disc follow the downward slope of the articular eminence. The mandible slides slightly downward during protrusion and slightly upward during retrusion. The path and extent of the movement usually vary depending on the degree of opening and closing of the mouth (described ahead).

LATERAL EXCURSION

Lateral excursion involves primarily a side-to-side translation of the condyle and disc within the fossa. Slight multiplanar rotations are typically combined with lateral excursion. For example, Fig. 11.14B shows lateral excursion combined with a slight horizontal plane rotation. The mandibular condyle on the side of the lateral excursion serves as a relatively fixed pivot point, allowing a slightly wider arc of rotation by the contralateral condyle.[108,112]

DEPRESSION AND ELEVATION

Opening and closing of the mouth occur by depression and elevation of the mandible, respectively. During these movements, each TMJ experiences a combination of rotation *and* translation among the mandibular condyle, articular disc, and fossa. No other joint in the body experiences such a large proportion of translation and rotation. These complex arthrokinematics are a necessary mechanical component of mastication (grinding and crushing of food) and for speaking. Because rotation and translation occur simultaneously, the axis of rotation is constantly moving. In the ideal case the movements within both TMJs result in a maximal range of mouth opening with minimal physical stress placed on the articular surfaces.

It is likely not possible to define a single rotation-to-translation ratio that describes the kinematics of the TMJ during opening and closing of the mouth.[96] This ratio varies based on the natural variability in one's movement strategy and cranial-dental anatomy, including the shape of the articular discs and articular surfaces. Data from the literature combined with fluoroscopic observations can, however, provide general insight into these arthrokinematics, at least for the early and late phase of opening the mouth (Fig. 11.16).[122,151] The *early phase,* constituting the first 35% to 50% of the range of motion, involves primarily *rotation* of the mandible relative to the cranium. As depicted in Fig. 11.16A, the condyle rolls posteriorly within the concave inferior surface of the disc. (The direction of the roll is described relative to the rotation of a point on the *ramus* of the mandible.) The rolling motion swings the body of the mandible inferiorly and posteriorly. The axis of rotation for this motion is not fixed but migrates within the vicinity of the mandibular neck and condyle.[48,108,114] The rolling motion of the condyle stretches the oblique portion of the lateral ligament, which helps initiate the late phase of opening the mouth.[108,110]

The *late phase* of opening the mouth consists of the final 50% to 65% of the total range of motion. This phase is marked by a *gradual transition from primary rotation to primary translation.* This transition can be readily appreciated by palpating the condyle of the mandible during the full opening of the mouth. The full amount of translation is large, about 1.5 to 2 cm in the adult.[27,93] During the translation, the condyle *and* disc slide together in a forward and inferior direction against the slope of the articular eminence (see Fig. 11.16B). At the end of opening, the axis of rotation shifts inferiorly. The exact point of the axis is difficult to define because it depends on the person's unique rotation-to-translation ratio. At the later phase of opening, the axis is usually located below the neck of the mandible.[48]

Full opening of the mouth maximally stretches and pulls the disc anteriorly. The extent of the forward translation (protrusion) is limited, in part, by tension in the stretched, elastic superior retrodiscal lamina. The intermediate region of the disc translates forward while remaining between the superior aspect of the condyle and the articular eminence. This placement of the disc maximizes joint congruency and reduces intra-articular contact pressure.[72]

The arthrokinematics of *closing the mouth* occur in the reverse order of that described for opening. When the mouth is fully opened and prepared to close, tension in the superior retrodiscal lamina starts to retrude the disc, helping to initiate the early translational phase of closing. The later phase is dominated by rotation of the condyle within the concavity of the disc, terminated when contact is made between the upper and lower teeth.

MUSCLE AND JOINT INTERACTION

Innervation of the Muscles and Joints

The muscles of mastication and their innervation are listed in Table 11.2. Based primarily on size and force potential, the muscles of mastication are divided into two groups: primary and secondary. The primary muscles are the masseter, temporalis, medial pterygoid, and lateral pterygoid. Many of the secondary muscles attach to the hyoid bone, located inferiorly to the mandible and lower teeth. The primary muscles of mastication are innervated by the mandibular nerve, a division of the *trigeminal nerve* (cranial

nerve V). This nerve exits the skull via the foramen ovale, which is just medial and slightly anterior to the mandibular fossa (see Fig. 11.5).

The central part of the disc within the TMJ lacks sensory innervation. The peripheries of the disc, capsule, lateral ligament, and retrodiscal tissues, however, possess pain fibers and mechanoreceptors.[135,150] In addition, mechanoreceptors and sensory nerves from oral mucosa, periodontal ligaments, and muscles provide the nervous system with a rich source of proprioception. This sensory information helps protect the soft oral tissues, such as the tongue and cheeks, from trauma caused by the teeth during chewing or speaking. Furthermore, the sensation helps coordinate the neuromuscular reflexes that synchronize the functional interaction among the muscles of the TMJ and in the craniocervical region. The sensory innervation from the TMJ is carried through two branches of the mandibular nerve: auriculotemporal and masseteric.[135]

Muscular Anatomy and Function

PRIMARY MUSCLES OF MASTICATION

The primary muscles of mastication are the masseter, temporalis, medial pterygoid, and lateral pterygoid. Refer to Appendix III, Part C for a summary of muscle attachments.

Masseter

The masseter is a thick, strong muscle, easily palpable just above the angle of the mandible (Fig. 11.17A). The muscle originates from the zygomatic arch and zygomatic bone (see Figs. 11.1 and 11.5) and inserts inferiorly on the external surface of the ramus of the mandible (see Fig. 11.2).

TABLE 11.2 Primary and Secondary Muscles of Mastication and Their Innervation	
Muscles	**Innervation**
Primary Muscles	
Masseter	Branch of the mandibular nerve, a division of cranial nerve V
Temporalis	Branch of the mandibular nerve, a division of cranial nerve V
Medial pterygoid	Branch of the mandibular nerve, a division of cranial nerve V
Lateral pterygoid	Branch of the mandibular nerve, a division of cranial nerve V
Secondary Muscles	
Suprahyoid Group	
Digastric (posterior belly)	Facial nerve (cranial nerve VII)
Digastric (anterior belly)	Inferior alveolar nerve (branch of the mandibular nerve, a division of cranial nerve V)
Geniohyoid	C^1 via the hypoglossal nerve (cranial nerve XII)
Mylohyoid	Inferior alveolar nerve (branch of the mandibular nerve, a division of cranial nerve V)
Stylohyoid	Facial nerve (cranial nerve VII)
Infrahyoid Group	
Omohyoid	Ventral rami of C^1–C^3
Sternohyoid	Ventral rami of C^1–C^3
Sternothyroid	Ventral rami of C^1–C^3
Thyrohyoid	Ventral rami of C^1 (via cranial nerve XII)

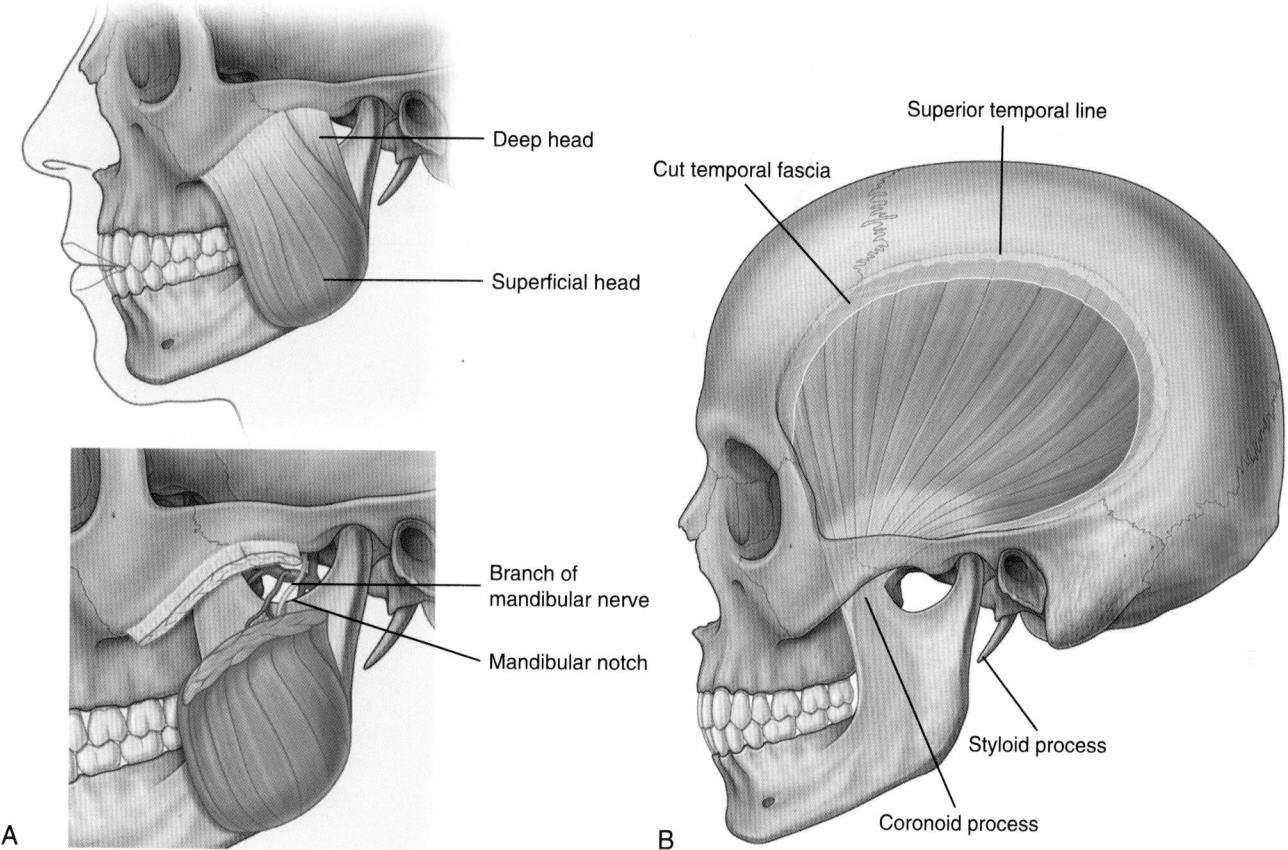

FIGURE 11.17 Illustration highlighting the left masseter (intact and cut specimens) (A) and left temporalis (B) muscles. (From Drake RL, Vogl W, Mitchell AWM: *Gray's anatomy for students,* ed 3, St Louis, 2015, Churchill Livingstone.)

The masseter has superficial and deep heads (see Fig. 11.17A). The fibers of the larger, more *superficial head* travel inferiorly and posteriorly, attaching inferiorly near the angle of the mandible. The fibers from the smaller *deep head* attach inferiorly to the upper region of the ramus of the mandible, close to the base of the coronoid process.

The actions of both heads of the masseter are essentially the same. Bilateral contraction *elevates* the mandible to bring the teeth into contact during mastication. The line of force of the muscle is nearly perpendicular to the biting surface of the molars. The primary function of the masseter, therefore, is to develop potentially large forces between the molars for effective crushing of food. Bilateral action of the masseters also *protrudes* the mandible slightly. Unilateral contraction of the masseter, however, causes slight *ipsilateral excursion* of the mandible (Fig. 11.18). The effectiveness of this ipsilateral action, however, is enhanced when the mandible is in a position of contralateral excursion at the time of the muscle contraction. This position stretches the muscle (presumably augmenting its activation) and likely increases its force potential within the horizontal plane. The masseter's ability to combine ipsilateral excursion with a strong biting force makes it very suitable for grinding food.

Temporalis

The temporalis is a flat, fan-shaped muscle that fills much of the concavity of the temporal fossa of the skull (see Fig. 11.17B). The superficial surface of the muscle is covered by and partially adhered to a relatively thick sheet of fascia, which limits the ease of palpating the belly of the muscle. From its cranial attachment, the temporalis forms a broad tendon that narrows distally as it passes through a space formed between the zygomatic arch and the lateral side of the skull (see Fig. 11.5). The muscle attaches distally to the coronoid process and to the anterior edge and medial surface of the ramus of the mandible (see Fig. 11.2). Bilateral contractions of the temporalis muscles *elevate the mandible,* producing a very effective biting force.[123] The more oblique posterior fibers *elevate and retrude* the mandible.

Like the masseter, the temporalis courses slightly medially as it approaches its distal attachment. Unilateral contraction of the temporalis, therefore, as when chewing in a side-to-side manner, causes slight *ipsilateral excursion* of the mandible (see Fig. 11.18). As explained for the masseter, the effectiveness of the temporalis for producing ipsilateral excursion is enhanced when the muscle is activated from a position of contralateral excursion—a natural, cyclic kinematic pattern used while chewing.

Medial Pterygoid

The medial pterygoid muscle arises from two disproportionately sized heads (Fig. 11.19A). The much larger *deep head* attaches on the medial surface of the lateral pterygoid plate of the sphenoid bone (see Figs. 11.5 and 11.6). The smaller *superficial head* attaches to a region of the posterior side of the maxilla, just above the third molar (compare perspectives of Figs. 11.6 and 11.7).[135] Both heads course nearly parallel with the masseter muscle and attach on the internal surface of the ramus, near the angle of the mandible (compare perspectives of Figs. 11.2 and 11.4).

The actions of the two heads of the medial pterygoid are essentially identical. Acting bilaterally, the medial pterygoid *elevates* and,

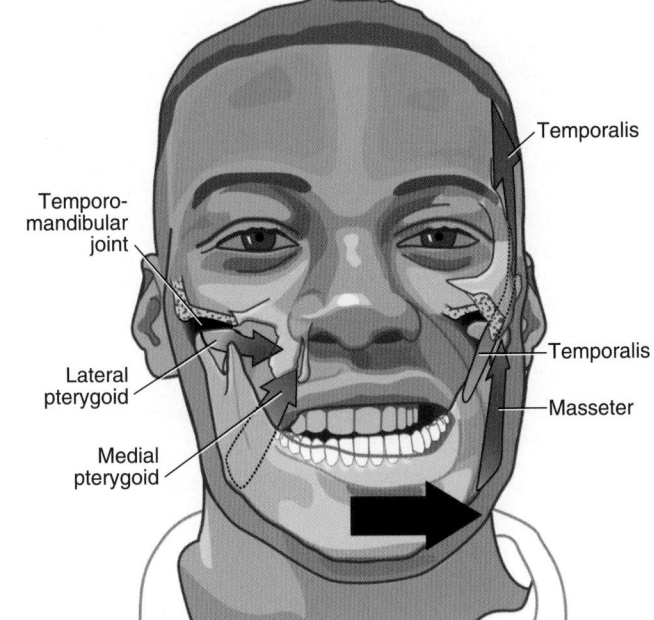

to a limited extent, *protrudes* the mandible. Because of the oblique line of force of the muscle, a unilateral contraction of the medial pterygoid produces a very effective *contralateral excursion* of the mandible (see Fig. 11.18).

Lateral Pterygoid

The lateral pterygoid muscle has two distinct heads (see Fig. 11.19B).[41,102,108,136] The *superior head* arises from the greater wing of the sphenoid bone (see Figs. 11.5 and 11.7). The considerably larger *inferior head* arises from the lateral surface of the lateral pterygoid plate and adjoining region of the maxilla (see Fig. 11.7).

FIGURE 11.18 Frontal plane view shows the muscular interaction during *left lateral excursion* of the mandible. This action may occur during a side-to-side grinding motion while chewing. The muscles producing the movement are indicated in red.

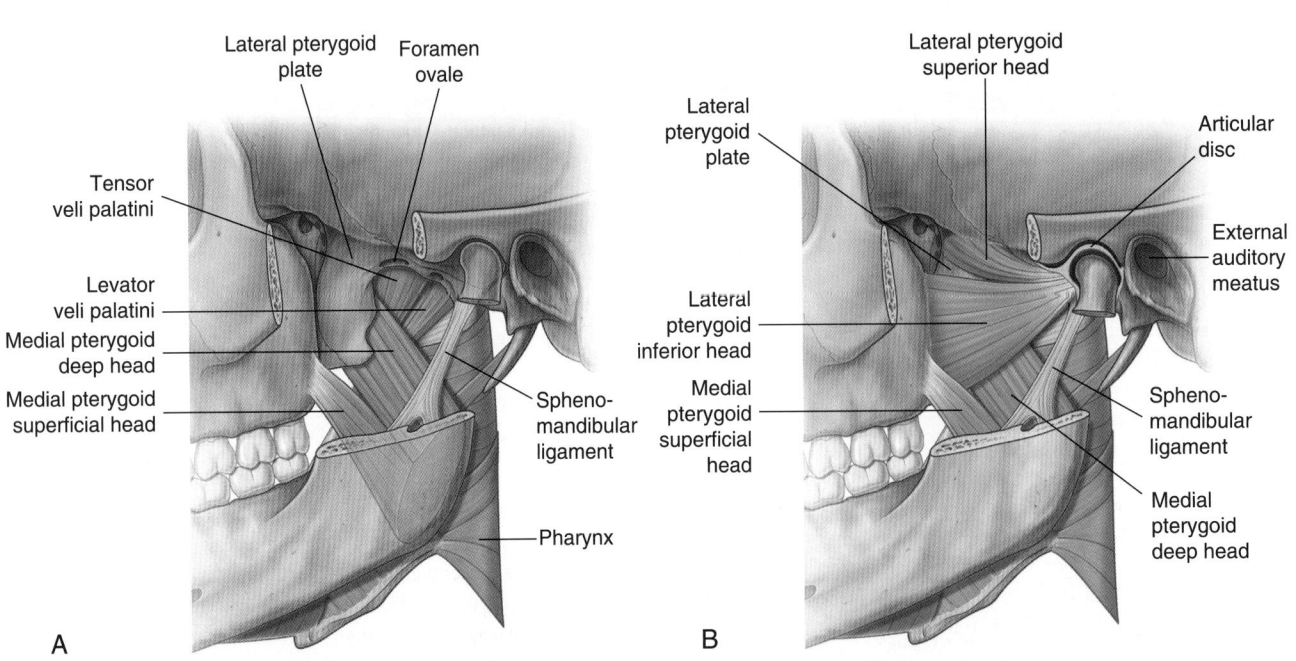

FIGURE 11.19 Illustration highlighting the left medial pterygoid (A) and lateral pterygoid (B) muscles. The mandible and zygomatic arch have been cut for better exposure of the pterygoid muscles. (From Drake RL, Vogl W, Mitchell AWM: *Gray's anatomy for students,* ed 3, St Louis, 2015, Churchill Livingstone.)

Both heads of the lateral pterygoid traverse nearly horizontally to insert into a region of the neck of the mandible, very near the joint (review Fig. 11.10).[7,41,135] Although the specific anatomic details are debated, the *superior head* of the lateral pterygoid shares attachments with the pterygoid fossa (see Fig. 11.2), the medial wall

of the capsule, and the medial side of the articular disc. The *inferior head* attaches within the pterygoid fossa and adjacent neck of the mandible.

The precise action and role of the two heads of the lateral pterygoid muscle during mastication is controversial and not completely understood.[108] The lack of understanding partially reflects the muscle's deep location and subsequent technical challenge to electromyographic (EMG) study. It is generally agreed, however, that unilateral contraction of both heads of the lateral pterygoid produces *contralateral excursion* of the mandible (see Fig. 11.18). Furthermore, unilateral muscle contraction rotates the ipsilateral condyle anterior-medially within the horizontal plane—a typical kinematic component of contralateral excursion (reviewed in Fig. 11.14B). A given right or left lateral pterygoid muscle typically contracts synergistically with other muscles during mastication. For example, as depicted in Fig. 11.18, a biting motion that involves left lateral excursion is controlled by the right lateral and medial pterygoid and, to a lesser extent, by the left masseter and temporalis.

Bilateral contraction of both heads of the lateral pterygoid produces a strong *protrusion* of the mandible.[81] As fully described ahead in the discussion of muscular control of opening and closing of the mouth, the two heads of the lateral pterygoid are active at different phases of opening and closing of the mouth. (For this and other morphologic considerations, some authors have argued that the two heads of the lateral pterygoid are actually separate muscles.[41]) Most sources suggest that the *inferior head* is the primary depressor of the mandible, especially during resisted opening of the mouth.[92,102,108,113] The *superior head,* in contrast, helps control the tension within the disc and its position during resisted closure of the jaw.[92,102] This action is especially important during resisted, unilateral closure of the jaw, such as when biting down on a hard piece of candy.

SPECIAL FOCUS 11.1

Functional Interactions between the Masseter and Medial Pterygoid Muscles

The medial pterygoid and masseter muscles form a *functional sling* around the angle of the mandible (Fig. 11.20). Simultaneous contractions of these muscles can exert a powerful biting force that is directed through the jaw and ultimately between the upper and lower molars. The maximal biting force in this region averages about 422 N (95 lb) in the adult, twice that generated between the incisors.[81]

Acting on the internal and external sides of the mandible, the medial pterygoid and the masseter also produce an important side-to-side force between the upper and lower molars. As shown in Fig. 11.18, simultaneous contraction of the right medial pterygoid and left masseter produces left lateral deviation. Contraction of these muscles in this synergistic fashion can produce a very effective shear force between the molars and food, on both sides of the mouth. The combined muscular action is very effective at grinding and crushing food before swallowing.

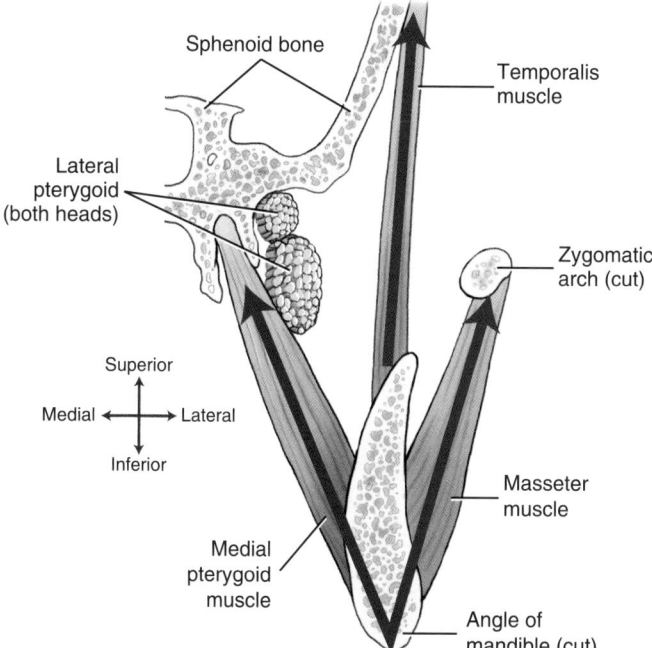

FIGURE 11.20 A frontal plane, cross-sectional perspective of the cranium is shown through the mid region of the zygomatic arch, as viewed from the front. This cross-sectional perspective includes the primary muscles of mastication (left side only). The lines of force are indicated for the primary muscles that close the mouth: masseter, temporalis, and medial pterygoid. Note the functional sling formed around the angle of the mandible by the masseter and medial pterygoid muscles.

SPECIAL FOCUS 11.2

Internal Derangement of the Disc

Mechanical dysfunction of the TMJ often causes joint popping sounds, along with painful, highly variable, and reduced and slowed movements of the jaw.[117] In addition, mechanical dysfunction may involve an abnormal position of the disc relative to the condyle and fossa, an impairment referred to as *internal derangement of the disc.*[108] The derangement can be caused by pathology, trauma, or other conditions within the joint, including altered disc shape, abnormal slope of the articular eminence, overstretched capsule, or loss of elasticity within the superior retrodiscal lamina.[55] In addition, internal derangement of the disc may be associated with hyperactivity of muscle, most notably the *superior head of the lateral pterygoid.* Based on the line of pull and attachments of these muscle fibers, excessive activation can pull and subsequently displace the disc in an anterior and medial direction relative to the joint.[7,40,139,140] The cause of the hyperactivity in this muscle is not known for certain, but it can be associated with chronic emotional stress and parafunctional habits, such as excessive tooth grinding or clenching of the teeth.[41,136] Once the disc is abnormally positioned, it is vulnerable to potentially large and damaging trauma.[108]

SECONDARY MUSCLES OF MASTICATION

The suprahyoid and infrahyoid muscles are considered secondary muscles of mastication (Fig. 11.21). These muscles are listed in Table 11.2. Forces produced by these muscles are transferred either directly or indirectly to the mandible. The *suprahyoid muscles* attach between the base of the cranium, hyoid bone, and mandible; the *infrahyoid muscles* attach superiorly to the hyoid and inferiorly to the thyroid cartilage, sternum, and scapula. The mandibular attachments of three of the suprahyoid muscles—anterior belly of the digastric, geniohyoid, and mylohyoid—are shown in Fig. 11.4. Appendix III, Part C includes the attachments of the suprahyoid and infrahyoid muscles.

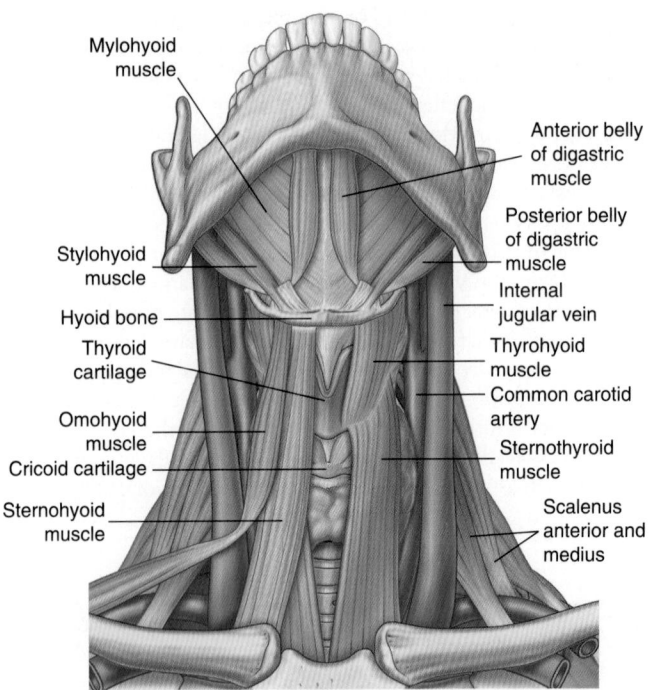

FIGURE 11.21 The suprahyoid and infrahyoid muscles are shown, attaching to the hyoid bone. The geniohyoid is deep to the mylohyoid and not visible. (From Drake RL, Vogl W, Mitchell AWM: *Gray's anatomy for students,* ed 3, St Louis, 2015, Churchill Livingstone.)

With the hyoid bone stabilized by sufficient activation of the infrahyoid muscles, the suprahyoid muscles can assist with depression of the mandible and thereby opening of the mouth.[23] The suprahyoid and infrahyoid muscles are also involved in speech, tongue movement, and swallowing and in controlling of boluses of food before swallowing.

SUMMARY OF INDIVIDUAL MUSCLE ACTION

Table 11.3 provides a summary of the individual actions of the muscles of mastication.

MUSCULAR CONTROL OF OPENING AND CLOSING OF THE MOUTH

Opening the Mouth

Opening the mouth is performed primarily through contraction of the *inferior head of the lateral pterygoid* and the *suprahyoid group of muscles.*[141] This action is depicted in Fig. 11.22A as the mouth opens in preparation to bite on a grape. The inferior head of the lateral pterygoid is primarily responsible for the forward translation (protrusion) of the mandibular condyle. This muscle is also involved in a force-couple with the contracting suprahyoid muscles. The force-couple rotates the mandible around its axis of rotation, shown as a green circle below the neck of the mandible. Although mandibular rotation is reduced during the late phase of opening the mouth, it does facilitate the extremes of this action. Although gravity assists slightly with opening the mouth, significant muscle activation is required to open it fully. Interestingly, and perhaps not expectedly, mathematical modeling indicates that during full opening of the mouth, the translating mandibular condyle makes firmer contact with the articular eminence than during nonresisitve closing of the mouth.[141] As expected, however, *resistive* closing of the mouth (as during chewing) generates much greater joint loading and disc compression compared with full opening, based primarily on the need for large muscular biting forces.

As described previously, the disc and condyle translate forward as a unit during the late phase of opening of the mouth. The disc is stretched and pulled anteriorly by (1) the translating condyle and (2) the increased intra-articular contact pressure created by

	TABLE 11.3 Actions of the Muscles of Mastication				
Muscle	**Elevation (Closing of the Mouth)**	**Depression (Opening of the Mouth)**	**Lateral Excursion**	**Protrusion**	**Retrusion**
Masseter	XXX	—	X (IL)	X	—
Medial pterygoid	XXX	—	XXX (CL)	X	—
Lateral pterygoid (superior head)	*	—	XXX (CL)	XXX	—
Lateral pterygoid (inferior head)	—	XXX	XXX (CL)	XXX	—
Temporalis	XXX	—	X (IL)	—	XXX (posterior fibers)
Suprahyoid muscle group	—	XXX	—	—	X†

CL, Contralateral excursion; *IL,* ipsilateral excursion. A muscle's relative potential to move the mandible is assigned one of three scores: X = minimal, XX = moderate, and XXX = maximum. A dash indicates no effective muscular action.

*Stabilizes or adjusts the position of the articular disc.

†By direct action of the geniohyoid, mylohyoid, and digastric (anterior belly) only.

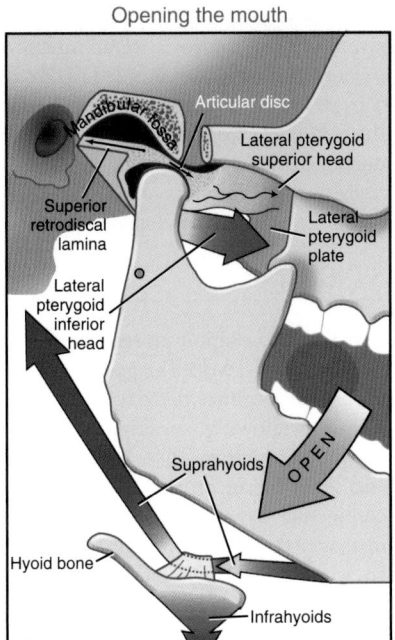

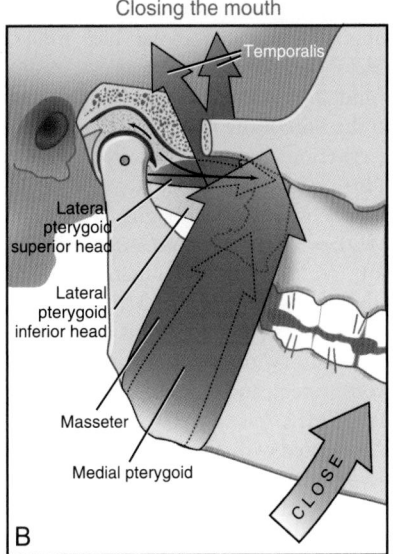

FIGURE 11.22 The muscle and joint interaction during opening (A) and closing (B) of the mouth. The relative degree of muscle activation is indicated by the different intensities of red. In (B), the superior head of the lateral pterygoid muscle is shown eccentrically active. The locations of the axes of rotation (shown as small green circles in panels A and B) are estimates only.

activation of the inferior head of the lateral pterygoid. Although the superior head of the lateral pterygoid attaches directly to the disc, most of the literature indicates that it is relatively inactive while the mouth is opening.

Closing the Mouth

Closing the mouth against resistance is performed primarily by contraction of the *masseter, medial pterygoid,* and *temporalis muscles* (see Fig. 11.22B).[141] These muscles all have a very favorable moment arm (leverage) for this action. The more oblique posterior fibers of the temporalis muscle also *retrude* the mandible. This action translates the mandible in a posterior-superior direction, helping to reseat the condyle within the fossa at the very end phase of closing the mouth.

Although the muscular action is not completely understood or agreed upon, the *superior head* of the lateral pterygoid is likely active *eccentrically* during closing of the mouth. Eccentric activation exerts a forward tension on the disc and neck of the mandible (see Fig. 11.22B). The tension helps to stabilize and optimally position the disc between the condyle and articular eminence. The muscle activation also helps balance the strong retrusion force generated by the posterior fibers of the temporalis.

TEMPOROMANDIBULAR DISORDERS

Temporomandibular disorders (TMDs) describe several complex and painful conditions associated with the TMJ.[87,120] TMDs pose a substantial public health problem, reported to occur in 5% to 20% of the population, with women affected at least twice as often as men.[17,91,99,128]

SPECIAL FOCUS 11.3

The Special Role of the Superior Head of the Lateral Pterygoid in Adjusting Disc Position

The specific position of the disc relative to the condyle during biting is strongly influenced by the type of resistance created by the objects being chewed. While the mouth is closing against a relatively low bite resistance, such as on a grape as depicted in Fig. 11.22B, the thin intermediate region of the disc is typically in its ideal position between the condyle and articular eminence. During the application of a large, asymmetric bite force, however, the position of the disc may need to be adjusted. Unilaterally biting on a hard piece of candy between the molars, for example, momentarily reduces the intra-articular contact pressure within the ipsilateral temporomandibular joint. Until the candy is crushed, it acts as a "spacer" between the upper and lower jaw, which reduces joint contact. During this event, a forceful *concentric contraction* of the superior head of the lateral pterygoid muscle can protrude the disc forward, thereby sliding its thicker, posterior region between the condyle and articular eminence. The thicker surface increases the congruency within the joint, helping to stabilize it against the uneven forces applied to the mandible as a whole.

Symptoms may include painful jaw movements, difficulty chewing, joint sounds ("popping"), reduced molar bite forces, reduced range in opening of the mouth, headache, tinnitus, painful or hyperactive masticatory and craniocervical muscles ("trigger points"), and pain referred to the skin of the face and scalp.[a] Based on a widely used diagnostic criterion, patients typically receive a TMD diagnosis that falls into one of two broad categories: 1) *painful disorder* (e.g., masticatory myalgia, arthralgia, myofascial pain, headache caused by TMD), or 2) *mechanical disruption of the joint* (e.g., disc derangement, subluxation, degenerative arthritis).[87,128,145] It is noteworthy that almost 80% of all TMD diagnoses are associated with muscle pain (myalgia), both local and referred.[129] Some research suggests that masticatory muscles serve as a primary nociceptive input to the nervous system, and may contribute to the often chronic nature of myalgic TMD.[99]

Many factors appear to be associated with TMD, including sensitization of the central nervous system, psychological stress or other emotional disturbances, daily oral parafunctional habits (e.g., grinding of teeth, repetitive biting of the lip or tongue), sleep bruxism, chronic forward head posturing, cervical spine pathology, and structural changes in muscle.[108] The often chronic and painful nature of TMD can lead to psychosocial problems such as stress, pain catastrophizing, and depression.[87] The amount to which the associated factors cause or result from TMD is not well understood. Although most cases of TMD are self-limiting, a small percentage may progress to osteoarthritis, which can lead to significant degenerative changes within the joint, remodeling of bone, and a marked loss of function.

No single mechanical or physiologic explanation can account for the myriad of symptoms associated with TMD. The pathomechanics involved with a particular set of symptoms may stem from excessive load placed on the joint due to abnormal anatomy, dentition, dental occlusion, internal derangement of the disc, or trauma, such as a fall, facial trauma, or cervical whiplash injury.[56,84]

The multiple symptoms associated with TMD often require collaborative treatments from a team of clinicians, which may include dentists, physical therapists, behavioral therapists, and psychologists.[b] Some of the more common conservative treatments are listed in the following box.

> **Common Conservative Treatments for Temporomandibular Disorders**
> - Muscle strengthening and mandibular mobility exercises
> - Manual therapy, soft tissue mobilization
> - Biophysical agents (e.g., iontophoresis, phonophoresis, transcutaneous electrical nerve stimulation, continuous ultrasound, interferential stimulation, cold, heat)
> - Dry needling
> - Biofeedback, relaxation techniques, stress management
> - Patient education (e.g., postural correction, ergonomics)
> - Behavioral therapies
> - Pharmacotherapy
> - Intra-articular injections (local anesthetics or corticosteroids)
> - Occlusal therapy (altering tooth structure or jaw position)
> - Oral appliances (splints)

Discussing the relative clinical effectiveness of the many approaches of physical therapy to TMD is beyond the scope of this chapter. Briefly, however, although some studies report conflicting data, many show some evidence that physical and manual therapy can reduce symptoms and improve overall function associated with TMD.[c]

Surgery for severe or chronic TMD may include arthrocentesis, arthroscopy to inspect the joint and remove adhesions, condylotomy to realign the mandibular condyle relative to the disc, arthrotomy (surgical procedures such as disc repositioning and discectomy), mandibular or maxillary realignment osteotomies, and TMJ replacement. Specific physical therapy programs have been developed following arthroscopic surgery.[1,28]

SYNOPSIS

Part 1 of this chapter presents the kinesiology of the temporomandibular joint (TMJ). The pair of joints is physically engaged literally thousands of times per day, not only during mastication, but also during swallowing, speaking, singing, and other nonspecific, subconscious activities. These activities invariably produce compression and shear forces on the joints' articular surfaces and periarticular connective tissues. Forces may range from being very small, for instance, during swallowing, to much larger as when vigorously chewing of food. These forces originate primarily from the actions of muscles. Muscles interact synergistically to open and close the mouth as well as to move the mandible in side-to-side and front-to-back fashions—actions that very effectively crush and grind food prior to being swallowed.

In addition to producing large and multidirectional forces, the TMJs must allow extensive motion of the mandible, from just a few millimeters during whispering, to perhaps 5 cm of depression while preparing to bite on a large apple. The unique functional demands placed on the TMJ are reflected by the joint's distinctive structure. The joint is loosely articulated to allow both rotation and translation of the mandibular condyle. This combined "sliding-and-hinge joint" increases the potential excursion of the mandible. To protect the joint from potentially large and repetitive forces, the bony articular surfaces are lined with a layer of fibrocartilage and are partially covered by a thick intra-articular disc. The primary functions of the disc are to guide the arthrokinematics, stabilize the joint, and, perhaps most importantly, reduce contact pressure on the joint's articular surfaces.

During movement of the mandible the disc is constantly repositioned to optimally reduce contact pressure—especially between the mandibular condyle and sloped articular eminence of the mandibular fossa. The positioning of the disc is guided by a combination of forces, including passive tension from the stretched capsule and retrodiscal laminae, compression from the mandibular condyle, and active forces from the superior head of the lateral pterygoid muscle. In some persons the disc becomes temporarily or permanently displaced, no longer able to protect the joint from potentially damaging force. In more severe and chronic cases, internal derangement (or displacement) of the disc may lead to painful and reduced motion of the mandible, often associated with chronic inflammation and degeneration of periarticular connective tissue.

Other painful chronic conditions exist at the TMJ, even when the disc is well aligned. Such conditions are often perplexing and difficult to treat. Treatment approaches vary considerably across disciplines. Regardless of approach, clinicians are challenged with understanding the complicated anatomy and kinesiology of the TMJ. This knowledge is the first step toward appreciating the varied clinical manifestations of temporomandibular disorders, as well as understanding the rationale for most conservative and surgical treatment interventions.

---

[a]5,42,58,60,67,108,118,144
[b]9,26,52,60,68,71,100,108,109,127

[c]8,11,39,50,71,80,87,97,130

PART 2: VENTILATION

Ventilation is the mechanical process by which air is inhaled and exhaled through the lungs and airways. This rhythmic process occurs 12 to 20 times per minute at rest and is essential to the maintenance of life. This part of the chapter focuses on the kinesiology of ventilation.

Ventilation allows for respiration, i.e., the exchange of oxygen and carbon dioxide between the alveoli of the lungs and the blood. This gas exchange is essential for oxidative metabolism within muscle fibers. This process uses oxygen to produce ATP to fuel the mechanical processes within muscle required to move and stabilize the joints of the body. Adequate ventilation, therefore, is a prerequisite to effective movement.

The relative intensity of ventilation can be described as "quiet" or "forced." In the healthy population, *quiet ventilation* occurs during relatively sedentary activities that have low metabolic demands. In contrast, *forced ventilation* occurs during activities that require rapid and voluminous movement of air, such as when exercising or coughing. A wide and continuous range of ventilation intensity exists between quiet and forced ventilation.

Fig. 11.23 shows the lung volumes and capacities in the normal adult. As depicted, the *total lung capacity* is about 5.5 to 6 L of air. *Vital capacity,* normally about 4.5 L, is the maximum volume of air that can be exhaled after a maximal inhalation. *Tidal volume* is the volume of air moved in and out of the lungs during each breath. At rest, tidal volume is about 0.5 L, approximately 10% of vital capacity.

Ventilation is driven by a combination of active and passive forces that alter the volume within the expandable and semielastic thorax. The change in intrathoracic volume causes a change in air pressure as described by *Boyle's law.* This law states that, given a fixed temperature and mass, the *volume* and *pressure* of a gas, such as air, are *inversely* proportional. Increasing the volume within the chamber of a piston, for example, lowers the pressure of the contained air. Because air flows spontaneously from high to low pressure, the

relatively high air pressure outside the piston forces air into an opening at the top of the piston. In other words, the negative pressure created within the piston sucks air into its chamber (Fig. 11.24A). This analogy between the thorax and the piston can be very helpful in understanding the mechanics of ventilation. It is also useful for understanding several clinical aspects of ventilation, such as the pathomechanics of a pneumothorax ("collapsed lung") which can result from a puncture wound of the thoracic wall, and the design of the "iron lung" used to ventilate some people with paralysis of their ventilatory muscles following infection with the polio virus.[103]

During *inspiration,* the intrathoracic volume is increased by contraction of the muscles that attach to the ribs and sternum (see Fig. 11.24B). As the thorax expands, the pressure within the interpleural space, which is already negative, is further reduced, creating a suction that expands the lungs. The resulting expansion of the lungs reduces alveolar pressure below atmospheric pressure, ultimately drawing air from the atmosphere into the lungs.

Expiration is the process of expiring (exhaling) air from the lungs into the environment. In accord with the analogy to the piston previously described, *decreasing* the volume within the chamber of a piston *increases* the pressure on the contained air, forcing it outward. Expiration in the human also occurs by a similar process. Reducing the

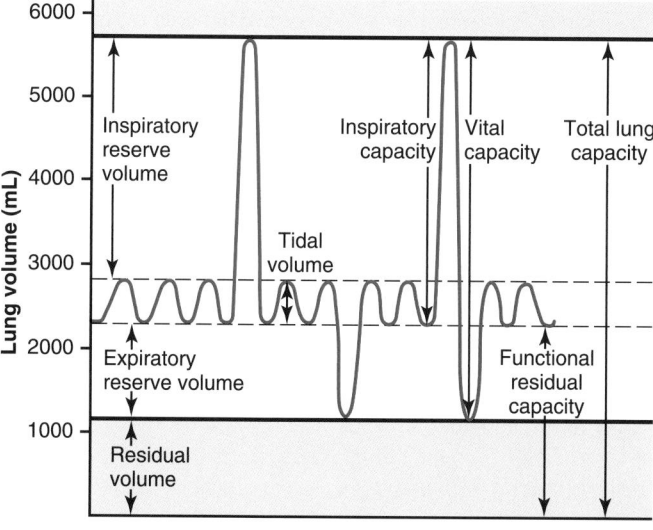

FIGURE 11.23 The lung volumes and capacities in the normal adult. Lung capacity is the sum of two or more volumes. (From Hall JE: *Guyton and Hall textbook of medical physiology,* ed 13, Philadelphia, 2015, Saunders.)

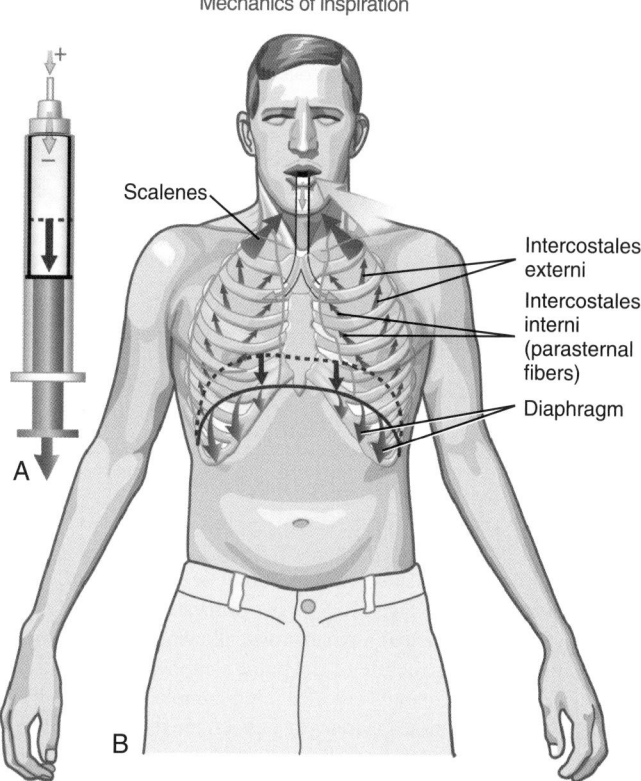

Mechanics of inspiration

FIGURE 11.24 The muscular mechanics of inspiration. (A) Using an expanding piston and air to show an analogy using Boyle's law. Increasing the volume within a piston reduces the air pressure within the chamber of the piston. The negative air pressure creates suction that draws the outside, higher-pressure air into the piston through an aperture at the top of the piston. (B) A healthy adult shows how contraction of the primary muscles of inspiration (diaphragm, scalenes, and intercostales) increases intrathoracic volume, which in turn expands the lungs and reduces alveolar pressure. The negative alveolar pressure draws air into the lungs. The descent of the diaphragm is indicated by the pair of thick, purple, vertical arrows.

intrathoracic volume increases the alveolar pressure, thereby driving air from the alveoli, out of the lungs, and to the atmosphere.

In healthy persons, *quiet expiration* is essentially a passive process that relies little on muscle activation.[2,69] When the muscles of inspiration relax after contraction, the intrathoracic volume is naturally decreased primarily by the elastic recoil of the lungs, rib cage, and connective tissues of stretched inspiratory muscles. *Forced expiration,* required during deeper or rapid breathing, coughing, or blowing out a candle, requires the active force produced by expiratory muscles, such as the abdominals.

ARTHROLOGY

Thorax

The thorax, or rib cage, is a closed system that functions as a mechanical bellows for ventilation. The internal aspect of the thorax is sealed from the outside by fascial membranes and several musculoskeletal tissues. Although this chapter focuses on how the thorax generates air movement, the thorax also protects cardiopulmonary organs and large vessels; serves as a structural base for the cervical spine; and provides a site for attachment of muscles that either directly or indirectly act on the head, neck, and extremities.

Articulations within the Thorax

Multiple articulations within the thorax contribute to the fluctuations in intrathoracic volume that occur during ventilation (see list in box below).

Articulations within the Thorax

- Manubriosternal joint
- Sternocostal joints (including the costochondral and chondrosternal junctions)
- Interchondral joints
- Costovertebral joints
  - Costocorporeal
  - Costotransverse
- Thoracic intervertebral joints

MANUBRIOSTERNAL JOINT

The manubrium articulates with the body of the sternum at the *manubriosternal joint* (Fig. 11.25). This fibrocartilaginous articulation is typically classified as a synarthrosis, allowing very little movement, similar to the structure of the pubic symphysis. A partial disc fills the cavity of the manubriosternal joint, completely ossifying late in life.[135] Although not apparent in Fig. 11.25, the manubrium is angled approximately 10 to 15 degrees posterior (within the sagittal plane) relative to the body of the sternum. This semirigid angle is often referred to as the *sternal angle* (or angle of Louis). Before ossification, the manubrium is pliable enough to rotate posteriorly about 4 degrees (relative to the sternum) during maximum inspiration.[12]

STERNOCOSTAL JOINTS

Bilaterally the anterior cartilaginous ends of the first seven ribs articulate with the lateral sides of the sternum. In a broad sense, these articulations are referred to as *sternocostal joints* (see Fig. 11.25).

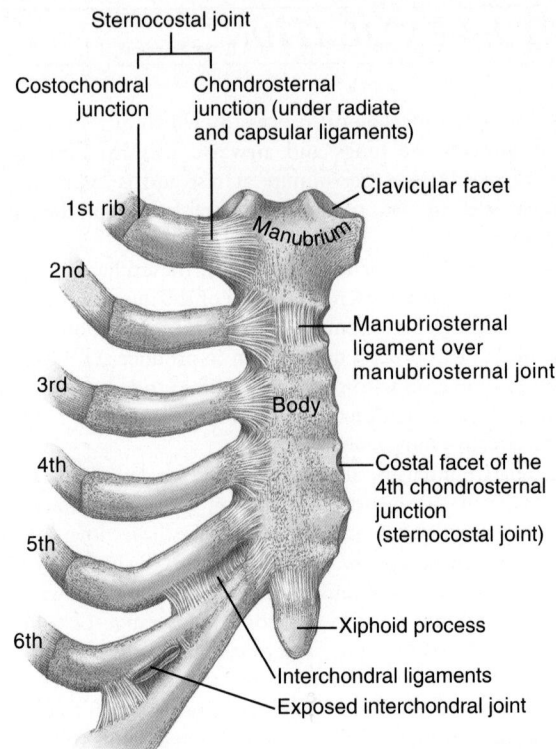

FIGURE 11.25 Anterior view of part of the thoracic wall highlights the manubriosternal joint, sternocostal joints (with costochondral and chondrosternal junctions), and interchondral joints. The ribs are removed on the left side to expose the costal facets.

Because of the intervening cartilage between the bones of the ribs and the sternum, however, each sternocostal joint is structurally divided into costochondral and chondrosternal junctions.

The chondrosternal *junctions* represent the transition between the bone and cartilage of the anterior ends of each rib. No capsule or ligament reinforces these junctions. The periosteum of the ribs gradually transforms into the perichondrium of the cartilage. Costochondral junctions permit little movement.

The *chondrosternal junctions* are formed between the medial ends of the cartilage of the ribs and the slightly concave costal facets on the sternum. All seven chondrosternal junctions contribute to rib movement during maximum-effort ventilation, most notable in the more cranial junctions.[12] The first chondrosternal junction is considered a flexible, fibrous synarthrosis. The second through the seventh joints, however, are more synovial in nature. Each synovial joint is surrounded by a capsule that is strengthened by *radiate ligaments*.

INTERCHONDRAL JOINTS

The opposed borders of the cartilages of ribs 5 through 10 form small, synovial-lined *interchondral joints,* strengthened by *interchondral ligaments* (see Fig. 11.25). Ribs 11 and 12 do not attach anteriorly to the sternum.

COSTOVERTEBRAL JOINTS

The posterior end of the ribs attaches to the vertebral column via a pair of costovertebral joints: costocorporeal and costotransverse. The *costocorporeal joints* connect the heads of each of the 12 ribs to the corresponding sides of the bodies of the thoracic vertebrae.

The *costotransverse joints* connect the articular tubercles of ribs 1 to 10 to the transverse processes of the corresponding thoracic vertebrae. Ribs 11 and 12 usually lack costotransverse joints. The anatomy and ligamentous structures of these joints are described and illustrated in Chapter 9 (see Fig. 9.51).

THORACIC INTERVERTEBRAL JOINTS

Movement within the thoracic vertebral column occurs primarily at the interbody and apophyseal joints within the region. The structure and function of these joints are described in Chapter 9.

Changes in Intrathoracic Volume during Ventilation

VERTICAL CHANGES

During inspiration, the vertical diameter of the thorax is increased primarily by contraction and subsequent lowering of the dome of the diaphragm muscle (see Fig. 11.24B). During quiet expiration the diaphragm relaxes, allowing the dome to recoil upward to its resting position.

ANTERIOR-POSTERIOR AND MEDIAL-LATERAL CHANGES

Elevation and depression of the ribs and sternum produce changes in the anterior-posterior and medial-lateral diameters of the thorax.[12] Although all articulations within the thorax may contribute to these changes in diameter, the costovertebral joints have a primary role in these kinematics.[13] Angular motions occur in all three degrees of freedom at the costovertebral joints, but, by far, the greatest freedom of rotation occurs in a path corresponding

with elevation and depression of the shaft of the ribs (described later).[46] On average, about 15 degrees of rotation occur about a given pair of costovertebral joints as the corresponding rib is fully raised and lowered.[46,85]

During *inspiration,* the shaft of the ribs elevates in a path perpendicular to the *axis of rotation* that lies generally parallel with the associated transverse processes. As depicted in Fig. 11.26, the axis of rotation lies nearly parallel with the costovertebral joints. Upon inspiration, the downward sloped ribs rotate upward and outward, increasing the intrathoracic volume in both anterior-posterior and medial-lateral diameters. This mechanism is somewhat like the rotation of a bucket handle. During *forced inspiration,* the movement of the ribs is typically combined with slight extension throughout the thoracic spine.

The specific path of movement of a given rib depends partially on its unique shape, but also on the spatial orientation of the axis of rotation and associated thoracic transverse process. In the *upper six ribs* the axis is displaced horizontally approximately 25 to 35 degrees from the frontal plane; in the *lower six ribs* the axis is displaced horizontally approximately 35 to 45 degrees from the frontal plane. (The anatomic specimen used to illustrate Fig. 11.26A shows an approximate 35-degree horizontal displacement from the frontal plane.) This slight difference in angulations causes the upper ribs to elevate slightly more in the anterior direction, thereby facilitating the forward and upward movement of the sternum.[86]

The elevating ribs and sternum create slight bending and twisting movements within the pliable cartilages associated with the joints of the thorax.[12] As depicted in Fig. 11.26B, torsion created in the twisted cartilage and other soft tissues within a sternocostal joint stores a component of the energy used to elevate the ribs. The energy

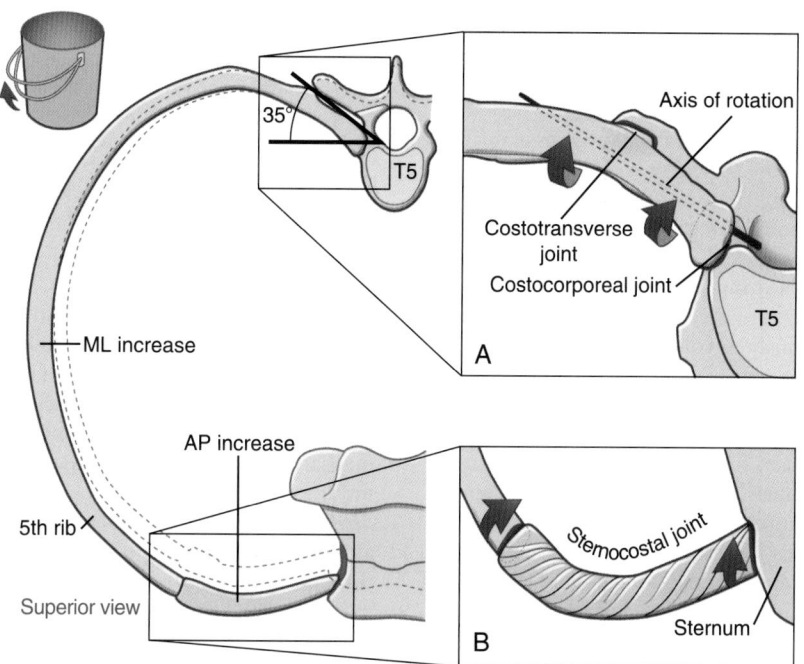

FIGURE 11.26 A top view of the fifth rib shows the "bucket-handle" mechanism of elevation of the ribs during inspiration. The ghosted outline of the rib indicates its position before inspiration. Elevation of the rib increases both the anterior-posterior *(AP)* and the medial-lateral *(ML)* diameters of the thorax. The rib connects to the vertebral column via the costovertebral joints (costotransverse and costocorporeal) (A) and to the sternum via the sternocostal joint (B). During elevation, the head-and-neck of the rib rotates around an axis of rotation that courses near the costovertebral joints—parallel with the associated transverse process. The elevating rib creates a twist or torsion in the cartilage associated with the sternocostal joint.

Factors That Can Oppose Expansion of the Thorax

The work performed by the muscles of inspiration must overcome the natural elastic recoil of the lung tissue and connective tissues that comprise the thorax. Additional work is also required to overcome the resistance of the inspired air as it passes through the extensive airways. The amount of air that reaches the alveoli depends on the generation of negative alveolar pressure, which is determined in part by the net effect of muscle contraction and the mechanical properties that oppose thoracic expansion.

Several factors can significantly oppose expansion of the thorax, including changes within lung tissue and the surrounding chest wall. Pulmonary fibrosis, for example, is a disease marked by excessive scarring and thickening of the lungs, causing increased pulmonary stiffness and reduced compliance. Compliance, in this context, is a measure of the extensibility of the lungs produced by a given drop in transpulmonary pressure. A greater reduction in pressure is therefore required to inspire a given volume of air. In effect, muscles must work harder during inspiration to move the same volume of air.

Rheumatoid arthritis (RA) is an example of a disease that alters the compliance of the chest wall. RA can increase the stiffness of the cartilage of the sternocostal joints, thereby resisting an increase in intrathoracic volume. Similarly, postsurgical adhesions, obesity, advanced age,[95] or abnormal musculoskeletal alignment can also oppose thoracic expansion. For example, postural abnormalities associated with severe scoliosis or kyphosis can physically limit the expansion of the thorax and interfere with the mechanics of ventilation.[137] Even in healthy persons, extreme changes in sitting posture within any of the three cardinal planes can have a significant influence on the kinematics of ventilation.[83]

---

is partially recaptured during expiration, as the rib cage recoils to its relatively constricted state.

During *expiration,* the muscles of inspiration relax, allowing the ribs and the sternum to return to their preinspiration position. The lowering of the body of the ribs combined with the inferior and posterior movements of the sternum decreases the anterior-posterior and medial-lateral diameters of the thorax. During *forced expiration,* the movement of the ribs is typically accompanied by slight flexion throughout the thoracic spine.

MUSCULAR ACTIONS DURING VENTILATION

The kinesiology of ventilation is complex and involves many muscular interactions, spread across the entire axial skeleton. Such a robust system is needed to precisely control the many different intensities of ventilation (from sitting at rest to a full sprint, for example), plus those nonventilatory behaviors such as speaking, singing, sniffing, laughing, yawning, or holding one's breath while underwater swimming. Furthermore, muscles of ventilation are frequently and simultaneously involved with the control of posture, movement, and stability of the trunk and craniocervical regions and, indirectly, the upper and lower extremities. Accordingly, reduced strength and endurance of the muscles of ventilation can negatively affect many functional activities. Fortunately, like other skeletal muscles, muscles of ventilation can be strengthened through exercise, resulting in a marked increase in their function.[3,43,124] Notably, this favorable therapeutic response has been shown for the diaphragm muscle—the primary muscle of inspiration, across a wide range of ages, including persons 60 to 80 years of age.[134]

A great deal is still to be learned about the specific functions of the muscles of ventilation. Some methods used to study this topic are listed in the following box.[d]

> **Common Measurements or Technology Used to Determine the Functions of Ventilatory Muscles**
>
> - Muscle mass, cross-sectional area, line of force relative to ribs, fiber type
> - Kinematics of the thoracic cage or abdominal cavity during ventilation (e.g., through optoelectronic plethysmography)
> - Standard pulmonary function measurements (such as forced vital capacity, forced expiratory volume per time, etc.)
> - Ventilatory pressures, including changes in pleural pressure per unit of normalized muscle force
> - Electromyography from human and animal subjects using surface, fine wire, or (for the diaphragm muscle) esophageal-based electrodes
> - Fluoroscopic, ultrasonic, computed tomography and magnetic resonance imaging
> - Effects of nerve and transcranial magnetic stimulation
> - Surface mechanomyography

In addition, clinical observations of the effects of muscle paralysis after spinal cord injury have helped considerably in the understanding of the normal function of the ventilatory muscles.[105,111,133]

As will be described, any muscle that attaches to the thorax can potentially alter intrathoracic volume and thereby assist with the mechanics of ventilation. More specifically, a muscle that *increases* intrathoracic volume is a muscle of *inspiration;* a muscle that *decreases* intrathoracic volume is a muscle of *expiration.* The detailed anatomy and innervation of the muscles of ventilation are found throughout Appendix III, Part C, in particular in the section on muscles related primarily to ventilation.

Muscles of Quiet Inspiration

The primary muscles of quiet inspiration are the diaphragm, scalenes, and intercostales (introduced in Fig. 11.24). These muscles are active even at rest, and their activation increases with greater work intensities. The mode of action and innervation of the primary muscles of inspiration are summarized in Table 11.4.

---

[d]15,44,45,82,88,89,90,98,105,138

DIAPHRAGM MUSCLE

The *diaphragm* is a dome-shaped, thin, musculotendinous sheet of tissue that separates the thoracic cavity from the abdominal cavity. Its convex upper surface is the floor of the thoracic cavity, and its concave lower surface is the roof of the abdominal cavity (Fig. 11.27).

The diaphragm has three parts based on the anatomy of bony attachments: the *costal part* arises from the upper margins of the lower six ribs and adjacent transversus abdominis muscle; the relatively small and variable *sternal part* arises from the posterior side of the xiphoid process; and the thicker *lumbar part* is attached to the bodies of the upper three lumbar vertebrae through two distinct tendinous attachments known as the *right* and *left crus*. The lumbar, or crural, part of the diaphragm contains the longest and most vertically oriented fibers. Some of these fibers blend with the anterior longitudinal ligament of the vertebral column.[135]

The three sets of attachments of the diaphragm converge to form a *central tendon* at the upper dome of the muscle. Each half of the diaphragm receives its innervation via the *phrenic nerve,* which is formed from nerve roots C^3–C^5, with a primarily contribution from C^4. The location of these nerve roots explains why irritation of the diaphragm or phrenic nerve can cause a referred pain to the shoulder region.

Because of the position of the liver within the abdomen, the right side of the resting diaphragm lies slightly higher than the left. During quiet inspiration while seated, the dome of the diaphragm drops an average of 1.8 cm in healthy adults.[14] During forced inspiration, however, the diaphragm flattens and descends on average of about 6 cm. At maximum inspiration, the right side descends to the level of the body of T11; the left side descends to the level of the body of T12.

The diaphragm is the most important muscle of inspiration, performing 60% to 80% of the work of the ventilatory process.[4,119] The muscle's predominant role in inspiration is largely a result of its ability to increase intrathoracic volume in *all* three diameters: vertical, medial-lateral, and anterior-posterior. A given level of muscle contraction therefore yields a relatively large drop in intrathoracic pressure.

The diaphragm is the first muscle to be activated by the nervous system during an inspiratory effort.[126] With the lower ribs stabilized, the initial contraction of the diaphragm causes a lowering and flattening of its dome (see Fig. 11.27). This lowering piston action substantially increases the *vertical diameter* of the thorax. This action is the primary method by which the diaphragm increases intrathoracic volume. An additional increase in volume requires resistance from within the abdomen. The descent of the diaphragm into the abdominal cavity is resisted by an increase in intra-abdominal pressure; by compressed abdominal contents; and by low-level activation (tone) and passive tension in stretched abdominal muscles, particularly the transversus abdominis.[69] At some point, this abdominal resistance stabilizes the position of the dome of the diaphragm, allowing its continued contraction to *elevate* the lower six ribs. The elevation can be visualized by reversing the direction of the arrowheads in Fig. 11.27. As described earlier, elevation of the ribs expands the thorax in the anterior-posterior and medial-lateral diameters.

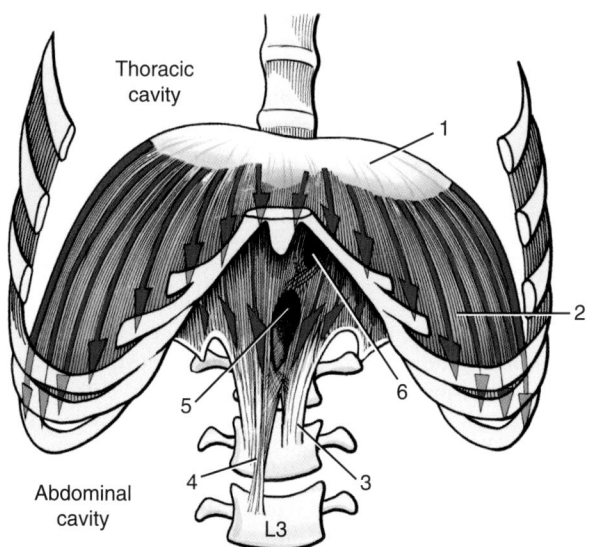

FIGURE 11.27 The action of the diaphragm muscle during the initiation phase of inspiration. *1,* Central tendon; *2,* muscle fibers (costal part); *3,* left crus; *4,* right crus; *5,* opening for the aorta; *6,* opening for the esophagus. (Modified from Kapandji IA: *The physiology of joints,* vol 3, New York, 1974, Churchill Livingstone.)

TABLE 11.4	Primary Muscles of Inspiration		
Muscle	**Mode of Action**	**Innervation**	**Location of Illustrations**
Diaphragm	*Primary:* The dome of the contracting diaphragm lowers and flattens during inspiration. This movement increases the vertical diameter of the thorax. *Secondary:* The descent of the diaphragm is resisted by the abdomen, which in turn stabilizes the position of the dome of the diaphragm. Further diaphragmatic contraction can *elevate* the lower ribs.	Phrenic nerve (C^3–C^5)	Chapter 11 (Fig. 11.27)
Scalenes	The scalene anterior, medius, and posterior increase intrathoracic volume by elevating the ribs and the sternum.	Ventral rami of spinal nerve roots (C^3–C^7)	Chapter 10
Intercostales	The parasternal fibers of the intercostales interni and the intercostales externi increase intrathoracic volume by elevating the ribs. During inspiration, the intercostales stabilize the intercostal spaces to prevent an inward collapse of the thoracic wall.	Intercostal nerves (T^2–T^{12})	Chapter 11 (Fig. 11.28)

The diaphragm muscle is one of the most continuously active muscles in the body. As such, the muscle is particularly sensitive to the withdrawal of neural influences.[116,131] During full-support mechanical ventilation, the diaphragm muscle is not required to support breathing. Consequently, the diaphragm undergoes rapid atrophy after just 8 to 12 hours of mechanical ventilation.[115] Interestingly, if even a small amount of diaphragm contraction can be maintained (e.g., spontaneous breathing trials or electrical stimulation), even intermittently, diaphragm dysfunction can be minimized,[54,75] which can facilitate weaning from ventilatory support.

The primary role of the diaphragm in driving the mechanics of inspiration has long been appreciated. More recent research, however, strongly suggests that this muscle is involved in many other physiologic functions, including providing postural stability to the trunk.[57,77] This stabilization function is based on the muscle's extensive attachments to the axial skeleton, combined with its ability to increase intra-abdominal pressure when coupled with a strong activation of the abdominal and pelvic floor muscles (reviewed in Chapter 10).[62,63,78] Activation of the diaphragm's crural fibers likely lends some mechanical support to the upper-and-middle regions of the lumbar spine. At least theoretically, weakness, fatigue, or abnormal function of the diaphragm muscle may be associated with the pathomechanics of low back pain.[73,74,79]

Interestingly, the relationship between the diaphragm and control of the axial skeleton has been exploited by some patients with tetraplegia, whereby they learn to activate their diaphragm muscle to assist rolling from supine to a prone position.[104]

SCALENE MUSCLES

The *scalenus anterior, medius,* and *posterior* muscles attach between the cervical spine and the upper two ribs (see Chapter 10). If the cervical spine is assumed to be well stabilized, bilateral contraction of the muscles increases intrathoracic volume by elevating the upper

ribs and attached sternum. The scalene muscles are active, along with the diaphragm, during every inspiration cycle.[33,66,126]

INTERCOSTALES MUSCLES

Anatomy

The *intercostales* are a thin, three-layer set of muscles that occupy the intercostal spaces. Each set of intercostal muscles within a given intercostal space is innervated by an adjacent intercostal nerve (Fig. 11.28).

The *intercostales externi* are most superficial, analogous in depth and fiber direction to the obliquus abdominis externus of the trunk (see Chapter 10). There are 11 per side, and each intercostalis externus arises from the lower border of a rib and inserts on the upper border of the rib below (see Fig. 11.28, inset). Fibers travel obliquely between ribs in an inferior and medial direction. The intercostales externi are most developed laterally. Anteriorly, within the region of the sternocostal joints, the intercostales externi are replaced by a thin external intercostal membrane.

The *intercostales interni* are deep to the externi and are analogous in depth and fiber direction to the obliquus abdominis internus of the trunk. There are also 11 per side, with each muscle occupying an intercostal space, in a manner similar to that in the intercostales externi. A major difference, however, is that the fibers of the intercostales interni travel almost perpendicular to the fibers of the intercostales externi (see Fig. 11.28, inset). The intercostales interni are most developed anteriorly within the region of the sternocostal joints; posteriorly, the muscles terminate as the internal intercostal membrane.

Primarily because of differences in function, the research literature typically refers to the intercostales interni as two different sets of muscle fibers: the *parasternal intercostals,* occupying the region of the sternocostal joints; and the *interosseous intercostals,* occupying the more lateral and posterior-lateral intercostal spaces.[35] This terminology will be used in subsequent discussions.

Finally, the *intercostales intimi* are the deepest and least developed of the intercostales. Often referred to as the "innermost intercostals," these muscles run parallel and deep to the intercostales interni (see Fig. 11.28, inset). Fibers of the intercostales intimi located near the angle of the ribs (often designated as *subcostales* muscles) may cross one or two intercostal spaces. The intercostales intimi are most developed in the lower thorax. The actions of these deep and relatively inaccessible muscles have not been extensively studied via EMG. It is tempting to speculate, however, that they have actions like those of the adjacent intercostales interni.[135]

Function of the Intercostales Externi and Interni Muscles

The intercostales externi and interni muscles are often informally referred to as the "external and internal intercostals," respectively. The specific actions of the intercostal muscles during ventilation are not well understood.[35] The conventional wisdom on this topic is that the external intercostals muscles drive *inspiration,* and the internal intercostals drive *forced expiration.* To a large extent these functions are based on the contrasting lines of force (fiber direction) of the muscles relative to the axis of rotation through the costotransverse joints. In theory, isolated contraction of an external intercostal muscle has greater leverage to elevate the lower rib than to depress the upper rib. Conversely, an isolated contraction of an internal intercostal muscle has greater leverage to depress the upper rib than to elevate the lower rib.

Although the proposed relatively simple reciprocal actions of the external and internal intercostals have generally been supported through EMG and other methods of research, the overall muscular kinesiology is much more complicated and variable.[18,32,61,65,154]

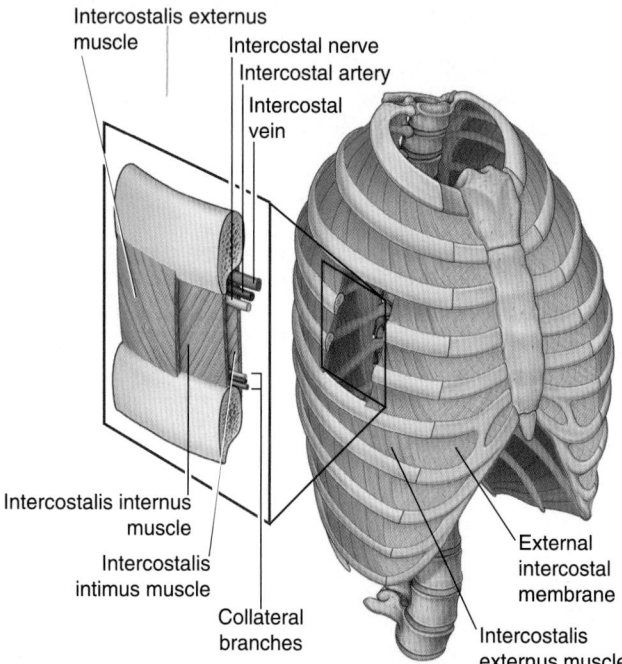

Intercostalis externus muscle
Intercostal nerve
Intercostal artery
Intercostal vein

Intercostalis internus muscle
Intercostalis intimus muscle
Collateral branches

External intercostal membrane
Intercostalis externus muscle

FIGURE 11.28 Illustration showing the three layers of intercostales muscles. (From Drake RL, Vogl W, Mitchell AWM: *Gray's anatomy for students,* ed 3, St Louis, 2015, Churchill Livingstone.)

Compelling arguments exist that the specific action of any given intercostal muscle is influenced not only by its fiber direction and line of pull, but also by factors associated with the specific intercostal space or region where the muscle resides.[35] Some of these regional-specific factors include: the local muscles' force- and torque-generating capability (based on cross-sectional areas and moment arm lengths, respectively) and proximity to the relatively deformable sternocostal end of the ribs, the stabilizing influence of other local muscles, curvature of the associated ribs, and (perhaps most importantly) differing neurologic strategies for the recruitment of motor units.[30,35,53,65,154] This neurologic strategy has been referred to as *neuromechanical matching*, where the neural drive is directed at the specific intercostal muscles that are most mechanically suited to meet the unique functional demands placed on a given intercostal space or region.[35,65] The mechanical demands may be complex, associated not only with ventilation but also with other simultaneously performed functions, such as controlling the posture of the trunk, or talking, sighing, and other actions that require control of airflow to the lungs.

Although there is still much to be learned about the specific actions of the intercostal muscles, the following summary statements reflect what is known on the topic based on a combination of animal and human research.

- The *external intercostal muscles* are primary muscles of *inspiration*.[30,34,35,126] The effectiveness of this action is greatest in the dorsal and upper (cranial) regions of the thorax and diminishes in a ventral-to-caudal direction.[34,149]
- The *parasternal fibers of the internal intercostal muscles* are primary muscles of *inspiration*.[30,35,64,65] The effectiveness of this action, however, diminishes in a cranial-to-caudal direction.[36,149]
- The *interosseous fibers of the internal intercostal muscles* are primary muscles of *forced expiration*.[19] The effectiveness of this action persists throughout the thorax.

In addition to functioning as muscles of inspiration or expiration, the lateral set of intercostal muscles (both external and internal) show considerable activation during axial rotation of the trunk. In a similar manner as the "oblique abdominals" (see Chapter 10), the *external* intercostals are most active during contralateral trunk rotation, and the more *internal* intercostals are most active during ipsilateral trunk rotation.[64,65] The relative contribution of these muscles to the overall biomechanics of axial rotation of the trunk is uncertain.

SPECIAL FOCUS 11.5

"Paradoxical Breathing" after Cervical Spinal Cord Injury

In the healthy person, ventilation typically involves a characteristic pattern of movement between the thorax and abdomen. During inspiration, the thorax expands outwardly because of the elevation of the ribs. The abdomen typically protrudes slightly because of the anterior displacement of the abdominal viscera, compressed by the descending diaphragm.

A complete cervical spinal cord injury below the C4 vertebra typically does not completely paralyze the diaphragm because its innervation is primarily from the C^4 spinal nerve root. The intercostal and abdominal muscles are, however, typically totally paralyzed. The person with this level of spinal cord injury often displays a "paradoxical breathing" pattern. The pathomechanics of this breathing pattern provide insight into the important functional interactions among the diaphragm, intercostals, and abdominal muscles during inspiration.

Without the splinting action of the intercostal muscles across the intercostal spaces, the lowering of the dome of the diaphragm creates an internal suction within the chest that constricts the upper thorax, especially in its anterior-posterior diameter.[47,142] The term *paradoxical* breathing describes the constriction, rather than the normal expansion, of the rib cage during inspiration. Video 11.1 shows a person with C^6 level tetraplegia (quadriplegia) demonstrating the described paradoxical breathing pattern while at rest and lying supine.

The paradoxical constriction of the thorax, as described earlier, can reduce the vital capacity of a person with an acute cervical spinal cord injury. In the healthy adult, vital capacity is about 4500 mL (review Fig. 11.23). About 3000 mL of this inspired volume is accounted for by contraction and full descent of the diaphragm. The vital capacity of a person immediately after a C^4 spinal cord injury may fall as low as 300 mL. Although the diaphragm may be operating at near-normal capacity, the constricting (rather than the normally expanding) thorax likely accounts for much of the

reduced volume of inhalation. Several weeks or months after a spinal injury, however, the atonic (flaccid) intercostals may become slightly hypertonic and therefore more rigid. The increased muscular rigidity can act as a splint to the thoracic wall, as evidenced by the fact that vital capacity in an average-size adult with an injury at C^4 or below often returns to near 3000 mL.

In addition to the constriction of the upper thorax during inspiration, a person with an acute cervical spinal cord injury often displays marked *forward protrusion* of the abdomen during inspiration. The atonic and paralyzed abdominal muscles offer little resistance to the forward migration of the abdominal contents. Without this resistance, the contracting diaphragm loses its effectiveness to expand the middle and lower ribs. These pathomechanics also contribute to the loss of vital capacity after a cervical spinal cord injury.

A person with an acute tetraplegia may be advised to wear an elastic abdominal binder for support when sitting upright. In the seated position, the dome of the diaphragm rests lower than in the supine position. By partially mimicking the tone of innervated abdominal muscles, an abdominal binder provides useful resistance against the descent of the diaphragm.[31] Research has indeed shown improvements in ventilatory function from wearing an abdominal binder in persons both with acute (1 year) and with long-standing (average of 10 years) tetraplegia.[69,147] Improvements varied but included significant increases in vital capacity, total inspiratory capacity, forced expiratory volume in 1 sec, and a decrease in functional residual capacity. The surrogate resistance offered by the binder may be especially useful in the time just following a spinal cord injury before the anticipated return of some of the firmness in the abdominal muscles. Practical reasons, such as comfort, skin irritation, and difficulty donning, may limit the long-term use of an abdominal binder.

In addition to expanding the intrathoracic volume during inspiration, contraction of the external and parasternal intercostal muscles also provide rigidity to the rib cage.[18,34,53] Although often overlooked, this stabilizing function is a very important component of ventilation. With the assistance of the scalene muscles, the splinting action on the ribs prevents the thoracic wall from being partially sucked inward by the reduced intrathoracic pressure caused by contraction of the diaphragm.

As the intercostal muscles contract to stiffen the thoracic cage during inspiration, muscles located in the pharyngeal region also contract to stiffen and dilate the upper airway. This action reduces the resistance to the inspired air. One of the main upper airway dilator muscles is the *genioglossus,* a dominant extrinsic muscle of the tongue. The neural control of this muscle during breathing has been extensively studied, primarily because of its possible role in obstructive sleep apnea.[18,125]

Muscles of Forced Inspiration

Forced inspiration requires additional muscles to assist the primary muscles of inspiration. As a group, the additional muscles are referred to as *muscles of forced inspiration,* or *accessory muscles of inspiration.* Table 11.5 lists a sample of several muscles of forced inspiration, including their possible mode of action. Each muscle has a line of action that can directly or indirectly increase intrathoracic volume. Most muscles listed in Table 11.5 are illustrated elsewhere in this textbook. The serratus posterior superior and serratus posterior inferior are illustrated in Fig. 11.29.

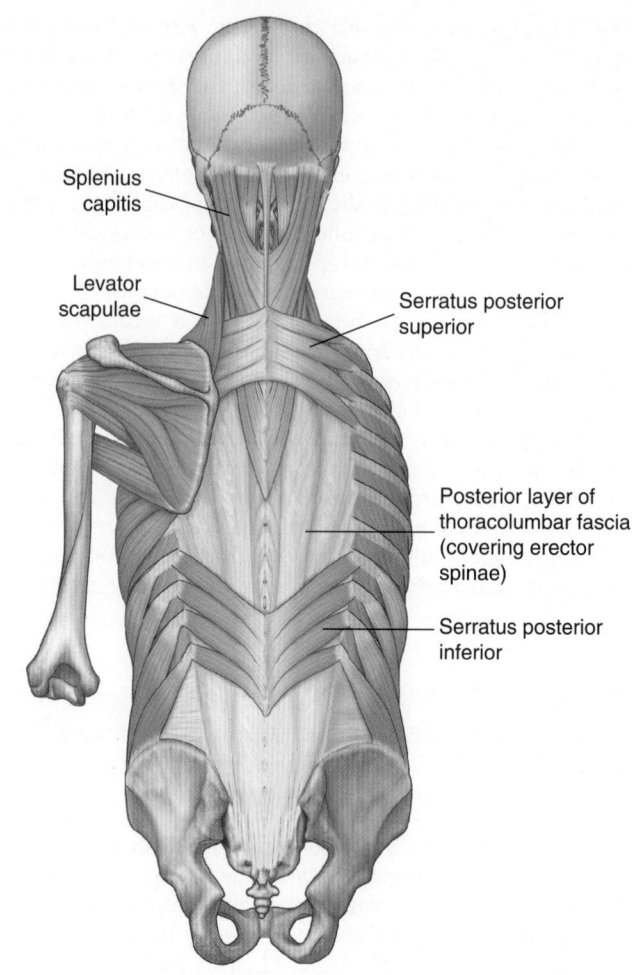

FIGURE 11.29 Illustration highlighting the serratus posterior superior and serratus posterior inferior muscles. These muscles are located within the intermediate layer of the posterior trunk muscles. (From Drake RL, Vogl W, Mitchell AWM: *Gray's anatomy for students,* ed 3, St Louis, 2015, Churchill Livingstone.)

TABLE 11.5 A Sample of Muscles of Forced Inspiration			
Muscle	**Mode of Action**	**Innervation**	**Location of Illustrations**
Serratus posterior superior	Increases intrathoracic volume by elevating the upper ribs.	Intercostal nerves (T^2–T^5)	Chapter 11 (Fig. 11.29)
Serratus posterior inferior	Stabilizes the lower ribs for initial contraction of the diaphragm.	Intercostal nerves (T^9–T^{12})	Chapter 11 (Fig. 11.29)
Levatores costarum (longi and breves)	Increase intrathoracic volume by elevating the ribs.	Dorsi rami of adjacent thoracic spinal nerve roots (C^7–T^{11})	Chapter 10
Sternocleidomastoid	Increases intrathoracic volume by elevating the sternum and upper ribs.	Primary source: spinal accessory nerve (cranial nerve XI)	Chapter 10
Latissimus dorsi	Increases intrathoracic volume by elevating the lower ribs; requires the arms to be fixed.	Thoracodorsal nerve (C^6–C^8)	Chapter 5
Iliocostalis thoracis and cervicis (erector spinae)	Increase intrathoracic volume by extending the trunk.	Adjacent dorsal rami of spinal nerve roots	Chapter 10
Pectoralis minor	Increases intrathoracic volume by elevating the upper ribs; requires activation from muscles such as trapezius and levator scapulae to stabilize the scapula.	Medial pectoral nerve (C^8–T^1)	Chapter 5
Pectoralis major (sternocostal head)	Increases intrathoracic volume by elevating the middle ribs and sternum; this action requires the arms to be held fixed and, ideally, in some degree of flexion or abduction.	Medial pectoral nerve (C^8–T^1)	Chapter 5
Quadratus lumborum	Stabilizes the lower ribs for contraction of the diaphragm during early forced inspiration.	Ventral rami of spinal nerve roots (T^{12}–L^3)	Chapter 10

The muscles of forced inspiration are typically used in healthy persons to increase the rate and volume of inspired air.[146] These muscles may also be recruited at rest to help compensate for the weakness, fatigue, or otherwise reduced function of one or more of the primary muscles of inspiration, such as the diaphragm.

Muscles of Forced Expiration

Quiet expiration is normally a passive process, driven primarily by the elastic recoil of the lungs, thorax, and relaxing diaphragm. In healthy lungs, this passive process is sufficient to exhale the approximately 500 mL of air normally released with quiet expiration.

During forced expiration, active muscle contraction is required to rapidly reduce intrathoracic volume. *Muscles of forced expiration* include the four abdominal muscles, the transversus thoracis, and the interosseous fibers of the intercostales interni (Fig. 11.30). The

mode of action of the muscles of forced expiration is summarized in Table 11.6.

ABDOMINAL MUSCLES

The "abdominal" muscles include the rectus abdominis, obliquus externus abdominis, obliquus internus abdominis, and transversus abdominis (see Chapter 10). Contraction of these muscles has a direct and indirect effect on forced expiration. By acting *directly,* contraction of the abdominal muscles flexes and compresses the thorax and depresses the ribs and sternum. These actions rapidly and forcefully reduce intrathoracic volume, such as when coughing, sneezing, or vigorously exhaling to the limits of the expiratory reserve volume. When acting *indirectly,* contraction of the abdominal muscles—especially the transversus abdominis—increases intra-abdominal pressure and compresses the abdominal viscera. The increased pressure forcefully pushes the relaxed diaphragm *upward,* well into the thoracic cavity (see Fig. 11.30). In this manner, active contraction of the abdominal muscles takes advantage of the parachute-shaped diaphragm to help expel air from the thorax. As described in Chapter 10, increased intra-abdominal pressure is a fundamental component of the Valsalva maneuver, which is functionally related to many functions including childbirth, defecation, and rigorous lifting and pulling.

Although the abdominal muscles are described here as muscles of forced expiration, their contraction also indirectly enhances inspiration. As the diaphragm is forced upward at maximal expiration, it is stretched to an optimal point on its length-tension curve. Therefore the muscle is more prepared to initiate a forceful contraction at the next inspiration cycle.

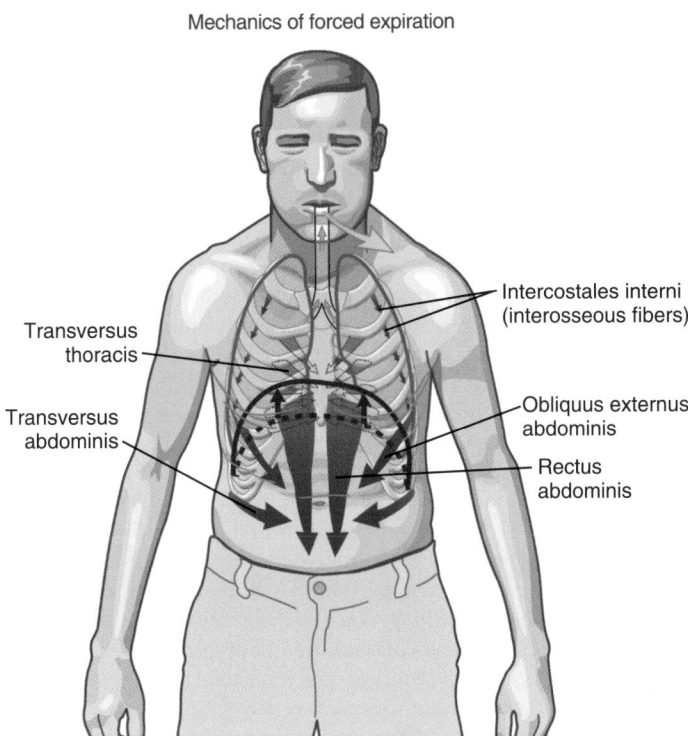

Mechanics of forced expiration

Transversus thoracis

Transversus abdominis

Intercostales interni (interosseous fibers)

Obliquus externus abdominis

Rectus abdominis

FIGURE 11.30 Muscle activation during forced expiration. Contraction of "abdominal" muscles, transversus thoracis, and intercostales interni (interosseous fibers) increases intrathoracic and intra-abdominal pressures. The passive recoil of the diaphragm is indicated by the pair of thick, purple, vertical arrows.

TABLE 11.6 Muscles of Forced Expiration

Muscle	Mode of Action	Innervation	Location of Illustrations
Abdominal muscles: Rectus abdominis Obliquus externus abdominis Obliquus internus abdominis Transversus abdominis	1. Decrease intrathoracic volume by flexing the trunk and depressing the ribs. 2. Compress the abdominal wall and contents, which increases intra-abdominal pressure; as a result, the relaxed diaphragm is pushed upward, decreasing intrathoracic volume.	Intercostal nerves (T^7–L^1)	Chapter 10
Transversus thoracis	Decreases intrathoracic volume by depressing the ribs and pulling them inward (constricting the thorax).	Adjacent intercostal nerves	Chapter 11 (Fig. 11.31)
Intercostales interni (interosseous fibers)	The interosseous fibers of the intercostales interni decrease intrathoracic volume by depressing the ribs.	Intercostal nerves (T^2–T^{12})	Chapter 11 (Fig. 11.28)

SPECIAL FOCUS 11.6

Important Physiologic Functions of the Abdominal Muscles

Forceful expiration is driven primarily by contraction of the abdominal muscles. These muscles are strongly involved in several ventilatory-related functions, including singing, laughing, coughing, and adequately responding to a "gag" reflex when one is choking. The latter two functions are particularly vital to one's health and safety. Coughing or vigorously "clearing the throat" is a natural way to remove secretions from the bronchial tree, thereby reducing the likelihood of lung infection. (Indeed, a leading cause of death among persons with a spinal cord injury is pneumonia.[106]) A strong contraction of the abdominal muscles is also used to dislodge objects lodged in the trachea.

Persons with weakened or completely paralyzed abdominal muscles must learn alternative methods of coughing or have others "manually" assist with this function. Consider, for example, a person with a complete spinal cord lesion at the T^4 level. Because of the innervation of the abdominal muscles (ventral rami of T^7–L^1), this person would likely have completely paralyzed abdominal muscles. Persons with paralyzed or very weakened abdominal muscles must exercise extra caution to prevent choking.

TRANSVERSUS THORACIS AND INTERCOSTALES INTERNI

The transversus thoracis (also referred to as the *triangularis sterni*) is a muscle of forced expiration.[36,69] The muscle is located on the internal side of the thorax, running horizontally and obliquely superiorly between the lower third of the sternum and the sternocostal joints of the adjacent four or five ribs (Fig. 11.31). The muscle's neural activation is synchronized with the abdominal muscles and interosseous fibers of the internal intercostals during forced expiration.[35,37]

SYNOPSIS

Ventilation produces the necessary intrathoracic pressure gradient that results in bulk flow of air in and out of the lungs. This air flow allows for the exchange of oxygen and carbon dioxide gas within the lungs. This process sustains oxidative cellular respiration, which, among other things, provides the energy required for active human movement. Part 2 of this chapter focuses almost exclusively on the muscle and joint interactions that drive the mechanics of ventilation.

Four phases of ventilation were studied: quiet inspiration, forced inspiration, quiet expiration, and forced expiration. In each phase but quiet expiration, muscle contraction provides the primary mechanism that changes the volume within the flexible thorax. Based on Boyle's law, changing intrathoracic volume has an inverse relationship on the contained intrathoracic pressure. Because air naturally flows away from high pressure and toward low pressure, a muscle force that increases intrathoracic volume will assist with inspiration. Conversely, a muscle force that reduces intrathoracic volume will assist in expiration.

Passive tension created within stretched connective tissues embedded within the lungs, muscle, ligaments, and the cartilage of the sternocostal joints also has an important role in ventilation, specifically expiration. Once stretched after inspiration, these connective tissues exhibit "elastic recoil" that assists with forcing air out of the lungs.

Internal view

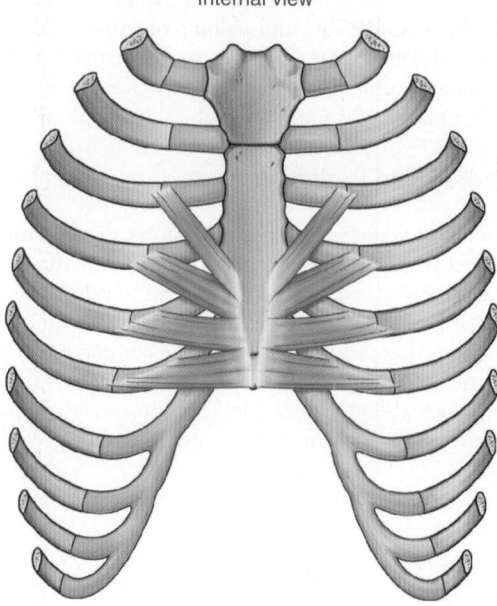

FIGURE 11.31 An internal view of the anterior thoracic wall shows the transversus thoracis muscle. (From Drake RL, Vogl W, Mitchell AWM: *Gray's anatomy for students,* ed 3, St Louis, 2015, Churchill Livingstone.)

Pathology, trauma, prolonged inactivity, and, in some persons, advanced age can significantly affect the mechanics of ventilation. Consider, for example, the effects of abnormal muscle function. An extreme example is a complete spinal cord injury above C^4, causing paralysis or at least marked weakness of most primary muscles of ventilation, most notably the diaphragm. Without sufficient force from the diaphragm muscle, attempts to expand the thorax during inspiration may generate only small or no change in intrathoracic pressure. As a result, inspiration draws in negligible amounts of air to the lungs, perhaps insufficient to sustain life without medical intervention. Typically, such intervention is furnished through a mechanical ventilator, an electrically powered device that forces pressurized air into the lungs (via a tracheotomy) at a preset volume, flow rate, humidity, and concentration of oxygen.

Another example of abnormal muscle function affecting ventilation may occur in some persons with cerebral palsy.[124] Although the person may have essentially full innervation of their muscles, the muscles may exhibit excessive tone. Hypertonicity of the abdominal muscles, for example, may result in a sustained and overbearing increase in intra-abdominal pressure, resisting the descent of the diaphragm during inspiration. If the diaphragm cannot overcome the resistance, the likely reduced vital capacity may limit the physical endurance of the person in other activities, including locomotion. This scenario may be particularly relevant if the person's ability to walk is already labored by increased tone, weakness, or poor control of muscles in the lower extremity.

In addition to abnormal functioning of muscle, pathology affecting the skeletal and other connective tissue systems of the thorax can also affect the mechanics of ventilation. Consider, for example, moderate-to-severe scoliosis, posttraumatic thoracic kyphosis, or advanced ankylosing spondylitis. All these conditions can oppose thoracic expansion and therefore reduce vital capacity. Often, a secondary effect of these conditions is reduced exercise tolerance and subsequent difficulty in maintaining a healthy level of aerobic fitness. Therapeutic interventions for these persons must, when feasible, incorporate creative strategies that appropriately challenge the cardiopulmonary system while simultaneously respecting the limitations imposed by the primary pathology.

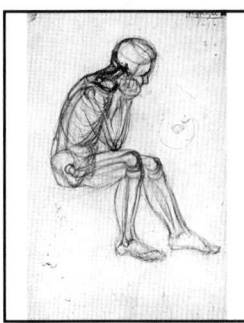

ADDITIONAL CLINICAL CONNECTIONS

CONTENTS

Clinical Connection 11.1: The Influence of Posture on the Potential Stress on the Temporomandibular Joint, 477

Clinical Connection 11.2: Chronic Obstructive Pulmonary Disease: Altered Muscle Mechanics, 478

CLINICAL CONNECTION 11.1

The Influence of Posture on the Potential Stress on the Temporomandibular Joint

Based on shared muscular attachments, it seems reasonable to assume that the posture of the head and neck can influence the resting posture of the mandible. Consider, for example, the chronic forward head posture described previously in Chapters 9 and 10. The person depicted in Fig. 11.32 shows a variant of this posture. Observe that the protracted (forward) head is combined with a flexed upper thoracic and lower cervical spine and with an extended upper craniocervical region. This posture stretches infrahyoid muscles, such as the sternohyoid and omohyoid, which can create an inferior and posterior pull on the hyoid bone. The traction is transferred to the mandible through suprahyoid muscles such as the anterior belly of the digastric. As a result, the mandible

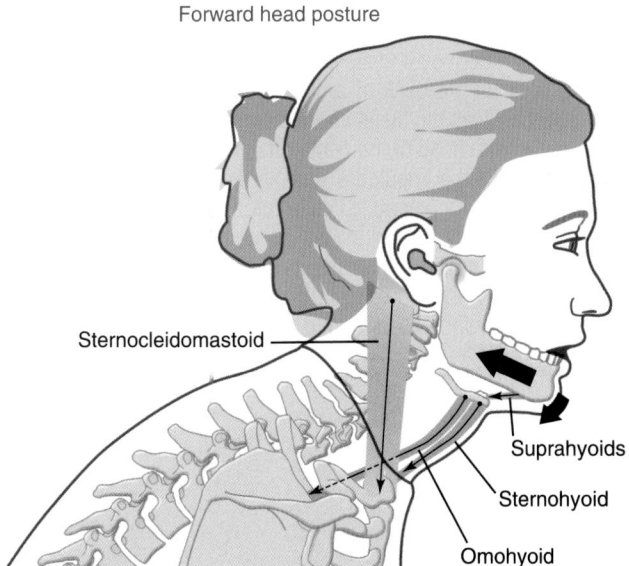

Forward head posture

FIGURE 11.32 A forward head posture shows one mechanism by which passive tension in selected suprahyoid and infrahyoid muscles could alter the resting posture of the mandible. The mandible is pulled inferiorly and posteriorly, changing the position of the condyle within the temporomandibular joint.

is pulled in a direction of retrusion and depression.[6] If chronic, the pull on the mandible may bias a partially opened posture of the mouth, creating additional force demands on muscles that close the mouth, such as the masseter and medial pterygoid. Because of the attachment of the omohyoid to the scapula, poor posture of the shoulder girdle (i.e., an excessively depressed, downwardly rotated, or protracted scapulothoracic joint) can place additional stretch on this muscle and therefore additional pull on the mandible.

Altering the resting posture of the mandible changes the position of its condyle within the mandibular fossa of the temporal bone. A posteriorly displaced condyle could, in theory, compress the delicate and sensitive retrodiscal tissues, creating significant pain and inflammation. Spasm or excessive activation in either head of the lateral pterygoid muscle may occur as a natural protective mechanism to *protrude* the mandible away from the compressed retrodiscal tissues.[21] Chronic spasm within the muscle's superior head may, however, abnormally displace the disc *anterior and medial* to the condyle.[7,9,139] This situation may predispose a person to a condition of internal derangement of the disc.

Some studies suggest a cause-and-effect relationship between abnormal craniocervical posture and disorders of the temporomandibular disorders (TMDs).[24,70,94,148] Other studies, however, are uncertain or inconclusive.[101] Studies on this topic, in general, tend to lack a design needed to unequivocally determine such a link, often lacking methods to objectively quantify posture, and relying on subjects that have mixed TMD diagnoses. More rigorous research is needed in this area to help guide treatment.

One underlying concept espoused in the preceding kinesiologic analysis is that one part of the axial skeleton can affect another. Usually, this kinesiologic interrelationship is positive in the sense that it optimizes the ease and physiologic efficiency of movement. Abnormal posture, however, can negatively affect this relationship. As described earlier, abnormal scapulothoracic posture likely affects mandibular posture, and ultimately increases the stress on the TMJ. An evaluation of a person with TMD should therefore include a thorough analysis of the posture of the entire trunk, from lumbar spine to craniocervical region.

ADDITIONAL CLINICAL CONNECTIONS

CLINICAL CONNECTION 11.2
Chronic Obstructive Pulmonary Disease: Altered Muscle Mechanics

Chronic obstructive pulmonary disease (COPD) is a disorder that typically incorporates both chronic bronchitis and emphysema. Symptoms include chronic inflammation and narrowing of the bronchioles, chronic cough, and mucus-filled airways, with overdistension and destruction of the alveoli. A significant complication of COPD is the loss of elastic recoil within the lungs and collapsed bronchioles. As a result, air remains trapped in the lungs at the end of expiration. In advanced cases the thorax remains in a chronic state of relative inflation, regardless of the actual phase of ventilation. This complication is called *hyperinflation of the lungs*.[38,49] The thorax of a person with advanced COPD, therefore, may develop a "barrel-shaped" appearance, describing a fixed expansion of the chest and rib cage, primarily in anterior-posterior directions.

The excessive air in the lungs at the end of expiration can alter the position and geometry of the muscles of inspiration, especially the diaphragm. In severe cases the diaphragm remains relatively low in the thorax, with a flattened dome. This change in position and shape could alter the muscle's *resting length* and *line of force*.[29,76] Operating at a chronically shortened length reduces the muscle's contractile excursion as well as efficiency—often measured as the ratio of power output per level of muscle activation.[49,51] Furthermore, the lowered position can redirect the line of force of the costal fibers to a more horizontal orientation (reviewed in Fig. 11.27). As a consequence, the muscle loses some of its effectiveness in elevating the ribs.[143] At a low enough position, the line of force of the muscle can paradoxically draw the lower ribs *inward* toward the midline of the body, thereby inhibiting lateral expansion of the ribs. These factors can significantly reduce the effectiveness of the diaphragm to fill the lungs during inspiration. Over time, reduced functioning of the diaphragm muscle can lead to respiratory distress and exercise intolerance, contributing to overall physical deconditioning and reduced mass of all the body's musculature.[29]

Because of the compromised function of the diaphragm and the increased resistance to airflow in the narrowed bronchioles, persons with advanced COPD often overuse both primary and accessory muscles of inspiration during quiet inspiration. The scalenes, sternocleidomastoid, and erector spinae appear to be overactive and in phase with inspiration, even at relatively low levels of exertion. Often, a person with COPD may stand or walk with the body partially bent over while placing one or both arms on a stable object, such as the back of a chair, grocery cart, or walker. This strategy stabilizes the distal attachments of arm muscles, such as the sternocostal head of the pectoralis major and latissimus dorsi. Especially with the shoulders partially flexed or abducted, these muscles possess a favorable line of force to assist with inspiration by elevating the sternum and ribs. Although this method increases the number of muscles available to assist with inspiration, it also increases the workload of standing and walking, often starting a vicious circle of increased fatigue and dyspnea.

REFERENCES

1. Abboud WA, Yarom N, Yahalom R, et al.: Comparison of two physiotherapy programmes for rehabilitation after temporomandibular joint arthroscopy, *Int J Oral Maxillofac Surg* 47(6):755–761, 2018.
2. Abe T, Kusuhara N, Yoshimura N, et al.: Differential respiratory activity of four abdominal muscles in humans, *J Appl Physiol* 80(4):1379–1389, 1996.
3. Ahmed S, Daniel Martin A, Smith BK: Inspiratory muscle training in patients with prolonged mechanical ventilation: narrative review, *Cardiopulm Phys Ther J* 30(1):44–50, 2019.
4. Aliverti A, Cala SJ, Duranti R, et al.: Human respiratory muscle actions and control during exercise, *J Appl Physiol* 83:1256–1269, 1997.
5. Alonso-Blanco C, Fernandez-de-las-Penas C, de-la Llave-Rincon AI, et al.: Characteristics of referred muscle pain to the head from active trigger points in women with myofascial temporomandibular pain and fibromyalgia syndrome, *J Headache Pain* 13(8):625–637, 2012.
6. An JS, Jeon DM, Jung WS, et al.: Influence of temporomandibular joint disc displacement on craniocervical posture and hyoid bone position, *Am J Orthod Dentofacial Orthop* 147(1):72–79, 2015.
7. Antonopoulou M, Iatrou I, Paraschos A, et al.: Variations of the attachment of the superior head of human lateral pterygoid muscle, *J Cranio-Maxillo-Fac Surg* 41(6):e91–e97, 2013.
8. Armijo-Olivo S, Pitance L, Singh V, et al.: Effectiveness of manual therapy and therapeutic exercise for temporomandibular disorders: systematic review and meta-analysis, *Phys Ther* 96(1):9–25, 2016.
9. Armijo-Olivo S, Silvestre R, Fuentes J, et al.: Electromyographic activity of the cervical flexor muscles in patients with temporomandibular disorders while performing the craniocervical flexion test: a cross-sectional study, *Phys Ther* 91(8):1184–1197, 2011.
10. Baeyens JP, Gilomen H, Erdmann B, et al.: In vivo measurement of the 3D kinematics of the temporomandibular joint using miniaturized electromagnetic trackers: technical report, *Med Biol Eng Comput* 51(4):479–484, 2013.
11. Barbosa MA, Tahara AK, Ferreira IC, et al.: Effects of 8 weeks of masticatory muscles focused endurance exercises on women with oro-facial pain and temporomandibular disorders: a placebo randomised controlled trial, *J Oral Rehabil* 46(10):885–894, 2019.
12. Beyer B, Feipel V, Sholukha V, et al.: In-Vivo analysis of sternal angle, sternal and sternocostal kinematics in supine humans during breathing, *J Biomech* 64:32–40, 2017.
13. Beyer B, Sholukha V, Dugailly PM, et al.: In vivo thorax 3D modelling from costovertebral joint complex kinematics, *Clin Biomech* 29(4):434–438, 2014.
14. Boussuges A, Finance J, Chaumet G, et al.: Diaphragmatic motion recorded by m-mode ultrasonography: limits of normality, *ERJ Open Res* 7(1), 2021.
15. Brown C, Tseng SC, Mitchell K, et al.: Body position affects ultrasonographic measurement of diaphragm contractility, *Cardiopulm Phys Ther J* 29(4):166–172, 2018.
16. Buschang PH, Throckmorton GS, Travers KH, et al.: Incisor and mandibular condylar movements of young adult females during maximum protrusion and lateratrusion of the jaw, *Arch Oral Biol* 46(1):39–48, 2001.
17. Bush F, Harkins S, Harrington W, et al.: Analysis of gender effects on pain perception and symptom presentation in temporomandibular pain, *Pain* 53(1):73–80, 1993.
18. Butler JE: Drive to the human respiratory muscles, *Respir Physiol Neurobiol* 159:115–126, 2007.
19. Butler JE, Gandevia SC: The output from human inspiratory motoneurone pools, *J Physiol* 586:1257–1264, 2008.
20. Butler JE, McKenzie DK, Gandevia SC: Discharge frequencies of single motor units in human diaphragm and parasternal muscles in lying and standing, *J Appl Physiol* 90:147–154, 2001.

21. Cabuk D, Etoz M, Akgun IE, et al.: The evaluation of lateral pterygoid signal intensity changes related to temporomandibular joint anterior disc displacement, *Oral Radiol* 37(1):74–79, 2021.
22. Cala SJ, Kenyon CM, Lee A, et al.: Respiratory ultrasonography of human parasternal intercostal muscle in vivo, *Ultrasound Med Biol* 24:313–326, 1998.
23. Castro HA, Resende LA, Bérzin F, et al.: Electromyographic analysis of superior belly of the omohyoid muscle and anterior belly of the digastric muscle in mandibular movements, *Electromyogr Clin Neurophysiol* 38:443–447, 1998.
24. Chaves TC, Turci AM, Pinheiro CF, et al.: Static body postural misalignment in individuals with temporomandibular disorders: a systematic review, *Braz J Phys Ther* 18(6):481–501, 2014.
25. Chuhuaicura P, Lezcano MF, Dias FJ, et al.: Mandibular border movements: the two envelopes of motion, *J Oral Rehabil* 48(4):384–391, 2021.
26. Craane B, Dijkstra PU, Stappaerts K, et al.: Randomized controlled trial on physical therapy for TMJ closed lock, *J Dent Res* 91(4):364–369, 2012.
27. De Felicio CM, Mapelli A, Sidequersky FV, et al.: Mandibular kinematics and masticatory muscles: EMG in patients with short lasting TMD of mild-moderate severity, *J Electromyogr Kinesiol* 23(3):627–633, 2013.
28. De Meurechy NKG, Loos PJ, Mommaerts MY: Postoperative physiotherapy after open temporomandibular joint surgery: a 3-step program, *J Oral Maxillofac Surg* 77(5):932–950, 2019.
29. de Sa RB, Pessoa MF, Cavalcanti AGL, et al.: Immediate effects of respiratory muscle stretching on chest wall kinematics and electromyography in COPD patients, *Respir Physiol Neurobiol* 242:1–7, 2017.
30. De Troyer A, Leduc D: Role of pleural pressure in the coupling between the intercostal muscles and the ribs, *J Appl Physiol* 102(6):2332–2337, 2007.
31. De Troyer A, Wilson TA: Mechanism of the increased rib cage expansion produced by the diaphragm with abdominal support, *J Appl Physiol* 118(8):989–995, 2015.
32. De Troyer A: Relationship between neural drive and mechanical effect in the respiratory system, *Adv Exp Med Biol* 508:507–514, 2002.
33. De Troyer A, Estenne M: Functional anatomy of the respiratory muscles, *Clin Chest Med* 9:175–193, 1988.
34. De Troyer A, Gorman RB, Gandevia SC: Distribution of inspiratory drive to the external intercostal muscles in humans, *J Physiol* 546:943–954, 2003.
35. De Troyer A, Kirkwood PA, Wilson TA: Respiratory action of the intercostal muscles, *Physiol Rev* 85:717–756, 2005.
36. De Troyer A, Legrand A, Gevenois PA, et al.: Mechanical advantage of the human parasternal intercostal and triangularis sterni muscles, *J Physiol* 513:915–925, 1998.
37. De Troyer A, Ninane V, Gilmartin JJ, et al.: Triangularis sterni muscle use in supine humans, *J Appl Physiol* 62:919–925, 1987.
38. Decramer M: Hyperinflation and respiratory muscle interaction, *Eur Respir J* 10:934–941, 1997.
39. Delgado de la Serna P, Plaza-Manzano G, Cleland J, et al.: Effects of cervico-mandibular manual therapy in patients with temporomandibular pain disorders and associated somatic tinnitus: a randomized clinical trial, *Pain Med* 21(3):613–624, 2020.
40. Dergin G, Kilic C, Gozneli R, et al.: Evaluating the correlation between the lateral pterygoid muscle attachment type and internal derangement of the temporomandibular joint with an emphasis on MR imaging findings, *J Cranio-Maxillo-Fac Surg* 40(5):459–463, 2012.
41. Desmons S, Graux F, Atassi M, et al.: The lateral pterygoid muscle, a heterogeneous unit implicated in temporomandibular disorder: a literature review, *Cranio* 25:283–291, 2007.

42. Dinsdale A, Liang Z, Thomas L, et al.: Is jaw muscle activity impaired in adults with persistent temporomandibular disorders? A systematic review and meta-analysis, *J Oral Rehabil* 48(4):487–516, 2021.
43. Dipp T, Macagnan FE, Schardong J, et al.: Short period of high-intensity inspiratory muscle training improves inspiratory muscle strength in patients with chronic kidney disease on hemodialysis: a randomized controlled Trial, *Braz J Phys Ther* 24(3):280–286, 2020.
44. Dong Z, Liu Y, Gai Y, et al.: Early rehabilitation relieves diaphragm dysfunction induced by prolonged mechanical ventilation: a randomised control study, *BMC Pulm Med* 21(1):106, 2021.
45. Dos Reis IMM, Ohara DG, Januário LB, et al.: Surface electromyography in inspiratory muscles in adults and elderly individuals: a systematic review, *J Electromyogr Kinesiol* 44:139–155, 2019.
46. Duprey S, Subit D, Guillemot H, et al.: Biomechanical properties of the costovertebral joint, *Med Eng Phys* 32(2):222–227, 2010.
47. Estenne M, De Troyer A: Relationship between respiratory muscle electromyogram and rib cage motion in tetraplegia, *Am Rev Respir Dis* 132:53–59, 1985.
48. Ferrario VF, Sforza C, Miani Jr A, et al.: Open-close movements in the human temporomandibular joint: does a pure rotation around the intercondylar hinge axis exist? *J Oral Rehabil* 23:401–408, 1996.
49. Finucane KE, Panizza JA, Singh B: Efficiency of the normal human diaphragm with hyperinflation, *J Appl Physiol* 99:1402–1411, 2005.
50. Fisch G, Finke A, Ragonese J, et al.: Outcomes of physical therapy in patients with temporomandibular disorder: a retrospective review, *Br J Oral Maxillofac Surg* 59(2):145–150, 2021.
51. Frazão M, Santos ADC, Araújo AA, et al.: Neuromuscular efficiency is impaired during exercise in COPD patients, *Respir Physiol Neurobiol* 290:103673, 2021.
52. Furto ES, Cleland JA, Whitman JM, et al.: Manual physical therapy interventions and exercise for patients with temporomandibular disorders, *Cranio* 24:283–291, 2006.
53. Gandevia SC, Hudson AL, Gorman RB, et al.: Spatial distribution of inspiratory drive to the parasternal intercostal muscles in humans, *J Physiol* 573:263–275, 2006.
54. Gayan-Ramirez G, Testelmans D, Maes K, et al.: Intermittent spontaneous breathing protects the rat diaphragm from mechanical ventilation effects, *Crit Care Med* 33:2804–2809, 2005.
55. Gokalp H, Turkkahraman H, Bzeizi N: Correlation between eminence steepness and condyle disc movements in temporomandibular joints with internal derangements on magnetic resonance imaging, *Eur J Orthod* 23:579–584, 2001.
56. Haggman-Henrikson B, Rezvani M, List T: Prevalence of whiplash trauma in TMD patients: a systematic review, *J Oral Rehabil* 41:59–68, 2014.
57. Hamaoui A, Hudson AL, Laviolette L, et al.: Postural disturbances resulting from unilateral and bilateral diaphragm contractions: a phrenic nerve stimulation study, *J Appl Physiol* 117(8):825–883, 2014.
58. Hansdottir R, Bakke M: Joint tenderness, jaw opening, chewing velocity, and bite force in patients with temporomandibular joint pain and matched healthy control subjects, *J Orofac Pain* 18:108–113, 2004.
59. Hansson T, Oberg T, Carlsson GE, et al.: Thickness of the soft tissue layers and the articular disk in the temporomandibular joint, *Acta Odontol Scand* 35:77–83, 1977.
60. Harrison AL, Thorp JN, Ritzline PD: A proposed diagnostic classification of patients with temporomandibular disorders: implications for physical therapists, *J Orthop Sports Phys Ther* 44(3):182–197, 2014.
61. Hawkes EZ, Nowicky AV, McConnell AK: Diaphragm and intercostal surface EMG and muscle performance after acute inspiratory muscle loading, *Respir Physiol Neurobiol* 155:213–219, 2007.

62. Hodges PW, Butler JE, McKenzie DK, et al.: Contraction of the human diaphragm during rapid postural adjustments, *J Physiol (Lond)* 505(Pt 2):539–548, 1997.

63. Hodges PW, Cresswell AG, Daggfeldt K, et al.: In vivo measurement of the effect of intra-abdominal pressure on the human spine, *J Biomech* 34:347–353, 2001.

64. Hudson AL, Butler JE, Gandevia SC, et al.: Interplay between the inspiratory and postural functions of the human parasternal intercostal muscles, *J Neurophysiol* 103(3):1622–1629, 2010.

65. Hudson AL, Gandevia SC, Butler JE: Task-Dependent output of human parasternal intercostal motor units across spinal levels, *J Physiol* 595(23):7081–7092, 2017.

66. Hudson AL, Gandevia SC, Butler JE: The effect of lung volume on the co-ordinated recruitment of scalene and sternomastoid muscles in humans, *J Physiol* 584:261–270, 2007.

67. Hugger S, Schindler HJ, Kordass B, et al.: Clinical relevance of surface EMG of the masticatory muscles. (Part 1): resting activity, maximal and submaximal voluntary contraction, symmetry of EMG activity [Review], *Int J Comput Dent* 15(4):297–314, 2012.

68. Hugger S, Schindler HJ, Kordass B, et al.: Surface EMG of the masticatory muscles. (Part 4): effects of occlusal splints and other treatment modalities [Review], *Int J Comput Dent* 16(3):225–239, 2013.

69. Iizuka M: Respiration-related control of abdominal motoneurons [Review], *Respir Physiol Neurobiol* 179(1):80–88, 2011.

70. Ioi H, Matsumoto R, Nishioka M, et al.: Relationship of TMJ osteoarthritis/osteoarthrosis to head posture and dentofacial morphology, *Orthod Craniofac Res* 11:8–16, 2008.

71. Ismail F, Demling A, Hessling K, et al.: Short-term efficacy of physical therapy compared to splint therapy in treatment of arthrogenous TMD, *J Oral Rehabil* 34:807–813, 2007.

72. Iwasaki LR, Crosby MJ, Marx DB, et al.: Human temporomandibular joint eminence shape and load minimization, *J Dent Res* 89(7):722–727, 2010.

73. Janssens L, Brumagne S, McConnell AK, et al.: Greater diaphragm fatigability in individuals with recurrent low back pain, *Respir Physiol Neurobiol* 188(2):119–123, 2013.

74. Janssens L, Brumagne S, Polspoel K, et al.: The effect of inspiratory muscles fatigue on postural control in people with and without recurrent low back pain, *Spine* 35(10):1088–1094, 2010.

75. Jung B, Constantin JM, Rossel N, et al.: Adaptive support ventilation prevents ventilator-induce diaphragmatic dysfunction in piglet: an in vivo and in vitro study, *Anesthesiology* 112:1435–1443, 2010.

76. Kasawara KT, Castellanos MM, Hanada M, et al.: Pathophysiology of muscle in pulmonary and cardiovascular conditions, *Cardiopulm Phys Ther J* 30:4–14, 2019.

77. Kocjan J, Adamek M, Gzik-Zroska B, et al.: Network of breathing. multifunctional role of the diaphragm: a Review, *Adv Respir Med* 85(4):224–232, 2017.

78. Kolar P, Sulc J, Kyncl M, et al.: Stabilizing function of the diaphragm: dynamic MRI and synchronized spirometric assessment, *J Appl Physiol* 109:1064–1071, 2010.

79. Kolar P, Sulc J, Kyncl M, et al.: Postural function of the diaphragm in persons with and without chronic low back pain, *J Orthop Sports Phys Ther* 42(4):352–362, 2012.

80. Kraus S, Prodoehl J: Outcomes and patient satisfaction following individualized physical therapy treatment for patients diagnosed with temporomandibular disc displacement without reduction with limited opening: a cross-sectional study, *Cranio* 37(1):20–27, 2019.

81. Lafreniere CM, Lamontagne M, el Sawy R: The role of the lateral pterygoid muscles in TMJ disorders during static conditions, *Cranio* 15:38–52, 1997.

82. Laveneziana P, Albuquerque A, Aliverti A, et al.: ERS statement on respiratory muscle testing at rest and during exercise, *Eur Respir J* 53(6):06, 2019.

83. Lee LJ, Chang AT, Coppieters MW, et al.: Changes in sitting posture induce multiplanar changes in chest wall shape and motion with breathing, *Respir Physiol Neurobiol* 170(3):236–245, 2010.

84. Lee YH, Lee KM, Auh QS, et al.: Sex-Related differences in symptoms of temporomandibular disorders and structural changes in the lateral pterygoid muscle after whiplash injury, *J Oral Rehabil* 46(12):1107–1120, 2019.

85. Lemosse D, Le Rue O, Diop A, et al.: Characterization of the mechanical behaviour parameters of the costovertebral joint, *Eur Spine J* 7:16–23, 1998.

86. Liebsch C, Graf N, Wilke HJ: In vitro analysis of kinematics and elastostatics of the human rib cage during thoracic spinal movement for the validation of numerical models, *J Biomech* 94:147–157, 2019.

87. List T, Jensen RH: Temporomandibular disorders: old ideas and new concepts, *Cephalalgia* 37(7):692–704, 2017.

88. Lozano-García M, Sarlabous L, Moxham J, et al.: Surface mechanomyography and electromyography provide non-invasive indices of inspiratory muscle force and activation in healthy subjects, *Sci Rep* 8(1):16921, 2018.

89. Luu BL, Saboisky JP, Taylor JL, et al.: Supraspinal fatigue in human inspiratory muscles with repeated sustained maximal efforts, *J Appl Physiol* 129(6):1365–1372, 2020.

90. MacBean V, Jolley CJ, Sutton TG, et al.: Parasternal intercostal electromyography: a novel tool to assess respiratory load in children, *Pediatr Res* 80(3):407–414, 2016.

91. Magnusson T, Egermark I, Carlsson GE: A longitudinal epidemiologic study of signs and symptoms of temporomandibular disorders from 15 to 35 years of age, *J Orofac Pain* 14(4):310–319, 2000.

92. Mahan PE, Wilkinson TM, Gibbs CH, et al.: Superior and inferior bellies of the lateral pterygoid muscle EMG activity at basic jaw positions, *J Prosthet Dent* 50:710–718, 1983.

93. Mapelli A, Galante D, Lovecchio N, et al.: Translation and rotation movements of the mandible during mouth opening and closing, *Clin Anat* 22(3):311–318, 2009.

94. McLean L: The effect of postural correction on muscle activation amplitudes recorded from the cervicobrachial region, *J Electromyogr Kinesiol* 15:527–535, 2005.

95. Mendes LPS, Vieira DSR, Gabriel LS, et al.: Influence of posture, sex, and age on breathing pattern and chest wall motion in healthy subjects, *Braz J Phys Ther* 24(3):240–248, 2020.

96. Mesnard M, Coutant JC, Aoun M, et al.: Relationships between geometry and kinematic characteristics in the temporomandibular joint, *Comput Methods Biomech Biomed Eng* 15(4):393–400, 2012.

97. Minakuchi H, Kuboki T, Matsuka Y, et al.: Randomized controlled evaluation of non-surgical treatments for temporomandibular joint anterior disk displacement without reduction, *J Dent Res* 80:924–928, 2001.

98. Mizuno M: Human respiratory muscles: fibre morphology and capillary supply, *Eur Respir J* 4:587–601, 1991.

99. Moayedi M, Krishnamoorthy G, He PT, et al.: Structural abnormalities in the temporalis musculoaponeurotic complex in chronic muscular temporomandibular disorders, *Pain* 161(8):1787–1797, 2020.

100. Moleirinho-Alves PMM, Almeida A, Exposto FG, et al.: Effects of therapeutic exercise and aerobic exercise programmes on pain, anxiety and oral health-related quality of life in patients with temporomandibular disorders, *J Oral Rehabil* 48(11):1201–1209, 2021.

101. Munhoz WC, Hsing WT: The inconclusiveness of research on functional pathologies of the temporomandibular system and body posture: paths followed, paths ahead: a critical review, *Cranio* 39(3):254–265, 2021.

102. Murray GM, Bhutada M, Peck CC, et al.: The human lateral pterygoid muscle, *Arch Oral Biol* 52:377–380, 2007.

103. Neumann DA: Polio: its impact on the people of the United States and the emerging profession of physical therapy, *J Orthop Sports Phys Ther* 34(8):479–492, 2004.

104. Neumann DA: Use of diaphragm to assist rolling for the patient with quadriplegia, *Phys Ther* 59(1):39, 1979.

105. Nguyen DAT, Lewis RHC, Boswell-Ruys CL, et al.: Increased diaphragm motor unit discharge frequencies during quiet breathing in people with chronic tetraplegia, *J Physiol* 598(11):2243–2256, 2020.

106. NSCISC: Spinal cord injury facts and figures at a glance, *J Spinal Cord Med* 36:1–2, 2013.

107. Oberg T, Carlsson GE, Fajers CM: The temporomandibular joint. A morphologic study on a human autopsy material, *Acta Odontol Scand* 29(3):349–384, 1971.

108. Okeson JP: *Management of temporomandibular disorders and occlusion*, ed 8, St Louis, 2020, Elsevier.

109. Orlando B, Manfredini D, Salvetti G, et al.: Evaluation of the effectiveness of biobehavioral therapy in the treatment of temporomandibular disorders: a literature review, *Behav Med* 33:101–118, 2007.

110. Osborn JW: The temporomandibular ligament and the articular eminence as constraints during jaw opening, *J Oral Rehabil* 16:323–333, 1989.

111. Ovechkin A, Vitaz T, de Paleville DT, et al.: Evaluation of respiratory muscle activation in individuals with chronic spinal cord injury, *Respir Physiol Neurobiol* 173(3):171–178, 2010.

112. Peck CC, Murray GM, Johnson CW, et al.: Trajectories of condylar points during working-side excursive movements of the mandible, *J Prosthet Dent* 81(4):444–452, 1999.

113. Phanachet I, Whittle T, Wanigaratne K, et al.: Functional properties of single motor units in the inferior head of human lateral pterygoid muscle: task firing rates, *J Neurophysiol* 88:751–760, 2002.

114. Piehslinger E, Celar AG, Celar RM, et al.: Computerized axiography: principles and methods, *Cranio* 9:344–355, 1991.

115. Powers SK, Kavazis AN, Levine S: Prolonged mechanical ventilation alters diaphragmatic structure and function, *Crit Care Med* 37:S347–353, 2009.

116. Powers SK, Smuder AJ, Fuller D, et al.: CrossTalk proposal: mechanical ventilation-induced diaphragm atrophy is primarily due to inactivity, *J Physiol* 591:5255–5257, 2013.

117. Radke JC, Kamyszek GJ, Kull RS, et al.: TMJ symptoms reduce chewing amplitude and velocity and increase variability, *Cranio* 37(1):12–19, 2019.

118. Radke JC, Kull RS, Sethi MS: Chewing movements altered in the presence of temporomandibular joint internal derangements, *Cranio* 32(3):187–192, 2014.

119. Ratnovsky A, Elad D: Anatomical model of the human trunk for analysis of respiratory muscles mechanics, *Respir Physiol Neurobiol* 148:245–262, 2005.

120. Reneker J, Paz J, Petrosino C, et al.: Diagnostic accuracy of clinical tests and signs of temporomandibular joint disorders: a systematic review of the literature [Review], *J Orthop Sports Phys Ther* 41(6):408–416, 2011.

121. Robinson PD: Articular cartilage of the temporomandibular joint: can it regenerate? *Ann R Coll Surg Engl* 75:231–236, 1993.

122. Rocabado M: Arthrokinematics of the temporomandibular joint, *Dent Clin North Am* 27:573–594, 1983.

123. Rues S, Lenz J, Turp JC, et al.: Muscle and joint forces under variable equilibrium states of the mandible, *Clin Oral Investig* 15(5):737–747, 2011.

124. Rutka M, Adamczyk WM, Linek P: Effects of physical therapist intervention on pulmonary function in children with cerebral palsy: a systematic review and meta-analysis, *Phys Ther* 101(8), 2021.

125. Saboisky JP, Butler JE, Fogel RB, et al.: Tonic and phasic respiratory drives to human genioglossus motoneurons during breathing, *J Neurophysiol* 95:2213–2221, 2006.

126. Saboisky JP, Gorman RB, De Troyer A, et al.: Differential activation among five human inspiratory

motoneuron pools during tidal breathing, *J Appl Physiol* 102:772–780, 2007.

127. Sakaguchi K, Taguchi N, Kobayashi R, et al.: Immediate curative effects of exercise therapy in patients with myalgia of the masticatory muscles, *J Oral Rehabil* 49(10):937–943, 2022.
128. Schiffman E, Ohrbach R, Truelove E, et al.: Diagnostic criteria for temporomandibular disorders (DC/TMD) for clinical and research applications: recommendations of the international RDC/TMD consortium network and orofacial pain special interest group, *J Oral Facial Pain Headache* 28(1):6–27, 2014.
129. Schiffman EL, Truelove EL, Ohrbach R, et al.: The research diagnostic criteria for temporomandibular disorders: overview and methodology for assessment of validity, *J Orofac Pain* 24(1):7–24, 2010.
130. Shimada A, Ishigaki S, Matsuka Y, et al.: Effects of exercise therapy on painful temporomandibular disorders, *J Oral Rehabil* 46(5):475–481, 2019.
131. Sieck GC, Mantilla CB: CrossTalk opposing view: the diaphragm muscle does not atrophy as a result of inactivity, *J Physiol* 591:5259–5262, 2013.
132. Sinn DP, de Assis EA, Throckmorton GS: Mandibular excursions and maximum bite forces in patients with temporomandibular joint disorders, *J Oral Maxillofac Surg* 54:671–679, 1996.
133. Sobreira M, Almeida MP, Gomes A, et al.: Minimal clinically important differences for measures of pain, lung function, fatigue, and functionality in spinal cord injury, *Phys Ther* 101(2), 2021.
134. Souza H, Rocha T, Pessoa M, et al.: Effects of inspiratory muscle training in elderly women on respiratory muscle strength, diaphragm thickness and mobility, *J Gerontol A Biol Sci Med Sci* 69(12):1545–1553, 2014.
135. Standring S: *Gray's anatomy: the anatomical basis of clinical practice*, ed 42, St Louis, 2021, Elsevier.
136. Stimmer H, Grill F, Goetz C, et al.: Lesions of the lateral pterygoid muscle-an overestimated reason for temporomandibular dysfunction: a 3T magnetic resonance imaging study, *Int J Oral Maxillofac Surg* 49(12):1611–1617, 2020.
137. Takahashi S, Suzuki N, Asazuma T, et al.: Factors of thoracic cage deformity that affect pulmonary function in adolescent idiopathic thoracic scoliosis, *Spine* 32:106–112, 2007.
138. Takazakura R, Takahashi M, Nitta N, et al.: Diaphragmatic motion in the sitting and supine positions: healthy subject study using a vertically open magnetic resonance system, *J Magn Reson Imaging* 19:605–609, 2004.
139. Tanaka E, Hirose M, Inubushi T, et al.: Effect of hyperactivity of the lateral pterygoid muscle on the temporomandibular joint disk, *J Biomech Eng* 129:890–897, 2007.
140. Taskaya-Yilmaz N, Ceylan G, Incesu L, et al.: A possible etiology of the internal derangement of the temporomandibular joint based on the MRI observations of the lateral pterygoid muscle, *Surg Radiol Anat* 27:19–24, 2005.
141. Tuijt M, Koolstra JH, Lobbezoo F, et al.: Differences in loading of the temporomandibular joint during opening and closing of the jaw, *J Biomech* 43(6):1048–1054, 2010.
142. Urmey W, Loring S, Mead J, et al.: Upper and lower rib cage deformation during breathing in quadriplegics, *J Appl Physiol* 60:618–622, 1986.
143. Vassilakopoulos T, Zakynthinos S, Roussos C: Respiratory muscles and weaning failure, *Eur Respir J* 9:2383–2400, 1996.
144. Villaca Avoglio JL: Dental occlusion as one cause of tinnitus, *Med Hypotheses* 130:109280, 2019.
145. von Piekartz H, Schwiddessen J, Reineke L, et al.: International consensus on the most useful assessments used by physical therapists to evaluate patients with temporomandibular disorders: a delphi study, *J Oral Rehabil* 47(6):685–702, 2020.
146. Washino S, Mankyu H, Kanehisa H, et al.: Effects of inspiratory muscle strength and inspiratory resistance on neck inspiratory muscle activation during controlled inspirations, *Exp Physiol* 104(4):556–567, 2019.
147. West CR, Campbell IG, Shave RE, et al.: Effects of abdominal binding on cardiorespiratory function in cervical spinal cord injury, *Respir Physiol Neurobiol* 180(2–3):275–282, 2012.
148. Westersund CD, Scholten J, Turner RJ: Relationship between craniocervical orientation and center of force of occlusion in adults, *Cranio* 35(5):283–289, 2017.
149. Wilson TA, Legrand A, Gevenois PA, et al.: Respiratory effects of the external and internal intercostal muscles in humans, *J Physiol* 530:319–330, 2001.
150. Wink CS, St OM, Zimny ML: Neural elements in the human temporomandibular articular disc, *J Oral Maxillofac Surg* 50:334–337, 1992.
151. Yustin DC, Rieger MR, McGuckin RS, et al.: Determination of the existence of hinge movements of the temporomandibular joint during normal opening by Cine-MRI and computer digital addition, *J Prosthodont* 2:190–195, 1993.
152. Zaugg M, Lucchinetti E: Respiratory function in the elderly, *Anesthesiol Clin North Am* 18:47–58, 2000.
153. Zeleznik J: Normative aging of the respiratory system, *Clin Geriatr Med* 19:1–18, 2003.
154. Zhang G, Chen X, Ohgi J, et al.: Effect of intercostal muscle contraction on rib motion in humans studied by finite element analysis, *J Appl Physiol* 125(4):1165–1170, 2018.

STUDY QUESTIONS

PART 1: MASTICATION

1. Explain the mechanism by which the intermediate region of the articular disc within the temporomandibular joints protects the joint throughout the late phase of opening the mouth.
2. Compare the distal attachments of the medial and lateral pterygoid muscles. Which attachments form a "functional sling" with the masseter muscle?
3. Explain, in theory, how an overly depressed scapulothoracic joint could predispose derangement of the articular disc of the TMJ.
4. Compare the different functional demands placed on the dome of the mandibular fossa and the articular eminence of the temporal bone while chewing.
5. Describe the functional role of the oblique fibers of the lateral ligament of the TMJ during opening the mouth.
6. Explain the function of the temporalis muscles in closing the mouth.
7. Describe the synergistic relationship between the masseter and contralateral medial pterygoid muscle during the production of shearing (grinding) force between the molars.
8. Using Fig. 11.22 as a guide, describe the specific function of the lateral pterygoid muscle during opening and closing of the mouth.
9. Describe how the inferior head of the lateral pterygoid muscle and the suprahyoid muscles act synergistically during a rapid opening of the mouth.
10. List the bones that make up temporal fossa of the cranium.

PART 2: VENTILATION

11. Describe the function of the diaphragm muscle during inspiration, and explain why it is considered the most important muscle of ventilation.
12. Explain how the sternal head of the pectoralis major could function as an effective muscle of forced inspiration.
13. How could a chronically lowered (flattened) diaphragm muscle negatively affect the mechanics of ventilation?
14. List the articulations that can alter the anterior-posterior and medial-lateral dimensions of the thorax during ventilation.
15. What structures seal the inferior and superior poles of the thoracic cavity?
16. Explain how the normal "tone" within the abdominal muscles contributes to the mechanics of inspiration.
17. How does paralysis of the intercostal muscles in a person with tetraplegia (quadriplegia) contribute to the pathomechanics of "paradoxical breathing"?
18. Describe the changes in intrathoracic and intra-abdominal pressure during forced expiration.
19. List factors explaining why quiet expiration is considered a "passive" process.
20. List the muscles most likely rendered fully paralyzed after a complete spinal cord lesion at the level of T4.

Answers to the study questions are available in the accompanying enhanced eBook version included with the print purchase of this textbook.

Additional Video Educational Content

- Videofluoroscopy of the Temporomandibular Joint (TMJ) in an Asymptomatic Adult Male while Opening and Closing the Mouth.

ALL VIDEOS in this chapter are available in the accompanying enhanced eBook version included with the print purchase of this textbook.

Reference Materials for the Cauda Equina, and Attachments, Innervations, and Selected Moment Arms of Muscles of the Axial Skeleton

Part A:
Formation of the Cauda Equina

Part B:
Thoracic Dermatomes of the Trunk

Part C:
Attachments and Innervation of the Muscles of the Axial Skeleton

  Muscles of the Trunk
   Set 1: Muscles of the Posterior Trunk
   Set 2: Muscles of the Anterior-Lateral Trunk: "Abdominal" Muscles
  Muscles of the Craniocervical Region
   Set 1: Muscles of the Anterior-Lateral Craniocervical Region
   Set 2: Muscles of the Posterior Craniocervical Region
  Miscellaneous: Quadratus Lumborum
  Primary Muscles of Mastication
  Suprahyoid Muscles
  Infrahyoid Muscles
  Muscles Related Primarily to Ventilation

Part D:
Moment Arm Data for Selected Craniocervical Muscles

Part A: Formation of the Cauda Equina

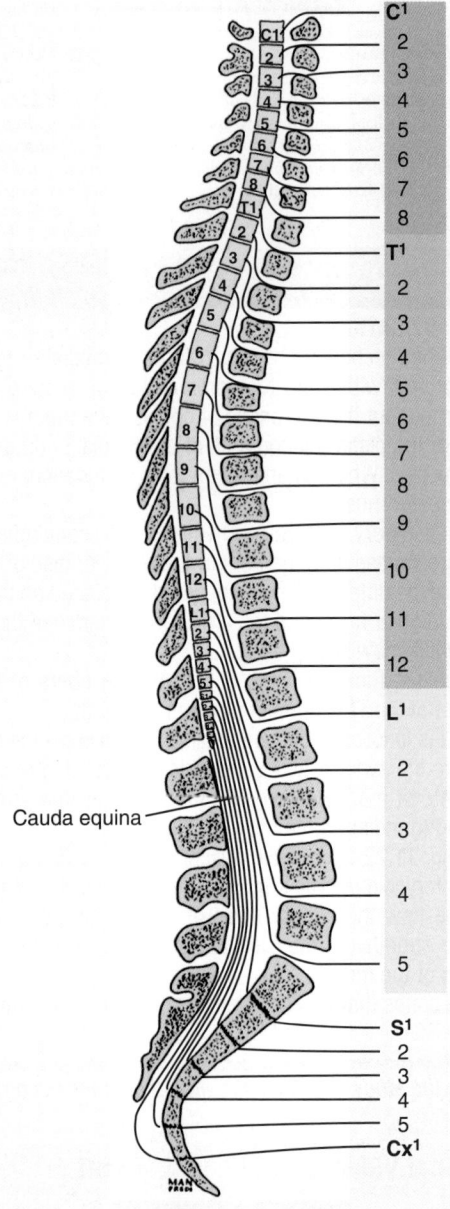

FIGURE III.1 The anatomic relationship of the spinal cord and spinal nerve roots to the bony elements of the vertebral column. The spinal cord is shown in yellow, and spinal nerve roots are shown in black. The intervertebral foramina through which the spinal nerve roots pass are shown in multiple colors on the right. In the adult, the spinal cord is shorter than the vertebral column. The lumbar and sacral nerve roots must therefore travel a considerable distance before each reaches its corresponding intervertebral foramen. These spinal nerve roots coursing through the vertebral canal of the lumbar and sacral vertebrae are called the *cauda equina*. Note that the spinal cord terminates at the L1–L2 intervertebral foramen, cranial to the cauda equina. (From Haymaker W, Woodhall B: *Peripheral nerve injuries,* ed 2, Philadelphia, 1953, Saunders.)

Part B: Thoracic Dermatomes of the Trunk

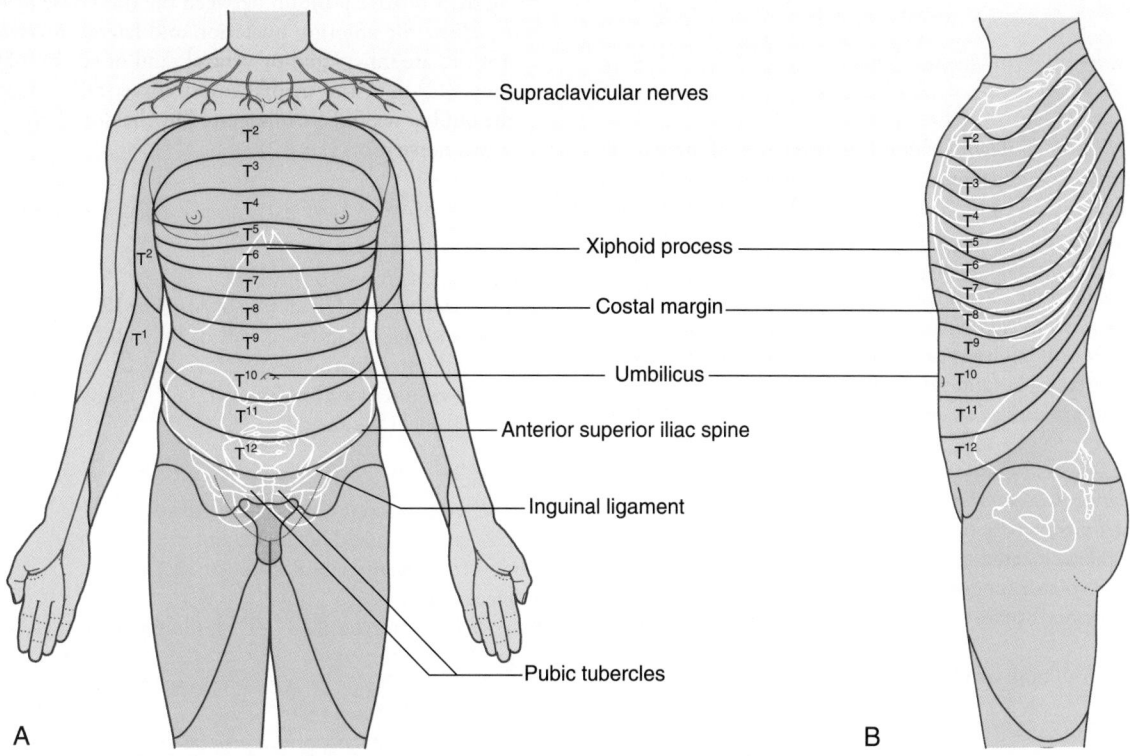

FIGURE III.2 The thoracic dermatomes of the trunk. (A) Anterior view. (B) Lateral view. T^1, First thoracic nerve root, and so on. (From Drake R, Vogl W, Mitchell A: *Gray's anatomy for students,* ed 3, Philadelphia, 2015, Churchill Livingstone.)

Part C: Attachments and Innervation of the Muscles of the Axial Skeleton

MUSCLES OF THE TRUNK

SET 1: MUSCLES OF THE POSTERIOR TRUNK

See Appendix II for attachments and innervations of the muscles in the superficial layer of the posterior trunk (trapezius, latissimus dorsi, serratus anterior, and so forth).

Erector Spinae Group (Iliocostalis, Longissimus, and Spinalis Muscles)

Iliocostalis Lumborum
Inferior attachment: common tendon*
Superior attachments: angle of ribs 6 to 12

Iliocostalis Thoracis
Inferior attachments: angle of ribs 6 to 12
Superior attachments: angle of ribs 1 to 6

---

*The broad common tendon connects the inferior end of most of the erector spinae to the base of the axial skeleton. The specific attachments of the tendon include the sacrum, spinous processes and supraspinous ligaments in the lower thoracic and entire lumbar region, iliac crest and tuberosities, sacrotuberous and sacroiliac ligaments, gluteus maximus, and multifidus muscle.

Iliocostalis Cervicis
Inferior attachments: angle of ribs 3 to 7
Superior attachments: posterior tubercles of the transverse processes of C4 to C6

Longissimus Thoracis
Inferior attachment: common tendon
Superior attachments: tubercle and angle of ribs 3 to 12; transverse processes of T1 to T12

Longissimus Cervicis
Inferior attachments: transverse processes of T1 to T4
Superior attachments: posterior tubercles of the transverse processes of C2 to C6

Longissimus Capitis
Inferior attachments: transverse processes of T1 to T5 and articular processes of C4 to C7
Superior attachments: posterior margin of the mastoid process of the temporal bone

Spinalis Thoracis
Inferior attachment: common tendon
Superior attachments: spinous processes of most thoracic vertebrae

Spinalis Cervicis
Inferior attachments: ligamentum nuchae and spinous processes of C7 to T1
Superior attachment: spinous process of C2

Spinalis Capitis (Blends with Semispinalis Capitis)

Innervation to the erector spinae: dorsal rami of adjacent spinal nerve roots (C^3–L^5)

Transversospinal Group (Multifidus, Rotatores, and Semispinalis Muscles)

Multifidus

Inferior attachments (lumbar): mammillary processes of lumbar vertebrae, lumbosacral ligaments, deep part of the common tendon of the erector spinae, posterior surface of the sacrum, posterior-superior iliac spine of the pelvis, and capsule of the lumbar and lumbosacral apophyseal joints
Inferior attachments (thoracic): transverse processes of T1 to T12
Inferior attachments (cervical): articular processes of C3 to C7
Superior attachments: spinous processes of vertebrae located two to four intervertebral junctions superior
Innervation: dorsal rami of adjacent spinal nerve roots (C^4–S^3)

Rotatores: Longus and Brevis

Inferior attachments: transverse processes of all vertebrae
Superior attachments: base of spinous processes and adjacent laminae of vertebrae located one or two segments superior
NOTE: The rotator longus crosses two intervertebral junctions; the more horizontal rotator brevis crosses only one intervertebral junction.
Innervation: dorsal rami of adjacent spinal nerve roots (C^4–L^4)

Semispinalis Thoracis

Inferior attachments: transverse processes of T6 to T10
Superior attachments: spinous processes of C6 to T4

Semispinalis Cervicis

Inferior attachments: transverse processes of T1 to T6
Superior attachments: spinous processes of C2 to C5, primarily C2

Semispinalis Capitis

Inferior attachments: transverse processes of C7 to T7
Superior attachments: articular processes of C4–C6; continuing cranially to attach between the superior and inferior nuchal lines of the occipital bone
Innervation to the semispinalis muscles: dorsal rami of adjacent spinal nerve roots (C^1–T^6)

Short Segmental Group (Interspinalis and Intertransversarius Muscles)

Interspinalis Muscles

These paired muscles attach regularly between adjacent spinous processes within the cervical vertebrae (except C1 and C2) and the lumbar vertebrae. In the thoracic spine, the interspinalis muscles exist only at the extreme upper and lower regions.
Innervation: dorsal rami of adjacent spinal nerve roots (C^3–L^5)

Intertransversarius Muscles

These paired right and left muscles attach between adjacent transverse processes of all cervical, lower thoracic, and lumbar vertebrae. In the cervical region, the intertransversarius muscles are subdivided into small anterior and posterior muscles, indicating their position relative to the anterior and posterior tubercles of the transverse processes, respectively. In the lumbar region the intertransversarius muscles are subdivided into small lateral and medial muscles, indicating their relative position between the transverse processes.
Innervation: the anterior, posterior, and lateral intertransversarius muscles are innervated by ventral rami of adjacent spinal nerve roots (C^3–L^5); the medial intertransversarius muscles, within the lumbar region, are innervated by the dorsal rami of adjacent spinal nerve roots (L^1–L^5)

SET 2: MUSCLES OF THE ANTERIOR-LATERAL TRUNK: "ABDOMINAL" MUSCLES

Obliquus Externus Abdominis

Lateral attachments: lateral side of ribs 5 to 12
Medial attachments: anterior half of the outer lip of the iliac crest, linea alba and contralateral rectus sheath
Innervation: intercostal nerves (T^8–T^{12}), iliohypogastric (L^1), and ilioinguinal (L^1) nerves

Obliquus Internus Abdominis

Lateral attachments: anterior two-thirds of the middle lip of the iliac crest, inguinal ligament, and the thoracolumbar fascia
Medial attachments: ribs 9 to 11 (or 12), linea alba and contralateral rectus sheath
Innervation: intercostal (T^8–T^{12}), iliohypogastric (L^1), and ilioinguinal (L^1) nerves

Rectus Abdominis

Superior attachments: xiphoid process and cartilages of ribs 5 to 7
Inferior attachments: crest of pubis and adjacent ligaments supporting the pubic symphysis joint
Innervation: intercostal nerves (T^7–T^{12})

Transversus Abdominis

Lateral attachments: anterior two-thirds of the inner lip of the iliac crest, thoracolumbar fascia, inner surface of the cartilages of ribs 6 to 12, and inguinal ligament
Medial attachments: linea alba and contralateral rectus sheath
Innervation: intercostal (T^7–T^{12}), iliohypogastric (L^1), and ilioinguinal (L^1) nerves

MUSCLES OF THE CRANIOCERVICAL REGION

SET 1: MUSCLES OF THE ANTERIOR-LATERAL CRANIOCERVICAL REGION

Longus Capitis

Inferior attachments: anterior tubercles of transverse processes of C3 to C6
Superior attachment: inferior surface of the basilar part of the occipital bone, immediately anterior to the attachment of the rectus capitis anterior
Innervation: ventral rami of spinal nerve roots C^1–C^3

Longus Colli

Superior Oblique Portion
Inferior attachments: anterior tubercles of transverse processes of C3 to C5
Superior attachment: tubercle on anterior arch of C1

Vertical Portion

Inferior attachments: anterior surface of the bodies of C5 to T3
Superior attachments: anterior surface of the bodies of C2 to C4

Inferior Oblique Portion

Inferior attachments: anterior surface of the bodies of T1 to T3
Superior attachments: anterior tubercles of transverse processes of C5 to C6
Innervation: ventral rami of adjacent spinal nerve roots (C^2–C^8)

Rectus Capitis Anterior

Inferior attachment: anterior surface of the transverse process of C1
Superior attachment: inferior surface of the basilar part of the occipital bone immediately anterior to the occipital condyle
Innervation: ventral rami of spinal nerve roots C^1–C^2

Rectus Capitis Lateralis

Inferior attachment: superior surface of the transverse process of C1
Superior attachment: inferior surface of the occipital bone immediately lateral to the occipital condyle
Innervation: ventral rami of spinal nerve roots C^1–C^2

Scalenes

Scalenus Anterior

Superior attachments: anterior tubercles of the transverse processes of C3 to C6
Inferior attachment: inner border of the anterior-lateral aspect of the first rib (scalene tubercle)

Scalenus Medius

Superior attachments: posterior tubercles of the transverse processes of C2 to C7
Inferior attachment: upper border of the first rib, near its angle; posterior to the attachment of the scalenus anterior

Scalenus Posterior

Superior attachments: posterior tubercles of the transverse processes of C5 to C7
Inferior attachment: external surface of the second rib, near its angle
Innervation to the scalene muscles: ventral rami of adjacent spinal nerve roots (C^3–C^7)

Sternocleidomastoid

Inferior attachments: sternal head, anterior surface of the upper aspect of the manubrium of the sternum; clavicular head; posterior-superior surface of the medial one-third of the clavicle
Superior attachments: lateral surface of the mastoid process of the temporal bone and lateral one-half of the superior nuchal line of the occipital bone
Innervation: spinal accessory nerve (cranial nerve XI); a secondary source of innervation is through the ventral rami of nerve roots from the mid-and-upper cervical plexus, which may carry sensory (proprioceptive) information

Splenius Capitis

Inferior attachments: inferior half of the ligamentum nuchae and spinous processes of C7 to T4
Superior attachments: mastoid process of the temporal bone and the lateral one-third of the superior nuchal line of the occipital bone
Innervation: dorsal rami of spinal nerve roots C^2–C^8

Splenius Cervicis

Inferior attachments: spinous processes of T3 to T6
Superior attachments: Transverse processes of C1-2 and posterior tubercle of the transverse process of C3
Innervation: dorsal rami of spinal nerve roots C^2–C^8

Suboccipital Muscles

Obliquus Capitis Inferior

Inferior attachment: apex of the spinous process of C2
Superior attachment: inferior margin of the transverse process of C1

Obliquus Capitis Superior

Inferior attachment: superior margin of the transverse process of C1
Superior attachments: between the lateral end of the inferior and superior nuchal lines

Rectus Capitis Posterior Major

Inferior attachment: spinous process of C2
Superior attachment: immediately anterior and medial to the lateral end of the inferior nuchal line

Rectus Capitis Posterior Minor

Inferior attachment: tubercle on the posterior arch of C1
Superior attachment: immediately anterior to the medial end of the inferior nuchal line, just posterior to the foramen magnum
Innervation to suboccipital muscles: suboccipital nerve (dorsal ramus of spinal nerve root C^1)

MISCELLANEOUS: QUADRATUS LUMBORUM

Quadratus Lumborum

Inferior attachments: iliolumbar ligament and crest of the ilium
Superior attachments: rib 12 and tips of the transverse processes of L1 to L4
Innervation: ventral ramus of spinal nerve roots T^{12}–L^3

PRIMARY MUSCLES OF MASTICATION

Masseter: Combined Superficial and Deep Heads

Proximal attachments: lateral-inferior surfaces of the zygomatic bone and inferior surfaces of the zygomatic arch
Distal attachment: external surface of the mandible, between the angle and just below the coronoid process
Innervation: branch of the mandibular nerve, a division of cranial nerve V

Temporalis
Proximal attachments: temporal fossa and deep surfaces of temporal fascia
Distal attachments: apex and medial surfaces of the coronoid process of the mandible and the entire anterior edge of the ramus of the mandible
Innervation: branch of the mandibular nerve, a division of cranial nerve V

Medial Pterygoid: Combined Superficial and Deep Heads
Proximal attachments: medial surface of the lateral pterygoid plate; small area on the posterior-lateral maxilla, just above the socket for the third molar
Distal attachment: internal surface of the mandible between the angle and mandibular foramen
Innervation: branch of the mandibular nerve, a division of cranial nerve V

Lateral Pterygoid (Superior Head)
Proximal attachment: greater wing of the sphenoid bone
Distal attachments: medial wall of the capsule of the temporomandibular joint (TMJ), medial side of the articular disc, and pterygoid fossa of the mandible

Lateral Pterygoid (Inferior Head)
Proximal attachments: lateral side of the lateral pterygoid plate and adjoining region of the maxilla
Distal attachments: pterygoid fossa and adjacent neck of the mandible
Innervation: branch of the mandibular nerve, a division of cranial nerve V

SUPRAHYOID MUSCLES
Digastric: Posterior Belly
Proximal attachment: mastoid notch of the temporal bone
Distal attachment: fascial sling attached to the lateral aspect of the hyoid bone
Innervation: facial nerve (cranial nerve VII)

Digastric: Anterior Belly
Proximal attachment: fascial sling attached to the lateral aspect of the hyoid bone
Distal attachment: base of the mandible near its midline (digastric fossa)
Innervation: inferior alveolar nerve (branch of the mandibular nerve, a division of cranial nerve V)

Geniohyoid
Proximal attachment: small region at the midline of the anterior aspect of the mandible's internal surface (symphysis menti)
Distal attachment: body of the hyoid bone
Innervation: C^1 via the hypoglossal nerve (cranial nerve XII)

Mylohyoid
Proximal attachment: the internal surface of the mandible, bilaterally on the mylohyoid line

Distal attachment: body of the hyoid bone
Innervation: inferior alveolar nerve (branch of the mandibular nerve, a division of cranial nerve V)

Stylohyoid
Proximal attachment: base of the styloid process of the temporal bone
Distal attachment: anterior edge of the greater horn of the hyoid bone
Innervation: facial nerve (cranial nerve VII)

INFRAHYOID MUSCLES
Omohyoid
Inferior attachment: upper border of the scapula near the scapular notch
Superior attachment: body of the hyoid bone
Innervation: ventral rami of spinal nerve roots C^1–C^3

Sternohyoid
Inferior attachments: posterior surface of the medial end of the clavicle, superior-posterior part of the manubrium sternum, and posterior sternoclavicular ligament
Superior attachment: body of the hyoid bone
Innervation: ventral rami of spinal nerve roots C^1–C^3

Sternothyroid
Inferior attachments: posterior part of the manubrium of the sternum and the cartilage of the first rib
Superior attachment: thyroid cartilage
Innervation: ventral rami of spinal nerve roots C^1–C^3

Thyrohyoid
Inferior attachment: thyroid cartilage
Superior attachment: junction of the body and greater horn of the hyoid bone
Innervation: ventral ramus of spinal nerve root C^1 (via cranial nerve XII)

MUSCLES RELATED PRIMARILY TO VENTILATION
Diaphragm
Inferior Attachments
Costal part: inner surfaces of the cartilages and adjacent bony regions of ribs 7 to 12; some fibers blend with the transversus abdominis
Sternal part: posterior side of the xiphoid process
Crural (lumbar) part: (1) two aponeurotic arches covering the external surfaces of the quadratus lumborum and psoas major muscles; (2) right and left crus, originating from the bodies of L1 to 3 and their intervertebral discs

Superior Attachment
Central tendon near the center of the dome of the muscle
Innervation: phrenic nerve (C^3–C^5)

Intercostales Externi

Attachments: Eleven per side; each muscle arises from the lower border of a rib and inserts on the upper border of the rib below. Fibers are the most superficial of the intercostales muscles, running in an inferior and medial direction. Fibers are most *developed laterally*

Intercostales Interni

Attachments: Eleven per side; each muscle arises from the lower border of a rib and inserts on the upper border of the rib below. Fibers run in a plane immediately deep to the intercostales externi. Fibers of the intercostales interni run in an inferior and slightly lateral direction, nearly perpendicular to the direction of the intercostales externi. Fibers of the intercostales interni are most developed adjacent to the sternum, parasternally

Intercostales Intimi

Attachments: Each muscle arises from the lower border of a rib near its angle and inserts on the upper border of the second or third rib below. Fibers run parallel and deep to the intercostales interni. Fibers of the intercostales intimi located near the angle of the ribs, often called *subcostales,* may cross two intercostal spaces. The intercostales intimi are most developed in the lower thorax

Innervation to the intercostales: intercostal nerves (T^2–T^{12})

Levatores Costarum (Longi and Breves)

Superior attachments: ends of the transverse processes of C7 to T11

Inferior attachments: external surfaces of ribs, between the tubercle and angle. Muscles may attach to the rib immediately inferior to its superior attachment (levatores costarum breves), or, most notably in the lower segments, to the rib two segments inferior to its superior attachment (levatores costarum longi)

Innervation: dorsal rami of adjacent thoracic spinal nerve roots (C^7–T^{11})

Serratus Posterior Inferior

Superior attachments: posterior surfaces of ribs 9 to 12, near their angles

Inferior attachments: spinous processes and supraspinous ligaments of T11 to L3

Innervation: intercostal nerves (T^9–T^{12})

Serratus Posterior Superior

Superior attachments: spinous processes of C6 to T3, including supraspinous ligaments and ligamentum nuchae

Inferior attachments: posterior surfaces of ribs 2 to 5, near their angles

Innervation: intercostal nerves (T^2–T^5)

Transversus Thoracis

Inferior (medial) attachments: inner surfaces of the lower third of the body of the sternum and adjacent surfaces of the xiphoid process

Superior (lateral) attachments: internal surfaces of the sternocostal joints associated with the second (or third) through the sixth ribs

Innervation: adjacent intercostal nerves

Part D: Moment Arm Data for Selected Craniocervical Muscles

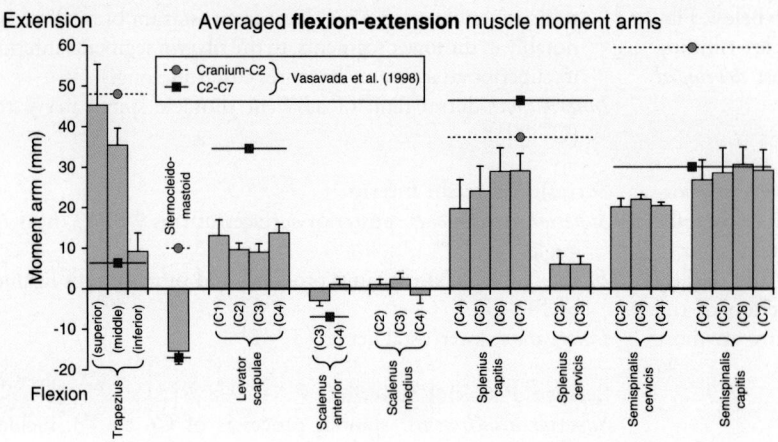

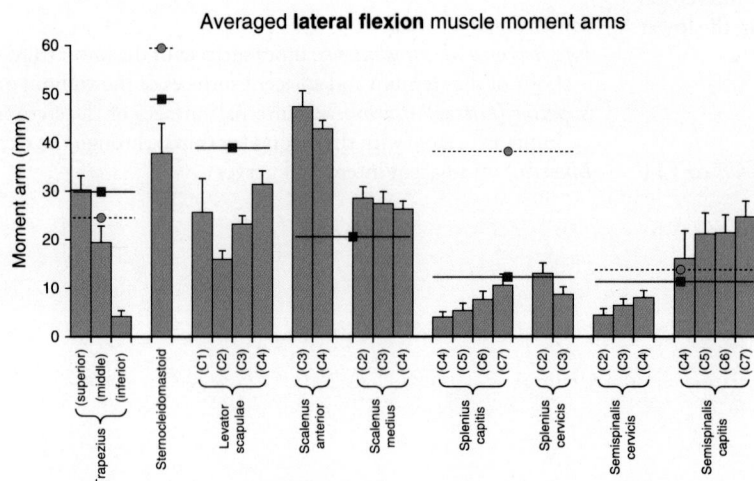

FIGURE III.3 Averaged moment arms (mm) of selected craniocervical muscles for (A) extension and flexion; (B) lateral flexion; and (C) axial rotation. Bar graph data (from Ackland and colleagues, 2011) are based on analysis of five adult cadaver specimens. The labels appearing parenthetically next to the muscle names (near horizontal axes) identify the subregion of the muscle group being studied; for example, scalenus anterior (C4) identifies the part of this muscle that attaches to C4. The illustration also shows moment arm data from Vasavada and colleagues (1998). These additional data show moment arms from muscles (or parts of muscles) crossing between *cranium–C2* (brown circles) and *C2–C7* (red squares). The horizontal lines associated with the squares or circles indicate the muscle under study. (Overall graph design and bar graph data from Ackland DC, Merritt JS, Pandy MG: Moment arms of the human neck muscles in flexion, bending and rotation, *J Biomech* 44[3]:475–486, 2011. Additional data from Vasavada AN, Li S, Delp SL: Influence of muscle morphometry and moment arms on the moment-generating capacity of human neck muscles, *Spine* 23:412–422, 1998.)

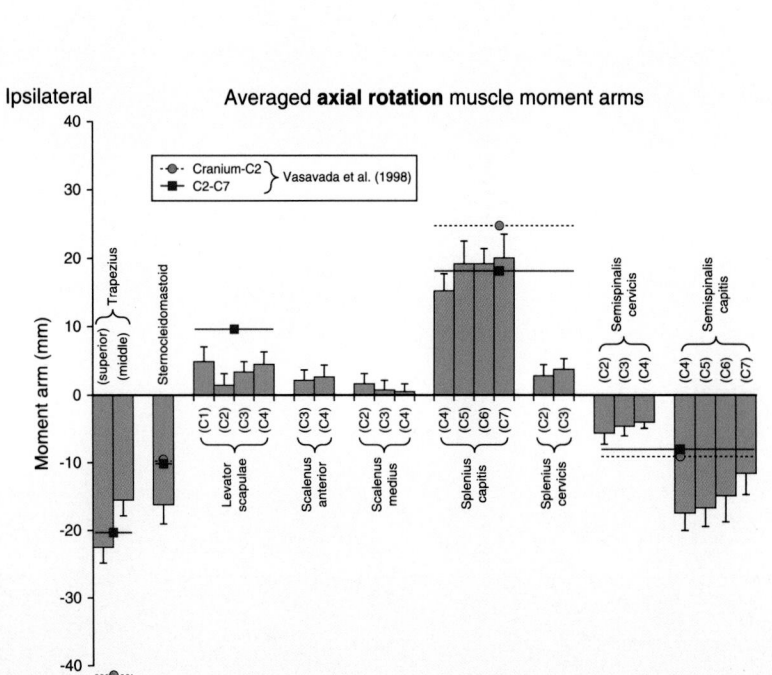

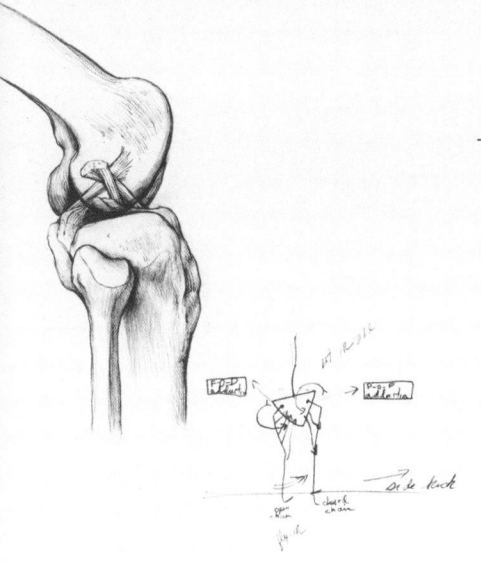

Section

IV

Lower Extremity

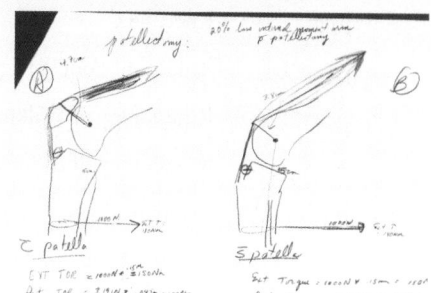

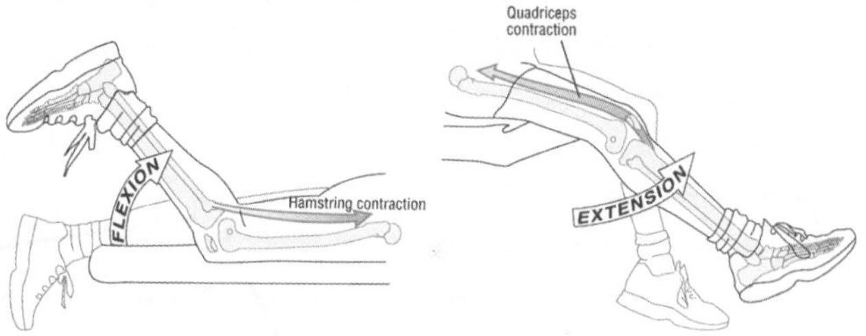

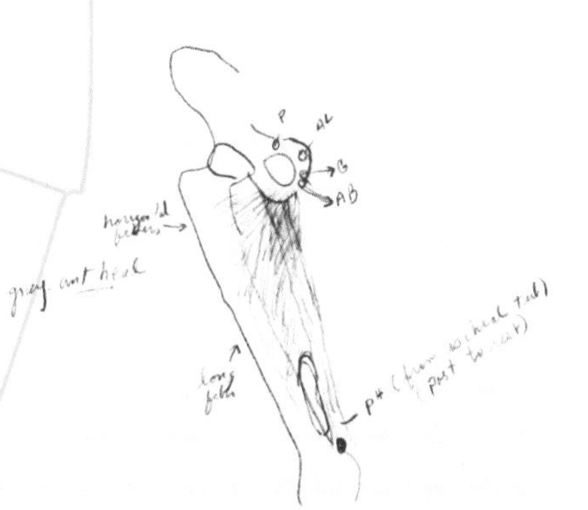

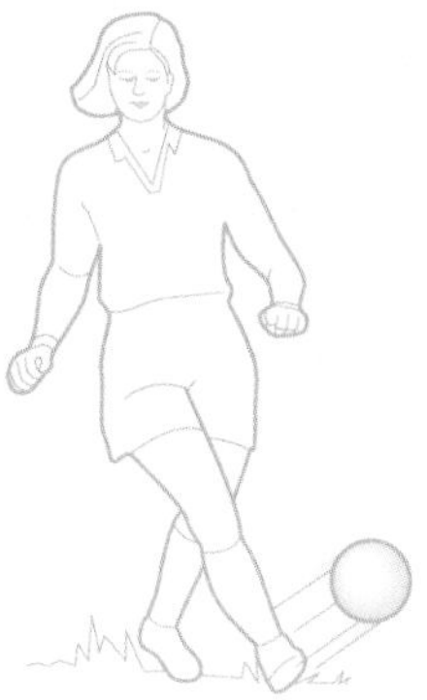

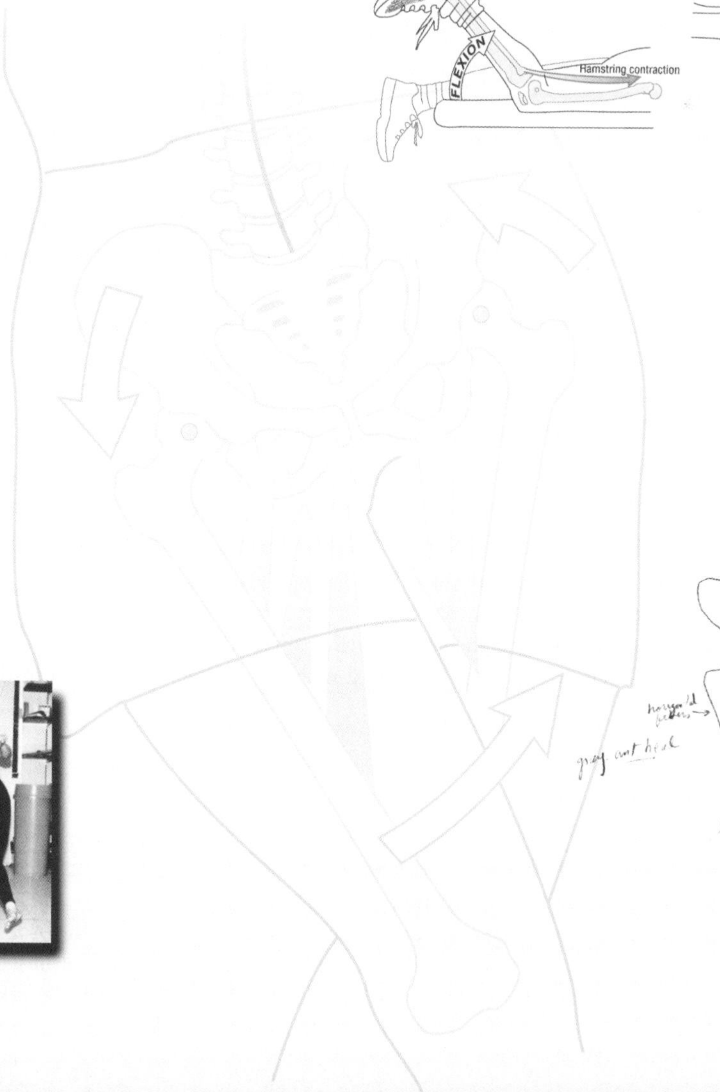

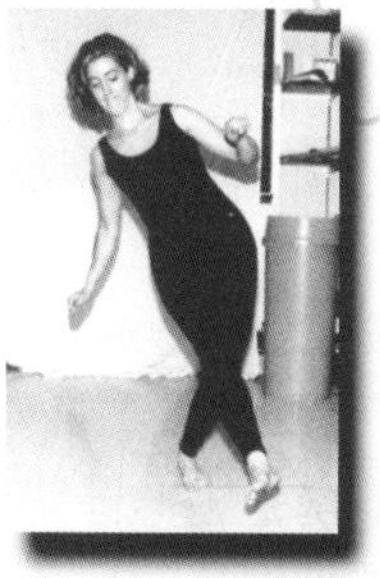

Section IV

Lower Extremity

Section IV is divided into five chapters. Chapters 12 to 14 describe the kinesiology of the articular regions within the lower extremity, that is, from the pelvis to the toes. Chapters 15 and 16 describe the kinesiology of walking and running—the ultimate functional expressions of the kinesiology of the lower extremity. Chapters 12 to 14 describe the function of the muscles and joints from two perspectives: when the distal end of the extremity is fixed, and when it is free. An understanding of both types of actions greatly increases the ability to appreciate the beauty and complexity of human movement, as well as to diagnose, treat, and prevent related impairments of the musculoskeletal system.

EDUCATIONAL eCONTENT

Chapters 12-16 contain several videos, e-figures, and e-tables that are designed to greatly enhance the understanding of the kinesiology presented within Section IV. Videos include fluoroscopy of joint movement, cadaver dissections and demonstrations, short lectures by authors or others, special teaching models, walking and running animated skeletal models demonstrating kinetics and kinematics, an EMG-based display of activated muscles as a healthy person walks and runs on a treadmill, and more.

Certain videos and other assets relate specifically to the text material. Other materials, referred to as *additional video educational content* are not indicated in the text but are listed at the very end of each chapter.

How to view? The videos and e-figures are available in the accompanying enhanced eBook version included with the print purchase of this textbook. Visit Elsevier eBooks+ (eBooks.Health.Elsevier.com) to access this content.

 ## ADDITIONAL CLINICAL CONNECTIONS

Additional Clinical Connections are included at the end of each chapter. This feature is intended to highlight or expand on a particular clinical concept associated with the kinesiology covered in the chapter.

 ## STUDY QUESTIONS

Study Questions are also included at the end of each chapter. These questions are designed to challenge the reader to review or reinforce some of the main concepts contained within the chapter. The process of answering these questions is an effective way for students to prepare for examinations. The answers to the questions are available in the accompanying enhanced eBook version included with the print purchase of this textbook.

The hip is the articulation between the large spherical head of the femur and the socket provided by the acetabulum of the pelvis (Fig. 12.1). Given the central location of the hips within the body, the question may arise: Do the hips serve as "base" joints for the lower extremities, or do they serve as basilar joints for the entire superimposed pelvis and trunk? As the chapter unfolds, it will become clear that the hips serve *both* roles. For this reason, the hips play a dominant kinesiologic role in movements of the lower extremities, trunk, and whole body. Pathology or trauma affecting the hips typically causes a wide range of functional limitations, including difficulty in walking, dressing, driving a car, lifting and carrying loads, and climbing stairs.

The hip joint has many anatomic features that contribute to stability during standing, climbing, walking, and running. The femoral head is stabilized by a relatively deep socket that is surrounded and sealed by an extensive set of connective tissues. Many large and forceful muscles generate substantial torques needed to accelerate the body upward and forward or to decelerate the body in a controlled manner. Weakness in these muscles can have a profound effect on the mobility and stability of the body as a whole.

Hip disease and injury are relatively frequent among very young and older adult populations. An abnormally or poorly developed (dysplastic) hip in an infant may be prone to dislocation. The aging hip is vulnerable to degenerative joint disease. Increased prevalence of osteoporosis coupled with increased risk of falling also predisposes older persons to a higher incidence of hip fracture.

Advances in hip arthroscopy and medical imaging have contributed to the recognition of additional pathologies of the hip across the adolescent and middle years of life as well. For example, subtle variations in the shape of the proximal femur or acetabulum, whether identified as a child or adult, can result in local tissues being impinged or otherwise stressed, especially when the joint repeatedly approaches relatively extreme positions. Over time, this impingement can cause pain or, in some people, trigger premature hip osteoarthritis. Accordingly, a central theme of surgical and nonsurgical interventions for stressed regions of relatively young hips is to limit further degeneration later in life.

This chapter describes the structure and function of the hip and its associated periarticular connective tissues as well as the actions of the surrounding musculature. This information helps form a basis for treatment and diagnosis of musculoskeletal problems in this important region of the body.

OSTEOLOGY

Innominate

Each *innominate* (from the Latin *innominatum*, meaning "nameless") is the union of three bones: the *ilium, pubis,* and *ischium* (Figs. 12.1 and 12.2). The right and left innominates connect with each other anteriorly at the pubic symphysis and posteriorly at the sacrum. These connections form a complete osteoligamentous ring, referred to as the *pelvis* (from the Latin, meaning "basin" or "bowl"). The pelvis is associated with three important and very different functions. First, the pelvis serves as a common attachment point for many muscles of the lower extremity and the trunk. The pelvis also transmits the weight of the upper body and trunk either to the ischial tuberosities during sitting or to the lower extremities during standing and walking. Last, with the aid of the muscles and connective tissues of the pelvic floor, the pelvis supports the organs involved with bowel, bladder, sexual, and reproductive functions.

The external surface of the pelvis has three striking features. The large fan-shaped *wing* (or *ala*) of the ilium forms the superior half of the innominate. Just below the wing is the deep, cup-shaped *acetabulum.* Just inferior and slightly medial to the acetabulum is the *obturator foramen*—the largest foramen in the body. This foramen is covered by an *obturator membrane* (Fig. 12.1).

Although highly variable, while a person stands the pelvis is typically oriented so that when viewed laterally, a vertical line passes generally between the anterior-superior iliac spine and the pubic tubercle (Fig. 12.2).

Osteologic Features of the Ilium

EXTERNAL SURFACE
- Posterior, anterior, and inferior gluteal lines
- Anterior-superior iliac spine
- Anterior-inferior iliac spine
- Iliac crest
- Posterior-superior iliac spine
- Posterior-inferior iliac spine
- Greater sciatic notch
- Greater sciatic foramen
- Sacrotuberous and sacrospinous ligaments

INTERNAL SURFACE
- Iliac fossa
- Auricular surface
- Iliac tuberosity

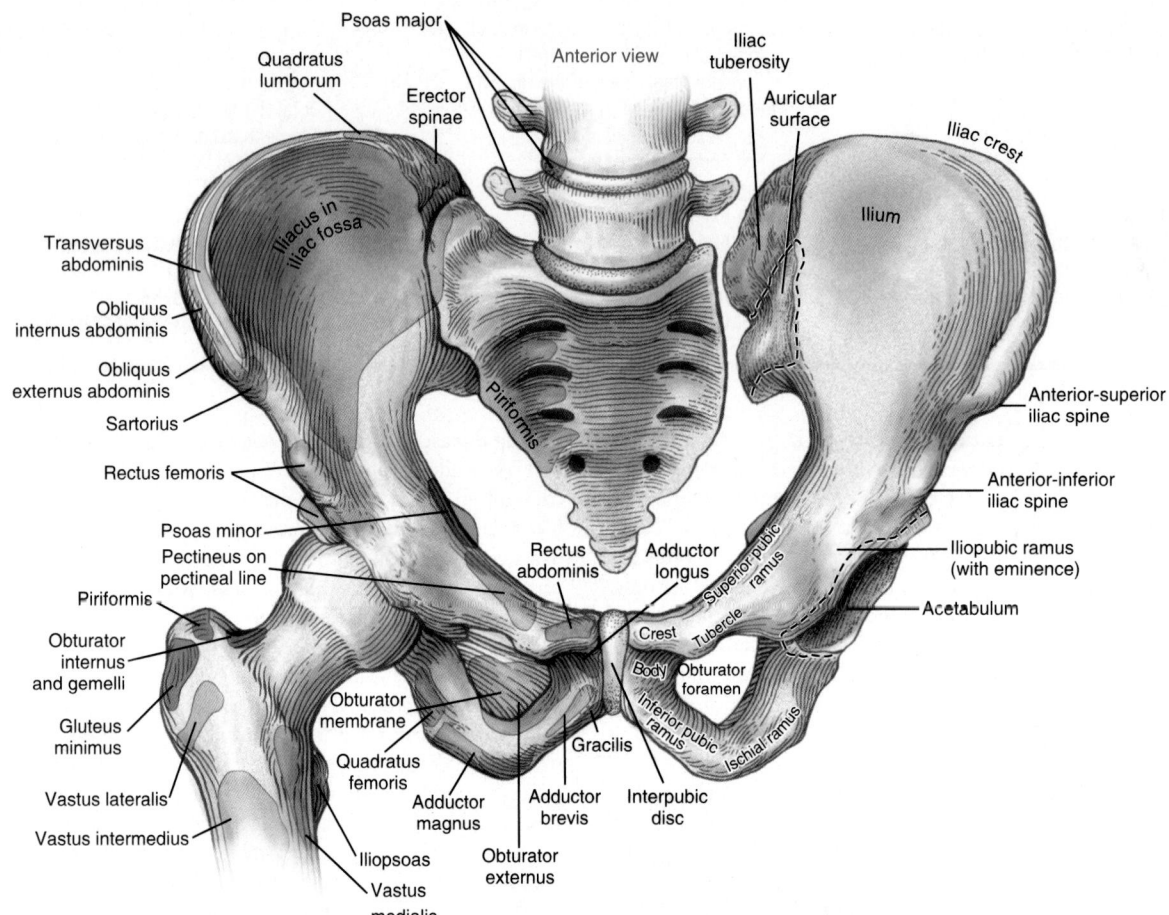

FIG. 12.1 The anterior aspect of the pelvis, sacrum, and right proximal femur. Proximal attachments are indicated in red, distal attachments in gray. A section of the left side of the sacrum is removed to expose the auricular surface of the sacroiliac joint. The pelvic attachments of the capsule around the sacroiliac joint are indicated by dashed lines.

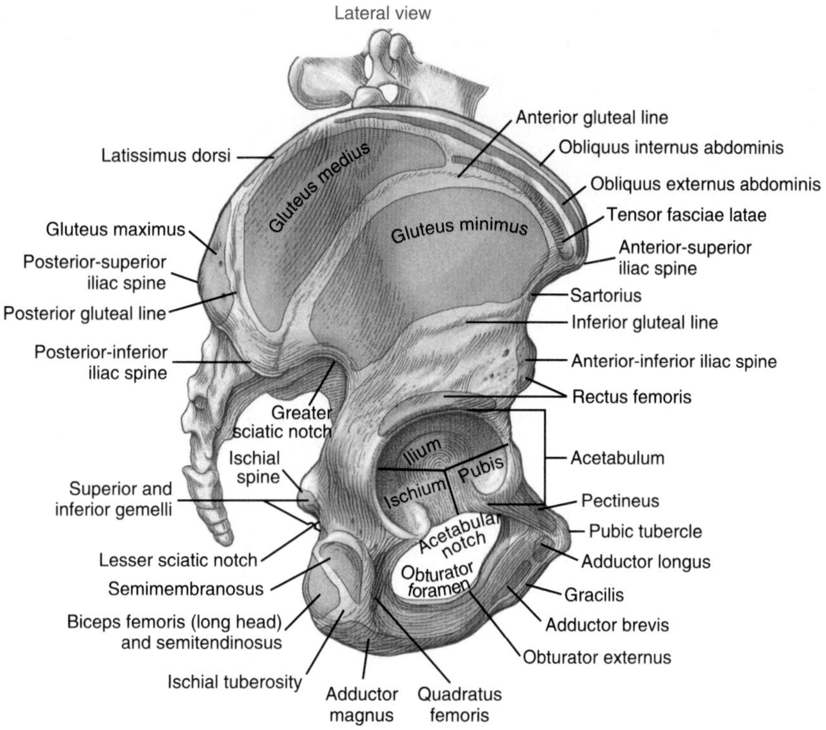

FIG. 12.2 A lateral view of the right innominate bone. As depicted, the pubis, ischium, and ilium each constitute a part of the acetabulum. Proximal attachments of muscle are indicated in red, distal attachments in gray.

ILIUM

The external surface of the ilium is marked by rather faint *posterior, anterior,* and *inferior gluteal lines* (Fig. 12.2). These lines help identify attachment sites of the gluteal muscles. At the most anterior extent of the ilium is the easily palpable *anterior-superior iliac spine* (see Figs. 12.1 and 12.2). Below this spine is the *anterior-inferior iliac spine.* The prominent *iliac crest,* the most superior rim of the ilium, continues posteriorly and ends at the *posterior-superior iliac spine* (see Fig. 12.3). The soft tissue superficial to the posterior-superior iliac spine is often marked by a dimple in the skin. The less prominent *posterior-inferior iliac spine* marks the superior rim of the *greater sciatic notch.* The opening of this notch is converted into the *greater sciatic foramen* by the *sacrospinous ligament* and the proximal part of the *sacrotuberous ligament.*

The internal aspect of the ilium has three notable features (Fig. 12.1). Anteriorly, the smooth concave *iliac fossa* is filled by the iliacus muscle. Posteriorly, the *auricular surface* articulates with the sacrum at the sacroiliac joint. Just posterior to the auricular surface is the large, rough *iliac tuberosity,* which marks the attachments of sacroiliac ligaments and caudal part of the erector spinae muscle group.

PUBIS

The *superior pubic ramus* extends medially from its origin at the *iliopubic ramus* (and associated raised *iliopubic eminence*) to the large, flattened *body* of the pubis (see Fig. 12.1). The upper border of the body of the pubis is the pubic *crest,* serving as an attachment for the rectus abdominis muscle. On the upper surface of the superior ramus is the *pectineal line* (or *pecten pubis*), marking the proximal attachment of the pectineus muscle. The *pubic tubercle*

projects anteriorly from the superior pubic ramus, serving as an attachment for the inguinal ligament. The *inferior pubic ramus* extends from the body of the pubis posteriorly to the junction of the ischium.

The two pubic bones articulate in the midline by way of the *pubic symphysis joint* (Fig. 12.1). This relatively immobile joint is typically classified as a synarthrosis. Hyaline cartilage lines the opposing surfaces of the articulation; the surfaces are not completely flat but possess small, raised ridges, likely helpful to resist shear. The joint is firmly bound by a fibrocartilaginous *interpubic disc* and ligaments. The interpubic disc is strengthened by an interlacing of collagen fibers, combined with distal attachments from the rectus abdominis muscles. Up to 2 mm of translation and very slight rotation occur at the pubic symphysis joint.[316] The pubic symphysis provides stress relief throughout the ring of the pelvis during walking and, in women, during pregnancy and childbirth. During pregnancy or just after giving birth, some women suffer pain attributable to instability of the symphysis pubis caused by the physiologic relaxation of the joint's supporting ligaments.

Osteologic Features of the Pubis

- Superior pubic ramus
- Iliopubic ramus (with iliopubic eminence)
- Body
- Crest
- Pectineal line (pectin pubis)
- Pubic tubercle
- Pubic symphysis joint and disc
- Inferior pubic ramus

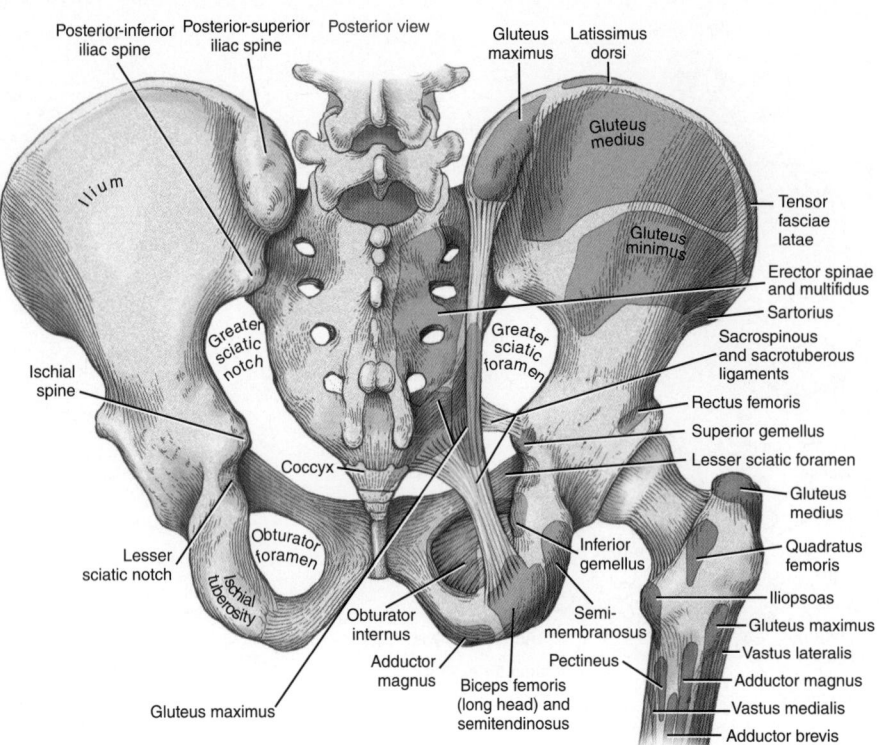

FIG. 12.3 The posterior aspect of the pelvis, sacrum, and right proximal femur. Proximal attachments of muscles are indicated in red, distal attachments in gray.

ISCHIUM

The sharp *ischial spine* projects from the posterior side of the ischium, just inferior to the greater sciatic notch (see Fig. 12.3). The *lesser sciatic notch* is located just inferior to the spine. The *sacrospinous ligament* and distal part of the *sacrotuberous ligament* convert the lesser sciatic notch into a *lesser sciatic foramen*.

Projecting posteriorly and inferiorly from the acetabulum is the large, stout *ischial tuberosity* (see Fig. 12.3). This palpable structure serves as the proximal attachment for many muscles of the lower extremity, most notably the hamstrings and part of the adductor magnus. The *ischial ramus* extends anteriorly from the ischial tuberosity, ending at the junction with the inferior pubic ramus (see Fig. 12.1).

Osteologic Features of the Ischium

- Ischial spine
- Lesser sciatic notch
- Lesser sciatic foramen
- Ischial tuberosity
- Ischial ramus

ACETABULUM

Located just above the obturator foramen is the large cup-shaped acetabulum (see Fig. 12.2). The acetabulum forms the socket of the hip. All three bones of the pelvis contribute to the formation of the acetabulum: the ilium and ischium contribute about 75%, and the pubis contributes the remaining approximately 25%. Specific features of the acetabulum are discussed in the section on arthrology.

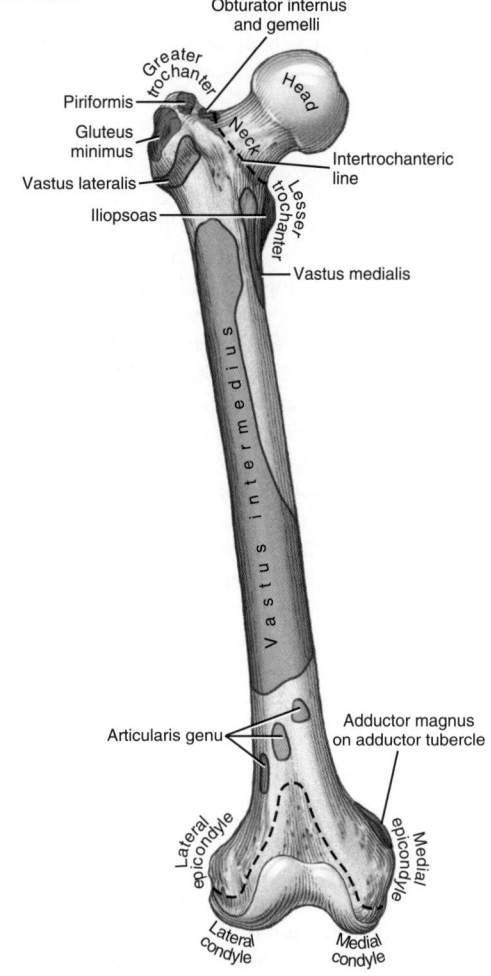

FIG. 12.4 The anterior aspect of the right femur. Proximal attachments of muscles are indicated in red, distal attachments in gray. The femoral attachments of the hip joint capsule and the knee joint capsule are indicated by dashed lines.

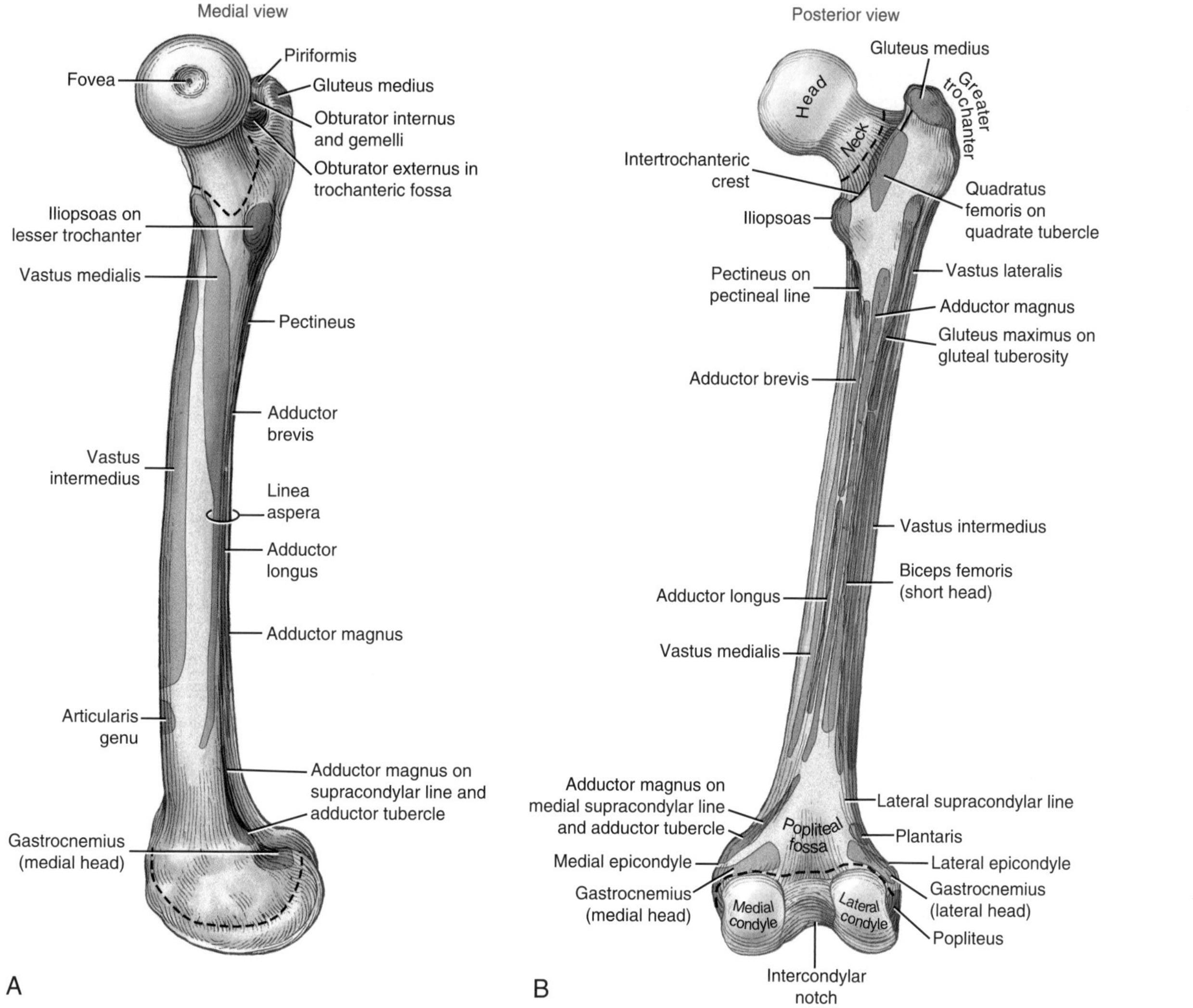

Medial view
Fovea
Piriformis
Gluteus medius
Obturator internus and gemelli
Obturator externus in trochanteric fossa
Iliopsoas on lesser trochanter
Vastus medialis
Pectineus
Adductor brevis
Vastus intermedius
Linea aspera
Adductor longus
Adductor magnus
Articularis genu
Adductor magnus on supracondylar line and adductor tubercle
Gastrocnemius (medial head)
A
Posterior view
Gluteus medius
Head
Greater trochanter
Neck
Intertrochanteric crest
Iliopsoas
Quadratus femoris on quadrate tubercle
Vastus lateralis
Pectineus on pectineal line
Adductor magnus
Gluteus maximus on gluteal tuberosity
Adductor brevis
Vastus intermedius
Biceps femoris (short head)
Adductor longus
Vastus medialis
Adductor magnus on medial supracondylar line and adductor tubercle
Popliteal fossa
Lateral supracondylar line
Plantaris
Medial epicondyle
Lateral epicondyle
Gastrocnemius (medial head)
Medial condyle
Lateral condyle
Gastrocnemius (lateral head)
Popliteus
Intercondylar notch
B

FIG. 12.5 The medial (A) and posterior (B) surfaces of the right femur. Proximal attachments of muscles are indicated in red, distal attachments in gray. The femoral attachments of the hip joint capsule and the knee joint capsule are indicated by dashed lines.

Femur

The femur is the longest bone of the human body (Fig. 12.4). Its shape and robust stature reflect the powerful action of muscles and contribute to the long stride length during walking and running. At the bone's proximal end, the femoral *head* projects medially and slightly anteriorly to articulate with the acetabulum. The femoral *neck* connects the femoral head to the shaft. The neck serves to displace the proximal shaft of the femur laterally away from the joint, thereby facilitating the clearance required between the femur and pelvis during locomotion. Distal to the neck, the shaft of the femur courses slightly medially, effectively placing the knees and feet closer to the midline of the body.

The shaft of the femur displays a slight anterior convexity (Fig. 12.5A). As a long, eccentrically loaded column, the femur bows slightly when subjected to the weight of the body. Consequently, stress along the bone is dissipated through compression along its posterior shaft and through tension along its anterior shaft. Ultimately this bowing allows the femur to bear a greater load than if the femur were perfectly straight.

Anteriorly, the *intertrochanteric line* marks the distal attachment of the capsular ligaments (see Fig. 12.4). The *greater trochanter* extends laterally and posteriorly from the junction of the femoral neck and shaft (Fig. 12.5B). This prominent and easily palpable structure serves as the distal attachment for many muscles. On the medial surface of the greater trochanter is a small pit called the *trochanteric fossa* (see Figs. 12.5A and 12.6). This fossa marks the distal attachment of the obturator externus muscle.

Anterior
Superior view
Acetabulum
Femoral head
Obturator externus in trochanteric fossa
Obturator internus and gemelli
Gluteus minimus (anterior facet)
Piriformis
Gluteus medius (superior-posterior and lateral facets)
Iliopsoas
Quadratus femoris

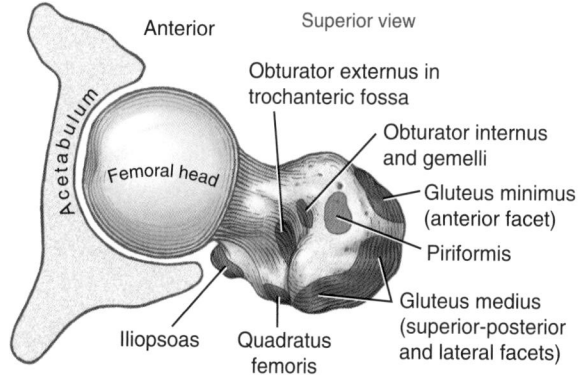

FIG. 12.6 The superior aspect of the right femur. Distal attachments of muscles are shown in gray.

Posteriorly, the femoral neck joins the femoral shaft at the raised *intertrochanteric crest* (Fig. 12.5B). The *quadrate tubercle*, the distal attachment of the quadratus femoris muscle, is a slightly raised area on the crest just inferior to the trochanteric fossa. The *lesser trochanter* projects sharply from the inferior end of the crest in a posterior-medial direction. The lesser trochanter serves as the primary distal attachment for the iliopsoas, a dominant hip flexor and effective vertical stabilizer of the lumbar spine (Chapter 10).

The middle third of the posterior side of the femoral shaft is clearly marked by a vertical ridge called the *linea aspera* (Latin words *linea*, line, and *aspera*, rough). The bone located on either side of the linea aspera is especially dense, owing to the concentration of compressive forces caused by the natural anterior convexity of the femoral shaft. The raised and irregular linea aspera serves as a partial attachment site for the vasti muscles of the quadriceps group, many of the adductor muscles, and the intermuscular fascia of the thigh. Proximally, the linea aspera splits into the *pectineal line* medially and the *gluteal tuberosity* laterally (see Fig. 12.5B). At the distal end of the femur, the linea aspera divides into the *lateral* and *medial supra-condylar lines*. The *adductor tubercle* is located at the extreme distal end of the medial supracondylar line.

Osteologic Features of the Femur

- Femoral head
- Femoral neck
- Intertrochanteric line
- Greater trochanter
- Trochanteric fossa
- Intertrochanteric crest
- Quadrate tubercle
- Lesser trochanter
- Linea aspera
- Pectineal line
- Gluteal tuberosity
- Lateral and medial supracondylar lines
- Adductor tubercle

SHAPE OF THE PROXIMAL FEMUR

The final shape and configuration of the developing proximal femur are determined by several factors, which may include differential growth of the bone's ossification centers, mechanical loading from the force of muscle activation and gravity, genetics, hormones, and blood supply. Abnormal growth resulting in a misshaped proximal femur is often categorized as a type of *dysplasia* (from the Greek *dys*, ill or bad, and *plasia*, growth).[270] (The specific term *developmental dysplasia* is used when the condition develops primarily in utero or

in early childhood; see Clinical Connection 12.4.) Trauma or other systemic factors, regardless of age, can also influence the overall shape of the proximal femur, which can affect the congruity, articular stability, and stress placed on the joint—variables that can increase the risk for developing hip osteoarthritis.[265] This topic will be revisited throughout this chapter.

Two specific angulations of the proximal femur help define its shape: the angle of inclination and the amount of torsion along its shaft.

Angle of Inclination

The *angle of inclination* of the proximal femur describes an angle in the frontal plane between the femoral neck and the medial side of the femoral shaft (Fig. 12.7). Although the angle of inclination is normally about 125 degrees in the adult, at birth the angle measures about 165 to 170 degrees. Primarily because of muscle forces and the associated loading across the femoral neck during walking, this angulation usually *decreases* by about 2 degrees per year between 2 and 8 years of age.[312] Although all hip muscles likely have a mechanical role in the progressive reduction in neck-shaft angle, the role of the hip abductors during walking is especially dominant.[332] The angle of inclination continues to decrease by varying rates until reaching its normal adulthood value of about 125 degrees.[231] As depicted by the pair of red dots in Fig. 12.7A, this angulation typically optimizes the alignment of the joint surfaces.

A change in the normal angle of inclination is referred to as either *coxa vara* or *coxa valga*. Coxa vara (Latin *coxa*, hip, and *vara*, to bend inward) describes an angle of inclination markedly *less than* 125 degrees; coxa valga (Latin *valga*, to bend outward) describes an angle of inclination markedly *greater than* about 125 degrees (see Fig. 12.7B–C for angles that may be considered abnormal). Abnormal neck-shaft angles can alter the articular fit between the femoral head and the acetabulum, thereby affecting hip biomechanics. Severe malalignment may lead to dislocation or stress-induced degeneration of the joint. Although variable, persons with cerebral palsy typically possess a coxa valga deformity that well exceeds that depicted in Fig. 12.7C.[312] The reduced or abnormal loading across the hips in this population apparently interferes with the gradual decline in the angle of inclination that is normally observed in active, ambulatory children with a typically developed neuromuscular system.

Femoral Torsion

Femoral torsion describes the relative rotation (twist) between the bone's shaft and neck. Typically, as viewed from above within the horizontal plane, the femoral neck projects several degrees *anterior* to a medial-lateral axis through the femoral condyles. Fig. 12.8A depicts a normal anteversion angle of about 15 degrees, although "normal" values reported in the literature vary from 8 to 20 degrees.[80,161] In conjunction with the normal angle of inclination

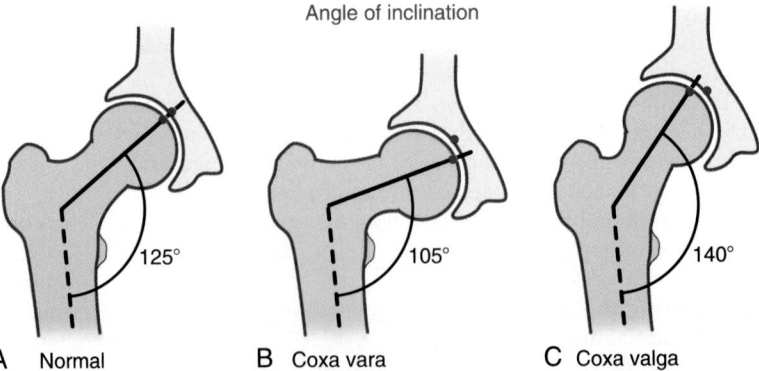

FIG. 12.7 The (frontal plane) neck-shaft angle of the proximal femur is shown: (A) normal angle of inclination; (B) coxa vara; (C) coxa valga. The pair of red dots in each figure indicates the different alignments of the hip joint surfaces. Optimal alignment is shown in (A).

Angle of inclination

125°   105°   140°

A Normal   B Coxa vara   C Coxa valga

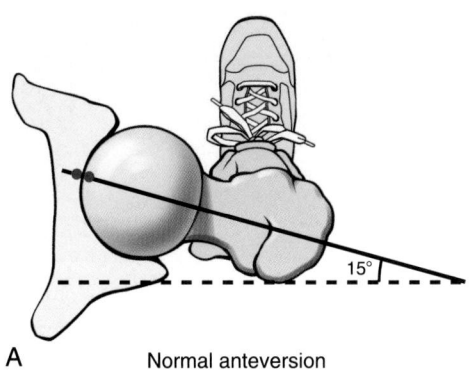

A   Normal anteversion

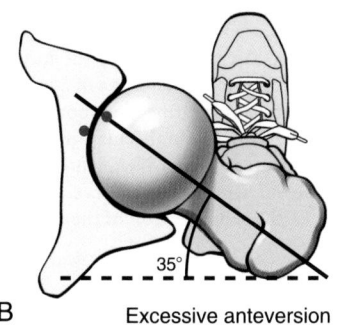

B   Excessive anteversion

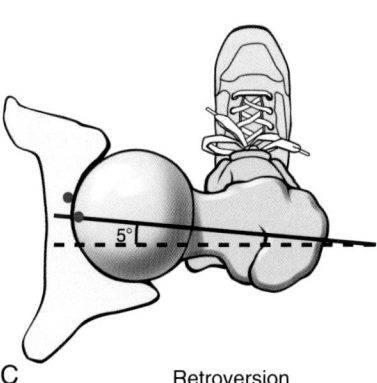

C   Retroversion

FIG. 12.8 The angle of torsion is shown between the neck and shaft of the femur. The angle is measured between the neck and a line running through the condyles at the knee (depicted as a *dashed line*); (A) normal anteversion; (B) excessive anteversion; (C) retroversion. The pair of red dots in each figure indicates the different alignments of the hip joint surfaces. Optimal alignment is shown in (A).

(described previously), an approximate 15-degree angle of anteversion affords optimal alignment and joint congruence (see alignment of red dots in Fig. 12.8A).

Femoral torsion may be considered abnormal if it markedly deviates from 15 degrees. Typically, torsion greatly beyond 15 degrees is referred to as *excessive anteversion* (Fig. 12.8B) and torsion significantly less than 15 degrees (i.e., approaching 0 degrees) is called *retroversion* (Fig. 12.8C). Because of the relatively large natural variability in femoral torsion across the population, the clinical distinction between what is "normal" and "abnormal" is often ambiguous. This uncertainty is also related to the lack of a precise, simple clinical method of measuring femoral torsion, other than that based on medical imaging, such as magnetic resonance imaging (MRI) or computed tomography (CT) scans.[288] Even measurements made through CT imaging can be difficult to interpret clinically because of the lack of universal standards in measurement protocol.[269]

Typically, a healthy infant is born with about 40 degrees of femoral anteversion.[84] With continued bone growth, increased weight-bearing across the joint, and muscle activity, this angle usually reduces (or "de-rotates") to about 15 degrees by 16 years of age. Excessive anteversion that persists into adulthood can alter the biomechanics of the hip (such as a change in moment arm lengths of muscles) and create gait deviations.[3,29] Depending on extent, excessive anteversion can also increase the loading profiles at the hip and patellofemoral joints.[126,236] The associated articular incongruence at the hip coupled with greater contact forces may, over time, damage the articular cartilage or acetabular labrum.

Excessive anteversion in children may be associated with an abnormal gait pattern called "in-toeing." In-toeing is a walking pattern with exaggerated posturing of lower limb internal rotation. Although this gait pattern can be the result of malalignment throughout the lower limb, in some children it may be a compensation to guide the femoral head of the excessively anteverted femur more directly into the acetabulum (Fig. 12.9).[51] In addition, Arnold and colleagues have shown that the exaggerated internally rotated position during walking serves to increase the moment arm of the important hip abductor muscles—leverage that is reduced with excessive femoral anteversion.[3,16] With this preference to walk with the hip internally rotated, some of the muscles and ligaments crossing the hip might eventually become structurally shortened, limiting the range of external rotation. The gait pattern typically improves with time because of a natural normalization of the anteversion of the femur or a combined structural compensation in other parts of the lower extremity, such as excessive external torsion of the

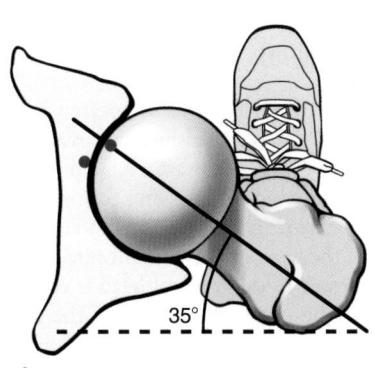

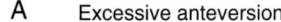

A   Excessive anteversion

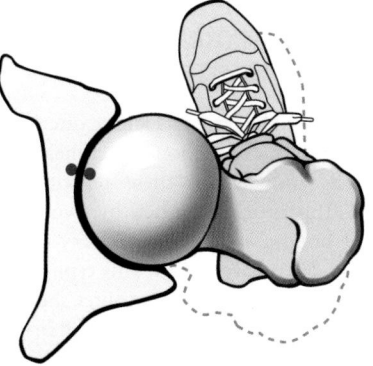

B   Excessive anteversion with "in-toeing"

FIG. 12.9 Two situations show the same individual with excessive anteversion of the proximal femur. (A) Offset red dots indicate malalignment of the hip while a subject stands in the anatomic position. (B) As evidenced by the alignment of the red dots, standing with the hip internally rotated ("in-toeing") improves the joint congruity.

SPECIAL FOCUS 12.1

Natural Anteversion of the Femur: A Reflection of the Prenatal Development of the Lower Limb

During prenatal development, both upper and lower extremities undergo significant axial rotation. By about 54 days after conception, the lower limbs have rotated *internally* (medially) about 90 degrees.[207] This rotation turns the kneecap region to its final anterior position. In essence, the lower limbs have become permanently "pronated." This helps to explain why the "extensor" muscles—such as the quadriceps and tibialis anterior—face anteriorly, and the "flexor" muscles—such as the hamstrings and gastrocnemius—face posteriorly after birth. The approximately 40 degrees of hip anteversion typically present at birth may be an indication of this lower limb medial rotation. As stated previously, as the newborn child typically develops, the shaft of the femur de-rotates (laterally or externally) until it reaches its final adult anteversion value of about 15 degrees. Interestingly, this de-rotation process of the femur is similar but in opposite directions to that which occurs in the humerus.[79] As reviewed in Chapter 5, prenatally the humerus undergoes ample *retroversion*, to about 60 degrees by birth, followed by a gradual postnatal (internal or medial) de-rotation that reaches its final 30-degree retroversion angle by 16 to 20 years of age.

A functional consequence of the medial rotation of the lower limbs is that the soles of the feet assume plantigrade positions, suitable for walking. This fixed pronation of the lower limb is evident by the medial position of the great toe of the lower limb, analogous to the thumb's orientation in a fully pronated forearm.

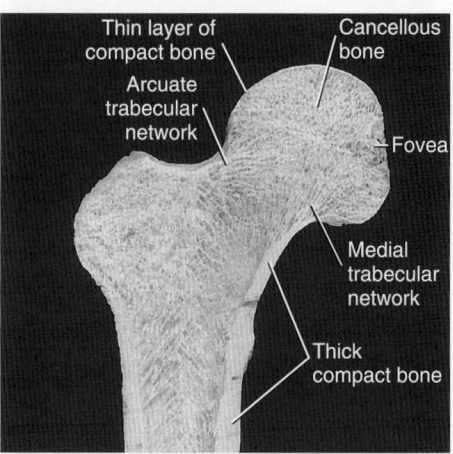

FIG. 12.10 A frontal plane cross-section showing the internal architecture of the proximal femur. Note the thicker areas of compact (external) bone around the neck and shaft, and the cancellous bone occupying most of the medullary (internal) region. Two trabecular networks within the cancellous bone are also indicated. (From Neumann DA: *An arthritis home study course. The synovial joint: anatomy, function, and dysfunction*, LaCrosse, WI, 1998, Orthopedic Section of the American Physical Therapy Association.)

much of the internal region of the proximal femur, as shown in Fig. 12.10. The relative elasticity of cancellous bone is ideal for repeatedly absorbing loads, especially important within and adjacent to the femoral head. Cancellous bone tends to concentrate along lines of stress, forming *trabecular networks*. A *medial trabecular network* and an *arcuate trabecular network* are visible within the femur shown in Fig. 12.10. The overall pattern of the trabecular network changes when the proximal femur is subjected to abnormal forces over an extended time.

ARTHROLOGY

Functional Anatomy of the Hip Joint

The hip is the classic ball-and-socket joint of the body, secured within the acetabulum by an extensive set of connective tissues and muscles. Thick layers of articular cartilage and the presence of cancellous bone in the proximal femur help dampen the large forces that routinely cross the hip. Failure of these protective mechanisms, especially in the presence of trauma or dysplasia and its associated malalignment, may, over time, lead to deterioration of the joint structure.

FEMORAL HEAD

The femoral head is typically located just inferior to the middle one-third of the inguinal ligament. On average, the centers of the two adult femoral heads are 17.5 cm (6.9 inches) apart from each other.[219] The head of the femur forms about two-thirds of a nearly perfect sphere (Fig. 12.11). Located slightly posterior-inferior to the center of the head is a prominent pit, or *fovea* (see Fig. 12.5A). The entire surface of the femoral head is covered by articular cartilage, except in the region of the fovea. The cartilage is thickest (about 3.5 mm) in a broad region above and slightly anterior to the fovea (see highlighted region in Fig. 12.11).[162]

The *ligamentum teres* (ligament to the head of the femur) is a tubular, synovial-lined connective tissue that arises proximally

tibia.[51,236,295] There is no evidence that nonoperative treatment can reduce excessive femoral anteversion.

Excessive femoral anteversion of 25 to 45 degrees is common in persons with cerebral palsy; in fact, anteversion as high as 60 to 80 degrees has been reported.[15,38] In-toeing, among other gait abnormalities, are common in children with cerebral palsy who are ambulatory.[255] Spasticity or tightness of hip internal rotator and adductor muscles along with excessive pelvic rotation may contribute to the in-toeing posturing. In select cases, a femoral de-rotational osteotomy may be considered as a way of reducing the excessive internal rotational posturing observed in gait.[249]

INTERNAL STRUCTURE OF THE PROXIMAL FEMUR

Compact and Cancellous Bone

Walking produces large forces on the proximal femur, often substantially exceeding one's body weight. Throughout a lifetime, the proximal femur typically resists and absorbs these repetitive forces without incurring injury. This is accomplished by two strikingly different compositions of bone. *Compact bone* is very dense and unyielding, able to withstand very large loads. This type of bone is particularly thick in and adjacent to the cortex (outer shell) of the posterior-medial surface of the lower femoral neck (often referred to as the femoral *calcar*) and the entire shaft (Fig. 12.10). These regions can rigidly withstand compression, shear, and torsion; this is in contrast to *cancellous bone*, which is relatively porous, consisting of a spongy, three-dimensional trabecular lattice located throughout

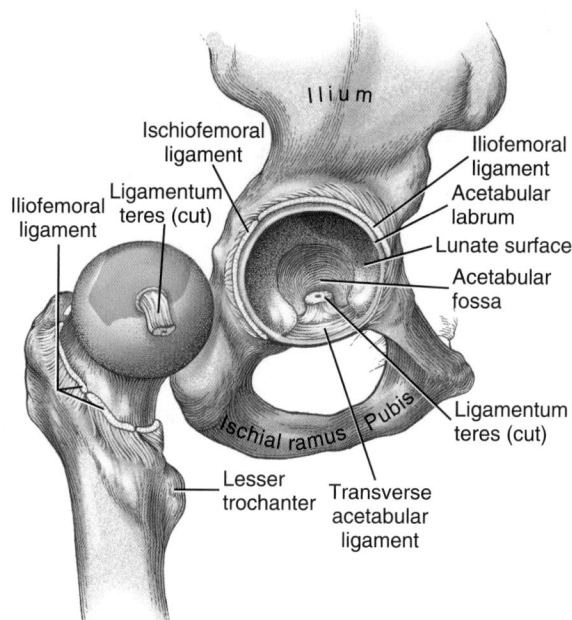

FIG. 12.11 The right hip joint is opened to expose its internal components. The regions of thickest cartilage are highlighted (in *blue*) on the articular surfaces of the femoral head and acetabulum.

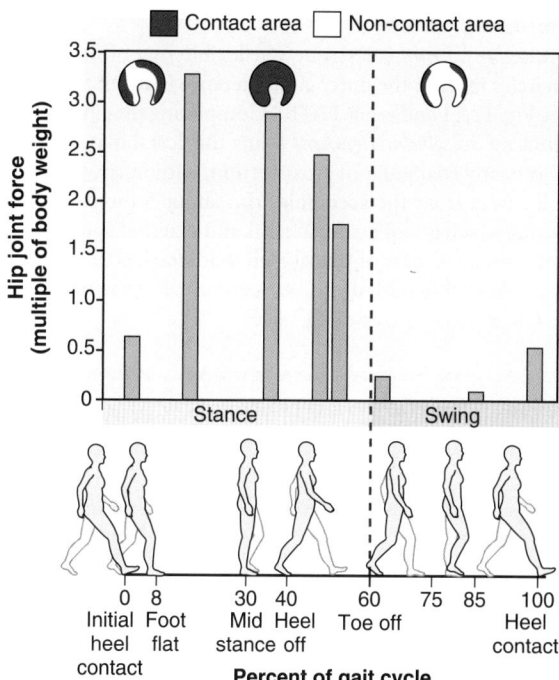

FIG. 12.12 Graph showing an estimate of the hip joint compression force as a multiple of body weight during the gait cycle (vertical stippled line separates the stance and swing phases of gait). The images above the graph indicate the approximate area of acetabular contact at three selected magnitudes of hip joint force, estimated by data published in the literature. The area of joint contact may increase from about 20% of the lunate surface during the swing phase to about 98% during mid stance phase.

from the transverse acetabular ligament and posterior edge of the acetabular notch and attaches distally to the fovea of the femoral head (Fig. 12.11).[226] The ligament serves as a protective sheath for the passage of blood through the small *acetabular artery* to the femoral head (e-Fig. 12.1A).[65,240] Although the acetabular artery appears to have a small role in vascularizing the developing proximal femur in the child, this role is likely even less or nonexistent later in life.[98,168,226,241] It has been speculated that the ligamentum teres may help stabilize the fetal hip at a time when the acetabulum is shallow and the hip is relatively vulnerable to dislocation.[27]

Traditionally, hip movements believed to stretch the ligamentum teres include the combination of flexion, adduction, and external rotation—a position where much of the capsular ligaments of the hip are relatively slackened (described ahead).[27,226] The ligamentum teres has also been described as acting like a sling or a cradle, supporting the inferior part of the femoral head when the hip is flexed and abducted, such as when assuming a squat position.[159,199] Although its mechanical role is uncertain, the ligamentum teres undoubtedly provides some functional stability to the hip, especially to motions that are relatively extreme. The relative amount of stability, however, is unclear and likely considerably less than that generated by healthy capsular ligaments and surrounding activated muscles.[226,260,310] The relative stabilizing role of the ligamentum teres likely increases when the more dominant stabilizers are weakened, or, in the case of hip dysplasia, when the abnormally shaped acetabulum fails to adequately contain the femoral head.[260,310] Because the ligamentum teres contains mechanoreceptors and free nerve endings, the ligament may lend indirect stability or protection to the hip by providing a means for additional proprioceptive or nociceptive sensory feedback.[241,260]

Medical interest in the ligamentum teres has paralleled the advancements in medical imaging and hip arthroscopy (e-Fig.12.2). Because

of its sensory innervation, the ligamentum teres can be a source of intra-articular hip pain if injured or mechanically stressed.[175,267]

ACETABULUM

The acetabulum (from Latin, meaning "vinegar cup") is a deep, hemispheric cuplike socket that accepts the femoral head. The bony rim of this socket is incomplete inferiorly, forming a 55-to-65-degree gap known as the *acetabular notch* (see Fig. 12.2).

The femoral head normally contacts the acetabulum only along its horseshoe-shaped *lunate surface* (Fig. 12.11). This surface is covered with articular cartilage, thickest along the superior-anterior region of its dome.[78,162] The region of thickest cartilage (about 3.5 mm) corresponds to approximately the same region as that of the highest joint force encountered during walking.[66] During walking, hip forces fluctuate from 13% of body weight during the mid swing phase to more than 300% of body weight during the mid stance phase. During the stance phase—when compressive forces are the greatest—the lunate surface deforms slightly, causing the transverse acetabular ligament to elongate and acetabular notch to widen slightly.[87,182] Such a natural deformation likely increases contact area (as depicted in Fig. 12.12), thereby reducing peak contact pressure while walking. This natural damping mechanism represents yet another design that limits the stress on the subchondral bone to within physiologically tolerable levels.

The *acetabular fossa* is a depression located deep within the floor of the acetabulum. Because the fossa does not normally contact the femoral head, it is devoid of cartilage. Instead, the fossa allows space for the ligamentum teres, fat, synovial membrane, and blood vessels.

ACETABULAR LABRUM

The *acetabular labrum* is a strong yet flexible ring of fibrocartilage that encircles most of the outer circumference (rim) of the acetabulum (see Fig. 12.11 and e-Fig.12.1B). Completing the ring inferiorly, the *transverse acetabular ligament* spans the acetabular notch. The labrum is nearly triangular in cross-section, with its *apex* projecting externally away from the acetabular rim about 5 mm. The *base* of the labrum attaches along the internal and external surfaces of the acetabular rim. The part of the labrum that attaches to the internal surface gradually blends with the articular cartilage at the so-called *chondrolabral junction* (see e-Fig.12.1B).

Anatomic Features of the Hip Joint

FEMORAL HEAD
- Fovea
- Ligamentum teres (ligament to the head of the femur)

ACETABULUM
- Acetabular notch
- Lunate surface
- Acetabular fossa
- Labrum and transverse acetabular ligament

The acetabular labrum provides structural stability to the hip joint by "gripping" the femoral head and by deepening the acetabular socket. The *mechanical seal* formed around the hip by an intact labrum helps maintain a negative intra-articular pressure, which is effective at resisting separation of the joint surfaces.[294] The resulting "suction seal" has been shown to be more effective than the capsule at resisting the first 1 to 2 mm of joint distraction (separation).[213] In addition, an intact labrum forms a *fluid seal* around the joint that helps prevent leakage of synovial fluid from the joint.[44,245] Maintaining the synovial fluid over weight-bearing surfaces enhances the lubrication of the articular cartilage and thereby reduces frictional resistance to movement.[287]

Because of an inherently poor vascularization, a torn labrum has only a limited ability to heal on its own accord.[151] The labrum is, however, well supplied by afferent nerves capable of providing proprioceptive feedback and sensation of pain.[157]

Because of its location, the acetabular labrum is subjected to compressive and tensile loads from virtually all movements between the pelvis and femurs, which typically also includes movements of the lumbopelvic region and trunk. Not surprisingly, therefore, the acetabular labrum is often involved with movement-associated pathology, which can include sport-related trauma, excessive loading associated with hip dysplasia, or the repeated microtrauma of femoroacetabular impingement (see Clinical Connection 12.3). Left unrepaired, a torn labrum reduces the mechanical integrity of the hip, subjecting it to excessive mechanical stress that can result in marked pain and associated functional impairments.

ACETABULAR ALIGNMENT

In the anatomic position, the acetabulum typically projects generally laterally from the body, with varying amounts of inferior and anterior inclination. Ideally, this orientation provides optimal coverage or containment of the femoral head, augmenting the joint's structural stability. However, a poorly developed or *dysplastic acetabulum*, typically diagnosed in infants, may fail to adequately cover the femoral head; this situation, when severe, can be associated with chronic dislocation and, later in life, premature hip osteoarthritis.[119,254,270]

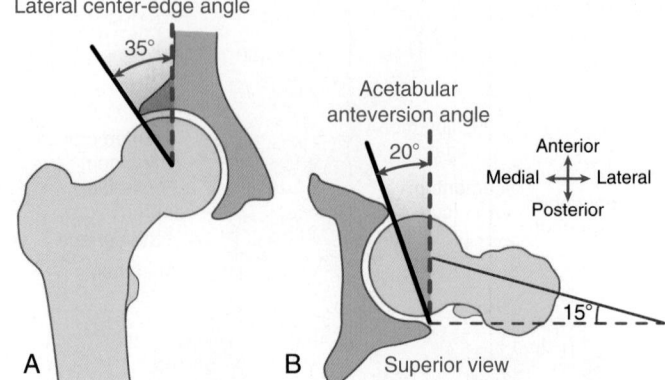

FIG. 12.13 (A) The *lateral center-edge (LCE) angle* is typically made from an anterior-posterior radiograph, measuring the frontal plane orientation of the acetabulum relative to the pelvis. The LCE angle is measured as the intersection of a vertical, *fixed reference line (stippled in red)* with the *acetabular reference line (bold black solid line)* that connects the upper lateral edge of the acetabulum with the center of the femoral head. A more vertical acetabular reference line would result in a smaller LCE angle, providing *less* lateral coverage over the femoral head. (B) The *acetabular anteversion angle*, as viewed from above within the horizontal plane, measures the orientation of the acetabulum relative to the pelvis. This measurement indicates the extent to which the acetabulum covers the *front* of the femoral head. The angle is formed by the intersection of a fixed *anterior-posterior reference line (stippled in red)* with an *acetabular reference line (bold black solid line)* that connects the anterior and posterior rim of the acetabulum. A larger acetabular anteversion angle creates *less* acetabular containment of the anterior side of the femoral head. (A normal *femoral* anteversion of 15 degrees is also shown.)

Medical imaging can provide measurements that help define the extent of acetabular dysplasia, thereby guiding appropriate medical intervention. Two of the many measurements used for this purpose are highlighted next: the lateral center-edge angle, and the acetabular anteversion angle.

Lateral Center-Edge Angle

The *lateral center-edge (LCE) angle* indicates the degree to which the acetabulum extends laterally over the femoral head, as viewed within the frontal plane (Fig. 12.13A).[119] An LCE angle of 25 to 40 degrees is generally considered normal, whereas a hip with an LCE angle less than 20 degrees may be considered "dysplastic."[254,270] A *low* LCE angle indicates abnormally *reduced* femoral head coverage by the acetabulum, indicating a greater risk of dislocation and, equally important, less contact area within the joint.[166] An LCE angle of only 15 degrees, for example, suggests as much as a 35% *decrease* in joint contact area.[102] During the single-limb–support phase of walking, this smaller interface would increase joint pressure (force/area) theoretically by about 50%, potentially predisposing the joint to premature degeneration.[120] Although the LCE angle is typically used to measure an inadequacy of femoral head coverage by the acetabulum, a *high* LCE angle (e.g., beyond 40–45 degrees) suggests *excessive coverage* of the femoral head.[299] Over-coverage, possibly from an excessively deep acetabulum, may result in a damaging femoroacetabular impingement.

Acetabular Anteversion Angle

The *acetabular anteversion angle* indicates the extent to which the acetabulum is oriented *anteriorly*, as viewed within the horizontal plane (Fig. 12.13B). Normally this angle measures about 15 to 20 degrees, which typically leaves part of the femoral head exposed anteriorly (Fig. 12.14).[8,253,268] The thick anterior capsular ligament and

Anterior view

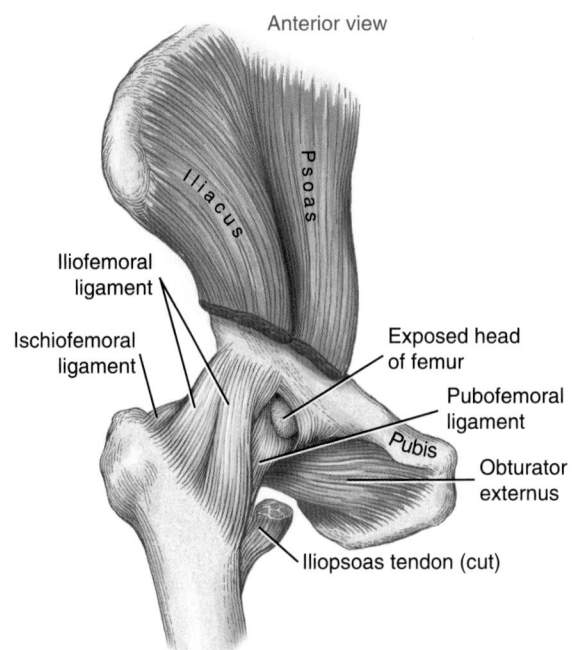

Iliacus

Psoas

Iliofemoral
ligament

Ischiofemoral
ligament

Exposed head
of femur

Pubofemoral
ligament

Pubis

Obturator
externus

Iliopsoas tendon (cut)

FIG. 12.14 The anterior capsule and ligaments of the right hip. The iliopsoas, consisting of the iliacus and psoas (major), has been cut away to expose the anterior side of the joint. Note that part of the femoral head protrudes just medial to the iliofemoral ligament. This region is covered by the joint capsule and, in some cases, also by a bursa.

Posterior view

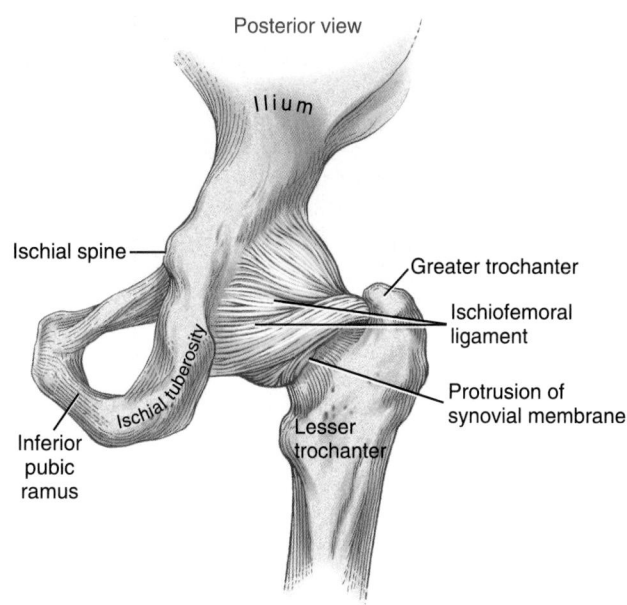

Ilium

Ischial spine

Greater trochanter

Ischiofemoral
ligament

Ischial tuberosity

Protrusion of
synovial membrane

Inferior
pubic
ramus

Lesser
trochanter

FIG. 12.15 The posterior capsule and ligaments of the right hip.

iliopsoas tendon cover and support this exposed portion, although the amount of exposure that needs to be covered becomes greater in a hip with *excessive acetabular anteversion.* If the anteversion is severe, the hip may become vulnerable to anterior dislocation if strongly externally rotated. If the hip has excesses of *both* femoral and acetabular anteversions, the amount of anterior exposure and instability may become greater. If instead the acetabular anteversion angle is close to zero (i.e., the acetabulum faces directly laterally) or is actually negative (i.e., the acetabulum faces posterior-laterally), the *retroverted* acetabulum can create abnormal stress on the joint's interface.

CAPSULAR LIGAMENTS OF THE HIP

The hip joint is surrounded by a robust *fibrous capsule* that is lined internally with a *synovial membrane.* The external surface of the capsule is reinforced by iliofemoral, pubofemoral, and ischiofemoral ligaments (Figs. 12.14 and 12.15). As described later in this chapter, the anterior capsule is further strengthened by attachments from three muscles: the iliocapsularis, the gluteus minimus, and the reflected head of the rectus femoris.[317] Along with a well-formed socket and intact acetabular labrum, the capsular ligamentous complex normally affords excellent stability to the joint. Passive tension in stretched capsular ligaments and the surrounding muscles help define the joint's end range of movement (see Table 12.1). Increasing the flexibility in an abnormally stiff or shortened capsule and muscle is an important component of physical therapy for improving the range of motion and function of the hip.

Each of the three capsular ligaments of the hip is named according to its specific proximal attachment to the bony circumference of the acetabulum. The *iliofemoral ligament,* resembling an inverted Y, is the strongest and stiffest ligament of the hip.[128,293] Proximally, the iliofemoral ligament attaches near the anterior-inferior iliac spine and along the adjacent rim of the acetabulum. Longitudinal running fibers

form distinct medial and lateral fasciculi that, side by side, attach along the entire length of the intertrochanteric line of the femur (see Fig. 12.14). Hip extension stretches the iliofemoral ligament and associated anterior capsule.[130] External rotation also elongates the iliofemoral ligament, especially the lateral fasciculus.[130,228,310]

When a person stands with the hips extended, the anterior surface of the femoral heads press firmly against the iliofemoral ligament, anterior capsule, and superimposed iliopsoas muscle. Passive tension in these structures forms an important stabilizing force that *resists further hip extension.* Some persons with paraplegia use this passive tension in the iliofemoral ligament and hip flexor muscles to assist with standing upright while ambulating with the assistance of braces (e-Fig. 12.3).

Although thinner than the fibers of the iliofemoral ligament, the pubofemoral and ischiofemoral ligaments blend with and strengthen adjacent aspects of the capsule. The *pubofemoral ligament* attaches along the anterior and inferior rim of the acetabulum and adjacent parts of the superior pubic ramus and obturator membrane (Fig. 12.14). The fibers blend with the medial fasciculus of the iliofemoral ligament, becoming taut in hip abduction and extension and, to a lesser degree, external rotation.[130,198,228]

The *ischiofemoral ligament* attaches from the posterior and inferior aspects of the acetabulum, primarily from the adjacent ischium (see Fig. 12.15). The more superficial fibers of this ligament spiral superiorly and laterally across the posterior neck of the femur to attach near the apex of the greater trochanter (see Fig. 12.14). Although these fibers are pulled only slightly taut in full extension, they are wound significantly taut in internal rotation,[228,310] most notably when combined with 10 to 20 degrees of abduction.[130] In general, internal rotation of the hip effectively increases the length (and subsequent passive tension) in the ischiofemoral ligament, in much of the posterior capsule, and in several of the closely anatomically aligned short external rotator muscles, such as the obturator internus.

Although not visible in Figs. 12.14 and 12.15, a separate set of deep, horizontal fibers of the capsule encircles the femoral neck. These deep capsular fibers, thickest posteriorly, are typically known as the *zona orbicularis.* By closely encircling the femoral neck, the zona orbicularis is believed to act as a "stability-inducing collar" to

TABLE 12.1 Connective Tissues and a Sample of Muscles That Are Significantly Stretched at the End Ranges of Passive Hip Motion

End Range Position	Stretched or Taut Tissue
Hip flexion (knee extended)	Hamstrings
Hip flexion (knee flexed)	Zona orbicularis*, gluteus maximus
Hip extension (knee extended)	Primarily iliofemoral ligament, anterior capsule; also, some fibers of the pubofemoral and ischiofemoral ligaments, zona orbicularis*; iliopsoas
Hip extension (knee flexed)	Rectus femoris
Abduction	Pubofemoral ligament; adductor muscles
Adduction	Iliotibial band; abductor muscles such as the tensor fasciae latae and gluteus medius
Internal rotation	Ischiofemoral ligament; short external rotator muscles, such as the obturator internus and piriformis; gluteus maximus
External rotation	Iliofemoral and pubofemoral ligaments; internal rotator muscles, such as the tensor fasciae latae and gluteus minimus

*At extremes of motion only.

the region that, along with the acetabular labrum, limits excessive distraction of the femoral head.[188,228] The zona orbicularis may also help "tighten" the capsule and stabilize the joint at the extremes of flexion and extension.[228]

In closing, the natural passive tension within the hip capsule and embedded ligaments has important functional consequences at the hip. Abnormally tight or stiff capsular ligaments can interfere with the ease and quality of many common activities or postures, especially those requiring the hip to be extended, such as when comfortably standing upright. Conversely (and likely less common), the capsular ligaments of the hip may be pathologically *lax or loose*, allowing hypermobility of the joint. In some people, such a condition is described as microinstability: a term used to draw attention to the *microtrauma* that can occur when an abnormally slackened joint is exposed to the cumulative effect of relatively small but repetitive contact stresses. Although typically not nearly as common as in the glenohumeral joint, microinstability of the hip can occur in young adults, causing pain and disability and even a potential predisposition to early hip osteoarthritis. Microinstability due to capsular laxity is often linked with mild or borderline hip dysplasia, labral tears, genetic abnormalities (such as those related to Ehlers-Danlos syndrome), history of dislocation or activities that place repeated stretch on the capsule, or incomplete closure or repair of the anterior capsule after hip surgery.[113,146]

Close-Packed Position of the Hip

Isolated movements that significantly elongate or stretch the capsular ligaments are listed in Table 12.1. From a slightly different perspective, it may be clinically useful to consider that the hip position that likely produces the greatest *simultaneous* elongation to most parts of the capsular ligaments combines full extension of the hip (i.e., about 20 degrees beyond the neutral position) with slight internal rotation and slight abduction (Fig. 12.16). This can be important therapeutically because this singular motion can be used to stretch the majority of the hip's capsule. Because this position spirals and tenses most of the capsular ligaments, it may be considered the close-packed position of the hip. The passive tension generated especially by full extension lends stability to the joint and reduces passive accessory movement or "joint play." The hip is one of very few joints in the body in which the close-packed position is *not* also associated with the position of maximal joint congruency. The hip joint surfaces fit most congruently in about 90 degrees of flexion with moderate abduction and external rotation—a position that a young child's dysplastic and unstable hip is often held with assistance of a harness to promote natural formation and stability of the joint.[333] In this position, much of the capsule and associated

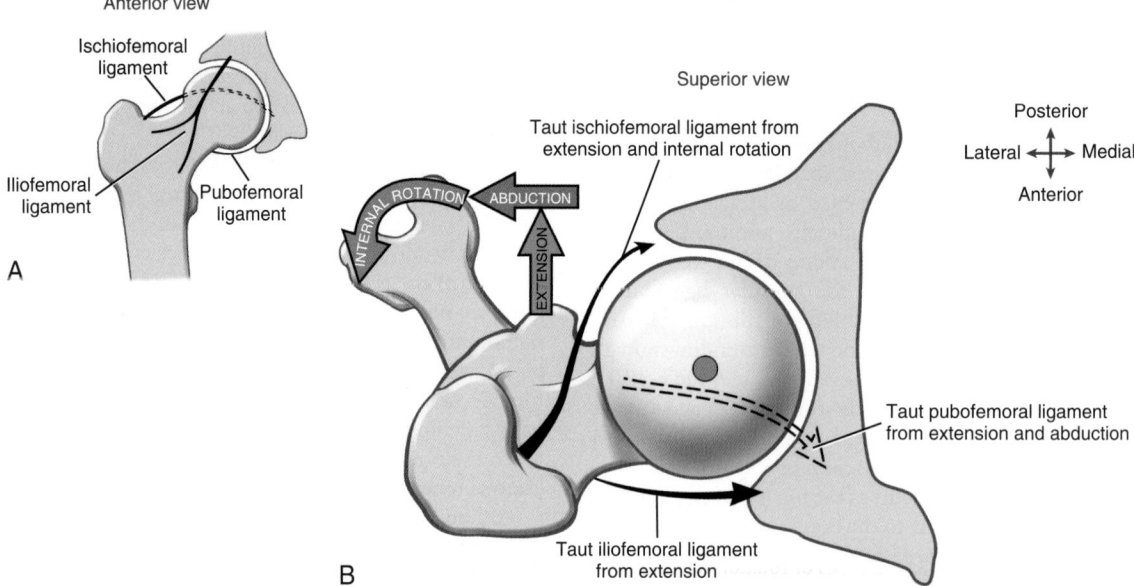

FIG. 12.16 (A) The hip is shown in a neutral position, with all three capsular ligaments identified. (B) Superior view of the hip in its close-packed position (i.e., fully extended with slight abduction and internal rotation). This position elongates at least some component of all three capsular ligaments.

ligaments have unraveled to a more relatively slackened state, providing only modest passive tension to the joint.

Osteokinematics

This section focuses on the range of motion allowed by the adult hip, including the factors that permit and restrict this motion. Reduced hip motion may be an early indicator of disease or trauma, at either the hip or elsewhere in the body. Limited hip motion can impose significant functional limitations in activities such as walking, dressing, standing upright comfortably, or picking up objects off the floor.

Two terms are used to describe the kinematics at the hip. *Femoral-on-pelvic* hip osteokinematics describes the rotation of the femur about a relatively fixed pelvis. *Pelvic-on-femoral* hip osteokinematics, in contrast, describes the rotation of the pelvis, and often the superimposed trunk, over relatively fixed femurs. Regardless of whether the femur or the pelvis is the moving segment, the osteokinematics are described from the anatomic position. The names of the movements are as follows: *flexion* and *extension* in the sagittal plane, *abduction* and *adduction* in the frontal plane, and *internal* and *external rotation* in the horizontal plane (Fig. 12.17).

Reporting the range of motion at the hip uses the anatomic position as the 0-degree or neutral reference point. Within the sagittal plane, for example, femoral-on-pelvic (hip) flexion occurs as the femur rotates anteriorly, whether toward or beyond the 0-degree reference position. Extension, the reverse movement, occurs as the

femur rotates posteriorly, toward or beyond the 0-degree reference position. The term hyperextension is *not* used in this chapter to describe normal range of motion at the hip.

As depicted in Fig. 12.17, each plane of motion is associated with a unique *axis of rotation*. The axis is assumed to pass through or near the center of the femoral head. Although this is only an estimate, it is usually acceptable for most common clinical purposes, such as manual goniometry or for proposing a likely action of a muscle. More in-depth and sophisticated analysis is required, however, when a more precise estimate of the axis of rotation is needed, such as when planning, performing, or revising a total hip arthroplasty (hip replacement).[145]

The axis of rotation for internal and external rotation at the hip is often referred to as a "longitudinal" or vertical axis. While standing, this axis of rotation extends vertically as a straight line between the center of the femoral head and the center of the knee joint. Because of the angle of inclination of the proximal femur and the anterior bowing of the femoral shaft, most of the longitudinal axis of rotation lies *outside* the femur itself (see Fig. 12.17A–B). This extramedullary axis has implications regarding some of the actions of hip muscles, a point discussed later in this chapter.

Unless otherwise specified, the following discussions refer to *passive* ranges of motion. Some of the connective tissues and muscles that limit passive motion are summarized in Table 12.1. The muscles used to produce and control hip motion are discussed in more detail later in this chapter. Although femoral-on-pelvic and pelvic-on-femoral movements often occur simultaneously, they are presented here separately.

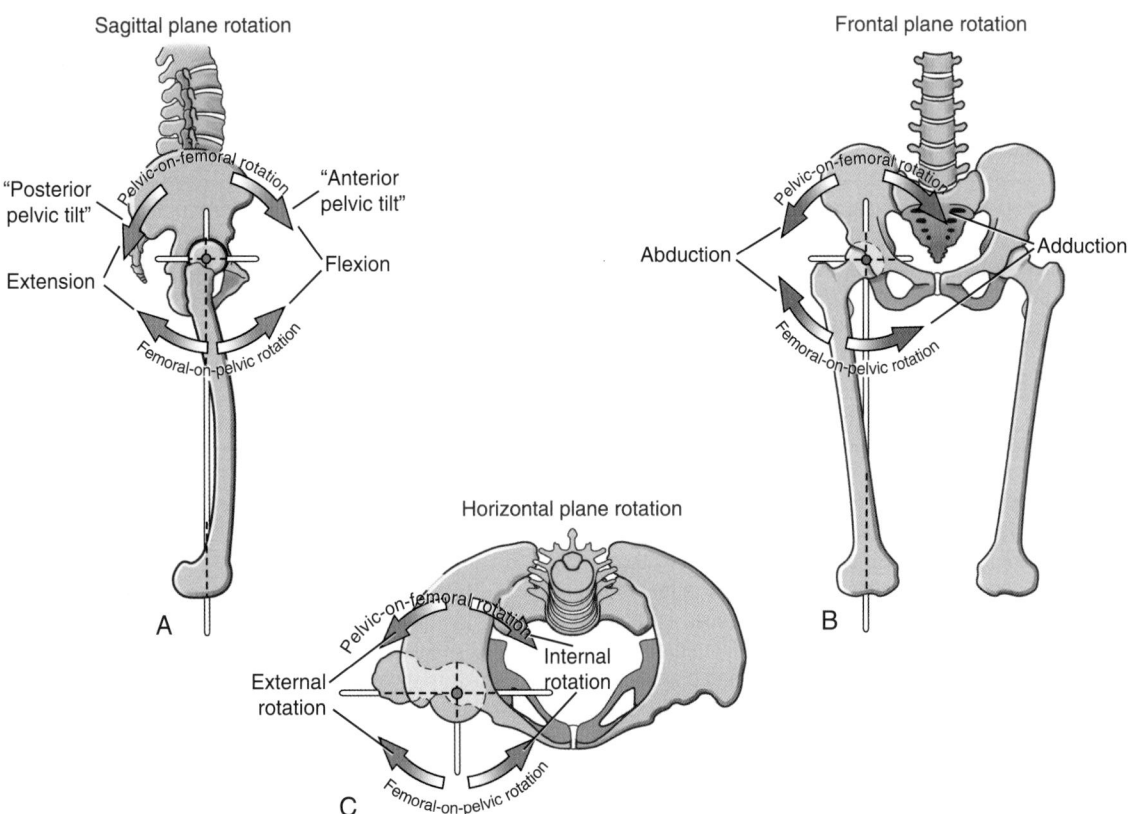

FIG. 12.17 The osteokinematics of the right hip. Femoral-on-pelvic and pelvic-on-femoral rotations occur in three planes. The axis of rotation for each plane of movement is shown as a colored dot, located at the center of the femoral head. (A) Side view shows *sagittal plane rotations* around a medial-lateral axis of rotation. (B) Front view shows *frontal plane rotations* around an anterior-posterior axis of rotation. (C) Top view shows *horizontal plane rotations* around a longitudinal, or vertical, axis of rotation.

FEMORAL-ON-PELVIC OSTEOKINEMATICS

Rotation of the Femur in the Sagittal Plane

On average, with the knee flexed, the hip *flexes* to about 120 degrees (Fig. 12.18A).[82,256] Activities such as squatting, sitting cross-legged, or tying a shoelace typically require close to this full amount of flexion.[114] Flexing the hip, in general, slackens most of the fibers within the three primary capsular ligaments. The extremes of full flexion, however, tighten the deeper (zona orbicularis) fibers of capsule. The last several degrees of full hip flexion, therefore, are typically the result of femoral rotation combined with modest but observable posterior tilting of the pelvis and associated flexion of the lumbar region.[165] In essence, when the hip approaches full passive flexion, the pelvis "follows" the rotation direction of the femur because of the tension exerted on the deep part of the capsule as well as hip extensor muscles such as the gluteus maximus. With the knee fully extended, hip flexion is typically limited to 70 to 80 degrees by increased tension in the hamstring muscles. The amount of this movement varies considerably because people have such different degrees of hamstring muscle flexibility.

The hip normally *extends* about 20 degrees beyond the neutral position.[256] Many activities routinely approach this amount of hip extension, such as just prior to the push off phase of walking at an average speed (see Fig. 15.13). For many adults, a loss of only about 10 degrees of hip extension would likely require an observable kinematic compensation by other joints within the lower limbs. Full hip extension increases the passive tension throughout much of the capsular ligaments, especially the iliofemoral ligament as well as the hip flexor muscles. When the knee is fully flexed during hip extension, passive tension in the stretched rectus femoris, which crosses both the hip and the knee, typically reduces hip extension to about the neutral position.

Rotation of the Femur in the Frontal Plane

The hip *abducts*, on average, about 40 to 45 degrees, limited primarily by the pubofemoral ligament and the adductor muscles (see Fig. 12.18B).[256] Some activities require supraphysiologic demands on this motion—as high as 70 degrees of abduction during some forms of ballet dance.[114] The hip *adducts* about 25 degrees beyond the neutral position. In addition to interference with the contralateral limb, adduction may be limited by passive tension in stretched hip abductor muscles, including the piriformis, and the iliotibial band.

Rotation of the Femur in the Horizontal Plane

The magnitude of internal and external rotation of the hip is particularly variable among subjects. On average, the hip *internally rotates* about 35 degrees from the neutral position (see Fig. 12.18C).[256,282] With the hip in extension, maximal internal rotation elongates the external rotator muscles, such as the piriformis, and parts of the ischiofemoral ligament.

The extended hip *externally rotates* on average about 45 degrees. Excessive tension in the lateral fasciculus of the iliofemoral ligament can limit full external rotation, as can heightened stiffness of any muscle that contributes to internal rotation.

SPECIAL FOCUS 12.2

Intracapsular Pressure within the Hip

As described earlier, the intracapsular pressure within the healthy hip is normally less than atmospheric pressure. Assuming an intact acetabular labrum, the relatively low pressure creates a partial suction that provides some stability to the hip.

Wingstrand and colleagues studied the effect of joint position and capsular swelling on the intracapsular pressure within cadaveric hips.[327] Except for the extremes of motion, pressures remained relatively low throughout most of flexion and extension. When fluid was injected into the joint to simulate capsular swelling, pressure rose dramatically throughout a greater portion of the range of motion (Fig. 12.19). Regardless of the amount of injected fluid, however, pressure always remained lowest in the *middle* of the range of motion. These data help explain why someone with capsulitis and swelling within the hip tends to feel most comfortable holding the hip in partial flexion. Reduced intracapsular pressure may decrease distension of the inflamed capsule. Unfortunately, over time, a maintained flexed position may lead to contracture caused by the adaptive shortening of the hip flexor muscles and capsular ligaments.

A person with capsular swelling associated with an inflamed synovium, capsule, or bursa of the hip is thus susceptible to developing hip flexion tightness. Reducing the inflammation and swelling through medicine and physical therapy can make activities that favor the extended position more tolerable. Exercises should be devised that strengthen hip extensor muscles while

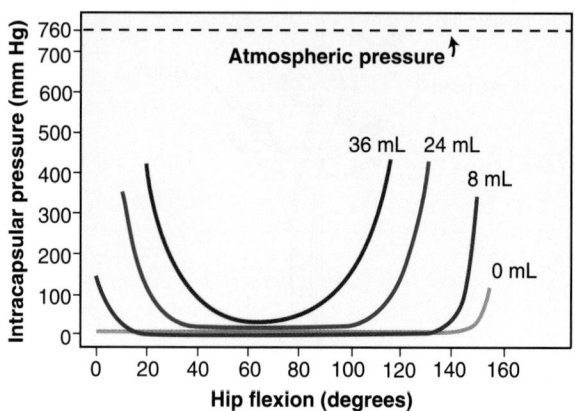

FIG. 12.19 The intracapsular pressure in the hip joints of cadavers as a function of hip flexion angle. The four curved lines indicate the pressure–angle relationships after the injection of different volumes of fluid into the capsule of the hip.[327]

also stretching the hip flexor muscles and anterior capsular structures. Research strongly suggests that the gluteus maximus (a primary hip extensor) is neurologically inhibited following simulated intracapsular effusion (swelling),[94] so therapeutic activities that encourage strong activation of the hip extensor muscles are especially important.

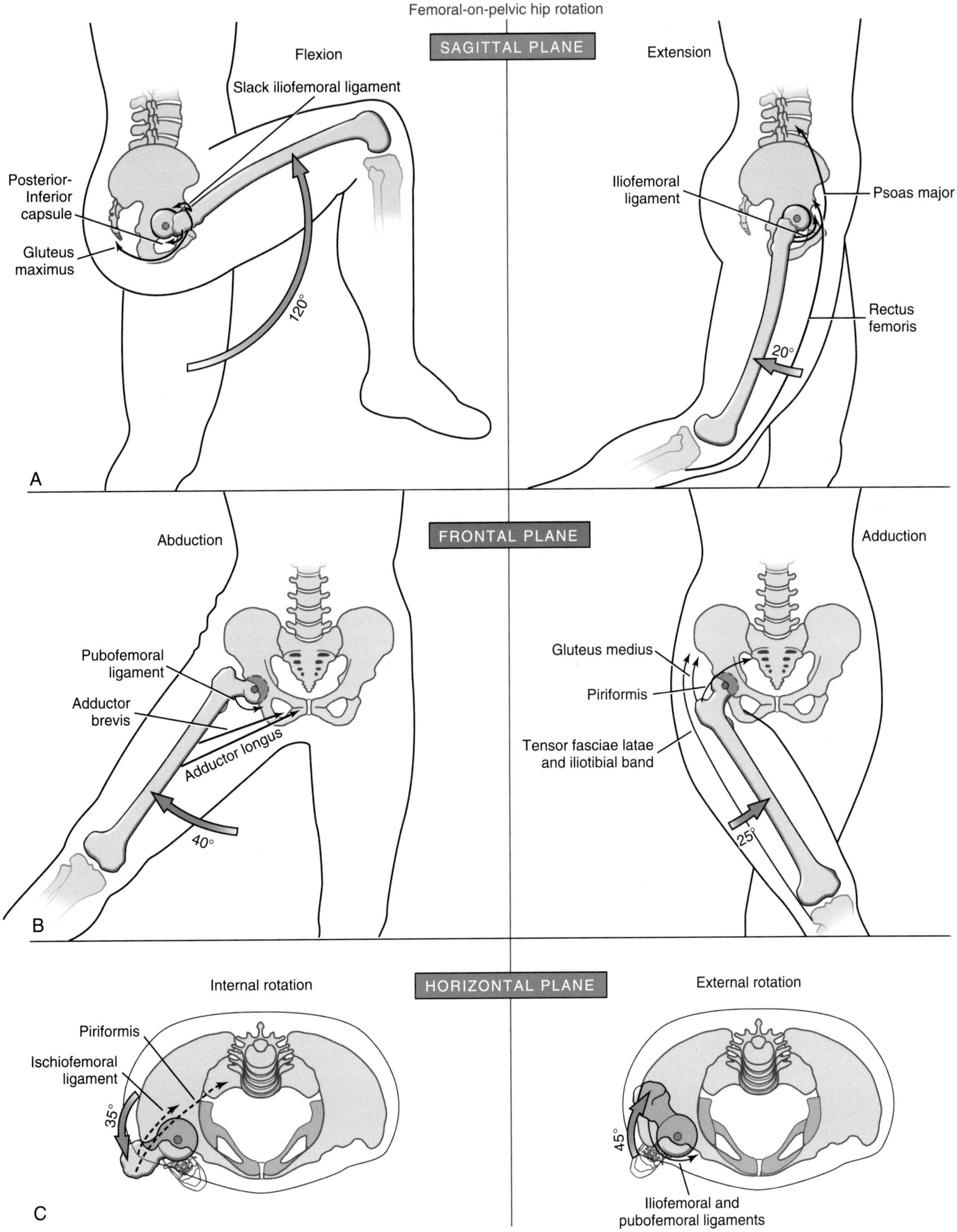

FIG. 12.18 The near maximal range of *femoral-on-pelvic* (hip) motion is depicted in the sagittal plane (A), frontal plane (B), and horizontal plane (C). Tissues that are elongated or pulled taut are indicated by straight black or dashed black arrows. Slackened tissue is indicated by a wavy black arrow.

PELVIC-ON-FEMORAL OSTEOKINEMATICS

Lumbopelvic Rhythm

The caudal end of the axial skeleton is normally firmly attached to the pelvis by way of the sacroiliac joints. As a consequence, rotation of the pelvis over the femoral heads changes the configuration of the lumbar spine. This important kinematic relationship is known as *lumbopelvic rhythm*, introduced in Chapter 9. This concept is revisited in this chapter with a focus on the kinesiology at the hip.

Fig. 12.20 shows two contrasting types of lumbopelvic rhythm frequently used during pelvic-on-femoral (hip) flexion. Although the kinematics depicted are limited to the sagittal plane, the concepts can also be applied to pelvic rotations in the frontal and horizontal planes. Fig. 12.20A shows an example of an *ipsidirectional lumbopelvic rhythm*, in which the pelvis and lumbar spine rotate in the *same* direction. The effect of this movement is to maximize the angular displacement of the *entire* trunk relative to the lower extremities—an effective strategy for increasing reach of the upper extremities. The kinematics of the ipsidirectional lumbopelvic rhythm are discussed in detail in Chapter 9. In contrast, during *contradirectional lumbopelvic rhythm* the pelvis rotates in one direction while the lumbar spine simultaneously rotates in the *opposite* direction (see Fig. 12.20B). The important consequence of this movement is that the supralumbar trunk (i.e., that part of the body located above the first lumbar vertebra) can remain nearly stationary as the pelvis rotates over the femurs. This type of rhythm is used during walking, for example, when the movement of the supralumbar trunk—including the head and eyes—need to be minimized and performed independently of the rotation of the pelvis. In this manner the lumbar spine functions as a mechanical "decoupler," allowing the pelvis and the supralumbar trunk to move independently. A person with a fused lumbar spine, therefore, is unable to freely rotate the pelvis about the hips without a similar rotation of parts of the supralumbar trunk, often observable when the individual walks.

Fig. 12.21 shows pelvic-on-femoral osteokinematics at the hip, organized by plane of motion. These kinematics are based on a *contradirectional* lumbopelvic rhythm. In many cases the amount of these pelvic-on-femoral rotations is restricted by natural limitations of movement within the lumbar spine.

Pelvic Rotation in the Sagittal Plane: Anterior and Posterior Pelvic Tilting

Hip flexion can occur through an *anterior pelvic tilt* (see Fig. 12.21A). (As defined in Chapter 9, a "pelvic tilt" is a short-arc, sagittal plane rotation of the pelvis relative to stationary femurs. The named direction of the tilt—*anterior* versus *posterior*—is based on the direction of the iliac crest as it moves around a medial-lateral axis passing through both femoral heads.) The associated increased lumbar lordosis that accompanies an anterior pelvic tilt offsets most of the tendency of the supralumbar trunk to follow the forward rotation of the pelvis. While sitting with 90 degrees of hip flexion, the normal adult can perform about 30 degrees of additional pelvic-on-femoral hip flexion before being restricted by a completely extended lumbar spine. Full anterior tilt of the pelvis slackens most of the ligaments of the hip, most notably the iliofemoral ligament. Marked tightness in any hip extensor muscle—such as the hamstrings—could theoretically limit the extremes of an anterior pelvic tilt. As depicted in Fig. 12.21A, however, because the knees are flexed, the partially slackened hamstring muscles would not generate noticeable resistance to an anterior pelvic tilt. For most people, however, sitting with knees fully extended would stretch the hamstrings to a point of limiting the total amount of anterior pelvic tilt.

As depicted in Fig. 12.21A, the hips can be *extended* about 10 to 20 degrees from the 90-degree sitting posture via a *posterior tilt* of the pelvis. During sitting, this short-arc pelvic rotation would increase the length (and therefore tension) only minimally in the iliofemoral ligament and rectus femoris muscle. With femurs fixed, the posterior tilting of the pelvis flexes the lumbar spine and reduces its lordosis.[125]

As described in Chapter 9 and highlighted in Fig. 9.63, changing the amount of lumbar lordosis through anterior and posterior tilting the pelvis effects many biomechanical features of the lumbar spine, including altering the diameter of the intervertebral foramen and influencing the direction of the pressure flow gradient of the nucleus pulposus. (These and several other effects on the lumbar spine can be reviewed in Table 9.10.) The aforementioned relationships between the hip and lumbar spine have important clinical implications when evaluating and treating pain or movement dysfunction in this area of the body. In addition, this region shares similar patterns of referred pain. The combination of these biomechanical and anatomic factors can make it very difficult to identify the primary source of a person's pathology or pathokinesiology: Is it the spine, hip, or both? Correct identification, however, can be critical to successful surgical and nonsurgical interventions. This clinical dilemma, first published in 1983, remains well addressed in the literature under the title Hip Spine Syndrome.[18,42,189,247,315]

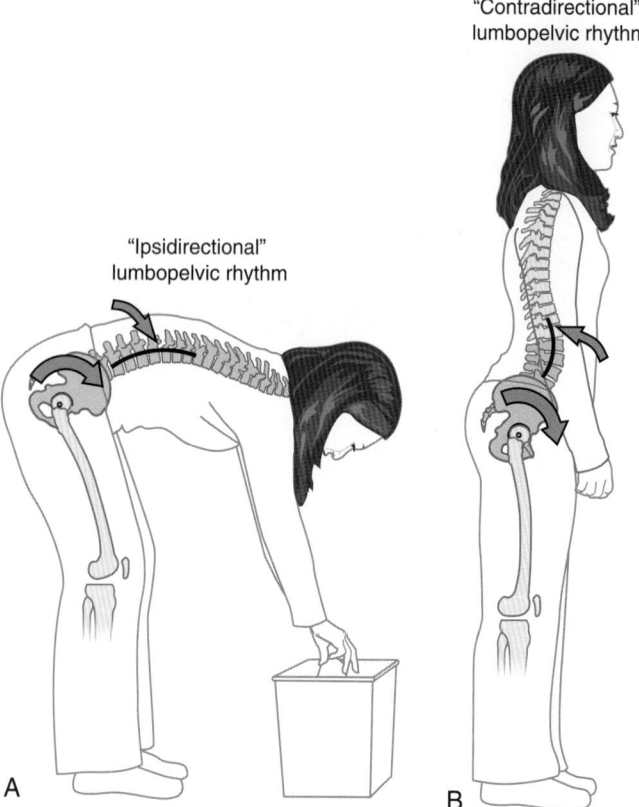

"Ipsidirectional" lumbopelvic rhythm

"Contradirectional" lumbopelvic rhythm

FIG. 12.20 Two contrasting types of lumbopelvic rhythms used to rotate the pelvis over fixed femurs. (A) An "ipsidirectional" rhythm describes a movement in which the lumbar spine and pelvis rotate in the *same* direction, thus amplifying overall trunk motion. (B) A "contradirectional" rhythm describes a movement in which the lumbar spine and pelvis rotate in *opposite* directions. See text for further explanation.

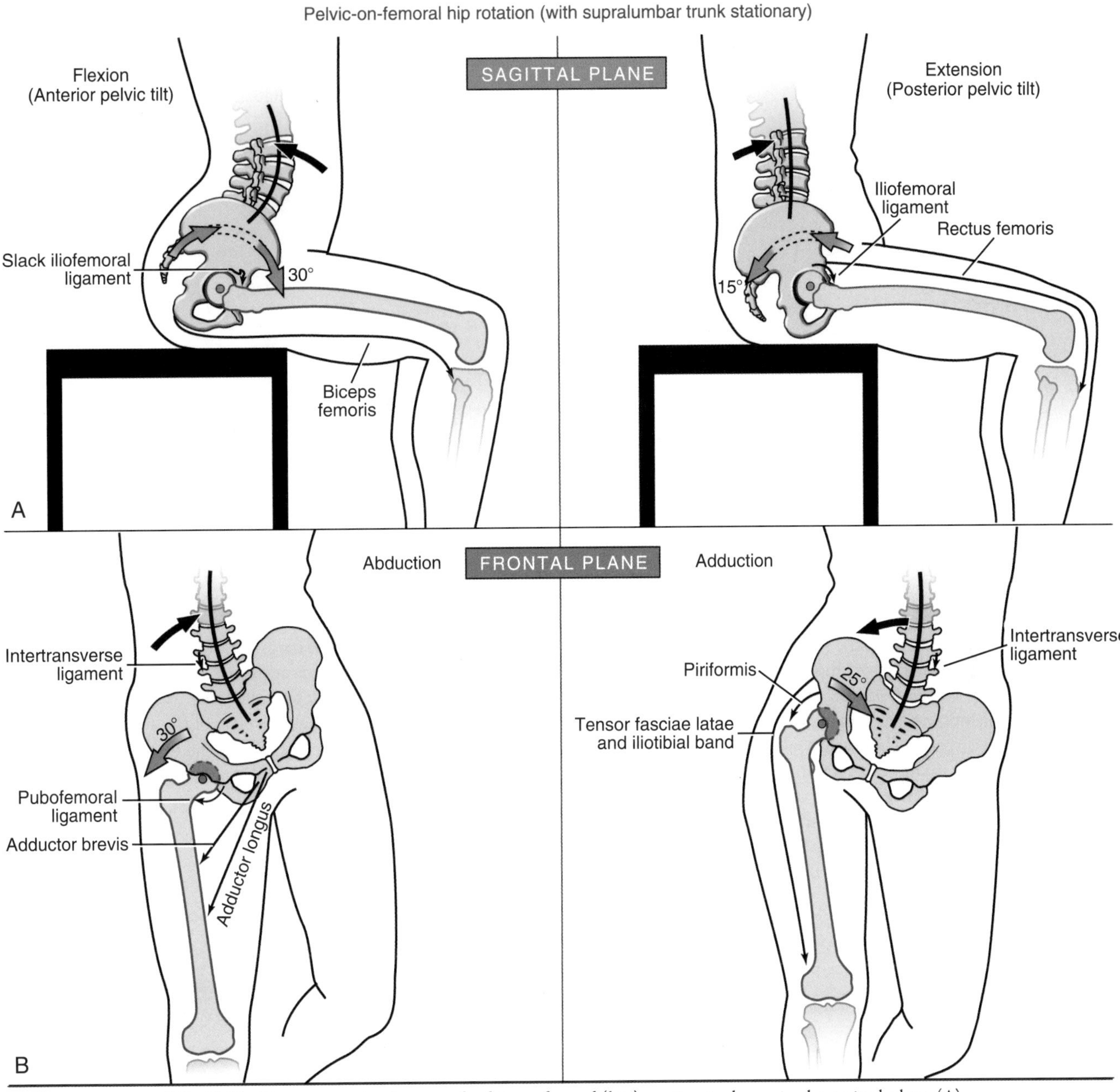

FIG. 12.21 The near maximal range of *pelvic-on-femoral* (hip) motion is shown in the sagittal plane (A) and frontal plane (B). The motion assumes that the supralumbar trunk remains nearly stationary during the hip motion (i.e., kinematics based on a *contradirectional* lumbopelvic rhythm). The large colored and black arrows depict pelvic rotation and the associated "offsetting" lumbar motion. Tissues that are elongated or pulled taut are indicated by thin, straight black arrows; tissue slackened is indicated by thin wavy black arrow.

Continued

Pelvic Rotation in the Frontal Plane

Pelvic-on-femoral rotation in the frontal and horizontal planes is aptly described by a person standing on one limb in the context of a contradirectional lumbopelvic rhythm. Within this context, the weight-bearing extremity is referred to as the "support hip" throughout this chapter.

Abduction of the support hip occurs by *raising* or "hiking" the iliac crest on the side of the nonsupport hip (see Fig. 12.21B). Such a movement could be driven, in part, by contraction of the gluteus medius and minimus on the side of the support hip. Assuming that the supralumbar trunk remains nearly stationary, the lumbar spine must bend in the direction opposite the rotating pelvis. The lumbar region thus forms a slight lateral convexity toward the side of the abducting support hip.

Pelvic-on-femoral hip abduction is restricted to about 30 degrees, primarily because of the natural limits of lateral bending in the lumbar

spine. Marked tightness in the ipsilateral adductor muscles or in the pubofemoral ligament can limit pelvic-on-femoral hip abduction. If a marked adductor tightness is present, the iliac crest on the side of the nonsupport hip may remain *lower* than the iliac crest of the support hip, which can interfere with the fluidity of walking.

Adduction of the support hip occurs by a *lowering* of the iliac crest on the side of the nonsupport hip. This movement can be partially controlled by an eccentric activation of the gluteus medius and minimus on the side of the support hip. This motion produces a slight lateral concavity within the lumbar region toward the side of the adducted support hip (see Fig. 12.21B). A hypomobile or painful lumbar spine and/or reduced extensibility in the iliotibial band or hip abductor muscles, such as the gluteus medius, piriformis, or tensor fasciae latae, may restrict the extremes of this motion.

Pelvic-on-femoral hip rotation (with supralumbar trunk stationary)

Internal rotation   HORIZONTAL PLANE   External rotation

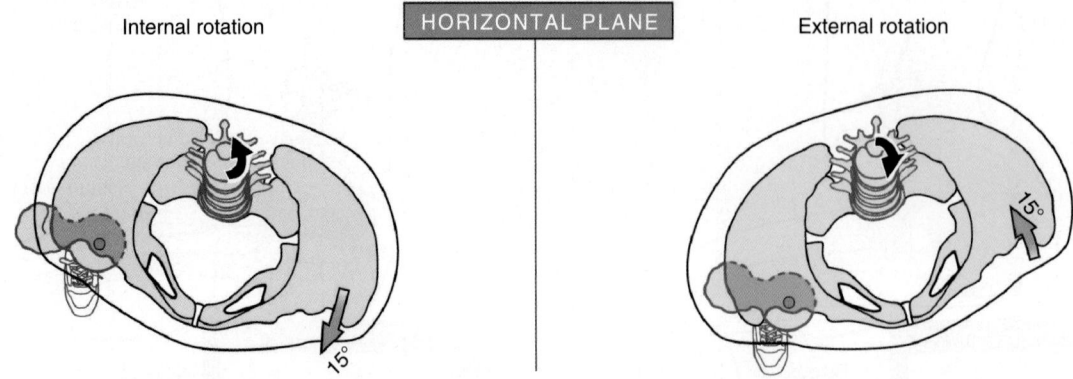

C

FIG. 12.21, cont'd. The near maximal range of *pelvic-on-femoral* (hip) internal and external is shown in the horizontal plane (C). The motion assumes that the supralumbar trunk remains nearly stationary during the hip motion (i.e., kinematics based on *contradirectional* lumbopelvic rhythm). The large colored and black arrows depict pelvic rotation and the associated "offsetting" lumbar motion.

Pelvic Rotation in the Horizontal Plane

Pelvic-on-femoral rotation occurs in the horizontal plane about a longitudinal axis of rotation (see green circle at femoral head in Fig. 12.21C). *Internal rotation* of the support hip occurs as the iliac crest on the side of the nonsupport hip rotates *forward* in the horizontal plane. During *external rotation*, in contrast, the iliac crest on the side of the nonsupport hip rotates *backward* in the horizontal plane. If the pelvis is rotating beneath a relatively stationary trunk, the lumbar spine must *rotate* (or twist) in the opposite direction as the rotating pelvis. The small amount of axial rotation normally permitted in the lumbar spine significantly limits the full expression of horizontal plane rotation of the support hip when attempting to maintain a forward-facing position of the trunk. The full potential of pelvic-on-femoral rotation requires that the lumbar spine *and* trunk follow the rotation of the pelvis—a movement strategy more consistent with an ipsidirectional lumbopelvic rhythm.

Arthrokinematics

During movement, the nearly spherical femoral head normally remains well seated within the confines of the acetabulum. As a result, the well-formed hip is typically inherently stable, allowing relatively minimal arthrokinematic translations. The steep walls and relative depth of the acetabulum, in conjunction with the capsular ligaments and tightly fitting acetabular labrum, restrict the average physiologic translation between articular surfaces during movement to about 2 mm or less.[148,186] This amount of joint "play" is naturally greater during movements that involve greater flexion, primarily because of the transient laxity placed within the capsular ligaments.[113] Compared with other articulations (such as the wrist or glenohumeral joints), however, the magnitude of translation within the hip during movement is relatively small. Nevertheless, the arthrokinematics at the hip follow the traditional convex-on-concave and concave-on-convex principles described in Chapter 1.

Fig. 12.22 shows a highly mechanical illustration of a hip opened to enable visualization of the paths of articular motion. Assuming motion starting in the anatomic position, *abduction* and *adduction* occur along the longitudinal diameter of the joint surfaces. *Internal rotation* and *external rotation* occur across the transverse diameter of the joint surfaces. *Flexion* and *extension* occur as a spin between the femoral head and the lunate surfaces of the acetabulum. The axis of rotation for this spin passes through the femoral head.

Articular paths of hip motion

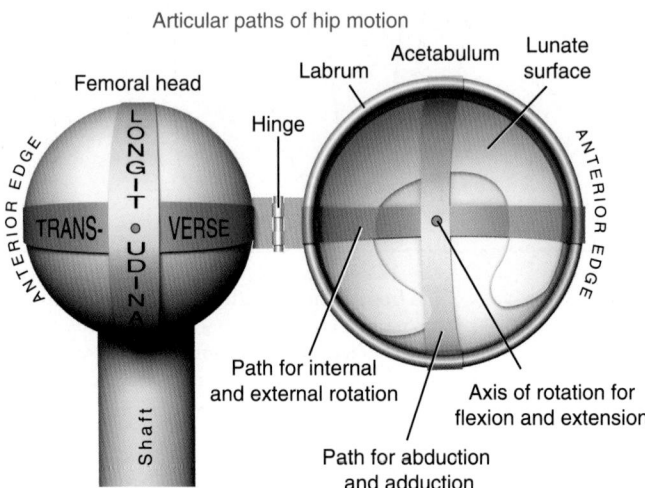

FIG. 12.22 A mechanical drawing of the right hip. The joint surfaces are exposed by swinging the femur open like a door on a hinge. The articular paths of hip frontal and horizontal plane motion occur along the longitudinal (*purple*) and transverse (*blue*) diameters, respectively. Consider these paths of motion for both femoral-on-pelvic and pelvic-on-femoral motions.

Norms for Range of Motion: What About the Hip of the Child?

The normative range of motion of the hip (or any joint) is often determined by using a goniometer. Typically, these normative measurements are made by experienced clinicians, using a relatively large sample of subjects, most often adults. These kinematic data serve many purposes, such as assessing an underlying pathology, determining the ability to perform self-care activities (such as reaching to don shoes), or designing medical equipment and prosthetic limbs. Although not as common, published normative values are also available to describe pediatric hip range of motion. As in the case with adults, these norms for children can help determine underlying medical problems. For example, a child with an inflammatory arthropathy of the hip typically exhibits limited internal rotation. Likewise, a child with a slipped capital femoral epiphysis (SCFE) often will have reduced internal rotation and

excessive external rotation because of the posterior-inferior slippage of the femoral epiphysis relative to the shaft of the femur.[181]

e-Table 12.1 lists average (passive) range of motion values measured from a sample of 252 young patients (2–17 years of age) who had no underlying pathology affecting their lower limbs.[266] Analysis of the data showed a *decreasing* trend in most ranges of hip motion as age advanced. The decline in range of motion, however, differed slightly by biological sex. Whereas no significant difference between boys and girls was detected in any range of motion among the 2-to-5-year-olds, the oldest group of boys had less range of motion than girls for sagittal and frontal plane movements as well as for external rotation with the hip extended. These considerations are important for clinicians who treat children across a wide range of ages.

MUSCLE AND JOINT INTERACTION

Innervation of the Muscles and Joint

INNERVATION OF MUSCLES

The lumbar plexus and the sacral plexus arise from the ventral rami of spinal nerve roots T^{12} through S^4. Nerves from the lumbar plexus innervate the muscles of the anterior and medial thigh, including the quadriceps femoris. Nerves from the sacral plexus innervate the muscles of the posterior and lateral hip, posterior thigh, and entire lower leg.

Lumbar Plexus

The lumbar plexus is formed from the ventral rami of spinal nerve roots T^{12} to L^4. This plexus gives rise to the femoral and obturator nerves (Fig. 12.23A). The *femoral nerve*, the largest branch of the lumbar plexus, is formed by L^2 to L^4 nerve roots. *Motor branches* innervate most hip flexors and all knee extensors. Within the pelvis, proximal to the inguinal ligament, the femoral nerve innervates the psoas major and iliacus. Distal to the inguinal ligament, the femoral nerve innervates the sartorius, part of the pectineus, and the quadriceps muscle group. The femoral nerve has an extensive *sensory distribution* covering much of the skin of the anterior-medial aspect of the thigh. The sensory branches of the femoral nerve innervate the skin of the anterior-medial aspect of the lower leg via the saphenous cutaneous nerve.

> **Motor Innervation of the Lower Extremity Originating from the Lumbar Plexus**
> - Femoral nerve (L^2–L^4)
> - Obturator nerve (L^2–L^4)

Like the femoral nerve, the *obturator nerve* is formed from L^2 to L^4 nerve roots. *Motor branches* innervate the hip adductor muscles.

The obturator nerve divides into anterior and posterior branches as it passes through the obturator foramen. The posterior branch innervates the obturator externus and anterior head of the adductor magnus. The anterior branch innervates part of the pectineus, the adductor brevis, the adductor longus, and the gracilis. The obturator nerve has a *sensory distribution* to the skin of the medial thigh.

Sacral Plexus

The sacral plexus, located on the posterior wall of the pelvis, is formed from the ventral rami of L^4 to S^4 spinal nerve roots. Most nerves from the sacral plexus exit the pelvis via the greater sciatic foramen to innervate the posterior hip muscles (see Fig. 12.23B).

> **Motor Innervation of the Lower Extremity Originating from the Sacral Plexus**
> - Nerve to the obturator internus and gemellus superior (L^5–S^2)
> - Nerve to the quadratus femoris and gemellus inferior (L^4–S^1)
> - Superior gluteal nerve (L^4–S^1)
> - Inferior gluteal nerve (L^5–S^2)
> - Sciatic nerve (L^4–S^3), including tibial and common fibular (peroneal) portions

Five of the six "short external rotators" of the hip are innervated through the sacral plexus. The *nerve to the obturator internus* and *gemellus superior* (L^5–S^2) and the *nerve to the quadratus femoris* and *gemellus inferior* (L^4–S^1) travel to and innervate their respective muscles.

The *superior* and *inferior gluteal nerves* are named according to their positions relative to the piriformis muscle as they exit the greater sciatic notch. The *superior gluteal nerve* (L^4–S^1) innervates the gluteus medius, gluteus minimus, tensor fasciae latae, and piriformis. (The piriformis also receives secondary innervation, within the pelvis, from ventral rami of S^1 and S^2.[143]) The *inferior gluteal nerve* (L^5–S^2) provides the sole innervation to the gluteus maximus.

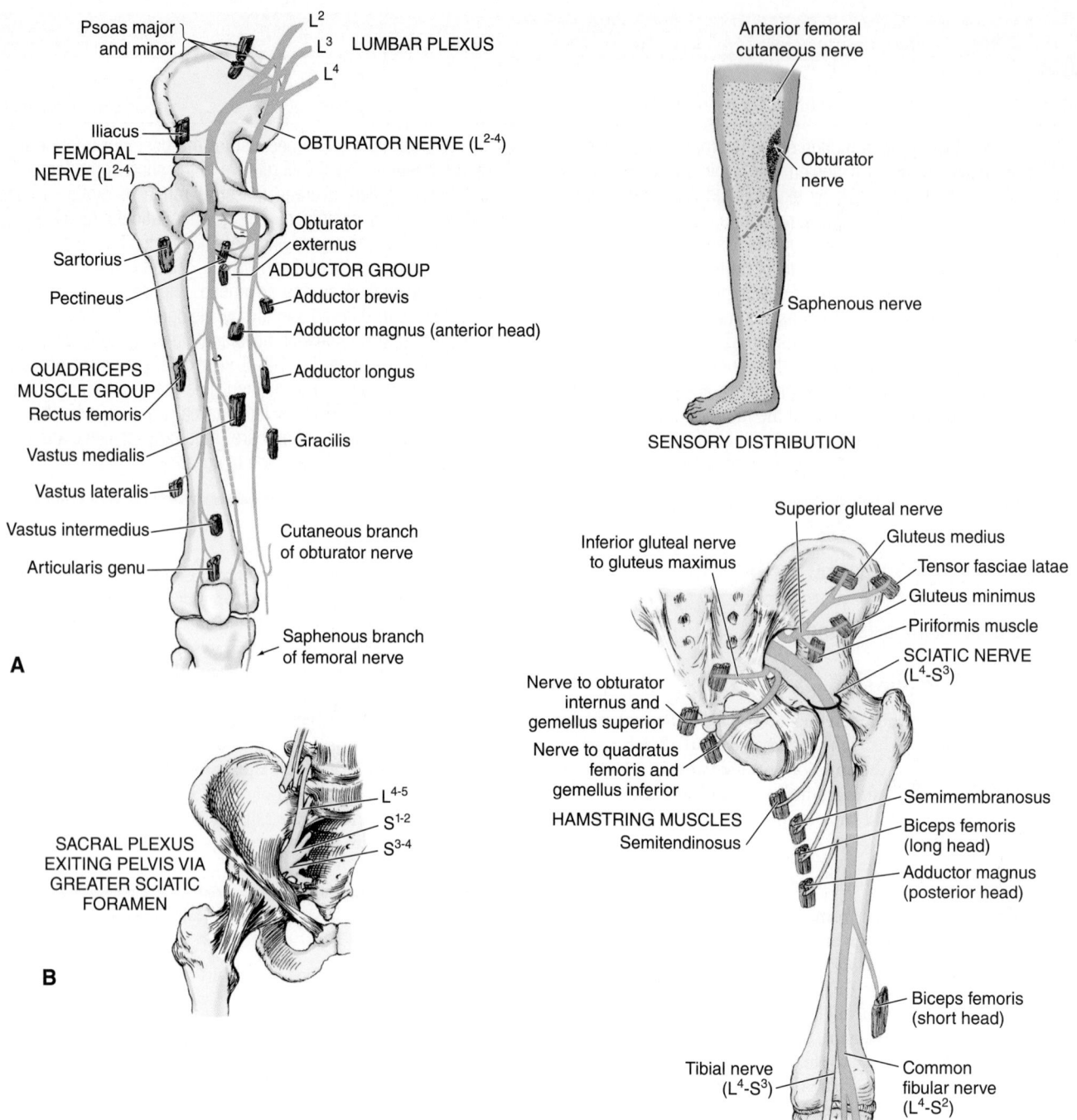

FIG. 12.23 The general path of muscle innervation from the lumbar plexus (A) and the sacral plexus (B). The spinal nerve roots for each nerve are shown in parentheses. The drawing on the right side of (A) shows the sensory branches of the femoral and obturator nerves. (Modified from deGroot J: *Correlative neuroanatomy,* ed 21, Norwalk, Conn, 1991, Appleton & Lange.)

The *sciatic nerve,* the widest and longest nerve in the body, is formed from L^4 to S^3 nerve roots. The sciatic nerve consists of the tibial and the common fibular (peroneal) nerves, typically both enveloped in one connective tissue sheath. In the posterior thigh, the *tibial portion* of the sciatic nerve innervates all the biarticular muscles within the hamstring group and the posterior head of the adductor magnus. The *common fibular portion* of the sciatic nerve innervates the short head of the biceps femoris.

In 85% of cases, the sciatic nerve exits the greater sciatic foramen as a single structure, passing *inferior* to the piriformis. If the sciatic nerve bifurcates proximal to the greater sciatic foramen, the common fibular nerve frequently *pierces* the piriformis as it exits the pelvis, potentially being a source of neurogenic pain from being compressed within the muscle.[308]

As a reference, the primary spinal nerve roots that supply the muscles of the lower extremity are listed in Appendix IV, Part A. In addition, Part B and Fig. IV.1 in Part C of Appendix IV include additional reference items to help guide the clinical assessment of the functional status of structures innervated by L^2 to S^3 nerve roots.

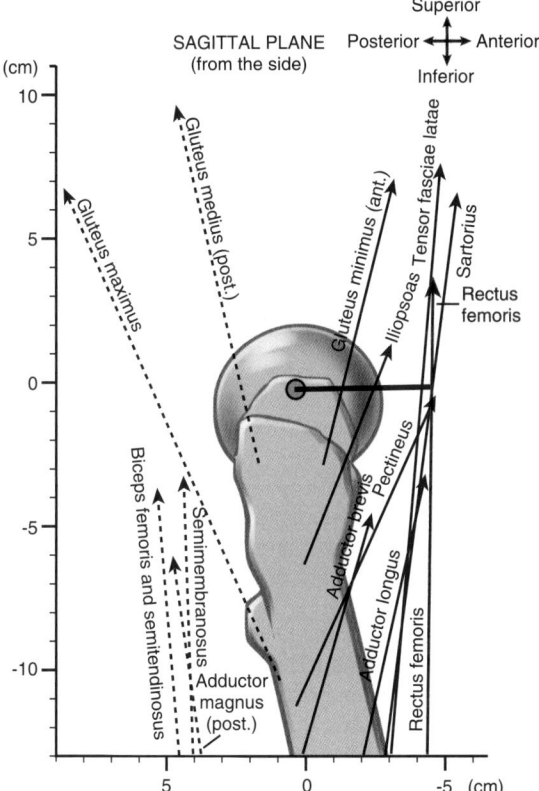

SAGITTAL PLANE
(from the side)

Superior
Posterior ← → Anterior
Inferior

FIG. 12.24 A view from the side that depicts the of lines of force of several hip muscles relative to the sagittal plane. The axis of rotation is directed in the medial-lateral direction through the femoral head. The flexors are indicated by solid lines and the extensors by dashed lines. The internal moment arm used by the rectus femoris is represented by the thick black line.

SENSORY INNERVATION OF THE HIP

The anterior capsule of the hip and acetabular labrum receive sensory innervation primarily from the femoral and obturator nerves.[31] The posterior capsule receives sensory fibers from nerve roots originating from the sacral plexus, carried primarily through the sciatic and superior gluteal nerves, as well as the nerve to the quadratus femoris.[31] The connective tissues of the anterior-medial aspects of the hip and medial part of the knee both receive sensory fibers from the obturator nerve, notably the L^3 nerve root. This may explain why inflammation of the hip may be perceived as pain in the medial knee region.[260]

Muscular Function at the Hip

Throughout this chapter, the lines of force of various muscles are illustrated relative to certain axes of rotation at the hip. Fig. 12.24, for example, shows a sagittal plane representation of the significant flexor and extensor muscles of the hip.[76,77] Although Fig. 12.24 provides useful insight into the potential function of several muscles, two limitations must be considered. First, the line of force of each muscle does *not* represent a force vector; rather it depicts the overall *direction* of the muscle's force that acts within the sagittal plane. The figure therefore does not provide the information needed to compare the "strength"—or torque—potential between the muscles. This comparison requires additional information, such as the muscle's three-dimensional orientation to the hip and its cross-sectional area. Second, the lines of force and subsequent lengths of the moment arms depicted in Fig. 12.24 apply only when the hip is in the anatomic position. Once the hip moves out of this position, the direction of action and the torque potential of each muscle can change considerably. This partially explains why the maximal-effort torque (or maximum strength) of a muscle group varies throughout the range of motion.

Also, throughout this chapter, a muscle's action is considered as either primary or secondary (Table 12.2). The designation of muscle action is based on data such as moment arm length, cross-sectional area, overall muscle fiber direction, and, when available, published reports from electromyography (EMG)-based and anatomic studies. Unless otherwise specified, muscle actions are based on a concentric

	Flexors	**Adductors**	**Internal Rotators**	**Extensors**	**Abductors**	**External Rotators**
Primary	Iliopsoas	Pectineus	Not applicable	Gluteus maximus	Gluteus medius	Gluteus maximus
	Sartorius	Adductor longus		Biceps femoris (long head)	Gluteus minimus	Piriformis
	Tensor fasciae latae	Gracilis		Semitendinosus	Tensor fasciae latae	Obturator internus
	Rectus femoris	Adductor brevis		Semimembranosus		Gemellus superior
	Adductor longus	Adductor magnus		Adductor magnus (posterior head)		Gemellus inferior
	Pectineus					Quadratus femoris
Secondary	Adductor brevis	Biceps femoris (long head)	Gluteus minimus and medius (anterior fibers)	Gluteus medius (middle and posterior fibers)	Piriformis	Gluteus medius and minimus (posterior fibers)
	Gracilis	Gluteus maximus (inferior/ posterior fibers)	Tensor fasciae latae	Adductor magnus (anterior head)	Sartorius	Obturator externus
	Gluteus minimus (anterior fibers)	Quadratus femoris	Adductor longus		Rectus femoris	Sartorius
		Obturator externus	Adductor brevis		Gluteus maximus (anterior/ superior) fibers	Biceps femoris (long head)
			Pectineus			

TABLE 12.2 Muscles of the Hip, Organized According to Primary or Secondary Actions*

*Each action assumes a muscle contraction that originates from the anatomic position. Several of these muscles may have a different action (or strength of action) when they contract from a position other than the anatomic position.

contraction originating from the anatomic position. Muscles with relatively insignificant or inherently weak actions, or actions that are substantial only outside of the anatomic position, are not included in Table 12.2. Refer to Appendix IV, Part D, for a listing of more detailed attachments and innervation of all muscles of the hip. Also, as a reference, cross-sectional areas of selected muscles of the hip are listed in Appendix IV, Part E.

HIP FLEXOR MUSCLES

The primary hip flexors are the iliopsoas, sartorius, tensor fasciae latae, rectus femoris, adductor longus, and pectineus (Fig. 12.25). Fig. 12.24 shows the excellent flexion leverage of many of these muscles. Secondary hip flexors include the adductor brevis, gracilis, and anterior fibers of the gluteus minimus. The psoas minor, although not a hip flexor on its own merit, is also discussed in this section.

Anatomy and Individual Actions
The Iliopsoas and Psoas Minor
The *iliopsoas* is large and long, spanning a considerable distance between the last thoracic vertebra and the proximal femur (see Fig. 12.25). Anatomically, the iliopsoas consists of two muscles: the iliacus and the psoas major. The *iliacus* attaches on the iliac fossa and extreme lateral edge of the sacrum, just over the sacroiliac joint. The *psoas major* attaches along the transverse processes of the last thoracic and all lumbar vertebrae, including the intervertebral discs. Some of the proximal fibers of the psoas major intermix with the adjacent exiting L^{1-4} nerve roots of the lumbar plexus.[226]

The iliacus and the psoas major muscles join just anterior to the femoral head, forming a united musculotendinous unit that flows distally to attach on and near the lesser trochanter of the femur (Fig. 12.26). As evident in the lateral view of Fig.12.26, en route to the

femur, the broad iliopsoas tendon is deflected *posteriorly* about 45 degrees as it crosses over the outer anterior brim of the pelvis (near the junction of the iliopubic ramus and superior pubic ramus; review Fig. 12.1). With the hip in extension, this deflection raises the tendon's angle-of-insertion to the femur, thereby increasing the muscle's leverage for hip flexion. As the hip flexes to 90 degrees, the moment arm increases even further, which may help compensate for the muscle's loss in force when in a significantly shortened state.[35]

Between the hip joint and the lesser trochanter, the iliopsoas tendon consists of an intermingling of several sets of muscle *and* tendinous strands of tissue.[243] The distal iliacus typically remains more muscular than the more tendinous distal psoas major.[36,300] Deep to and separate from the distal iliacus is a slender, poorly defined "streak" of muscle fibers known as the *iliocapsularis*. Measuring on average 117 mm long by 13 mm wide, the fibers blend with the anterior-medial capsule of the hip.[187] When activated, the iliocapsularis may prevent the capsule from excessive slackening during hip flexion, thereby preventing the capsule from being impinged between the femoral head and edge of the acetabulum (Video 12.1).[41,169] In some cases of developmental hip dysplasia, the iliocapsularis appears hypertrophied, conceivably as a compensation for a chronically weakened and subsequently lax anterior capsule.[23,111,228]

Video 12.2 highlights the musculotendinous anatomy of the distal iliopsoas as it crosses the hip joint toward the lesser trochanter. This area of the hip is clinically important as the distal iliopsoas may become mechanically abraded or impinged as it courses over the iliopubic eminence (review Fig. 12.1), acetabular labrum, femoral head, or anterior brim of the pelvis. In some cases, the repetitive mechanical stress to the undersurface of the iliopsoas leads to iliopsoas tendonitis or tendinopathy (IPT), often associated with anterior hip or groin pain that is aggravated by muscle activation or stretch. IPT has also been reported to occur as a postoperative

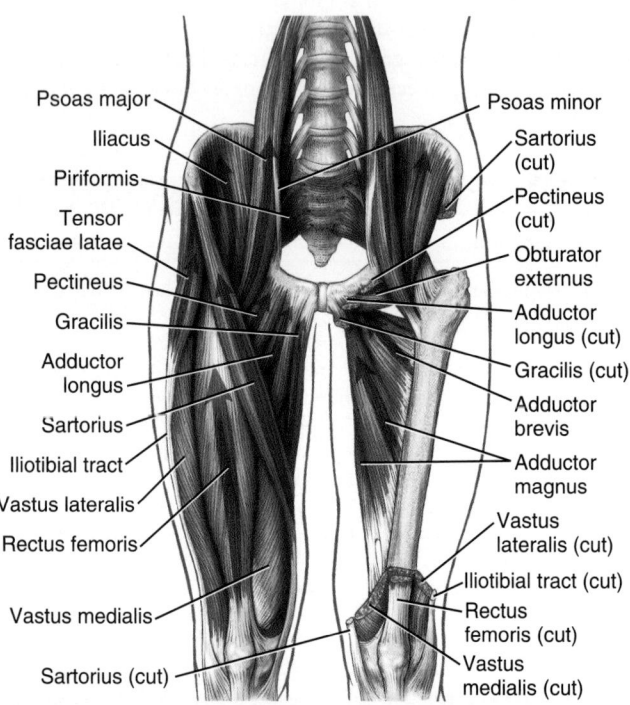

FIG. 12.25 Muscles of the anterior hip region. The right side of the body shows flexors and adductor muscles. Many muscles on the left side are cut away to expose the adductor brevis and adductor magnus.

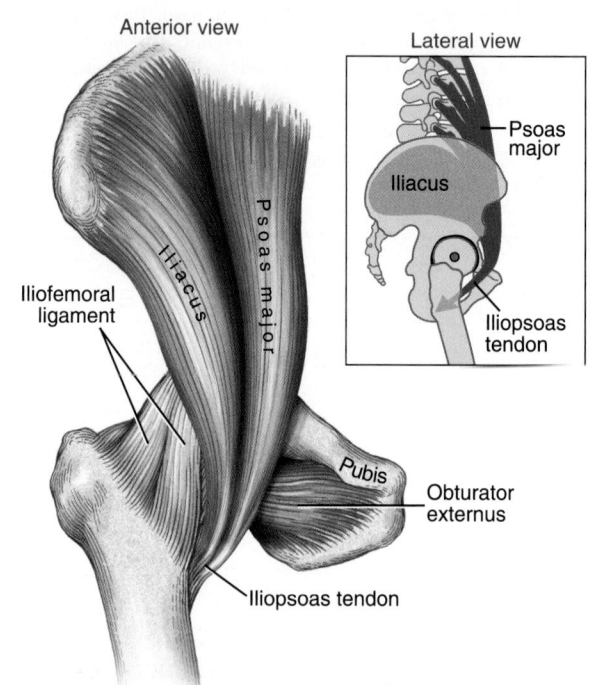

FIG. 12.26 Anterior and lateral views of the right iliacus and psoas major, flowing into the iliopsoas tendon en route to the lesser trochanter.

complication in 7% of hip arthroscopic procedures.[46] Although less common, IPT may also occur after a total hip replacement, possibly because of the tendon being repeatedly abraded against an oversized or malpositioned prosthetic hip implant.[137,185]

Another recognized but relatively rare manifestation of mechanical abrasion of the iliopsoas tendon is referred to as "internal snapping hip" syndrome.[106,185] This syndrome is named for the audible click of the tendon as it abruptly crosses over structures such as the anterior labrum or iliopectineal eminence, often as the flexed and externally rotated hip is moved into full extension and internal rotation. The snapping condition, which may not be painful, tends to occur more often in relatively younger, active populations. As with all forms of mechanically based IPT, the first course of treatment should consist of conservative measures, including physical therapy, activity modification, anti-inflammatory medication, or ultrasound-guided corticosteroid injection.[185] If the painful snapping condition persists, in select cases, a partial surgical release or lengthening of the tendinous parts of the distal iliopsoas may be indicated.[106,137,239] A tenotomy that spares the more muscular fibers of the musculotendinous complex is typically desired as a way to limit loss of hip flexion strength, a possible complication of this procedure.[239]

Kinesiologically, the iliopsoas is a prominent femoral-on-pelvic hip flexor. This action is expressed to varying degrees during late stance and the swing phase of walking and running (Chapters 15–16). Based on the muscle's spatial orientation and tendon's angle-of-insertion to the femur, the iliopsoas generates most of the anterior-directed joint reaction force against the femoral head as the limb is advanced forward while walking.[64] From the anatomic position, the iliopsoas is not an effective rotator, although with the hip abducted the iliopsoas tendon changes its approach to the femur and thereby may assist with external rotation.[285]

The extensive psoas major imparts a dominant kinetic impact across the entire midsection of the body, from thoracolumbar junction to the hips. In addition to being a dominant flexor of the trunk-and-pelvis over fixed thighs, the psoas major, when active bilaterally, also contributes significant frontal plane stability to the lumbar spine. This contribution to lumbar spine stability is evident based on EMG observations of strong *bilateral* activation of the psoas major muscles as healthy subjects performed a resisted *unilateral* straight-leg-raise effort.[139] Without this bilateral activation, the lumbar spine would theoretically be pulled unilaterally to the side of the strongly contracting psoas major performing the resisted hip flexion.

The *psoas minor* lies directly anterior to the muscle belly of the psoas major, although it may be present only in about 60% to 65% of people.[226] This slender, typically bilateral muscle attaches proximally on the lateral bodies of the twelfth thoracic and first lumbar vertebrae and distally to the inner brim of the pelvis, just medial to the acetabulum and iliopubic eminence (see Fig. 12.1). The muscle belly occupies just the proximal 35% to 40% of the entire musculotendinous structure.[217] (Other muscles with a somewhat similar morphology include the palmaris longus and the plantaris.) In addition to its bony attachment to the pelvis, the relatively long tendon of the psoas minor also attaches distally into a broad band of *iliac fascia* that drapes over the distal iliopsoas and femoral nerve.[217] As illustrated in e-Fig. 12.4, by connecting to the iliac fascia, contraction of the psoas minor may stabilize the position of the underlying iliopsoas as it crosses the hip and anterior brim of the pelvis.[223] Such stabilization might protect the iliopsoas from injury by preventing it from freely sliding across the underlying pelvis during hip motion. By adjusting the active tension within the iliac fascia, the psoas minor may also limit "bowstringing" of the iliopsoas away from the hip joint during high degrees of hip flexion[217] (Video 12.3).

The Remaining Primary Hip Flexors

The *sartorius*, the longest muscle in the body, originates at the anterior-superior iliac spine (see Fig. 12.25). This fusiform muscle courses distally and medially across the thigh to attach on the medial surface of the proximal tibia (see Fig. 13.7). The name *sartorius* is based on the Latin root *sartor*, referring to a tailor's position of cross-legged sitting while sewing, which happens to describe the muscle's combined action of hip flexion, external rotation, and abduction.

The *tensor fasciae latae* attaches to the ilium just lateral to the sartorius (see Fig. 12.25). This relatively short muscle attaches distally to the proximal part of the iliotibial band. The naturally stiff and relatively thick band extends distally across the knee to attach to the lateral side of the lateral condyle of the tibia.

The iliotibial band is a component of a more extensive connective tissue known as the *fascia lata of the thigh*. Laterally, the fascia lata is thickened by attachments from the tensor fasciae latae and the gluteus maximus. The remainder of the fascia lata encircles the thigh, located within a plane deep to subcutaneous fat. At multiple locations, the fascia lata of the thigh turns inward between muscles, forming distinct fascial sheets known as *intermuscular septa*. These septa partition the main muscle groups of the thigh according to innervation. The intermuscular septa of the thigh ultimately attach to the linea aspera on the posterior surface of the femur, along with partial attachments of most of the adductor muscles and several of the vasti muscles (components of the quadriceps).

From the anatomic position, the tensor fascia latae is a primary flexor and abductor of the hip. The muscle is often considered a secondary internal rotator,[77,227,234] although its leverage for this action is likely only functionally significant when activated from a position of external rotation. As suggested by its name, the tensor fasciae latae increases tension in the fascia lata. Although it is speculation, activation of the tensor fasciae latae (and theoretically the gluteus maximus and to a lesser extent the psoas minor [217]) can transmit a force around the thigh and between muscle groups. In some manner, this tensional force within the fascia lata may influence the function of the underlying thigh muscles. Tension in the fascia lata is most certainly transmitted inferiorly through the iliotibial band and may help stabilize the extended knee. Repetitive tension within the iliotibial band may cause inflammation at its insertion site near the lateral side of the lateral condyle of the tibia: a painful condition relatively common in distance runners.[97] Maneuvers intended to stretch a tightened tensor fascia latae (which may include the iliotibial band and adjacent tissues) are often performed with the knee extended combined with various combinations of hip adduction and extension. The degree to which the naturally stiff iliotibial band can actually be elongated through manual stretch is not known.[97]

The proximal part of the *rectus femoris* emerges between the limbs of an inverted V formed by the sartorius and tensor fasciae latae (see Fig. 12.25). This large bipennate-shaped muscle has its proximal attachments on the anterior-inferior iliac spine, along the superior rim of the acetabulum, and in the adjacent joint capsule. The relatively robust capsular attachment made by the "reflected" tendon of the rectus femoris has been described as an important stabilizer of the anterior capsule.[317]

Along with the other members of the quadriceps, the rectus femoris attaches to the tibia via the patellar tendon. The rectus femoris is responsible for about one-third of the total isometric flexion torque at the hip.[196] In addition, the rectus femoris is a primary knee extensor. The combined two-joint actions of this important muscle are considered in Chapter 13. The anatomy and function of the pectineus and adductor longus are described in the section on the adductors of the hip.

The Functional Importance of the Fully Extendable Hip

Hips that remain flexed for a prolonged time are more prone to develop flexion tightness or contractures. This situation may be associated with spasticity of the hip flexors, weakness of the hip extensors, a painful or inflamed hip joint capsule, or excessive time spent in the seated position. Over time, adaptive shortening occurs in the flexor muscles and capsular ligaments, thereby limiting full hip extension.

One consequence of limited hip extension is a disruption in the normal biomechanics and thus metabolic efficiency of walking and standing.[52] Upright standing in healthy people can usually be maintained with relatively little muscular activation across the hips. The extended hip can be passively stabilized through an interaction of two opposing torques: body weight and passive tension from stretched capsular ligaments, especially the iliofemoral ligament (Fig. 12.27A). As illustrated, standing with the hips near full extension typically directs the force of body weight through or more typically just *posterior* to the medial-lateral axis of rotation at the hip (small green circle). When posterior to the axis, the force of body weight gives rise to a small, but nevertheless useful, hip extension torque. The hip is prevented from further extension by a passive flexion torque created by the stretched capsular ligaments, such as the iliofemoral ligament, and by hip flexor muscles. The normal upright posture tends to align the acetabulum and femoral head such that their thicker regions of articular cartilage partially overlap. This overlap, indicated by the pair of red dots in Fig. 12.27A, maximizes the protection of the subchondral bone.

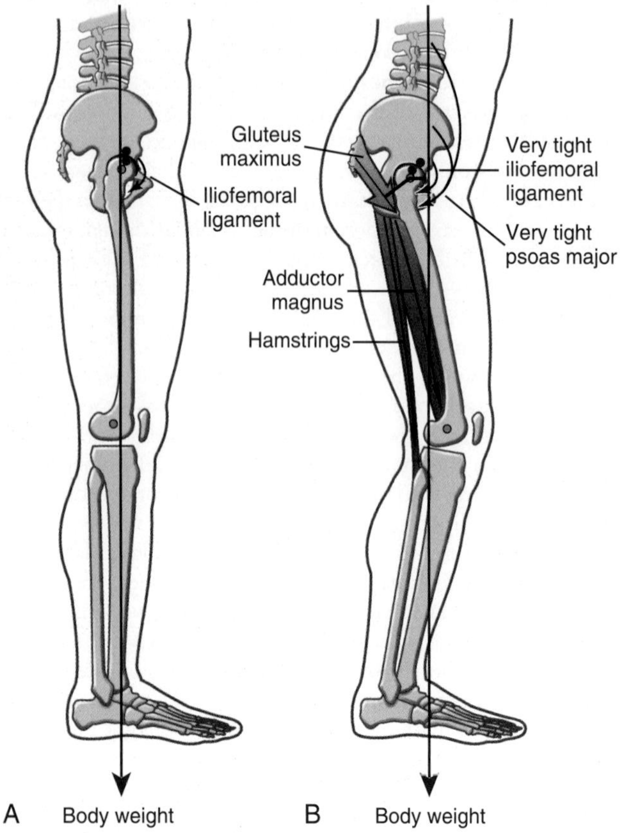

The static equilibrium formed between the forces of gravity and of stretched tissues minimizes the need for metabolically "expensive" muscle activation during quiet standing. Of course, when needed, the muscles of the hip are very capable of generating large forces, such as when the pelvis must be strongly fixed to form a stable base for the trunk.

With limited hip extension, the hip remains partially flexed while the person attempts to stand upright. This posture redirects the force of body weight *anterior* to the hip's axis of rotation, creating a hip flexion torque (see Fig. 12.27B). Whereas gravity normally extends the hip during standing, *gravity now acts to flex the hip.* To prevent a collapse into greater hip and knee flexion, active forces are required from hip extensor muscles because the hip's capsular ligaments, as a whole, are unable to generate significant resistance to a flexing hip. The increased muscular demands, in turn, increase the metabolic cost of standing, and in some people, over time, this increases the desire to sit. Prolonged sitting may perpetuate the circumstances that initiated the hip flexion tightness.[40]

Prolonged standing with hip flexion tightness also interferes with the ability to optimally dissipate compression loads across the joint. Hip joint forces increase in response to the greater muscular demand to support the flexed posture. Furthermore, as indicated by the pair of red dots in Fig. 12.27B, standing with partially flexed hips aligns the joint surfaces in a way that their regions of thickest articular cartilage no longer optimally overlap. This arrangement theoretically increases the stress across the hip, which over time may increase the wear on the joint surfaces.

Therapeutic goals for many impairments of the hip should include, when appropriate, maximizing activation of the hip extensor muscles. This may be particularly relevant for the aged population based on a study showing that healthy individuals between 75 and 86 years old walk with, on average, 30% less hip extension than a much younger group.[10] Therapeutic strategies should include strengthening the hip extensor muscles and stretching the hip flexor muscles as well as the capsular ligaments, especially the iliofemoral ligament. Activation of the abdominal muscles through posterior tilting of the pelvis may also encourage extension of the hip joint. A significant portion of the capsular ligaments of the hip may be further stretched when extension is combined with slight abduction and internal rotation—the close-packed position of the hip.

FIG. 12.27 The effect of hip flexion tightness (or contracture) on the biomechanics of standing. (A) Ideal standing posture. (B) Attempts at standing upright with hip flexion tightness. Hip extensor muscles are shown active (in *red*) to varying magnitudes to prevent further hip flexion. The moment arms used by the muscles and body weight are indicated as short black lines originating at the hip's axis of rotation (shown as *green circle* at the center of the femoral head). The pair of red circles denotes the overlap of the relatively thicker areas of articular cartilage.

Overall Function

Pelvic-on-Femoral Hip Flexion: Anterior Pelvic Tilt

An anterior pelvic tilt is performed by a force-couple formed between the hip flexors and low back extensor muscles (Fig. 12.28). With the femurs fixed, hip flexors rotate the pelvis about a medial-lateral axis that passes through both hip joints. Although Fig. 12.28 illustrates only the iliopsoas and sartorius as hip flexors, *any muscle capable of femoral-on-pelvic flexion is equally capable of tilting the pelvis anteriorly*. Clinically, an important aspect of the anterior tilt is related to the increase in lordosis at the lumbar spine. Greater lordosis increases the compressive loads on the lumbar apophyseal joints and increases anterior shear force at the lumbosacral junction. Normally, these internal forces are well tolerated; however, if excessive and chronic, they can over stress the local bony tissues.

A lumbopelvic posture with a normal or typical amount of lumbar lordosis optimizes the alignment of the entire spine (review Chapter 9). Some people, however, have difficulty achieving or maintaining lumbar lordosis and thus have relatively flat (i.e., slightly flexed) lumbar spines. This abnormal posture may be associated with several interrelated factors, including pain avoidance, prolonged or habitual "slumped" sitting posture, compensation from another poorly aligned region of the body, increased stiffness in connective tissue around the lumbar spine, and, in extreme cases, excessive tension emanating from hip extensor muscles.

Femoral-on-Pelvic Hip Flexion

Femoral-on-pelvic hip flexion often occurs simultaneously with knee flexion as a means to shorten the functional length of the lower extremity during walking or running. Moderate to high-power hip flexion requires coactivation of the hip flexor and abdominal muscles. This intermuscular cooperation is particularly apparent when the leg is lifted while the knee is held in extension (i.e., a "straight-leg–raise" movement). This action requires that the rectus

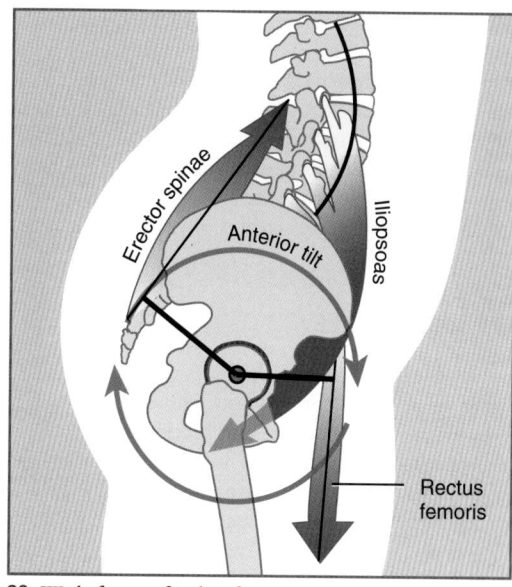

FIG. 12.28 With femurs fixed, a force couple is shown between two hip flexor muscles and the erector spinae to anteriorly tilt the pelvis. The moment arms for the erector spinae and sartorius are indicated by the dark black lines. Note the increased lordosis at the lumbar spine.

abdominis (a representative "abdominal" muscle) generates a strong enough *posterior* pelvic tilt to neutralize the strong *anterior* pelvic tilt exerted by the hip flexor muscles (Fig. 12.29A).[133] The degree to which the abdominal muscles actually neutralize the anterior pelvic tilt depends on the demands of the activity and the relative forces produced by the contributing muscle groups. Without sufficient stabilization from the abdominal muscles, however, contraction of the hip flexor muscles is inefficiently spent tilting the pelvis *anteriorly* (see Fig. 12.29B).

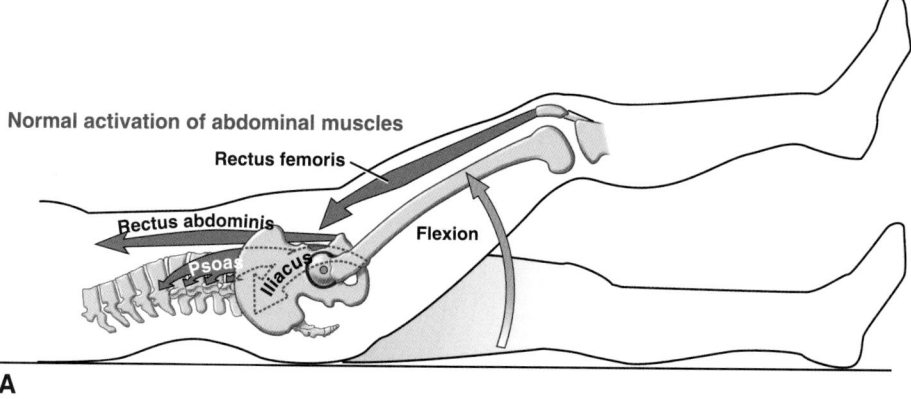

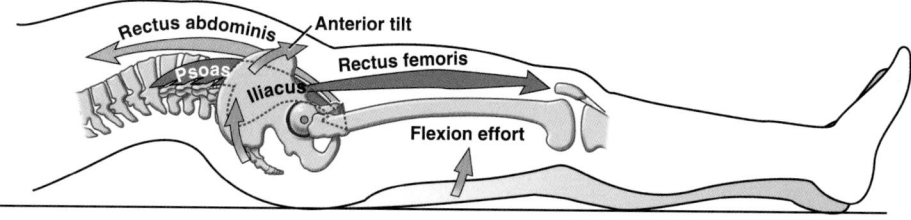

FIG. 12.29 The stabilizing role of the abdominal muscles is shown during a unilateral straight-leg raise. (A) With normal activation of the abdominal muscles (such as the rectus abdominis), the pelvis is stabilized and prevented from anterior tilting by the strong inferior pull of the hip flexor muscles. (B) With reduced activation of the rectus abdominis, contraction of the hip flexor muscles causes a marked anterior tilt of the pelvis. Note the increase in lumbar lordosis that accompanies the anterior tilt of the pelvis. The reduced activation in the abdominal muscle is indicated by the lighter red.

The pathomechanics depicted in Fig. 12.29B are most severe in situations when the abdominal muscles are markedly weakened but the hip flexors remain relatively strong. This may result from a host of reasons—from disuse atrophy of the abdominal muscles to a more serious pathology, such as poliomyelitis or muscular dystrophy. In this situation the unopposed force of the hip flexors pulls the lumbar spine further into lordosis; low back pain may develop if the excessive lumbar lordosis creates physiologically large regions of articular stress.

HIP ADDUCTOR MUSCLES

The primary adductors of the hip are the pectineus, adductor longus, gracilis, adductor brevis, and adductor magnus (see Fig. 12.25). Secondary adductors are the biceps femoris (long head), the gluteus maximus, especially the inferior (posterior) fibers, the quadratus femoris, and the obturator externus. The lines of force and relatively large moment arm lengths available to many of the hip adductors are shown in Fig. 12.30.[227] Although this leverage may be a functional advantage in augmenting adduction torque (strength), it can be a functional disadvantage in cases where the adductor muscle force is significantly increased resulting from spasticity and/or atypical recruitment, which, for example, can interfere with walking in persons with cerebral palsy or incomplete spinal cord injury.

Functional Anatomy

Topographically, the adductor muscles are organized into three layers (Fig. 12.31). The pectineus, adductor longus, and gracilis occupy the *superficial layer*. Proximally, these muscles attach along the superior and inferior pubic ramus and adjacent body of the pubis. Distally, the pectineus and the adductor longus attach to the posterior surface of the femur—near and along regions of the linea aspera. The long and slender gracilis attaches distally to the medial side of the proximal tibia (see Fig. 13.7). The *middle layer* of the adductor group is occupied by the triangular-shaped *adductor brevis*. The adductor brevis attaches to the pelvis on the inferior pubic ramus and to the femur near and along the proximal one-third of the linea aspera.

The *deep layer* of the adductor group is occupied by the massive, triangular *adductor magnus* (see Fig. 12.25, left side; and Fig. 12.38, right side). As its name implies, the adductor magnus is the largest of the adductor muscles, accounting for 60% of the total cross-sectional area of the entire adductor muscle group.[297] As a whole, the adductor magnus attaches proximally to the pelvis from two heads: an anterior head from the ischial ramus and a posterior head from the ischial tuberosity. The *anterior head of the adductor magnus* has two sets of fibers: horizontal and oblique. The relatively small (and often poorly defined) set of horizontally directed fibers crosses from the inferior pubic ramus to the extreme proximal end of the linea aspera, often called the adductor minimus.[226] The larger obliquely directed fibers run from the ischial ramus to nearly the entire length of the linea aspera, as far distally as the medial supracondylar line. Both parts of the anterior head are innervated by the obturator nerve, which is typical of the adductor muscles.

The *posterior head of the adductor magnus* consists of a thick mass of the fibers arising from the region of the pelvis adjacent to the ischial tuberosity. From this posterior attachment, the fibers run vertically and attach as a tendon on the adductor tubercle on the medial side of the distal femur. The posterior head of the adductor magnus is innervated by the tibial branch of the sciatic nerve, as are most of the hamstring muscles. Because location, innervation, and action are similar to those of the hamstring muscles, the posterior head may also be referred to as the *extensor head* of the adductor magnus.

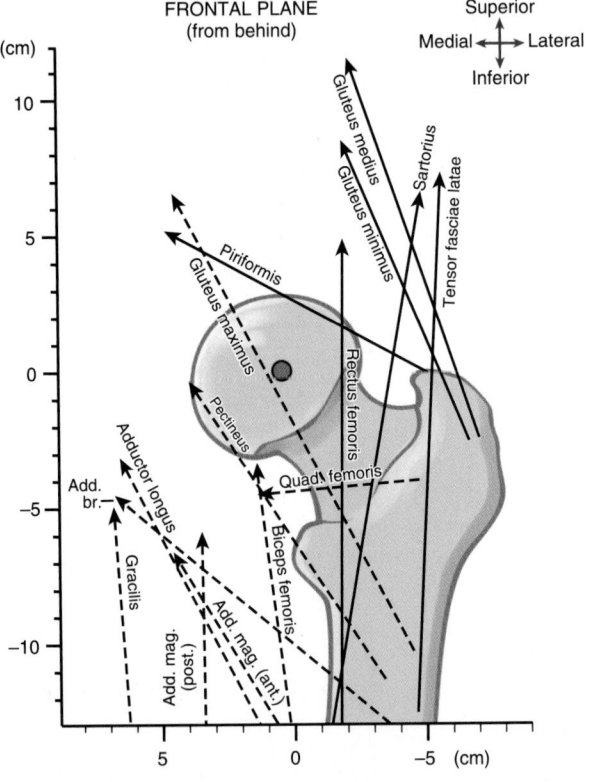

FIG. 12.30 A posterior view depicts the lines of force of several hip muscles relative to the frontal plane. The axis of rotation is directed in the anterior-posterior direction through the femoral head. The abductors are indicated by solid lines and the adductors by dashed lines.

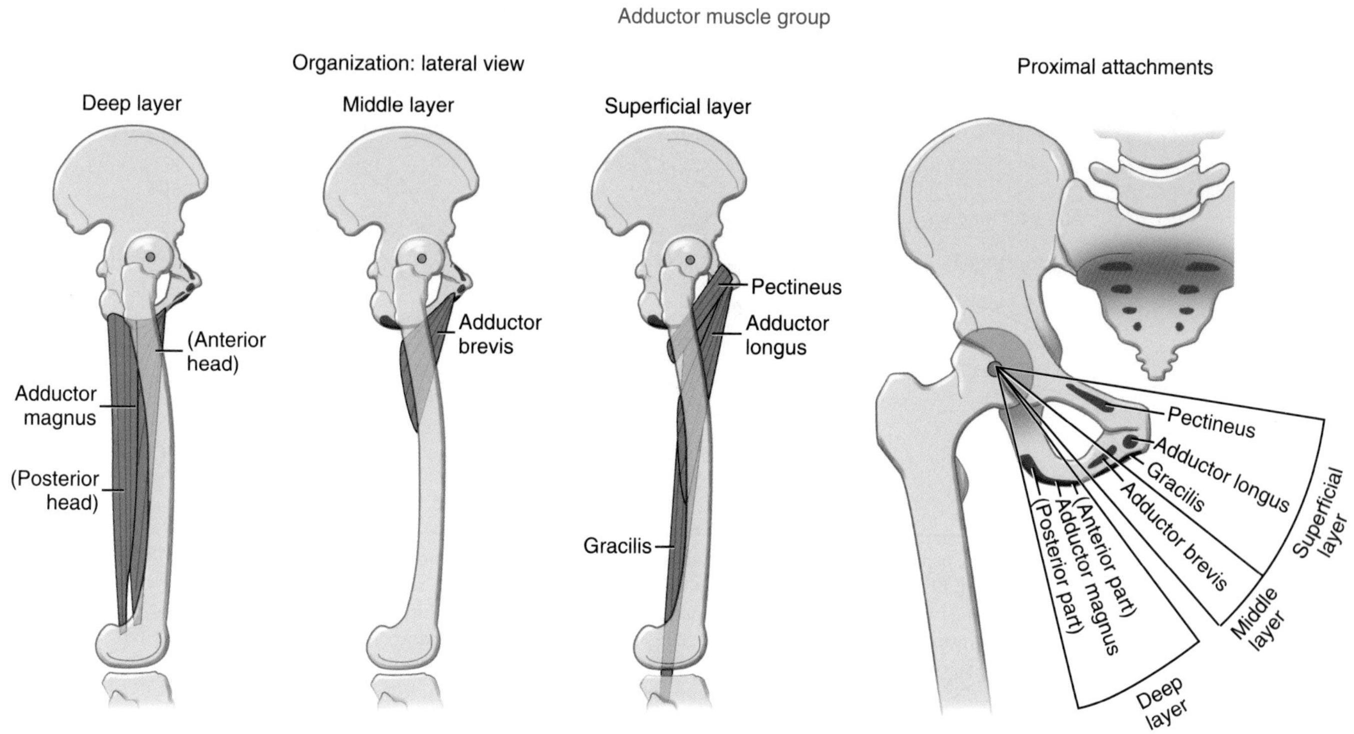

Adductor muscle group

Organization: lateral view

Deep layer

(Anterior head)

Adductor magnus

(Posterior head)

Middle layer

Adductor brevis

Superficial layer

Pectineus

Adductor longus

Gracilis

Proximal attachments

Pectineus

Adductor longus

Gracilis

Adductor brevis

(Anterior part) Adductor magnus (Posterior part)

Superficial layer

Middle layer

Deep layer

FIG. 12.31 The anatomic organization and proximal attachments of the adductor muscle group.

Overall Function

The lines of force of the adductors approach the hip from many different orientations. Functionally, therefore, the adductor muscles produce torques in all three planes at the hip.[77,105,211,297] The following section considers the primary actions of the adductors in the frontal and sagittal planes. The action of these muscles as secondary internal rotators is discussed later in this chapter. Understanding that the adductor muscles produce torques in *all* three planes of motion helps justify their large size and possibly their vulnerability to strain-related injury.

Frontal Plane Function

The most obvious function of the adductor muscles is production of adduction torque. This torque controls the kinematics of both femoral-on-pelvic and pelvic-on-femoral hip adduction. Fig. 12.32 shows an example of selected adductor muscles contracting bilaterally to control both forms of motion. On the right side, several adductors are shown accelerating the femur to strike the soccer ball. Adding to the forcefulness of this action is the downward rotation or lowering of the right iliac crest—a motion occurring by pelvic-on-femoral adduction of the left hip. Although only the adductor magnus is shown on the left side, other adductor muscles assist in this action.[319] The overall adduction of the planted left hip typically incorporates *eccentric* activation of the gluteus medius to help decelerate and thus help control the kinematics of pelvic-on-femoral motion.

Sagittal Plane Function

Regardless of hip position, the posterior fibers of the adductor magnus are powerful extensors of the hip, similar to the hamstring muscles.[297] Of interest, however, is that within an arc of about 40 to 70 degrees of hip flexion, the lines of force of most of the other adductor muscles runs *directly through or close to* the medial-lateral axis of rotation of the hip. At this point, the adductor muscles, as a

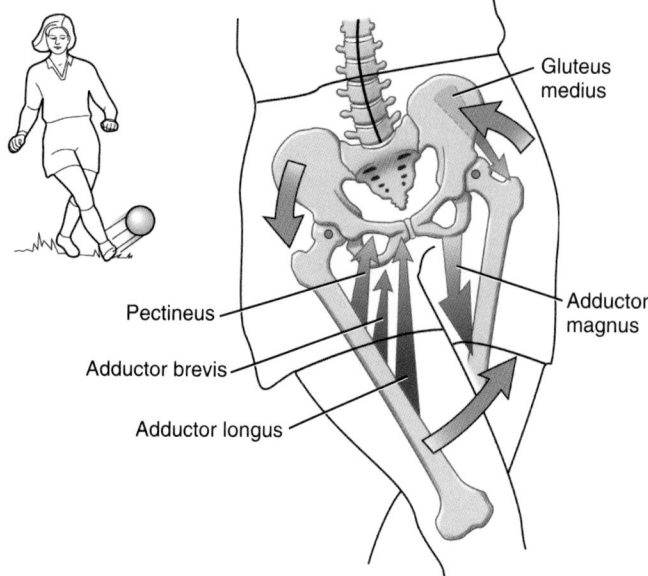

FIG. 12.32 The bilateral cooperative action of selected adductor muscles during one style of kicking a soccer ball. The left adductor magnus is shown actively producing *pelvic-on-femoral adduction*. Several right adductor muscles are shown actively producing *femoral-on-pelvic adduction*, needed to accelerate the ball. Note the eccentric activation of the left gluteus medius to help control the velocity and extent of drop of the adducting left hip.

group, lose much of their potential to produce torque in the sagittal plane.[138] When *outside* the 40-to-70-degree flexed position, however, the individual adductor muscles regain leverage as

Adductor longus as a hip extensor   Adductor longus as a hip flexor

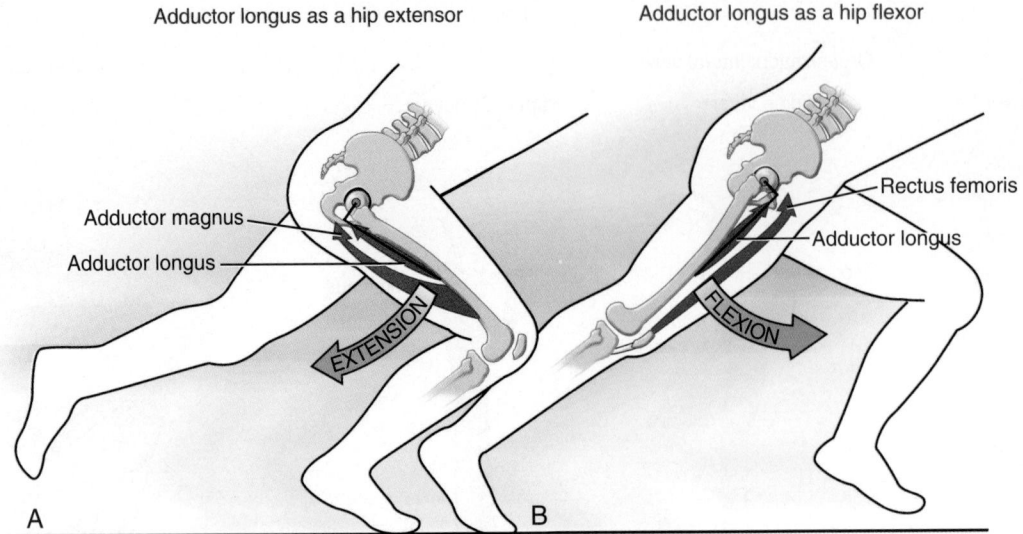

FIG. 12.33 The dual sagittal plane action of the adductor longus muscle is demonstrated during sprinting. (A) With the hip flexed, the adductor longus is in position to extend the hip, along with the adductor magnus. (B) With the hip extended, the adductor longus is in position to flex the hip, along with the rectus femoris. These contrasting actions are based on the change in line of force of the adductor longus, relative to the medial-lateral axis of rotation at the hip.

significant flexors *or* extensors of the hip.[77,138] Consider, for example, the adductor longus as a representative adductor muscle during a fast sprint (Fig. 12.33A). From a position of about 100 degrees of hip flexion, the line of force of the adductor longus is well *posterior* to the medial-lateral axis of the joint. At this position the adductor longus has an extensor moment arm and is capable of generating an extension torque—similar to the posterior head of the adductor magnus. From a hip position of near extension, however, the line of force of the adductor longus is well *anterior* to the medial-lateral axis of rotation (see Fig. 12.33B). The adductor longus now has a flexor moment arm and generates a flexion torque qualitatively similar to that of the rectus femoris, for example. The adductor muscles therefore provide a useful source of flexion *and* extension torque at the hip.[149] The bidirectional torques are useful during high-power, cyclic motions such as sprinting, cycling, running up a steep hill, and descending and rising from a deep squat. When the hip is near full flexion, the adductors are most mechanically prepared to augment the extensors. In contrast, when the hip is near full extension, the adductors (with the exception of the adductor magnus) are most mechanically prepared to augment the flexors. This utilitarian function of the adductors may partially explain their relatively high susceptibility to soreness, inflammation, or strain injury during running and jumping, especially while quickly changing directions. This condition may involve the adductor longus tendon along with its shared pelvic attachments with the rectus abdominis (often part of a groin-related pain condition reported in athletes).[92,323]

HIP INTERNAL ROTATOR MUSCLES

Function

An "ideal" primary internal rotator muscle of the hip would theoretically be oriented entirely within the horizontal plane while standing upright, acting with a moment arm relative to the vertical axis of rotation. From the anatomic position, however, there are *no* primary internal rotators because no muscle is oriented even close to the horizontal plane. Several secondary internal rotators exist, however, including the anterior fibers of the gluteus minimus and gluteus medius, tensor fasciae latae, adductor longus, adductor

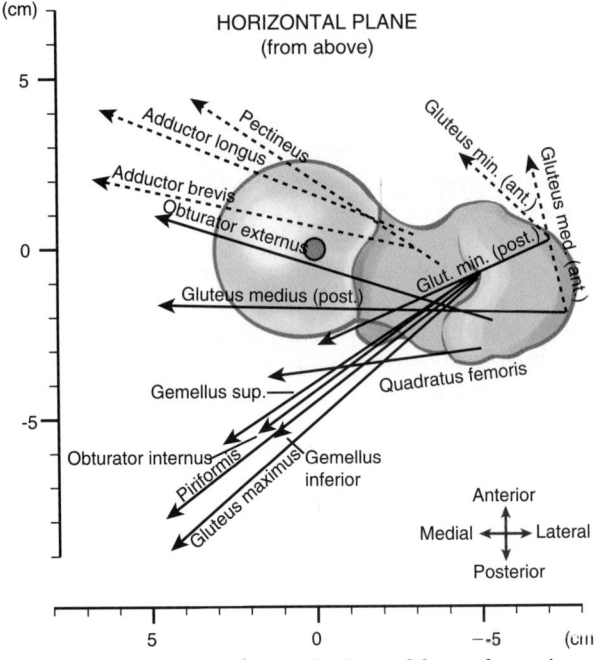

FIG. 12.34 A superior view depicts the lines of force of several muscles relative to the horizontal plane. The longitudinal axis of rotation is in the superior-inferior direction through the femoral head. The external rotators are indicated by solid lines and the internal rotators by dashed lines.

brevis, and pectineus. The relatively small horizontal line of force component of several of these muscles are depicted in Fig. 12.34.[77,172] The combined torque potential of the many secondary internal rotators adequately meets the typical functional demands placed on the hip. The anatomy of each of the internal rotators is described in other sections (see Figs. 12.25 and 12.42).

Like all muscles of the lower extremity, the internal rotators have a unique function during locomotion. During the stance phase of gait, the internal rotators rotate the pelvis in the horizontal plane over a relatively fixed femur. These pelvic-on-femoral kinematics are

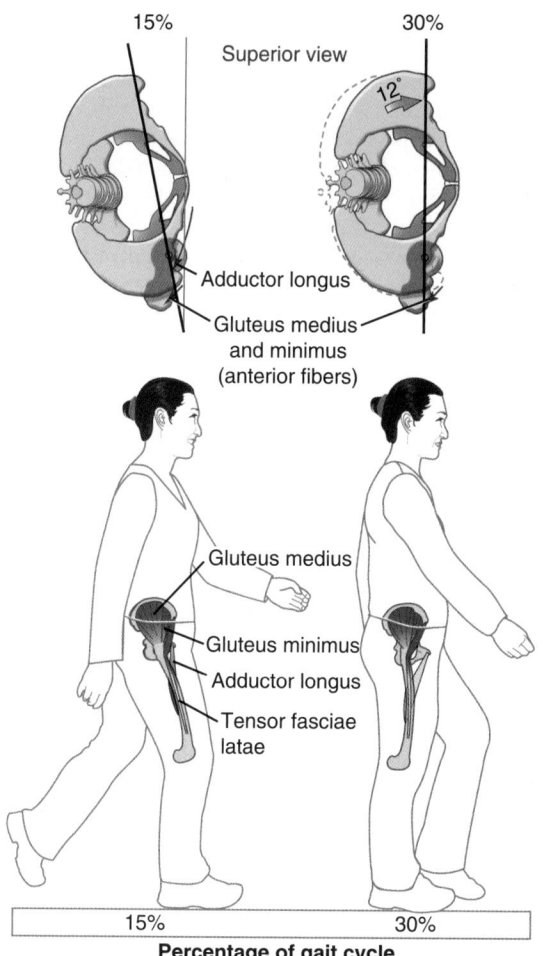

FIG. 12.35 The activation pattern of several internal rotator muscles of the right hip is depicted during the first 30% of the gait cycle. (*Brighter red* indicates greater muscle activation.) Specifically, the tensor fasciae latae, anterior fibers of the gluteus minimus and gluteus medius, and adductor longus are shown rotating the pelvis in the horizontal plane over a relatively fixed right femur. (Compare the bottom and top views.)

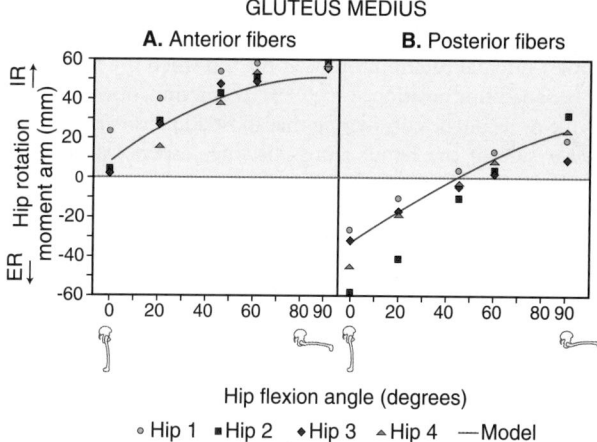

FIG. 12.36 Horizontal plane rotational moment arms for the anterior and posterior fibers of the gluteus medius, plotted as functions of hip flexion: (A) anterior fibers; (B) posterior fibers. *IR*, Internal rotation moment arm; *ER*, external rotation moment arm. The 0-degree flexion angle on the horizontal (X) axis marks the anatomic (neutral) position of the hip. (Modified with permission from Neumann DA: Kinesiology of the hip: a focus on muscular actions, *J Orthop Sports Phys Ther* 40:82–94, 2010. Data are based on a study originally published by Delp SL, et al.[73])

illustrated for the first 30% of the gait cycle in Fig. 12.35. The pelvic rotation about the right hip is shown by the forward rotation of the *left* iliac crest (seen from above). The right internal rotator muscles therefore can provide some of the drive to the contralateral (left) swinging limb, especially useful while walking uphill or increasing stride length. As described later in this chapter, the tensor fasciae latae and the gluteus minimus and gluteus medius are also functioning as hip abductors during this part of the gait cycle. Activation of these muscles is necessary to stabilize the pelvis in the frontal plane during this part of the gait cycle.

Active Internal Rotation Torque Increases with Hip Flexion

With the hip approaching 90 degrees of flexion, the internal rotation torque potential of the internal rotator muscles significantly increases.[73,76,77,194,227] This becomes clear with the help of a skeleton model and a piece of string to mimic the line of force of a muscle, such as the anterior fibers of the gluteus minimus or the gluteus medius. Flexing the hip close to 90 degrees reorients the lines of force of these muscles from nearly parallel to nearly perpendicular to the longitudinal axis of rotation of the femur. This occurs because the longitudinal axis of rotation remains parallel with the shaft of the repositioned femur. Delp and co-workers have reported that the internal rotation moment arm of the anterior

fibers of the gluteus medius, for example, increases eightfold between 0 and 90 degrees of flexion (Fig. 12.36A).[73] Even some of the external rotator muscles, such as the posterior fibers of the gluteus medius (depicted in Fig. 12.36B), piriformis, anterior (superior) fibers of the gluteus maximus, and posterior fibers of the gluteus minimus, switch actions and become internal rotators when the hip is flexed to about 60 degrees or beyond.[73,227] The altered biomechanics of many of the hip rotator muscles with increased hip flexion may partially explain why maximal-effort internal rotation torque in healthy people is about 35% to 55% greater with the hip flexed to about 90 degrees compared with when it is extended.[26,37,56,180] The augmented torque potential of the anterior fibers of the gluteus medius, for example, may be naturally advantageous for stabilizing the pelvis in the frontal plane during demanding activities associated with a unilaterally supported squat, such as ascending a very steep step.

Although the greater internal rotation torque potential with hip flexion may have some functional advantages for the general population, this may be disadvantageous for people with a compromised neuromuscular system. Consider, for example, how the kinesiologic phenomenon described in the previous paragraph could partially explain the excessively internally rotated and flexed ("crouched") gait pattern often observed in persons with cerebral palsy.[129,251,303] With poor active control of hip extension (especially if combined with excessive tightness of the hip flexor muscles), the flexed hip posture boosts the internal rotation torque potential of many muscles of the hip.[13,14,73] Although it is speculation, the crouched gait (and associated increased tension in hip adductor and internal rotator muscles) may contribute to the persistence of excessive femoral anteversion in ambulatory persons with cerebral palsy. Theoretically, the crouched gait pattern may be better controlled by heightened activation or strength of the gluteus maximus, a potent extensor and external rotator. For example, exercises such as the single-limb bridge and step-up have been shown to significantly activate the gluteus maximus in a sample of ambulatory persons with cerebral palsy.[67] It is not known whether targeting this muscle can make a meaningful improvement in the altered gait pattern, although it warrants further investigation.

Biomechanics of the Adductor Muscles as Internal Rotators of the Hip

In general, most of the adductor muscles are capable of producing a modest internal rotation torque at the hip when the body is in or near the anatomic position.[77,172,194,227] This action, however, may be difficult to reconcile considering that most adductors attach to the *posterior* side of the femur along the linea aspera. With normal anatomy of the hip, a shortening of these muscles would appear to rotate the femur *externally* instead of internally. What must be considered, however, is the effect that the natural anterior bowing of the femoral shaft has on the lines of force of the muscles. The bowing places much of the linea aspera *anterior* to the longitudinal axis of rotation at the hip (Fig. 12.37A). As depicted in Fig. 12.37B, the horizontal force component of an adductor muscle, such as the adductor longus, lies *anterior* to the axis of rotation. Force from this muscle therefore acts with a moment arm to produce internal rotation (Video 12.4).

HIP EXTENSOR MUSCLES

Anatomy and Individual Actions

The primary hip extensors are the gluteus maximus, the hamstrings (i.e., the long head of the biceps femoris, the semitendinosus, and the semimembranosus), and the posterior head of the adductor magnus (Fig. 12.38).[77] The middle and posterior fibers of the gluteus medius and the anterior fibers of the adductor magnus are secondary extensors.[227] With the hip flexed to at least about 70 degrees and beyond, the adductor muscles (with the possible exception of the pectineus) are capable of assisting with hip extension.

The *gluteus maximus* has numerous proximal attachments from the posterior side of the ilium, sacrum, coccyx, sacrotuberous and posterior sacroiliac ligaments, and adjacent thoracolumbar fascia. The muscle attaches into the iliotibial band of the fascia lata (along with the tensor fasciae latae) and the gluteal tuberosity on the femur. At the hip, the gluteus maximus is a primary extensor and external

rotator as well as a secondary abductor. As described in Chapters 9 and 10, the gluteus maximus is also an important muscle for stabilizing the sacroiliac joint and the lumbar region via its extensive ligamentous and fascial attachments in the region.[28,326]

The three biarticular *hamstring muscles* have their proximal attachment on the ischial tuberosity and attach distally to the tibia and fibula. Based on these attachments, the hamstrings extend the hip *and* flex the knee. The anatomy and function of the posterior head of the *adductor magnus*, an often-underappreciated hip extensor muscle, is described in the section on adductors of the hip.

Fig. 12.24 depicts the lines of force of the primary hip extensors. In the extended position the posterior head of the adductor magnus has the greatest moment arm for extension. The adductor magnus and the gluteus maximus have the greatest cross-sectional areas of all the extensors.[328]

Overall Function

Pelvic-on-Femoral Hip Extension

The following sections describe two different situations in which the hip extensor muscles control pelvic-on-femoral extension.

Hip Extensors Performing a Posterior Pelvic Tilt. With the supralumbar trunk held relatively stationary, the hip extensor and abdominal muscles act as a force-couple to posteriorly tilt the pelvis (Fig. 12.39). The posterior tilt extends the hip joints slightly and reduces the lumbar lordosis.

The muscular mechanics involved with posterior tilting of the pelvis are generally similar to those described for the anterior tilting of the pelvis (compare Figs. 12.28 and 12.39). In both tilting actions, the hip and trunk muscles form a force-couple for rotating the pelvis through a relatively short arc around the femoral heads. During standing, tensions exerted by the hip's capsular ligaments and by hip flexor muscles normally determine the end range of the posterior pelvic tilt, in contrast to how the lumbar spine typically restricts the end range of an anterior pelvic tilt.

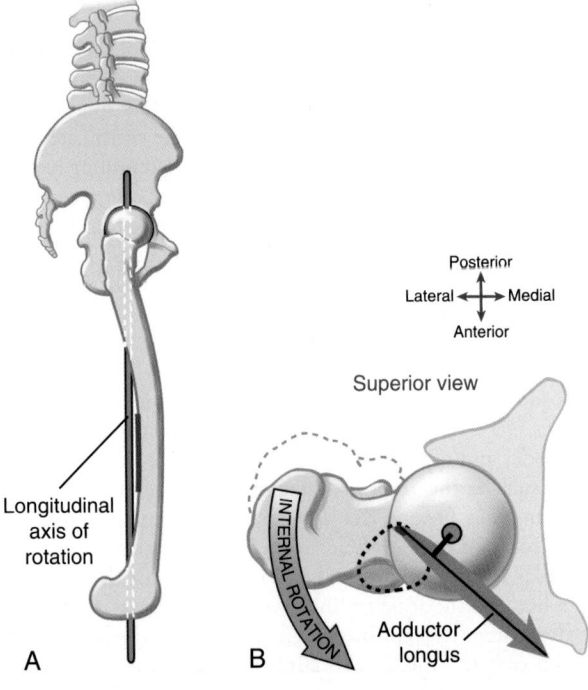

FIG. 12.37 The adductor muscles as secondary internal rotators of the hip. (A) Because of the anterior bowing of the femoral shaft, a segment of the linea aspera (*short red line*) runs *anterior* to the longitudinal axis of rotation (*blue rod*). (B) A superior view of the right hip shows the horizontal line of force of the adductor longus. The muscle causes an internal rotation torque by producing a force that passes anterior to the axis of rotation (*small blue circle at femoral head*). The moment arm used by the adductor longus is indicated by the thick dark line. The oval set of dashed black lines represents the outline of the midshaft of the femur at the region of the distal attachment of the adductor longus.

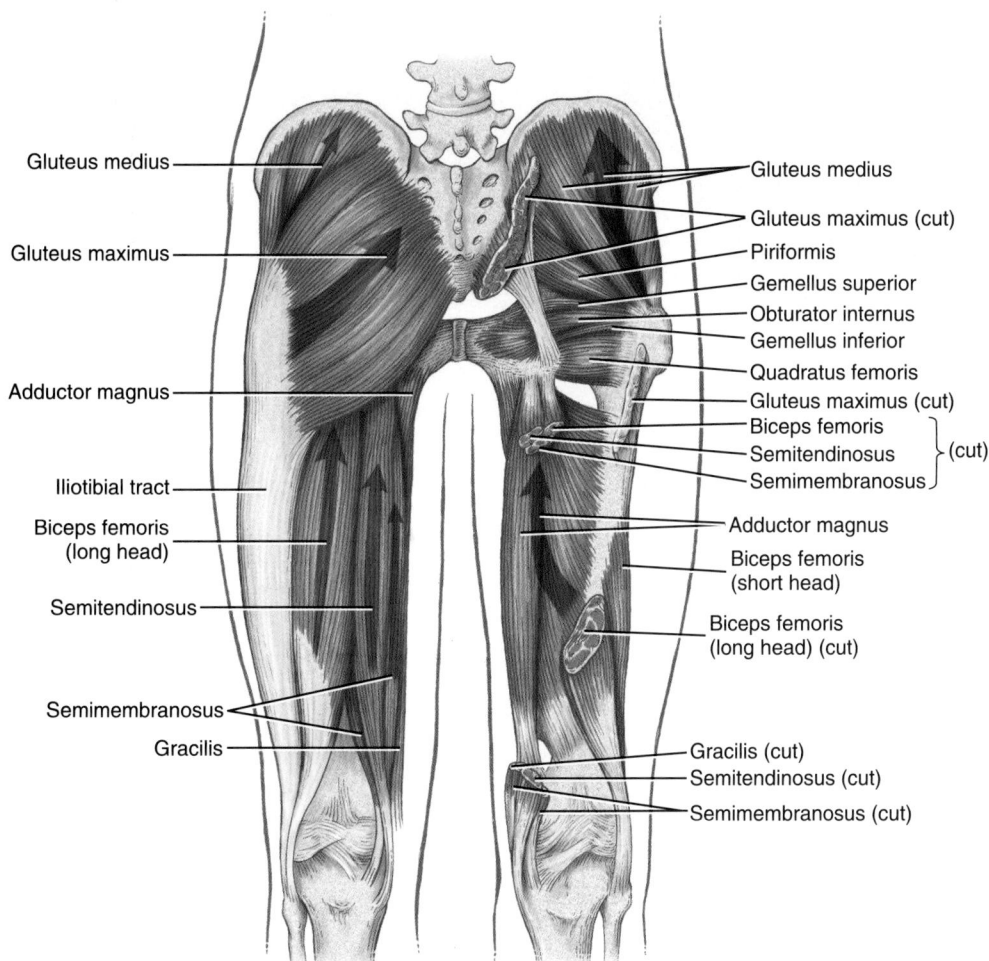

Gluteus medius

Gluteus maximus

Adductor magnus

Iliotibial tract

Biceps femoris
(long head)

Semitendinosus

Semimembranosus

Gracilis

Gluteus medius

Gluteus maximus (cut)

Piriformis

Gemellus superior

Obturator internus

Gemellus inferior

Quadratus femoris

Gluteus maximus (cut)

Biceps femoris
Semitendinosus } (cut)
Semimembranosus

Adductor magnus

Biceps femoris
(short head)

Biceps femoris
(long head) (cut)

Gracilis (cut)

Semitendinosus (cut)

Semimembranosus (cut)

FIG. 12.38 The posterior muscles of the hip. The left side highlights the gluteus maximus and hamstring muscles (long head of the biceps femoris, semitendinosus, and semimembranosus). The right side shows the gluteus maximus and hamstring muscles cut away to expose the gluteus medius, five of the six short external rotators (i.e., piriformis, gemellus superior and inferior, obturator internus, and quadratus femoris), adductor magnus, and short head of the biceps femoris.

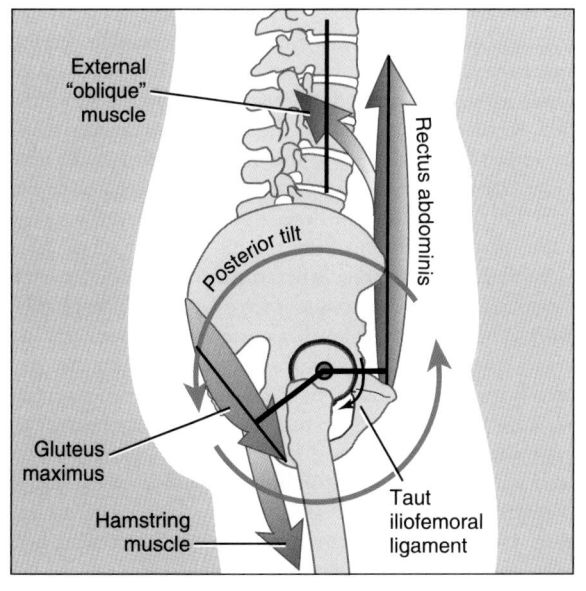

External "oblique" muscle

Rectus abdominis

Posterior tilt

Gluteus maximus

Hamstring muscle

Taut iliofemoral ligament

FIG. 12.39 With femurs fixed, a force couple is shown between representative hip extensors (gluteus maximus and hamstrings) and abdominal muscles (rectus abdominis and obliquus externus abdominis) to posteriorly tilt the pelvis. The moment arms for each muscle group are indicated by dark black lines. The extension at the hip stretches the iliofemoral ligament.

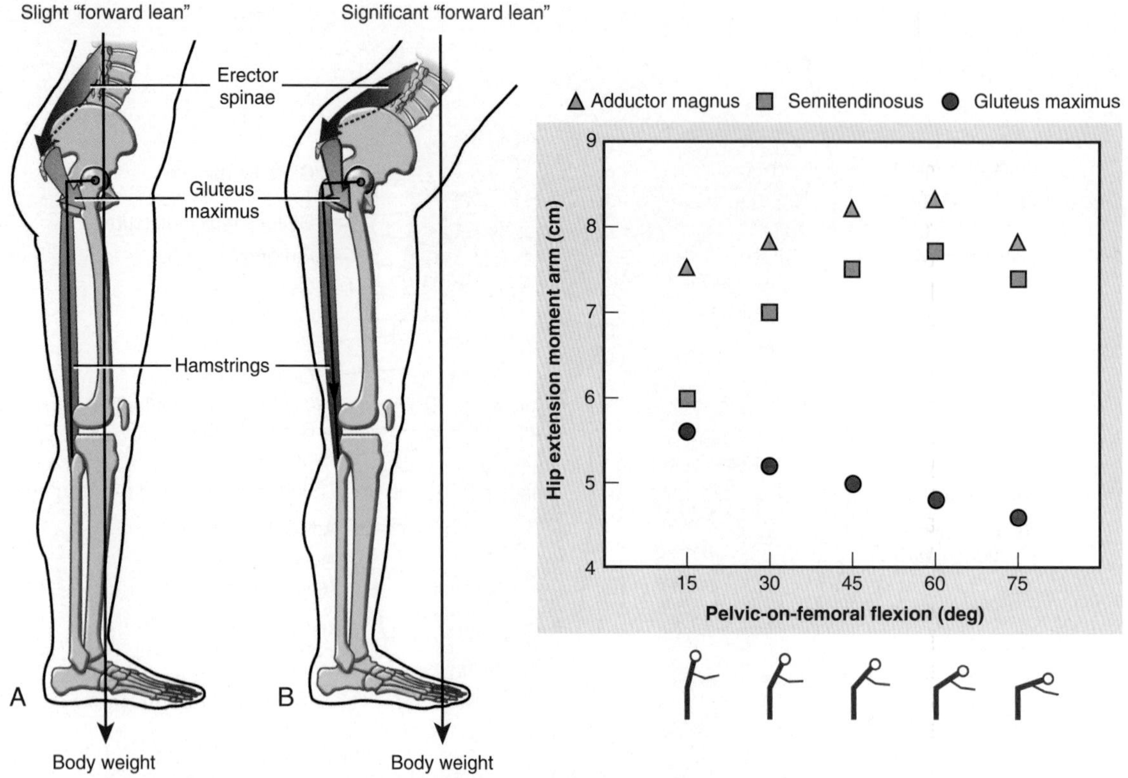

FIG. 12.40 The hip extensor muscles are shown controlling a forward lean of the pelvis over the thighs. (A) Slight forward lean of the upper body displaces the body weight force slightly anterior to the medial-lateral axis of rotation at the hip. (B) A more significant forward lean displaces the body weight force even farther anteriorly. The greater flexion of the hips rotates the ischial tuberosities posteriorly, thereby increasing the hip extension moment arm of the hamstrings. The taut line (with arrowhead within the stretched hamstring muscles) indicates the increased passive tension. In both (A) and (B), the relative activation demands placed on the muscles are shown by relative shades of red. The graph shows the lengths of hip extension moment arms of selected hip extensors as functions of forward lean.[246]

Hip Extensors Controlling a Forward Lean of the Body. Leaning forward while standing is a very common activity. Consider, for example, the forward lean used when brushing teeth over a sink. The muscular support at the hip for this near static posture is primarily the responsibility of the hamstring muscles. Consider two phases of a forward lean shown in Fig. 12.40. During a slight forward lean (see Fig. 12.40A), body weight is displaced just anterior to the medial-lateral axis of rotation at the hips. This slightly flexed posture is restrained by minimal activation from the gluteus maximus and hamstring muscles. A more significant forward lean, however, displaces body weight farther in front of the hips (see Fig. 12.40B). Supporting this markedly flexed posture requires greater muscle activation from the hamstring muscles. The gluteus maximus, however, remains relatively inactive in this position—a point verifiable by palpation and inferred from electromyographic data.[88] The apparent increased responsibility of the hamstrings (in contrast to the gluteus maximus) can be explained biomechanically and physiologically. Forward leaning *increases* the hip extension moment arm of the hamstring muscles, mechanically optimizing the muscle's hip extensor torque potential,[138] whereas it *decreases* the hip extensor moment arm of the gluteus maximus.[246] (Compare the 15-degree and 30-degree points in the graph in Fig. 12.40.) Therefore, for a given hip extensor torque demand resulting from forward trunk leaning, the required force production is less for the hamstrings than it is for the gluteus maximus. A significant forward lean also elongates the hamstring muscles across the hip *and* the knee joints. The resulting increased passive tension in these elongated biarticular

muscles helps support the partially flexed position of the hips. For these reasons, the hamstrings appear uniquely equipped to support the hip during a forward lean. The nervous system may strive to optimize energy efficiency by recruiting the elongated hamstrings to support the forward trunk lean while reserving the gluteus maximus for more powerful hip extension activities, such as rapidly climbing a flight of stairs.

Femoral-on-Pelvic Hip Extension

As a group, the hip extensor muscles are frequently required to produce large and powerful femoral-on-pelvic hip extension torque to rapidly accelerate the body forward and upward. Consider, for example, the demands placed on the right hip extensors while one climbs a steep hill (Fig. 12.41). The flexed position of the right hip while the climber is carrying a heavy pack imposes a large *external* (flexion) torque at the hip. The flexed position, however, favors greater extension torque generation from the hip extensor muscles.[320] Furthermore, with the hip markedly flexed, many of the adductor muscles can produce an extension torque, thereby assisting the primary hip extensors. Activation of the low back extensor muscles helps support the flexed trunk and also stabilizes the pelvis so that the strongly activated hip extensor muscles have a secure proximal attachment.

Fig. 12.41 underscores the functional interdependence among many of the muscles of the lower extremity, particularly those involved with activities that combine hip-and-knee extension and ankle plantar flexion, such as climbing, sprinting, cycling, or jumping. Consider, for instance, the kinetic interaction between the rectus femoris and the gluteus maximus—two essential muscles

Maximizing Gluteus Maximus Activation to Reach Its Functional and Therapeutic Potential: How and Why?

The demands placed on the gluteus maximus during a multi-joint motion as described in Fig. 12.41 are indeed surprisingly large. Weakness or poor control of this dominant muscle can disrupt the quality and strength of movements throughout the lower limb.[47,50,135] Exercises that purportedly strengthen or improve the control of the gluteus maximus have been used to treat and prevent a broad spectrum of movement-associated pathologies, including non-contact anterior cruciate ligament injury, femoroacetabular impingement, abnormal tracking of the patellofemoral joint, iliotibial band syndrome, and a crouched or flexed gait often associated with cerebral palsy.[19,48,50,67,275] Exercises designed to challenge the gluteus maximus typically include hip (and often knee) extension, external rotation, and abduction. These movements can be performed individually or in combination, while in an upright, weight-bearing position; reclined; or a combination thereof. Specific and relatively demanding exercises often include variations of step-ups, squats, lunges, barbell hip thrusts, dead lifts, and the use of a Roman chair or seated back extension machine. Because the gluteus maximus is difficult to isolate from other primary hip extensor muscles, strategies have been proposed that aim to more specifically target this muscle.[9,20,62,214,261] Cannon et al, for instance, have shown that a relatively simple but focused "gluteus maximus activation program" can increase the neuromuscular recruitment of this muscle when performing more challenging weight-bearing-based exercises (such as double-leg or single-leg squats).[50] The activation program, performed twice daily for 7 consecutive days, consisted of three isometric exercises using band resistance: side-lying clam, side-lying hip abduction, and quadruped "fire-hydrant." (Note these exercises represent a triplanar sampling of actions that significantly activate the versatile gluteus maximus.) Evidence using transcranial magnetic stimulation (TMS) strongly suggests that a focused gluteus maximus activation program actually increases the muscle's corticomotor excitability.[50,89] Is it possible that a focused, short-duration, and action-specific program for the gluteus maximus can "prime" the central nervous system such that subsequent and more challenging exercises can be more effective for increasing strength or improving neuromuscular control? Through increased availability of TMS, perhaps these and other clinically important questions can be further addressed.

necessary to perform the climbing activity depicted in Fig. 12.41. Large knee extension torque is required from the rectus femoris to offset the large knee flexion torques produced not only by body weight (and the supported external load) but also by large active knee flexion torques generated by the simultaneously activated hamstring and gastrocnemius muscles. Because of the biarticular arrangement of the rectus femoris, large forces produced by this muscle to extend the knee will, by necessity, also contribute to a large *hip flexion* torque: a torque that appears mechanically counterproductive to the movement of hip extension. Muscles such as the gluteus maximus and adductor magnus must thus *match and exceed* the hip flexion torque created by the active rectus femoris. Only then will the hip extensors accelerate the body upward and forward.

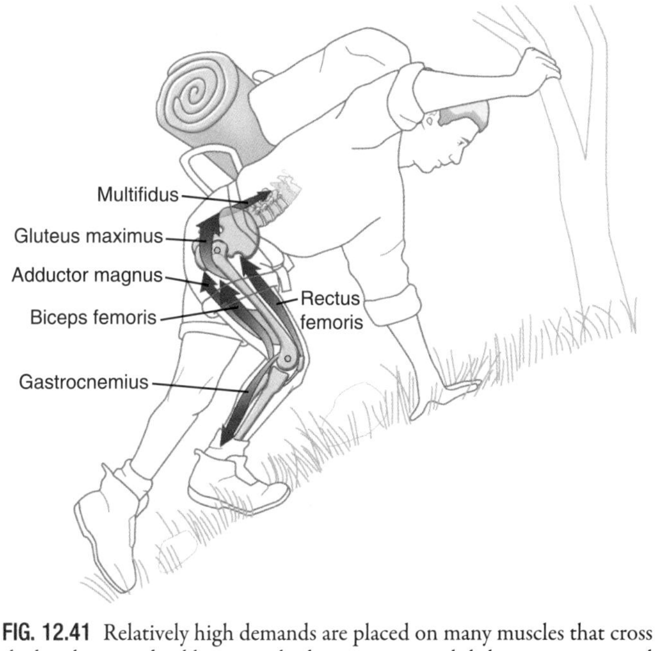

HIP ABDUCTOR MUSCLES

Anatomy and Individual Actions

The primary hip abductor muscles include the gluteus medius, gluteus minimus, and tensor fasciae latae—often simply referred to as the "hip abductors." As will be described, the main function of the primary hip abductors is in providing frontal plane stability of the pelvis while in the stance phase of walking. The piriformis, sartorius, rectus femoris, and anterior (or superior) fibers of the gluteus maximus are considered secondary hip abductors.[227]

The *gluteus medius* is a broad muscle that attaches on the external surface of the ilium above the anterior gluteal line. The distal, more tendinous part of the muscle attaches to the greater trochanter (see Fig. 12.38), more specifically to its superior-posterior and lateral facets (see Fig. 12.6).[134,257] The distal attachment to the laterally projected greater trochanter provides the gluteus medius with excellent leverage to perform hip abduction (see Fig. 12.30).[286] The gluteus medius is the largest of the hip abductor muscles, occupying about 60% to 65% of the cross-sectional area of the primary abductors.[59,90] The broad and fan-shaped gluteus medius has been considered as having three functional sets of fibers: anterior, middle, and posterior.[277] All fibers contribute to abduction of the hip; however, from the anatomic position, the anterior fibers and posterior fibers are antagonists in respect to their horizontal plane actions.

FIG. 12.41 Relatively high demands are placed on many muscles that cross the hip, knee, and ankle as one climbs a mountain while bearing an external load. Activation is also required in low back extensor muscles (such as, for example, the lower multifidus) to stabilize the position of the pelvis. Note the medial-lateral axis of rotation at the hip and knee.

The *gluteus minimus* lies deep and slightly anterior to the gluteus medius (Fig. 12.42). The gluteus minimus attaches proximally on the ilium—between the anterior and inferior gluteal lines—and distally on anterior facet of the greater trochanter (see Fig. 12.6).[90] The distal attachment also blends with the capsule of the hip joint.[134,317] These muscular attachments may retract this part of the capsule away from the joint during motion—a mechanism that may prevent capsular impingement.

The gluteus minimus is smaller than the gluteus medius, occupying about 20% to 30% of the cross-sectional area of the primary hip abductors.[59,90] All fibers of the gluteus minimus contribute to abduction. The more anterior fibers also contribute to internal rotation and flexion, and the most posterior fibers contribute to external rotation. Fine-wire EMG analysis of the gluteus minimus shows that the anterior and posterior fibers are most active at slightly different times in the stance phase of walking, suggesting that they have slightly different roles in stabilizing the hip.[276]

The *tensor fascia latae* is the smallest of the three primary hip abductors, occupying only about 4% to 10% of the primary abductor cross-sectional area.[59,90] The anatomy of the tensor fasciae latae was discussed previously in this chapter.

It is worth noting that the primary hip abductors are capable of either internally or externally rotating the hip. Theoretically, therefore, active *pure* abduction requires that the abductors neutralize (or offset) one another's undesired horizontal plane torque potential.

Hip Abductor Mechanism: Control of Frontal Plane Stability of the Pelvis during Walking

The primary function of the hip abductors is to produce a torque that kinetically stabilizes the pelvis in the frontal plane while walking. Throughout much of the stance phase, therefore, the hip abductors are actively performing this function (see Fig. 12.35 and Fig. 15.29A). The hip abductor muscles play a dominant role in controlling the pelvis in both frontal and, as discussed previously, horizontal planes.

The abduction torque produced by the hip abductor muscles is particularly important during the *single-limb–support phase* of gait. During this phase the opposite leg is off the ground and swinging forward. Without adequate abduction torque on the stance limb, the pelvis may become mechanically unstable and drop uncontrollably toward the side of the swinging limb. The activation of the hip abductor muscles can be readily appreciated by palpating the gluteus medius just superior to the greater trochanter. The right gluteus medius, for example, becomes firm as the left leg lifts off the ground.

Hip Abductor Mechanism: Dominant Role in the Production of Compression Force at the Hip

Fig. 12.43 shows the major factors involved with maintaining frontal plane stability of the right hip during single-limb support, similar to that required during the mid stance phase of walking. The forces created by active hip abductors and body weight create opposing torques that control the position and stability of the pelvis (within the frontal plane) over the femoral head. During single-limb support, the pelvis is comparable to a seesaw, with its fulcrum represented by the femoral head. When the seesaw is balanced, the counterclockwise (internal) torque produced by the right hip abductor force (HAF) equals the clockwise (external) torque caused by body weight (BW). This balance of opposing torques is called *static rotary equilibrium.*

During single-limb support, the hip abductor muscles—in particular the gluteus medius—produce most of the vertical compression force across the hip.[64] This important point is demonstrated by

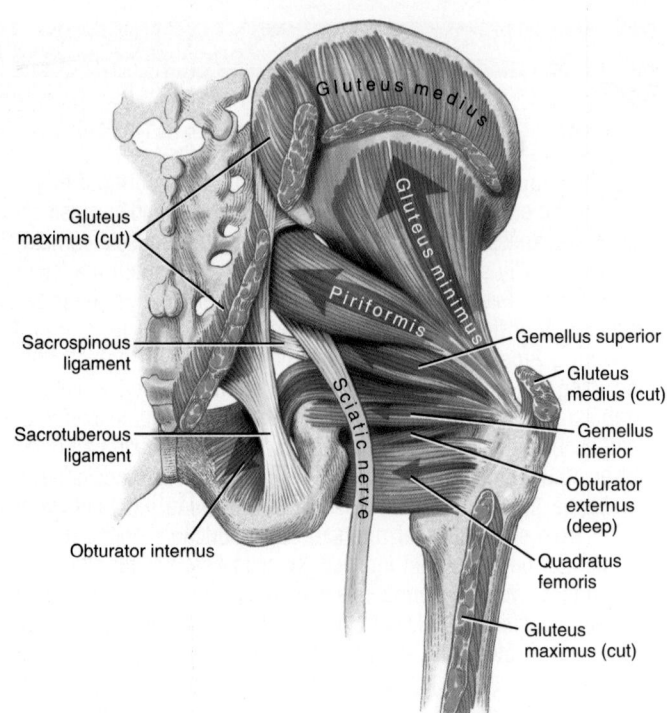

FIG. 12.42 Deep muscles of the posterior and lateral hip region. The gluteus medius and the gluteus maximus are cut away to expose deeper muscles.

the model in Fig. 12.43.[222,225] Note that the internal moment arm (D) used by the hip abductor muscles is about half the length of the external moment arm (D_1) used by BW.[219] Given this length disparity, the hip abductor muscles must produce a force *twice* that of BW in order to achieve stability during single-limb support. On every step, therefore, the acetabulum is pulled against the femoral head by the combined forces produced by the hip abductor muscles *and* the gravitational pull of BW. To achieve static linear equilibrium, this downward force is counteracted by a joint reaction force (JRF) of equal magnitude but oriented in nearly the opposite direction (see Fig. 12.43). The JRF is directed 10 to 15 degrees from vertical—an angle that is strongly influenced by the orientation of the hip abductor muscle force vector.[142]

The sample data supplied in Fig. 12.43 show how to estimate the approximate magnitude of the HAF and corresponding hip JRF during single-limb support. (For simplicity, all forces are assumed to act vertically, as shown in the seesaw model.) As shown in the calculations, an upward-directed JRF of 1873.8 N (421.3 lb) occurs when a person weighing 760.6 N (171 lb) is in single-limb support over the right limb. This reaction force is about 2.5 times BW, *66% of which comes from the hip abductor muscles.* During walking, the JRF is even greater because of the acceleration of the pelvis over the femoral head. Data based on three-dimensional computer modeling or direct measurements from strain gauges implanted into a hip prosthesis show that joint compression forces reach three to almost four times BW during walking.[53,64,291] These forces can increase to at least five or six times BW while running or ascending and descending stairs or ramps.[263] JRFs increase with increasing walking speed or when associated with significant gait deviations.[53,64]

Although the hip abductor muscles contribute significantly to compression force while in single-limb support, these and other muscles also contribute significantly to hip joint forces during non-ambulatory activities performed outside the frontal plane. For

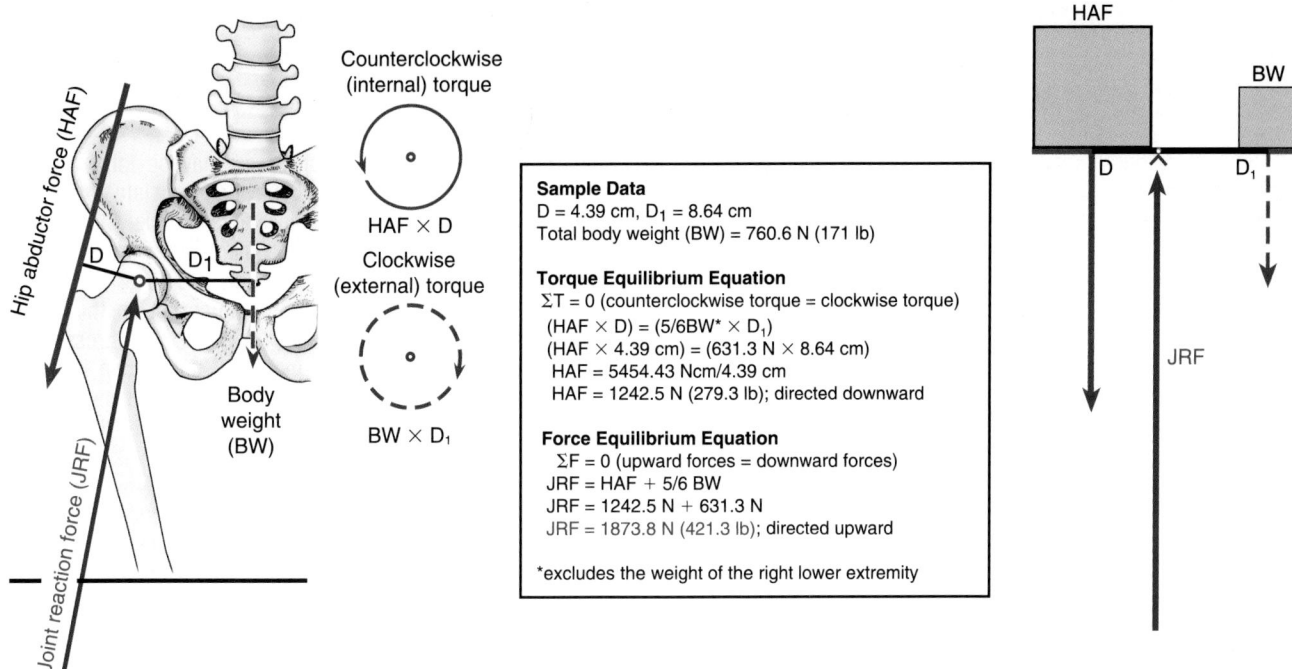

Sample Data
D = 4.39 cm, D_1 = 8.64 cm
Total body weight (BW) = 760.6 N (171 lb)

Torque Equilibrium Equation
$\Sigma T = 0$ (counterclockwise torque = clockwise torque)
$(HAF \times D) = (5/6 BW^* \times D_1)$
$(HAF \times 4.39\ cm) = (631.3\ N \times 8.64\ cm)$
HAF = 5454.43 Ncm/4.39 cm
HAF = 1242.5 N (279.3 lb); directed downward

Force Equilibrium Equation
$\Sigma F = 0$ (upward forces = downward forces)
JRF = HAF + 5/6 BW
JRF = 1242.5 N + 631.3 N
JRF = 1873.8 N (421.3 lb); directed upward

*excludes the weight of the right lower extremity

FIG. 12.43 A frontal plane diagram shows the function of the right hip abductor muscles during single-limb support on the right hip. The illustration on the left assumes that the pelvis and trunk are in static (linear and rotary) equilibrium about the right hip. The *counterclockwise torque* (*solid circle*) is the product of the right hip abductor force (HAF) times internal moment arm (*D*); the *clockwise torque* (*dashed circle*) is the product of body weight (BW) times external moment arm (*D_1*). Because the system is assumed to be in equilibrium, the torques in the frontal plane are equal in magnitude and opposite in direction: $HAF \times D = BW \times D_1$. The see-saw model (*right*) simplifies the major kinetic events during single-limb support. A joint reaction force (JRF) is directed through the fulcrum of the seesaw (hip joint). The sample data in the box are used in the torque and force equilibrium equations. These equations allow an estimate of the approximate magnitude of the hip abductor force and joint reaction force generated during single-limb support. (To simplify the mathematics, the calculations assume that all forces are acting in a vertical direction. This assumption introduces modest error in the results. Again, for simplicity, all moment arm directions are assigned positive values.)

example, actively performing a "straight-leg raise" while lying supine generates hip JRFs of about 1.4 times BW or about 50% of the joint force naturally produced while walking on a level surface.[271] Furthermore, performing a unilateral (supine) hip "bridging" exercise generates a hip JRF of about three times BW, similar to forces produced while walking. The magnitudes of these forces must be kept in mind when prescribing exercises for patients after hip surgery, such as a total hip arthroplasty or fracture repair.

In most situations, forces acting on the healthy or well-developed hip by hip abductors or other muscles serve important physiologic functions, such as stabilizing the femoral head within the acetabulum, assisting in the nutrition of the articular cartilage, and providing stimuli for normal development and shaping of joint structure in the growing child. The articular cartilage and trabecular bone normally protect the joint by safely dispersing large forces. A hip with arthritis or otherwise damaged articular cartilage, however, may no longer be able to provide this protection.

Maximal Abduction Torque Varies According to Hip Joint Angle

The unique relationship between a muscle group's internal torque and joint angle provides insight into the functional demands naturally placed on the muscles. The shape of the plot depicted in Fig. 12.44, for example, clearly shows that the abductor muscles produce their peak torque (greatest strength) when elongated.[219] The maximal torque is produced when the hip is *adducted* just beyond the neutral (0-degree) hip position. This frontal plane hip angle

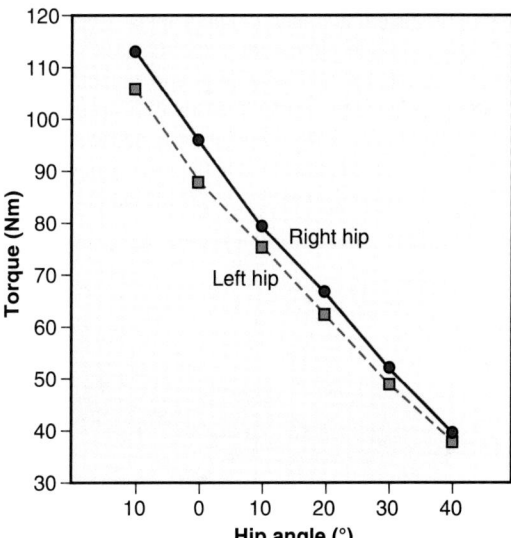

FIG. 12.44 This plot shows the effect of frontal plane range of hip motion on the maximal-effort, isometric hip abduction torque in 30 healthy persons.[219] The −10-degree hip angle represents the adducted position at which the muscles are at their longest. Data are shown for both right and left sides.

Greater Trochanteric Pain Syndrome

Greater trochanteric pain syndrome (GTPS) involves degenerative changes or tears of the distal tendinous attachments of the gluteus medius and minimus and, in some cases, associated bursitis.[85] GTPS can be a primary cause of lateral hip pain, most commonly affecting women approximately 40 to 50 years of age.[109,201] Classic signs include point tenderness near or on the greater trochanter (where the gluteal muscles attach), weakened hip abduction, and a gait deviation consistent with weak or painful hip abductor muscles (described later in this chapter).[4] Symptoms are often exacerbated by activities that demand high, sustained, or repetitive forces from the hip abductors, such as standing on one limb, climbing stairs or hills, or prolonged walking. As with all pain in the hip region, associated comorbidities must be ruled out as well as pain referred from the low back region.

The primarily pathology underlying GTPS is tendinopathy of the gluteus medius and minimus. MRI often shows a thickening or a thinning of the affected tendons as well as partial- or full-thickness tears.[5,57,109] Tears occur more frequently in the tendon of the gluteus medius as it attaches to the lateral and superior-posterior facets of the greater trochanter.[5] In up to 20% of cases, bursitis may be associated with GTPS, either in the bursa beneath the distal attachments of the gluteus medius and minimus or, more frequently, in the bursa over the posterior-inferior aspect of the greater trochanter and just under the gluteus maximus.[109,184,329]

The pathology associated with tendinopathy of the gluteus medius or gluteus minimus has features similar to rotator cuff pathology.[69] For this reason, GTPS has been loosely referred to as the "rotator cuff syndrome of the hip." The supraspinatus and gluteal tendons both tend to show degenerative changes on the undersurface of the tendon as it abuts against bone. Pain is usually insidious and chronic in both GTPS and rotator cuff syndrome, typically involving attritional degeneration or tears rather than acute rupture from an isolated event. The degenerative changes that occur in these muscles are, in some way, related to a failure of the tissues to absorb and tolerate mechanical stress. Forces from the strongly activated gluteal muscles, required at every stance phase of gait, impose relatively large and repetitive stresses on their respective tendons. These stresses may occur as *tension* as the tendons are pulled *away* from the bone; however, stresses may also occur as *compression* as the undersurface of distal aspect of the tendons are pulled inward *against* the bone and bursa. The

magnitude of the compressional stress may be influenced by simultaneous forces acting on the overlying fascia lata of the thigh exerted in part by the tensor fasciae latae muscle. Stiffening of this complex could create an inward push against the underlying gluteal tendons as they wrap superior-medially over the greater trochanter, amplifying the localized compression on the gluteal tendons.[109] Over time, the repeated compressional stress might degrade and weaken the tissue matrix of the tendon insertion. Subsequent small tears or abrasions in the tendon theoretically place greater stress on the intact, healthy parts of the tendon, thereby predisposing these tissues to degeneration as well.

Although theoretical, one factor leading to GTPS may be related to a prior history of weakness or otherwise reduced abduction torque potential of the gluteus medius and minimus. A scenario of weakened gluteal muscles could increase the compensatory demands on the more superficial hip abductor mechanism (i.e., the tensor fasciae latae muscle and associated lateral fascia of the thigh). Such compensation, if occurring during every gait cycle, could plausibly abrade the gluteal tendons to the point that they undergo attritional degeneration or even failure. More biomechanical and histologic research is needed to better understand the pathogenesis of GTPS in order to better treat this condition.

Conservative treatment has been described for GTPS, including use of anti-inflammatory medication, corticosteroid or platelet-rich plasma injections, use of a cane in the hand contralateral to the affected hip, activity modification, patient education, and exercise.[109,201,204] Grimaldi and Fearon have proposed a physical therapy approach that limits activities or exercises involving hip *adduction* (both pelvic-on-femoral and vice versa).[109] This precaution is based on the likelihood that greater hip adduction would increase compressional stress on the insertions of the gluteal tendons as the tensor fasciae latae and associated lateral fascia are stretched across the lateral side of the hip. In addition, initial physical therapy sessions may incorporate non–pain-provoking *isometric* abduction exercises in positions that *limit hip adduction*. As thoroughly outlined by Grimaldi and Fearon,[109] methods of applying greater resistance with non–isometric-type exercises may be judiciously incorporated when tolerated.

When conservative treatment is unsuccessful, surgical repair of the tendons may be indicated. Both open and endoscopic surgical approaches have been shown to produce favorable results.[5,57,201]

Hip Abductor Muscle Weakness

The demands placed on the hip abductor muscles to simply stand on one limb while maintaining frontal plane stability are surprisingly high—likely, on average, at least about 50% to 60% of an adult's maximal isometric abduction strength. This is a very general estimate based on comparing the muscle group's maximal internal torque potential (Fig. 12.44) with the approximate external torque required to stand on one limb (Fig. 12.43). This muscle demand is typically greater while walking. A wide range of pathologic conditions can involve major weakness of the hip abductors, thereby significantly altering the quality of walking.[4,93,121,200] These conditions may range from cerebral palsy or muscular dystrophy to a host of hip-related pathologies, such as chronic hip pain, developmental hip dysplasia, postoperative hip replacement, and greater trochanter pain syndrome. Furthermore, people with a painful or unstable hip, regardless of underlying pathology, may develop disuse-related muscle weakness by purposely limiting their abductor activation while walking. This strategy is often employed subconsciously as a way to minimize the associated myogenic hip force, typically to avoid pain. Unfortunately, however, if this strategy becomes chronic, the disuse weakness may ultimately exacerbate the hip pain and instability. Hip muscles with only secondary hip abductor potential may be strongly recruited to compensate for the primary abductor muscle weakness. Recruiting this secondary subset of hip abductors may result in less control of the pelvis, ultimately creating unnecessarily high and poorly dissipated *peak* loads across the hip.[209] Improving the functional strength of the primary hip abductors is therefore an important therapeutic goal, not only to improve overall functional mobility but to limit large, repetitive, and potentially damaging peak loads across the joint.

The classic indicator of hip abductor weakness is the *Trendelenburg sign*.[118] The patient is asked to stand in single-limb support over the suspected weak hip. The sign is positive if the pelvis drops to the side of the unsupported limb; in other words, the weak hip "falls" into pelvic-on-femoral adduction (see Fig. 12.21B). The clinician needs to be cautious, however, in interpreting and documenting the results of this test. The patient with a weak right hip abductor muscle, for example, may indeed drop the left side of the pelvis when asked to stand only on the right limb. The weakness may be masked, however, by a compensatory lean of the *trunk* to the right, especially if the weakness is marked. Leaning the trunk *to the side of the weakness* can significantly reduce the external torque demand on the abductor muscles by reducing the length of the external moment arm (see Fig. 12.43, D_1). When observed while a person is walking, this compensatory lean to the side of weakness may be referred to as a "gluteus medius limp" or "compensated Trendelenburg gait," although other more descriptive

terminology is described in the clinical literature.[67] As described later in this chapter, using a cane in the hand opposite the weakened hip abductors can significantly improve this abnormal gait pattern.[224]

Weakness of the hip abductor muscles often persists longer than in other muscle groups. Regardless of the cause, the functional and pathomechanical implications of prolonged hip abductor weakness can be wide-reaching, especially considering their important kinesiologic significance in upright, weight-bearing activities.[311] In addition to disruptions in walking and local hip kinesiology, prolonged weakness of the hip abductor muscles has been associated with patellofemoral pain syndrome, low back pain, increased risk of ankle sprain, knee stability, and falling in older adults.[154,170,264,292]

Based on the pathomechanical ramifications of weak hip abductors, considerable EMG research has studied which exercises most specifically target and thereby potentially strengthen the hip abductors. Data show that exercises placing a high demand on the gluteus medius are those that specifically involve straight frontal plane hip *abduction* (from femoral-on-pelvic or pelvic-on-femoral perspectives) performed in extension, internal, or external rotation.[100,242,275] These results are expected based on the primary or secondary actions of the various fibers of the gluteus medius listed in Table 12.2. Note, however, that Philippon and colleagues reported that a *single-leg* "bridging exercise" (with contralateral lower limb held in a "straight-leg raised" position) generated slightly higher EMG levels from the gluteus medius than any exercise involving side-lying hip abduction.[242] The surprisingly high demands placed on the gluteus medius during the single-leg bridging exercise may provide insight into the muscular complexity of performing this seemingly simple, single-plane exercise. Assume for the sake of discussion that the single-leg bridging exercise is powered by the *right* hip while the left lower extremity is held in a "straight-leg-raised" position. This exercise challenges the middle and posterior fibers of the right gluteus medius for extension support while the middle fibers offset the strong adduction action of the right adductor magnus. Furthermore, the anterior fibers of the right gluteus medius are challenged to help offset *both* the external rotation potential of the right gluteus maximus and the external rotation (pelvic-on-femoral) gravitation torque placed on the right hip. Interestingly, this same EMG study reported far less gluteus medius activation during a *bilateral* bridging exercise. Dividing the hip extension torque across both hips reduces the demand on each individual gluteus medius to only 11% of maximum voluntary contraction (compared with 35% for a unilateral bridging exercise).

naturally occurs when the body is in or close to the single-limb support phase of walking: precisely when these muscles are needed to provide frontal plane stability to the hip. In essence, the abductor muscles have their greatest torque reserve at a muscle length (and joint angle) that corresponds to their greatest functional demands.

The adducted position of the hip also increases the passive tension in the naturally stiff iliotibial band. This passive tension, although likely relatively small, can nevertheless augment the abduction torque required during the single-limb–support phase of walking.[220]

In contrast, hip abduction torque potential is *least* at the near fully shortened muscle length that corresponds to 40 degrees of abduction (see Fig. 12.44). Interestingly, even though the internal (abduction) moment arm of the gluteus medius is relatively large in full abduction (compared with the adducted position), the much-shortened length of the muscle in this position significantly reduces its active force (and therefore torque) output.[127] Ironically, the near maximally abducted hip is in the position traditionally suggested for manually testing the "maximal" strength of the hip abductor muscles.[152]

HIP EXTERNAL ROTATOR MUSCLES

The primary external rotator muscles of the hip include the gluteus maximus and five of the six "short external rotators." In the anatomic position, secondary external rotators include the posterior fibers of the gluteus medius and minimus, obturator externus, sartorius, and long head of the biceps femoris.[227] The obturator externus is considered a secondary rotator because its line of force lies only a few millimeters posterior to the longitudinal axis of rotation (see Fig. 12.34).

The attachments of the gluteus maximus and sartorius were previously described under the topics of hip extensors and hip flexors, respectively.

Functional Anatomy of the "Short External Rotators"

The six "short external rotators" of the hip are the piriformis, obturator internus, gemellus superior, gemellus inferior, quadratus femoris, and obturator externus (see Figs. 12.14, 12.38, and 12.42). The lines

of force of these muscles are oriented primarily in the horizontal plane. This orientation is optimal for producing external rotation torque because the majority of the force of each muscle has a perpendicular intersection with the vertical axis of rotation.[235] In a manner similar to the infraspinatus and teres minor at the shoulder, the short external rotators are well aligned to compress and thereby stabilize the articulation. Although the physiologic cross-sectional area of each short external rotator is relatively small, the total area of the group is notable— similar to the size of the gluteus minimus (see Appendix IV, Part E).[235]

The *piriformis* attaches proximally on the anterior surface of the sacrum, between the most cranial ventral sacral foramina (see Figs. 12.1 and 12.25). Exiting the pelvis posteriorly through the greater sciatic foramen, the piriformis attaches via a tendon to the superior aspect of the greater trochanter (see Fig. 12.42).

In addition to the action of external rotation, the piriformis is a secondary hip abductor. Both actions are apparent by the muscle's line of force relative to the axes of rotation at the hip (see Figs. 12.30 and 12.34).

The *obturator internus* originates from the internal surface of the obturator membrane and from the adjacent bone surrounding the obturator foramen (see Fig. 12.42). Although not visible in Fig. 12.42, much of the muscle's proximal attachment extends superiorly and slightly posteriorly on the internal surface of the ischium, about 2 to 3 cm above the ischial spine. From this extensive origin, muscle fibers converge to a tendon after exiting the pelvis through the lesser sciatic foramen. The lesser sciatic notch, which is lined with hyaline cartilage, functions as a pulley by deflecting the tendon of the obturator internus by about 130 degrees on its approach to the medial surface of the greater trochanter (Fig. 12.45A). With the femur firmly fixed during standing, strong contraction of a *right* obturator internus, for example, can rotate the pelvis (and superimposed trunk) contralaterally to the *left* relative to the femoral head (Fig. 12.45B). In addition to rotating the pelvis, the force produced by the nearly horizontally running obturator internus likely compresses and stabilizes the joint. A fine wire ultrasound-guided EMG analysis suggests that this muscle plays a special role in adjusting the positional stability of the joint just before the activation of the other muscles.[132] Although it is speculation, the obturator internus,

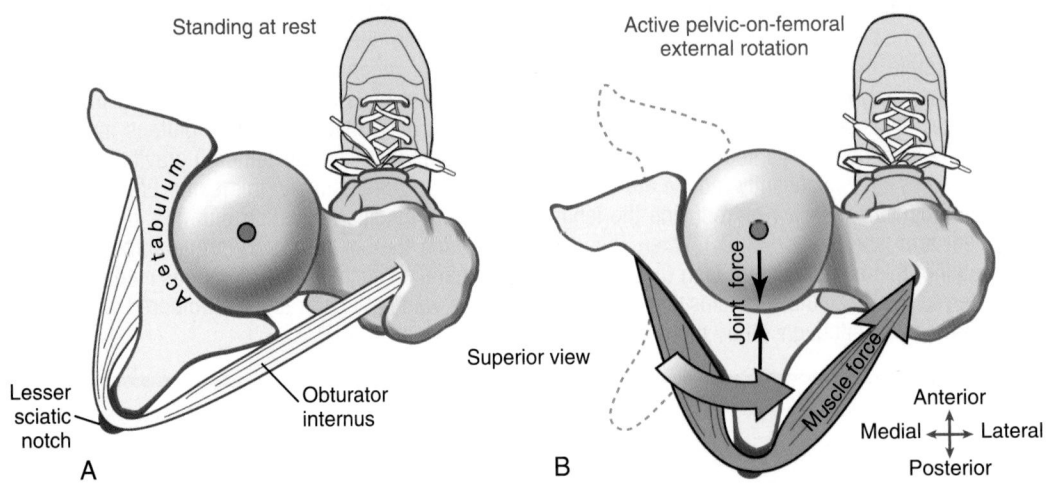

FIG. 12.45 Superior view depicts the orientation and action of the obturator internus muscle. (A) Standing at rest, the course of the obturator internus muscle is shown as it passes through the pulley formed by the lesser sciatic notch. (B) With the femur fixed during standing, contraction of this muscle causes pelvic-on-femoral (hip) external rotation. The opposing black arrows indicate the compression force generated into the joint as a result of the muscle contraction.

along with other short external rotators, may also have a role in directing the compression forces within the joint toward the center of the acetabulum, away from the regions that often show degeneration.[203]

A relatively dense layer of connective tissue covers and adheres to part of the medial (intrapelvic) surface of the obturator internus muscle, often described as the *obturator fascia*.[226] This fascia serves as part of the attachment of the levator ani, the main muscle of the pelvic floor. (Refer to Appendix IV, Part F, for attachments, innervation, and actions of the muscles of the pelvic floor.) Because of this direct anatomic connection, some treatments for *pelvic floor pain syndrome or dysfunction* incorporate methods that alter the active or passive tension in the obturator internus.[63,237,248,309]

The *gemellus superior* and *inferior* (from the Latin root *geminus*, meaning "twins") are two small, nearly identically shaped muscles with proximal attachments on either side of the lesser sciatic notch (see Fig. 12.42). Each muscle blends in with the central tendon of the obturator internus, forming a common tricipital attachment to the femur.[226,278] Immediately below the gemellus inferior is the thicker *quadratus femoris* muscle. This muscle arises from the external side of the ischial tuberosity and inserts on the posterior side of the proximal femur. In cases of abnormal bony morphology, this muscle may become impinged between the lesser trochanter and ischium, typically during motions that involve the extremes of external rotation.[283] If chronic and repetitive, this clinically termed "ischiofemoral impingement" may cause groin and buttock pain along with abnormal magnetic resonance (MR) signaling from the quadratus femoris muscle.[289]

The *obturator externus* muscle arises from the external side of the obturator membrane and adjacent ilium (see Fig. 12.14). The belly of this muscle is visible from the anterior side of the pelvis after removal of the adductor longus and pectineus muscles (see Fig. 12.25, left side). The muscle attaches posteriorly on the femur at the trochanteric fossa (see Fig. 12.6). (Based on its leverage to produce adduction, location, and innervation, the obturator externus is more anatomically associated with the *adductor group* of muscles than with the other five short external rotators. The obturator externus is innervated by nerve roots that originate from the lumbar plexus [via the obturator nerve], as are most of the other adductor muscles. The other small external rotators, in contrast, are innervated through the sacral plexus, with nerve roots as low as S^2.)

Overall Function

The gluteus maximus is a potent external rotator of the hip. In addition to its dominant size, the muscle's approximate 45-degree line of force (with respect to the frontal plane) suggests that about 70% of its force (i.e., cosine of 45 degrees) is dedicated exclusively within the horizontal plane while standing. Such an orientation favors the production of external rotation torque. The deeper and near horizontally oriented short external rotators augment this rotational torque and likely excel as simultaneous stabilizers and intrinsic controllers of the articulation. Accordingly, surgical repair of incised short external rotators during a posterior-lateral approach to a total hip arthroplasty is considered an important step in preventing subsequent dislocation of the implanted hip.[290]

The horizontal plane action of the external rotators of the hip is particularly evident during pelvic-on-femoral rotation. Consider, for example, the external rotator muscles contracting to rotate the pelvis over the femur (Fig. 12.46). With the right lower extremity firmly in contact with the ground, contraction of the right external rotators accelerates the anterior side of the pelvis and attached trunk to the left—*contralateral* to the fixed femur. This action of planting a foot and "cutting" to the opposite side is the natural way to abruptly change direction while running. As indicated in Fig. 12.46, activation of the right gluteus maximus, for instance, is very capable of imparting both the extension and the external rotation thrust to the hip during this action. If needed, the external rotation torque can be decelerated by eccentric action of internal rotator muscles. Sudden eccentric activation of the adductor longus or brevis, for example, might occur to decelerate the pelvis as it swings to face contralaterally—an action that may cause "strain" injury to these muscles. The mechanism of injury may partially explain the relatively high incidence of adductor muscle strain during many sporting activities that involve rapid rotation of the pelvis and trunk while running.

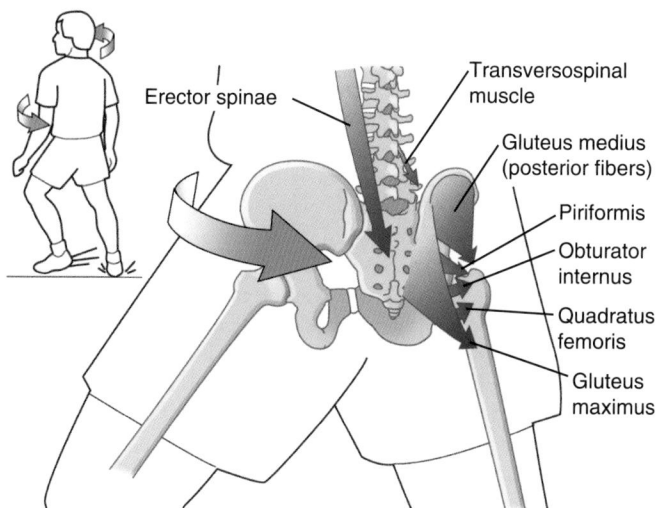

FIG. 12.46 Action of the right external rotator muscles during pelvic-on-femoral external rotation of the right hip. Back extensor muscles are also shown rotating the lower trunk to the left.

Erector spinae

Transversospinal muscle

Gluteus medius (posterior fibers)

Piriformis

Obturator internus

Quadratus femoris

Gluteus maximus

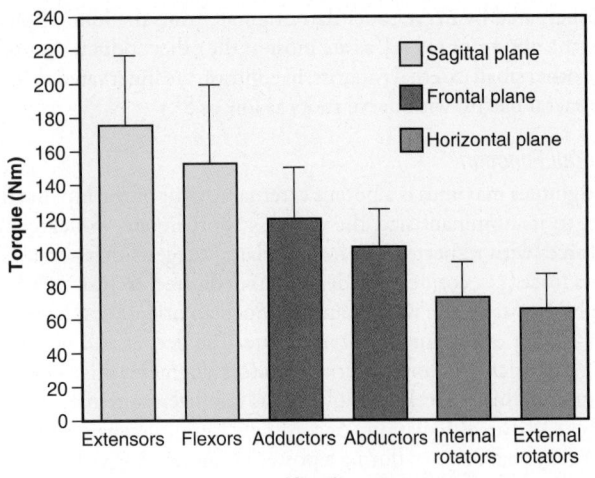

FIG. 12.47 Average maximal-effort torque (Nm) produced by the six major muscle groups of the hip (standard deviations indicated by brackets). See text for source. Data were measured isokinetically at 30 degrees/sec in 35 healthy males (average age 28 years) and were averaged over the full range of motion. Data for sagittal and frontal planes torques were obtained with subjects standing with hip in extension. Data for horizontal plane torques were obtained with subjects sitting, with hip flexed 60 degrees and knee flexed 90 degrees.

MAXIMAL TORQUE PRODUCED BY THE HIP MUSCLES

Normative data on the maximal-effort torque (strength) production of the hip muscles may be useful for assessing progress and setting of goals for people involved in rehabilitation and training programs. Fig. 12.47 depicts the average, maximal internal torque produced by a sample of healthy males.[45] It is interesting to observe the ranking of the torques across the three planes of motion. The *greatest* torque is produced in the sagittal plane, with extension torque slightly exceeding flexion torque. The predominant strength of the hip extensors compared with all other muscle groups is not surprising: these muscles must lift or propel the body upward (and often forward) against gravity or control the descent of the body. The relatively high strength of the hip flexor muscles reflects the need to rapidly accelerate the lower limb during running, in addition to controlling the entire trunk and pelvis relative to fixed lower extremities. Consider in the latter case the forceful iliopsoas, for example—a muscle that likely accounts for a significant proportion of the flexion torque potential at the hip.

The adductor and abductor muscles generate similar magnitudes of peak torque within the frontal plane, although less than the flexor and extensor muscles.[45,304] The internal and external rotator muscles produce the *least* magnitude of torque of all muscle groups of the hip. Such a ranking likely results from the fact that, in the upright position, these muscles produce a rotary torque between the femur and pelvis in a plane that does *not* typically directly oppose the force of gravity.

EXAMPLE OF HIP PATHOLOGY AND SELECTED THERAPEUTIC AND SURGICAL INTERVENTIONS

One of the most common causes of hip pain and associated impairment is osteoarthritis. This section introduces this often-disabling condition, followed by a discussion of clinical biomechanics associated with selected therapeutic and surgical interventions for a few examples of hip pathology.

Osteoarthritis of the Hip

Hip osteoarthritis is a disease manifested by deterioration of the joint's articular cartilage and a loss of joint space, thickening and stiffening of the joint capsule, varying amounts of soft tissue inflammation, presence of osteophytes, and sclerosis of subchondral bone. The resulting reduced damping mechanism at the joint can increase local contact pressure, thereby contributing to marked degeneration and change in shape of the joint.[150] Several years ago, the American College of Rheumatology recommended the following criteria for diagnosing hip osteoarthritis *without* the use of radiography: hip pain, less than 115 degrees of hip flexion, and less than 15 degrees of internal rotation.[7] The reduced range of motion may be caused by restrictions in soft tissue (such as posterior and inferior capsule or parts of the ischiofemoral ligament) and, in more severe cases, articular malalignment and osteophyte formation. Additional symptoms may include atrophy and weakness of hip muscles, morning stiffness, crepitus, and modified gait (such as a compensated Trendelenburg gait) or altered step length.[17,205] The impairments associated with advanced hip osteoarthritis can cause a significant loss in overall function, including difficulty climbing stairs, walking, bathing, dressing the lower extremities, getting in and out of a car, and rising from a low chair.

Hip osteoarthritis may be classified as either a primary (idiopathic) or a secondary disease. *Primary hip osteoarthritis* is an arthritic condition without a known or obvious cause. *Secondary hip osteoarthritis*, in contrast, is an arthritic condition resulting from a known or relatively obvious mechanical disruption of the joint. This may occur from trauma or exposure to high repetitive loads; structural failure, such as a slipped capital femoral epiphysis or avascular necrosis of the femoral head (e.g., Legg-Calvé-Perthes disease); significant anatomic asymmetry or dysplasia, such as excessive acetabular or femoral anteversion; or repeated dislocations and chronic instability.[32,55,123,273]

Often the source of the mechanical disruption is not so obvious, and relatively subtle anatomic variations in bony structure can be a precursor to osteoarthritis. The resulting joint incongruity (even when relatively slight and asymptomatic), especially if combined with certain habitual and near full range movements, can lead to repeated and stressful femoroacetabular impingement that can potentially trigger osteoarthritis.[101,313]

Despite decades of clinical and basic science research, the exact underlying cause of primary hip osteoarthritis remains unclear.[150,265] Although the frequency of osteoarthritis at any joint increases with age, the disease is not triggered solely by the aging process. If that were true, then all older people would eventually develop this disease. The causes of primary osteoarthritis are complicated and not exclusively based on a simple wear-and-tear phenomenon. Although physical stress can increase the rate and amount of wear at the hip, this does not always lead to the disease of osteoarthritis.[179,252] Other factors possibly associated with the development of osteoarthritis include altered metabolism and loosening of the ground matrix of the cartilage, increased body mass index, genetics, female sex, immune system and molecular inflammatory factors, neuromuscular disorders, and biochemical factors.[115,131,150,183,229]

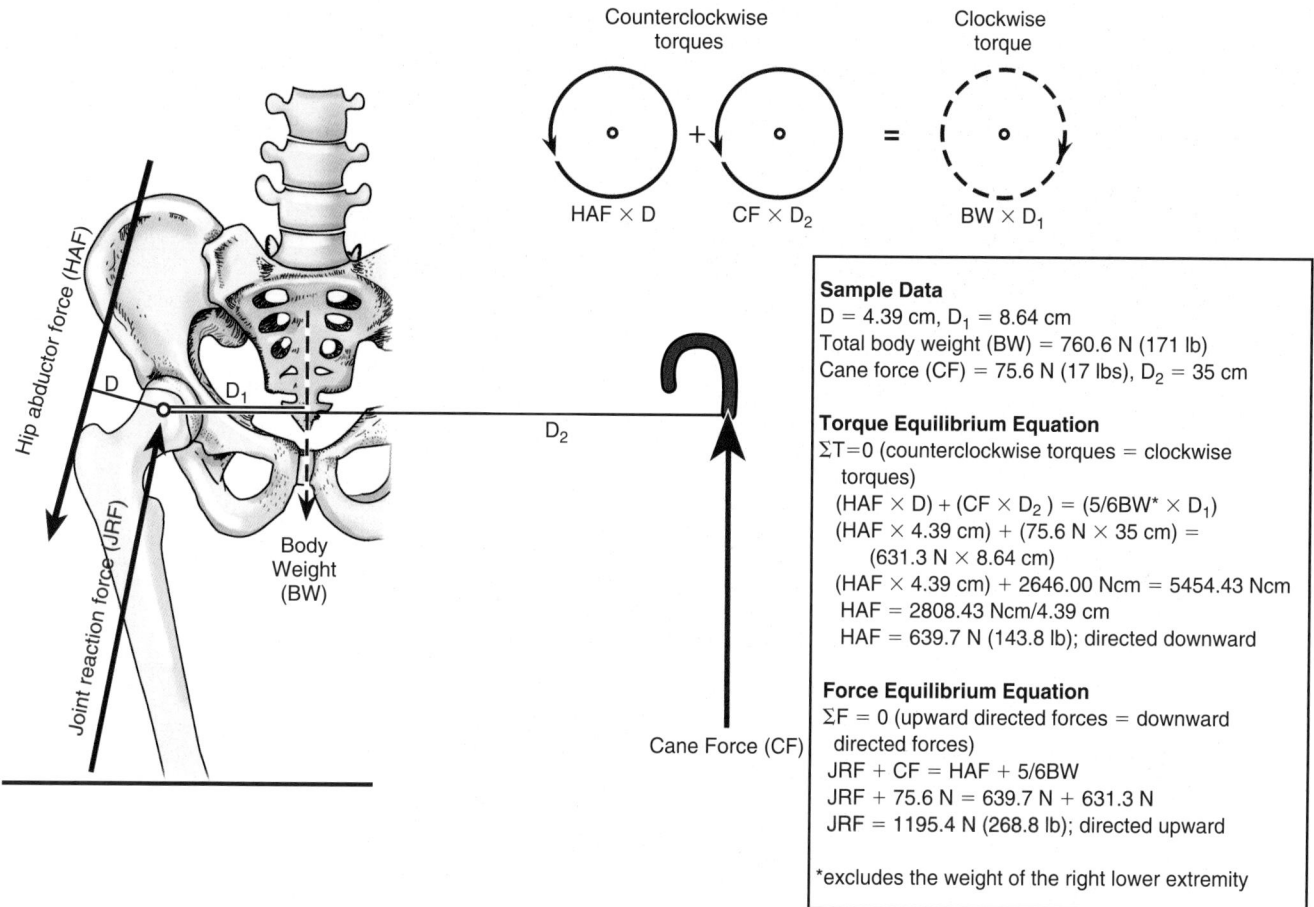

Sample Data
D = 4.39 cm, D_1 = 8.64 cm
Total body weight (BW) = 760.6 N (171 lb)
Cane force (CF) = 75.6 N (17 lbs), D_2 = 35 cm

Torque Equilibrium Equation
$\Sigma T = 0$ (counterclockwise torques = clockwise torques)
(HAF × D) + (CF × D_2) = (5/6BW* × D_1)
(HAF × 4.39 cm) + (75.6 N × 35 cm) =
    (631.3 N × 8.64 cm)
(HAF × 4.39 cm) + 2646.00 Ncm = 5454.43 Ncm
HAF 2808.43 Ncm/4.39 cm
HAF = 639.7 N (143.8 lb); directed downward

Force Equilibrium Equation
$\Sigma F = 0$ (upward directed forces = downward directed forces)
JRF + CF = HAF + 5/6BW
JRF + 75.6 N = 639.7 N + 631.3 N
JRF = 1195.4 N (268.8 lb); directed upward

*excludes the weight of the right lower extremity

FIG. 12.48 A frontal plane diagram shows how a cane force (CF) applied by the left hand produces a frontal plane torque about the right hip in single-limb support. The pelvis and trunk are assumed to be in static (linear and rotary) equilibrium about the right hip. The cane-produced torque minimizes the torque and force demands on the right hip abductor muscles. Note that the *clockwise torque* (*dashed circle*) resulting from body weight (*BW × D₁*) is balanced by the *counterclockwise torques* (*solid circles*) resulting from the hip abductor force (*HAF × D*) *and* the cane force (*CF × D₂*). The data shown in the box are used in the torque and force equilibrium equations to estimate the approximate magnitude of hip abductor force and joint reaction force (JRF). The moment arm used by cane force is represented by D_2. See Fig. 12.43 for additional abbreviations and background. (To simplify the mathematics, the calculations assume that all forces are acting in a vertical direction. This assumption introduces modest error in the results. All moment arm directions are assigned positive values.) (From Neumann DA: Hip abductor muscle activity as subjects with hip prosthesis walk with different methods of using a cane, *Phys Ther* 78:490, 1998. With permission of the American Physical Therapy Association.)

Selected Therapeutic and Surgical Interventions for a Painful, Degenerated, or Mechanically Unstable Hip

EXERCISE, ACTIVITY MODIFICATION, USING A CANE, AND ADVISED METHODS FOR CARRYING EXTERNAL LOADS

Osteoarthritis of the hip can lead to chronic pain and reduced functional mobility. These potentially disabling impairments can also occur in a hip after a fracture or a hip that is acutely inflamed, brittle because of severe osteoporosis, or mechanically unstable from marked dysplasia. Conservative treatment for such conditions may include patient education, modalities for relieving pain, and, when appropriate, graded aerobic conditioning, physical activity, general exercise with or without manual therapy, and muscle-specific resistive exercise—both on land and in water.[a] In addition, clinicians frequently provide advice on how to limit the magnitude of potentially large forces that may exacerbate or further complicate the

[a]96,144,160,163,258,261,262,284,301

underlying degenerative pathology. Such advice on hip "joint protection" may include instructions on how to modify daily activities, such as lifting; reducing excess body weight; walking with reduced speed, cadence, and stride length; using assistive devices while walking; and using specific methods of carrying loads.[30,64,68,221,233]

One of the most practical and effective methods of reducing compression forces on the hip during walking is to use a *cane* held in the hand *opposite* the affected hip. Use of the cane in this fashion reduces joint reaction force (JRF) primarily by reducing the activation of the hip abductor muscles.[224] Fig. 12.48 shows that applying a cane force by the left hand results in a JRF at the right hip of 1195.4 N (268.8 lb).[224] This is 36% lower than when a cane is not used (see Fig. 12.43 for comparison). In essence, the force applied to the cane (held in the left hand) produces a torque about the right hip that is in the *same rotary direction* as that produced by the overlying hip abductor muscles. Pushing on the cane, therefore, can substitute for part of the force that is normally required by the hip abductor muscles: reduced demands placed on the hip abductor muscles during single-limb support equates to reduced compression force on the hip joint.

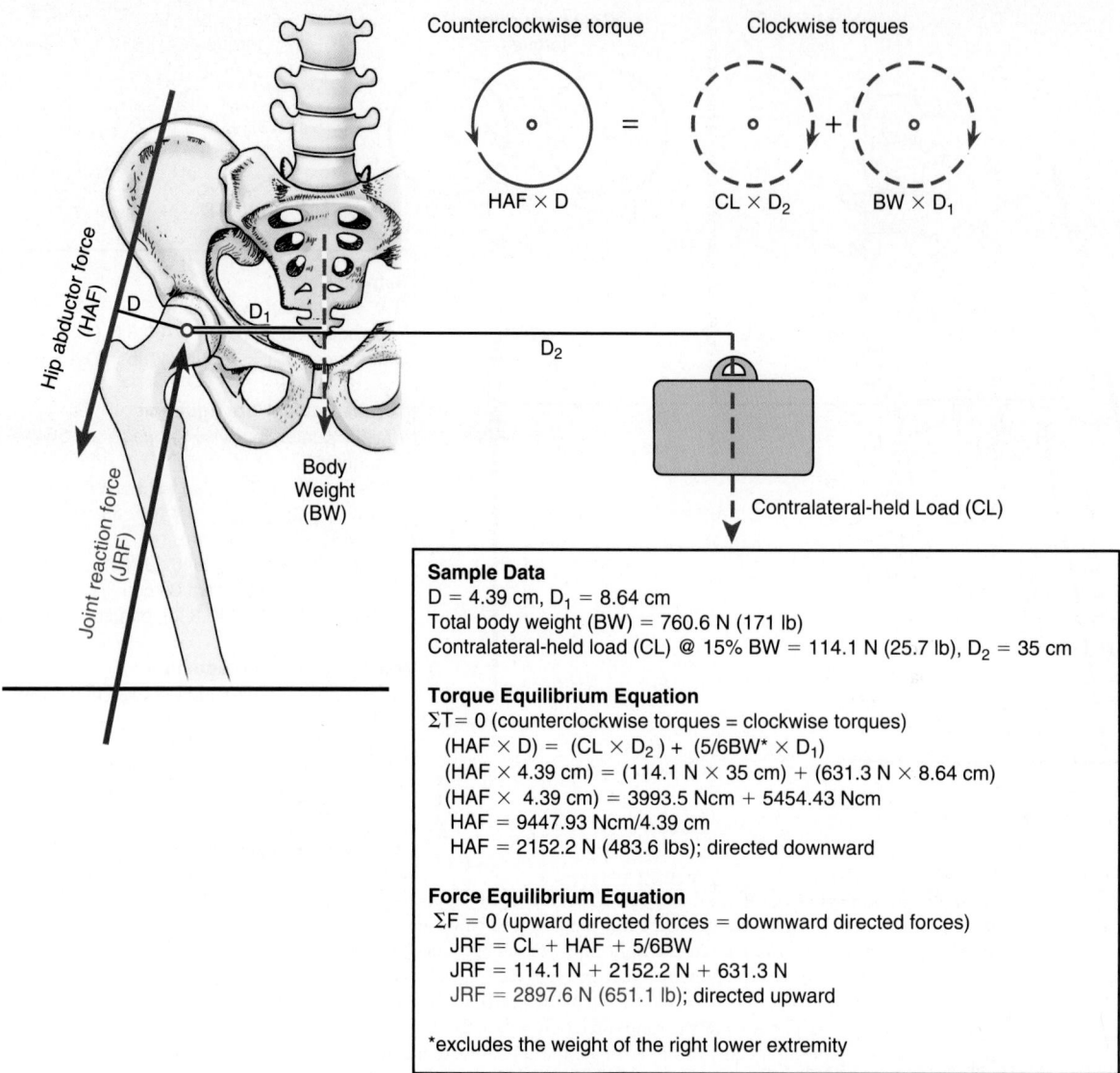

Counterclockwise torque

Clockwise torques

$$HAF \times D = CL \times D_2 + BW \times D_1$$

Hip abductor force (HAF)

Joint reaction force (JRF)

D   D₁

D₂

Body Weight (BW)

Contralateral-held Load (CL)

Sample Data
D = 4.39 cm, D_1 = 8.64 cm
Total body weight (BW) = 760.6 N (171 lb)
Contralateral-held load (CL) @ 15% BW = 114.1 N (25.7 lb), D_2 = 35 cm

Torque Equilibrium Equation
ΣT = 0 (counterclockwise torques = clockwise torques)
(HAF × D) = (CL × D_2) + (5/6BW* × D_1)
(HAF × 4.39 cm) = (114.1 N × 35 cm) + (631.3 N × 8.64 cm)
(HAF × 4.39 cm) = 3993.5 Ncm + 5454.43 Ncm
HAF = 9447.93 Ncm/4.39 cm
HAF = 2152.2 N (483.6 lbs); directed downward

Force Equilibrium Equation
ΣF = 0 (upward directed forces = downward directed forces)
JRF = CL + HAF + 5/6BW
JRF = 114.1 N + 2152.2 N + 631.3 N
JRF = 2897.6 N (651.1 lb); directed upward

*excludes the weight of the right lower extremity

FIG. 12.49 A frontal plane diagram shows how a load held in the left hand significantly increases the right hip abductor force (HAF) during single-limb support. Two clockwise torques (*dashed circles*) are produced about the right hip because of the contralateral-held load ($CL \times D_2$) *and* body weight ($BW \times D_1$). For equilibrium about the right hip, the clockwise torques must be balanced by a counterclockwise torque (*solid circle*) produced by the hip abductor force ($HAF \times D$). The data shown in the box are used in the torque and force equilibrium equations to estimate the approximate magnitude of HAF and joint reaction force (JRF). D_2 designates the moment arm used by the contralateral-held load (*CL*). Refer to Fig. 12.43 for background and other abbreviations. (To simplify the mathematics, the calculations assume that all force vectors are acting in a vertical direction. This assumption introduces modest error in the results. All moment arm directions are assigned positive values.) (From Neumann DA: Hip abductor muscle activity in persons with a hip prosthesis while carrying loads in one hand, *Phys Ther* 76:1320, 1996. With permission of the American Physical Therapy Association.)

Methods of *carrying external loads* significantly influence the demands placed on the hip abductor muscles and thus on the underlying hip joint. People with painful, unstable, or surgically replaced hips are to be cautioned about the consequences of carrying relatively large hand-held loads *opposite*, or contralateral to, the affected hip.[30,216,218,225] As shown in Fig. 12.49, the contralateral load has a very large external moment arm (D_2), creating a substantial clockwise torque about the right hip. For frontal plane stability, the right hip abductors must create a counterclockwise torque large enough to balance the clockwise torques caused by the external load (CL × D_2) *and* body weight (BW × D_1). As a result of the relatively small moment arm available to the hip abductor muscles (D), the hip abductor force (HAF) during single-limb support is very large. As shown by the calculations in Fig. 12.49, carrying a contralaterally held load of 15% of body weight (114.1 N or 25.7 lb) produces a joint reaction force (JRF) of 2897.6 N (651.1 lb). A healthy hip can usually tolerate this amount of force without difficulty. Caution must be exercised, however, if structural stability of the hip is compromised.

As a general principle, someone with a mechanically unstable or painful hip should be advised to avoid or limit carrying any external loads. For most ambulatory people, however, this advice is impractical. More practically, when loads *must* be carried, they should be as light as possible, carried in a backpack or by hand ipsilateral to the affected hip, or divided in half and carried bilaterally.[215,221,222] Research has shown that a strategy of *combining* the use of a contralaterally held cane with an ipsilaterally held load (equal to or less than 15% of body weight) reduces the demands on the hip abductor muscles to a greater degree than either method implemented separately.[221]

The previous discussion focuses on methods that reduce the force demands on the hip abductor muscles as a means to reduce the joint reaction force on a painful or an unstable hip. The same methods also apply to protecting an unstable hip associated with a total hip arthroplasty. Although these methods may have their desired effect, the reduced functional demand placed on the hip may also perpetuate prolonged weakness in the hip abductor muscles, which, in turn, can increase peak levels of damaging contact pressure on the joint. Clinicians must often confront a paradox. How does one protect a vulnerable hip from excessive and potentially damaging forces from the abductor muscles while simultaneously increasing the functional strength and endurance of these same muscles? This requires knowledge of the normal and abnormal frontal plane biomechanics of the hip, the pathology and specialized care that is specific to the patient's unique condition, and the symptoms indicating that the hip is being subjected to potentially damaging forces. These signs and symptoms include excessive pain, sudden and marked gait deviation, and abnormal positioning of the lower limb.

TOTAL HIP ARTHROPLASTY

A *total hip arthroplasty* is often performed when a person with hip disease, most often osteoarthritis, has pain or immobility that significantly limits function and quality of life. This regularly performed operation replaces the diseased or degenerated acetabulum and/or femoral head with relatively biologically inert materials, typically some combination of ceramic, metal, or polyethylene (e-Fig. 12.5). A prosthetic hip may be secured by cement or through biological fixation provided by bone growth into the surface of the implanted components. Although the total hip arthroplasty is typically a very successful procedure, a small percentage of patients experience premature loosening, failure, or dislocation of the femoral and/or acetabular components.[39,153,158,208,331] Large torsional loads between the prosthetic implant and the bony interface may contribute to the loss of fixation. Additionally, complications may arise from debris shed from worn implanted components, resulting in osteolysis and a weakening of the surrounding bone.

Despite potential complications, total hip arthroplasty remains a highly regarded surgery in terms of reducing pain and improving function.[193,195] Research continues in earnest, however, to determine the most durable and safe materials, effective methods of fixation and implantation, and optimal and least anatomically invasive surgical approach (e.g., anterior versus posterior to the hip).[21,72,91,136,202] Furthermore, an improved awareness of the interrelated biomechanics between the lumbar spine and hip may lead to better functional outcomes for certain patient populations receiving a hip replacement. For example, people with a fused or overly stiff lumbar spine have a higher rate of prosthetic hip dislocation compared with those with a healthy and flexible lumbar spine.[193] Reduced lumbar mobility reduces pelvic-on-femoral mobility, consequently preventing the prosthetic cup from optimally covering the prosthetic femoral head.[306] This optimal coverage is particularly important for hip stability as the body changes postural positions, like moving from sit to stand, for example.[141] This biomechanical scenario serves as a reminder of the importance of respecting the lumbar spine as an important functional biomechanical component of the hip.

BIOMECHANICAL CONSEQUENCES OF COXA VARA AND COXA VALGA

As previously described in this chapter, the average angle of inclination of the femoral neck is approximately 125 degrees (see Fig. 12.7A). The angle may be changed as a result of a surgical repair of a fractured hip or the specific design of a prosthetic hip. In addition, a surgical operation known as a *coxa vara* (or *valga*) *osteotomy* intentionally alters a preexisting angle of inclination. This operation involves cutting a wedge of bone from the proximal femur, thereby changing the orientation of the femoral head to the acetabulum. A goal of this operation is often to improve the congruency of the weight-bearing surfaces of the hip.

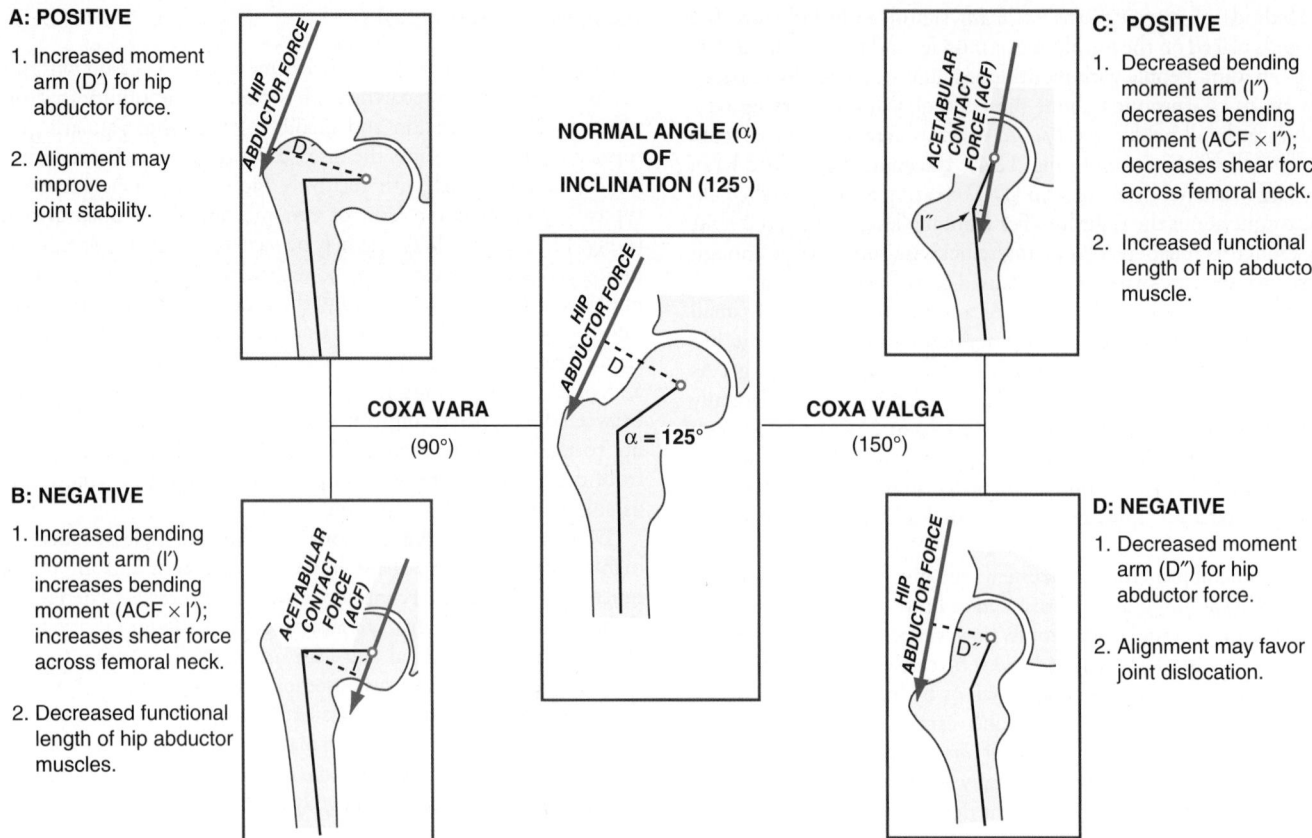

A: POSITIVE

1. Increased moment arm (D′) for hip abductor force.

2. Alignment may improve joint stability.

NORMAL ANGLE (α) OF INCLINATION (125°)

C: POSITIVE

1. Decreased bending moment arm (I″) decreases bending moment (ACF × I″); decreases shear force across femoral neck.

2. Increased functional length of hip abductor muscle.

COXA VARA
(90°)

COXA VALGA
(150°)

B: NEGATIVE

1. Increased bending moment arm (I′) increases bending moment (ACF × I′); increases shear force across femoral neck.

2. Decreased functional length of hip abductor muscles.

D: NEGATIVE

1. Decreased moment arm (D″) for hip abductor force.

2. Alignment may favor joint dislocation.

FIG. 12.50 The negative and positive biomechanical effects of coxa vara and coxa valga are contrasted. As a reference, a hip with a normal angle of inclination (α = 125 degrees) is shown in the center of the display. D is the internal moment arm used by hip abductor force; I is the bending moment arm across the femoral neck.

Regardless of the type of and rationale for the hip surgery, changing the angle of inclination of the proximal femur can alter the biomechanics of the joint. These alterations, especially if significant, can have positive or negative biomechanical effects. Fig. 12.50A shows two potentially positive biomechanical effects of coxa vara. The varus position increases the moment arm of the hip abductor force (indicated by D′). The greater leverage increases the abduction torque produced per unit of hip abductor muscle force. This situation may benefit people with hip abductor weakness. Also, increasing the leverage of the abductor muscles may allow a given level of abduction torque required during the stance phase of walking to be generated by less muscle force. Such reduction of muscular-based joint forces can help protect an arthritic or unstable prosthetic hip from excessive wear during walking. A varus osteotomy may in some patients improve the stability of the joint by aligning the femoral head more directly into the acetabulum.

A potentially negative effect of coxa vara is an increased bending moment (or torque) generated across the femoral neck (see Fig. 12.50B). The bending moment arm (dashed line indicated by I′) increases as the angle of inclination approaches 90 degrees. Increasing the bending moment raises the tension across the superior aspect of the femoral neck. This situation may cause a fracture of the femoral neck or a structural failure of a prosthesis. Marked coxa vara increases the vertical shear between the femoral head and the adjacent epiphysis. In children this situation may lead to a condition known as a *slipped capital femoral epiphysis*. Coxa vara may also decrease the functional length of the hip abductor muscles, thereby reducing their force-generating capability and increasing the likelihood of a "gluteus medius limp." The loss in muscle force may offset the increased abduction torque potential gained by the increased hip abductor moment arm.

Coxa valga may result from a surgical intervention or from such pathology as hip dysplasia. A potentially positive effect of the valgus position is a decrease in bending moment arm across the femoral neck (see I″ in Fig. 12.50C). This situation also decreases the vertical shear across the femoral neck. The valgus position may also increase the functional length of the hip abductor muscles, thus improving their force-generating ability. In contrast, a potentially negative effect of coxa valga is the decreased moment arm available to the hip abductor force (indicated by D″ in Fig. 12.50D). In extreme coxa valga, the femoral head may be positioned more laterally in the acetabulum, possibly increasing the risk of dislocation.

SYNOPSIS

The hip joints function as basilar joints for both the axial skeleton and the lower extremities. As such, the hips form the central pivot point for common movements of the body as a whole, especially those involving flexion and extension. Consider, for instance, lifting the leg to ascend a steep stair, or bending down at the waist to pick up an object from the floor. Both motions demand a significant amount of movement and muscular force between the proximal femurs and the pelvis. Weakness, instability, or pain in the hips therefore typically causes marked difficulty in performing a wide range of activities across a lifespan—learning how to walk, getting in and out of a chair, engaging in high-level sport, or just engaging in moderate aerobic exercise.

The osteology and arthrology of the hip joint are designed more for ensuring stability than for providing ample mobility, a condition essentially the opposite of that for the glenohumeral joint—the analogous proximal joint of the upper extremity. The deep-seated and well-contained femoral head, surrounded by thick capsular ligaments and muscles, ensures hip stability especially in the weight-bearing phase of walking—a phase that occupies about 60% of a given gait cycle.

A surprisingly small amount of muscle activity is required to stabilize the hips while one stands in an upright relaxed posture, assuming that one or both of the hips are extended. Such a posture typically orients the body's line of gravity just posterior to the medial-lateral axis of rotation at the hips. The force of gravity thus can help keep the hips passively extended. The ligaments of the hip, relatively taut in hip extension, create useful tension that further stabilizes the extended hips. Muscle forces may occasionally be required to augment or readjust stability of the hips while one stands at ease, but this active mechanism is normally used as a reserve or secondary source. This is not the case, however, with a hip flexion contracture of significant tightness; stability while one stands in partial flexion demands significant and constant activation from the hip extensor muscles. Such a condition not only is metabolically "expensive" but also imposes unnecessarily larger muscular-based forces across the hip joints. These forces, acting over time, may be harmful in a malaligned joint that cannot properly dissipate stress.

The full extent to which the hip joints contribute to full body movement requires an understanding of both femoral-on-pelvic and pelvic-on-femoral kinematics. Femoral-on-pelvic movements are often associated with changing location of lower limbs, such as when stepping up a step or advancing the body forward while walking. Pelvic-on-femoral movements, on the other hand, are often performed to change the position of the pelvis—and often the entire superimposed trunk—relative to fixed lower extremities. Pelvic-on-femoral movements are expressed in many forms, from subtle oscillations of the pelvis during the stance phase of each gait cycle to more obvious large-arc rotations of the pelvis (and trunk) as a figure skater spins on the ice while bending forward at the waist. Adding to the complexity of pelvic-on-femoral movements is the strong association with the kinematics of the lumbar spine. Clinical evaluation of the causes of reduced or abnormal motions at the hip must therefore include an evaluation of the flexibility and prevailing posture of the lumbar region. Limitations of movement at *either* the lumbar spine or the hips alter the kinematic sequencing throughout the trunk and proximal end of the lower kinematic chain. Being able to localize the source of abnormal kinematics within this broad area of the body certainly improves the likelihood of successful clinical diagnosis and intervention.

Nearly one-third of muscles that cross the hip joint attach proximally to the pelvis and distally to either the tibia or the fibula. An imbalance of forces among these muscles—whether generated actively or passively by any one of them—can thus influence posture and range of motion across multiple segments, especially the lumbar spine, hips, and knees. Clinicians regularly evaluate and treat functional limitations that may arise from impairments in and among these and other synergistic muscles. Treatment requires thoroughly understanding of how muscles interact across a very mechanically interrelated region of the body.

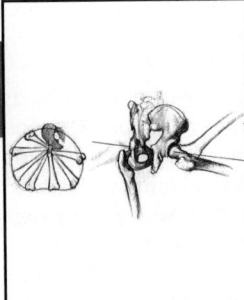

ADDITIONAL CLINICAL CONNECTIONS

CLINICAL CONNECTION 12.1
Augmenting the Therapeutic Stretch of Selected Biarticular Muscles of the Hip

Clinicians frequently employ methods of stretching muscles to treat or prevent musculoskeletal disorders. Biarticular muscles of the hip receive specific clinical attention, especially the poly-articular hamstrings and rectus femoris. Reduced extensibility of these muscles can alter the posture, range of motion, and fluidity (or ease) of movement across multiple segments, including the lumbar spine, hip, and knee.[83,104,112,152] Because these muscles cross so many joints, different combinations of active movements and static positions can be used to stretch them. This Clinical Connection explores a method of how a person may augment self-stretching of some of these biarticular muscles.

As the first of two examples, consider how one may stretch the *hamstring* muscles. One of the more traditional methods incorporates a static position of near full knee extension with varying amounts of hip flexion (Fig. 12.51A). As depicted in this figure, the increased muscular tension in the stretched hamstrings typically pulls the ischial tuberosity *forward*, thereby increasing the posterior tilt of the pelvis and reducing the lordosis in the subject's lumbar spine. This posterior pelvic tilt would theoretically reduce the effectiveness of the stretch on the hamstring muscles. As a way to augment the extent of this stretch, the subject can be instructed to *actively contract* muscles that are antagonists to the tightened hamstring group, such as the rectus femoris and multifidus (see Fig. 12.51B). These muscles are considered antagonists to the hamstrings because of their ability to perform *pelvic-on-femoral (hip) flexion* by rotating the pelvis anteriorly relative to the fixed femurs. Active contraction of this pair of muscles elongates the right hamstrings, which, as noted in Fig. 12.51B, is evidenced by the increased lumbar lordosis.

By actively contracting the quadriceps, the rectus femoris can flex the hip (via a pelvic-on-femoral perspective) while also stabilizing the knee in extension. This stabilizing action of the quadriceps can resist a possible knee flexion response created by the taut hamstrings, which would also reduce the effectiveness of the stretch.

Consider a second example, involving a similar strategy, for augmenting the self-stretch of the *rectus femoris* muscle. Fig. 12.52A shows a woman positioned to stretch her rectus femoris muscle by maintaining the combined position of hip extension and knee flexion. The increased passive tension in the stretched biarticular rectus femoris typically rotates the pelvis anteriorly, thus increasing the anterior pelvic tilt and lumbar lordosis. As depicted in Fig. 12.52B, active contraction of the subject's abdominal muscles and gluteus maximus (among other hip extensors) can be used to stretch all hip flexor muscles, including the rectus femoris. Both of these activated muscles are antagonists to the rectus femoris because of their ability to perform *pelvic-on-femoral (hip) extension* by rotating the pelvis posteriorly relative to fixed femurs. This posterior pelvic tilt would also assist in stretching much of the capsule of the hip, especially in the region of the iliofemoral ligament. (Although not depicted in Fig. 12.52B, instructing the person to also manually push her right hip further into *adduction* would theoretically add to the stretch of the rectus femoris. This is based on the *abduction* moment arm of this muscle; see Fig. 12.30.)

This Clinical Connection has demonstrated methods of stretching selected biarticular muscles of the hip. In each case, the standard stretching procedure was augmented by a *volitional contraction* of a muscle group considered antagonistic to the tight muscle. This therapeutic approach requires a sound understanding of how multiple muscles can affect the hip, either directly or indirectly. It is not certain whether activating these antagonist muscles in the manner described produces greater or more prolonged flexibility in tightened biarticular hip muscles than a more standard passive stretch, although it presents an interesting question. The underlying answer may transcend simple mechanics. Strong contraction of an antagonistic muscle might inhibit resistance in the tightened muscle through *reciprocal inhibition*. A more certain benefit of this therapeutic approach is that the patient or client is more actively involved in the treatment, which may enhance his or her ability to learn and thereby better control the biomechanics of this and other regions of the body.

In closing, the primary intent of Figs. 12.51 and 12.52 is to show how a thorough understanding of muscular kinesiology can provide creative ideas for augmenting the effectiveness of stretching or elongating biarticular muscles associated with the hip. Although the stretching activities illustrated are relatively basic, the factors underlying muscle tightness can be complex, including but not limited to neuromuscular control, weakness, coordination, balance, and other important factors of motor capacity and behavior. This complexity means that stretching exercises are rarely effective in isolation and compels clinicians to consider a multifactorial approach to the treatment, perhaps by including meaningful and functional-specific challenges to the stability, balance, and strength of the body as a whole.

ADDITIONAL CLINICAL CONNECTIONS

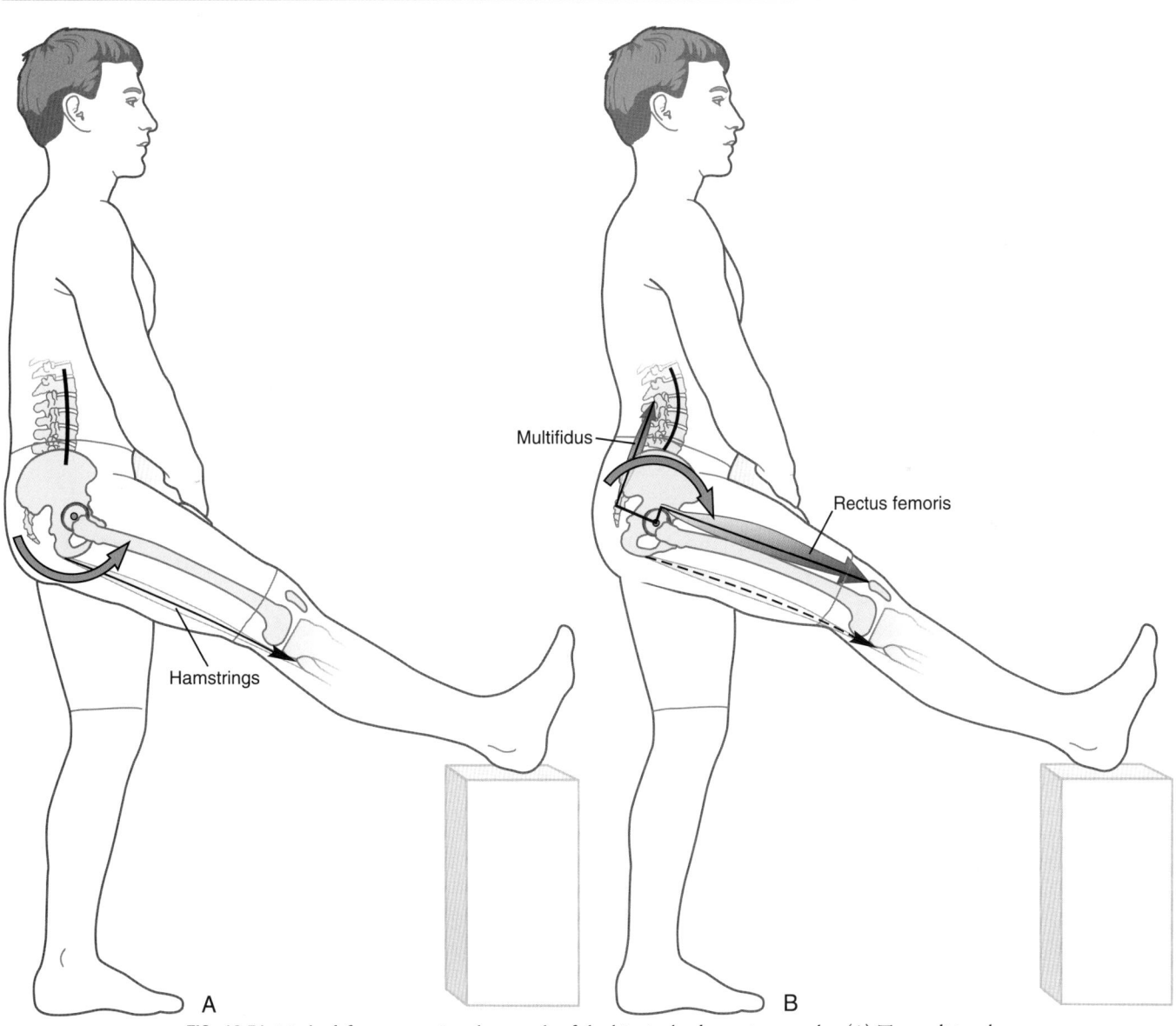

FIG. 12.51 Method for augmenting the stretch of the biarticular *hamstring* muscles. (A) The traditional starting position for stretching hamstring muscles combines hip flexion and knee extension. The green counterclockwise arrow depicts the passive, posterior pelvic tilt caused by the tension in the stretched hamstrings. (B) Active contraction of the multifidus and rectus femoris creates an anterior tilt of the pelvis (*green clockwise arrow*), increasing the elongation and subsequent stretch within the hamstring muscles (*dashed arrow*). The moment arms of the activated muscles are shown as black lines, originating at the axis of rotation of the hip (*small green circle* at the femoral head).

Continued

ADDITIONAL CLINICAL CONNECTIONS

CLINICAL CONNECTION 12.1
Augmenting the Therapeutic Stretch of Selected Biarticular Muscles of the Hip—cont'd

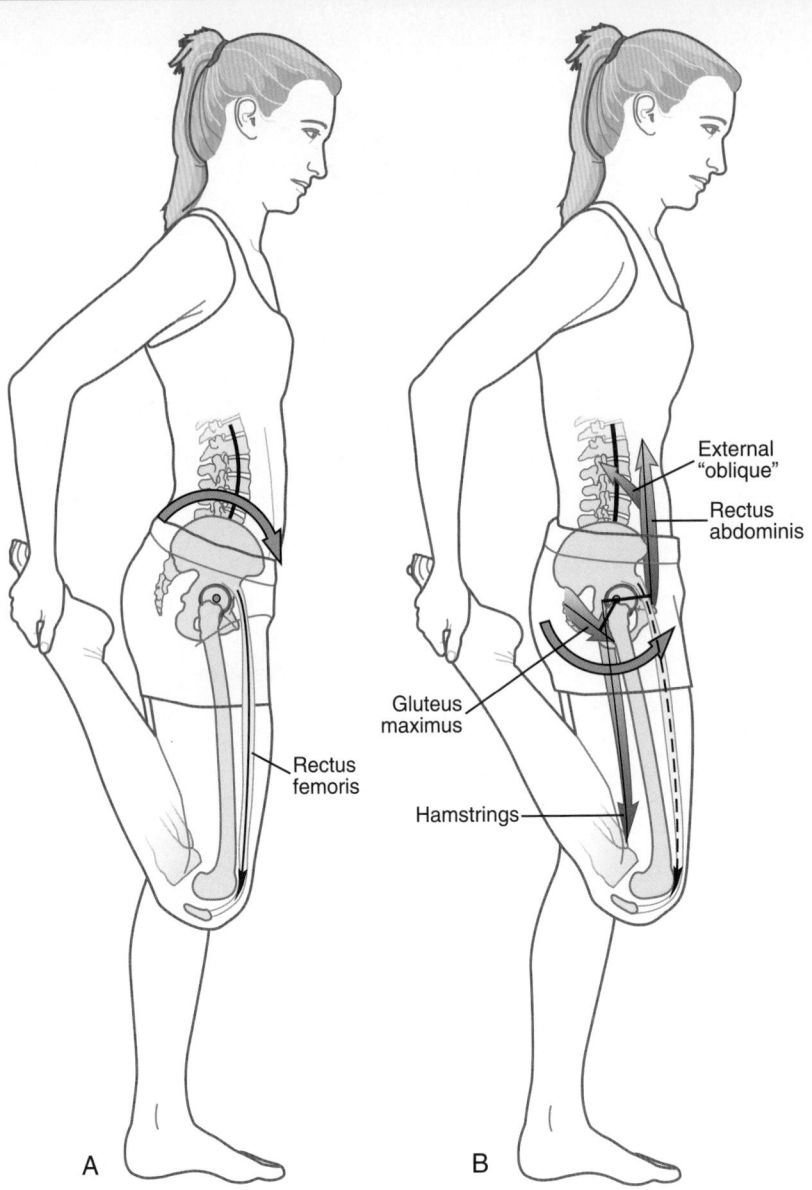

FIG. 12.52 Method for augmenting the self-stretch of the *rectus femoris* muscle. (A) A position typically used to stretch the rectus femoris combines hip extension with knee flexion. The green clockwise arrow depicts the passive, anterior pelvic tilt caused by the tension in the stretched rectus femoris. (B) Active contraction of representative hip extensors and abdominal muscles causes a posterior tilt of the pelvis (*green counterclockwise arrow*), increasing the stretch within the rectus femoris (*dashed arrow*). The moment arms of the activated muscles are shown as black lines, originating at the axis of rotation of the hip (*small green circle* at the femoral head).

ADDITIONAL CLINICAL CONNECTIONS

CLINICAL CONNECTION 12.2
Justifying a Standard Method of Stretching the Piriformis Muscle

Restrictions in the extensibility of the piriformis muscle may limit hip internal rotation, compress the sciatic nerve, or produce abnormal stress on the sacroiliac joint. Some clinicians believe that an inflamed and tight piriformis may also create a painful "trigger" point deep in the buttock region. The buttock pain often radiates into the hip, posterior thigh, or proximal lower leg. This poorly defined condition is often referred to as "piriformis syndrome."[305]

Treatment of a tightened piriformis muscle may involve stretching. Among the many ways to stretch this muscle, one common theme is to combine full flexion and *external rotation* of the hip, typically with the knee flexed to reduce tension from the biarticular hamstring muscles. At first thought, the external rotation component of the piriformis stretch position appears counterintuitive,

based on the muscle's action as a primary *external* rotator of the hip. Further kinesiologic consideration, however, can help justify this method of stretch.[73,110,307] As described previously in this chapter, with the hip flexed the piriformis switches its action from an external rotator (in neutral hip extension) to an internal rotator. This can be visualized nicely with a skeleton model and a piece of flexible cord that mimics the muscle's line of force (Fig. 12.53A). Flexing the hip beyond 90 degrees, therefore, allows external rotation of the hip to cause *further elongation* of the piriformis (Fig. 12.53B).

In closing, even though the piriformis switches its rotary action in flexion, the principle used to stretch this muscle is not violated: stretching a muscle requires that the muscle be placed in a position *opposite* to its primary actions.

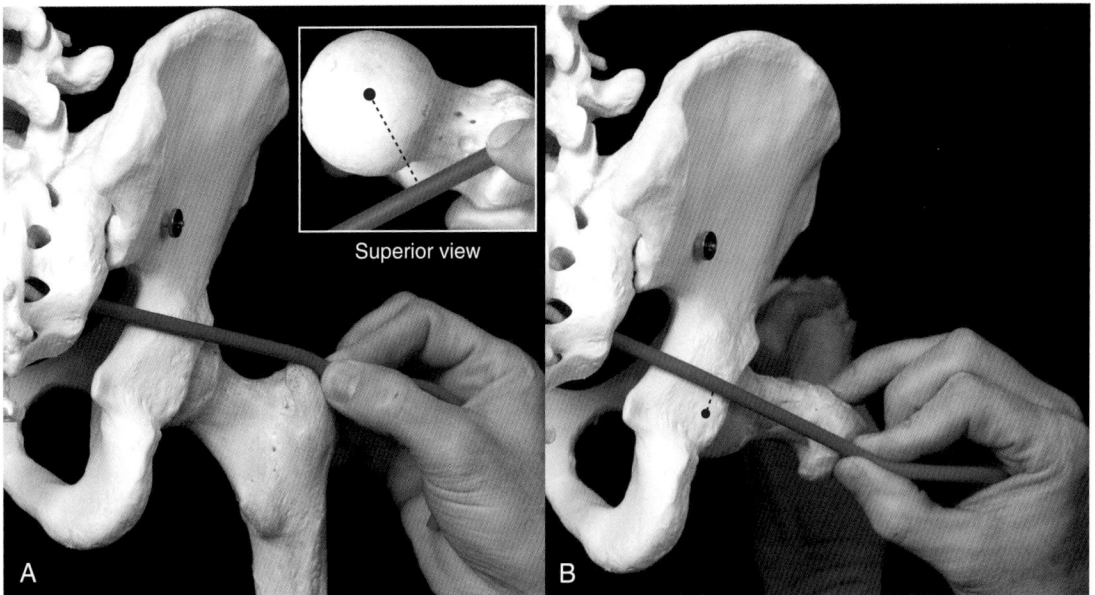

Superior view

A   B

FIG. 12.53 The changing action of the piriformis is shown with hip flexion. (A) With the hip extended, the piriformis (*red cord*) has a line of force to externally rotate the hip. As shown from a superior view in the inset, the muscle's line of pull is posterior to the vertical axis of rotation. The muscle's moment arm for this action is shown as a dashed line. (B) With the hip flexed, the line of force of the piriformis shifts its position to the opposite side of the longitudinal axis of rotation. Although acting with a relatively small moment arm, the muscle is now an internal rotator of the hip.

ADDITIONAL CLINICAL CONNECTIONS

CLINICAL CONNECTION 12.3
Vulnerability of the Acetabular Labrum to Injury: Pathomechanic and Treatment Considerations

MECHANICALLY VULNERABLE ACETABULAR LABRUM

Most movements involving the trunk and lower limbs produce at least some compressive, tensile, or shearing force against the acetabular labrum, rendering it particularly vulnerable to mechanical-based pathology. Coupled with the tissue's poor healing potential, an injured labrum can become a chronic and painful condition. Clinical awareness and treatment of acetabular labral pathology has increased dramatically over the last few decades, paralleling technical advances in arthroscopic surgery and imaging techniques such as magnetic resonance arthrography (Fig. 12.54).

Acetabular labral pathology may be linked to several incidents, such as trauma, typically associated with rotational, repetitive, or near–end range movements of the hip; excessive wear associated with reaching advanced age; developmental hip dysplasia or other childhood hip disease; or, as described in the remainder of the Clinical Connection, to repeated impingement related to an often subtle malformation of the acetabulum or proximal femur.[32,58,123,176] Mechanical symptoms associated with labral

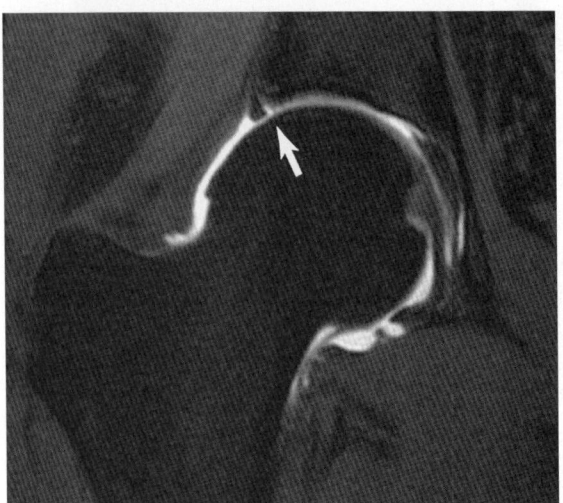

FIG. 12.54 Frontal plane (T¹ fat-saturated) magnetic resonance (MR) arthrogram showing a torn acetabular labrum (*arrow*). The MR arthrogram involves an intra-articular injection of gadolinium contrast. The labral tear was confirmed and excised during arthroscopic surgery. (Courtesy Michael O'Brien, MD, Wisconsin Radiology Specialists, Milwaukee, WI).

tears often include a clicking, "catching," or buckling sensation. Pain is typically reported in the anterior hip or groin area.

BONY PATHOMORPHOLOGY AND ASSOCIATED LABRAL DAMAGE

The normal skeletal configuration of the hip usually minimizes stressful contact between the proximal end of the femur and the rim of the acetabulum, providing protection that is particularly important near end range movements. Relatively slight deviations in the bones' morphology, however, can compromise the dynamic clearance between these two regions. Without adequate clearance, cyclic and continued abutment of the proximal femur against the acetabular rim (or vice versa) can damage the relatively delicate acetabular labrum and adjacent cartilage—leading to a well-recognized painful condition described as *femoroacetabular impingement (FAI) syndrome*.[108,259] Repeated and forceful contact within the joint can traumatize not only the labrum but also the articular cartilage and subchondral bone. FAI syndrome has been recognized as a key risk factor for developing hip osteoarthritis, likely accounting for many cases of early-onset hip osteoarthritis that would have been diagnosed as "idiopathic" in previous decades.[101,115,279]

Three types of bony morphologic patterns of the hip have been associated with FAI: cam-type, pincer-type, and a mixed variety.[49,61,117] The most common *cam-type morphology* presents with extra bone formed at the anterior-superior region of the femoral head-and-neck junction (Fig. 12.55A). The malformation, even if slight, alters the spherical shape of the femoral head, resulting in a loss of the natural tapering of the femoral head–neck junction (often referred to as a reduced *femoral head-neck offset*). A *cam-type impingement* occurs by movements that force the incongruent bulge of the femoral head against or into the acetabulum. Over time, this impingement traumatizes the labrum, most often its anterior-superior circumference. Damage may extend inward toward the chondrolabral junction. The combination of flexion beyond 90 degrees along with internal rotation and adduction tends to maximize the contact stress associated with the impingement.[25,147] For this reason, this deep flexion pattern of movement is often painful and purposely avoided.[24,173] Although exceptions exist, cam-type impingement is frequently found in athletic younger males, especially those who regularly engage in sports that combine hip flexion and internal rotation, such as football, soccer, and ice hockey.[164] Young athletic males therefore tend to be at a higher risk for developing FAI syndrome, although

ADDITIONAL CLINICAL CONNECTIONS

this disorder can occur outside this typical demographic profile. A universal and predicable causal mechanism behind FAI syndrome is not fully understood.[61]

Whereas a cam-type morphology involves the proximal femur, the less common *pincer-type morphology* involves an abnormal shape of the acetabulum (Fig. 12.55B). A pincer-type morphology is defined as an abnormal bony extension of the anterior-lateral rim of acetabulum; in essence, the acetabulum *overcovers* the femoral head. A pincer-type morphology is often quantified by a center-edge angle of at least 45 to 50 degrees (see a normal center-edge angle in Fig. 12.13A). An acetabulum that is unusually deep (*acetabular profunda*) or overly *retroverted* may, in certain cases, mimic or amplify excessive anterior-lateral coverage of the femoral head and proximal neck regions.[117,156,174] Regardless of cause, flexing and internally rotating the hip tends to cause premature abutment of the proximal femur against the protruding acetabular rim and labrum. Such potentially damaging pathomechanics are often referred to as *pincertype impingement*, reflecting the pincerlike manner with which the acetabular rim and labrum "embrace" the femoral head and proximal neck region. Whereas cam-type impingement is seen more often in males, pincer-type impingement occurs more often in females, plausibly because of differing pelvic anthropometrics.[177,280] Actually, both men and women with FAI syndrome frequently demonstrate elements of both cam- and pincer-type impingement.[318]

PATHOMECHANICAL LINK BETWEEN FAI SYNDROME AND OSTEOARTHRITIS

The link between FAI syndrome and osteoarthritis of the hip is not completely understood. The following series of events may, however, offer a glimpse into the pathologic complexity of the process. First, and perhaps most obvious, is that the initial chondrolabral damage and subsequent joint inflammation associated with FAI syndrome may stem from a repeated "outside-in" mechanical trauma, originating by the force of the bony impingement. Trauma to the articular cartilage may be exaggerated by altered and stressful arthrokinematics, caused by repetitive attempts at moving the joint against an abnormal bony morphology. Although the arthrokinematic stress is likely greater during near end range movements, an in vivo study using biplanar fluoroscopy suggests that even moderate range of hip movement associated with normal walking can potentially alter the arthrokinematics in someone with cam-type impingement.[178] Additionally, as part of an inflammatory process, an acquired capsular thickening may further distort the joint's active arthrokinematics, thereby creating additional stress to the articular cartilage.[49] And finally, as described previously in this chapter,[213] degenerative lesions of the articular cartilage may result from failure of the damaged labrum to provide a sufficient mechanical and fluid seal to the joint.

The processes described above focused on articular stress caused primarily through biomechanical factors. Although unclear, recent evidence suggests that *neuromuscular factors* may also have a role in the pathogenesis of FAI syndrome.[178] Multiple studies have reported that people with FAI syndrome demonstrate three-dimensional lower limb movement impairments that are generally consistent with hip postures that likely predispose FAI, often evident while performing unilateral or bilateral squat maneuvers.[330] The impairments appear associated with reduced neuromuscular control, abnormal lower limb osteokinematics, decreased dynamic single-leg and standing balance, and reduced activation of dominant hip muscles.[b] Impaired muscle function with preferential atrophy appears particularly evident in dominant muscles such as the gluteal maximus.[192,274] Perhaps arthrogenic neural inhibition of the gluteus maximus is caused by pain and inflammation of the hip's capsule.[49] Furthermore, reduced motor control of the hip may be related to reduced proprioception caused by damaged mechanoreceptors within the traumatized labrum. Reduced motor

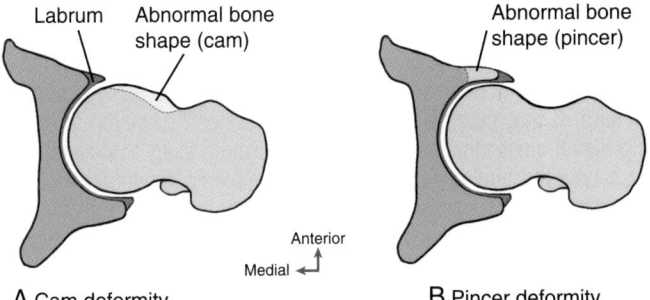

FIG. 12.55 A superior view of a drawing of (A) a cam deformity and (B) a pincer deformity of the right hip.

[b]6,48,49,95,103,122,191

Continued

ADDITIONAL CLINICAL CONNECTIONS

Alpha angle (α) to quantify cam deformity

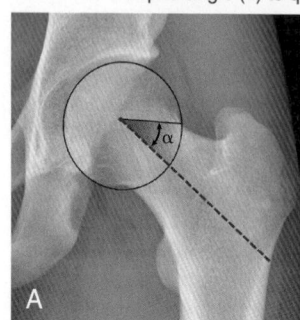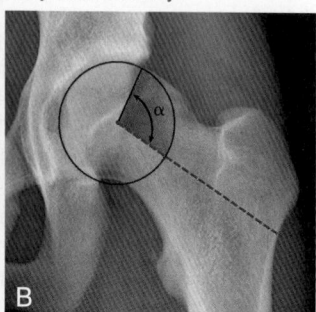

FIG. 12.56 Alpha angle (α) used to measure a cam-type morphology, based on an anterior-posterior (AP) pelvis radiograph. The alpha angle of 41 degrees shown in (A) is considered to be within normal limits. The 98-degree alpha angle depicted in (B) is excessive and considered to be a pathologic cam-type morphology (see text). The alpha angle is the angle formed between a line that extends from the center of the femoral head (center of circle) and through the neck of the femur (*red, dashed line*) and a line starting at the center of the femoral head to a point where the head–neck junction deviates from the circle. (Modified with permission from Agricola R, Waarsing JH, Thomas GE, et al: Cam impingement: defining the presence of a cam deformity by the alpha angle: data from the CHECK cohort and Chingford cohort, *Osteoarthr Cartilage* 22[2]:218–225, 2014.)

control and diminished muscular strength likely create higher focal loading on the articular structures. To what degree, however, do these neuromuscular control factors have in the often-cascading events that cause more severe FAI or potentially predispose osteoarthritis? A better understanding of this topic may help improve interventions that strive to reduce the likelihood of FAI syndrome (or other pre-arthritic hip conditions) from progressing to premature osteoarthritis and need for a total hip arthroplasty.[49,117]

POSSIBLE GENESIS OF THE COMMON CAM-TYPE MALFORMATION

Most of the biomechanical research on FAI syndrome has focused on the *cam-type* impingement, perhaps because of its relatively strong correlation with chondrolabral lesions and osteoarthritis. A cam-type morphology or deformity is typically diagnosed with the aid of MRI or radiography (x-ray), by measuring the degree to which the shape of the femoral head deviates from being spherical. The amount of deviation can be measured via an anterior-posterior

(AP) pelvis radiograph by what is described as an *alpha angle* (Fig. 12.56).[230] Although definitions vary, a hip with an alpha angle equal to or greater than 55 to 60 degrees has been designated as having a *true* cam-type morphology, whereas a hip with an alpha angle equal to or greater than about 80 degrees has been designated as a *pathologic* cam-type morphology. The latter of these has a high statistical risk of developing chondrolabral lesions and potentially osteoarthritis.[2] Although data on the exact prevalence of cam-type morphology is mixed, it is reported to be fairly common: occurring naturally in 15% to 54% of men and 5% to 36% of women.[2,74,325] Certainly not every person with a cam-type morphology necessarily develops a labral lesion, hip pain, or hip osteoarthritis.[155] A diagnosis of FAI and associated labral lesion typically requires additional information, such as history of pain and aggravating activities, provocative manual-based testing that reproduces the impingement-based pain (often involving significant flexion, combined with adduction and internal rotation), and diagnostic imaging.

Causes of idiopathic cam-type morphology in the general population is not clear, although several factors have been implicated, including past trauma or infection, genetics, an unresolved or partially slipped capital femoral epiphysis (SCFE), or, most likely, excessive bone formation attributable to current or previous overloading of the proximal femur (i.e., based on Wolff's Law).[280] The overload factor is based on studies that have shown that the frequency of cam-type morphology is much greater in higher-level athletic males compared with controls.[167,244,281] The frequency of cam morphology in this often elite subgroup has been reported to be as high as 50% to 90%.[1] The unusually high frequency of this malformation is believed to be related to the proximal femur's hypertrophic response to high-impact sports (such as ice hockey, soccer, gymnastics, and football) performed during young adolescence, at a critical time of skeletal maturation.[1,54,86,325] The period of high loading may also alter the physiology of growth plate closure of the proximal femur.[116] What is clear, however, is that high-level male athletes, as a group, are more likely to develop a cam-type morphology and more likely to sustain significant labral damage.[43,197,212] This active population is not only more likely to have an underlying developmental cam-type morphology but also more likely to engage in extreme and repetitive movements that might provoke more stressful impingement. Better knowledge of the chronology and factors associated with excessive cam-type development in adolescence may provide useful guidelines for

ADDITIONAL CLINICAL CONNECTIONS

parents and coaches for adjusting the intensity of certain high-impact sporting activities during a critical time of skeletal maturation.[1,232]

TREATMENT OPTIONS FOR FAI SYNDROME

Conservative treatment for FAI syndrome often includes nonsteroidal anti-inflammatory medication, intra-articular steroid injections, and physical therapy. The focus of physical therapy often consist of improving neuromuscular control of the lumbopelvic region, challenging dynamic upright posturing, increasing functional range of motion and flexibility, mobilizing appropriate soft tissues, and providing instructions on modifying or avoiding movements that may have caused or exacerbate the impingement condition.[81,140,206,298,334] Specialized strengthening exercises target muscles that would reduce the likelihood of creating FAI; for example, muscles that posteriorly tilt the pelvis, such as the abdominal muscles and hip extensors (review Fig. 12.39). A posterior pelvic tilt rotates the anterior-superior rim of the acetabulum (and labrum) *away* from the proximal femur, thereby allowing greater range of femoral flexion (combined with internal rotation and adduction) before actual bony impingement.[238] An activated gluteus maximus may be particularly effective at minimizing FAI because of its ability to combine hip extension *and* external rotation. Preliminary study on a group of people with cam-type FAI syndrome indicates that a modest increase in "cued" activation of the gluteus maximus during a deep squat *reduced* accompanying internal rotation

by 5 degrees, resulting in a 32% reduction in acetabular contact pressure.[49] These results may be therapeutically significant because the acetabular pressure (force/area) *decreased* even as the total acetabular compressive force *increased* due to muscle contraction. Such results provide a solid foundation for developing exercises that may help limit the development or progression of FAI syndrome.

Arthroscopic surgery is often used to treat FAI syndrome, especially when conservative approaches are unsuccessful or not appropriate based on the severity of the FAI symptoms, magnitude of the alpha angle, or willingness of the patient to modify activities that likely provoked the impingement (such as an elite or professional athlete). The mainstay of the surgery involves an arthroscopic osteoplasty to reshape or realign the malformed bones.[11,22,75,117] e-Fig. 12.6 shows preoperative and postoperative radiographs of an arthroscopic femoral osteoplasty to trim excessive bone from the femoral neck-head junction in a person with a cam-type morphology and FAI syndrome. If needed, the surgery may involve debridement or repair of the fragmented labrum and use of a microfracture technique to stimulate growth of damaged cartilage. The arthroscopic surgery is often promoted as a "hip preservation" procedure based on the promising likelihood that the intervention prevents eventual development of significant osteoarthritis. Physical therapy after surgical intervention plays a major role in the rehabilitation process.[190,298,302]

ADDITIONAL CLINICAL CONNECTIONS

Developmental dysplasia of the hip (DDH) is one of the most common orthopedic disorders to affect the hip; it often manifests at birth or within the first few years of life.[270] DDH can involve both the acetabulum and femoral head, although the primary focus of the condition is usually placed on the shallow acetabulum. The condition involves a continuum of disorders associated primarily with abnormal structural development and growth (i.e., *dysplasia*) of the bones that constitute the hip. Because the hip naturally continues to develop after birth and throughout childhood, a specific diagnosis and prognosis of DDH is not always made in the newborn child. The presence of a shallow, dislocated, or abnormally unstable hip in the neonate indicates the possibility of DDH.

Many symptoms associated with mild DDH in an otherwise healthy child may spontaneously resolve with little or no treatment.[321] Unfortunately, trying to predict at an early age which child's symptoms will resolve and which will not is not very feasible. Those whose symptoms continue or worsen may present an evolving clinical picture that can persist throughout adolescence. The more pronounced cases of DDH can lead to permanent physical impairments in the younger adult if not properly treated. Ideally, DDH is diagnosed at birth by physical examination and, when appropriate, by such imaging techniques as ultrasonography.[33] If the original diagnosis is missed, the condition may surface later in childhood, adolescence, or adulthood—often because of unexplained hip pain or gait deviation.

Depending on diagnostic criteria, the prevalence of DDH varies between 2% and 8%.[171,296] The underlying and constant feature of fully manifested DDH is an abnormally formed and poorly articulated hip joint.[171,322] The primary pathomechanics typically start on the acetabular side of the joint but could also involve the proximal femur. A poorly developed acetabulum provides a short and shallow "roof" over the femoral head, preventing a natural congruent articulation with the femoral head. (Typically, a diagnosis of DDH is associated with an LCE angle of 20 degrees or less; values of 20 to 25 degrees are often referred to as "borderline" DDH; review Fig. 12.13A.[171]) If a true and stable joint fails to form, the proximal femur loses its primary mechanical stimulus to develop normally, typically exhibiting a slightly flattened head, excessive anteversion, or coxa varus or coxa valgus.

Although the precise causes of DDH are not universally agreed upon, family history, breech delivery, and female sex have been cited as leading risks for developing the condition.[60,70] The overall propensity for DDH in humans may be indirectly associated with the natural course of fetal development of the hip. In the 12-week-old human fetus the developing femoral head is completely covered and secured within the developing acetabulum. The percentage of coverage, however, naturally *diminishes* until birth and then gradually begins to increase with normal postnatal development.[250] In the perinatal period, therefore, the hip is potentially unstable, consisting of a shallow and relatively flat acetabulum and a partially exposed femoral head, both of which are composed chiefly of soft cartilage. Subsequent normal growth and development of the hip are strongly influenced by the contact forces made by a well-centered femoral head. Such contact helps mold the concavity of the pliable acetabulum to the spherical shape of the femoral head and vice versa, eventually facilitating the formation of a normal and stable joint.

Abnormally applied forces and contact patterns at the hip in the very plastic and vulnerable perinatal phase of development can directly affect the ultimate morphology of the joint. Sources of some of these potentially deforming forces early in life are further described in the following paragraphs.

EXCESSIVE JOINT LAXITY
Excessive laxity in the capsule and ligaments of the hip can lead to increased shear between the joint surfaces. In cases of severe laxity, the unstable hip demonstrates increased translation and joint "play," often resulting in a greater risk of dislocation and subluxation. An abnormally aligned or dislocated hip lacks the normal kinetic stimulus to guide its growth and development.

Increased laxity in the child's connective tissues is often associated with genetic predisposition.[124] The increased laxity may also be caused by an exaggerated response to the maternal hormone *relaxin*, normally intended to induce pelvic laxity in the mother during childbirth. Females are more responsive to the effects of relaxin, which may partially explain the higher incidence of DDH in female infants.[60]

ABNORMAL INTRAUTERINE POSITIONING
Abnormal positioning of the fetus within the uterus may place abnormal forces on the developing hip. This relationship is suggested by the fact that DDH occurs with increased frequency in children born by breech delivery. Some evidence also suggests that firstborn children have a higher risk of DDH, presumably because of larger forces placed on the child from the mother's uterus that is yet to be stretched.[34] Furthermore, children with DDH may have

ADDITIONAL CLINICAL CONNECTIONS

CLINICAL CONNECTION 12.4
Developmental Dysplasia of the Hip: Often an Evolving Disorder—cont'd

a slightly higher incidence of torticollis (see Chapter 10), also thought to be associated with abnormal prenatal positioning.[322]

POSTNATAL POSITIONING
Postnatal positioning may also have some influence on the structural development of the infant's hip. Some evidence of this relationship may be found in cultures in which infants are traditionally swaddled in a manner that maintains the hips relatively immobile and in extension and adduction,[33,34,107] which over a long period may create abnormal stress on hips that are naturally flexed in the "fetal position." Thus, some have suggested that the hips of the swaddled child be allowed to move naturally into flexion and abduction.[314]

ABNORMAL NEUROMUSCULAR DEVELOPMENT
Children with pathology involving the neuromuscular system have a higher-than-normal incidence of DDH. This association exists, for example, in children with cerebral palsy and may be explained by abnormal muscle tone, retained primitive reflexes, and lack of normal weight-bearing activities. Fig. 12.57 shows significant hip dysplasia in an adolescent girl with severe cerebral palsy.

Persisting or severe cases of untreated DDH can create significant functional problems in the maturing child, especially related to walking.[322] If the hip joint is unstable, the femoral head may "drift" superiorly and posterior-laterally from the acetabulum.

This migration of the femoral head may reduce the hip abduction moment arm of the gluteus medius.[121] Pelvic stability is therefore lost during the mid stance phase of walking, causing the characteristic compensated Trendelenburg gait pattern.

The specific treatment for DDH depends on the age of the patient, the functional limitations of the patient, and the natural progression of the disease. In the very young child, splinting the hip in flexion and abduction using a *Pavlik harness* is often performed in an attempt to "seat" the femoral head more directly into the acetabulum.[12,33,210,322] Over time, this position stimulates the formation of a more normally formed acetabulum. When used correctly and in a timely fashion, the Pavlik harness has been reported to have an 85% to 90% success rate.[12,107]

Surgical realignment of the pelvis and/or the proximal femur may be required to improve stability and increase the hip's surface area for weight-bearing activities.[119,270,324] The underlying goal of both surgical and nonsurgical treatment is to restore a stable articulation and facilitate optimum growth and development of the joint. Residual bony abnormalities associated with untreated or undetected DDH are a leading cause of premature hip osteoarthritis later in life[270,322] (Fig. 12.58), often necessitating a total hip replacement.

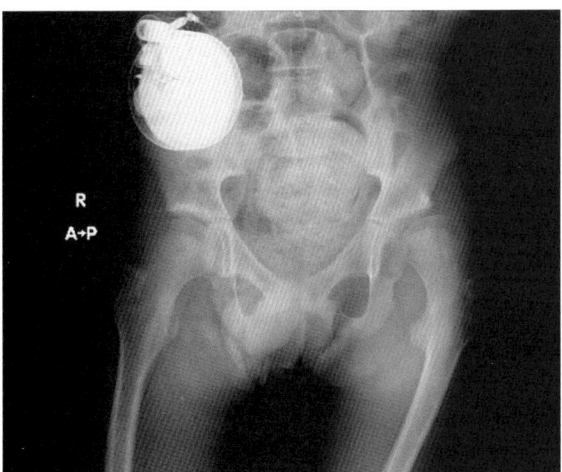

FIG. 12.57 Pelvic radiograph of a dysplastic and subluxed left hip of an adolescent girl with severe cerebral palsy. The subject is non-ambulatory. (Courtesy Jeffrey P. Schwab, MD, Department of Orthopaedic Surgery, Medical College of Wisconsin.)

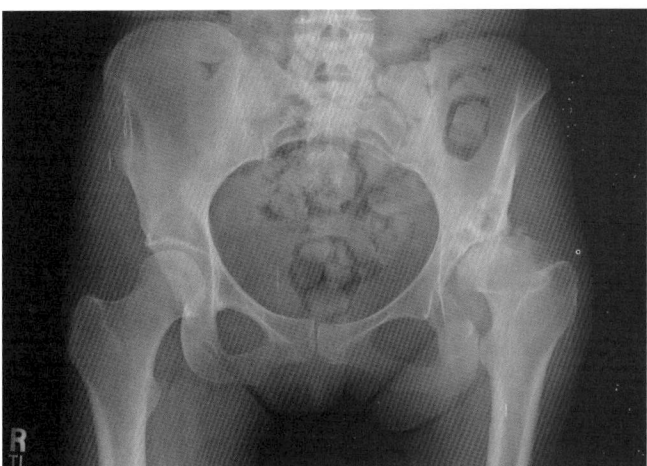

FIG. 12.58 Pelvic radiograph showing degenerative arthritis of the left hip in a 38-year-old woman, secondary to the residual effects of hip dysplasia as an infant. Note the laterally displaced and flattened femoral head as well as inadequate coverage provided by the acetabulum. The right hip is normal and asymptomatic. (Courtesy Michael O'Brien, MD, Wisconsin Radiology Specialists, Milwaukee, WI.)

REFERENCES

1. Agricola R, Heijboer MP, Ginai AZ, et al.: A cam deformity is gradually acquired during skeletal maturation in adolescent and young male soccer players: a prospective study with minimum 2-year follow-up, *Am J Sports Med* 42(4):798–806, 2014.

2. Agricola R, Waarsing JH, Thomas GE, et al.: Cam impingement: defining the presence of a cam deformity by the alpha angle: data from the CHECK cohort and Chingford cohort, *Osteoarthritis Cartilage* 22(2):218–225, 2014.

3. Alexander N, Studer K, Lengnick H, et al.: The impact of increased femoral antetorsion on gait deviations in healthy adolescents, *J Biomech* 86:167–174, 2019.

4. Allison K, Vicenzino B, Wrigley TV, et al.: Hip abductor muscle weakness in individuals with gluteal tendinopathy, *Med Sci Sports Exerc* 48(3):346–352, 2016.

5. Alpaugh K, Chilelli BJ, Xu S, et al.: Outcomes after primary open or endoscopic abductor tendon repair in the hip: a systematic review of the literature [Review], *Arthroscopy* 31(3):530–540, 2015.

6. Alrashdi NZ, Brown-Taylor L, Bell MM, et al.: Movement patterns and their associations with pain, function, and hip morphology in individuals with femoroacetabular impingement syndrome: a scoping review, *Phys Ther* 101(11), 2021.

7. Altman R, Alarcón G, Appelrouth D, et al.: The American College of Rheumatology criteria for the classification and reporting of osteoarthritis of the hip, *Arthritis Rheum* 34:505–514, 1991.

8. Anda S, Svenningsen S, Dale LG, et al.: The acetabular sector angle of the adult hip determined by computed tomography, *Acta Radiol Diagn* 27:443–447, 1986.

9. Andersen V, Pedersen H, Fimland MS, et al.: Comparison of muscle activity in three single-joint, hip extension exercises in resistance-trained women, *J Sports Sci Med* 20(2):181–187, 2021.

10. Anderson DE, Madigan ML: Healthy older adults have insufficient hip range of motion and plantar flexor strength to walk like healthy young adults, *J Biomech* 47(5):1104–1109, 2014.

11. Arciero E, Kakazu R, Garvin P, et al.: Favorable patient-reported outcomes and high return to sport rates following hip arthroscopy in adolescent athletes: a systematic review, *Arthroscopy* 38(9):2730–2740, 2022.

12. Ardila OJ, Divo EA, Moslehy FA, et al.: Mechanics of hip dysplasia reductions in infants using the Pavlik harness: a physics-based computational model, *J Biomech* 46(9):1501–1507, 2013.

13. Arnold AS, Anderson FC, Pandy MG, et al.: Muscular contributions to hip and knee extension during the single limb stance phase of normal gait: a framework for investigating the causes of crouch gait, *J Biomech* 38:2181–2189, 2005.

14. Arnold AS, Asakawa DJ, Delp SL: Do the hamstrings and adductors contribute to excessive internal rotation of the hip in persons with cerebral palsy? *Gait Posture* 11:181–190, 2000.

15. Arnold AS, Delp SL: Rotational moment arms of the medial hamstrings and adductors vary with femoral geometry and limb position: implications for the treatment of internally rotated gait, *J Biomech* 34:437–447, 2001.

16. Arnold AS, Komattu AV, Delp SL: Internal rotation gait: a compensatory mechanism to restore abduction capacity decreased by bone deformity, *Dev Med Child Neurol* 39:40–44, 1997.

17. Arokoski MH, Arokoski JP, Haara M, et al.: Hip muscle strength and muscle cross sectional area in men with and without hip osteoarthritis, *J Rheumatol* 29:2187–2195, 2002.

18. Ashberg L, Close MR, Perets I, et al.: The hip-spine connection: how to differentiate hip conditions from spine pathology, *Orthopedics* 44(6):e699–e706, 2021.

19. Atkins LT, James CR, Yang HS, et al.: Immediate improvements in patellofemoral pain are associated with sagittal plane movement training to improve use of gluteus maximus muscle during single limb landing, *Phys Ther* 101(10), 2021.

20. Atkins LT, Reid J, Zink D: The effects of increased forward trunk lean during stair ascent on hip adduction and internal rotation in asymptomatic females, *Gait Posture* 97:147–151, 2022.

21. Awad ME, Farley BJ, Mostafa G, et al.: Direct anterior approach has short-term functional benefit and higher resource requirements compared with the posterior approach in primary total hip arthroplasty: a meta-analysis of functional outcomes and cost, *Bone Joint J* 103-B(6):1078–1087, 2021.

22. Ayeni OR, Karlsson J, Heels-Ansdell D, et al.: Osteochondroplasty and labral repair for the treatment of young adults with femoroacetabular impingement: a randomized controlled Trial, *Am J Sports Med* 49(1):25–34, 2021.

23. Babst D, Steppacher SD, Ganz R, et al.: The iliocapsularis muscle: an important stabilizer in the dysplastic hip, *Clin Orthop Relat Res* 469(6):1728–1734, 2011.

24. Bagwell JJ, Fukuda TY, Powers CM: Sagittal plane pelvis motion influences transverse plane motion of the femur: kinematic coupling at the hip joint, *Gait Posture* 43:120–124, 2016.

25. Bagwell JJ, Powers CM: The influence of squat kinematics and cam morphology on acetabular stress, *Arthrosc J Arthrosc Relat Surg* 33(10):1797–1803, 2017.

26. Baldon RM, Furlan L, Serrao FV: Influence of the hip flexion angle on isokinetic hip rotator torque and acceleration time of the hip rotator muscles, *J Appl Biomech* 29(5):593–599, 2013.

27. Bardakos NV, Villar RN: The ligamentum teres of the adult hip, *J Bone Joint Surg Br* 91(1):8–15, 2009.

28. Barker PJ, Hapuarachchi KS, Ross JA, et al.: Anatomy and biomechanics of gluteus maximus and the thoracolumbar fascia at the sacroiliac joint, *Clin Anat* 27(2):234–240, 2014.

29. Batailler C, Weidner J, Wyatt M, et al.: Position of the greater trochanter and functional femoral antetorsion, *Bone Joint J* 100-B(6):712–719, 2018.

30. Bergmann G, Graichen F, Rohlmann A, et al.: Hip joint forces during load carrying, *Clin Orthop Relat Res* 335:190–201, 1997.

31. Birnbaum K, Prescher A, Hessler S, et al.: The sensory innervation of the hip joint—an anatomical study, *Surg Radiol Anat* 19(6):371–375, 1997.

32. Bittersohl B, Benedikter C, Franz A, et al.: Elite rowers demonstrate consistent patterns of hip cartilage damage compared with matched controls: a T2 mapping study, *Clin Orthop Relat Res* 477(5):1007–1018, 2019.

33. Blankespoor M, Ferrell K, Reuter A, et al.: Developmental dysplasia of the hip in infants - a review for providers, *S D Med* 73(5):223–227, 2020.

34. Blatt SH: To swaddle, or not to swaddle? Paleoepidemiology of developmental dysplasia of the hip and the swaddling dilemma among the indigenous populations of North America, *Am J Hum Biol* 27(1):116–128, 2015.

35. Blemker SS, Delp SL: Three-dimensional representation of complex muscle architectures and geometries, *Ann Biomed Eng* 33:661–673, 2005.

36. Blomberg JR, Zellner BS, Keene JS: Cross-sectional analysis of iliopsoas muscle-tendon units at the sites of arthroscopic tenotomies: an anatomic study, *Am J Sports Med* 39(Suppl-63S), 2011.

37. Bloom N, Cornbleet SL: Hip rotator strength in healthy young adults measured in hip flexion and extension by using a hand-held dynamometer, *PMR* 6(12):1137–1142, 2014.

38. Bobroff ED, Chambers HG, Sartoris DJ, et al.: Femoral anteversion and neck-shaft angle in children with cerebral palsy, *Clin Orthop Relat Res* 364:194–204, 1999.

39. Bordini B, Stea S, De CM, et al.: Factors affecting aseptic loosening of 4750 total hip arthroplasties: multivariate survival analysis, *BMC Musculoskelet Disord* 8:69, 2007.

40. Boukabache A, Preece SJ, Brookes N: Prolonged sitting and physical inactivity are associated with limited hip extension: a cross-sectional study, *Musculoskelet Sci Pract* 51:102282, 2021.

41. Breckling ACM, Katrikh AZ, Jones MW, et al.: Iliocapsularis: an exploration of the muscle and its omission in education, *J Morphol* 283(7):899–907, 2022.

42. Burns SA, Cleland JA, Rivett DA, et al.: When treating coexisting low back pain and hip impairments, focus on the back: adding specific hip treatment does not yield additional benefits-a randomized controlled trial, *J Orthop Sports Phys Ther* 51(12):581–601, 2021.

43. Byrd JW: Femoroacetabular impingement in athletes: current concepts, *Am J Sports Med* 42(3):737–751, 2014.

44. Cadet ER, Chan AK, Vorys GC, et al.: Investigation of the preservation of the fluid seal effect in the repaired, partially resected, and reconstructed acetabular labrum in a cadaveric hip model, *Am J Sports Med* 40(10):2218–2223, 2012.

45. Cahalan TD, Johnson ME, Liu S, et al.: Quantitative measurements of hip strength in different age groups, *Clin Orthop Relat Res* 246:136–145, 1989.

46. Campbell A, Thompson K, Pham H, et al.: The incidence and pattern of iliopsoas tendinitis following hip arthroscopy, *Hip Int* 31(4):542–547, 2021.

47. Cannon J, Cambridge EDJ, McGill SM: Anterior cruciate ligament injury mechanisms and the kinetic chain linkage: the effect of proximal joint stiffness on distal knee control during bilateral landings, *J Orthop Sports Phys Ther* 49(8):601–610, 2019.

48. Cannon J, Kulig K, Weber AE, et al.: Gluteal activation during squatting reduces acetabular contact pressure in persons with femoroacetabular impingement syndrome: a patient-specific finite element analysis, *Clin Biomech* 101:105849, 2022.

49. Cannon J, Weber AE, Park S, et al.: Pathomechanics underlying femoroacetabular impingement syndrome: theoretical framework to inform clinical practice, *Phys Ther* 100(5):788–797, 2020.

50. Cannon J, Weithman BA, Powers CM: Activation training facilitates gluteus maximus recruitment during weight-bearing strengthening exercises, *J Electromyogr Kinesiol* 63:102643, 2022.

51. Cao LA, Wimberly L: When to be concerned about abnormal gait: toe walking, in-toeing, out-toeing, bowlegs, and knock-knees, *Pediatr Ann* 51(9):e340–e345, 2022.

52. Carey TS, Crompton RH: The metabolic costs of "bent-hip, bent-knee" walking in humans, *J Hum Evol* 48:25–44, 2005.

53. Carriero A, Zavatsky A, Stebbins J, et al.: Influence of altered gait patterns on the hip joint contact forces, *Comput Methods Biomech Biomed Engin* 17(4):352–359, 2014.

54. Carsen S, Moroz PJ, Rakhra K, et al.: The Otto Aufranc Award. On the etiology of the cam deformity: a cross-sectional pediatric MRI study, *Clin Orthop Relat Res* 472(2):430–436, 2014.

55. Castano-Betancourt MC, Van Meurs JB, Bierma-Zeinstra S, et al.: The contribution of hip geometry to the prediction of hip osteoarthritis, *Osteoarthritis Cartilage* 21(10):1530–1536, 2013.

56. Castro MP, Ruschel C, Santos GM, et al.: Isokinetic hip muscle strength: a systematic review of normative data, *Sports BioMech* 19(1):26–54, 2020.

57. Chandrasekaran S, Gui C, Hutchinson MR, et al.: Outcomes of endoscopic gluteus medius repair: study of thirty-four patients with minimum 2-year follow-up, *J Bone Joint Surg Am* 97(16):1340–1347, 2015.

58. Charbonnier C, Kolo FC, Duthon VB, et al.: Assessment of congruence and impingement of the hip joint in professional ballet dancers: a motion capture study, *Am J Sports Med* 39(3):557–566, 2011.

59. Clark JM, Haynor DR: Anatomy of the abductor muscles of the hip as studied by computed tomography, *J Bone Joint Surg Am* 69:1021–1031, 1987.

60. Clarke NM: Developmental dysplasia of the hip: diagnosis and management to 18 months, *Instr Course Lect* 63:307–311, 2014.

61. Clohisy JC, Baca G, Beaulé PE, et al.: Descriptive epidemiology of femoroacetabular impingement, *Am J Sports Med* 41:1348–1356, 2013.

62. Contreras B, Vigotsky AD, Schoenfeld BJ, et al.: A comparison of gluteus maximus, biceps femoris, and vastus lateralis electromyographic activity in the back squat and barbell hip thrust exercises, *J Appl Biomech* 31(6):452–458, 2015.

63. Cook MS, Bou-Malham L, Esparza MC, et al.: Age-related alterations in female obturator internus muscle, *Int Urogynecol J* 28(5):729–734, 2017.

64. Correa TA, Crossley KM, Kim HJ, et al.: Contributions of individual muscles to hip joint contact force in normal walking, *J Biomech* 43(8):1618–1622, 2010.

65. Crock HV: An atlas of the arterial supply of the head and neck of the femur in man, *Clin Orthop Relat Res* 152:17–27, 1980.

66. Dalstra M, Huiskes R: Load transfer across the pelvic bone, *J Biomech* 28:715–724, 1995.

67. Daly C, Lafferty E, Joyce M, et al.: Determining the most effective exercise for gluteal muscle activation in children with cerebral palsy using surface electromyography, *Gait Posture* 70:270–274, 2019.

68. Damm P, Reitmaier S, Hahn S, et al.: In vivo hip and lumbar spine implant loads during activities in forward bent Postures, *J Biomech* 102:109517, 2020.

69. Davies JF, Stiehl JB, Davies JA, et al.: Surgical treatment of hip abductor tendon tears, *J Bone Joint Surg Am* 95(15):1420–1425, 2013.

70. de Hundt M, Vlemmix F, Bais JM, et al.: Risk factors for developmental dysplasia of the hip: a meta-analysis [Review], *Eur J Obstet Gynecol Reprod Biol* 165(1):8–17, 2012.

71. de SA D, Phillips M, Philippon MJ, et al.: Ligamentum teres injuries of the hip: a systematic review examining surgical indications, treatment options, and outcomes [Review], *Arthroscopy* 30(12):1634–1641, 2014.

72. de Steiger RN, Lorimer M, Solomon M: What is the learning curve for the anterior approach for total hip arthroplasty? *Clin Orthop Relat Res* 473(12):3860–3866, 2015.

73. Delp SL, Hess WE, Hungerford DS, et al.: Variation of rotation moment arms with hip flexion, *J Biomech* 32:493–501, 1999.

74. Dickenson EJ, Wall PDH, Hutchinson CE, et al.: The prevalence of cam morphology in a general population sample, *Osteoarthritis Cartilage* 27(3):444–448, 2019.

75. Domb BG, Martin TJ, Gui C, et al.: Predictors of clinical outcomes after hip arthroscopy: a prospective analysis of 1038 patients with 2-year follow-up, *Am J Sports Med* 46(6):1324–1330, 2018.

76. Dostal WF, Andrews JG: A three-dimensional biomechanical model of hip musculature, *J Biomech* 14:803–812, 1981.

77. Dostal WF, Soderberg GL, Andrews JG: Actions of hip muscles, *Phys Ther* 66:351–361, 1986.

78. Eckstein F, von Eisenhart-Rothe R, Landgraf J, et al.: Quantitative analysis of incongruity, contact areas and cartilage thickness in the human hip joint, *Acta Anat* 158:192–204, 1997.

79. Edelson G: The development of humeral head retroversion, *J Shoulder Elbow Surg* 9(4):316–318, 2000.

80. Ejnisman L, Philippon MJ, Lertwanich P, et al.: Relationship between femoral anteversion and findings in hips with femoroacetabular impingement, *Orthopedics* 36(3):e293–e300, 2013.

81. Enseki KR, Martin RL, Draovitch P, et al.: The hip joint: arthroscopic procedures and postoperative rehabilitation, *J Orthop Sports Phys Ther* 36:516–525, 2006.

82. Escalante A, Lichtenstein MJ, Dhanda R, et al.: Determinants of hip and knee flexion range: results from the san antonio longitudinal study of aging, *Arthritis Care Res* 12:8–18, 1999.

83. Esola MA, McClure PW, Fitzgerald GK, et al.: Analysis of lumbar spine and hip motion during forward bending in subjects with and without a history of low back pain, *Spine* 21:71–78, 1996.

84. Fabry G, MacEwen GD, Shands Jr AR: Torsion of the femur. A follow-up study in normal and abnormal conditions, *J Bone Joint Surg Am* 55:1726–1738, 1973.

85. Fearon A, Stephens S, Cook J, et al.: The relationship of femoral neck shaft angle and adiposity to greater trochanteric pain syndrome in women. A case control morphology and anthropometric study, *Br J Sports Med* 46:888–892, 2012.

86. Fernquest S, Palmer A, Gimpel M, et al.: A longitudinal cohort study of adolescent elite footballers and controls investigating the development of cam morphology, *Sci Rep* 11(1):18567, 2021.

87. Field RE, Rajakulendran K: The labro-acetabular complex [Review], *J Bone Joint Surg Am* 93(Suppl-7), 2011.

88. Fischer FJ, Houtz SJ: Evaluation of the function of the gluteus maximus muscle. An electromyographic study, *Am J Phys Med* 47:182–191, 1968.

89. Fisher BE, Southam AC, Kuo YL: Evidence of altered corticomotor excitability following targeted activation of gluteus maximus training in healthy individuals, *Neuroreport* 27(6):415–421, 2016.

90. Flack NA, Nicholson HD, Woodley SJ: The anatomy of the hip abductor muscles, *Clin Anat* 27(2):241–253, 2014.

91. Flevas DA, Tsantes AG, Mavrogenis AF: Direct anterior approach total hip arthroplasty revisited, *JBJS Rev* 8(4):e0144, 2020.

92. Forlizzi JM, Ward MB, Whalen J, et al.: Core muscle injury: evaluation and treatment in the athlete, *Am J Sports Med*, 2022. 3635465211063890.

93. Foucher KC, Cinnamon CC, Ryan CA, et al.: Hip abductor strength and fatigue are associated with activity levels more than 1 Year after total hip replacement, *J Orthop Res* 36(5):1519–1525, 2018.

94. Freeman S, Mascia A, McGill S: Arthrogenic neuromusculature inhibition: a foundational investigation of existence in the hip joint, *Clin Biomech* 28(2):171–177, 2013.

95. Freke M, Kemp J, Semciw A, et al.: Hip strength and range of movement are associated with dynamic postural control performance in individuals scheduled for arthroscopic hip surgery, *J Orthop Sports Phys Ther* 48(4):280–288, 2018.

96. French HP, Cusack T, Brennan A, et al.: Exercise and manual physiotherapy arthritis research trial (EMPART) for osteoarthritis of the hip: a multicenter randomized controlled trial, *Arch Phys Med Rehabil* 94(2):302–314, 2013.

97. Friede MC, Innerhofer G, Fink C, et al.: Conservative treatment of iliotibial band syndrome in runners: are we targeting the right goals? *Phys Ther Sport* 54:44–52, 2022.

98. Gadinsky NE, Klinger CE, Sculco PK, et al.: Femoral head vascularity: implications following trauma and surgery about the hip, *Orthopedics* 42(5):250–257, 2019.

99. Gafner SC, Bastiaenen CHG, Ferrari S, et al.: The role of hip abductor strength in identifying older persons at risk of falls: a diagnostic accuracy study, *Clin Interv Aging* 15:645–654, 2020.

100. Ganderton C, Pizzari T, Cook J, et al.: Gluteus minimus and gluteus medius muscle activity during common rehabilitation exercises in healthy postmenopausal women, *J Orthop Sports Phys Ther* 47(12):914–922, 2017.

101. Ganz R, Parvizi J, Beck M, et al.: Femoroacetabular impingement: a cause for osteoarthritis of the hip, *Clin Orthop Relat Res* 417:112–120, 2003.

102. Genda E, Iwasaki N, Li G, et al.: Normal hip joint contact pressure distribution in single-leg standing—effect of gender and anatomic parameters, *J Biomech* 34:895–905, 2001.

103. Gomes D, Ribeiro DC, Ferreira T, et al.: Knee and hip dynamic muscle strength in individuals with femoroacetabular impingement syndrome scheduled for hip arthroscopy: a case-control study, *Clin Biomech* 93:105584, 2022.

104. Gonzalez-Galvez N, Marcos-Pardo PJ, Trejo-Alfaro H, et al.: Effect of 9-month Pilates program on sagittal spinal curvatures and hamstring extensibility in adolescents: randomised controlled trial, *Sci Rep* 10(1):9977, 2020.

105. Gottschall JS, Okita N, Sheehan RC: Muscle activity patterns of the tensor fascia latae and adductor longus for ramp and stair walking, *J Electromyogr Kinesiol* 22(1):67–73, 2012. 79.

106. Gouveia K, Shah A, Kay J, et al.: Iliopsoas tenotomy during hip arthroscopy: a systematic review of postoperative outcomes, *Am J Sports Med* 49(3):817–829, 2021.

107. Graham SM, Manara J, Chokotho L, et al.: Back-carrying infants to prevent developmental hip dysplasia and its sequelae: is a new public health initiative needed? *J Pediatr Orthop* 35(1):57–61, 2015.

108. Griffin DR, Dickenson EJ, O'Donnell J, et al.: The Warwick agreement on femoroacetabular impingement syndrome (FAI syndrome): an international consensus statement, *Br J Sports Med* 50:1169–1176, 2016.

109. Grimaldi A, Fearon A: Gluteal tendinopathy: integrating pathomechanics and clinical features in its management, *J Orthop Sports Phys Ther* 45:910–922, 2015.

110. Gulledge BM, Marcellin-Little DJ, Levine D, et al.: Comparison of two stretching methods and optimization of stretching protocol for the piriformis muscle, *Med Eng Phys* 36(2):212–218, 2014.

111. Haefeli PC, Steppacher SD, Babst D, et al.: An increased iliocapsularis-to-rectus-femoris ratio is suggestive for instability in borderline hips, *Clin Orthop Relat Res* 473(12):3725–3734, 2015.

112. Halbertsma JP, Göeken LN, Hof AL, et al.: Extensibility and stiffness of the hamstrings in patients with nonspecific low back pain, *Arch Phys Med Rehabil* 82:232–238, 2001.

113. Han S, Alexander JW, Thomas VS, et al.: Does capsular laxity lead to microinstability of the native hip? *Am J Sports Med* 46(6):1315–1323, 2018.

114. Han S, Kim RS, Harris JD, et al.: The envelope of active hip motion in different sporting, recreational, and daily living activities: a systematic review, *Gait Posture* 71:227–233, 2019.

115. Haneda M, Rai MF, O'Keefe RJ, et al.: Inflammatory response of articular cartilage to femoroacetabular impingement in the hip, *Am J Sports Med* 48(7):1647–1656, 2020.

116. Hanke MS, Schmaranzer F, Steppacher SD, et al.: A cam morphology develops in the early phase of the final growth spurt in adolescent ice hockey players: results of a prospective MRI-based Study, *Clin Orthop Relat Res* 479(5):906–918, 2021.

117. Hankins DA, Korcek L, Richter DL: Femoroacetabular impingement and management of labral tears in the athlete, *Clin Sports Med* 40(2):259–270, 2021.

118. Hardcastle P, Nade S: The significance of the Trendelenburg test, *J Bone Joint Surg Br* 67:741–746, 1985.

119. Harris JD, Lewis BD, Park KJ: Hip dysplasia, *Clin Sports Med* 40(2):271–288, 2021.

120. Harris MD, Anderson AE, Henak CR, et al.: Finite element prediction of cartilage contact stresses in normal human hips, *J Orthop Res* 30(7):1133–1139, 2012.

121. Harris MD, Shepherd MC, Song K, et al.: The biomechanical disadvantage of dysplastic hips, *J Orthop Res* 40(6):1387–1396, 2022.

122. Harris-Hayes M, Hillen TJ, Commean PK, et al.: Hip kinematics during single-leg tasks in people with and without hip-related groin pain and the association among kinematics, hip muscle strength, and bony morphology, *J Orthop Sports Phys Ther* 50(5):243–251, 2020.

123. Harris-Hayes M, Royer NK: Relationship of acetabular dysplasia and femoroacetabular impingement to hip osteoarthritis: a focused review [Review], *Pharm Manag PM R* 3(11):1055–1067, 2011.

124. Harsanyi S, Zamborsky R, Kokavec M, et al.: Genetics of developmental dysplasia of the hip, *Eur J Med Genet* 63(9):103990, 2020.

125. Hayden AM, Hayes AM, Brechbuhler JL, et al.: The effect of pelvic motion on spinopelvic parameters, *Spine J* 18(1):173–178, 2018.

126. Heller MO, Bergmann G, Deuretzbacher G, et al.: Influence of femoral anteversion on proximal femoral loading: measurement and simulation in four patients, *Clin Biomech* 16:644–649, 2001.

127. Henderson ER, Marulanda GA, Cheong D, et al.: Hip abductor moment arm—a mathematical analysis for proximal femoral replacement, *J Orthop Surg* 6(6), 2011.

128. Hewitt JD, Glisson RR, Guilak F, et al.: The mechanical properties of the human hip capsule ligaments, *J Arthroplasty* 17:82–89, 2002.

129. Hicks JL, Schwartz MH, Arnold AS, et al.: Crouched postures reduce the capacity of muscles to extend the hip and knee during the single-limb stance phase of gait, *J Biomech* 41:960–967, 2008.

130. Hidaka E, Aoki M, Izumi T, et al.: Ligament strain on the iliofemoral, pubofemoral, and ischiofemoral ligaments in cadaver specimens: biomechanical measurement and anatomical observation, *Clin Anat* 27(7):1068–1075, 2014.

131. Hoaglund FT, Steinbach LS: Primary osteoarthritis of the hip: etiology and epidemiology, *J Am Acad Orthop Surg* 9:320–327, 2001.

132. Hodges PW, McLean L, Hodder J: Insight into the function of the obturator internus muscle in humans: observations with development and validation of an electromyography recording technique, *J Electromyogr Kinesiol* 24(4):489–496, 2014.

133. Hodges PW, Richardson CA: Contraction of the abdominal muscles associated with movement of the lower limb, *Phys Ther* 77:132–142, 1997.

134. Hoffmann A, Pfirrmann CW: The hip abductors at MR imaging, *Eur J Radiol* 81(12):3755–3762, 2012.

135. Hollman JH, Beise NJ, Fischer ML, et al.: Coupled gluteus maximus and gluteus medius recruitment patterns modulate hip adduction variability during single-limb step-downs: a cross-sectional study, *J Sport Rehabil* 30(4):625–630, 2020.

136. Hoskins W, Bingham R, Lorimer M, et al.: Early rate of revision of total hip arthroplasty related to surgical approach: an analysis of 122,345 primary total hip arthroplasties, *J Bone Joint Surg Am* 102(21):1874–1882, 2020.

137. Howell M, Rae FJ, Khan A, et al.: Iliopsoas pathology after total hip arthroplasty: a young person's complication, *Bone Joint J* 103-B(2):305–308, 2021.

138. Hoy MG, Zajac FE, Gordon ME: A musculoskeletal model of the human lower extremity: the effect of muscle, tendon, and moment arm on the moment-angle relationship of musculotendon actuators at the hip, knee, and ankle, *J Biomech* 23:157–169, 1990.

139. Hu H, Meijer OG, van Dieen JH, et al.: Is the psoas a hip flexor in the active straight leg raise? *Eur Spine J* 20(5):759–765, 2011.

140. Hunter DJ, Eyles J, Murphy NJ, et al.: Multi-centre randomised controlled trial comparing arthroscopic hip surgery to physiotherapist-led care for femoroacetabular impingement (FAI) syndrome on hip cartilage metabolism: the Australian fashion trial, *BMC Muscoskel Disord* 22(1):697, 2021.

141. Ike H, Dorr LD, Trasolini N, et al.: Spine-pelvis-hip relationship in the functioning of a total hip replacement, *J Bone Joint Surg Am* 100(18):1606–1615, 2018.

142. Inman VT, Saunders JB: Referred pain from skeletal structures, *J Nerv Ment Dis* 99:660–667, 1944.

143. Iwanaga J, Eid S, Simonds E, et al.: The majority of piriformis muscles are innervated by the superior gluteal nerve, *Clin Anat* 32(2):282–286, 2019.

144. Jacobsen JS, Thorborg K, Nielsen R, et al.: Comparing exercise and patient education with usual care in the treatment of hip dysplasia: a protocol for a randomised controlled trial with 6-month follow-up (Movethehip Trial), *BMJ Open* 12(9):e064242, 2022.

145. Jang SJ, Kunze KN, Vigdorchik JM, et al.: John Charnley Award: Deep learning prediction of hip joint center on standard pelvis radiographs, *J Arthroplasty* 37(7s):S400–S407.e1, 2022.

146. Johannsen AM, Behn AW, Shibata K, et al.: The role of anterior capsular laxity in hip microinstability: a novel biomechanical model, *Am J Sports Med* 47(5):1151–1158, 2019.

147. Jorge JP, Simoes FM, Pires EB, et al.: Finite element simulations of a hip joint with femoroacetabular impingement, *Comput Methods Biomech Biomed Engin* 17(11):1275–1284, 2014.

148. Kapron AL, Aoki SK, Peters CL, et al.: In-vivo hip arthrokinematics during supine clinical exams: application to the study of femoroacetabular impingement, *J Biomech* 48(11):2879–2886, 2015.

149. Kato T, Taniguchi K, Akima H, et al.: Effect of hip angle on neuromuscular activation of the adductor longus and adductor magnus muscles during isometric hip flexion and extension, *Eur J Appl Physiol* 119(7):1611–1617, 2019.

150. Katz JN, Arant KR, Loeser RF: Diagnosis and treatment of hip and knee osteoarthritis: a review, *JAMA* 325(6):568–578, 2021.

151. Kelly BT, Shapiro GS, Digiovanni CW, et al.: Vascularity of the hip labrum: a cadaveric investigation, *Arthroscopy* 21(1):3–11, 2005.

152. Kendall FP, McCreary AK, Provance PG: *Muscles: testing and function*, ed 4, Baltimore, 1993, Williams & Wilkins.

153. Keurentjes JC, Pijls BG, Van Tol FR, et al.: Which implant should we use for primary total hip replacement? A systematic review and meta-analysis [Review], *J Bone Joint Surg Am* 96:Suppl–97, 2014.

154. Khalaj N, Vicenzino B, Heales LJ, et al.: Is chronic ankle instability associated with impaired muscle strength? Ankle, knee and hip muscle strength in individuals with chronic ankle instability: a systematic review with meta-analysis, *Br J Sports Med* 54(14):839–847, 2020.

155. Khan AZ, Abu-Amer W, Thapa S, et al.: Factors associated with disease progression in the contralateral hip of patients with symptomatic femoroacetabular impingement: a minimum 5-year analysis, *Am J Sports Med* 50(12):3174–3183, 2022.

156. Kim WY, Hutchinson CE, Andrew JG, et al.: The relationship between acetabular retroversion and osteoarthritis of the hip, *J Bone Joint Surg Br* 88:727–729, 2006.

157. Kim YT, Azuma H: The nerve endings of the acetabular labrum, *Clin Orthop Relat Res* 320:176–181, 1995.

158. Kinov P, Leithner A, Radl R, et al.: Role of free radicals in aseptic loosening of hip arthroplasty, *J Orthop Res* 24:55–62, 2006.

159. Kivlan BR, Richard CF, Martin RL, et al.: Function of the ligamentum teres during multi-planar movement of the hip joint, *Knee Surg Sports Traumatol Arthrosc* 21(7):1664–1668, 2013.

160. Kraus VB, Sprow K, Powell KE, et al.: Effects of physical activity in knee and hip osteoarthritis: a systematic umbrella review, *Med Sci Sports Exerc* 51(6):1324–1339, 2019.

161. Kulig K, Harper-Hanigan K, Souza RB, et al.: Measurement of femoral torsion by ultrasound and magnetic resonance imaging: concurrent validity, *Phys Ther* 90(11):1641–1648, 2010.

162. Kurrat HJ, Oberlander W: The thickness of the cartilage in the hip joint, *J Anat* 126:145–155, 1978.

163. Kutzner I, Richter A, Gordt K, et al.: Does aquatic exercise reduce hip and knee joint loading? In vivo load measurements with instrumented implants, *PLoS One* 12(3):e0171972, 2017.

164. Laborie LB, Lehmann TG, Engesaeter IO, et al.: Is a positive femoroacetabular impingement test a common finding in healthy young adults? *Clin Orthop Relat Res* 471(7):2267–2277, 2013.

165. Larkin B, van Holsbeeck M, Koueiter D, et al.: What is the impingement-free range of motion of the asymptomatic hip in young adult males? *Clin Orthop Relat Res* 473(4):1284–1288, 2015.

166. Larson CM, Moreau-Gaudry A, Kelly BT, et al.: Are normal hips being labeled as pathologic? A CT-based method for defining normal acetabular coverage, *Clin Orthop Relat Res* 473(4):1247–1254, 2015.

167. Larson CM, Sikka RS, Sardelli MC, et al.: Increasing alpha angle is predictive of athletic-related "hip" and "groin" pain in collegiate National Football League prospects, *Arthroscopy* 29(3):405–410, 2013.

168. Lauritzen J: The arterial supply to the femoral head in children, *Acta Orthop Scand* 45(5):724–736, 1974.

169. Lawrenson P, Hodges P, Crossley K, et al.: The effect of altered stride length on iliocapsularis and pericapsular muscles of the anterior hip: an electromyography investigation during asymptomatic gait, *Gait Posture* 71:26–31, 2019.

170. Lee SP, Souza RB, Powers CM: The influence of hip abductor muscle performance on dynamic postural stability in females with patellofemoral pain, *Gait Posture* 36(3):425–429, 2012.

171. Leide R, Bohman A, Wenger D, et al.: Hip dysplasia is not uncommon but frequently overlooked: a cross-sectional study based on radiographic examination of 1870 adults, *Acta Orthop* 92(5):575–580, 2021.

172. Lengsfeld M, Pressel T, Stammberger U: Lengths and lever arms of hip joint muscles: geometrical analyses using a human multibody model, *Gait Posture* 6:18–26, 1997.

173. Lerch TD, Antioco T, Boschung A, et al.: Hip impingement location in maximal hip flexion in patients with femoroacetabular impingement with and without femoral retroversion, *Am J Sports Med* 50(11):2989–2997, 2022.

174. Lerch TD, Siegfried M, Schmaranzer F, et al.: Location of intra- and extra-articular hip impingement is different in patients with pincer-type and mixed-type femoroacetabular impingement due to acetabular retroversion or protrusio acetabuli on 3D CT-based impingement simulation, *Am J Sports Med* 48(3):661–672, 2020.

175. Leunig M, Beck M, Stauffer E, et al.: Free nerve endings in the ligamentum capitis femoris, *Acta Orthop Scand* 71(5):452–454, 2000.

176. Leunig M, Beck M, Woo A, et al.: Acetabular rim degeneration: a constant finding in the aged hip, *Clin Orthop Relat Res* 413:201–207, 2003.

177. Leunig M, Juni P, Werlen S, et al.: Prevalence of cam and pincer-type deformities on hip MRI in an asymptomatic young Swiss female population: a cross-sectional study, *Osteoarthritis Cartilage* 21(4):544–550, 2013.

178. Lewis CL, Uemura K, Atkins PR, et al.: Patients with cam-type femoroacetabular impingement demonstrate increased change in bone-to-bone distance during walking: a dual fluoroscopy study, *J Orthop Res* 41(1):161–169, 2023.

179. Lievense AM, Bierma-Zeinstra SM, Verhagen AP, et al.: Influence of sporting activities on the development of osteoarthritis of the hip: a systematic review, *Arthritis Rheum* 49:228–236, 2003.

180. Lindsay DM, Maitland ME, Lowe RC: Comparison of isokinetic internal and external hip rotation torques using different testing positions, *J Orthop Sports Phys Ther* 16:43–50, 1992.

181. Loder RT, Aronsson DD, Weinstein SL, et al.: Slipped capital femoral epiphysis, *Instr Course Lect* 57:473–498, 2008.

182. Löhe F, Eckstein F, Sauer T, et al.: Structure, strain and function of the transverse acetabular ligament, *Acta Anat* 157:315–323, 1996.

183. Lohmander LS: Articular cartilage and osteoarthrosis. The role of molecular markers to monitor breakdown, repair and disease, *J Anat* 184:477–492, 1994.

184. Long SS, Surrey DE, Nazarian LN: Sonography of greater trochanteric pain syndrome and the rarity of primary bursitis, *AJR Am J Roentgenol* 201(5):1083–1086, 2013.

185. Longstaffe R, Hendrikx S, Naudie D, et al.: Iliopsoas release: a systematic review of clinical efficacy and associated complications, *Clin J Sport Med* 31(6):522–529, 2021.

186. Loubert PV, Zipple JT, Klobucher MJ, et al.: In vivo ultrasound measurement of posterior femoral glide during hip joint mobilization in healthy college students, *J Orthop Sports Phys Ther* 43(8):534–541, 2013.

187. Mac Dermott KD, Venter RG, Bergsteedt BJ, et al.: Anatomical features of the iliocapsularis muscle: a dissection study, *Surg Radiol Anat* 44(4):599–608, 2022.

188. Malagelada F, Tayar R, Barke S, et al.: Anatomy of the zona orbicularis of the hip: a magnetic resonance study, *Surg Radiol Anat* 37(1):11–18, 2015.

189. Maldonado DR, Mu BH, Ornelas J, et al.: Hip-spine syndrome: the diagnostic utility of guided intra-articular hip injections, *Orthopedics* 43(2):e65–e71, 2020.

190. Malloy P, Malloy M, Draovitch P: Guidelines and pitfalls for the rehabilitation following hip arthroscopy, *Curr Rev Musculoskelet Med* 6:235–241, 2013.

191. Malloy P, Neumann DA, Kipp K: Hip biomechanics during a single-leg squat: 5 key differences between people with femoroacetabular impingement syndrome and those without hip Pain, *J Orthop Sports Phys Ther* 49(12):908–916, 2019.

192. Malloy P, Stone AV, Kunze KN, et al.: Patients with unilateral femoroacetabular impingement syndrome have asymmetrical hip muscle cross-sectional area and compensatory muscle changes associated with preoperative pain level, *Arthroscopy* 35(5):1445–1453, 2019.

193. Mancino F, Cacciola G, Di Matteo V, et al.: Surgical implications of the hip-spine relationship in total hip arthroplasty, *Orthop Rev* 12(Suppl 1):8656, 2020.

194. Mansour JM, Pereira JM: Quantitative functional anatomy of the lower limb with application to human gait, *J Biomech* 20:51–58, 1987.

195. Maradit KH, Larson DR, Crowson CS, et al.: Prevalence of total hip and knee replacement in the United States, *J Bone Joint Surg Am* 97(17):1386–1397, 2015.

196. Markhede G, Stener B: Function after removal of various hip and thigh muscles for extirpation of tumors, *Acta Orthop Scand* 52:373–395, 1981.

197. Marom N, Dooley MS, Burger JA, et al.: Characteristics of soccer players undergoing primary hip arthroscopy for femoroacetabular impingement: a sex- and competitive level-specific analysis, *Am J Sports Med* 1(13):3255–3264, 2020.

198. Martin HD, Savage A, Braly BA, et al.: The function of the hip capsular ligaments: a quantitative report, *Arthroscopy* 24:188–195, 2008.

199. Martin RL, Palmer I, Martin HD: Ligamentum Teres: a functional description and potential clinical relevance, *Knee Surg Sports Traumatol Arthrosc* 20(6):1209–1214, 2012.

200. Mastenbrook MJ, Commean PK, Hillen TJ, et al.: Hip abductor muscle volume and strength differences between women with chronic hip joint pain and asymptomatic controls, *J Orthop Sports Phys Ther* 47(12):923–930, 2017.

201. Meghpara MB, Bheem R, Shah S, et al.: Prevalence of gluteus medius pathology on magnetic resonance imaging in patients undergoing hip arthroscopy for femoroacetabular impingement: asymptomatic tears are rare, whereas tendinosis is common, *Am J Sports Med* 48(12):2933–2938, 2020.

202. Mehmood S, Jinnah RH, Pandit H: Review on ceramic-on-ceramic total hip arthroplasty, *J Surg Orthop Adv* 17:45–50, 2008.

203. Meinders E, Pizzolato C, Goncalves B, et al.: Activation of the deep hip muscles can change the direction of loading at the hip, *J Biomech* 135:111019, 2022.

204. Mellor R, Kasza J, Grimaldi A, et al.: Mediators and moderators of education plus exercise on perceived improvement in individuals with gluteal tendinopathy: an exploratory analysis of a 3-arm randomized trial, *J Orthop Sports Phys Ther* 52(12):826–836, 2022.

205. Meyer CAG, Wesseling M, Corten K, et al.: Hip movement pathomechanics of patients with hip osteoarthritis aim at reducing hip joint loading on the osteoarthritic side, *Gait Posture* 59:11–17, 2018.

206. Monn S, Maffiuletti NA, Bizzini M, et al.: Midterm outcomes of exercise therapy for the non-surgical management of femoroacetabular impingement syndrome: are short-term effects persisting? *Phys Ther Sport* 55:168–175, 2022.

207. Moore KL, Persaud TVN: *The developing human: clinically oriented embryology*, ed 7, St Louis, 2003, Elsevier.

208. Münger P, Röder C, Ackermann-Liebrich U, et al.: Patient-related risk factors leading to aseptic stem loosening in total hip arthroplasty: a case-control study of 5035 patients, *Acta Orthop* 77:567–574, 2006.

209. Myers CA, Laz PJ, Shelburne KB, et al.: Simulated hip abductor strengthening reduces peak joint contact forces in patients with total hip arthroplasty, *J Biomech* 93:18–27, 2019.

210. Nakamura J, Kamegaya M, Saisu T, et al.: Treatment for developmental dysplasia of the hip using the Pavlik harness: long-term results, *J Bone Joint Surg Br* 89:230–235, 2007.

211. Nemeth G, Ohlsen H: Moment arms of the hip abductor and adductor muscles measured in vivo by computed tomography, *Clin Biomech* 4:133–136, 1989.

212. Nepple JJ, Brophy RH, Matava MJ, et al.: Radiographic findings of femoroacetabular impingement in National Football League combine athletes undergoing radiographs for previous hip or groin pain, *Arthroscopy* 28:1396–1403, 2012.

213. Nepple JJ, Philippon MJ, Campbell KJ, et al.: The hip fluid seal—Part II: the effect of an acetabular labral tear, repair, resection, and reconstruction on hip stability to distraction, *Knee Surg Sports Traumatol Arthrosc* 22(4):730–736, 2014.

214. Neto WK, Soares EG, Vieira TL, et al.: Gluteus maximus activation during common strength and hypertrophy exercises: a systematic review, *J Sports Sci Med* 19(1):195–203, 2020.

215. Neumann DA, Cook TM, Sholty RL, et al.: An electromyographic analysis of hip abductor muscle activity when subjects are carrying loads in one or both hands, *Phys Ther* 72:207–217, 1992.

216. Neumann DA, Cook TM: Effect of load and carrying position on the electromyographic activity of the gluteus medius muscle during walking, *Phys Ther* 65:305–311, 1985.

217. Neumann DA, Garceau LR: A proposed novel function of the psoas minor revealed through cadaver dissection, *Clin Anat* 28:243–252, 2015.

218. Neumann DA, Hase AD: An electromyographic analysis of the hip abductors during load carriage: implications for hip joint protection, *J Orthop Sports Phys Ther* 19:296–304, 1994.

219. Neumann DA, Soderberg GL, Cook TM: Comparison of maximal isometric hip abductor muscle torques between hip sides, *Phys Ther* 68:496–502, 1988.

220. Neumann DA, Soderberg GL, Cook TM: Electromyographic analysis of hip abductor musculature in healthy right-handed persons, *Phys Ther* 69:431–440, 1989.

221. Neumann DA: An electromyographic study of the hip abductor muscles as subjects with a hip prosthesis walked with different methods of using a cane and carrying a load, *Phys Ther* 79:1163–1173, 1999.

222. Neumann DA: Biomechanical analysis of selected principles of hip joint protection, *Arthritis Care Res* 2:146–155, 1989.

223. Neumann DA: Commentary 9.2: a proposed novel action of the psoas Minor. In Standring S, editor: *Pelvic girdle, hip and thigh (chapter 77), Gray's anatomy (British edition): the anatomical basis of clinical practice*, 42nd ed, St Louis, 2021, Elsevier.

224. Neumann DA: Hip abductor muscle activity as subjects with hip prostheses walk with different methods of using a cane, *Phys Ther* 78:490–501, 1998.

225. Neumann DA: Hip abductor muscle activity in persons with a hip prosthesis while carrying loads in one hand, *Phys Ther* 76:1320–1330, 1996.

226. Neumann DA: Lead contributor to pelvic girdle, hip and thigh. In Standring S, editor: *Gray's Anatomy (British edition): the anatomical basis of clinical practice*, 42sd ed, St Louis, 2021, Elsevier.

227. Neumann DA: The actions of hip muscles, *J Orthop Sports Phys Ther* 40:82–94, 2010.

228. Ng KCG, Jeffers JRT, Beaulé PE: Hip joint capsular anatomy, mechanics, and surgical management, *J Bone Joint Surg Am* 101(23):2141–2151, 2019.

229. Nho SJ, Kymes SM, Callaghan JJ, et al.: The burden of hip osteoarthritis in the United States: epidemiologic and economic considerations, *J Am Acad Orthop Surg* 21(Suppl-6), 2013.

230. Notzli HP, Wyss TF, Stoecklin CH, et al.: The contour of the femoral head-neck junction as a predictor for the risk of anterior impingement, *J Bone Joint Surg Br* 84:556–560, 2002.

231. Oguz O: Measurement and relationship of the inclination angle, Alsberg angle and the angle between the anatomical and mechanical axes of the femur in males, *Surg Radiol Anat* 18:29–31, 1996.

232. Palmer A, Fernquest S, Gimpel M, et al.: Physical activity during adolescence and the development of cam morphology: a cross-sectional cohort study of 210 individuals, *Br J Sports Med* 52(9):601–610, 2018.

233. Palmowski Y, Popovic S, Schuster SG, et al.: In vivo analysis of hip joint loading on Nordic walking novices, *J* 16(1):596, 2021.

234. Pare EB, Stern Jr JT, Schwartz JM: Functional differentiation within the tensor fasciae latae. A telemetered electromyographic analysis of its locomotor roles, *J Bone Joint Surg Am* 63:1457–1471, 1981.

235. Parvaresh KC, Chang C, Patel A, et al.: Architecture of the short external rotator muscles of the hip, *BMC Muscoskel Disord* 20(1):611, 2019.

236. Passmore E, Graham HK, Pandy MG, et al.: Hip- and patellofemoral-joint loading during gait are increased in children with idiopathic torsional deformities, *Gait Posture* 63:228–235, 2018.

237. Pastore EA, Katzman WB: Recognizing myofascial pelvic pain in the female patient with chronic pelvic pain [Review], *J Obstet Gynecol Neonatal Nurs* 41(5):680–691, 2012.

238. Patel RV, Han S, Lenherr C, et al.: Pelvic tilt and range of motion in hips with femoroacetabular impingement syndrome, *J Am Acad Orthop Surg* 28(10):e427–e432, 2020.

239. Perets I, Chaharbakhshi EO, Mansor Y, et al.: Midterm outcomes of iliopsoas fractional lengthening for internal snapping as a part of hip arthroscopy for femoroacetabular impingement and labral tear: a matched control study, *Arthroscopy* 35(5):1432–1440, 2019.

240. Perumal V, Techataweewan N, Woodley SJ, et al.: Clinical anatomy of the ligament of the head of femur, *Clin Anat* 32(1):90–98, 2019.

241. Perumal V, Woodley SJ, Nicholson HD: Neurovascular structures of the ligament of the head of femur, *J Anat* 234(6):778–786, 2019.

242. Philippon MJ, Decker MJ, Giphart JE, et al.: Rehabilitation exercise progression for the gluteus medius muscle with consideration for iliopsoas tendinitis: an in vivo electromyography study, *Am J Sports Med* 39(8):1777–1785, 2011.

243. Philippon MJ, Devitt BM, Campbell KJ, et al.: Anatomic variance of the iliopsoas tendon, *Am J Sports Med* 42:807–811, 2014.

244. Philippon MJ, Ho CP, Briggs KK, et al.: Prevalence of increased alpha angles as a measure of cam-type femoroacetabular impingement in youth ice hockey players, *Am J Sports Med* 41(6):1357–1362, 2013.

245. Philippon MJ, Nepple JJ, Campbell KJ, et al.: The hip fluid seal—Part I: the effect of an acetabular labral tear, repair, resection, and reconstruction on hip fluid pressurization, *Knee Surg Sports Traumatol Arthrosc* 22(4):722–729, 2014.

246. Pohtilla JF: Kinesiology of hip extension at selected angles of pelvifemoral extension, *Arch Phys Med Rehabil* 50:241–250, 1969.

247. Prather H, van Dillen L: Links between the hip and the lumbar spine (hip spine syndrome) as they relate to clinical decision making for patients with lumbopelvic pain, *PM R* 11(Suppl 1):S64–s72, 2019.

248. Prather H, Dugan S, Fitzgerald C, et al.: Review of anatomy, evaluation, and treatment of musculoskeletal pelvic floor pain in women [Review, 63 refs], *Pharm Manag PM R* 1(4):346–358, 2009.

249. Putz C, Wolf SI, Geisbusch A, et al.: Femoral derotation osteotomy in adults with cerebral palsy, *Gait Posture* 49:290–296, 2016.

250. Ralis Z, McKibbin B: Changes in shape of the human hip joint during its development and their relation to its stability, *J Bone Joint Surg Br* 55:780–785, 1973.

251. Ravera EP, Crespo MJ, Rozumalski A: Individual muscle force-energy rate is altered during crouch gait: a neuro-musculoskeletal evaluation, *J Biomech* 139:111141, 2022.

252. Recnik G, Kralj-Iglic V, Iglic A, et al.: Higher peak contact hip stress predetermines the side of hip involved in idiopathic osteoarthritis, *Clin Biomech* 22:1119–1124, 2007.

253. Reikeras O, Bjerkreim I, Kolbenstvedt A: Anteversion of the acetabulum and femoral neck in normals and in patients with osteoarthritis of the hip, *Acta Orthop Scand* 54:18–23, 1983.

254. Reiman MP, Décary S, Mathew B, et al.: Accuracy of clinical and imaging tests for the diagnosis of hip dysplasia and instability: a systematic review, *J Orthop Sports Phys Ther* 49(2):87–97, 2019.

255. Rethlefsen SA, Healy BS, Wren TA, et al.: Causes of intoeing gait in children with cerebral palsy, *J Bone Joint Surg Am* 88:2175–2180, 2006.

256. Roach KE, Miles TP: Normal hip and knee active range of motion: the relationship to age, *Phys Ther* 71:656–665, 1991.

257. Robertson WJ, Gardner MJ, Barker JU, et al.: Anatomy and dimensions of the gluteus medius tendon insertion, *Arthroscopy* 24(2):130–136, 2008.

258. Roddy E, Zhang W, Doherty M, et al.: Evidence-based recommendations for the role of exercise in the management of osteoarthritis of the hip or knee—the MOVE consensus, *Rheumatology* 44:67–73, 2005.

259. Rogers MJ, Sato EH, LaBelle MW, et al.: Association of cam deformity on anteroposterior pelvic radiographs and more severe chondral damage in femoroacetabular impingement syndrome, *Am J Sports Med* 50(11):2980–2988, 2022.

260. Rosinsky PJ, Shapira J, Lall AC, et al.: All about the ligamentum teres: from biomechanical role to surgical reconstruction, *J Am Acad Orthop Surg* 28(8):e328–e339, 2020.

261. ZPJ R, Zacharias A, Semciw AI, et al.: Effects of a targeted resistance intervention compared to a sham intervention on gluteal muscle hypertrophy, fatty infiltration and strength in people with hip osteoarthritis: analysis of secondary outcomes from a randomised clinical trial, *BMC Musculoskelet Disord* 23(1):944, 2022.

262. Runge N, Aina A, May S: The benefits of adding manual therapy to exercise therapy for improving pain and function in patients with knee or hip osteoarthritis: a systematic review with meta-analysis, *J Orthop Sports Phys Ther* 52(10), 2022. 675-a13.

263. Rydell N: Biomechanics of the hip-joint, *Clin Orthop Relat Res* 92:6–15, 1973.

264. Sadler S, Cassidy S, Peterson B, et al.: Gluteus medius muscle function in people with and without low back pain: a systematic review, *BMC Musculoskelet Disord* 20(1):463, 2019.

265. Sanchez Egea AJ, Valera M, Parraga Quiroga JM, et al.: Impact of hip anatomical variations on the cartilage stress: a finite element analysis toward the biomechanical exploration of the factors that may explain primary hip arthritis in morphologically normal subjects, *Clin Biomech* 29(4):444–450, 2014.

266. Sankar WN, Laird CT, Baldwin KD: Hip range of motion in children: what is the norm? *J Pediatr Orthop* 32(4):399–405, 2012.

267. Sarban S, Baba F, Kocabey Y, et al.: Free nerve endings and morphological features of the ligamentum capitis femoris in developmental dysplasia of the hip, *J Pediatr Orthop B* 16(5):351–356, 2007.

268. Sarban S, Ozturk A, Tabur H, et al.: Anteversion of the acetabulum and femoral neck in early walking age patients with developmental dysplasia of the hip, *J Pediatr Orthop B* 14(6):410–414, 2005.

269. Schmaranzer F, Lerch TD, Siebenrock KA, et al.: Differences in femoral torsion among various measurement methods increase in hips with excessive femoral torsion, *Clin Orthop Relat Res* 477(5):1073–1083, 2019.

270. Schmitz MR, Murtha AS, Clohisy JC, et al.: Developmental dysplasia of the hip in adolescents and young adults, *J Am Acad Orthop Surg* 28(3):91–101, 2020.

271. Schwachmeyer V, Damm P, Bender A, et al.: In vivo hip joint loading during post-operative physiotherapeutic exercises, *PLoS One* 8(10):e77807, 2013.

272. Seeley MA, Georgiadis AG, Sankar WN: Hip Vascularity: a review of the anatomy and clinical implications, *J Am Acad Orthop Surg* 24(8):515–526, 2016.

273. Seidler A, Luben L, Hegewald J, et al.: Dose-response relationship between cumulative physical workload and osteoarthritis of the hip - a meta-analysis applying an external reference population for exposure assignment, *BMC Musculoskelet Disord* 19(1):182, 2018.

274. Seijas R, Alentorn-Geli E, AAlvarez-Díaz P, et al.: Gluteus maximus impairment in femoroacetabular impingement: a tensiomyographic evaluation of a clinical fact, *Arch Orthop Trauma Surg* 136(6):785–789, 2016.

275. Selkowitz DM, Beneck GJ, Powers CM: Which exercises target the gluteal muscles while minimizing activation of the tensor fascia lata? Electromyographic assessment using fine-wire electrodes, *J Orthop Sports Phys Ther* 43(2):54–64, 2013.

276. Semciw AI, Green RA, Murley GS, et al.: Gluteus minimus: an intramuscular EMG investigation of anterior and posterior segments during gait, *Gait Posture* 39(2):822–826, 2014.

277. Semciw AI, Pizzari T, Murley GS, et al.: Gluteus medius: an intramuscular EMG investigation of anterior, middle and posterior segments during gait, *J Electromyogr Kinesiol* 23(4):858–864, 2013.

278. Shinohara H: Gemelli and obturator internus muscles: different heads of one muscle? *Anat Rec* 243(1):145–150, 1995.

279. Siebenrock KA, Schoeniger R, Ganz R: Anterior femoro-acetabular impingement due to acetabular retroversion. Treatment with periacetabular osteotomy, *J Bone Joint Surg Am* 85-A:278–286, 2003.

280. Siebenrock KA: Femoroacetabular impingement: a cause for osteoarthritis of the hip, *Clin Orthop Relat Res* 417:112–120, 2003.

281. Silvis ML, Mosher TJ, Smetana BS, et al.: High prevalence of pelvic and hip magnetic resonance imaging findings in asymptomatic collegiate and professional hockey players, *Am J Sports Med* 39(4):715–721, 2011.

282. Simoneau GG, Hoenig KJ, Lepley JE, et al.: Influence of hip position and gender on active hip internal and external rotation, *J Orthop Sports Phys Ther* 28:158–164, 1998.

283. Singer AD, Subhawong TK, Jose J, et al.: Ischiofemoral impingement syndrome: a meta-analysis [Review], *Skeletal Radiol* 44(6):831–837, 2015.

284. Skou ST, Pedersen BK, Abbott JH, et al.: Physical activity and exercise therapy benefit more than just symptoms and impairments in people with hip and knee osteoarthritis, *J Orthop Sports Phys Ther* 48(6):439–447, 2018.

285. Skyrme AD, Cahill DJ, Marsh HP, et al.: Psoas major and its controversial rotational action, *Clin Anat* 12:264–265, 1999.

286. Song K, Gaffney BMM, Shelburne KB, et al.: Dysplastic hip anatomy alters muscle moment arm lengths, lines of action, and contributions to joint reaction forces during gait, *J Biomech* 110:109968, 2020.

287. Song Y, Ito H, Kourtis L, et al.: Articular cartilage friction increases in hip joints after the removal of acetabular labrum, *J Biomech* 45(3):524–530, 2012.

288. Souza RB, Powers CM: Concurrent criterion-related validity and reliability of a clinical test to measure femoral anteversion, *J Orthop Sports Phys Ther* 39(8):586–592, 2009.

289. Stafford GH, Villar RN: Ischiofemoral impingement. [Review], *J Bone Joint Surg Br* 93(10):1300–1302, 2011.

290. Stangl-Correa P, Stangl-Herrera W, Correa-Valderrama A, et al.: Postoperative failure frequency of short external rotator and posterior capsule with successful reinsertion after primary total hip arthroplasty: an ultrasound assessment, *J Arthroplasty* 35(12):3607–3612, 2020.

291. Stansfield BW, Nicol AC: Hip joint contact forces in normal subjects and subjects with total hip prostheses: walking and stair and ramp negotiation, *Clin Biomech* 17:130–139, 2002.

292. Stearns KM, Powers CM: Improvements in hip muscle performance result in increased use of the hip extensors and abductors during a landing task, *Am J Sports Med* 42(3):602–609, 2014.

293. Stewart K, Edmonds-Wilson R, Brand R, et al.: Spatial distribution of hip capsule structural and material properties, *J Biomech* 35:1491–1498, 2002.

294. Storaci HW, Utsunomiya H, Kemler BR, et al.: The hip suction seal, part I: the role of acetabular labral height on hip distractive stability, *Am J Sports Med,* 1(11):2726–2732, 2020.

295. Svenningsen S, Apalset K, Terjesen T, et al.: Regression of femoral anteversion. A prospective study of intoeing children, *Acta Orthop Scand* 60:170–173, 1989.

296. Swarup I, Penny CL, Dodwell ER: Developmental dysplasia of the hip: an update on diagnosis and management from birth to 6 months, *Curr Opin Pediatr* 30(1):84–92, 2018.

297. Takizawa M, Suzuki D, Ito H, et al.: Why adductor magnus muscle is large: the function based on muscle morphology in cadavers, *Scand J Med Sci Sports* 24(1):197–203, 2014.

298. Takla A, O'Donnell J, Voight M, et al.: The 2019 international society of hip preservation (ISHA) physiotherapy agreement on assessment and treatment of femoroacetabular impingement syndrome (FAIS): an international consensus statement, *J Hip Preserv Surg* 7(4):631–642, 2020.

299. Tannast M, Hanke MS, Zheng G, et al.: What are the radiographic reference values for acetabular under- and overcoverage? *Clin Orthop Relat Res* 473(4):1234–1246, 2015.

300. Tatu L, Parratte B, Vuillier F, et al.: Descriptive anatomy of the femoral portion of the iliopsoas muscle. Anatomical basis of anterior snapping of the hip, *Surg Radiol Anat* 23(6):371–374, 2001.

301. Teo PL, Hinman RS, Egerton T, et al.: Identifying and prioritizing clinical guideline recommendations most relevant to physical therapy practice for hip and/or knee osteoarthritis, *J Orthop Sports Phys Ther* 49(7):501–512, 2019.

302. Terrell SL, Olson GE, Lynch J: Therapeutic exercise approaches to nonoperative and postoperative management of femoroacetabular impingement syndrome, *J Athl Train* 56(1):31–45, 2021.

303. Thelen DD, Riewald SA, Asakawa DS, et al.: Abnormal coupling of knee and hip moments during maximal exertions in persons with cerebral palsy, *Muscle Nerve* 27:486–493, 2003.

304. Thorborg K, Serner A, Petersen J, et al.: Hip adduction and abduction strength profiles in elite soccer players: implications for clinical evaluation of hip adductor muscle recovery after injury, *Am J Sports Med* 39(1):121–126, 2011.

305. Tonley JC, Yun SM, Kochevar RJ, et al.: Treatment of an individual with piriformis syndrome focusing on hip muscle strengthening and movement reeducation: a case report, *J Orthop Sports Phys Ther* 40(2):103–111, 2010.

306. Uemura K, Atkins PR, Peters CL, et al.: The effect of pelvic tilt on three-dimensional coverage of the femoral head: a computational simulation study using patient-specific anatomy, *Anat Rec* 304(2):258–265, 2021.

307. Vaarbakken K, Steen H, Samuelsen G, et al.: Lengths of the external hip rotators in mobilized cadavers indicate the quadriceps coxa as a primary abductor and extensor of the flexed hip, *Clin Biomech* 29(7):794–802, 2014.

308. Vajapey SP, Morris J, Lynch D, et al.: Nerve injuries with the direct anterior approach to total hip arthroplasty, *JBJS Rev* 8(2):e0109, 2020.

309. Van Alstyne LS, Harrington KL, Haskvitz EM: Physical therapist management of chronic prostatitis/chronic pelvic pain syndrome, *Phys Ther* 90(12):1795–1806, 2010.

310. van Arkel RJ, Amis AA, Cobb JP, et al.: The capsular ligaments provide more hip rotational restraint than the acetabular labrum and the ligamentum teres: an experimental study, *Bone Joint Lett J* 97-B(4):484–491, 2015.

311. Van der Krogt MM, Delp SL, Schwartz MH: How robust is human gait to muscle weakness? *Gait Posture* 36(1).113–119, 2012.

312. van der List JP, Witbreuk MM, Buizer AI, et al.: The head-shaft angle of the hip in early childhood: a comparison of reference values for children with cerebral palsy and normally developing hips, *Bone Joint Lett J* 97-B(9):1291–1295, 2015.

313. van Klij P, Heerey J, Waarsing JH, et al.: The prevalence of cam and pincer morphology and its association with development of hip osteoarthritis, *J Orthop Sports Phys Ther* 48(4):230–238, 2018.

314. van Sleuwen BE, Engelberts AC, Boere-Boonekamp MM, et al.: Swaddling: a systematic review [Review, 82 refs], *Pediatrics* 120(4):e1097–e1106, 2007.

315. Vaswani R, White AE, Feingold J, et al.: Hip-spine syndrome in the nonarthritic patient, *Arthroscopy,* 2022.

316. Walheim GG, Selvik G: Mobility of the pubic symphysis. In vivo measurements with an electromechanic method and a roentgen stereophotogrammetric method, *Clin Orthop Relat Res* 191:129–135, 1984.

317. Walters BL, Cooper JH, Rodriguez JA: New findings in hip capsular anatomy: dimensions of capsular thickness and pericapsular contributions, *Arthroscopy* 30(10):1235–1245, 2014.

318. Wassilew GI, Janz V, Heller MO, et al.: Real time visualization of femoroacetabular impingement and subluxation using 320-slice computed tomography, *J Orthop Res* 31(2):275–281, 2013.

319. Watanabe K, Nunome H, Inoue K, et al.: Electromyographic analysis of hip adductor muscles in soccer instep and side-foot kicking, *Sports BioMech* 19(3):295–306, 2020.

320. Waters RL, Perry J, McDaniels JM, et al.: The relative strength of the hamstrings during hip extension, *J Bone Joint Surg Am* 56(8):1592–1597, 1974.

321. Weinstein SL, Mubarak SJ, Wenger DR: Developmental hip dysplasia and dislocation: Part I, *Instr Course Lect* 53:523–530, 2004.

322. Weinstein SL, Mubarak SJ, Wenger DR: Fundamental concepts of developmental dysplasia of the hip, *Instr Course Lect* 63:299–305, 2014.

323. Weir A, Brukner P, Delahunt E, et al.: Doha agreement meeting on terminology and definitions in groin pain in athletes, *Br J Sports Med* 49(12):768–774, 2015.

324. Wenger DR: Surgical treatment of developmental dysplasia of the hip, *Instr Course Lect* 63:313–323, 2014.

325. Westermann RW, Scott EJ, Schaver AL, et al.: Activity level and sport type in adolescents correlate with the development of cam morphology, *JB JS Open Access* 6(4), 2021.

326. Willard FH, Vleeming A, Schuenke MD, et al.: The thoracolumbar fascia: anatomy, function and clinical considerations [Review], *J Anat* 221(6):507–536, 2012.

327. Wingstrand H, Wingstrand A, Krantz P: Intracapsular and atmospheric pressure in the dynamics and stability of the hip. A biomechanical study, *Acta Orthop Scand* 61:231–235, 1990.

328. Winter DA: *Biomechanics and motor control of human movement*, Hoboken, NJ, 2005, John Wiley & Sons.

329. Woodley SJ, Nicholson HD, Livingstone V, et al.: Lateral hip pain: findings from magnetic resonance imaging and clinical examination, *J Orthop Sports Phys Ther* 38:313–328, 2008.

330. Wright AA, Tarara DT, Gisselman AS, et al.: Do currently prescribed exercises reflect contributing pathomechanics associated with femoroacetabular impingement syndrome? A scoping review, *Phys Ther Sport* 47:127–133, 2021.

331. Wright-Chisem J, Elbuluk AM, Mayman DJ, et al.: The journey to preventing dislocation after total hip arthroplasty: how did we get here? *Bone Joint J* 104-B(1):8–11, 2022.

332. Yadav P, Shefelbine SJ, Ponten E, et al.: Influence of muscle groups' activation on proximal femoral growth tendency, *Biomech Model Mechanobiol* 16(6):1869–1883, 2017.

333. Young JR, Anderson MJ, O'Connor CM, et al.: Team approach: developmental dysplasia of the hip, *JBJS Rev* 8(9), 2020. e20.00030.

334. Zogby AM, Bomar JD, Johnson KP, et al.: Nonoperative management of femoroacetabular impingement in adolescents: clinical outcomes at a mean of 5 years: a prospective study, *Am J Sports Med* 49(11):2960–2967, 2021.

STUDY QUESTIONS

1. What structures convert the greater sciatic notch to a foramen? List three structures (nerves or muscles) that pass through this foramen.

2. What characteristics define the close-packed position of the hip? How do these characteristics differ from most other synovial joints of the body?

3. Explain why a patient with an inflamed capsule of the hip joint may be susceptible to a hip flexion contracture.

4. Describe how the ischiofemoral ligament becomes taut in full internal rotation and extension of the hip. Include both femoral-on-pelvic and pelvic-on-femoral perspectives in your description.

5. While standing, a person performs a full posterior pelvic tilt while keeping the trunk essentially stationary. Describe how this movement could alter the tension in the anterior longitudinal ligament and the ligamentum flavum in the lumbar region.

6. Based on Fig. 12.34, which muscle has (a) the least leverage and (b) the greatest leverage for producing internal rotation torque?

7. A patient sustained a severe fracture of the femoral head and the acetabulum, with marked reduction in contact area between the articular surfaces of the joint. As part of the reconstructive surgery, the surgeon decides to slightly increase the internal moment arm of the hip abductor muscles. What is the likely rationale for this procedure?

8. Explain how a reduced center-edge angle of the acetabulum could favor a dislocation of the hip.

9. Contrast the arthrokinematics of (femoral-on-pelvic) hip flexion and extension with those of internal and external rotation.

10. As indicated in Fig. 12.12, during the swing phase of walking the hip experiences (compression) forces of about 10%–20% of body weight. What causes this force?

11. Fig. 12.21A shows a seated person performing a 30-degree anterior pelvic tilt. What structure(s) is/are most likely responsible for determining the end range of this motion?

12. A person sustained an injury of the cauda equina resulting in reduced function of spinal nerve roots L^3 and below. What pattern of muscular tightness may develop without adequate physical therapy intervention? (Consult Appendix IV, Part A, for assistance in responding to this question.)

13. Justify how bilateral tightness in the adductor longus and brevis could contribute to excessive lumbar lordosis while standing.

14. A standard way for persons to stretch their own rectus femoris is to simultaneously flex the knee while extending the hip. When performing this stretch, some persons with a "tight" rectus femoris purposely hold their extended hip slightly abducted. Why might this be?

15. Estimate the approximate change in joint reaction force at the hip as a healthy, asymptomatic person moves from standing at ease on both legs (i.e., double-limb support) to standing at ease on one leg (i.e., single-limb support). Hint: Approach your estimate based on the role of the hip abductor muscles in providing single-limb support within the frontal plane, as described in Fig. 12.43.

Answers to the study questions are available in the accompanying enhanced eBook version included with the print purchase of this textbook.

Additional Video Educational Content

- Anterior Hip Joint Region of a Cadaver Specimen
  Key features: Anterior hip muscles and adjacent capsular region, ligamentum teres (ligament to the head of the femur), and obturator externus

- Fascia Lata of the Thigh in a Cadaver Specimen
  Key features: Extensive anatomy of the fascia lata, tensor fasciae latae and gluteus maximus attaching into the fascia lata, iliotibial band as it crosses and blends with lateral patellar retinacular fibers of the knee

- Fluoroscopic Observations of Selected Arthrokinematics of the Lower Extremity

ALL VIDEOS in this chapter are available in the accompanying enhanced eBook version included with the print purchase of this textbook.

C h a p t e r

13

Knee

DONALD A. NEUMANN, PT, PhD, FAPTA

CHAPTER AT A GLANCE

The knee consists of the lateral and medial compartments of the tibiofemoral joint and the patellofemoral joint (Fig. 13.1). Motion at the knee occurs in two planes, allowing flexion, extension, and internal and external rotation. Functionally, however, these movements rarely occur independent of movement at other joints within the lower limb. Consider, for example, the interaction among the hip, knee, and ankle during running, climbing, or standing from a seated position. The strong functional association within the joints of the lower limb is reflected by the fact that about two-thirds of the muscles that cross the knee also cross either the hip or the ankle.

The knee has important biomechanical functions, many of which are expressed during walking and running (covered in Chapters 15 and 16). During the "swing phase" of walking, the knee flexes to shorten the functional length of the lower limb; otherwise, the foot would not easily clear the ground. During the "stance phase," the knee flexes slightly, providing shock absorption, conservation of energy, and transmission of forces through the lower limb. Running requires that the knee move through a greater range of motion than walking, especially in the sagittal plane. In addition, rapidly changing direction during walking or running demands adequate internal and external rotation of the knee.

Stability of the knee is based primarily on its soft-tissue constraints rather than on its bony configuration. The massively convex femoral condyles articulate against the only slightly concave articular surfaces of the tibia, held in place by extensive ligaments, joint capsule, menisci, and large muscles. With the foot firmly in contact with the ground, these soft tissues are often subjected to large forces, from both muscles and external sources. Injuries to ligaments, menisci, and articular cartilage are unfortunately common consequences of the large functional demands often placed on the anatomically vulnerable knee. Knowledge of the anatomy and kinesiology of the knee is an essential prerequisite to the understanding of most mechanisms of injury and effective therapeutic intervention.

OSTEOLOGY

Distal Femur

At the distal end of the femur are the large *lateral* and *medial condyles* (from the Greek *kondylos,* knuckle) (Fig. 13.2). *Lateral* and *medial epicondyles* provide elevated attachment sites for the collateral ligaments. A large *intercondylar notch* separates the lateral

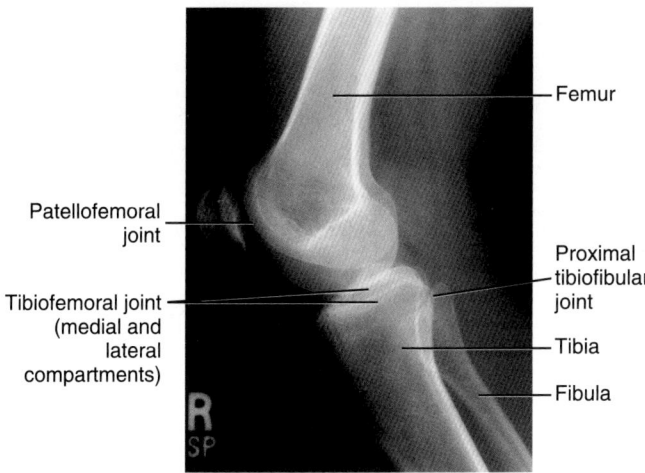

Patellofemoral joint

Femur

Tibiofemoral joint (medial and lateral compartments)

Proximal tibiofibular joint

Tibia

Fibula

FIGURE 13.1 Radiograph showing the bones and associated articulations of the knee.

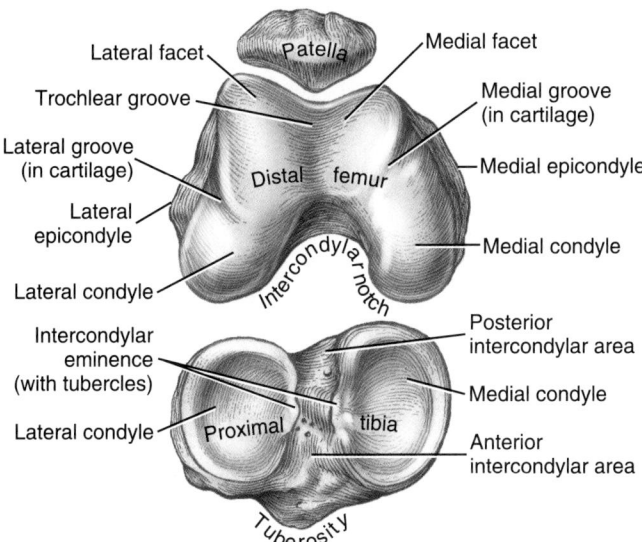

Lateral facet — **Patella** — Medial facet

Trochlear groove — — Medial groove (in cartilage)

Lateral groove (in cartilage) — **Distal   femur** — Medial epicondyle

Lateral epicondyle — — Medial condyle

Lateral condyle — *Intercondylar notch*

Intercondylar eminence (with tubercles) — — Posterior intercondylar area

Lateral condyle — **Proximal   tibia** — Medial condyle

— Anterior intercondylar area

Tuberosity

FIGURE 13.2 Osteology of the right patella, articular surfaces of the distal femur, and proximal tibia.

and medial condyles, forming a passageway for the cruciate ligaments.

The femoral condyles join anteriorly to form the *trochlear (intercondylar) groove* (Fig. 13.2). This groove articulates with the posterior side of the patella, forming the patellofemoral joint. The trochlear groove is concave from side to side and slightly convex from front to back. The sloping sides of the trochlear groove form *lateral* and *medial facets*. The more pronounced lateral facet extends more proximally and anteriorly than the medial facet. The steeper slope of the lateral facet helps to stabilize the patella within the groove during knee movement.

Lateral and *medial grooves* are etched faintly in the cartilage that covers much of the articular surface of the femoral condyles (Fig. 13.2). When the knee is fully extended, the anterior edge of the tibia is aligned with these grooves. The position of the grooves highlights the asymmetry in the shape of the medial and lateral articular surfaces of the distal femur. As explained later, the asymmetry in the shape of the condyles affects the sagittal plane kinematics of the knee, especially near full extension.

Osteologic Features of the Distal Femur
- Lateral and medial condyles
- Lateral and medial epicondyles
- Intercondylar notch
- Trochlear (intercondylar) groove
- Lateral and medial facets (for the patella)
- Lateral and medial grooves (etched in the cartilage of the femoral condyles)
- Popliteal surface

The articular capsule of the knee extends across all sides of the tibiofemoral joint and the patellofemoral joint (see dashed lines in Fig. 13.3). Posteriorly, the capsule attaches just proximal to the femoral condyles, immediately distal to the *popliteal surface* of the femur.

Proximal Tibia and Fibula

Although the fibula has no direct function at the knee, the slender bone splints the lateral side of the tibia and helps maintain its relative vertical alignment. The *head* of the fibula serves as an attachment for the biceps femoris and the lateral collateral ligament. The fibula is attached to the lateral side of the tibia by proximal and distal tibiofibular joints (Fig. 13.3). The structure and function of these joints are discussed in Chapter 14.

Osteologic Features of the Proximal Tibia and Fibula
PROXIMAL FIBULA
- Head

PROXIMAL TIBIA
- Medial and lateral condyles
- Intercondylar eminence (with tubercles)
- Anterior intercondylar area
- Posterior intercondylar area
- Tibial tuberosity
- Soleal line

The tibia transfers a majority of the load between the knee and foot. The proximal end of the tibia flares into *medial* and *lateral condyles,* which form articular surfaces with the distal femur (Fig. 13.3). The superior surfaces of the condyles form a broad flattened region, often referred to as the *tibial plateau.* The plateau supports two smooth articular surfaces that accept the large femoral condyles, forming medial and lateral compartments of the tibiofemoral joint. With menisci removed, the slightly larger, medial articular surface is slightly concave, whereas the lateral articular surface is generally flat, although it undulates slightly between being marginally concave and convex. The articular surfaces are separated down the midline by an *intercondylar eminence,* formed by irregularly shaped medial and lateral tubercles (Fig. 13.2). Shallow anterior and posterior *intercondylar areas* flank both ends of the eminence. The cruciate ligaments and menisci attach along the intercondylar region of the tibia.

The prominent *tibial tuberosity* is located on the anterior surface of the proximal shaft of the tibia (Fig. 13.3A). The tibial tuberosity serves as the distal attachment for the quadriceps femoris muscle, via the patellar tendon. Strong activation of the quadriceps muscle during running and jumping activities can produce large tension at the insertion site of the patellar tendon. In some cases, particularly

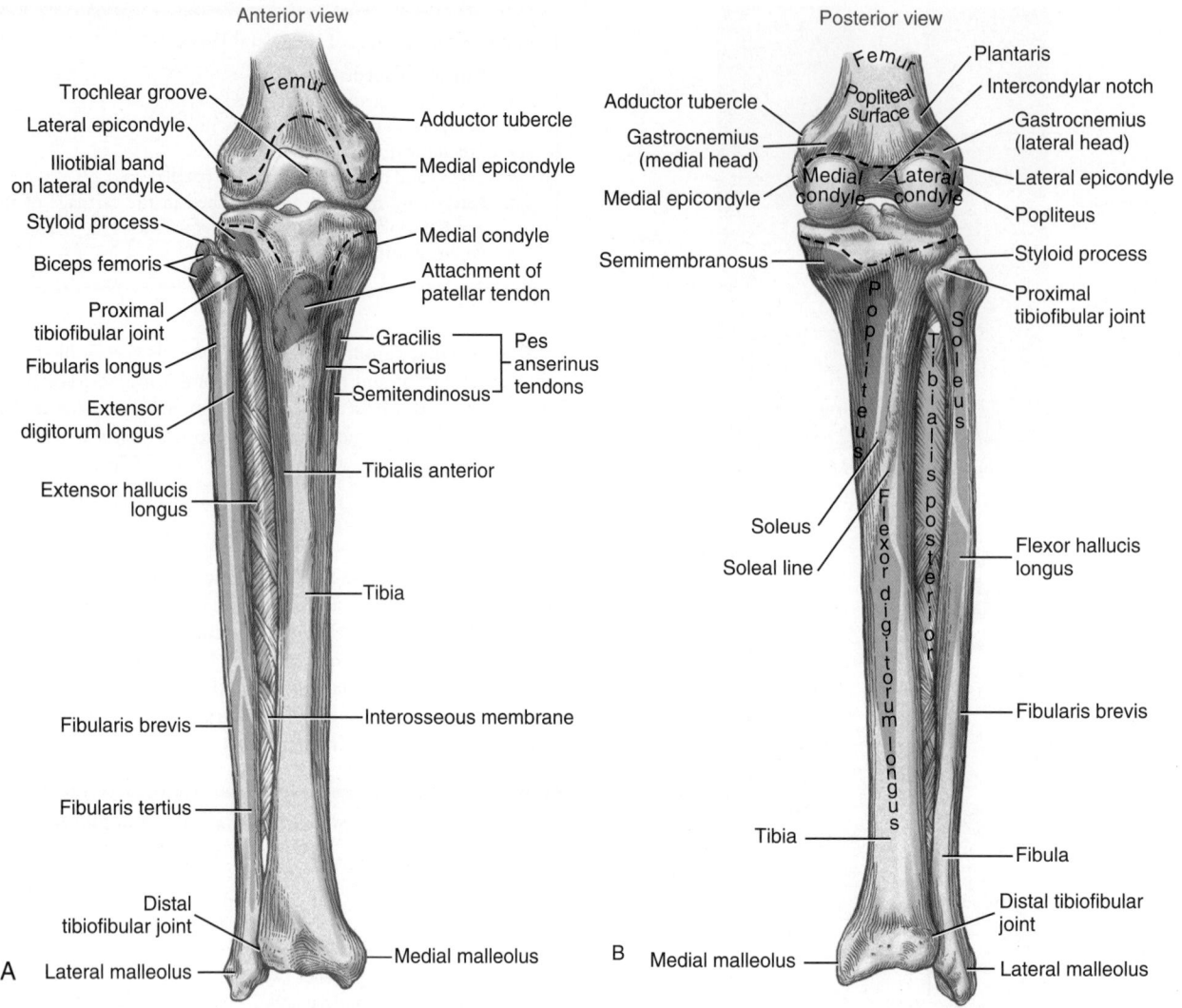

FIGURE 13.3 Right distal femur, tibia, and fibula. (A) Anterior view. (B) Posterior view. Proximal attachments of muscles are shown in red, distal attachments in gray. The dashed lines show the attachment of the joint capsule of the knee.

in rapidly growing adolescents, the tension can create local inflammation and a hypertrophy of the tibial tuberosity, creating an obvious lump, just distal to the patella. This condition is often referred to as *Osgood-Schlatter disease.*

On the posterior side of the proximal tibia is a roughened *soleal line,* coursing diagonally in a distal-to-medial direction (see Fig. 13.3B).

Patella

The patella (from the Latin, "small plate") is a nearly triangular bone embedded within the quadriceps tendon. It is the largest sesamoid bone in the body. The patella has a curved *base* superiorly and a pointed *apex* inferiorly (Figs. 13.4 and 13.5). The thick patellar tendon attaches proximally to the apex of the patella and distally to the tibial tuberosity. In a relaxed standing position, the apex of the patella lies just proximal to the knee joint line. The subcutaneous *anterior surface* of the patella is convex in all directions.

> **Osteologic Features of the Patella**
> - Base
> - Apex
> - Anterior surface
> - Posterior articular surface
> - Vertical ridge
> - Lateral, medial, and "odd" facets

The *posterior articular surface* of the patella is covered by a thick layer of articular cartilage, often cited as the thickest in the body (Fig. 13.5).[343] This thickness is required to help disperse the large contact pressure typically encountered at the patellofemoral joint. A rounded *vertical ridge* runs longitudinally from top to bottom across the posterior surface of the patella. On either side of this ridge is a lateral or medial facet. The larger and slightly concave *lateral facet* matches the general contour of the lateral facet on the trochlear

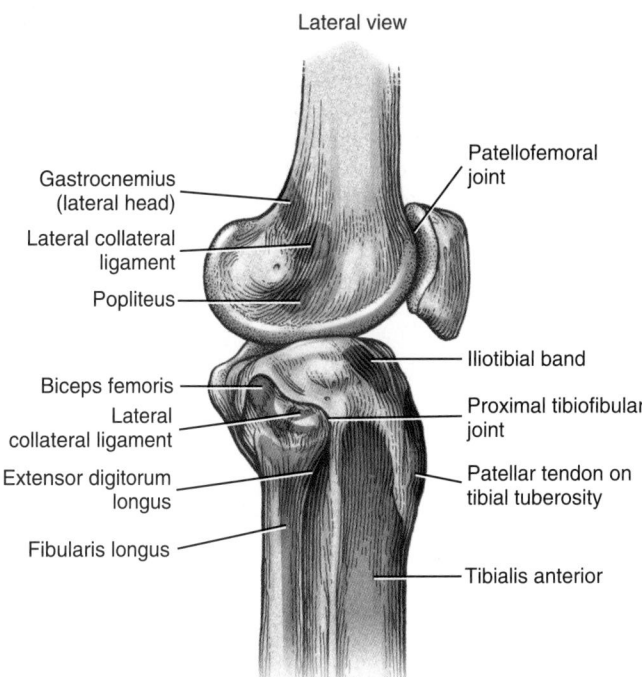

Lateral view

Gastrocnemius (lateral head)
Lateral collateral ligament
Popliteus
Biceps femoris
Lateral collateral ligament
Extensor digitorum longus
Fibularis longus

Patellofemoral joint
Iliotibial band
Proximal tibiofibular joint
Patellar tendon on tibial tuberosity
Tibialis anterior

FIGURE 13.4 Lateral view of the right knee. Note the curved articular surface of the lateral femoral condyle. Proximal attachments of muscles and ligaments are shown in red, distal attachments in gray.

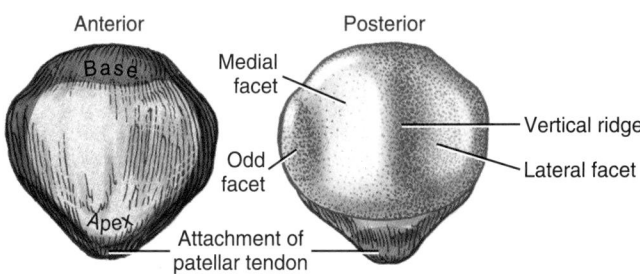

Anterior   Posterior
Base
Medial facet
Vertical ridge
Odd facet
Lateral facet
Apex
Attachment of patellar tendon

FIGURE 13.5 Anterior and posterior surfaces of the right patella. The attachment of the tendon of the quadriceps muscle is indicated in gray; the proximal attachment of the patellar tendon is indicated in red. Note the smooth articular cartilage covering the posterior articular surface of the patella.

groove of the femur (see Fig. 13.2). The *medial facet* shows significant anatomic variation. A third *"odd" facet* exists along the extreme medial border of the medial facet.

ARTHROLOGY

General Anatomic and Alignment Considerations

The shaft of the femur slants slightly medially as it descends toward the knee. This oblique orientation is a result of the approximate 125-degree angle of inclination typically present at the proximal femur (Fig. 13.6A). Because the articular surface of the proximal tibia is oriented nearly horizontally, the knee forms an angle on its lateral side of about 170 to 175 degrees. This normal alignment of the knee within the frontal plane is referred to as *genu valgum.*

Variation in normal frontal plane alignment at the knee is not uncommon. A lateral angle less than about 170 degrees is called

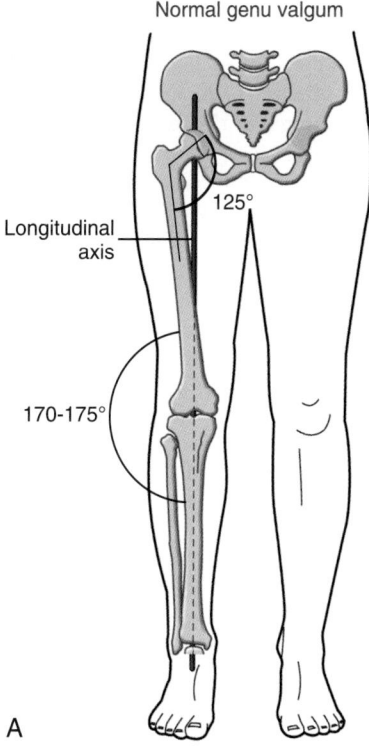

Normal genu valgum

Longitudinal axis
125°
170-175°

A

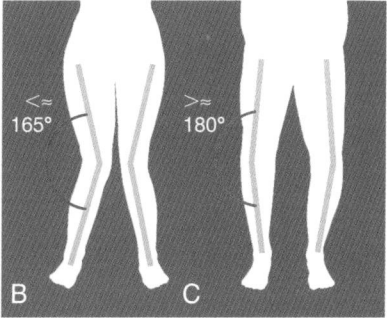

Excessive frontal plane deviation

Excessive genu valgum (knock-knee)   Genu varum (bow-leg)

<≈ 165°   >≈ 180°

B   C

FIGURE 13.6 Frontal plane deviations of the knee. (A) Normal genu valgum. The normal 125-degree angle of inclination of the proximal femur and the longitudinal axis of rotation throughout the entire lower extremity are also shown. (B) and (C) illustrate excessive frontal plane deviations.

excessive genu valgum, or "knock-knee" (Fig. 13.6B). In contrast, a lateral angle that exceeds about 180 degrees is called *genu varum,* or "bow-leg" (Fig. 13.6C).

The longitudinal or vertical axis of rotation at the hip is defined in Chapter 12 as a line connecting the femoral head with the center of the knee joint. As depicted in Fig. 13.6A, this longitudinal axis can be extended inferiorly through the knee to the ankle and foot. The axis mechanically links the horizontal plane movements of the major joints of the entire lower limb. In a weight-bearing position, horizontal plane rotations that occur in the hip, for example, affect the posture of the joints throughout the lower limb as far distal as those in the foot, and vice versa.

Capsule and Reinforcing Ligaments

The fibrous capsule of the knee encloses both the tibiofemoral and patellofemoral joints. The proximal and distal attachments of the capsule to bone are indicated by the dashed lines in Fig. 13.3A and B. The capsule of the knee is significantly reinforced by muscles, ligaments, and fascia. Five reinforced regions of the capsule are described next and are summarized in Table 13.1 below.

The *anterior capsule* of the knee attaches to the margins of the patella and the patellar tendon and is reinforced by the quadriceps muscle and *medial* and *lateral patellar retinacular fibers* (Fig. 13.7). The retinacular fibers are extensions of connective tissues that cover or blend with the vastus lateralis, vastus medialis, and iliotibial band. These fibers form a thin, netlike veil that drapes and interconnects parts of the patella, femur, tibia, quadriceps and patellar tendons, collateral ligaments, and menisci.

The *anterior-lateral capsule* of the knee is reinforced by superficial and deep layers of the iliotibial band, the lateral (fibular) collateral ligament, and the lateral patellar retinacular fibers (Fig. 13.8).[184,343] Deep to the iliotibial band, the capsule thickens and forms the variably described, obliquely running, *anterior-lateral ligament*.[127,185,396] This ligament arises from near the lateral epicondyle of the femur and inserts on the lateral-proximal region of the lateral condyle of the tibia, just anterior and superior to the fibular head. Muscular stability of the anterior-lateral capsule is supplied by the biceps femoris, the tendon of the popliteus, and the lateral head of the gastrocnemius.

The *posterior capsule* is reinforced by the oblique popliteal ligament and the arcuate popliteal ligament (Fig. 13.9). The *oblique popliteal ligament* originates medially from the posterior-medial capsule and the semimembranosus tendon. Laterally and superiorly, the fibers blend with the capsule adjacent to the lateral femoral condyle. This ligament is pulled taut in full knee extension, a position that naturally includes slight external rotation of the tibia relative to the femur. The *arcuate popliteal ligament* originates from the fibular head and divides into two limbs. The larger and more prominent limb arches (hence the term "arcuate") across the tendon of the popliteus muscle to attach to the posterior intercondylar area of the tibia. An inconsistent and smaller limb attaches to the posterior side of the lateral femoral condyle and often to a sesamoid bone (or *fabella*, meaning "little bean") embedded within the lateral head of the

gastrocnemius. The posterior capsule is further reinforced by the popliteus, gastrocnemius, and hamstring muscles, especially by fibrous extensions of the semimembranosus tendon. Unlike the elbow, the knee has no direct bony block against hyperextension. The muscles, ligaments, and posterior capsule limit hyperextension.

The *posterior-lateral capsule* of the knee is reinforced by the arcuate popliteal ligament, the lateral collateral ligament, and the

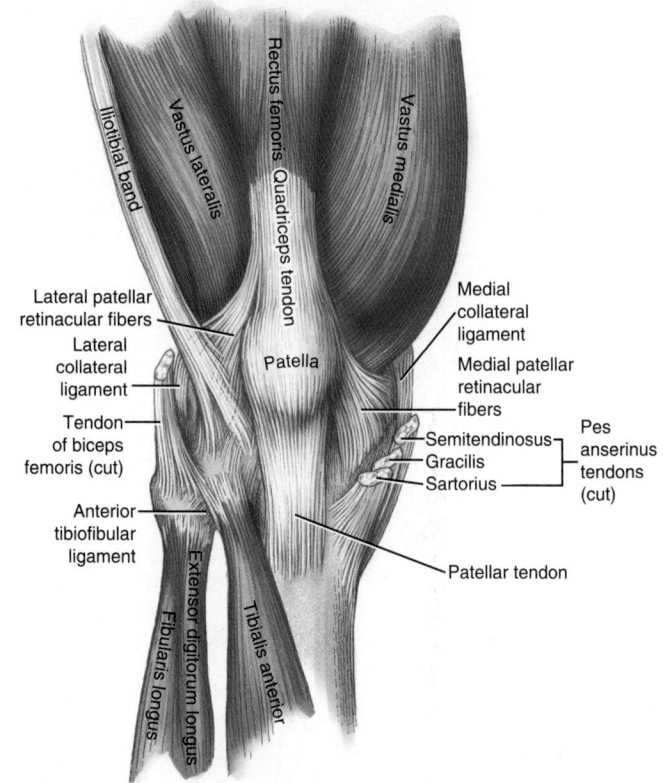

FIGURE 13.7 Anterior view of the right knee, highlighting many muscles and connective tissues. The pes anserinus tendons are cut to expose the medial collateral ligament and the medial patellar retinaculum.

Region of the Capsule	Connective Tissue Reinforcement	Muscular-Tendinous Reinforcement
Anterior	Patellar tendon Patellar retinacular fibers	Quadriceps
Anterior-lateral	Lateral collateral ligament Lateral patellar retinacular fibers Iliotibial band Anterior-lateral ligament	Biceps femoris Tendon of the popliteus Lateral head of the gastrocnemius
Posterior	Oblique popliteal ligament Arcuate popliteal ligament	Popliteus Gastrocnemius Hamstrings, especially the tendon of the semimembranosus
Posterior-lateral	Arcuate popliteal ligament Lateral collateral ligament Popliteofibular ligament	Tendon of the popliteus
Medial	Medial patellar retinacular fibers* Medial collateral ligament Posterior-medial capsule†	Expansions from the tendon of the semimembranosus Tendons of the sartorius, gracilis, and semitendinosus

TABLE 13.1 Ligaments, Fascia, and Muscles That Reinforce the Capsule of the Knee

*Often includes the medial patellofemoral ligament.
†Often formally referred to as the *posterior oblique ligament*.

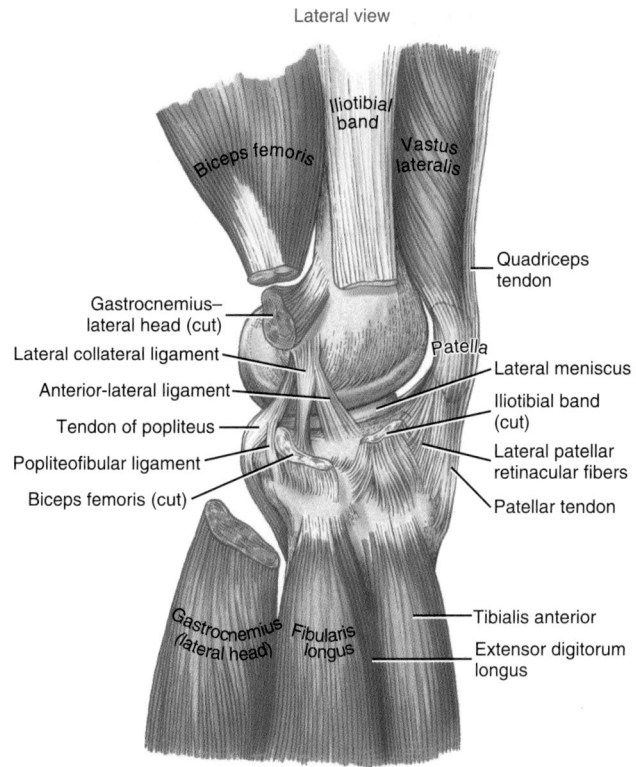

Lateral view

FIGURE 13.8 Lateral view of the right knee shows many muscles and connective tissues, with much of the lateral capsule removed for clarity. The iliotibial band, lateral head of the gastrocnemius, and biceps femoris are cut to better expose the lateral collateral ligament, anterior-lateral ligament, popliteofibular ligament, popliteus tendon, and lateral meniscus.

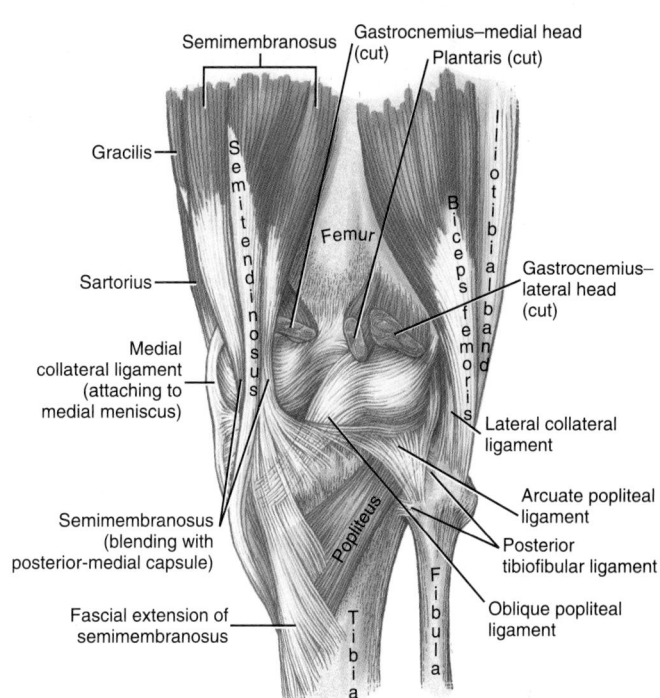

Posterior view

FIGURE 13.9 Posterior view of the right knee that emphasizes the major parts of the posterior capsule: the oblique popliteal and arcuate popliteal ligaments. The lateral and medial heads of the gastrocnemius and plantaris muscles are cut to expose the posterior capsule. Note the popliteus muscle deep in the popliteal fossa, lying partially covered by the fascial extension of the semimembranosus.

tendon of the popliteus. Furthermore, the variable-sized *popliteofibular ligament,* attaching between the tendon of the popliteus and the head of the fibula (Fig. 13.8), provides significant stability to this region of the knee.[155,221,387] The posterior-lateral capsule and associated tendinous-and-ligamentous stabilizers constitute what is often referred to as the *posterior-lateral corner* of the knee. LaPrade and colleagues have estimated that the structures within the posterior-lateral corner of the knee are involved in 16% of all knee injuries, often associated with injuries to other ligaments, such as the medial collateral or cruciate ligaments.[198]

The *medial capsule* of the knee extends in varying thickness from the patellar tendon to the medial edge of the posterior capsule.[307,343] Its anterior one-third consists of a thin layer of fascia reinforced by the medial patellar retinacular fibers (Fig. 13.10). The middle one-third of the capsule is reinforced by a continuation of the medial patellar retinacular fibers and, more substantially, by the superficial and deep fibers of the medial collateral ligament (the deep fibers are not exposed in Fig. 13.10). The posterior one-third of the capsule is relatively thick, originating near the adductor tubercle and blending with tendinous expansions of the semimembranosus and the adjacent posterior capsule. The posterior one-third of the medial capsule is relatively well-defined, referred to generally as the *posterior-medial capsule* as labeled in Fig. 13.10, or, often more formally, as the *posterior oblique ligament.*[34,307] The posterior-medial capsule is reinforced by the flat conjoined tendons of the sartorius, gracilis, and semitendinosus—collectively referred to as the *pes anserinus* (from the Latin, "goose's foot") *tendons.* The posterior two-thirds of the medial capsule and its associated structures provide an important source of stabilization to the knee.[177,306]

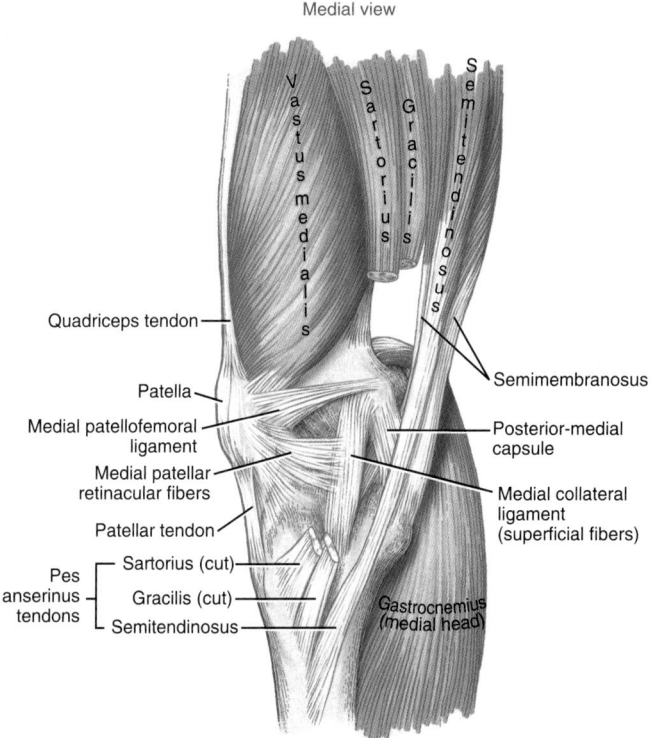

Medial view

FIGURE 13.10 Medial view of the right knee shows many muscles and connective tissues. The tendons of the sartorius and gracilis are cut to better expose the superficial part of the medial collateral ligament, the posterior-medial capsule, and the medial patellofemoral ligament.

Synovial Membrane, Bursae, and Fat Pads

The internal surface of the capsule of the knee is lined with a synovial membrane. The anatomic organization of this membrane is complicated, in part, by the knee's convoluted embryonic development.[343]

The knee may contain as many as 14 bursae, which typically form at inter-tissue junctions that encounter friction during movement. These inter-tissue junctions involve tendon, ligament, skin, bone, capsule, and muscle (Table 13.2). Although some bursae are simply extensions of the synovial membrane, others are formed external to the capsule. Activities that involve excessive and repetitive forces at these inter-tissue junctions potentially lead to bursitis, which involves inflammation of the bursa.

Fat pads are often associated with bursae around the knee. Fat and synovial fluid reduce friction between moving parts. At the knee, the most extensive fat pads are associated with the suprapatellar and deep infrapatellar bursae.

Tibiofemoral Joint

The tibiofemoral joint consists of the articulations between the large, convex femoral condyles and the nearly flat and smaller tibial condyles (see Fig. 13.4). The large articular surface area of the femoral condyles permits extensive knee motion in the sagittal plane for activities such as running, squatting, and climbing. Joint stability is provided not by virtue of bony fit, but by forces and physical containment provided by muscles, ligaments, capsule, menisci, and body weight. For this reason, trauma to the knee often involves injuries to multiple soft tissues.

MENISCI

Anatomic Considerations

The medial and lateral menisci are crescent-shaped, fibrocartilaginous structures located within the knee joint (Fig. 13.11). Acting as gaskets, the menisci transform the articular surfaces of the tibia into smooth, shallow seats for the much larger convex femoral condyles. This transformation is particularly important on the tibia's lateral articular surface because of its more irregular surface contour.

The menisci are anchored to the intercondylar region of the tibia by their free ends, known as *anterior* and *posterior horns* (Fig. 13.11B). The external edge of each meniscus is attached to the tibia and the adjacent capsule by *coronary* (or *meniscotibial*) *ligaments* (Fig. 13.11A). The coronary ligaments are relatively loose, thereby

---

TABLE 13.2 Examples of Bursae at Various Inter-tissue Junctions

Inter-tissue Junction	Examples
Ligament and tendon	Bursa between the lateral collateral ligament and the tendon of the biceps femoris
	Bursa between the medial collateral ligament and tendons of the pes anserinus (i.e., gracilis, semitendinosus, and sartorius)
Muscle and capsule	Unnamed bursa between the medial head of the gastrocnemius and the medial side of the capsule
Bone and skin	*Subcutaneous prepatellar bursa* between the inferior border of the patella and the skin
Tendon and bone	*Semimembranosus bursa* between the tendon of the semimembranosus and the medial condyle of the tibia
Bone and muscle	*Suprapatellar bursa* between the femur and the quadriceps femoris (largest of the knee)
Bone and ligament	*Deep infrapatellar bursa* between the tibia and patellar tendon

---

SPECIAL FOCUS 13.1

Development of Knee Synovial Plicae

During embryonic development, the knee experiences significant physical transformation. Mesenchymal tissues thicken and then reabsorb, forming primitive joint cavities or compartments. Incomplete resorption of the mesenchymal boundaries between the cavities forms vestigial tissues known as *plicae*.[390] Plicae, or synovial pleats, appear as folds in the synovial membranes. Plicae may be very small and unrecognizable, or so large that they nearly separate the knee into different compartments. The literature reports a wide range in the presence of plicae within the knee, ranging from 20% to 70%.[273] Plicae may serve to reinforce the synovial membrane of the knee, although this is only speculation. Plicae exist in other joints to lesser degrees, including the elbow and hip.[390]

The three most described plicae in the knee are named by their position relative to the patella: (1) suprapatellar plica; (2) infrapatellar plica, first called the ligamentum mucosum by Vesalius in the sixteenth century; and (3) mediopatellar plica. Lateral plicae exist in the knee but are rare. The most prominent *mediopatellar plica* is known by many names, including *alar ligament, synovialis patellaris,* and *intra-articular medial band.* Plicae that are unusually large or thickened owing to mechanical irritation or trauma can cause knee pain. Because this pathology occurs most often in the mediopatellar plica, pain is often reported in the anterior-medial region of the knee. If particularly large, some medial plicae are visible or palpable under the skin. Observations during arthroscopy suggest that an enlarged mediopatellar plica can cause abrasion of the facing articular cartilage of the medial femoral condyle.[225] Inflammation and pain of the mediopatellar plica may be easily confused with patellar tendonitis, a torn medial meniscus, or patellofemoral joint pain. Treatment includes rest, anti-inflammatory medication, physical therapy, and, in some cases, arthroscopic resection.

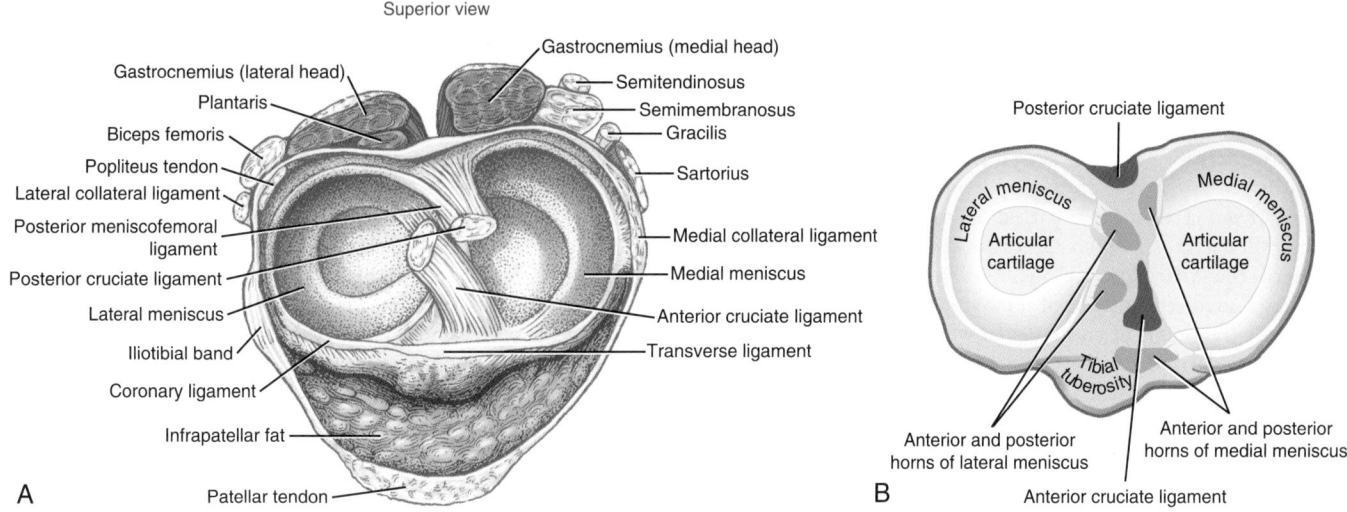

FIGURE 13.11 (A) The superior surface of the right tibia shows the menisci and other cut structures: collateral, cruciate, and posterior meniscofemoral ligaments, as well as muscles and tendons. (This specimen does not have an anterior meniscofemoral ligament.) (B) The superior view of the right tibia marks the attachment points of the menisci and cruciate ligaments within the intercondylar region.

allowing the menisci, especially the lateral meniscus, to pivot freely during movement. A slender *transverse ligament* connects the two menisci anteriorly.

Several muscles have secondary attachments into the menisci. The quadriceps and semimembranosus attach to both menisci,[174] whereas the popliteus attaches to the lateral meniscus.[89] Through these attachments, the muscles help stabilize the menisci in a position that maximizes joint congruency.

The peripheral (external) one-third of the menisci receives a direct source of blood from a series of anastomosing genicular arteries (branches of the popliteal artery) that pierce the surrounding capsule. This region of both menisci is therefore often referred to by surgeons as the "red zone." In contrast, the inner (deeper) two-thirds of the menisci is essentially avascular; this so-called "white zone" receives its nourishment only from synovial fluid. The narrow junction between red and white zones is often referred to as the "pink zone," because of its significantly reduced vascularity compared with the "red zone." The potential for the menisci to heal after injury is directly related to its vascularity as well as to the severity of injury.

The two menisci have different shapes and methods of attaching to the tibia. The medial meniscus has an oval shape, with its external border attaching to the deep surface of the medial collateral ligament and adjacent capsule; the lateral meniscus has more of a circular shape, with its external border attaching only to the anterior-lateral capsule. The tendon of the popliteus passes between the lateral collateral ligament and the external border of the lateral meniscus (Fig. 13.12).

Functional Considerations

The primary function of the menisci is to reduce points of high compressive stress across the tibiofemoral joint.[146] Other functions of the menisci include stabilizing the joint during motion, lubricating the articular cartilage, providing proprioception,[398] and helping to guide the knee's arthrokinematics.

By nearly tripling the area of joint contact, the menisci significantly reduce contact pressure (i.e., force per unit area) on the

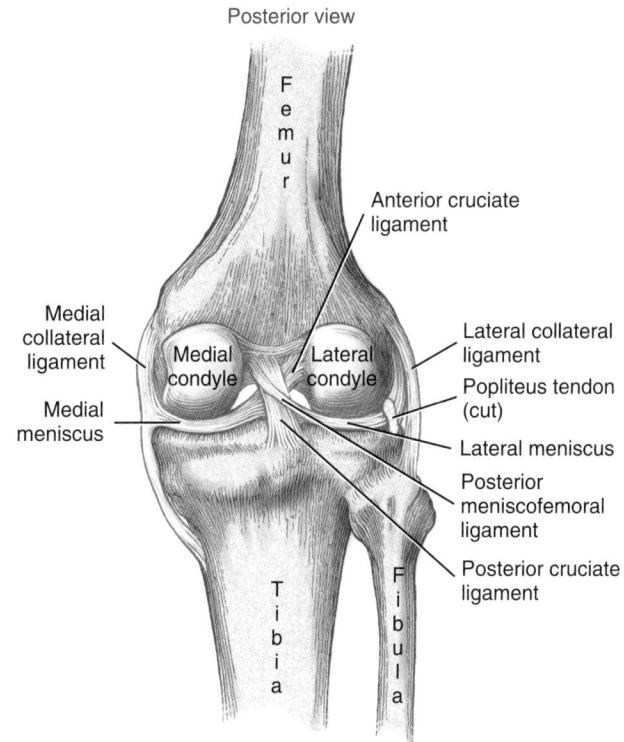

FIGURE 13.12 Posterior view of the deep structures of the right knee after all muscles and the posterior capsule have been removed. Observe the menisci, collateral ligaments, and cruciate ligaments. Note the popliteus tendon, which courses between the lateral meniscus and lateral collateral ligament.

articular cartilage. This method of attenuating peak contact pressure is essential to the health and protection of the knee joint, especially when considering the relatively large and repetitive forces experienced over a lifetime. Compression forces at the knee joint, for example, routinely reach two to three times one's body weight while walking and more than four times one's body weight while landing from a single-limb hop.[61,365,397] A non–weight-bearing activity such as cycling on a stationary bicycle at moderate power produces a knee joint force of almost 1.2 times one's body weight.[193] A complete lateral meniscectomy has been shown to increase peak contact pressures at the knee by 230%, which increases the risk of development of stress-related arthritis.[83,234] Even a tear or a partial meniscectomy significantly increases local stress, which can cause excessive wear and breakdown of the articular cartilage.[245] When possible, surgically repairing a meniscus instead of removing the damaged regions is clearly the treatment of choice, even when the tear extends into the less vascularized regions.[261] In certain cases after a complete meniscectomy, a meniscal allograft transplantation may be indicated (i.e., a meniscus from a genetically nonidentical donor of the same species), with goals of limiting the degeneration of the articular cartilage.

As the knee is loaded while walking or running, the menisci deform in a radial (outward) direction as they are compressed between the femur and tibia. This radial deformation allows part of the compressive load to be absorbed by circumferential tension generated in each meniscus. This load attenuating function, known formally in engineering terms as "hoop stress," requires a structurally intact meniscus. Experiments show that a torn medial meniscus, most notably with an avulsion tear of its posterior horn, loses its ability to optimally incorporate the hoop stress principle,

thereby reducing the capacity for protecting the underlying articular cartilage and bone.[233]

Common Mechanisms of Injury

Tears of the meniscus are the most common injury of the knee, occurring relatively frequently in both the athletic and the general population.[216] According to research cited by Lohmander and colleagues, 50% of all acute injuries of the anterior cruciate ligaments are associated with a concurrent injury to a meniscus.[217] In general, meniscal tears are often associated with a forceful, axial (horizontal plane) rotation of the femoral condyles over a flexed and weight-bearing knee. The axial torsion within the compressed knee can pinch and dislodge the meniscus. A dislodged or folded flap of meniscus (often referred to as a "bucket-handle tear") can mechanically block knee movement.

The medial meniscus is injured twice as frequently as the lateral meniscus.[46] The mechanism of injury for a medial meniscus tear often involves axial rotation and may also involve an external force applied to the lateral aspect of the knee. This force—typically described as a "valgus force"—can cause an excessive valgus position of the knee and subsequent large stress on other structures such as the medial collateral ligament and posterior-medial capsule. Because of the anatomic connections between the medial meniscus and these connective tissues, a significant valgus force delivered to the knee can indirectly strain and thereby injure the medial meniscus.

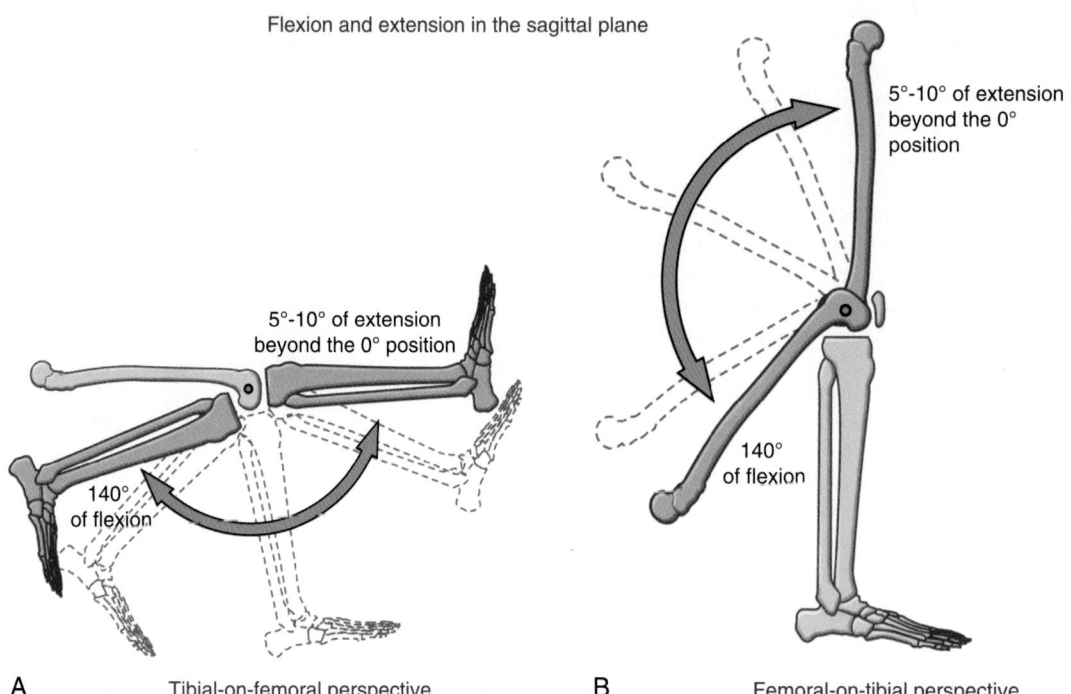

FIGURE 13.13 Sagittal plane motion at the knee. (A) Tibial-on-femoral perspective (femur is stationary). (B) Femoral-on-tibial perspective (tibia is stationary). In each case, the axis of rotation is shown as a small circle through the femoral condyle.

SPECIAL FOCUS 13.2

Meniscofemoral Ligaments

The posterior horn of the lateral meniscus is usually attached to the lateral aspect of the medial condyle of the femur by anterior or posterior *meniscofemoral ligaments.* The meniscofemoral ligaments are named for their position relative to the posterior cruciate ligament (PCL), with which they share similar femoral attachments. Only the posterior meniscofemoral ligament is present in the specimen illustrated in Fig. 13.11A.

Cadaveric studies reveal that at least one of the meniscofemoral ligaments is present in 92% of knees, and both are present in 32% of knees.[120] The posterior meniscofemoral ligament is usually the more substantial of the two structures. After arising

from the posterior horn of the lateral meniscus, the posterior meniscofemoral ligament attaches to the femur just posterior and slightly medial to the PCL (see Fig. 13.12). The meniscofemoral ligaments sometimes serve as the only bony attachment of the posterior horn of the lateral meniscus. The exact functions of the meniscofemoral ligaments are uncertain, although they may offer a secondary restraint to posterior translation of the tibia, especially with the knee flexed 90 degrees.[3] Acting in concert with the popliteus muscle, the ligaments may also help stabilize the posterior horn of the lateral meniscus during movement.[294]

OSTEOKINEMATICS AT THE TIBIOFEMORAL JOINT

The tibiofemoral (knee) joint possesses two degrees of freedom: flexion and extension in the sagittal plane and, provided the knee is at least slightly flexed, internal and external rotation. Frontal plane motion at the knee occurs passively only, limited to about 6 to 7 degrees.[231]

Flexion and Extension

Flexion and extension at the knee occur about a medial-lateral axis of rotation for both tibial-on-femoral and femoral-on-tibial situations (Fig. 13.13). Range of motion varies with age and sex, but in general the healthy knee moves from 130 to 150 degrees of flexion to about 5 to 10 degrees beyond the 0-degree (straight) position.[128,305]

The medial-lateral axis of rotation for flexion and extension is not fixed but migrates within the femoral condyles. The curved path of the axis is known as an "evolute" (Fig. 13.14). The path of the axis of rotation is influenced by the eccentric (out-of-round) curvature of the femoral condyles.[140] As described in Chapter 2, a slightly moveable or migrating axis of rotation is more the rule than the exception for most joints in the body. Chapter 2 also illustrates a method for estimating the axis of rotation at the knee using a series of radiographs.

The migrating axis of rotation has biomechanical and clinical implications. Biomechanically, the migrating axis alters the length of the internal moment arm of the flexor and extensor muscles of the knee. This fact may explain, in part, why maximal-effort internal torque varies across the range of motion. Clinically, many external devices that attach to the knee, such as a goniometer, an isokinetic testing device, or a hinged knee orthosis, rotate about a *fixed* axis of rotation. During knee motion, therefore, the external devices may rotate in a slightly dissimilar arc than the leg. Consequently, a hinged orthosis, for example, may act as a piston relative to the leg, causing rubbing against and abrasion to the skin. To minimize this consequence, care must be taken to align the fixed axis of the external device as close as possible to the "average" axis

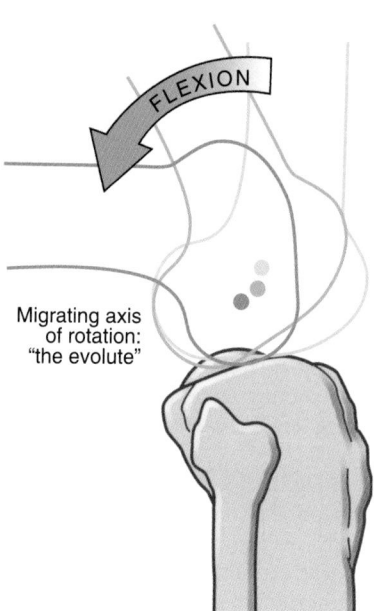

FIGURE 13.14 The flexing knee generates a migrating medial-lateral axis of rotation (shown as *three small circles*).

of rotation of the knee, which is close to the lateral epicondyle of the femur.

Internal and External (Axial) Rotation

Internal and external rotation of the knee will be described for both tibial-on-femoral and femoral-on-tibial perspectives (Fig. 13.15). These kinematics occur as a rotation in a plane perpendicular to the longitudinal axis that courses within the length of the tibial shaft. This "intramedullary" tibial axis is assumed to remain in place, regardless of knee position or relative kinematics (i.e., proximal-on-distal or distal-on-proximal kinematics).

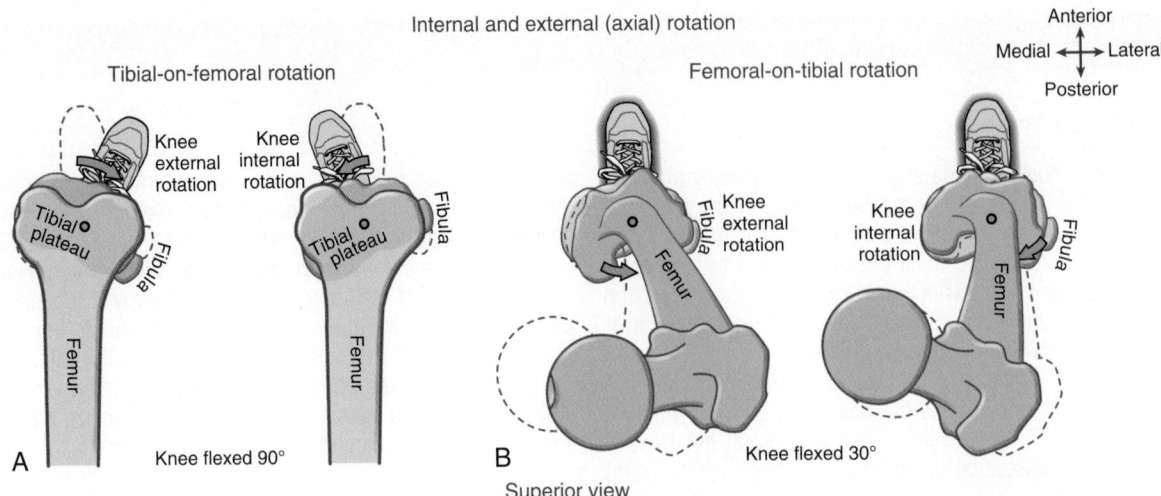

FIGURE 13.15 Internal and external (axial) rotation of the right knee. The axes of rotation are shown as small circles near the center of the joint. (A) Tibial-on-femoral (knee) rotation. In this case the direction of the knee rotation (internal or external) is the same as the motion of the tibia; the femur is stationary. (B) Femoral-on-tibial rotation. In this case the tibia is stationary and the femur is rotating (over a partially flexed knee). The direction of the knee rotation (external or internal) is the opposite of the motion of the moving femur: *external rotation* of the knee occurs by internal rotation of the femur; *internal rotation* of the knee occurs by external rotation of the femur.

The term "axial rotation" is often used to describe the "rotary" osteokinematics illustrated in Fig. 13.15. Little, if any, significant axial rotation occurs between the tibia and femur with the knee fully extended. The rotation is resisted by passive tension in taut ligaments and capsular tissues, and by increased bony congruity within the joint. The freedom of axial rotation significantly increases, however, as the knee is progressively flexed. A knee flexed to 90 degrees, for example, can perform about 40 to 45 degrees of total axial rotation.[246,264] External rotation range of motion generally exceeds internal rotation by a ratio of nearly 2:1.

As depicted in Fig. 13.15, axial rotation of the knee occurs by either tibial-on-femoral or femoral-on-tibial rotation. Axial rotation of the knee provides an important functional element of mobility to the lower extremity as a whole. The terminology used to describe axial rotation of the knee is important to understand. As a rule, the naming of axial rotation of the knee is based on the position of *the tibial tuberosity relative to the anterior distal femur.* External rotation of the knee, for example, occurs when the tibial tuberosity is located lateral to the distal anterior femur. This rule, however, does *not* stipulate whether the femur or tibia is the moving bone; it only stipulates the relative articular orientation of the rotated knee. To demonstrate, compare external rotation of the knee in parts A and B of Fig. 13.15. Tibial-on-femoral external rotation of the knee occurs as the tibia rotates *externally* relative to a stationary femur. On the other hand, femoral-on-tibial external rotation of the knee occurs as the *femur rotates internally* relative to a stationary tibia (and foot). Both examples fit the definition of external rotation of the knee because both motions result in a similar articular orientation: the tibial tuberosity is located lateral to the anterior distal femur. The distinction between *bony* rotation (tibial or femoral) and *knee joint* rotation must always be clear to avoid misinterpretation. This point is particularly important in describing femoral-on-tibial osteokinematics.

ARTHROKINEMATICS AT THE TIBIOFEMORAL JOINT

Extension of the Knee

Fig. 13.16 depicts the arthrokinematics of the last 90 degrees of active knee extension. During *tibial-on-femoral extension,* the articular surface of the tibia rolls and slides anteriorly on the femoral condyles (Fig. 13.16A).

During *femoral-on-tibial extension,* as in standing up from a seated position, the femoral condyles simultaneously roll anteriorly and slide posteriorly on the articular surface of the tibia (Fig. 13.16B). These "offsetting" arthrokinematics limit the magnitude of anterior translation of the femur on the tibia. The quadriceps muscle directs the roll of the femoral condyles and stabilizes the menisci against the horizontal shear caused by the sliding femur.

"Screw-Home" Rotation of the Knee

Locking the knee in full extension requires about 10 degrees of external rotation.[152] The rotary locking action has historically been referred to as the *"screw-home" rotation,* based on the observable twisting of the knee during the last 30 or so degrees of extension. The external rotation described here is fundamentally different from the axial rotation illustrated in Fig. 13.15. Screw-home (external) rotation is described as a *conjunct rotation,* emphasizing the fact that it is mechanically linked (or coupled) to the flexion and extension kinematics and cannot be performed independently. The combined external rotation and knee extension maximizes the overall joint contact area and congruence within the knee.[275] Furthermore, this stable, close-packed position provides maximum overlap of the thickest layers of articular cartilage at the femoral tibial joint interface.[10] This overlap naturally protects the underlying subchondral bone, protection that is lost in a knee that lacks full extension.

To observe the screw-home rotation at the knee, have a partner sit with the knee flexed to about 90 degrees. Draw a line on the skin between the tibial tuberosity and the apex of the patella. After the partner completes full tibial-on-femoral extension, redraw this line between the same landmarks and note the change in position of the externally rotated tibia. A similar but less obvious locking mechanism also functions during femoral-on-tibial extension (compare parts A and B of Fig. 13.16). When one rises from a seated position, for example, the knee locks into extension as the femur internally rotates relative to the fixed tibia. Regardless of whether the thigh or leg is the moving segment, both knee extension movements depicted in Fig. 13.16A and B show a knee *joint* that is relatively *externally* rotated when fully extended.

The screw-home rotation mechanics are driven by at least three factors: the shape of the medial femoral condyle, the passive tension in the anterior cruciate ligament, and the slight lateral pull of the quadriceps muscle (Fig. 13.17). The most important (or at least obvious) factor is the shape of the medial femoral condyle. As depicted in Fig. 13.17B, the articular surface of the medial femoral condyle curves about 30 degrees laterally as it approaches the trochlear groove. Because the articular surface of the medial condyle extends farther anteriorly than the lateral condyle, the tibia is obliged to "follow" the laterally curved path into full tibial-on-femoral extension. During femoral-on-tibial extension, the femur follows a medially curved path on the tibia. In either case, the result is external rotation of the knee at full extension (Video 13.1).

Flexion of the Knee

The arthrokinematics of knee flexion between full extension and 90 degrees of flexion would likely occur in essentially a reverse fashion as that depicted in Fig. 13.16. Unlocking a fully extended knee requires that the joint first internally rotate slightly.[25,275] This rotation is driven primarily by the popliteus muscle. The muscle can rotate the femur externally to initiate femoral-on-tibial flexion or can rotate the tibia internally to initiate tibial-on-femoral flexion.

Internal and External (Axial) Rotation of the Knee

As described earlier, the knee must be flexed to maximize independent axial rotation between the tibia and femur. Once the knee is flexed, the arthrokinematics of internal and external rotation involve primarily a *spin* between the menisci and the articular surfaces of the tibia and femur. Axial rotation of the femur over the tibia causes the menisci to deform slightly, as they are compressed by the spinning femoral condyles. The menisci are stabilized by connections from active musculature such as the popliteus and semimembranosus muscles.

MEDIAL AND LATERAL COLLATERAL LIGAMENTS

Anatomic Considerations

The *medial (tibial) collateral ligament* (MCL) is a flat, broad structure that spans the medial side of the joint. Although different terminology exists, this chapter describes the MCL as having superficial and deep parts.[34,197] The larger *superficial part* consists of a relatively well-defined set of parallel running fibers about 10 cm in length (see Fig. 13.10). After arising from the medial epicondyle of the femur, the superficial fibers course distally to blend with medial patellar retinacular fibers before attaching to the medial-proximal aspect of the tibia. The fibers attach just posterior to the distal attachments of the closely aligned tendons of the sartorius and the gracilis.

The *deep part* of the MCL consists of a shorter and more oblique set of fibers, lying immediately deep and slightly posterior and distal to the proximal attachment of the superficial fibers. Although not visible in Fig. 13.10, the deep fibers attach distally to the

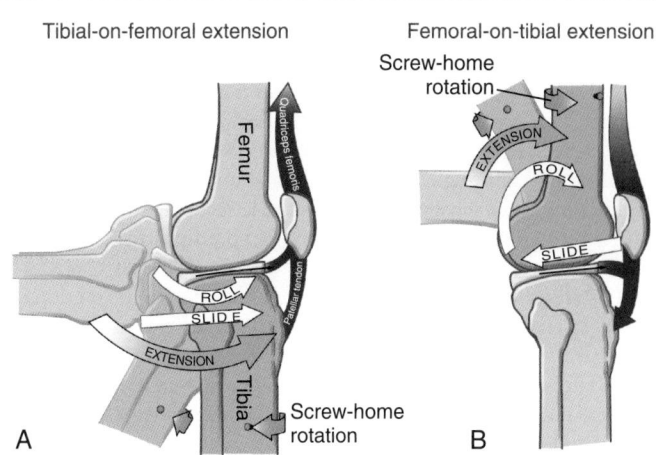

FIGURE 13.16 The active arthrokinematics of knee extension. (A) Tibial-on-femoral perspective. (B) Femoral-on-tibial perspective. In both (A) and (B), the menisci are shown pulled anteriorly by the contracting quadriceps muscle.

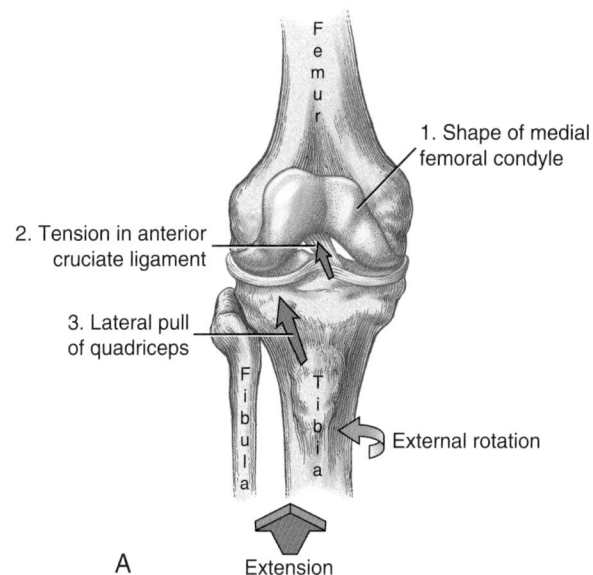

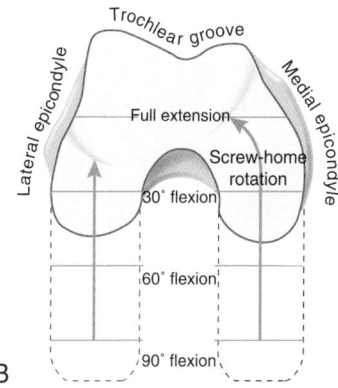

FIGURE 13.17 The "screw-home" rotation locking mechanism of the knee. (A) During terminal tibial-on-femoral extension, three factors contribute to the locking mechanism of the knee. Each factor contributes bias to external rotation of the tibia, relative to the femur. (B) The two arrows depict the path of the tibia across the femoral condyles during the last 90 degrees of extension. Note that the curved medial femoral condyle helps to direct the tibia to its externally rotated and locked position.

posterior-medial joint capsule, medial meniscus, and tendon of the semimembranosus muscle.

The *lateral (fibular) collateral ligament* is a relatively short, cord-like structure that runs nearly vertically between the lateral epicondyle of the femur and the head of the fibula (see Fig. 13.8).[312] Interestingly, although the MCL has about twice the ultimate failure point (i.e., tensile strength) as the lateral collateral ligament, the two structures exhibit nearly equivalent prerupture stiffness (i.e., resistance to elongation).[387]

Distally, the lateral collateral ligament blends with the tendon of the biceps femoris muscle. Unlike its medial counterpart, the MCL, the lateral collateral ligament typically does *not* attach to the adjacent (lateral) meniscus (see Fig. 13.12). As mentioned earlier, the tendon of the popliteus courses *between* the lateral meniscus and the lateral collateral ligament.

Functional Considerations

The primary function of the collateral ligaments is to limit excessive knee motion within the *frontal* plane. With the knee nearly or fully extended, the MCL provides a primary resistance against a valgus (abduction) force.[24,117,197] The lateral collateral ligament, on the other hand, provides a primary resistance against a

varus-producing (adduction) force.[387] Table 13.3 lists several other tissues that provide restraint against valgus and varus forces producing to the knee.

A secondary function of the medial and lateral collateral ligaments is to produce a generalized stabilizing tension to the near or fully extended knee. Although some of the fibers that constitute the very broad MCL are taut throughout a wide arc of knee flexion and extension, most are positioned slightly posterior to the medial-lateral axis of rotation of the knee and therefore are pulled most taut in or *near full extension*.[271,306,363] This natural tensioning of much of the MCL near full extension provides some protective stability to the knee, such as during the early load acceptance phase of walking.[214] Other structures that become more taut in full extension are the posterior-medial capsule, the oblique popliteal ligament (representative of the posterior capsule), the knee flexor muscles, and components of the anterior cruciate ligament.[271,281] Fig. 13.18 demonstrates these tissues as being relatively slack in flexion (A) and more taut as the knee assumes the locked position of full femoral-on-tibial extension (B). Full extension—which includes the kinematics of the screw-home rotation—elongates the collateral ligaments approximately 20% beyond their length at full flexion.[371] Although a valuable stabilizer in full extension, a taut MCL and posterior-medial

TABLE 13.3	**Tissues That Provide Primary and Secondary Restraints Against Valgus- and Varus-Directed Forces to the Knee***	
	Resists a Valgus-directed Force	**Resists a Varus-directed Force**
Primary restraint:	Medial collateral ligament: • *superficial fibers* especially with knee flexed 20–30 degrees • *deep fibers* especially with knee in full extension Anterior cruciate ligament	Lateral collateral ligament
Secondary restraint:	Posterior-medial capsule† (includes semimembranosus tendon) Posterior cruciate ligament Joint contact laterally Compression of the lateral meniscus Medial retinacular fibers Pes anserinus (i.e., tendons of the sartorius, gracilis, and semitendinous) Gastrocnemius (medial head)	Posterior-lateral corner of the knee (includes posterior-lateral capsule, arcuate popliteal ligament, lateral collateral ligament, popliteofibular ligament, and the popliteus tendon) Iliotibial band Biceps femoris tendon Joint contact medially Compression of the medial meniscus Anterior and posterior cruciate ligaments Gastrocnemius (lateral head)

*Assumes a near or fully extended knee.
†Also referred to as the *posterior oblique ligament*.

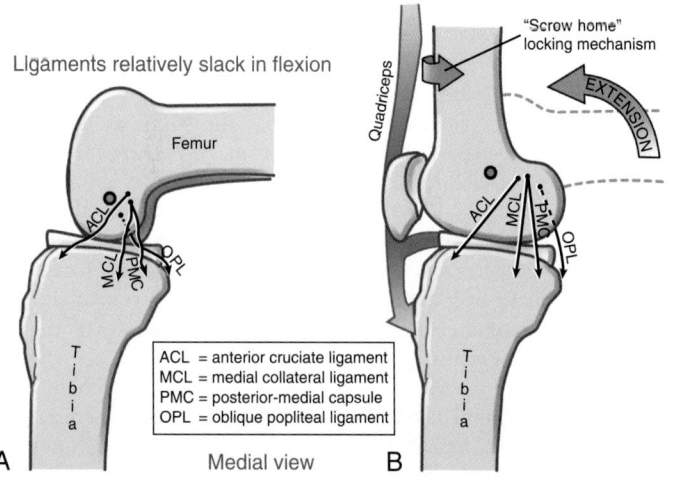

FIGURE 13.18 Medial view of the knee depicts the relative elongation of some fibers of the medial collateral ligament, oblique popliteal ligament, posterior capsule, and components of the anterior cruciate ligament *(ACL)* during active femoral-on-tibial extension. (A) In knee flexion the structures are shown in a relatively slackened (or least taut) state. (B) The structures are pulled relatively taut as the knee actively extends by contraction of the quadriceps. Note the "screw-home" rotation of the knee during end-range extension. The combined external rotation and extension on the knee specifically elongate the posterior-medial capsule and oblique popliteal ligament (within the posterior capsule).

Ligaments relatively slack in flexion

Ligaments pulled taut in extension

"Screw home" locking mechanism

EXTENSION

Quadriceps

Femur

Tibia

ACL

MCL

PMC

OPL

Tibia

ACL = anterior cruciate ligament
MCL = medial collateral ligament
PMC = posterior-medial capsule
OPL = oblique popliteal ligament

A   Medial view   B

capsule in extension are especially vulnerable to injury from a valgus-producing external load delivered over a planted foot. This is a common mechanism of injury to the medial knee structures as well as the anterior cruciate ligament from a "clipping" infraction in American football.

The collateral ligaments and adjacent capsule also provide resistance to the extremes of internal and external rotation of the knee.[312,320,371] Most notable in this regard are the elongation and subsequent increased passive tension in fibers of the MCL at the extremes of external rotation of the knee.[34,117,306] Planting the right foot securely on the ground and vigorously rotating the superimposed femur (and entire body) to the left, for example, may damage the superficial fibers of the right MCL. This potential for injury increases if the externally rotating knee (i.e., internally rotating femur) is simultaneously experiencing a substantial valgus-producing external load.

Table 13.4 provides a summary of the functions and common mechanisms of injury for the major ligaments of the knee, including the posterior-medial and posterior capsule. Although the different tissues are organized as separate anatomic entities, the restraining function of each is based on the combined action of all. The integrity of the MCL, for example, helps protect the anterior cruciate ligament, and vice versa. This co-dependency in function partially explains why a single-plane traumatic event can injure multiple structures.

ANTERIOR AND POSTERIOR CRUCIATE LIGAMENTS

General Considerations

Cruciate, meaning cross-shaped, describes the spatial relation of the anterior and posterior cruciate ligaments as they cross within the intercondylar notch of the femur (see ahead Fig. 13.19). The cruciate ligaments are intracapsular and mostly surrounded by an extensive synovial membrane. The ligaments have a relatively poor blood supply, originating primarily from the medial genicular artery, a branch of the popliteal artery. Most of the blood that reaches the ligaments flows through very small vessels embedded within an extensive synovial membrane that lines the ligaments. As with the menisci, the scant blood supply to the cruciates limits their ability to heal after injury.

The cruciate ligaments are named according to their relative attachments to the tibia (see Fig. 13.11). Both ligaments are thick and strong, reflecting their important role in providing stability to the knee. The anterior cruciate ligament in younger adults, for example, can tolerate tensile loads of about 1800 N (405 lb) before rupture, with failure occurring either within the ligament or within the ligament-bone interface.[51,391]

Acting together, the anterior and posterior cruciate ligaments resist the extremes of essentially *all* knee movements (review Table 13.4). Most important, however, the cruciate ligaments provide most of the resistance to anterior-posterior shear forces created between the tibia and femur. These shear forces are inherent to the natural sagittal plane kinematics associated with walking, running, squatting, and landing from a jump. Furthermore, the oblique and crossed orientation of the ligaments also allow them to stabilize the knee within the frontal and horizontal planes, such as those that may occur during twisting and lateral "cutting" maneuvers.

In addition to providing essential dynamic stability to the knee, tension in the anterior and posterior cruciate ligaments helps guide the knee's arthrokinematics. Furthermore, because the cruciates contain mechanoreceptors, they provide the nervous system with proprioceptive feedback.[300,317] In addition to

TABLE 13.4 Function of Ligaments at the Knee and Common Mechanisms of Injury		
Structure	**Function**	**Common Mechanisms of Injury**
Medial collateral ligament (and posterior-medial capsule)	1. Resists valgus (abduction) 2. Resists knee extension 3. Resists extremes of axial rotation (especially knee external rotation)	1. Valgus force with foot planted (e.g., "clip" in football) 2. Severe hyperextension of the knee
Lateral collateral ligament	1. Resists varus (adduction) 2. Resists knee extension 3. Resists extremes of axial rotation	1. Varus-producing force with foot planted 2. Severe hyperextension of the knee
Posterior capsule	1. Resists knee extension 2. Oblique popliteal ligament resists knee external rotation 3. Posterior-lateral capsule resists varus	1. Hyperextension or combined hyperextension with external rotation of the knee
Anterior cruciate ligament	1. Most fibers resist extension (either excessive anterior translation of the tibia, posterior translation of the femur, or a combination thereof) 2. Resists extremes of valgus, varus, and axial rotation	1. Large valgus force with the foot firmly planted 2. Large axial rotation torque applied to the knee (in either rotation direction), with the foot firmly planted 3. Any combination of 1 and 2 (listed directly above), especially involving strong quadriceps contraction with the knee biased toward extension 4. Severe hyperextension of the knee
Posterior cruciate ligament	1. Most fibers resist knee flexion (either excessive posterior translation of the tibia or anterior translation of the femur, or a combination thereof) 2. Resists extremes of varus or valgus, or axial rotation especially with the knee flexed to or beyond 90 degrees	1. Falling on a fully flexed knee (with ankle fully plantar flexed) such that the proximal tibia first strikes the ground 2. Any event that causes a forceful posterior translation of the tibia (i.e., "dashboard" injury) or anterior translation of the femur, especially while the knee is flexed 3. Large axial rotation or valgus-varus-directed torque to the knee with the foot firmly planted, especially when the knee is flexed 4. Severe hyperextension of the knee causing a large gapping of the posterior side of the joint

helping control movement, these sensory receptors may also have a protective role by reflexively limiting muscle activation that could create large and potentially damaging strain on the ligaments.[361]

General Functions of the Anterior and Posterior Cruciate Ligaments

- Provide multiple planar dynamic stability to the knee, most notably to shear forces in the sagittal plane
- Guide the natural arthrokinematics, especially those related to the restraint of anterior-posterior translation between the tibia and femur
- Contribute to proprioception of the knee

ANTERIOR CRUCIATE LIGAMENT

Anatomy and Function

The anterior cruciate ligament (ACL) inserts along an impression on the anterior intercondylar area of the tibial plateau. From this attachment, the ligament twists on itself as it courses obliquely in a posterior, superior, and lateral direction to attach on the medial side of the lateral femoral condyle (Fig. 13.19). The collagen fibers within the ACL form discrete sets of spiraling bundles, made primarily of type I collagen. Although different numbers and descriptions have been reported, most authors cite *two* sets of fiber bundles within the ACL: *anterior-medial* and *posterior-lateral,* named according to their relative attachments to the tibia.[57,82] Although the individual fiber bundles are not obvious to the naked eye, they are discernable through microdissection.

The tension, twist, and overall spatial orientation of the fiber bundles within the ACL change as the knee flexes and extends.[7] At any given point throughout the sagittal plane range of motion, it is likely that some fibers of the ACL are relatively taut. Most fibers, however, especially those within the posterior-lateral bundle, become *increasingly taut as the knee approaches and reaches full extension.*[7,81,82,251] These same fibers slacken as the knee is progressively flexed. In addition to most fibers of the ACL, the posterior

capsule, parts of the collateral ligaments, and all knee flexor muscles become relatively taut in extension, thereby helping to stabilize the knee especially during weight-bearing activities (reviewed in Fig. 13.18B). Extending the knee well beyond the neutral anatomic position further elongates and stretches these tissues, increasing the likelihood of tissue failure.

During the last approximately 50 to 60 degrees of full knee extension, the active force generated by the contracting quadriceps pulls the tibia *anteriorly,* thereby driving the anterior slide arthrokinematics (Fig. 13.20A).[80,232] The resulting tension in the stretched fibers of the ACL helps limit the extent of this anterior slide. Clinically, it is useful to appreciate the general similarity between the anterior force placed on the ACL by quadriceps contraction and the anterior-directed pull applied to the tibia as a clinician performs an *anterior drawer* test (see Fig. 13.20B). This test is one of several used by clinicians to assess the anterior laxity in a knee with a suspected injured ACL. The basic component of this test involves pulling the proximal end of the tibia (leg) forward with the knee flexed to about 90 degrees. In the normal knee the ACL provides about 85% of the total passive resistance to the anterior translation of the tibia.[42] An anterior translation of 8 mm (⅓ inch) greater than the contralateral knee suggests a possible tear of the ACL. As illustrated in Fig. 13.20B, protective spasm in the hamstring muscles may limit anterior translation of the tibia, thereby masking a torn ACL.

Clinically, the quadriceps muscle has been referred to as an "ACL antagonist." This naming reflects the fact that the contraction force from the quadriceps at relatively low flexion angles stretches (or antagonizes) most fibers of the ACL.[81,104,238] Studies have reported a 4.4% strain (relative elongation) of the ACL after a maximal-effort, isometric activation of the quadriceps at 15 degrees of flexion.[27] Theoretically, this level of strain would increase from a very forceful contraction of the quadriceps that abruptly brings the tibia into full knee extension. The ability of the quadriceps to strain the ACL is greatest at full extension because this position maximizes the angle-of-insertion of the patellar tendon relative to the tibia (see α in Fig. 13.20A).[80] The greater this angle-of-insertion, the greater the proportion of quadriceps force is available to translate the tibia *anteriorly* relative to the femur. The

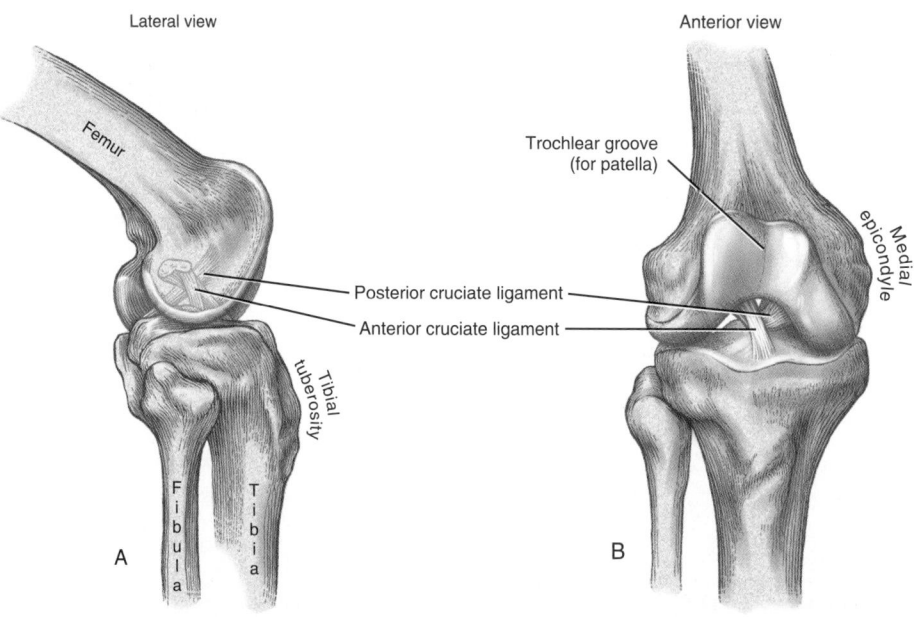

FIGURE 13.19 The anterior and posterior cruciate ligaments of the right knee. (A) Lateral view. (B) Anterior view. The two fiber bundles within the anterior cruciate ligament are evident in (A).

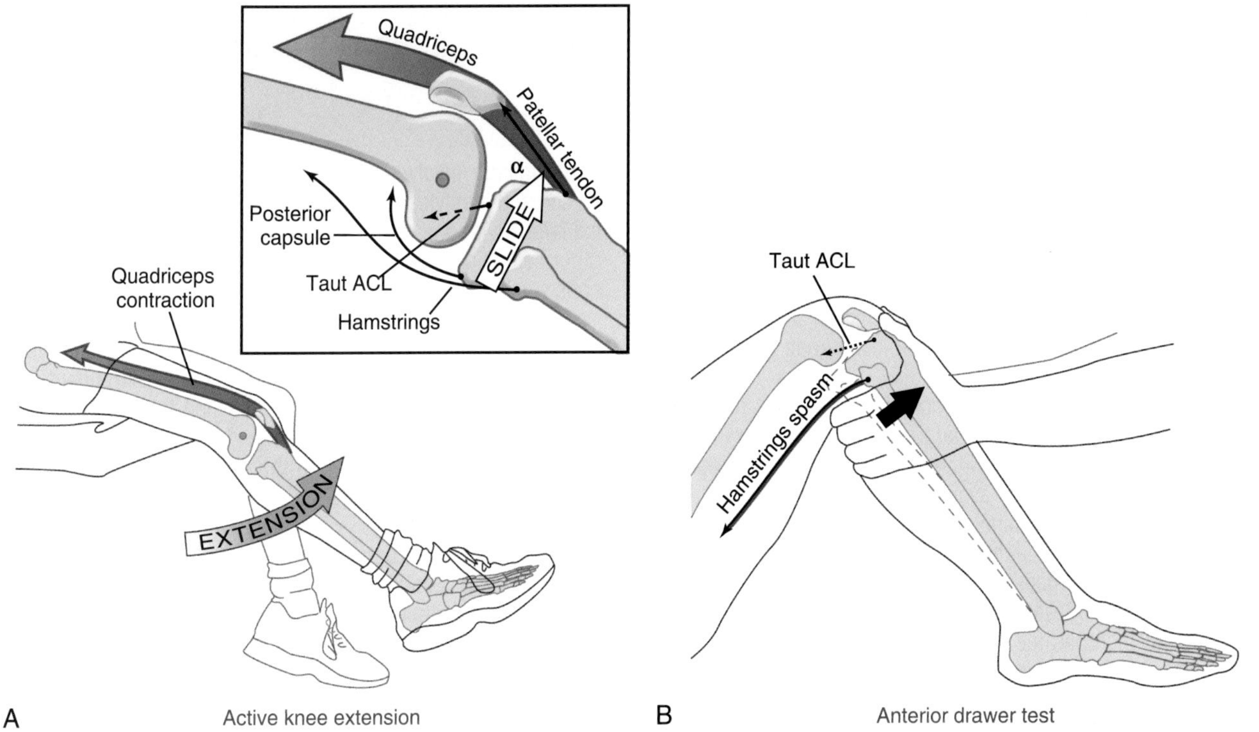

FIGURE 13.20 The interaction between muscle contraction and tension within the anterior cruciate ligaments. (A) Contraction of the quadriceps muscle extends the knee and slides the tibia anterior relative to the femur. Knee extension also elongates most of the anterior cruciate ligament *(ACL)*, posterior capsule, hamstring muscles, collateral ligaments, and adjacent capsule (the last two structures not depicted). Note that the quadriceps and ACL have an antagonistic relationship throughout most of the terminal range of extension. (The angle-of-insertion between the patellar tendon and the anterior-superior tibia is indicated by α.) (B) The anterior drawer test evaluates the integrity of the ACL. Note that spasm in the hamstring muscles places a posterior force on the tibia, which can limit the tension on the ACL.

angle-of-insertion is progressively reduced with greater knee flexion, thereby reducing the muscle's ability to translate the tibia anteriorly and stretch the ACL.[104] Understanding how these factors affect the strain on the ACL helps explain some of the mechanisms of injury and how to design effective and prudent strategies for strengthening the quadriceps after ACL injury or reconstruction.[81] This issue will be further explored in Clinical Connection 13.3.

Common Mechanisms of Injury

The oblique spatial orientation and multiple fiber bundles within the ACL allow for at least a part of its structure to resist the extremes of essentially all movements of the knee. Although this anatomic arrangement is ideal for providing a wide range of stability, it also renders the ligament vulnerable to injury from many combinations of extreme movements.[96,212,295] As with any ligament, the structural integrity of the ACL fails when an applied tensile load or strain exceeds the tissues' physiologic strength or length. To put this into perspective, consider that the ultimate failure point of the ACL has been estimated to occur at strain lengths of 11% to 19%.[41,212] However, most common activities like climbing stairs, pedaling a stationary bicycle, or squatting produce strain on the ACL of less than 4%.[87,92,187] Clearly, a movement situation that ruptures a healthy ACL must involve extreme acute loading and/or a combination of factors that renders the ACL susceptible to injury. Interestingly, experimental work on human cadaver knees has shown that the tension required to rupture the ACL is reduced after the ligament has been subjected to repetitive and rapidly applied strains.[212] This suggests that movement

mechanics that sufficiently strain the ACL to sub-failure magnitudes may lower the tolerance of the tissue over time. Considerable research tries to better understand the specific movement combinations and associated loads that render an ACL most vulnerable to injury. This type of research provides essential insight into programs or recommendations aimed at preventing ACL injuries.

Biomechanical factors associated with the amount of tension or strain in the ACL at any given instant are indeed interrelated and exceedingly complex. These factors include: the direction and magnitude of the ground reaction force; the amount and direction of compression and shear at the tibiofemoral joint; the amount, control, and precise sequencing of muscular forces; the integrity and strength of the surrounding connective tissues; and the alignment and position of the knee and other joints in the lower limb and trunk.[24,47,133,187,369]

The ACL is the most frequently totally ruptured ligament of the knee. Approximately half of all injuries occur in active persons between 15 and 25 years of age, often during high-velocity sporting activities such as American football, downhill skiing, lacrosse, basketball, and soccer. Females within this group are several times more likely of sustaining an ACL injury than males.[347] This issue is further covered in Clinical Connection 13.1.

Most ACL tears involve a transient subluxation of the knee, potentially causing secondary trauma to other tissues, including bone, articular cartilage, or the menisci.[274,277,314] Injury to the ACL can lead to chronic instability of the knee, altering the kinematics of walking and adding further stress to other tissues, especially the menisci and ultimately the articular cartilage.[84,217]

SPECIAL FOCUS 13.3

Treatment Options Following ACL Injury for the Young Athlete: "One Size Does *Not* Fit All"

Rupture of the ACL is a serious event that can result in significant knee instability (i.e., uncontrolled joint laxity), persistent quadriceps weakness, and, for many, an apprehension about returning to their previous level of physical activity. Importantly, this persistent quadriceps weakness and ongoing functional instability can alter the loading pattern on the menisci and articular cartilage, thereby predisposing the ACL deficient knee to early-onset osteoarthritis.[2,59,124,277,383]

There are several treatment options for the young athlete with an ACL injury. Although most undergo ACL reconstructive surgery, many choose a more conservative, exercise-based approach to treatment, and subsequently avoid or delay surgery. To add clarity to this topic, a useful terminology has evolved that conveniently describes the patient as either being a coper, adapter, or noncoper.[163,243] A *coper* foregoes, or at least delays, surgery, and instead pursues a structured and progressive exercise program. Ideally, this program incorporates neuromuscular, resistive, perturbative and balance exercises, as well as high-level dynamic tasks that are specific to the patient's sport or other needs. The primary intent of the program is to build sufficient strength and stability in the athlete's ACL-deficient knee to allow them to safely return to their pre-injury activity level.[73,77,354] Surgery is typically avoided if frequent assessment of the patient's function continues to demonstrate an adequately strong and stable knee. An *adapter* avoids the need for surgery by significantly modifying or lowering their future activity level, which may involve continued structured exercise. And finally, a *noncoper* ultimately chooses surgery followed by formal postoperative rehabilitation. Many factors may influence this choice, including an inadequate response to an initial structured exercise program, or other practical considerations, such as time constraints imposed by school or work, or the desire of the athlete to more quickly return to their pre-injury level of physical activity.[69,163]

Extensive research shows that, on average, there are no clear and consistent functional and health benefits of undergoing immediate ACL surgery versus avoiding surgery and pursuing a structured exercise program.[91,163,250] Most studies and meta-analysis conclude that both treatment options have similar medium- and long-term outcomes for measures of joint laxity, quadriceps strength, development of osteoarthritis, pain, physical function, activity level, and overall patient satisfaction.[100,101,125,244,376] Some limited level evidence suggests that surgery results in less chronic joint laxity compared with exercise as a primary treatment.[250,366] A caveat of this literature is that conclusions are often drawn from studies that lack a high-quality, randomly controlled design.[91,250]

Recommendations from health professionals on the most appropriate treatment for ACL injury ideally are highly individualized and, when available, based on scientific evidence.[69,91,354,366]

Some factors involved in specific recommendations are patient choice and lifestyle, desired timeline for returning to sport, physical intensity and pivoting demands of the sport, extent of injury to other secondary knee stabilizers, degree of joint laxity or quadriceps weakness, and history of previous knee injury.[69,91]

By far, the most frequent first-line treatment for a torn ACL in North America for young and active persons is reconstructive surgery, followed by postoperative rehabilitation. This frequent choice is usually not primarily driven by published long-term functional outcomes, rather, in part, by a likely quicker return to high-level physical activity, combined with the probability of having a more stable knee that can tolerate strenuous activities such as pivoting or jumping.[49,69,91,366]

Most ACL reconstructive surgeries use the person's own patellar, quadriceps, semitendinosus, or gracilis tendon to replace their damaged ACL, either with or without reconstructing other native capsular tissues, such as the anterior-lateral ligament.[142,247] Regardless of which grafted material is used, surgery is reasonably successful at restoring basic stability and function to the knee, however the natural kinematics and pre-injury quadriceps strength are typically not fully restored.[84,113,183,250,395] Even after surgical ACL reconstruction, persons are at significantly higher risk for developing knee osteoarthritis.[84,125] The increased risk is associated with the degree of trauma to other structures at the time of injury, most notably the menisci.[217,256,277]

A large body of research strives to improve the effectiveness of ACL reconstruction, especially in restoring the ACL-deficient knee's pre-injury kinematics and stability.[367] Some factors of interest are optimal tensioning and fixation, position, and type of the ACL graft material. In addition, attempts are made to match the anatomic configuration of the grafted material more precisely with the natural ACL.[7,82] The prevailing logic is that a closer anatomic match in terms of fiber bundle orientation will allow the grafted material to better control the knee's kinematics. As mentioned earlier, the native ACL is typically described as having two separate fiber bundles: anterior-medial and posterior-lateral. Although the bundles share similar length changes during flexion and extension, they exhibit different magnitudes of stiffness throughout knee motion which may help guide the joints' natural arthrokinematics.[7,82,180] Most ACL surgeries performed in the United States currently use a single-bundle technique when attaching the grafted material, however, there is interest in using a two-bundle grafting technique in selected patients in hopes to better mimic the complex anatomy and biomechanics of the ACL.[57,249,364] To date, similar favorable outcomes have been reported for using single- or double-bundle reconstructions. Research continues worldwide aimed at matching the biomechanical and structural properties of grafted material with the native ACL.

Approximately 56% to 70% of all ACL sporting-related injuries occur through noncontact, or at least minimal contact, situations.[119,161,187,241] Many noncontact injuries occur while landing from a jump, or while quickly and forcefully decelerating, cutting, or pivoting over a single planted lower limb.[119,161,274,326] The

mechanisms causing the injury are often unpredictable and occur very rapidly—within 30 to 50 ms of landing;[187] therefore the precise position and prevailing direction of the forces applied to the knee at the time of injury are not always certain. Much of what is known about the biomechanics of noncontact ACL injuries is learned from research using video analysis of the injury, mechanical injury simulators on cadaver limbs, strain gauges implanted within the ACL, and computer-based biomechanical models. Research frequently points to at least three overlapping biomechanical factors associated with a noncontact ACL injury, often involving single-limb landing: (1) strong activation of the quadriceps muscle over a knee that is biased toward extension (i.e., flexed about 30 degrees or less), (2) excessive frontal plane "valgus collapse" of the knee, and (3) forceful horizontal plane rotation of the knee. As depicted in Fig. 13.21, all three of these events typically occur nearly simultaneously, with the valgus collapse of the knee being most potentially injurious to the ACL.[a] Realize that in a weight-bearing position, the instantaneous horizontal plane position of the knee is based on the concomitant kinematics of the femur (from the hip) and the tibia (from the subtalar joint). The illustration in Fig. 13.21 describes the position of the *knee* as being *externally* rotated, given that the femur has rotated internally over an *assumed stationary tibia*. (Review definitions of horizontal plane femoral-on-tibial knee kinematics associated with Fig. 13.15B.) Although not depicted in Fig. 13.21, excessive knee *internal* rotation (when combined with relative extension and extreme valgus) is also a mechanism of excessive ACL strain and injury.[23,254,262,326,327]

Another common mechanism for injuring the ACL involves excessive hyperextension of the knee while the foot is firmly planted on the ground.[31,240] From a femoral-on-tibial perspective, normal extension kinematics would, in theory, involve an excessive posterior slide of the femur relative to the tibia (review Fig. 13.16B). During a forceful hyperextension, however, the posterior femoral slide relative to the fixed tibia may overstretch and rupture the ACL. A large

***

[a]24,68,79,132,137,187,262,314,326,356

concurrent activation of the quadriceps muscle may pull the tibia forward relative to the posterior sliding femur, thereby adding to the likelihood of injury. Often, hyperextension-related ACL injuries are associated with large axial rotation or valgus-producing forces, thereby further increasing the tension on the ACL. In addition to injuring the ACL, marked hyperextension may also injure the posterior capsule and components of the MCL. Table 13.4 summarizes many of the common mechanisms of injury that may be associated with the ACL.

POSTERIOR CRUCIATE LIGAMENT

Anatomy and Function

Thicker and stiffer than the ACL, the posterior cruciate ligament (PCL) attaches from the posterior intercondylar area of the tibia to the lateral side of the medial femoral condyle (see Figs. 13.11, 13.12, and 13.19). The PCL is typically described as having two primary bundles, named according to their relative attachments to the femur: a *six-fold* stronger *anterior set* (anterior-lateral), forming the bulk of the ligament, and a smaller *posterior set* (posterior-medial).[296,368]

As the knee flexes, the PCL undergoes a complex twisting and changing in length and orientation. The precise mechanical effect of this dynamic deformation is not completely understood. Because of the relative low incidence of PCL injury, research regarding its specific function has lagged that of the ACL. What is known, however, is that although some fibers within the PCL remain taut throughout most of flexion and extension, the majority of the ligament (including both fiber bundles) *becomes increasingly taut with greater flexion*.[168,270,373] Between full extension and approximately 30 to 40 degrees of flexion, most of the PCL is relatively slackened; tension peaks between 90 and 120 degrees of flexion.[58,168,204,270]

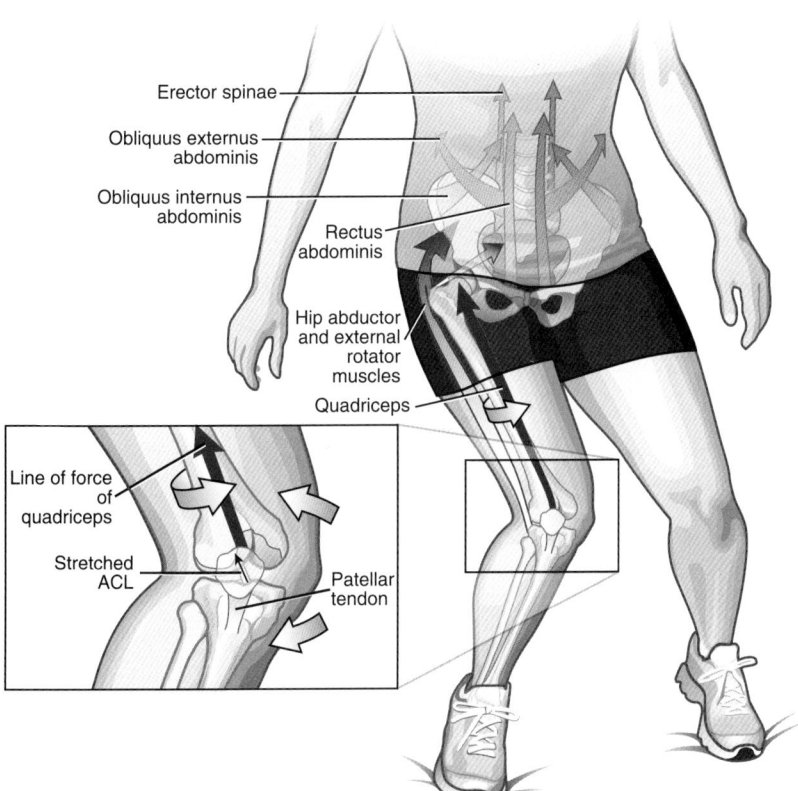

Erector spinae
Obliquus externus abdominis
Obliquus internus abdominis
Rectus abdominis
Hip abductor and external rotator muscles
Quadriceps

Line of force of quadriceps
Stretched ACL
Patellar tendon

FIGURE 13.21 A drawing of a young person immediately after landing from a jump. Note the combined and excessive valgus and externally rotated position of the right knee (via internal femoral rotation over a fixed tibia). In a weight-bearing position, the positions of the right hip and foot strongly influence the positions of the femur and tibia, respectively. In particular, the right hip is adducted and internally rotated, which strongly contributes to the exaggerated valgus and externally rotated position of the knee. Reduced activation of the hip abductors and external rotators of the hip and various trunk musculature could all contribute to the poor control of the hip. The inset on the left shows the increased tension in the ACL and the line of force of the quadriceps muscle. Note the relative lateral displacement of the patella relative to the trochlear groove of the femur. (Purple arrows depict excessive valgus alignment; blue arrows depict the excessive internal rotation of the femur.)

In vivo analysis through magnetic resonance imaging (MRI) shows that, on average, the bulk of the PCL elongates approximately 30% of its length between full extension and 90 degrees of flexion; this correlates to an approximate 3% increase in length per 10 degrees of flexion.[270] This relative sharp increase in tension explains, in part, why many PCL injuries involve significant knee flexion. In addition to becoming increasingly taut in flexion, the PCL provides a secondary restraint to both varus-and-valgus-directed forces, as well as excessive axial rotation especially with knee flexed to or beyond 90 degrees.[168]

While a person actively flexes the knee against gravity, such as when lying prone, the knee flexor muscles (such as the hamstrings) actively slide the tibia (along with the fibula) posteriorly relative to the femur. The extent of the posterior slide arthrokinematics is limited, in part, by passive tension in the PCL (Fig. 13.22A). For this reason, the hamstrings are often referred to as a "PCL antagonist," especially at flexion angles closer to a 90-degree position, which aligns the hamstrings nearly perpendicular to the long axis of the tibia. Adding a forceful contraction of the quadriceps to an existing hamstring contraction reduces the strain on the PCL.[112,138]

One of the most performed tests to evaluate the integrity of the PCL is the *"posterior drawer" test.* This test involves pushing the proximal end of the tibia (leg) posteriorly with the knee flexed to about 90 degrees (see Fig. 13.22B). In this position the PCL provides about 95% of the total passive resistance to the posterior translation of the tibia.[9] With the knee held between 0 and about 30 degrees of flexion, the PCL provides only negligible passive resistance to posterior translation of the tibia; most of the resistance is furnished by the posterior capsule and most of the fibers within the collateral ligaments—tissues that are naturally stretched in near extension.[58]

Another function of the PCL is to limit the extent of anterior translation of the *femur* relative to the fixed lower leg. Activities such

as rapid descent into a deep squat can create a potential anterior translation of the *femur relative to the tibia.* The femur is prevented from sliding off the anterior edge of the tibia by tension in the PCL as well as the surrounding capsule and compression forces within the tibiofemoral joint caused by gravity and muscular coactivation. As apparent in Fig. 13.8, the stout tendon of the popliteus, by crossing obliquely across the posterior-lateral side of the knee, can resist anterior translation of the femur relative to the tibia (or conversely, posterior translation of the tibia relative to the femur). From a clinical perspective, it is believed that the restraining function of the popliteus is particularly noteworthy in persons with a PCL-deficient knee.[312]

Common Mechanisms of Injury

Most PCL injuries are associated with high-energy trauma, such as being in an automobile accident or playing contact sports like American football. Isolated sports-related PCL injuries are relatively rare, generally 2% to 10% of all knee injuries.[56,230,282] A significant number of PCL injuries involve other structures, including the meniscus, articular cartilage, MCL, ACL, and posterior-lateral capsule.[215,316]

Several mechanisms have been described for injury to the PCL.[182,240,282] One relatively frequent mechanism involves *falling onto a fully flexed knee* (with the ankle plantar flexed) such that the proximal tibia first strikes the ground. One of the most common high-energy injuries to the PCL is the *"dashboard" injury,* in which the knee of a passenger in an automobile strikes the dashboard during a front-end collision, driving the tibia posteriorly relative to the femur. Other mechanisms of injury are listed in Table 13.4.

Often after a PCL injury, an observable posterior sag of the proximal tibia relative to the femur is evident when the lower leg is subjected to the pull of gravity, such as in the supine hook-lying position shown in Fig. 13.22B. This observation, in conjunction

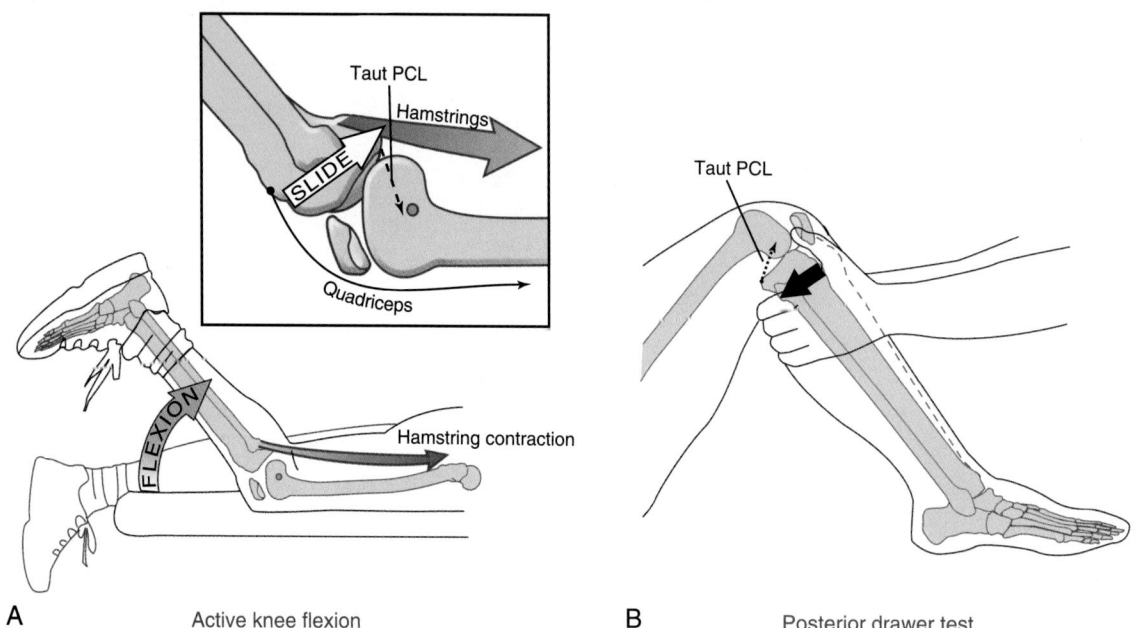

A   Active knee flexion

B   Posterior drawer test

FIGURE 13.22 (A) Contraction of the hamstring muscles flexes the knee and slides the tibia posterior relative to the femur. Knee flexion elongates the quadriceps muscle and most of the fibers within the posterior cruciate ligament *(PCL).* (B) The posterior drawer test evaluates the integrity of the PCL. Tissues pulled taut are indicated by thin black arrows.

with a positive posterior drawer sign, suggests a ruptured PCL. Often, isolated PCL injuries can be managed conservatively without tendon graft reconstructive surgery. Surgical reconstruction is often recommended, however, if marked posterior instability or subluxation is evident and (as frequently is the case) the PCL is injured along with other ligaments.[368] Data on long-term function of the knee after PCL injury or reconstruction are lacking.[171] Most studies suggest that the PCL-deficient knee has an increased likelihood of developing knee osteoarthritis.[50,303,323]

Patellofemoral Joint

The patellofemoral joint is the interface between the articular side of the patella and the trochlear groove of the femur. Local stabilizers of this joint include forces produced by the quadriceps muscle, the fit of the articular surfaces, and passive restraint from the surrounding anatomic soft tissues. Abnormal kinematics and associated instability of the patellofemoral joint are common clinical issues, often implicated with pain and joint degeneration. These pathomechanics are fully addressed later in this chapter. As a background to this topic, the following sections describe the normal kinematics at the patellofemoral joint.

As the knee cycles through flexion and extension, a sliding motion occurs between the articular surface of the patella and the trochlear groove of the femur. During *tibial-on-femoral movements,* the patella slides relative to the fixed trochlear groove of the femur. Because of the firm attachment of the patellar tendon into the tibial tuberosity, the patella is pulled in the direction of the moving tibia during knee flexion. During *femoral-on-tibial movements* (such as during descent into a squat position), the trochlear groove of the femur slides relative to the fixed patella. The patella is held relatively stationary by the balance of forces between the pull of eccentrically active quadriceps and the relatively unyielding patellar tendon.

PATELLOFEMORAL JOINT KINEMATICS

Path and Area of Patellar Contact on the Femur

Data from in vivo and in vitro studies have provided reasonably consistent descriptions of the kinematics and contact areas within the patellofemoral joint during both weight-bearing and non–weight-bearing flexion and extension movements.[b] Historically, data have been collected using MRI, biplanar fluoroscopy and videoradiography, placement of intracortical pins, pressure-sensitive film or specialized dye, optical, magnetic, or video tracking systems, and simulated muscular rigs using cadaver specimens.[5,377]

---

[b]36,178,179,195,208,257,265,321,348

SPECIAL FOCUS 13.4

Accessory Patellar Kinematics

Technological advances in MRI and biplanar fluoroscopy have provided researchers the ability to measure in vivo patellofemoral joint kinematics in far greater detail than the relative global patellar movements depicted in Fig. 13.23.[321,348] The more detailed *accessory patellar kinematics* include patellar *tilt* (near horizontal plane rotation about a near vertical axis), *spin*[*] (frontal plane rotation about an anterior-posterior axis), and lateral-medial *shift* (translation). Other kinematic terms have also been used.[227,257,321,377] These relatively slight and often overlooked accessory patellar kinematics accompany all patellofemoral movements. Several factors cause accessory patellar kinematics. Consider, for example, active tibial-on-femoral knee flexion, starting from full extension. The moving tibia pulls the patellar tendon and patella distally relative to the femur, causing the patella to undulate slightly within the irregular contours of the patellofemoral joint. In addition, accessory patellar kinematics are caused by concurrent axial rotation of the tibia (related to the unlocking of the knee), as well as the fluctuating passive tension in the patellofemoral retinacular fibers (including a subset of fibers often called the medial patellofemoral ligament; described ahead), iliotibial band, and stretched quadriceps.

The amount and direction of the accessory patellar kinematics vary considerably among persons, types of movement (tibia fixed versus femur fixed), types of muscle activation or coactivation (eccentric, isometric, etc.), bony anatomy, and the magnitude of the external load placed on the muscles.[36,195,226,352] The reported high variability also reflects the different methodology used to measure these elusive kinematics. It is difficult, therefore, to make

meaningful comparisons of accessory kinematics across research studies or loading conditions.

Perhaps the most consistently described accessory patellar kinematics during flexion and extension of the knee are medial or lateral *shifts* of the patella within the trochlear groove.[6,226,386] As the asymptomatic knee initially flexes from full extension, the patella first shifts medially slightly, then switches to a lateral shift (and tilt) as flexion continues to 90 degrees.[36,257,348,377] The net lateral patellar shift throughout flexion is small, generally about 3 mm. MacIntyre and co-workers compared patellar kinematics in healthy subjects to those with chronic anterior knee pain.[226,227] The trends in the patellar kinematic data were similar in the two groups except for the symptomatic (painful) group showed a statistically greater *lateral* shift of the patella compared with the control group, most notably at about 20 degrees of flexion. As explored further in this chapter, excessive lateral shift of the patella during knee movement may contribute to stress-related pathology and pain at the patellofemoral joint.

In summary, accessory patellar kinematics normally accompany all knee motions. Although not well understood or predictable, there is likely an optimal amount and pattern of patellar accessory kinematics that help minimize the stress within the patellofemoral joint. Much more clinical and basic research is needed to better define and recognize the pattern of accessory patellar kinematics, both in asymptomatic persons and in those with a painful, eroded, or an unstable patellofemoral joint. A better understanding of this topic may provide a clearer picture of the underlying stress-related pathology at the patellofemoral joint as well as improve treatment.

---

[*]Also referred to as "rotation."

A measurement technique used by Goodfellow and colleagues helped construct the model illustrated in Fig. 13.23.[115] At 135 degrees of flexion, the patella contacts the femur primarily near its base, or superior pole (Fig. 13.23A). At this near fully flexed position, the patella rests well below the trochlear groove, bridging the intercondylar notch of the femur (Fig. 13.23D).[115,178] In this position, the lateral edge of the lateral facet and the "odd" facet of the patella share articular contact with the femur (Fig. 13.23E). As the knee extends toward 90 degrees of flexion, the primary contact region on the patella starts to migrate toward its apex, or inferior pole (Fig. 13.23B).[178,311] Between about 90 and 60 degrees of flexion, the patella is usually well engaged within the trochlear groove of the femur. Within this arc of motion, the contact area between the patella and femur is therefore greatest (Fig. 13.23D and E).[60,148] Even at its maximum, however, the contact area is only about one-third of the total surface area of the posterior side of the patella. Joint contact pressure (i.e., compression force per unit area), therefore, can rise to very large levels within the patellofemoral joint, given strong activation of the quadriceps muscle.

As the knee extends through the last 20 to 30 degrees of flexion, the primary contact point on the patella migrates to its inferior pole (Fig. 13.23C). Within this arc of movement, the patella loses much of its mechanical engagement within the trochlear groove. Consequently, the contact area between the patella and trochlear groove reduces to about 45% of that occurring at 60 degrees of knee flexion.[26,36] Once in full extension, the patella rests completely proximal to the trochlear groove and against the suprapatellar fat pad. In this position, with the quadriceps relaxed, the patella can be moved freely relative to the femur. The overall reduced fit of the patella within the trochlear groove of the femur near and in extension explains, in part, why most chronic lateral dislocations (or subluxations) of the patella occur in this position.[6] The reason why the patella typically dislocates *laterally* is based primarily on the overall lateral line of force of the quadriceps muscle relative to the long axis of the patellar tendon—a topic that is covered in the upcoming sections that describe the structure and function of the quadriceps muscle.

MUSCLE AND JOINT INTERACTION

Innervation of the Muscles

The quadriceps femoris is innervated by the *femoral nerve* (see Fig. 12.23A). Like the triceps at the elbow, the knee's sole extensor group is innervated by just one nerve. A complete femoral nerve lesion, therefore, can cause total paralysis of the knee extensors. The flexors and rotators of the knee are innervated by several nerves from both the lumbar and the sacral plexus, but primarily by the *tibial portion of the sciatic nerve* (see Fig. 12.23B). Table 13.5 lists the motor innervation and actions of all muscles that cross the knee.

As an additional reference, the primary spinal nerve roots that supply the muscles of the lower extremity are listed in Appendix IV, Part A. In addition, Part B and Fig. IV.1 in Part C include additional reference items to help guide the clinical assessment of the functional status of the L^2–S^3 spinal nerve roots.

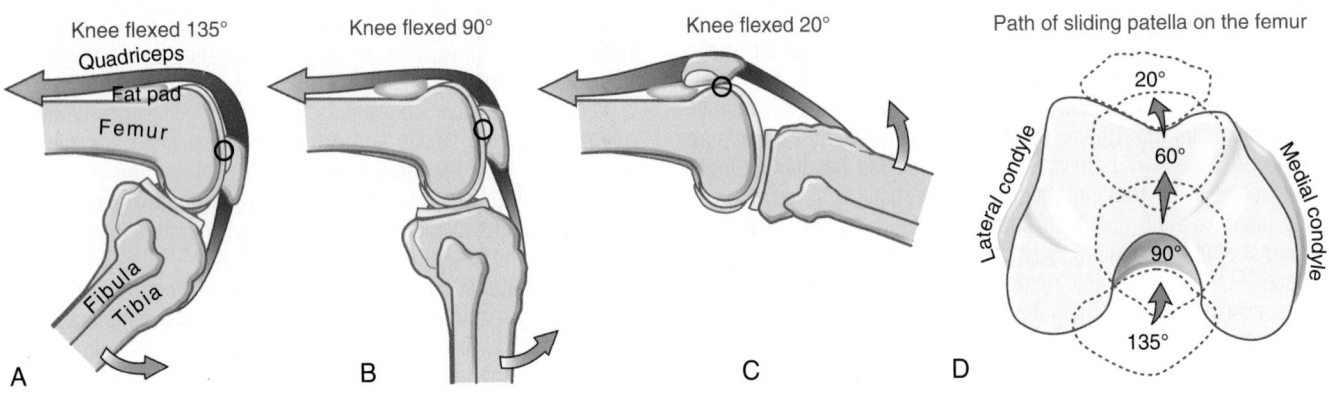

FIGURE 13.23 The kinematics at the patellofemoral joint during active tibial-on-femoral extension. The circles depicted in (A) through (C) indicate the point of maximal contact between the patella and the femur. As the knee extends, the contact point on the patella migrates from its superior pole to its inferior pole. Note the suprapatellar fat pad deep to the quadriceps. (D) and (E) show the path and contact areas of the patella on the trochlear groove of the femur. The values 135, 90, 60, and 20 degrees indicate flexed positions of the knee.

TABLE 13.5 Actions and Innervation of Muscles That Cross the Knee*

Muscle	Action	Innervation	Plexus
Sartorius	Hip flexion, external rotation, and abduction **Knee flexion and internal rotation**	Femoral nerve	Lumbar
Gracilis	Hip flexion and adduction **Knee flexion and internal rotation**	Obturator nerve	Lumbar
Quadriceps femoris		Femoral nerve	Lumbar
Rectus femoris	**Knee extension** and hip flexion		
Vastus group	**Knee extension**		
Popliteus	**Knee flexion and internal rotation**	Tibial nerve	Sacral
Semimembranosus	Hip extension **Knee flexion and internal rotation**	Sciatic nerve (tibial portion)	Sacral
Semitendinosus	Hip extension **Knee flexion and internal rotation**	Sciatic nerve (tibial portion)	Sacral
Biceps femoris (short head)	**Knee flexion and external rotation**	Sciatic nerve (common fibular portion)	Sacral
Biceps femoris (long head)	Hip extension **Knee flexion and external rotation**	Sciatic nerve (tibial portion)	Sacral
Gastrocnemius	**Knee flexion** Ankle plantar flexion	Tibial nerve	Sacral
Plantaris	**Knee flexion** Ankle plantar flexion	Tibial nerve	Sacral

*The actions involving the knee are shown in boldface type. Muscles are listed in descending order of nerve root innervations.

Sensory Innervation of the Knee Joint

Sensory innervation of the knee and associated ligaments is supplied primarily from the L[3] through L[5] spinal nerve roots, which travel to the spinal cord primarily in the posterior tibial, obturator, and femoral nerves.[151,167] The *posterior tibial nerve* (a branch of the tibial portion of the sciatic nerve) is the largest afferent supply to the knee joint. It supplies sensation to the posterior capsule and associated ligaments and most of the internal structures of the knee as far anterior as the infrapatellar fat pad. Afferent fibers within the *obturator nerve* carry sensation from the skin over the medial aspect of the knee and parts of the posterior and posterior-medial capsule. Afferent fibers from the *femoral nerve* supply most of the anterior-medial and anterior-lateral capsule.

Muscular Function at the Knee

Muscles of the knee are described as two groups: the *knee extensors* (i.e., quadriceps femoris) and the *knee flexor-rotators*. The attachments of many of these muscles are presented in Chapter 12. Consult Appendix IV, Part D for a summary of the attachments and nerve supply to the muscles of the knee. Also, as a reference, a list of cross-sectional areas of selected muscles of the knee is presented in Appendix IV, Part E.

EXTENSORS OF THE KNEE: QUADRICEPS FEMORIS MUSCLE

Anatomic Considerations

The *quadriceps femoris* is a large extensor muscle, with a cross-sectional area up to 2.8 times larger than the hamstring muscles.[192] The quadriceps consists of the rectus femoris, vastus lateralis, vastus medialis, and deeper vastus intermedius (see Figs. 13.7 and 13.24).[d] The large vastus group produces about 80% of the total extension

torque at the knee, and the rectus femoris produces about 20%.[145] Contraction of the vastus muscles extends the knee only. Contraction of the rectus femoris, however, causes hip flexion and knee extension.

All heads of the quadriceps unite distally to form a strong *quadriceps tendon* that attaches to the base (top) and sides of the patella. The *patellar tendon* connects the apex of the patella to the tibial tuberosity. The vastus lateralis and vastus medialis muscles also attach distally into the capsule and menisci via patellar retinacular fibers (see Fig. 13.7). Together, the quadriceps muscle, patella, and patellar tendon are referred to as the *knee extensor mechanism*.

The knee extensor mechanism in a healthy and active person can generate surprisingly large forces. Although perhaps an extreme example, the quadriceps in trained young males can theoretically produce maximal-effort forces of up to 6000 N (almost 1350 lb).[70] Certainly much less force is required by any given individual to perform most ordinary functional activities. Nevertheless, substantially large forces produced by the extensor mechanism are routinely transferred across the tibiofemoral and patellofemoral joints, and through certain ligaments and opposing muscles. This realization is important clinically, whether for providing advice on injury prevention or for designing exercises after injury or pathology.

The *rectus femoris* attaches to the pelvis near the anterior-inferior iliac spine and immediately superior to the acetabulum. The vastus muscles, however, have their proximal attachments to parts of the anterior, lateral, and medial sides of the proximal three-fourths of the femur, from near the femoral neck and greater trochanter to alongside the linea aspera, as far distal as the proximal medial supracondylar line (see Figs. 12.4 and 12.5). Although the *vastus lateralis* has the largest cross-sectional area of the quadriceps muscles, the vastus medialis extends farther distally toward the knee.[17,389]

---

[d]A fifth head of the quadriceps, the *tensor vastus intermedius*, may exist. When present, this muscle shares its proximal attachments with fascia associated with the vastus lateralis and vastus intermedius.

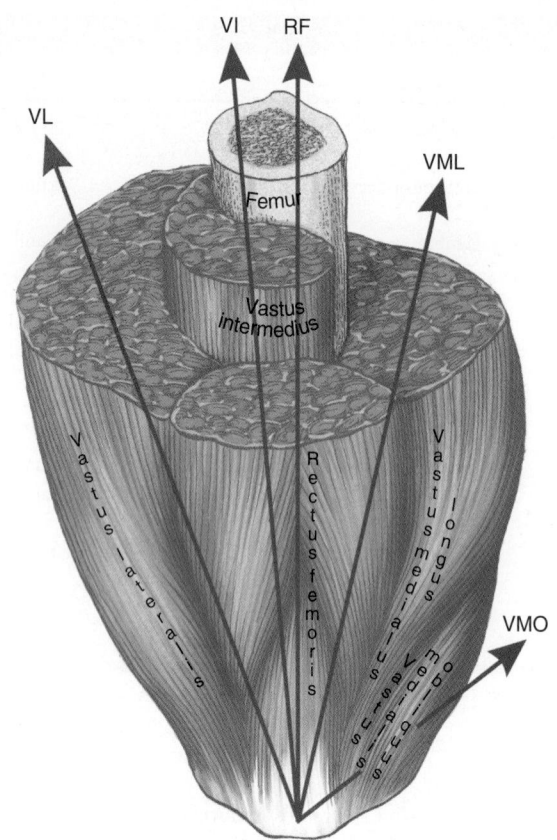

FIGURE 13.24 A cross-section through the right quadriceps muscle. The arrows depict the approximate line of force of each part of the quadriceps: vastus lateralis *(VL),* vastus intermedius *(VI),* rectus femoris *(RF),* vastus medialis longus *(VML),* and vastus medialis obliquus *(VMO).* Much of the vastus medialis and vastus lateralis muscles originate on the posterior side of the femur, at the linea aspera.

The *vastus medialis* consists of fibers that form two distinct fiber directions. The more distal oblique fibers (the vastus medialis "obliquus") approach the patella at 50 to 55 degrees medial to the quadriceps tendon (see Fig. 13.24). The remaining more longitudinal fibers (the vastus medialis "longus") approach the patella at 15 to 18 degrees medial to the quadriceps tendon.[209] The oblique fibers of the vastus medialis extend farther distally than other muscular components of the quadriceps. Although the oblique fibers account for only 30% of the cross-sectional area of the entire vastus medialis muscle,[297] the oblique pull on the patella has important implications for the stabilization and orientation of the patella as it slides (tracks) through the trochlear groove of the femur.[278]

The deepest quadriceps muscle, the *vastus intermedius,* is located deep to the rectus femoris and vastus lateralis. Deep to the vastus intermedius is the poorly defined *articularis genu.* This muscle contains a few slips of fibers that attach proximally to the anterior side of the distal femur, and then distally into the anterior capsule. This muscle pulls the capsule and synovial membrane proximally during active knee extension.[343] The articularis genu is analogous to the poorly defined *articularis cubiti* at the elbow.

Functional Considerations

On average, the knee extensor muscles produce a torque about two-thirds greater than that produced by the knee flexor muscles.[44,116] Through their isometric, eccentric, and concentric activations, this extensor torque is used to perform multiple functions at the knee. Through *isometric activation,* the quadriceps stabilizes and helps to protect the knee; through *eccentric activation,* the quadriceps controls the rate of descent of the body's center of mass, such as when sitting, squatting, or landing from a jump. Eccentric activation of these muscles also provides shock absorption to the knee. At the heel contact phase of walking, the knee flexes slightly in response to the ground reaction force. Eccentrically active quadriceps control the extent of the knee flexion. Acting as a spring, the muscle helps dampen the impact of loading on the joint. This protection is especially useful during high-impact loading, such as during landing from a jump, when making the initial foot contact phase of running, or when descending from a high step. A person whose knee is braced or unnaturally held in extension lacks this natural shock absorption mechanism.

In the previous examples, eccentric activation of the quadriceps is employed to decelerate knee flexion. *Concentric contraction* of this muscle, in contrast, accelerates the tibia or femur toward knee extension. This action is often used to raise the body's center of mass, such as during running uphill, jumping, or standing from a seated position.

Quadriceps Action at the Knee: Understanding the Biomechanical Interactions between External and Internal Torques

In many upright activities, an *external* (flexor) torque is acting on the knee. This external torque is equal to the external load being moved or supported, multiplied by its external moment arm. The external (flexor) torque must often be met or exceeded by an opposing *internal* (extensor) torque, which is the product of quadriceps force multiplied by its internal moment arm. An understanding of how these opposing torques are produced and functionally interact is the focus of this section. This topic is an important component of many aspects of strengthening the quadriceps as part of a rehabilitation program.

External Torque Demands Placed against the Quadriceps: Contrasting "Tibial-on-Femoral" with "Femoral-on-Tibial" Methods of Knee Extension

Many strengthening exercises designed to challenge the quadriceps rely on resistive, external torques generated only by gravity acting on the body. The magnitude of the external torque is highly dependent on the specific way the knee is being extended. These differences are illustrated in Fig. 13.25. During *tibial-on-femoral* knee extension, the external moment arm of the weight of the lower leg *increases* from 90 to 0 degrees of knee flexion (see Fig. 13.25A–C). In contrast, during *femoral-on-tibial* knee extension (as in rising from a squat position), the external moment arm of the upper body weight *decreases* from 90 to 0 degrees of knee flexion (see Fig. 13.25D–F). The graph included in Fig. 13.25 contrasts the external torque–knee angle relationships for the two methods of extending the knee between 90 degrees of flexion and full extension.

Information contained in the graph in Fig. 13.25 is useful for designing quadriceps strengthening exercises. By necessity, exercises that significantly challenge the quadriceps also stress the knee joint, patellofemoral joint, and periarticular connective tissues, such as the ACL. Clinically, this stress may be considered potentially damaging or therapeutic, depending on the underlying, if any, pathology of the person performing the exercise. A person with acute or marked patellofemoral joint pain or painful knee arthritis, for example, is typically advised against producing large muscular-based stresses on the knee. An asymptomatic person or a high-level

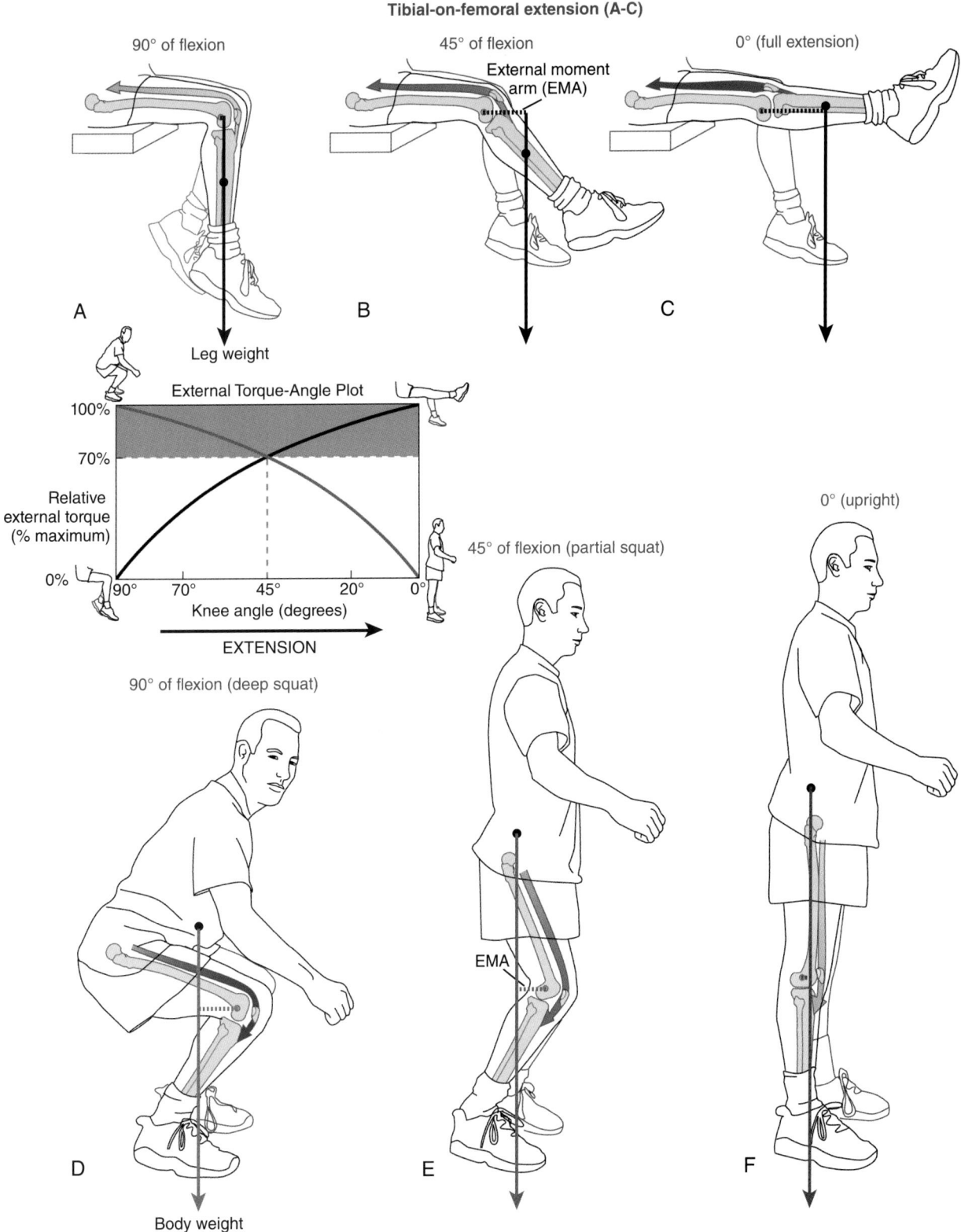

FIGURE 13.25 The external (flexion) torques are shown imposed on the knee between flexion (90 degrees) and full extension (0 degrees). *Tibial-on-femoral* extension is shown in (A) to (C), and *femoral-on-tibial* extension is shown in (D) to (F). The external torques are equal to the product of body or leg weight times the external moment arm *(EMA).* The increasing red color of the quadriceps muscle denotes the increasing demand on the muscle and underlying joint, in response to the increasing external torque. The graph shows the relationship between the external torque—normalized to a maximum (100%) torque for each method of extending the knee—for selected knee joint angles. (Tibial-on-femoral extension is shown in black; femoral-on-tibial extension is shown in gray.) External torques greater than 70% for each method of extension are shaded in red.

Patellar Tendinopathy, or "Jumpers" Knee: Some Etiologic and Biomechanic Considerations

*P*atellar tendinopathy is an overuse condition of the patellar tendon characterized by persistent tendon pain.[318] Its precise pathology is poorly understood.[37] In about two-thirds of cases, the pain is localized near the distal pole of the patella.[62] This condition is often referred to as "jumper's knee," although this term may be ambiguous because it could also infer *quadriceps tendinopathy*— possibly a different pathology.[341] Nevertheless, patellar tendinopathy most often afflicts young athletes who regularly participate in sports involving explosive and repetitive jumping, such as basketball and volleyball. Over time, these vigorous activities can cause a gradual structural degeneration within the patellar tendon, often at a pace that exceeds natural healing. Some evidence suggests an epigenetic alteration of selected genes in persons with patellar tendinopathy.[304] Regardless of cause, this debilitating and sometimes career-ending condition has been reported in up to 40% to 50% of elite volleyball players.[170,205]

In tendons diagnosed with patellar tendinopathy, ultrasound, MRI, and histologic sampling commonly reveal classic signs of overload and wear, including tendon thickening and micro-tears, collagen disorganization, and neovascularization.[62,172,191] Because the pathology typically lacks signs of inflammation, the term *tendinopathy* is the preferred term to describe this condition.[37]

A few risk factors have shown moderate levels of evidence for developing patellar tendinopathy. These include reduced passive ankle dorsiflexion, restricted flexibility in quadriceps and hamstring muscles, impairments at the hip and foot, and large volume of training.[16,237,342] Large patellar tendon forces associated with specific landing or jumping techniques have also been implicated as a risk factor for patellar tendinopathy.[76,301] These tendon forces have been reported to be as high as seven times one's body weight.[76] The pathogenesis of patellar tendinopathy is likely associated with the magnitude and repetitive nature of the tendon forces produced during jumping and landing, especially when combined with the risk factors cited earlier.

One line of research on the causes of patellar tendinopathy has focused on the biomechanics of landing from a jump.[156] Two important factors normally involved with dissipating the kinetic energy of landing from a jump are the rate and amount of ankle dorsiflexion and the eccentric activation of lower limb muscles, particularly the quadriceps and plantar flexors. It has been theorized that limited ankle dorsiflexion would reduce the load absorption capability of the plantar flexors muscles. As a consequence, a greater percentage of the total load absorption would shift to the quadriceps mechanism. Over many repetitions of landing, the additional eccentrically activated force within the quadriceps may lead to microtrauma within the tendon, thereby contributing to the pathogenesis of patellar tendinopathy. This theory has received some support from a longitudinal study on 90 junior elite Swedish basketball players between the ages of 14 and 20 years.[16] This study suggests that exercises that *increase* dorsiflexion of the ankle in athletes with relatively reduced motion may help prevent or reduce the severity of patellar tendinopathy.

Research has also shown that landing from a jump in *greater trunk flexion* significantly *reduces* the force demands on the quadriceps and therefore the patellar tendon.[313] Landing with greater trunk flexion allows the hip extensor muscles to accept more of the kinetic demands of the landing, thereby shielding the patellar ligament from large loads. (The specific biomechanics describing how greater trunk flexion partially unloads the quadriceps while landing is described further in Clinical Connection 13.1 within the context of "safe landing" to protect other structures of the knee.) This Special Focus provides two examples of how practical biomechanics can provide useful clues for improving the treatment and prevention of a stress-related musculoskeletal condition.

---

athlete in the later phases of postsurgical ACL rehabilitation, in contrast, may benefit from such judiciously applied muscular stresses to the knee.

External torques applied to the knee by a constant load vary in a predictable fashion, based on knee angle and orientation of the limb segments. As depicted by the red shading in the graph in Fig. 13.25, external torques are relatively large from 90 to 45 degrees of flexion via femoral-on-tibial extension, and from 45 to 0 degrees of flexion via tibial-on-femoral extension. Reducing these external torques can be accomplished by several strategies. For example, the knee can be extended through tibial-on-femoral kinematics through a limited arc of between 90 and 45 degrees of flexion. This activity could be followed by an exercise that involves rising from a partial squat position, a motion that may incorporate femoral-on-tibial extension between 45 and 0 degrees of flexion. Combining both exercises in the manner described provides only moderate to minimal external torques against the quadriceps, throughout a continuous range of motion. This strategy of applying relatively low and predictable external torques to the knee may be particularly useful when attempting to strengthen the quadriceps yet minimize the stress on the patellar tendon or underlying patellofemoral joint.

Internal Torque–Joint Angle Relationship of the Quadriceps Muscle
Maximal knee extension (internal) torque typically occurs between 45 and 70 degrees of knee flexion, with less torque produced near the extremes of flexion and extension.[122,149,188,286,298] The shape of this torque-angle curve varies considerably however, based on the type and speed of activation and position of the hip. A representative maximal-effort torque versus joint angle curve obtained from healthy male subjects is displayed in Fig. 13.26.[333] As depicted by the red line in Fig. 13.26, maximal-effort knee extension torque remains at least 90% of maximum between 80 and 30 degrees of flexion. This high-torque potential of the quadriceps within this arc of motion is used during many functional activities that incorporate *femoral-on-tibial* kinematics, such as ascending a high step, rising from a chair, or holding a partial squat position while participating in sports, such as basketball or speed skating. Note the rapid decline in internal torque potential as the knee angle

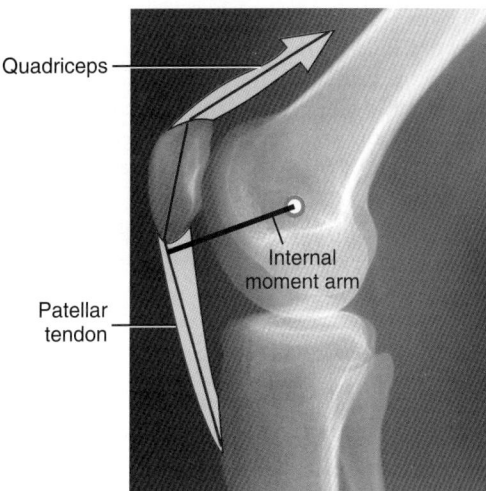

FIGURE 13.27 The quadriceps uses the patella to increase its internal moment arm (*thick black line*). The axis of rotation is shown as the open circle near the lateral epicondyle of the femur.

SPECIAL FOCUS 13.6

Quadriceps Weakness: Pathomechanics of "Extensor Lag"

Persons with significant weakness in the quadriceps often show considerable difficulty completing the full range of tibial-on-femoral extension of the knee, commonly displayed while sitting. This difficulty persists even when the external load is limited to just the weight of the lower leg. Although the knee can be fully extended passively, efforts at active extension often fail to produce the last 15 to 20 degrees of extension. Clinically, this characteristic demonstration of quadriceps weakness is referred to as an "extensor lag."

Extensor lag at the knee is often a persistent and perplexing problem during rehabilitation of the postsurgical or posttraumatized knee. The mechanics that create this condition during the seated position can be explained as follows. As the knee approaches terminal extension, the maximal internal torque potential of the quadriceps is *least* while the opposing external (flexor) torque is *greatest* (compare graphs in Figs. 13.25 and 13.26). This natural disparity is not observed in persons with normal quadriceps strength. With significant muscle weakness, however, the disparity often results in extensor lag.

Swelling or effusion of the knee increases the likelihood of an extensor lag. Swelling increases intra-articular volumetric pressure, which can physically impede full knee extension.[393] Increased intra-articular pressure can also reflexively inhibit the neural activation of the quadriceps muscle.[64,235,268] Methods that reduce swelling of the knee, therefore, can have an important role in a therapeutic exercise program of the knee. Passive resistance from hamstring muscles that are stretched across a flexed hip in a seated position can also play a role in limiting full extension.

The plot (Figure 13.26) shows knee flexion angle (degrees) on the x-axis from 90 to 5, and maximal knee extension torque (Nm) on the y-axis from 60 to 130. A note reads: "Red line indicates torques that are at least 90% of maximum." The bar labeled "Maximal leverage" spans approximately 60 to 20 degrees.

FIGURE 13.26 A plot showing the maximal-effort, knee extension torques produced between about 90 and 5 degrees of flexion. The internal moment arm (leverage) used by the quadriceps is greatest between about 60 and 20 degrees of knee flexion. Knee extensor torques are produced isometrically by maximal effort, with the hip held in extension. Data from 26 healthy males, average age 28 years old.[333]

approaches full extension. Most studies report a 50% to 70% reduction in maximal internal torque as the knee approaches full extension.[99,149,190,286] Of interest, the *external torque* applied against the knee during femoral-on-tibial extension also declines rapidly during this same range of motion (see Fig. 13.25, graph). There appears to be a general biomechanical match between the internal torque potential of the quadriceps and the external torque applied against the quadriceps during the last approximately 45 to 70 degrees of complete femoral-on-tibial knee extension. This match accounts, in part, for the popularity of "closed-kinematic chain" exercises that focus on applying resistance to the quadriceps while the upright person moves the body through this arc of femoral-on-tibial knee extension.

Functional Role of the Patella. The patella functions as a "spacer" between the femur and quadriceps muscle, which increases the internal moment arm of the knee extensor mechanism (Fig. 13.27). By definition, the knee extensor internal moment arm is the perpendicular distance between the medial-lateral axis of rotation and the line of force of the muscle. Because torque is the product of force and its moment arm, the presence of the patella augments the extension torque at the knee.

Research has shown that the knee extensor internal moment arm changes considerably across the full arc of knee flexion and extension.[186,333,340] Although the data published on this topic differ considerably based on methodology and natural variability, most studies report that the knee extensor moment arm is greatest between about 60 and 20 degrees of knee flexion (see bar on horizontal axis in graph of Fig. 13.26).[17,39,186,333] This range of relatively high leverage partially explains why knee extension torques are typically highest across a significant part of this same range of motion. Maximal-effort knee extension torque typically falls off dramatically in the last 30 degrees of extension, likely because of a combination of reduced extension leverage and shortened muscle length.

At least three factors affect the length of the knee extension moment arm across the sagittal plane range of motion. These include (1) the shape and changing position of the patella, (2) the shape of the distal femur (including the depth and slope of the trochlear groove), and (3) the migrating medial-lateral axis of rotation at the knee (referred to as the *evolute* earlier in this chapter).[378] Exactly how the changing length of the internal moment arm influences the shape of the extensor torque–joint angle curve, such as that depicted in Fig. 13.26, is uncertain. It is technically difficult to isolate the effects of leverage from those of changing muscle length: both factors simultaneously change throughout the range of motion, and both directly or indirectly affect knee extension torque.

PATELLOFEMORAL JOINT KINETICS

The patellofemoral joint is routinely exposed to high magnitudes of compression force. A sampling of these forces includes 1.3 times one's body weight during walking on level surfaces, 2.6 times one's body weight during performance of a straight leg raise, 3.3 times one's body weight during climbing of stairs, and up to 7.8 times one's body weight during performance of deep "knee bends" or squats.[199,299,324] Although these compression forces originate primarily from active forces produced from the overlying quadriceps, their magnitude is strongly influenced by the amount of knee flexion at the time of muscle activation.[54,290] To illustrate this important interaction, consider the compression force on the patellofemoral joint in a partial squat position (Fig. 13.28A). Forces within the extensor mechanism are transmitted proximally and distally through the quadriceps tendon (QT) and patellar tendon (PT), much like a cable crossing a pulley. The resultant, or combined, effect of these forces is directed toward the trochlear groove

of the femur as a joint compression force (CF). Increasing knee flexion by descending into a deeper squat significantly raises the force demands throughout the extensor mechanism, and ultimately on the patellofemoral joint (see Fig. 13.28B). The increased knee flexion associated with the deeper squat also reduces the angle formed by the intersection of force vectors QT and PT. As shown by vector addition, reducing the angle of these force *increases* the magnitude of the CF directed between the patella and the femur. In theory, if the QT and PT vectors were collinear and oriented in opposite directions, the muscular-based compression force on the patellofemoral joint would be zero. In reality, however, this situation would not normally occur; even in full knee extension, a significant portion of the distal fibers of the quadriceps remain angulated somewhat posteriorly, thereby still capable of exerting a compressive force through the patellofemoral joint. This angulation can be appreciated by reviewing Figs. 13.8 and 13.10.

When in a weight-bearing position depicted in Fig. 13.28, *both* the compression force and the area of articular contact at the patellofemoral joint increase with greater femoral-on-tibial knee flexion, reaching a maximum between about 60 and 90 degrees.[148,223,311] The relative increase of these two variables, however, is not the same: increasing knee flexion increases the quadriceps-driven compression force to a greater relative extent than it increases articular surface contact area. As a result, the contact *pressure* (force/area) increases at the patellofemoral joint as the knee approaches 60 to 90 degrees of knee femoral-on-tibial flexion.[54,288] An important point to consider, however, is that without the relatively large contact area to disperse the large compression force produced by the quadriceps, the contact

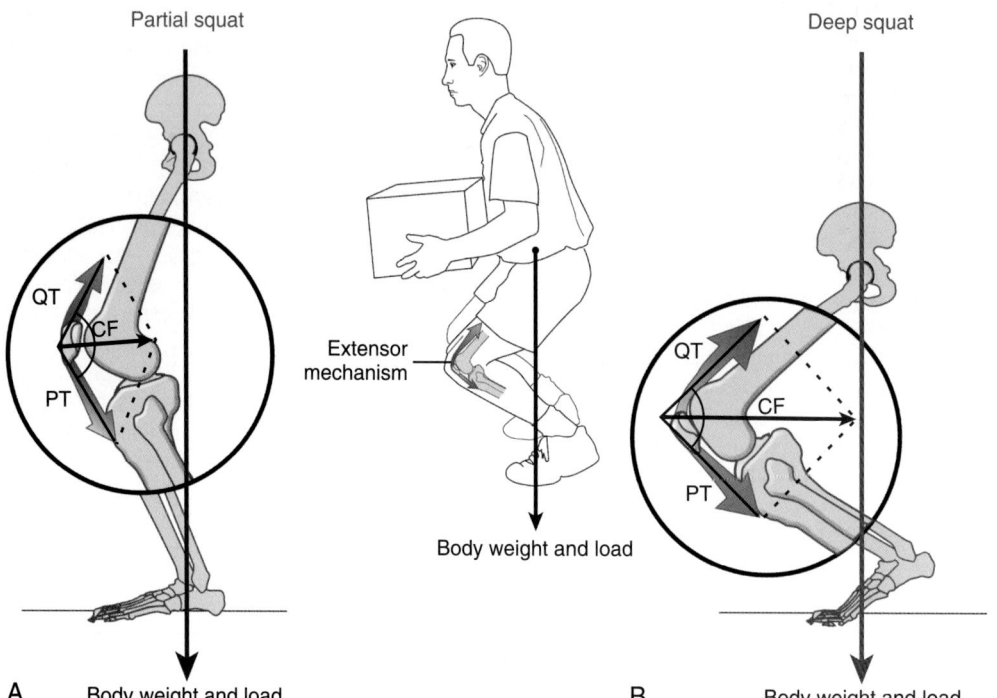

FIGURE 13.28 The relationship between quadriceps activation, depth of a squat, and the compression force within the patellofemoral joint is shown as a person lifts a box. (A) Maintaining a partial squat requires that the quadriceps transmit a force through the quadriceps tendon *(QT)* and the patellar tendon *(PT)*. The vector addition of QT and PT provides an estimation of the patellofemoral joint compression force *(CF)*. (B) A deeper squat requires greater force from the quadriceps because of the greater external (flexion) torque on the knee. Furthermore, the greater knee flexion (B) decreases the angle between QT and PT and consequently produces a greater joint force between the patella and femur.

pressure-based stress on the joint would likely rise to intolerable physiologic levels.[38,118] Having the area of joint contact greatest at positions that are generally associated with the largest muscular-based compression force naturally protects the joint against stress-induced cartilage degeneration. This is especially relevant considering how frequently the quadriceps are challenged to control activities like stair climbing, landing from a jump, or lowering to a seated position. This natural ability of the patellofemoral joint to dissipate large muscular-based forces allows most healthy and normally aligned patellofemoral joints to function relatively well over a lifetime, often with little appreciable discomfort or degeneration of the articular cartilage or subchondral bone. As will be explained, for many persons, however, the natural high-force environment within the patellofemoral joint can be a major contributing factor to the development of *patellofemoral pain syndrome.*

FACTORS AFFECTING THE TRACKING OF THE PATELLA ACROSS THE PATELLOFEMORAL JOINT

The large compression forces that naturally occur at the patellofemoral joint are typically well tolerated, provided they are well dispersed across the largest possible area of articular surface. A joint with less-than-optimal congruity, or one with structural anomalies, will likely experience abnormal "tracking" of the patella during movement. Consequently, the patellofemoral joint is exposed to altered, and typically higher, contact pressures, thereby increasing its risk of degeneration and chronic knee pain.[290]

Role of the Quadriceps Muscle in Patellar Tracking

Among the most important influences on patellofemoral joint biomechanics are the magnitude and direction of force produced by the quadriceps muscle. As the knee is extending via tibial-on-femoral kinematics, the contracting quadriceps pulls the patella not only superiorly within the trochlear groove of the femur, but also slightly *laterally and posteriorly.* The slight but omnipresent lateral line of force exerted by the quadriceps is caused, in part, by the larger cross-sectional area and force potential of the vastus lateralis. Because of the purported association between patellofemoral joint pain and excessive *lateral* tracking (and possible dislocation) of the patella, assessing the overall line of pull of the quadriceps relative to the patella is a meaningful clinical measure. Such a measure is referred to as the *quadriceps angle,* or more commonly the *Q-angle* (Fig. 13.29A).[98,269] Clinically, the Q-angle is estimated first by constructing a line representing the resultant force vector produced by the different heads of the quadriceps. On average, this line runs between the midpoint of the patella and the femoral neck.[350] (Due to ease of palpation, the anterior-superior iliac spine is typically used clinically as a reasonably close proxy to the less palpable femoral neck.) A second line represents the long axis of the patellar tendon, made by connecting a point on the tibial tuberosity with the midpoint of the patella. The Q-angle is formed at the intersection of these two lines, typically measuring about 13 to 15 degrees (±4.5 degrees) within a healthy adult population.[269] The Q-angle assessment has been criticized for its poor association with pathology at the patellofemoral joint, inadequate standardized measurement protocol, and inability to measure dynamic alignment.[129,194,290,293] Nevertheless, the Q-angle remains a general and relatively simple clinical index for estimating the relative lateral pull of the quadriceps on the patella. Factors that naturally offset or limit the lateral pull of the patella are described in the next section. If these factors fail to operate in a coordinated fashion, the patella

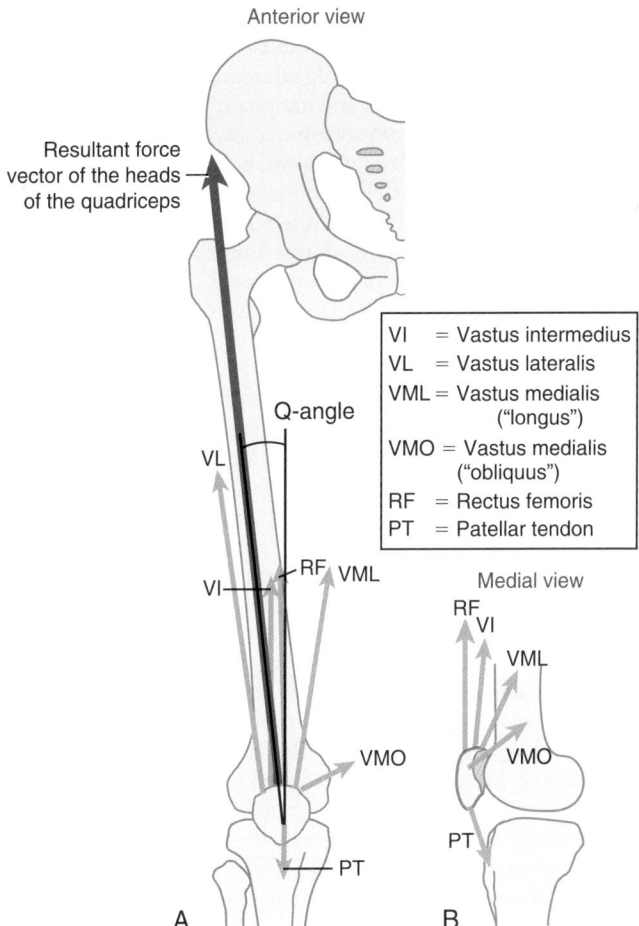

FIGURE 13.29 (A) The overall line of force of the quadriceps is shown as well as the separate lines of force of each muscular component. The vastus medialis is divided into its two predominant fiber groups: the obliquus and the longus. The net lateral pull exerted on the patella by the quadriceps is indicated by the Q-angle. The larger the Q-angle, the greater the lateral muscle pull on the patella. (B) The lines of force of several of the muscular components are observed from a medial view, emphasizing the posterior pull of the oblique fibers of the vastus medialis.

may track (shift and/or tilt) more laterally within the trochlear groove—kinematics that may reduce contact area and increase patellofemoral joint contact pressure.[36,208,290,292,337]

Activation of the quadriceps, as a whole, pulls and compresses the patella *posteriorly* against the femur, thereby stabilizing its path of movement. This stabilization effect increases with the knee in greater flexion (review Fig. 13.28). However as described earlier, even in full knee extension some fibers of the quadriceps are aligned to compress the patellofemoral joint, most notably the oblique fibers of the vastus medialis.[321] (See side view of VMO in Fig. 13.29B.) The posterior stabilizing effect of this muscle on the patella is especially useful in the last 20 to 30 degrees of extension, at a point when (1) the patella is no longer fully engaged within the trochlear groove of the femur and (2) the resultant patellofemoral joint compression (stabilizing) force produced by the activated quadriceps as a whole is least.[6]

Factors That Naturally Oppose the Lateral Pull of the Quadriceps on the Patella

Several factors throughout the lower extremity naturally oppose and thereby limit the lateral bias in pull of the quadriceps relative to the patellofemoral joint. These factors are important to optimal tracking. In this context, *optimal tracking* is defined as movement between the patella and femur across the greatest possible area of articular surface with the least possible stress. Understanding the factors that favor optimal tracking often provides insight into the underlying pathomechanics and rationale for many traditional treatments for pain and other dysfunctions of the patellofemoral joint. Both local and global factors will be described. *Local factors* are those that act directly on the patellofemoral joint. *Global factors,* on the other hand, are those related to the alignment of the bones and joints of the lower limb. Although extensive research supports many of the proposed pathomechanics of abnormal tracking, a full understanding of the topic remains elusive.[290,331,377]

Local Factors

As previously introduced, the overall line of force of the quadriceps is often estimated by the Q-angle (see Fig. 13.29A). Biomechanically, the overall lateral pull of the quadriceps produces a lateral "bowstringing" force on the patella (Fig. 13.30). As apparent by the vector addition in Fig. 13.30, a larger Q-angle creates a larger lateral bowstringing force.[148,292] A large lateral bowstringing force has the tendency to pull the patella laterally over a region of reduced contact area, thereby increasing the contact pressure on its articular surfaces as well as potentially increasing the likelihood of lateral dislocation.[162]

As indicated in Fig. 13.30, excessive tension in the iliotibial band or interconnected lateral patellar retinacular fibers can add to the natural lateral pull on the patella. This lateral pull may be exaggerated if connective tissues associated with the medial capsule of the knee are weakened or lax (review list in Table 13.1).

Structures that *oppose* the lateral bowstringing force on the patella are shown on the right side of Fig. 13.30. The *lateral facet of the trochlear groove* of the femur is normally steeper than the medial facet (compare facets depicted in Fig. 13.23D). This steeper slope naturally blocks, or at least resists, an approaching patella and thereby limits its excessive lateral shift.[53,352] For a patella to laterally dislocate, it must traverse completely "up and over" this relatively steep slope. Researchers who experimentally flattened the lateral facet of the trochlear groove on cadaver specimens report an average 55% loss of medial patellar stability across the tested knee range of motion; in other words, the patella could be shifted laterally with 55% *less* force than before the facet was flattened.[319] The normally steep slope of the lateral facet of the trochlear groove of the femur provides an essential local resistance to excessive lateral translation of the patella. A dysplastic, "flattened" trochlear groove may occur in otherwise healthy persons and is one of several recognized risk factors for excessive lateral tracking or chronic dislocation of the patella. In addition, an abnormally high riding patella ("patella alta") is also associated with excessive lateral tracking of the patella.[53,352] As the knee extends through its final 30 to 40 degrees, a high patella is prematurely pulled proximal to the trochlear groove and thereby loses an element of bony stability.

The *oblique fibers of the vastus medialis* (frequently abbreviated as VMO) are uniquely oriented to help offset at least part of the lateral pull exerted on the patella by the quadriceps muscle as a whole (review Fig. 13.24).[114,218,321,322] Selectively removing the force attributable to the VMO in cadaver specimens produces an average 27% loss of medial patellar stability across the tested knee range of motion.[319] This finding may be difficult to apply to clinical settings because it is extremely rare for a person to have isolated paralysis of the VMO. For decades, however, anecdotal evidence has suggested a preferential *atrophy* in the VMO in persons with chronic patellofemoral pain or history of chronic dislocation, apparently from disuse or neurogenic inhibition. Although some

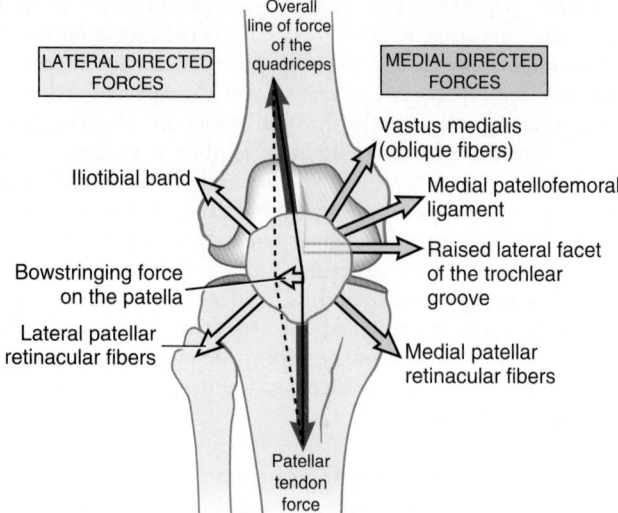

Major guiding forces acting on the patella

FIGURE 13.30 Highly diagrammatic and conceptualized model showing the interaction of locally produced forces acting on the patella as it moves through the trochlear groove of the femur. Each force tends to pull (or push) the patella generally laterally *or* medially. Ideally, the opposing forces counteract one another so that the patella tracks optimally during flexion and extension of the knee. Note that the magnitude of the lateral bowstringing force is determined by the parallelogram method of vector addition (see Chapter 4). Vectors are not drawn to scale.

studies support this notion, others have shown that atrophy of the VMO is no more extreme than the atrophy often observed in other parts of the quadriceps muscle.[110,111,135,331] Research that clearly supports the contention that abnormal neuromuscular activation of the VMO is a *cause* of patellofemoral pain syndrome or chronic lateral dislocation is mixed and controversial.[108,194,266,331] Nevertheless, the suspicion of preferential atrophy, inhibition, or delayed or reduced activation of the VMO has historically led to the development of treatment approaches designed to selectively recruit, strengthen, or otherwise augment the action of this portion of the quadriceps. Although the rationale for this treatment approach is biomechanically sound, the ability to selectively alter the control, activation timing, or strength of only one component of the quadriceps remains a controversial topic.[e]

Finally, the *medial patellar retinacular fibers* flow broadly from the medial edge of the patella toward the medial tibiofemoral articulation. The clinical and research literature often refers to a thickened subset of these fibers as the *medial patellofemoral ligament* (see Fig. 13.10).[147,339] This narrow fan-shaped ligament reinforces the medial side of the knee, primarily by connections between the patella and the femur, medial meniscus, and VMO. The medial patellofemoral ligament is well-known medically because of its high likelihood of being ruptured after a complete lateral dislocation of the patella. Biomechanically, the ligament is well respected for its ability to limit a lateral shift of the patella. Selectively cutting the medial patellofemoral ligament in cadaver specimens produces an average 25% loss in medial patellar stability across the tested knee range of motion.[319] It is noteworthy that the loss of medial patellar stability increases sharply to 50% when the knee is in full extension. The medial patellofemoral ligament is drawn most taut in the last 20 to 30 degrees of extension.[4,285] Bicos and colleagues suggest that the ligament is pulled taut in extension with the aid of the activated

---

[e] 181,200,219,266,279,291,335

VMO, to which the ligament partially attaches.[29] These combined active and passive actions provide an important source of medial stability to the patella at a point in the knee's range of motion at which the patella is least stable because, in part, it is relatively disengaged from the bony "grip" of the trochlear groove of the femur.

Global Factors

The magnitude of the lateral bowstringing force applied to the patella is strongly influenced by the frontal and horizontal plane alignment of the bones associated with the knee extensor mechanism. As a general principle, *factors that resist an excessive valgus position or the extremes of axial rotation of the tibiofemoral joint favor optimal tracking of the patellofemoral joint.* These factors are referred to as "global" in the sense that they are associated with joints distant to the patellofemoral joint, as far removed as the trunk, hip, and joints of the foot.

Excessive genu valgus as a result of dynamic weight-bearing activities can increase the Q-angle and thereby increase the lateral bowstringing force on the patella (Fig. 13.31). If persistent, the lateral force on the patella can alter its alignment and thereby increase the stress on the patellofemoral joint, especially laterally.[208,290] Increased valgus position of the knee can occur from ligamentous laxity or injury, but also indirectly from a dynamic posture of the hip that involves increased *adduction* of the femur (hip) in a weight-bearing position, such as when landing from a jump.[260,293] Weakness or reduced activation of the hip abductor muscles (including trunk muscles that stabilize the lumbopelvic region) can allow the femur to slant excessively medially toward the midline, thereby placing excessive tension on the medial structures of the knee—often a precursor to excessive valgus position of the knee.[48,252,255,260,290] Furthermore, during relatively demanding activities such as a single limb squat, persons with weak hip abductors may lean their trunk *toward* the side of the weakened muscle group (i.e., compensated Trendelenburg sign described in Chapter 12). This ipsilateral trunk lean can shift body weight (and thus the ground reaction force) *lateral* to the stance knee,

thereby creating a genu valgus-directed torque.[252] Lastly, excessive pronation (eversion) of the subtalar joint, especially while landing from a jump, may create excessive valgus posturing at the knee. The kinematic relationship between the subtalar joint and the knee is described in greater detail in Chapter 14.

As depicted by the woman's knee in Fig. 13.31B, excessive *external rotation of the knee* (via femoral internal rotation) often occurs in conjunction with an excessive valgus deviation at the knee.[208] External rotation of the knee places the tibial tuberosity and attached patellar tendon in a more lateral position relative to the distal femur. As shown in Fig. 13.31, excessive external rotation of the knee can also increase the Q-angle and thereby amplify the lateral bowstringing force on the patella.[199,310] As indicated by the pair of blue arrows in Fig. 13.31, external rotation of the knee can occur as a combination of femoral-on-tibial and tibial-on-femoral perspectives. Often, however, excessive external rotation of the knee is expressed in a weight-bearing position, as the *femur is internally rotated* relative to a fixed or nearly fixed lower leg.[206,208] Persistent internal rotation posturing of the femur during weight-bearing activities may occur from reduced strength or neuromuscular control of the external rotator muscles of the hip, tightness of the hip internal rotator muscles, reduced activation of lumbopelvic stabilizer muscles, or as a compensation for excessive femoral anteversion (see Chapter 12) or excessive external tibial torsion (Chapter 14).[f] When weakness or poor control of the hip muscles is present, the posture of excessive hip internal rotation is often combined with varying amounts of hip adduction.[21,30,260] Although this postural weakness can be subtle, it is often observed when a person is asked to slowly descend a step or assume a partial single-leg squat position. During this maneuver, the distal femur may be observed to "roll" inward slightly, despite conscious effort to resist this motion by activation of hip muscles.

---

[f]48,173,175,272,292,293,310,338,388

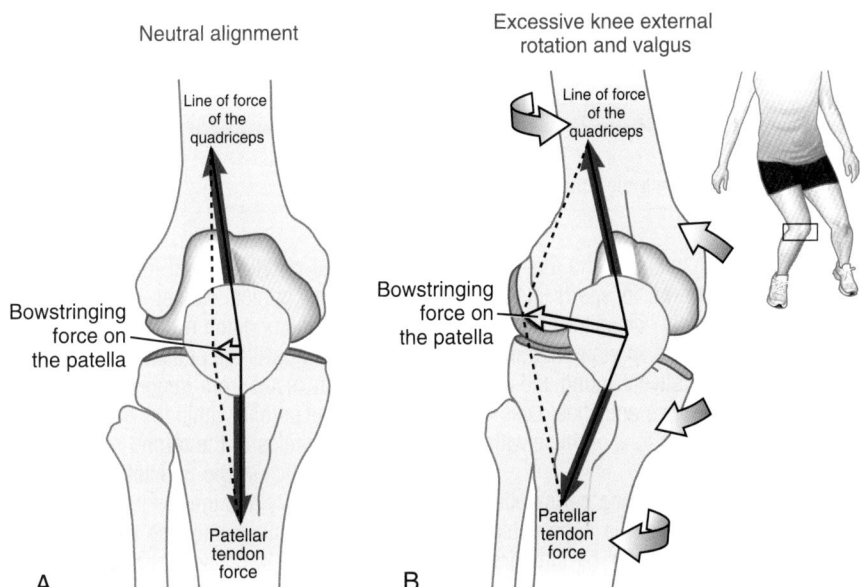

FIGURE 13.31 (A) Neutral alignment of the knee, showing the lateral bowstringing force acting on the patella. (B) Excessive knee valgus and knee external rotation can increase the Q-angle and thereby increase the lateral bowstringing force. Blue arrows indicate bone movement that can increase knee external rotation, and purple arrows indicate an increased valgus positioning of the knee. Note that the increased external rotation of the knee can occur as a combination of excessive internal rotation of the femur and external rotation of the tibia.

According to many sources in the literature, weakness or reduced control of the hip external rotator and abductor muscles is more pronounced in women and may increase the risk for developing patellofemoral joint pain or being predisposed to lateral dislocation of the patella.[g] To explore this association, Powers and colleagues used kinematic MRI to evaluate the patellofemoral kinematics in a group of young females with a history of patellofemoral joint pain.[289] One component of the study instructed subjects to actively rise from a partial one-legged squat position, from 45 degrees of flexion to full knee extension. On average, the femurs of the extending hips rotated *internally* rather sharply throughout the last 20 degrees of full knee extension. On close individual analysis, images showed that the trochlear groove of the femur rotated *medially under the patella,* which was held fixed by the strong contraction of the quadriceps. Such *femoral-on-patellar* kinematics aligned the extensor mechanism and embedded patella more laterally and closer to the raised lateral facet of the trochlear groove of the femur. This precarious alignment may place the patella closer to a point of lateral dislocation. Furthermore, these observations suggest that the pathomechanics of excessive lateral tracking can result from the femur being displaced medially under the patella, as well as from the patella being displaced laterally over the femur, as is generally described.

Excessive *internal rotation of the knee* while walking has also been suggested as a predisposing factor to patellofemoral joint pain.[21,224,293] Clinically, excessive internal rotation of the tibia is most often associated with excessive *pronation* of the subtalar joint in the early and mid stance phase of walking (Chapter 14). Although excessive internal rotation of the tibia (at the knee) would theoretically *decrease* the Q-angle and associated lateral bowstringing force on the patella, it has been theorized that a compensatory excessive *internal rotation of the femur* would result, thereby increasing the stress at the patellofemoral joint.[224,357] For this reason, the use of foot orthotics to control the subtalar joint may be an appropriate treatment strategy for some people with patellofemoral pain syndrome.[35,370,385]

[g]176,228,252,308,310,338,384

As alluded to earlier, data show that females experience a greater incidence of abnormal kinematics and related pathology at the patellofemoral joint than males. Data collected at a large sports medicine clinic, for example, showed that recurrent lateral dislocation of the patella accounted for 58.4% of all joint dislocations in women, compared with only 14% in men.[65] It has been speculated that the sex bias in chronic patellar dislocation may in some persons be biomechanically associated with the 3 to 4 degrees of greater Q-angle often measured in females.[143] A greater Q-angle may reflect a greater pelvic width–to–femoral length ratio in females.[269] Whether the apparent greater Q-angle in females (and assumed greater lateral bowstringing force on the patella) alters patellar tracking to a point of *causing* an increased incidence in dislocation and stress-related pain is difficult to prove, although this is a reasonable point to consider.

Summary

Abnormal tracking of the patella is a complicated topic for several reasons. First, tracking kinematics are subtle, highly variable, and difficult to measure. Second, the link between abnormal tracking and pathology is not well established or universally agreed upon. Although it is generally believed that abnormal tracking can contribute to stress-related cartilage injury and ultimately patellofemoral pain syndrome (PFPS), its role in chronic patellar lateral dislocation is not as clear. It is relatively common for a person with classic symptoms of PFPS to have no history of acute or chronic patellar dislocation. Likewise, a person with chronic patellar instability (i.e., history of multiple dislocations) may be relatively pain-free except during and immediately after a dislocation. Often, patellar instability with a history of multiple dislocations stems from an initial, traumatic event where the patellar dislocation was severe enough to injure soft-tissue stabilizers of the patellofemoral joint, such as the medial patellofemoral ligament. Such an injury may predispose a person to multiple dislocations, each rendering the patellofemoral joint more unstable. Adding to the complicated clinical picture is that it is not uncommon for a person to show the classic signs of PFPS and to have a history of chronic dislocations.

SPECIAL FOCUS 13.7

Patellofemoral Pain Syndrome: An All-Too-Common Condition Affecting the Knee

Patellofemoral pain syndrome (PFPS) is one of the most common orthopedic conditions encountered in sports medicine outpatient settings.[351,355] This potentially disabling condition accounts for about 30% of all knee disorders in women and 20% in men.[65] PFPS most frequently affects relatively young and active persons and is often associated with overuse activities. Less frequently, however, PFPS affects sedentary persons or those with no history of overuse or trauma.

Persons with PFPS typically experience diffuse peripatellar or retropatellar pain with an insidious onset. Pain is aggravated by excessive squatting, climbing stairs, running, or by sitting with knees flexed for a prolonged period. Cases of PFPS may be mild, involving only a generalized aching about the anterior knee, or they may be so severe it limits participation in some daily activities.

The exact pathogenesis of PFPS is unknown and may involve an interaction among anatomic, neuromuscular, and biomechanical factors.[290,331,377,385] Chronic pain may also be driven by amplified responsiveness of nociceptors located near and within

a stressed patellofemoral joint.[329] This chapter focuses on possible biomechanical causes of PFPS, with an underlying assumption that the condition results primarily from stress intolerance of the articular cartilage and innervated subchondral bone. Excessive stress can result from abnormal movement (tracking) and alignment of the patella within the trochlear groove. Complicating these pathomechanics is the strong relationship between the kinematics and kinetics of the patellofemoral joint with other joints of the lower extremity and the trunk, especially in a weight-bearing situation. Furthermore, knowing whether the pathomechanics are the primary cause *or* consequence of increased stress and associated pain within the patellofemoral joint is not always certain. The lack of understanding of the exact cause and underlying pathology of PFPS can make this condition one of the most difficult treatment challenges in physical and sports medicine. The biomechanical rationale behind many of the traditional treatment approaches to PFPS are addressed within this chapter.[370]

Although the pathomechanical relationships between PFPS and patellar instability are not clear, factors associated with abnormal tracking of the patella need to be at least suspected as part of the underlying cause. Table 13.6 provides a list of potential indirect and direct causes of excessive lateral tracking of the patella. Although many of the causes listed in Table 13.6 are described as separate entities, many occur in combinations. Clinical evaluation of persons with patellofemoral joint pathology must therefore consider several potential interrelated factors that can contribute to the problem. Much more clinical research is needed in this area to improve the conservative and surgical treatment of patellofemoral joint pain and chronic dislocation.

TABLE 13.6 Potential Indirect and Direct Causes of Excessive Lateral Tracking of the Patella

Structural or Functional Causes	Specific Examples
Bony dysplasia or other anomaly	Dysplastic lateral facet of the trochlear groove of the femur ("flattened" groove) "High" patella (patella alta)
Excessive laxity in periarticular connective tissue	Laxity of the medial patellar retinacular fibers (medial patellofemoral ligament) Laxity or attrition of the medial collateral ligament of the knee Laxity and reduced height of the medial longitudinal arch of the foot (related to overpronation of the subtalar joint)
Excessive stiffness or tightness in periarticular connective tissue and muscle	Increased tightness in the lateral patellar retinacular fibers or iliotibial band Increased tightness of the internal rotator or adductor muscles of the hip
Extremes of bony or joint alignment	Coxa varus Excessive hip internal rotation as a compensation for excessive anteversion of the proximal femur (Chapter 12) or excessive external tibial torsion (Chapter 14) Large Q-angle Excessive genu valgum
Muscle weakness	Weakness or poor control of • hip external rotator and abductor muscles • the vastus medialis (oblique fibers) • the tibialis posterior muscle (related to overpronation of the foot)

SPECIAL FOCUS 13.8

Traditional Treatment Principles for Abnormal Tracking and Chronic Dislocation of the Patellofemoral Joint

Much of the orthopedic treatment and physical therapy for abnormal tracking of the patella and chronic lateral dislocation focus on addressing the underlying pathomechanics described in this chapter. Unfortunately, there is no universally accepted gold standard approach to treatment.[290,385] Generally, treatments strive to alter, when feasible, the alignment of the tibiofemoral and patellofemoral joints to reduce the magnitude of the lateral bowstringing force on the patella. To achieve this goal, exercises are often prescribed with the intention of strengthening and challenging the motor control of the hip abductor and external rotator muscles (including the gluteus maximus), trunk muscles, quadriceps, and other muscles capable of supporting the medial longitudinal arch of the foot.[h] As an adjunct to these exercises, treatment may also include stretching tight periarticular connective tissues and muscles of the lower limb, manual therapy, taping of the patella, or using a foot orthosis to reduce excessive pronation of the foot.[74,219,224,385]

Another treatment intervention involves teaching patients how to modify their movements to reduce the likelihood of encountering unnecessarily large patellofemoral stress. Gait retraining, for example, may focus on teaching patients how to run while avoiding hip movements that promote excessive valgus positioning at the knee, such as excessive hip adduction or internal rotation.[63] (Other gait retraining methods employed to reduce demands on the patellofemoral joint are described in Chapter 16.) In addition, while performing any type of partial squat movement, patients should also be encouraged to avoid excessive hip adduction and internal rotation by giving reminders to "keep their knees in line with their second toe," or similar verbal cueing.[78] This advice can be very useful, as Liao et al. calculated that only 5 degrees of femur internal rotation while weight-bearing increases the contact pressure on the patellar cartilage by 26%, primarily over the lateral facet.[207] Teaching patients how to control their knee posturing through active control of the hip is an essential training point.

Other topics of patient education focus on the natural link between quadriceps force and patellofemoral stress. For example, when significant anterior knee pain is present, it is typically advised to avoid placing unnecessarily large demands on the quadriceps, for example, by limiting activities such as climbing steep stairs, especially while carrying a substantial load. Furthermore, ascending a step with a slight forward lean of the trunk significantly reduces the force on the patellofemoral joint.[15] As described elsewhere in this chapter, a forward lean of the trunk partially shifts the muscular forces from the quadriceps to the hip extensor muscles.

Clinicians also need to consider the relative force (or load) placed on the patellofemoral joint when advising patients on quadriceps strengthening exercises. Ample data on this topic are available in the research literature. For example, Van Rossom et al report that a sideward lunge produces about 80% greater average contact force on the patellofemoral joint as a forward lunge, or a bilateral squat produces about 85% greater average contact force as ascending a 16 cm (about 6 inches) step.[365]

Continued

Traditional Treatment Principles for Abnormal Tracking and Chronic Dislocation of the Patellofemoral Joint—cont'd

Surgeries have been designed to lessen the effect of exaggerated lateral forces on the patella, especially in cases of chronic lateral dislocation. Examples include lateral retinacular release, trochleoplasty, repair of a torn or lax medial patellofemoral ligament, realignment of the extensor mechanism (in particular the oblique fibers of the vastus medialis), and a medial transfer or elevation of the tibial tuberosity.[150,196,334] In extreme cases of excessive femoral anteversion, de-rotation osteotomies may be considered to reduce the internal rotation posturing. Just as there are many conservative approaches to treatment of impairments of the patellofemoral joint, there are also many surgical approaches to this problem—many of which remain controversial. The myriad treatment approaches reflect, in part, the difficulty in understanding the potentially complex pathogenesis of the problem.

[h]18,105,139,181,253,385

KNEE FLEXOR-ROTATOR MUSCLES

Except for the gastrocnemius, all muscles that cross posterior to the knee can flex and rotate the knee internally or externally. The so-called *flexor-rotator group* includes the hamstrings, sartorius, gracilis, and popliteus. Unlike the knee extensor group, which is innervated by the femoral nerve, the flexor-rotator muscles have three sources of innervation: femoral, obturator, and sciatic.

Functional Anatomy

The *hamstring muscles* (i.e., semimembranosus, semitendinosus, and long head of the biceps femoris) have their proximal attachment on the ischial tuberosity. The short head of the biceps has its proximal attachment on the lateral lip of the linea aspera of the femur. Distally, the hamstrings cross the knee joint and attach to the tibia and fibula (see Figs. 13.9 and 13.10).

The *semimembranosus* attaches distally to the posterior side of the medial condyle of the tibia. Additional distal attachments include the MCL, both menisci, the oblique popliteal ligament, and fascia covering the popliteus muscle. These extensive attachments provide significant support to the posterior-medial corner of the knee.[177]

For most of its course, the sinewy *semitendinosus* tendon lies posterior to the semimembranosus muscle. Just proximal to the knee, however, the tendon of the semitendinosus courses anteriorly toward its distal attachment on the anterior-medial aspect of tibia. Both heads of the *biceps femoris* attach primarily to the head of the fibula, with lesser insertions to the lateral collateral ligament, the capsule of the proximal tibiofibular joint, and the lateral side of the lateral condyle of the tibia.

All hamstring muscles, except the short head of the biceps femoris, cross the hip and knee. As described in Chapter 12, the three biarticular hamstrings are very effective hip extensors, especially in the control of the position of the pelvis and trunk over the femur.

In addition to flexing the knee, the medial hamstrings (i.e., semimembranosus and semitendinosus) internally rotate the knee. The biceps femoris flexes and externally rotates the knee. Active axial rotation in either direction is greatest when the knee is partially flexed. This can be appreciated by palpating the tendons of the semitendinosus and biceps femoris behind the knee as the leg is actively internally and externally rotated repeatedly. This is performed while the subject sits with the knee flexed 70 to 90 degrees. As the knee is gradually extended, the pivot point of the rotating lower leg shifts from the knee to the hip. At full extension, active rotation at the knee is restricted because the knee is mechanically locked, and most ligaments are pulled taut. Furthermore, the moment arm of the hamstrings for internal and external rotation of the knee is reduced significantly in full extension.[40]

The *sartorius* and *gracilis* have their proximal attachments on different parts of the pelvis (see Chapter 12). Distally, however, the tendons travel side by side across the medial side of the knee to attach to the proximal anterior-medial shaft of the tibia, near the semitendinosus (see Fig. 13.10). The three conjoined tendons of the sartorius, gracilis, and semitendinosus attach to the tibia through a common broad sheet of connective tissue known as the *pes anserinus* (e-Fig. 13.1). As a group the "pes muscles" are effective internal rotators of the knee. Connective tissues hold the tendons of the pes group just *posterior* to the medial-lateral axis of rotation of the knee. The three pes muscles therefore flex as well as internally rotate the knee.

The pes anserinus group adds significant dynamic stability to the medial side of the knee. Along with the MCL, posterior-medial capsule, and oblique popliteal ligament, active tension in the pes muscles resists knee *external* rotation and excessive valgus of the knee.

The *popliteus* is a triangular muscle located deep to the gastrocnemius within the popliteal fossa (see Fig. 13.9). By a strong intracapsular tendon, the popliteus attaches proximally to the lateral condyle of the femur, between the lateral collateral ligament and the lateral meniscus (see Figs. 13.8 and 13.12).[392] Just inferior to the knee joint, fibers from the tendon of the popliteus connect to the adjacent posterior edge of the lateral meniscus and to the head of the fibula (via the popliteofibular ligament; see Fig. 13.8).[221] More distally, the popliteus has an extensive attachment to the posterior side of the tibia, under cover of a fascial extension from the semimembranosus (Fig. 13.9). In conjunction with the arcuate popliteal ligament, this dense fascial extension prevents the muscle from bowstringing outward during flexion.

The anatomy and action of the gastrocnemius and plantaris are considered in Chapter 14.

Group Action of Flexor-Rotator Muscles

Many of the functions of the flexor-rotator muscles of the knee are expressed during walking and running activities. Examples of these functions are considered separately for tibial-on-femoral and femoral-on-tibial movements of the knee.

Control of Tibial-on-Femoral Osteokinematics

An important function of the knee flexor-rotator muscles is to decelerate the advancing lower leg while brisk walking and while running. This action is clearly demonstrated by the biarticular hamstring muscles. During the late part of the swing phase, the hamstrings produce relatively low-to-moderate forces but at relatively high lengthening velocities. Through their eccentric action, the muscles can dampen the potentially large joint impact of reaching full knee extension, thereby reducing strain on tissues such as the ACL and posterior capsule of the knee. The deceleration demand on the hamstrings during the late swing phase of sprinting can be especially large. The combination of large force produced at long muscle length may account, in part, for the hamstring's increased vulnerability to strain-related injury at this phase of running.[55,166] The mechanics of hamstring strain injury while sprinting is discussed further in Chapter 16.

Control of Femoral-on-Tibial Osteokinematics

The muscular demand needed to control femoral-on-tibial motions is generally larger and more complex than that needed to control most ordinary tibial-on-femoral knee motions. A muscle such as the sartorius, for example, may have to simultaneously control up to 5 degrees of freedom (i.e., 2 degrees at the knee and 3 degrees at the hip). Consider the action of several knee flexor-rotator muscles while one runs and turns to catch a ball (Fig. 13.32A). While the right foot is firmly fixed to the ground, the right femur, pelvis, trunk, neck, head, and eyes all rotate to the left. Note the diagonal flow of activated muscles between the right fibula and left side of the neck. The muscle action epitomizes intermuscular synergy. In this case the short head of the biceps femoris helps to anchor the bottom of the diagonal kinetic chain to the fibula. The fibula, in turn, is anchored to the tibia primarily by the interosseous membrane and the proximal and distal tibiofibular joints.

Stability and control at the rotating knee require interaction of forces produced by surrounding muscles and ligaments, especially during high-velocity movements. To illustrate, refer to Fig. 13.32B. With the right foot planted, the short head of the biceps femoris accelerates the femur internally. By way of eccentric activation, the pes anserinus muscles help decelerate the internal rotation of the femur over the tibia. The pes anserinus group may be regarded as a "dynamic medial collateral ligament" by resisting not only the external rotation of the knee but also concurrent valgus-producing forces. The pes group of muscles may help compensate for a weak or lax MCL or posterior-medial capsule. Although not depicted in Fig. 13.32B, eccentric activation of the popliteus and semimembranosus can also assist the pes group with decelerating external rotation of the knee.[177]

Maximal Torque Production of the Knee Flexor-Rotator Muscles

Studies indicate that maximal-effort, isometrically-generated knee flexion torque is generally greatest with the knee in the last 20 to 30 degrees of full extension, then declines steadily as the knee is progressively flexed.[8,99,190,362,394] A representative plot of published

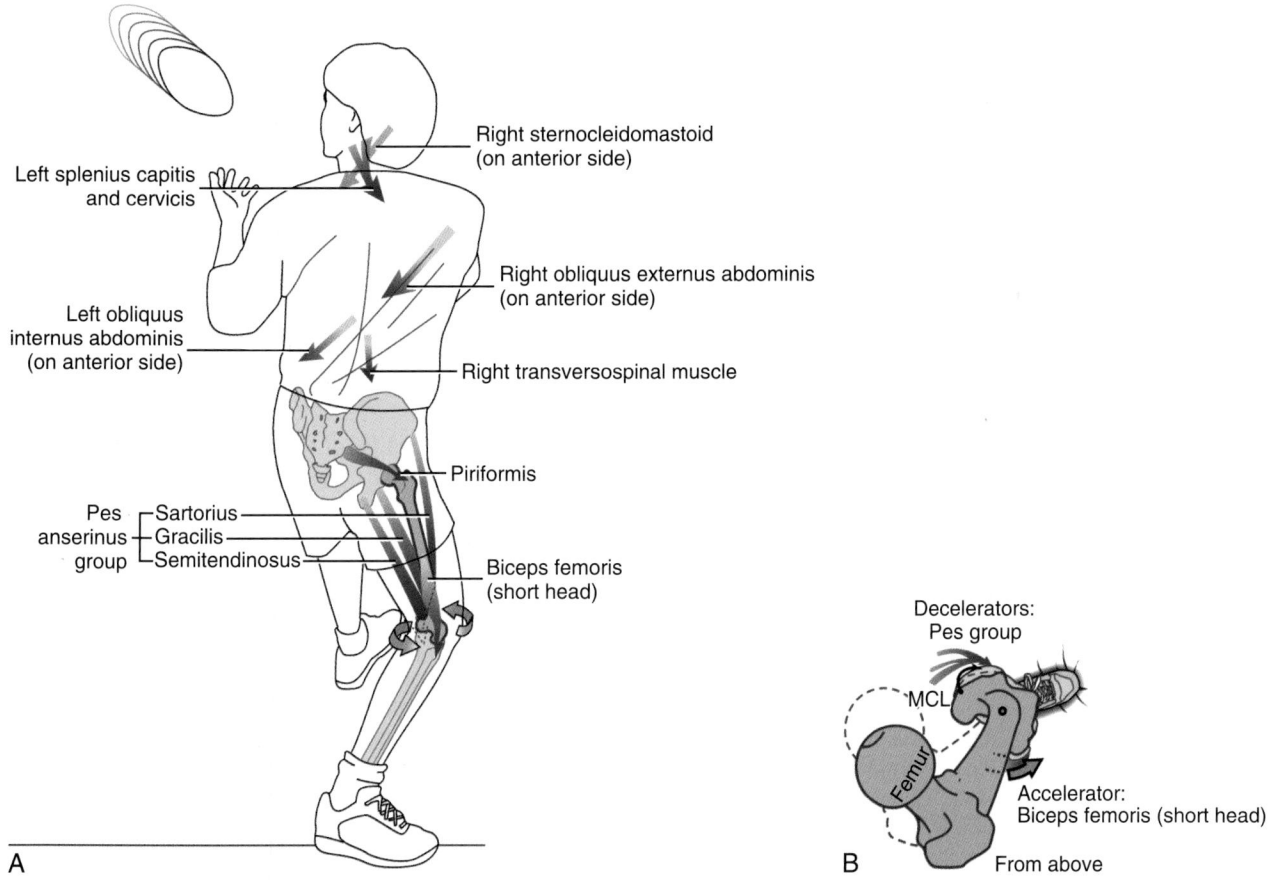

FIGURE 13.32 (A) Several muscles are shown controlling the rotation of the head, neck, trunk, pelvis, and femur toward the approaching ball. Because the right foot is fixed to the ground, the right knee functions as an important pivot point. (B) Control of axial rotation of the right knee is illustrated from above. The short head of the biceps femoris contracts to accelerate the femur internally (i.e., the knee joint moves into external rotation). Active force from the pes anserinus muscles in conjunction with a passive force from the stretched medial collateral ligament *(MCL)* and oblique popliteal ligament (not shown) helps to decelerate, or limit, the external rotation at the knee.

torque data from healthy males is shown in Fig. 13.33.[333] Subjects produced maximal-effort isometric knee flexion torque with hips held in extension. Although a wide range of values have been reported, overall, the hamstrings have their greatest flexor moment

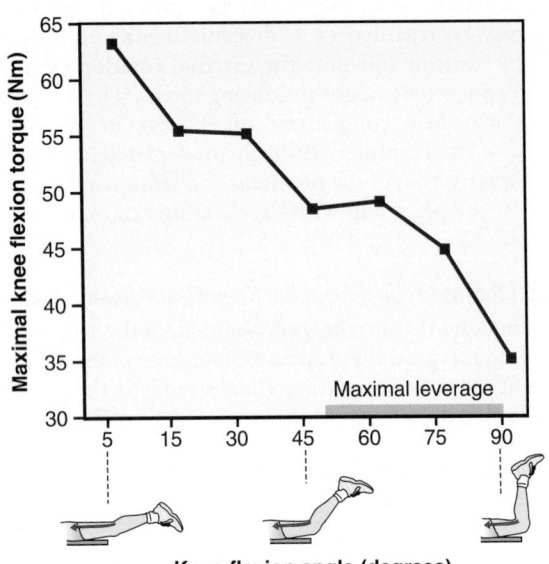

Knee flexion angle (degrees)

FIGURE 13.33 A plot showing the maximal-effort knee flexor torques produced between 5 degrees and about 90 degrees of flexion. The internal moment arm (leverage) used by the knee flexors (hamstrings) is greatest between about 50 and 90 degrees of knee flexion. Knee flexor torques are produced isometrically by maximal effort, with the hip held in extension. Data from 26 healthy males, average age 28 years old.[333]

arm (leverage) at 50 to 90 degrees of knee flexion (see bar on horizontal axis in graph of Fig. 13.33).[39,165,220,267,333] The torque-angle data depicted in Fig. 13.33 clearly indicate that the knee flexors generate their greatest torque at knee angles that coincide with relative elongated muscle length, rather than high leverage. (As noted in Fig. 13.26, this is in slight contrast to the quadriceps, where maximal-effort knee extensor torque partially overlaps the arc in the range of motion where leverage is greatest.) Flexing the hip to elongate the hamstrings promotes even greater knee flexion torque.[33] The length-tension relationship appears to be a very influential factor in determining the flexion torque potential of the hamstring muscles.

Few data are available on the maximal torque potential of the internal and external rotator muscles of the knee. When tested isokinetically with the knee flexed to 90 degrees, the internal and external rotators at the knee have been shown to produce nearly equal peak torques.[12] At first thought, these results may be surprising considering the far greater number of internal rotator muscles compared with just one external rotator muscle at the knee (i.e., the biceps femoris). The apparent conflict may be partially reconciled by the fact that, with the knee flexed to 90 degrees, the biceps femoris muscle has a threefold greater axial rotation moment arm than the average of all the internal rotators.[40] The laterally displaced distal attachment of the biceps femoris to the head of the fibula apparently augments this muscle's rotational leverage.

The average axial rotation leverage for virtually all rotators of the knee is greatest between 70 and 90 degrees of knee flexion, where the muscles' lines of force are nearly perpendicular to the longitudinal (vertical) axis of rotation through the tibia.[40] The only exception to this design is the popliteus muscle, which has its greatest moment arm to internally rotate the knee at about 40 degrees of flexion.

SPECIAL FOCUS 13.9

Popliteus Muscle: The "Key to the Knee," and More

The exact functions of the popliteus muscle are still not fully recognized, despite research dating back many decades.[22] The muscle has received more recent orthopedic interest in the context of surgically reconstructing the posterior-lateral corner of the knee.[392] The deep location of the popliteus makes it difficult to study via surface EMG electrodes, although this has been done.[315] Many of the proposed functions of this muscle described herein are based on anatomic location and line of force.

The popliteus is an internal rotator and flexor of the knee. As the extended and locked knee prepares to flex, the popliteus provides an important *internal rotation* torque that helps mechanically *unlock* the knee.[4] (Recall that the knee is mechanically locked by a combination of extension and external rotation of the joint.) From a standing position, unlocking the knee to prepare to flex into a squat position, for example, requires that the *femur* externally rotates slightly over a relatively fixed tibia. The ability of the popliteus to externally rotate the femur (and hence internally rotate the knee) is apparent by observing the muscle's oblique line of force as it crosses behind the knee (see Fig. 13.9).[392]

The popliteus muscle's oblique line of pull is particularly favorable for producing axial rotation on an extended knee. The lines of force of the other knee flexor muscles are nearly vertical when the knee is extended, which greatly minimizes their potential to produce axial rotation. Because of the popliteus muscle's favorable mechanical ability to initiate internal rotation of the locked knee, it has been referred to as the "key to the knee."

Another function of the popliteus is to help dynamically stabilize both the lateral and the medial sides of the knee. Along with other tissues within the posterior-lateral corner of the knee, the popliteus, by way of its strong intracapsular tendon, provides a significant resistance against a *varus-producing* torque to the knee. The popliteus also stabilizes the medial side of the knee by decelerating and limiting excessive *external rotation* of the knee. This action, performed through eccentric activation, may reduce the stress placed on the medial collateral ligament, posterior-medial capsule, and anterior cruciate ligament.

The popliteus has been long recognized as a static stabilizer of the knee in a partial squat position. This proposed action, which has been advanced by studies using indwelling and surface EMG electrodes, may assist the posterior cruciate ligament in resisting a forward slide of the femur relative to the tibia when holding a partial-squat position.[22,315]

Abnormal Alignment of the Knee

FRONTAL PLANE

The knee is normally aligned in the frontal plane in about 5 to 10 degrees of valgus. Deviation from this alignment is referred to as excessive genu valgum or genu varum.

Genu Varum with Unicompartmental Osteoarthritis of the Knee

During walking at normal speeds across level terrain, the joint reaction force at the knee routinely reaches about two to three times one's body weight.[123] These forces peak at about 15% and again at 45% of the gait cycle (relatively early and late stance phase).[67] The force is created primarily by the interaction of the forces generated by muscles throughout the lower limb and by the ground reaction force. During virtually the entire stance phase of walking, the ground reaction force normally passes just lateral to the heel, then upward and *medial* to the knee as it continues toward the center of gravity of the body as a whole. As depicted in Fig. 13.34, by passing medial to an anterior-posterior axis at the knee, the ground reaction force causes a *varus torque* (and associated 2–3 degrees of knee adduction) with each step.[1] As a result, joint reaction force during walking is normally several times greater on the *medial* joint compartment than on the lateral compartment.[123,325] Throughout one's lifetime, this repetitive varus (adduction) torque is partially absorbed through structures such as the lateral collateral ligament, iliotibial band, and the articular cartilage and meniscus within the medial compartment of the knee.

Most persons tolerate the asymmetric loading of the medial side of the knee while walking with little or no difficulty. The articular cartilage in some persons, however, does not tolerate the asymmetry and associated excessive wear, and ultimately develops (medial) unicompartmental osteoarthritis.[75,284] A 20% increase in peak varus torque at the knee during walking has been shown to be associated with a sixfold increase in the risk of developing medial compartment osteoarthritis.[242] Thinning of the articular cartilage on the medial side can tilt the knee into genu varum, or a bow-legged deformity (Fig. 13.35A). This deformity can initiate a vicious cycle: the varus deformity increases medial joint compartment loading, resulting in greater loss of medial joint space, greater knee adduction movement, increased strain on the lateral collateral ligament, further increased medial joint loading, and so on. Fig. 13.35B shows an x-ray film of bilateral genu varum. Both knees show signs of medial joint osteoarthritis (i.e., loss of medial joint space and hypertrophic reactive bone around the medial compartment). Management of relatively severe genu varum often involves surgery, such as a total knee replacement or, as shown in Fig. 13.35C, a high tibial (wedge) osteotomy. The ultimate goals of the osteotomy are to correct the varus deformity and reduce the potentially damaging stress over the medial joint compartment of the knee.

In addition to surgery, other more conservative measures have been proposed to reduce the compression forces on the medial articular surface of the knee in persons with medial compartment arthritis. Although studies are mixed regarding their clinical efficacy, the more common nonsurgical interventions include valgus-*inducing* knee bracing, laterally wedged insoles worn within the shoe, gait modification, reducing walking velocity, and strengthening of the gluteus maximus and tensor fascia lata to transmit a genu *valgus*–directed torque to the knee via tension through the iliotibial band.[i]

---

[i]20,72,106,123,134,154,248,302,328,349

Joint reaction forces through the normal knee

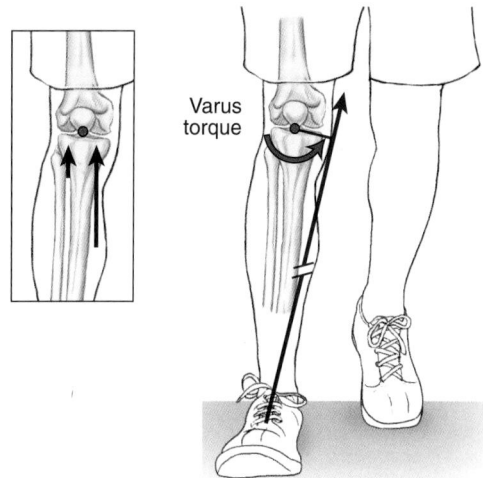

FIGURE 13.34 The ground reaction force (*long straight arrow* originating from the ground) passes medial to the knee joint, creating a varus-directed torque at the knee with every step. The moment arm available to the ground reaction force is shown, extending between the anterior-posterior axis at the knee (*small purple circle*) and the ground reaction force. As depicted by the pair of arrows in the inset to the left, greater compression force is generated over the medial articular surface of the joint.

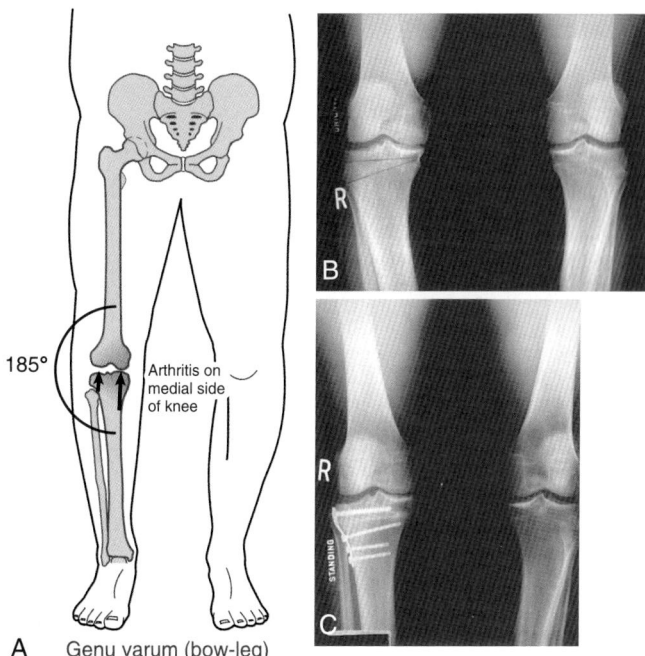

A   Genu varum (bow-leg)

FIGURE 13.35 Bilateral genu varum with osteoarthritis in the medial compartment of the right knee. (A) The varus deformity of the right knee is shown with greater joint reaction force on the medial compartment. (B) An anterior x-ray view with the subject (a 43-year-old man) standing, showing bilateral genu varum and medial joint osteoarthritis. Both knees have a loss of medial joint space and hypertrophic bone around the medial compartment. To correct the deformity on the right (R) knee, a wedge of bone will be surgically removed by a procedure known as a *high tibial osteotomy*. (C) The x-ray film shows the right knee after the removal of the wedge of bone. Note the change in joint alignment compared with the same knee in (B). (Courtesy Joseph Davies, MD, Aurora Advanced Orthopedics, Milwaukee, WI.)

In closing, although joint forces are normally higher on the medial compartment while walking, research shows that some weight-bearing exercises or activities create slightly higher forces across the lateral compartment, such as during squatting or lowering to a seated position.[365] Consulting this research literature allows the clinician to better personalize exercise prescriptions to limit large loads over a particular region of the knee that may be involved with acute degeneration or inflammation.

Excessive Genu Valgum

Several factors can lead to excessive genu valgum, or knock-knee. These include previous injury, genetic predisposition, high body mass index, and laxity of ligaments. Genu valgum may also result from or be exacerbated by abnormal alignment or muscle weakness at either end of the lower extremity. As indicated in Fig. 13.36A, reduced strength of the hip abductors can, at least in theory, increase the valgus load on the knee. In some cases excessive foot pronation may increase the valgus load on the knee by allowing the distal end of the tibia to slant ("abduct") farther away from the midline of the body. Over time, the tensional stress placed on the MCL and adjacent capsule may weaken the tissue. As described earlier in this chapter, excessive valgus of the knee may negatively affect patellofemoral joint tracking and create additional stress on the ACL.

Standing with a valgus deformity of approximately 10 degrees greater than normal alignment directs most of the joint compression force to the lateral joint compartment.[158] This increased regional stress may lead to lateral unicompartmental tibiofemoral osteoarthritis which is more common in women.[75,90] A total knee replacement may be performed to correct a valgus deformity associated with osteoarthritis, especially if it is progressive, is painful, or causes loss of function (Fig. 13.36B and C).

SAGITTAL PLANE

Genu Recurvatum

Full extension with slight external rotation is the knee's close-packed, most stable position. The knee may be extended beyond neutral an additional 5 to 10 degrees, although this is highly variable among persons. Standing with the knee in full extension usually directs the line of gravity from body weight slightly *anterior* to the medial-lateral axis of rotation at the knee. Gravity, therefore, produces a slight knee extension torque that can naturally assist with locking of the knee, allowing the quadriceps to relax intermittently during standing. Normally this gravity-assisted extension torque is resisted primarily by passive tension in stretched tissues such as the posterior capsule and flexor muscles of the knee, including the gastrocnemius.

Hyperextension beyond 10 degrees of neutral is frequently called *genu recurvatum* (from the Latin *genu,* knee, + *recurvare,* to bend backward). Mild cases of recurvatum may occur in otherwise healthy persons, often because of generalized laxity of the posterior structures of the knee. The primary cause of more severe genu recurvatum is a chronic, overpowering (net) knee extensor torque that eventually overstretches the posterior structures of the knee. The overpowering knee extension torque may stem from poor postural control or from neuromuscular disease that causes spasticity of the quadriceps muscles and/or paralysis of the knee flexors.

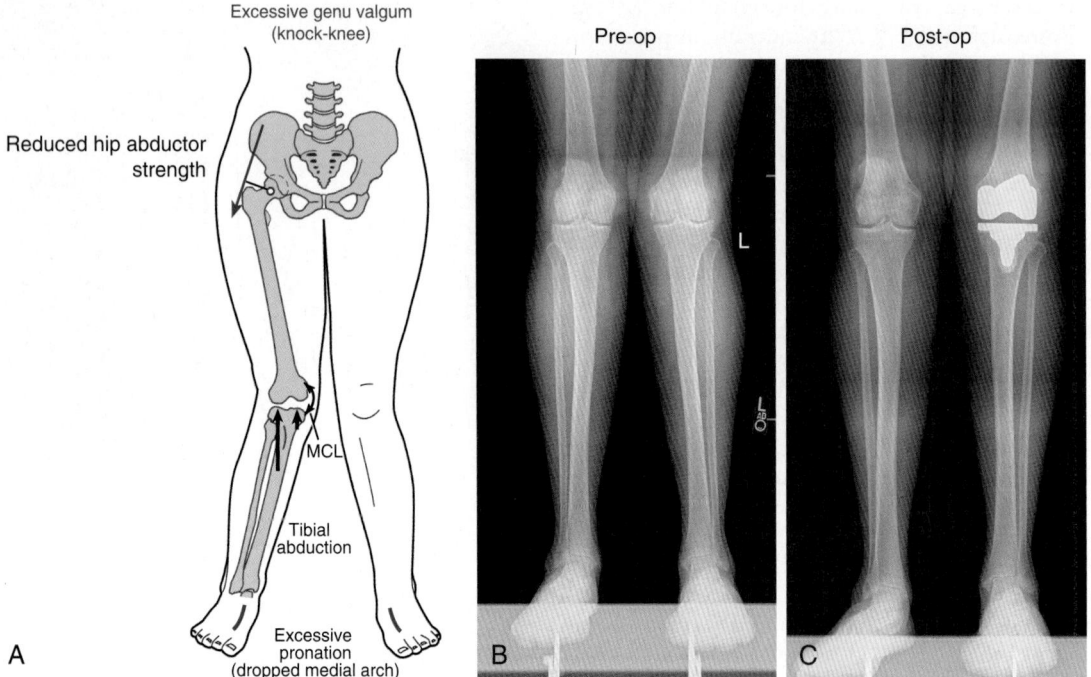

FIGURE 13.36 (A) Excessive genu valgum of the right knee. In this example, the valgus deformity could occur because of abnormal alignment or reduced muscle strength at either end of the lower limb. The pair of vertical arrows representing force vectors at the knee indicates greater compression force on the lateral compartment. (B) Pre-operative x-ray of a female with left knee osteoarthritis, associated with left excessive genu valgum. Note greater left femoral adduction. (C) Post-operative x-ray of same patient after total knee replacement. (x-rays courtesy Jacob Capin, PT, PhD; Michael Bade, PT, PhD; and Jennifer Stevens-Lapsley, PT, PhD, University of Colorado Denver, Anschutz Medical Campus, Aurora, CO.)

SPECIAL FOCUS 13.10

Case Report: Pathomechanics and Treatment of Severe Genu Recurvatum

Fig. 13.37A shows a case of severe genu recurvatum of the left knee caused by a flaccid muscle paralysis from polio, contracted 30 years earlier. The deformity progressed slowly over the previous 20 years as the individual continued to walk without a knee brace. She has partial paralysis of the left quadriceps and hip flexors but complete paralysis of all left knee flexors. Her completely paralyzed left ankle joint was previously fused surgically in about 25 degrees of plantar flexion.

Several interrelated factors are responsible for the development of the severe deformity depicted in Fig. 13.37A. Because of the fixed plantar flexion position of the fused ankle, the tibia must be tilted *posteriorly* so that the bottom of the foot makes full contact with the ground. This surgical fusion had been designed 30 years earlier to provide the knee with greater stability in extension. Over the years, however, the posterior tilted position of the tibia led to an overstretching of the posterior structures of the knee, which ultimately led to the hyperextension deformity. Of particular importance is the fact that total paralysis of the knee's flexor muscles provided no direct muscular resistance against the knee's ensuing hyperextension deformity. Furthermore, the greater the hyperextension deformity, the longer the external moment arm (EMA)

available to body weight to perpetuate the deformity. Without bracing of the knee, the hyperextension deformity produced a vicious circle, allowing continuous stretching of the posterior structures of the knee, increased length of the external moment arm, greater extension external torque, and a continuous progression of the deformity.

A recurring theme in this chapter is the fact that the knee functions as the middle link of the lower limb, and it is therefore vulnerable to deforming loads from musculoskeletal pathology at either end of the lower extremity. This case report demonstrates how an excessive and fixed plantar flexed ankle can, over the years, predispose a person to genu recurvatum.[203] As depicted in Fig. 13.37B, a relatively simple and inexpensive modification in footwear was used to treat the hyperextension deformity. Wearing tennis shoes with "built-up" heels provided excellent reduction in the severity of the genu recurvatum. The raised heel tilted the tibia and knee *anteriorly,* thereby significantly reducing the length of the deforming external moment arm at the knee. Body weight now produced less hyperextension torque at the knee, held in check by the anteriorly tilted tibia and the rigidity provided by the fused ankle joint.

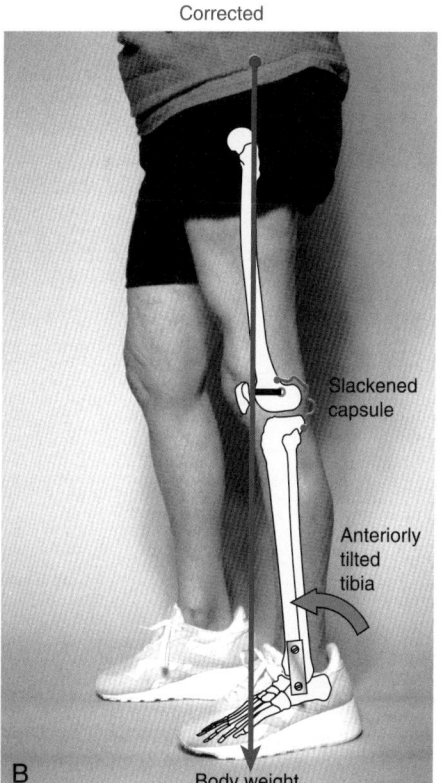

Genu recurvatum

FIGURE 13.37 Subject showing severe genu recurvatum of the left knee secondary to polio. In addition to sporadic muscle weakness throughout the left lower extremity, the left ankle was surgically fused in 25 degrees of plantar flexion. (A) When the subject stands barefoot, body weight acts with an abnormally large external moment arm *(EMA)* at the knee. The resulting large extensor torque amplifies the magnitude of the knee hyperextension deformity. (B) Subject can reduce the severity of the recurvatum deformity by wearing tennis shoes with a built-up heel. The shoe tilts her tibia and knee forward (indicated by the *green arrow*), thereby reducing the length of the deforming external moment arm at the knee.

SYNOPSIS

The unique movements allowed at the knee can be observed during many activities that involve the lower limb as a whole. Consider, for example, a person jumping high into the air. During the preparatory phase of the jump, the body lowers as the hips and knees flex and the ankles dorsiflex. This action stretches the appropriate biarticular muscles to augment their propulsive action as hip-and-knee extensors and ankle plantar flexors. When optimally timed, these actions propel and functionally elongate the body, maximizing the distance of the jump. A person with limited motion, pain, or significant weakness of the hip, knee, or ankle muscles would naturally have great difficulty in performing this activity.

Although axial rotation of the knee is essential to a normal gait pattern, the full expression of this motion is most apparent during femoral-on-tibial activities, in which the femur (and the rest of the upper body) rotates relative to a fixed lower leg. This movement is fundamental to running and rapidly changing directions, as well as many sporting activities, including dance. This femoral-on-tibial motion is guided and stabilized by muscle activation, body weight, articular fit between the femoral condyles and the menisci, and tension in several ligaments. As will be described in the next chapter, the tibia and talus typically participate in this activity by rotating relative to a fixed calcaneus. Pain, muscle weakness, or reduced motion in any single joint in the lower limb will require some musculoskeletal compensation at one or several other joints. Such compensations often give important clues to the underlying cause of the origin of the pathomechanics.

In contrast to other joints of the lower limb, the stability of the knee is dependent less on its bony fit and more on the surrounding muscles and periarticular connective tissues. The lack of bony restraint to most knee motions enhances its range of motion, but at the expense of increasing the vulnerability of the knee to injury. The MCL, posterior-medial capsule, and ACL are particularly vulnerable to injury from large valgus and axial rotation loads delivered to a weight-bearing lower limb, especially if the knee is in or near full extension. The extended knee, the joint's close-packed position, renders most tissues taut. Although this ligamentous pretension offers greater protection to the knee, the ligaments are closer to their mechanical failure point and therefore more vulnerable to injury when further strained. And finally, any closing discussion on mechanisms of knee injury should include the notion that the loss of restraining function of any single ligament increases the vulnerability of all the remaining structures.

Prevention of knee injuries is an important topic within sports medicine and demands continued attention and research. Although it may be possible to reduce the incidence of knee injuries during some noncontact sports, completely avoiding knee injury may be virtually impossible in certain high-velocity contact sports, such as American football or rugby. Protection may be maximized, however, by improving the athlete's ability to absorb or, when feasible, avoid the full effect of such an impact. This may be accomplished through better design of equipment and playing environment, and establishment of training programs that sufficiently strengthen and condition muscles, increase control and agility of the sport-specific movements, and improve the athlete's proprioception and ability to better perceive situations when the knee is particularly vulnerable to injury. Determining how and if these preventative approaches are successful requires systematic and controlled research performed by a wide range of health, physical education, and medical professionals.

As described previously in this chapter, the biomechanics of the knee are strongly influenced by its intermediate location between the hip and foot. During weight-bearing, the position of the hip directly affects the position of the knee. This strong kinematic dependency has important clinical implications. Consider, for example, that contraction of the gluteus maximus can indirectly assist with knee extension provided that the foot is firmly planted on the ground. This concept is important when teaching a person with a transfemoral amputation to ascend a step while wearing an above-the-knee prosthesis. Many other clinical examples relate to the role of the hip abductor and external rotator muscles in controlling the frontal and horizontal plane alignment of the knee. This concept is heavily embedded within the treatment or prevention of ACL injury and abnormal tracking of the patella. The next chapter will describe how the bones and joints of the ankle and foot influence the alignment of the lower leg, which ultimately affects the tension and stress within the structures of the knee.

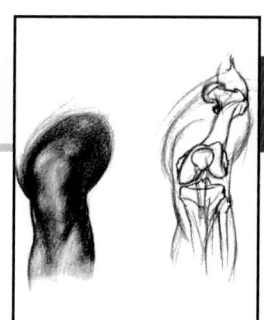

ADDITIONAL CLINICAL CONNECTIONS

CONTENTS

CLINICAL CONNECTION 13.1

Female Athletes Are at a Greater Risk for Anterior Cruciate Ligament Injury: Can This Be Changed?

Younger female athletes are at least three to five times more likely to experience an ACL injury compared with their male counterparts.[88,119,121,347] The risk is greatest in noncontact sports that involve jumping, landing, and pivoting motions, such as in basketball and soccer.[119] The elevated risk of injury, combined with the growing popularity of young women participating in high-school and collegiate sports, has led to a significant increase in the number of ACL injuries in this population.[276] This increase is concerning given the potential negative long-term health consequences that may result from an ACL injury at such a young age, including premature knee osteoarthritis, increased risk of a second ACL injury, loss of self-confidence, and the possibility of not returning to their previous level of sporting activity.[66,91,250,332,356]

Considerable research has focused on the underlying causes for the sex bias in ACL injuries. Understanding the causes are an essential step in developing effective preventative measures. Several risk factors have been cited, many of which are listed in Table 13.7.[j] Risk factors associated with reduced neuromuscular control and strength are of particular interest, in part because they are likely modifiable through training.[356] Several studies have reported that females typically land from a jump with their knees in greater valgus alignment than males.[52,211,330,356] An example of this type of landing was previously highlighted in Fig. 13.21. Landing in this manner, particularly if unexpected and unprotected by

[j]28,32,119,144,160,250,330,346,372,380

specific muscular activation, can place large and potentially damaging strain on the ACL.[283,356] This potentially deleterious knee alignment while landing or performing cutting maneuvers appears to be related to reduced muscular control or strength, at least in some athletes. As discussed in reference to Fig. 13.21, weakness or poor control of the hip abductors and external rotator muscles (notably the gluteus medius and gluteus maximus), coupled with reduced activation of trunk muscles, could allow the hip (femur) to assume a relative adducted and internally rotated position—kinematics believed to predispose a valgus "collapse" of the knee.[47,48,141,380]

Furthermore, research has shown that females typically land from a jump with trunk, hip, and knees held in slightly greater *extension* (less flexed) than males—frequently referred to as a "stiffer" or "erect" landing.[52,95,96] Electromyographic (EMG) studies have also shown that females, on average, display a reduced hamstring-to-quadriceps activation ratio compared with males at or near the time of landing.[94,95,379] It has been theorized that the greater relative quadriceps activation in females increases the anterior translation of the tibia and thereby increases the potential for causing excessive strain to the ACL, especially when landing with the knees biased more toward extension.[79,80,81,292]

Prevention programs have been developed that aim to reduce the frequency of ACL injury in female athletes, most commonly involving the sport of soccer. In addition to the traditional focus on enhancing strength of hip and trunk muscles, flexibility,

TABLE 13.7 **Studied Risk Factors Associated with Greater Incidence of ACL Injury in Female Athletes**

Environmental	Anatomic/Alignment	Biomechanical/Neuromuscular	Physiologic
• Practice or game setting • Playing position and surface • Time in season (late, early)	• Joint alignment (e.g., Q-angle, foot position at landing, knee hyperextension) • Body mass index • Femoral intercondylar notch width • Posterior-inferior directed slope of the lateral condyle of the tibia	• Muscular strength, control, or endurance (especially about the hip and trunk) • Hamstring/quadriceps strength or activation ratios • Control of the lower limb during landing from a jump and cutting maneuvers • Strength and volume of the ACL	• Physical maturation, age • Hormonal fluctuations • Proprioception or kinesthesis • Overall joint laxity • Genetic predisposition

Continued

Additional Clinical Connections

balance, aerobic conditioning, and sport-specific skills, many programs incorporate proprioceptive and "neuromuscular" coordination components within the training and warm-up activities.[13,157,159,263,287] These components include more complex and rigorous agility and plyometric training, in addition to educating the athletes about safer landing, pivoting, and side-stepping techniques.[13,71,97,356] Attention has focused on teaching the athlete to land from a jump in a "softer" fashion, incorporating slightly greater trunk-and-hip flexion. One purported benefit of this landing strategy is to favor an *increased* hamstring-to-quadriceps activation or force pattern.[95,189,380] This is further explained with the help of Fig. 13.38 that shows two contrasting ways of landing from a jump. In general, the different ways of landing may be considered relatively unsafe (A) or safe (B) for creating muscular responses that could potentially overstrain the ACL. In Fig. 13.38A, the athlete lands with her trunk more vertical, with relatively moderate amounts of hip flexion. Note how the resulting body configuration affects the length of the (flexion) external moment arms of body weight at the hip and knee. Specifically, the body weight vector generates a (i) relatively large knee flexion torque and (ii) a relatively small hip flexion torque (see difference in external moment arms in figure). Hip and knee muscles respond accordingly to the magnitude and direction of these external torques.[47] Landing with a more erect trunk, therefore, requires relatively high activation (and presumed force) from the quadriceps (as knee extensors) while only relatively moderate activation from the hamstrings and gluteus maximus (as hip extensors).[95,189] This so-called "quadriceps dominant" response demonstrated in Fig. 13.38A, observed more often in females, has the potential to create a biomechanical situation that favors anterior tibial shear at the knee with associated strain on the ACL. The lower demands and therefore reduced activation of the hamstring muscles limit their ability to resist a quadriceps-induced strain on the ACL. Realize that a quadriceps-dominant landing likely only *lowers the threshold* for an ACL injury to occur, rather than directly causing it.[80,119] The level of strain required to rupture an ACL typically requires other concurrent biomechanical events, such as landing on a single leg with the knee held closer toward extension (i.e., <30 degrees of flexion), coupled with a large and uncontrolled valgus-producing torque.[24,32]

In general, to minimize the risk of ACL injury, athletes are often instructed to *avoid* landing with the relatively erect trunk illustrated in Fig. 13.38A. One clue of this unsafe landing is apparent by the knees falling *in front of the toes*.[87] This alignment reflects the

excessive forward rotation of the lower legs relative to the feet (i.e., excessive ankle dorsiflexion)—a necessity for maintaining the body weight vector over the base of support (feet) to preserve landing balance. The excessive dorsiflexion typically increases tension in the Achilles tendon, which tends to raise the heels off the floor slightly.

A more preferred and assumed safer landing for the knee is depicted in Fig. 13.38B. Note that the athlete lands with her trunk and hips in greater flexion than that depicted in Fig. 13.38A. This softer, more flexed, and more "giving" landing alters the relative lengths of the external moment arms so that body weight generates (i) a relatively small knee flexion torque and (ii) a relatively large hip flexion torque (compared with Fig. 13.38A). (Note how the knees land directly over or behind the toes—often a clue of a safer landing.) Muscles typically respond accordingly with *less* quadriceps activation and *greater* hamstring or gluteal muscle activation. A greater hamstrings-to-quadriceps activation (or force ratio) theoretically limits the potential for inducing strain on the bulk of the ACL.[189] The more "balanced" muscular coactivation and strength at the knee may also guard against excessive valgus collapse at the knee.[95,157,375,380] Additional frontal plane stability at the knee may also be indirectly gained by greater gluteus maximus activation (a dominant hip extensor and external rotator).[48]

These biomechanical benefits described for landing with increased trunk flexion were directed at reducing strain on the ACL. This same principle, however, can be applied to reducing the force on the patellofemoral joint during landing and during other weight-bearing activities, such as performing squats.[14,15,169,189,313] The overriding principle is based on shifting the muscular demands *from the quadriceps to the hip extensor muscles*. Teng and colleagues analyzed 24 asymptomatic recreational runners and estimated that a 10-degree increase beyond their self-selected trunk angle while running resulted in a 13.4% *reduction* in peak patellofemoral stress.[353]

Fortunately, many ACL prevention programs for female athletes have been shown to markedly decrease the number of injuries.[k] Although the results are promising, the overall rate of ACL injuries in females remains high. More rigorous research is needed to better understand the neuromuscular and biomechanical mechanisms behind the proposed interventions. This should lead to further improvement of prevention strategies, and hopefully allow them to be directed toward a wide range of sporting activities, for the entire population of active persons, regardless of sex or age.

[k]107,109,119,131,229,263,345,374

ADDITIONAL CLINICAL CONNECTIONS

Landing from a jump

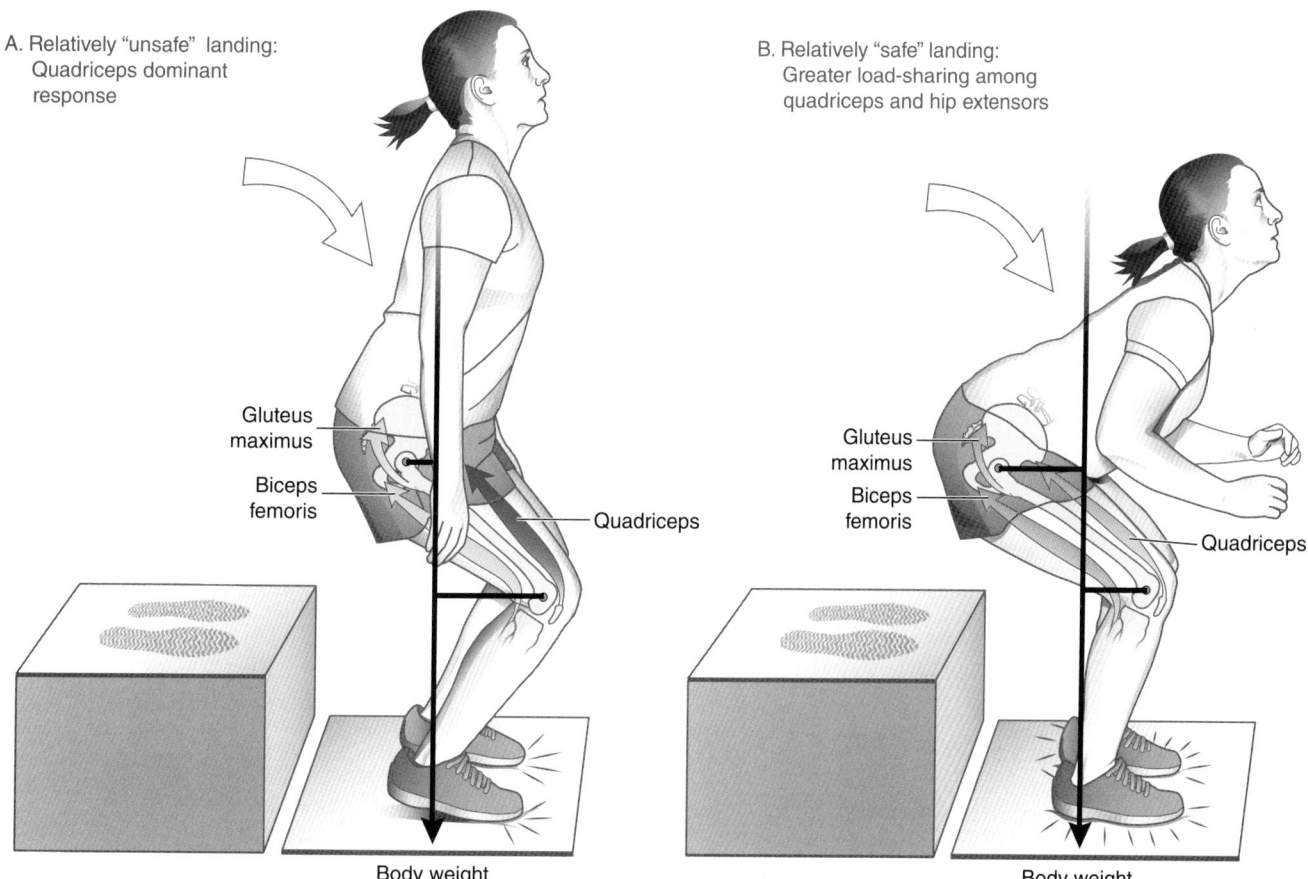

A. Relatively "unsafe" landing:
Quadriceps dominant
response

Gluteus
maximus

Biceps
femoris

Quadriceps

Body weight

B. Relatively "safe" landing:
Greater load-sharing among
quadriceps and hip extensors

Gluteus
maximus

Biceps
femoris

Quadriceps

Body weight

FIGURE 13.38 Two contrasting landing patterns from a jump that could be considered relatively "*unsafe*" (A) or "*safe*" (B) in terms of muscular responses that could harm the knee in certain situations. The landing pattern in (A) is associated with a smaller hip external (flexion) moment arm and a larger knee external (flexion) moment arm (see *black lines* originating at the medial-lateral axis of rotation at the hip and knee). The landing pattern in (B), in contrast, results in a reversal of the relative lengths of the hip and knee external moment arms. The relative activation of the muscles is indicated by different shades of red; see disproportionately high activation of the quadriceps in (A). Body weight vectors are shown intersecting with the various external moment arms. NOTE: Biceps femoris is shown as only one representative of the hamstring muscle group.

ADDITIONAL CLINICAL CONNECTIONS

CLINICAL CONNECTION 13.2
Further Biomechanical Considerations on the Function of the Patella

As described in the text, the patella displaces the tendon of the quadriceps anteriorly, thereby increasing the internal moment arm used by the knee extensor mechanism. In this way the patella can augment the torque potential of the quadriceps. Fig. 13.39 shows an analogy between a mechanical crane and the human knee. Both use a "spacer" to increase the distance between the axis of rotation and the "lifting force": the quadriceps or the crane's cable. The larger the internal moment arm, the greater the internal torque produced per level of force generated by the quadriceps muscle of the human knee (or transferred by the cable in the crane).

In cases of disease or trauma, the patella may need to be surgically removed. One study measured that the internal moment arm of a patellectomized knee reduced from 4.7 cm to 3.8 cm, when averaged across the full range of motion.[164] Depending on the patient, the clinician may consider the functional effect of this reduced moment arm (leverage) in one of two ways. First,

the reduced leverage suggests that, in theory, the maximal knee extensor torque potential may be reduced by about 19%, although muscle hypertrophy or other neuromuscular adaptations may minimize this torque deficit. A second consideration, however, may be that without a patella a person would need to generate 23.5% *more force* to produce an equivalent pre-patellectomized extensor torque. The increased muscle force is required to compensate for the proportional loss in leverage. Therefore greater muscular-based compression force is generated on the tibiofemoral joint, creating greater wear on the articular cartilage (Fig. 13.40). A subtle but important function of the patella, therefore, is to reduce the magnitude of the quadriceps force needed to perform ordinary submaximal efforts, such as ascending a step. This reduced demand indirectly lowers the compressive load across the articular cartilage and menisci at the knee. When considered over many years, this reduction would limit mechanical wear on the knee.

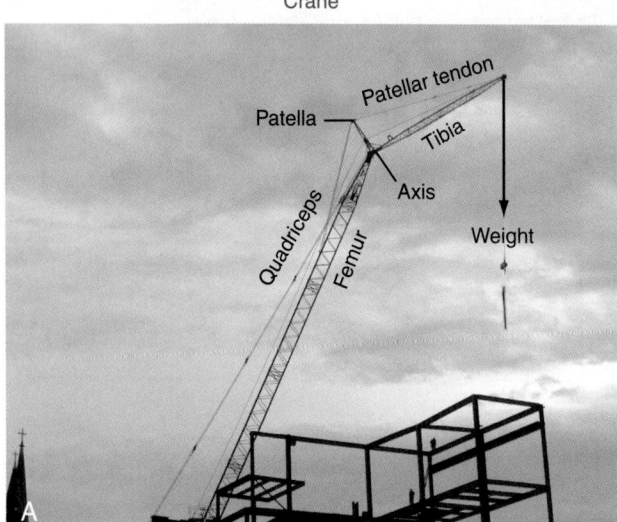

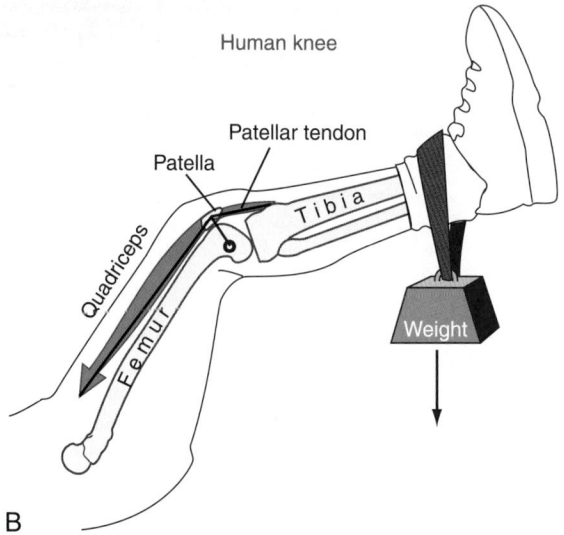

FIGURE 13.39 An analogy is made between a mechanical crane (A) and the human knee (B). In the human knee, the moment arm is the distance between the axis of rotation (circle in distal femur) and quadriceps mechanism. In the crane, the moment arm is the distance between the axis and the tip of the metal piece that functions in a similar manner as a patella.

ADDITIONAL CLINICAL CONNECTIONS

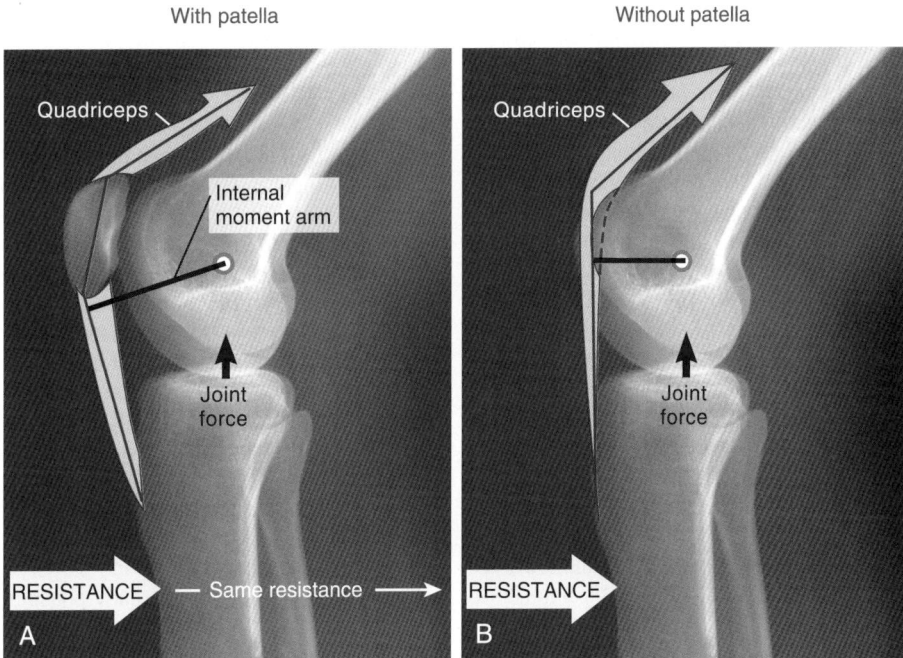

FIGURE 13.40 The quadriceps is shown contracting with a patella (A) and without a patella (B). In each case the quadriceps muscle maintains static rotary equilibrium at the knee by responding to an external resistance (torque). The magnitude of the external resistance (torque) is assumed to be equal in (A) and (B). The moment arm *(black line)* is reduced in (B) because of the patellectomy. As a consequence, the quadriceps in (B) must produce a proportional greater force to match the external resistance. The greater force of the quadriceps creates a greater joint (reaction) force, which must cross the tibiofemoral joint.

ADDITIONAL CLINICAL CONNECTIONS

CLINICAL CONNECTION 13.3
Rebuilding Quadriceps Strength is an Essential Component of Rehabilitation After ACL Reconstruction: Some Biomechanical and Practical Matters

AN OVERVIEW OF THE PROBLEM
Approximately 200,000 persons undergo anterior cruciate ligament reconstruction (ACLR) each year in the United States.[103] Athletes facing ACLR may spend up to 6 to 12 months of physical rehabilitation preparing themselves to return to their previous level of sport. Goals of rehabilitation typically include restoring the knee's strength, kinematics, and mechanical stability to pre-injury levels. Unfortunately, many athletes fall short of these goals. For example, according to a meta-analysis involving 7000 athletes, only 55% of participants actually returned to competitive level sport.[11] Other negative outcomes of ACLR may include a subsequent ACL injury, chronic knee instability, abnormal walking, running, and jumping-and-landing kinematics, fear of re-injury, reduced quality of life, and, over time, a higher risk of premature osteoarthritis.[66,103,201,213,276] Clearly, an ACL injury for a competitive athlete can be a life-changing event—on many levels.

Remarkably, most negative functional outcomes of ACLR are strongly associated with persistent weakness and atrophy of the quadriceps muscle on the side of injury.[19,66,201,213] Even after 6 months of rehabilitation, studies show that, on average, athletes planning to return to sport had a 23% deficit in quadriceps strength compared with pre-operative levels.[201] To put this strength deficit into perspective, Toole et al. reported that fewer than 50% of post-ACLR athletes met their quadriceps strength goals at the time they were cleared to return to sport.[359] Deficits in knee extensor strength and associated limb-loading tasks may persist for at least 2 years after ACLR.[201]

The exact pathogenesis of prolonged quadriceps weakness after ACLR is not clear, although it appears to be related to an *incomplete voluntary activation* and associated reduced recruitment of motor units.[309] The diminished motor recruitment may be associated with "arthrogenic inhibition" caused by reduced sensory feedback resulting from the loss of mechanoreceptors in the native ACL. Alterations in both spinal-reflex and supraspinal excitability suggest inhibition across multiple levels of the nervous system.[202,213,309] Local changes are also apparent in the quadriceps muscle, including observable loss of volume (atrophy), the switching of some fiber types, and reduced number of satellite cells.[102,259] Some data also suggest that an increase in the atrophy-inducing cytokine myostatin may be involved in the chronic weakness.[236]

From a biomechanical perspective, it is not surprising that prolonged weakness of a muscle as dominant as the quadriceps would disrupt the natural kinematics, kinetics, and motor-and-sensory integration in the knee of an active athlete, especially those who engage in sports with high amounts of jumping and pivoting.[153] These disruptions could explain the often suboptimal physical performance and, in some athletes, the damaging stress placed on secondary knee stabilizers and articular cartilage.[359] It is paramount, therefore, that rehabilitation specialists strive to develop strategies that better counteract this prolonged weakness of the quadriceps after ACL injury, with or without reconstruction.[213]

A THERAPEUTIC DILEMMA?
Any exercise strategy designed to strengthen the quadriceps must involve the application of large resistance forces, equivalent to at least 60% to 70% of a one-repetition maximum. This premise cannot be circumvented. However, as described in this chapter, strong contraction of the quadriceps at relatively low knee flexion angles naturally translates the tibia anteriorly, placing a strain on the ACL (review inset box discussed previously in Fig. 13.20). In certain situations, this strain may be considered harmful to either the graft used in a ACLR (typically either a hamstring tendon or using part of the patellar tendon) or to a partially torn native ACL (i.e., an ACL-deficient knee). As reviewed by Escamilla and colleagues,[87] excessive (or moderate but repetitive) strain on the ACL can result in permanent deformation of the graft or disruption of the graft fixation to the bone, thereby affecting the stability of the knee and the effectiveness of the surgery. This concern is usually most relevant during the early phase of rehabilitation, when the grafted ACL—especially a hamstring tendon—is most vulnerable to injury or to being overstretched.[259] Clinicians often face an apparent "dilemma" of needing to apply large resistance against the quadriceps (sufficient to increase strength) while simultaneously limiting unnecessarily large strain on the ACL graft.[87] From a therapeutic perspective, this dilemma can be reconciled through a sound biomechanical understanding of the functional interactions between three factors: (1) activation of the quadriceps and hamstrings, (2) knee flexion angle, and (3) strain potential on the ACL.

RELEVANT BIOMECHANICS
With the knee in full extension, the line of force of the quadriceps (patellar tendon) is oriented approximately 20 degrees anterior to the long axis of the tibia (Fig. 13.41A).[80,130] Therefore, at full knee extension, approximately 34% of the force produced by the quadriceps (based on the sine of 20 degrees) would pull the tibia anteriorly (dashed arrow), opposing the primary action of the ACL. A mathematic-based computerized model expands this concept across 80 degrees of flexion by plotting the tension in the ACL caused by forces generated by *isolated,* submaximal contraction of the quadriceps, and by the *combined* submaximal coactivation

ADDITIONAL CLINICAL CONNECTIONS

CLINICAL CONNECTION 13.3
Rebuilding Quadriceps Strength is an Essential Component of Rehabilitation After ACL Reconstruction: Some Biomechanical and Practical Matters—cont'd

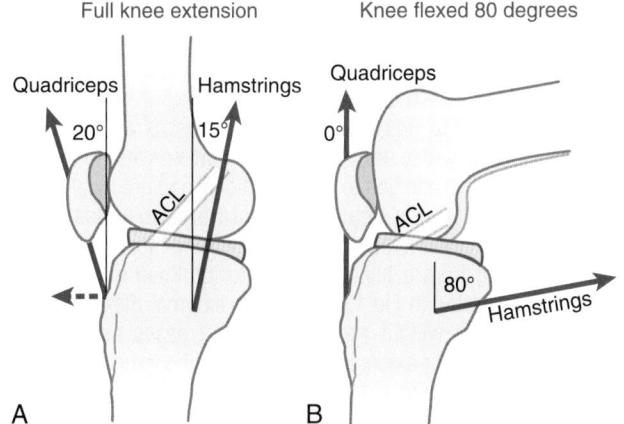

FIGURE 13.41 Lines of force of the quadriceps and hamstring muscles relative to the anterior cruciate ligament *(ACL)* for a knee in full extension (A) and in 80 degrees of flexion (B). Dashed red arrow in A shows the force that translates the tibia anteriorly. Drawing is based on work from Herzog and Read.[130] Note that the change in joint angle significantly alters the line of forces of the muscles and the orientation of the ACL. Angles-of-insertion of the muscles are indicated relative to the long axis of the tibia. Angles are approximate, and vectors are not drawn to scale.

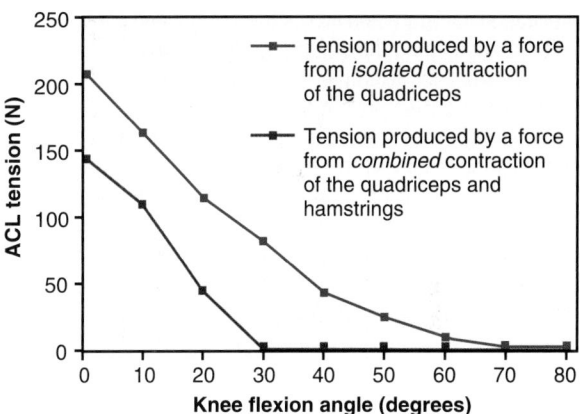

FIGURE 13.42 Relationship between the tension in the anterior cruciate ligament *(ACL)* and the knee joint angle during a submaximal force produced by (1) isolated contraction of the quadriceps and (2) a combined contraction from the quadriceps and hamstrings. The combined muscle force was designed to simulate co-contraction of the two sets of muscles. (Data based on the work of Mesfar and Shirazi-Adl.[239])

of both the quadriceps and hamstring muscles (Fig. 13.42).[239] Note that the computerized model predicts a relatively sharp increase in ACL tension during an *isolated* contraction of the quadriceps between 40 degrees of flexion and full knee extension. Tension in the ACL is greatest during isolated quadriceps contraction with the knee in extension because this posture creates the greatest angle-of-insertion of the patellar tendon into the tibial tuberosity (shown as 20 degrees in Fig. 13.41A). Although not shown in the graph in Fig. 13.42, it should be apparent that the tension in the ACL would increase proportionally to the increase in the magnitude of the contractile force in the quadriceps muscle. Theoretically, in the absence of quadriceps activity, regardless of knee angle, most of the fibers in the ACL would *not* be subjected to a significant tensile load. It is important to note in Fig. 13.42 that although coactivation of the quadriceps and the hamstrings in the last 20 to 30 degrees of extension reduces ACL tension by about 25%, the coactivation does *not* completely eliminate the tension. At these low flexion knee joint angles, the line of pull of the hamstrings has a relatively large component of force aligned parallel with the long axis of the tibia, thereby reducing the muscle's ability to completely offset the strong anterior pull of the quadriceps on the ACL.[189,380]

The biomechanics of quadriceps-induced tension in the ACL change considerably when analyzed in greater knee flexion. With

the knee flexed to 80 degrees, for example, the line of force of the quadriceps is approximately parallel with the long axis of the tibia (see Fig. 13.41B). Most of the force generated by the quadriceps would pull the tibia superiorly against the femur; very little, if any, of this force would pull the tibia anteriorly against the ACL. As noted in Fig. 13.42, at knee angles greater than 60 to 70 degrees of flexion, ACL tension resulting from *isolated* quadriceps contraction is very low or zero. Moreover, *co-contraction* of the quadriceps and the hamstrings at knee angles greater than 30 degrees of flexion theoretically eliminates tension in the ACL. *Hamstring activation generally unloads the ACL, most notably in the flexed knee.* The explanation for this is apparent in the 80-degree flexed knee depicted in Fig. 13.41B. The line of force of the hamstring muscles at 80 degrees of knee flexion is approximately 80 degrees to the long axis of the tibia. At this amount of knee flexion, 98% of the force in the hamstrings (based on the sine of 80 degrees) would pull the tibia posteriorly, very effectively unloading (relatively slackening) the ACL.

Applying the Biomechanics to Exercise Strategies for Strengthening the Quadriceps

The "ideal" exercise for strengthening the quadriceps after ACLR is one that *maximizes the resistance against the muscle while minimizing the risk of unnecessarily large strain on the ACL.* Such an exercise may involve knee movements performed by either *open kinematic chain* (OKC) or *closed kinematic chain* (CKC) methods. This terminology, described in Chapter 1, is often used in the knee

Continued

ADDITIONAL CLINICAL CONNECTIONS

CLINICAL CONNECTION 13.3

Rebuilding Quadriceps Strength is an Essential Component of Rehabilitation After ACL Reconstruction: Some Biomechanical and Practical Matters—cont'd

rehabilitation literature and clinics to describe and contrast strategies for strengthening the quadriceps after ACLR.[93,258,280,381] OKC knee extension, for example, typically refers to a non–weight-bearing, tibial-on-femoral movement, such as seated "leg" extension. CKC knee extension, in contrast, usually refers to a weight-bearing, femoral-on-tibial movement, such as squats or lunges. The following discussion will compare the potential pros and cons of how selected OKC- and CKC-based quadriceps exercises match up to the "ideal" exercise definition stated earlier. This comparison will provide a format to hopefully clarify this often debated and, at times, misunderstood topic.[258,381]

OKC KNEE EXTENSION

Two classic examples of this method of strengthening the quadriceps are seated leg extension with weight attached to the ankle and using an electromechanical dynamometer (isokinetic device). The overwhelming benefit of these exercises is their ability to target resistance exclusively against the quadriceps muscle. This targeted resistance is very relevant considering the paramount need to strengthen this muscle after ACLR.

The OKC-type exercise has the obvious benefit of isolating the mechanical resistance to the quadriceps, however it may predispose the ACL to excessive strain, especially during the last 40 degrees of extension.[87,381] To understand this concern, consider a seated exercise involving complete (tibial-on-femoral) knee extension with a relatively large weight applied to the ankle. This exercise challenges the quadriceps with a flexion (external) torque that progressively *increases* as the knee moves toward greater extension (review Fig. 13.25A-C). Depending on the amount and location of the applied resistance and level of volitional effort, this exercise could place large force demands on the quadriceps and, as explained earlier, cause a relatively large strain on the ACL graft. This strain occurs as the ligament is stretched with little, if any, protective restraint provided by hamstrings.[382] Because typically the therapeutic intent is to avoid large strain on the graft or bony fixation during the early phase of ACLR rehabilitation, it seems reasonable that resistive OKC knee extension exercises should *avoid the last 40 degrees of extension*. Not only would avoiding this arc of motion limit the larger strains on the healing ACL graft, but may also reduce the probability of developing *anterior knee pain*—a problem that plagues some persons during ACLR rehabilitation.[43] Anterior knee pain may be caused by irritation of the patellar ligament graft site or from inflammation of the patellofemoral joint (PFJ). As described earlier in this chapter, because the articular contact area within the PFJ is smallest as the knee approaches full extension, the joint is less able to disperse quadriceps-based compression forces. Under heavy resistance, PFJ contact pressure can therefore rise to very high levels as the knee approaches full extension.[86,344]

CKC KNEE EXTENSION

Squats, lunges, step-ups/downs, and leg presses are frequently chosen CKC exercises to strengthen the quadriceps during rehabilitation after ACLR. In addition to their functional and practical nature, these exercises place the greatest external (resistive) torque against the quadriceps as *the knees are flexed*. Consider, for example, the motion of rising from a bilateral squat to full knee extension, as previously illustrated in Fig.13.25D-F. The external (flexion) torque imposed by body weight progressively *decreases* as the knee moves toward greater extension. Even though the length of the ACL is increasing as the knee extends, the parallel reduction in demand on the quadriceps likely limits the magnitude of a quadriceps-based strain on the ACL. Furthermore, CKC knee exercises require simultaneous motions of the hip and knee, and therefore can promote greater co-activation of the quadriceps and hamstring muscles. Increased coactivation would help limit the anterior translation that may strain the ACL.[189] As suggested in Fig. 13.42, exercises that demand coactivation of quadriceps *and* hamstrings (rather than isolated quadriceps contraction) likely result in lower strain on the ACL between 20 to 30 degrees of flexion and full extension, and virtually none at angles that exceed 30 degrees of flexion.

Although there are many therapeutic advantages proposed for CKC exercises after ACLR, there may be one notable drawback. Because these exercises excel at sharing the work between the knee and hip extensors, they may have the unintended consequence of limiting resistance against the quadriceps to a point that may interfere with optimal strength development. Although research on this topic is mixed and inconclusive,[280] this potential drawback ironically opposes a primary goal espoused for ACLR rehabilitation: that is to specifically challenge and strengthen the quadriceps to prcinjury levels.

SUMMARY OF RELATED ACL STRAIN RESEARCH

Figs. 13.41 and 13.42 provide fundamental background to help understand much of the research data on ACL strain behavior while performing OKC and CKC exercises to strengthen the quadriceps. For example, Fleming et al. summarized the strain measured directly in intact ACLs from 18 common OKC and CKC quadriceps loading conditions.[93] Samples of these data are presented here: The highest strain value reported from any OKC condition was 4.4%, produced by 30 Nm of quadriceps-produced torque at 15 degrees of knee flexion. Under the same OKC loading conditions, strains were reduced to 2.7% at 30 degrees of flexion and 0% at

ADDITIONAL CLINICAL CONNECTIONS

CLINICAL CONNECTION 13.3
Rebuilding Quadriceps Strength is an Essential Component of Rehabilitation After ACL Reconstruction: Some Biomechanical and Practical Matters—cont'd

60 and 90 degrees of flexion. A strain of 0.4% was measured in an OKC condition involving coactivation of quadriceps and hamstrings at 30 degrees of flexion. Peak strain measured from *CKC*-performed squats and lunges were 3.7% and 1.9%, respectively. For perspective, Fleming et al. also reported that a 90 N (20 lb) forward pull on the tibia from a Lachman test (anterior draw test performed at 30 degrees of flexion) caused an ACL strain of 3.6%. From a physiologic perspective, regardless of the method of exercise, the amount of ACL strains reported here are relatively low when considering that an intact ACL typically fails at a strain of 11% to 19%.[41,212] It is important to note that Fleming et al.'s data were based on intact healthy ACLs, so extending these values to ACL graft material must be done with caution.

The data reported by Fleming et al. (and other reports) show that the magnitude of ACL strain produced while performing common OKC and CKC knee extension are relatively low and fall within a relatively similar range.[93,222] Nevertheless, a consistent theme emerges when looking closely at the trends within the data. In general, ACL strains are generally higher for OKC knee extension compared with CKC knee extension, most notably when the OKC exercise is performed at the end ranges of knee extension under high resistance. Furthermore, strains on the ACL from OKC extension tend to rise sharper from increased resistance compared with CKC exercise. It appears, therefore, that the quadriceps can tolerate greater loading with less ACL strain through CKC exercise.

Understanding how OKC and CKC quadriceps exercises affect ACL strain can provide valuable information for exercise selection. More importantly, however, is how the different exercises actually influence patient outcomes. Perriman et al. published a systematic review and meta-analyses which included 10 studies with 485 young participants (average age 24–33 years) undergoing rehabilitation for ACLR.[280] Interestingly, the study concluded that there was no significant difference in physical function (measured or patient reported), anterior tibial laxity, or quadriceps strength from rehabilitation using OKC or CKC type of quadriceps exercises, across multiple points in time. Because the studies evaluated in Perriman et al.'s work showed only limited to moderate levels of evidence, the authors suggested that because of the trends in previous reported ACL strain data, clinicians should use caution when prescribing OKC quadriceps exercises within the first 12 weeks after ACLR.[280]

SUMMARY AND CLOSING COMMENTS
More effective strengthening of the quadriceps is needed to improve the long-term success of persons with ACLR. A fundamental requirement to build muscle strength is to offer appropriately high levels of resistance. This Clinical Connection posed the question whether clinicians face a therapeutic dilemma by needing to place high loads on the quadriceps while simultaneously respecting the vulnerability of the ACL graft. Based on information provided within this Clinical Connection, the answer to this rhetorical question is a resounding "no!"

Clinicians must thoughtfully challenge the quadriceps through exercise, while maintaining a healthy respect for the vulnerability of a constructed ACL graft, especially in the first 6 to 12 weeks after surgery.[280] Armed with this respect and knowledge of the biomechanics of ACL strain during different forms of exercise, clinicians should feel comfortable, within appropriate time frames and individualized patient circumstances, prescribing a mix of demanding exercises for the quadriceps. In general, large resistive loads can be safely applied through multiple types of CKC exercises, across a full range of motion.[222] Exercise strategies should demand strong activation of both the quadriceps and the hamstring muscles. This form of exercise can provide a mix of creative and functional activities that can also challenge balance, coordination, sport specific activities, and aerobic capacity.

Many types of OKC quadriceps exercises can also be safely employed by avoiding the last 40 degrees of knee extension. This modified-range OKC exercise option can effectively isolate the quadriceps, thereby allowing the muscle to be loaded to near its maximum physiologic capacity. As with essentially all CKC exercises, the modified OKC approach may limit the likelihood of causing anterior knee pain.

Combining CKC and modified OKC quadriceps exercises can offer a range of therapeutic benefits across most of the knee's range of motion. Consider, for example, alternating OKC type exercises between 90 and 40 degrees of flexion and CKC type exercises between approximately 70 degrees and near full extension.

An important theme of this Clinical Connection is the importance of protecting the ACL graft from large and potentially damaging quadriceps-induced ACL strain. Although this is important, it should also be recognized that at some time point in the rehabilitation process, tension in the ACL (or grafted material) facilitates healing and is considered therapeutic.[45,358] The exact window of time of this protective-to-therapeutic transition is not known and likely depends significantly on the unique characteristics of the patient and the type of graft material used in the ACLR.

In closing, the clinician must continually be aware of emerging research on effective interventions to improve strength building strategies for the quadriceps after ACLR. Some interventions may serve as useful adjuncts to existing progressive resistive exercise programs, such as neuromuscular electrical stimulation, blood flow restriction therapy, and techniques intended to enhance motor neuron excitability during exercise.[85,126,136,336,360]

ADDITIONAL CLINICAL CONNECTIONS

TYPICAL MOVEMENT COMBINATIONS: HIP-AND-KNEE EXTENSION OR HIP-AND-KNEE FLEXION

Many movements performed by the lower extremities involve the cyclic actions of hip-and-knee extension or hip-and-knee flexion. These patterns of movement are fundamental components of walking, running, jumping, and climbing. Hip-and-knee extension propels the body forward or upward. Conversely, hip-and-knee flexion advances or swings the lower limb or is used to slowly lower the body toward the ground. These movements are controlled, in part, through a synergy among monoarticular and polyarticular muscles, many of which cross the hip and knee.

Fig. 13.43 shows an interaction of muscles during the hip-and-knee extension phase of running. The vastus group and gluteus maximus—two monoarticular muscles—are active synergistically, along with the biarticular semitendinosus and rectus femoris muscles. The vastus group of the quadriceps and the semitendinosus are both electrically active, yet their net torque at the knee favors *extension*. This occurs because the contracting vastus muscles overpower the contraction efforts of the semitendinosus. Consequently, the tension stored in the forced lengthening of the

semitendinosus across the knee is used to assist with active extension at the hip. In the combined movement of hip-and-knee extension, therefore, the semitendinosus muscle (when considered as a whole) extends the hip but actually contracts or shortens a relatively short distance. Because the contraction excursion is low, so is the contraction velocity when considered over a similar time span.

The action of the semitendinosus muscle as described favors relatively high force production per level of neural drive or effort. The physiologic basis for this efficient muscular action rests on the force-velocity and length-tension relationships of muscle (see Chapter 3). Consider first the effect of muscle contraction velocity on muscle force production. Muscle force per level of effort increases sharply as the contraction velocity is reduced. As an example, a muscle contracting at 6.3% of its maximum shortening velocity produces a force of about 75% of its maximum. Slowing the contraction velocity to only 2.2% of maximal (i.e., very near isometric) raises force output to 90% of maximum.[210] In the movement of hip-and-knee extension, the vastus muscles, by extending the knee, indirectly augment hip extension force by reducing the contraction velocity of the semitendinosus.

FIGURE 13.43 The actions of several monoarticular and biarticular muscles are depicted during the hip-and-knee extension phase of running. Observe that the vastus muscles extend the knee, which then stretches the distal end of the semitendinosus. The gluteus maximus extends the hip, which stretches the proximal end of the rectus femoris. The stretched biarticular muscles are depicted by thin black arrows. The stretch placed on the active biarticular muscles reduces the rate and amount of their overall contraction. Note: Semitendinosus is shown as only one representative of the hamstring muscle group. (See text for further details.)

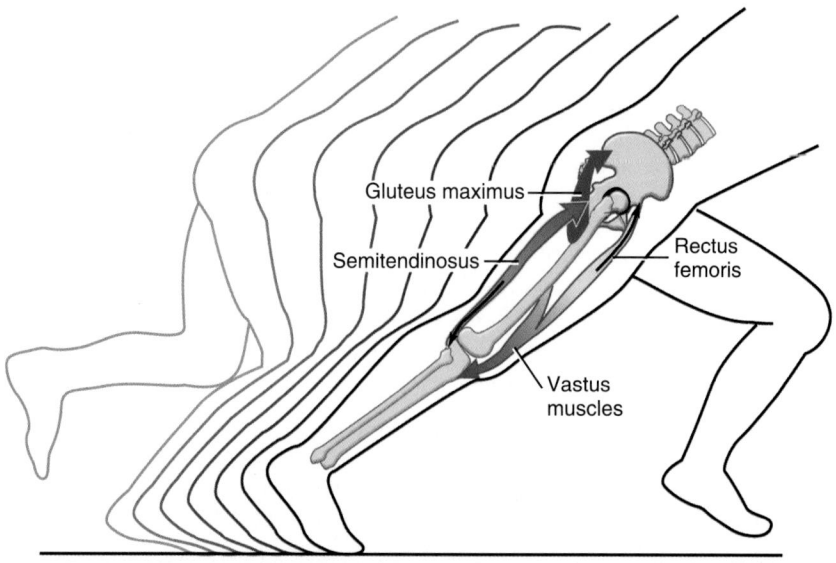

Gluteus maximus

Semitendinosus

Rectus femoris

Vastus muscles

ADDITIONAL CLINICAL CONNECTIONS

Consider next the effect of muscle length on the *passive* force produced within a biarticular muscle. Based on a muscle's passive length-tension relationship, the internal resistance or force within a muscle, such as the semitendinosus, increases as it is stretched. The passive force created within the stretched semitendinosus across the extending knee, in this particular example, is "recycled" and used to help extend the hip. In this manner the semitendinosus—as well as all biarticular hamstrings—functions as a "transducer" by transferring force ultimately produced by the contracting vastus muscles to the extending hip.

During active hip-and-knee extension, the gluteus maximus and rectus femoris have a relationship like that described between the vastus muscles and the semitendinosus. In essence, the monoarticular gluteus maximus augments knee extension force by its dominating influence over hip extension. This dominance, in turn, stretches the activated rectus femoris. In this example the rectus femoris is the biarticular transducer, transferring force from the gluteus maximus to knee extension. A summary of these and other muscular interactions used during hip-and-knee flexion is listed in Table 13.8.

The functional interdependence among the hip-and-knee extensor muscles and among the hip-and-knee flexor muscles should be considered in evaluation of functional activities that require these active movement combinations. Consider, for example, the combined movements of hip-and-knee extension required to stand from a seated position. Weakness of the vastus muscles could indirectly cause difficulty in extending the hip, whereas weakness of the gluteus maximus could indirectly cause difficulty in extending the knee. Strengthening programs may benefit by designing resistive challenges that incorporate this natural synergy between these muscles.

ATYPICAL MOVEMENT COMBINATIONS: HIP FLEXION AND KNEE EXTENSION, OR HIP EXTENSION AND KNEE FLEXION

Consider active movement patterns of the hip and knee that are "out of phase" with the more typical movement patterns described earlier. Hip flexion can occur with knee extension (Fig. 13.44A), or hip extension can occur with knee flexion (Fig. 13.44B). The physiologic consequences of these movements are very different from those described in Fig. 13.43. In Fig. 13.44A, the biarticular rectus femoris must shorten a great distance, and with relatively high velocity, to simultaneously flex the hip and extend the knee. Even with maximal effort, active knee extension is usually limited during this action. Based on the length-tension and force-velocity relationships of muscle, the rectus femoris is likely not able to develop maximal knee extensor force. The biarticular hamstrings are also overstretched across both the hip and knee, thereby passively resisting knee extension.

The situation described in Fig. 13.44A also applies to the movement depicted in Fig. 13.44B. The biarticular hamstrings must contract to a very short length—a movement that is often accompanied by cramping. Furthermore, the biarticular rectus femoris is overstretched across both the hip and the knee, thereby passively resisting knee flexion. For both reasons, knee flexion force and range of motion are usually limited by the out-of-phase movement.

The atypical movements depicted in Fig. 13.44 may have a useful purpose. Consider the action of kicking a ball. Elastic energy is stored in the stretched rectus femoris by the preparatory

TABLE 13.8 Examples of Muscle Synergies at the Hip and Knee

	Monoarticular Muscle(s)	Action	Biarticular Transducer(s)	Action Augmented
Active hip *and* knee *extension*	Vasti	Knee *extension*	Two-joint hamstrings	Hip *extension*
	Gluteus maximus	Hip *extension*	Rectus femoris	Knee *extension*
Active hip *and* knee *flexion*	Iliopsoas	Hip *flexion*	Two-joint hamstrings	Knee *flexion*
	Biceps femoris (short head), popliteus	Knee *flexion*	Rectus femoris	Hip *flexion*

Modified from Leiber RL: *Skeletal muscle: structure and function*, Baltimore, 1992, Williams & Wilkins.

Continued

ADDITIONAL CLINICAL CONNECTIONS

Hip flexion
and knee extension

Rectus femoris actively
"overshortened"

Hamstrings passively
"overstretched"

Hip extension
and knee flexion

Hamstrings actively
"overshortened"

A

Rectus femoris passively
"overstretched"

B

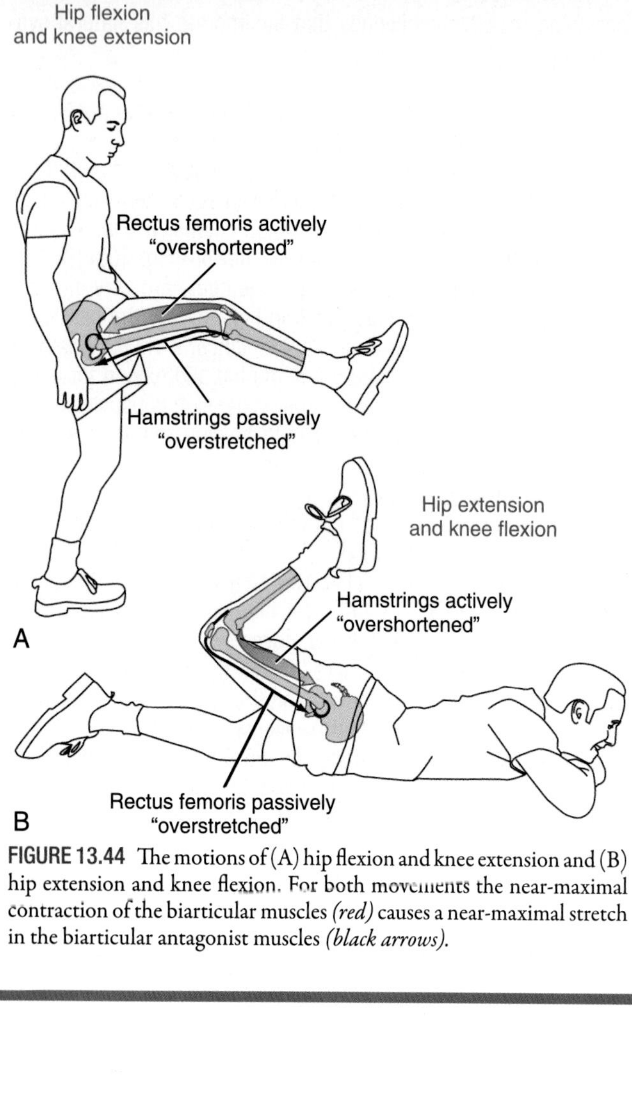

FIGURE 13.44 The motions of (A) hip flexion and knee extension and (B) hip extension and knee flexion. For both movements the near-maximal contraction of the biarticular muscles *(red)* causes a near-maximal stretch in the biarticular antagonist muscles *(black arrows)*.

movement of combined hip extension and knee flexion. The action of kicking the ball involves a rapid and near full contraction of the rectus femoris to simultaneously flex the hip and extend the knee. The goal of this action is to dissipate *all* force in the rectus femoris as quickly as possible. In contrast, activities such as walking, jogging, or cycling use biarticular muscles in a manner that forces are developed more slowly and in a repetitive or cyclic fashion. In these examples, the length changes in the rectus femoris and semitendinosus, for example, are relatively small throughout much of the activation cycle (as shown in Fig. 13.43). In this way, muscles avoid repetitive cycles of storing and immediately releasing relatively large amounts of energy. More moderate levels of active and passive forces are cooperatively shared between muscles, thereby optimizing the metabolic efficiency of the movement.

REFERENCES

1. Adouni M, Shirazi-Adl A: Partitioning of knee joint internal forces in gait is dictated by the knee adduction angle and not by the knee adduction moment, *J Biomech* 47(7):1696–1703, 2014.

2. Alonso B, Bravo B, Mediavilla L, et al.: Osteoarthritis-related biomarkers profile in chronic anterior cruciate ligament injured knee, *Knee* 27(1):51–60, 2020.

3. Amis AA, Bull AM, Gupte CM, et al.: Biomechanics of the PCL and related structures: posterolateral, posteromedial and meniscofemoral ligaments, *Knee Surg Sports Traumatol Arthrosc* 11:271–281, 2003.

4. Amis AA, Firer P, Mountney J, et al.: Anatomy and biomechanics of the medial patellofemoral ligament, *Knee* 10:215–220, 2003.

5. Amis AA, Senavongse W: Bull AM: patellofemoral kinematics during knee flexion-extension: an in vitro study, *J Orthop Res* 24:2201–2211, 2006.

6. Amis AA: Current concepts on anatomy and biomechanics of patellar stability, *Sports Med Arthrosc* 15:48–56, 2007.

7. Amis AA: The functions of the fibre bundles of the anterior cruciate ligament in anterior drawer, rotational laxity and the pivot shift [Review], *Knee Surg Sports Traumatol Arthrosc* 20(4):613–620, 2012.

8. Anderson DE, Madigan ML, Nussbaum MA: Maximum voluntary joint torque as a function of joint angle and angular velocity: model development and application to the lower limb, *J Biomech* 40(14):3105–3113, 2007.

9. Andriacchi TP, Birac D: Functional testing in the anterior cruciate ligament–deficient knee, *Clin Orthop Relat Res* 288:40–47, 1993.

10. Andriacchi TP, Mündermann A, Smith RL, et al.: A framework for the in vivo pathomechanics of osteoarthritis at the knee, *Ann Biomed Eng* 32(3):447–457, 2004.

11. Ardern CL, Taylor NF, Feller JA, et al.: Fifty-five per cent return to competitive sport following anterior cruciate ligament reconstruction surgery: an updated systematic review and meta-analysis including aspects of physical functioning and contextual factors, *Br J Sports Med* 48(21):1543–1552, 2014.

12. Armour T, Forwell L, Litchfield R, et al.: Isokinetic evaluation of internal/external tibial rotation strength after the use of hamstring tendons for anterior cruciate ligament reconstruction, *Am J Sports Med* 32:1639–1643, 2004.

13. Arundale AJH, Bizzini M, Giordano A, et al.: Exercise-based knee and anterior cruciate ligament injury prevention, *J Orthop Sports Phys Ther* 48(9):A1–A42, 2018.

14. Atkins LT, James CR, Yang HS, et al.: Immediate improvements in patellofemoral pain are associated with sagittal plane movement training to improve use of gluteus maximus muscle during single limb Landing, *Phys Ther* 101(10), 2021.

15. Atkins LT, Smithson C, Grimes D, et al.: The influence of sagittal trunk posture on the magnitude and rate of patellofemoral joint stress during stair ascent in asymptomatic females, *Gait Posture* 74:121–127, 2019.

16. Backman LJ, Danielson P: Low range of ankle dorsiflexion predisposes for patellar tendinopathy in junior elite basketball players: a 1-year prospective study, *Am J Sports Med* 39(12):2626–2633, 2011.

17. Bakenecker P, Raiteri B, Hahn D: Patella tendon moment arm function considerations for human vastus lateralis force estimates, *J Biomech* 86:225–231, 2019.

18. Baldon Rde M, Serrão FV, Scattone Silva R, et al.: Effects of functional stabilization training on pain, function, and lower extremity biomechanics in women with patellofemoral pain: a randomized clinical trial, *J Orthop Sports Phys Ther* 44(4):240–A800, 2014.

19. Baron JE, Parker EA, Duchman KR, et al.: Perioperative and postoperative factors influence quadriceps atrophy and strength after ACL reconstruction: a systematic review, *Orthop J Sports Med* 8(6), 2020. 2325967120930296.

20. Barrios JA, Butler RJ, Crenshaw JR, et al.: Mechanical effectiveness of lateral foot wedging in medial knee osteoarthritis after 1 year of wear, *J Orthop Res* 31(5):659–664, 2013.

21. Barton CJ, Levinger P, Crossley KM, et al.: The relationship between rearfoot, tibial and hip kinematics in individuals with patellofemoral pain syndrome, *Clin Biomech* 27(7):702–705, 2012.

22. Basmajian JV: *Muscles alive: their functions revealed by electromyography*, ed 3, Baltimore, 1974, Williams & Wilkins.

23. Bates NA, Myer GD, Shearn JT, et al.: Anterior cruciate ligament biomechanics during robotic and mechanical simulations of physiologic and clinical motion tasks: a systematic review and meta-analysis, *Clin Biomech* 30(1):1–13, 2015.

24. Bates NA, Schilaty ND, Nagelli CV, et al.: Multiplanar loading of the knee and its influence on anterior cruciate ligament and medial collateral ligament strain during simulated landings and noncontact tears, *Am J Sports Med* 47(8):1844–1853, 2019.

25. Belvedere C, Leardini A, Giannini S, et al.: Does medio-lateral motion occur in the normal knee? An in-vitro study in passive motion, *J Biomech* 44(5):877–884, 2011.

26. Besier TF, Draper CE, Gold GE, et al.: Patellofemoral joint contact area increases with knee flexion and weight-bearing, *J Orthop Res* 23:345–350, 2005.

27. Beynnon BD, Fleming BC: Anterior cruciate ligament strain in-vivo: a review of previous work, *J Biomech* 31:519–525, 1998.

28. Beynnon BD, Hall JS, Sturnick DR, et al.: Increased slope of the lateral tibial plateau subchondral bone is associated with greater risk of noncontact ACL injury in females but not in males: a prospective cohort study with a nested, matched case-control analysis, *Am J Sports Med* 42(5):1039–1048, 2014.

29. Bicos J, Fulkerson JP, Amis A: Current concepts review: the medial patellofemoral ligament, *Am J Sports Med* 35:484–492, 2007.

30. Bittencourt NF, Ocarino JM, Mendonca LD, et al.: Foot and hip contributions to high frontal plane knee projection angle in athletes: a classification and regression tree approach, *J Orthop Sports Phys Ther* 42(12):996–1004, 2012.

31. Boden BP, Dean GS, Feagin JA Jr, et al.: Mechanisms of anterior cruciate ligament injury, *Orthopedics* 23:573–578, 2000.

32. Boden BP, Sheehan FT, Torg JS, et al.: Noncontact anterior cruciate ligament injuries: mechanisms and risk factors. [Review], *J Am Acad Orthop Surg* 18(9):520–527, 2010.

33. Bohannon RW, Gajdosik RL, LeVeau BF: Isokinetic knee flexion and extension torque in the upright sitting and semireclined sitting positions, *Phys Ther* 66:1083–1086, 1986.

34. Bollier M, Smith PA: Anterior cruciate ligament and medial collateral ligament injuries [Review], *J Knee Surg* 27(5):359–368, 2014.

35. Bonifácio D, Richards J, Selfe J, et al.: Influence and benefits of foot orthoses on kinematics, kinetics and muscle activation during step descent task, *Gait Posture* 65:106–111, 2018.

36. Borotikar BS, Sheehan FT: In vivo patellofemoral contact mechanics during active extension using a novel dynamic MRI-based methodology, *Osteoarthritis Cartilage* 21(12):1886–1894, 2013.

37. Breda SJ, Oei EHG, Zwerver J, et al.: Effectiveness of progressive tendon-loading exercise therapy in patients with patellar tendinopathy: a randomised clinical trial, *Br J Sports Med* 55(9):501–509, 2021.

38. Buckwalter JA, Mankin HJ, Grodzinsky AJ: Articular cartilage and osteoarthritis, *Instr Course Lect* 54:465–480, 2005.

39. Buford WL Jr, Ivey FM Jr, Malone JD, et al.: Muscle balance at the knee—moment arms for the normal knee and the ACL-minus knee, *IEEE Trans Rehabil Eng* 5:367–379, 1997.

40. Buford WL Jr, Ivey FM Jr, Nakamura T, et al.: Internal/external rotation moment arms of muscles at the knee: moment arms for the normal knee and the ACL-deficient knee, *Knee* 8:293–303, 2001.

41. Butler DL, Guan Y, Kay MD, et al.: Location-dependent variations in the material properties of the anterior cruciate ligament, *J Biomech* 25(5):511–518, 1992.

42. Butler DL, Noyes FR, Grood ES: Ligamentous restraints to anterior-posterior drawer in the human knee. A biomechanical study, *J Bone Joint Surg Am* 62:259–270, 1980.

43. Bynum EB, Barrack RL, Alexander AH: Open versus closed chain kinetic exercises after anterior cruciate ligament reconstruction. A prospective randomized study, *Am J Sports Med* 23:401–406, 1995.

44. Calmels PM, Nellen M, van dB I, et al.: Concentric and eccentric isokinetic assessment of flexor-extensor torque ratios at the hip, knee, and ankle in a sample population of healthy subjects, *Arch Phys Med Rehabil* 78:1224–1230, 1997.

45. Camp CL, Lebaschi A, Cong GT, et al.: Timing of postoperative mechanical loading affects healing following anterior cruciate ligament reconstruction: analysis in a murine model, *J Bone Joint Surg Am* 99(16):1382–1391, 2017.

46. Campbell SE, Sanders TG, Morrison WB: MR imaging of meniscal cysts: incidence, location, and clinical significance, *AJR Am J Roentgenol* 177:409–413, 2001.

47. Cannon J, Cambridge EDJ, McGill SM: Anterior cruciate ligament injury mechanisms and the kinetic chain linkage: the effect of proximal joint stiffness on distal knee control during bilateral landings, *J Orthop Sports Phys Ther* 49(8):601–610, 2019.

48. Cannon J, Cambridge EDJ, McGill SM: Increased core stability is associated with reduced knee valgus during single-leg landing tasks: investigating lumbar spine and hip joint rotational stiffness, *J Biomech* 116:110240, 2021.

49. Chalmers PN, Mall NA, Moric M, et al.: Does ACL Reconstruction alter natural history?: a systematic literature review of long-term outcomes, *J Bone Joint Surg Am* 96(4):292–300, 2014.

50. Chandrasekaran S, Ma D, Scarvell JM, et al.: A review of the anatomical, biomechanical and kinematic findings of posterior cruciate ligament injury with respect to non-operative management [Review], *Knee* 19(6):738–745, 2012.

51. Chandrashekar N, Mansouri H, Slauterbeck J, et al.: Sex-based differences in the tensile properties of the human anterior cruciate ligament, *J Biomech* 39:2943–2950, 2006.

52. Chappell JD, Creighton RA, Giuliani C, et al.: Kinematics and electromyography of landing preparation in vertical stop-jump: risks for noncontact anterior cruciate ligament injury, *Am J Sports Med* 35:235–241, 2007.

53. Charles MD, Haloman S, Chen L, et al.: Magnetic resonance imaging-based topographical differences between control and recurrent patellofemoral instability patients, *Am J Sports Med* 41(2):374–384, 2013.

54. Chinkulprasert C, Vachalathiti R, Powers CM: Patellofemoral joint forces and stress during forward step-up, lateral step-up, and forward step-down exercises, *J Orthop Sports Phys Ther* 41(4):241–248, 2011.

55. Chumanov ES, Heiderscheit BC, Thelen DG: The effect of speed and influence of individual muscles on hamstring mechanics during the swing phase of sprinting, *J Biomech* 40(16):3555–3562, 2007.

56. Clancy WG Jr, Sutherland TB: Combined posterior cruciate ligament injuries, *Clin Sports Med* 13:629–647, 1994.

57. Cone SG, Howe D, Fisher MB: Size and shape of the human anterior cruciate ligament and the impact of sex and skeletal growth: a Systematic Review, *JBJS Rev* 7(6):e8, 2019.

58. Covey DC, Sapega AA, Riffenburgh RH: The effects of sequential sectioning of defined posterior cruciate

ligament fiber regions on translational knee motion, *Am J Sports Med* 36:480–486, 2008.

59. Crook BS, Collins AT, Lad NK, et al.: Effect of walking on in vivo tibiofemoral cartilage strain in ACL-deficient versus intact knees, *J Biomech* 116:110210, 2020.

60. Csintalan RP, Schulz MM, Woo J, et al.: Gender differences in patellofemoral joint biomechanics, *Clin Orthop Relat Res* 402:260–269, 2002.

61. Damm P, Kutzner I, Bergmann G, et al.: Comparison of in vivo measured loads in knee, hip and spinal implants during level walking, *J Biomech* 51:128–132, 2017.

62. Dan M, Parr W, Broe D, et al.: Biomechanics of the knee extensor mechanism and its relationship to patella tendinopathy: a review, *J Orthop Res* 36(12):3105–3112, 2018.

63. Davis IS, Tenforde AS, Neal BS, et al.: Gait retraining as an intervention for patellofemoral pain, *Curr Rev Musculoskelet Med* 13(1):103–114, 2020.

64. deAndrade JR, Grant C, Dixon ASJ: Joint distension and reflex muscle inhibition in the knee, *J Bone Joint Surg Am* 47:313–322, 1965.

65. DeHaven KE, Lintner DM: Athletic injuries: comparison by age, sport, and gender, *Am J Sports Med* 14:218–224, 1986.

66. Della Villa F, Straub RK, Mandelbaum B, et al.: Confidence to return to play after anterior cruciate ligament reconstruction is influenced by quadriceps strength symmetry and injury mechanism, *Sports Health*, 2021. 1941738120976377.

67. Demers MS, Pal S, Delp SL: Changes in tibiofemoral forces due to variations in muscle activity during walking, *J Orthop Res* 32(6):769–776, 2014.

68. DeMorat G, Weinhold P, Blackburn T, et al.: Aggressive quadriceps loading can induce noncontact anterior cruciate ligament injury, *Am J Sports Med* 32:477–483, 2004.

69. Diermeier T, Rothrauff BB, Engebretsen L, et al.: Treatment after anterior cruciate ligament injury: panther symposium ACL treatment consensus group, *Knee Surg Sports Traumatol Arthrosc* 28(8):2390–2402, 2020.

70. Domire ZJ, Boros RL, Hashemi J: An examination of possible quadriceps force at the time of anterior cruciate ligament injury during landing: a simulation study, *J Biomech* 44(8):1630–1632, 2011.

71. Donnelly CJ, Lloyd DG, Elliott BC, et al.: Optimizing whole-body kinematics to minimize valgus knee loading during sidestepping: implications for ACL injury risk, *J Biomech* 45(8):1491–1497, 2012.

72. Duivenvoorden T, van Raaij TM, Horemans HL, et al.: Do laterally wedged insoles or valgus braces unload the medial compartment of the knee in patients with osteoarthritis? *Clin Orthop Relat Res* 473(1):265–274, 2015.

73. Eastlack ME, Axe MJ, Snyder-Mackler L: Laxity, instability, and functional outcome after ACL injury: copers versus noncopers, *Med Sci Sports Exerc* 31(2):210–215, 1999.

74. Eckenrode BJ, Kietrys DM, Parrott JS: Effectiveness of manual therapy for pain and self-reported function in individuals with patellofemoral pain: systematic review and meta-analysis, *J Orthop Sports Phys Ther* 48(5):358–371, 2018.

75. Eckstein F, Wirth W, Hudelmaier M, et al.: Patterns of femorotibial cartilage loss in knees with neutral, varus, and valgus alignment, *Arthritis Rheum* 59:1563–1570, 2008.

76. Edwards S, Steele JR, McGhee DE, et al.: Landing strategies of athletes with an asymptomatic patellar tendon abnormality, *Med Sci Sports Exerc* 42(11):2072–2080, 2010.

77. Eitzen I, Moksnes H, Snyder-Mackler L, et al.: A progressive 5-week exercise therapy program leads to significant improvement in knee function early after anterior cruciate ligament injury, *J Orthop Sports Phys Ther* 40(11):705–721, 2010.

78. Emamvirdi M, Letafatkar A, Khaleghi Tazji M: The effect of valgus control instruction exercises on pain, strength, and functionality in active females with patellofemoral pain syndrome, *Sports Health* 11(3):223–237, 2019.

79. Englander ZA, Baldwin EL, Smith WAR, et al.: In Vivo anterior cruciate ligament deformation during a single-legged jump measured by magnetic resonance imaging and high-speed biplanar radiography, *Am J Sports Med* 47(13):3166–3172, 2019.

80. Englander ZA, Cutcliffe HC, Utturkar GM, et al.: In vivo assessment of the interaction of patellar tendon tibial shaft angle and anterior cruciate ligament elongation during flexion, *J Biomech* 90:123–127, 2019.

81. Englander ZA, Garrett WE, Spritzer CE, et al.: In vivo attachment site to attachment site length and strain of the ACL and its bundles during the full gait cycle measured by MRI and high-speed biplanar radiography, *J Biomech* 98:109443, 2020.

82. Englander ZA, Wittstein JR, Goode AP, et al.: Reconsidering reciprocal length patterns of the anteromedial and posterolateral bundles of the anterior cruciate ligament during in vivo gait, *Am J Sports Med* 48(8):1893–1899, 2020.

83. Englund M, Roos EM, Lohmander LS: Impact of type of meniscal tear on radiographic and symptomatic knee osteoarthritis: a sixteen-year followup of meniscectomy with matched controls, *Arthritis Rheum* 48:2178–2187, 2003.

84. Erhart-Hledik J, Chu C, Asay J, et al.: Longitudinal changes in the total knee joint moment after anterior cruciate ligament reconstruction correlate with cartilage thickness changes, *J Orthop Res* 37(7):1546–1554, 2019.

85. Erickson LN, Lucas KCH, Davis KA, et al.: Effect of blood flow restriction training on quadriceps muscle strength, morphology, physiology, and knee biomechanics before and after anterior cruciate ligament reconstruction: protocol for a randomized clinical trial, *Phys Ther* 99(8):1010–1019, 2019.

86. Escamilla RF, Fleisig GS, Zheng N, et al.: Biomechanics of the knee during closed kinetic chain and open kinetic chain exercises, *Med Sci Sports Exerc* 30(4):556–569, 1998.

87. Escamilla RF, MacLeod TD, Wilk KE, et al.: Anterior cruciate ligament strain and tensile forces for weight-bearing and non-weight-bearing exercises: a guide to exercise selection [Review], *J Orthop Sports Phys Ther* 42(3):208–220, 2012.

88. Evans KN, Kilcoyne KG, Dickens JF, et al.: Predisposing risk factors for non-contact ACL injuries in military subjects, *Knee Surg Sports Traumatol Arthrosc* 20(8):1554–1559, 2012.

89. Feipel V, Simonnet ML, Rooze M: The proximal attachments of the popliteus muscle: a quantitative study and clinical significance, *Surg Radiol Anat* 25:58–63, 2003.

90. Felson DT, Nevitt MC, Zhang Y, et al.: High prevalence of lateral knee osteoarthritis in Beijing Chinese compared with Framingham Caucasian subjects, *Arthritis Rheum* 46(5):1217–1222, 2002.

91. Filbay SR, Grindem H: Evidence-based recommendations for the management of anterior cruciate ligament (ACL) rupture, *Best Pract Res Clin Rheumatol* 33(1):33–47, 2019.

92. Fleming BC, Beynnon BD, Renstrom PA, et al.: The strain behavior of the anterior cruciate ligament during bicycling. An in vivo study, *Am J Sports Med* 26:109–118, 1998.

93. Fleming BC, Oksendahl H, Beynnon BD: Open- or closed-kinetic chain exercises after anterior cruciate ligament reconstruction? *Exerc Sport Sci Rev* 33(3):134–140, 2005.

94. Ford KR, Myer GD, Hewett TE: Valgus knee motion during landing in high school female and male basketball players, *Med Sci Sports Exerc* 35:1745–1750, 2003.

95. Ford KR, Myer GD, Schmitt LC, et al.: Preferential quadriceps activation in female athletes with incremental increases in landing intensity, *J Appl Biomech* 27(3):215–222, 2011.

96. Fox AS, Bonacci J, McLean SG, et al.: What is normal? Female lower limb kinematic profiles during athletic tasks used to examine anterior cruciate ligament injury risk: a systematic review [Review], *Sports Med* 44(6):815–832, 2014.

97. Frank B, Bell DR, Norcross MF, et al.: Trunk and hip biomechanics influence anterior cruciate loading mechanisms in physically active participants, *Am J Sports Med* 41(11):2676–2683, 2013.

98. Fredericson M, Yoon K: Physical examination and patellofemoral pain syndrome, *Am J Phys Med Rehabil* 85:234–243, 2006.

99. Frey-Law LA, Laake A, Avin KG, et al.: Knee and elbow 3D strength surfaces: peak torque-angle-velocity relationships, *J Appl Biomech* 28(6):726–737, 2012.

100. Frobell RB, Roos EM, Roos HP, et al.: A Randomized trial of treatment for acute anterior cruciate ligament tears, *N Engl J Med* 363(4):331–342, 2010.

101. Frobell RB, Roos HP, Roos EM, et al.: Treatment for acute anterior cruciate ligament tear: five year outcome of randomised trial, *BMJ* 346:f232, 2013.

102. Fry CS, Johnson DL, Ireland ML, et al.: ACL injury reduces satellite cell abundance and promotes fibrogenic cell expansion within skeletal muscle, *J Orthop Res* 35(9):1876–1885, 2017.

103. Fryer C, Ithurburn MP, McNally MP, et al.: The relationship between frontal plane trunk control during landing and lower extremity muscle strength in young athletes after anterior cruciate ligament reconstruction, *Clin Biomech* 62:58–65, 2019.

104. Fujiya H, Kousa P, Fleming BC, et al.: Effect of muscle loads and torque applied to the tibia on the strain behavior of the anterior cruciate ligament: an in vitro investigation, *Clin Biomech* 26(10):1005–1011, 2011.

105. Fukuda TY, Melo WP, Zaffalon BM, et al.: Hip posterolateral musculature strengthening in sedentary women with patellofemoral pain syndrome: a randomized controlled clinical trial with 1-year follow-up, *J Orthop Sports Phys Ther* 42(10):823–830, 2012.

106. Gadikota HR, Kikuta S, Qi W, et al.: Effect of increased iliotibial band load on tibiofemoral kinematics and force distributions: a direct measurement in cadaveric knees, *J Orthop Sports Phys Ther* 43(7):478–485, 2013.

107. Gagnier JJ, Morgenstern H, Chess L: Interventions designed to prevent anterior cruciate ligament injuries in adolescents and adults: a systematic review and meta-analysis [Review], *Am J Sports Med* 41(8):1952–1962, 2013.

108. Gallina A, Wakeling JM, Hodges PW, et al.: Regional vastus medialis and vastus lateralis activation in females with patellofemoral pain, *Med Sci Sports Exerc* 51(3):411–420, 2019.

109. Gilchrist J, Mandelbaum BR, Melancon H, et al.: A randomized controlled trial to prevent noncontact anterior cruciate ligament injury in female collegiate soccer players, *Am J Sports Med* 36:1476–1483, 2008.

110. Giles LS, Webster KE, McClelland JA, et al.: Atrophy of the quadriceps is not isolated to the vastus medialis oblique in individuals with patellofemoral pain, *J Orthop Sports Phys Ther* 45(8):613–619, 2015.

111. Giles LS, Webster KE, McClelland JA, et al.: Does quadriceps atrophy exist in individuals with patellofemoral pain? A systematic literature review with meta-analysis, *J Orthop Sports Phys Ther* 43(11):766–776, 2013.

112. Gill TJ, DeFrate LE, Wang C, et al.: The biomechanical effect of posterior cruciate ligament reconstruction on knee joint function. Kinematic response to simulated muscle loads, *Am J Sports Med* 31:530–536, 2003.

113. Goerger BM, Marshall SW, Beutler AI, et al.: Anterior cruciate ligament injury alters preinjury lower extremity biomechanics in the injured and uninjured leg: the jump-ACL study, *Br J Sports Med* 49(3):188–195, 2015.

114. Goh JC, Lee PY, Bose K: A cadaver study of the function of the oblique part of vastus medialis, *J Bone Joint Surg Br* 77(2):225–231, 1995.

115. Goodfellow J, Hungerford DS, Zindel M: Patello-femoral joint mechanics and pathology. 1. Functional anatomy of the patello-femoral joint, *J Bone Joint Surg Br* 58:287–290, 1976.

116. Grace TG, Sweetser ER, Nelson MA, et al.: Isokinetic muscle imbalance and knee-joint injuries. A prospective blind study, *J Bone Joint Surg Am* 66:734–740, 1984.

117. Griffith CJ, Wijdicks CA, LaPrade RF, et al.: Force measurements on the posterior oblique ligament and superficial medial collateral ligament proximal and distal divisions to applied loads, *Am J Sports Med* 37:140–148, 2009.

118. Guilak F: Biomechanical factors in osteoarthritis, *Best Pract Res Clin Rheumatol* 25:815–823, 2011.

119. Gupta AS, Pierpoint LA, Comstock RD, et al.: Sex-based differences in anterior cruciate ligament injuries among United States high school soccer players: an epidemiological study, *Orthop J Sports Med* 8(5), 2020. 2325967120919178.

120. Gupte CM, Bull AM, Thomas RD, et al.: A review of the function and biomechanics of the meniscofemoral ligaments, *Arthroscopy* 19:161–171, 2003.

121. Gwinn DE, Wilckens JH, McDevitt ER, et al.: The relative incidence of anterior cruciate ligament injury in men and women at the United States Naval Academy, *Am J Sports Med* 28:98–102, 2000.

122. Hahn D, Olvermann M, Richtberg J, et al.: Knee and ankle joint torque-angle relationships of multi-joint leg extension, *J Biomech* 44(11):2059–2065, 2011.

123. Hall M, Diamond LE, Lenton GK, et al.: Immediate effects of valgus knee bracing on tibiofemoral contact forces and knee muscle forces, *Gait Posture* 68:55–62, 2019.

124. Harlaar J, Macri EM, Wesseling M: Osteoarthritis year in review 2021: mechanics, Osteoarthritis Cartilage, 2022.

125. Harris KP, Driban JB, Sitler MR, et al.: Tibiofemoral osteoarthritis after surgical or nonsurgical treatment of anterior cruciate ligament rupture: a systematic review, *J Athl Train* 52(6):507–517, 2017.

126. Hart JM, Kuenze CM, Diduch DR, et al.: Quadriceps muscle function after rehabilitation with cryotherapy in patients with anterior cruciate ligament reconstruction, *J Athl Train* 49(6):733–739, 2014.

127. Helito CP, do Prado Torres JA, Bonadio MB, et al.: Anterolateral ligament of the fetal knee: an anatomic and histological study, *Am J Sports Med* 45(1):91–96, 2017.

128. Hemmerich A, Brown H, Smith S, et al.: Hip, knee, and ankle kinematics of high range of motion activities of daily living, *J Orthop Res* 24:770–781, 2006.

129. Herrington L, Nester C: Q-angle undervalued? The relationship between Q-angle and medio-lateral position of the patella, *Clin Biomech* 19:1070–1073, 2004.

130. Herzog W, Read LJ: Lines of action and moment arms of the major force-carrying structures crossing the human knee joint, *J Anat* 182:213–230, 1993.

131. Hewett TE, Ford KR, Myer GD: Anterior cruciate ligament injuries in female athletes: Part 2, a meta-analysis of neuromuscular interventions aimed at injury prevention, *Am J Sports Med* 34:490–498, 2006.

132. Hewett TE, Myer GD, Ford KR, et al.: Biomechanical measures of neuromuscular control and valgus loading of the knee predict anterior cruciate ligament injury risk in female athletes: a prospective study, *Am J Sports Med* 33:492–501, 2005.

133. Hewett TE, Zazulak BT, Myer GD, et al.: A review of electromyographic activation levels, timing differences, and increased anterior cruciate ligament injury incidence in female athletes, *Br J Sports Med* 39:347–350, 2005.

134. Hinman RS, Payne C, Metcalf BR, et al.: Lateral wedges in knee osteoarthritis: what are their immediate clinical and biomechanical effects and can these predict a three-month clinical outcome? *Arthritis Rheum* 59:408–415, 2008.

135. Ho KY, Chen YJ, Farrokhi S, et al.: Selective atrophy of the vastus medialis: does it exist in women with nontraumatic patellofemoral pain? *Am J Sports Med* 49(3):700–705, 2021.

136. Hoch JM, Perkins WO, Hartman JR, et al.: Somatosensory deficits in post-ACL reconstruction patients: a case-control study, *Muscle Nerve* 55(1):5–8, 2017.

137. Hogg JA, Vanrenterghem J, Ackerman T, et al.: Temporal kinematic differences throughout single and double-leg forward landings, *J Biomech* 99:109559, 2020.

138. Höher J, Vogrin TM, Woo SL, et al.: In situ forces in the human posterior cruciate ligament in response to muscle loads: a cadaveric study, *J Orthop Res* 17:763–768, 1999.

139. Holden S, Matthews M, Rathleff MS, et al.: How do hip exercises improve pain in individuals with patellofemoral pain? Secondary mediation analysis of strength and psychological factors as mechanisms, *J Orthop Sports Phys Ther* 51(12):602–610, 2021.

140. Hollister AM, Jatana S, Singh AK, et al.: The axes of rotation of the knee, *Clin Orthop Relat Res* 290:259–268, 1993.

141. Hollman JH, Ginos BE, Kozuchowski J, et al.: Relationships between knee valgus, hip-muscle strength, and hip-muscle recruitment during a single-limb step-down, *J Sport Rehabil* 18:104–117, 2009.

142. Hopper GP, Pioger C, Philippe C, et al.: Risk factors for anterior cruciate ligament graft failure in professional athletes: an analysis of 342 patients with a mean follow-up of 100 months from the SANTI study group, *Am J Sports Med* 50(12):3218–3227, 2022.

143. Horton MG, Hall TL: Quadriceps femoris muscle angle: normal values and relationships with gender and selected skeletal measures, *Phys Ther* 69:897–901, 1989.

144. Hosseinzadeh S, Kiapour AM: Sex differences in anatomic features linked to anterior cruciate ligament injuries during skeletal growth and maturation, *Am J Sports Med* 48(9):2205–2212, 2020.

145. Hoy MG, Zajac FE, Gordon ME: A musculoskeletal model of the human lower extremity: the effect of muscle, tendon, and moment arm on the moment-angle relationship of musculotendon actuators at the hip, knee, and ankle, *J Biomech* 23:157–169, 1990.

146. Hu J, Xin H, Chen Z, et al.: The role of menisci in knee contact mechanics and secondary kinematics during human walking, *Clin Biomech* 61:58–63, 2019.

147. Huber C, Zhang Q, Taylor WR, et al.: Properties and function of the medial patellofemoral ligament: a systematic review, *Am J Sports Med* 48(3):754–766, 2020.

148. Huberti HH, Hayes WC: Patellofemoral contact pressures. The influence of Q-angle and tibiofemoral contact, *J Bone Joint Surg Am* 66:715–724, 1984.

149. Hume DR, Navacchia A, Ali AA, et al.: The interaction of muscle moment arm, knee laxity, and torque in a multi-scale musculoskeletal model of the lower limb, *J Biomech* 76:173–180, 2018.

150. Inderhaug E, Stephen JM, Williams A, et al.: Effect of anterolateral complex sectioning and tenodesis on patellar kinematics and patellofemoral joint contact pressures, *Am J Sports Med* 46(12):2922–2928, 2018.

151. Inman VT, Saunders JB: Referred pain from skeletal structures, *J Nerv Ment Dis* 99:660–667, 1944.

152. Ishii Y, Terajima K, Terashima S, et al.: Three-dimensional kinematics of the human knee with intracortical pin fixation, *Clin Orthop Relat Res* 343:144–150, 1997.

153. Ithurburn MP, Altenburger AR, Thomas S, et al.: Young athletes after ACL reconstruction with quadriceps strength asymmetry at the time of return-to-sport demonstrate decreased knee function 1 year later, *Knee Surg Sports Traumatol Arthrosc* 26(2):426–433, 2018.

154. Jafarnezhadgero AA, Oliveira AS, Mousavi SH, et al.: Combining valgus knee brace and lateral foot wedges reduces external forces and moments in osteoarthritis patients, *Gait Posture* 59:104–110, 2018.

155. James EW, LaPrade CM, LaPrade RF: Anatomy and biomechanics of the lateral side of the knee and surgical implications [Review], *Sports Med Arthrosc* 23(1):2–9, 2015.

156. Janssen I, Steele JR, Munro BJ, et al.: Predicting the patellar tendon force generated when landing from a jump, *Med Sci Sports Exerc* 45(5):927–934, 2013.

157. Jeong J, Choi DH, Shin CS: Core strength training can alter neuromuscular and biomechanical risk factors for anterior cruciate ligament injury, *Am J Sports Med* 49(1):183–192, 2021.

158. Johnson F, Leitl S, Waugh W: The distribution of load across the knee. A comparison of static and dynamic measurements, *J Bone Joint Surg Br* 62:346–349, 1980.

159. Johnson JL, Capin JJ, Arundale AJH, et al.: A secondary injury prevention program may decrease contralateral anterior cruciate ligament injuries in female athletes: 2-year injury rates in the ACL-sports randomized controlled trial, *J Orthop Sports Phys Ther* 50(9):523–530, 2020.

160. Johnson JS, Morscher MA, Jones KC, et al.: Gene expression differences between ruptured anterior cruciate ligaments in young male and female subjects, *J Bone Joint Surg Am* 97(1):71–79, 2015.

161. Kaeding CC, Léger-St-Jean B, Magnussen RA: Epidemiology and diagnosis of anterior cruciate ligament injuries, *Clin Sports Med* 36(1):1–8, 2017.

162. Kan JH, Heemskerk AM, Ding Z, et al.: DTI-based muscle fiber tracking of the quadriceps mechanism in lateral patellar dislocation, *J Magn Reson Imaging* 29:663–670, 2009.

163. Kaplan Y: Identifying individuals with an anterior cruciate ligament-deficient knee as copers and noncopers: a narrative literature review. [Review], *J Orthop Sports Phys Ther* 41(10):758–766, 2011.

164. Kaufer H: Mechanical function of the patella, *J Bone Joint Surg Am* 53:1551–1560, 1971.

165. Kellis E, Baltzopoulos V: In vivo determination of the patella tendon and hamstrings moment arms in adult males using videofluoroscopy during submaximal knee extension and flexion, *Clin Biomech* 14:118–124, 1999.

166. Kenneally-Dabrowski CJB, Brown NAT, Lai AKM, et al.: Late swing or early stance? A narrative review of hamstring injury mechanisms during high-speed running, *Scand J Med Sci Sports* 29(8):1083–1091, 2019.

167. Kennedy JC, Alexander IJ, Hayes KC: Nerve supply of the human knee and its functional importance, *Am J Sports Med* 10:329–335, 1982.

168. Kennedy NI, Wijdicks CA, Goldsmith MT, et al.: Kinematic analysis of the posterior cruciate ligament, part 1: the individual and collective function of the anterolateral and posteromedial bundles, *Am J Sports Med* 41(12):2828–2838, 2013.

169. Kernozek T, Schiller M, Rutherford D, et al.: Real-Time visual feedback reduces patellofemoral joint forces during squatting in individuals with patellofemoral pain, *Clin Biomech* 77:105050, 2020.

170. Kettunen JA, Kvist M, Alanen E, et al.: Long-term prognosis for jumper's knee in male athletes: a prospective follow-up study, *Am J Sports Med* 30(5):689–692, 2002.

171. Kew ME, Miller MD: Posterior cruciate ligament reconstruction in the multiple ligament injured knee, *J Knee Surg* 33(5):421–430, 2020.

172. Khan KM, Bonar F, Desmond PM, et al.: Patellar tendinosis (jumper's knee): findings at histopathologic examination, US, and MR imaging–Victorian Institute of Sport Tendon Study Group, *Radiology* 200(3):821–827, 1996.

173. Khayambashi K, Fallah A, Movahedi A, et al.: Posterolateral hip muscle strengthening versus quadriceps strengthening for patellofemoral pain: a comparative control trial, *Arch Phys Med Rehabil* 95(5):900–907, 2014.

174. Kim YC, Yoo WK, Chung IH, et al.: Tendinous insertion of semimembranosus muscle into the lateral meniscus, *Surg Radiol Anat* 19:365–369, 1997.

175. Kindel C, Challis J: Joint moment-angle properties of the hip extensors in subjects with and without patellofemoral pain, *J Appl Biomech* 34(2):159–166, 2018.

176. Kiriyama S, Sato H, Takahira N: Gender differences in rotation of the shank during single-legged drop landing and its relation to rotational muscle strength of the knee, *Am J Sports Med* 37:168–174, 2009.

177. Kittl C, Becker DK, Raschke MJ, et al.: Dynamic restraints of the medial side of the knee: the semimembranosus corner revisited, *Am J Sports Med* 47(4):863–869, 2019.

178. Kobayashi K, Hosseini A, Sakamoto M, et al.: In vivo kinematics of the extensor mechanism of the knee during deep flexion, *J Biomech Eng* 135(8):81002, 2013.

179. Koh TJ, Grabiner MD, De Swart RJ: In vivo tracking of the human patella, *J Biomech* 25:637–643, 1992.

180. Komzak M, Hart R, Okal F, et al.: AM bundle controls the anterior-posterior and rotational stability to a greater extent than the PL bundle - a cadaver study, *Knee* 20(6):551–555, 2013.

181. Kooiker L, Van De Port IG, Weir A, et al.: Effects of physical therapist-guided quadriceps-strengthening exercises for the treatment of patellofemoral pain syndrome: a systematic review [Review], *J Orthop Sports Phys Ther* 44(6), 2014. 391–B1.

182. Kopkow C, Freiberg A, Kirschner S, et al.: Physical examination tests for the diagnosis of posterior cruciate ligament rupture: a systematic review [Review], *J Orthop Sports Phys Ther* 43(11):804–813, 2013.

183. Kotsifaki A, Korakakis V, Whiteley R, et al.: Measuring only hop distance during single leg hop testing is insufficient to detect deficits in knee function after ACL reconstruction: a systematic review and meta-analysis, *Br J Sports Med* 54(3):139–153, 2020.

184. Kowalczuk M, Herbst E, Burnham JM, et al.: A layered anatomic description of the anterolateral complex of the knee, *Clin Sports Med* 37(1):1–8, 2018.

185. Kraeutler MJ, Welton KL, Chahla J, et al.: Current concepts of the anterolateral ligament of the knee: anatomy, biomechanics, and reconstruction, *Am J Sports Med* 46(5):1235–1242, 2018.

186. Krevolin JL, Pandy MG, Pearce JC: Moment arm of the patellar tendon in the human knee, *J Biomech* 37:785–788, 2004.

187. Krosshaug T, Nakamae A, Boden BP, et al.: Mechanisms of anterior cruciate ligament injury in basketball: video analysis of 39 cases, *Am J Sports Med* 35:359–367, 2007.

188. Kubo K, Ohgo K, Takeishi R, et al.: Effects of series elasticity on the human knee extension torque-angle relationship in vivo, *Res Q Exerc Sport* 77:408–416, 2006.

189. Kulas AS, Hortobagyi T, DeVita P: Trunk position modulates anterior cruciate ligament forces and strains during a single-leg squat, *Clin Biomech* 27(1):16–21, 2012.

190. Kulig K, Andrews JG, Hay JG: Human strength curves, *Exerc Sport Sci Rev* 12:417–466, 1984.

191. Kulig K, Landel R, Chang YJ, et al.: Patellar tendon morphology in volleyball athletes with and without patellar tendinopathy, *Scand J Med Sci Sports* 23(2):e81–e88, 2013.

192. Kumar D, Subburaj K, Lin W, et al.: Quadriceps and hamstrings morphology is related to walking mechanics and knee cartilage MRI relaxation times in young adults, *J Orthop Sports Phys Ther* 43(12):881–890, 2013.

193. Kutzner I, Heinlein B, Graichen F, et al.: Loading of the knee joint during ergometer cycling: telemetric in vivo data, *J Orthop Sports Phys Ther* 42(12):103, 2012.

194. Lankhorst NE, Bierma-Zeinstra SM, van Middelkoop M: Risk factors for patellofemoral pain syndrome: a systematic review, *J Orthop Sports Phys Ther* 42(2):81–94, 2012.

195. Laprade J, Lee R: Real-time measurement of patellofemoral kinematics in asymptomatic subjects, *Knee* 12:63–72, 2005.

196. LaPrade MD, Kallenbach SL, Aman ZS, et al.: Biomechanical evaluation of the medial stabilizers of the patella, *Am J Sports Med* 46(7):1575–1582, 2018.

197. LaPrade RF, Bernhardson AS, Griffith CJ, et al.: Correlation of valgus stress radiographs with medial knee ligament injuries: an in vitro biomechanical study, *Am J Sports Med* 38(2):330–338, 2010.

198. LaPrade RF, Wentorf FA, Fritts H, et al.: A prospective magnetic resonance imaging study of the incidence of posterolateral and multiple ligament injuries in acute knee injuries presenting with a hemarthrosis, *Arthroscopy* 23(12):1341–1347, 2007.

199. Lee TQ, Morris G, Csintalan RP: The influence of tibial and femoral rotation on patellofemoral contact area and pressure, *J Orthop Sports Phys Ther* 33:686–693, 2003.

200. Lenhart RL, Smith CR, Vignos MF, et al.: Influence of step rate and quadriceps load distribution on patellofemoral cartilage contact pressures during running, *J Biomech* 48(11):2871–2878, 2015.

201. Lepley AS, Gribble PA, Thomas AC, et al.: Quadriceps neural alterations in anterior cruciate ligament reconstructed patients: a 6-month longitudinal investigation, *Scand J Med Sci Sports* 25(6):828–839, 2015.

202. Lepley AS, Grooms DR, Burland JP, et al.: Quadriceps muscle function following anterior cruciate ligament reconstruction: systemic differences in neural and morphological characteristics, *Exp Brain Res* 237(5):1267–1278, 2019.

203. Leung J, Smith R, Harvey LA, et al.: The impact of simulated ankle plantarflexion contracture on the knee joint during stance phase of gait: a within-subject study, *Clin Biomech* 29(4):423–428, 2014.

204. Li G, Most E, DeFrate LE, et al.: Effect of the posterior cruciate ligament on posterior stability of the knee in high flexion, *J Biomech* 37:779–783, 2004.

205. Lian OB, Engebretsen L, Bahr R: Prevalence of jumper's knee among elite athletes from different sports: a cross-sectional study, *Am J Sports Med* 33(4):561–567, 2005.

206. Liao TC, Neal BS, Barton CJ, Birn-Jeffery A, et al.: Increased hip adduction during running is associated with patellofemoral pain and differs between males and females: a case-control study, *J Biomech* 91:133–139, 2019.

207. Liao TC, Yang N, Ho KY, et al.: Femur rotation increases patella cartilage stress in females with patellofemoral pain, *Med Sci Sports Exerc* 47(9):1775–1780, 2015.

208. Liao TC, Yin L, Powers CM: The influence of isolated femur and tibia rotations on patella cartilage stress: a sensitivity analysis, *Clin Biomech* 54:125–131, 2018.

209. Lieb FJ, Perry J: Quadriceps function. An anatomical and mechanical study using amputated limbs, *J Bone Joint Surg Am* 50:1535–1548, 1968.

210. Lieber RL: *Skeletal muscle structure, function and plasticity*, ed 3, Baltimore, 2010, Lippincott Williams & Wilkins.

211. Liederbach M, Kremenic IJ, Orishimo KF, et al.: Comparison of landing biomechanics between male and female dancers and athletes, part 2: influence of fatigue and implications for anterior cruciate ligament injury, *Am J Sports Med* 42(5):1089–1095, 2014.

212. Lipps DB, Wojtys EM, Ashton-Miller JA: Anterior cruciate ligament fatigue failures in knees subjected to repeated simulated pivot landings, *Am J Sports Med* 41(5):1058–1066, 2013.

213. Lisee C, Lepley AS, Birchmeier T, et al.: Quadriceps strength and volitional activation after anterior cruciate ligament reconstruction: a systematic review and meta-analysis, *Sports Health* 11(2):163–179, 2019.

214. Liu F, Gadikota HR, Kozanek M, et al.: In vivo length patterns of the medial collateral ligament during the stance phase of gait, *Knee Surg Sports Traumatol Arthrosc* 19(5):719–727, 2011.

215. Logan CA, Beaulieu-Jones BR, Sanchez G, et al.: Posterior cruciate ligament injuries of the knee at the national football league combine: an imaging and epidemiology study, *Arthroscopy* 34(3):681–686, 2018.

216. Logerstedt DS, Scalzitti DA, Bennell KL, et al.: Knee pain and mobility impairments: meniscal and articular cartilage lesions revision 2018, *J Orthop Sports Phys Ther* 48(2):A1–a50, 2018.

217. Lohmander LS, Englund PM, Dahl LL, et al.: The long-term consequence of anterior cruciate ligament and meniscus injuries: osteoarthritis, *Am J Sports Med* 35:1756–1769, 2007.

218. Lorenz A, Muller O, Kohler P, et al.: The influence of asymmetric quadriceps loading on patellar tracking—an in vitro study, *Knee* 19(6):818–822, 2012.

219. Lowry CD, Cleland JA, Dyke K: Management of patients with patellofemoral pain syndrome using a multimodal approach: a case series, *J Orthop Sports Phys Ther* 38:691–702, 2008.

220. Lu TW, O'Connor JJ: Lines of action and moment arms of the major force-bearing structures crossing the human knee joint: comparison between theory and experiment, *J Anat* 189:575–585, 1996.

221. Lunden JB, Bzdusek PJ, Monson JK, et al.: Current concepts in the recognition and treatment of posterolateral corner injuries of the knee, *J Orthop Sports Phys Ther* 40(8):502–516, 2010.

222. Luque-Seron JA, Medina-Porqueres I: Anterior cruciate ligament strain in vivo: S systematic review, *Sports Health* 8(5):451–455, 2016.

223. Luyckx T, Didden K, Vandenneucker H, et al.: Is there a biomechanical explanation for anterior knee pain in patients with patella alta? Influence of patellar height on patellofemoral contact force, contact area and contact pressure, *J Bone Joint Surg Br* 91:344–350, 2009.

224. Luz BC, Dos Santos AF, de Souza MC, et al.: Relationship between rearfoot, tibia and femur kinematics in runners with and without patellofemoral pain, *Gait Posture* 61:416–422, 2018.

225. Lyu SR: Relationship of medial plica and medial femoral condyle during flexion, *Clin Biomech* 22:1013–1016, 2007.

226. MacIntyre NJ, Hill NA, Fellows RA, et al.: Patellofemoral joint kinematics in individuals with and without patellofemoral pain syndrome, *J Bone Joint Surg Am* 88:2596–2605, 2006.

227. MacIntyre NJ, McKnight EK, Day A, et al.: Consistency of patellar spin, tilt and lateral translation side-to-side and over a 1 year period in healthy young males, *J Biomech* 41:3094–3096, 2008.

228. Magalhaes E, Fukuda TY, Sacramento SN, et al.: A comparison of hip strength between sedentary females with and without patellofemoral pain syndrome, *J Orthop Sports Phys Ther* 40:641–647, 2010.

229. Mandelbaum BR, Silvers HJ, Watanabe DS, et al.: Effectiveness of a neuromuscular and proprioceptive training program in preventing anterior cruciate ligament injuries in female athletes: 2-year follow-up, *Am J Sports Med* 33:1003–1010, 2005.

230. Margheritini F, Rihn J, Musahl V, et al.: Posterior cruciate ligament injuries in the athlete: an anatomical, biomechanical and clinical review, *Sports Med* 32:393–408, 2002.

231. Markolf KL, Graff-Radford A, Amstutz HC: In vivo knee stability. A quantitative assessment using an instrumented clinical testing apparatus, *J Bone Joint Surg Am* 60:664–674, 1978.

232. Markolf KL, O'Neill G, Jackson SR, et al.: Effects of applied quadriceps and hamstrings muscle loads on forces in the anterior and posterior cruciate ligaments, *Am J Sports Med* 32:1144–1149, 2004.

233. Marzo JM, Gurske-DePerio J: Effects of medial meniscus posterior horn avulsion and repair on tibiofemoral contact area and peak contact pressure with clinical implications, *Am J Sports Med* 37:124–129, 2009.

234. McDermott ID, Amis AA: The consequences of meniscectomy, *J Bone Joint Surg Br* 88:1549–1556, 2006.

235. McNair PJ, Marshall RN, Maguire K: Swelling of the knee joint: effects of exercise on quadriceps muscle strength, *Arch Phys Med Rehabil* 77:896–899, 1996.

236. Mendias CL, Lynch EB, Davis ME, et al.: Changes in circulating biomarkers of muscle atrophy, inflammation, and cartilage turnover in patients undergoing anterior cruciate ligament reconstruction and rehabilitation, *Am J Sports Med* 41(8):1819–1826, 2013.

237. Mendonca LD, Ocarino JM, Bittencourt NFN, et al.: Association of hip and foot factors with patellar tendinopathy (jumper's knee) in Athletes, *J Orthop Sports Phys Ther* 48(9):676–684, 2018.

238. Mesfar W, Shirazi-Adl A: Biomechanics of changes in ACL and PCL material properties or prestrains in flexion under muscle force-implications in ligament reconstruction, *Comput Methods Biomech Biomed Eng* 9:201–209, 2006.

239. Mesfar W, Shirazi-Adl A: Knee joint mechanics under quadriceps—hamstrings muscle forces are influenced by tibial restraint, *Clin Biomech* 21:841–848, 2006.

240. Meyer EG, Baumer TG, Haut RC: Pure passive hyper-extension of the human cadaver knee generates simultaneous bicruciate ligament rupture, *J Biomech Eng* 133(1):011012, 2011.

241. Mihata LC, Beutler AI, Boden BP: Comparing the incidence of anterior cruciate ligament injury in collegiate lacrosse, soccer, and basketball players: implications for anterior cruciate ligament mechanism and prevention, *Am J Sports Med* 34:899–904, 2006.

242. Miyazaki T, Wada M, Kawahara H, et al.: Dynamic load at baseline can predict radiographic disease progression in medial compartment knee osteoarthritis, *Ann Rheum Dis* 61:617–622, 2002.

243. Moksnes H, Snyder-Mackler L, Risberg MA: Individuals with an anterior cruciate ligament-deficient knee classified as noncopers may be candidates for nonsurgical rehabilitation, *J Orthop Sports Phys Ther* 38(10):586–595, 2008.

244. Monk AP, Davies LJ, Hopewell S, et al.: Surgical versus conservative interventions for treating anterior cruciate ligament injuries, *Cochrane Database Syst Rev* 4(4), 2016. Cd011166.

245. Mononen ME, Jurvelin JS, Korhonen RK: Effects of radial tears and partial meniscectomy of lateral meniscus on the knee joint mechanics during the stance phase of the gait cycle—a 3D finite element study, *J Orthop Res* 31(8):1208–1217, 2013.

246. Mossber KA, Smith LK: Axial rotation of the knee in women, *J Orthop Sports Phys Ther* 4:236–240, 1983.

247. Mouarbes D, Menetrey J, Marot V, et al.: Anterior cruciate ligament reconstruction: a systematic review and meta-analysis of outcomes for quadriceps tendon autograft versus bone-patellar tendon-bone and hamstring-tendon autografts, *Am J Sports Med* 47(14):3531–3540, 2019.

248. Moyer RF, Birmingham TB, Bryant DM, et al.: Biomechanical effects of valgus knee bracing: a systematic review and meta-analysis [Review], *Osteoarthritis Cartilage* 23(2):178–188, 2015.

249. Murawski CD, van Eck CF, Irrgang JJ, et al.: Operative treatment of primary anterior cruciate ligament rupture in adults [Review], *J Bone Joint Surg Am* 96(8):685–694, 2014.

250. Musahl V, Karlsson J: Anterior cruciate ligament tear, *N Engl J Med* 380(24):2341–2348, 2019.

251. Nagai K, Gale T, Chiba D, et al.: The complex relationship between in vivo ACL elongation and knee kinematics during walking and running, *J Orthop Res* 37(9):1920–1928, 2019.

252. Nakagawa TH, Moriya ET, Maciel CD, et al.: Frontal plane biomechanics in males and females with and without patellofemoral pain, *Med Sci Sports Exerc* 44(9):1747–1755, 2012.

253. Nascimento LR, Teixeira-Salmela LF, Souza RB, et al.: Hip and knee strengthening is more effective than knee strengthening alone for reducing pain and improving activity in individuals with patellofemoral pain: a systematic review with meta-analysis, *J Orthop Sports Phys Ther* 48(1):19–31, 2018.

254. Navacchia A, Bates NA, Schilaty ND, et al.: Knee abduction and internal rotation moments increase ACL force during landing through the posterior slope of the tibia, *J Orthop Res* 37(8):1730–1742, 2019.

255. Neal BS, Barton CJ, Birn-Jeffery A, et al.: Increased hip adduction during running is associated with patellofemoral pain and differs between males and females: a case-control study, *J Biomech* 91:133–139, 2019.

256. Nebelung W, Wuschech H: Thirty-five years of follow-up of anterior cruciate ligament-deficient knees in high-level athletes, *Arthroscopy* 21:696–702, 2005.

257. Nha KW, Papannagari R, Gill TJ, et al.: In vivo patellar tracking: clinical motions and patellofemoral indices, *J Orthop Res* 26:1067–1074, 2008.

258. Noehren B, Snyder-Mackler L: Who's afraid of the big bad wolf? Open-chain exercises after anterior cruciate ligament reconstruction, *J Orthop Sports Phys Ther* 50(9):473–475, 2020.

259. Noehren B, Andersen A, Hardy P, et al.: Cellular and morphological alterations in the vastus lateralis muscle as the result of ACL injury and reconstruction, *J Bone Joint Surg Am* 98(18):1541–1547, 2016.

260. Noehren B, Hamill J, Davis I: Prospective evidence for a hip etiology in patellofemoral pain, *Med Sci Sports Exerc* 45(6):1120–1124, 2013.

261. Noyes FR, Heckmann TP, Barber-Westin SD: Meniscus repair and transplantation: a comprehensive update, *J Orthop Sports Phys Ther* 42(3):274–290, 2012.

262. Oh YK, Lipps DB, Ashton-Miller JA, et al.: What strains the anterior cruciate ligament during a pivot landing? *Am J Sports Med* 40(3):574–583, 2012.

263. Omi Y, Sugimoto D, Kuriyama S, et al.: Effect of hip-focused injury prevention training for anterior cruciate ligament injury reduction in female basketball players: a 12-year prospective intervention study, *Am J Sports Med* 46(4):852–861, 2018.

264. Osternig LR, Bates BT, James SL: Patterns of tibial rotary torque in knees of healthy subjects, *Med Sci Sports Exerc* 12:195–199, 1980.

265. Pal S, Besier TF, Beaupre GS, et al.: Patellar maltracking is prevalent among patellofemoral pain subjects with patella alta: an upright, weightbearing MRI study, *J Orthop Res* 31(3):448–457, 2013.

266. Pal S, Besier TF, Gold GE, et al.: Patellofemoral cartilage stresses are most sensitive to variations in vastus medialis muscle forces, *Comput Methods Biomech Biomed Eng* 22(2):206–216, 2019.

267. Pal S, Langenderfer JE, Stowe JQ, et al.: Probabilistic modeling of knee muscle moment arms: effects of methods, origin-insertion, and kinematic variability, *Ann Biomed Eng* 35:1632–1642, 2007.

268. Palmieri-Smith RM, Kreinbrink J, Ashton-Miller JA, et al.: Quadriceps inhibition induced by an experimental knee joint effusion affects knee joint mechanics during a single-legged drop landing, *Am J Sports Med* 35:1269–1275, 2007.

269. Pantano KJ, White SC, Gilchrist LA, et al.: Differences in peak knee valgus angles between individuals with high and low Q-angles during a single limb squat, *Clin Biomech* 20:966–972, 2005.

270. Papannagari R, DeFrate LE, Nha KW, et al.: Function of posterior cruciate ligament bundles during in vivo knee flexion, *Am J Sports Med* 35:1507–1512, 2007.

271. Park SE, DeFrate LE, Suggs JF, et al.: The change in length of the medial and lateral collateral ligaments during in vivo knee flexion, *Knee* 12:377–382, 2005.

272. Passmore E, Graham HK, Pandy MG, et al.: Hip- and patellofemoral-joint loading during gait are increased in children with idiopathic torsional deformities, *Gait Posture* 63:228–235, 2018.

273. Patel D: Arthroscopy of the plicae—synovial folds and their significance, *Am J Sports Med* 6:217–225, 1978.

274. Patel SA, Hageman J, Quatman CE, et al.: Prevalence and location of bone bruises associated with anterior cruciate ligament injury and implications for mechanism of injury: a systematic review. [Review], *Sports Med* 44(2):281–293, 2014.

275. Patel VV, Hall K, Ries M, et al.: A three-dimensional MRI analysis of knee kinematics, *J Orthop Res* 22:283–292, 2004.

276. Paterno MV, Rauh MJ, Schmitt LC, et al.: Incidence of second ACL injuries 2 years after primary ACL reconstruction and return to sport, *Am J Sports Med* 42:1567–1573, 2014.

277. Pedersen M, Johnson JL, Grindem H, et al.: Meniscus or cartilage injury at the time of anterior cruciate ligament tear is associated with worse prognosis for patient-reported outcome 2 to 10 years after anterior cruciate ligament injury: a systematic review, *J Orthop Sports Phys Ther* 50(9):490–502, 2020.

278. Peng YL, Tenan MS, Griffin L: Hip position and sex differences in motor unit firing patterns of the vastus medialis and vastus medialis oblique in healthy individuals, *J Appl Physiol* 124(6):1438–1446, 2018.

279. Peng HT, Kernozek TW, Song CY: Muscle activation of vastus medialis obliquus and vastus lateralis during a dynamic leg press exercise with and without isometric hip adduction, *Phys Ther Sport* 14(1):44–49, 2013.

280. Perriman A, Leahy E, Semciw AI: The effect of open-versus closed-kinetic-chain exercises on anterior tibial laxity, strength, and function following anterior cruciate ligament reconstruction: a systematic review and meta-analysis, *J Orthop Sports Phys Ther* 48(7):552–566, 2018.

281. Petersen W, Loerch S, Schanz S, et al.: The role of the posterior oblique ligament in controlling posterior tibial translation in the posterior cruciate ligament-deficient knee, *Am J Sports Med* 36:495–501, 2008.

282. Petrigliano FA, McAllister DR: Isolated posterior cruciate ligament injuries of the knee, *Sports Med Arthrosc* 14:206–212, 2006.

283. Petrovic M, Sigurðsson HB, Sigurðsson HJ, et al.: Effect of sex on anterior cruciate ligament injury-related biomechanics during the cutting maneuver in preadolescent athletes, *Orthop J Sports Med* 8(7), 2020. 2325967120936980.

284. Pfeiffer SJ, Valentine JA, Goodwin JS, et al.: Effects of a knee valgus unloader brace on medial femoral articular cartilage deformation following walking in varus-aligned individuals, *Knee* 26(5):1067–1072, 2019.

285. Philippot R, Boyer B, Testa R, et al.: Study of patellar kinematics after reconstruction of the medial patellofemoral ligament, *Clin Biomech* 27(1):22–26, 2012.

286. Pincivero DM, Salfetnikov Y, Campy RM, et al.: Angle- and gender-specific quadriceps femoris muscle recruitment and knee extensor torque, *J Biomech* 37:1689–1697, 2004.

287. Postma WF, West RV: Anterior cruciate ligament injury-prevention programs [Review], *J Bone Joint Surg Am* 95(7):661–669, 2013.

288. Powers CM, Ho KY, Chen YJ, et al.: Patellofemoral joint stress during weight-bearing and non-weight-bearing quadriceps exercises, *J Orthop Sports Phys Ther* 44(5):320–327, 2014.

289. Powers CM, Ward SR, Fredericson M, et al.: Patellofemoral kinematics during weight-bearing and non-weight-bearing knee extension in persons with lateral subluxation of the patella: a preliminary study, *J Orthop Sports Phys Ther* 33:677–685, 2003.

290. Powers CM, Witvrouw E, Davis IS, et al.: Evidence-Based framework for a pathomechanical model of patellofemoral pain: 2017 patellofemoral pain consensus statement from the 4th international patellofemoral pain research retreat, Manchester, UK: Part 3, *Br J Sports Med* 51(24):1713–1723, 2017.

291. Powers CM: Patellar kinematics, part I: the influence of vastus muscle activity in subjects with and without patellofemoral pain, *Phys Ther* 80:956–964, 2000.

292. Powers CM: The influence of abnormal hip mechanics on knee injury: a biomechanical perspective [Review, 86 refs], *J Orthop Sports Phys Ther* 40(2):42–51, 2010.

293. Powers CM: The influence of altered lower-extremity kinematics on patellofemoral joint dysfunction: a theoretical perspective, *J Orthop Sports Phys Ther* 33:639–646, 2003.

294. Poynton A, Moran CJ, Moran R, et al.: The meniscofemoral ligaments influence lateral meniscal motion at the human knee joint, *Arthroscopy* 27(3):365–371, 2011.

295. Quatman CE, Kiapour AM, Demetropoulos CK, et al.: Preferential loading of the ACL compared with the MCL during landing: a novel in sim approach yields the multiplanar mechanism of dynamic valgus during ACL injuries, *Am J Sports Med* 42(1):177–186, 2014.

296. Race A, Amis AA: The mechanical properties of the two bundles of the human posterior cruciate ligament, *J Biomech* 27(1):13–24, 1994.

297. Raimondo RA, Ahmad CS, Blankevoort L, et al.: Patellar stabilization: a quantitative evaluation of the vastus medialis obliquus muscle, *Orthopedics* 21:791–795, 1998.

298. Rajala GM, Neumann DA, Foster C: Quadriceps muscle performance in male speed skaters, *J Strength Condit Res* 8:48–52, 1994.

299. Reilly DT, Martens M: Experimental analysis of the quadriceps muscle force and patello-femoral joint reaction force for various activities, *Acta Orthop Scand* 43:126–137, 1972.

300. Relph N, Herrington L, Tyson S: The effects of ACL injury on knee proprioception: a meta-analysis, *Physiotherapy* 100(3):187–195, 2014.

301. Richards DP, Ajemian SV, Wiley JP, et al.: Knee joint dynamics predict patellar tendinitis in elite volleyball players, *Am J Sports Med* 24(5):676–683, 1996.

302. Richards Pfeiffer SJ, Valentine JA, Goodwin JS, et al.: Effects of a knee valgus unloader brace on medial femoral articular cartilage deformation following walking in varus-aligned individuals, *Knee* 26(5):1067–1072, 2019.

303. Richter M, Kiefer H, Hehl G, et al.: Primary repair for posterior cruciate ligament injuries. An eight-year followup of fifty-three patients, *Am J Sports Med* 24:298–305, 1996.

304. Rickaby R, El Khoury LY, Samiric T, et al.: Epigenetic status of the human MMP11 gene promoter is altered in patellar tendinopathy, *J Sports Sci Med* 18(1):155–159, 2019.

305. Roach KE, Miles TP: Normal hip and knee active range of motion: the relationship to age, *Phys Ther* 71:656–665, 1991.

306. Robinson JR, Bull AM, Thomas RR, et al.: The role of the medial collateral ligament and posteromedial capsule in controlling knee laxity, *Am J Sports Med* 34:1815–1823, 2006.

307. Robinson JR, Sanchez-Ballester J, Bull AM, et al.: The posteromedial corner revisited. An anatomical description of the passive restraining structures of the medial aspect of the human knee, *J Bone Joint Surg Br* 86:674–681, 2004.

308. Robinson RL, Nee RJ: Analysis of hip strength in females seeking physical therapy treatment for unilateral patellofemoral pain syndrome, *J Orthop Sports Phys Ther* 37:232–238, 2007.

309. Rodriguez KM, Palmieri-Smith RM, Krishnan C: How does anterior cruciate ligament reconstruction affect the functioning of the brain and spinal cord? a systematic review with meta-analysis, *J Sport Health Sci* 10(2):172–181, 2021.

310. Salsich GB, Graci V, Maxam DE: The effects of movement pattern modification on lower extremity kinematics and pain in women with patellofemoral pain, *J Orthop Sports Phys Ther* 42(12):1017–1024, 2012.

311. Salsich GB, Perman WH: Patellofemoral joint contact area is influenced by tibiofemoral rotation alignment in individuals who have patellofemoral pain, *J Orthop Sports Phys Ther* 37:521–528, 2007.

312. Sanchez 2nd AR, Sugalski MT, LaPrade RF: Anatomy and biomechanics of the lateral side of the knee, *Sports Med Arthrosc* 14:2–11, 2006.

313. Scattone SR, Purdam CR, Fearon AM, et al.: Effects of altering trunk position during landings on patellar tendon force and pain, *Med Sci Sports Exerc* 49(12):2517–2527, 2017.

314. Schilaty ND, Bates NA, Krych AJ, et al.: Frontal plane loading characteristics of medial collateral ligament strain concurrent with anterior cruciate ligament failure, *Am J Sports Med* 47(9):2143–2150, 2019.

315. Schinhan M, Bijak M, Unger E, et al.: Electromyographic study of the popliteus muscle in the dynamic stabilization of the posterolateral corner structures of the knee, *Am J Sports Med* 39(1):173–179, 2011.

316. Schulz MS, Russe K, Weiler A, et al.: Epidemiology of posterior cruciate ligament injuries, *Arch Orthop Trauma Surg* 123:186–191, 2003.

317. Schutte MJ, Dabezies EJ, Zimny ML, et al.: Neural anatomy of the human anterior cruciate ligament, *J Bone Joint Surg Am* 69:243–247, 1987.

318. Scott A, Squier K, Alfredson H, et al.: ICON 2019: international scientific tendinopathy symposium consensus: clinical terminology, *Br J Sports Med* 54(5):260–262, 2020.

319. Senavongse W, Amis AA: The effects of articular, retinacular, or muscular deficiencies on patellofemoral joint stability, *J Bone Joint Surg Br* 87:577–582, 2005.

320. Shahane SA, Ibbotson C, Strachan R, et al.: The popliteofibular ligament. An anatomical study of the posterolateral corner of the knee, *J Bone Joint Surg Br* 81(4):636–642, 1999.

321. Shalhoub S, Maletsky LP: Variation in patellofemoral kinematics due to changes in quadriceps loading configuration during in vitro testing, *J Biomech* 47(1):130–136, 2014.

322. Sheehan FT, Borotikar BS, Behnam AJ, et al.: Alterations in in vivo knee joint kinematics following a femoral nerve branch block of the vastus medialis: implications for patellofemoral pain syndrome, *Clin Biomech* 27(6):525–531, 2012.

323. Shelbourne KD, Davis TJ, Patel DV: The natural history of acute, isolated, nonoperatively treated posterior cruciate ligament injuries. A prospective study, *Am J Sports Med* 27:276–283, 1999.

324. Shelburne KB, Pandy MG, Torry MR: Comparison of shear forces and ligament loading in the healthy and ACL-deficient knee during gait, *J Biomech* 37:313–319, 2004.

325. Shelburne KB, Torry MR, Steadman JR, et al.: Effects of foot orthoses and valgus bracing on the knee adduction moment and medial joint load during gait, *Clin Biomech* 23:814–821, 2008.

326. Shimokochi Y, Shultz SJ: Mechanisms of noncontact anterior cruciate ligament injury, *J Athl Train* 43:396–408, 2008.

327. Shin CS, Chaudhari AM, Andriacchi TP: Valgus plus internal rotation moments increase anterior cruciate ligament strain more than either alone, *Med Sci Sports Exerc* 43(8):1484–1491, 2011.

328. Shull PB, Silder A, Shultz R, et al.: Six-week gait retraining program reduces knee adduction moment, reduces pain, and improves function for individuals with medial compartment knee osteoarthritis, *J Orthop Res* 31(7):1020–1025, 2013.

329. Sigmund KJ, Hoeger Bement MK, Earl-Boehm JE: Exploring the pain in patellofemoral pain: a systematic review and meta-analysis examining signs of central sensitization, *J Athl Train*, 2020.

330. Sigward SM, Pollard CD, Havens KL, et al.: Influence of sex and maturation on knee mechanics during side-step cutting, *Med Sci Sports Exerc* 44(8):1497–1503, 2012.

331. Sisk D, Fredericson M: Update of risk factors, diagnosis, and management of patellofemoral pain, *Curr Rev Musculoskelet Med* 12(4):534–541, 2019.

332. Slater LV, Blemker SS, Hertel J, et al.: Sex affects gait adaptations after exercise in individuals with anterior cruciate ligament reconstruction, *Clin Biomech* 71:189–195, 2020.

333. Smidt GL: Biomechanical analysis of knee flexion and extension, *J Biomech* 6:79–92, 1973.

334. Smith TO, Donell S, Song F, et al.: Surgical versus non-surgical interventions for treating patellar dislocation, *Cochrane Database Syst Rev* 2, 2015. Cd008106.

335. Song CY, Lin YF, Wei TC, et al.: Surplus value of hip adduction in leg-press exercise in patients with patellofemoral pain syndrome: a randomized controlled trial, *Phys Ther* 89:409–418, 2009.

336. Sonnery-Cottet B, Saithna A, Quelard B, et al.: Arthrogenic muscle inhibition after ACL reconstruction: a scoping review of the efficacy of interventions, *Br J Sports Med* 53(5):289–298, 2019.

337. Souza RB, Draper CE, Fredericson M, et al.: Femur rotation and patellofemoral joint kinematics: a weight-bearing magnetic resonance imaging analysis, *J Orthop Sports Phys Ther* 40(5):277–285, 2010.

338. Souza RB, Powers CM: Differences in hip kinematics, muscle strength, and muscle activation between subjects with and without patellofemoral pain, *J Orthop Sports Phys Ther* 39:12–19, 2009.

339. Spang R, Egan J, Hanna P, et al.: Comparison of patellofemoral kinematics and stability after medial patellofemoral ligament and medial quadriceps tendon-femoral ligament reconstruction, *Am J Sports Med* 48(9):2252–2259, 2020.

340. Spoor CW, van Leeuwen JL: Knee muscle moment arms from MRI and from tendon travel, *J Biomech* 25:201–206, 1992.

341. Sprague A, Epsley S, Silbernagel KG: Distinguishing quadriceps tendinopathy and patellar tendinopathy: semantics or significant? *J Orthop Sports Phys Ther* 49(9):627–630, 2019.

342. Sprague AL, Smith AH, Knox P, et al.: Modifiable risk factors for patellar tendinopathy in athletes: a systematic review and meta-analysis, *Br J Sports Med* 52(24):1575–1585, 2018.

343. Standring S: *Gray's anatomy: the anatomical basis of clinical practice*, ed 42, St Louis, 2021, Elsevier.

344. Steinkamp LA, Dillingham MF, Markel MD, et al.: Biomechanical considerations in patellofemoral joint rehabilitation, *Am J Sports Med* 21(3):438–444, 1993.

345. Stevenson JH, Beattie CS, Schwartz JB, et al.: Assessing the effectiveness of neuromuscular training programs in reducing the incidence of anterior cruciate ligament injuries in female athletes: a systematic review [Review], *Am J Sports Med* 43(2):482–490, 2015.

346. Sturnick DR, Vacek PM, Desarno MJ, et al.: Combined anatomic factors predicting risk of anterior cruciate ligament injury for males and females, *Am J Sports Med* 43(4):839–847, 2015.

347. Sutton KM, Bullock JM: Anterior cruciate ligament rupture: differences between males and females, *J Am Acad Orthop Surg* 21(1):41–50, 2013.

348. Suzuki T, Hosseini A, Li JS, et al.: In vivo patellar tracking and patellofemoral cartilage contacts during dynamic stair ascending, *J Biomech* 45(14):2432–2437, 2012.

349. Takacs J, Hunt MA: The effect of contralateral pelvic drop and trunk lean on frontal plane knee biomechanics during single limb standing, *J Biomech* 45(16):2791–2796, 2012.

350. Tanifuji O, Blaha JD, Kai S: The vector of quadriceps pull is directed from the patella to the femoral neck, *Clin Orthop Relat Res* 471(3):1014–1020, 2013.

351. Taunton JE, Ryan MB, Clement DB, et al.: A retrospective case-control analysis of 2002 running injuries, *Br J Sports Med* 36:95–101, 2002.

352. Teng HL, Chen YJ, Powers CM: Predictors of patellar alignment during weight bearing: an examination of patellar height and trochlear geometry, *Knee* 21(1):142–146, 2014.

353. Teng HL, Powers CM: Sagittal plane trunk posture influences patellofemoral joint stress during running, *J Orthop Sports Phys Ther* 44(10):785–792, 2014.

354. Thoma LM, Grindem H, Logerstedt D, et al.: Coper classification early after anterior cruciate ligament rupture changes with progressive neuromuscular and strength training and is associated with 2-year success: the Delaware-Oslo ACL cohort study, *Am J Sports Med* 47(4):807–814, 2019.

355. Thomeé R, Renström P, Karlsson J, et al.: Patellofemoral pain syndrome in young women. II. Muscle function in patients and healthy controls, *Scand J Med Sci Sports* 5:245–251, 1995.

356. Thompson JA, Tran AA, Gatewood CT, et al.: Biomechanical effects of an injury prevention program in preadolescent female soccer athletes, *Am J Sports Med* 45(2):294–301, 2017.

357. Tiberio D: The effect of excessive subtalar joint pronation on patellofemoral mechanics: a theoretical model, *J Orthop Sports Phys Ther* 9:160–165, 1987.

358. Tipton CM, Vailas AC, Matthes RD: Experimental studies on the influences of physical activity on ligaments, tendons and joints: a brief review, *Acta Med Scand Suppl* 711:157–168, 1986.

359. Toole AR, Ithurburn MP, Rauh MJ, et al.: Young athletes cleared for sports participation after anterior cruciate ligament reconstruction: how many actually meet recommended return-to-sport criterion cutoffs? *J Orthop Sports Phys Ther* 47(11):825–833, 2017.

360. Toth MJ, Tourville TW, Voigt TB, et al.: Utility of neuromuscular electrical stimulation to preserve quadriceps muscle fiber size and contractility after anterior cruciate ligament injuries and reconstruction: a randomized, sham-controlled, blinded trial, *Am J Sports Med* 48(10):2429–2437, 2020.

361. Tsuda E, Okamura Y, Otsuka H, et al.: Direct evidence of the anterior cruciate ligament-hamstring reflex arc in humans, *Am J Sports Med* 29:83–87, 2001.

362. Ullrich B, Brueggemann GP: Moment-Knee angle relation in well trained athletes, *Int J Sports Med* 29(8):639–645, 2008.

363. Van de Velde SK, DeFrate LE, Gill TJ, et al.: The effect of anterior cruciate ligament deficiency on the in vivo elongation of the medial and lateral collateral ligaments, *Am J Sports Med* 35:294–300, 2007.

364. van Eck CF, Lesniak BP, Schreiber VM, et al.: Anatomic single- and double bundle anterior cruciate ligament reconstruction flowchart, *Arthroscopy* 26(2):258–268, 2010.

365. Van Rossom S, Smith CR, Thelen DG, et al.: Knee joint loading in healthy adults during functional exercises: implications for rehabilitation guidelines, *J Orthop Sports Phys Ther* 48(3):162–173, 2018.

366. van Yperen DT, Reijman M, van Es EM, et al.: Twenty-year follow-up study comparing operative versus nonoperative treatment of anterior cruciate ligament ruptures in high-level athletes, *Am J Sports Med* 46(5):1129–1136, 2018.

367. Voleti PB, Tjoumakaris FP, Rotmil G, et al.: Fifty most-cited articles in anterior cruciate ligament research, *Orthopedics* 38(4):e297–e304, 2015.

368. Voos JE, Mauro CS, Wente T, et al.: Posterior cruciate ligament: anatomy, biomechanics, and outcomes [Review], *Am J Sports Med* 40(1):222–231, 2012.

369. Wall SJ, Rose DM, Sutter EG, et al.: The role of axial compressive and quadriceps forces in noncontact anterior cruciate ligament injury: a cadaveric study, *Am J Sports Med* 40(3):568–573, 2012.

370. Wallis JA, Roddy L, Bottrell J, et al.: A systematic review of clinical practice guidelines for physical therapist management of patellofemoral pain, *Phys Ther* 101(3), 2021.

371. Wang CJ, Walker PS: The effects of flexion and rotation on the length patterns of the ligaments of the knee, *J Biomech* 6:587–596, 1973.

372. Wang HM, Shultz SJ, Ross SE, et al.: Sex comparisons of in vivo anterior cruciate ligament morphometry, *J Athlet Train* 54(5):513–518, 2019.

373. Wang JH, Kato Y, Ingham SJ, et al.: Effects of knee flexion angle and loading conditions on the end-to-end distance of the posterior cruciate ligament: a comparison of the roles of the anterolateral and posteromedial bundles, *Am J Sports Med* 42(12):2972–2978, 2014.

374. Webster KE, Hewett TE: Meta-Analysis of meta-analyses of anterior cruciate ligament injury reduction training programs, *J Orthop Res* 36(10):2696–2708, 2018.

375. Weinhandl JT, Earl-Boehm JE, Ebersole KT, et al.: Reduced hamstring strength increases anterior cruciate ligament loading during anticipated sidestep cutting, *Clin Biomech* 29(7):752–759, 2014.

376. Wellsandt E, Khandha A, Capin J, et al.: Operative and nonoperative management of anterior cruciate ligament injury: differences in gait biomechanics at 5 years, *J Orthop Res* 38(12):2675–2684, 2020.

377. Wheatley MGA, Rainbow MJ, Clouthier AL: Patellofemoral mechanics: a review of pathomechanics and research approaches, *Curr Rev Musculoskelet Med* 13(3):326–337, 2020.

378. Wheatley MGA, Thelen DG, Deluzio KJ, et al.: Knee extension moment arm variations relate to mechanical function in walking and running, *J R Soc Interface* 18(181):20210326, 2021.

379. White KK, Lee SS, Cutuk A, et al.: EMG power spectra of intercollegiate athletes and anterior cruciate ligament injury risk in females, *Med Sci Sports Exerc* 35:371–376, 2003.

380. Wild CY, Steele JR, Munro BJ: Insufficient hamstring strength compromises landing technique in adolescent girls, *Med Sci Sports Exerc* 45(3):497–505, 2013.

381. Wilk KE, Arrigo CA, Bagwell MS, et al.: Considerations with open kinetic chain knee extension exercise following ACL reconstruction, *Int J Sports Phys Ther* 16(1):282–284, 2021.

382. Wilk KE, Escamilla RF, Fleisig GS, et al.: A comparison of tibiofemoral joint forces and electromyographic activity during open and closed kinetic chain exercises, *Am J Sports Med* 24(4):518–527, 1996.

383. Williams GN, Barrance PJ, Snyder-Mackler L, et al.: Altered quadriceps control in people with anterior cruciate ligament deficiency, *Med Sci Sports Exerc* 36(7):1089–1097, 2004.

384. Willson JD, Davis IS: Lower extremity strength and mechanics during jumping in women with patellofemoral pain, *J Sport Rehabil* 18:76–90, 2009.

385. Willy RW, Hoglund LT, Barton CJ, et al.: Patellofemoral pain, *J Orthop Sports Phys Ther* 49(9):Cpg1–cpg95, 2019.

386. Wilson NA, Press JM, Koh JL, et al.: In vivo noninvasive evaluation of abnormal patellar tracking during squatting in patients with patellofemoral pain, *J Bone Joint Surg Am* 91:558–566, 2009.

387. Wilson WT, Deakin AH, Payne AP, et al.: Comparative analysis of the structural properties of the collateral ligaments of the human knee, *J Orthop Sports Phys Ther* 42(4):345–351, 2012.

388. Winkler PW, Lutz PM, Rupp MC, et al.: Increased external tibial torsion is an infratuberositary deformity and is not correlated with a lateralized position of the tibial tuberosity, *Knee Surg Sports Traumatol Arthrosc* 29(5):1678–1685, 2021.

389. Winter DA: *Biomechanics and motor control of human movement*, Hoboken, New Jersey, 2005, John Wiley & Sons.

390. Wong JS, Lalam R: Plicae: where do they come from and when are they relevant? *Semin Musculoskelet Radiol* 23(5):547–568, 2019.

391. Woo SL, Hollis JM, Adams DJ, et al.: Tensile properties of the human femur-anterior cruciate ligament-tibia complex. The effects of specimen age and orientation, *Am J Sports Med* 19:217–225, 1991.

392. Wood A, Boren M, Dodgen T, et al.: Muscular architecture of the popliteus muscle and the basic science implications, *Knee* 27(2):308–314, 2020.

393. Wood L, Ferrell WR, Baxendale RH: Pressures in normal and acutely distended human knee joints and effects on quadriceps maximal voluntary contractions, *Q J Exp Physiol* 73:305–314, 1988.

394. Worrell TW, Karst G, Adamczyk D, et al.: Influence of joint position on electromyographic and torque generation during maximal voluntary isometric contractions of the hamstrings and gluteus maximus muscles, *J Orthop Sports Phys Ther* 31(12):730–740, 2001.

395. Yapali G, Kürklü GB: Effects of the graft type used for anterior cruciate ligament reconstruction on isokinetic muscle strength and quality of life, *J Knee Surg* 35(8):2858–2861, 2022.

396. Zaffagnini S, Grassi A, Marcheggiani Muccioli GM, et al.: The anterolateral ligament does exist: an anatomic description, *Clin Sports Med* 37(1):9–19, 2018.

397. Zhao D, Banks SA, Mitchell KH, et al.: Correlation between the knee adduction torque and medial contact force for a variety of gait patterns, *J Orthop Res* 25:789–797, 2007.

398. Zimny ML, Albright DJ, Dabezies E: Mechanoreceptors in the human medial meniscus, *Acta Anat* 133:35–40, 1988.

STUDY QUESTIONS

1. As described in this chapter, the maximum-effort torques produced by the internal and external rotator muscles of the knee (when tested at 90 degrees of flexion) are of about equal magnitudes. How can this fact be justified given the disparity in the number of internal and external rotator muscles?

2. How can severe hyperextension of the knee (while in a weight-bearing position) cause injury to both the ACL and the PCL?

3. Explain why the patellofemoral joint is least mechanically stable in the last 20 to 30 degrees of knee extension.

4. Why do most persons have slightly greater active knee flexion range of motion with the hip fully flexed as compared to fully extended?

5. List muscles and ligaments capable of resisting external rotation of the knee. Why would this function be especially important from a femoral-on-tibial (weight-bearing) perspective?

6. Which of the following activities create greater compression stress (pressure) on the articular surfaces of the patellofemoral joint: (a) maintain holding a partial squat with knees flexed to 10–20 degrees or (b) holding a deeper squat with knees flexed to 60–90 degrees? Why?

7. Why do the medial collateral ligament and the medial meniscus often become traumatized by a similar mechanism of injury?

8. Describe how contraction of the quadriceps muscle could elongate (strain) the anterior cruciate ligament. How is the strain on the ligament affected by (a) the knee joint angle and (b) the magnitude of quadriceps and hamstring muscle coactivation?

9. Describe the timing and type of muscular activity of the quadriceps muscle during the early part of the stance phase of gait.

10. At about what arc of knee motion does the quadriceps muscle produce its largest internal torque? What factor(s) most likely account for this?

11. Justify (a) why the popliteus is called the "key to the knee" and (b) how the popliteus can provide both medial and lateral stability to the knee.

12. With the knee resting in complete extension, does an active, isometric "quad set" generate compression force across the patellofemoral joint? Please justify your answer.

13. Describe the type of muscle activation (i.e., eccentric, concentric, etc.) that occurs within the vastus and hamstring muscles while slowly lowering into a chair.

14. Polio affecting the L^2–L^4 spinal nerve roots would theoretically cause paralysis of what muscle group of the knee? (Hint: Consult Appendix IV, Part A.)

15. List factors that could limit full (active or passive) knee extension.

16. Referring to Figure 13.38, how does increasing forward trunk lean while landing from a jump alter the magnitude of the muscular response of the quadriceps and hamstring muscles? What are the clinical implications of this alteration?

Answers to the study questions are available in the accompanying enhanced eBook version included with the print purchase of this textbook.

Additional Video Educational Content

- Fluoroscopic Observations of Selected Arthrokinematics of the Lower Extremity

- Cadaver Dissection Showing Advanced Arthritis at the Patellofemoral Joint with Excessive Wear and Structural Changes at and Around the Joint Surfaces

ALL VIDEOS in this chapter are available in the accompanying enhanced eBook version included with the print purchase of this textbook.

Ankle and Foot

DONALD A. NEUMANN, PT, PhD, FAPTA

CHAPTER AT A GLANCE

Walking and running require the foot to be sufficiently pliable to store and recycle elastic energy and to conform to the countless spatial configurations between it and the ground. Walking and running also require the foot to be relatively rigid in order to transfer large propulsive forces through the ground. The healthy foot satisfies the seemingly paradoxical requirements of shock absorption, pliability, and strength through a complex functional and structural interaction among its joints, connective tissues, and muscles. Although not emphasized enough in this chapter, normal sensation of the foot protects the region from injury and provides the central nervous system with information needed for proprioception and to monitor the precise actions of muscle.

This chapter sets forth a firm basis for an understanding of the evaluation and treatment of several disorders that affect the ankle and foot, many of which are kinesiologically related to the movement of the entire lower extremity. Several of the kinesiologic issues addressed in this chapter are related specifically to

the process of walking and running, topics that are covered in detail in Chapters 15 and 16. Figs. 15.10 or 15.11 should be consulted as a reference to the terminology used throughout Chapter 14 to describe the different phases of the walking or gait cycle.

OSTEOLOGY

Basic Terms and Concepts

INTRODUCTION TO JOINTS AND REGIONS OF THE ANKLE AND FOOT

Fig. 14.1 presents a pictorial overview of the organization of the bones, major joints, and regions within the ankle and foot. The *ankle* includes the distal tibia and fibula and the talus. The *foot* includes all tarsal bones, metatarsals, and phalanges, which are

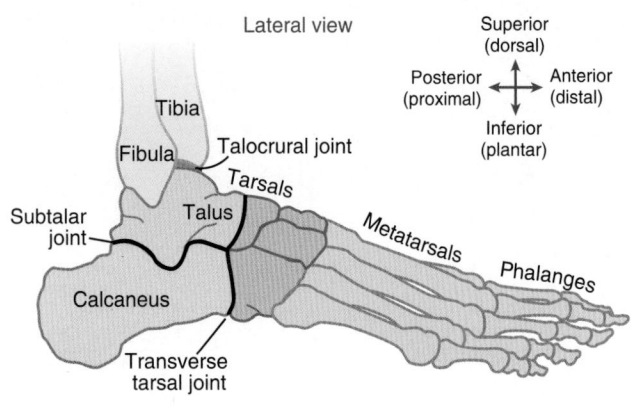

FIG. 14.1 Pictorial overview of the organization of the bones, major joints, and regions of the foot and ankle.

TABLE 14.1 **Listing of the Bones and Associated Joints within the Ankle and Foot**

	Ankle	Foot
Bones	Distal tibia Distal fibula Talus	Calcaneus and talus* (rearfoot) Navicular, cuboid, and cuneiforms (midfoot) Metatarsals and phalanges (forefoot)
Associated Joints	Talocrural Proximal tibiofibular Distal tibiofibular	Subtalar Transverse tarsal Distal intertarsal Tarsometatarsal Intermetatarsal Metatarsophalangeal Interphalangeal (proximal and distal)

*Talus is included as a bone of the ankle and of the foot.

further divided into three regions: the *rearfoot* contains the talus and calcaneus; the *midfoot* contains the navicular, cuboid, and three cuneiforms; and the *forefoot* contains the metatarsals and phalanges. Table 14.1 lists the bones and their associated joints within the ankle and foot.

The terms *anterior* and *posterior* have their conventional meanings with reference to the tibia and fibula (i.e., the leg). When describing the ankle and foot, however, these terms are often used interchangeably with *distal* and *proximal*, respectively. The terms *dorsal* and *plantar* describe the superior (top) and inferior aspects of the foot, respectively.

OSTEOLOGIC SIMILARITIES BETWEEN THE DISTAL LEG AND THE DISTAL ARM

The ankle and foot have several features that are structurally like the wrist and hand. The radius in the forearm and the tibia in the leg are both principal weight-bearing bones, each articulating with a set

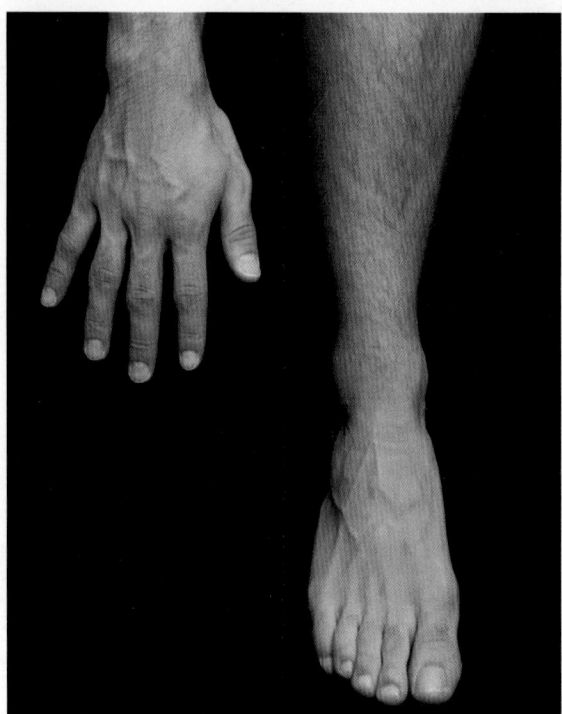

FIG. 14.2 Topographic similarities between a pronated forearm and the ankle and foot. Note that the thumb and great toe are both located on the medial side of their respective extremity.

of small bones—the carpus and tarsus, respectively. Also, the general anatomic plan of the metatarsus and metacarpus, as well as the more distal phalanges, is remarkably similar. A notable exception is that the first (great) toe in the foot is not as functionally developed as the thumb in the hand.

As described in Chapter 12, the long bones of the lower extremity progressively rotate internally (or medially) during embryologic development. As a result, the great toe is positioned on the medial side of the foot, and the top of the foot is actually its dorsal surface. This orientation is similar to that of the hand when the forearm is fully pronated (Fig. 14.2). This plantigrade position of the foot is necessary for walking and standing. With the forearm held pronated, flexion and extension of the wrist are similar to plantar flexion and dorsiflexion of the ankle, respectively.

Individual Bones

FIBULA

The long and thin fibula is located lateral and parallel to the tibia (Figs. 14.3). The fibular *head* can be palpated just lateral to the lateral condyle of the tibia. While standing, the slender shaft of the fibula transfers only about 6% to 17% of body weight through the leg; the remaining weight is transferred through the thicker tibia.[102] The shaft of the fibula continues distally to form the easily palpable *lateral malleolus* (from the Latin root *malleus*, hammer). The lateral malleolus functions as a pulley for the tendons of the fibularis (peroneus) longus and brevis. On the medial surface of the lateral malleolus is a prominent *articular facet for the talus* (see ahead Fig. 14.11).

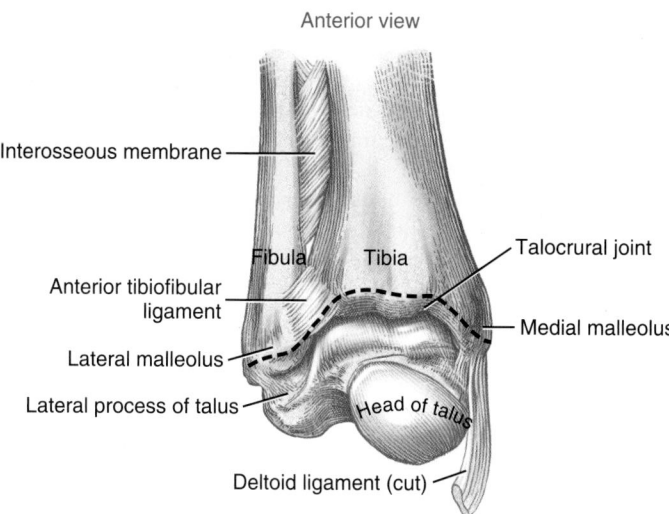

Anterior view

Interosseous membrane

Fibula   Tibia

Talocrural joint

Anterior tibiofibular ligament

Medial malleolus

Lateral malleolus

Lateral process of talus

Head of talus

Deltoid ligament (cut)

FIG. 14.3 An anterior view of the distal end of the right tibia and fibula and the talus. The articulation of the three bones forms the talocrural (ankle) joint. The dashed line shows the proximal attachment of the capsule of the ankle joint.

In the articulated ankle, this facet forms part of the talocrural joint (Fig. 14.3).

DISTAL TIBIA

The distal end of the tibia broadens to allow greater contact area for transferring loads across the ankle. On its medial side is the prominent *medial malleolus*. On the lateral surface of the medial malleolus is the *articular facet for the talus* (see ahead Fig. 14.11). In the articulated ankle, this facet forms a small part of the talocrural joint. On the lateral side of the distal tibia is the triangular and slightly concave *fibular notch* (with its triangular base oriented distally). The fibular notch (often called the *incisura fibularis*) accepts the distal end of the fibula at the distal tibiofibular joint (Fig. 14.11).

In the adult, the distal end of the tibia is twisted externally around its long axis approximately 30 degrees relative to its proximal end.[271] This natural torsion is evident by the slight externally rotated position of the foot during standing. This twist of the lower leg is referred to as *external (lateral) tibial torsion*, based on the orientation of the bone's distal end relative to its proximal end.

Osteologic Features of the Fibula and Distal Tibia
FIBULA
- Head
- Lateral malleolus
- Articular facet (for the talus)

DISTAL TIBIA
- Medial malleolus
- Articular facet (for the talus)
- Fibular notch

TARSAL BONES

The seven tarsal bones are shown in four different perspectives in Figs. 14.4 through 14.8.

Osteologic Features of the Tarsal Bones
TALUS
- Body, neck, and head
- Trochlear surface (dome)
- Lateral process
- Tibial and fibular facets
- Anterior, middle, and posterior facets
- Talar sulcus
- Lateral and medial tubercles

CALCANEUS
- Tuberosity
- Lateral and medial processes
- Anterior, middle, and posterior facets
- Calcaneal sulcus
- Sustentaculum tali

NAVICULAR
- Proximal articular surface
- Tuberosity

MEDIAL, INTERMEDIATE, AND LATERAL CUNEIFORMS
- Transverse arch

CUBOID
- Groove (for the tendon of the fibularis longus)

Talus

The dominant features of the talus include its *body, neck,* and *head,* all evident from a superior view (Fig. 14.4). The prominent head of the talus projects forward and slightly medially toward the navicular (Fig. 14.3). In the adult, the long axis of the neck of the talus positions the head of this bone about 30 degrees medial to the sagittal plane. In small children, the head is projected medially about 40 to 50 degrees, partially accounting for the often-inverted appearance of their feet. The body's dorsal or *trochlear surface* is a rounded dome: convex anterior-posteriorly and slightly concave medial-laterally. The body's lateral surface has a dominant *lateral process*, which widens the bone considerably. A continuous layer of articular cartilage covers the bone's trochlear surface and adjacent *tibial* and *fibular facets*, providing smooth articular surfaces for the malleoli within the talocrural joint (Figs. 14.6 and 14.7).

Fig. 14.8 shows three articular facets on the plantar (inferior) surface of the talus. The flat *anterior* and *middle facets* are often continuous and may blend with the adjacent articular cartilage on the head of the talus.[122] The oval, concave *posterior facet* is the largest facet. As a set, the three facets articulate with the three facets on the dorsal (superior) surface of the calcaneus, forming the subtalar joint. The *talar sulcus* is an obliquely running groove between the anterior-middle and posterior facets.

Lateral and *medial tubercles* are located on the posterior-medial surface of the talus (Fig. 14.4). A groove formed between these tubercles serves as a pulley for the tendon of the flexor hallucis longus (see ahead Fig. 14.12).

Calcaneus

The calcaneus, the largest of the tarsal bones, is well suited to accept the impact of heel strike during walking. The large and rough *calcaneal tuberosity* receives the attachment of the Achilles tendon. The plantar surface of the tuberosity has *lateral* and *medial processes* that serve as attachments for many of the intrinsic muscles and the deep plantar fascia of the foot (Fig. 14.5).

The calcaneus articulates with other tarsal bones on its anterior and dorsal surfaces. The relatively small, curved anterior surface of the calcaneus joins the cuboid at the calcaneocuboid joint (Fig. 14.7).

The more extensive dorsal surface contains three facets that join the matching facets on the talus (Fig. 14.8). The *anterior* and *middle facets* are relatively small and nearly flat. The *posterior facet* is large and convex, conforming to the concave shape of the equally large posterior facet on the talus. Between the posterior and middle facets is a wide oblique groove called the *calcaneal sulcus*. Located within this sulcus are the attachments of strong ligaments that bind the subtalar joint. With the subtalar joint articulated, the sulci of the calcaneus and talus form the *tarsal sinus* within the

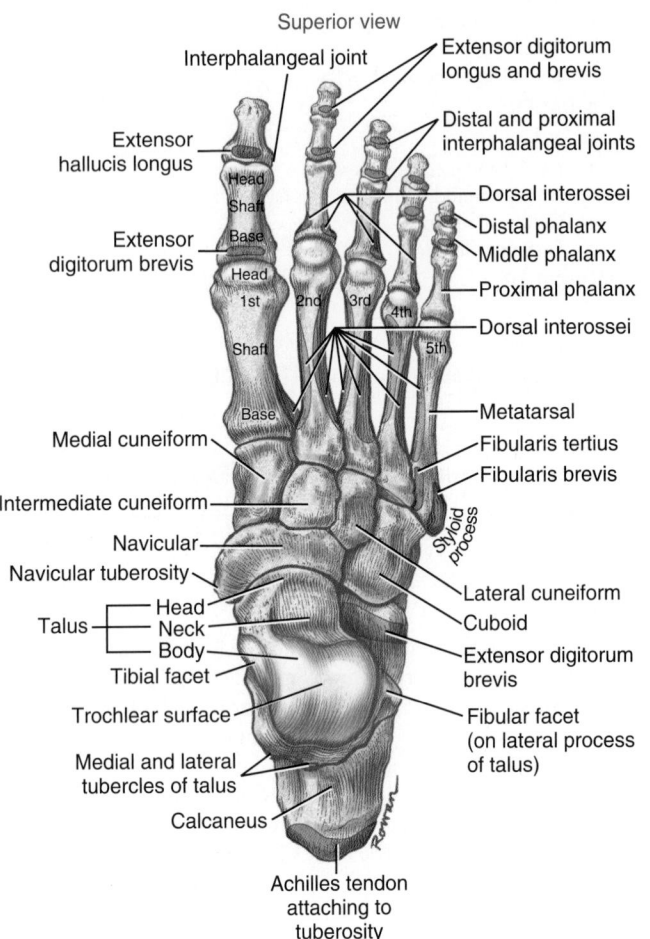

FIG. 14.4 A superior (dorsal) view of the bones of the right foot. Proximal attachments of muscles are indicated in red, distal attachments in gray.

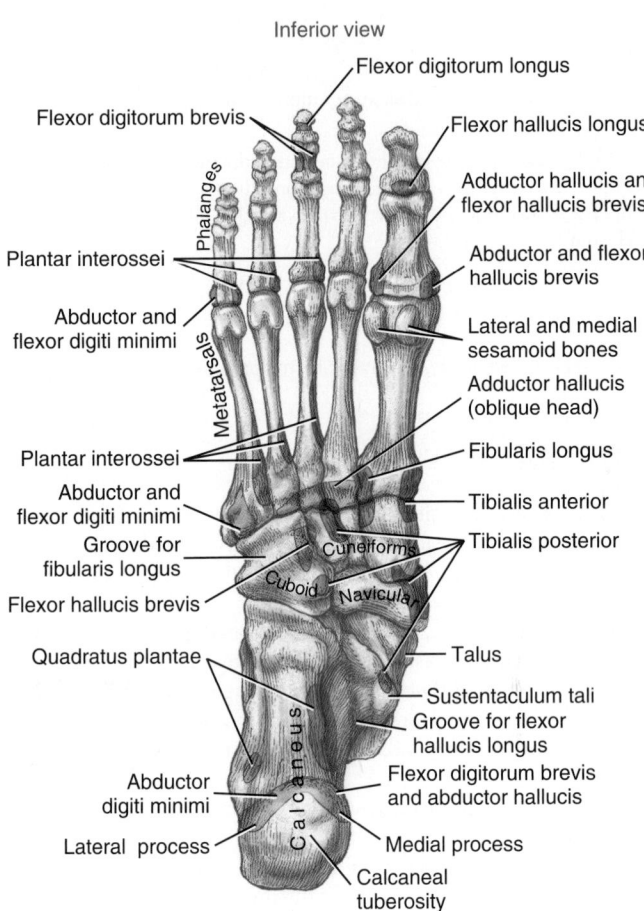

FIG. 14.5 An inferior (plantar) view of the bones of the right foot. Proximal attachments of muscles are indicated in red, distal attachments in gray.

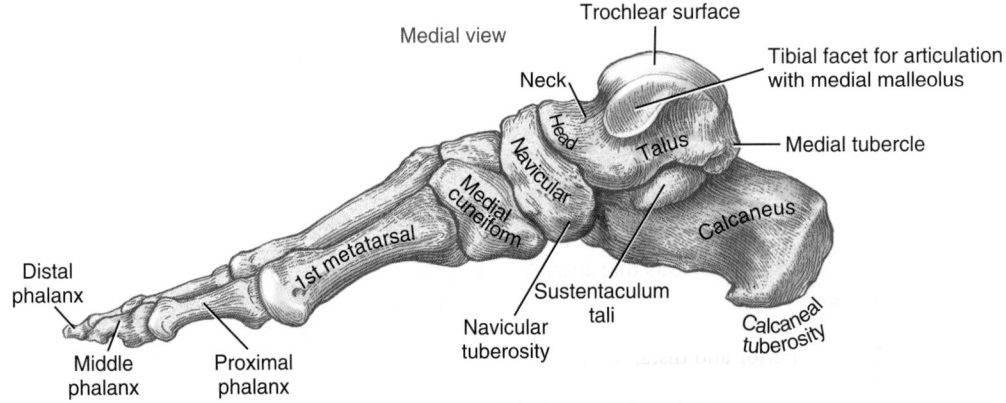

FIG. 14.6 A medial view of the bones of the right foot.

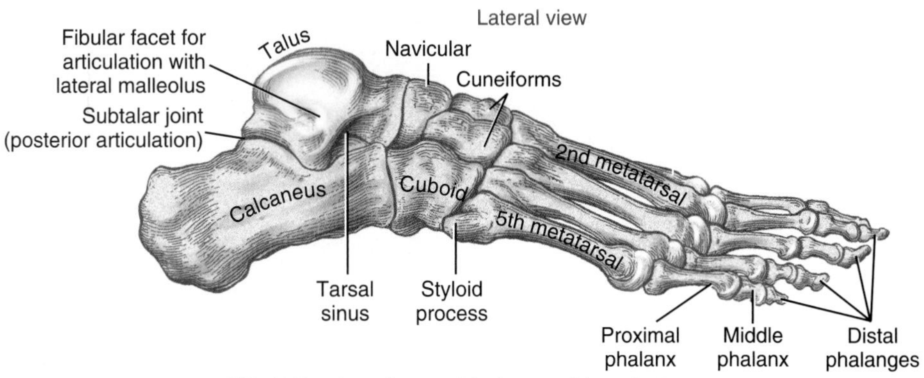

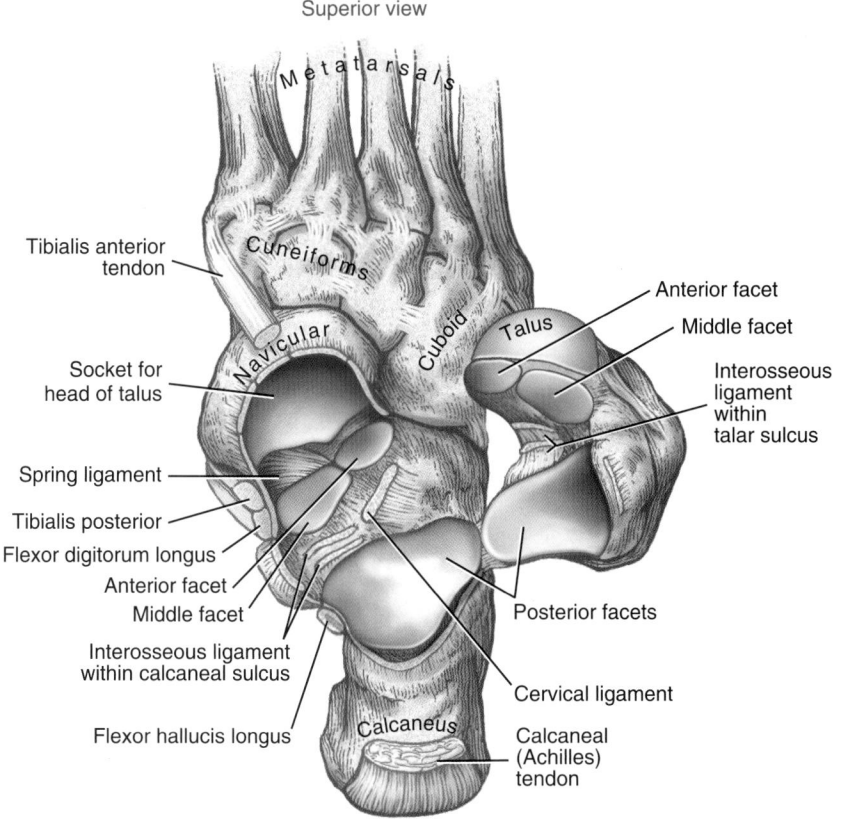

FIG. 14.7 A lateral view of the bones of the right foot.

FIG. 14.8 A superior view of the talus flipped laterally to reveal its plantar surface as well as the dorsal surface of the calcaneus. With the talus reflected, it is possible to observe the three articular facets on the talus and on the calcaneus. Note also the deep, continuous concavity formed by the proximal side of the navicular and the spring ligament. This concavity accepts the head of the talus, forming the talonavicular joint. (The interosseous and cervical ligaments and multiple tendons have been cut.)

subtalar joint. The lateral opening of the tarsal sinus is evident in Fig. 14.7.

The *sustentaculum tali* projects medially as a horizontal shelf from the dorsal surface of the calcaneus (Fig. 14.6). The sustentaculum tali lies under and supports the middle facet of the talus. (Sustentaculum tali literally means a "shelf for the talus.")

Navicular

The navicular is named for its resemblance to a ship (i.e., referring to "navy"). Its *proximal* (concave) *articular surface* accepts the head of the talus at the talonavicular joint (Fig. 14.4). The distal surface of the navicular bone contains three relatively flat facets that articulate with the three cuneiform bones.

The medial surface of the navicular has a prominent *tuberosity*, palpable in the adult at about 2.5 cm inferior and distal (anterior) to the tip of the medial malleolus (Fig. 14.6). This tuberosity serves as one of several distal attachments of the tibialis posterior muscle.

A small, accessory navicular bone (os naviculare) may be present in about 20% to 30% of feet, typically located near the navicular tuberosity, often within the tendon of the tibialis posterior.[138]

Medial, Intermediate, and Lateral Cuneiforms

The cuneiform bones (from the Latin root meaning "wedge") act as a spacer between the navicular and bases of the three medial metatarsal bones (Fig. 14.4). The cuneiforms contribute to the *transverse arch* of the foot, accounting, in part, for the transverse convexity of the dorsal aspect of the midfoot.

Cuboid

As its name indicates, the cuboid has six surfaces, three of which articulate with adjacent tarsal bones (Figs. 14.4, 14.5, and 14.7). The distal surface articulates with the bases of both the fourth and the fifth metatarsals. The cuboid is therefore homologous to the hamate bone in the wrist.

The entire, curved proximal surface of the cuboid articulates with the calcaneus (Fig. 14.4). The medial surface has an oval facet for articulation with the lateral cuneiform and a small facet for articulation with the navicular. A distinct *groove* runs across the plantar surface of the cuboid, occupied by the tendon of the fibularis longus muscle (Fig. 14.5).

RAYS OF THE FOOT

A *ray* of the forefoot is functionally defined as one metatarsal and its associated set of phalanges.

Metatarsals

The five metatarsal bones link the distal row of tarsal bones with the proximal phalanges (see Fig. 14.4). Metatarsals are numbered 1 through 5, starting on the medial side. The first metatarsal is the shortest and thickest, and the second is usually the longest. The second and usually the third metatarsals are the most rigidly attached to the distal row of tarsal bones. These morphologic characteristics generally reflect the larger forces that pass through this region of the forefoot during the push off phase of gait. Each metatarsal has a *base* at its proximal end, a *shaft*, and a convex *head* at its distal end (Fig. 14.4, first metatarsal). The bases of the metatarsals have small *articular facets* that mark the site of articulation with the bases of the adjacent metatarsals.

Longitudinally, the shafts of the metatarsals are slightly concave on their plantar side (Fig. 14.6). This arched shape of the metatarsals enhances their load-supporting ability and provides additional space for muscles and tendons. The plantar surface of the first metatarsal head has two small facets for articulation with two *sesamoid bones* that are imbedded within the tendon of the flexor hallucis brevis (Fig. 14.5). The fifth metatarsal has a prominent *styloid process* just lateral to its base, marking the attachment of the fibularis brevis muscle (Fig. 14.7).

Osteologic Features of a Metatarsal

- Base (with articular facets for articulation with the bases of adjacent metatarsals)
- Shaft
- Head
- Styloid process (on the fifth metatarsal only)

Phalanges

As in the hand, the foot has 14 phalanges. Each of the four lateral toes contains a proximal, middle, and distal phalanx (see Fig. 14.4). The first toe—more commonly called the *great toe* or *hallux*—has two phalanges, designated as proximal and distal. In general, each phalanx has a concave *base* at its proximal end, a *shaft,* and a convex *head* at its distal end.

Osteologic Features of a Phalanx

- Base
- Shaft
- Head

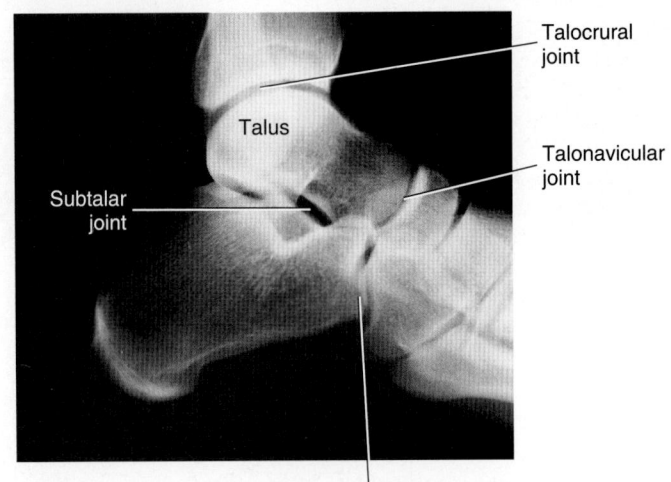

FIG. 14.9 A radiograph from a healthy person showing the major joints of the ankle and foot: talocrural, subtalar, talonavicular, and calcaneocuboid. The talonavicular and calcaneocuboid joints are part of the larger transverse tarsal joint. Note the central location of the talus.

ARTHROLOGY

Depending on the chosen nomenclature, one could argue that up to 14 joints or joint complexes are structurally or functionally associated with the ankle and foot. Although all the joints contribute to the kinesiologic function of the region, this chapter spends considerable attention to the interaction of three major joints: *talocrural, subtalar, and transverse tarsal* (Fig. 14.9). As will be described, the talus is mechanically integrated with all three of these joints. The multiple articulations made by the talus help explain the bone's complex shape, with nearly 70% of its surface covered with articular cartilage. *An understanding of the shape of the talus is crucial to understanding much of the kinesiology of the ankle and foot.*

Terminology Used to Describe Movements

The terminology used to describe movements of the ankle and foot incorporates two sets of definitions: a fundamental set and an applied set. The *fundamental terminology* defines movement of the foot or ankle as occurring at right angles to the three standard axes of rotation (Fig. 14.10A). *Dorsiflexion* (extension) and *plantar flexion* describe motion that is parallel to the sagittal plane, around a medial-lateral axis of rotation. *Eversion and inversion* describe motion that is parallel to the frontal plane, around an anterior-posterior axis of rotation. *Abduction and adduction* describe motion that is parallel to the horizontal (transverse) plane, around a vertical (superior-inferior) axis of rotation. For at least the three major joints of the ankle and foot, these fundamental definitions are inadequate because most movements at these joints occur about an *oblique axis* rather than about the three standard orthogonal axes of rotation depicted in Fig. 14.10A.

A second and more *applied terminology* has therefore evolved in the attempt to define the movements that occur perpendicular to the prevailing oblique axes of rotation at the ankle and foot (Fig. 14.10B). *Pronation* is defined as a motion that has elements of eversion, abduction, and dorsiflexion. *Supination*, in contrast, is defined as a motion that has elements of inversion, adduction, and plantar flexion. The orientation of the oblique axis of rotation depicted in Fig. 14.10B varies across the major joints but, in general, has a pitch that is roughly similar to that illustrated. The exact pitch of each major joint's axis of rotation is described in subsequent sections.

Pronation and supination motions have been called "triplanar" motions. Unfortunately, this description is misleading. The term *triplanar* implies only that the movements "cut through" each of the three cardinal planes, not that the joint exhibiting this movement possesses three degrees of freedom. *Pronation and supination share a given plane.* Table 14.2 summarizes the terminology used to describe the movements of the ankle and foot, including the terminology that describes abnormal posture or deformity.

Structure and Function of the Joints Associated with the Ankle

From an anatomic perspective, the ankle includes one functional articulation: *the talocrural joint.* An important structural component of this joint is the articulation formed between the tibia and fibula—an articulation reinforced by the *proximal* and *distal tibiofibular joints* and the *interosseous membrane* of the leg (see Fig. 13.3). Because of this structural association, the proximal and distal tibiofibular joints are described before proceeding to the talocrural joint.

PROXIMAL TIBIOFIBULAR JOINT

The proximal tibiofibular joint is a synovial joint formed between the head of the fibula and the posterior-lateral aspect of the lateral condyle of the tibia (see Fig. 13.4). The surfaces of the joint are covered with articular cartilage and vary in shape between being flat to slightly oval.[233] The joint is reinforced primarily by anterior

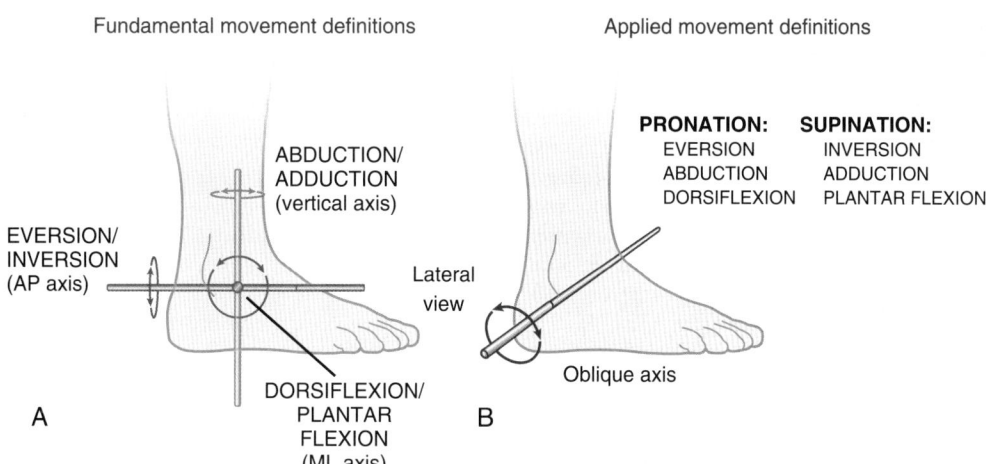

FIG. 14.10 (A) *Fundamental movement definitions* are based on the movement of any part of the ankle or foot in a plane perpendicular to the three standard axes of rotation: vertical, anterior-posterior *(AP)*, and medial-lateral *(ML)*. (B) *Applied movement definitions* are based on the movements that occur at right angles to one of several oblique axes of rotation within the foot and ankle. The two main movements are defined as either pronation or supination.

TABLE 14.2 Terms That Describe Movements and Deformities of the Ankle and Foot

Motion	Axis of Rotation	Plane of Motion	Example of Fixed Deformity or Abnormal Posture
Plantar flexion / Dorsiflexion	Medial-lateral	Sagittal	Pes equinus / Pes calcaneus
Inversion / Eversion	Anterior-posterior	Frontal	Varus / Valgus
Abduction / Adduction	Vertical	Horizontal	Abductus / Adductus
Supination	Oblique (varies by joint)	Varying elements of inversion, adduction, and plantar flexion	Inconsistent terminology—usually implies one or more of the components of supination
Pronation		Varying elements of eversion, abduction, and dorsiflexion	Inconsistent terminology—usually implies one or more of the components of pronation

and posterior ligaments.[3] When subjected to forces equivalent to those experienced while walking, 1 to 3 mm of anterior and posterior fibular translations have been measured at the proximal tibiofibular joint in cadaver specimens.[218] Stability is needed at the joint to ensure that muscular and ligamentous forces applied to the fibula are transferred effectively to the tibia. Although relatively rare, dislocations of the proximal tibiofibular joint may occur most often in an anterior-lateral direction.[3]

DISTAL TIBIOFIBULAR JOINT

The distal tibiofibular joint is formed by the junction of the concave, triangular *fibular notch of the tibia* and the corresponding flat-to-convex triangular-shaped region of the medial surface of the distal fibula. Fig. 14.11 shows the joint opened anteriorly to display the surface morphology and cut remains of the pyramidal-shaped interosseous (tibiofibular) ligament.[96,268] The distal tibiofibular joint is often referred to as the tibiofibular *syndesmosis*, which is a type of synarthrodial joint that allows limited movement and partially bound by fibrous connective tissue. As will be described, the design for stability at the tibiofibular syndesmosis is necessary to secure the shape and therefore congruity of the talocrural (ankle) joint.

The primary stabilizers of the distal tibiofibular joint are the relatively thick *anterior* and *posterior (distal) tibiofibular ligaments* (Figs. 14.11 and 14.12).[223] Secondary stability is provided through the *interosseous ligament*, which is a thickened but usually separate extension of the interosseous membrane of the leg.[96,271] The interosseous ligament of the distal tibiofibular joint is a mix of collagen fibers and fat, filling most of the articulation. The fatty-fibrous consistency of the ligament usually limits direct bony contact within the joint, with the frequent exception of a small area near the anterior base (bottom) of the joint, just posterior to the anterior tibiofibular ligament (and therefore obscured from view in Fig. 14.11).[14,96,271] When present, this area of direct contact is between 3 and 9 mm in length and 2 and 5 mm in height and is covered by a thin layer of articular cartilage, flanked by a strip of fat and synovial plica.[14,96]

When the ankle region is subjected to physiologic loading, slight fibular movements occur at the distal tibiofibular joint. Although studies vary, most report fibular motions from 0.5 to 3

mm of translation and 2 to 5 degrees of rotation.[102,261] These micro-kinematics will be further described in the upcoming section on the talocrural joint.

TALOCRURAL JOINT

Articular Structure

The talocrural joint, or ankle, is the articulation of the trochlear surface (dome) and sides of the talus with the rectangular cavity formed by the distal end of the tibia and both malleoli (see Figs. 14.3 and 14.9). The talocrural joint is often referred to as the "mortise" because of its resemblance to the wood joint used by carpenters (Fig. 14.13). The concave shape of the tibiofibular side of the mortise is maintained by ligaments that bind the distal tibiofibular joint. The confining shape of the talocrural joint provides a major source of stability to the ankle.[262]

The structure of the mortise must be sufficiently strong to accept the forces that pass between the leg and foot. Roughly 80% to 90% of the compressive force that crosses the ankle passes through the central dome of the talus and the tibia;[29] most of the remaining force passes through the lateral aspect of the talus and the fibula. The talocrural joint is lined with about 3 mm of articular cartilage, which can be compressed by 30% to 40% in response to peak physiologic loads.[260] This load-absorption mechanism protects the intra-articular subchondral bone from damaging stress.

Ligaments

The *articular capsule* of the talocrural joint is reinforced by collateral ligaments that help maintain the stability and alignment between the talus and the rectangular "socket" of the mortise. In addition to adding structural strength to the mortise, ligaments possess mechanoreceptors (primarily *free nerve* and *Ruffini endings*) that ultimately enhance the ability of muscles to subconsciously stabilize the region.[202]

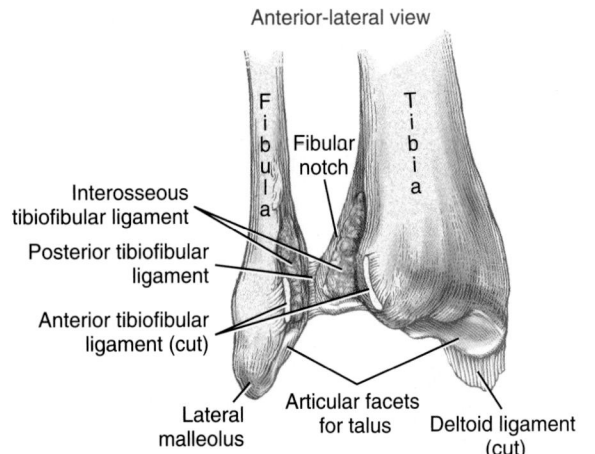

Anterior-lateral view

FIG. 14.11 An anterior view of the right distal tibiofibular joint with the fibula reflected to show the articular surfaces. To open the joint, the anterior (distal) tibiofibular and interosseous (tibiofibular) ligaments were cut. The fatty interosseous ligament was shaved close to bone to better expose the triangular articular surfaces.

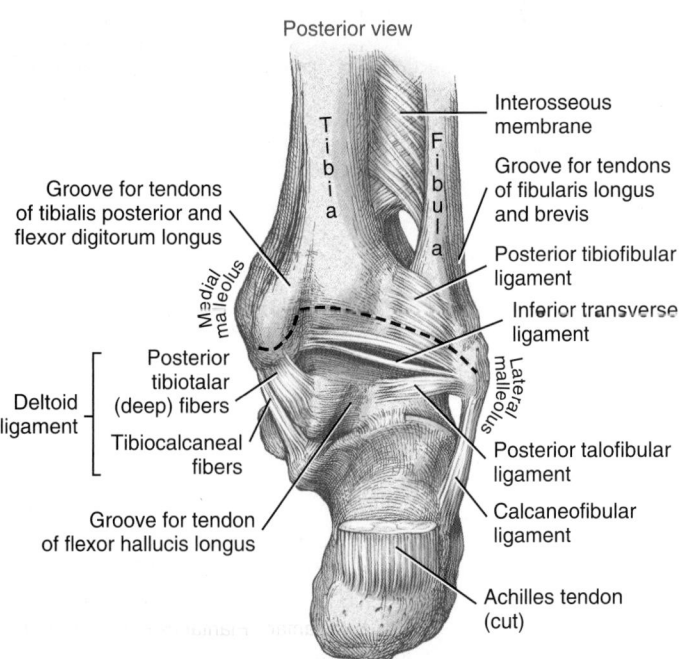

Posterior view

FIG. 14.12 Posterior view of the right ankle region shows several ligaments of the distal tibiofibular, talocrural, and subtalar joints. The dashed line indicates the proximal attachments of the capsule of the talocrural (ankle) joint.

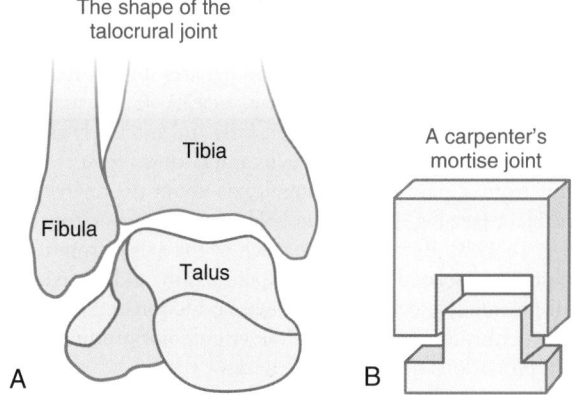

FIG. 14.13 The similarity in shape of the talocrural joint (A) and a carpenter's mortise joint (B) is demonstrated. Note the extensive area of the talus that is lined with articular cartilage (*blue*).

The medial collateral ligament of the talocrural joint is often referred to as the *deltoid ligament*, named based on its triangular shape. The apex of this ligament attaches along the distal medial malleolus, with its base thickening and expanding to include a *superficial set* of four bands of fibers.[30] The distal attachments of the superficial fibers are highlighted in Fig. 14.14 and listed in the box to the right. Although obscured from view in Fig. 14.14, a shorter and more vertical *deep set* of anterior and posterior tibiotalar fibers attach between the medial malleolus and medial side of the talus, immediately inferior to the talocrural joint line. The deep posterior tibiotalar fibers are the largest and thickest fibers of the entire deltoid ligament (Fig. 14.12).[30]

The primary function of the deltoid ligament is to reinforce the medial side of the ankle. Taken as a group, the ligament's fibers are oriented to limit the extremes of eversion across the talocrural, subtalar, and talonavicular joints. Fibers also provide multidirectional rotatory stability to the mortise, a function shared by the lateral collateral ligaments and ligaments that stabilize the distal tibiofibular joint.[30,262] Isolated injury to the deltoid ligament is rare; typically it is associated with trauma to other structures, including the distal tibiofibular joint syndesmosis, lateral collateral ligaments, spring ligament (formally described ahead), and fracture or bruising of the distal fibula or tibia.[112,211] This cluster of associated injuries may be

severe, frequently occurring when landing awkwardly from a jump or from extreme twisting of the loaded lower limb, often when combining the extremes of eversion and abduction (external rotation) of the ankle. (The literature often uses the terms *abduction* and *external rotation* of the ankle interchangeably. While weight-bearing over the foot, excessive abduction of the ankle occurs by way of excessive *internal* rotation of the lower leg relative to the fixed talus.)

The *lateral collateral ligaments* of the ankle include the anterior and posterior talofibular and the calcaneofibular ligaments. After sharing a common origin from the lateral malleolus, each ligament courses in different directions toward its distal attachment (Fig. 14.15).[50] The mechanics of the typical "sprained ankle" usually involve a component of excessive *inversion*. Not surprisingly therefore, about 80% of all ankle sprains are associated with injury to one or more of the lateral collateral ligaments.[113,265]

The *anterior talofibular ligament* attaches to the anterior and medial aspects of the lateral malleolus, then courses anteriorly and medially to the neck of the talus (see Fig. 14.15). This ligament is the most frequently injured of the lateral ligaments.[76] Injury is typically caused by excessive inversion or by horizontal plane adduction (internal rotation) of the ankle, often combined with excessive

> **Distal Attachments of the Fibers Comprising the Deltoid Ligament**
> **SUPERFICIAL SET**
> Tibionavicular fibers attach to the navicular, above its tuberosity just distal to the talonavicular joint line.
> Tibiospring fibers blend with the plantar calcaneonavicular ("spring") ligament.
> Tibiocalcaneal fibers attach to the sustentaculum tali of the calcaneus.
> Tibiotalar fibers attach anterior to the medial tubercle of the talus.
> **DEEP SET**
> Anterior and posterior tibiotalar fibers attach along much of the medial surface of the talus, close to and along the talocrural joint line.

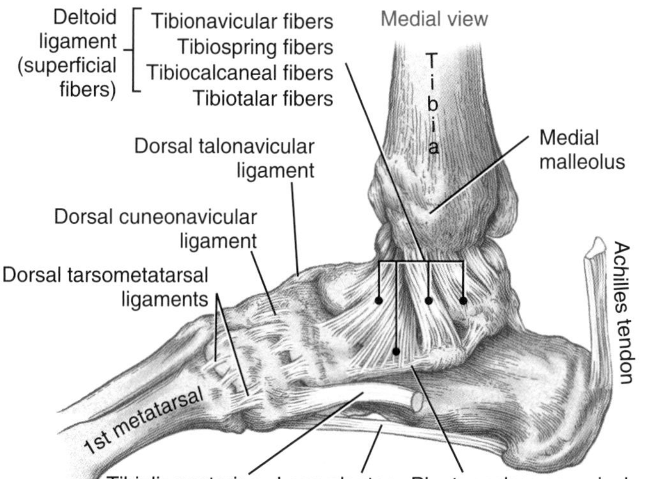

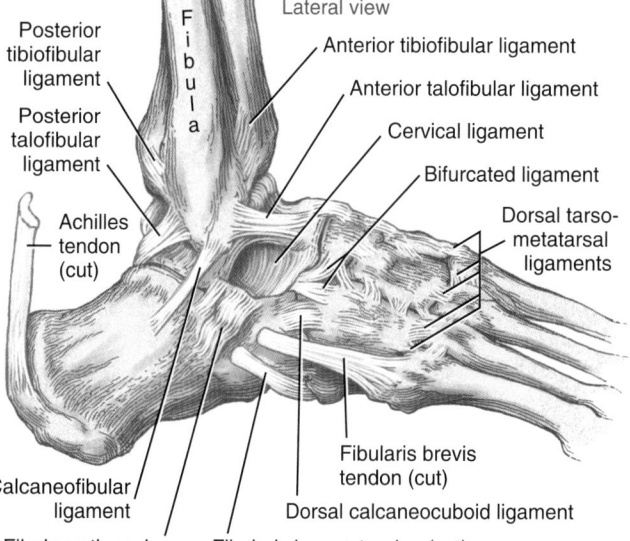

FIG. 14.14 Medial view of the right ankle region highlights the deltoid (medial collateral) ligament. The distal attachment points of the four sets of superficial fibers are indicated by black dots.

FIG. 14.15 Lateral view of the right ankle region highlights the lateral collateral ligaments.

plantar flexion—for example, when inadvertently stepping into a hole or onto someone's foot while landing from a jump. The *calcaneofibular ligament* courses inferiorly and posteriorly from the distal and medial aspects of the lateral malleolus to the lateral surface of the calcaneus (see Fig. 14.15). This ligament primarily resists inversion across the talocrural joint (especially when fully dorsiflexed) and the subtalar joint. As a pair, the calcaneofibular and anterior talofibular ligaments provide resistance to inversion throughout most of the range of ankle dorsiflexion and plantar flexion. Although the calcaneofibular ligament is considerably stronger than the anterior talofibular ligament, both are involved in about two-thirds of all lateral ankle ligament injuries.[107]

> **Three Major Components of the Lateral Collateral Ligaments of the Ankle**
> - Anterior talofibular ligament
> - Calcaneofibular ligament
> - Posterior talofibular ligament

The *posterior talofibular ligament* originates on the posterior and medial aspects of the lateral malleolus and attaches to the lateral tubercle of the talus (review Figs. 14.12 and 14.15). Its fibers run nearly horizontally across the posterior side of the talocrural joint, in an oblique anterior-lateral to posterior-medial direction (Fig. 14.16). The primary function of the posterior talofibular ligament is to provide horizontal plane stability within the mortise. In particular, the ligament limits excessive abduction (external rotation) of the talus, especially when the ankle is fully dorsiflexed.[40,82]

The *inferior transverse ligament* is a small thick strand of fibers considered part of the posterior talofibular ligament (see Fig. 14.12). The fibers attach medially to the posterior aspect of the medial malleolus, forming part of the posterior wall of the talocrural joint.

In summary, the medial and lateral collateral ligaments of the ankle primarily limit excessive eversion and inversion of the ankle, respectively. Furthermore, because most of the ligaments course obliquely in varying anterior or posterior directions, most also limit the extremes of anterior or posterior translations of the talus within the mortise.[82,262] As described in the section on arthrokinematics, the movements of plantar flexion and dorsiflexion are kinematically linked to anterior and posterior translation of the talus, respectively. For these reasons, several of the collateral ligaments are stretched at the extremes of dorsiflexion or plantar flexion of the talocrural joint.

As described, many of the ligaments that cross the talocrural joint also cross other joints of the foot, such as the subtalar and talonavicular joints. These ligaments therefore provide stability across multiple joints. Table 14.3 provides a summary of selected movements that stretch the major ligaments of the ankle. This information helps explain several aspects of clinical practice, including the mechanisms by which ligaments are injured, the reasoning for how certain stress tests can assess the integrity of ligaments, and the rationale behind some forms of manual therapy performed to increase the extent of movement.

This section described the anatomy, function, and primary mechanism of acute injury of the ligaments at the talocrural joint. Mechanisms associated with repeated or chronic ligament injury are described in Clinical Connection 14.2.

Osteokinematics

The talocrural joint possesses one degree of freedom. Although more complex biomechanical descriptions have been published,[228] this chapter assumes that rotation at the talocrural joint occurs around an axis of rotation that passes through the body of the talus and through the tips of both malleoli. Because the lateral malleolus is inferior and posterior to the medial malleolus (which can be verified by palpation), the axis of rotation departs slightly from a pure medial-lateral axis. As depicted in Fig. 14.17A–C, the axis of rotation (in red) is inclined slightly superiorly and anteriorly as it passes laterally to medially through the talus and both malleoli.[153] The axis deviates from a pure medial-lateral axis about 10 degrees in the frontal plane (see Fig. 14.17A) and 6 degrees in the horizontal plane (see Fig. 14.17B). Because of the pitch of the axis of rotation, dorsiflexion is associated with slight abduction and eversion, and plantar flexion is associated with slight adduction and inversion.[224] By strict definition, therefore, the talocrural joint produces a movement of pronation and supination. Because the axis of rotation deviates only minimally from the pure medial-lateral axis, the main components of pronation and supination at the talocrural joint are *overwhelmingly dorsiflexion and plantar flexion* (Fig. 14.17D–E).[146,227] The horizontal and frontal plane components of pronation and supination are indeed small and ignored in most clinical situations.

The 0-degree (neutral) position at the talocrural joint is defined by the foot held at 90 degrees to the leg. From this position, the talocrural joint permits about 15 to 30 degrees of dorsiflexion and 40 to 60 degrees of plantar flexion; about a 2:1 ratio in favor of plantar flexion.[23,87,161,224] Studies have shown that joints located distal to the talocrural joint can contribute 8% to 30% of the total reported "ankle" motion.[215,229]

Finally, the kinematics of dorsiflexion and plantar flexion at the talocrural joint need to be visualized when the foot is free to move, and, as shown in Video 14.1, when the foot is held relatively fixed, such as during the stance phase of walking.

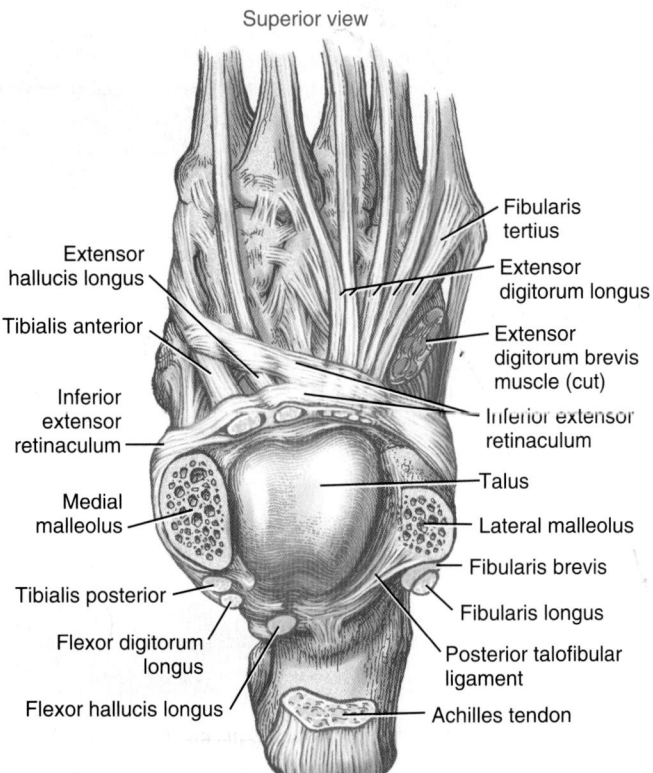

Superior view

Fibularis tertius

Extensor hallucis longus

Tibialis anterior

Inferior extensor retinaculum

Medial malleolus

Tibialis posterior

Flexor digitorum longus

Flexor hallucis longus

Extensor digitorum longus

Extensor digitorum brevis muscle (cut)

Inferior extensor retinaculum

Talus

Lateral malleolus

Fibularis brevis

Fibularis longus

Posterior talofibular ligament

Achilles tendon

FIG. 14.16 A superior view displays a cross-section through the right talocrural joint. The talus remains intact, but the lateral and medial malleolus and all the tendons are cut.

TABLE 14.3 **Selected Full Movements That Stretch the Ligaments of the Ankle***

Ligaments	Crossed Joints	Selected Full Movements That Stretch Ligaments
Deltoid ligament (tibiotalar fibers)	Talocrural joint	Eversion, dorsiflexion with associated posterior slide of talus within the mortise (posterior fibers)
Deltoid ligament (tibionavicular fibers)	Talocrural joint	Eversion, abduction, plantar flexion with associated anterior slide of talus within the mortise
	Talonavicular joint	Eversion, abduction
Deltoid ligament (tibiocalcaneal fibers)	Talocrural joint and subtalar joint	Eversion
Anterior talofibular ligament	Talocrural joint	Inversion, adduction, plantar flexion with associated anterior slide of talus within the mortise
Calcaneofibular ligament	Talocrural joint	Inversion, dorsiflexion with associated posterior slide of talus within the mortise
	Subtalar joint	Inversion
Posterior talofibular ligament	Talocrural joint	Abduction, inversion, dorsiflexion with associated posterior slide of talus within the mortise

*The information is based on movements of the unloaded foot relative to a stationary leg.

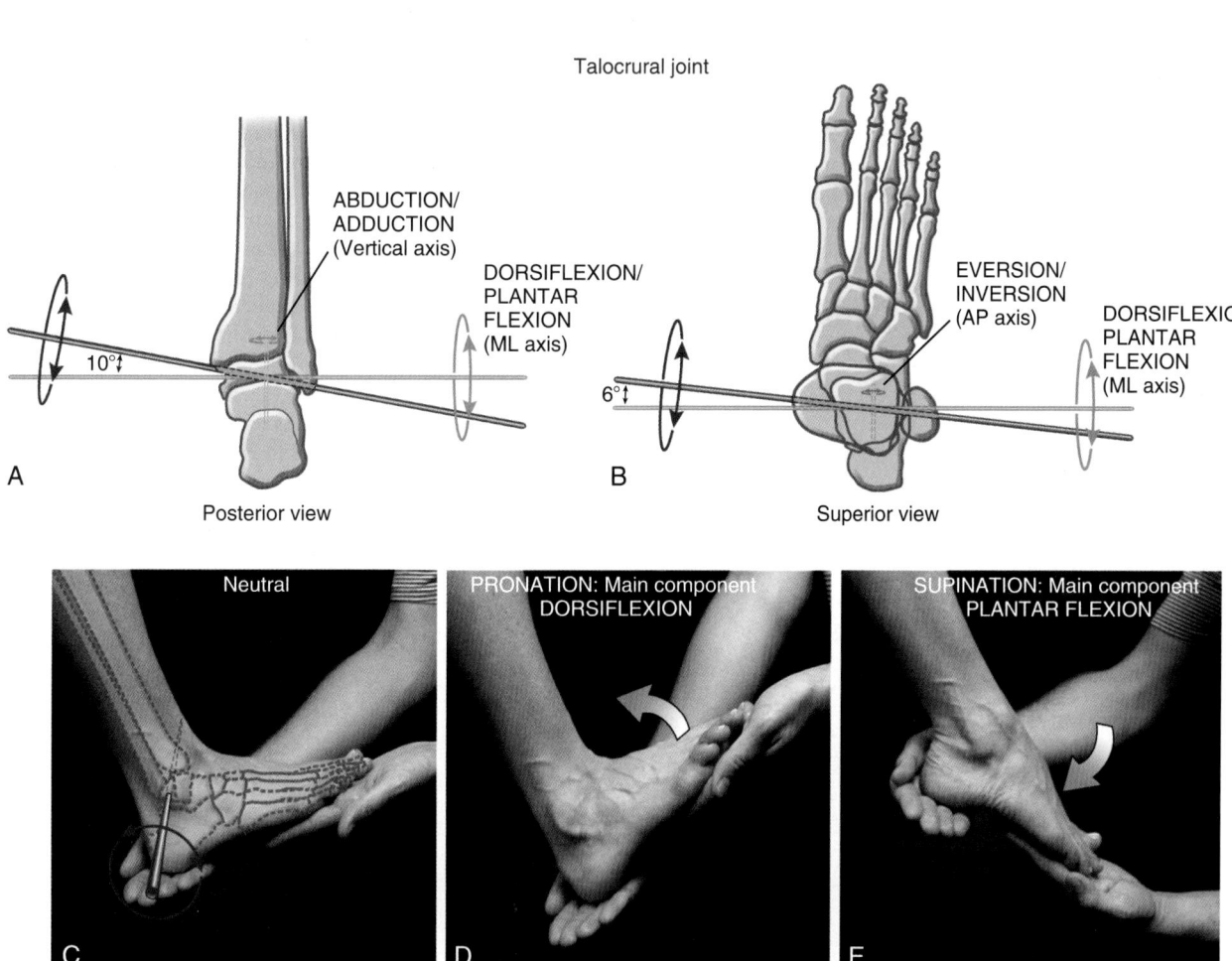

FIG. 14.17 The axis of rotation and osteokinematics at the talocrural joint. The slightly oblique axis of rotation (*red*) is shown from behind (A) and from above (B); this axis is shown again in (C). The component axes [vertical, medial-lateral (ML), and anterior-posterior (AP)] and associated osteokinematics are also depicted in (A) and (B). Although subtle, dorsiflexion (D) is combined with slight abduction and eversion, which are components of pronation; plantar flexion (E) is combined with slight adduction and inversion, which are components of supination.

Arthrokinematics
Dorsiflexion

The following discussion assumes that the foot is unloaded and free to rotate. During *dorsiflexion* the talus rolls forward relative to the leg as it simultaneously slides *posteriorly* (Fig. 14.18A). The simultaneous posterior slide allows the talus to rotate with only limited net anterior translation.[41,259] Fig. 14.18A shows the calcaneofibular ligament becoming taut in response to the posterior sliding tendency of the talus-and-calcaneal segment. Generally, *any collateral ligament that becomes increasingly taut from posterior translation of the talus also becomes increasingly taut during dorsiflexion.* In addition to the calcaneofibular ligament, full dorsiflexion also elongates the posterior talofibular ligament and posterior tibiotalar fibers of the deltoid ligament.[31,82] Although the magnitude of the resistance produced by these collateral ligaments may be relatively small compared with a tissue like the Achilles tendon, in certain clinical situations the mechanical stiffness exerted by these and other ligaments may be abnormally large and may restrict full dorsiflexion. Restricted dorsiflexion can significantly interfere with the ease of performing many daily functions, especially those involving weight-bearing. Consider, for example, the large amount of ankle dorsiflexion that naturally accompanies a motion such as bilaterally squatting to the floor. To achieve this functionally important motion, someone with reduced dorsiflexion may habitually seek alternative biomechanical strategies which can overburden other regions. For example, one compensation strategy is to overly *pronate* at the more distal, transverse tarsal joint. As will be explained later in this chapter, dorsiflexion is a significant component of the overall pronation motion at the transverse tarsal joint. Although the person may functionally benefit from the additional global dorsiflexion of the foot, the greater pronation can, over time, create an irritating stress on structures such as the tibialis posterior tendon or, indirectly, the patellofemoral joint.

Conservative measures aimed at restoring full dorsiflexion at the talocrural joint often aim to increase the length or flexibility of excessively tightened tissues, which may include musculotendinous, capsular, or ligamentous structures. Specific mobilization applied to the talocrural joint can be particularly effective at increasing dorsiflexion.[97] For example, the clinician may apply a *posterior-directed* translation of the talus-and-foot segment relative to the leg.[259] An appropriately applied posterior slide is designed to stretch connective tissues that naturally limit dorsiflexion, which includes many of the collateral ligaments. The posterior slide also mimics the natural arthrokinematics of dorsiflexion. As an adjunct to this (or any) treatment, clinicians need to encourage exercises or functional activities that maintain adequate length in the tissues that, if allowed to tighten, can restrict dorsiflexion, such as the Achilles tendon or most collateral ligaments of the ankle.

Plantar Flexion

During plantar flexion, the talus rolls posteriorly as the bone simultaneously slides anteriorly (Fig. 14.18B). Generally, *any collateral ligament that becomes increasingly taut from anterior translation of the talus also becomes increasingly taut during plantar flexion.* As depicted in Fig. 14.18B, the anterior talofibular ligament is stretched in full plantar flexion. (Although not depicted, the tibionavicular fibers of the deltoid ligament would also become taut at full plantar flexion [review Table 14.3].)[31] Plantar flexion also stretches the dorsiflexor muscles and the anterior capsule of the joint. The extremes of plantar flexion can cause an impingement between the distal tibia and the posterior talus or calcaneus, especially in the presence of an os trigonum (a small and relatively rare accessory bone located near the posterior-lateral talus).

Progressive Stabilization of the Talocrural Joint Throughout the Stance Phase of Gait

At initial heel contact during walking, the ankle rapidly plantar flexes to lower the foot to the ground (Fig. 14.19; from 0% to 5% of the gait cycle).[195] As soon as the foot flat phase of gait is reached, the leg starts to rotate forward (dorsiflex) over the grounded foot. Dorsiflexion continues until just after heel off phase. At this point in the gait cycle, the ankle becomes increasingly stable because of increased tension in many stretched collateral ligaments and plantar flexor muscles (Fig. 14.20A). The dorsiflexed ankle is further stabilized as the tibiofibular component of the mortise moves over the irregular-shaped talus. Careful inspection of the talus reveals two pertinent aspects of its morphology, both appreciated by comparing the red lines in Fig. 14.20B–C.[90,250] First and foremost, the *trochlear surface* of the talus is about 25% wider at its anterior end compared with its posterior end. Second, the *lateral process of the talus* significantly expands the bone's lateral dimension. As the tibiofibular component of the mortise rolls and slides over the wider part of the talus, the fibula is forced *away* from the tibia (see path of green arrows in Fig. 14.20C). Although

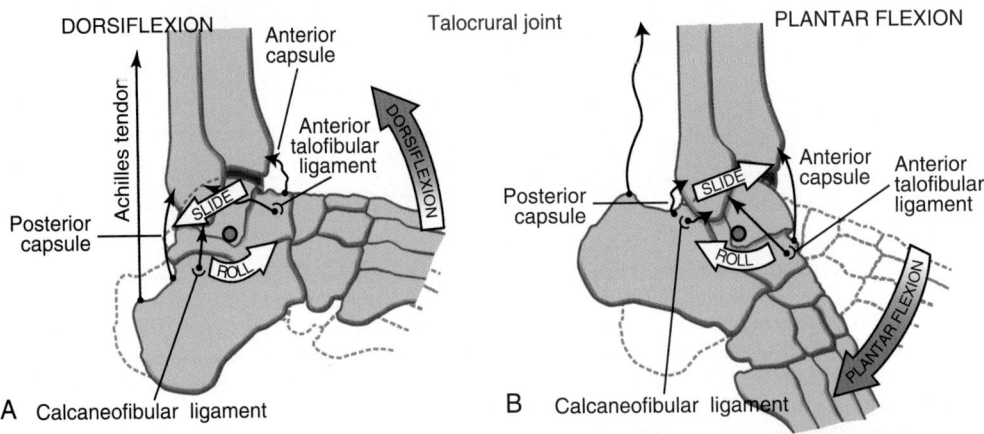

FIG. 14.18 A lateral view depicts the arthrokinematics at the talocrural joint during passive dorsiflexion (A) and plantar flexion (B). Stretched (taut) structures are shown as thin elongated arrows; slackened structures are shown as wavy arrows.

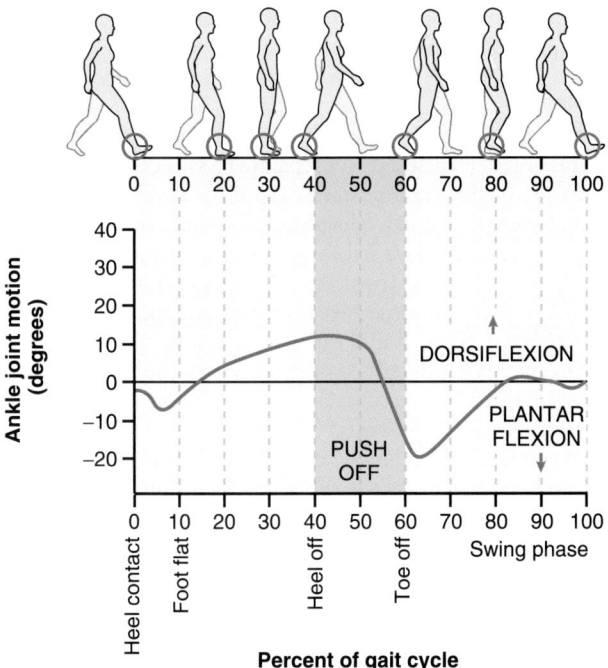

FIG. 14.19 The range of motion of the right ankle (talocrural) joint is depicted during the major phases of the gait cycle. The push off (propulsion) phase (about 40%–60% of the gait cycle) is indicated in the darker shade of green.

the resulting movement of the distal tibiofibular joint is slight and inconsistently reported, weight-bearing dorsiflexion causes the fibula to translate *laterally and posteriorly* a few millimeters and to rotate *externally* a few degrees.[102,105,194,261] As depicted in Fig. 14.20A, the fibular movement is naturally resisted by tension within stretched ligaments, such as the anterior tibiofibular

ligament.[20,96] As a result of the ligamentous tension and tight fit of the mortise, the dorsiflexed ankle is secured within its stable, close-packed position.

At the initiation of the push off phase of walking (just after about 40% of the gait cycle; see Fig. 14.19), the near fully dorsiflexed and optimally "tightened" talocrural joint is well prepared to accept ensuing compression forces that may reach four times body weight.[234] The inherent congruity of the joint during push off phase may partially account for the relatively low frequency of natural "wear-and-tear" (primary) osteoarthritis at the talocrural joint.[217] Remarkably, primary osteoarthritis of the talocrural joint occurs nine times *less* frequently than at the hip or knee.[244] This relatively low incidence of ankle osteoarthritis is *not* the case, however, when the mortise is misaligned after ankle trauma, such as an injury to the distal tibiofibular joint (i.e., a syndesmotic or "high ankle" sprain).[4] A misaligned mortise can create excessive contact pressure that is typically not well tolerated by the articular cartilage and subchondral bone.[28] The mechanisms that commonly cause a syndesmosis injury are discussed in Clinical Connection 14.1.

Structure and Function of the Joints Associated with the Foot

SUBTALAR JOINT

The subtalar joint, as its name indicates, resides under the talus (see Fig. 14.9). To appreciate the extent of subtalar joint motion, one need only firmly grasp the unloaded calcaneus (heel) and twist it in a side-to-side and rotary fashion. During this motion, the talus should remain nearly stationary within the tight-fitting talocrural joint. Pronation and supination during non–weight-bearing activities occur as the calcaneus moves relative to the fixed talus. During weight-bearing activities, such as when in the stance

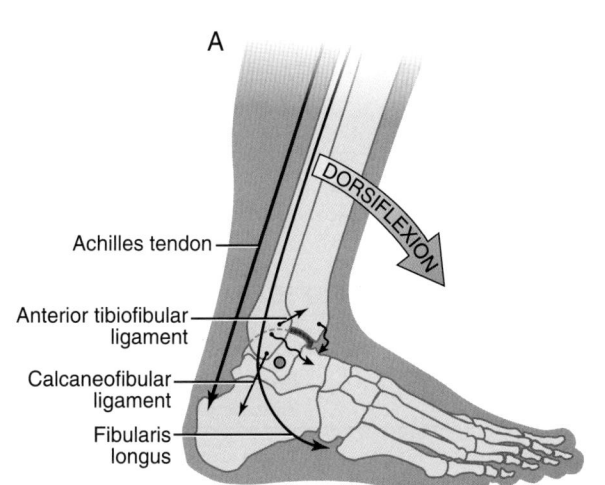

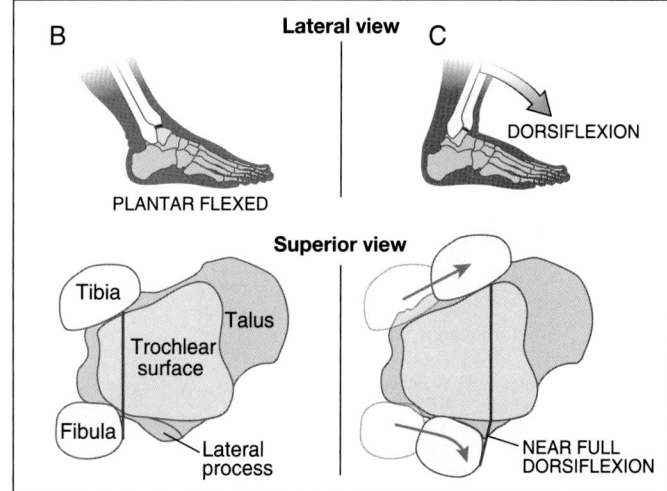

FIG. 14.20 Factors that increase the mechanical stability of the dorsiflexed talocrural joint. (A) Dorsiflexion stretches and increases tension in several tissues (depicted by *elongated arrows*). The two wavy thin arrows represent the slackened anterior capsule and anterior talofibular ligament. (B) The ankle is shown plantar flexed, with the red line indicating the relative narrow (posterior) width of the talus. (C) The path of dorsiflexion (indicated by *green arrows*) places the tibiofibular component (of the mortise) in contact with (1) the wider anterior dimension of the trochlear surface and (2) the outwardly flared lateral process of the talus; depicted by the red line. This dynamic contact within the lateral mortise forces the fibula to rotate and translate slightly in a generalized external rotation direction (indicated by the *curved green arrow*). See text for more details.

phase of walking, however, pronation and supination occur as the leg-and-talus (as a common unit) rotate *over* a relatively stationary (fixed) calcaneus. These weight-bearing–based kinematics of the subtalar joint are essential to understanding of the kinesiology of the foot. These kinematics allow the foot to assume positions that are independent of the orientation of the superimposed ankle and leg. This function is required during activities such as walking across a steep hill, standing with the feet held wide apart, changing directions while walking or running, and keeping one's balance on a rocking boat.

Articular Structure

The large, complex subtalar joint consists of three articulations between the posterior, middle, and anterior facets of the calcaneus and the talus. These articulations are depicted in yellow in Fig. 14.21.

The prominent *posterior articulation* of the subtalar joint occupies about 70% of the total articular surface area. This articulation consists of the concave posterior facet of the talus joining the reciprocally convex posterior facet of the calcaneus. The articulation is held tightly opposed by its interlocking shape, ligaments, body weight, and activated muscle. The closely aligned *anterior* and *middle articulations* consist of smaller, nearly flat joint surfaces. Although all three articulations contribute to movement at the subtalar joint, clinicians typically focus on the more

prominent posterior articulation when performing mobilization techniques to increase the mobility of the rearfoot.[a]

Ligaments

The posterior and anterior-middle articulations within the subtalar joint are each enclosed by a separate fibrous capsule. The external margin of the larger posterior capsule is reinforced by slender and indistinctly named talocalcaneal ligaments. The ligaments that provide the primary stability to the subtalar joint are listed in Table 14.4. Located extrinsic to the subtalar joint, the *calcaneofibular ligament* limits excessive inversion, and the *deltoid ligament* (*tibiocalcaneal fibers*) limits excessive eversion. (The anatomy of these ligaments was described previously with the talocrural joint.) Located intrinsic to the subtalar joint are the *interosseous* (*talocalcaneal*) and *cervical ligaments*.[61,169] Because these ligaments attach directly between the talus and calcaneus, they provide the greatest direct reinforcement of the subtalar joint. These broad and flat ligaments cross obliquely within the tarsal sinus and therefore are difficult to view unless the joint is disarticulated (as depicted in Figs. 14.8 and 14.21). The *interosseous ligament* consists of differently shaped bands that arise from the medial-posterior end of the calcaneal sulcus, then course superiorly to attach between the middle and posterior facets within talar sulcus (Fig. 14.21). The larger and often multi-fascicled *cervical ligament* has an oblique fiber arrangement like the interosseous ligament but, most often, arises closer to the lateral-anterior end of the calcaneal sulcus.[169] From this attachment, the cervical ligament courses superiormedially to attach to the inferior-lateral surface of the neck of the talus (hence the name "cervical") (see Fig. 14.15). As a pair, the interosseous and cervical ligaments limit the extremes of frontal plane motions—most notably inversion.[123,169,233,247]

Although the ligaments within the tarsal sinus are recognized as primary stabilizers of the subtalar joint, a full understanding of their function remains unclear.[169] This lack of understanding has limited the development of standard clinical "stress tests" to aid in the diagnosis of ligamentous injury. Cadaveric studies suggest that a lateral-to-medial translational force applied to the calcaneus specifically stresses the interosseous ligament.[247] This finding is consistent with the ligament's proposed function of resisting inversion at the subtalar joint.

Kinematics

The arthrokinematics at the subtalar joint involve a sliding motion among the three sets of articulated facets, yielding a curvilinear arc of movement between the calcaneus and the talus. The literature is in general agreement that, although variable, the axis of rotation

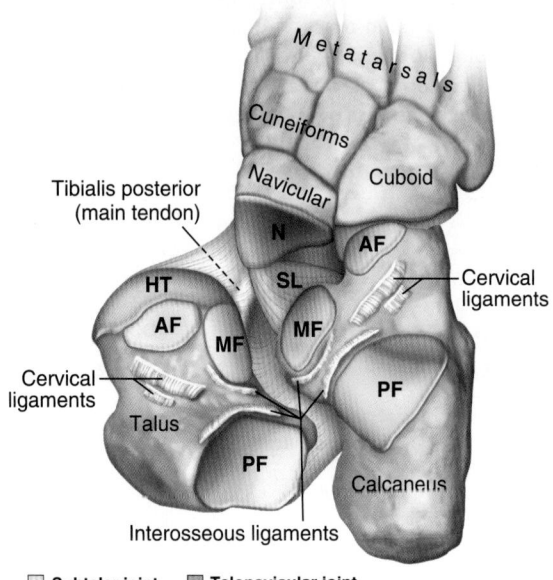

Superior view

FIG. 14.21 A superior view of the right foot is shown with the talus flipped medially, exposing most of its plantar surface. The talus is suspended from other tarsal bones by parts of the deltoid ligament. The articular surfaces of the *subtalar joint* are shown in yellow; the nearby articular surfaces of the *talonavicular joint* are shown in light purple. Exposing the subtalar joint reveals the cervical and interosseous ligaments. Replacing the talus to its natural position joins the three sets of articular facets within the subtalar joint—anterior facet *(AF)*, middle facet *(MF)*, and posterior facet *(PF)*. Replacing the talus also rearticulates the talonavicular joint by joining the head of the talus *(HT)* within the concavity formed by the concave surfaces of the navicular *(N)* and the spring ligament *(SL)*. The thick, main tendon of the tibialis posterior is evident as it courses medial to the deltoid ligament, toward the navicular tuberosity.

TABLE 14.4 Primary Functions of the Ligaments of the Subtalar Joint	
Ligament	**Primary Function at the Subtalar Joint**
Calcaneofibular	Limits excessive inversion
Tibiocalcaneal fibers of the deltoid ligament	Limits excessive eversion
Interosseous (talocalcaneal) Cervical	Both ligaments bind the talus with the calcaneus; limit the extremes of all motions, especially inversion

[a]Because the subtalar joint is the only joint within the rearfoot, the literature often uses the terms *subtalar joint* and *rearfoot* interchangeably. This terminology will be followed in this chapter as well.

for subtalar joint motion pierces the lateral-posterior heel and courses through the subtalar joint in anterior, medial, and superior directions (Fig. 14.22A–C, red).[38,192] The axis of rotation depicted in this chapter is based on the classic work of Close et al: an axis oriented 42 degrees from the horizontal plane (see Fig. 14.22A) and 16 degrees from the sagittal plane (see Fig. 14.22B).[38]

Pronation and supination of the subtalar joint occur as the calcaneus moves relative to the talus (or vice versa when the foot is planted) in an arc that is perpendicular to the axis of rotation (see the red circular arrows in Fig. 14.22A–C). Given the general pitch to the axis, only two of the three main components of pronation and supination are strongly evident: inversion and eversion, and abduction and adduction (see Fig. 14.22A–B). *Pronation*, therefore, has main components of *eversion* and *abduction* (see Fig. 14.22D); *supination* has main components of *inversion* and *adduction* (see Fig. 14.22E). The calcaneus does dorsiflex and plantar flex slightly relative to the talus; however, this motion is small and usually ignored clinically. Interestingly, however, the amount of sagittal plane mobility at the subtalar joint is significant in persons who have had a complete surgical fusion of their talocrural joint.[140] Although this compensation likely satisfies the important functional need to dorsiflex and plantar flex the foot while walking, the increased demand on the subtalar joint likely explains its high incidence of osteoarthritis in the years after the fused talocrural joint.

For simplicity, the osteokinematics of the subtalar joint have been pictorially demonstrated (in Fig. 14.22) as the calcaneus moving relative to a fixed and essentially immobile talus. During walking, however, because the calcaneus is relatively fixed under the load of body weight, a significant portion of pronation and supination at the subtalar joint occurs by *horizontal plane rotation of the talus*. Because of the inherent stability and fit provided by the mortise, the horizontal plane rotation of the talus is strongly mechanically linked to the rotation of the entire lower leg.

Range of Motion

Grimston and colleagues reported active range of inversion and eversion at the subtalar joint across 120 healthy subjects (aged 9 through 79 years).[87] Results showed that inversion exceeds eversion by nearly double: inversion, 22.6 degrees; eversion, 12.5 degrees. Although these data include accessory motions at the talocrural joint, the much greater ratio of inversion to eversion is typical of that reported for the subtalar joint alone.[18,242] Studies that measure passive (in contrast to active) range of motion usually report greater magnitudes of motion, with inversion-to-eversion ratios approaching 3:1.[274] Regardless of active or passive motion, the distally projecting lateral malleolus and the relatively thick deltoid ligament naturally limit eversion.

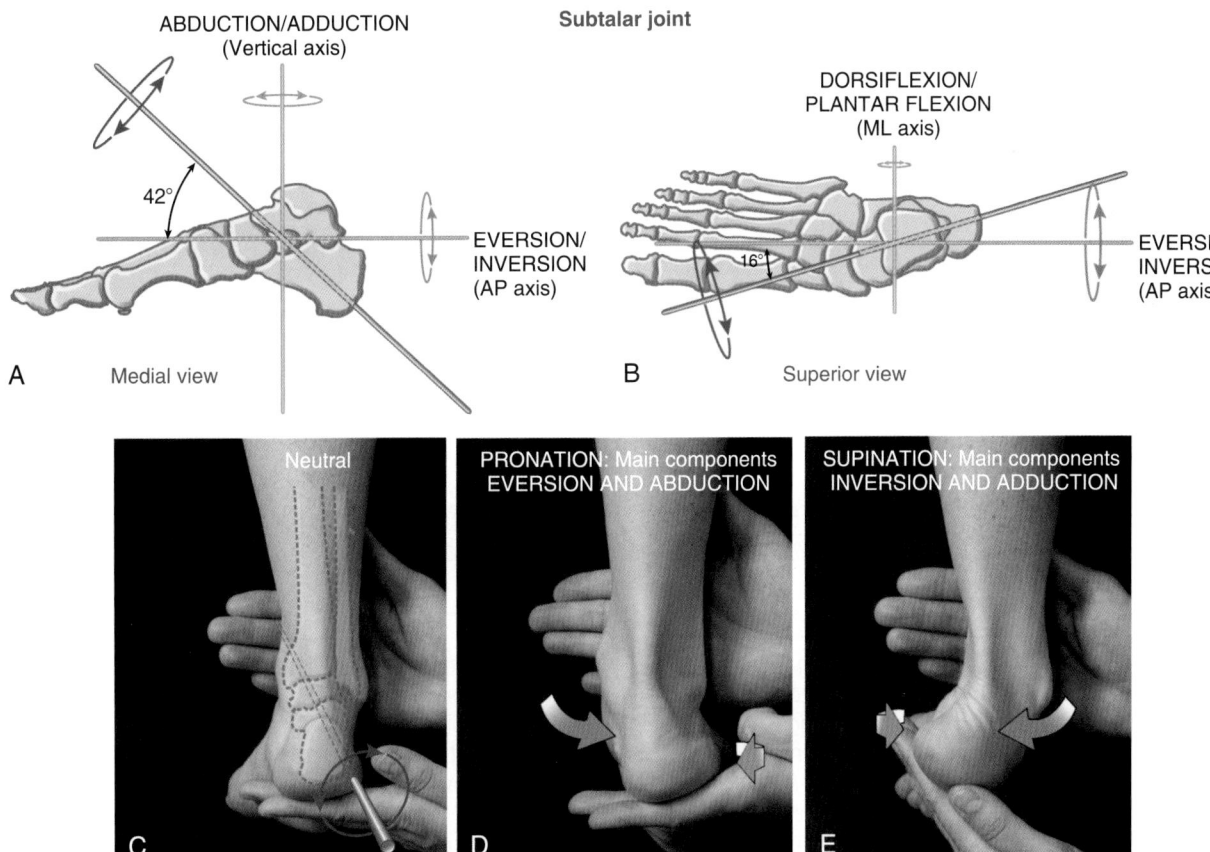

FIG. 14.22 The axis of rotation and osteokinematics at the subtalar joint. The axis of rotation (*red*) is shown from the side (A) and above (B); this axis is shown again in (C). The component axes [vertical, anterior-posterior (AP), and medial-lateral (ML)] and associated osteokinematics are also depicted in (A) and (B). The movement of pronation, with the main components of eversion and abduction, is demonstrated in (D). The movement of supination, with the main components of inversion and adduction, is demonstrated in (E). In (D) and (E), blue arrows indicate abduction and adduction, and purple arrows indicate eversion and inversion.

TRANSVERSE TARSAL JOINT (TALONAVICULAR AND CALCANEOCUBOID JOINTS)

The transverse tarsal joint, also known as the *midtarsal or Chopart's joint*, consists of two anatomically distinct articulations: the *talonavicular joint* and the *calcaneocuboid joint*. As shown in Fig. 14.23, these joints connect the rearfoot with the midfoot.

At this point in this chapter, it may be instructive to consider the functional characteristics of the transverse tarsal joint within the context of the other major joints of the ankle and foot. As described earlier, the talocrural (ankle) joint permits motion primarily in the sagittal plane: dorsiflexion and plantar flexion. The subtalar joint, however, permits a more oblique path of motion consisting of two primary components: inversion-eversion and abduction-adduction. This section now describes how the transverse tarsal joint, the most versatile joint of the foot, moves through a more oblique path of motion, coursing nearly equally through all three cardinal planes. Among other important functions, the path of pronation and supination at the transverse tarsal joint allows the weight-bearing foot to adapt to a variety of surface contours (Fig. 14.24).

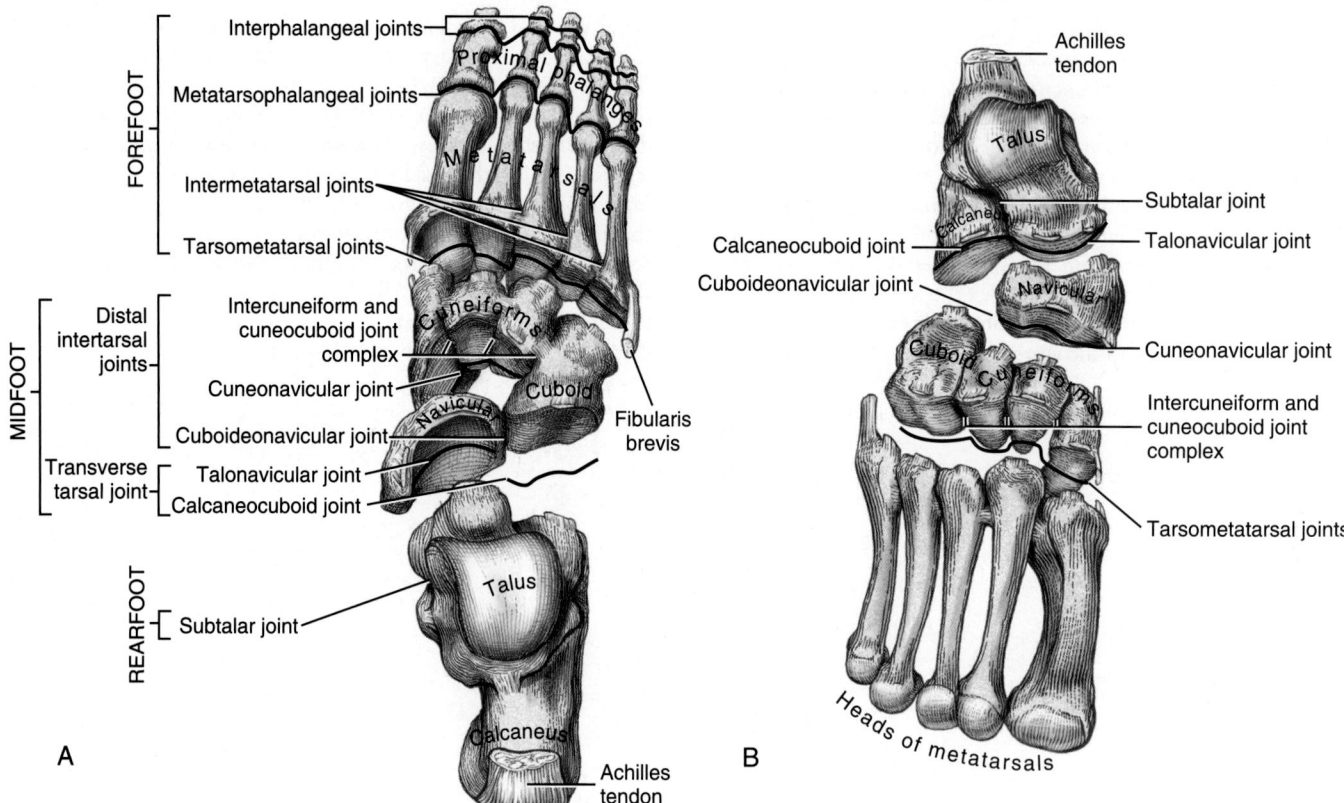

FIG. 14.23 (A) The bones and disarticulated joints of the right foot are shown from two perspectives: superior-posterior (A) and superior-anterior (B). The rearfoot, midfoot, and forefoot regions are indicated in (A).

SPECIAL FOCUS 14.1

Clinical Assessment of Subtalar Joint Motion

It is difficult to accurately measure the extent of pronation and supination at the subtalar joint through standard goniometry. This difficulty reflects the inability of a standard, rigid goniometer to follow the oblique arc of pronation and supination, compounded by simultaneous movements in surrounding joints. As a method to circumvent this problem, clinicians and researchers often measure subtalar joint motion solely by the amount of inversion and eversion of the rearfoot (calcaneus). This shortcut is valid provided that it is understood that the frontal plane movements of inversion and eversion are only *components* of supination and pronation, not identical substitutes.

The expression "subtalar joint neutral" is often used clinically to describe a baseline posture of the resting foot, typically to aid in the fabrication of an orthotic device.[119,143] The neutral position of the subtalar joint is defined by placing the subject's calcaneus in a position that allows both lateral and medial sides of the talus to be equally exposed for palpation within the mortise. In this "neutral" position, the joint is approximately one-third the distance from full eversion and two-thirds the distance from full inversion. Although the measurement's clinical usefulness has been questioned,[92] it remains a convenient method to approximate the neutral, frontal plane position of the subtalar joint.

The transverse tarsal joint has a strong functional relationship with the subtalar joint. As will be described, these two joints function cooperatively to control most of the pronation and supination posturing of the entire foot.

Articular Structure and Ligamentous Support

Talonavicular Joint

The talonavicular joint (the medial compartment of the transverse tarsal joint) resembles a ball-and-socket type of articulation, providing substantial mobility to the medial (longitudinal) column of the foot. Much of this mobility is expressed as a twisting (inverting and everting) and bending (flexing and extending) of the midfoot-and-forefoot relative to the rearfoot. The talonavicular joint consists of the articulation between the convex head of the talus and the continuous, deep concavity formed by the proximal side of the navicular bone and the spring ligament (see Fig. 14.8). The convex-concave relationship of the talonavicular joint is evident in Fig. 14.21. The *spring ligament* (labeled as *SL* in Fig. 14.21) is a thick and wide band of fibrocartilage, spanning the gap between the sustentaculum tali of the calcaneus and the medial-plantar surface of the navicular bone.[51,166,240] The tibiospring fibers of the deltoid ligament blend with and reinforce the spring ligament.[30] By directly supporting the medial and plantar convexity of the head of the talus, the spring ligament forms the structural "floor and medial wall" of the talonavicular joint. Considerable support is required in this region of the foot because while standing the weight of the body depresses the head of the talus in plantar and medial directions—toward the earth. Tears or laxity in the spring ligament therefore can contribute to a flatfoot deformity.[270] (The more formal and precise name of the spring ligament is the *plantar calcaneonavicular ligament*. The term "spring" is actually a misnomer because it has little, if any, elasticity; its highly fibrocartilaginous consistency offers considerable strength and resistance to elongation. Nevertheless, the term *spring* remains well established in the clinical and research literature.[166])

An irregularly shaped capsule surrounds the talonavicular joint. The ligaments reinforcing this capsule are included in the box.

Summary of Ligaments That Support or Reinforce the Talonavicular Joint

- Spring (plantar calcaneonavicular) ligament forms a fibrocartilaginous sling for the head of the talus (see Figs. 14.8 and 14.21).
- Dorsal talonavicular ligament reinforces the capsule *dorsally* (see Fig. 14.14).
- Bifurcated ligament (calcaneonavicular fibers) reinforces the capsule *laterally* (see Fig. 14.15).
- Tibionavicular and tibiospring fibers of the deltoid ligament reinforce the capsule *medially* (see Fig. 14.14).

Calcaneocuboid Joint

The calcaneocuboid joint is the lateral component of the transverse tarsal joint, formed by the junction of the anterior (distal) surface of the calcaneus with the proximal surface of the cuboid (Fig. 14.23). Each articular surface has a concave and convex curvature. The joint surfaces form an interlocking wedge that resists sliding. The relative inflexibility of the calcaneocuboid joint (compared with the talonavicular joint) provides stability to the lateral (longitudinal) column of the foot.

The dorsal and lateral parts of the capsule of the calcaneocuboid joint are thickened by the *dorsal calcaneocuboid ligament* (see Fig. 14.15). Three additional ligaments further stabilize the joint. The *bifurcated ligament* is a Y-shaped band of tissue with its stem attached to the calcaneus, just proximal to the dorsal surface of the calcaneocuboid joint. The stem of the ligament flares into lateral and medial fiber bundles. The aforementioned medial (calcaneonavicular) fibers reinforce the lateral side of the talonavicular joint. The lateral (calcaneocuboid) fibers cross the dorsal side of the calcaneocuboid joint, forming the primary bond between the two bones.[233]

The long and short plantar ligaments reinforce the plantar side of the calcaneocuboid joint (Fig. 14.25). The *long plantar ligament*, the longest ligament in the foot, arises from the plantar surface of the calcaneus, just anterior to the calcaneal tuberosity.[233] The ligament inserts on the plantar surface of the bases of the lateral three or four metatarsal bones. The *short plantar ligament*, also called the *plantar calcaneocuboid ligament*, arises just anterior and deep to the long plantar ligament and inserts on the plantar surface of the cuboid bone. By passing perpendicularly to the calcaneocuboid joint, the plantar ligaments provide excellent structural stability to the lateral column of the foot.[139]

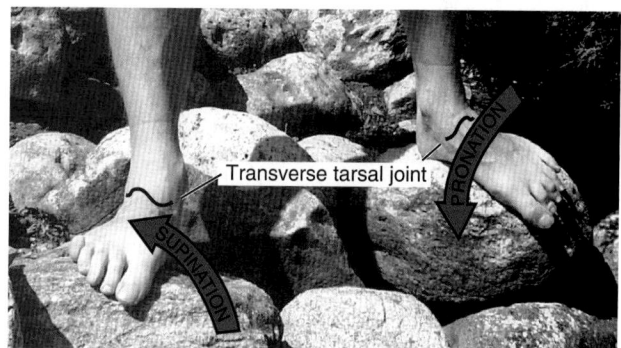

FIG. 14.24 The transverse tarsal joints allow for pronation and supination of the midfoot while one stands on uneven surfaces.

Plantar view

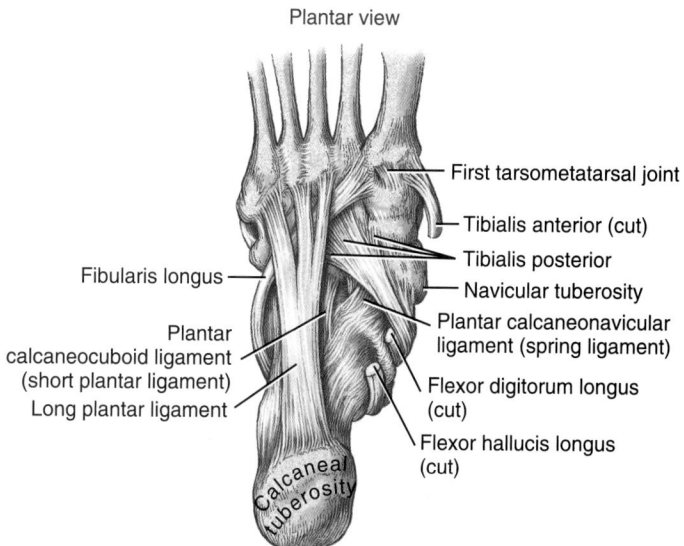

First tarsometatarsal joint
Tibialis anterior (cut)
Tibialis posterior
Navicular tuberosity
Plantar calcaneonavicular ligament (spring ligament)
Flexor digitorum longus (cut)
Flexor hallucis longus (cut)

Fibularis longus

Plantar calcaneocuboid ligament (short plantar ligament)
Long plantar ligament

Calcaneal tuberosity

FIG. 14.25 Ligaments and tendons deep within the plantar aspect of the right foot. Note the course of the tendons of the fibularis longus and tibialis posterior.

Summary of Ligaments That Reinforce the Calcaneocuboid Joint

- Dorsal calcaneocuboid ligament reinforces the capsule *dorsal-laterally* (see Fig. 14.15).
- Bifurcated ligament (calcaneocuboid fibers) reinforces the calcaneocuboid joint *dorsally* (see Fig. 14.15).
- Long and short plantar ligaments (see Fig. 14.25) reinforce the *plantar side* of the calcaneocuboid joint.

Kinematics

The transverse tarsal joint rarely moves without associated movements at nearby joints, especially the subtalar joint. To appreciate the mobility that occurs primarily at the transverse tarsal joint, hold the calcaneus firmly fixed while maximally pronating and supinating the midfoot (Fig. 14.26A and C, respectively). During these motions, the navicular spins within the talonavicular joint. Combining motions across *both* the subtalar and the transverse tarsal joints accounts for most of the pronation and supination throughout the foot (see Fig. 14.26B and D, respectively). As evident throughout Fig. 14.26, mobility of the *forefoot* (especially the first ray) also contributes to the pronation and supination posturing of the entire foot.

Three noteworthy points should be made when studying the kinematics of the transverse tarsal joint. First, two separate axes of rotation have been described. Second, the amplitude and direction of movement is typically different during weight-bearing compared with non–weight-bearing activities. Third, the kinematics of the transverse tarsal joint are functionally influenced by the position of the subtalar joint. The upcoming sections discuss each of these factors.

Axes of Rotation and Corresponding Movements

Manter originally described two axes of rotation for movement at the transverse tarsal joint: *longitudinal* and *oblique*.[154] Based on this description, movement therefore occurs naturally in two unique planes, each oriented perpendicular to a specific axis of rotation. Although this concept has not been fully biomechanically validated, it nevertheless provides a useful way to conceptualize the movements allowed across this complex joint. The *longitudinal axis* at the transverse tarsal joint is nearly coincident with the straight anterior-posterior axis (Fig. 14.27A–C), with the primary component motions of *eversion* and *inversion* (see Fig. 14.27D–E). The *oblique axis*, in contrast, has a strong vertical *and* medial-lateral pitch (see Fig. 14.27F–H). Motion around this axis, therefore, occurs freely as a *combination of abduction and dorsiflexion* (see Fig. 14.27I) and *adduction and plantar flexion* (see Fig. 14.27J).

The transverse tarsal joint was just described as possessing two separate axes of rotation, with each axis producing a unique kinematic pattern. Although this may be technically correct, the functional kinematics associated with most weight-bearing activities occur as a blending of movements across *both* axes—a blend that yields the purest form of pronation and supination (i.e., movement that maximally expresses components of *all three* cardinal planes).[146] Pronation and supination at the transverse tarsal joint allow the midfoot (and ultimately the forefoot) to adapt to many varied shapes and contours.

Range of motion at the transverse tarsal joint is difficult to measure and isolate from adjacent joints. By visual and manual inspection, however, it is evident that the midfoot allows about twice as much supination as pronation. The amount of pure inversion and eversion of the midfoot occurs in a pattern similar to that observed at the subtalar joint: about 20 to 25 degrees of inversion and 10 to 15 degrees of eversion.

Arthrokinematics

From a functional perspective, it may be useful to describe the arthrokinematics at the transverse tarsal joint in context with motion across both the rearfoot and the midfoot. Consider the movement of active *supination* of the unloaded foot in Fig. 14.26D. The tibialis posterior muscle, with its multiple attachments, is the prime supinator of the foot. Because of the relative rigidity of the calcaneocuboid joint, an inverting and adducting calcaneus draws the lateral column of the foot "under" the medial column of the foot. The important pivot point for this motion is the talonavicular joint. The pull of the tibialis posterior contributes to the spin of the navicular, and to the raising of the medial longitudinal arch (instep) of the foot. During this motion, the concave proximal surface of the navicular and the spring ligament both spin around the convex head of the talus.

Pronation of the unloaded foot occurs by similar but reverse kinematics as those described. The pull of the fibularis longus helps lower the medial side and raise the lateral side of the foot.

SPECIAL FOCUS 14.2

Position of the Subtalar Joint Affecting Stability of the Transverse Tarsal Joint

In addition to controlling the posture of the rearfoot, the subtalar joint also indirectly controls the stability of the more distal joints, especially the transverse tarsal joint. Although the relevance of this concept is discussed later in this chapter, *full supination at the subtalar joint restricts the overall flexibility of the midfoot.* A very loosely articulated skeletal model helps to demonstrate this principle. With one hand stabilizing the talus, firmly "swing" the calcaneus (heel) into full inversion and note that the lateral aspect of the midfoot "drops" relative to the medial aspect. As a result, the talonavicular and calcaneocuboid joints (components of the transverse tarsal joint) become twisted longitudinally, thereby increasing the relative rigidity of the midfoot. *Full pronation of the subtalar joint, in contrast, increases the overall flexibility of the midfoot.* Again, returning to a loosely articulated skeleton model, maximal eversion of the calcaneus untwists the medial and lateral aspects of the midfoot, placing them in a nearly parallel position. As a result, the talonavicular and calcaneocuboid joints untwist longitudinally, thereby increasing the flexibility of the midfoot. Make the effort to "feel" on a partner the *increased* multiplanar flexibility of the midfoot (and forefoot) as the calcaneus is gradually moved from full inversion to full eversion.[21] As described in subsequent sections, the ability of the midfoot to change its flexibility has important mechanical implications during the stance phase of gait.

PRONATION of the foot (dorsal-medial view)

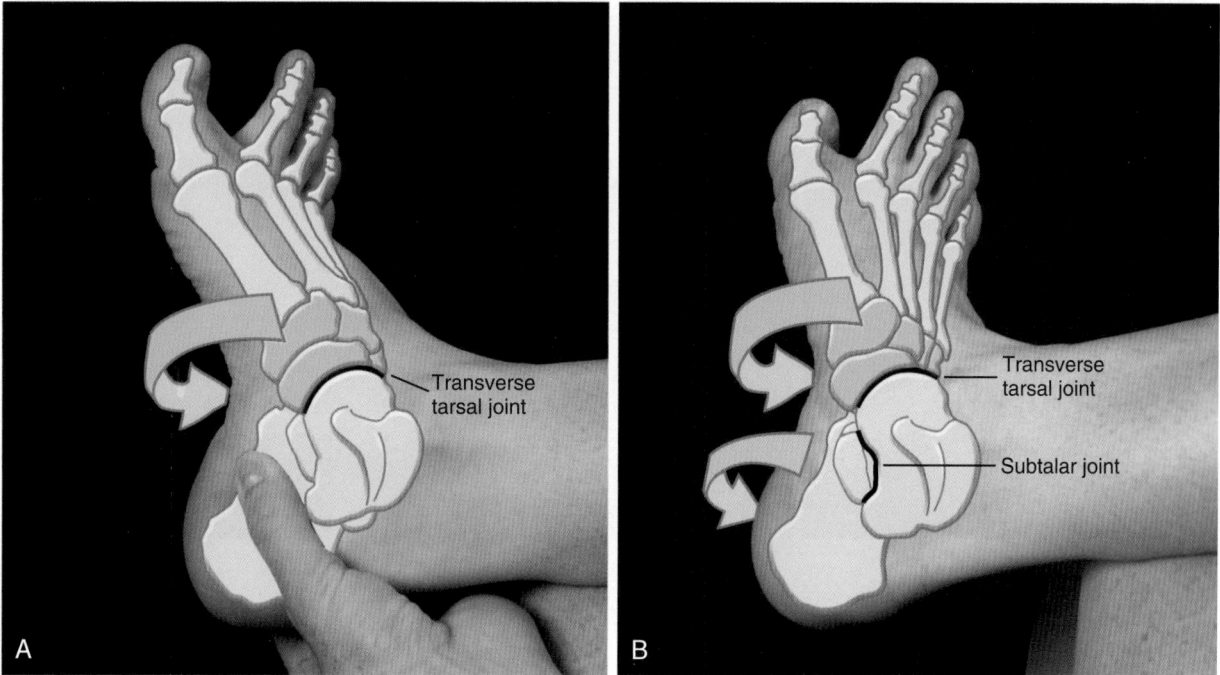

SUPINATION of the foot (plantar-medial view)

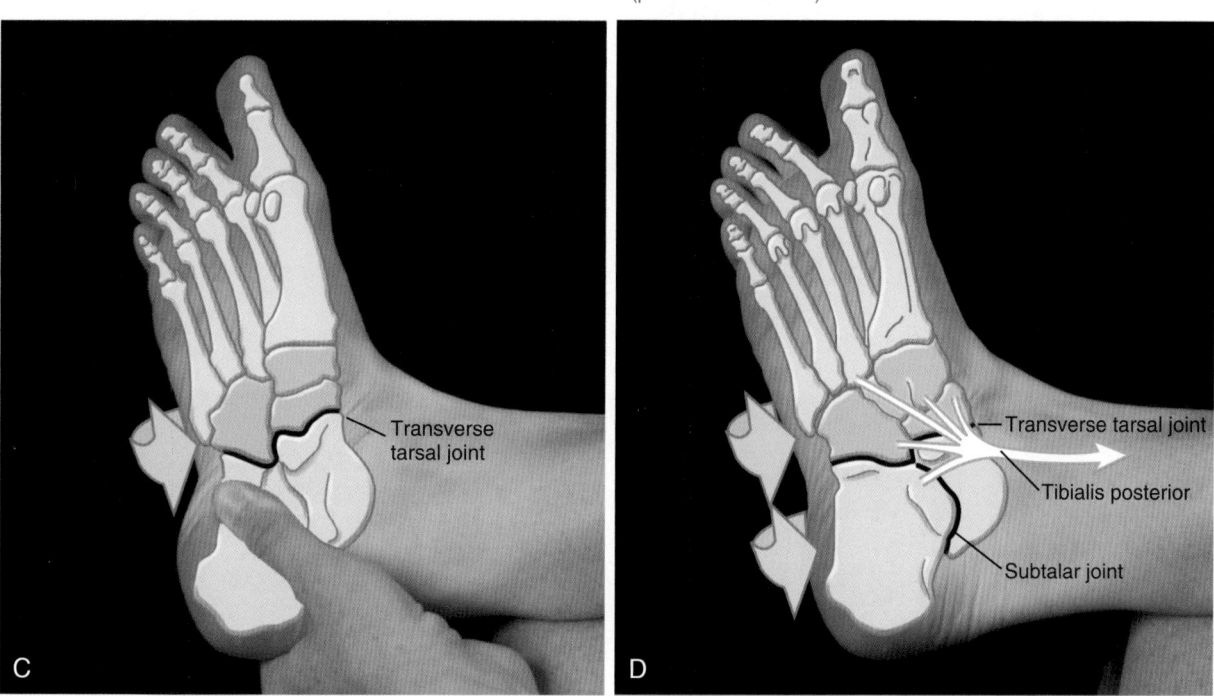

FIG. 14.26 Pronation and supination of the unloaded right foot demonstrate the interplay of the subtalar and transverse tarsal joints. With the calcaneus held fixed, pronation and supination occur primarily at the midfoot (A and C). When the calcaneus is free, pronation and supination occur as a summation across both the rearfoot and the midfoot (B and D). Rearfoot movement is indicated by pink arrows; midfoot movement is indicated by blue arrows. The pull of the tibialis posterior muscle is shown in (D) as it directs active supination over both the rearfoot and the midfoot.

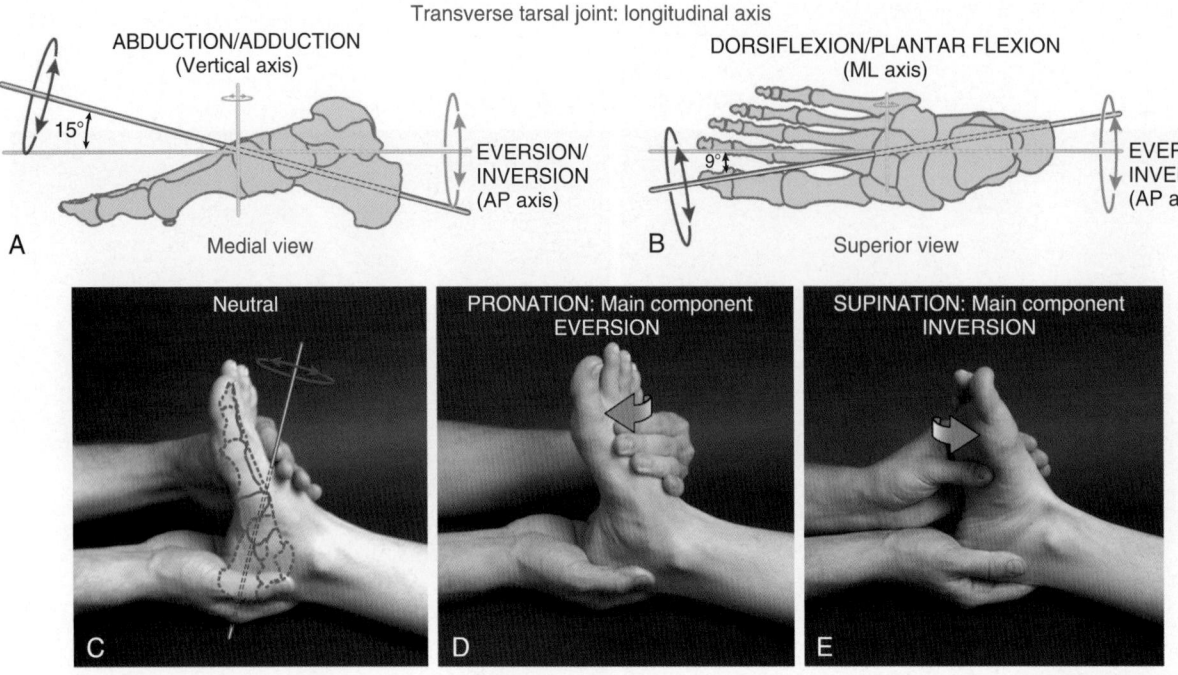

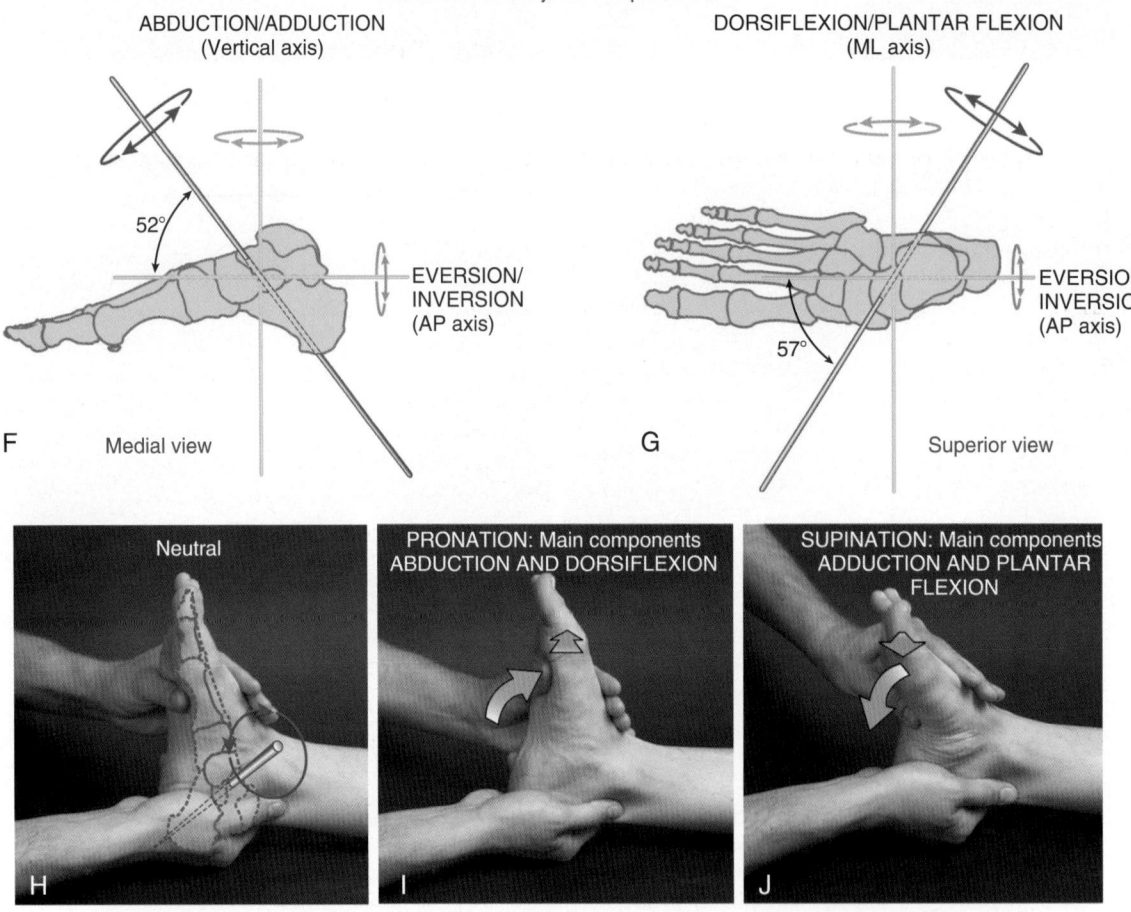

FIG. 14.27 The axes of rotation and osteokinematics at the transverse tarsal joint. The *longitudinal axis of rotation* is shown in red from the side (A and C) and from above (B). (The component axes and associated osteokinematics are also depicted in panels A and B.) Movements that occur around the longitudinal axis are (D) *pronation* (with the main component of eversion) and (E) *supination* (with the main component of inversion). The *oblique axis of rotation* is shown in red from the side (F and H) and from above (G). (The component axes and associated osteokinematics are also depicted in panels F and G.) Movements that occur around the oblique axis are (I) *pronation* (with main components of abduction and dorsiflexion) and (J) *supination* (with main components of adduction and plantar flexion). In (I) and (J), blue arrows indicate abduction and adduction, and green arrows indicate dorsiflexion and plantar flexion.

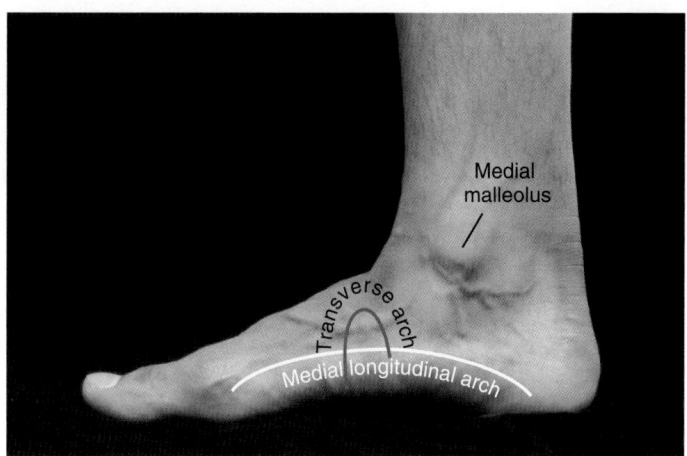

FIG. 14.28 The medial side of a normal foot shows the medial longitudinal arch (*white*) and the transverse arch (*red*).

The previously described arthrokinematics of supination and pronation assume that the foot is unloaded, or off the ground. The challenge is to understand these arthrokinematics when the foot is *on* the ground, typically during the walking process. This topic is addressed later in this chapter.

Medial Longitudinal Arch of the Foot

Fig. 14.28 shows the locations of the medial longitudinal and transverse arches of the foot. Both arches lend crucial elements of stability and resiliency to the loaded foot. The structure and function of the medial longitudinal arch is addressed in this section. The transverse arch is described later during the study of the distal intertarsal joints.

The *medial longitudinal arch* follows the characteristic concave "instep" of the medial side of the foot. This arch is the primary load-bearing and shock-absorbing structure of the foot.[248] The bones that contribute structurally to the medial longitudinal arch include the calcaneus, talus, navicular, cuneiforms, and associated three medial metatarsals. Several connective tissues help maintain the shape of the medial arch (described later in the chapter). Without this arched configuration, the large and rapidly produced forces applied against the foot during running and marching, for examples, would likely exceed the physiologic weight-bearing capacity of the bones. Additional structures that assist the arch in absorbing loads are the plantar fat pads, sesamoid bones located at the plantar base of the great toe, and superficial plantar fascia (which attaches primarily to the overlying thick dermis, functioning primarily to minimize shear forces). As will be described, the medial longitudinal arch and associated connective tissues are the primary sources of support for the foot during relatively low-stress or near-static conditions—for example, while standing at ease. Although variable, relaxed standing typically requires relatively small amounts of *active* muscular support to maintain the shape of the healthy arch, at least compared with the dominant support provided by the connective tissues.[b] Significantly higher levels of active muscular support are required when the arch is naturally stressed while walking, or by larger loading scenarios that involve standing on one foot only, or on tiptoes, jumping, or running. The role of muscles in providing active support

is described later in this chapter, in the study of muscles of the ankle and foot.

The following section describes the passive support mechanism provided by the medial longitudinal arch.

Passive Support Mechanism of the Medial Longitudinal Arch

The talonavicular joint and associated connective tissues form the *keystone* of the medial longitudinal arch. Additional nonmuscular structures responsible for maintaining the height and shape of the arch are the plantar fascia, spring ligament, and first tarsometatarsal joint. The *plantar fascia of the foot* provides the primary passive support to the medial longitudinal arch.[7,63,103] This dense connective tissue covers the sole and sides of the foot and is organized into superficial and deep fibers. The *superficial* fibers, introduced earlier, blend primarily with the overlying thick dermis of the plantar surface of the foot. The more extensive and thicker *deep* plantar fascia (or aponeurosis) attaches posteriorly to the medial process of the calcaneal tuberosity (e-Fig. 14.1). This tissue, 2 to 2.5 mm thick, consists of a series of longitudinal and transverse bands of collagen-rich tissue.[120,191] The fascia is extremely strong, capable of resisting approximately 810 N (more than 180 lb) of tension before permanent elongation.[191,273] From the tissue's firm attachment to the calcaneus, lateral, medial, and central sets of fibers course anteriorly, blending with and covering the first layer of the intrinsic muscles of the foot. The main, larger, central set of fibers extends toward the metatarsal heads, where they eventually blend with the plantar plates (ligaments) of the metatarsophalangeal joints, fibrous sheaths of the flexor tendons of the digits, and fascia covering the plantar aspect of the toes. Extension of the toes therefore stretches the central fibers of the deep fascia, adding tension to the medial longitudinal arch. This mechanism is useful because it increases tension in the arch when one stands on tiptoes or during the late push off phase of gait.[128,145]

When one stands normally, the weight of the body falls through the foot near the region of the talonavicular joint.[19] This load is distributed anteriorly and posteriorly throughout the medial longitudinal arch, passing to the fat pads and the thick dermis over the heel and ball (metatarsal head region) of the foot. Normally the rearfoot receives about twice the compressive load as the forefoot.[33] The mean pressure under the forefoot is usually greatest in the region of the heads of the second and third metatarsal bones.

---

[b] 15,16,67,86,95,117,152

During standing, body weight normally pushes the talus inferiorly, slightly lowering the medial longitudinal arch (Fig 14.29A). The amount of depression of the arch while weight-bearing can be measured clinically by the distance between the ground and the navicular tuberosity, a static measurement referred to as the "navicular drop test."[119] The drop of the arch (on average about 7 mm in healthy adult males) increases the distance between the calcaneus and metatarsal heads.[19] Tension in stretched connective tissues, especially the deep plantar fascia, acts as a semi-elastic tie-rod that "gives" slightly under load,[191] allowing only a slight drop in the arch (see stretched spring in Fig. 14.29A). Acting like a truss, the tie-rod supports body weight.[128] Experiments on cadaveric specimens indicate that the deep plantar fascia is the major structure that maintains the height of the medial longitudinal arch, selectively cutting (or releasing) the fascia decreased arch stiffness by 25%.[103]

As the arch is depressed, the subtalar joint normally pronates a few degrees. This is most evident from a posterior view as the calcaneus everts slightly relative to the tibia. As the foot is unloaded, such as when shifting body weight to the other leg during walking, the naturally elastic and flexible arch returns to its preloaded raised height. The calcaneus inverts slightly back to its neutral position, allowing the mechanism to repeat its shock absorption function once again.

As stated earlier, the height and shape of the medial longitudinal arch are controlled primarily by passive restraints from the connective tissues depicted by the spring in Fig. 14.29A. Active muscle support while quiet standing is relatively small and variable and may be considered as a "secondary line of support"—for example, for controlling postural sway, for switching from double to single limb support, for supporting relatively heavy loads, or when the arch lacks inherent support because of overstretched or weakened connective tissues.[117,246]

Pes Planus—"Abnormally Dropped" Medial Longitudinal Arch

Pes planus or "flatfoot" describes a chronically dropped or abnormally low medial longitudinal arch. This condition is often the result of laxity within the talonavicular joint, distal intertarsal joints, and the first tarsometatarsal joint, typically combined with an overstretched, torn, or weakened plantar fascia, spring ligament, or tibialis posterior tendon.[11,189,270,275] As a consequence, the subtalar joint is excessively pronated causing the rearfoot to assume an exaggerated valgus posture (calcaneus everted away from the midline). In addition, the forefoot is often in excessive abduction. Often the depressed talus and navicular rub against the inside of the footwear, forming a callus on the adjacent skin.

Fig. 14.29B shows the foot of a person with pes planus. The abnormally wide midfoot region evident in the footprint is indicative of excessive laxity within the joints that normally support the arch. A person with moderate or severe pes planus typically has a compromised ability to optimally support and dissipate loads through the foot. Significant active forces from intrinsic and extrinsic muscles may be required to partially compensate for the lack of tension produced in overstretched or weakened connective tissues. Significant muscular activity may be needed even during quiet standing, which may contribute to fatigue and various overuse symptoms, including general foot and leg pain or bone spurs.

Pes planus is often described as being either a rigid or a flexible deformity, although many conditions are not as literal as these terms imply. By definition, the foot with *rigid pes planus* (as shown in Fig. 14.29B) demonstrates a dropped arch even in non–weight-bearing positions. This deformity is often congenital, secondary to joint malformation, such as a tarsal coalition (i.e., partial fusion of the calcaneus with the talus fixed in eversion), or abnormally shape

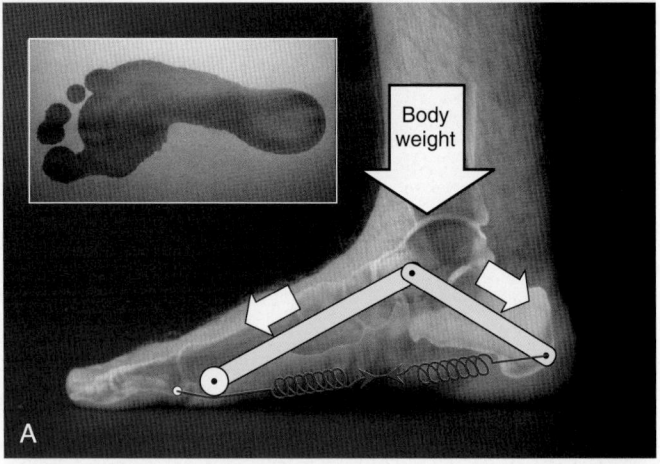

Normal arch

A

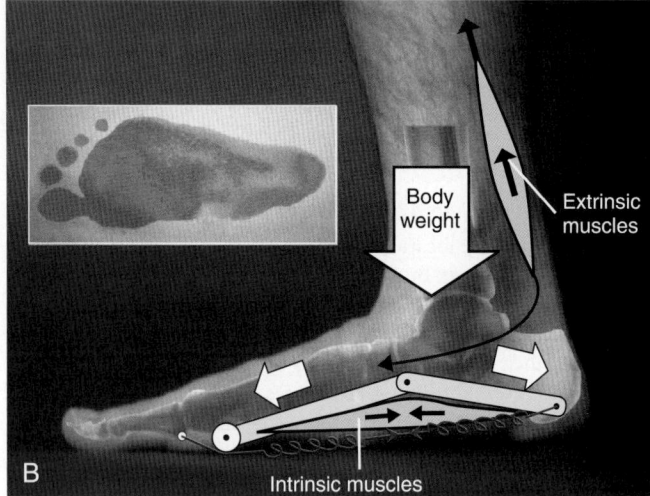

Dropped arch

Body weight

Extrinsic muscles

Body weight

Intrinsic muscles

B

FIG. 14.29 Models of the foot show a mechanism of accepting body weight during standing. (A) With a normal medial longitudinal arch, body weight is accepted and dissipated primarily through elongation of the plantar fascia, depicted as a red spring. The footprint illustrates the concavity of the normal arch. (B) With an abnormally dropped medial longitudinal arch, an overstretched or weakened plantar fascia, depicted as an overstretched red spring, may be unable to adequately accept or dissipate body weight. Consequently, various extrinsic and intrinsic muscles may be activated as a secondary source of support to the arch. The footprint illustrates the dropped arch and loss of a characteristic instep.

bones.[178] Pes planus may also occur from spastic paralysis and the resultant overpull from certain muscles. Because of the fixed nature and potential for producing painful symptoms, rigid pes planus in the child may require surgical correction.

Flexible pes planus is the more common form of a dropped arch. The medial longitudinal arch appears essentially normal when unloaded but drops excessively on weight-bearing. Flexible pes planus may be associated with laxity of local supporting connective tissues, generalized weakness or pain in muscles that can support the arch, or compensatory mechanisms that cause excessive pronation of the foot. Surgical intervention is rarely indicated for flexible pes planus. Treatment is usually in the form of providing orthoses using specialized footwear, and performing strengthening exercises of muscles in the foot and throughout the lower limb.[6,135,151,267]

SPECIAL FOCUS 14.3

Pes Cavus—Abnormally Raised Medial Longitudinal Arch

The alignment and height of the medial longitudinal arch can be broadly categorized as either pes planus, pes rectus (normal or optimal alignment), or pes cavus. This categorization can be determined through several non-radiographic measures, including navicular height, *Foot Posture Index*, goniometry (e.g., standing rearfoot varus), height and flexibility of the medial longitudinal arch, footprints, or static or dynamic plantar loading patterns.[119,249] *Pes cavus* is less common than pes planus.[99] In its least complicated form, pes cavus describes an abnormally *raised* medial longitudinal arch, typically associated with excessive rearfoot varus (calcaneal inversion) (Fig. 14.30).[132] Excessive forefoot valgus (eversion) may also be present, often as a compensation used to keep the medial forefoot firmly in contact with the ground while standing or walking.

Pes cavus may be fixed or progressive and may manifest in infancy, early childhood, or later in life. Many relatively mild forms of pes cavus are considered *idiopathic* with a strong genetic predisposition, such as the subject depicted in Fig. 14.30. Functional limitations associated with mild or subtle pes cavus vary from nonexistent to marked. The chronically raised arch reduces the area of contact between the plantar surface of the foot and the floor[65] and, in some cases, shifts the center of plantar pressure *laterally* while walking.[168] As depicted in Fig. 14.30, the abnormally high arch also places the metatarsal bones at a greater angle with the ground. When combined with the reduced area of plantar contact, plantar pressures typically rise and shift anteriorly over the forefoot (compared with pes rectus or planus). For this reason, persons with marked pes cavus may have pain (metatarsalgia) and callous formation over the region of the metatarsal heads. Furthermore, a foot with a chronically raised (and relatively rigid) arch cannot, in theory, optimally absorb the repeated impacts of walking and

running. A person with significant pes cavus may therefore be at a higher risk of developing stress-related injuries within the foot and lower limb.[249]

More severe cases of pes cavus also exist—many of which are associated with a known cause.[24] Pes cavus may be *posttraumatic*, caused by, for example, severe fracture, crush injury, or burn. An unresolved congenital *clubfoot* in childhood may persist later in life as pes cavus.[179] The most debilitating causes of pes cavus, however, have a *neurologic* origin, often caused by an imbalance of forces resulting from paralysis or contracture of the muscles of the foot. These neurologic pathologies can include idiopathic or diabetic peripheral neuropathy, Charcot-Marie-Tooth disease, poliomyelitis, myelomeningocele, spinal cord injury, and cerebral palsy. Because muscle weakness can affect the entire foot, a neurogenic pes cavus is often combined with other deformities.[24] For example, spastic or otherwise overpowering tibialis posterior and fibularis longus muscles combined with a weakened tibialis anterior muscle favor development of a rearfoot varus and forefoot valgus deformity. The weakened tibialis anterior may also allow the unopposed (stronger) fibularis longus to overpull the first metatarsal into excessive plantar flexion. A combined rearfoot varus, forefoot valgus, and excessively plantar flexed first metatarsal are often the more prominent features of a neurogenic pes cavus. Mechanical-based treatment options vary based on age and the organic cause and degree of involvement, but may combine physical therapy, the use of braces, or tendon transfer surgery.

THE PONSETI METHOD

Conservative management of non-neurogenic, congenital pes cavus (clubfoot) may include using physical therapy, stretching of tight muscles (including the typically tight gastrocnemius and soleus), and using specialized footwear or orthotic devices. In infants and children, these methods have been used in conjunction with the *Ponseti method*,[52,62,159,179,231] based on the original work of Ignacio V. Ponseti, a Spanish orthopedic surgeon who did much of his work at the University of Iowa. This highly respected method of treatment typically requires a series of five to seven plaster casts applied to the relatively malleable clubfoot of the infant, with each successive cast holding the foot in a position closer to a neutral position.[12] The application of the casts and the gentle (and very specific) manipulation of the foot need to be performed by a trained individual because this process requires knowledge of the anatomy and basic pathokinesiology of the clubfoot.[9,111,276] In addition, a percutaneous tenotomy of the tightened Achilles tendon is typically required. The success of this relatively conservative method of treatment is predicated on the prolonged nightly use of an "external rotation" (Denis Browne type) brace to maintain the correction. In more severe or complicated cases, extensive surgery may be indicated if the conservative approaches by trained personal are unsuccessful.

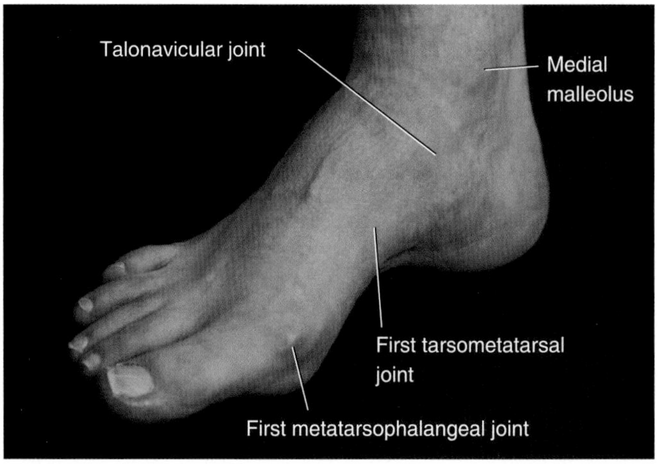

Pes cavus

Talonavicular joint

Medial malleolus

First tarsometatarsal joint

First metatarsophalangeal joint

FIG. 14.30 A photograph of a right foot of a man with idiopathic pes cavus.

Clinicians have developed a host of relatively simple measurements to help determine the structural severity of pes planus. In addition to the navicular drop test described earlier, other measures include the medial longitudinal arch angle, the Achilles tendon angle, rearfoot angle, and the popular 6-item *Foot Posture Index*.[17,119,277] Although clinically very useful, these static measurements lack the accuracy and sophistication to fully capture the three-dimensional and dynamic mechanics of the foot during locomotion. Such measurements typically require a gait laboratory equipped to measure the ambulating person's "center of pressure" across the plantar surface of the foot (Chapter 15), ground reaction force, instantaneous height of the medial longitudinal arch, and the eversion and inversion kinematics at the subtalar joint as well as kinematics in other regions of the lower limb. This information can help determine the functional impact that different severities of pes planus may have on the local tissues in the foot and, indirectly, on other regions of the body. Although such an elaborate gait measurement system is typically not available in most clinical settings, the data produced in laboratory settings may be very enlightening. For example, the medial longitudinal arch may appear flat while standing, but certain muscular or kinematic adjustments made while walking may compensate for some of the potential deleterious effects of the pes planus. These natural compensations may partially explain why some healthy persons with pes planus exhibit no painful symptoms while walking.[99] The compensations may, however, be exceptions rather than the rule; when studied across a very large population, pes planus and excessive foot pronation while walking are considered risk factors for developing stress-related, painful conditions in the low back and lower limb.[130,167,199,277]

COMBINED ACTION OF THE SUBTALAR AND TRANSVERSE TARSAL JOINTS

When the foot is *unloaded* (i.e., not bearing weight), pronation twists the sole of the foot outward, whereas supination twists the sole of the foot inward. While the foot is under load during the stance phase of walking, however, pronation and supination permit the *leg-and-talus* to rotate in all three planes relative to a comparatively fixed calcaneus. This important mechanism is orchestrated primarily through an interaction among the subtalar joint, transverse tarsal joint, and medial longitudinal arch.

In the healthy foot, the medial longitudinal arch rises and lowers cyclically throughout the gait cycle. During most of the stance phase, the arch *lowers slightly* in response to the progressive loading of body weight (Fig. 14.31A).[19] Structures that resist the lowering of the arch absorb stress as the foot is progressively compressed by body weight. This load attenuation mechanism offers essential protection to the foot and lower limb against stress-related, overuse injury.[83,269]

During the first 30% to 35% of the gait cycle, the subtalar joint pronates (everts), adding an element of flexibility to the midfoot (see Fig. 14.31B).[44] By late stance, the arch rises sharply as the now supinating subtalar joint adds rigidity to the midfoot.[19] The rigidity prepares the foot to support the large load produced at the peak of the push off phase. The ability of the foot to repeatedly transform from a flexible and shock-absorbent structure to a more rigid lever during each gait cycle is one of the most important and clinically relevant actions of the foot. As subsequently described, the subtalar joint is the principal joint that directs the pronation and supination kinematics of the foot.

Early to Mid Stance Phase of Gait: Kinematics of Pronation at the Subtalar Joint

Immediately after the heel contact phase of gait, the dorsiflexed talocrural joint and slightly supinated subtalar joint rapidly plantar flex and pronate, respectively (see Figs. 14.19 and 14.31B).[44,195] Although the data plotted in Fig. 14.31B show only about 4 degrees of movement toward eversion (pronation) between 0% and 30% of the gait cycle, other data sources using asymptomatic subjects (with normal medial arch heights) report values in the range of 5 to 9 degrees.[32,106,248,263] Differences in defining the 0-degree position of the subtalar joint, dissimilar sample sizes and foot types, and the varying measurement techniques account for much of this inconsistency within the literature. For this reason, it is often difficult to specifically define "abnormal" eversion (pronation) during walking.

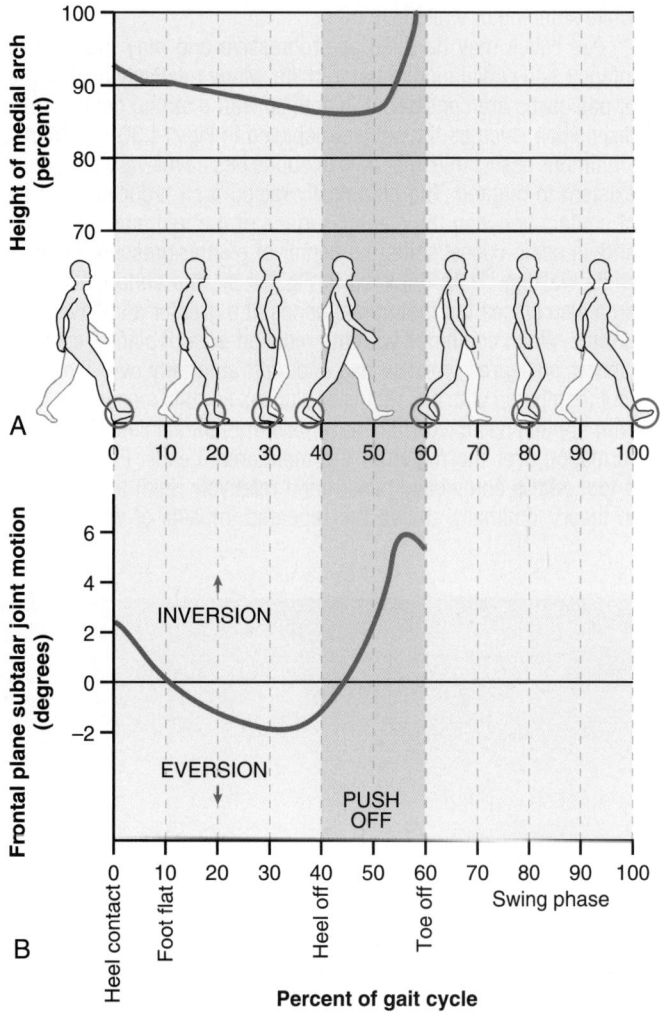

FIG. 14.31 (A) The percent change in height of the medial longitudinal arch throughout the stance phase (0%–60%) of the gait cycle. On the vertical axis, the 100% value is the height of the arch when the foot is unloaded during the swing phase. (B) Plot of frontal plane range of motion at the subtalar joint (i.e., inversion and eversion of the calcaneus) throughout the stance phase. The 0-degree reference for frontal plane motions is defined as the position of the calcaneus (observed posteriorly) while a subject stands at rest. The push off phase of walking is indicated by the darker shade of purple.

The pronation (eversion) at the subtalar joint during stance occurs primarily by two mechanisms. First, the calcaneus tips into slight eversion in response to the ground reaction force passing upward and just lateral to the midpoint of the posterior calcaneus. The simultaneous impact of heel contact also pushes the head of the talus medially in the horizontal plane and inferiorly in the sagittal plane. Relative to the calcaneus, this motion of the talus abducts and (slightly) dorsiflexes the subtalar joint. These motions are consistent with the formal definition of pronation. A loosely articulated skeletal model aids in the visualization of this motion. Second, during the early to mid stance phase, the tibia and fibula, and to a lesser extent the femur, internally rotate after initial heel contact.[203,205] Because of the embracing configuration of the talocrural joint, *the internally rotating lower leg steers the subtalar joint into further pronation.* An argument may be made that with the calcaneus in contact with the ground, pronation at the subtalar joint causes, rather than follows, internal rotation of the leg; either perspective is valid.

The amplitude of pronation at the subtalar joint during the early to mid stance phase of walking is indeed relatively small, occurring for only one-quarter of a second during average-speed walking. The amount and the speed of the pronation nevertheless influence the kinematics of the more proximal joints of the lower extremity, especially the hip.[131] These effects can be readily appreciated by exaggerating and dramatically slowing the pronation action of the rearfoot during the initial loading phase of gait. Consider the demonstration depicted in Fig. 14.32. While standing over a loaded and fixed foot, forcefully but slowly *internally rotate* the entire lower limb and observe the associated pronation at the subtalar joint and simultaneous lowering of the medial longitudinal arch. If sufficiently forceful, this action also tends to internally rotate, slightly flex, and adduct the hip and create a valgus stress on the knee (Table 14.5). These mechanical events are indeed exaggerated and do not all occur to this degree and pattern during walking at normal speed. Nevertheless, because of the linkages throughout the lower limb, excessive or uncontrolled pronation of the subtalar joint could exaggerate one or more of these mechanically related joint actions. Clinically, a person who excessively pronates during early stance, for example, may complain of medial knee pain, possibly from excessive valgus stress placed on the knee. This type of inter-joint relationship is important because it can aid in the design of strengthening exercises for the lower limb and for the use of orthotics to limit excessive or poorly controlled subtalar joint pronation.[66,267]

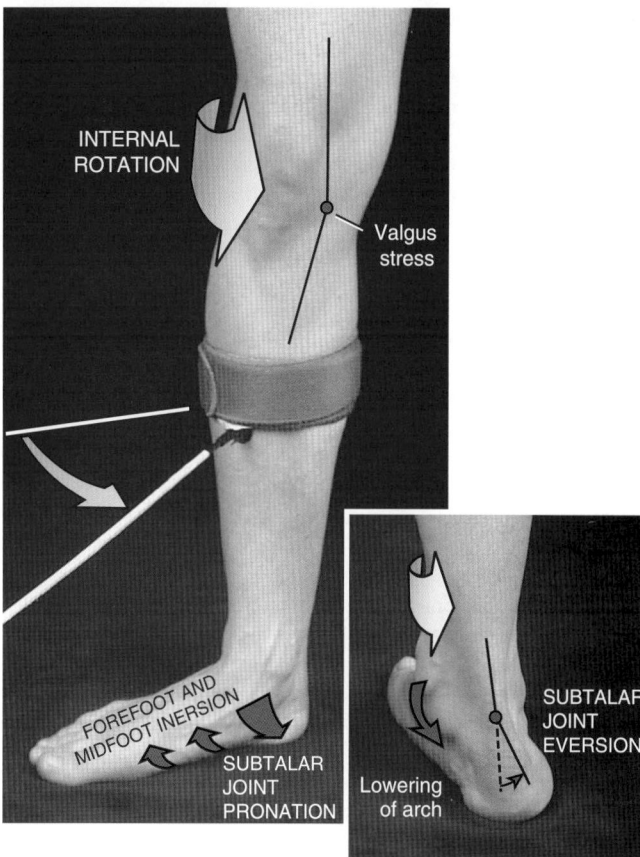

FIG. 14.32 With the foot firmly planted to the ground, full and vigorous *internal rotation* of the lower limb is mechanically associated with subtalar joint pronation (eversion as seen from behind), lowering of the medial longitudinal arch, and valgus stress at the knee. Note that as the subtalar joint strongly pronates, the floor "pushes" parts of the forefoot and midfoot upwards towards inversion.

 SPECIAL FOCUS 14.4

Example of the Kinematic Versatility of the Foot

Earlier in this section, the point was made that pronation of the *unloaded* foot occurs primarily as a summation of pronation across both the subtalar and the transverse tarsal joints (see Fig. 14.26B). This kinematic summation changes, however, when the foot is under the load of body weight. In this case the pronating subtalar joint causes components of the midfoot and forefoot, when receiving firm upward counterforce from the floor, to ultimately twist toward *inversion* (see Fig. 14.32). This reciprocal kinematic relationship between the rearfoot and the more anterior region of the foot demonstrates the versatility of the foot, either amplifying the other region's action when the foot is partially or fully unloaded (as shown in Fig. 14.26B) or counteracting the other region's action when the foot is firmly loaded (see Fig. 14.32). The exact details of these reciprocal kinematics are variable and may depend on several factors, including the firmness of the walking surface (e.g., pavement versus soft sand), walking velocity, and the natural resting posture of the foot (i.e., pes planus, cavus, or rectus).

Joint or Region	Action
Hip	Internal rotation, flexion, and adduction
Knee	Increased valgus stress
Subtalar joint	Pronation (eversion) with a lowering of medial longitudinal arch
Midfoot and forefoot	Inversion as a response to the upward counterforce from the ground

TABLE 14.5   **Selected Actions Associated with Exaggerated Pronation of the Subtalar Joint during Weight-Bearing**

Biomechanical Benefits of Controlling Pronation during the Stance Phase

A controlled and limited amount of pronation of the subtalar joint through the mid stance phase of walking has useful biomechanical effects. Pronation at the subtalar joint permits the talus and entire lower extremity to rotate internally slightly *after* the calcaneus has contacted the ground.[32] The strong horizontal orientation of the facets at the subtalar joint certainly facilitates this action. Without such a joint mechanism, the plantar surface of the calcaneus would otherwise "spin" like a child's top against the walking surface, along with the internally rotating leg. Eccentric activation of supinator muscles, mainly the tibialis posterior, can help decelerate the pronation and resist the lowering of the medial longitudinal arch. Controlled pronation of the subtalar joint favors relative flexibility of the midfoot, allowing the foot to accommodate to the varied shapes and contours of walking surfaces.

Biomechanical Consequences of Excessive Pronation during the Stance Phase

Innumerable examples exist on how malalignment within the foot affects the kinematics of walking. One common scenario results from excessive, prolonged, or poorly controlled pronation at the subtalar joint (rearfoot) during the stance phase. As a consequence, the path of the center of plantar pressure falls more medially on the sole of the foot than in a normal arch.[99] After many repetitions of the gait cycle, cumulative stress may build within the medial foot resulting in local inflammation and pain. Stressed local regions of the foot include the plantar fascia, talonavicular joint (keystone of the medial arch), and tibialis posterior tendon.[167]

The pathomechanics of pes planus may include weakness of muscles throughout the lower extremity, laxity or weakness in the mechanisms that normally support and control the medial longitudinal arch, or abnormal shape or mobility of the tarsal bones.[178]

Regardless of cause, the rearfoot falls into excessive valgus (eversion) after heel contact, in some cases doubling the normal amount.[263] Excessive subtalar joint pronation may be a compensation for excessive or restricted motion throughout the lower extremity, particularly in the frontal and horizontal planes.

Paradoxically, one of the most common structural deformities within an overpronated foot is a relatively fixed *rearfoot varus*. (Varus describes a segment of the foot that is *inverted* toward the midline.) As a response to rearfoot varus, the subtalar joint often overcompensates by excessively pronating, in speed and/or magnitude, to ensure that the medial aspect of the forefoot contacts the ground during the stance phase.[164,205] Similar compensations may occur with a *forefoot varus* deformity. Whether the forefoot varus deformity causes or results from excessive pronation of the rearfoot is not always clear.

As described previously, excessive rearfoot pronation is typically associated with excessive (horizontal plane) internal rotation of the talus-and-leg during walking.[205] Such a movement may create a "chain reaction" of kinematic disturbances and compensations throughout the entire limb, such as those depicted in Fig. 14.32.[241] For example, as described in Chapter 13, an abnormal kinematic sequence between the tibia and femur may alter the contact area at the patellofemoral joint, potentially increasing contact pressure at this joint.[267] For these reasons, clinicians often note the position of the subtalar joint while the patient stands and walks as part of an evaluation for a mechanical cause of patellofemoral joint pain or other overuse syndromes throughout the lower limb, including the hip and spine.[72,241]

The underlying pathomechanics of excessively pronated feet are a concern for both running and non–running populations. Repetitive impact from high-intensity and high-volume running and marching is a risk factor for sustaining a stress fracture, most often

SPECIAL FOCUS 14.5

The Use of a Foot Orthosis for Controlling Excessive Pronation

Varying levels of evidence exist that support the therapeutic value of using a foot orthosis for persons with pes planus or other conditions that cause excessive pronation during walking or running.[6,71,133,181,210] Evidence is even stronger for using a foot orthosis as a preventive measure, such as to reduce the frequency of overuse injuries in the lower limb from high-intensity physical training, typically experienced by military recruits.[39,72] Overuse injuries often reported to be associated with excessive rearfoot pronation include inflammation of the iliotibial tract, medial tibial stress syndrome, patellofemoral pain syndrome, plantar fasciitis, tibial posterior tendinopathy, stress fractures, and Achilles and patellar tendinopathy.[13,36,72,267,277]

In its basic form, a pronation-controlling orthosis incorporates medial wedging (or posting) in specific regions of the foot and a contoured in-step that fits inside of a shoe. In simple terms, the orthosis "brings the floor up to the foot." Orthoses may be prefabricated or highly customized to accommodate the unique shape of the foot, body weight, and arch dynamics.[72,157] It is not possible to unequivocally state which type of orthosis is most effective given its many design options and clinical uses.[39,72,184,220,243] Each type likely has its advantages and disadvantages as far as cost and function.

A properly fit and well-designed foot orthosis can reduce peak subtalar joint pronation during standing, walking, and running by an average of about 2 degrees.[37] This kinematic change does not however necessarily explain *how* the orthosis moderates existing painful syndromes or prevents overuse injuries throughout the lower limb. Perhaps a foot orthosis reduces the force or strain demands on muscles or tendons (such as the tibialis posterior or Achilles tendon), optimizes the alignment of the bones and joints, produces a subtle change in the kinematic sequencing in the joints proximal to the foot, or simply provides physical support to the plantar medial aspect of the foot.[26,60,183] Although not thoroughly understood, it is likely that the therapeutic benefit arises as a combination of these and other unidentified factors.[22,64,147,151,209]

As an adjunct to using a foot orthosis to control excessive pronation, clinicians typically advocate for increasing the strength and control of the intrinsic and extrinsic muscles of the foot.[6] Greater control over the muscles that decelerate pronation and other associated motions mechanically linked to pronation (such as those listed in Table 14.5) may reduce the rate of loading of tissues throughout the lower limb. Some of these extrinsic muscles include the supinators of the foot (notably the tibialis posterior) and the more proximal external rotators and abductors of the hip.

involving the navicular and tibia.[27,94,172] Research on civilian female distance runners has shown that those with a history of a previous tibial stress fracture exhibit greater rearfoot eversion during the stance phase while running compared with a control group.[173] Whether the excessive eversion at heel contact ultimately caused the increased likelihood of having a stress fracture cannot be stated with certainty, although the possibility should be considered.

In summary, the pathomechanics of overpronation can involve many dynamic kinematic relationships within the joints of the foot and between the foot and the joints in the lower limb and low back region.[168,176] The origin of the pathomechanics may be related to interactions between the hip and knee (described in Chapter 13) and expressed distally as impairments at the subtalar joint. Even if the pathomechanics are obviously located within the foot, abnormal motion in the forefoot may be compensated by abnormal motion in the rearfoot and vice versa. Furthermore, extrinsic factors, such as footwear, orthotics, terrain, and speed or cadence of walking and running alter the kinematic relationships within the foot and lower extremity. An understanding of the complex kinesiology of the entire lower extremity is a definite prerequisite for the effective treatment of the painful or misaligned foot.

Mid-to-Late Stance Phase of Gait: Kinematics of Supination at the Subtalar Joint

At about 15% to 20% into the gait cycle, the entire stance limb begins to gradually reverse its direction of motion from internal to external rotation.[109,203,205] The external rotation commences roughly at the beginning of the swing phase of the contralateral lower extremity. With the stance foot securely planted, external rotation of the femur, followed by the tibia, gradually reverses the horizontal plane direction of the talus from *internal to external* rotation. As a result, at about 30% to 35% into the gait cycle, the pronated (everted) subtalar joint starts to move sharply toward supination (inversion) (see Fig. 14.31B). As demonstrated by the exaggerated movement depicted in Fig. 14.33, with the subtalar joint supinating, parts of the midfoot and forefoot twist toward eversion to ensure that the medial side of the foot remains in contact with the ground. By late stance, the supinated subtalar joint and the elevated and tensed medial longitudinal arch help convert the midfoot (and ultimately the forefoot) into a more rigid lever. Muscles such as the gastrocnemius and soleus use this stability to transfer forces from the Achilles tendon, through the midfoot, to the metatarsal heads during the push off phase of walking or running.

A person who, for whatever reason, remains excessively pronated late into stance phase may have difficulty stabilizing the midfoot at a time when it is naturally required.[165] Consequently, excessive activity may be required from extrinsic and intrinsic muscles of the foot to reinforce the medial longitudinal arch. Over time, hyperactivity may lead to generalized muscle fatigue and painful "overuse" syndromes throughout the lower limb and foot.

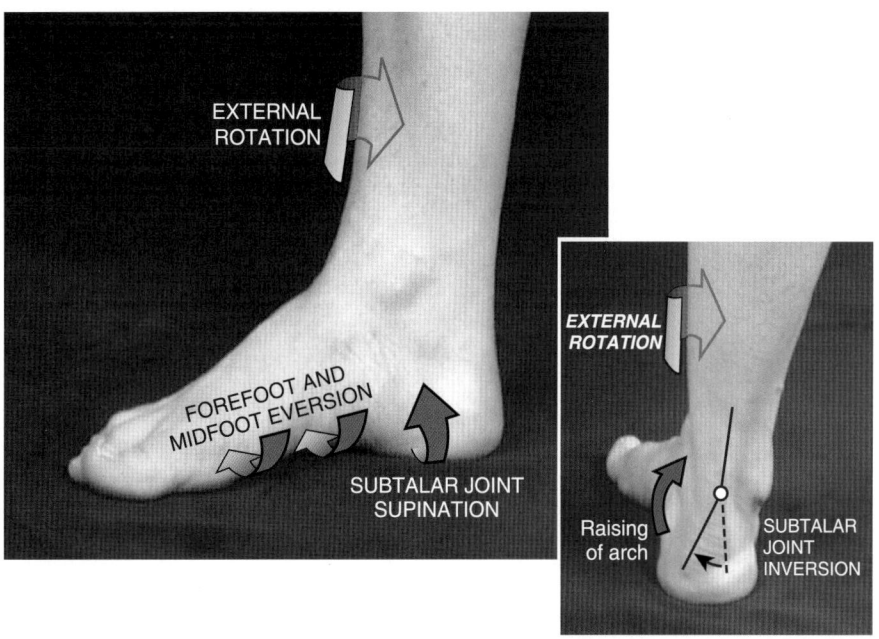

FIG. 14.33 With the foot firmly planted to the ground, an exaggerated and full *external rotation* of the weight-bearing lower limb demonstrates the kinematic association between subtalar joint supination (inversion as seen from behind) and a raising of the medial longitudinal arch. Note that as the subtalar joint supinates, the forefoot and midfoot region twist toward eversion to keep the medial side of the foot in contact with the ground.

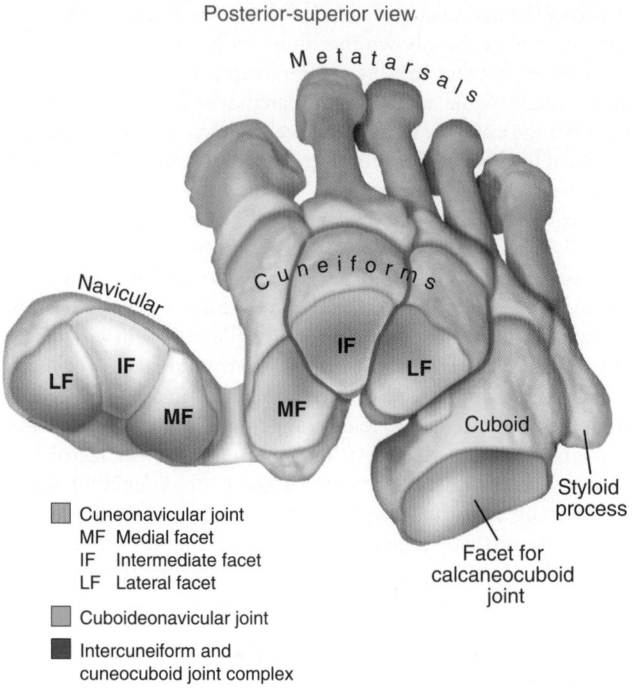

Posterior-superior view

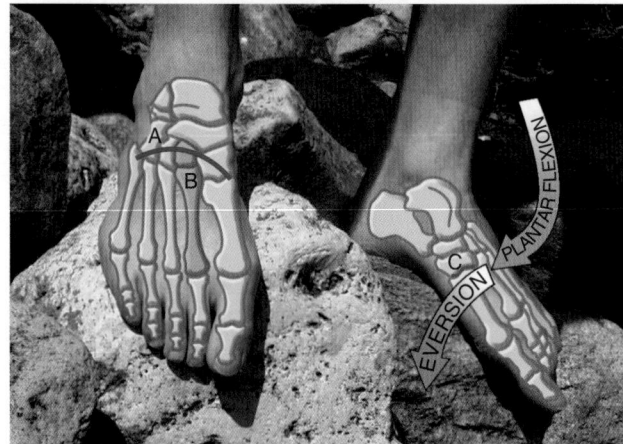

FIG. 14.34 A posterior-superior view of the right foot is shown with the talus and calcaneus removed. The navicular bone has been flipped medially, exposing its anterior surface and the many articulations within the *distal intertarsal joints*. Articular surfaces have been color coded as follows: *cuneonavicular joint in light purple*, the small *cuboideonavicular joint in green*, and the *intercuneiform and cuneocuboid joint complex in blue*. Replacing the navicular to its natural position would join the three sets of articular facets within the cuneonavicular joint—medial facet *(MF)*, intermediate facet *(IF)*, and lateral facet *(LF)*. Replacing the navicular would also rearticulate the cuboideonavicular joint *(green)*.

DISTAL INTERTARSAL JOINTS

The distal intertarsal joints are a collection of three joints or joint complexes, each located within the midfoot (review Fig. 14.23). The articular surfaces of the distal intertarsal joints are shown exposed and color coded in Fig. 14.34.

Basic Structure and Function

As a group, the distal intertarsal joints (1) assist the transverse tarsal joint in pronating and supinating the midfoot and (2) provide stability across the midfoot by forming the transverse arch of the foot. Motions at these joints are small and typically not specifically measured clinically.

Cuneonavicular Joint

Three articulations are formed between the anterior side of the navicular and the posterior surfaces of the three cuneiform bones (see Fig. 14.34, purple). Plantar and dorsal ligaments surround these articulations. The slightly concave facets (lateral, intermediate, and medial) on each of the three cuneiforms fit into one of three slightly convex facets on the anterior side of the navicular. The major function of the cuneonavicular joint is to help transfer components of pronation and supination distally from the talonavicular toward the forefoot.

Cuboideonavicular Joint

The small synarthrodial (fibrous) or sometimes synovial cuboideonavicular joint is located between the lateral side of the navicular and a proximal region of the medial side of the cuboid (see Fig. 14.34, green). This joint provides a smooth contact point between the lateral and medial longitudinal columns of the foot. Observations on cadaver specimens show that the articular surfaces slide slightly against each other during movements of the midfoot, most notably during inversion and eversion.

Intercuneiform and Cuneocuboid Joint Complex

The intercuneiform and cuneocuboid joint complex consists of three articulations: two between the set of three cuneiforms and one between the lateral cuneiform and medial surface of the cuboid (see Fig. 14.34, blue). Articular surfaces are nearly flat and aligned nearly parallel with the long axis of the metatarsals. Plantar, dorsal, and interosseous ligaments strengthen this set of articulations.

The intercuneiform and cuneocuboid joint complex forms the *transverse arch* of the foot (Fig. 14.35A). This arch provides direct transverse stability to the midfoot. Under the load of body weight, the transverse arch depresses slightly, allowing body weight to be shared across all five metatarsal heads. Theoretical experiments suggest that the transverse arch also indirectly provides longitudinal stability to the foot, similar to the way slightly curling a sheet of paper in its transverse direction increases its longitudinal stiffness.[257]

The transverse arch receives support from intrinsic muscles, extrinsic muscles such as the tibialis posterior and fibularis longus, connective tissues, and the keystone of the transverse arch: the intermediate cuneiform (see *IF* in Fig. 14.34).

FIG. 14.35 Structural and functional features of the midfoot and forefoot. (A) The transverse arch is formed by the intercuneiform and cuneocuboid joint complex. (B) The stable second ray is reinforced by the recessed second tarsometatarsal joint. (C) Combined plantar flexion and eversion of the left tarsometatarsal joint of the first ray allow the forefoot to better conform to the surface of the rock.

TARSOMETATARSAL JOINTS

Anatomic Considerations

The tarsometatarsal joints are frequently called *Lisfranc's joints*, after Jacques Lisfranc, a French field surgeon in Napoleon's army who described an amputation in this region of the foot. As a group, the five tarsometatarsal joints separate the midfoot from the forefoot (review Fig. 14.23). The joints consist of the articulation between the bases of the metatarsals and the distal surfaces of the three cuneiforms and cuboid. Specifically, the first (most medial) metatarsal articulates with the medial cuneiform, the second with the intermediate cuneiform, and the third with the lateral cuneiform. The bases of the fourth and fifth metatarsals both articulate with the distal surface of the cuboid.

The articular surfaces of the tarsometatarsal joints are generally flat, although the medial two show slight, irregular curvatures. Dorsal, plantar, and interosseous ligaments add stability to these articulations. Only the first tarsometatarsal joint has a well-developed capsule.[233]

Kinematic Considerations

The tarsometatarsal joints form the base of the forefoot. Mobility is least at the second and third tarsometatarsal joints, in part because of strong ligaments and the wedged position of the base of the second ray between the medial and lateral cuneiforms (see Fig. 14.35B). Consequently, the second and third rays produce an element of longitudinal stability throughout the foot, similar to the second and third rays in the hand. This stability is useful in late stance as the forefoot prepares for the dynamics of push off.

Overall mobility is greatest in the first, fourth, and fifth tarsometatarsal joints, most notably in the first (most medial) joint.[46,74] During the early to mid stance phase of walking, the first tarsometatarsal joint (base of the forefoot) *dorsiflexes* about 5 degrees.[43,54] This motion occurs as body weight depresses the cuneiform region downward as the ground simultaneously pushes the distal end of the first ray upward. This movement is associated with a gradual lowering of the medial longitudinal arch—a previously described mechanism that absorbs part of the stress of body weight acting on the foot. At the late stance (push off) phase of gait, however, the first tarsometatarsal joint rapidly *plantar flexes* about 5 to 15 degrees.[36,43] The plantar flexion of the first ray, controlled in part by pull of the fibularis longus, effectively "shortens" the medial forefoot slightly, thereby helping to raise the medial longitudinal arch. This mechanism increases the stability of the arch (and medial column of the foot) at a time in the gait cycle when the midfoot and forefoot are under higher loads.

Most literature describes a natural mechanical coupling of the kinematics at the first tarsometatarsal joint: specifically, *plantar flexion occurs with slight eversion* and *dorsiflexion with slight inversion*.[84,85,137] Such passive mobility does indeed occur naturally when assessed in a non–weight-bearing condition (Fig. 14.36). Although these movement combinations do not fit the standard definitions of pronation or supination, they nevertheless provide useful functions. Combining plantar flexion and eversion, for example, allows the medial side of the foot to better conform around irregular surfaces on the ground (see Fig. 14.35C). (This motion of the first metatarsal is generally similar to the movement of the thumb metacarpal as the pronated hand grasps a large spherical object.)

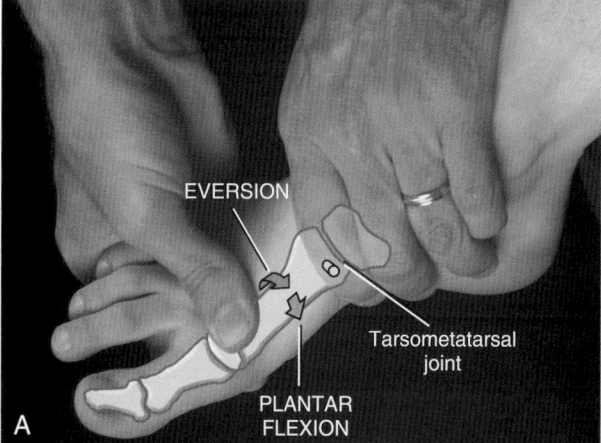

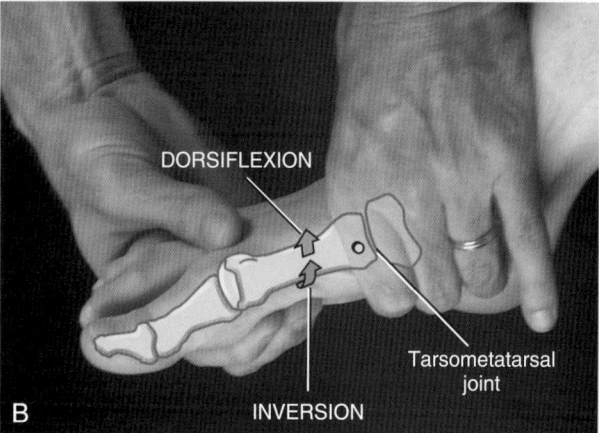

FIG. 14.36 The osteokinematics of the first tarsometatarsal joint. Plantar flexion occurs with slight eversion (A), and dorsiflexion occurs with slight inversion (B).

INTERMETATARSAL JOINTS

Structure and Function

Plantar, dorsal, and interosseous ligaments interconnect the bases of the four lateral metatarsals. These points of contact form three small intermetatarsal synovial joints. Although interconnected by ligaments, a true joint does not typically form between the bases of the first and second metatarsals. This lack of articulation increases the relative movement of the first ray, in a manner like the hand. Unlike in the hand, however, the deep transverse metatarsal ligaments interconnect the distal end of all five metatarsals. Slight motion at the intermetatarsal joints augments the flexibility at the tarsometatarsal joints.

METATARSOPHALANGEAL JOINTS

Anatomic Considerations

Five metatarsophalangeal joints are formed between the convex head of each metatarsal and the shallow concavity of the proximal end of each proximal phalanx (see Fig. 14.23). These joints are located about 2.5 cm proximal to the "web spaces" of the toes. With the joints flexed, the prominent heads of the metatarsals are easily palpable on the dorsum of the distal foot.

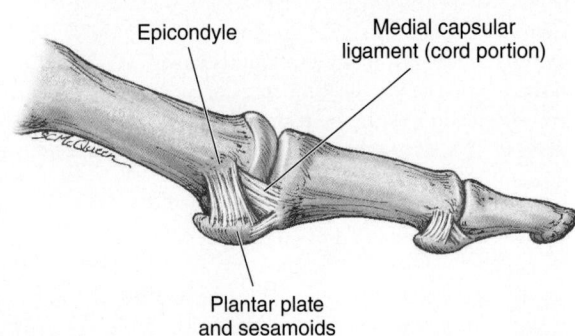

Epicondyle

Medial capsular
ligament (cord portion)

Plantar plate
and sesamoids

FIG. 14.37 A medial view of the first metatarsophalangeal joint showing the cord and accessory portions of the medial (collateral) capsular ligament. The accessory portion attaches to the plantar plate and sesamoid bones. (Redrawn from Haines R, McDougall A: Anatomy of hallux valgus, *J Bone Joint Surg Br* 36:272, 1954.)

Articular cartilage covers the distal end of each metatarsal head (Fig. 14.37). A pair of *collateral ligaments* spans each metatarsophalangeal joint, blending with and reinforcing the capsule. As in the hand, each collateral ligament courses obliquely from a dorsal-proximal to a plantar-distal direction, forming a thick cord portion and a fanlike accessory portion.

The accessory portion attaches to the thick, dense *plantar plate* located on the plantar side of the joint. The plate, or ligament, is grooved for the passage of flexor tendons. Fibers from the deep plantar fascia attach to the plantar plates and sheaths of the flexor tendons. Two *sesamoid bones* located within the tendon of the flexor hallucis brevis rest against the plantar plate of the first metatarsophalangeal joint (Fig. 14.38). Connective tissue attachments between the sesamoid bones and the collateral ligaments help stabilize the position of the pair of bones relative to the head of the first metatarsal bone. Although not depicted in Fig. 14.38, four deep *transverse metatarsal ligaments* blend with and join the adjacent plantar plates of all five metatarsophalangeal joints. By interconnecting all five plates, the transverse metatarsal ligaments help maintain the first ray in a similar plane as the lesser rays, thereby adapting the foot for propulsion and weight-bearing rather than manipulation. In the hand, the deep transverse metacarpal ligament connects only the fingers, freeing the thumb for opposition.

A *fibrous capsule* encloses each metatarsophalangeal joint and blends with the collateral ligaments and plantar plates. A poorly defined *dorsal digital expansion* covers the dorsal side of each metatarsophalangeal joint. This structure (analogous to the extensor mechanism in the digits of the hand) consists of a thin layer of connective tissue that is essentially inseparable from the dorsal capsule and extensor tendons.

Kinematic Considerations

Movement at the metatarsophalangeal joints occurs in two degrees of freedom. *Extension* (dorsiflexion) and *flexion* (plantar flexion) occur approximately in the sagittal plane about a medial-lateral axis; *abduction* and *adduction* occur in the horizontal plane about a vertical axis. The second digit serves as the reference digit for naming the movements of abduction and adduction of the toes. (The reference digit for naming abduction and adduction in the hand is the third or middle digit.) The axes of rotation for all volitional movements of the metatarsophalangeal joints pass through the center of each metatarsal head.

Superior view

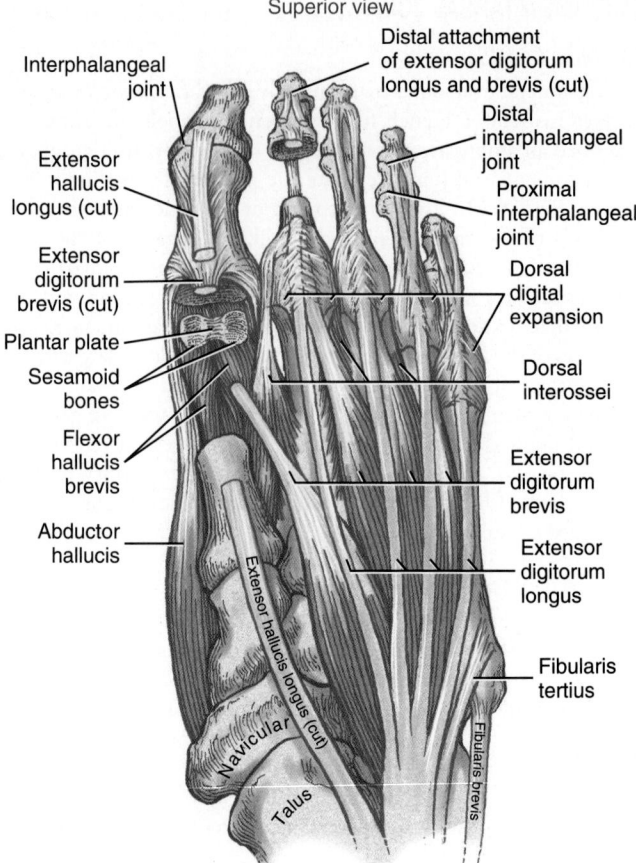

Interphalangeal joint

Extensor hallucis longus (cut)

Extensor digitorum brevis (cut)

Plantar plate

Sesamoid bones

Flexor hallucis brevis

Abductor hallucis

Distal attachment of extensor digitorum longus and brevis (cut)

Distal interphalangeal joint

Proximal interphalangeal joint

Dorsal digital expansion

Dorsal interossei

Extensor digitorum brevis

Extensor digitorum longus

Fibularis tertius

Extensor hallucis longus (cut)

Fibularis brevis

Navicular

Talus

FIG. 14.38 Muscles and joints of the dorsal surface of the right forefoot. The distal half of the first metatarsal is removed to expose the concave surface of the first metatarsophalangeal joint. A pair of sesamoid bones is located deep within the first metatarsophalangeal joint. The proximal phalanx of the second toe is removed to expose the concave side of the proximal interphalangeal joint.

Most people demonstrate limited dexterity in active movements at the metatarsophalangeal joints, especially in abduction and adduction. From a neutral position, the toes can be passively extended about 65 degrees and flexed about 30 to 40 degrees. The great toe typically allows greater extension, to near 85 degrees.[255] This magnitude of extension is readily apparent as one stands up on "tiptoes."

Arthritis, Trauma, and Deformities Involving the Metatarsophalangeal Joint of the Great Toe
Hallux Rigidus

Hallux rigidus, or "limitus" in its less severe form, describes a chronic, degenerative condition of the great toe with marked restrictions in passive extension of the metatarsophalangeal joint.[45,79] The disorder typically presents with degenerative changes on x-ray (e.g., osteophytes, subchondral sclerosis, and reduced joint space), swelling, and pain with movement. Although the condition is associated with osteoarthritis and advanced age, the pathophysiology remains poorly understood.

The reduced and painful extension of the great toe can significantly impact walking. Normally, walking requires about 40 to 50 degrees of extension at the first metatarsophalangeal joint as the heel rises at late stance phase.[36] A person with hallux rigidus may not have this amount of toe extension and therefore may attempt to avoid extending their toe by walking on the outer surface of the affected foot or by walking with the foot pointed outward and "rolling over" the medial arch of the foot. Without this gait modification, plantar pressure and associated discomfort may increase considerably under the hallux.[255] Other modifications used to "protect" this potentially sensitive region include wearing stiff-soled shoes (or stiff inserts placed within the shoes) and avoiding inclines or declines. Physical therapy has been shown to be effective in restoring range of motion and reducing pain.[222]

Turf Toe

Turf toe describes an acute injury to the plantar aspect of the metatarsophalangeal joint of the great toe, typically involving athletes participating in cutting and pivoting contact sports.[156] The term *turf toe* originated in the 1960s after an increase in toe injuries in American football players resulting from the replacement of natural grass with artificial turf and the use of lighter-weight shoes.[25] In American football, running backs, quarterbacks, and receivers are most affected because of their need to accelerate while rapidly changing running directions.[81]

The most common mechanism of injury for turf toe involves severe *hyperextension* of the metatarsophalangeal joint of the great toe, often involving contact with another player. When severe, the forceful hyperextension may tear the plantar plate, intrinsic muscles, or tendon of the flexor hallucis longus; dorsally dislocate the joint; and fracture the sesamoid bones.[156,188] A severe injury can be career ending for an elite athlete. Painful or limited extension of the great toe after injury significantly interferes with walking and running, and limits the effectiveness of the windlass mechanism (described ahead) to stabilize the medial longitudinal arch. If unresolved and chronic, the injury may progress to posttraumatic osteoarthritis and hallux rigidus.[79,81]

Hallux Valgus

The central feature of *hallux valgus* (or bunion) is a progressive lateral deviation of the great toe relative to the midline of the body. Although the deformity appears to involve primarily the metatarsophalangeal joint, the pathomechanics of hallux valgus usually involve the entire first ray (Fig. 14.39A–B). As depicted in the radiograph, hallux valgus is typically associated with excessive *adduction* of the first metatarsal (defined in this case relative to the *body* and not the second digit) about its tarsometatarsal joint.[84] The adducted position of the first metatarsal can eventually lead to lateral dislocation of the metatarsophalangeal joint, thereby completely exposing the metatarsal head as a lump or "bunion." The deformed metatarsophalangeal joint often becomes inflamed and painful, and potentially osteoarthritic.[193] If the proximal phalanx laterally deviates more than about 30 degrees, the proximal phalanx often begins to evert about its long axis. The bunion deformity is also referred to as "hallux abducto-valgus" to account for the deviations in both horizontal and frontal planes.

The progressive medial deviation (adduction) of the first metatarsal coupled with the axial rotation of the laterally deviated proximal phalanx of the hallux creates a muscular imbalance in the forces that normally align the metatarsophalangeal joint.[8,193] The abductor hallucis muscle (normally located *medial* to the first metatarsophalangeal joint) may gradually shift toward the plantar side of the joint. The subsequent unopposed pull of the adductor hallucis and lateral head of the flexor hallucis brevis progressively increases the lateral deviation posture of the proximal phalanx. As the lateral deviation of the hallux progresses, the tendons of the flexor and extensor hallucis longus may become displaced lateral to the vertical axis at the metatarsophalangeal joint. Forces in these tendons therefore create an additional valgus torque to the underlying joint. In time, the overstretched medial collateral ligament and capsule may weaken or rupture, removing the primary source of reinforcement to the medial side of the joint. The deformity also positions the pair of sesamoids laterally relative the metatarsophalangeal joint (see Fig. 14.39B).

Persons with marked hallux valgus typically limit placing weight over the first metatarsophalangeal joint while walking, causing the lateral metatarsal bones to accept a greater proportion of the load.[127] The pathomechanics of marked hallux valgus involve a zigzag-like collapse of the first ray, like the "ulnar drift" of the metacarpophalangeal joint in the hand with rheumatoid arthritis (see Chapter 8).

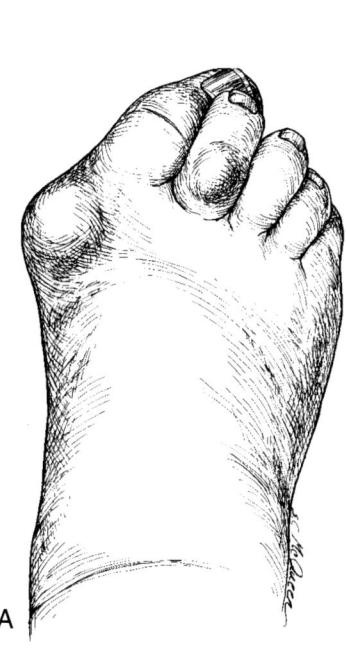
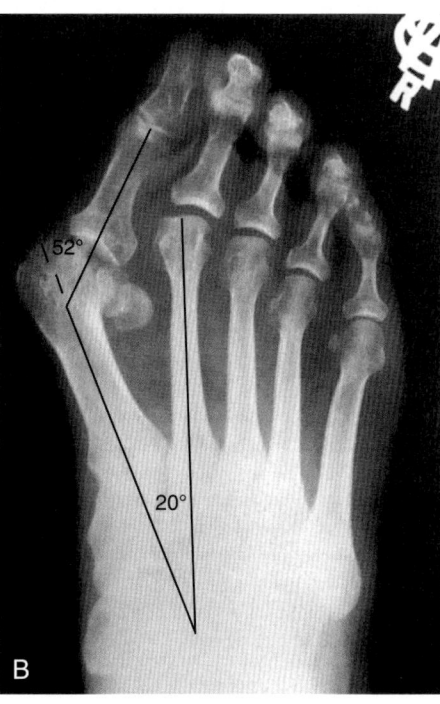

FIG. 14.39 Hallux valgus. (A) Multiple features of hallux valgus (bunion) and associated deformities. (B) Radiograph shows the following pathomechanics often associated with hallux valgus: (1) adduction of the first metatarsal (toward the midline of the body), evidenced by the increased angle between the first and second metatarsal bones (normally 11 degrees[84]); (2) lateral deviation of the proximal phalanx (normally <15 degrees[84]) with dislocation or subluxation of the first metatarsophalangeal joint; (3) visible lateral sesamoid between first and second metatarsals; (4) displacement of the lateral sesamoid; (5) rotation (eversion) of the phalanges of the great toe; and (6) exposed first metatarsal head, forming the so-called bunion. (A, From Richardson EG: Disorders of the hallux. In Canale ST, Beaty JH: *Campbell's operative orthopaedics,* vol 4, ed 11, St Louis, 2008, Mosby; B, From Richardson EG: Disorders of the hallux. In Canale ST, Beaty JH: *Campbell's operative orthopaedics,* vol 4, ed 12, St Louis, 2012, Mosby.)

Although the cause and underlying pathomechanics of hallux valgus are not completely understood, several factors appear to be associated with either the initiation or the progression of the disorder. Some of these factors include genetics, sexual dimorphism, incorrect footwear,[193] abnormal alignment of the lower limb,[235] excessive rearfoot valgus and associated altered axis of rotation at the base of the first ray,[84] excessive pronation (eversion) of the first ray,[49] tightness of the Achilles tendon,[193] pes planus,[10] and instability of the base of the first ray.[46] The full spectrum of severe hallux valgus often includes dislocation and osteoarthritis of the metatarsophalangeal joint, metatarsus varus, valgus (lateral deviation) of the great toe, bunion formation (and bursitis) over the medial metatarsophalangeal joint, hammer toe of the second digit, calluses, and metatarsalgia.

A meta-analysis indicates moderate level evidence that wearing a foot orthosis can reduce pain and that Botox injections can reduce the magnitude of the hallux valgus deformity.[108] Surgical intervention is often indicated in cases of marked deformity with continued pain.

INTERPHALANGEAL JOINTS

As in the fingers, each toe has a *proximal interphalangeal* and a *distal interphalangeal joint*. The great toe, being analogous to the thumb, has only one *interphalangeal joint*.

All interphalangeal joints of the foot possess similar anatomic features. The joint consists of the convex head of the more proximal phalanx articulating with the concave base of the more distal

phalanx. The proximal phalanx of the second toe is removed in Fig. 14.38 to expose the concave side of the proximal interphalangeal joint. The structure and function of the connective tissues at the interphalangeal joints are generally like those described for the metatarsophalangeal joints. Collateral ligaments, plantar plates, and capsules are present but smaller and less defined.

Mobility at the interphalangeal joints is limited primarily to flexion and extension. The amplitude of flexion generally exceeds extension, and motion tends to be greater at the proximal than the distal joints. Extension is limited primarily by passive tension in the toe flexor muscles and plantar ligaments.

ACTION OF THE JOINTS ASSOCIATED WITH THE FOREFOOT DURING THE LATE STANCE PHASE OF GAIT

The joints of the forefoot include all articulations associated with each ray, from the tarsometatarsal joint to the distal interphalangeal joints of the toe. Depending on the phase of gait, these joints provide an element of flexibility or stability to the foot.

At the end of stance phase, the midfoot and forefoot must become relatively stable to accept the relative stress associated with the push off phase of walking. In addition to activation of the intrinsic and extrinsic muscles (notably the tibialis posterior), a rising of the medial longitudinal arch further stabilizes the foot.[115,128] One of the primary mechanisms used to lift the arch has been historically described as the "windlass mechanism" which can be demonstrated by standing on tiptoes (Fig. 14.40A).[10] Because of the attachments between the deep plantar

Normal foot
Foot with pes planus

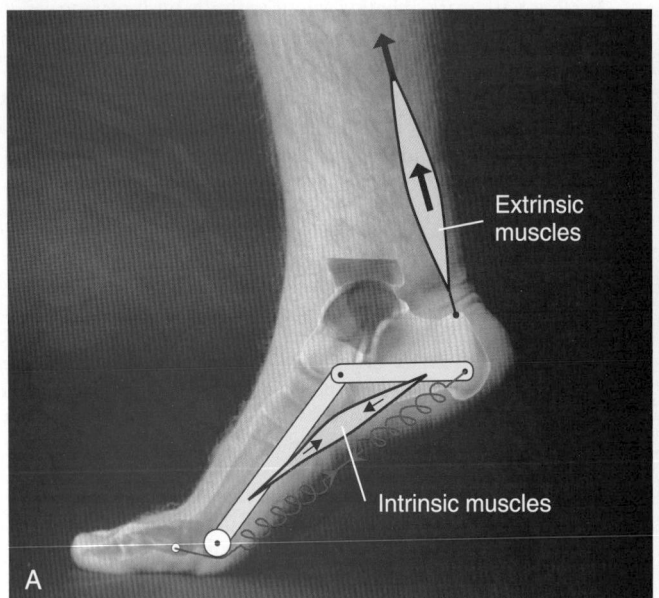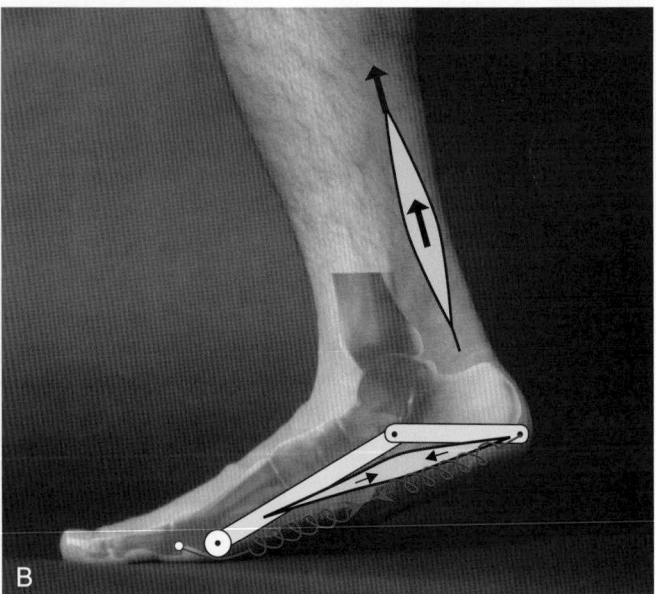

FIG. 14.40 The windlass mechanism of the plantar fascia is demonstrated while a subject stands on tiptoes. (A windlass is a hauling or lifting device consisting of a rope wound around a cylinder that is turned by a crank. The rope is analogous to the plantar fascia, and the cylinder is analogous to the metatarsophalangeal joint.) (A) In the normal foot, contraction of the extrinsic plantar flexor muscles lifts the calcaneus, thereby transferring body weight forward over the metatarsal heads. The resulting extension of the metatarsophalangeal joints (shown collectively as the white disk) stretches (or winds up) the plantar fascia within the medial longitudinal arch (red spring). The increased tension from the stretch raises the arch and strengthens the midfoot and forefoot. Contraction of the intrinsic muscles provides additional reinforcement to the arch. (B) The foot with pes planus (flat foot) typically has a poorly supported medial longitudinal arch. During an attempt to stand up on tiptoes, the forefoot sags under the load of body weight. The reduced extension of the metatarsophalangeal joints limits the usefulness of the windlass mechanism. Even with strong activation of the intrinsic muscles, the arch remains flattened with an unstable midfoot and forefoot.

fascia and the toes, extension of the metatarsophalangeal joints increases the tension throughout the medial longitudinal arch. The increased tension is used to stabilize the arch as the metatarsophalangeal joints are naturally extended during the push off phase of walking.[128] As the heel and most of the foot are lifted by contraction of the plantar flexor muscles, body weight shifts anteriorly toward the more medial metatarsal heads. Local fat pads reduce potentially damaging stress to the bone, and the sesamoid bones protect the long flexor tendon of the great toe. Once stabilized by the stretched plantar fascia and reinforced arch, the second and third rays function as relatively rigid levers capable of withstanding the large bending moments created by the contracting gastrocnemius and soleus muscles. The tensile force within the stretched plantar fascia during very late stance has been estimated to be near 100% of body weight.[63] Failure of the plantar fascia to transmit this force from the calcaneus to the base of the toes would limit the effectiveness of the windlass mechanism in raising the arch. This, indeed, is often observed by noting the guarded or ineffective manner of "push off" in a person who has had a plantar fasciotomy or is experiencing painful plantar fasciitis.

In contrast to the healthy foot, consider the pathomechanics that may be involved as a person with pes planus attempts to stand up on "tiptoes" (see Fig. 14.40B). Although the individual has no neuromuscular pathology, there is significant loss in the lift of the heel, even on maximal muscular effort. With a structurally weakened medial longitudinal arch, the unstable, unlocked midfoot and forefoot sag under body weight. The lack of "lift" of the metatarsals (relative to the toes) reduces the extension at the metatarsophalangeal joints, lessening the ability to fully engage the windlass mechanism. Supporting the arch through appropriate anti-pronation orthotics, footwear, or taping may allow greater metatarsophalangeal joint extension during push off, therefore enhancing the ability of the windlass mechanism to stiffen the plantar fascia. This mechanism may partially explain how this intervention may reduce the risk of injuries associated with overpronation.[26,72,145,267]

This concluding section on kinematics closes with Table 14.6, which summarizes important kinematics of the ankle and foot across the entire stance phase.

MUSCLE AND JOINT INTERACTION

Innervation of Muscles and Joints

INNERVATION OF MUSCLES

Extrinsic muscles of the ankle and foot have their proximal attachments in the leg, and a few extend as far proximal as the femur. Intrinsic muscles, in contrast, have both their proximal and distal attachments within the foot.

TABLE 14.6 Important Actions of the Ankle and Foot During the Stance Phase of Walking

Joint or Region	Early Stance Action	Desired Function	Mid to Late Stance Action	Desired Function
Talocrural joint	Plantar flexion	Allows rapid foot contact with the ground	Continued dorsiflexion followed by rapid plantar flexion	Produces a stable mortise (ankle) to accept body weight, followed by thrust needed for push off
Subtalar joint	Pronation and lowering of the medial longitudinal arch	Permits internal rotation of lower limb; Allows the foot to function as a shock absorber; Produces a pliable midfoot	Continued pronation changing to supination, followed by a raising of the medial longitudinal arch	Permits external rotation of lower limb; Converts the midfoot to a rigid lever for push off
Midfoot and Forefoot	Inversion as a response to an upward counterforce from the ground	Allows full extent of pronation at the subtalar joint	Eversion	Allows the medial side of the foot to maintain contact with the ground
Metatarsophalangeal joint	Insignificant	—	Extension	Through the windlass mechanism, raises the medial longitudinal arch and stabilizes the midfoot and forefoot for push off

The extrinsic muscles are arranged in three compartments of the leg: anterior, lateral, and posterior. A different motor nerve innervates the muscles within each compartment (see cross-sections in Figs. 14.41 and 14.42). Each motor nerve is a branch of the sciatic nerve, formed from the L^4–S^3 spinal nerve roots of the sacral plexus.

Lateral to the head of the fibula, the common fibular (peroneal) nerve (L^4–S^2) divides into a deep and a superficial branch (see Fig. 14.41). The *deep branch of the fibular nerve* innervates the muscles within the *anterior compartment*: the tibialis anterior, extensor digitorum longus, extensor hallucis longus, and fibularis (peroneus) tertius. The deep branch continues distally to innervate the extensor digitorum brevis (an intrinsic muscle located within the dorsum of the foot). It also supplies sensory innervation to a triangular area of skin in the web space between the first and second toes. The *superficial branch of the fibular nerve* innervates the fibularis longus and fibularis brevis within the lateral compartment. The nerve then continues distally as a sensory nerve to much of the skin on the dorsal and lateral aspects of the leg and foot.

The *tibial nerve* (L^4–S^3) and its terminal branches innervate the remainder of the extrinsic and intrinsic muscles of the foot and ankle (see Fig. 14.42). The muscles within the *posterior compartment* are divided into superficial and deep sets. The *superficial* set includes the calf muscles: the gastrocnemius and soleus (together known as the *triceps surae*) and the small plantaris. The *deep* set includes the tibialis posterior, flexor hallucis longus, and flexor digitorum longus. As the tibial nerve approaches the medial side of the ankle, it sends a sensory branch to the skin over the heel.

Just posterior to the medial malleolus, the tibial nerve bifurcates into the *medial plantar nerve* (L^4–S^2) and the *lateral plantar nerve* (L^5–S^3). The plantar nerves supply sensation to the skin on most of the plantar surface of the foot and motor innervation to all intrinsic muscles, except the extensor digitorum brevis. The general organization of the innervation of the intrinsic muscles of the foot is similar to that in the hand. The medial plantar nerve is analogous to the median nerve, whereas the lateral plantar nerve is analogous to the ulnar nerve.

The spinal nerve roots that supply the muscles of the lower extremity are listed in Appendix IV, Part A. Part B of this appendix

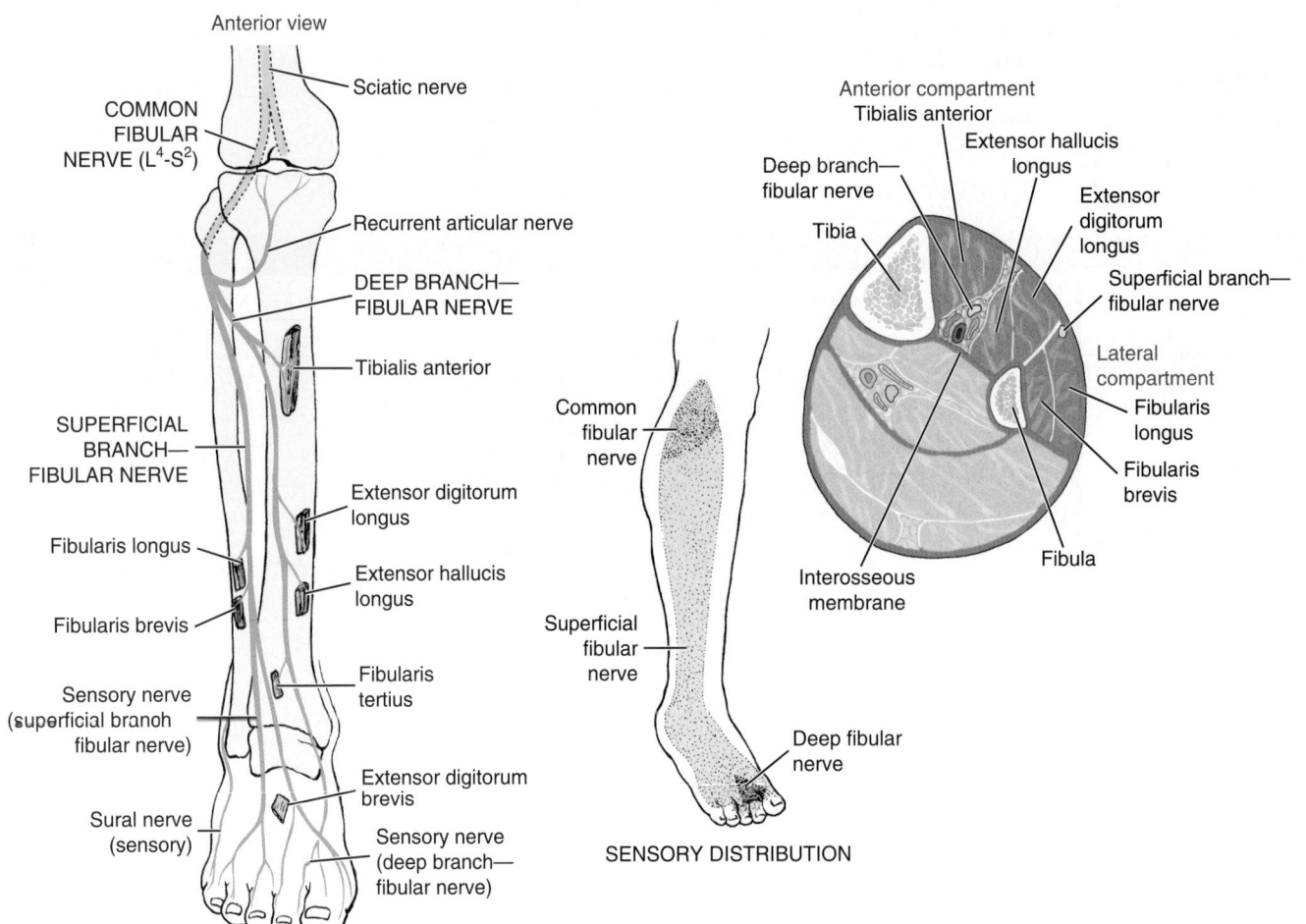

FIG. 14.41 The path and general proximal-to-distal order of muscle innervation for the deep and superficial branches of the *common fibular (peroneal) nerve*. The primary spinal nerve roots are in parentheses. The sensory distribution of this nerve (and its branches) is highlighted along the dorsal-lateral aspect of the leg and foot. The dorsal "web space" of the foot is innervated solely by sensory branches of the deep branch of the fibular nerve. The cross-section highlights the muscles and nerves located within the anterior and lateral compartments of the leg. (Modified with permission from deGroot J: *Correlative neuroanatomy*, ed 21, Norwalk, Conn, 1991, Appleton & Lange.)

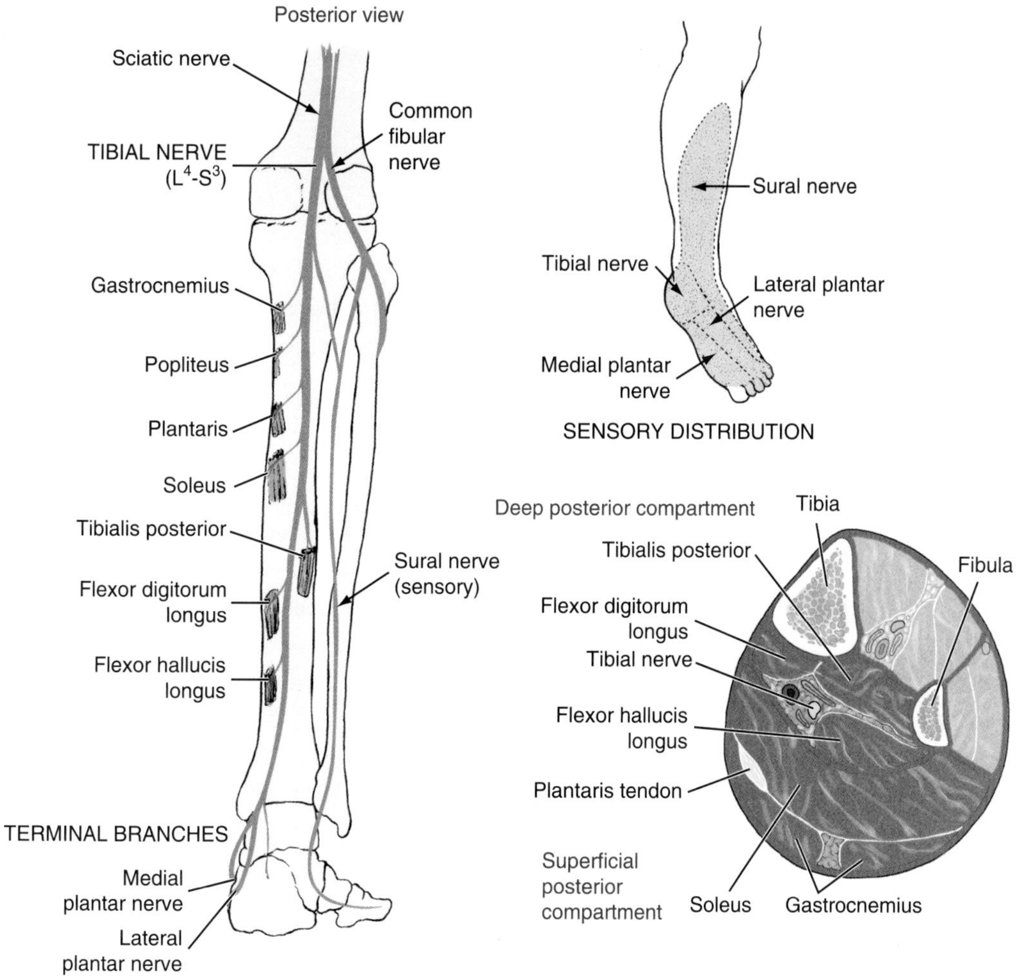

FIG. 14.42 The path and general proximal-to-distal order of muscle innervation for the *tibial nerve* and its branches. The primary spinal nerve roots are in parentheses. The sensory distribution of this nerve is highlighted along the lateral and plantar aspects of the leg and foot. The cross-section highlights the muscles and nerves located within the deep and superficial parts of the posterior compartment of the leg. (Modified with permission from deGroot J: *Correlative neuroanatomy*, ed 21, Norwalk, Conn, 1991, Appleton & Lange.)

lists key muscles typically used to test the functional status of the L^2–S^3 spinal nerve roots. Part C shows a dermatome map of the lower extremity.

SENSORY INNERVATION OF THE JOINTS

The *talocrural joint* receives sensory innervation from the deep branch of the fibular nerve. In general, the sensory innervation to the other joints of the foot is supplied by nerve branches that cross the region. Each major joint receives multiple sources of sensory innervation, traveling to the spinal cord primarily through S^1 and S^2 nerve roots.[233]

Anatomy and Function of the Muscles

The muscles of the ankle and foot not only control the specific actions of the underlying joints but also provide the stability, thrust,

and shock absorption necessary for locomotion. Additional discussion of the muscular interactions during walking and running follows in Chapters 15 and 16.

Because all extrinsic muscles cross multiple joints, they possess multiple actions. Many of these actions are evident by noting where the tendons cross the axes of rotation at the talocrural and subtalar joints (see ahead in Fig. 14.43). Although Fig. 14.43 is oversimplified (by lacking the transverse tarsal joint as well as other components of pronation and supination of the foot), it nevertheless is a useful guide for understanding the actions of the extrinsic muscles.

Throughout the remainder of this chapter, it may be helpful to consult Appendix IV, Part D for a summary of the attachments and nerve supply to the muscles of the ankle and foot. Also, as a reference, a list of cross-sectional areas of selected muscles of these regions is provided in Appendix IV, Part E.

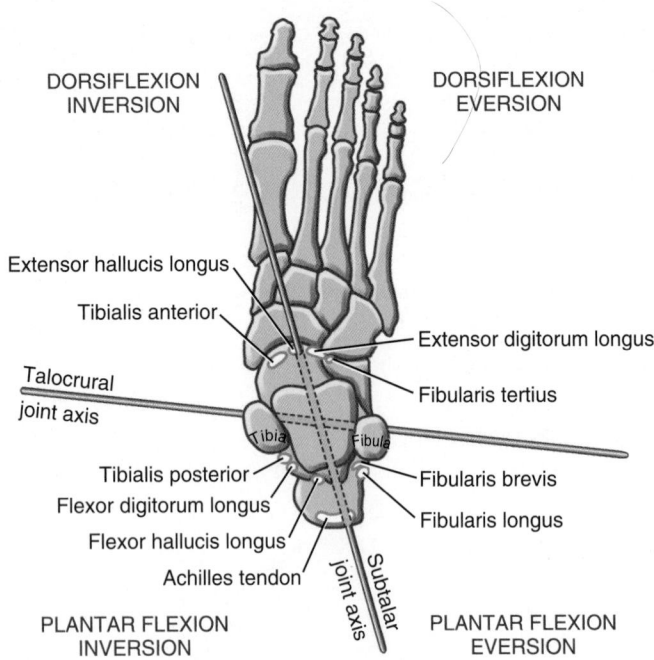

FIG. 14.43 The multiple actions of muscles that cross the talocrural and subtalar joints, as viewed from above. The actions of each muscle are based on its position relative to the axes of rotation at the joints. Note that the muscles have multiple actions.

EXTRINSIC MUSCLES

Anterior Compartment Muscles
Anatomy

The four muscles of the anterior compartment are listed in the box. As a group, these "pretibial" muscles have their proximal attachments on the anterior and lateral aspects of the proximal half of the tibia, the adjacent fibula, and the interosseous membrane (Fig. 14.44). The tendons of these muscles cross the dorsal side of the ankle, restrained by a synovial-lined *superior and inferior extensor retinaculum.* Located most medially is the prominent tendon of the *tibialis anterior,* coursing distally to attach to the medial-plantar surface of the first tarsometatarsal joint (Fig. 14.45). The tendon of the *extensor hallucis longus* passes just lateral to the tendon of the tibialis anterior as it courses toward the dorsal surface of the great toe (see Fig. 14.44). Progressing laterally across the dorsum of the ankle are the tendons of the *extensor digitorum longus* and the *fibularis tertius* (or "third" fibularis muscle). The four tendons of the *extensor digitorum longus* attach to the dorsal surface of the middle and distal phalanges via the dorsal digital expansion. The *fibularis tertius* is part of the extensor digitorum longus muscle and may be considered as this muscle's fifth tendon. The fibularis tertius attaches to the base of the fifth metatarsal bone.

Muscles of the Anterior Compartment of the Leg (Pretibial "Dorsiflexors")

MUSCLES
- Tibialis anterior
- Extensor digitorum longus
- Extensor hallucis longus
- Fibularis tertius

INNERVATION
- Deep branch of the fibular nerve

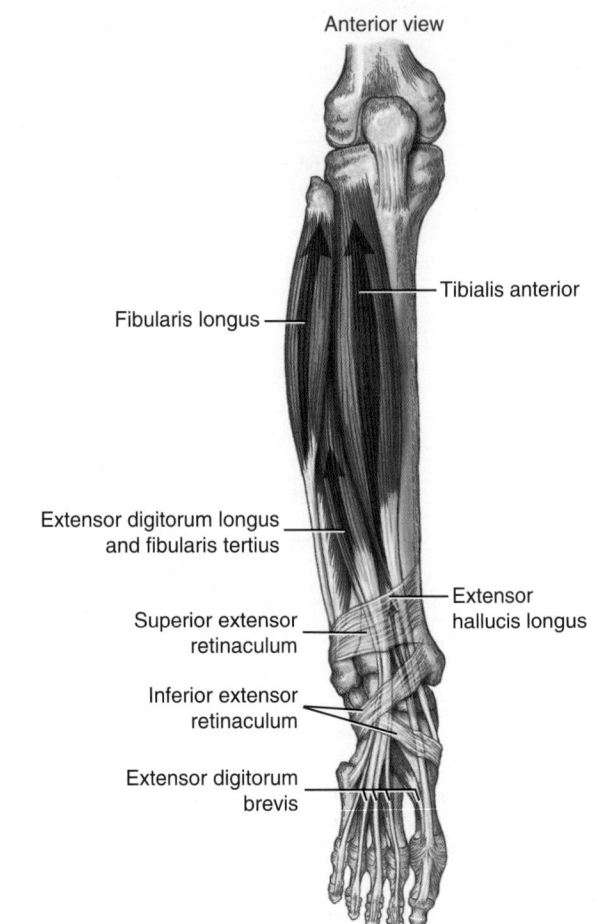

FIG. 14.44 The pretibial muscles of the leg: tibialis anterior, extensor digitorum longus, extensor hallucis longus, and fibularis tertius. All four muscles dorsiflex the ankle.

Joint Action

All four pretibial muscles are dorsiflexors because they cross anterior to the axis of rotation at the talocrural joint (see Fig. 14.43). From the anatomic position, the *tibialis anterior* also inverts the subtalar joint by passing medial to the axis of rotation. The tibialis anterior inverts and adducts the talonavicular joint, and, when the demand arises, supports the medial longitudinal arch.

The primary actions of the *extensor hallucis longus* are dorsiflexion at the talocrural joint and extension of the great toe. Inversion at the subtalar joint is negligible because of its small moment arm, at least when analyzed from the anatomic position. In addition to dorsiflexion of the ankle, the *extensor digitorum longus* and *fibularis tertius* evert the foot.

The previously stated muscular actions of the pretibial muscles assume that the muscles are activated while the joints in question are in the anatomic, or neutral, position. It is likely, however, that the potential torque (or possibly even action) of some of the muscles changes when the joints are positioned well *outside* the anatomic position. This change may have important functional implications. Consider, for example, that the inversion moment arms of the tibialis anterior or extensor hallucis longus would progressively increase with greater inversion (consult Fig. 14.43 as a visual guide).[196] Such a biomechanical scenario may at times be counterproductive, theoretically increasing the muscle's inversion torque potential at a time when evertor muscles (the fibularis longus and brevis) are attempting to resist this primary component of the classic inversion ankle sprain.[80,101]

Plantar view

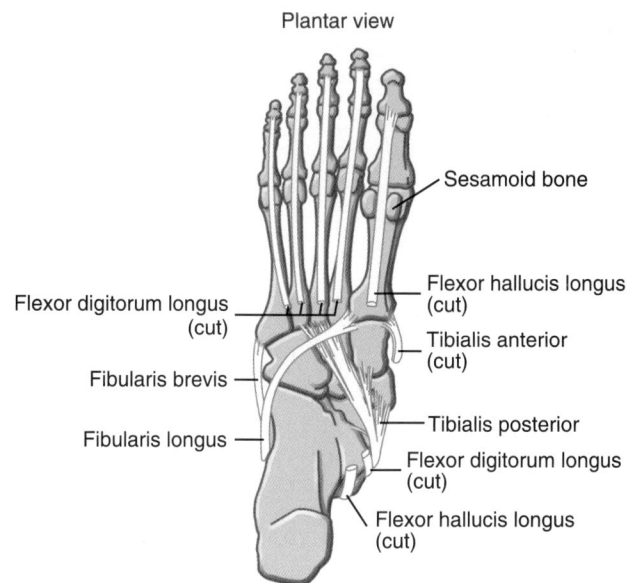

Sesamoid bone

Flexor digitorum longus
(cut)

Flexor hallucis longus
(cut)

Tibialis anterior
(cut)

Fibularis brevis

Fibularis longus

Tibialis posterior

Flexor digitorum longus
(cut)

Flexor hallucis longus
(cut)

FIG. 14.45 A plantar view of the right foot shows the distal course of the tendons of the fibularis longus, fibularis brevis, and tibialis posterior. The tendons of the tibialis anterior, flexor digitorum longus, and flexor hallucis longus are cut.

The pretibial muscles are most active during the early stance phase and again throughout the entire swing phase of gait (see Fig. 15.29, tibialis anterior). During early stance, the muscles are eccentrically active to control the rate of plantar flexion (i.e., the period between heel contact and foot flat; see Fig. 14.19). Controlled plantar flexion is necessary for a soft landing of the foot. Through continued eccentric activation, the tibialis anterior helps decelerate the lowering of the medial longitudinal arch and therefore indirectly helps to control pronation (eversion) of the subtalar rearfoot (review Fig. 14.31). During the swing phase, the pretibial muscles actively dorsiflex the ankle and extend the toes to ensure that the foot clears the ground.

The ability to actively dorsiflex the foot in the near sagittal plane requires an exacting balance of forces from the pretibial muscles. The eversion and/or abduction influence of the extensor digitorum longus and fibularis tertius must counterbalance the inversion and adduction influence of the tibialis anterior. With isolated paralysis of the tibialis anterior muscle, the ankle can still actively dorsiflex but would do so with an eversion-and-abduction bias.

Lateral Compartment Muscles
Anatomy
The fibularis longus and the fibularis brevis muscles (formerly called the *peroneus longus* and *peroneus brevis*, respectively) occupy the lateral compartment of the leg muscles (Fig. 14.46). Both muscles attach proximally along the lateral fibula. The tendon of the *fibularis longus*, the more superficial of the two, courses distally a remarkable distance. After wrapping around the posterior side of the lateral malleolus, the tendon enters the plantar side of the foot through a groove in the cuboid bone. The tendon then travels between the long and short plantar ligaments to its final distal attachment on the plantar-lateral aspect of the first tarsometatarsal joint (see Fig. 14.45). It is noteworthy that the fibularis longus and tibialis anterior attach on either side of the plantar surface first tarsometatarsal joint. This pair of muscles therefore provides a balanced kinetic stability to the base of the first ray.

Lateral view

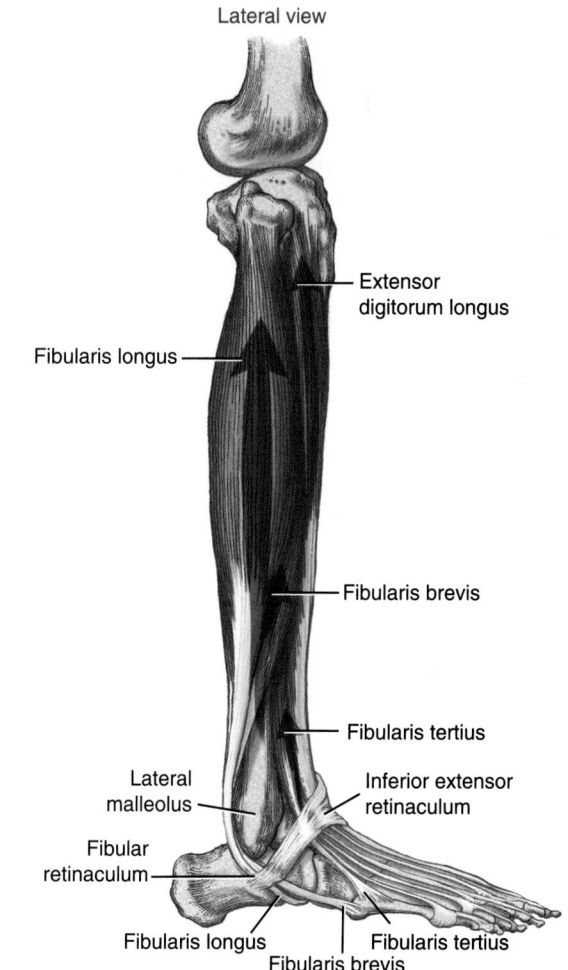

Extensor
digitorum longus

Fibularis longus

Fibularis brevis

Fibularis tertius

Lateral
malleolus

Inferior extensor
retinaculum

Fibular
retinaculum

Fibularis longus

Fibularis tertius

Fibularis brevis

FIG. 14.46 A lateral view of the muscles of the leg is shown. Note how both the fibularis longus and fibularis brevis (primary evertors) use the lateral malleolus as a pulley to change direction of muscular pull across the ankle.

Lateral Compartment of the Leg ("Evertors")
MUSCLES
- Fibularis longus
- Fibularis brevis

INNERVATION
- Superficial branch of the fibular nerve

The tendon of the *fibularis brevis* courses alongside the fibularis longus in a shallow groove on the posterior side of the distal fibula. More distally, both fibular tendons occupy the same synovial sheath as they pass under the *fibular retinaculum* (see Fig. 14.46). Just distal to the retinaculum, the tendon of the fibularis brevis separates from the fibularis longus tendon and courses toward its distal attachment on the styloid process of the fifth metatarsal. Frequently observed in dancers, the styloid process may experience an avulsion fracture after a very strong contraction of the fibularis brevis, often in response to a sudden and extreme inversion movement of the ankle or foot.

Joint Action

The *fibularis longus* and *fibularis brevis* muscles are the primary evertors of the foot (see Fig. 14.43).[160] These muscles provide the main source of active stability to the lateral side of the ankle. Reduced activation of these muscles has been reported as a risk factor for developing or perpetuating chronic ankle (inversion) instability.[58] For this reason, strengthening, conditioning, and coordination exercises involving these muscles are often designed for persons who may be vulnerable to inversion sprains, such as those who participate in playing basketball or volleyball.[101] Of interest, although the evertor muscles are very effective at resisting inversion, a purely reflexive muscular contraction in response to an unexpected inversion movement is typically too slow to prevent injury.[129] Other, more complex whole-body neuromuscular mechanisms are also required for this protection, likely those involving feed-forward or anticipatory responses to an impending inversion injury.

The fibularis longus and brevis have substantial moment arms for eversion across the subtalar joint—more than 2 cm.[121] The lateral malleolus, serving as a fixed pulley, routes the fibular tendons posterior to the axis of rotation at the talocrural joint. Both muscles therefore are also plantar flexors of the talocrural joint. Although not evident in Fig. 14.43, the fibularis longus and brevis also abduct the subtalar and transverse tarsal joints.

The distal attachment of the fibularis longus generates eversion torque as far anterior as the base of the medial forefoot. This is evident as the base of the first ray everts and depresses (plantar flexes) slightly during maximal-effort pronation of the unloaded foot. In addition, the fibularis longus stabilizes the first tarsometatarsal joint against the potent medial pull of the tibialis anterior. Without this stability, the first ray may migrate medially, potentially predisposing a person to a hallux valgus deformity.[193]

The fibularis longus and brevis are active throughout much of the stance phase of walking (see Fig. 15.29).[201,216] Although relatively small, the concentric activation of the fibularis longus at and immediately after heel contact may help control the kinematics of the pronating rearfoot, which are being simultaneously further controlled by the eccentric activation of the tibialis posterior and tibialis anterior. The fibularis muscles are at their highest level of activation throughout mid stance and push off, a time when the subtalar joint is supinating (inverting) and the dorsiflexing talocrural joint is changing its direction of movement toward plantar flexion (review Figs. 14.19 and 14.31).[182,201] An important function of the fibularis muscles during this phase of walking is to decelerate, and thus control, the rate and extent of the supinating subtalar joint. Furthermore, the active force within the fibularis longus helps to fixate the first ray securely to the ground, an action demonstrated by the everting forefoot in Fig. 14.33. With weakness, paralysis, or inhibition of the fibularis longus, the potent supination pull of the tibialis posterior on the forefoot is unopposed. As a result, the forefoot follows the rearfoot into supination, causing the person to walk on the lateral border of the foot, possibly increasing the likelihood of an inversion sprain.[101]

At very late stance phase, during push off, the fibularis longus and brevis muscles assist other muscles with plantar flexion at the talocrural joint. The lateral position of the fibularis muscles helps neutralize the strong inversion (supination) bias of the remaining active plantar flexors, including the tibialis posterior, and, to a limited degree, the gastrocnemius (and soleus). The necessity for

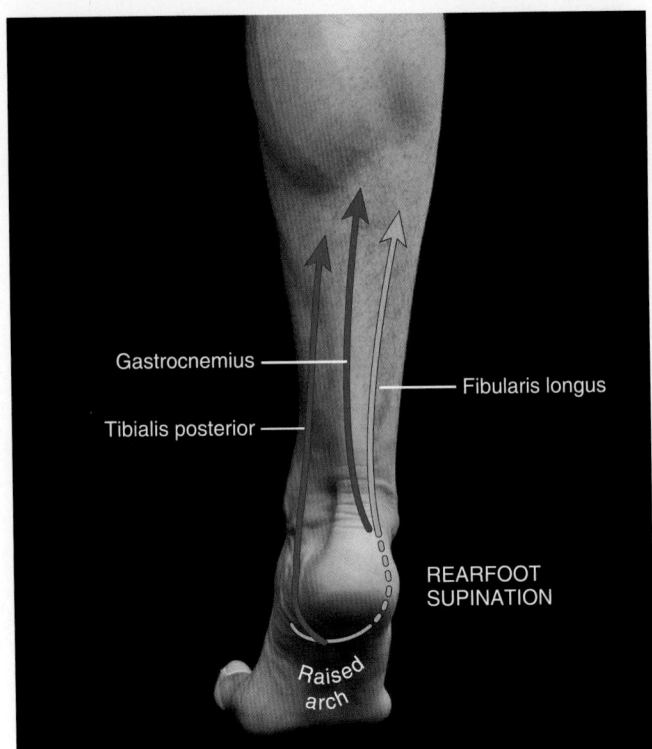

FIG. 14.47 The lines of force of several plantar flexor muscles while a subject rises on tiptoes. Note that the fibularis longus and tibialis posterior form a sling that supports the transverse and medial longitudinal arches. The pull of the gastrocnemius and tibialis posterior muscles causes a slight supination of the rearfoot, which adds further stability to the foot. (Invertor muscles are indicated by the *red arrows;* evertor muscle by the *green arrow.*)

balance of these muscle forces is shown as a person stands on tiptoes in Fig. 14.47. As the heel rises, the strongly activated fibularis longus and tibialis posterior muscles neutralize each other as they form a functional "sling" that supports the transverse and medial longitudinal arches. Usually, the net effect of this muscle interaction slightly supinates the unloaded rearfoot, which provides further stability to the medial longitudinal arch and more distal regions of the foot. This stability ensures that the plantar flexion torque required to stand on tiptoes (or propel the body upward and forward) is effectively transferred distally through the foot, toward the metatarsal heads.

Furthermore, as the heel is raised during the push off phase of walking, contraction of the fibularis muscles, especially the longus, helps transfer body weight from the lateral to the medial side of the forefoot. This action shifts body weight toward the opposite foot, which has just entered its early stance phase of gait.

Posterior Compartment Muscles

Anatomy

The muscles of the posterior compartment are divided into two groups. The *superficial group* includes the gastrocnemius, soleus (together known as the *triceps surae*), and plantaris (Fig. 14.48). The *deep group* includes the tibialis posterior, flexor digitorum longus, and flexor hallucis longus (see ahead Fig. 14.49).

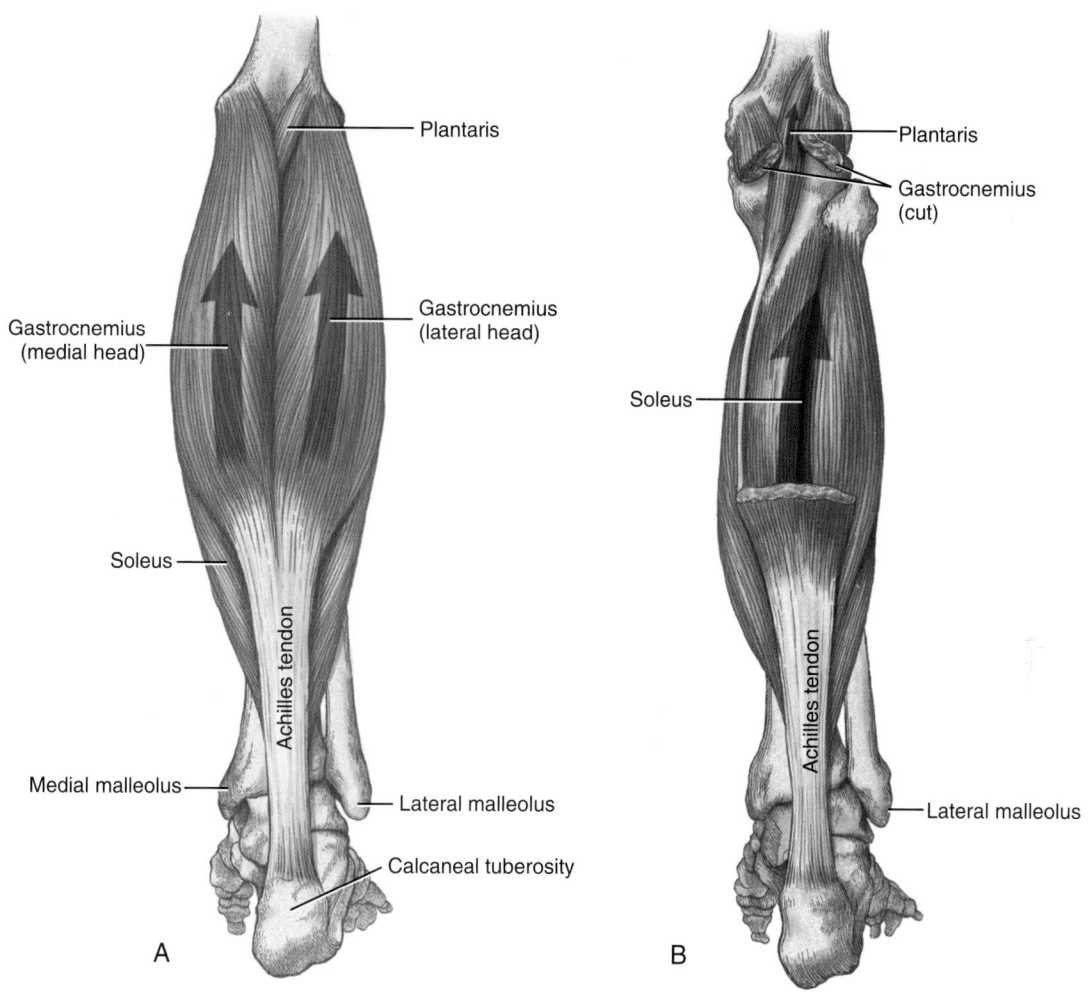

FIG. 14.48 The superficial muscles of the posterior compartment of the right leg are shown: (A) gastrocnemius; (B) soleus and plantaris.

<table><tr><td>

Muscles of the Posterior Compartment of the Leg
SUPERFICIAL GROUP ("PLANTAR FLEXORS")
- Gastrocnemius
- Soleus
- Plantaris

DEEP GROUP ("INVERTORS")
- Tibialis posterior
- Flexor digitorum longus
- Flexor hallucis longus

INNERVATION
- Tibial nerve
</td></tr></table>

Superficial Group. The *gastrocnemius* muscle forms the prominent belly of the calf. The medial and lateral heads of this muscle arise from the posterior sides of the medial and lateral femoral condyles. The larger, medial head joins the lateral head midway down the leg, blending with the *Achilles tendon*. The broad and thick *soleus* lies deep to the gastrocnemius, arising primarily from the posterior side of the proximal fibula and middle tibia. Although not immediately apparent through causal observation, the soleus has twice the cross-sectional area as the overlying gastrocnemius.[272] Like both heads of the gastrocnemius, the soleus blends with the Achilles tendon for a distal attachment to the calcaneal tuberosity. Each muscle within the triceps surae forms separate, twisted subtendons within the internal structure of the Achilles tendon.[239] Computational modeling suggests that the twisting of the subtendons is ideal for distributing stress through the Achilles tendon and for increasing its tensile strength.[91]

Realize that the gastrocnemius crosses the knee, but the soleus does not. For this reason, a more effective stretch can be applied to the gastrocnemius by combining knee *extension* with dorsiflexion.

The *plantaris* muscle arises from the lateral supracondylar line of the femur. The fusiform muscle belly is only 7 to 10 cm long, unusually small compared with the other muscles in the area. The plantaris has a very long, slender tendon that courses between the gastrocnemius and soleus, eventually fusing with the medial margin of the Achilles tendon.

Deep Group. The tibialis posterior, flexor hallucis longus, and flexor digitorum longus muscles are located deep to the soleus muscle (Fig. 14.49). As a group, these muscles arise from the posterior side of the tibia, fibula, and interosseous membrane. The more centrally located tibialis posterior muscle is framed and partially covered by the flexor hallucis longus laterally and the flexor digitorum longus medially. At their distal musculotendinous junctions, all

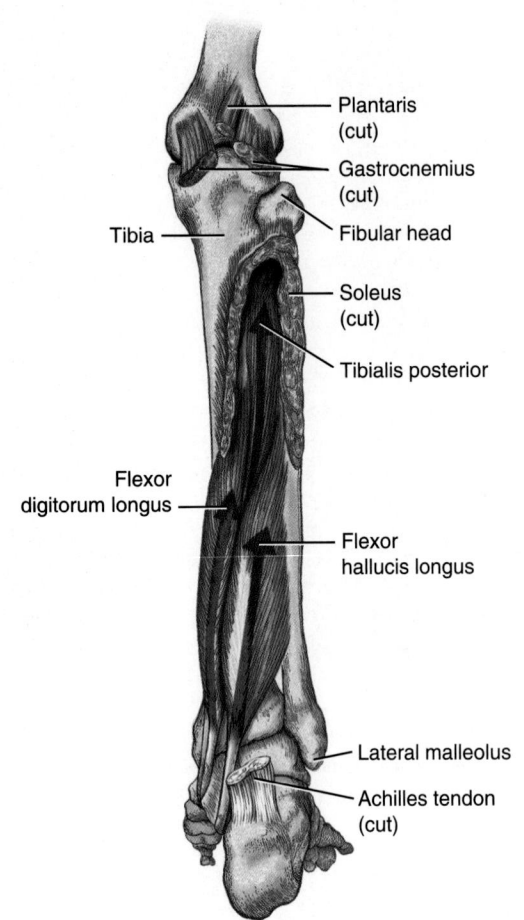

FIG. 14.49 The deep muscles of the posterior compartment of the right leg: the tibialis posterior, flexor digitorum longus, and flexor hallucis longus.

three muscles enter the plantar aspect of the foot from its medial side (see Fig. 14.45). The position of the tendons as they cross the ankle and foot explains the strong supination (inversion) component of these muscles, most notably the tibialis posterior (see Fig. 14.43).[121,196] The tibialis posterior, flexor digitorum longus, and tibial neurovascular bundle course through the *tarsal tunnel*, located just deep to the flexor retinaculum (Fig. 14.50). The tarsal tunnel is analogous to the carpal tunnel in the wrist. "Tarsal tunnel syndrome" (analogous to carpal tunnel syndrome) is characterized by entrapment of the tibial nerve beneath the flexor retinaculum and subsequent paresthesia over the plantar aspect of the foot.

The tendon of the *flexor hallucis longus* courses distally through the ankle in a groove formed between the tubercles of the talus and the inferior edge of the sustentaculum tali (see Fig. 14.12). Fibrous bands convert this groove into a synovial-lined sleeve, anchoring the position of the tendon. The deeper (lateral) position of the tendon relative to the tibialis posterior and flexor digitorum longus explains why the flexor hallucis longus is *not* a structure within the tarsal tunnel. Once in the plantar aspect of the foot, the tendon of the flexor hallucis longus eventually courses between the two sesamoid bones of the first metatarsophalangeal joint, finally attaching to the plantar side of the base of the distal phalanx of the great toe (see Fig. 14.45).

The tendon of the *flexor digitorum longus* courses distally across the ankle posterior to the medial malleolus. At about the level of the base of the metatarsals, the main tendon of the flexor digitorum longus divides into four smaller tendons, each attaching to the base of the distal phalanx of the lesser toes (see Fig. 14.45).

The tendon of the *tibialis posterior* muscle lies just anterior to the tendon of the flexor digitorum longus in a shared groove on the posterior side of the medial malleolus (see Fig. 14.50). The tendon of the tibialis posterior continues distally and passes deep to the flexor retinaculum but immediately superficial to the deltoid and spring ligaments. At this point, the main tendon divides into superficial and deep parts, attaching *to every tarsal bone except the talus*, and the bases of the more central metatarsal bones (see Fig. 14.45). The most prominent distal attachment of the tibialis posterior is on the plantar aspect of the navicular tuberosity. The main tendon is usually palpable for several centimeters just proximal to the navicular tuberosity during resisted adduction and inversion of the foot. The widespread netlike distal attachments of the tibialis posterior form a kinetic sling for supporting both the adjacent spring ligament and the medial longitudinal arch.[125]

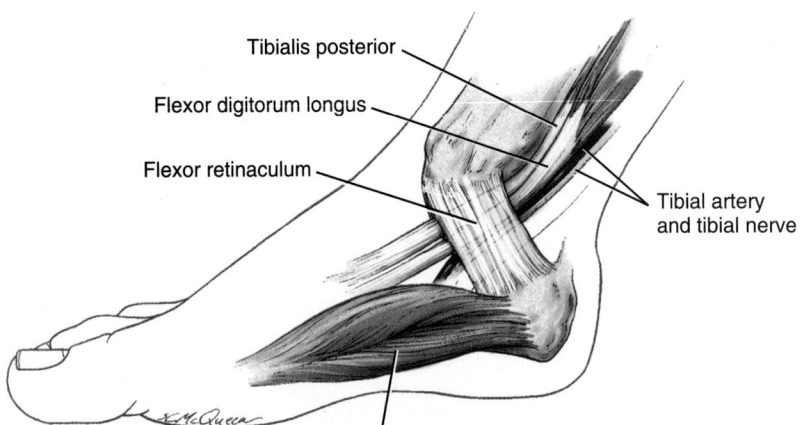

FIG. 14.50 A medial view of the flexor retinaculum that covers the tendons of the tibialis posterior, flexor digitorum longus, and tibial neurovascular bundle. (From Richardson EG: Neurogenic disorders. In Canale ST, Beaty JH, editors: *Campbell's operative orthopaedics*, vol 4, ed 12, St Louis, 2012, Mosby.)

The tendons of both the tibialis posterior and the flexor digitorum longus use the medial malleolus as a fixed pulley to direct their force posterior to the axis of rotation at the talocrural joint. An analogous pulley exists for the fibularis longus and brevis tendons, as these structures pass posterior to the lateral malleolus (see Fig. 14.46). Tendons of the tibialis posterior and flexor digitorum longus are positioned posterior to the medial malleolus by the flexor retinaculum. The flexor hallucis longus uses a different plantar flexion pulley system, formed proximally by the medial and lateral tubercles of the talus and distally by the sustentaculum tali of the calcaneus.

Joint Action

Except for the fibularis longus and brevis, all muscles that plantar flex the talocrural joint also supinate (invert) the subtalar or transverse tarsal joints. This strong inversion bias is apparent by the position of all muscles within the posterior compartment of the leg relative to the subtalar joint (see Fig. 14.43). From the anatomic and inverted positions, even the triceps surae inverts slightly, as the Achilles tendon passes just medial to the subtalar joint's axis of rotation.[121,160]

The tibialis posterior, flexor hallucis longus, and flexor digitorum longus are the primary supinators of the foot. The tibialis posterior produces the greatest supination torque (especially in the direction of adduction) across the subtalar and transverse tarsal joints.[121,134,206] The muscle's extensive distal attachments, especially to the navicular, provide an effective inversion "twist" of the midfoot (see Fig. 14.26D). In addition to plantar flexion and supination, the flexor digitorum longus and flexor hallucis longus have additional actions at the more distal joints of the foot, especially at the metatarsophalangeal and interphalangeal joints.

Activation of the Plantar Flexor and Supinator Muscles during Walking. The plantar flexor and supinator muscles are active throughout most of the stance phase of gait, (see electromyographic activation in Fig. 15.29).[236,237] The gastrocnemius and soleus become active immediately after the dorsiflexor muscles relax. From foot flat to just prior to heel off, the plantar flexors act eccentrically to decelerate the forward rotation (dorsiflexion) of the leg over the fixed talus.[70,185] During this period, the stretching of the Achilles tendon stores considerable elastic energy.[1,136] During the heel off and toe off phases of walking, the stored energy augments the now concentrically-activated force produced by the muscles, providing the necessary plantar flexion thrust for push off phase. In addition, forces in the flexor hallucis longus, flexor digitorum longus, and intrinsic foot muscles (e.g., flexor digitorum brevis, lumbricals, and interossei) hold the plantar surface of the extending toes firmly against the ground. This action expands the weight-bearing surfaces of the toes, thereby minimizing contact pressures.

The tibialis posterior, flexor hallucis longus, and flexor digitorum longus muscles are all capable of resisting pronation and assisting with supination during the stance phase of walking. Of the three muscles, however, the tibialis posterior is most designed for this function. The tibialis posterior is active throughout the majority of the stance phase, longer than any other supinator muscle.[182,236] As the foot contacts the ground in early stance, the tibialis posterior decelerates the pronating subtalar joint, which assists with a gradual and controlled lowering of the medial longitudinal arch (review Fig. 14.31). This load absorption mechanism is driven largely by *eccentric* activation of the tibialis posterior. Data suggest, however, that most of the actual lengthening of the tibialis posterior during early stance comes from the muscle's extensive tendinous network. In theory, the muscle fibers may, at times, be active in a near-isometric state.[150] Like a pretensioned spring, the tendinous elongation can effectively

store energy for use later in the gait cycle. Persons who excessively and/or rapidly pronate during the stance phase of walking or running may place excessive "eccentric" demands on the tibialis posterior's entire musculotendinous apparatus. Over many cycles, this large demand may lead to painful tendinopathy, muscle fatigue, or stress on the muscle's proximal attachments, possibly associated with medial tibial stress syndrome (formally known as "shin splints").[214,225,266] Reluctance or failure to fully activate the tibialis posterior limits an important shock absorption mechanism across the entire foot.

Throughout mid to late stance, contraction of the healthy tibialis posterior helps guide the rearfoot *toward* supination. This same muscular force may assist with the concurrent external rotation of the lower leg-and-talus, as well as reestablishing the height of the medial longitudinal arch. Concurrent activation of the fibularis muscles helps control the speed and amount of the supination motion, while adding medial-lateral stability to the mortise.

Plantar Flexion Torque Generated for Propulsion. At the very end of the stance phase, the muscles within the posterior compartment contract to plantar flex the talocrural joint. The fibularis longus and brevis (within the lateral compartment) also contribute to this torque. Although the plantar flexors provide the primary propulsive force to advance the body while walking, secondary energy sources may include the hip extensors, especially when walking at a relatively high cadence.[204,264]

In healthy persons, maximal isometric plantar flexion torque exceeds the torque potential of all other movements about the ankle and foot combined (Fig. 14.51).[221,238] Large plantar flexion torque is needed to rapidly accelerate the body up and forward during running, jumping, and climbing. Plantar flexion torque is greatest when the ankle approaches full dorsiflexion (i.e., when plantar flexor muscles are elongated) and is least when the ankle is fully plantar flexed.[73,88,190] The ankle is typically dorsiflexed to prepare to sprint or jump. Of interest, as the ankle vigorously plantar flexes at the "take off" of a sprint or jump, the contracting gastrocnemius is simultaneously elongated by the action of the quadriceps extending the knee. This biarticular arrangement prevents the gastrocnemius from over shortening, allowing greater plantar flexion torque throughout a larger range of ankle motion.[88,109] Because the soleus muscle does not cross the knee, its length-tension relationship is relatively unaffected by the position of the knee. Perhaps the relative slow-twitch muscle characteristics of the soleus are optimally suited

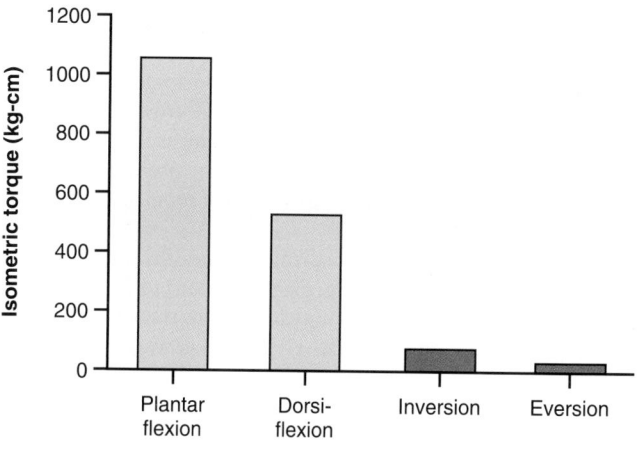

FIG. 14.51 The magnitude of maximal-effort isometric torque is shown for four actions of the ankle and foot. (N = 86 healthy men and women.[221])

Adult Acquired Flatfoot Deformity: Consequence of Loss of Support from the Tibialis Posterior

As described, a large demand is placed on the tibialis posterior during the stance phase of walking. Within the approximate 600 ms of a typical stance phase, the muscle and its tendon must rapidly switch from actively lowering the medial longitudinal arch through mid stance to lifting the arch (and superimposed body weight) through late stance. These repetitive and demanding events may naturally predispose the tendon to excessive strain-related injury. Trauma, chronic inflammation, or degenerative pathology within the muscle's tendon or associated sheath can result in its eventual attrition or rupture, leading to a complete collapse of the medial longitudinal arch. This often progressive condition in the adult has been referred to as *adult acquired flatfoot deformity* (AAFD), although several others names have been proposed.[187,232,275] Structural failure of the tibialis posterior tendon is typically associated with a dropped navicular, pain during or inability to perform a single-leg heel raise, and marked eversion of the rearfoot with a splaying of the forefoot into excessive abduction.[212,263] In addition to the rupture of the tendon, the juxtaposed spring (plantar calcaneonavicular) ligament may also experience excessive attrition, evidenced by a drop in height of the head of the talus and an associated subluxation of the talonavicular joint.[198]

Four stages of AAFD have been described.[68] Stage 1, its mildest form, involves tibialis posterior tendonitis without deformity. At the other end of the spectrum, Stage 4, the most severe form, is associated with complete rupture or severe attenuation of the tibialis posterior tendon along with a fixed rearfoot (eversion) valgus deformity and an overstretched or torn deltoid ligament. Without adequate support of the medial ankle, the talus typically tilts sharply within the mortise toward valgus. The excessive tilt of the talus often predisposes the ankle to high "point loading" and eventual osteoarthritis. Marked eversion and lateral instability of the mortise can also strain the tibial nerve within the tarsal tunnel, potentially causing a neuropathy and associated weakness of intrinsic muscles of the foot along with sensory disturbances.

Rupture or pain in the tibialis posterior tendon can initiate a series of events that perpetuates a severe rearfoot valgus deformity, often in conjunction with an adaptive and fixed forefoot varus. With loss of the dominant invertor force at the rearfoot, the eversion forces produced by the fibularis longus and brevis are left significantly unopposed, thereby strongly biasing rearfoot eversion. Consequently, the overly everted calcaneus may shift the line of force of the gastrocnemius-soleus (Achilles tendon) slightly to the lateral side of the axis of rotation at the subtalar joint (refer to Fig. 14.43 for visual guide).[160,232] Although the leverage for eversion may be slight, the large force potential carried within the Achilles tendon may produce a significant (and relentless) eversion torque. An underlying tightness of the Achilles tendon may even increase the severity of a rearfoot eversion deformity.

AAFD can be painful and disabling, occurring in varying severities in up to 10% of older women.[124] The chronically and severely pronated foot fails to lock in late stance, which significantly reduces the stability needed during push off. The early stages of AAFD may respond well to physical therapy and orthotics; however, surgery is often necessary in the later stages. The tendons of either the flexor hallucis longus or the flexor digitorum longus may be surgically transferred to augment support to the medial longitudinal arch and talonavicular joint region.[232]

---

to control the subtle postural sway movements of the leg (and body) over the talus during standing. The faster-twitch characteristics of the gastrocnemius, on the other hand, may be better suited for providing a propulsive plantar flexion torque for activities that also involve dynamic knee extension, such as jumping and sprinting.

Of all the plantar flexor muscles, the gastrocnemius and soleus are by far the strongest, theoretically capable of producing about 80% of the total plantar flexion torque at the ankle.[185] This large torque potential results from the muscles' large cross-sectional area and relatively long moment arm. The protruding calcaneal tuberosity provides the triceps surae with a moment arm of about 5 cm from the talocrural joint, nearly twice the average moment arm of the other plantar flexor muscles.[93,121]

Executing push off during walking in a healthy adult requires about 70% of the maximal-effort (plantar flexion) torque capability of the gastrocnemius and soleus muscles.[252] This is surprisingly high for a task as common and relatively "easy" as walking. The low "torque reserve" of the plantar flexors may explain why only moderate weakness of the gastrocnemius-soleus muscles typically results in an obvious disturbance in one's gait or locomotive pattern. This may explain some of the natural changes in kinematics and reduced metabolic efficiency of walking in healthy older persons as they continue to walk while naturally losing plantar flexion strength with age.[5,197] Although the ipsilateral hip extensors may serve as an indirect source of power to assist with propulsion of walking, these proximal muscles lack the biomechanical specificity for this task compared with the plantar flexor muscles. Maintaining optimal strength of the primary plantar flexor muscles while walking is important biomechanically and physiologically, especially in older persons.

The Achilles tendon, the strongest in the body, must routinely transmit large forces between the calf muscles and the calcaneal tuberosity. These forces can be extreme, especially during rapid and explosive acceleration or deceleration motions of the ankle, often associated with running, jumping, or landing. Although normally strong, rupture of the Achilles tendon is not uncommon. In the United States, 75% of ruptures occur in persons less than 55 years of age, most frequently associated with participation in basketball, football, and tennis.[200]

As with many periarticular connective tissues, the Achilles tendon is relatively *compliant* (i.e., the inverse of stiffness) and elastic. During walking and running, for example, the tendon experiences a strain (i.e., relative elongation) of about 5% to 6%.[142] The relative compliance and elasticity of the Achilles tendon may serve useful biomechanical functions. As eluded to earlier, the Achilles tendon stores a considerable amount of passive energy when stretched during most of the stance phase of gait, only to be used to augment active plantar flexion during propulsion.[110,148] Although the natural compliance of the Achilles tendon has several benefits during locomotion, certain activities involving repetitive overload may lead to Achilles tendinopathy.[55,149,171] The primary location of the tendinopathy may be at the tendon's insertion site to the calcaneus, or at the mid portion of the tendon.[254]

INTRINSIC MUSCLES

Anatomic Considerations

Intrinsic muscles are those that originate and insert within the foot. Most of these muscles of the foot are anatomically analogous to an intrinsic muscle of the hand. One exception, however, is that the foot does *not* contain muscles that perform opposition of the first and fifth digits. Understanding these analogies should help with learning the anatomy, innervation, and specific actions of these muscles. Table 14.7 summarizes the relevant information on the intrinsic muscles of the foot. More detailed attachments of these muscles are presented in Appendix IV, Part D.

The dorsum of the foot has one intrinsic muscle, the extensor digitorum brevis, which is innervated by the deep branch of the fibular nerve. The *extensor digitorum brevis* originates on the dorsal-lateral surface of the calcaneus, just proximal to the calcaneocuboid articulation. The muscle belly sends four tendons: one to the dorsal surface of the great toe (often designated as the extensor hallucis brevis) and three that join the tendons of the extensor digitorum longus of the second through the fourth toes (see Fig. 14.44). The extensor digitorum brevis assists the extensor hallucis longus and extensor digitorum longus in extension of the toes.

The remaining intrinsic muscles originate and insert within the plantar aspect of the foot. These muscles are organized into four layers (Fig. 14.52). The plantar fascia runs parallel and superficial to the first layer of muscles.

TABLE 14.7 Summary of the Relevant Information on the Intrinsic Muscles of the Foot

Intrinsic Muscle	Location	Isolated Action	Innervation	Analogous Muscle in the Hand
Extensor digitorum brevis	Dorsum of the foot	Extension of the toes	Deep branch of the fibular nerve	None
Flexor digitorum brevis	Layer 1	Flexion of the proximal interphalangeal and metatarsophalangeal joints of the lesser toes	Medial plantar nerve	Flexor digitorum superficialis
Abductor hallucis	Layer 1	Abduction and (assistance with) flexion of the metatarsophalangeal joint of the great toe	Medial plantar nerve	Abductor pollicis brevis
Abductor digiti minimi	Layer 1	Abduction and (assistance with) flexion of the metatarsophalangeal joint of the fifth digit	Lateral plantar nerve	Abductor digiti minimi
Quadratus plantae	Layer 2	Provides medial stabilization to the common tendons of the flexor digitorum longus	Lateral plantar nerve	None
Lumbricals	Layer 2	Flexion of the metatarsophalangeal joints and extension of the interphalangeal joints of the lesser toes	*Second digit:* Medial plantar nerve *Third through fifth digits:* Lateral plantar nerve	Lumbricals
Adductor hallucis	Layer 3	Adduction and (assistance with) flexion of the metatarsophalangeal joint of the great toe	Lateral plantar nerve	Adductor pollicis
Flexor hallucis brevis	Layer 3	Flexion of the metatarsophalangeal joint of the great toe	Medial plantar nerve	Flexor pollicis brevis
Flexor digiti minimi	Layer 3	Flexion of the metatarsophalangeal joint of the fifth digit	Lateral plantar nerve	Flexor digiti minimi
Plantar interossei (three)	Layer 4	Adduction of the metatarsophalangeal joints of the third, fourth, and fifth digits (relative to a reference in line through the second digit)	Lateral plantar nerve	Palmar interossei
Dorsal interossei (four)	Layer 4	Abduction of the metatarsophalangeal joints of the second, third, and fourth digits (relative to a reference in line through the second digit)	Lateral plantar nerve	Dorsal interossei

Layer 1

The intrinsic muscles in the first layer of the foot are the flexor digitorum brevis, abductor hallucis, and abductor digiti minimi (Fig. 14.52A). As a group, these muscles originate on the lateral and medial processes of the calcaneal tuberosity and nearby connective tissues. The *flexor digitorum brevis* attaches to both sides of the plantar aspect of the middle phalanges of the four lesser toes. Proximal to this distal attachment, each tendon divides to allow passage of the tendons of the flexor digitorum longus. (Note the similar relationship between the flexor digitorum superficialis and profundus of the hand.) The flexor digitorum brevis assists the flexor digitorum longus with flexing the toes. The *abductor hallucis*, the largest of the intrinsic muscles, forms the medial border of the foot, providing a covered passage for the nerves that enter the plantar aspect of the foot. The abductor muscle attaches distally to the medial border of the proximal phalanx of the great toe, sharing an attachment with the medial head of the flexor hallucis brevis (see Fig. 14.52C). The *abductor digiti minimi* helps form the lateral-plantar margin of the foot, attaching distally to the lateral border of the base of the proximal phalanx of the fifth toe. Each muscle abducts and assists with flexion of its respective digit.

Intrinsic Muscles of the Foot, Layer 1
- Flexor digitorum brevis
- Abductor hallucis
- Abductor digiti minimi

Layer 2

The intrinsic muscles in the second layer are the quadratus plantae and the lumbricals (Fig. 14.52B). Both muscles are anatomically related to the tendons of the flexor digitorum longus. The *quadratus plantae* attaches by two heads to the plantar aspect of the calcaneus. Both heads attach distally to the lateral edge of the common tendon of the flexor digitorum longus. The quadratus plantae helps to stabilize the tendons of the flexor digitorum longus, preventing them from migrating medially.[141] The four *lumbricals* have their proximal attachment from the tendons of the flexor digitorum longus. These small fleshy muscles pass on the medial side of the lesser toes to attach into the extensor digital expansion. The lumbricals flex the metatarsophalangeal joints and extend the interphalangeal joints—actions that are functionally equivalent to the actions performed by the lumbricals of the hand.

Intrinsic Muscles of the Foot, Layer 2
- Quadratus plantae
- Lumbricals

Layer 3

The intrinsic muscles in the third layer are the adductor hallucis, flexor hallucis brevis, and flexor digiti minimi (Fig. 14.52C). As a group, these muscles arise from the plantar aspect of the cuboid, cuneiforms, and bases of more central metatarsal bones, and from local connective tissues. Like the adductor pollicis in the hand, the *adductor hallucis* arises from two heads: oblique and transverse. Both heads attach to the lateral base of the proximal phalanx of the great toe and adjacent lateral sesamoid bone. The muscle adducts and assists with flexion of the metatarsophalangeal joint of the great toe. The *flexor hallucis brevis* has two heads that attach distally to the medial and lateral sides of the base of the proximal phalanx of the great toe. Medial and lateral sesamoid bones are located within the two tendons of this muscle, possibly providing greater leverage to produce toe flexion torque. The *flexor digiti minimi* attaches to the lateral base of the proximal phalanx of the fifth toe, sharing a common attachment with the abductor digiti minimi. Both short flexor muscles flex the metatarsophalangeal joint of their respective toes.

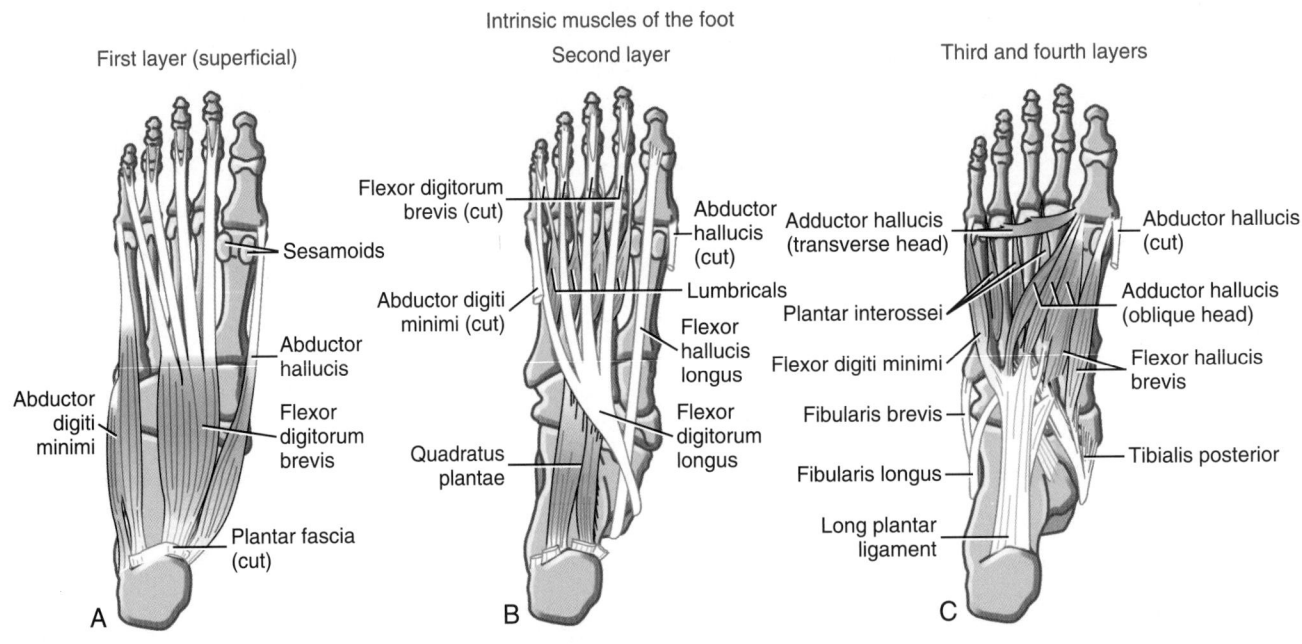

FIG. 14.52 The intrinsic muscles of the plantar aspect of the foot are organized into four layers.

Layer 4

The fourth layer of intrinsic muscles contains three plantar and four dorsal interossei muscles. The *plantar interossei* are shown in Fig. 14.52C, along with the muscles of the third layer. The dorsal interossei are illustrated in Fig. 14.38. The general anatomic plan of the interossei is similar to that of the hand, except that the "reference digit" for abduction and adduction of the toes is the second instead of the third digit as in the hand.

┌───┐
Intrinsic Muscles of the Foot, Layer 4
- Plantar interossei (three)
- Dorsal interossei (four)
└───┘

The *dorsal interossei* are two-headed, bipennate muscles. The second digit contains two dorsal interossei, whereas the third and fourth digits contain one each. All dorsal interossei insert on the base of the proximal phalanges; the first and second interossei insert on the medial and lateral side of the second digit, respectively, and the third and fourth dorsal interossei insert on the lateral side of the third and fourth digit (review attachments in Fig. 14.4). Each dorsal interosseus muscle abducts the metatarsophalangeal joint. Each of the third, fourth, and fifth digits contains a *plantar interosseus* muscle. Each muscle consists of one head and inserts on the medial side of the base of the corresponding proximal phalanx (review attachments in Fig. 14.5). These muscles adduct their respective metatarsophalangeal joint.

Functional Considerations

Table 14.7 assigns actions to the intrinsic muscles assuming the foot is unloaded, and the toes are free to move. Although this information allows clinicians to test the strength and dexterity of the individual muscles, it does not reveal the muscles' more global and routine functions. Unlike the intrinsic muscles of the hand, which are designed for precise manual dexterity, the intrinsic muscles of the foot are designed to accept loads associated with walking and to assist with standing balance and postural sway.[115,117,180] Most notably, the intrinsic muscles stiffen the medial longitudinal arch as the foot moves from the mid stance to the push off phase of walking.[115,208] This function explains why most of the intrinsic muscles are maximally active during this part of the stance cycle (e.g., see EMG of flexor hallucis brevis in Fig. 15.29).

As a group, the intrinsic muscles run parallel with and immediately deep to the plantar fascia. These parallel structures stiffen the medial longitudinal arch using slightly different mechanisms. Prior to and throughout push off, the plantar fascia stiffens the arch through the action of the extending toes and the previously described windlass mechanism. At the same time, the activated intrinsic muscles are also being stretched distally by the extending toes. Study shows that the activated muscle fibers within the flexor digitorum brevis, a centrally located intrinsic muscle, are held in a near isometric length as the tendons are pulled distally.[116] Although speculation, this type of activation may occur in several other intrinsic muscles during the late stance. Such an actively controlled springlike mechanism is ideal for generating and storing longitudinal stiffness

within the foot as it progresses through the push off phase of walking.

The intrinsic muscles are normally surprisingly thick, as a group having a cross-sectional area comparable to the tibialis posterior.[35] The relatively large strength potential of the intrinsic muscles reflects their important role in dynamically stabilizing the medial longitudinal arch during locomotion. As such, these muscles have been referred to as "foot core," comparable to the abdominal muscles being referred to as "core" stabilizers in the lumbo-pelvic region.[162]

Weakness of the intrinsic muscles can have significant negative functional consequences, often readily apparent in persons with advanced peripheral neuropathy. Significant atrophy of the intrinsic muscles can reduce some of the natural padding over local bones, thereby increasing the likelihood of pressure-related ulceration to the adjacent skin. Even in the healthy foot, the strength of the intrinsic muscles naturally declines with aging and is considered a risk factor for balance-related falls.[170,174] In addition to safety concerns, weakness of the intrinsic muscles at any age places greater demands on structures that dynamically support the arch, such as the plantar fascia and tibialis posterior. Strengthening the intrinsic muscles, therefore, is often suggested as a treatment for plantar fasciitis or posterior tibialis tendinopathy.[162] In addition to strengthening exercises, the wearing of minimalist shoes has shown to hypertrophy the intrinsic muscles.[207] For some people, the reduced support offered by this style of footwear may provide a therapeutic supplement to strengthening exercises for the intrinsic muscles.

MUSCULAR PARALYSIS AFTER INJURY TO THE FIBULAR OR TIBIAL NERVE

Injury to the Common Fibular Nerve and Its Branches

The *common fibular nerve* is injured relatively frequently from trauma that involves a fractured proximal fibula. Injury to the *deep branch of the fibular nerve* can result in paralysis of *all* the dorsiflexor (pretibial) muscles (see Fig. 14.41). With paralysis of the dorsiflexor muscles, the foot rapidly and uncontrollably plantar flexes immediately after the heel contact phase of walking. During the swing phase, the hip must excessively flex to ensure that the toes clear the ground.

Paralysis of the dorsiflexor muscles dramatically increases the likelihood of developing a plantar flexion contracture at the talocrural joint. This deformity is referred to as a *drop-foot* or *pes equinus*. In a surprisingly short period, a plantar flexed posture may lead to adaptive shortening and tightening of the Achilles tendon as well as other collateral ligaments of the ankle. The relentless pull of gravity can also contribute to a plantar flexion contracture, often requiring an ankle-foot orthosis to maintain adequate dorsiflexion during walking.

An injury to the *superficial branch of the fibular nerve* may result in paralysis of the fibularis longus and fibularis brevis (see Fig. 14.41). Over time, paralysis may lead to a supinated or inverted posture of the foot, a condition called *pes varus*. An injury to the *common fibular nerve* may involve both deep and superficial nerve branches. The resulting paralysis of all dorsiflexor *and* evertor muscles strongly predisposes a person to a deformity of combined plantar flexion of the ankle and supination of the foot, a condition referred to as *pes equinovarus*.

Injury to the Tibial Nerve and Its Branches

Injury to the tibial nerve may cause varying levels of weakness or paralysis in the muscles of the posterior compartment (see Fig. 14.42). Isolated paralysis of the gastrocnemius and soleus because of tibial nerve injury is rare. Nevertheless, regardless of underlying pathology, paralysis of these muscles results in profound loss of plantar flexion torque. Over time, a fixed dorsiflexion posture may

SPECIAL FOCUS 14.7

Biomechanics of Raising Up on Tiptoes

The functional strength of the plantar flexor muscles is often evaluated by requiring a subject to repeatedly rise on tiptoes. As shown in Fig. 14.53, maximally raising the body requires an interaction of two concurrent internal plantar flexion torques: one at the talocrural joint and one at the metatarsophalangeal joints. The plantar flexor muscles, represented by the gastrocnemius, plantar flex the *talocrural joint* by rotating the calcaneus and talus within the mortise. The primary torque used to raise the body, however, occurs through extension across the *metatarsophalangeal joints*. Acting about the medial-lateral axes of rotation at the toes, the gastrocnemius has an internal moment arm that greatly exceeds the external moment arm of body weight (compare panels B and C in Fig. 14.53). Such a large mechanical advantage is rare in the musculoskeletal system. Acting as a second-class lever with the pivot point at the metatarsophalangeal joints, the gastrocnemius lifts the body using mechanics analogous to those of a person lifting a load with a wheelbarrow. If, for instance, the gastrocnemius functions with a mechanical advantage of 3:1 (i.e., ratio of the internal-to-external moment arms, or B and C in Fig. 14.53), the muscle needs to produce a lifting force of only one-third, or 33%, of body weight to support the plantar flexed position. Rarely in the body does a muscle produce a force less than the load it is supporting. As a biomechanical trade-off, however, the gastrocnemius, in theory, needs to shorten a distance three times *greater* than the vertical displacement of the body's center of mass (see Chapter 1). (A more precise estimate of the vertical displacement requires knowledge of the average angle of pennation of all the plantar flexor muscles.) Nevertheless, the nature of this mechanical trade-off allows one to stand up on tiptoes with relative ease.

Fig. 14.53 shows the importance of ample extension range of motion at the metatarsophalangeal joints. Not only do the plantar flexor muscles use these joints to augment their internal moment arm, but also, as described previously, full extension of these joints pulls the plantar fascia taut via the windlass mechanism. This action helps the intrinsic muscles support the medial longitudinal arch and maintain a rigid forefoot, thereby allowing the foot to accept the load imposed by body weight.

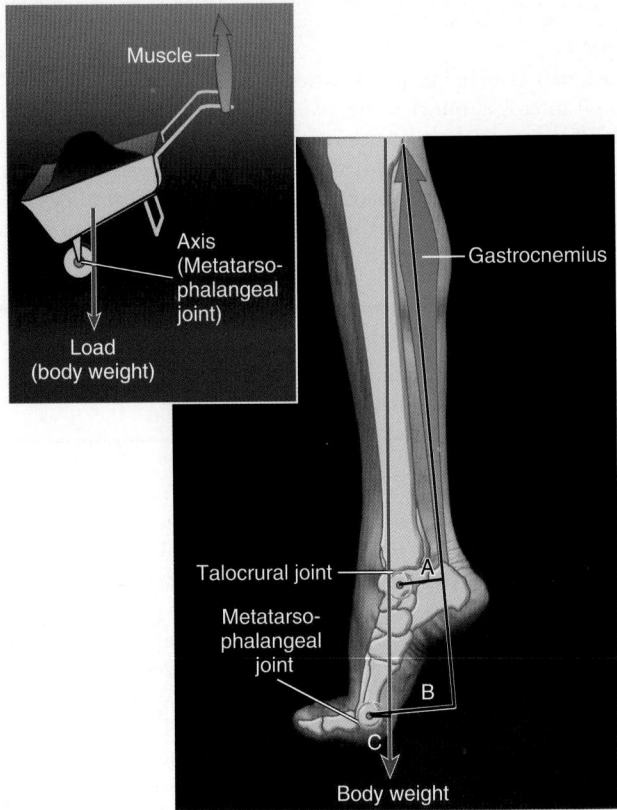

FIG. 14.53 A mechanical model shows the biomechanics of standing on tiptoes. The force of a contracting gastrocnemius muscle acts with a relatively short internal moment arm from the talocrural joint (A), and a relatively long internal moment arm from the metatarsophalangeal joints (B). Once on tiptoes, the line of gravity from body weight falls just posterior to the axis of rotation at the metatarsophalangeal joints. As a result, body weight acts with a relatively small external moment arm (C), originating from the metatarsophalangeal joints.

---

result at the talocrural joint, a condition known as *pes calcaneus*. The term *calcaneus* is used to describe the often-prominent heel pad that forms in response to the heel of the chronically dorsiflexed ankle sharply striking the ground at the initiation of the stance phase.

Paralysis involving primarily the supinator muscles of the foot may result in a fixed pronated deformity, primarily the result of the unopposed action of the fibularis longus and brevis muscles. The term *pes valgus* typically describes both eversion and abduction components of the pronation deformity. Paralysis involving *all* the muscles of the posterior compartment increases the potential for a fixed deformity called *pes calcaneovalgus*.

Injury or pathology involving the distal tibial nerve may involve the *medial and lateral plantar nerves* (see Fig. 14.42). Depending on severity, weakness of the intrinsic muscles within the foot can cause "clawing" of the toes: hyperextension of the metatarsophalangeal joints with flexion of the interphalangeal joints. (This deformity results primarily from an unopposed pull of the extrinsic toe extensor muscles across the metatarsophalangeal joints, like that described in

the hand after a combined ulnar and median nerve injury.) In some severe and chronic cases, hyperextension of the metatarsophalangeal joints pulls the intrinsic muscles and plantar fascia in a distal direction. The resulting tension draws the forefoot and rearfoot closer together, thereby pathologically raising the medial longitudinal arch and possibly contributing to a pes cavus deformity. The resulting high medial arch may appear exaggerated when combined with marked atrophy of the abductor hallucis and flexor hallucis brevis muscles.

The common fixed deformities or abnormal postures of the ankle, foot, and toes are summarized according to nerve injury in Table 14.8.

SYNOPSIS

As an integrated complex, the ankle and foot function as the dynamic interface between the lower extremity and the earth's surface. This interface is amazingly adaptable: pliable enough to

TABLE 14.8 Nerve Injury and Common Resulting Deformities or Abnormal Postures throughout the Ankle, Foot,* and Toes

Nerve Injury and Associated Muscle Paralysis	Possible Ensuing Deformity or Abnormal Posture	Common Clinical Name	Examples of Structures Likely to Experience Adaptive Shortening and Subsequent Tightness
Injury to the *deep branch of the fibular nerve* with paralysis of pretibial muscles	Plantar flexion of the talocrural joint	Drop-foot or pes equinus	Achilles tendon, posterior capsule of the talocrural joint
Injury to the *superficial branch of the fibular nerve* with paralysis of the fibularis longus and brevis	Inversion of the foot	Pes varus	Tibialis posterior, tibiocalcaneal fibers of the deltoid ligament and adjacent capsule of the subtalar joint
Injury to the *common fibular nerve* with paralysis of all dorsiflexor and evertor muscles	Plantar flexion of the talocrural joint and inversion of the foot	Pes equinovarus	Achilles tendon, tibialis posterior muscle
Injury to the *proximal portion of the tibial nerve* with paralysis of *all* plantar flexor and supinator muscles	Dorsiflexion† of the talocrural joint and eversion of the foot	Pes calcaneovalgus	Dorsiflexor and evertor muscles, anterior talofibular ligament and adjacent capsule of the subtalar joint
Injury to the *middle portion of the tibial nerve* with paralysis of supinator muscles	Eversion of the foot	Pes valgus	Fibularis muscles
Injury or pathology involving the *medial and lateral plantar nerves*	Hyperextension of the metatarsophalangeal joints, and flexion of the interphalangeal joints	Clawing of the toes	Extensor digitorum longus and brevis

*The *foot* refers primarily to the subtalar and transverse tarsal joints.
†Severity depends on the influence of gravity.

absorb repetitive loading and to accommodate to irregular ground surfaces, yet sufficiently rigid to support body weight and the muscular thrust of walking and running.

Twenty-eight individual muscles, acting across 32 joints or joint complexes, control the kinesiology of the ankle and foot. To organize the anatomy, the foot is conveniently divided into three regions: the rearfoot, midfoot, and forefoot. The kinesiology of the foot, however, is based on a functional interaction among or between these regions.

The most effective way to summarize the kinesiology of the ankle and foot is to follow the main events of the stance phase of walking. At *early stance* phase, the ankle rapidly plantar flexes as the rearfoot (subtalar joint) pronates. During this so-called *load-acceptance phase of gait* the dorsiflexor and supinator (invertor) muscles act mostly eccentrically to decelerate the prevailing kinematics, as well as to absorb the impact of the foot striking the ground.

As part of this load-acceptance and shock-absorption mechanism, the medial longitudinal arch depresses slowly in response to body weight. Several tissues help support and decelerate the lowering of the arch, including the spring ligament, capsule of the talonavicular joint, plantar fascia, and muscles such as the tibialis posterior and tibialis anterior. Tissues that slow the lowering of the arch absorb energy and therefore protect the foot. Failure to control the extent or rate of the combined rearfoot pronation and associated lowering of the medial longitudinal arch may, over time, lead to damaging stress and associated pain in local tissues. Treatment for this problem may involve orthotics, taping, activity modification, and selected stretching, strengthening, and reeducation of lower extremity muscles that directly or indirectly control the ankle and foot.

During the *middle and late stance phases* of gait, the entire lower limb (which was previously internally rotating) sharply changes its rotation direction. The now externally rotating lower limb, although the movement is slight and barely perceptible, helps initiate the gradual transition from an everting to an inverting rearfoot. Mechanically coupled with an impending rising of the medial

longitudinal arch, the foot, ideally, becomes increasingly rigid. The increased rigidity acts to stabilize the foot—both longitudinally and transversely—during the push off phase of walking. The rising of the arch during this latter part of the stance phase is driven primarily through the contraction of invertor muscles (notably the tibialis posterior), coupled with strong activation of the intrinsic muscles. As the heel rises, just before the toe off phase, body weight is transferred forward toward the metatarsal heads. The continued coactivation of intrinsic and extrinsic muscles, in conjunction with the windlass mechanism across the extending metatarsophalangeal joints, provides the final elements of stability to the propelling foot.

Impairments of the ankle and foot have multiple causes, including pathology or trauma affecting the connective tissues, muscles, peripheral nerves, or the central nervous system. Acute trauma may occur from an isolated event, such as an inversion sprain, fracture of the styloid process of the fifth metatarsal, or severe hyperextension of the great toe. Chronic trauma may result from an accumulation of lower magnitude stress over an extended time, leading to plantar fasciitis, displacement of the tendon of the fibularis longus relative to the fibula, tibialis posterior tendinopathy, "heel spurs," or metatarsalgia. Often, stress caused by microtrauma is associated with abnormal alignment within the joints of the foot or in proximal parts of the lower extremity. Abnormal alignment may lead to excessive kinematic compensations that stress or induce fatigue in muscles and supporting connective tissues. Because of the frequency and regular necessity of using the foot, many stress-related conditions involve inflammation and associated pain.

Knowledge of the anatomy and kinesiology of the ankle and foot is a prerequisite to understanding the associated pathomechanics. Muscle and joint interactions must be understood both when the foot is unloaded and when the foot is fixed to the ground. Furthermore, the clinician must appreciate the mechanical interdependence between the kinematics of the ankle and foot and more proximal regions of the lower limb.

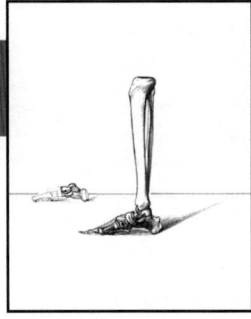

ADDITIONAL CLINICAL CONNECTIONS

CLINICAL CONNECTION 14.1

Ankle Injury Resulting from the Extremes of Dorsiflexion or Plantar Flexion

The ligaments of the distal tibiofibular joint and the interosseous membrane have a close structural relationship with the talocrural joint. An important component of this relationship was depicted previously in this chapter when describing the biomechanics of talocrural joint dorsiflexion during the stance phase of walking; review Fig. 14.20. Although the dorsiflexed ankle adds stability to the mortise, excessive and violent dorsiflexion can traumatize the region. Consider extreme *dorsiflexion* of the ankle (leg over the foot) while landing from a jump or a fall. If forceful enough, the dorsiflexion can cause the mortise to "explode" outward, injuring several tissues. This traumatic widening of the mortise and associated displacement of the fibula at the distal tibiofibular joint is often referred to as a *high ankle or syndesmotic sprain.*[230,265]

Isolated syndesmotic sprains account for approximately 10% of all ankle sprains; however, the risk of injury increases in athletic populations, especially those participating in contact/collision sports.[158,265] In combination with extreme dorsiflexion, the mechanism of injury of high ankle sprains often involves an excessive *abduction* (external rotation) torque applied to the mortise. From a weight-bearing perspective, this extreme motion could occur while landing from a jump on the right dorsiflexed ankle as the body and lower leg simultaneously rotate sharply to the *left*. (Such a motion forcefully *internally* rotates the right tibia and fibula relative to the grounded talus-and-foot segment.) This stressful movement often involves excessive *eversion* of the talus within the mortise.[265] Research simulating the classic mechanism of injury for high ankle sprains has reported that the highest ligamentous strains occurred in the anterior (distal) tibiofibular ligament, followed closely by the anterior fibers of the deltoid ligament. Strain values of 8% to 9% were measured in these ligaments—a stretch theoretically capable of causing injury. These two ligaments act as a force-couple that directly or indirectly resists excessive abduction (external rotation) torque applied to the dorsiflexed mortise. The proposed mechanism of injury partially clarifies why serious syndesmotic injuries can involve fractures of the lateral or medial malleolus, or tears of the entire set of distal tibiofibular ligaments (including the interosseous membrane) and the deltoid ligament.[144,211,230]

Because of the likelihood of trauma to multiple tissues, the time to return to sports after a high ankle sprain typically exceeds that required for the more common inversion sprain.[158] Furthermore, high ankle sprains, particularly if severe and not appropriately treated, can cause long-term functional impairments of the ankle.[230] Surgical repair is often required to repair a syndesmotic injury, especially if the joint shows persistent instability. An unstable syndesmosis is typically surgically stabilized by using screws or a suture-button technique. The suture-button technique fixates the joint by inserting a braided polyethylene cord tightly between the distal tibia and fibula. This flexible method of fixation has the advantage of allowing physiologic motion while still maintaining proper alignment. The literature reports favorable outcomes for the suture-button method.[226]

In contrast to ankle dorsiflexion, full *plantar flexion*—the loose packed position of the talocrural joint—slackens many collateral ligaments of the ankle and all plantar flexor muscles. In addition, plantar flexion places the *narrower* width of the talus between the malleoli, thereby releasing tension within the mortise. Consequently, full plantar flexion causes the distal tibia and fibula to "loosen their grip" on the talus. Bearing body weight over a fully plantar flexed ankle, therefore, places the talocrural joint in a relatively unstable position.[76,262] Wearing high heels or landing from a jump in a plantar flexed (and usually inverted) position increases the likelihood of destabilizing the mortise and potentially injuring the lateral ligaments of the ankle, notably the anterior tibiofibular ligament.[69,75]

ADDITIONAL CLINICAL CONNECTIONS

CLINICAL CONNECTION 14.2
Lateral Ankle Sprains and the Potential for Chronic Ankle Instability

Lateral ankle or "inversion" sprains are the most common injuries in sports and represent a large percentage of orthopedic injuries in the general population. Most of these injuries involve excessive *inversion* of the ankle or foot. In vivo electromyography (EMG) and kinematic data have been obtained during an actual (unexpected) inversion ankle sprain as a healthy athlete performed an experiment involving sharp "cutting" movements.[80] The ankle sprain consisted of the classic combination of excessive ankle inversion, adduction (internal rotation), and plantar flexion. Maximum inversion of 45 degrees occurred 60 ms after heel contact with the ground, at a peak angular velocity of 1290 degrees per second. The enhanced and prolonged EMG response from the tibialis anterior and fibular longus during the injury suggests these muscles have a subconscious role in protecting the ankle by reflexively decelerating and thus limiting the extremes of some of the damaging movements. Interestingly, however, although activation of the tibialis anterior could limit the extremes of plantar flexion, it may contribute to excessive inversion.

If severe, inversion sprains may cause significant injury to several tissues, most frequently involving the anterior talofibular and calcaneofibular ligaments. Perhaps less appreciated, inversion sprains involving excessive plantar flexion and other excessive rotations and translations within the mortise could theoretically overstretch and damage various fibers of the deltoid ligament.[47] Furthermore, excessive inversion may cause a compression and subsequent bruising of the talus and medial malleolus.[34] The concurrent trauma to the medial side of the ankle may explain why some severe "inversion" sprains show swelling, ecchymosis, and tenderness on lateral *and* medial sides of the ankle.

About 40% of persons who experience an isolated and significant inversion sprain may later develop *chronic ankle instability* (CAI), a condition typically characterized by recurrent ankle sprains to the same foot, chronic pain, generalized joint instability, and, in some, lifelong physical activity limitations.[2,56,256] In addition to loss of function, persons with CAI may also be at a higher risk for developing ankle osteoarthritis.[163,251]

Generally speaking, CAI may possess both mechanical and functional characteristics. *Mechanical characteristics* include excessive anterior laxity of the talus within the mortise (possibly reflecting a torn or lax anterior talofibular ligament), restrictions in posterior slide (or glide) of the talus with associated reduced dorsiflexion at the talocrural joint, and degenerative changes within the ankle.[48,100] *Functional characteristics* include chronic pain, weakness, subjective feelings of the ankle "giving away," reduced balance, and altered sense of ankle joint position or proprioception. Why certain persons develop CAI and others do not is poorly understood. A considerable amount of evidence suggests that the pathogenesis of CAI may involve diminished sensation caused by prior or repeated injury to mechanoreceptors embedded within the injured ligaments and capsule of the ankle.[129,253] A distorted

flow of sensory input reduces the body's ability to generate an effective and timely defensive muscular response to protect the ankle, especially after an unexpected inversion perturbation. Indeed, research has shown that persons with CAI have altered ankle proprioception (positional awareness), increased postural unsteadiness or reduced balance (most notably while standing on one limb), delayed or reduced reaction times in local muscles (notably the fibularis longus and brevis), altered kinematic coupling between the leg and foot during stance, and altered recruitment patterns and strength of muscles throughout the lower limb.[a] Gait analysis has revealed that persons with CAI tend to walk with greater subtalar joint inversion and talocrural joint adduction (internal rotation) compared with normal controls.[78,177] This inversion/adduction bias during walking may reflect the subjects' inability to control ankle position, a delay in activation of the fibularis muscles, or a combination thereof.[101] These abnormal responses may be the result of damage to the mechanoreceptors located within the injured ligaments.[177,245] Biomechanically, greater inversion at heel contact increases the likelihood that the upward-directed ground forces at heel contact would create a large and often unexpected inversion torque.

Hubbard and colleagues reported that persons with CAI, on average, have an excessively anteriorly aligned distal fibula relative to the tibia at the distal tibiofibular joint.[104] More research is needed, however, to determine the universality of this association. Nevertheless, an altered position of the fibula may result from excessive anterior tension from repeated overstretching of the anterior talofibular ligament, or from increased "tone" in the fibularis muscles secondary to increased activity in the gamma motoneuron system. This increased neural activity may be a response to abnormal afferent impulses from the damaged mechanoreceptors embedded within the injured lateral ankle ligaments.[186] Regardless of cause, excessive anterior migration of the distal fibula will alter the kinematics and likely increase the stress within the distal tibiofibular and talocrural joints.

In summary, the specific pathogenesis of CAI is unclear and likely involves several factors. Research consistently implicates diminished proprioception about the ankle, which reduces overall postural steadiness as well as the body's dynamic response to protecting the ankle from injury. It remains uncertain, however, whether the postural unsteadiness or lack of muscular control often associated with CAI is more the cause or the effect of repeated ankle sprains.

Treatment and evaluation of persons with CAI should address not only the instability at the ankle but also balance and strength deficits across the body as a whole. Some recommended treatments include whole-body neuromuscular and proprioception-based exercise, balance board training, graded joint mobilization to improve dorsiflexion, trigger point dry needling in conjunction with proprioceptive training, and visual biofeedback during gait training to limit the amount of foot inversion at heel strike.[b]

[a]42,53,57,58,59,114,118,175,216
[b]89,126,155,213,219,258

ADDITIONAL CLINICAL CONNECTIONS

CLINICAL CONNECTION 14.3
Palpation of Selected Anatomy of the Ankle and Foot

The ability to palpate and thus identify the bones and joints of the body is an essential clinical skill, routinely used in both evaluation and treatment of musculoskeletal disorders. Such a skill allows the clinician a "window" into the anatomy (and ultimately the kinesiology) of the region. Skill with palpation (1) facilitates clinical communication and documentation, (2) improves the ability to identify key tissues often for the purpose of diagnosing or monitoring a patient's condition, (3) improves the implementation of manually based treatment, and (4) helps with the assessment of normal and abnormal movement and posture.

The following section provides examples of bony regions of the ankle and foot that are routinely palpated as part of the assessment or treatment of common musculoskeletal disorders. These bony regions or joints are highlighted in medial and lateral perspectives using a radiograph and photograph of a healthy 23-year-old man (Figs. 14.54 and 14.55). Each figure is associated with a table that describes (1) a method for palpating the structure and (2) examples of why clinicians may be interested in the region.

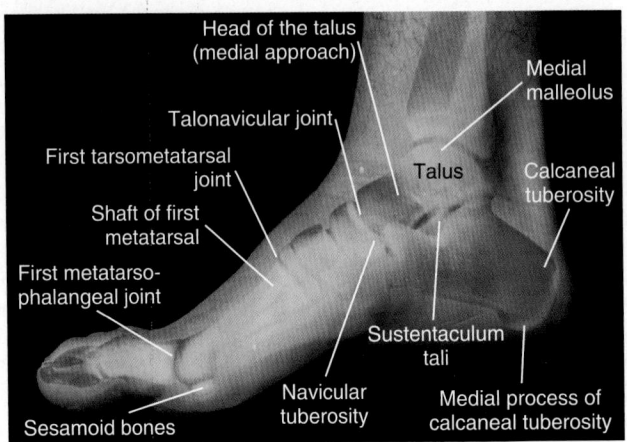

Medial perspective

Structure	Where to Palpate	Possible Reasons for Palpation

Medial malleolus	Extreme distal end of medial tibia	• Assess tenderness of the proximal attachment of the deltoid ligament
		• Assess leg length
		• Estimate medial-lateral axis of rotation at the talocrural joint
		• Anatomic reference for locating structures in the tarsal tunnel, such as:
		  o tendon of the tibialis posterior
		  o flexor digitorum longus
		  o tibial nerve and terminal branches (medial and lateral plantar nerves)

Calcaneal tuberosity	Posterior-plantar heel region	• Evaluate for Achilles tendinopathy • Check for abnormal bone formation (possibly related to excessive stress placed on the Achilles tendon)
Medial process of calcaneal tuberosity	Plantar-medial heel region	• Evaluate for plantar fasciitis, heel spurs, or inflamed proximal attachment of many intrinsic muscles of the foot
Sustentaculum tali	Approximately 2-3 cm inferior to the tip of the medial malleolus	• Anatomic reference for locating medial surface of the subtalar joint • Evaluate tenderness of (a) distal attachment of tibiocalcaneal fibers of the deltoid ligament, (b) proximal attachment of the "spring" ligament

FIG. 14.54 Medial perspective using a radiograph and photograph of a healthy 23-year-old man.

Continued

ADDITIONAL CLINICAL CONNECTIONS

Structure	Where to Palpate	Possible Reasons for Palpation
Navicular tuberosity	As a relatively sharp projection, located approximately 4 cm inferior-and-anterior to the tip of the medial malleolus	• General reference for locating the navicular bone, including the nearby talonavicular and first cuneonavicular joints • Assess height of medial longitudinal arch • Assess tibialis posterior tendinopathy
Sesamoid bones	Plantar aspect of metatarsophalangeal joint of great toe (typically difficult to distinguish from flexor tendons crossing the joint)	• Evaluate for tenderness associated with sesamoiditis or fracture (common in dancers)
First metatarsophalangeal joint	Dorsal or medially; immediately distal to the head of the first metatarsal bone	• Evaluate severity of hallux valgus or "turf toe"
Shaft of the first metatarsal	Dorsal or medial aspect of forefoot	• Assess alignment (e.g., valgus or varus) and overall flexibility of the forefoot • Evaluate plantar flexed first ray, such as that often associated with pes cavus, or increased tension in the fibularis longus
Tarsometatarsal joint	Immediately proximal to the base of the metatarsal	• Evaluate laxity or alignment of the joint of the first digit • Assess Lisfranc's dislocation (typically second digit)
Talonavicular joint	Immediately posterior (and slightly superior) to the navicular tuberosity	• Evaluate for sprain, tenderness, and general mobility of the medial component of the transverse tarsal joint • Check stability of the keystone of the medial longitudinal arch
Head of the talus	Medial approach: About midway between the anterior-distal edge of the medial malleolus and the navicular tuberosity	• Assess height of medial longitudinal arch

FIG. 14.54, cont'd

Continued

ADDITIONAL CLINICAL CONNECTIONS

CLINICAL CONNECTION 14.3
Palpation of Selected Anatomy of the Ankle and Foot—cont'd

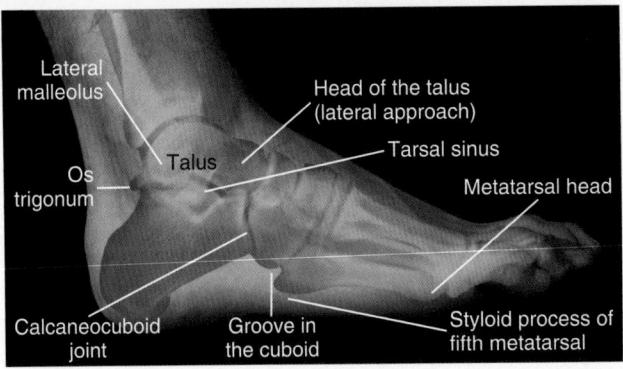

Lateral malleolus

Head of the talus (lateral approach)

Talus

Tarsal sinus

Os trigonum

Metatarsal head

Calcaneocuboid joint

Groove in the cuboid

Styloid process of fifth metatarsal

Lateral perspective

Structure	Where to Palpate	Possible Reasons for Palpation
Lateral malleolus	Extreme distal end of fibula	• Estimate medial-lateral axis of rotation at the talocrural joint • Reference for locating the tendons (and sheaths) of the fibularis longus and brevis • Testing the stability or alignment of the distal tibiofibular joint
Tarsal sinus	As a slight depression, just anterior to the extreme distal aspect of the lateral malleolus. This sinus (or canal) courses obliquely through the subtalar joint	• Assess tenderness in the anterior talofibular ligament • Evaluate swelling possibly from injury to the cervical (talocalcaneal) ligament, located within the tarsal sinus
Head of the talus	Lateral approach: Immediately superior to the tarsal sinus	• In conjunction with a medial palpation approach, used to determine "subtalar neutral position"
Metatarsal head	Plantar aspect of the distal end of the metatarsal bone	• Assess severity of metatarsalgia (frequently on second or third digits)
Styloid process of fifth metatarsal	As a sharp projection, located at the approximate midpoint of the lateral side of the foot	• Assess possible avulsion fracture and tear of the fibularis brevis tendon
Groove in the cuboid	Immediately proximal to the styloid process of the fifth metatarsal	• Assess tenderness of the tendon of the fibularis longus
Calcaneocuboid joint	About 2 cm proximal to the styloid process of the fifth metatarsal	• Evaluate subluxation or other trauma associated with the cuboid
Os trigonum (infrequent appearance of an accessory bone, usually located posterior-lateral to the talus)	On the posterior aspect of the ankle, posterior to the lateral malleolus; depending on its size, however, this structure may not be readily palpable	• Evaluate possible impingement of the Os trigonum within the talocrural joint, usually at the extremes of plantar flexion

FIG. 14.55 Lateral perspective using a radiograph and photograph of a healthy 23-year-old man.

ADDITIONAL CLINICAL CONNECTIONS

An important function of the plantar flexor muscles is to stabilize the knee in extension while in an upright and weight-bearing position. This function becomes evident while observing the gait of a person with weakened or poorly activated plantar flexor muscles. Normally the plantar flexor muscles "brake" or decelerate ankle dorsiflexion (leg moving forward on foot) during the mid-to-late stance phase of gait. Excessive dorsiflexion at this time in the gait cycle can contribute to knee instability. Fig. 14.56A shows a hypothetical case of a person with a weakened soleus muscle unable to control forward rotation of the leg. The excessively dorsiflexed ankle shifts the force of body weight well *posterior* to the medial-lateral axis of rotation at the knee. This shift can create a sudden and often unexpected knee flexion torque. (Indeed, persons with weakened plantar flexors often describe a sensation of their knee "giving away" or buckling during mid stance phase or while standing on one leg.) The dorsiflexed ankle, in this case, biases flexion of the knee. Normally the soleus muscle can resist excessive forward rotation of the leg, thereby maintaining body weight closer to the knee's medial-lateral axis of rotation.

With the foot fixed to the ground, active contraction of the plantar flexion muscles can assist in extending the knee (see Fig. 14.56B). In this example, contraction of the soleus muscle rotates the leg posteriorly about the talocrural joint's axis of rotation.

Although any plantar flexor muscle is theoretically capable of this action, the soleus is particularly well suited to stabilize the knee in extension. As a predominantly slow-twitch muscle, the soleus can produce forces over a relatively long duration before fatiguing. Marked spasticity in the soleus muscle can exert a potent and chronic knee extension bias that, over time, can contribute to genu recurvatum deformity.

The ability of the plantar flexor muscles to assist indirectly with knee extension is a potentially important clinical phenomenon. Equally important in this regard is the ability of the *hip extensor muscles* to assist indirectly with knee extension. With the foot planted to the ground, strong activation of a hip extensor (such as that depicted in Fig. 14.56B) can pull the femur posteriorly. If the femur is pulled into full hip extension, body weight can help mechanically lock the knee into extension. A hip or knee flexion contracture would reduce the effectiveness of this mechanical locking.

By far, the most direct and effective knee extensor muscle is the quadriceps. In cases of quadriceps weakness, however, it is clinically useful to know how other muscles can assist (even if slightly) with knee extension when standing. Even persons with strong quadriceps can benefit from recruiting hip extensor and plantar flexor muscles as indirect extensors of the knee. Reducing local demands on the quadriceps can minimize forces at the patellofemoral joint, which is often a desired strategy (at least in the short term) for someone with pain, instability, or arthritis at this joint.

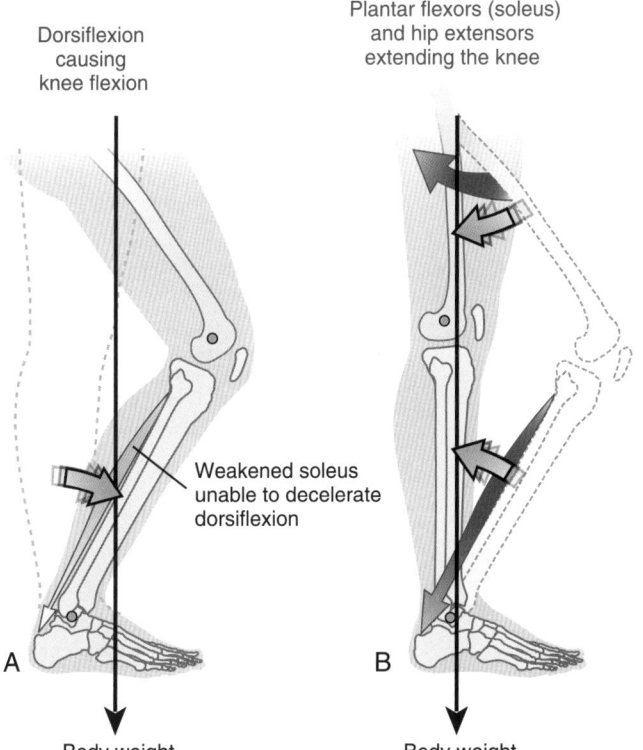

Dorsiflexion causing knee flexion

Plantar flexors (soleus) and hip extensors extending the knee

Weakened soleus unable to decelerate dorsiflexion

A

B

Body weight

Body weight

FIG. 14.56 Two examples of how the ankle affects the position and stability of the knee during standing. (A) The weakened soleus muscle is unable to decelerate ankle dorsiflexion. With the foot fixed to the ground, ankle dorsiflexion occurs as a forward rotation of the leg over the talus. The forward position of the leg shifts the force of body weight well posterior to the knee, potentially causing it to "buckle" into flexion. (B) Normal strength and control of the soleus muscle can cause the ankle to plantar flex. With the foot fixed to the ground, plantar flexion rotates the leg posteriorly, bringing the knee toward extension. The contraction of a hip extensor muscle (such as the gluteus maximus) is also shown helping to extend the knee by pulling the femur posteriorly. (NOTE: The downward-directed body weight vectors could be considered as acting upward as ground reaction forces; either assumption is valid.)

REFERENCES

1. Alexander RM, Bennet-Clark HC: Storage of elastic strain energy in muscle and other tissues, *Nature* 265(5590):114–117, 1977.
2. Anandacoomarasamy A, Barnsley L: Long term outcomes of inversion ankle injuries, *Br J Sports Med* 39:e14, 2005.
3. Anavian J, Marchetti DC, Moatshe G, et al.: The forgotten joint: quantifying the anatomy of the proximal tibiofibular joint, *Knee Surg Sports Traumatol Arthrosc* 26(4):1096–1103, 2018.
4. Anderson DD, Chubinskaya S, Guilak F, et al.: Post-traumatic osteoarthritis: improved understanding and opportunities for early intervention [Review], *J Orthop Res* 29(6):802–809, 2011.
5. Anderson DE, Madigan ML: Healthy older adults have insufficient hip range of motion and plantar flexor strength to walk like healthy young adults, *J Biomech* 47:1104–1109, 2014.
6. Andreasen J, Molgaard CM, Christensen M, et al.: Exercise therapy and custom-made insoles are effective in patients with excessive pronation and chronic foot pain–a randomized controlled trial, *Foot (Edinb)* 23(1):22–28, 2013.
7. Angin S, Mickle KJ, Nester CJ: Contributions of foot muscles and plantar fascia morphology to foot posture, *Gait Posture* 61:238–242, 2018.
8. Arinci Incel N, Genc H, Erdem HR, et al.: Muscle imbalance in hallux valgus: an electromyographic study, *Am J Phys Med Rehabil* 82:345–349, 2003.
9. Asitha J, Zionts LE, Morcuende JA: Management of idiopathic clubfoot after formal training in the Ponseti method: a multi-year, international survey, *Iowa Orthop J* 33:136–141, 2013.
10. Atbasi Z, Erdem Y, Kose O, et al.: Relationship between hallux valgus and pes planus: real or fiction? *J Foot Ankle Surg* 59:513–517, 2020.
11. Aynardi MC, Saloky K, Roush EP, et al.: Biomechanical evaluation of spring ligament augmentation with the fibertape device in a cadaveric flatfoot model, *Foot Ankle Int* 40(5):596–602, 2019.
12. Banskota B, Banskota AK, Regmi R, et al.: The Ponseti method in the treatment of children with idiopathic clubfoot presenting between five and ten years of age, *Bone Joint Lett J* 95-B(12):1721–1725, 2013.
13. Barton CJ, Menz HB, Levinger P, et al.: Greater peak rearfoot eversion predicts foot orthoses efficacy in individuals with patellofemoral pain syndrome, *Br J Sports Med* 45(9):697–701, 2011.
14. Bartoníček J: Anatomy of the tibiofibular syndesmosis and its clinical relevance, *Surg Radiol Anat* 25(5-6):379–386, 2003.
15. Basmajian JV, Bentzon JW: An electromyographic study of certain muscles of the foot in the standing position, *Surg Gynecol Obstet* V98:662–666, 1954.
16. Basmajian JV, Stecko G: The role of muscles in arch support of the foot, *J Bone Joint Surg Am* 45:1184–1190, 1963.
17. Behling AV, Nigg BM: Relationships between the foot posture index and static as well as dynamic rear foot and arch variables, *J Biomech* 98:109448, 2020.
18. Beimers L, Tuijthof GJ, Blankevoort L, et al.: In-vivo range of motion of the subtalar joint using computed tomography, *J Biomech* 41:1390–1397, 2008.
19. Bencke J, Christiansen D, Jensen K, et al.: Measuring medial longitudinal arch deformation during gait. A reliability study, *Gait Posture* 35(3):400–404, 2012.
20. Beumer A, van Hemert WL, Swierstra BA, et al.: A biomechanical evaluation of the tibiofibular and tibiotalar ligaments of the ankle, *Foot Ankle Int* 24:426–429, 2003.
21. Blackwood CB, Yuen TJ, Sangeorzan BJ, et al.: The midtarsal joint locking mechanism, *Foot Ankle Int* 26:1074–1080, 2005.
22. Boldt AR, Willson JD, Barrios JA, et al.: Effects of medially wedged foot orthoses on knee and hip joint running mechanics in females with and without patellofemoral pain syndrome, *J Appl Biomech* 29(1):68–77, 2013.
23. Boone DC, Azen SP: Normal range of motion of joints in male subjects, *J Bone Joint Surg Am* 61:756–759, 1979.
24. Bouchard M: Assessment and management of the pediatric cavovarus foot, *Instr Course Lect* 69:381–390, 2020.
25. Bowers Jr KD, Martin RB: Turf-toe: a shoe-surface related football injury, *Med Sci Sports* 8:81–83, 1976.
26. Braga UM, Mendonca LD, Mascarenhas RO, et al.: Effects of medially wedged insoles on the biomechanics of the lower limbs of runners with excessive foot pronation and foot varus alignment, *Gait Posture* 74:242–249, 2019.
27. Brukner P, Bradshaw C, Khan KM, et al.: Stress fractures: a review of 180 cases, *Clin J Sport Med* 6:85–89, 1996.
28. Buckwalter JA, Brown TD: Joint injury, repair and remodeling: roles in post-traumatic osteoarthritis, *Clin Orthop Relat Res* 423:7–16, 2004.
29. Calhoun JH, Li F, Ledbetter BR, et al.: A comprehensive study of pressure distribution in the ankle joint with inversion and eversion, *Foot Ankle Int* 15:125–133, 1994.
30. Campbell KJ, Michalski MP, Wilson KJ, et al.: The ligament anatomy of the deltoid complex of the ankle: a qualitative and quantitative anatomical study, *J Bone Joint Surg Am* 96(8):e62, 2014. 1–10.
31. Cao S, Wang C, Zhang C, et al.: Length change pattern of the ankle deltoid ligament during physiological ankle motion, *Foot Ankle Surg* 28(7):950–955, 2022.
32. Cardoso TB, Ocarino JM, Fajardo CC, et al.: Hip external rotation stiffness and midfoot passive mechanical resistance are associated with lower limb movement in the frontal and transverse planes during gait, *Gait Posture* 76:305–310, 2020.
33. Cavanagh PR, Rodgers MM, Iiboshi A: Pressure distribution under symptom-free feet during barefoot standing, *Foot Ankle* 7:262–276, 1987.
34. Chan VO, Moran DE, Shine S, et al.: Medial joint line bone bruising at MRI complicating acute ankle inversion injury: what is its clinical significance? *Clin Radiol* 68(10):e519–e523, 2013.
35. Chang R, Kent-Braun JA, Hamill J: Use of MRI for volume estimation of tibialis posterior and plantar intrinsic foot muscles in healthy and chronic plantar fasciitis limbs, *Clin Biomech (Bristol, Avon)* 27(5):500–505, 2012.
36. Chang R, Rodrigues PA, Van Emmerik RE, et al.: Multi-segment foot kinematics and ground reaction forces during gait of individuals with plantar fasciitis, *J Biomech* 47(11):2571–2577, 2014.
37. Cheung RT, Chung RC, Ng GY: Efficacies of different external controls for excessive foot pronation: a meta analysis, *Br J Sports Med* 45:743–751, 2011.
38. Close JR, Inman VT, Poor PM, et al.: The function of the subtalar joint, *Clin Orthop Relat Res* 50:159–179, 1967.
39. Collins N, Bisset L, McPoil T, et al.: Foot orthoses in lower limb overuse conditions: a systematic review and meta-analysis, *Foot Ankle Int* 28(3):396–412, 2007.
40. Colville MR, Marder RA, Boyle JJ, et al.: Strain measurement in lateral ankle ligaments, *Am J Sports Med* 18:196–200, 1990.
41. Corazza F, Stagni R, Castelli VP, et al.: Articular contact at the tibiotalar joint in passive flexion, *J Biomech* 38:1205–1212, 2005.
42. Cornwall MW, Jain T, Hagel T: Tibial and calcaneal coupling during walking in those with chronic ankle instability, *Gait Posture* 70:130–135, 2019.
43. Cornwall MW, McPoil TG: Motion of the calcaneus, navicular, and first metatarsal during the stance phase of walking, *J Am Podiatr Med Assoc* 92:67–76, 2002.
44. Cornwall MW, McPoil TG: Three-dimensional movement of the foot during the stance phase of walking, *J Am Podiatr Med Assoc* 89:56–66, 1999.
45. Coughlin MJ, Kemp TJ, Hirose CB: Turf toe: soft tissue and osteocartilaginous injury to the first metatarsophalangeal joint, *Phys Sportsmed* 38(1):91–100, 2010.
46. Cowie S, Parsons S, Scammell B, et al.: Hypermobility of the first ray in patients with planovalgus feet and tarsometatarsal osteoarthritis, *J Foot Ankle Surg* 18(4):237–240, 2012.
47. Crim JR, Beals TC, Nickisch F, et al.: Deltoid ligament abnormalities in chronic lateral ankle instability, *Foot Ankle Int* 32(9):873–878, 2011.
48. Croy T, Saliba SA, Saliba E, et al.: Differences in lateral ankle laxity measured via stress ultrasonography in individuals with chronic ankle instability, ankle sprain copers, and healthy individuals, *J Orthop Sports Phys Ther* 42(7):593–600, 2012.
49. Cruz EP, Wagner FV, Henning C, et al.: Does hallux valgus exhibit a deformity inherent to the first metatarsal bone? *J Foot Ankle Surg* 58(6):1210–1214, 2019.
50. Dalmau-Pastor M, Malagelada F, Calder J, et al.: The lateral ankle ligaments are interconnected: the medial connecting fibres between the anterior talofibular, calcaneofibular and posterior talofibular ligaments, *Knee Surg Sports Traumatol Arthrosc* 28(1):34–39, 2020.
51. Davis WH, Sobel M, DiCarlo EF, et al.: Gross, histological, and microvascular anatomy and biomechanical testing of the spring ligament complex, *Foot Ankle Int* 17:95–102, 1996.
52. de Podesta Haje D, Maranho DA, Ferreira GF, et al.: Ponseti method after walking age - a multi-centric study of 429 feet: results, possible treatment modifications and outcomes according to age groups, *Iowa Orthop J* 40(2):1–12, 2020.
53. Dejong AF, Koldenhoven RM, Hertel J: Proximal adaptations in chronic ankle instability: systematic review and meta-analysis, *Med Sci Sports Exerc* 52(7):1563–1575, 2020.
54. Dietze A, Bahlke U, Martin H, et al.: First ray instability in hallux valgus deformity: a radiokinematic and pedobarographic analysis, *Foot Ankle Int* 34(1):124–130, 2013.
55. Docking SI, Hart HF, Rio E, et al.: Explaining variability in the prevalence of Aachilles tendon abnormalities: a systematic review with meta-analysis of imaging studies in asymptomatic individuals, *J Orthop Sports Phys Ther* 51(5):232–252, 2021.
56. Doherty C, Bleakley C, Hertel J, et al.: Recovery from a first-time lateral ankle sprain and the predictors of chronic ankle instability: a prospective cohort analysis, *Am J Sports Med* 44(4):995–1003, 2016.
57. Doherty C, Bleakley C, Hertel J, et al.: Dynamic balance deficits 6 months following first-time acute lateral ankle sprain: a laboratory analysis, *J Orthop Sports Phys Ther* 45(8):626–633, 2015.
58. Donahue MS, Docherty CL, Riley ZA: Decreased fibularis reflex response during inversion perturbations in FAI subjects, *J Electromyogr Kinesiol* 24(1):84–89, 2014.
59. Dury J, Michel F, Ravier G: Fatigue of hip abductor muscles implies neuromuscular and kinematic adaptations of the ankle during dynamic balance, *Scand J Med Sci Sports* 32(9):1324–1334, 2022.
60. Edama M, Takabayashi T, Inai T, et al.: Differences in the strain applied to Achilles tendon fibers when the subtalar joint is overpronated: a simulation study, *Surg Radiol Anat* 41(5):595–599, 2019.
61. Edama M, Takabayashi T, Inai T, et al.: Morphological features of the cervical ligament, *Surg Radiol Anat* 42(2):215–218, 2020.
62. Elbaum R, Noel B, Degueldre V, et al.: 20 years of functional treatment for clubfoot: advantages and limitations compared with the Ponseti method, *J Pediatr Orthop B*, 2021.
63. Erdemir A, Hamel AJ, Fauth AR, et al.: Dynamic loading of the plantar aponeurosis in walking, *J Bone Joint Surg Am* 86:546–552, 2004.
64. Ferber R, Davis IM, Williams III DS: Effect of foot orthotics on rearfoot and tibia joint coupling patterns and variability, *J Biomech* 38:477–483, 2005.
65. Fernandez-Seguin LM, Diaz Mancha JA, Sanchez RR, et al.: Comparison of plantar pressures and contact

area between normal and cavus foot, *Gait Posture* 39(2):789–792, 2014.

66. Ferreira AS, de Oliveira Silva D, Briani RV, et al.: Which is the best predictor of excessive hip internal rotation in women with patellofemoral pain: rearfoot eversion or hip muscle strength? Exploring subgroups, *Gait Posture* 62:366–371, 2018.

67. Fiolkowski P, Brunt D, Bishop M, et al.: Intrinsic pedal musculature support of the medial longitudinal arch: an electromyography study, *J Foot Ankle Surg* 42(6):327–333, 2003.

68. Flores DV, Mejia Gomez C, Fernandez Hernando M, et al.: Adult acquired flatfoot deformity: anatomy, biomechanics, staging, and imaging findings, *Radiographics* 39(5):1437–1460, 2019.

69. Foster A, Blanchette MG, Chou YC, et al.: The influence of heel height on frontal plane ankle biomechanics: implications for lateral ankle sprains, *Foot Ankle Int* 33(1):64–69, 2012.

70. Francis CA, Lenz AL, Lenhart RL, et al.: The modulation of forward propulsion, vertical support, and center of pressure by the plantar flexors during human walking, *Gait Posture* 38(4):993–997, 2013.

71. Franettovich M, Chapman A, Blanch P, et al.: A physiological and psychological basis for anti-pronation taping from a critical review of the literature, *Sports Med* 38:617–631, 2008.

72. Franklyn-Miller A, Wilson C, Bilzon J, et al.: Foot orthoses in the prevention of injury in initial military training: a randomized controlled trial, *Am J Sports Med* 39(1):30–37, 2011.

73. Frisk RF, Lorentzen J, Barber L, et al.: Characterization of torque generating properties of ankle plantar flexor muscles in ambulant adults with cerebral palsy, *Eur J Appl Physiol* 119(5):1127–1136, 2019.

74. Fritz GR, Prieskorn D: First metatarsocuneiform motion: a radiographic and statistical analysis, *Foot Ankle Int* 16:117–123, 1995.

75. Fujii T, Kitaoka HB, Luo ZP, et al.: Analysis of ankle-hindfoot stability in multiple planes: an in vitro study, *Foot Ankle Int* 26:633–637, 2005.

76. Fujii T, Kitaoka HB, Watanabe K, et al.: Ankle stability in simulated lateral ankle ligament injuries, *Foot Ankle Int* 31(6):531–537, 2010.

77. Fujii T, Luo ZP, Kitaoka HB, et al.: The manual stress test may not be sufficient to differentiate ankle ligament injuries, *Clin Biomech* 15:619–623, 2000.

78. Fukano M, Fukubayashi T, Kumai T: In vivo talocrural and subtalar kinematics during the stance phase of walking in individuals with repetitive ankle sprains, *J Biomech* 101:109651, 2020.

79. Fung J, Sherman A, Stachura S, et al.: Nonoperative management of hallux limitus using a novel forefoot orthosis, *J Foot Ankle Surg* 59(6):1192–1196, 2020.

80. Gehring D, Wissler S, Mornieux G, et al.: How to sprain your ankle—a biomechanical case report of an inversion trauma, *J Biomech* 46(1):175–178, 2013.

81. George E, Harris AH, Dragoo JL, et al.: Incidence and risk factors for turf toe injuries in intercollegiate football: data from the national collegiate athletic association injury surveillance system, *Foot Ankle Int* 35(2):108–115, 2014.

82. Gerard R, Unno-Veith F, Fasel J, et al.: The effect of collateral ligament release on ankle dorsiflexion: an anatomical study, *J Foot Ankle Surg* 17(3):193–196, 2011.

83. Ghani Zadeh Hesar N, Van Ginckel A, Cools A, et al.: A prospective study on gait-related intrinsic risk factors for lower leg overuse injuries, *Br J Sports Med* 43(13):1057–1061, 2009.

84. Glasoe WM, Phadke V, Pena FA, et al.: An image-based gait simulation study of tarsal kinematics in women with hallux valgus, *Phys Ther* 93(11):1551–1562, 2013.

85. Glasoe WM, Yack HJ, Saltzman CL: Anatomy and biomechanics of the first ray, *Phys Ther* 79:854–859, 1999.

86. Gray EG, Basmajian JV: Electromyography and cinematography of leg and foot ("normal" and flat) during walking, *Anat Rec* 161:1–15, 1968.

87. Grimston SK, Nigg BM, Hanley DA, et al.: Differences in ankle joint complex range of motion as a function of age, *Foot Ankle* 14:215–222, 1993.

88. Hahn D, Olvermann M, Richtberg J, et al.: Knee and ankle joint torque-angle relationships of multi-joint leg extension, *J Biomech* 44(11):2059–2065, 2011.

89. Hale SA, Hertel J, Olmsted-Kramer LC: The effect of a 4-week comprehensive rehabilitation program on postural control and lower extremity function in individuals with chronic ankle instability, *J Orthop Sports Phys Ther* 37:303–311, 2007.

90. Han Q, Liu Y, Chang F, et al.: Measurement of talar morphology in northeast Chinese population based on three-dimensional computed tomography, *Medicine (Baltim)* 98(37):e17142, 2019.

91. Handsfield GG, Greiner J, Madl J, et al.: Achilles subtendon structure and behavior as evidenced from tendon imaging and computational modeling, *Front Sports Act Living* 2:70, 2020.

92. Harradine P, Gates L, Bowen C: If it doesn't work, why do we still do it? The continuing use of subtalar joint neutral theory in the face of overpowering critical research, *J Orthop Sports Phys Ther* 48(3):130–132, 2018.

93. Hashizume S, Iwanuma S, Akagi R, et al.: In vivo determination of the Achilles tendon moment arm in three-dimensions, *J Biomech* 45(2):409–413, 2012.

94. Hauret KG, Shippey DL, Knapik JJ: The physical training and rehabilitation program: duration of rehabilitation and final outcome of injuries in basic combat training, *Mil Med* 166:820–826, 2001.

95. Headlee DL, Leonard JL, Hart JM, et al.: Fatigue of the plantar intrinsic foot muscles increases navicular drop, *J Electromyogr Kinesiol* 18(3):420–425, 2008.

96. Hermans JJ, Beumer A, de Jong TA, et al.: Anatomy of the distal tibiofibular syndesmosis in adults: a pictorial essay with a multimodality approach. [Review], *J Anat* 217(6):633–645, 2010.

97. Hernandez-Guillen D, Blasco JM: A randomized controlled trial assessing the evolution of the weight-bearing ankle dorsiflexion range of motion over 6 sessions of talus mobilizations in older adults, *Phys Ther* 100(4):645–652, 2020.

98. Hicks JH: The mechanics of the foot. II. The plantar aponeurosis and the arch, *J Anat* 88(1):25–30, 1954.

99. Hillstrom HJ, Song J, Kraszewski AP, et al.: Foot type biomechanics part 1: structure and function of the asymptomatic foot, *Gait Posture* 37(3):445–451, 2013.

100. Hoch MC, Andreatta RD, Mullineaux DR, et al.: Two-week joint mobilization intervention improves self-reported function, range of motion, and dynamic balance in those with chronic ankle instability, *J Orthop Res* 30(11):1798–1804, 2012.

101. Hopkins JT, Coglianese M, Glasgow P, et al.: Alterations in evertor/invertor muscle activation and center of pressure trajectory in participants with functional ankle instability, *J Electromyogr Kinesiol* 22(2):280–285, 2012.

102. Hu WK, Chen DW, Li B, et al.: Motion of the distal tibiofibular syndesmosis under different loading patterns: a biomechanical study, *J Ortho Surg* 27(2):1–6, 2019.

103. Huang CK, Kitaoka HB, An KN, et al.: Biomechanical evaluation of longitudinal arch stability, *Foot Ankle* 14:353–357, 1993.

104. Hubbard TJ, Hertel J, Sherbondy P: Fibular position in individuals with self-reported chronic ankle instability, *J Orthop Sports Phys Ther* 36:3–9, 2006.

105. Huber T, Schmoelz W, Bölderl A: Motion of the fibula relative to the tibia and its alterations with syndesmosis screws: a cadaver study, *Foot Ankle Surg* 18(3):203–209, 2012.

106. Hunt AE, Smith RM: Mechanics and control of the flat versus normal foot during the stance phase of walking, *Clin Biomech (Bristol, Avon)* 19:391–397, 2004.

107. Hunt KJ, Pereira H, Kelley J, et al.: The role of calcaneofibular ligament injury in ankle instability: implications for surgical management, *Am J Sports Med* 47(2):431–437, 2019.

108. Hurn SE, Matthews BG, Munteanu SE, et al.: Effectiveness of nonsurgical interventions for hallux valgus: S systematic review and meta-analysis, *Arthritis Care Res (Hoboken)* 74(10):1676–1688, 2022.

109. Inman VT, Ralston HJ, Todd F: *Human walking*, Baltimore, 1981, Williams & Wilkins.

110. Ishikawa M, Komi PV, Grey MJ, et al.: Muscle–tendon interaction and elastic energy usage in human walking, *J Appl Physiol* 99(2):603–608, 2005.

111. Jayawardena A, Wijayasinghe SR, Tennakoon D, et al.: Early effects of a 'train the trainer' approach to Ponseti method dissemination: a case study of Sri Lanka, *Iowa Orthop J* 33:153–160, 2013.

112. Jeong MS, Choi YS, Kim YJ, et al.: Deltoid ligament in acute ankle injury: MR imaging analysis, *Skeletal Radiol* 43(5):655–663, 2014.

113. Jones MH, Amendola AS: Acute treatment of inversion ankle sprains: immobilization versus functional treatment, *Clin Orthop Relat Res* 455:169–172, 2007.

114. Kavanagh JJ, Bisset LM, Tsao H: Deficits in reaction time due to increased motor time of peroneus longus in people with chronic ankle instability, *J Biomech* 45(3):605–608, 2012.

115. Kelly LA, Cresswell AG, Racinais S, et al.: Intrinsic foot muscles have the capacity to control deformation of the longitudinal arch, *J R Soc Interface* 11(93):20131188, 2014.

116. Kelly LA, Farris DJ, Cresswell AG, et al.: Intrinsic foot muscles contribute to elastic energy storage and return in the human foot, *J Appl Physiol* 126(1):231–238, 2019.

117. Kelly LA, Kuitunen S, Racinais S, et al.: Recruitment of the plantar intrinsic foot muscles with increasing postural demand, *Clin Biomech* 27(1):46–51, 2012.

118. Khalaj N, Vicenzino B, Heales LJ, et al.: Is chronic ankle instability associated with impaired muscle strength? Ankle, knee and hip muscle strength in individuals with chronic ankle instability: a systematic review with meta-Analysis, *Br J Sports Med* 54(14):839–847, 2020.

119. Kirmizi M, Cakiroglu MA, Elvan A, et al.: Reliability of different clinical techniques for assessing foot posture, *J Manip Physiol Ther* 43(9):901–908, 2020.

120. Kitaoka HB, Luo ZP, Growney ES, et al.: Material properties of the plantar aponeurosis, *Foot Ankle Int* 15:557–560, 1994.

121. Klein P, Mattys S, Rooze M: Moment arm length variations of selected muscles acting on talocrural and subtalar joints during movement: an in vitro study, *J Biomech* 29:21–30, 1996.

122. Kleipool RP, Vuurberg G, Stufkens SAS, et al.: Bilateral symmetry of the subtalar joint facets and the relationship between the morphology and osteoarthritic changes, *Clin Anat* 33(7):997–1006, 2020.

123. Knudson GA, Kitaoka HB, Lu CL, et al.: Subtalar joint stability. Talocalcaneal interosseous ligament function studied in cadaver specimens, *Acta Orthop Scand* 68:442–446, 1997.

124. Kohls-Gatzoulis J, Angel JC, Singh D, et al.: Tibialis posterior dysfunction: a common and treatable cause of adult acquired flatfoot, *Br Med J* 329:1328–1333, 2004.

125. Kokubo T, Hashimoto T, Nagura T, et al.: Effect of the posterior tibial and peroneal longus on the mechanical properties of the foot arch, *Foot Ankle Int* 33(4):320–325, 2012.

126. Koldenhoven RM, Jaffri AH, DeJong AF, et al.: Gait biofeedback and impairment-based rehabilitation for chronic ankle instability, *Scand J Med Sci Sports* 31(1):193–204, 2021.

127. Koller U, Willegger M, Windhager R, et al.: Plantar pressure characteristics in hallux valgus feet, *J Orthop Res* 32(12):1688–1693, 2014.

128. Kondo M, Iwamoto Y, Kito N: Relationship between forward propulsion and foot motion during gait in healthy young adults, *J Biomech* 121:110431, 2021.

129. Konradsen L: Sensori-motor control of the uninjured and injured human ankle, *J Electromyogr Kinesiol* 12:199–203, 2002.

130. Kosashvili Y, Fridman T, Backstein D, et al.: The correlation between pes planus and anterior knee or intermittent low back pain, *Foot Ankle Int* 29:910–913, 2008.

131. Koshino Y, Yamanaka M, Ezawa Y, et al.: Coupling motion between rearfoot and hip and knee joints during walking and single-leg landing, *J Electromyogr Kinesiol* 37:75–83, 2017.

132. Kruger KM, Graf A, Flanagan A, et al.: Segmental foot and ankle kinematic differences between rectus, planus, and cavus foot types, *J Biomech* 94:180–186, 2019.

133. Kulig K, Burnfield JM, Reischl S, et al.: Effect of foot orthoses on tibialis posterior activation in persons with pes planus, *Med Sci Sports Exerc* 37:24–29, 2005.

134. Kulig K, Burnfield JM, Requejo SM, et al.: Selective activation of tibialis posterior: evaluation by magnetic resonance imaging, *Med Sci Sports Exerc* 36:862–867, 2004.

135. Kulig K, Reischl SF, Pomrantz AB, et al.: Nonsurgical management of posterior tibial tendon dysfunction with orthoses and resistive exercise: a randomized controlled trial, *Phys Ther* 89:26–37, 2009.

136. Lai A, Lichtwark GA, Schache AG, et al.: In vivo behavior of the human soleus muscle with increasing walking and running speeds, *J Appl Physiol* 118(10):1266–1275, 2015.

137. Leardini A, Benedetti MG, Berti L, et al.: Rear-foot, mid-foot and fore-foot motion during the stance phase of gait, *Gait Posture* 25:453–462, 2007.

138. Lee JH, Kyung MG, Cho YJ, et al.: Prevalence of accessory bones and tarsal coalitions based on radiographic findings in a healthy, asymptomatic population, *Clin Orthop Surg* 12(2):245–251, 2020.

139. Leland RH, Marymont JV, Trevino SG, et al.: Calcaneocuboid stability: a clinical and anatomic study, *Foot Ankle Int* 22:880–884, 2001.

140. Lenz AL, Nichols JA, Roach KE, et al.: Compensatory motion of the subtalar joint following tibiotalar arthrodesis: an in vivo dual-fluoroscopy imaging study, *J Bone Joint Surg Am* 102(7):600–608, 2020.

141. Lewis OJ: The comparative morphology of M. flexor accessorius and the associated long flexor tendons, *J Anat* 96:321–333, 1962.

142. Lichtwark GA, Wilson AM: Interactions between the human gastrocnemius muscle and the Achilles tendon during incline, level and decline locomotion, *J Exp Biol* 209(21):4379–4388, 2006.

143. Lin KW, Hu CJ, Yang WW, et al.: Biomechanical evaluation and strength test of 3D-printed foot orthoses, *Appl Bionics Biomech* 2019:4989534, 2019.

144. Longo UG, Loppini M, Fumo C, et al.: Deep deltoid ligament injury is related to rotational instability of the ankle joint: a biomechanical study, *Knee Surg Sports Traumatol Arthrosc*, 2020.

145. Lucas R, Cornwall M: Influence of foot posture on the functioning of the windlass mechanism, *Foot* 30:38–42, 2017.

146. Lundgren P, Nester C, Liu A, et al.: Invasive in vivo measurement of rear-, mid- and forefoot motion during walking, *Gait Posture* 28:93–100, 2008.

147. MacLean C, Davis IM, Hamill J: Influence of a custom foot orthotic intervention on lower extremity dynamics in healthy runners, *Clin Biomech* 21:623–630, 2006.

148. Maganaris CN, Paul JP: Tensile properties of the in vivo human gastrocnemius tendon, *J Biomech* 35(12):1639–1646, 2002.

149. Magnan B, Bondi M, Pierantoni S, et al.: The pathogenesis of Achilles tendinopathy: a systematic review, *Foot Ankle Surg* 20(3):154–159, 2014.

150. Maharaj JN, Cresswell AG, Lichtwark GA: Subtalar joint pronation and energy absorption requirements during walking are related to tibialis posterior tendinous tissue strain, *Sci Rep* 7(1):17958, 2017.

151. Maharaj JN, Cresswell AG, Lichtwark GA: The immediate effect of foot orthoses on subtalar joint mechanics and energetics, *Med Sci Sports Exerc* 50(7):1449–1456, 2018.

152. Mann R, Inman V: Phasic activity of intrinsic muscles of the foot, *J Bone Joint Surg* 46A:469–481, 1964.

153. Mann RA: Biomechanics of the foot. In American academy of orthopedic surgeons. In *Atlas of orthotics: biomechanical principles and application*, St Louis, 1975, Mosby.

154. Manter JT: Movements of the subtalar joint and transverse tarsal joint, *Anat Rec* 80:397–410, 1941.

155. Martin RL, Davenport TE, Fraser JJ, et al.: Ankle stability and movement coordination impairments: lateral ankle ligament sprains revision 2021, *J Orthop Sports Phys Ther* 51(4):Cpg1–cpg80, 2021.

156. Mason LW, Molloy AP: Turf toe and disorders of the sesamoid complex, *Clin Sports Med* 34(4):725–739, 2015.

157. Matthews M, Rathleff MS, Claus A, et al.: The foot orthoses versus hip exercises (Fohx) trial for patellofemoral pain: a protocol for a randomized clinical trial to determine if foot mobility is associated with better outcomes with foot Orthoses, *J Foot Ankle Res* 10:5, 2017.

158. Mauntel TC, Wikstrom EA, Roos KG, et al.: The epidemiology of high ankle sprains in national collegiate athletic association sports, *Am J Sports Med* 45(9):2156–2163, 2017.

159. Mayne AI, Bidwai AS, Beirne P, et al.: The effect of a dedicated Ponseti service on the outcome of idiopathic clubfoot treatment, *Bone Joint Lett J* 96B(10):1424–1426, 2014.

160. McCullough MB, Ringleb SI, Arai K, et al.: Moment arms of the ankle throughout the range of motion in three planes, *Foot Ankle Int* 32(3):300–306, 2011.

161. McKay MJ, Baldwin JN, Ferreira P, et al.: Normative reference values for strength and flexibility of 1,000 children and adults, *Neurology* 88(1):36–43, 2017.

162. McKeon PO, Hertel J, Bramble D, et al.: The Foot Core System: a new paradigm for understanding intrinsic foot muscle function, *Br J Sports Med* 49(5):290, 2015.

163. McKinley TO, Rudert MJ, Koos DC, et al.: Incongruity versus instability in the etiology of posttraumatic arthritis, *Clin Orthop Relat Res* 423:44–51, 2004.

164. McPoil TG, Knecht HG, Schuit D: A survey of foot types in normal females between ages of 18 and 30 years, *J Orthop Sports Phys Ther* 9:406–409, 1988.

165. McPoil TG, Warren M, Vicenzino B, et al.: Variations in foot posture and mobility between individuals with patellofemoral pain and those in a control group, *J Am Podiatr Med Assoc* 101(4):289–296, 2011.

166. Mengiardi B, Zanetti M, Schöttle PB, et al.: Spring ligament complex: MR imaging–anatomic correlation and findings in asymptomatic subjects, *Radiology* 237:242–249, 2005.

167. Menz HB, Dufour AB, Riskowski JL, et al.: Association of planus foot posture and pronated foot function with foot pain: the Framingham foot study, *Arthritis Care Res* 65(12):1991–1999, 2013.

168. Menz HB, Dufour AB, Riskowski JL, et al.: Foot posture, foot function and low back pain: the Framingham Foot Study, *Rheumatology* 52(12):2275–2282, 2013.

169. Michels F, Matricali G, Vereecke E, et al.: The Intrinsic subtalar ligaments have a consistent presence, location and morphology, *Foot Ankle Surg* 27(1):101–109, 2021.

170. Mickle KJ, Angin S, Crofts G, et al.: Effects of age on strength and morphology of toe flexor muscles, *J Orthop Sports Phys Ther* 46(12):1065–1070, 2016.

171. Millar N, Silbernagel K, Thorborg K, et al.: Tendinopathy, *Nat Rev Dis Primers* 7:1–21, 2021.

172. Milner CE, Ferber R, Pollard CD, et al.: Biomechanical factors associated with tibial stress fracture in female runners, *Med Sci Sports Exerc* 38:323–328, 2006.

173. Milner CE, Hamill J, Davis IS: Distinct hip and rearfoot kinematics in female runners with a history of tibial stress fracture, *J Orthop Sports Phys Ther* 40(2):59–66, 2010.

174. Miura S, Seko T, Himuro N, et al.: Toe grip strength declines earlier than hand grip strength and knee

extension strength in community-dwelling older men: a cross sectional study, *J Foot Ankle Res* 15(1):79, 2022.

175. Moisan G, Mainville C, Descarreaux M, et al.: Unilateral jump landing neuromechanics of individuals with chronic ankle instability, *J Sci Med Sport* 23(5):430–436, 2020.

176. Monaghan GM, Lewis CL, Hsu WH, et al.: Forefoot angle determines duration and amplitude of pronation during walking, *Gait Posture* 38(1):8–13, 2013.

177. Monaghan K, Delahunt E, Caulfield B: Ankle function during gait in patients with chronic ankle instability compared to controls, *Clin Biomech* 21:168–174, 2006.

178. Moore ES, Kindig MW, McKearney DA, et al.: Hind-and midfoot bone morphology varies with foot type and sex, *J Orthop Res* 37(3):744–759, 2019.

179. Morcuende JA, Dolan LA, Dietz FR, et al.: Radical reduction in the rate of extensive corrective surgery for clubfoot using the Ponseti method, *Pediatrics* 113(2):376–380, 2004.

180. Mulligan EP, Cook PG: Effect of plantar intrinsic muscle training on medial longitudinal arch morphology and dynamic function, *Man Ther* 18(5):425–430, 2013.

181. Mundermann A, Nigg BM, Neil HR, et al.: Foot orthotics affect lower extremity kinematics and kinetics during running, *Clin Biomech* 18:254–262, 2003.

182. Murley GS, Buldt AK, Trump PJ, et al.: Tibialis posterior EMG activity during barefoot walking in people with neutral foot posture, *J Electromyogr Kinesiol* 19:e69–e77, 2009a.

183. Murley GS, Landorf KB, Menz HB: Do foot orthoses change lower limb muscle activity in flat-arched feet towards a pattern observed in normal-arched feet? *Clin Biomech* 25(7):728–736, 2010.

184. Murley GS, Menz HB, Landorf KB: The effect of three levels of foot orthotic wedging on the electromyographic activity of selected lower limb muscles during gait, *Clin Biomech* 21(10):1074–1080, 2006.

185. Murray MP, Guten GN, Sepic SB, et al.: Function of the triceps surae during gait. Compensatory mechanisms for unilateral loss, *J Bone Joint Surg Am* 60:473–476, 1978.

186. Myers JB, Riemann BL, Hwang JH, et al.: Effect of peripheral afferent alteration of the lateral ankle ligaments on dynamic stability, *Am J Sports Med* 31:498–506, 2003.

187. Myerson MS, Thordarson DB, Johnson JE, et al.: Classification and nomenclature: progressive collapsing foot deformity, *Foot Ankle Int* 41(10):1271–1276, 2020.

188. Nery C, Fonseca LF, Goncalves JP, et al.: First MTP Joint instability - expanding the concept of "turf-toe" injuries, *J Foot Ankle Surg* 26(1):47–53, 2020.

189. Neville C, Flemister A, Tome J, et al.: Comparison of changes in posterior tibialis muscle length between subjects with posterior tibial tendon dysfunction and healthy controls during walking, *J Orthop Sports Phys Ther* 37:661–669, 2007.

190. Nistor L, Markhede G, Grimby G: A technique for measurements of plantar flexion torque with the Cybex II dynamometer, *Scand J Rehabil Med* 14:163–166, 1982.

191. Pavan PG, Stecco C, Darwish S, et al.: Investigation of the mechanical properties of the plantar aponeurosis, *Surg Radiol Anat* 33(10):905–911, 2011.

192. Peña Fernández M, Hoxha D, Chan O, et al.: Centre of rotation of the human subtalar joint using weight-bearing clinical computed tomography, *Sci Rep* 10(1):1035, 2020.

193. Perera AM, Mason L, Stephens MM: The pathogenesis of hallux valgus [Review], *J Bone Joint Surg Am* 93(17):1650–1661, 2011.

194. Peter RE, Harrington RM, Henley MB, et al.: Biomechanical effects of internal fixation of the distal tibiofibular syndesmotic joint: comparison of two fixation techniques, *J Orthop Trauma* 8(3):215–219, 1994.

195. Phan CB, Nguyen DP, Lee KM, et al.: Relative movement on the articular surfaces of the tibiotalar and subtalar joints during walking, *Bone Joint Res* 7(8):501–507, 2018.

196. Piazza SJ, Adamson RL, Moran MF, et al.: Effects of tensioning errors in split transfers of tibialis anterior and posterior tendons, *J Bone Joint Surg Am* 85(5):858–865, 2003.

197. Pieper NL, Baudendistel ST, Hass CJ, et al.: The metabolic and mechanical consequences of altered propulsive force generation in walking, *J Biomech* 122:110447, 2021.

198. Piraino JA, Theodoulou MH, Ortiz J, et al.: American college of foot and ankle surgeons clinical consensus statement: appropriate clinical management of adult-acquired flatfoot deformity, *J Foot Ankle Surg* 59(2):347–355, 2020.

199. Pohl MB, Hamill J, Davis IS: Biomechanical and anatomic factors associated with a history of plantar fasciitis in female runners, *Clin J Sport Med* 19(5):372–376, 2009.

200. Raikin SM, Garras DN, Krapchev PV: Achilles tendon injuries in a United States population, *Foot Ankle Int* 34(4):475–480, 2013.

201. Reeves J, Jones R, Liu A, et al.: The Between-day reliability of peroneus longus EMG during walking, *J Biomech* 86:243–246, 2019.

202. Rein S, Hagert E, Hanisch U, et al.: Immunohistochemical analysis of sensory nerve endings in ankle ligaments: a cadaver study, *Cells Tissues Organs* 197(1):64–76, 2013.

203. Reischl SF, Powers CM, Rao S, et al.: Relationship between foot pronation and rotation of the tibia and femur during walking, *Foot Ankle Int* 20:513–520, 1999.

204. Requião LF, Nadeau S, Milot MH, et al.: Quantification of level of effort at the plantar flexors and hip extensors and flexor muscles in healthy subjects walking at different cadences, *J Electromyogr Kinesiol* 15:393–405, 2005.

205. Resende RA, Deluzio KJ, Kirkwood RN, et al.: Increased unilateral foot pronation affects lower limbs and pelvic biomechanics during walking, *Gait Posture* 41(2):395–401, 2015.

206. Richie D: Biomechanics and orthotic treatment of the adult acquired flatfoot, *Clin Podiatr Med Surg* 37(1):71–89, 2020.

207. Ridge ST, Olsen MT, Bruening DA, et al.: Walking in minimalist shoes is effective for strengthening foot muscles, *Med Sci Sports Exerc* 51(1):104–113, 2019.

208. Robb KA, Melady HD, Perry SD: Fine-Wire electromyography of the transverse head of adductor hallucis during locomotion, *Gait Posture* 85:7–13, 2021.

209. Rodrigues P, Chang R, TenBroek T, et al.: Medially posted insoles consistently influence foot pronation in runners with and without anterior knee pain, *Gait Posture* 37(4):526–531, 2013.

210. Root ML: Development of the functional orthosis, *Clin Podiatr Med Surg* 11:183–210, 1994.

211. Rosa I, Rodeia J, Fernandes PX, et al.: Ultrasonographic assessment of deltoid ligament integrity in ankle fractures, *Foot Ankle Int* 41(2):147–153, 2020.

212. Ross MH, Smith MD, Mellor R, et al.: Clinical tests of tibialis posterior tendinopathy: are they reliable, and how well are they reflected in structural changes on imaging? *J Orthop Sports Phys Ther* 51(5):253–260, 2021.

213. Rotem-Lehrer N, Laufer Y: Effect of focus of attention on transfer of a postural control task following an ankle sprain, *J Orthop Sports Phys Ther* 37:564–569, 2007.

214. Ruohola JP, Kiuru MJ, Pihlajamaki HK: Fatigue bone injuries causing anterior lower leg pain, *Clin Orthop Relat Res* 444:216–223, 2006.

215. Russell JA, Shave RM, Kruse DW, et al.: Ankle and foot contributions to extreme plantar- and dorsiflexion in female ballet dancers, *Foot Ankle Int* 32(2):183–188, 2011.

216. Santilli V, Frascarelli MA, Paoloni M, et al.: Peroneus longus muscle activation pattern during gait cycle in athletes affected by functional ankle instability: a surface electromyographic study, *Am J Sports Med* 33:1183–1187, 2005.

217. Schaefer KL, Sangeorzan BJ, Fassbind MJ, et al.: The comparative morphology of idiopathic ankle osteoarthritis, *J Bone Joint Surg Am* 94(24):e181, 2012.

218. Scott J, Lee H, Barsoum W, et al.: The effect of tibiofemoral loading on proximal tibiofibular joint motion, *J Anat* 211(5):647–653, 2007.

219. Sefton JM, Yarar C, Hicks-Little CA, et al.: Six weeks of balance training improves sensorimotor function in individuals with chronic ankle instability, *J Orthop Sports Phys Ther* 41(2):81–89, 2011.

220. Seligman DAR, Dawson D, Streiner DL, et al.: Treating heel pain in adults: a randomized controlled trial of hard vs modified soft custom orthotics and heel pads, *Arch Phys Med Rehabil*(3)363–370, 2021.

221. Sepic SB, Murray MP, Mollinger LA, et al.: Strength and range of motion in the ankle in two age groups of men and women, *Am J Phys Med* 65:75–84, 1986.

222. Shamus J, Shamus E, Gugel RN, et al.: The effect of sesamoid mobilization, flexor hallucis strengthening, and gait training on reducing pain and restoring function in individuals with hallux limitus: a clinical trial, *J Orthop Sports Phys Ther* 34:368–376, 2004.

223. Sharif B, Welck M, Saifuddin A: MRI of the distal tibiofibular joint, *Skeletal Radiol* 49(1):1–17, 2020.

224. Sheehan FT, Seisler AR, Siegel KL: In vivo talocrural and subtalar kinematics: a non-invasive 3D dynamic MRI study, *Foot Ankle Int* 28:323–335, 2007.

225. Shibuya N, Kitterman RT, LaFontaine J, et al.: Demographic, physical, and radiographic factors associated with functional flatfoot deformity, *J Foot Ankle Surg* 53(2):168–172, 2014.

226. Shimozono Y, Hurley ET, Myerson CL, et al.: Suture button versus syndesmotic screw for syndesmosis injuries: a meta-analysis of randomized controlled trials, *Am J Sports Med* 47(11):2764–2771, 2019.

227. Siegler S, Chen J, Schneck CD: The three-dimensional kinematics and flexibility characteristics of the human ankle and subtalar joints—Part I: kinematics, *J Biomech Eng* 110:364–373, 1988.

228. Siegler S, Toy J, Seale D, et al.: The Clinical Biomechanics Award 2013—presented by the International Society of Biomechanics: new observations on the morphology of the talar dome and its relationship to ankle kinematics, *Clin Biomech* 29(1):1–6, 2014.

229. Smith MD, Lee D, Russell T, et al.: How much does the talocrural joint contribute to ankle dorsiflexion range of motion during the weight-bearing lunge test? Q cross-sectional radiographic validity study, *J Orthop Sports Phys Ther* 49(12):934–941, 2019.

230. Spennacchio P, Seil R, Gathen M, et al.: Diagnosing instability of ligamentous syndesmotic injuries: a biomechanical perspective, *Clin Biomech* 84:105312, 2021.

231. Spiegel DA: CORR Insights: results of clubfoot management using the Ponseti method: do the details matter? A systematic review, *Clin Orthop Relat Res* 472(5):1617–1618, 2014.

232. Spratley EM, Arnold JM, Owen JR, et al.: Plantar forces in flexor hallucis longus versus flexor digitorum longus transfer in adult acquired flatfoot deformity, *Foot Ankle Int* 34(9):1286–1293, 2013.

233. Standring S: *Gray's Anatomy: the anatomical basis of clinical practice*, ed 42, St Louis, 2021, Elsevier.

234. Stauffer RN, Chao EY, Brewster RC: Force and motion analysis of the normal, diseased, and prosthetic ankle joint, *Clin Orthop Relat Res* 127:189–196, 1977.

235. Steinberg N, Finestone A, Noff M, et al.: Relationship between lower extremity alignment and hallux valgus in women, *Foot Ankle Int* 34(6):824–831, 2013.

236. Sutherland DH: An electromyographic study of the plantar flexors of the ankle in normal walking on the level, *J Bone Joint Surg Am* 48:66–71, 1966.

237. Sutherland DH: The evolution of clinical gait analysis. Part 1: kinesiological EMG, *Gait Posture* 14:61–70, 2001.

238. Svoboda Z, Bizovska L, Gonosova Z, et al.: Effect of aging on the association between ankle muscle strength and the control of bipedal stance, *PLoS One* 14(10):e0223434, 2019.

239. Szaro P, Cifuentes Ramirez W, Borkmann S, et al.: Distribution of the subtendons in the midportion of the Achilles tendon revealed in vivo on MRI, *Sci Rep* 10(1):16348, 2020.

240. Taniguchi A, Tanaka Y, Takakura Y, et al.: Anatomy of the spring ligament, *J Bone Joint Surg* 85-A:2174–2179, 2003.

241. Tateuchi H, Wada O, Ichihashi N: Effects of calcaneal eversion on three-dimensional kinematics of the hip, pelvis and thorax in unilateral weight bearing, *Hum Mov Sci* 30(3):566–573, 2011.

242. Taylor KF, Bojescul JA, Howard RS, et al.: Measurement of isolated subtalar range of motion: a cadaver study, *Foot Ankle Int* 22:426–432, 2001.

243. Telfer S, Abbott M, Steultjens MP, et al.: Dose-response effects of customised foot orthoses on lower limb kinematics and kinetics in pronated foot type, *J Biomech* 46(9):1489–1495, 2013.

244. Thomas RH, Daniels TR: Ankle arthritis, *J Bone Joint Surg Am* 85-A(5):923–936, 2003.

245. Thompson CS, Hiller CE, Schabrun SM: Altered spinal-level sensorimotor control related to pain and perceived instability in people with chronic ankle instability, *J Sci Med Sport* 22(4):425–429, 2019.

246. Thordarson DB, Schmotzer H, Chon J, et al.: Dynamic support of the human longitudinal arch. A biomechanical evaluation, *Clin Orthop Relat Res* 316:165–172, 1995.

247. Tochigi Y, Amendola A, Rudert MJ, et al.: The role of the interosseous talocalcaneal ligament in subtalar joint stability, *Foot Ankle Int* 25:588–596, 2004.

248. Tome J, Nawoczenski DA, Flemister A, et al.: Comparison of foot kinematics between subjects with posterior tibialis tendon dysfunction and healthy controls, *J Orthop Sports Phys Ther* 36:635–644, 2006.

249. Tong JW, Kong PW: Association between foot type and lower extremity injuries: systematic literature review with meta-analysis, *J Orthop Sports Phys Ther* 43(10):700–714, 2013.

250. Tumer N, Vuurberg G, Blankevoort L, et al.: Typical shape differences in the subtalar joint bones between subjects with chronic ankle instability and controls, *J Orthop Res* 37(9):1892–1902, 2019.

251. Valderrabano V, Hintermann B, Horisberger M, et al.: Ligamentous posttraumatic ankle osteoarthritis, *Am J Sports Med* 34:612–620, 2006.

252. Van der Krogt MM, Delp SL, Schwartz MH: How robust is human gait to muscle weakness? *Gait Posture* 36(1):113–119, 2012.

253. Van Deun S, Staes FF, Stappaerts KH, et al.: Relationship of chronic ankle instability to muscle activation patterns during the transition from double-leg to single-leg stance, *Am J Sports Med* 35:274–281, 2007.

254. van Dijk CN, van Sterkenburg MN, Wiegerinck JI, et al.: Terminology for Achilles tendon related disorders, *Knee Surg Sports Traumatol Arthrosc* 19(5):835–841, 2011.

255. Van Gheluwe B, Dananberg HJ, Hagman F, et al.: Effects of hallux limitus on plantar foot pressure and foot kinematics during walking, *J Am Podiatr Med Assoc* 96(5):428–436, 2006.

256. van Rijn RM, van Os AG, Bernsen RM, et al.: What is the clinical course of acute ankle sprains? A systematic literature review, *Am J Med* 121(4):324–331 e326, 2008.

257. Venkadesan M, Yawar A, Eng CM, et al.: Stiffness of the human foot and evolution of the transverse arch, *Nature* 579(7797):97–100, 2020.

258. Verhagen E, van der Beek A, Twisk J, et al.: The effect of a proprioceptive balance board training program for the prevention of ankle sprains: a prospective controlled trial, *Am J Sports Med* 32:1385–1393, 2004.

259. Vicenzino B, Branjerdporn M, Teys P, et al.: Initial changes in posterior talar glide and dorsiflexion of the ankle after mobilization with movement in individuals with recurrent ankle sprain, *J Orthop Sports Phys Ther* 36:464–471, 2006.

260. Wan L, de Asla RJ, Rubash HE, et al.: In vivo cartilage contact deformation of human ankle joints under full body weight, *J Orthop Res* 26:1081–1089, 2008.

261. Wang C, Yang J, Wang S, et al.: Three-Dimensional motions of distal syndesmosis during walking, *J Orthop Surg Res* 10:166, 2015.
262. Watanabe K, Kitaoka HB, Berglund LJ, et al.: The role of ankle ligaments and articular geometry in stabilizing the ankle, *Clin Biomech* 27(2):189–195, 2012.
263. Watanabe K, Kitaoka HB, Fujii T, et al.: Posterior tibial tendon dysfunction and flatfoot: analysis with simulated walking, *Gait Posture* 37(2):264–268, 2013.
264. Waterval NFJ, Brehm MA, Ploeger HE, et al.: Compensations in lower limb joint work during walking in response to unilateral calf muscle weakness, *Gait Posture* 66:38–44, 2018.
265. Wei F, Braman JE, Weaver BT, et al.: Determination of dynamic ankle ligament strains from a computational model driven by motion analysis based kinematic data, *J Biomech* 44(15):2636–2641, 2011.
266. Willems TM, De Clercq D, Delbaere K, et al.: A prospective study of gait related risk factors for exercise-related lower leg pain, *Gait Posture* 23(1):91–98, 2006.
267. Willems TM, Ley C, Goetghebeur E, et al.: Motion-control shoes reduce the risk of pronation-related pathologies in recreational runners: a secondary analysis of a randomized controlled trial, *J Orthop Sports Phys Ther* 51(3):135–143, 2021.
268. Williams BT, Ahrberg AB, Goldsmith MT, et al.: Ankle syndesmosis: a qualitative and quantitative anatomic analysis, *Am J Sports Med* 43(1):88–97, 2015.
269. Williams III DS, McClay IS, Hamill J: Arch structure and injury patterns in runners, *Clin Biomech* 16:341–347, 2001.
270. Williams G, Widnall J, Evans P, et al.: Could failure of the spring ligament complex be the driving force behind the development of the adult flatfoot deformity? *J Foot Ankle Surg* 53(2):152–155, 2014.
271. Winkler PW, Lutz PM, Rupp MC, et al.: Increased external tibial torsion is an infratuberosity deformity and is not correlated with a lateralized position of the tibial tuberosity, *Knee Surg Sports Traumatol Arthrosc* 29:1678–1685, 2021.
272. Winter DA: *Biomechanics and motor control of human movement*, Hoboken, NJ, 2005, John Wiley & Sons.
273. Wright DG, Rennels DC: A study of elastic properties of plantar fascia, *J Bone Joint Surg Am* 46:482–492, 1964.
274. Youberg LD, Cornwall MW, McPoil TG, et al.: The amount of rearfoot motion used during the stance phase of walking, *J Am Podiatr Med Assoc* 95:376–382, 2005.
275. Zhang YJ, Du JY, Chen B, et al.: Correlation between three-dimensional medial longitudinal arch joint complex mobility and medial arch angle in stage II posterior tibial tendon dysfunction, *J Foot Ankle Surg* 25(6):721–726, 2019.
276. Zhao D, Li H, Zhao L, et al.: Results of clubfoot management using the Ponseti method: do the details matter? A systematic review [Review], *Clin Orthop Relat Res* 472(4):1329–1336, 2014.
277. Zuil-Escobar JC, Martinez-Cepa CB, Martin-Urrialde JA, et al.: Evaluating the medial longitudinal arch of the foot: correlations, reliability, and accuracy in people with a low arch, *Phys Ther* 99(3):364–372, 2019.

STUDY QUESTIONS

1. List the bones that make up (a) the ankle and (b) the rearfoot. Which bone is common to both regions?
2. Explain how excessive tibial torsion could mask the functional expression of excessive femoral anteversion.
3. Describe the path of the tendon of the flexor hallucis longus, from its belly to its insertion on the great toe.
4. Why does maximal plantarflexion place the talocrural joint in its least mechanically stable position?
5. Describe how the first tarsometatarsal joint is frequently involved with the development of hallux valgus (bunion).
6. Using Fig. 14.43 as a reference, contrast the inversion torque potential of the tibialis anterior and the extensor hallucis longus (at the subtalar joint).
7. Explain why a person with a weak calf muscle may complain of "buckling" of the knee before the push off phase of walking.
8. Compare the distal attachments of the fibularis brevis and fibularis tertius. Justify how these muscles have different actions within the sagittal plane but similar actions in the frontal plane.
9. Which structures (joints and connective tissues) bind the fibula to the tibia?
10. Describe the roll-and-slide arthrokinematics of dorsiflexion at the talocrural joint with the foot free (Fig. 14.18A) and with the foot fixed (Fig. 14.20A).
11. Which part of the gait cycle requires greater dorsiflexion at the talocrural joint: the stance phase or the swing phase?
12. What factors contribute to the stability of the talocrural joint in full dorsiflexion?
13. Considering the first tarsometatarsal joint, which muscle is considered the most direct antagonist to the fibularis longus?
14. Propose a mechanism that could explain why active plantar flexion torque at the ankle is about 20% to 30% greater with the knee extended than when flexed.
15. Which deformity would most likely develop after weakness of the invertor muscles? Which muscles would you stretch? Which muscles would you attempt to strengthen?
16. Describe two possible consequences that may result from long-term weakness of the fibularis longus muscle.

Answers to the study questions are available in the enhanced eBook version included with the print purchase of this textbook.

Additional Video Educational Content

- Fluoroscopic Observations of Selected Arthrokinematics of the Lower Extremity
- Defining and Demonstrating the Motions of Pronation and Supination at the Ankle and Foot
- Demonstration of the Kinematics and Axes of Rotation at the Talocrural, Subtalar, and Transverse Tarsal Joints

ALL VIDEOS in this chapter are available in the enhanced eBook version included with the print purchase of this textbook.

C h a p t e r

15

Kinesiology of Walking

GUY G. SIMONEAU, PT, PhD, FAPTA
BRYAN C. HEIDERSCHEIT, PT, PhD, FAPTA

CHAPTER AT A GLANCE

Walking, often referred to as ambulation or gait, serves an individual's basic need to move from place to place and is therefore one of the most common activities that people do on a daily basis. Ideally, walking is performed both efficiently, to minimize fatigue, and safely, to prevent falls and associated injuries. Years of practice provide a healthy person with the control needed to walk while carrying on a conversation, looking in various directions, and even handling obstacles and other destabilizing forces with minimal effort.

Although a healthy person makes walking seem effortless, the challenge can be appreciated by looking at individuals at both ends of the lifespan (Fig. 15.1). Early in life, the young child typically needs 11 to 15 months to learn how to stand and walk.[78] Once on their feet, children will refine how they move to visually resemble a mature adult's walking pattern by 4 to 5 years of age,[42,218] with further refinement taking place over possibly several more years.[87,91,96,135,245] Late in life, walking often becomes an

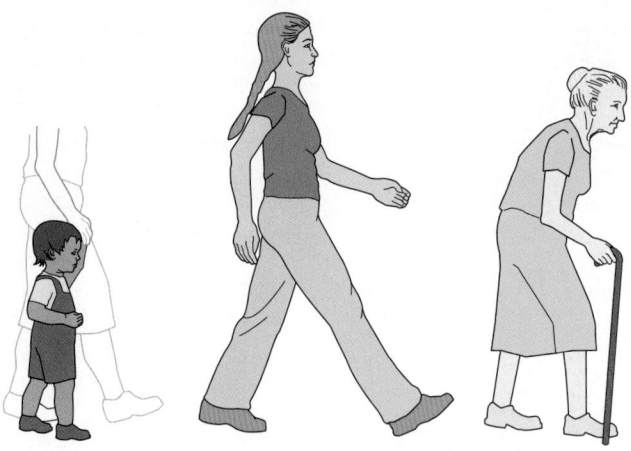

FIGURE 15.1 Walking at various stages in life.

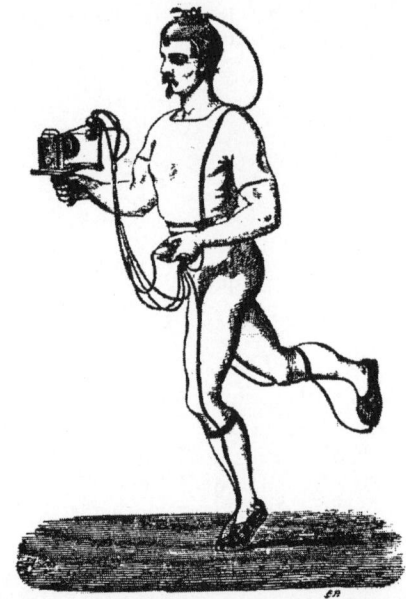

FIGURE 15.2 Marey's instrumented shoes used for the measurement of gait. (From Marey EJ: *La machine animal,* Paris, 1873, Librairie Germer Baillière.)

increasingly greater challenge. Because of decreased strength, decreased balance, or disease, the elderly may require a cane or walker to walk safely. Patla[176] eloquently expressed the importance of walking in our lives: "Nothing epitomizes a level of independence and our perception of a good quality of life more than the ability to travel independently under our own power from one place to another. We celebrate the development of this ability in children and try to nurture and sustain it throughout the lifespan."

This chapter provides a description of the fundamental kinesiologic characteristics of walking. Unless indicated otherwise, the information provided refers to individuals with a normal and mature gait pattern walking on level surfaces at a steady average speed. Although this chapter provides enough details to be read independently of the rest of this book, reading Chapters 12 to 14 will facilitate an even greater understanding of walking. Chapter 16 further builds on the information from this chapter to provide a description of the kinesiology of running.

Major Topics
- Spatial and temporal descriptors
- Joint kinematics
- Control of the body's center of mass
- Energy expenditure
- Muscle activity
- Walking kinetics
- Gait dysfunctions

The observation of walking, which is the focus of this chapter, provides information on the outcome of a complex set of "behind the scenes" interactions between sensory and motor functions. For a person to walk, the central nervous system must generate appropriate motor actions from the integration of visual, proprioceptive, and vestibular sensory inputs. Although this chapter covers the intricacy of limb and muscular actions performed during walking, it does not cover the concept of motor control. To gain a greater understanding of the complexity of the motor control of walking, the reader is advised to examine other sources on the topic.[53,97,119,170]

HISTORICAL PERSPECTIVE OF GAIT ANALYSIS

"If a man were to walk on the ground alongside a wall with a reed dipped in ink attached to his head, the line traced by the reed would not be straight but zig-zag, because it goes lower when he bends and

higher when he stands upright and raises himself."[12] This early written record by Aristotle (384–322 BC) and numerous earlier paintings and sculptures of individuals engaged in the process of walking are testament that both the casual and the detailed observation of walking has been of interest throughout history.

Despite this earlier interest, it was not until 1836 that the Weber brothers[250] published the first notable scientific work on walking, having benefited from the advances in science provided by individuals such as Galileo Galilei (1564–1642), Giovanni Borelli (1608–1679), and Isaac Newton (1642–1727), to name only a few. Willhelm, a physicist and electrician, and Eduard, an anatomist and physiologist, using instruments such as a stopwatch and a tape measure, described and measured elements of walking, such as step length, cadence, foot-to-ground clearance, and vertical excursion of the body. They also defined basic elements of the gait cycle, such as swing phase, stance phase, and double-limb support periods. Many of the terms they introduced remain in use today.[248,249] The Weber brothers hypothesized that the basic principle of walking is one of least muscular effort—a concept known to be true today, although the exact methods by which the body minimizes energy expenditure are still being studied.[40,122,169]

In the nineteenth century, other researchers, such as Marey, Carlet, and Vierordt, made use of ingenious technology to expand our knowledge of gait. Most often cited among Marey and Carlet's many novel methods of measurement are shoes that had air chambers attached to a recorder to indicate the swing and stance phase of gait (Fig. 15.2).[139-141] Another clever idea, by Vierordt, was the use of ink in small spray nozzles attached to the shoes and limbs.[243] The ink sprayed on the floor and wall as the individual walked, providing a permanent record of movement.

Concurrently, advances in the field of cinematography created a powerful medium to study and record the kinematic patterns of humans and animals walking. Muybridge may be the most recognized individual of his time to use cinematography to document sequence of movements. Muybridge is perhaps most famous for settling an old controversy regarding a trotting horse. In 1872, using sequence photography, he showed that all four feet of a trotting horse are indeed simultaneously off the ground for very brief periods of time. Muybridge created an impressive collection of photographs on human and animal gait.[164,165]

Initially, the description of walking was limited to planar analyses; the motion was typically recorded in the sagittal plane and less frequently in the frontal plane. Braune and Fisher[26,27] are credited as being the first, from 1895 to 1904, to perform a comprehensive three-dimensional analysis of a walking individual. By using four cameras and a number of light tubes attached to various body segments, they documented joint kinematics in three dimensions. They were also the first to use the principles of mechanics to measure dynamic quantities such as segmental acceleration, segmental inertial properties, and intersegmental loads (e.g., joint torques and forces). Their analysis of joint torques, limited to the swing phase of walking, refuted the earlier concept, suggested by Weber and Weber in 1836, that lower extremity motion during the swing phase could be explained solely by a passive pendulum theory.[252]

Throughout the twentieth century, the understanding of walking was greatly enhanced by many scientific advances. Instrumentation to document kinematics evolved from simple video cameras, with film

that required painstaking analysis with a ruler and protractor, to highly sophisticated computerized systems providing real-time coordinate data of limb segments. Recent evolution of this technology includes reliable "markerless" motion analysis systems,[99] wearable inertial measurement units,[234] and virtual reality/biofeedback systems.[240]

Notable researchers who contributed to the description of the kinematics of walking using a variety of imaging techniques include Eberhart,[62] Murray,[159] Inman,[94] Winter,[257] and Perry.[179] Murray, a physical therapist and researcher, published several papers in the 1960s, 1970s, and 1980s describing the kinematics of many aspects of normal and abnormal gait (Fig. 15.3).[159,161,162] Among other accomplishments, data from her research—on the kinematics of walking in individuals with disabilities—influenced the design of artificial joints and lower extremity prosthetic limbs.

Simultaneously, a more extensive understanding of the kinetics of walking was made possible through the development of devices to measure the forces taking place at the foot-ground interface. Amar,[8] Elftman,[64] Bresler and Frankel,[28] and Cunningham and Brown [51] all made significant contributions to this field. The ability to measure the forces between the foot and the ground led to computational methods to calculate the forces and torques taking place at the joints of the lower extremities during the stance phase of walking.[185,211]

The development of surface and intramuscular electrodes provided the opportunity to record the electrical activity of muscles during walking. When this information is integrated with the kinematics and kinetics of walking, the role that each muscle plays can be better appreciated and more objectively described. Many researchers, including Sutherland,[228] Perry,[179] Inman,[94] and Winter,[257] have made notable contributions to the study of electromyography (EMG) during walking.

Today, a detailed gait analysis is routinely performed in specialized biomechanics laboratories (Fig. 15.4 and Videos 15.1 and 15.2). Three-dimensional kinematic data are obtained by using two or more synchronized high-speed cameras. Ground reaction forces are measured using force platforms embedded in the floor or

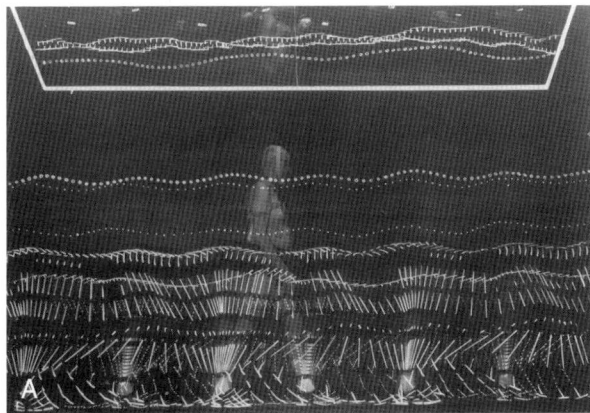

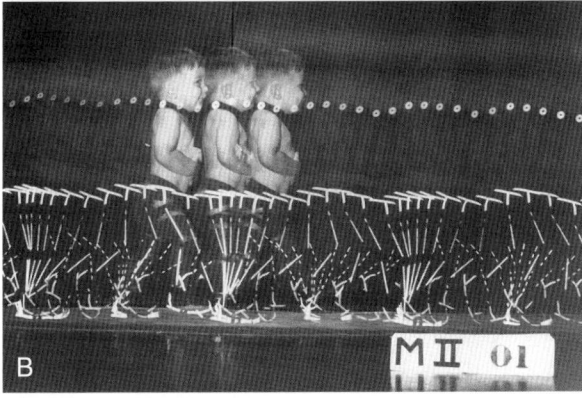

FIGURE 15.3 A sample of the technology used by Murray to record the basic kinematics of gait. An older man (A) and a young boy (B) wear reflective targets while walking in a semidark hallway. A camera was used with the shutter open, and light was flashed 20 times per second to track the location of the markers. An additional brighter flash of light was used to photograph the man or boy while walking. This early technique allowed the visualization of an entire gait cycle with a single photograph. A ceiling-mounted mirror was also employed to observe horizontal plane motion. (A, From Murray MP, Gore DR: Gait of patients with hip pain or loss of hip joint motion. In Black J, Dumbleton JH, editors: *Clinical biomechanics: a case history approach,* New York, 1981, Churchill Livingstone. B, From Stratham L, Murray MP: Early walking patterns of normal children, *Clin Orthop Relat Res* 79:8, 1971.)

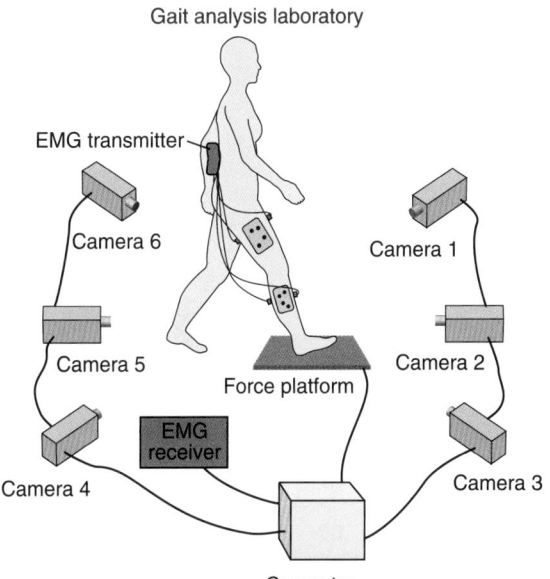

FIGURE 15.4 Instrumentation used in a typical gait laboratory to study walking (also see Videos 15.1 and 15.2).

treadmill. Muscle activity patterns are recorded by multichannel, often telemetered, electromyographic systems. Ultimately, lower extremity joint forces, torques, and powers are calculated with a combination of kinematic data, ground reaction forces, and anthropometric characteristics of the individual (Fig. 15.5). These data are then used to describe and study normal and abnormal walking patterns.

Individuals with a variety of pathologies can potentially benefit from instrumented gait analyses.[220,259] Currently, the primary beneficiaries of this technology, however, are often children with cerebral palsy. In this population, instrumented gait analysis is often used before surgery to help determine the proper intervention. It is employed again after surgery to objectively evaluate the outcome.[77] More comprehensive descriptions of the history, tools, and methods used for gait analysis can be found in other sources.[16,211]

Sophisticated technology, such as that described earlier, provides detailed information that can enhance the ability to describe and understand walking. Because such technology is rarely available in the typical clinical setting, clinicians must routinely rely on direct visual observation to evaluate the walking characteristics of their patients. Two-dimensional video-based assessment of walking and running using a high-speed camera is a common clinical approach, given the space, time, and cost burdens present with instrumented gait analysis.[253] Such observational analysis requires a thorough knowledge and understanding of normal walking and should not be

considered a replacement for instrumented gait analysis as that remains the gold standard. Learning about walking, as presented here, is a more dynamic and rewarding experience if the study of this chapter is combined with the observations of walking patterns of relatives, friends, neighbors, and patients in the clinical setting.

SPATIAL AND TEMPORAL DESCRIPTORS

This section describes measurements of distance and time as they relate to walking.

Gait Cycle

Walking is the result of a cyclic series of movements. As such, it can be conveniently characterized by a detailed description of its most fundamental unit: a *gait cycle* (Fig. 15.6). The gait cycle, by convention, is most often described as starting when the foot contacts the ground.[58] Because foot contact is normally made with the heel, the 0% point or beginning of the gait cycle is often referred to as *heel contact* or *heel strike*. The 100% point or completion of the gait cycle occurs as soon as the same foot once again makes contact with the ground. *Initial contact* is often used as a substitute term for heel contact when an individual makes first contact with the ground with a part of the foot other than the heel, but for the purpose of this chapter, focusing on normal walking, the term *heel contact* will be used.

A *stride* (synonymous with a gait cycle) is the sequence of events taking place between successive heel contacts of the same foot. In comparison, a *step* is the sequence of events that occurs within successive heel contacts of opposite feet, for example, between right and left heel contacts. A gait cycle, therefore, has two steps—a left step and a right step.

The most basic spatial descriptors of walking include the length of a stride and the length of a step (Fig. 15.7). *Stride length* is the distance between two successive heel contacts of the same foot. *Step length,* in contrast, is the distance between successive heel contacts of the two different feet. Comparing right with left step lengths can help evaluate the symmetry of walking between the lower extremities (Fig. 15.8). *Step width* is the lateral distance between the heel centers of two consecutive foot contacts and is on average around 8 to 10 cm (see Fig. 15.7).[145] *Foot angle,* the amount of "toe-out," is the angle between the line of progression of the body and the long

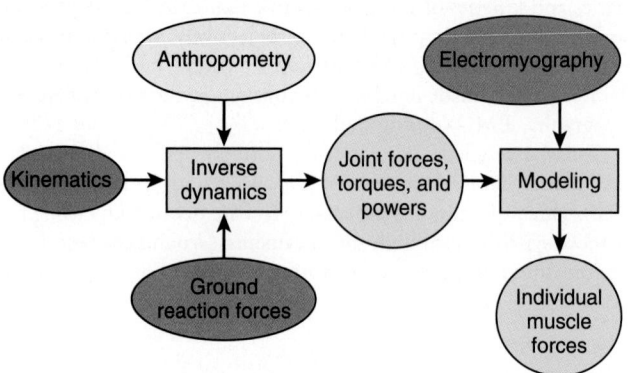

FIGURE 15.5 Typical approach used for the analysis of human motion. Variables in the colored ovals can be precisely measured. Computational methods, in the rectangles, are used to calculate the variables in the green circles.

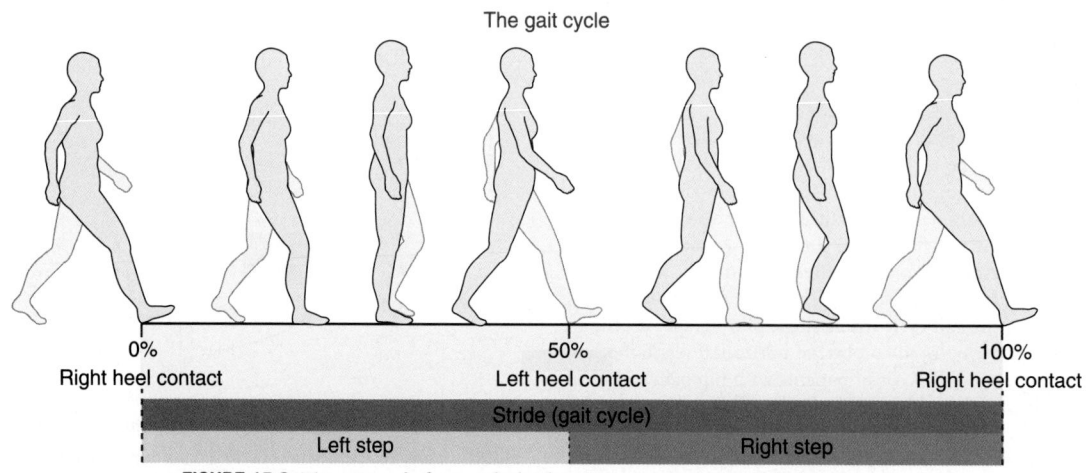

FIGURE 15.6 The gait cycle from right heel contact to subsequent right heel contact.

Spatial descriptors of gait

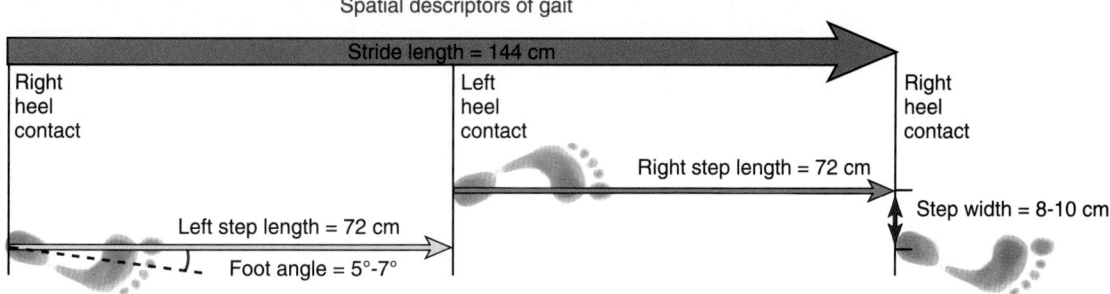

Stride length = 144 cm

Right heel contact

Left heel contact

Right step length = 72 cm

Right heel contact

Step width = 8-10 cm

Left step length = 72 cm

Foot angle = 5°-7°

FIGURE 15.7 Spatial descriptors of gait and their typical values for a right gait cycle.

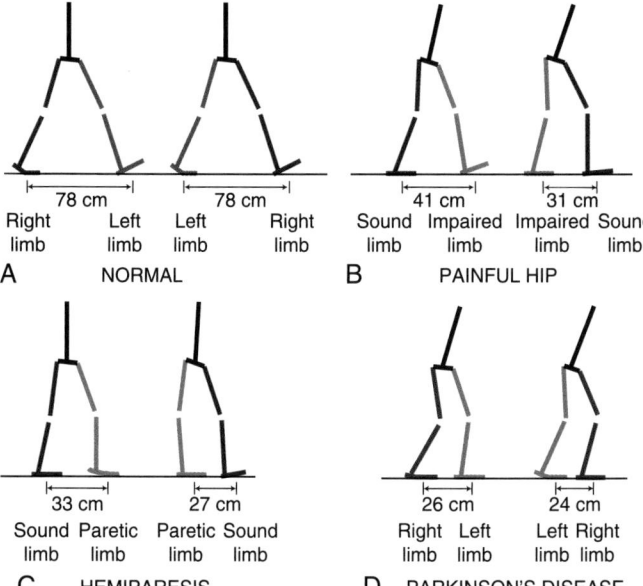

78 cm   78 cm

Right   Left   Left   Right
limb   limb   limb   limb

A   NORMAL

41 cm   31 cm

Sound Impaired   Impaired Sound
limb   limb   limb   limb

B   PAINFUL HIP

33 cm   27 cm

Sound Paretic   Paretic Sound
limb   limb   limb   limb

C   HEMIPARESIS

26 cm   24 cm

Right Left   Left Right
limb limb   limb limb

D   PARKINSON'S DISEASE

FIGURE 15.8 Influence of impairment and pathology on step length. (A) illustrates the symmetric step length expected in a healthy individual. (B) and (C) are examples of step length asymmetry often seen in those with an impairment or pathology that affects a single lower extremity. Note the bilateral shortening of the normal step length in both instances, demonstrating the interdependence of the lower extremities during gait. (D) illustrates a relatively symmetric bilateral reduction in step length secondary to Parkinson's disease, a pathology that affects both lower extremities. (Modified with permission from Murray MP: Gait as a total pattern of movement, *Am J Phys Med* 46:290, 1967.)

axis of the foot. About 5 to 7 degrees is considered average.[145] Data collected from 360 children 7 to 12 years of age indicate step width and foot angle values that are relatively similar to those in healthy young adults.[91]

Spatial Descriptors of Walking

- Stride length
- Step length
- Step width
- Foot angle

The most basic temporal descriptor of walking is *cadence,* the number of steps per minute, which is also called *step rate.* Other temporal descriptors of walking are *stride time* (the time for a full

gait cycle) and *step time* (the time for the completion of a right or a left step). Note that with symmetric walking, step time can be derived from cadence (i.e., step time is the reciprocal of cadence).

Walking speed combines both spatial and temporal measurements by providing information on the distance covered in a given amount of time. The units of measure are typically meters per second (m/sec) or miles per hour (mph). Speed can be calculated by measuring the time it takes to cover a given distance, the distance covered in a given amount of time, or by multiplying the step rate by the step length. Walking speed varies considerably among individuals based on factors such as age and physical characteristics (e.g., height and weight). Of all spatial and temporal measurements of walking, speed may be the best and most functional measure of an individual's walking ability.[201]

Temporal Descriptors of Walking

- Cadence
- Stride time
- Step time

Spatial-Temporal Descriptor of Walking

- Walking speed

For healthy adults, a gait cycle (i.e., two consecutive steps) takes slightly more than 1 second and covers approximately 1.44 m (4.5 feet), resulting in a walking speed of 1.37 m/sec. Data in Table 15.1 indicate that, at a freely chosen walking speed, women exhibit a slower walking speed, shorter step length, and faster cadence than men.[151,196] Even when anthropometrically matched with men, women still demonstrate a higher cadence and shorter step length than men when walking at the same speed.[29,161]

The classic data in Table 15.1 were derived from more than 2300 pedestrians walking outdoors in a large city and who were unaware that their walking characteristics were being measured. For comparison, Table 15.2 provides data from a small number of individuals who walked indoors on an instrumented walkway used to measure spatial and temporal characteristics of walking precisely and reliably. Unlike the pedestrians in the studies in Table 15.1, these individuals were aware that their walking characteristics were being measured, which may account in part for the small differences noted between the data in the two tables. A summary of a large data set stratified by age and sex from 23,111 healthy individuals walking over a short distance indicates an average walking velocity of 1.43 m/sec for men between the ages of 30 and 60 and an average walking velocity varying between 1.31 and 1.39 m/sec for women

TABLE 15.1 **Normative Data for Walking Speed, Step Rate, and Step Length**

	Drillis (1961)[61] (New York City)	**Molen (1973)[154] (Amsterdam)**	**Finley and Cody (1970)[69] (Philadelphia)**	**Average of Both Sexes and 3 Cities**
Walking speed (m/sec)	1.46*	1.39 (males) 1.27 (females)	1.37 (males) 1.24 (females)	1.37
Step rate (steps/sec)	1.9*	1.79 (males) 1.88 (females)	1.84 (males) 1.94 (females)	1.87
Step length (m)	0.76*	0.77 (males) 0.67 (females)	0.74 (males) 0.63 (females)	0.72

Data obtained from more than 2300 pedestrians unaware of being observed as they walked.
*Males and females are averaged together for these data.

TABLE 15.2 **Selected Data for Temporal and Spatial Gait Parameters Derived from Individuals Walking in a Laboratory Setting on an Instrumented Walkway***

	Walking Speed (m/sec)	**Cadence[†] (steps/min)**	**Stride Length[†] (m)**	**Step Width (cm)**	**Foot Angle (degrees)**
Marchetti et al (2008)[138]	1.43 (1.35–1.51)	119.1 (115.1–123.1)	0.707 (0.678–0.742) 0.726 (0.691–0.761)	8.1 (7.0–9.2)	
Hollman et al (2007)[90]	1.48 ± 0.15				
Youdas et al (2006)[260]	1.40 ± 0.13	119.6 ± 7.6	1.42 ± 0.13		
Menz et al (2004)[145]	1.43 ± 0.14	110.8 ± 6.9	0.77 ± 0.06	8.6 ± 3.2	6.7 ± 5.0
Bilney et al (2003)[22]	1.46 ± 0.16	114.7 ± 6.4	1.53 ± 0.14		
Grabiner et al (2001)[81]§				10.8 ± 2.7 8.7 ± 2.3	

*Data are means ± standard deviations, with the exception of Marchetti and colleagues, for whom data are means and 95% confidence intervals. All data are for healthy adults, and all groups include both males and females.
†Divide cadence by 60 to obtain step rate in steps per second.
‡The data by Marchetti and colleagues are for left and right step length, and the data by Menz and colleagues are for step length.
§Data for two different groups of individuals.

in the same age groups. For both men and women, walking velocity progressively decreased after 60 years of age (see full data set in e-Table 15.1).[24,215]

Normal Values for Walking Based on Data from Table 15.1
- Walking speed: 1.37 m/sec (3 mph)
- Step rate: 1.87 steps/sec (110 steps/min)
- Step length: 72 cm (28 inches)

The data in Tables 15.1 and 15.2 were collected from individuals walking at their freely chosen speed, which may not always be fast enough to reach a destination in the desired amount of time. When an increase in walking speed is needed, two strategies are available: increasing the stride (or step) length and increasing the cadence (Fig. 15.9). Typically, an individual combines both strategies until the longest practical step length is reached. From that point on, a further increase in walking speed is solely related to an increase in cadence. *It must be reemphasized, therefore, that all values (spatial, temporal, kinematic, and kinetic variables) obtained from the measurements of walking vary based on walking speed.*[75] Consequently, for proper reference and interpretation, reports of walking characteristics should always include the walking speed at which the data were collected. In addition, as walking characteristics also differ slightly between sexes and across age groups, ideal reporting should account for these factors as well.[32,195]

SPECIAL FOCUS 15.1

Simple Clinical Measurements of Walking

Sophisticated instrumentation, such as walkways and foot switches, exists to make spatial and temporal measurements of foot placement during walking.[198] For most clinical applications, this information can, however, be measured with readily available tools and a little imagination. Average walking speed can be measured using a stopwatch and a known distance. Step length and step width can be measured by the use of ink marks made by shoes or feet on a roll of paper covering the floor. This technique works especially well to document abnormal walking patterns, including asymmetry in step length.

Clinically, simple measurements of walking speed and distance can be helpful in monitoring functional progress or documenting functional limitations. Results obtained from a patient can be compared with normal values provided in Tables 15.1 and 15.2 or with minimum standards required to perform a specific task, such as crossing a street within the time allowed by the stoplights.[63,123] The following are two proposed minimum standards based on community-living activities: the ability to walk 300 m (1000 feet) in less than 11.5 minutes (walking speed of 0.45 m/sec or 1 mph) and the ability to walk at a speed of 1.2–1.3 m/sec (2.7–2.9 mph) for 13 to 27 m (42–85 feet) to safely cross a street.

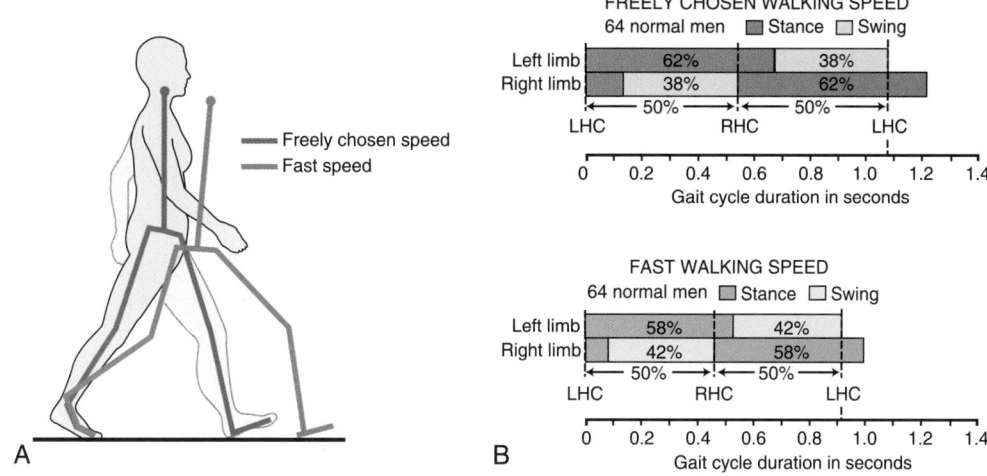

FIGURE 15.9 Methods to increase walking speed. (A) illustrates the longer step length used to increase walking speed. (B) illustrates the shorter gait cycle duration (faster walking cadence) used to increase walking speed. It also illustrates that at the faster walking speed, a smaller percentage of the gait cycle is spent in double-limb support (16% at fast speed compared with 24% at free speed walking). (Data from Murray MP, Kory RC, Clarkson BH, et al: Comparison of free and fast speed walking patterns of normal men, *Am J Phys Med* 45:8, 1966.)

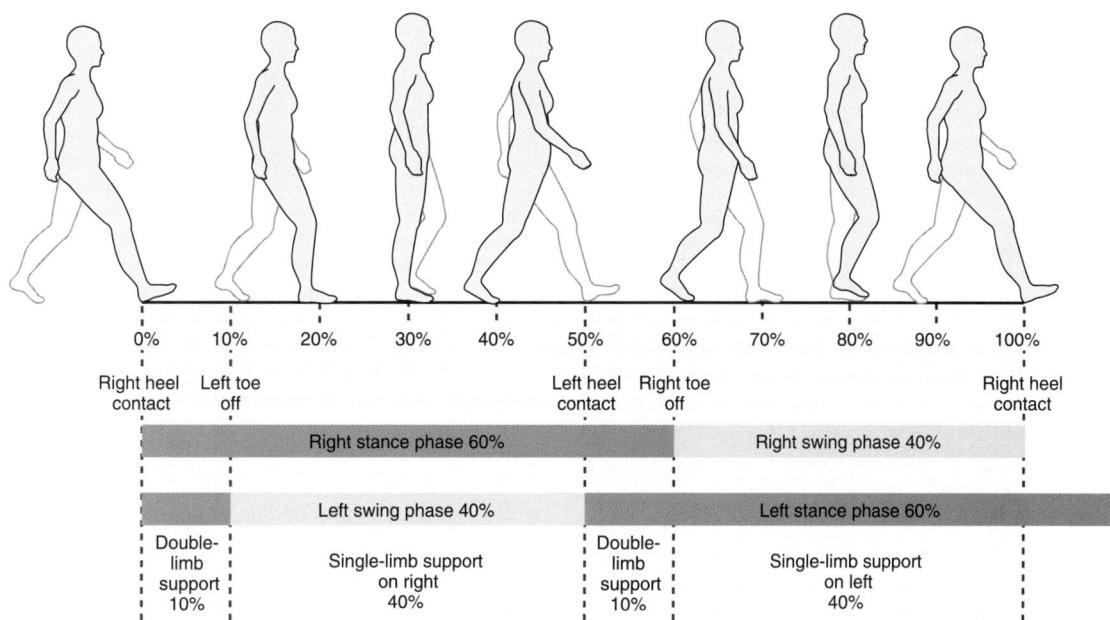

FIGURE 15.10 Subdivision of the gait cycle illustrating the phases of stance and swing and periods of single- and double-limb support.

Stance and Swing Phases

To help describe events taking place when walking, it is customary to subdivide the gait cycle from 0% to 100%. As stated earlier, heel or foot contact with the ground is usually considered the start of the gait cycle (0%) and the next ground contact made by the same foot is considered the end of the gait cycle (100%). Throughout this chapter, walking is described using the right lower extremity as a reference. A full gait cycle for the right lower extremity can be divided into two major phases: stance and swing (Fig. 15.10). *Stance phase* (from right heel contact to right toe off) occurs as the right foot is on the ground, supporting the body's weight. *Swing phase* (from right toe off to the next right heel contact) occurs as the right foot is in the

air, being advanced forward for the next contact with the ground. At normal walking speed, the stance phase occupies approximately 60% of the gait cycle, and the swing phase occupies the remaining 40%.

> **Gait Cycle**
> - Stance phase = 60% of gait cycle
> - Swing phase = 40% of gait cycle

Within a gait cycle, the body experiences two periods of *double-limb support* (when both feet are in contact with the ground simultaneously) and two periods of *single-limb support* (when only one

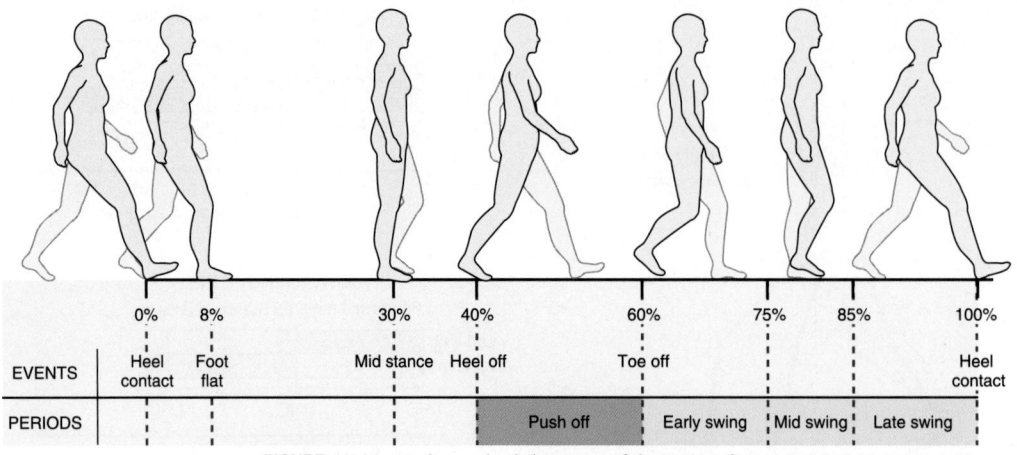

FIGURE 15.11 Traditional subdivisions of the gait cycle.

foot is on the ground) (see Fig. 15.10). We observe the first period of double-limb support at 0% to 10% of the gait cycle. During that time period, the body's weight is being transferred from the left to the right lower extremity. The right lower extremity is then in single-limb support until 50% of the gait cycle has been reached. During that time, the left lower extremity is in its swing phase, being advanced forward. The second period of double-limb support takes place at 50% to 60% of the gait cycle and serves the purpose of transferring the weight of the body from the right to the left lower extremity. Finally, at 60% to 100% of the gait cycle, the body is again in single-limb support, this time on the left lower extremity. This period of left single-limb support corresponds to the swing phase of the right lower extremity.

As walking speed increases, the percentage of the gait cycle spent in periods of double-limb support becomes shorter (see Fig. 15.9). Race walkers aim to walk as fast as possible while always keeping one foot in contact with the ground. For these athletes, greater speeds are achieved by increasing cadence and stride length and by minimizing periods of double-limb support to the point at which stance and swing phase times are about equal. Whereas maximum walking speed in adults 20 to 50 years of age is approximately 2.4 to 2.5 m/sec (5.5–5.7 mph),[25] walking speed during race walking can be in excess of 3.3 m/sec (7.5 mph).[160]

During running, the periods of double-limb support disappear altogether to be replaced by periods when both feet are off the ground simultaneously. The preferred transition speed from walking to running, triggered by the body's desire to optimize mechanical efficiency and load, normally occurs at a speed around 2.0 m/sec (4.5 mph)[115] or stride frequency of approximately 71 strides per minute.[85,244] The greater mechanical efficiency achieved with this transition means that at a speed above 2.0 m/sec, it is more energy efficient to run than to walk.

Conversely, at a slow walking speed, the periods of double-limb support occupy an increasingly greater percentage of the gait cycle. Walking slower provides greater stability because both feet are on the ground simultaneously for a greater percentage of the time. In fact, the reduced speed, shorter step length, and slower cadence commonly seen in the elderly with fear of falling or strength deficits serve to improve walking stability and prevent falls.[113]

SUBDIVISION OF STANCE AND SWING PHASES

Five specific events are typically described during stance phase: heel contact, foot flat, mid stance, heel off (or heel rise), and toe off (Fig. 15.11

TABLE 15.3 Common Terminology Defining the Subdivisions of the Gait Cycle

Phases	Events	Percentage of Cycle	Events of Opposite Limb
Stance	Heel contact	0	
	Foot flat	8	
		10	Toe off
	Mid stance	30	Mid swing (25–35%)
	Heel off	30–40	
		50	Heel contact
	Toe off	60	
Swing	Early swing	60–75	
	Mid swing	75–85	Mid stance (80%)
	Late swing	85–100	
		90	Heel off (80–90%)
	Heel contact	100	

and Table 15.3). *Heel contact* is defined as the instant the heel comes in contact with the ground, at 0% of the gait cycle. *Foot flat* corresponds to the instant the entire plantar surface of the foot comes in contact with the ground. This event occurs at approximately 8% of the gait cycle. *Mid stance* is most often defined as the point at which the body's weight passes directly over the supporting lower extremity. It is also defined as the time when the foot of the lower extremity in the swing phase passes the lower extremity in the stance phase (i.e., the feet are side by side). A third definition of mid stance is the time when the greater trochanter of the femur is vertically above the midpoint of the supporting foot in the sagittal plane. In reality, these three definitions all correspond to about 30% of the gait cycle or 50% of the stance phase. *Heel off*, the timing of which varies appreciably among individuals, occurs at somewhere between 30% and 40% of the gait cycle. It corresponds to the instant the heel comes off the ground. *Toe off*, which occurs at 60% of the gait cycle, is defined as the instant the toes come off the ground.

A period referred to as *push off* is also often used. This period roughly corresponds to the movement of ankle plantar flexion at 40% to 60% of the gait cycle.

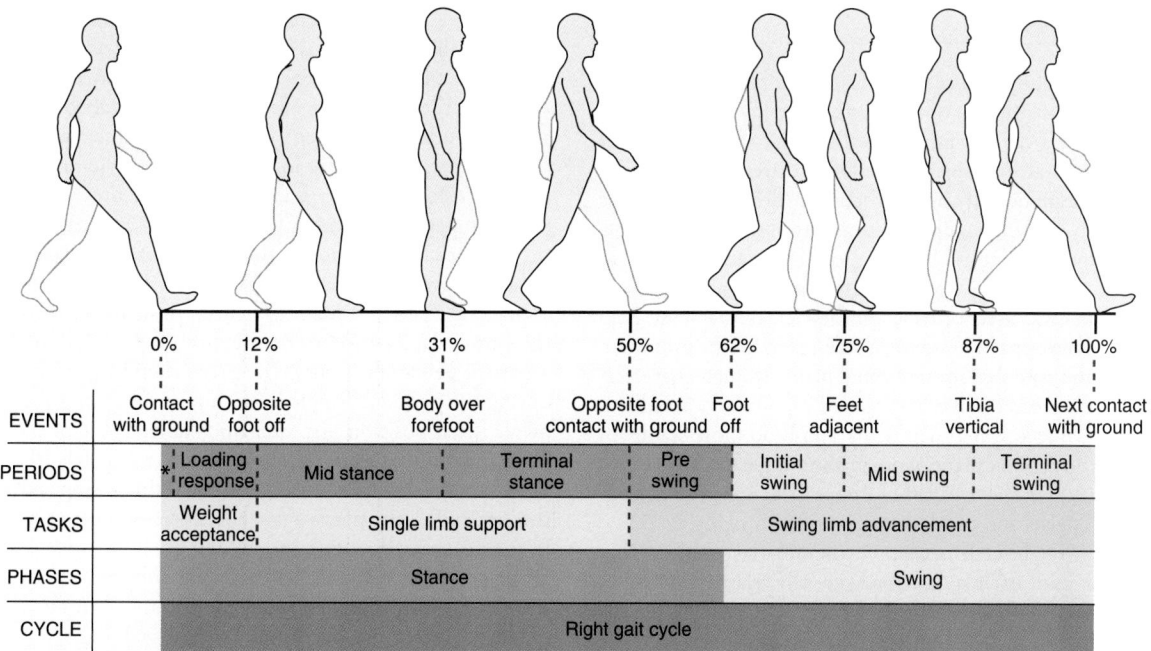

	0%	12%	31%	50%	62%	75%	87%	100%
EVENTS	Contact with ground	Opposite foot off	Body over forefoot	Opposite foot contact with ground	Foot off	Feet adjacent	Tibia vertical	Next contact with ground
PERIODS	*Loading response	Mid stance	Terminal stance		Pre swing	Initial swing	Mid swing	Terminal swing
TASKS	Weight acceptance	Single limb support			Swing limb advancement			
PHASES	Stance				Swing			
CYCLE	Right gait cycle							

*The first period of the gait cycle, called initial contact, takes place from 0 to 2% of the gait cycle

FIGURE 15.12 Terminology proposed by Perry and Burnfield. The gait cycle is divided into eight periods.[†] *Initial contact* (from 0% to 2% of the gait cycle), *loading response* (from 2% to 12% [opposite toe off] of the gait cycle), *mid stance* (from 12% to 31% [heel rise] of the gait cycle), *terminal stance* (from 31% to 50% [initial contact from opposite foot] of the gait cycle), *preswing* (from 50% to 62% [toe off] of the gait cycle), *initial swing* (from 62% to 75% [when the foot of the swing limb is next to the foot of the stance limb] of the gait cycle), *mid swing* (from 75% to 87% [tibia of the swing limb is vertical] of the gait cycle), and *terminal swing* (from 87% to 100% [immediately before the next initial contact] of the gait cycle). The first 12% of the gait cycle corresponds to a task of weight acceptance—when body mass is transferred from one lower extremity to the other while in double-limb support. Single-limb support, from 12% to 50% of the gait cycle, serves to support the weight of the body as the opposite limb swings forward. The last 12% of the stance phase, which corresponds to the second time in double-limb support, and the entire swing phase serve to advance the limb forward to a new location. Finally, note that in this figure, the stance phase occupies 62% of the gait cycle, with swing occupying the remaining 38%. ([†]The terminology in Fig. 15.12 and the text was modified from the original terminology by switching the terms "periods" and "phases.")

Although there is a significant amount of variation in the description of the swing phase of gait, this phase is traditionally subdivided into three sections: early, mid, and late swing (see Fig. 15.11). *Early swing* is the period from the time of toe off to mid swing (60% to 75% of the gait cycle). *Mid swing* corresponds to the time from slightly before to slightly after the mid stance event of the opposite lower extremity, when the foot of the swing limb passes next to the foot of the stance limb (75% to 85% of the gait cycle). *Late swing* is the period from the end of mid swing to foot contact with the ground (85% to 100% of the gait cycle).

An alternate terminology, proposed by Perry and Burnfield,[178] consists of eight periods (Fig. 15.12). The five periods included in the stance phase are *initial contact, loading response, mid stance, terminal stance,* and *pre swing.* The swing phase has three periods: *initial swing, mid swing,* and *terminal swing.* Perry and Burnfield further divide the gait cycle based on three *tasks:* weight acceptance (which includes initial contact and loading response), single-limb support (which includes mid stance and terminal stance), and swing limb advancement (which includes pre swing as well as initial, mid, and terminal swing).

SPECIAL FOCUS 15.2

Take Time to Develop Your Observation Skills

The events of the gait cycle can be observed by watching people walking in normal surroundings (streets, malls, airports). Like any clinical skill, observational gait analysis improves with practice. Repeated observation of individuals with normal walking patterns sharpens the ability to recognize normal walking variations and identify abnormal walking deviations. When appropriate, filming a person walk with an easily accessible smartphone can allow a more careful observation at a later time. Opportunities to practice this skill with a person already trained in observational gait analysis further sharpen these skills.

The existence of different terminologies can be confusing, especially when used interchangeably. In this chapter, to eliminate confusion, the terminology used to describe the gait cycle is most often supplemented with the timing of events as a percentage of the gait cycle.

JOINT KINEMATICS

When walking, the body is displaced linearly as a result of the summation of the angular rotation of the joints of the lower extremities, which is not unlike a car moving forward owing to the rotation of its tires. Movements at the joints of the lower extremities therefore are described as a function of angular rotation. Although walking is achieved primarily by joint angular rotation within the sagittal plane, other smaller (and often subtle) but important rotations occur in frontal and horizontal planes as well.[152] Interestingly, subtle nonsagittal plane kinematics often provide the best clues that may help distinguish the walking pattern between sexes, even for the untrained observers. Data indicate that in the frontal plane, women characteristically walk with greater pelvis and related hip abduction/adduction movement while keeping their trunk and head more stable. In addition, in the horizontal plane, women show a greater amount of hip internal rotation in the first half of stance as well as greater magnitude of overall pelvis and trunk rotation and arm swing.[29,195]

Most often throughout this chapter, the angular rotation that takes place at the joint itself is described (i.e., the relative motion of one bone compared with another). In some instances (e.g., for the sagittal plane motion of the pelvis), the movement of the bones in space is described *without* regard to movement at the joint. The reader must therefore be careful to recognize when a discussion pertains to joint kinematics and when it pertains to bone kinematics.

Finally, while the data presented in the following sections are most often expressed as a single value (single tracing in the graph-based figures), it should be recognized that these values reflect a grand average across several persons. Although it may not always be reported, it should be clear that a significant amount of normal variation exists among individuals. Normal variations between consecutive gait cycles also occur within individuals, each gait cycle not being exactly the same as the previous, with small variations continuously occurring in timing and/or amplitude of movement.[194] The amount of stride-to-stride gait variability is reflective of the quality of the neuromuscular system and is also influenced by a decline in cognitive function.[92] There is growing literature on the documentation of gait variability in young and older individuals across a variety of health conditions, in part in an attempt to identify the most relevant gait parameters that may have therapeutic value or that may predict individuals at greater risks of future falls and loss in function.[229,232,258]

Sagittal Plane Kinematics

Sagittal plane movement of the pelvis is small and is described here as movement of the bony structure itself. Conversely, the sagittal plane kinematics of the hip, knee, ankle, tarsometatarsal, and first metatarsophalangeal joints are of larger magnitude and are described as joint motion. In this section, as in the entire chapter, the gait cycle is described from right heel contact to subsequent right heel contact.

PELVIS

Movement of the pelvis in the sagittal plane is described as short-arc rotations in anterior and posterior directions about a medial-lateral axis through the hip joints (see Chapter 12). (The direction of the pelvic tilt is based on movement of the iliac crests.) The neutral position (0 degree of pelvic tilt) is defined as the orientation of the pelvis in relaxed stance. Because the pelvis is a relatively rigid

structure,[237] both iliac crests are considered as moving together. During walking at normal speed, the amount of anterior and posterior pelvic tilt is small (i.e., a total of approximately 2–4 degrees). Although the movement of the pelvis is described as movement of an independent "detached" structure, the kinematics actually take place primarily at the hip joints (through pelvic-on-femoral flexion and extension) and, to a lesser extent, at the lumbosacral joints (through pelvic-on-lumbar flexion and extension).

The pattern of motion of the pelvis over the full gait cycle resembles a sine wave with two full cycles (Fig. 15.13A). At right heel contact, the pelvis is in a near neutral position. From 0% to 10% of the gait cycle, a period of double-limb support, a small amount of posterior pelvic tilt occurs. The pelvis then begins tilting anteriorly during the period of single-limb support, reaching a slight anterior pelvic tilted position just after mid stance (30% of the gait cycle). In the second half of the stance phase, the pelvis tilts posteriorly until just after toe off. During early and mid swing (60% to 85% of the gait cycle), the pelvis again tilts anteriorly before starting to tilt in the posterior direction in late swing.

In general, pelvic tilting increases with the speed of ambulation.[94] Significant variability in the amount, timing, and direction of tilt, however, has been noted across walking speed and among individuals. The generally noted greater magnitude of pelvic tilt with faster walking speed serves to increase functional limb length, which in turn serves to increase step length.

The sagittal plane tilt of the pelvis during walking is caused by the sum of the passive and active forces produced by the hip joint capsule and the hip flexor and extensor muscles. In pathologic situations, persons with marked hip flexion contractures show an exaggerated anterior tilt of the pelvis in the second half of the stance phase (i.e., at 30% to 60% of the gait cycle). This is attributed to increased passive tension in the shortened anterior hip structures, creating an anterior tilting tendency of the pelvis as full hip extension is attempted. An excessive anterior pelvic tilt can, to some extent, compensate for the lack of passive hip extension in the latter part of stance and is typically associated with increased lumbar lordosis.

HIP

At a typical walking speed, the hip is flexed approximately 30 degrees at heel contact (Fig. 15.13B and Video 15.3). As the body moves forward over the fixed foot, the hip extends. Maximum hip extension of approximately 10 degrees is achieved before toe off. Flexion of the hip is initiated during push off, and the hip is at about 0 degrees of flexion by toe off (60% of gait). During the swing phase, the hip further flexes to bring the lower extremity forward for the next foot placement. Maximum flexion (slightly more than 30 degrees) is achieved just before heel contact. Note that at heel contact the hip has already started to extend in preparation for weight acceptance. Overall, approximately 30 degrees of flexion and 10 degrees of extension (from the anatomic neutral position) are needed at the hip for normal walking.[84,206] As for all of the joints of the lower extremities, the magnitude of hip movement is proportional to walking speed.

Individuals with limited sagittal plane hip mobility may appear to walk without a gait deviation as the movement of the pelvis and lumbar spine, compensating for reduced hip motion, may be initially unnoticed. Apparent hip extension, detectable with good visual observational skills, can be achieved through an anterior pelvic tilt

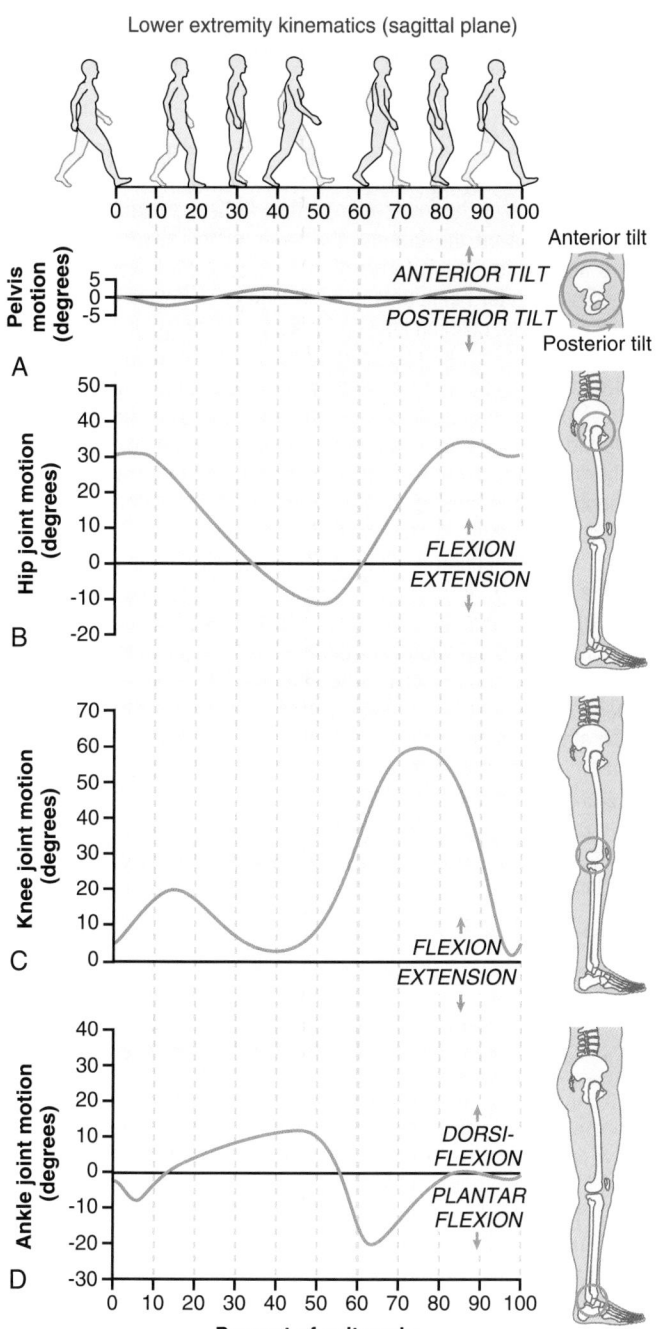

FIGURE 15.13 Sagittal plane angular rotation of the pelvis (A), hip (B), knee (C), and ankle (D) during a gait cycle (also see Video 15.3).

KNEE

The kinematic pattern of the knee in the sagittal plane is slightly more complex than that of the hip (Fig. 15.13C and Video 15.3).[206] At heel contact, the knee is flexed approximately 5 degrees, and it continues to flex an additional 10 to 15 degrees during the initial 15% of the gait cycle. This slight knee flexion, controlled by eccentric action of the quadriceps, serves the purpose of shock absorption and weight acceptance as body weight is progressively transferred to this lower extremity. Following initial flexion, the knee approaches near full extension until about heel off (occurring at 30% to 40% of the gait cycle). At this point the knee starts flexing, reaching approximately 35 degrees of flexion by the time of toe off (60% of the gait cycle). Maximum knee flexion of approximately 60 degrees is assumed by the beginning of mid swing (75% of the gait cycle). Knee flexion during early swing serves to shorten the length of the lower extremity, facilitating toe clearance. In mid and late swing, the knee extends to just short of full extension before starting to flex slightly in preparation for heel contact.

Normal function of the knee when walking on a level surface requires range of motion from nearly full extension to approximately 60 degrees of flexion. A limitation of knee extension (i.e., knee flexion contracture) results in a functionally shorter limb, affecting the kinematics of both the stance limb and the swing limb. The stance limb, lacking full knee extension, must assume a partially "crouched" position (often expressed in some persons with cerebral palsy), involving the hip, knee, and ankle, and the normal swing limb needs greater hip and possibly knee flexion to clear the toes from the ground. The flexed knee posture increases the muscular demand on the knee extensors and the uneven functional limb length leads to excessive trunk movement, both increasing the metabolic demands of walking.

A lack of sufficient knee flexion during the swing phase of gait interferes with toe clearance as the foot moves forward. To compensate, the hip must flex excessively. If the knee is immobilized in full extension with an orthosis or a cast, more noticeable compensations, such as hip "hiking" and hip circumduction, are required.[3]

ANKLE (TALOCRURAL JOINT)

At the ankle, heel contact occurs with the talocrural joint in a slightly plantar flexed position (between 0 and 5 degrees) (Fig. 15.13D and Video 15.3). Shortly after heel contact (the first 8% of the gait cycle), the foot is positioned flat on the ground by a movement of plantar flexion controlled through eccentric activation of the ankle dorsiflexors. Then, during stance, up to 10 degrees of ankle dorsiflexion occurs as the tibia moves forward over the foot, which is in firm contact with the ground (from 8% to 45% of the gait cycle). Shortly after heel off (occurring at 30% to 40% of the gait cycle), the ankle begins to plantar flex, reaching a maximum of 15 to 20 degrees of plantar flexion just after toe off. During the swing phase, the ankle is again dorsiflexed to a neutral position to allow the toes to clear the ground.[206]

Average walking speed requires approximately 10 degrees of dorsiflexion and 20 degrees of plantar flexion. It is of note that greater dorsiflexion is needed during the stance phase than during the swing phase of gait. As at the knee and the hip, limitation of motion at the ankle leads to an abnormal walking pattern. For example, limited ankle plantar flexion may result in a decreased push off, possibly leading to a shorter step length.

and associated increase in lumbar lordosis. Conversely, a posterior pelvic tilt accompanied by a flattening of the lumbar spine provides apparent hip flexion. To ambulate, individuals with a fused (i.e., ankylosed) hip use an exaggerated posterior and anterior pelvic tilt as a means to compensate for the absence of sagittal plane hip mobility (Fig. 15.14).[235] Because the pelvis and lumbar spine motions are mechanically linked at the sacroiliac joint, exaggerated pelvic tilting during walking may increase the stress at the lumbar spine. These stresses, repeated over many gait cycles, could eventually irritate the structures within this region, resulting in low back pain.

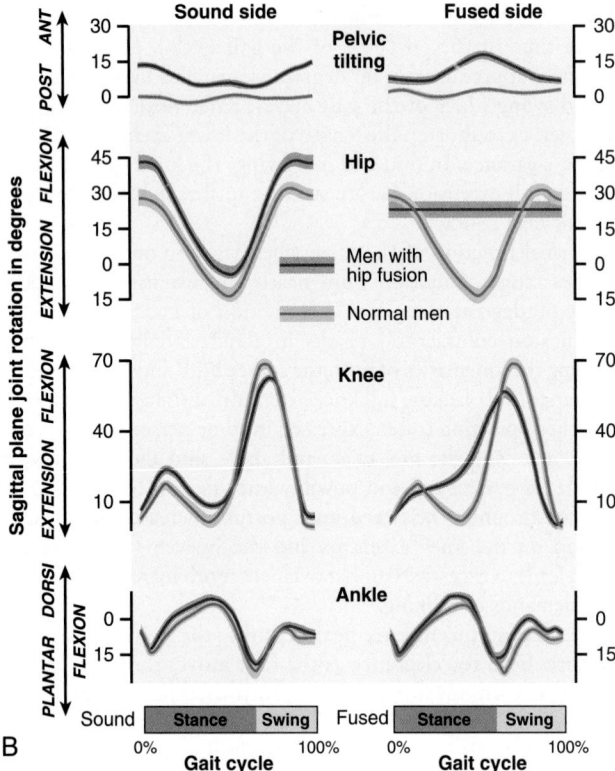

FIGURE 15.14 Body diagram (A) and average sagittal plane kinematic patterns (B) of men with unilateral hip fusion *(red lines)* compared with men with normal hip motion *(green lines).* The lack of mobility of one hip drastically affects motion of the pelvis, the ipsilateral knee, and the contralateral hip. Less significant effects are noted at the contralateral knee and at both ankles. This figure illustrates how impairment (i.e., reduced mobility of the hip) that affects a single joint will affect motion of the other joints. (Modified from Gore DR, Murray MP, Sepic SB, et al: Walking patterns of men with unilateral surgical hip fusion, *J Bone Joint Surg Am* 57:759, 1975.)

Conversely, a lack of adequate dorsiflexion mobility during stance, for example from a "tight" Achilles tendon, may cause a premature heel off, resulting in a "bouncing" type of walking pattern. Alternatively, a "toeing-out" walking pattern is often employed to partially compensate for limited ankle dorsiflexion. With excessive toeing-out of the foot, the individual rolls off the medial aspect of the foot in the second half of stance phase. Another commonly accepted compensation for a mild lack of ankle dorsiflexion is increased foot pronation. With or without toeing-out, excessive foot pronation can lead to greater stresses applied to the supporting soft-tissue structures of the plantar aspect of the foot.

Summary of Sagittal Plane Kinematics

Several underlying principles govern sagittal plane motion of the joints of the lower extremities. At heel contact, to position the foot on the ground, the joints of the lower extremity are aligned to "reach forward" or elongate the lower extremity. Shortly after heel contact, controlled knee flexion and ankle plantar flexion cushion loading for a smooth weight acceptance. All the joints of the supporting lower extremity then extend to support the weight of the body at the necessary height so that the foot of the contralateral swing limb can clear the ground. During swing, all the joints of the advancing limb participate in shortening the lower extremity to bring the foot forward without tripping on the ground. In late swing, the lower extremity again "reaches forward" for the next heel contact.

The level of control of the lower extremities when walking is remarkable. During swing, typical toe clearance (the minimum distance between the toes and the floor) varies between 1 and 3 cm within and between individuals.[20,39,149] This minimum clearance occurs at mid swing, when the foot has its greatest linear horizontal speed (4.5 m/sec). The transition from the swing to the stance phase is also amazingly well controlled. To provide smooth contact with the ground, vertical heel speed slows just before heel contact to only 0.05 m/sec. This level of control is the basis of the argument against using the term heel "strike" to describe the typically well-controlled heel contact with the ground.

A significant lack of ankle dorsiflexion may also affect knee motion, resulting in reduced knee flexion during stance. In more severe cases of reduced dorsiflexion, the knee may be forced into end range extension/hyperextension, especially in the second half of stance phase.[173] In extreme cases in which there is a pes equinus deformity (i.e., fixed plantar flexion of the ankle), the individual may walk on the forefoot (metatarsal heads) with extended toes, with the heel never coming in contact with the ground and the knee remaining in excessive flexion throughout stance. This condition is most commonly observed in individuals with cerebral palsy and serves as another reminder of how impairment at one joint may affect other joints of the ipsilateral lower extremity.

Limited ankle dorsiflexion also interferes with clearing the toes during swing phase. To compensate, increased hip flexion of the swing limb is needed. Limited dorsiflexion in swing may result from plantar flexor tightness, calf spasticity, or ankle dorsiflexor weakness.

FIRST TARSOMETATARSAL JOINT

The first tarsometatarsal joint, the function of which is described in Chapter 14, has a slight amount of plantar flexion and dorsiflexion contributing to height adjustments of the foot's medial longitudinal arch when walking.[17]

FIRST METATARSOPHALANGEAL JOINT

The metatarsophalangeal (MTP) joint of the hallux (great toe) is crucial to normal walking. At heel contact, the MTP joint is slightly extended. From shortly after heel contact to heel off, the MTP joint is in a relatively neutral position. Between heel off to just before toe off, the MTP joint extends approximately 45 degrees beyond neutral position. (This is the angle measured between the long axis of the first metatarsal and the proximal phalanx of the hallux.) During the late part of stance phase and early swing, the joint flexes and returns to a near neutral position.

Limited MTP joint extension because of a soft-tissue injury, such as a joint sprain (turf toe), or degeneration of the joint (hallux rigidus) typically results in a combination of rearfoot supination and forefoot abduction to avoid painful first MTP dorsiflexion during push off.[35] One consequence of this abnormal walking pattern is a shift of the weight bearing forces from the medial to the lateral aspect of the plantar surface of the foot, leading to a less efficient push off as well as a decrease in stride length. Potential interventions for hallux rigidus, with differing walking pattern outcomes, are MTP joint replacement [186] and MTP joint arthrodesis.[181]

Frontal Plane Kinematics

Joint rotations within the frontal plane (Video 15.4) are of smaller amplitude compared with those in the sagittal plane. These rotations are important, however, especially at the hip and subtalar joints.

PELVIS

Frontal plane motion of the pelvis during walking is best observed from either in front of or behind the individual, watching the iliac crests rise and fall in relationship to the horizontal plane. The pelvis rotates through a total excursion of about 10 to 15 degrees as a result of pelvic-on-femoral (hip) adduction and abduction on the stance limb. During weight acceptance on the right lower extremity (i.e., the first 15%–20% of the gait cycle), the left iliac crest drops slightly below the height of the right iliac crest (Fig. 15.15A); this drop of the left iliac crest reflects pelvic-on-femoral adduction of the right stance hip (see Fig. 15.15B). This initial downward motion of the left side of the pelvis is the result of gravity acting on the trunk and is controlled to a great extent by eccentric activation of the right hip abductors. From approximately 20% to 60% of the gait cycle, the left iliac crest is elevated by concentric activation of the right hip abductors, assisted by a slight shift of the trunk toward the right side. This shift brings the mass of the trunk over the right hip, thereby reducing the external torque demands on the right hip abductors. The elevation of the left iliac crest (on the swing limb) is effectively the result of pelvic-on-femoral abduction of the right stance hip. Throughout the swing phase on the right (stance phase on the left), a similar pattern occurs of initial controlled lowering of the right iliac crest followed by its progressive elevation.[45]

HIP

The pattern of elevation and depression of the iliac crests reflects the frontal plane motion of the hips (see Fig. 15.15B). During the stance phase, this frontal plane motion occurs primarily from pelvic-on-femoral kinematics (see Chapter 12). A much smaller and variable amount of hip frontal plane motion likely occurs during stance by way of femoral-on-pelvic kinematics, visually observed through

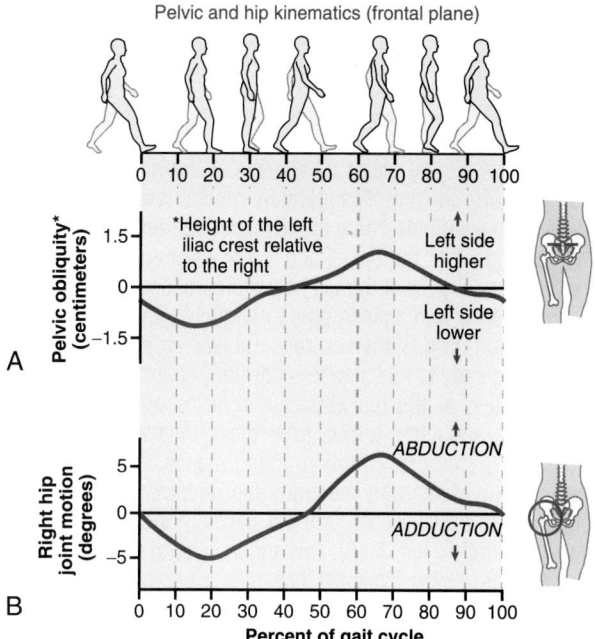

FIGURE 15.15 Frontal plane pelvis and hip motion for a full gait cycle starting with right heel contact (also see Video 15.4). (A) Illustrates the alignment of the pelvis itself considering the height of the left iliac crest in relationship to the right iliac crest. During right stance phase, the left iliac crest initially drops slightly before progressively moving upward. This small drop of the contralateral pelvis during early stance is considered normal. In the second half of the gait cycle, the relatively higher left iliac crest during the initial part of right swing phase reflects the controlled lowering of the right iliac crest by the left hip abductors when a person initially stands on the left lower extremity. (B) Illustrates frontal plane hip motion. When considering the movement of the pelvis (described earlier) in relationship to the femur, in the early part of stance on the right, the drop of the left iliac crest contributes to right hip adduction. As the left iliac crest is elevated in the latter part of the right stance phase and the right iliac crest is lowered in the early part of the right swing phase, right hip abduction is created. (Data from Ounpuu S: Clinical gait analysis. In Spivack BS, editor: *Evaluation and management of gait disorders,* New York, 1995, Marcel Dekker.)

medial-lateral movement of the knee. During the swing phase, the motion of the pelvis (about the stance limb) combines with motion of the advancing femur to return the hip to its neutral frontal plane position.[45,206]

KNEE

Because of its articular geometry and strong collateral ligaments, the knee is relatively stable in the frontal plane, allowing only a very small amount of angular movement.[21,120] Benoit et al[21] studied the kinematics at the tibiofemoral joints of six healthy individuals by recording the movement of reflective markers attached to the pins inserted in the cortexes of each person's femur and tibia. While study participants walked at a self-selected speed, knee movements were measured in three dimensions through the use of four infrared cameras. Overall, the authors found a minimal and inconsistent pattern of abduction-adduction movement (less than 3 degrees) at the knee during the first 80% of stance phase. In the last 20% of stance, just before toe off, approximately 5 degrees of knee adduction took place in most individuals. These data are generally consistent with those of a previously published study by Lafortune et al,

Possible Causes for Excessive Hip Frontal Plane Motion during Walking

Excessive frontal plane movement of the stance hip is quite common, causing exaggerated medial-lateral shifts in the center of mass (CoM). There are at least three reasons why excessive movement of the pelvis and hip in the frontal plane may be observed: weakness of the hip abductors, reduced "shortening" of the swing limb, and a discrepancy in limb length.

The slight drop of the contralateral iliac crest (i.e., hip adduction) during early to mid stance is normally controlled by an eccentric activation of the hip abductor muscles of the stance limb. Inadequate abduction torque from these muscles often leads to excessive frontal plane motion during stance. While standing on one limb, a person with moderate hip abductor weakness demonstrates an excessive drop of the pelvis to the side of the lifted lower extremity (Fig. 15.16). This action is referred to as a *positive Trendelenburg sign.* Typically, however, a person with weakened hip abductors, especially if severe, compensates by leaning the trunk to the *same side* as the weakened muscle during any single-limb support activities, whether standing or walking. During walking, this is called a "compensated" Trendelenburg gait or gluteus medius limp. Leaning of the trunk to the side of weakness minimizes the external torque demands resulting from body weight on the abductor muscles of the stance limb. This characteristic gait has been studied in individuals with cerebral palsy, with some variations noted in the leaning pattern shown by either the trunk or the pelvis.[108]

Another deviation that is observed by looking at the movement of the pelvis in the frontal plane is called hip "hiking." Hip hiking on the side of the swing lower extremity compensates for the inability of the knee and/or ankle of the lower extremity to sufficiently shorten the limb for clearance of the foot. The classic example is walking with a knee brace, keeping the knee in full extension.[3] Hip hiking is more accurately described as the excessive elevation of the iliac crest on the side of the swing limb. Elevation results from

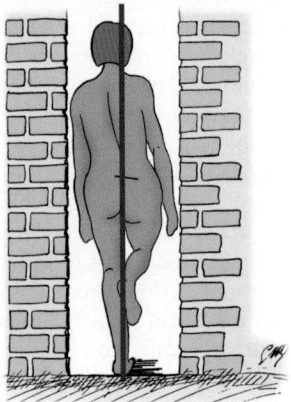

FIGURE 15.16 Excessive drop of the right (non–weight-bearing side) iliac crest resulting from a weak gluteus medius on the weight-bearing side. (Modified from Calvé J, Galland M, De Cagny R: Pathogenesis of the limp due to coxalgia: the antalgic gait, *J Bone Joint Surg Am* 21:12, 1939.)

pelvic-on-femoral abduction of the stance limb. Muscles involved in this movement include the primary abductors of the stance limb, the quadratus lumborum of the swing limb, and possibly the abdominals and back extensors on the side of the swing limb.

A significant limb length difference also affects movement of the pelvis in the frontal plane.[107] Limb length discrepancy can be severe, secondary to a fracture of the femur or a unilateral coxa vara or valga, or it can be slight (<5 mm) owing to natural variability. During periods of double-limb support, the iliac crest of the longer lower extremity is positioned higher than the iliac crest of the shorter lower extremity. This pelvic obliquity, which occurs for every gait cycle, results in increased cyclic side bending of the lumbar spine.

---

who used similar invasive methods on five individuals walking at 1.2 m/sec.[120] Lafortune et al reported the knee to be in an average of 1.2 degrees of abduction (valgus) at the time of heel contact (Fig. 15.17).[120] This alignment remained unchanged throughout the stance phase.

Lafortune et al also reported data for the swing phase of gait, indicating that the knee typically abducted an additional 5 degrees during initial swing phase.[120] Maximum abduction occurred when the knee was near its maximum flexion angle. The knee returned to its slightly abducted position before the next heel contact. The data from both studies provide a unique contribution to the literature. Most other published data on these kinematics are from studies using skin-mounted markers, which generally are associated with greater error.

ANKLE (TALOCRURAL JOINT)

The primary motion of the talocrural joint is dorsiflexion–plantar flexion. Although, as described in Chapter 14, the ankle everts and abducts slightly with dorsiflexion, and inverts and adducts

slightly with plantar flexion, these secondary frontal and horizontal plane motions are very small and are not discussed in this chapter.

FOOT AND SUBTALAR JOINT

The triplanar motions of pronation and supination occur through interaction of the subtalar and transverse tarsal joints. Pronation combines components of eversion, abduction, and dorsiflexion; supination combines inversion, adduction, and plantar flexion. This chapter considers the frontal plane motions of eversion and inversion at the subtalar joint to represent the more global motions of foot pronation and supination, respectively. Subtalar joint motions are typically measured as the angle made between the posterior aspect of the calcaneus and the posterior aspect of the lower leg (Fig. 15.18).

The subtalar joint is inverted approximately 2 to 3 degrees at the time of heel contact (Fig. 15.19). Immediately after heel contact, rapid eversion of the calcaneus begins and continues until mid stance (30%–35% of the gait cycle), where a maximally everted

Knee kinematics (frontal plane)

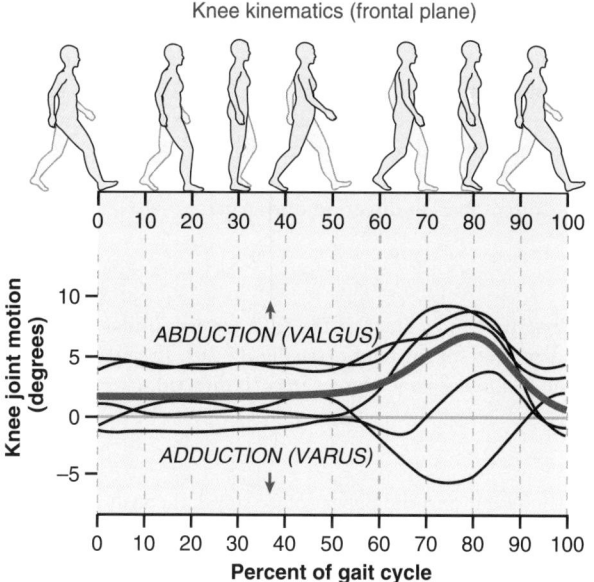

FIGURE 15.17 Frontal plane angular motion of the knee is illustrated. The purple line is the average of four of the five study participants. The smaller black lines are each participant's individual data. (Data from Lafortune MA, Cavanagh PR, Sommer HJ III, et al: Three-dimensional kinematics of the human knee during walking, *J Biomech* 25:347, 1992.)

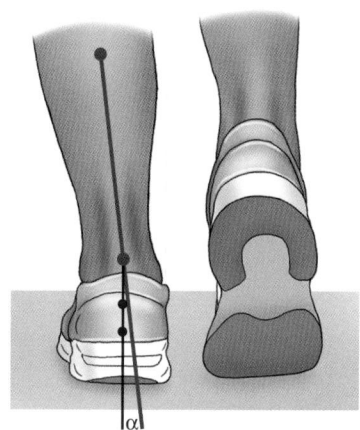

α = Frontal plane subtalar joint angle

FIGURE 15.18 Method to measure rear foot (subtalar joint) motion. The inversion or eversion angle, made by the lines bisecting the lower leg *(purple line)* and the calcaneus *(black line),* is measured as a simplified indicator of the amount of foot pronation or supination. This measurement can be made at a single point or throughout the gait cycle by the analysis of individual images recorded using a video system.

position of approximately 2 to 4 degrees is reached. At that time, the subtalar joint reverses its direction of movement and starts toward inversion. Normally, a relatively neutral position of the calcaneus is reached at about 40% to 45% of the gait cycle, which corresponds to approximately heel off. Between heel off and toe off, calcaneal inversion continues until it reaches a value of approximately 6 degrees of inversion. During swing, the calcaneus returns to a slightly inverted position in preparation for the next heel contact. This pattern of motion is generally agreed on in the literature; however, the reported amount of foot pronation when

Subtalar joint kinematics (frontal plane)

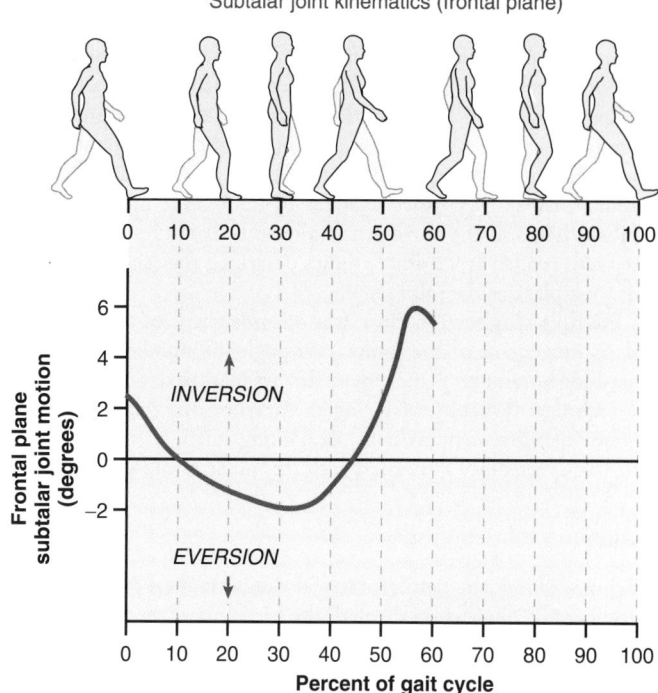

FIGURE 15.19 Frontal plane inversion and eversion of the calcaneus as an indicator of subtalar joint motion during walking. (Data from Cornwall MW, McPoil TG: Three-dimensional movement of the foot during the stance phase of walking, *J Am Podiatr Med Assoc* 89:56, 1999.)

walking varies considerably in the literature based on the techniques and preferences for measurement. For example, Reischl et al,[189] using a three-dimensional model of the foot, report a mean peak pronation of 10.5 ± 3.4 degrees, occurring at 26.8% ± 8.7% of the gait cycle.

The movement of foot pronation or supination during walking is accompanied by changes in height of the foot's medial longitudinal arch.[132,142,180] As thoroughly described in Chapter 14, individuals with "flat-arched" feet (pes planus) typically demonstrate a greater amount of rearfoot pronation when walking.[33,124] A detailed review of this associated kinesiology is provided in Chapter 14.

SPECIAL FOCUS 15.5

Summary of Frontal Plane Kinematics

The best location from which to observe frontal plane kinematics of the joints of the lower extremities is behind the individual. Hip motion plays an important role in reducing the vertical displacement of the body's center of mass (CoM). The rapid pronation (calcaneal eversion) of the foot after heel contact participates in the process of weight acceptance and provides a flexible and adaptable foot structure for making contact with the ground. Later in the stance phase, including between heel off and toe off, the inversion of the calcaneus associated with supination of the foot provides a more rigid foot structure, which helps propel the body forward.[132,142,180]

Horizontal Plane Kinematics

Information currently available about lower extremity kinematics in the horizontal plane during walking is provided by only a limited number of studies. To improve the accuracy of these measurements, some investigators fixed rigid metal pins in the pelvis, femur, and tibia of their study participants. Attached to these metal pins were markers that allowed video cameras to track bone movement. In some studies, only the movement of the bony structures in space was observed; reports from other studies described the relative motion that took place at the joint itself.[93,120]

The following section cites data on movement of the bones as well as movement of the joints. Although the number of studies describing horizontal plane kinematics has increased in recent years, the technical difficulty of trying to measure this relatively small amount of movement remains, explaining much of the reported kinematic variability associated with this plane of movement.

PELVIS

During walking, the pelvis rotates in the horizontal plane around a vertical axis of rotation through the hip joint of the stance limb. The following description of pelvic rotation is based on a *top view for a right gait cycle.* At right heel contact, the right anterior-superior iliac spine (ASIS) is forward compared with the left ASIS. For the initial 15% to 20% of the gait cycle, the pelvis rotates in an internal (counterclockwise) rotation, as viewed from above in Fig. 15.20. Throughout the rest of stance on the right lower extremity, an external (clockwise) rotation of the pelvis occurs as the left ASIS progressively moves forward along with the advancing left swing limb. At right toe off, the right ASIS is now behind the left. During swing of the right lower extremity, the right ASIS progressively moves forward. Throughout the gait cycle, the pelvis rotates 3 to 4 degrees in each direction. A greater amount of rotation of the pelvis occurs with increasing walking speed to increase step length.[127]

FEMUR

After heel contact, the femur rotates internally for the first 15% to 20% of the gait cycle (Fig. 15.20). At about 20% of the gait cycle, the femur reverses its direction and rotates externally until shortly after toe off. Internal rotation of the femur takes place throughout most of the swing phase. Overall, the femur rotates approximately 6 to 7 degrees in each direction during gait.

TIBIA

The pattern of movement of the tibia is very similar to the movement described for the femur (see Fig. 15.20). The magnitude of the rotation is about 8 to 9 degrees in each direction.

HIP

Both the femur and the pelvis rotate simultaneously. At right heel contact, the right hip is in slight external rotation based on the relative posterior position of the contralateral (left) ASIS (Fig. 15.21). A net internal rotation movement of the right hip occurs during most of stance on the right lower extremity, as the contralateral (left) ASIS is brought forward. A maximum internally rotated position is achieved by approximately 50% of the gait cycle. External rotation of the right hip occurs from 50% of gait until mid swing, as the right lower extremity is advanced forward. From mid swing to right heel contact, a slight amount of right hip internal rotation takes place.[45,206]

KNEE

There are two studies of particular interest that used intracortical pins attached to the femur and tibia as a means to precisely document horizontal plane rotation of the knee during

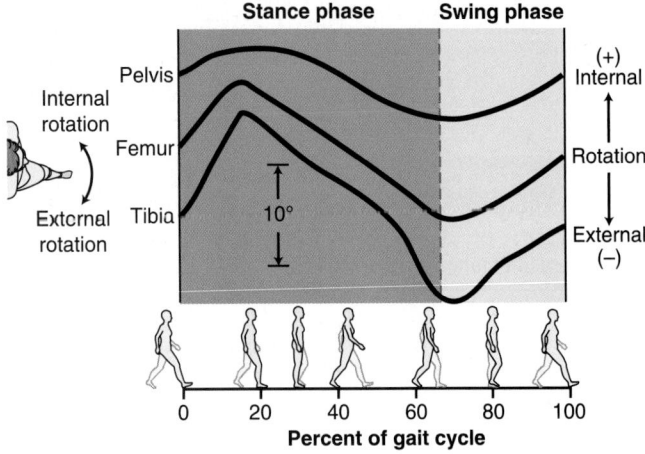

FIGURE 15.20 Pattern of horizontal plane motion of the pelvis, femur, and tibia as viewed from above. The pattern of motion is similar for the three bony structures, with progressively larger amplitude of movement for the more distal structures. View from above, for the right lower extremity, internal rotation of the pelvis, femur, and tibia, all corresponds with a counterclockwise motion. (From Mann RA: Biomechanics of the foot. In American Academy of Orthopedic Surgeons, editors: *Atlas of orthotics: biomechanical principles and application,* St Louis, 1975, Mosby.)

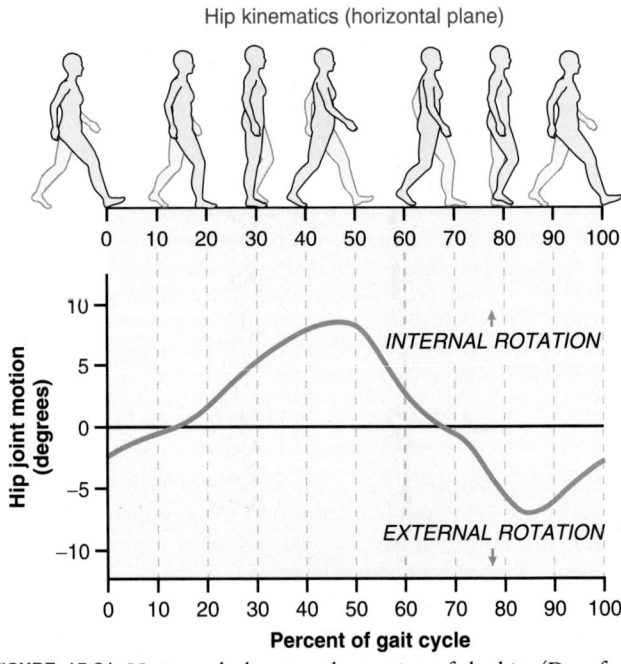

FIGURE 15.21 Horizontal plane angular motion of the hip. (Data from Sutherland DH, Kaufman KR, Moitoza JR: Kinematics of normal human walking. In Rose J, Gamble JG, editors: *Human walking,* ed 2, Philadelphia, 1994, Williams & Wilkins.)

Knee kinematics (horizontal plane)

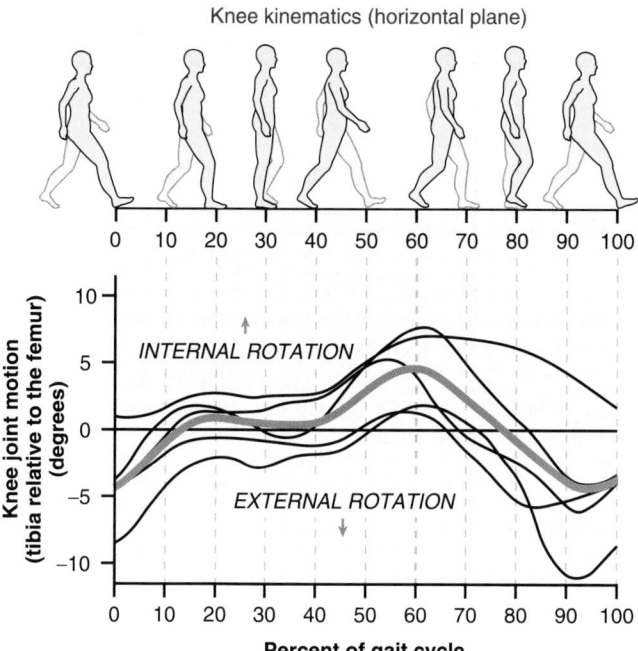

FIGURE 15.22 Horizontal plane angular motion of the knee. The blue line is the average of the five study participants. The smaller black lines are each participant's individual data. (Data from Lafortune MA, Cavanagh PR, Sommer HJ III, et al: Three-dimensional kinematics of the human knee during walking, *J Biomech* 25:347, 1992.)

walking.[21,120] Fig. 15.22 illustrates data from a study by Lafortune et al for each study participant, along with the group average.[120] Clearly, and consistent with data from Benoit et al,[21] the amount and direction of the horizontal plane rotation of the knee is highly variable. Much of this variability is masked by the process of averaging the data across individuals, as performed in Fig. 15.22 and in many descriptive and research reports. In fact, although Fig. 15.22 shows an overall trend toward internal rotation during the stance phase, data by Benoit et al[21] indicate an average overall pattern of knee external rotation motion. This variability makes it difficult to interpret many of the studies that have proposed a biomechanical link between knee pain and abnormal horizontal plane kinematics at this joint during walking and running.

ANKLE AND FOOT

Horizontal plane rotation of the talocrural joint is slight and not considered here. The primary movements of the subtalar joint (inversion and eversion) are in the frontal plane and are described earlier in this chapter.

Trunk and Upper Extremity Kinematics

The trunk and upper extremities play an important role in maintaining balance and minimizing energy expenditure during walking. In addition, small intricate spinal movements and muscular actions at the trunk serve to dampen the gait-related oscillations and accelerations produced by the movement of the lower extremities.[101,146] As a result, accelerations of the head segment are 10% to 40% less than those of the lower portion of the trunk. This dampening effect, keeping the head more stable, serves an important role in optimizing visual and vestibular function during walking.

TRUNK

During walking, translation of the head and trunk follows the general pattern of translation of the body's center of mass (CoM) as discussed and illustrated in the next section of this chapter. In addition, the trunk rotates in the horizontal plane around its vertical axis with the shoulder girdle rotating in the opposite direction as the pelvis. The average total rotational excursion of the shoulder girdle is about 7 to 9 degrees.[30,163] This pattern of motion of the trunk makes a small contribution to the overall efficiency of gait.[30] Restriction of trunk motion increases energy expenditure during walking by as much as 10%.[187]

Although the preceding paragraph briefly describes the horizontal plane motion of the trunk, Rozumalski and colleagues[197] published data in 2008 on segmental motion throughout the lumbar spine when walking. The uniqueness of this study is related to the methods of data collection, which included three-dimensional video analysis of markers rigidly fixed to the spinous processes of all lumbar segments using surgically inserted Kirshner wires. The data indicate complex intervertebral lumbar motion of up to 3 to 5 degrees in each direction, in all three planes.[197] These kinematics, although modest, are likely necessary to allow the previously described small triplanar pelvic motions to occur while the trunk is kept in a relatively erect posture. Individuals with pelvic girdle and low back pain have shown both an increase in horizontal plane range of motion of the pelvis and altered phase relationship between the rotation of the pelvis and thorax while walking. Such findings reinforce the potential for altered trunk/pelvis motor coordination in persons with chronic low back pain.[183]

SHOULDER

In the sagittal plane, the shoulder exhibits a sinusoidal pattern of movement that is out of phase with hip flexion and extension. As the hip (femur) moves toward extension, the ipsilateral shoulder (humerus) moves toward flexion, and vice versa.[224] At heel contact, the shoulder is in its maximally extended position of approximately 25 degrees beyond the neutral position. The shoulder then progressively rotates forward to reach a maximum of 10 degrees of flexion by 50% of the gait cycle. In the second half of the gait cycle, as the ipsilateral hip moves forward toward flexion, the shoulder extends to return to 25 degrees of extension by the next heel contact.

The pattern of movement of the shoulder is consistent across individuals, although the magnitude of movement varies greatly. In general, the amplitude of shoulder movement increases with greater speed.[192] Arm swing is partly active, rather than fully passive, with low level (less than 5% maximal voluntary isometric contraction) cyclical activation of namely the anterior and posterior deltoid muscles.[114,147] The major function of arm swing appears to be balancing the rotational forces in the trunk, stabilizing body motion about a vertical axis, and reducing energy expenditure.[147,175] Recent work showed that walking with arm swing, compared with no arm swing, reduced energy cost by 7% to 13% when walking at speeds greater than 1.00 m/sec.[236] Restriction of arm motion for one arm, as often used post injury or surgery also induced changes in spatiotemporal parameters of gait.[15]

ELBOW

The elbow is normally in approximately 20 degrees of flexion at heel contact. As the shoulder flexes in the first 50% of the gait cycle, the elbow also flexes to a maximum of approximately 45 degrees. In the second half of the gait cycle, as the shoulder extends, the elbow extends to return to 20 degrees of flexion.[163]

SPECIAL FOCUS 15.6

Summary of Horizontal Plane Kinematics

Fig. 15.23 summarizes the direction of horizontal plane rotation of the major bones of the lower extremity and subtalar joint during walking. The pelvis, femur, and tibia rotate internally, well after heel contact (i.e., through about 15%–20% of the gait cycle). This mass internal rotation is accompanied by subtalar joint eversion. As described in Chapter 14, an everting subtalar joint tends to increase the pliability of the midfoot region, including the transverse tarsal joint. A pliable midfoot serves to cushion the impact of limb loading. After about 15% to 20% of the gait cycle, the pelvis, femur, and tibia all begin to externally rotate until toe off. Simultaneously to this external rotation of the pelvis, femur, and tibia the subtalar joint begins moving toward inversion, which tends to increase the stability of the midfoot region. This stability enables the midfoot to serve as a rigid lever during the later part of stance phase (push off), allowing the plantar flexors to lift the calcaneus without the midfoot collapsing under the body's weight. Further investigation, such as that performed by Reischl et al,[189] is needed to clearly elucidate the exact relationship that exists between the timing and magnitude of pronation of the foot and rotation of the tibia and femur.

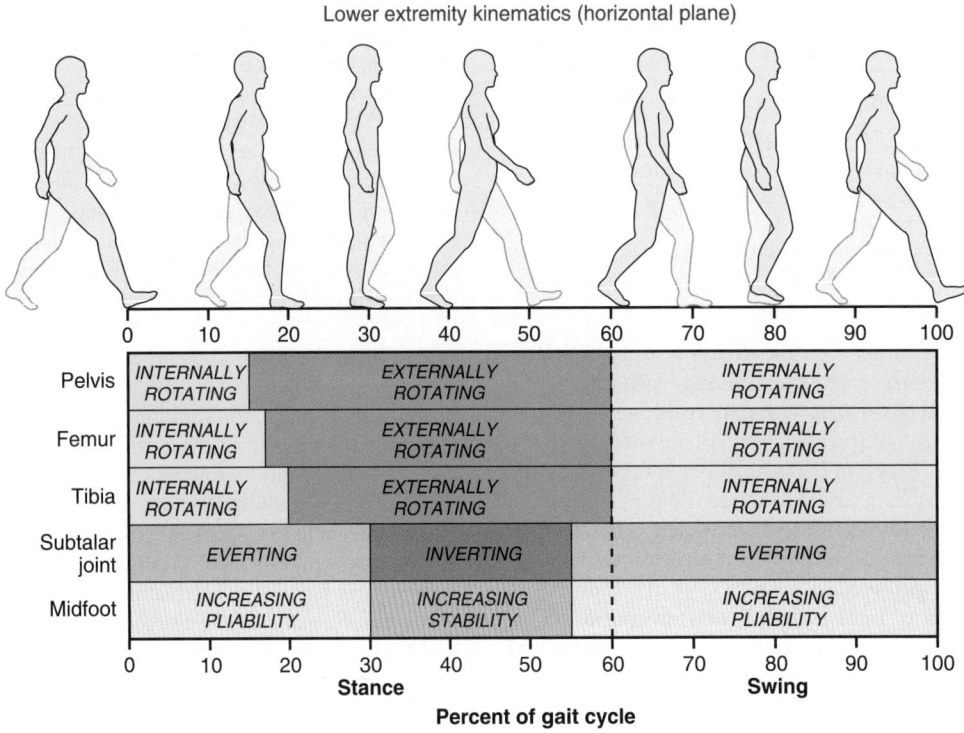

FIGURE 15.23 Horizontal plane rotation of the major bones of the lower extremity and subtalar joint during walking. View from above, for the right lower extremity, internal rotation of the pelvis, femur, and tibia, all corresponds with a counterclockwise motion. The graph shows the direction of rotation, which is not necessarily the same as the absolute joint position.

DISPLACEMENT AND CONTROL OF THE BODY'S CENTER OF MASS

Walking can be defined as a series of losses and recoveries of balance. Ambulation is initiated by allowing the body to lean forward. For a fall to be prevented, momentary recovery of balance is achieved by moving either foot forward to a new location. Once gait is initiated, the body's forward momentum carries the CoM of the body beyond the foot's new location, necessitating a step forward with the other foot. Forward progression is then achieved by the successive and alternate relocations of the feet. The smooth, controlled transition between loss and recovery of balance continues as long as forward displacement of the body is desired. Walking stops when foot placement stops the forward momentum of the body and balance is regained over the static base of support. Although this description provides a very simplified but useful and relatively accurate explanation of walking, it must be pointed out that walking also requires active participation of the musculature of the lower extremities and consequently energy expenditure.

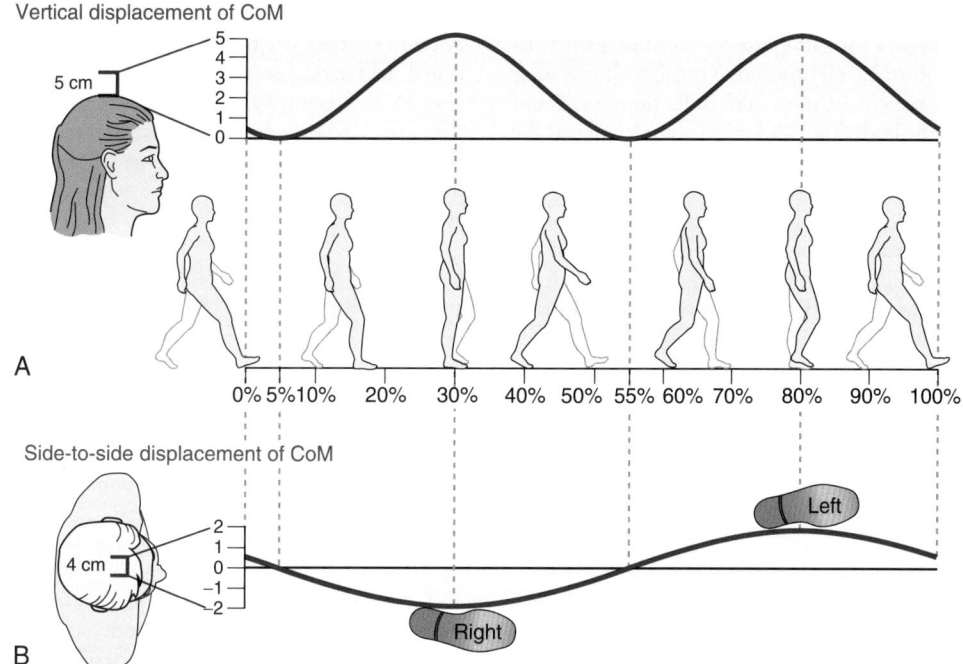

FIGURE 15.24 Vertical (A) and side-to-side (B) displacements of the center of mass (CoM) for a full gait cycle. The CoM is at its lowest and most central position in the side-to-side direction in the middle of double-limb support (5% and 55% of the gait cycle)—a position of relative stability with both feet on the ground. Conversely, the CoM is at its highest and most lateral position at mid stance (30% and 80% of the gait cycle)—a position of relative instability. During single-limb support, the trajectory of the CoM is never directly over the base of support. This fact is illustrated in (B) with the vertical projection of the CoM always located between the footprints.

Displacement of the Center of Mass

The body's CoM is located just anterior to the second sacral vertebra, but the best visualization of the movement of the CoM is obtained by tracking the displacement of the head or torso. Clearly, the most notable displacement of the body during walking is in the forward direction (Fig. 15.24). Superimposed on this forward displacement, however, are two sinusoidal patterns of movement that correspond to the movement of the CoM in the vertical and side-to-side directions.[233]

In the vertical direction, the CoM oscillates up and down to describe two full sine waves per gait cycle (see Fig. 15.24A). This movement of the CoM is best understood by looking at the individual from the side. Minimum height of the CoM occurs at the midpoint of both periods of double-limb support (5% and 55% of the gait cycle). Maximum height of the CoM occurs at the midpoint of both periods of single-limb support (30% and 80% of the gait cycle). A total vertical displacement of approximately 5 cm is noted at the average walking speed in the adult male.

During walking, the CoM is also alternately shifted from the right to the left lower extremity, creating a single side-to-side (right-to-left) sinusoidal pattern per gait cycle (see Fig. 15.24B). Maximum position of the CoM to the right occurs at the midpoint of the stance phase on the right lower extremity (30% of the gait cycle), and maximum position of the CoM to the left occurs at the midpoint of the stance phase on the left lower extremity (80% of the gait cycle). A total side-to-side displacement of approximately 4 cm occurs during normal walking.[94] The amount of displacement

increases when the individual has a wider base of support (i.e., walking with the feet wider apart) and decreases with a narrower base of support (i.e., walking with the feet closer together).

> **Displacement of the Center of Mass**
> - Total vertical displacement: 5 cm
> - Total side-to-side displacement: 4 cm

Let's next consider the total pattern of motion of the CoM during a full gait cycle (see Fig. 15.24). Starting shortly after right heel contact, the CoM is moving forward, upward, and toward the right foot. This general direction of movement continues for the first 30% of the gait cycle—the body is essentially "climbing and shifting its mass" over the supporting lower extremity. At right mid stance, the CoM reaches its highest and most lateral position toward the right. Just after right mid stance, the CoM continues forward but starts moving in a downward direction and toward the left side of the body—the body is essentially "falling away" from the supporting lower extremity. This is a critical moment in the gait cycle. With the left limb in its swing phase, the body depends on the left lower extremity to make secure contact with the ground to accept the weight transfer and to prevent a fall. Shortly after left heel contact, during the double-limb support phase, the CoM is located midway between the feet and reaches its lowest position as it continues to move forward and toward the left lower extremity. From right toe off to mid stance on the left lower extremity (80% of the gait cycle), the CoM moves forward, upward, and toward the left lower extremity, which is now providing support. At 80% of the gait cycle, the CoM is again at its highest point, but in its most lateral position to the left. Shortly after left mid stance, the movement of the CoM shifts downward and toward the right side of the body. The gait cycle is completed, and the process repeated when the right heel contacts the ground.

Noteworthy is the fact that the body's CoM is never directly located over the body's base of support during single-limb support (see Fig. 15.24B). This fact illustrates the relative imbalance of the body when walking, especially during single-limb support, when the foot must be positioned just slightly lateral to the vertical projection of the body's CoM to control its side-to-side movement. Proper location of the foot by hip motion in the frontal plane (i.e., hip abduction and adduction) is crucial considering the limited ability of the muscles of the subtalar joint to control the side-to-side motion of the CoM.[191,226]

Kinetic and Potential Energy Considerations

Although walking appears to take place at a steady forward speed, the body actually speeds up and slows down slightly with each step. When the supporting lower extremity is in front of the body's CoM, the body slows down. Conversely, when the supporting lower extremity is behind the body's CoM, the body speeds up. The body reaches its lowest velocity, therefore, at mid stance, once it has "climbed" on the supporting lower extremity, and its highest velocity during double-limb support, once it has "fallen away" from the supporting lower extremity and before "climbing" on the opposite limb. Because kinetic energy of the body during walking is a direct function of its velocity (Eq. 15.1), minimum kinetic energy is present at mid stance (30% and 80% of the gait cycle) and maximum kinetic energy is reached at double-limb support (5% and 55% of the gait cycle) (Fig. 15.25).

$$\text{Kinetic energy} = 0.5 \, mv^2 \qquad \text{(Eq. 15.1)}$$

where *m* is the mass of the body and *v* is the velocity of the body's CoM.

Kinetic energy is complemented by potential energy (Fig. 15.25). Potential energy is a function of the mass of the body, the gravitational field acting on the body, and the height of the body's CoM (Eq. 15.2). During walking, maximum potential energy is achieved when the CoM reaches its highest points (30% and 80% of the gait cycle). Minimum potential energy of the body occurs at double-limb support (5% and 55% of the gait cycle), when the body's CoM is at its lowest points.

$$\text{Potential energy} = mgh \qquad \text{(Eq. 15.2)}$$

where *m* is the mass of the body, *g* is the potential downward acceleration of the body resulting from gravity, and *h* is the height of the body's CoM.

In an "idealized" graphic representation of the changes in kinetic and potential energy during walking, a relationship between the curves is readily observed (see Fig. 15.25).[40] The times of maximum potential energy correspond to the times of minimum kinetic energy and vice versa. As potential energy is lost from mid stance to double-limb support (the CoM of the body going from its highest to its lowest location), kinetic energy is gained (the CoM of the body going from its minimum to maximum speed). Conversely, as kinetic energy is lost from double-limb support to mid stance, potential energy is gained. Therefore the body, acting to a great extent as an inverted pendulum, appears to use an optimal magnitude of vertical oscillation to transfer mechanical energy most effectively between its potential and kinetic forms. Deviation from this optimal vertical oscillation, by adoption of either a "bouncy" or a "flat" gait, has been demonstrated to increase energy expenditure.[5,143,172]

In closing, it must be noted that although the cyclic transfer between kinetic and potential energy minimizes the metabolic cost of walking, this process alone is not sufficient to sustain steady-speed ambulation.[31] Consequently, unlike the movement of a perfect pendulum, walking is dependent on the energy generated by muscles. Muscles of the lower extremity must generate forces to assist with forward propulsion of the body during the stance phase and help with the advancement of the lower limb during the swing phase.[252]

FIGURE 15.25 Transfer between potential and kinetic energy during gait. The minimum potential energy exists when the center of mass (CoM) is at its lowest points (5% and 55% of the gait cycle). The maximum potential energy occurs when the CoM is at its highest points (30% and 80% of the gait cycle). The reverse occurs for kinetic energy. This transfer between potential and kinetic energy is analogous to riding a bicycle that gains speed while going down a hill and loses speed while climbing up the next hill.

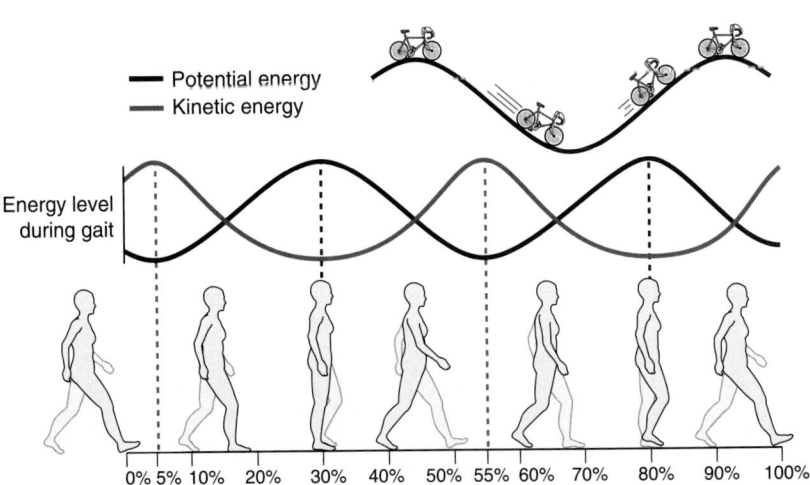

ENERGY EXPENDITURE

Energy expenditure during gait is measured by the amount of energy used in calories per meter walked per kilogram of body weight. Typically, energy expenditure is measured indirectly by quantifying oxygen consumption.[193] When walking, the body strives to minimize energy cost. Conservation of energy is achieved by optimizing the excursion of the CoM, controlling the body momentum, and taking advantage of intersegmental transfers of energy.[252]

The metabolic efficiency of walking is greatest at a walking speed of approximately 1.33 m/sec (3 mph).[193] Not surprisingly, this walking speed roughly corresponds to that freely adopted by

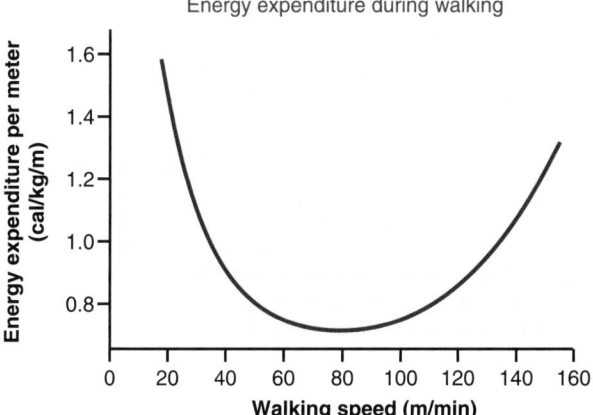

FIGURE 15.26 Energy expenditure as a function of walking speed. The lowest energy expenditure per meter walked is at a speed of approximately 1.33 m/sec (80 m/min). (Data from Ralston HJ: Effects of immobilization of various body segments on energy cost of human locomotion, *Ergon Suppl* 53, 1965.)

TABLE 15.4 Increased Energy Cost of Walking Associated with Specific Conditions

Conditions	Increased Energy Cost (%)*
Immobilization of one ankle, arthrodesis[247]	3
Immobilization of one knee in full extension[125]	17–37
Immobilization of one hip, arthrodesis[247]	32
Unilateral nonvascular (vascular) transtibial amputation, walking with prosthesis[67]	12 (36)
Unilateral nonvascular (vascular) transfemoral amputation, walking with prosthesis[67]	41 (102)
Postcerebrovascular accident, more (less) impaired[23]	100 (27)
Parkinson disease (mild to moderate severity)[98]	17
Cerebral palsy (heterogeneous severity and age)[166]	32
Aging[83]	12–17

*Percentage increase based on energy cost of normal gait.

individuals ambulating on the street (see Table 15.1). Walking faster or slower than that optimal speed increases the energy cost of walking (Fig. 15.26).

Walking speed is equal to the product of step length and cadence (step rate). Maximum energy efficiency of walking is achieved by the body's innate ability to adopt an ideal combination of step length and step rate. This combination is demonstrated across all walking speeds. Although the energy cost of walking increases with walking speed, the efficiency of walking is greatest at the maintained step length–step rate ratio of 0.0072 m/steps/min for men and 0.0064 m/steps/min for women across all walking speeds.[261] At any given walking speed, imposition of a different step length or step rate increases energy expenditure.[199]

With abnormal gait the energy cost of walking increases (Table 15.4). As a consequence, individuals with abnormal gait patterns tend to walk more slowly as a means to keep the rate of energy consumption at a comfortable aerobic level. Further discussion of the energetics of walking in individuals with pathologic gaits can be found in the textbook by Perry and Burnfield.[178]

Energy-Saving Strategies of Walking

When walking, five kinematic strategies serve to reduce the displacement of the CoM which, in turn, has long been believed to decrease energy cost. Vertical displacement of the CoM is reduced by the combined actions of the first four strategies. The fifth strategy serves to reduce the side-to-side displacement of the CoM (Table 15.5). The strategies detailed in this chapter are based on the work of Saunders and colleagues in 1953, originally referred to as the *determinants of gait*.[203] A detailed account of these determinants is found in the more classic publications of Inman and colleagues[93,94] and have been revisited in more recent publications.[116,129]

To appreciate the effects of the first four kinematic strategies used to optimize the vertical displacement of the CoM, envision walking without such mechanisms. This can be achieved by using two pencils connected at the eraser ends (Fig. 15.27A). During walking, a large vertical oscillation of the eraser end of the pencils (representing the pelvis and therefore the body's CoM) is readily observed. The eraser end is highest when the pencils are side by side in a vertically oriented position (i.e., mid stance). Conversely, the eraser end is lowest when the pencils are maximally angled (i.e., double-limb support).

Saunders and colleagues,[203] in their classic manuscript, suggested that the goal of these four strategies is to reduce the displacement of the CoM so as to decrease the energy expenditure related to the muscular effort needed to cyclically lift the body. This view has since been challenged in favor of a model in which the vertical displacement of the body acts more like an inverted pendulum, taking advantage of the transfer between potential and kinetic energy.[117] More recent data actually suggest that an optimal amount of vertical oscillation of the CoM exists, one that is neither too "flat" nor too "bouncy," which minimizes energy cost.[5,79,117,143,172] These data provide a new perspective on the interpretation of the goal of the original determinants of gait, possibly from "minimizing" to "optimizing" the CoM displacement. Additional work is needed to better understand the relationship among lower extremity kinematics, CoM excursion, and energy cost of walking.

TABLE 15.5 Kinematic Strategies to Optimize Energy Expenditure during Gait

Direction of Action	Name of Strategy	Action
Vertical	Horizontal plane pelvic rotation	Reduces the downward displacement of the center of mass (CoM)
Vertical	Sagittal plane ankle rotation	Reduces the downward displacement of the CoM
Vertical	Stance phase knee flexion	Reduces the upward displacement of the CoM
Vertical	Frontal plane pelvic rotation	Reduces the upward displacement of the CoM
Side to side	Frontal plane hip rotation (step width)	Reduces the side-to-side excursion of the CoM

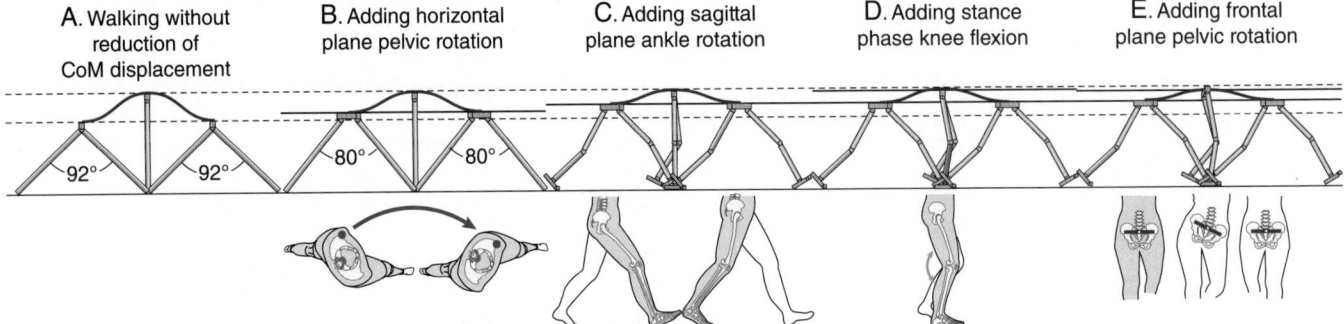

FIGURE 15.27 This series illustrates the individual and additive effects of four kinematic strategies to reduce vertical center of mass (CoM) excursion. (A) illustrates the large vertical oscillation of the CoM while a person walks *without* the strategies. (B) illustrates that rotation of the pelvis in the horizontal plane functionally lengthens the lower extremities and reduces the magnitude of the hip flexion-extension angle required for a given step length, thereby reducing the downward displacement of the CoM. (C) illustrates that further reduction of the downward displacement of the CoM is achieved by rotation of the ankle in the sagittal plane. (D) illustrates that the small amount of knee flexion present during stance reduces the functional length of the lower extremity and therefore the upward displacement of the CoM. (E) shows that the contralateral pelvic drop during stance also reduces the net overall elevation of the CoM. The angle values in (A) and (B) are for illustrative purposes only and do not represent the actual hip angles during walking.

VERTICAL DISPLACEMENT OF THE CENTER OF MASS

Reducing the downward displacement of the CoM is achieved by horizontal plane pelvic rotation and sagittal plane ankle rotation. Horizontal plane rotation of the pelvis advances the entire swing lower extremity forward, thereby minimizing the amount of hip flexion and extension needed for a given step length (compare Fig. 15.27A with Fig. 15.27B). As a consequence of the lower extremities remaining closer to a vertical orientation throughout the gait cycle, the lowest points of the CoM trajectory are raised, which reduces the downward displacement of the CoM. Sagittal plane ankle rotation makes use of the configuration of the ankle-foot complex (see Fig. 15.27C). At heel contact the alignment of the ankle places the large protruding calcaneus in contact with the ground, functionally elongating the lower extremity. Near the end of stance, as the hip extends and the knee begins to flex, the lower extremity is elongated by plantar flexion of the ankle (i.e., heel rise). This functional elongation of the lower extremity at both ends of stance phase further reduces the downward displacement of the CoM (compare Fig. 15.27B with Fig. 15.27C).[54,105,106]

Limiting the upward displacement of the CoM is partially achieved by stance phase knee flexion when the lower extremity is in its most vertical orientation (see Fig. 15.27D). Frontal plane pelvic rotation further assists in reducing upward displacement of the CoM (see Fig. 15.27E). During stance phase, the contralateral iliac crest falls as the ipsilateral iliac crest rises. Throughout a complete gait cycle, therefore, the iliac crests alternately rise and fall like the ends of a seesaw, but the point just anterior to the second sacral vertebra (i.e., the point representing the body's CoM) remains relatively stationary, as would the pivot point of a seesaw.[54,106]

As shown in Fig. 15.28, the combination of the four aforementioned strategies reduces the total net vertical displacement of the CoM. The downward displacement of the CoM is reduced by horizontal plane pelvic rotation and sagittal plane ankle rotation. The upward displacement of the CoM is reduced by stance phase knee flexion and frontal plane pelvic rotation. The work by Della Croce and colleagues[54] suggests that sagittal plane ankle rotation has the largest influence on CoM vertical displacement, followed by pelvic obliquity, stance phase knee flexion, and horizontal plane pelvic rotation. Not all research agrees with the functional importance or relevance of the determinants of gait. More recent work by Lin and colleagues,[129] for example, suggests that pelvic sagittal or horizontal plane rotation have a limited role in reducing vertical displacement of the CoM. Even after 60 years following the initial paper by Saunders and colleagues[203] about the determinants of gait, and despite the advances in technology since that time, there is still no complete agreement on the precise biomechanical role of each of these determinants. The determinants, nevertheless, hold an important historic foundation in the formal study of walking.

SIDE-TO-SIDE DISPLACEMENT OF THE CENTER OF MASS

While a person walks, their CoM shifts side-to-side and remains within the dynamic base of support provided by the feet (see Fig. 15.24). The amplitude of this lateral displacement, partially reflected

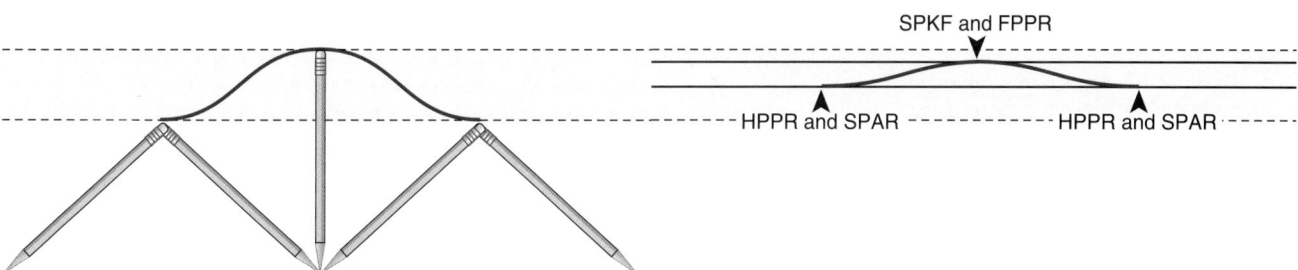

A. Walking without reduction of CoM displacement

B. Walking with reduction of CoM displacement

SPKF and FPPR

HPPR and SPAR   HPPR and SPAR

FIGURE 15.28 Combined action of the four kinematic strategies to reduce vertical center of mass (CoM) excursion. Without these strategies, a large vertical displacement of the body's CoM *(red)* would occur during walking (A). (B) illustrates the combined action of horizontal plane pelvic rotation *(HPPR)* and sagittal plane ankle rotation *(SPAR)* to reduce the downward displacement of the CoM during double-limb support. It also shows the action of stance phase knee flexion *(SPKF)* and frontal plane pelvic rotation *(FPPR)* to reduce the upward displacement of the CoM at mid stance.

by step width, is largely a function of frontal plane hip motion (i.e., hip abduction and adduction). The nervous system inherently adopts an 8- to 10-cm step width during walking (i.e., the fifth strategy, or determinant, of gait listed in Table 15.5) to optimize metabolic energy cost.[1,59,223] Wider steps require greater mechanical work to slow down and redirect the movement of the CoM in the other direction at each step, while narrower steps increase energy costs due to the greater muscular demand for stability and avoiding a loss of balance. An individual's self-selected step width could therefore also be regarded as a mechanical compromise between energy conservation and stability of the body as a whole. Persons with balance disorders, for example, often choose to walk with a wider base of support as a means to improve their stability. Although this strategy increases the energy cost of walking, the tradeoff is likely worthwhile, considering the often catastrophic consequences of falling, especially in the frail elderly.

But, as discussed earlier with regard to vertical displacement of the CoM, the normally adopted step width of 8 to 10 cm seems to reflect the inherent ability of the body to naturally use kinematic strategies to minimize energy expenditure. It has been demonstrated that walking with either a smaller or a larger step width increases energy cost in young healthy individuals.[1,59]

MUSCLE ACTIVITY

During a gait cycle, virtually all muscles of the lower extremities exhibit one or two short bursts of electrical activity, lasting from generally 100 to 400 msec (about 10%–40% of the gait cycle). Like all other elements of walking, this phasic muscular activation is repeated during each stride. Knowledge of when muscles are active when walking provides insight into their specific kinesiologic function. This knowledge allows gait deviations to be more easily understood and treated.

Activity of the lower extremity and trunk musculature has been studied extensively using EMG. In its simplest interpretation, muscular activity can be determined on a temporal basis; the muscle is simply considered "on" or "off." The muscle is considered "on" when the amplitude of its EMG signal reaches a predetermined value above the resting level. Otherwise, the muscle is considered to be "off," or electrically silent. As examples, the red horizontal bars in Fig. 15.29 illustrate when selected muscles are "on" during the gait cycle.[110]

Another method of reporting muscular activity during walking is to express the relative amount of EMG signal compared with a reference standard (review topic of EMG in Chapter 3). In many studies, the reference is the maximum signal recorded during a gait cycle for that same muscle, which explains why there are no units on the Y axis in Fig. 15.29 and why the EMG signal representation for each muscle takes full advantage of the graph's vertical dimension. This type of analysis provides insight into the relative level of activation of the muscle (i.e., an index of muscular effort) throughout the gait cycle.

Finally, the reader is reminded that the timing and especially relative activation of muscles during walking vary based on parameters such as walking velocity,[10,36,56,242] age,[128,238] additional loading,[242] and inclination[121] of the walking surface. Unless otherwise stated, the EMG data presented and discussed throughout this chapter are based on an average walking velocity of approximately 1.37 m/sec.

Trunk

Only the actions of the erector spinae and the rectus abdominis are discussed here. It is noteworthy that these muscles show near simultaneous activation on the right and the left sides of the body.

ERECTOR SPINAE

The erector spinae, at the level of the lumbar region, show two well-defined periods of activity. The first period is from slightly before heel contact to about 20% of the gait cycle. The second period is from 45% to 70% of the gait cycle, which corresponds to opposite heel contact.[9,36,43] These two bursts of activity, from both the right and the left erector spinae, control the forward angular momentum of the trunk relative to the hips shortly after heel contact (a braking force) for each step.

RECTUS ABDOMINIS

This muscle has very low and variable activity throughout the gait cycle.[9,50] Nevertheless, increased activity occurs at between 20% and 40% and again at between 70% and 90% of the gait cycle. This small increase in activity coincides with the time the hip flexors are actively flexing the hip. Increased activity of the rectus abdominis

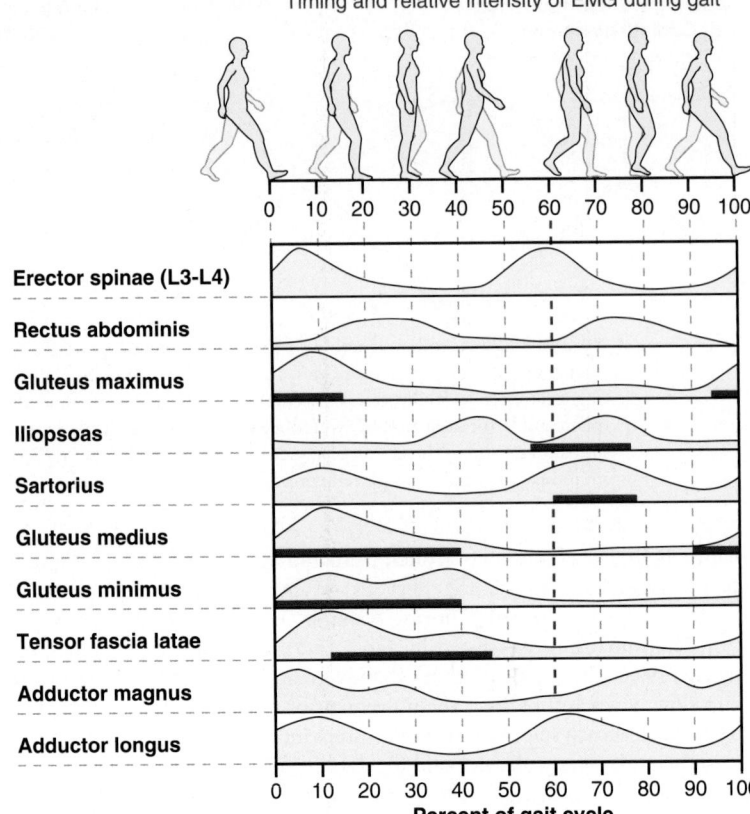

Timing and relative intensity of EMG during gait

FIGURE 15.29 (A,B) An electromyographic illustration showing the timing *(dark red bars)* and relative intensity *(light brown shading)* of muscle activation during walking. (Muscle timing data are from Knutson and Soderberg, 1995;[110] relative intensity of muscle activation data are from a compilation of several sources;[19,37,257] the general patterns of muscle activations are consistent with data reported in several other studies.[36,56,121,242]) The Y axis depicts the relative intensity of muscle activation for each muscle as a proportion of their maximum value obtained during the gait cycle. Based on this scaling, all muscles nearly fill the full vertical dimension of their respective graph, therefore precluding direct comparison of magnitude of muscle activation across muscles. Some muscles, such as the rectus abdominis, are only minimally active during gait in contrast to other muscles, such as the gluteus medius, where the peak in activation represents a more significant effort.

Figure continued on p. 694.

A

bilaterally therefore potentially helps stabilize the pelvis and lumbar spine and provides a more stable fixation point for the hip flexor muscles, principally the iliopsoas and rectus femoris.

Hip

Three muscle groups at the hip have been extensively studied during normal walking: the hip extensors, such as the gluteus maximus and the hamstrings; the hip flexors, such as the iliacus and the psoas; and the hip abductors, such as the gluteus medius and minimus.[10,36,121,242] Less well documented is the role of the hip adductors and rotators.[36,208]

HIP EXTENSORS

Activation of the gluteus maximus begins at late swing and serves two purposes—initiating hip extension and preparing the musculature for weight acceptance at the beginning of stance (see Fig. 15.13). At heel contact, the gluteus maximus is therefore already activated to extend the hip and prevent forward "jackknifing," or uncontrolled trunk flexion, over the femur. This "jackknifing" would occur if the forward displacement of the trunk were to continue at a steady velocity while the forward translation of the pelvis were suddenly slowed at heel contact. The gluteus maximus remains active from heel contact to mid stance (i.e., first 30% of the gait cycle) to support the weight of the body and produce hip extension. This relatively strong activation may also assist indirectly with knee

extension. In contrast, the gluteus maximus is relatively quiet during the second half of stance phase. During the swing phase, the gluteus maximus is largely inactive until late swing, when a modest activation is needed to first decelerate the flexing hip and then initiate its extension.

The hamstring muscles are active during the first 10% of the gait cycle, likely for similar reasons as the gluteus maximus to extend the hip and support the weight of the body (see Fig. 15.29B).

HIP FLEXORS

Electromyographic data on the hip flexors are relatively sparse in the literature, likely reflecting the need to use intramuscular electrodes for data collection. Available data indicate that the iliopsoas becomes active well before toe off and remains so through early swing.[10] The activation at between 30% and 50% of the gait cycle is likely initially eccentric, as the hip is extending at that time, followed by a concentric action to initiate hip flexion just before toe off. Despite the continued hip flexion into late swing, the hip flexor muscles are active only in the first 50% of the swing phase. Hip flexion in the second half of the swing phase is a result of the forward momentum that the thigh gains in early swing. The rectus femoris also acts as a hip flexor and therefore assists with the aforementioned actions.[10,168] The key roles of the hip flexors are to advance the lower extremity forward during swing in preparation for the next step and to lift the lower extremity to allow for toe clearance during swing.

The sartorius, another anterior muscle of the hip, is also active as a hip flexor from toe off until mid swing. The activation during early stance phase, as illustrated in Fig. 15.29A, has not been consistently reported by other studies, especially those using intramuscular EMG electrodes.[10] Studies reporting activation of this muscle in early stance typically used surface EMG electrodes, which raises the possibility that the increase in EMG signal is the result of "cross-talk" (see discussion of EMG in Chapter 3), the EMG signal effectively originating from the underlying vasti muscles.

HIP ABDUCTORS

Whereas hip flexors and extensors have their primary role in the sagittal plane, the hip abductors—gluteus medius, gluteus minimus, and tensor fascia latae—stabilize the pelvis in the frontal plane. The gluteus medius is active toward the very end of the swing phase in preparation for heel contact. The gluteus medius and minimus, the two primary hip abductors, are most active during the first 40% of the gait cycle, especially during single-limb support.[209,210] The primary function of the abductors is to control the slight lowering of the contralateral pelvis on the side of the swing limb (see Fig. 15.15). After this eccentric action, these muscles act concentrically to initiate the relative abduction of the hip that occurs in later stance. As described earlier in this chapter and extensively in Chapter 12, adequate frontal plane torque from the hip abductor muscles is crucial for frontal plane stability during gait. A cane used in the hand contralateral to the weak hip abductors is an effective way to reduce the demands placed on the weakened abductors, thereby reducing excessive frontal plane movement of the pelvis resulting from body weight (see Chapter 12).

The hip abductors also control the alignment of the femur in the frontal plane. Inadequate muscular activation may result in excessive adduction of the femur, causing poor alignment of the lower extremity and excessive valgus torque at the knee during the stance phase. Other accessory roles of the gluteus medius and minimus include assisting with hip flexion and internal rotation, using anterior fibers, and assisting with hip extension and external rotation, using posterior fibers. Accordingly, there is evidence of slightly different roles of the separate portions of these two muscles during gait, with the anterior fibers of both glutei being active later in stance than their respective posterior fibers. This selective anterior fiber activation may help with the forward contralateral (horizontal plane) rotation of the pelvis.[157,210]

HIP ADDUCTORS AND HIP ROTATORS

The hip adductors show two bursts of activity during walking.[257] The first burst occurs at heel contact and the second just after toe off. The initial burst of activity most likely serves to stabilize the hip through coactivation with the hip extensors and hip abductors. It is also probable that the adductor magnus and other adductors assist with hip extension at this time in the gait cycle. The second burst of activity, after toe off, likely assists with initiating hip flexion. As discussed in Chapter 12, the adductors have a moment arm to extend the hip when it is flexed (i.e., the hip position at heel contact) and a moment arm to flex the hip when it is in extension (i.e., the hip position at toe off). The adductor muscles therefore provide a useful source of flexion and extension torque at the hip.[100]

The hip internal rotators (tensor fascia latae, gluteus minimus, and anterior fibers of the gluteus medius) are active throughout much of the stance phase. During this time, these internal rotators move the contralateral side of the pelvis forward in the horizontal plane, thereby assisting with advancement of the swing limb (Fig. 12.35).

The hip external rotators, consisting of the six short external rotators, the posterior fibers of the gluteus medius, and the gluteus maximus, are most active during early stance. These muscles, in conjunction with the hip internal rotators, control the alignment of the hip in the horizontal plane. In particular, they control pelvic rotation while the lower limb is fixed to the ground. Consider the important action of these rotators in the rapid change of direction during walking or running.

Eccentric activation of the external rotators may be especially important to the control of the internal rotation of the lower limb in early stance (see Fig. 15.23). Inadequate strength or control of the external rotators may result in excessive internal rotation of the femur, often seen in conjunction with excessive foot pronation.

Knee

Two muscle groups play a critical role at the knee during ambulation: the knee extensors and knee flexors.[36,56,121,242]

KNEE EXTENSORS

As a group, the quadriceps is active in the very late stage of the swing phase in preparation for heel contact (see Fig. 15.29B). The major burst of activity, however, occurs shortly after heel contact. The function of the quadriceps at this time is to control the knee flexion that takes place in the first 10% of the gait cycle. Eccentric activation serves to cushion the rate of weight acceptance on the lower extremity (i.e., shock absorption) and to prevent excessive knee flexion. The quadriceps then acts concentrically to extend the knee and support the weight of the body during mid stance.

Nene and colleagues[168] critically compared the muscular activation of the rectus femoris and vasti components of the quadriceps during walking. They established that the rectus femoris was *not* active at heel contact as traditionally thought but only before and after toe off. The function of the rectus femoris at toe off is likely to control the extent of knee flexion. By using both surface and intramuscular electrodes in this study, Nene and co-workers[168] concluded that the burst of rectus femoris EMG signal typically reported at heel contact in the literature (and shown in Fig. 15.29B) is a result of cross-talk from the underlying vastus intermedius muscle.

In summary, it appears that the muscular components within the quadriceps have different functions during walking, at least as expressed during normal walking speed. Being active at heel contact, the vasti function primarily as shock absorbers. According to Andersson and colleagues[10] the rectus femoris may assist with this action during walking at speeds that exceed 2 m/sec and during running. The primary function of the rectus femoris in gait occurs in the transition from stance to swing phase and appears directed at assisting with initiating hip flexion as well as controlling knee flexion.

Timing and relative intensity of EMG during gait

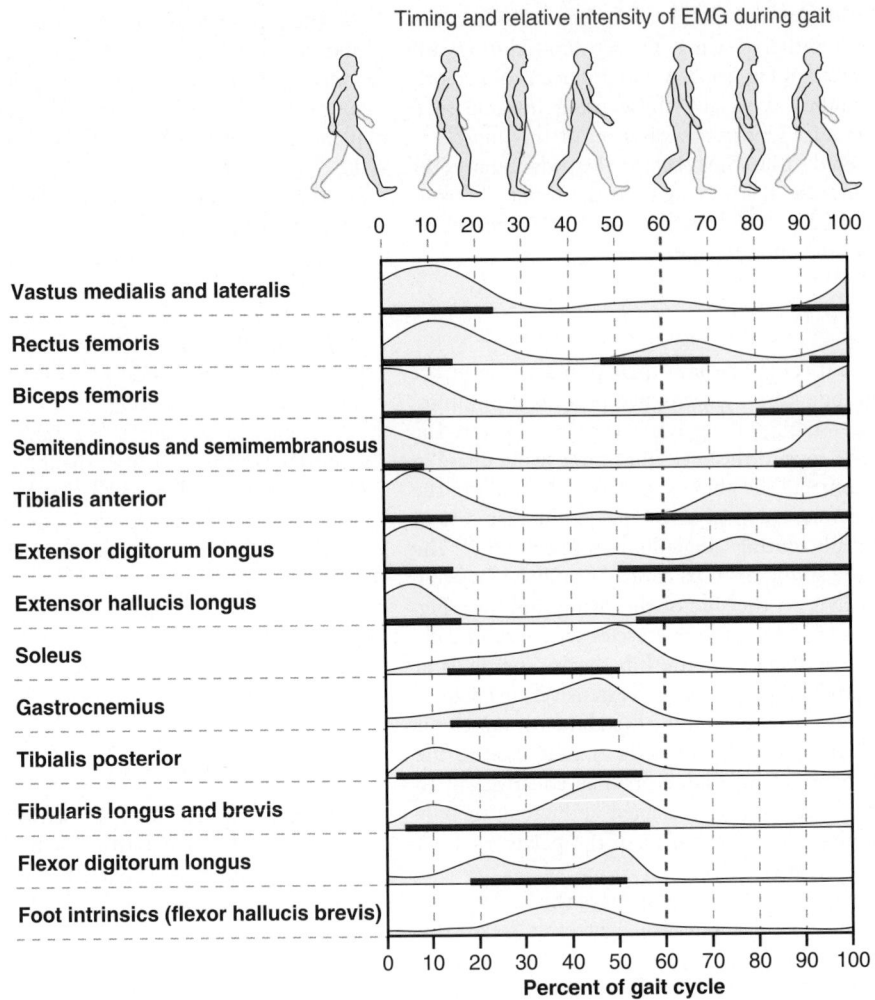

B

FIGURE 15.29, cont'd

KNEE FLEXORS

The hamstrings are most active from a period just before to just after heel contact. Before heel contact, the hamstrings decelerate knee extension in preparation for the placement of the foot on the ground. During the initial 10% of stance, the hamstrings are active to assist with hip extension and to provide stability to the knee through coactivation. The short head of the biceps femoris may also assist with knee flexion during the swing phase. Most of the knee flexion prior to toe off and during the swing phase of gait is performed passively as a result of the flexing hip and a small amount of gastrocnemius activation.[212]

Ankle and Foot

At the ankle and foot, several muscles play a crucial role in normal gait: the tibialis anterior, extensor digitorum longus, extensor hallucis longus, gastrocnemius, soleus, tibialis posterior, and fibularis longus and brevis.[36,56,156,242]

TIBIALIS ANTERIOR

The tibialis anterior has two periods of activity.[157] At heel contact, a strong eccentric activation is present to decelerate the passive plantar flexion of the ankle caused by the weight of the body being applied on the most posterior section of the calcaneus. If unopposed by the eccentric activation of the tibialis anterior and other ankle dorsiflexors, this large, passive plantar flexion torque results in the gait deviation referred to as "foot slap." This term is derived from the characteristic sound made by the foot slapping the ground just after heel contact. From heel contact to foot flat, the tibialis anterior may also assist with decelerating foot pronation, also through eccentric activation. The relatively poor mechanical advantage of the muscle to invert the foot, however, raises some doubt with regard to the effectiveness of the tibialis anterior in strongly controlling foot pronation.

The second period of activation of the tibialis anterior occurs during the swing phase. The purpose of this activation is to produce sufficient dorsiflexion of the ankle to clear the toes from the ground. Extreme weakness of the tibialis anterior and the other ankle dorsiflexors typically results in a "drop foot" during the swing phase. As a mechanism of compensation, along with a slower gait speed and shorter stride length, the individual typically excessively flexes the hip during swing.[148] Other compensatory maneuvers, such as vaulting, hip circumduction, and hip hiking (illustrated later in this chapter), may also be adopted to clear the toes from the ground. A common remedy for a drop-foot is a posterior ankle-foot orthosis that passively maintains ankle dorsiflexion during swing.

EXTENSOR DIGITORUM LONGUS AND EXTENSOR HALLUCIS LONGUS

Similar to the tibialis anterior, the extensor digitorum longus and extensor hallucis longus decelerate plantar flexion of the ankle at heel contact. These muscles, however, lack the line of force to decelerate foot pronation during the early part of stance phase (refer to Fig. 14.43 in the ankle and foot chapter). During swing, the toe extensors assist with dorsiflexion of the ankle and extend the toes to ensure that the toes clear the ground. Minor activity of the extensor digitorum longus and extensor hallucis longus during push off may provide stability to the ankle through coactivation with the ankle plantar flexors.

ANKLE PLANTAR FLEXORS

The soleus and gastrocnemius (triceps surae) are active throughout most of the stance phase, with the notable exception of the first 10% of the gait cycle. During this period, plantar flexion of the foot is controlled by an eccentric action of the ankle dorsiflexors. From about 10% of the gait cycle to heel off (approximately 30%–40% of the gait cycle), the ankle plantar flexors are active eccentrically to control the forward movement of the tibia and fibula relative to the talus (i.e., ankle dorsiflexion). Excessive or uncontrolled forward movement of the leg results in exaggerated ankle dorsiflexion and possibly uncontrolled knee flexion.

The major burst of activity of the ankle plantar flexors occurs near heel off and decreases rapidly to near zero at toe off. During this brief period, shortening of the muscles creates an ankle plantar flexion torque that participates in the forward propulsion of the body. This action is referred to as *push off*.

The gastrocnemius also generates low-level muscular activity in early swing, presumably to help with knee flexion. Because the rectus femoris is also active during early swing, a small amount of coactivation of the knee flexors and extensors is taking place.

The other plantar flexors of the ankle (tibialis posterior, flexor hallucis longus, flexor digitorum longus, and fibularis longus and brevis) assist the gastrocnemius-soleus group in the previously described actions. Additional actions of some of these muscles are noteworthy and discussed ahead.

SPECIAL FOCUS 15.7

Role of Triceps Surae

Work by Stewart and colleagues[225] provides some interesting additional insight into the functional role of the triceps surae in the stance phase of walking. In a healthy group of individuals, electrical stimulation of the soleus during the stance phase led to a reduced amount of knee flexion during this part of the gait cycle. In contrast, electrical stimulation of the biarticular gastrocnemius during the stance phase produced greater than normal knee flexion, as well as an increased ankle dorsiflexion. These findings suggest a complex biomechanical link between the sagittal plane control of the knee and ankle during the stance phase. Such a disruption in control of these two joints is often seen in individuals with certain neuromuscular diseases.

TIBIALIS POSTERIOR

The tibialis posterior, a potent supinator muscle of the foot, is active essentially throughout the entire stance phase. The tibialis posterior decelerates pronation of the foot from immediately after heel contact to about 35% of the gait cycle and supinates the foot from 35% to 55% (mid stance to toe off) of the gait cycle.[155,157,158]

The tibialis posterior muscle acts on both the foot and the tibia throughout the stance phase. Based on its line of pull, shortening of this muscle could supinate the rearfoot (and raise the arch of the foot) as it *simultaneously* externally rotates the lower leg relative to the foot. Indeed, both of these coupled kinematics occur as the tibialis posterior is active. Although speculation, it is interesting to consider how dorsiflexion of the talocrural joint (which occurs through 50% of the gait cycle) may serve to stretch the tibialis posterior at a time when it may be overshortening during its coupled external rotation-supination action on the lower leg and foot. Maintaining adequate length (and tension) in this muscle at this time may assist in raising the medial longitudinal arch and adding the necessary rigidity to the foot to prepare for its impending push off. The near simultaneous and combined concentric and eccentric muscular activation within the tibialis posterior across multiple joints may partially explain its relative vulnerability to painful tendinopathy or degeneration.[246,254] Such a cause and effect relationship is strengthened considering the large load placed on the muscle, spring ligament, and medial longitudinal arch during the countless gait cycles in a lifetime.

There is evidence in the literature that individuals with excessively pronated (flat) feet exhibit greater activation of supinator muscles such as the tibialis posterior, tibialis anterior, and flexor hallucis longus.[156] Active individuals with overly pronated feet may develop overuse and subsequent strain of the supinator muscles as they attempt to control the excessive pronation bias of the foot during early stance.

The tibialis posterior receives special attention in the treatment of people with cerebral palsy. The often hyperactive tibialis posterior, along with the soleus muscle, may cause an equinovarus deformity of the foot and ankle, resulting in the individual's walking on a foot that is plantar flexed and supinated.

FIBULARIS MUSCLES

The fibularis (peroneus) brevis and longus are active from about 5% of the gait cycle to just before toe off.[157] In addition to their function as plantar flexors, these pronator (evertor) muscles help counteract the strong inversion effect caused by activation of the tibialis posterior and other deep posterior muscles. The fibularis longus also assists in the kinematics of the foot by holding the first ray rigidly to the ground, which provides a firm base of support for the action of the foot as a rigid lever during the second half of the stance phase of gait.

INTRINSIC MUSCLES OF THE FOOT

The intrinsic muscles of the foot are typically active from mid stance to toe off (30% to 60% of the gait cycle). These muscles stabilize the forefoot and raise the medial longitudinal arch, thereby providing a rigid lever for ankle plantar flexion during the second half of the stance phase. They also likely help with control of balance during single-limb support [184] and controlling toe extension between heel off and toe off.

"Bottom-up" or "Top-down" Control of the Global "Pronation" of the Lower Extremity during Early Stance

As described earlier in the chapter and textbook, an important kinesiologic component of the loading response period of the gait cycle is a global internal rotation of the lower extremity in conjunction with pronation of the foot. This motion is often loosely described clinically as global "pronation" of the entire lower extremity. Such motion, when controlled, provides at least two useful biomechanical functions. First, the pronation at the subtalar joint (in particular its horizontal component) allows for dissipation of the residual internal rotation of the lower limb after heel contact. Second, pronation at the subtalar joint acts in concert with a controlled lowering of the medial longitudinal arch—both movements designed to help absorb some of the impact of loading. To be most effective, the overall "pronation response" of the lower limb must be performed within limited amplitude and prescribed duration. In worst-case scenarios, excessive lower limb pronation, especially during participation in sports that involve running and jumping, may result in a "medial collapse" of the knee, potentially leading to a variety of lower extremity pathologies, including patellofemoral pain and noncontact injury of the anterior cruciate ligament.[182]

A fundamental clinically relevant question relates to the source of the initiation and control of the global pronation of the lower extremity during the early part of the stance phase of walking and running.[82,182] Because of the weight-bearing nature of the stance phase, it has long been presumed that internal rotation of the lower extremity occurs *in response* to the overall pronation pattern of the foot. Pronation of the foot causes internal rotation of the tibia, which in turn leads to internal rotation of the femur. This view suggests a "bottom-up" kinesiologic control of global pronation of the lower extremity and is the basis for prescribing specialized footwear and foot orthoses for persons who demonstrate excessive (and pain-producing) global pronation of the entire lower extremity.[82]

Conversely, a more recent view advocating a "top-down" control of global lower limb pronation has been proposed. Based on this perspective, excessive pronation of the entire lower extremity primarily results from too much internal rotation and adduction of the femur secondary to inadequate activation or strength of the hip external rotator and abductor muscles throughout but especially during early stance.[150,216] This poorly controlled femoral motion would lead to excessive internal rotation of the tibia and ultimately excessive pronation of the foot. Proponents of this top-down perspective infer that correction of excessive pronation of the lower limb and the associated "medial collapse" of the knee is best achieved through therapeutic efforts that improve the control and strength of the musculature of the hip.

It is likely that both the bottom-up and top-down kinesiologic perspectives are complementary as opposed to exclusionary.[18] Continued clinical and biomechanical research is required to further refine diagnostic and treatment approaches for individuals with lower extremity pathologies related to excessive or poorly controlled global pronation of the lower extremity.

KINETICS

Understanding the forces that are responsible for movement when walking plays a critical role in understanding normal and pathologic movement. Although the kinetics (study of forces) of walking are not visually observable, they are ultimately responsible for the observed kinematics.

Ground Reaction Forces

When walking, forces are applied under the surface of the foot every time a person takes a step. The forces applied to the ground by the foot are called *foot forces*. Conversely, the forces applied to the foot by the ground are called *ground* (or *floor*) *reaction forces*. These forces are of equal magnitude but opposite direction. (Newton's Third Law—the law of action and reaction—states that forces are always present in pairs, equal in magnitude and opposite in direction.) This chapter focuses primarily on ground reaction forces because of the impact they potentially have on the body.

The description of the ground reaction forces follows a Cartesian coordinate system, with the forces being expressed along three orthogonal axes: vertical, anterior-posterior, and medial-lateral. The vector summation of the three forces gives a single resultant force vector between the foot and the ground. Such vector summation performed for the vertical and anterior-posterior components of the ground reaction forces leads to the classic "butterfly" representation of the ground reaction forces for a single step (Fig. 15.30).

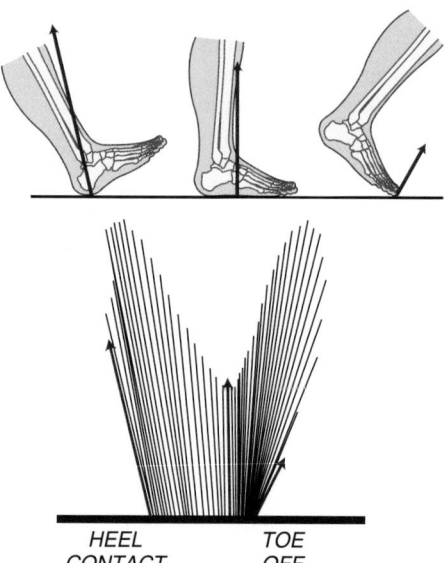

FIGURE 15.30 The bottom portion of the figure illustrates the classic "butterfly" representation of the ground reaction forces for a step. Each line represents the resultant force from the vector addition of the vertical and anterior-posterior forces at regular time intervals (i.e., every 10 msec in this case). The top portion of the figure represents how the successive lines from the "butterfly" reflect the progression of force application under the foot from heel contact to toe off. The vectors in red indicate heel contact, mid stance, and toe off. (Data from Whittle M: *Gait analysis: an introduction,* ed 4, Oxford, 2007, Butterworth-Heinemann.)

VERTICAL FORCES

The vertical forces are those directed perpendicular to the supporting surface. These vertical ground reaction forces peak twice in a given gait cycle. Forces are slightly greater than body weight at the time of early stance and again after heel off (Fig. 15.31A,C and Video 15.5). During mid stance, the ground reaction forces are slightly less than body weight. This fluctuation in force is a result of the vertical acceleration of the body's CoM. (Force is a function of mass and acceleration: $F = ma$.) In the early part of stance, the body's CoM is moving downward (see Fig. 15.24). A vertical ground reaction force greater than one's body weight, therefore, is needed to initially decelerate the downward movement of the body and then accelerate it upward. (This is similar to jumping on a bathroom scale and briefly reading a weight that is higher than static body weight.) At mid stance, the vertical ground reaction force is less than body weight as a result of a relative "unweighting" caused by the upward momentum of the body gained during the early part of stance. The higher ground reaction force at push off reflects the combined push provided by the plantar flexors and the need to reverse the downward movement of the body that occurs in late stance.

Peak Ground Reaction Forces (as a Percent of Body Weight)

- Vertical: 120% body weight (BW)
- Anterior-posterior: 20% BW
- Medial-lateral: 5% BW

ANTERIOR-POSTERIOR FORCES

In the anterior-posterior direction, shear forces are applied parallel to the supporting surface. At heel contact the ground reaction force is in the *posterior* direction (i.e., the foot applies an anteriorly directed force to the ground) (Fig. 15.31D and Video 15.5). At that time, sufficient friction is required between the foot and the ground to prevent the foot from slipping forward (picture the classic cartoon of a person falling to the ground after slipping on a banana peel). As the magnitude of the ground reaction force in the horizontal direction increases with longer steps and a faster walking speed, requirements for friction between the foot and the ground to prevent the foot from slipping increase.[48,86,131] Accordingly, the required coefficient of friction for ambulation is calculated as the ratio of the resultant shear force (which is the vector addition of the combined horizontal forces in the anterior-posterior and medial-lateral directions) divided by the vertical force applied under the foot.[34,48] Strategies to prevent slipping are minimizing the distance between foot location and the CoM of the body and reducing walking speed. This is why people often take shorter and narrower steps when walking on an icy surface—they are decreasing the demand for friction by keeping the feet nearly directly under the CoM.

During the second half of stance phase, the ground reaction force is directed *anteriorly,* with the foot applying a posteriorly directed force to the ground to propel the body forward. The magnitude of the propulsive force depends on walking speed and, especially, attempts to accelerate. Inadequate friction between the foot and the ground at this time often causes the foot to slide backward without propelling the body forward. This explains the difficulty experienced when one accelerates quickly while walking on a slippery surface.

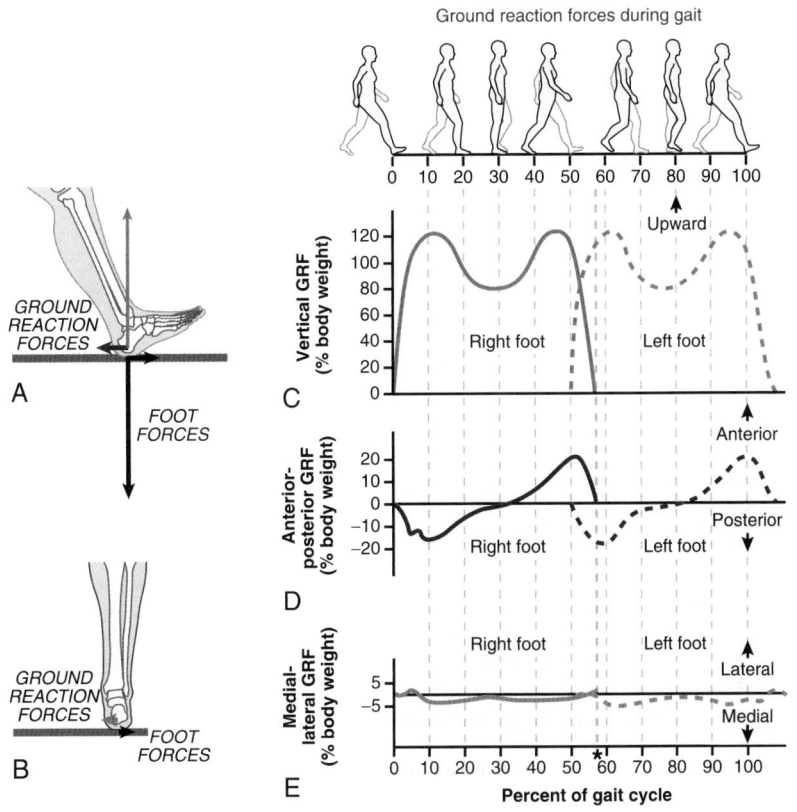

FIGURE 15.31 Ground reaction forces (GRFs) during gait (also see Videos 15.5 and 15.6). (A) illustrates the vertical *(orange arrows)* and anterior-posterior GRFs *(red arrows)* and foot forces *(black arrows)* at 10% of gait cycle. (B) illustrates the medial-lateral forces at 10% of gait cycle. (C–E) show the GRFs for a gait cycle. Dashed lines are data for the stance phase on the left foot.

* Toe off is at 57%

The peak anterior-posterior ground reaction force is typically equal to about 20% of body weight. These shear forces are in large part the result of the CoM of the body being either posterior (at heel contact) or anterior (second half of stance) to the foot. The larger the step length, the greater the shear forces because of the greater angle between the lower extremity and the floor. Inertial properties of the body, such as momentum, also contribute to anterior-posterior ground reaction forces.

The posteriorly directed ground reaction force at heel contact momentarily slows the forward progression of the body. Conversely, the body is momentarily accelerated forward at toe off as a result of an anteriorly directed ground reaction force. Note that the propulsive force of one lower extremity is applied simultaneously with the braking force of the opposite lower extremity during the times of double-limb support (see Fig. 15.31D). When one walks at a constant velocity, the propulsive force occurring late in stance balances the braking force occurring early in stance. Because these forces are of relatively equal magnitude but of opposite direction, they provide balance to the body when the weight is transferred from one lower extremity to the other at the time of double-limb support. Slowing down requires a greater braking force than propulsive force, and speeding up requires the opposite.

MEDIAL-LATERAL FORCES

The magnitude of the ground reaction force in the medial-lateral direction is relatively small (i.e., less than 5% of body weight) and more variable across individuals (see Fig. 15.31B,E and Video 15.6). As with anterior-posterior shear force, the magnitude and direction of this shear force depends mostly on the relationship between the position of the body's CoM and the location of the foot.[188] During the initial 5% or so of the gait cycle, a small, laterally directed ground reaction shear force is produced to stop the small lateral-to-medial velocity of the foot that is typically present at the time of heel contact. During the rest of stance phase, however, the CoM of the body is located medial to the foot (see Fig. 15.24), causing a laterally directed force to be applied to the ground by the foot and therefore a medially directed ground reaction force. These medially directed ground reaction forces throughout stance phase initially decelerate the lateral movement of the CoM. Then, these ground reaction forces accelerate the CoM medially toward the contralateral lower extremity, which is swinging forward and preparing to make the next foot contact with the ground.

Although the action of the medial-lateral ground reaction forces may not be easily felt during normal gait, they can be readily felt during walking while taking very large steps or when jumping from side to side. In fact, greater peak values in medial-lateral ground reaction forces are often seen in individuals with wider step widths. The need for friction can again be appreciated by observing someone walking on ice. Individuals walking on icy surfaces reduce their step widths almost as if they were walking on a tightrope. This learned adaptation is intended to keep the body's CoM directly over the feet to minimize the medial-lateral ground reaction forces and therefore the need for friction. Ice skaters make use of these medial-lateral ground reaction forces to propel their bodies forward. This is achieved by using a blade that digs into the ice, providing an adequate resistance for propulsion.

Path of the Center of Pressure

The path of the center of pressure (CoP) under the foot throughout stance follows a relatively reproducible pattern (Fig. 15.32). (The term *pressure* is used to describe the ground reaction force related to its specific area of application.) At heel contact, the CoP is located just lateral to the midpoint of the heel. It then moves progressively to the lateral midfoot region at mid stance, and to the medial forefoot region (under the first or second metatarsal head) during heel off to toe off. The location of the CoP helps to explain the tendency for the ankle and foot to plantar flex and evert, respectively, at heel contact (Fig. 15.33). Both tendencies are partially controlled by eccentric activation of ankle muscles, namely the ankle dorsiflexors, including the tibialis anterior.

Path of the center of pressure on the plantar surface of the foot

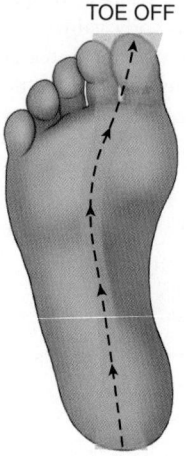

TOE OFF

HEEL CONTACT

FIGURE 15.32 Path of the center of pressure (CoP) under the foot from heel contact to toe off. The shaded area is representative of individual variability of the path of the CoP.

Torques generated by ground reaction forces at heel contact

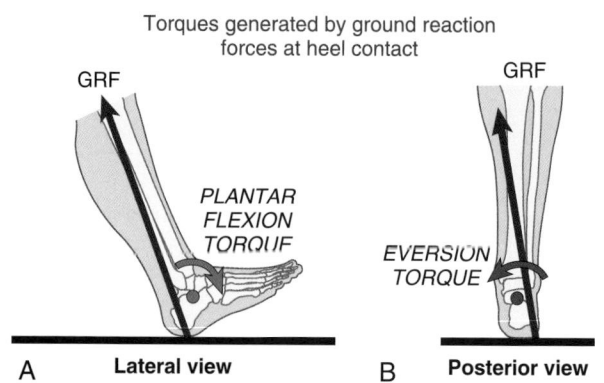

FIGURE 15.33 At heel contact, the point and direction of application of the ground reaction force *(GRF)* on the calcaneus falls posterior to the axis of rotation of the talocrural joint *(green circle)*, thereby creating a plantar flexion torque at the ankle (A). This external torque requires the generation of an opposing dorsiflexion internal torque by the ankle dorsiflexors. In (B), the lateral location of the ground reaction force on the calcaneus (relative to its near midpoint depicted as a purple circle) produces an eversion torque at the subtalar joint. This tendency is partially controlled by action of the tibialis anterior.

Joint Torques and Powers

When walking, the ground reaction forces applied under the foot generate an *external torque* on the joints of the lower extremities. This fact is illustrated in Fig. 15.34. During the loading response on the right limb, the line of action of the ground reaction force is located behind the ankle and knee but anterior to the hip. As a consequence, the ground reaction forces at heel contact produce ankle plantar flexion, knee flexion, and hip flexion. To prevent collapse of the lower extremity, these external torques are resisted by *internal torques* created by the activation of the ankle dorsiflexors, the knee extensors, and the hip extensors.

A simplified analysis of the magnitude of the internal (muscular) torques, as could be derived from a body diagram similar to Fig. 15.34, assumes a condition of static equilibrium. A more accurate calculation, however, requires the use of the inverse dynamics approach, which considers the dynamic nature of the action.[11] This approach requires the knowledge of the anthropometric characteristics of the individual's segment masses, location of the segments' CoM, segments' mass center inertia matrix, precise magnitude of body position and motion (each segment's linear and angular velocity), and ground reaction forces during the gait cycle (review Fig. 15.5). In this chapter, much of the data on internal torques during walking are based on the inverse dynamics approach.

As stated previously, the activation of muscles creates most of the internal torques that control joint motion, especially in midrange positions. This internal torque is associated with concentric muscle activation when the joint moves in the direction of the muscle's action; in contrast, internal torque is associated with eccentric muscle activation when the joint moves in the direction opposite the muscle's action. In either case, the magnitude of the internal torque reasonably matches the description of muscular activation provided earlier in this chapter.

Internal torques can also be created by passive forces generated by the deformation and recoil of connective tissues, such as the capsule, tendons, and ligaments.[112] It is not always possible to state with certainty the relative contribution of active and passive forces to the prevailing internal torque across a joint. In some cases, however, such as in the middle of the range of motion, it may be a fairly simple deductive process to identify the structures responsible (likely active muscles), but in other cases, such as near the end of the range of motion, contributions of both active and passive structures

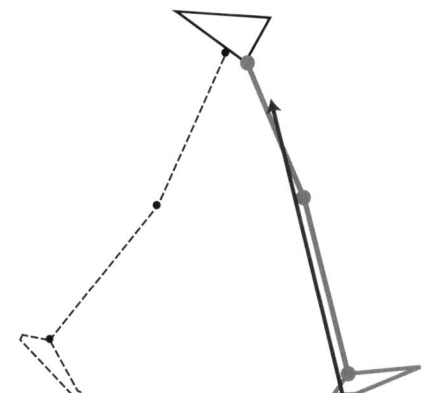

FIGURE 15.34 During the early part of stance the line of action of the ground reaction forces (posterior to the ankle, posterior to the knee, and anterior to the hip) promotes ankle plantar flexion, knee flexion, and hip flexion. (Modified from Whittle M: *Gait analysis: an introduction,* ed 4, Oxford, 2007, Butterworth-Heinemann.)

may need to be considered.[112,252] Many gait deviations associated with muscle weakness rely heavily on passive tensions created at the end range of a joint's position for the internal torques required for walking.

The literature often uses the term *net* internal joint torque in attempts to account for coactivation of agonist-antagonist muscle groups. For example, the flexion torque produced by the hip flexor muscles during the swing phase may be associated with slight (eccentric) activation of muscles that extend the hip. In theory, this extensor torque subtracts from the hip flexion torque, thereby yielding a net flexion torque. Although during walking this antagonistic torque is likely small, it is something to consider, especially in pathology such as stroke or Parkinson's disease. This chapter does not consistently use the modifying term *net,* although it is implied.

The concept of internal torque provides valuable insight into the role of particular muscles and connective tissues in controlling a joint during walking. Internal torque does not, however, describe the *rate* of work performed by the muscles or passive deformation of connective tissues; this requires knowledge of *power.* Joint power is the product of the net internal joint torque and the joint angular velocity. Joint power reflects the net rate of generating or absorbing energy by all muscles and other connective tissues crossing a joint. A positive value indicates power *generation,* which reflects concentric muscle activation and a release of energy from previously stretched connective tissues. A negative value, in contrast, indicates power *absorption,* which reflects eccentric muscle activation and the stretching of passive connective tissues.[252] The concept of power generation and absorption may be better understood with the example of performing a jump. During the initial squatting movement preceding a jump, most muscles of the lower extremities work eccentrically, absorbing energy. The reversal of movement direction is achieved by concentric muscle activation and release of energy from stretched connective tissues during the upward movement of the body. Application of this concept in the field of strength building is known as *plyometric training.*

It must be reemphasized that power generation and absorption are based on the *product* of angular velocity and internal torque. Consider, for example, that even a large internal torque may create only a small amount of power if the angular velocity is very low. Alternatively, the same torque creates a very large power if the angular velocity is large. This concept is important to consider when interpreting the data provided in Figs. 15.35, 15.36, 15.38, and 15.42.[256]

The following sections highlight the primary torques and powers generated during walking. These sections also provide figures that summarize the kinematics and kinetics of the hip, knee, and ankle in the sagittal plane, and the hip in the frontal plane. Careful study of these figures should provide an increased understanding of the relationships among joint motion, torque, power, and muscle activation during walking. There is overall strong agreement in the literature on the pattern and magnitude of the torque and power data in the sagittal plane during walking. But as with the kinematic data, as torque and power are partially derived from the kinematic data, there is more variation in the literature for frontal and especially horizontal plane torque and power data.[68,80,144,206]

Analysis of joint torques and powers gives a more complete picture of the biomechanics of walking.[57,252] These variables help establish the relative contribution of various joints and muscle groups to provide support and propulsion of the body.[31,130] The understanding of pathologic gait benefits from this type of information.

HIP

In the early part of stance phase, in the *sagittal plane,* the hip musculature generates a hip extension torque that serves to accept the weight of the body, control the forward momentum of the trunk, and extend the hip (Fig. 15.35A,B and Video 15.7). In the second half of stance, a flexion torque is generated to initially decelerate hip extension and then initiate hip flexion before toe off. This hip flexion torque is the result of a combination of passive forces from structures anterior to the hip joint, including the joint capsule, and activation of the hip flexors.[252] In early swing, a small hip flexion torque, corresponding to the concentric activation of the hip flexors, further assists hip flexion. In the second half of swing (at about 80% of the gait cycle), an extensor torque is needed to initially decelerate the movement of hip flexion, and then initiate hip extension.

Fig. 15.35C shows the power curve for the hip in the sagittal plane. In the first 35% of the gait cycle, power is generated to support the body, raise the CoM, control the trunk, and propel the body forward.[256] Power is then absorbed until approximately 50% of the gait cycle is reached, reflecting the deceleration of hip extension secondary to resistance provided by the anterior hip structures and the eccentric activation of the hip flexors. In late stance and early swing, power is generated to flex the hip.[252] A small amount of energy fluctuation takes place during the second half of swing, reflecting the combination of change in hip angular velocity and torque needed to first decelerate hip flexion then to initiate hip extension.

To complete the description of sagittal plane hip movement during gait, Fig. 15.35D illustrates the relative intensity and type of muscle activation of two primary antagonistic muscles of the hip. The areas of the EMG curve are coded to represent the muscles' presumed eccentric activation (shaded area) and concentric activation (hatched area) based on the direction of hip angular motion. In general, muscular activations correlate with power absorption (eccentric action) and power generation (concentric action).

In the *frontal plane,* a large abduction torque occurs throughout the stance phase to support the mass of the body that is located medial to the hip joint (Fig. 15.36A,B and Video 15.8). Power absorption occurs in the early part of stance (see Fig. 15.36C) as the opposite side of the pelvis is initially lowered (see Fig. 15.36A). These kinematics are controlled through eccentric activation of the hip abductors (see Fig. 15.36D). Two bursts of power generation are seen at approximately 20% and 50% of the gait cycle, as the contralateral pelvis is raised (see Fig. 15.36C).

In the *horizontal plane,* an external rotation torque is used to decelerate the internal rotation of the femur in the first 20% of the gait cycle (see Fig. 15.37A). This torque is followed by an internal rotation torque that advances the contralateral side of the pelvis forward during the remainder of stance. Note the small magnitude of these torques, approximately 15% of those in the sagittal and frontal planes. The eccentric activation of the hip external rotators in the initial 20% of the gait cycle accounts for the power absorption noted at that time in Fig. 15.37B. However, as stated earlier, variability exists in the reporting of these horizontal plane data for the hip, partially attributed to their smaller magnitude, the difficulties in making accurate kinematic measurements in the horizontal plane, and various methods of data processing.[205,206]

KNEE

In the *sagittal plane,* at heel contact, a very brief and early (within first 4% of the gait cycle) knee flexion torque presumably ensures

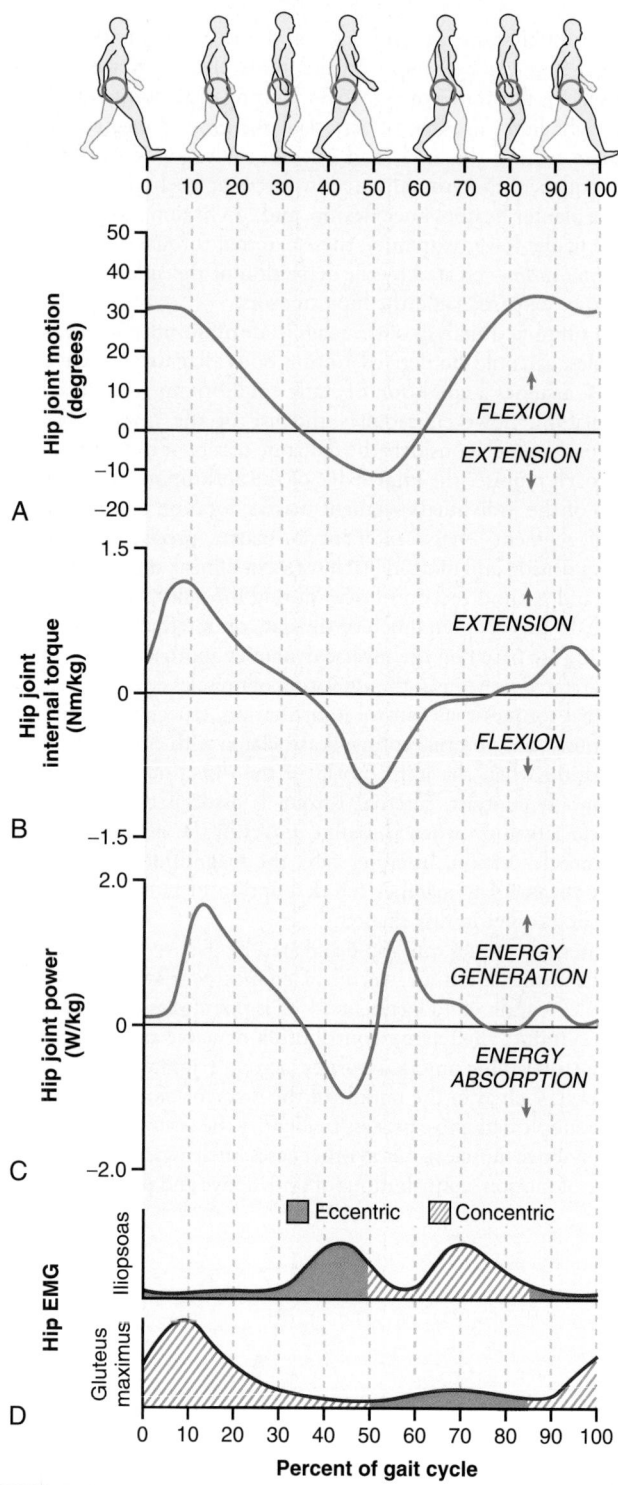

FIGURE 15.35 Sagittal plane hip motion (A), internal torques (B), powers (C), and electromyographic signal (D) for a gait cycle (also see Video 15.7). The electromyographic curves represent the relative intensity of the muscle activation during the gait cycle. (Torque and power data normalized to body mass from Winter and colleagues, 1996;[256] and electromyographic data from Winter, 1991,[257] and Bechtol, 1975.[19]) As in Fig. 15.29, note that electromyographic signal amplitude is illustrated so that its maximum value during the gait cycle fills the vertical dimension of the graphs. The signal is therefore normalized to the maximum value obtained during the gait cycle, not to its maximum capability to generate force.

Hip kinematics and kinetics (frontal plane)

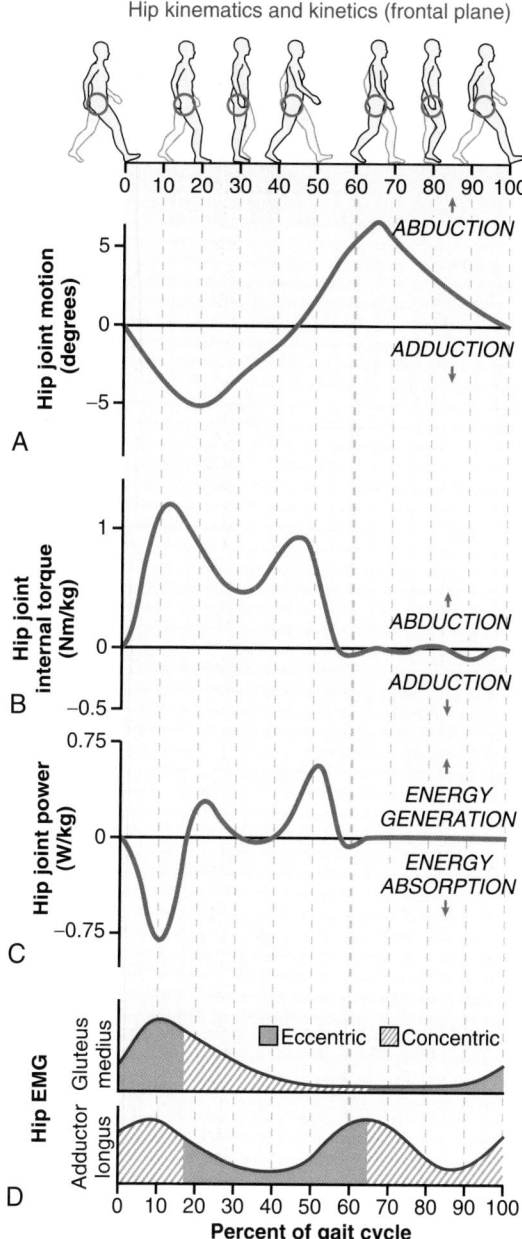

FIGURE 15.36 Frontal plane hip motion (A), internal torques (B), powers (C), and electromyographic signal (D) for a gait cycle (also see Video 15.8). The electromyographic curves represent the relative intensity of the muscle activation during the gait cycle. (Torque and power data normalized to body mass from Winter and colleagues, 1996,[256] and electromyographic data from Winter, 1991.[257]) See legend in Fig. 15.35 for additional comments on the normalization of the electromyographic data. *EMG,* electromyography.

Hip kinetics (horizontal plane)

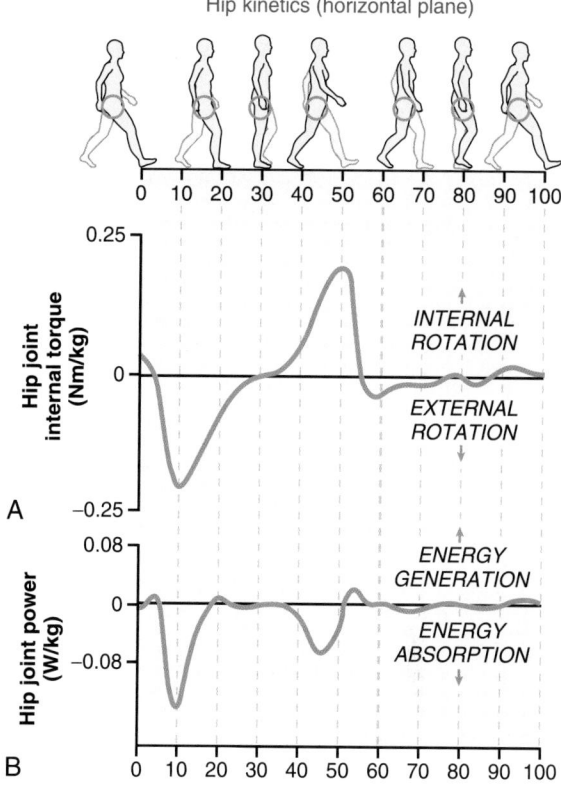

FIGURE 15.37 Horizontal plane internal torques (A) and powers (B) for the hip. (Data normalized to body mass from Winter DA, Eng JJ, Ishac M: Three-dimensional moments, powers and work in normal gait: implications for clinical assessments. In Harris GF, Smith PA, editors: *Human motion analysis: current applications and future directions,* New York, 1996, IEEE Press.)

phase, starts at 40% of the gait cycle, which matches the direction of the internal flexion torque at the knee at 40% to 50% of the gait cycle. Just before toe off, however, a small internal extension torque occurs to control knee flexion. In late swing, an internal flexion torque is generated to decelerate knee extension.

The power curve for the sagittal plane reflects the action of the musculature surrounding the knee (Fig. 15.38C,D). The short-duration power generation at early stance shows that the knee flexion torque creates flexion of the knee. Then power absorption momentarily takes place, reflecting the eccentric action of the quadriceps at 5% to 15% of the gait cycle. This is followed by another brief instant of power generation, indicating the start of knee extension produced by the continued knee extension torque. Just before toe off, at 50% to 60% of the gait cycle, power is absorbed by the knee extensors to control knee flexion. In the second half of the swing phase, the hamstrings absorb energy as the swing limb is decelerated (see Fig. 15.38C,D), until initiating knee flexion just before the next heel contact.

In the *frontal plane* (Fig. 15.39A), during stance, with the exclusion of heel contact when a brief external abduction torque occurs (Video 15.8), an internal abduction torque at the knee counters the external adduction (varus) torque created by the resultant ground reaction force passing medial to the knee (Fig. 15.40, Video 15.9).[2,174] The internal abduction torque is created by a combination of active and passive structures, including the vasti, gastrocnemius, lateral hamstrings, and potentially the tensor fascia latae and the posterolateral ligaments of the knee.[174] Despite the large torques (see Fig. 15.39A), power values in this plane are very low because of

that the knee is flexed to provide an adequate knee alignment for shock absorption (Fig. 15.38A,B and Video 15.7). A large extension torque needed for the loading response quickly follows this brief flexion torque. This extensor torque continues until 20% of gait has been reached, initially to control knee flexion, then to extend the knee. From 20% to 50% of the gait cycle, an internal flexion torque is present at the knee despite the knee extending at 20% to 40% of the gait cycle. Because little activity of the hamstrings is present at that time, the internal flexion torque likely results from passive tension in the posterior knee structures, including the capsule, that are being elongated. Knee flexion, in preparation for the swing

Knee kinematics and kinetics (sagittal plane)

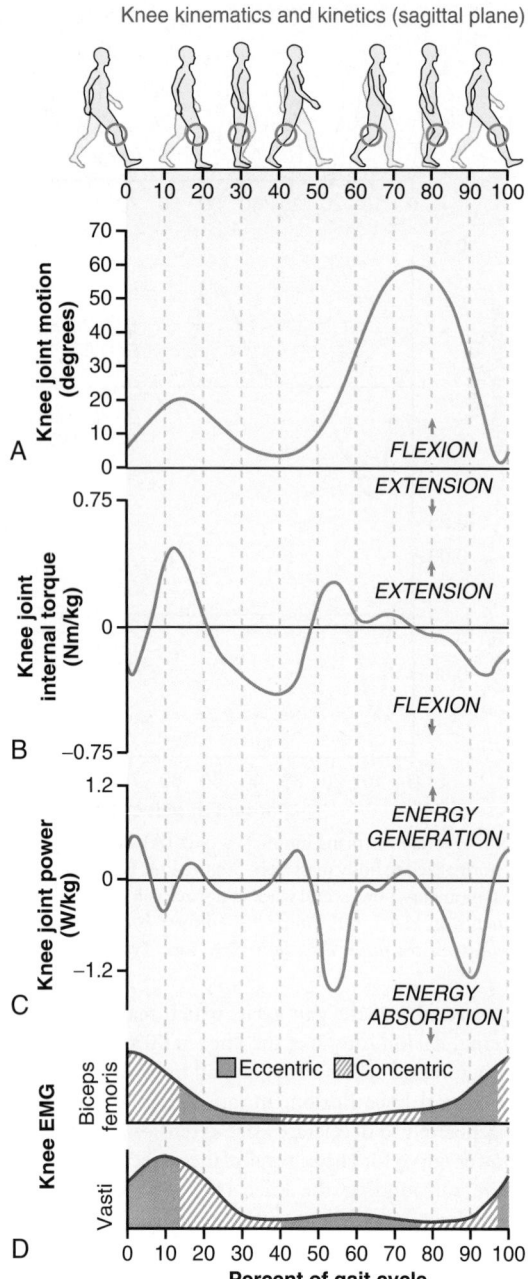

FIGURE 15.38 Sagittal plane knee motion (A), internal torques (B), powers (C), and electromyographic signal (D) for a gait cycle (also see Video 15.7). The electromyographic curves represent the relative intensity of the muscle activation during the gait cycle. (Torque and power data normalized to body mass from Winter and colleagues, 1996,[256] and electromyographic data from Winter, 1991.[257]) See legend in Fig. 15.35 for additional comments on normalization of the electromyographic data. *EMG,* electromyography.

the very small amount of knee movement and hence low angular velocity during stance (see Fig. 15.39B). Nevertheless, the pattern of initial energy generation followed by energy absorption suggests a small movement of knee abduction (valgus) initially followed by a small amount of knee adduction (varus).

In the *horizontal plane,* the joint torques at the knee are similar to those at the hip, with an external rotation torque in the first half of stance and an internal rotation torque in the second half (Fig. 15.41A). These torques are likely passive, being generated by knee ligaments in response to the active hip torques created in the horizontal plane.[66]

Knee kinetics (frontal plane)

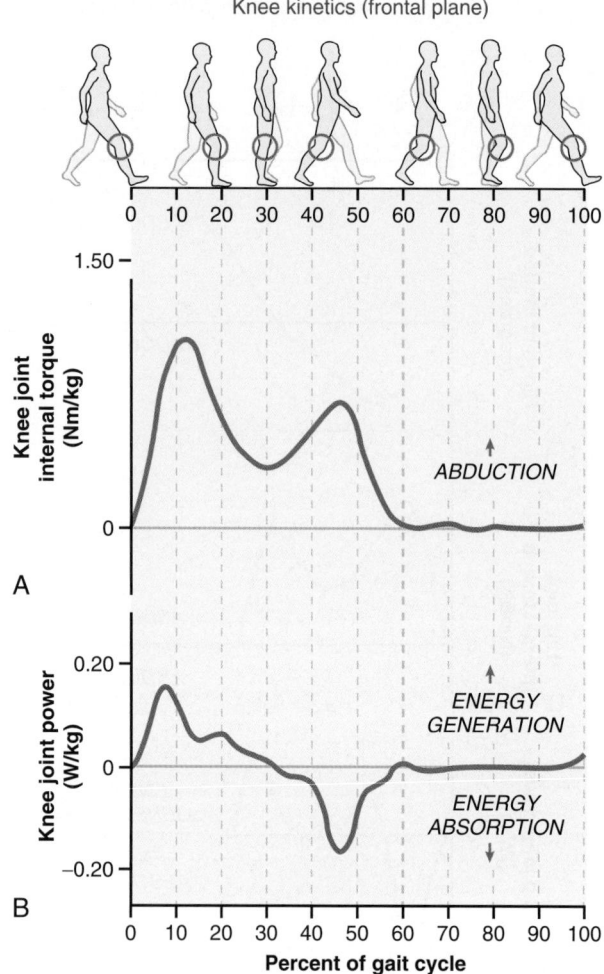

FIGURE 15.39 Frontal plane internal torques (A) and powers (B) for the knee. (Data normalized to body mass from Winter DA, Eng JJ, Ishac M: Three-dimensional moments, powers and work in normal gait: implications for clinical assessments. In Harris GF, Smith PA, editors: *Human motion analysis: current applications and future directions,* New York, 1996, IEEE Press.)

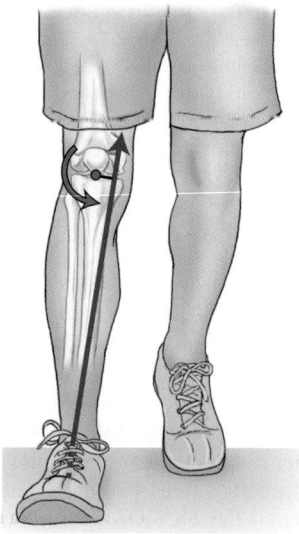

FIGURE 15.40 Throughout most of the stance phase, the ground reaction forces (red arrow) create a varus torque at the knee (also see Video 15.9).

Knee kinetics (horizontal plane)

Ankle kinematics and kinetics (sagittal plane)

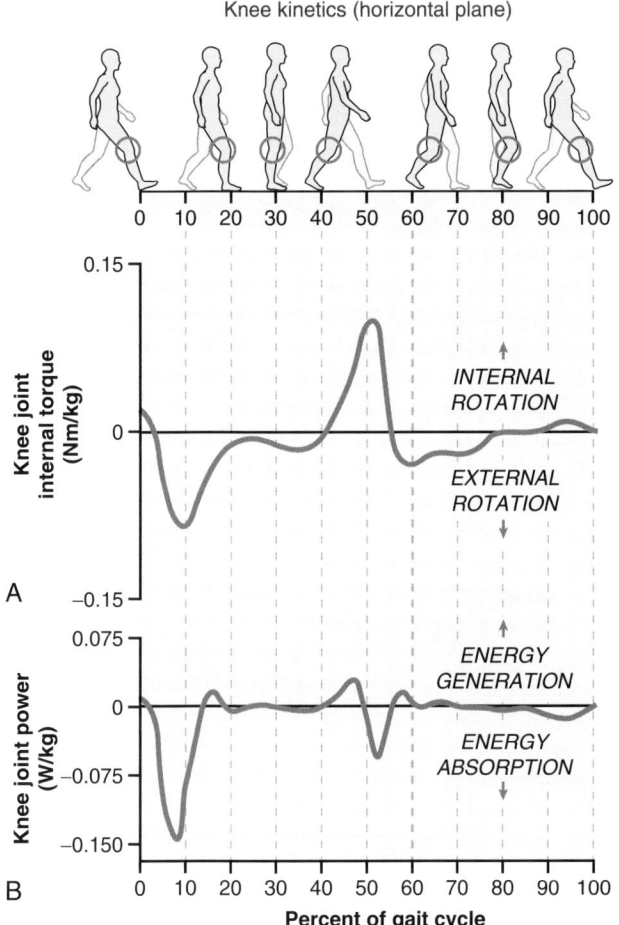

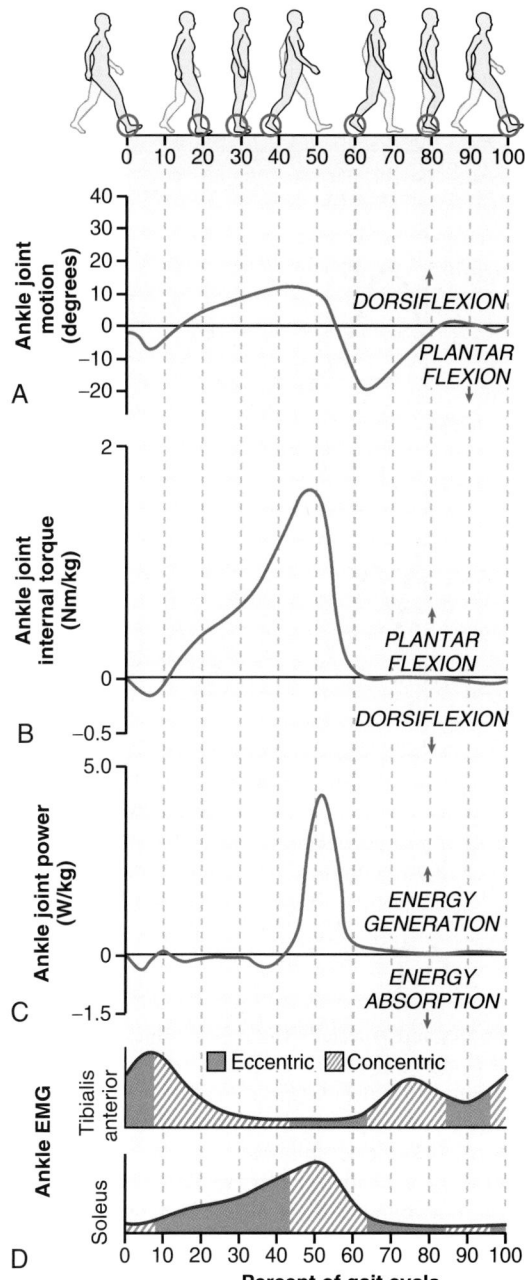

FIGURE 15.41 Horizontal plane internal torques (A) and powers (B) for the knee. (Data normalized to body mass from Winter DA, Eng JJ, Ishac M: Three-dimensional moments, powers and work in normal gait: implications for clinical assessments. In Harris GF, Smith PA, editors: *Human motion analysis: current applications and future directions,* New York, 1996, IEEE Press.)

During loading response, a small amount of power is absorbed as the knee's capsular and ligamentous structures resist the internal rotation motion of the femur on the tibia (or external rotation of the knee) (see Fig. 15.41B). Again, these torque and power values are of small magnitude in contrast to those in the sagittal and frontal planes.

ANKLE-AND-FOOT

In the *sagittal plane,* a small dorsiflexion torque is generated at the ankle immediately after heel contact (Fig. 15.42A,B and Video 15.7). This torque serves to control the movement of plantar flexion generated by the application of body weight on the calcaneus (review Fig. 15.33). A plantar flexion torque prevails throughout the rest of stance, initially to control the tibia advancing over the foot, and then to plantar flex the ankle at push off. A very small dorsiflexion torque is present during swing to keep the ankle dorsiflexed to clear the toes from the ground.

In the sagittal plane, power is absorbed just after heel contact as a result of the muscular deceleration of ankle plantar flexion (see Fig. 15.42C). Then some energy absorption occurs until push off, reflecting the eccentric activation of the plantar flexors at 10% to 40% of the gait cycle (see Fig. 15.42D), as the tibia is slowly advanced over the foot. The relatively slow ankle angular displacement (and assumed velocity) at 10% to 40% of the gait cycle explains the small power values (see Fig. 15.42C). A large generation of energy occurs

FIGURE 15.42 Sagittal plane ankle motion (A), internal torques (B), powers (C), and electromyographic signal (D) for a gait cycle (also see Video 15.7). The electromyographic curves represent the relative intensity of the muscle activation during the gait cycle. (Torque and power data normalized to body mass from Winter and colleagues, 1996,[256] and electromyographic data from Winter, 1991.[257]) See legend in Fig. 15.35 for additional comments on normalization of the electromyographic data. *EMG,* electromyography.

at push off (from 40% to 60% of the gait cycle) primarily as a result of a concentric action of the ankle plantar flexors, but with some contribution (approximately 10%–15% of the power burst) from a return of the energy absorbed through stretching of the ankle plantar flexors before heel off. This power generation noted at push off is considered the primary contributor to the forward propulsion of the body during normal gait.[31,104,190] Although debated, part of this forward propulsion may also be generated by the hip extensors, despite their relatively low-level activation (EMG) during the second half of stance phase.[65]

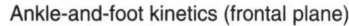

Ankle-and-foot kinetics (frontal plane)

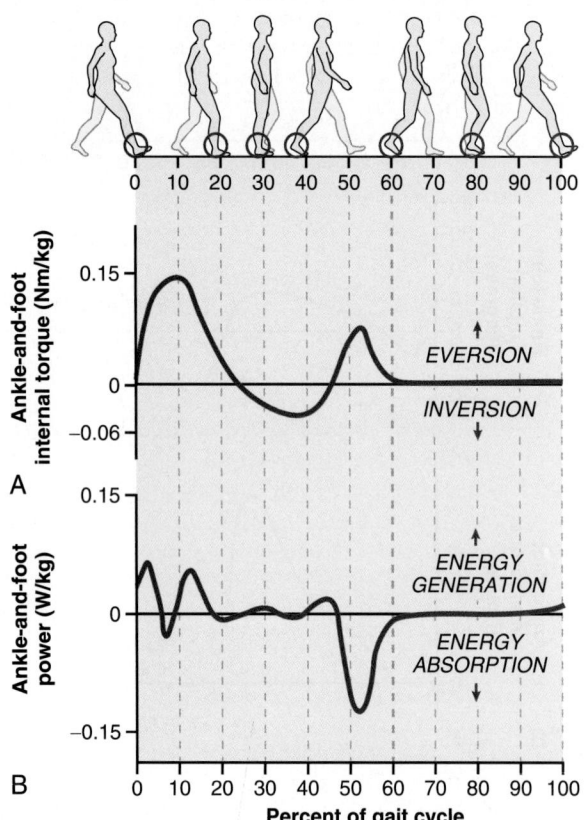

FIGURE 15.43 Frontal plane internal torques (A) and powers (B) for the ankle-and-foot. (Data normalized to body mass from Winter DA, Eng JJ, Ishac M: Three-dimensional moments, powers, and work in normal gait: implications for clinical assessments. In Harris GF, Smith PA, editors: *Human motion analysis: current applications and future directions,* New York, 1996, IEEE Press.)

The torques and especially the power values in the *frontal* and *horizontal planes* at the ankle-and-foot are very small and exhibit large variation among people (Figs. 15.43 and 15.44). In the frontal plane, stance phase is characterized by a small initial eversion torque (from 0% to 20% of gait) followed by an inversion torque (from 20% to 45% of gait) and a smaller eversion torque just before toe off.[256] In the horizontal plane, an external rotation torque is present during the stance phase. This external rotation torque should in fact be called an *abduction torque* based on the description of ankle and foot movements provided in Chapter 14.

Joint and Tendon Forces

Joint surfaces, ligaments, and tendons are all subjected to large compressive, tensile, or shear forces during walking.[109,126,204,231] Knowledge of the magnitude of these forces is of interest, especially to the clinician, orthopedic surgeon, and bioengineer.[55,74,118,219] The design of surgical joint implants, in particular, requires these types of data. Direct measurements in men and women are obviously not readily obtainable except through instrumented joint implants;[7,52] therefore these forces are typically calculated indirectly through biomechanical analysis including modeling and optimization techniques.[13,153]

Forces applied to various structures of the lower extremities during ambulation are presented in e-Table 15.2. These forces can be surprisingly large. Consider, for example, that the compressive force at the hip when walking at 1.4 m/sec has been measured to be 3 to as high as 6.4 times body weight.[4,214,251] It is of interest to

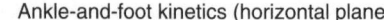

Ankle-and-foot kinetics (horizontal plane)

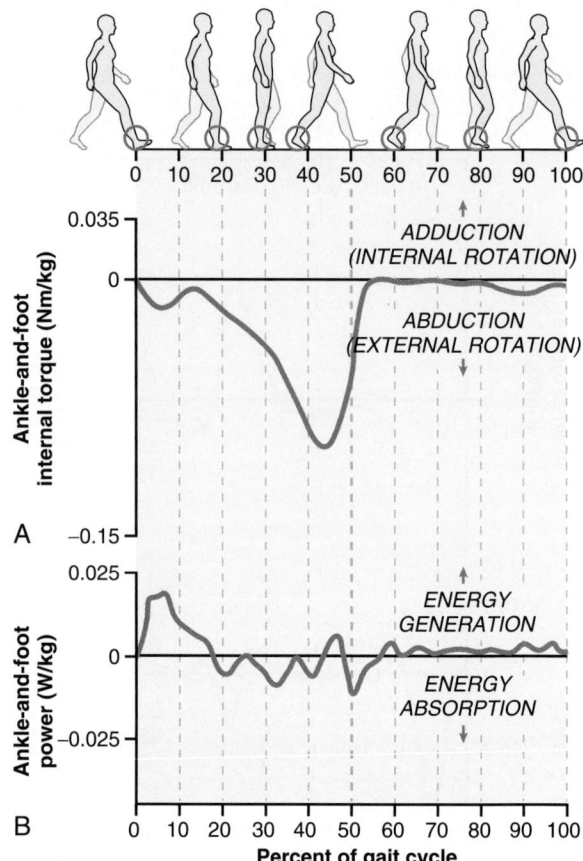

FIGURE 15.44 Horizontal plane internal torques (A) and powers (B) for the ankle-and-foot. (Data normalized to body mass from Winter DA, Eng JJ, Ishac M: Three-dimensional moments, powers, and work in normal gait: implications for clinical assessments. In Harris GF, Smith PA, editors: *Human motion analysis: current applications and future directions,* New York, 1996, IEEE Press.)

consider once more (see the discussion of hip joint compressive forces in Chapter 12) that muscle actions, from both those crossing and those not crossing the joint, and not body mass, are the largest contributors to lower extremity joint compressive forces when walking.[49,217] Therefore effective strategies to reduce these muscular actions, for example the use of a cane in the contralateral hand or reducing walking velocity, can potentially be key to alleviate forces to a painful hip joint associated with advanced osteoarthritic changes. Similarly, due consideration of how these forces are affected in the presence of pathologic gait is warranted in the planning of prevention and/or intervention strategies.[38,72,222]

GAIT DYSFUNCTIONS

Most of us take for granted our ability to walk. The fact is, unless we have personally experienced an injury or a physical impairment, we do not think of walking as a difficult task. The information provided thus far in this chapter, however, reminds us of the complexity of walking. Many actions must occur simultaneously at each part of the gait cycle for walking to take place with maximum efficiency.

Normal walking requires sufficient range of motion and strength at each participating joint. Walking also requires sophisticated control of movement through the central nervous system. The complexity of walking creates many opportunities for the normal gait pattern to be affected by impairment. The adaptability of the system, however, creates many opportunities to modify the gait pattern to preserve "walking," despite even severe impairments. In these cases, a normal gait pattern is sacrificed for the ability to move from one location to another independently. We have all used this ability to adapt how we walk, even if only for a painful blister under the foot or for walking on hot sand at the beach. In essence, an abnormal or a pathologic gait pattern reflects an effort to preserve walking through adaptation.[14] Typically, a deviation in one's normal gait comes at the expense of increased energy expenditure and greater physical stresses applied to the body.

Three common causes of pathologic gait patterns are listed in the box. Each includes specific and general pathologies. The observed deviations may be the direct reflection of the specific impairment, or they may be a biomechanical compensation for some aspect of the impairment. The features of pathologic gait therefore depend on the nature of the impairment as well as the ability of the individual to compensate for that impairment.

Causes of Pathologic Gait Patterns
- Pain
- Central nervous system disorders
- Musculoskeletal and peripheral nervous system impairments

Pain can cause an abnormal gait pattern that is often referred to as an *antalgic gait*. The pattern of weight avoidance on the painful limb often leads to characteristic features. The primary findings are a shorter step length, in conjunction with decreased stance time on the painful side. If the pain is related to hip joint compression from hip abductor muscle activation, lateral displacement of the head and trunk toward the painful weight-bearing lower extremity occurs (see Chapter 12). If the source of pain is other than the hip, the trunk may lean slightly toward the swing limb in an attempt to alleviate weight bearing on the injured stance limb.

Many neurologic disorders, such as cerebrovascular accidents (CVAs), Parkinson's disease, and cerebral palsy, can cause abnormal gait patterns.[227] Spasticity of muscles, defined as increased tone and resistance to stretch, results in inappropriate muscle activity and increased stiffness. It often affects the extensor musculature of individuals with cerebral palsy and CVA, resulting in a gait pattern that appears stiff-legged, accompanied by a tendency to circumduct and scuff the toes. Hyperactive hip adductors may contribute to a scissoring gait pattern. Parkinson's disease is associated with a lack of arm swing, flexed trunk, and short accelerating steps, also called *festinating gait*. Cerebellar lesions are associated with an *ataxic gait* pattern characterized by unsteady uncoordinated steps and a wide base of support. Individuals with impaired sensory function and balance may show an unsteady gait pattern.[213] With neurologic disorders, the primary cause of gait dysfunction is an inability to generate and control appropriate levels of muscle force.

Deficits in the musculoskeletal and peripheral nervous system, such as excessive or limited joint range of motion and/or limited muscle strength, can cause a wide variety of gait deviations. Abnormal joint range of motion may occur secondary to injury, tightness, or contracture of connective tissues and muscles; abnormal joint structure; joint instability; or congenital connective tissue laxity. In most cases, abnormal range of motion in one joint leads to some form of compensation in one or more surrounding joints.[14] Muscular weakness may result from disuse atrophy after an injury or a limited neural drive secondary to a peripheral neural injury. Whatever the cause, weakness ultimately leads to modification of the gait pattern. An interesting simulation study by van der Krogt and co-workers[239] attempted to study the adaptability of the locomotion system by measuring how robust human gait was to progressive weakness of a variety of muscle groups. Their work suggests that up to 40% overall muscle weakness in the lower limbs could be tolerated while still maintaining a relatively normal gait. When weakness was limited to single muscle groups, walking was found to be least tolerant to weakness of the ankle plantar flexors, hip abductors, and hip flexors. Conversely, and maybe surprisingly, walking was found to be quite robust (or functionally tolerant) to weakness of the hip and knee extensors. These findings, which apply to normal gait only, and not pathologic gait for which different strength requirements likely exist, could give implications for which muscle groups to target in rehabilitation.

Tables 15.6 through 15.11 and Figs. 15.45 through 15.50 present some of the more common gait deviations observed in the general population.

TABLE 15.6 Gait Deviations at the Ankle and Foot Secondary to Specific Ankle and Foot Impairments*

Observed Gait Deviation at the Ankle or Foot	Likely Impairment	Selected Pathologic Precursors	Mechanical Rationale and/or Associated Compensations
"Foot slap": rapid ankle plantar flexion occurs after **heel contact.**[†] The name *foot slap* is derived from the characteristic noise made by the forefoot hitting the ground.	Mild weakness of ankle dorsiflexors	Common fibular (peroneal) nerve palsy and distal peripheral neuropathy	Ankle dorsiflexors have sufficient strength to dorsiflex the ankle during swing but not enough to control ankle plantar flexion after heel contact. No other gait deviations.
"Foot flat": Entire plantar aspect of the foot touches the ground at **initial contact,**[‡] followed by normal, passive ankle dorsiflexion during the rest of stance.	Marked weakness of ankle dorsiflexors	Common fibular nerve palsy and distal peripheral neuropathy	Sufficient strength of the dorsiflexors to partially, but not completely, dorsiflex the ankle during swing. Normal dorsiflexion occurs during stance as long as the ankle has normal range of motion. No other gait deviations.
Initial contact with the ground is made by the forefoot followed by the heel region. Normal passive ankle dorsiflexion occurs during stance.	Severe weakness of ankle dorsiflexors	Common fibular nerve palsy and distal peripheral neuropathy	No active ankle dorsiflexion is possible during swing. Normal dorsiflexion occurs during stance as long as the ankle has normal range of motion. Likely requires excessive knee and hip flexion during swing to avoid catching the toes on the ground.

Continued

TABLE 15.6 Gait Deviations at the Ankle and Foot Secondary to Specific Ankle and Foot Impairments*—cont'd

Observed Gait Deviation at the Ankle or Foot	Likely Impairment	Selected Pathologic Precursors	Mechanical Rationale and/or Associated Compensations
Initial contact is made with the forefoot, but the heel never makes contact with the ground during stance.	Heel pain Plantar flexion contracture (pes equinus deformity) or spasticity of ankle plantar flexors	Calcaneal fracture, plantar fasciopathy Upper motor neuron lesion, cerebral palsy, cerebrovascular accident (CVA)	Purposeful strategy to avoid weight bearing on the heel. To maintain the weight over the forefoot, the knee and hip are kept in flexion throughout stance, leading to a "crouched gait." Requires short steps.
Initial contact is made with the forefoot, and the heel is brought to the ground by a posterior displacement of the tibia at midstance (see Fig. 15.45).	Plantar flexion contracture (pes equinus deformity) or spasticity of ankle plantar flexors	Upper motor neuron lesion (cerebral palsy, CVA) Ankle fusion in a plantar flexed position	Knee hyperextension occurs during stance owing to the inability of the tibia to move forward over the foot. Hip flexion and excessive forward trunk lean during terminal stance occur to shift the weight of the body over the foot.
Premature elevation of the heel in mid or terminal stance.	Lack of ankle dorsiflexion	Congenital or acquired muscular tightness of ankle plantar flexors	Characteristic bouncing gait pattern.
Heel remains in contact with the ground late in terminal stance.	Weakness or flaccid paralysis of plantar flexors with or without a fixed dorsiflexed position of the ankle (pes calcaneus deformity)	Peripheral or central nervous system disorders Excessive surgical lengthening of the Achilles tendon	Excessive ankle dorsiflexion results in prolonged heel contact, reduced push off, and a shorter step length.
Supinated foot position and weight bearing on the lateral aspect of the foot during stance.	Pes cavus deformity	Congenital structural deformity	A high medial longitudinal arch is noted with reduced midfoot mobility throughout swing and stance.
Excessive foot pronation occurs during stance, with failure of the foot to supinate in mid stance. Normal medial longitudinal arch noted during swing.	Rearfoot varus and/or forefoot varus	Congenital or acquired structural deformity	Excessive foot pronation and associated flattening of the medial longitudinal arch may be accompanied by a general internal rotation of the lower extremity during stance.
Excessive foot pronation with weight bearing on the medial portion of the foot during stance. The medial longitudinal arch remains absent during swing.	Weakness (paralysis) of ankle invertors Pes planus deformity	Upper motor neuron lesion Congenital structural deformity	An overall excessive internal rotation of the lower extremity during stance is possible.
Excessive inversion and plantar flexion of the foot and ankle occur during swing and at initial contact.	Pes equinovarus deformity caused by spasticity of the plantar flexors and invertors	Upper motor neuron lesion (cerebral palsy, CVA)	Contact with the ground is made with the lateral border of the forefoot. Weight bearing on the lateral border of the foot during stance.
Ankle remains plantar flexed during swing and can be associated with dragging of the toes, typically called *drop foot* (see Fig. 15.46).	Weakness of dorsiflexors and/or pes equinus deformity	Common fibular nerve palsy	Hip hiking, hip circumduction, or excessive hip flexion of the swing lower extremity or vaulting of the stance limb may be noted to lift the toes off the ground and prevent the toes from dragging during swing.

*Within this context, an impairment is a loss or an abnormality in physiologic or anatomic structure or function.

†The terms in boldface indicate when in the gait cycle the gait deviation is expressed.

‡*Initial contact* is often used instead of *heel contact* to reflect the fact that with many gait deviations the heel is not the section of the foot that makes initial contact with the ground. Accordingly, in this table, the terminology from Fig. 15.12 is used as it lends itself well to the description of gait deviations.

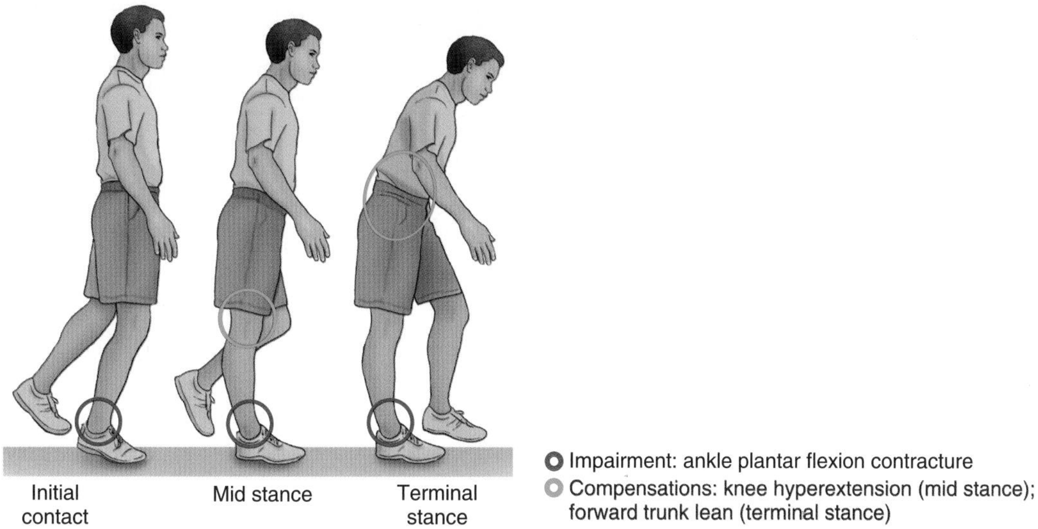

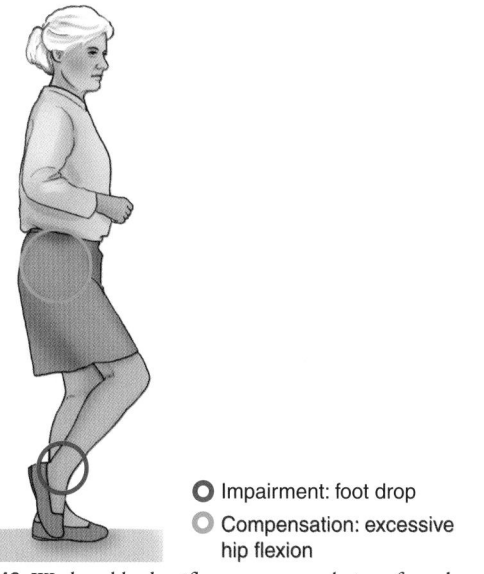

○ Impairment: ankle plantar flexion contracture
◐ Compensations: knee hyperextension (mid stance); forward trunk lean (terminal stance)

| Initial contact | Mid stance | Terminal stance |

FIGURE 15.45 Individuals with an ankle plantar flexion contracture will make initial contact with the ground with the forefoot region. At mid stance, bringing the heel to the ground will result in knee hyperextension.[173] Forward lean of the trunk occurs in terminal stance as a strategy to maintain forward progression of the center of mass.

○ Impairment: foot drop
◐ Compensation: excessive hip flexion

FIGURE 15.46 Weak ankle dorsiflexors may result in a foot drop during swing phase, requiring excessive hip flexion for the toes to clear the ground as the limb is advanced forward during swing.

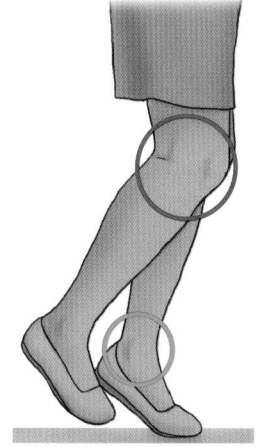

○ Impairment: reduced knee flexion
◐ Compensation: vaulting

FIGURE 15.47 Vaulting through excessive ankle plantar flexion of the unaffected stance limb is used to compensate for limited functional shortening of the affected swing limb.

TABLE 15.7 Gait Deviations Seen at the Ankle and Foot as a Compensation for an Impairment of the Ipsilateral Knee, Ipsilateral Hip, or Contralateral Lower Extremity

Observed Gait Deviation at the Ankle or Foot	Likely Impairment	Mechanical Rationale
Vaulting: compensatory mechanism demonstrated by exaggerated ankle plantar flexion during **mid stance**;* leads to excessive vertical movement of the body (see Fig. 15.47)	Any impairment of the contralateral lower extremity that reduces hip flexion, knee flexion, or ankle dorsiflexion during swing	Strategy used to allow the foot of a functionally long contralateral lower extremity to clear the ground during swing.
Excessive foot angle during **stance** that is called *toeing-out*	Femoral retroversion or tight hip external rotators	Foot is in excessive toeing-out because of excessive external rotation of the lower extremity.
Reduction of the normal foot angle during **stance** that is called *toeing-in*	Excessive femoral anteversion or spasticity of the hip adductors and/or hip internal rotators	General internal rotation of the lower extremity.

*Boldface terms indicate when in the gait cycle the gait deviation is expressed. In this table, the terminology from Fig. 15.12 is used as it lends itself well to the description of gait deviations.

TABLE 15.8 Gait Deviations at the Knee Secondary to Specific Knee Impairments

Observed Gait Deviation at the Knee	Likely Impairment	Selected Pathologic Precursors	Mechanical Rationale and/or Associated Compensations
Rapid extension of the knee (knee extensor thrust) after **initial contact***	Spasticity of the quadriceps	Upper motor neuron lesion	Depending on the status of the posterior structures of the knee, may occur with or without knee hyperextension.
Knee remains extended during the **loading response,** but there is no extensor thrust	Weak quadriceps	Femoral nerve palsy, L³–L⁴ compression neuropathy	Knee remains fully extended throughout stance. An associated anterior trunk lean in the early part of stance moves the line of gravity of the trunk slightly anterior to the axis of rotation of the knee (see Fig. 15.48). This keeps the knee extended without action of the knee extensors. This gait deviation may lead to an excessive stretching of the posterior capsule of the knee and eventual knee hyperextension (genu recurvatum) during stance.
	Knee pain	Arthritis	Knee is kept in extension to reduce the need for quadriceps activity and associated compressive forces. It may be accompanied by an antalgic gait pattern characterized by a reduced stance time and shorter step length.
Genu recurvatum during **stance**	Knee extensor weakness	Poliomyelitis	Secondary to progressive stretching of the posterior capsule of the knee.
Varus thrust during **stance**	Laxity of the posterior and lateral ligamentous joint structures of the knee	Traumatic injury or progressive laxity	Rapid varus deviation of the knee during mid stance, typically accompanied by knee hyperextension.
Flexed position of the knee during **stance** (see Fig. 15.49) and lack of knee extension in **terminal swing**	Knee flexion contracture >10 degrees (genu flexum), hamstring overactivity (spasticity)	Upper motor neuron lesion	Associated increase in hip flexion and ankle dorsiflexion during stance.
	Knee pain and joint effusion	Trauma or arthritis	Knee is kept in flexion because this is the position of lowest intraarticular pressure.
Reduced or absent knee flexion during **swing**	Spasticity of knee extensors	Upper motor neuron lesion	Compensatory hip hiking and/or hip circumduction could be noted.
	Knee extension contracture	Immobilization or surgical fusion	

*The terms in boldface indicate when in the gait cycle the gait deviation is expressed. In this table, the terminology from Fig. 15.12 is used as it lends itself well to the description of gait deviations.

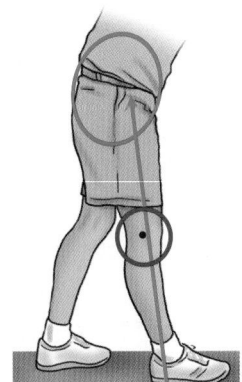

○ Impairment: weak quadriceps
○ Compensation: forward trunk lean

FIGURE 15.48 Weak quadriceps leading to anterior trunk lean to move the center of mass of the body anterior to the axis of rotation of the knee.

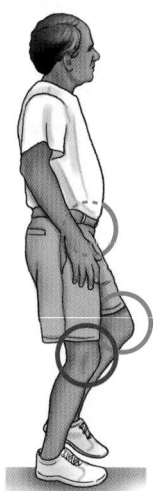

○ Impairment: knee flexion contracture
○ Compensations: exaggerated knee and hip flexion

FIGURE 15.49 Knee flexion contracture resulting in a crouched gait of the stance limb. To clear the toes during swing, the unaffected contralateral side must compensate with exaggerated knee and hip flexion.

TABLE 15.9 Gait Deviations Seen at the Knee as a Compensation for an Impairment of the Ipsilateral Ankle, Ipsilateral Hip, or Contralateral Lower Extremity

Observed Gait Deviation at the Knee	Likely Impairment	Mechanical Rationale
Knee is kept in flexion during **stance*** despite the knee having normal range of motion on examination	Impairments at the ankle or the hip including a pes calcaneus deformity, plantar flexor weakness, and hip flexion contracture	Exaggerated ankle dorsiflexion or hip flexion during stance forces the knee in a flexed position. The contralateral (healthy) swing limb shows exaggerated hip and knee flexion to clear the toes owing to the functionally shorter stance limb.
Hyperextension of the knee (genu recurvatum) from **initial contact to preswing**	Ankle plantar flexion contracture (pes equinus deformity) or spasticity of ankle plantar flexors	Knee must hyperextend to compensate for the lack of forward displacement of the tibia during mid stance (see Fig. 15.45).
Antalgic gait	Painful stance lower extremity	Characterized by a shorter step length and stance time on the side of the painful lower extremity; it may be accompanied by ipsilateral trunk lean with hip pain or a contralateral trunk lean with knee and foot pain.
Excessive knee flexion in **swing**	Lack of ankle dorsiflexion of the swing limb or a short stance limb	Strategy to increase toe clearance of the swing limb; is typically accompanied by increased hip flexion.

*The terms in boldface indicate when in the gait cycle the gait deviation is expressed. In this table, the terminology from Fig. 15.12 is used as it lends itself well to the description of gait deviations.

TABLE 15.10 Gait Deviations at the Hip, Pelvis, and Trunk Secondary to Specific Hip, Pelvis, or Trunk Impairments

Observed Gait Deviation at the Hip, Pelvis, or Trunk	Likely Impairment	Selected Pathologic Precursors	Mechanical Rationale and/or Associated Compensations
Backward trunk lean during **loading response.***	Weak hip extensors	Poliomyelitis	This action moves the line of gravity of the trunk behind the hip and reduces the need for hip extension torque.
Lateral trunk lean toward the **stance** lower extremity; because this movement compensates for a weakness, it is often called *compensated Trendelenburg gait* and is referred to as a *waddling gait* if bilateral.	Marked weakness of the hip abductors	Guillain-Barré or poliomyelitis	Shifting the trunk over the supporting limb reduces the demand on the hip abductors.
	Hip pain	Arthritis	Shifting the trunk over the supporting lower extremity reduces compressive joint forces associated with the action of hip abductors (see Fig. 15.16).
Excessive downward drop of the contralateral pelvis during **stance.** (Referred to as *positive Trendelenburg sign* if present during single-limb standing.)	Mild weakness of the gluteus medius of the stance limb	Guillain-Barré or poliomyelitis	Although the Trendelenburg sign may be seen in single-limb standing, a compensated Trendelenburg gait is often seen in severe weakness of the hip abductors.
Forward bending of the trunk during **mid** and **terminal stance,** as the hip is moved over the foot.	Hip flexion contracture	Hip osteoarthritis	Forward trunk lean is used to compensate for lack of hip extension. An alternative adaptation could be excessive lumbar lordosis.
	Hip pain	Hip osteoarthritis	Keeping the hip at 30 degrees of flexion minimizes intraarticular pressure.
Excessive lumbar lordosis in **terminal stance.**	Hip flexion contracture	Arthritis	Lack of hip extension in terminal stance is compensated for by increased lordosis.
Trunk lurches backward and toward the unaffected stance limb from **heel off** to **mid swing.**	Hip flexor weakness	L^2–L^3 nerve compression	Hip flexion is passively generated by a backward movement of the trunk.
Posterior tilt of the pelvis during **initial swing.**	Hip flexor weakness	L^2–L^3 nerve compression	Abdominals are used during initial swing to advance the swing lower extremity.
Hip circumduction: semicircle movement of the hip during **swing** (see Fig. 15.50).	Hip flexor weakness	L^2–L^3 nerve compression	Semicircle movement combining hip flexion, hip abduction, and forward rotation of the pelvis.

*The terms in boldface indicate when in the gait cycle the gait deviation is expressed. In this table, the terminology from Fig. 15.12 is used as it lends itself well to the description of gait deviations.

TABLE 15.11 **Gait Deviations Seen at the Hip, Pelvis, and Trunk as a Compensation for an Impairment of the Ipsilateral Ankle, Ipsilateral Knee, or Contralateral Lower Extremity**

Observed Gait Deviation at the Hip, Pelvis, or Trunk	Likely Impairment	Mechanical Rationale
Forward bending of the trunk during the **loading response***	Weak quadriceps	Trunk is brought forward to move the line of gravity anterior to the axis of rotation of the knee, thereby reducing the need for knee extensors (see Fig. 15.48).
Forward bending of the trunk during **mid** and **terminal stance**	Pes equinus deformity	Lack of ankle dorsiflexion during stance results in knee hyperextension at mid stance and forward trunk lean during terminal stance to move the weight of the body over the stance foot (see Fig. 15.45).
Excessive hip flexion during **swing** (see Fig. 15.46)	Often caused by lack of ankle dorsiflexion of the swing limb; may also be caused by a functionally or anatomically short contralateral stance lower extremity	Used to clear the toes of the swing limb
Hip circumduction during **swing** (see Fig. 15.50)	Lack of shortening of the swing limb secondary to reduced hip flexion, reduced knee flexion, and/or lack of ankle dorsiflexion	Used to lift the foot of the swing limb off the ground and provide toe clearance
Hip hiking (elevation of the ipsilateral pelvis during **swing**)	Lack of shortening of the swing limb secondary to reduced hip flexion, reduced knee flexion, and/or lack of ankle dorsiflexion Functionally or anatomically short stance limb	Used to lift the foot of the swing lower extremity off the ground and provide toe clearance.
Excessive backward horizontal rotation of the pelvis on the side of the stance lower extremity in **terminal stance**	Ankle plantar flexor weakness	Ankle plantar flexor weakness leads to prolonged heel contact and lack of push off. An increased pelvic horizontal rotation is used to lengthen the limb and maintain adequate step length.

*The terms in bold indicate when in the gait cycle the gait deviation is expressed. In this table, the terminology from Fig. 15.12 is used as it lends itself well to the description of gait deviations.

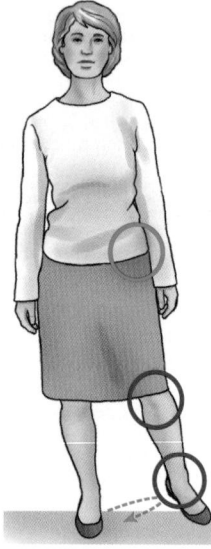
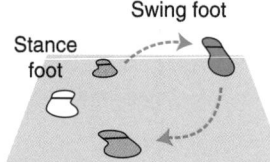

Swing foot

Stance foot

○ Impairment: reduced knee flexion and/or lack of ankle dorsiflexion

◯ Compensation: hip circumduction

FIGURE 15.50 Hip circumduction during swing is used to compensate for the inability to shorten the swing limb because of inadequate knee flexion or ankle dorsiflexion.

SYNOPSIS

Walking integrates the functions of all regions of the lower extremities. To fully understand the kinesiology of walking, the reader must consider the near simultaneous and relatively rapid musculoskeletal interactions that occur among multiple joints and planes, across both lower limbs and, to some extent, the trunk and upper extremities. In addition, the internal and external forces that act on each lower limb must be considered, both when the limb is freely moving (swing phase) and when it is fixed to the ground (stance phase).

A study of such a complex activity as human walking requires several terms and conventions to be defined. One of the first conventions discussed in this chapter is the description of walking based on a single gait cycle. The gait cycle consists of all events that occur between consecutive heel contacts of the same limb; walking at steady velocity is simply a repetition of that gait cycle. In its simplest subdivision, a gait cycle consists of a stance phase (heel contact to toe off) that encompasses approximately the first 60% of the gait cycle, and a swing phase that encompasses the remainder of the cycle (toe off to the next heel contact).

Throughout the gait cycle, the major joints of the lower limb rotate as a way to advance the body while also providing support against the external torques imposed by gravity. As the body is propelled forward, its CoM is also displaced slightly in both the medial-lateral and vertical directions. The natural cyclic displacement of the body gives walking the quality of an inverted pendulum, allowing a cyclic and smooth transfer of potential and kinetic mechanical energy. Such a mechanism minimizes the energy cost of walking.

In this chapter the biomechanics associated with the forward translation of the body as a whole are focused on the rotation of the joints of the lower limbs—most specifically the hip, knee, ankle, and foot. The greatest range of joint motion occurs within the sagittal plane, which reflects the primary forward direction of movement of the body. Less obvious, but equally important, are the frontal and horizontal plane rotations of the joints of the lower limbs. In addition to their modest contribution to the forward progression of the body, these extrasagittal plane motions help optimize the vertical and medial-lateral displacements of the body's CoM.

During walking, a limitation of motion at any one joint can have a profound effect on the quality and efficiency of movement of the body as a whole. Consider, for example, the disrupted walking pattern with a loss of the last 15 degrees of knee extension. Walking is still possible but only with significant kinematic compensations made by other joints and at a cost of an increased expenditure of energy.

Approximately 50 muscles operate each lower limb. No muscle has identical actions, and all are active to a varied extent at one time or another during the gait cycle. Many of these muscles express their specific actions in multiple ways: eccentrically, concentrically, or isometrically; across one or multiple joints; or as movers of either the distal or proximal segment of a joint, or a combination thereof. Consider the complex action of the tibialis posterior for example. During stance, this muscle first decelerates the pronation of the foot prior to reversing its action to help with foot supination. This is done all while assisting with controlling the advance of the tibia over the foot in the first half of stance, followed by a concentric activation that contributes to ankle plantar flexion during push off. Inhibition of this muscle action as a result of weakness or pain could significantly interfere with the natural transformation of the foot from a pliable platform at loading response to a more rigid lever at push off. Understanding this level of detail of each muscle's action is essential to recognizing as well as treating associated underlying pathomechanics.

A noticeable gait deviation will likely result if a muscle or muscle group fails to activate at an appropriate time and magnitude of effort. The deviation can often be minimized through biomechanical compensations naturally learned by the individual. Often, however, it is the role of the clinician to devise strategies that can either compensate for or eliminate the gait deviation. These strategies typically include exercises that aim to increase the control, strength, or flexibility of targeted muscles. In addition, strategies often include patient education, endurance and gait retraining activities, and the use of bracing, orthoses, electrical stimulators, biofeedback, or other assistive devices such as a cane or walker.

Walking may be considered the ultimate kinesiologic expression of the neuromuscular and musculoskeletal interactions of the lower body. Although the kinesiology of walking is complex, a thorough understanding of the subject serves as the direct or indirect basis for the evaluation and treatment of most disorders involving the lower limb. These disorders vary considerably and include local muscle injury or overuse, painful or replaced joints, neurologic trauma or disease, reduced endurance after bed rest or surgery, and the actual amputation, paralysis, or loss of control of a lower limb. The kinesiology presented in this chapter is intended to be a starting point for a study that lasts a lifetime.

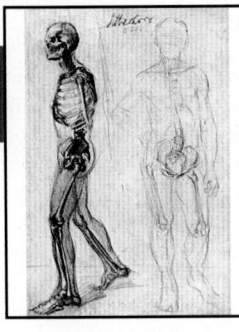

ADDITIONAL CLINICAL CONNECTIONS

CONTENTS

CLINICAL CONNECTION 15.1

Eccentric, Isometric, or Concentric Muscle Activation: Is It Really Always Known for Certain?

Much attention has been paid in this chapter to the type of activation of a muscle or muscle group during the different parts of the gait cycle. In a broad sense, isometric activation occurs when an activated muscle does not change length. Concentric activation occurs as the activated muscle is actually shortening (contracting), whereas eccentric activation occurs as the activated muscle is being elongated by some other more dominant force. As described in Chapter 3, the force output of a muscle is dependent on its type of activation, given a constant effort. This issue is therefore very relevant to the study of gait.

In most clinical or laboratory settings, the specific type of activation of a muscle can be estimated only by comparing its established action against the rotation direction of the joint that the muscle is crossing.[13] For example, the tibialis anterior is assumed to experience an eccentric activation after heel contact based on the fact that the ankle is plantar flexing at the time this primary dorsiflexor muscle is active. This clinical connection considers variables that may interfere with the logic of this practical method of analysis.

First, consider an activated pluri-articular muscle of the lower extremity. It is not unusual for such a muscle to contract across one joint while at the same time being elongated across a more proximal or distal joint.[89] The joint kinematics illustrated in Fig. 15.13 provide an opportunity to consider such a situation for pluri-articular muscles acting principally in the sagittal plane. For example, it may not be possible to determine with absolute certainty the net change in length of the activated rectus femoris as it is being elongated through hip extension and simultaneously shortened as a result of knee extension at 15% to 40% of the gait cycle. Similarly, the actual net change in length of the gastrocnemius may be quite challenging to determine when one considers the combination of ankle and knee movements during gait.[76,95]

To add to the complexity of the process of estimating the type of activation a muscle is experiencing during walking is the fact that net change in length of the muscle is affected by *both* the change in length of the activated muscle fibers and the stretch in its related tendon. Based on its stiffness, a tendon may elongate a significant amount when under load. The Achilles tendon, for example, elongates up to 8% of its resting length after a maximal contraction of the calf muscles.[133] The magnitude of elongation is dependent on the specific architecture of the muscle-tendon unit, but also on the amount and rate of the application of the force.

This physiologic property of a tendon may obscure the actual length change in the entire muscle-tendon unit during activation. It is possible that in some kinematic conditions, depending on the muscle, the overall contraction of the muscle fibers may be offset by a similar elongation of the tendon. In this example, an activation previously thought to be isometric for the entire muscle-tendon unit (based on no change in joint angle) may, in fact, be slightly concentric at the level of the muscle fibers.

Real-time ultrasonography now provides the ability to make direct measurements of the lengths of muscle fibers during dynamic movement.[44,134] This technique was used to study the specific function of the vastus lateralis during walking shortly after heel contact, a time when this muscle is known to be strongly activated and assumed to be active eccentrically. Despite the knee moving toward flexion, the length of the muscle fibers actually remained relatively constant—the load placed on the muscle caused significant lengthening of the tendon of the vastus lateralis. The authors of the same study also observed similar results when analyzing the muscle fibers of the tibialis anterior immediately after heel contact—a time when the muscle is strongly activated while the ankle moves toward plantar flexion. In both scenarios, an activation previously thought to be eccentric for the entire muscle-tendon unit was observed to be essentially isometric in nature at the level of the muscle fibers. The lengthening of the tendon is likely being used to dampen the impact on the overall muscle and for storage of elastic energy.[44,103,136,137]

These data expose the oversimplification of interpreting a muscle's type of action based on EMG and kinematic data alone. In some muscles, especially during short-arc movements as those described earlier, the compliance within the tendon (and other connective tissue) may account for some or all of the changes in joint motion. It is interesting to consider that the two factors highlighted in this clinical connection—pluri-articular muscles and tendon compliance—may minimize muscle fiber length changes during movement and thereby help maintain the muscle in a more optimal portion of its length-tension curve.

This clinical connection is not intended to negate the standard empiric method for inferring if a muscle is active isometrically, concentrically, or eccentrically, but rather highlights the potential limitation of this method in assessment of all muscles over a wide range of function.

ADDITIONAL CLINICAL CONNECTIONS

As illustrated throughout this chapter and in Fig.15.51A, the gait cycle is described from heel contact to heel contact of the same limb. The origin of this traditional perspective likely reflects the fact that heel contact represents such a clear and visually distinct demarcation of the walking process. Heel contact denotes the instant of transition from swing phase to stance phase, with the start of the loading response. Such a transition requires high muscular activity before, during, and after heel contact; in part, to prepare for and generate relatively large joint torques that are associated with the loading response. This important transition may not be immediately apparent by looking at the traditional graphic representation of the gait cycle that starts and ends at heel contact. An alternative visual representation may be to start and end the gait cycle at *toe off*—effectively placing heel contact and associated loading response toward the center (at 40%) of the gait cycle (contrast Fig. 15.51B with 15.51A).

The alternative representation of the gait cycle allows the pre–heel contact preparatory muscular activity of the gluteus maximus and biceps femoris to be better appreciated. These muscles act eccentrically to slow hip flexion and knee extension, respectively, prior to their strong concentric activation during the loading response following heel contact (at the 40% mark in Fig.15.51B).

Fig. 15.51B also clearly shows the initial rise in activation of the vastus medialis and lateralis in preparation for their action post–heel contact, despite knee extension actually decelerating in late swing. Similarly, for muscles like the gluteus medius and tibialis anterior, their pre–heel contact activation is quasi-isometric in nature, in preparation for a strong eccentric action at post–heel contact. In the previous examples, the alternative illustration of the gait cycle allows a better appreciation for how several muscles use the swing phase to prime (or ramp up) their activation to meet the high kinetic demands of the stance phase. In contrast, the gastrocnemius muscle, while relatively silent prior to heel contact, starts to slowly increase its activation post–heel contact, initially eccentrically to control tibial advancement and then concentrically for propulsion.

Reduced magnitude of muscle activation during the swing phase may impact the kinematics of the lower extremity during the subsequent loading response. This may potentially produce a gait that can lead to painful conditions. Alternatively, *enhanced* magnitude of muscle activation prior to loading response may offer a therapeutic benefit. For example, increased gluteus medius activation in late swing likely reduces peak hip adduction in early stance.[46,255] This may be beneficial assuming that excessive hip adduction in early stance may be associated with patellofemoral pain.

The alternative representation of the gait cycle offered in this Clinical Connection should be considered for other key muscles of gait, thereby providing additional insight into the muscular kinesiology of walking.

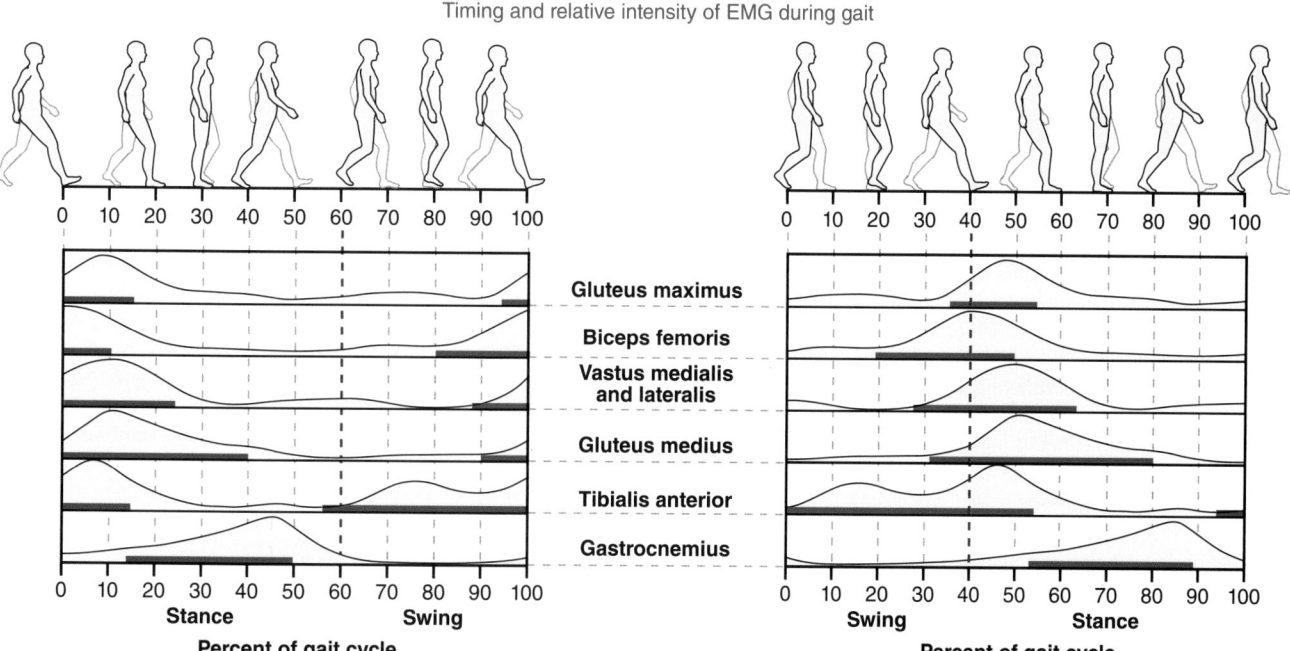

FIGURE 15.51 Muscle activation for selected muscles for a gait cycle from heel contact to the subsequent heel contact (A). Muscle activation for the same muscles for a gait cycle from toe off to the subsequent toe off, positioning heel contact toward the center (40%) of the gait cycle (B).

ADDITIONAL CLINICAL CONNECTIONS

CLINICAL CONNECTION 15.3
Walking and Running—A Kinesiologic Continuum

As will be described in Chapter 16, running, a natural progression of speeding up bipedal locomotion, shares many of the same fundamental kinesiologic principles as walking. However, notable differences need to be considered to provide optimal assessment and interventions for those seeking care for running-related injuries,[167] because it is not uncommon for individuals with impairments in the lower limbs to have pain when running and not while walking.

Similar to walking, running is a cyclic action that can be summarized through the description of a full cycle—from foot contact of one limb to the next foot contact of the same limb. Also as with walking, running can be described by patterns of movement, joint kinematics and kinetics, and the intensity and timing of muscle activation. Furthermore, as with walking, these variables differ substantially across the spectrum of running velocity, from slow jogging to sprinting. This speed-dependent kinesiology of running is often implicated in running-related injuries, as running faster typically requires greater movement amplitude, movement velocity, and generation of forces. A lack of progressive accommodations to these greater demands on the musculoskeletal system has the potential to lead to injuries such as tendinopathies and stress fractures.[241]

An individual transitions from walking to running, usually not because of the inability to walk faster, but because of the greater energy efficiency of running compared with walking when reaching a speed of approximately 2.1 to 2.2 m/sec.[202] By definition, running occurs when the two periods of double-limb support during walking are replaced by two "flight" periods—when both feet are off the ground at the same time. When transitioning from walking to running, the duration of stance phase for each limb drops suddenly from 60% to 40% of the cycle. The faster the running velocity, the shorter the duration of the running cycle and the lower the percentage of the stance phase in the total running cycle (Fig. 15.52).[60] Mechanically, when switching from walking to running, the body has transitioned from a mode of locomotion resembling an inverted pendulum to one resembling a "spring."[36,200] The cyclic transfer of potential and kinetic energy taking place over a relatively extended stance limb during walking has been replaced by a strategy taking advantage of elastic energy initially stored and then released by muscles, tendons, and other connective tissues on a relatively flexed stance limb during running (Fig. 15.53).

Through visual observation, it should be readily apparent that the movements of the joints of the lower extremities occur much more rapidly during running compared with walking. This is primarily because of the shorter duration of the running gait cycle but also, although to a lesser extent, the greater magnitude of joint movement used for running.[41] A detailed description of joint kinematics during running is provided in Chapter 16.

As would be suspected, Fig. 15.54 shows that the vertical ground reaction force during running is of greater magnitude than during walking. In this illustration the smooth single peak shape of

the curve is characteristic of a runner making initial contact with the forefoot.[6] If the runner makes initial contact with the rearfoot, then the vertical ground reaction force would exhibit an additional, highly characteristic, initial impact peak within the first 10% of the stance phase (see Chapter 16). Vertical ground reaction forces during running can be as high as three to four times body weight, being progressively larger as running speed increases.[41,102]

The larger ground reaction forces combined with the often-larger joint angular movements during running are associated with larger internal joint torques. As described in this chapter, the power across a

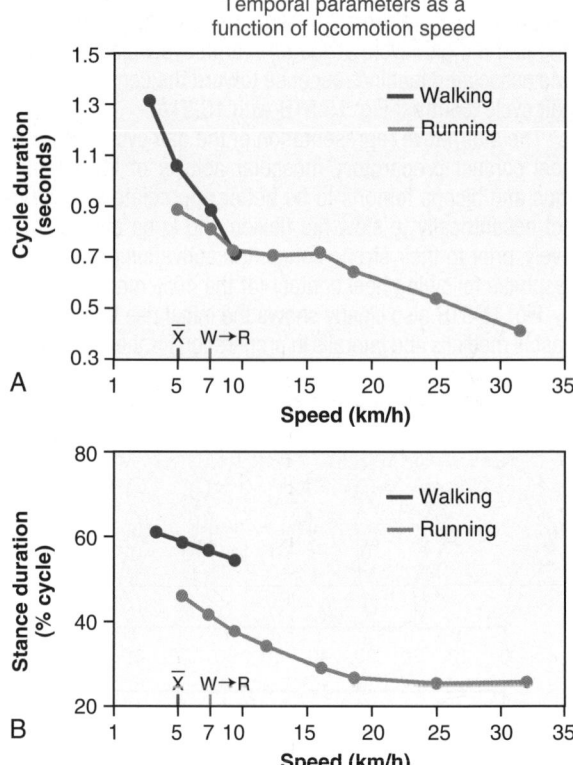

FIGURE 15.52 Time-duration of a gait and running cycle over a range of walking and running speeds (A). Stance phase duration over a range of walking and running speeds (B). NOTE: 5 km/hr (1.3 m/sec) is reflective of an average walking velocity (indicated by $\overline{X}$), and 7 km/hr (2 m/sec) is reflective of the speed when individuals transition from walking to running (indicated by W→R). (Data from Cappellini G, Ivanenko YP, Poppele RE, et al: Motor patterns in human walking and running, *J Neurophysiol* 95:3426, 2006; Swanson SC, Caldwell GE: An integrated biomechanical analysis of high speed incline and level treadmill running, *Med Sci Sports Exerc* 32:1146, 2000; Dorn TW, Schache AG, Pandy MG: Muscular strategy shift in human running: dependence of running speed on hip and ankle muscle performance, *J Exp Biol* 215:1944, 2012.)

ADDITIONAL CLINICAL CONNECTIONS

joint is the product of torque and angular velocity. It is therefore not surprising that the power generated or absorbed across the joints of the lower extremity during running is several times the magnitude of that experienced during walking (Fig. 15.55).[171] The presence of greater power and torque is expressed through the significant increase in muscular activation measured during running compared with walking (see Cappellini and colleagues [36] for the muscle activation profiles of 32 muscles across a spectrum of walking and running speeds).

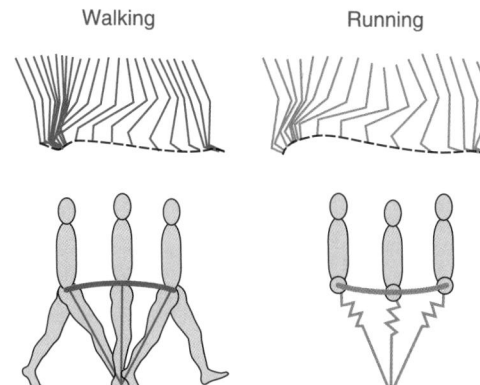

FIGURE 15.53 Top images illustrate stick diagrams representing the walking and running cycles, showing the slightly more flexed attitude of the lower extremity during stance and swing phases of running. Bottom images depict the trajectory of the center of mass during walking and running. The center of mass trajectory resembles an inverted pendulum during walking, indicating the transfer between the "out-of-phase" potential and kinetic energy (compare with Fig. 15.25). This is in contrast to running, which takes advantage of a transfer between "in-phase" potential and kinetic energy of the body and elastic energy from the muscles, tendons, and other connective tissues of the lower extremities. (Data from Cappellini G, Ivanenko YP, Poppele RE, et al: Motor patterns in human walking and running, *J Neurophysiol* 95:3426, 2006.)

From an injury and prevention perspective, one of the most important differences between walking and running is the magnitude of the forces applied to the musculoskeletal system (see e-Table 15.2). The magnitude and repetitive nature of these forces require adequate strength and endurance of the lower extremity musculature as well as progressive tissue adaptation over time. Furthermore, it is important to consider the influence of factors such as running speed and surface incline, which modify the running kinematics and kinetics and the demands on the system in a manner that potentially lead to injuries. Clinically, "training errors," leading to injuries during running, are more readily identified and understood with a better knowledge of how kinematics and kinetics change over a continuum of walking and running velocities. Much more information on the kinesiology of running is covered in Chapter 16.

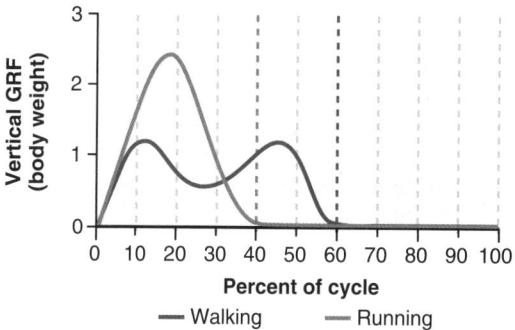

FIGURE 15.54 Vertical ground reaction forces *(GRFs)* for a walking (5.4 km/hr) and running (9.4 km/hr) cycle for one individual. Vertical dashed blue and orange lines indicate transition between stance and swing phases. (Data from Cappellini G, Ivanenko YP, Poppele RE, et al: Motor patterns in human walking and running, *J Neurophysiol* 95:3426, 2006.)

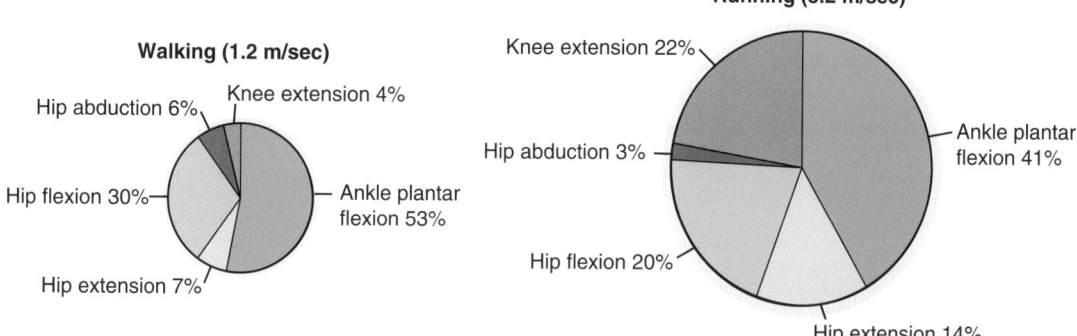

FIGURE 15.55 Power generation measured for the lower extremity joints during walking (1.2 m/sec) and running (3.2 m/sec). The surface area of each pie chart corresponds to the total amount of power generated, while the size of each portion of the pie chart corresponds to the percentage contribution from each joint source. (Data from Novacheck TF: The biomechanics of running, *Gait Posture* 7:77, 1998.)

REFERENCES

1. Abram SJ, Selinger JC, Donelan JM: Energy optimization is a major objective in the real-time control of step width in human walking, *J Biomech* 91:85–91, 2019.

2. Adouni M, Shirazi-Adl A: Partitioning of knee joint internal forces in gait is dictated by the knee adduction angle and not by the knee adduction moment, *J Biomech* 47:1696–1703, 2014.

3. Akbas T, Prajapati S, Ziemnicki D, et al.: Hip circumduction is not a compensation for reduced knee flexion angle during gait, *J Biomech* 87:150–156, 2019.

4. Alexander N, Schwameder H: Lower limb joint forces during walking on the level and slopes at different inclinations, *Gait Posture* 45:137–142, 2016.

5. Alexander RM: Flat and bouncy walking, *J Physiol* 582(2):474, 2007.

6. Almeida MO, Davis IS, Lopes AD: Biomechanical differences of foot-strike patterns during running: a systematic review with meta-analysis, *J Orthop Sports Phys Ther* 45:738–755, 2015.

7. Alves SA, Polzehl J, Brisson NM, et al.: Ground reaction forces and external hip joint moments predict in vivo hip contact forces during gait, *J Biomech* 135:111037–111045, 2022.

8. Amar J: Trottoir dynamographique, *C R Hebdomadaires des Séances de l'Acad des Sci* 163:130–133, 1916.

9. Anders C, Wagner H, Puta C, et al.: Trunk muscle activation patterns during walking at different speeds, *J Electromyogr Kinesiol* 17:245–252, 2007.

10. Andersson EA, Nilsson J, Thorstensson A: Intramuscular EMG from the hip flexor muscles during human locomotion, *Acta Physiol Scand* 161:361–370, 1997.

11. Andrews JG: Euler's and Lagranges equations for linked rigid-body models of three-dimensional human motion. In Allard P, Stokes IAF, Blanchi JP, editors: *Three-dimensional analysis of human movement*, Champaign, Ill, 1995, Human Kinetics.

12. Translated by Peck AL and Forster ES. *Aristotle: parts of animals: movement of animals, Progression of animals*, Cambridge, Mass, 1968, Harvard University Press.

13. Arnold EM, Hamner SR, Seth A, et al.: How muscle fiber lengths and velocities affect muscle force generation as humans walk and run at different speeds, *J Exp Biol* 216:2150–2160, 2013.

14. Attias M, Chevalley O, Bonnefoy-Mazure A, et al.: Effects of contracture on gait kinematics: a systematic review, *Clin Biomech* 33:103–110, 2016.

15. Bahrilli T, Topuz S: Does immobilization of the shoulder in different positions affect gait? *Gait Posture* 91:254–259, 2022.

16. Baker R: The history of gait analysis before the advent of modern computers, *Gait Posture* 26:331–342, 2007.

17. Bandholm T, Bousen L, Haugaard S, et al.: Foot medial longitudinal-arch deformation during quiet standing and gait in subjects with medial tibial stress syndrome, *J Foot Ankle Surg* 47(2):89–95, 2008.

18. Barwick A, Smith J, Chuter V: The relationship between foot motion and lumbopelvic-hip function: a review of literature, *Foot* 22:224–231, 2012.

19. Bechtol CO: Normal human gait. In Bowker JH, Hall CB, editors: *Atlas of orthotics: American academy of orthopaedic surgeons*, St Louis, 1975, Mosby.

20. Begg R, Best R, Del'Oro L, et al.: Minimum foot clearance during walking: strategies for the minimization of trip-related falls, *Gait Posture* 25:191–198, 2007.

21. Benoit DL, Ramsey DK, Lamontagne M, et al.: In vivo knee kinematics during gait reveals new rotation profiles and smaller translations, *Clin Orthop Relat Res* 454:81–88, 2007.

22. Bilney B, Morris M, Webster K: Concurrent related validity of the GAITRite walkway system for quantification of the spatial and temporal parameters of gait, *Gait Posture* 17:68–74, 2003.

23. Blokland I, Gravesteijn A, Busse M, et al.: The relationship between relative aerobic load, energy cost, and speed of walking in individuals post-stroke, *Gait Posture* 89:193–199, 2021.

24. Bohannon RW, Andrews AW: Normal walking speed: a descriptive meta-analysis, *Physiotherapy* 97:182–189, 2011.

25. Bohannon RW: Comfortable and maximum walking speed of adults aged 20-79 years: reference values and determinants, *Age Ageing* 26:15–19, 1997.

26. Braune W, Fisher O: *Der Gang des Menschen [The human gait]*, Leipzig, Germany, 1895-1904, BG Teubner.

27. Braune W, Fisher O: *The human gait (translation by Maquet P, Furlong R)*, Berlin, 1987, Springer-Verlag (Original work published 1895-1904.).

28. Bresler B, Frankel JP: Forces and moments in the leg during walking, *Trans Am Soc Mech Eng* 72:27, 1950.

29. Bruening DA, Frimenko RE, Goodyear CD, et al.: Sex differences in whole body gait kinematics at preferred speeds, *Gait Posture* 41:540–545, 2015.

30. Bruijn SM, Meijer OG, van Dieen JH, et al.: Coordination of leg swing, thorax rotations, and pelvis rotations during gait: the organization of total body angular momentum, *Gait Posture* 27:455–462, 2008.

31. Buczek FL, Cooney KM, Walker MR, et al.: Performance of an inverted pendulum model directly applied to normal human gait, *Clin Biomech* 21:288–296, 2006.

32. Buddhadev HH, Martin PE: Effects of age and physical activity status on redistribution of joint work during walking, *Gait Posture* 50:131–136, 2016.

33. Buldt AK, Murley GS, Butterworth P, et al.: The relationship between foot posture and lower limb kinematics during walking: a systematic review, *Gait Posture* 38:363–372, 2013.

34. Burnfield JM, Powers CM: The role of center of mass kinematics in predicting peak utilized coefficient of friction during walking, *J Forensic Sci* 52:1328–1333, 2007.

35. Cansel AJM, Stevens J, Bijnens W, et al.: Hallux rigidus affects lower limb kinematics assessed with the gait profile score, *Gait Posture* 84:273–279, 2021.

36. Cappellini G, Ivanenko YP, Poppele RE, et al.: Motor patterns in human walking and running, *J Neurophysiol* 95:3426–3437, 2006.

37. Carlsoo S: *How man moves: kinesiological methods and studies*, New York, 1972, Crane, Russak & Company.

38. Carriero A, Zavatsky A, Stebbins J, et al.: Influence of altered gait patterns on the hip joint contact forces, *Comput Methods Biomech Biomed Engin* 17:352–359, 2014.

39. Carter SC, Batavia MZ, Guterriez GM, et al.: Joint movements associated with minimum toe clearance variability in older adults during level overground walking, *Gait Posture* 75:14–21, 2020.

40. Cavagna GA, Legramandi MA: The phase shift between potential and kinetic energy in human walking, *J Exp Biol* 223:jeb232645–jeb232650, 2020.

41. Cavanagh PR: The biomechanics of lower extremity action in distance running, *Foot Ankle* 7:197–217, 1987.

42. Chester VL, Tingley M, Biden EN: A comparison of kinetic gait parameters for 3-13 year olds, *Clin Biomech* 21:726–732, 2006.

43. Chevutschi A, Lensel G, Vaast D, et al.: An electromyographic study of human gait both in water and on dry ground, *J Physiol Anthropol* 26:467–473, 2007.

44. Chleboun GS, Busic AB, Graham KK, et al.: Fascicle length change of the human tibialis anterior and vastus lateralis during walking, *J Orthop Sports Phys Ther* 37:372–379, 2007.

45. Chumanov ES, Wall-Scheffler C, Heiderscheit BC: Gender differences in walking and running on level and inclined surfaces, *Clin Biomech* 23:1260–1268, 2008.

46. Chumanov ES, Wille CM, Michalski MP, et al.: Changes in muscle activation patterns when running step rate is increased, *Gait Posture* 36:231–235, 2012.

47. Collins JJ: The redundant nature of locomotor optimization laws, *J Biomech* 28:251, 1995.

48. Cooper RC, Prebeau-Menezes LM, Butcher MT, et al.: Step length and required friction in walking, *Gait Posture* 27:547–551, 2008.

49. Correa TA, Crossley KM, Kim HJ, et al.: Contributions of individual muscles to hip joint contact force in normal walking, *J Biomech* 43:1618–1622, 2010.

50. Cromwell RL, Aadland-Monahan TK, Nelson AT, et al.: Sagittal plane analysis of head, neck, and trunk kinematics and electromyographic activity during locomotion, *J Orthop Sports Phys Ther* 31:255–262, 2001.

51. Cunningham D, Brown G: Two devices for measuring the forces acting on the human body during walking, *Exp Stress Anal* 75–90, 1952.

52. Damm P, Kutzner I, Bergmann G, et al.: Comparison of in vivo measured loads in knee, hip and spinal implants during level walking, *J Biomech* 51:128–132, 2017.

53. De Groote F, Falisse A: Perspective on musculoskeletal modelling and predictive simulations of human movement to assess the neuromechanics of gait, *Proc R Soc A B* 288:20202432–20202442, 2021.

54. Della Croce U, Riley PO, Lelas JL, et al.: A refined view of the determinants of gait, *Gait Posture* 14:79–84, 2001.

55. DeMers MS, Pal S, Delp SL: Changes in tibiofemoral forces due to variations during walking, *J Orthop Res* 32:769–776, 2014.

56. Den Otter AR, Geurts ACH, Mulder T, et al.: Speed related changes in muscle activity from normal to very slow walking speeds, *Gait Posture* 19:270–278, 2004.

57. DeVita P, Helseth J, Hortobagyi T: Muscles do more positive than negative work in human locomotion, *J Exp Biol* 210:3361–3373, 2007.

58. Devita P: The selection of a standard convention for analyzing gait data based on the analysis of relevant biomechanical factors, *J. Biomech* 27:501–508, 1994.

59. Donelan JM, Kram R, Kuo AD: Mechanical and metabolic determinants of the preferred step width in human walking, *Proc Biol Sci* 268:1985–1992, 2001.

60. Dorn TW, Schache AG, Pandy MG: Muscular strategy shift in human running: dependence of running speed on hip and ankle muscle performance, *J Exp Biol* 215(Pt 11):1944–1956, 2012.

61. Drillis R: The influence of aging on the kinematics of gait. In *Geriatric amputee (NAS-NRC pub. No. 919)*, Washington, DC, 1961, NAS-NRC.

62. Eberhart H: *Fundamental studies of human locomotion and other information relating to design of artificial limbs. Report to U.S. Veterans' Association*, Berkeley, 1947, University of California.

63. Eggenberger P, Tomovic S, Munzer T, et al.: Older adults must hurry at pedestrian lights! A cross-sectional analysis of preferred and fast walking speed under single- and dual-task conditions, *PLoS One* 12:e0182180–e0182197, 2017.

64. Elftman H: The measurement of the external force in walking, *Science* 88:152–153, 1938.

65. Ellis RG, Sumner BJ, Kram R: Muscle contributions to propulsion and braking during walking and running: insight from external force perturbations, *Gait Posture* 40:594–599, 2014.

66. Eng JJ, Winter DA: Kinetic analysis of the lower limbs during walking: what information can be gained from a three-dimensional model? *J Biomech* 28:753, 1995.

67. Ettema S, Kal E, Houdijk H: General estimates of the energy cost of walking in people with different levels and causes of lower-limb amputation: a systematic review and meta-analysis, *Prosthet Orthot Int* 45:417–427, 2021.

68. Ferrari A, Benedetti MG, Pavan E, et al.: Quantitative comparison of five current protocols in gait analysis, *Gait Posture* 28:207–216, 2008.

69. Finley F, Cody K: Locomotive characteristics of urban pedestrians, *Arch Phys Med Rehabil* 51:423, 1970.

70. Finni T, Komi PV, Lukkariniemi J: Achilles tendon loading during walking: application of a novel optic fiber technique, *Eur J Appl Physiol* 77:289, 1998.

71. Finni T, Lepola V, Komi PV: Tendomuscular loading in normal locomotion conditions. In Kyrolainen H, Avela J, Takala T, editors: *Limiting factors of human neuromuscular performance, Jyvaskyla, Finland*, University of Jyvaskyla, 1999.

72. Foster AD, Raichlen DA, Pontzer H: Muscle force production during bent-knee, bent-hip walking in humans, *J Hum Evol* 65:294–302, 2013.

73. Foster AD, Raichlen DA, Pontzer H: Muscle force production during bent-knee, bent-hip walking in humans, *J Hum Evol* 65:294–302, 2013.

74. Fregly BJ, Besier TF, Lloyd DG, et al.: Grand challenge competition to predict in vivo knee loads, *J Orthop Res* 30(4):503–513, 2012.

75. Fukuchi CA, Fukuchi RK, Duarte M: Effect of walking speed on gait biomechanics in healthy participants: a systematic review and meta-analysis, *Syst Rev* 8:153–163, 2019.

76. Fukunaga T, Kubo K, Kawakami Y, et al.: In vivo behaviour of human muscle tendon during walking, *Proc Biol Sci* 268:229–233, 2001.

77. Gage JR: Gait analysis in cerebral palsy. In *Clinic in developmental medicine*, London, 1991, Mac Keith Press.

78. Garrett M, McElroy AM, Staines A: Locomotor milestones and babywalkers: cross sectional study, *BMJ* 324:1494, 2002.

79. Gordon KE, Ferris DP, Kuo AD: Metabolic and mechanical costs of reducing vertical center of mass movement during gait, *Arch Phys Med Rehabil* 90:136–144, 2009.

80. Gorton GE, Hebert DA, Gannotti ME: Assessment of the kinematic variability among 12 motion analysis laboratories, *Gait Posture* 29:398–402, 2009.

81. Grabiner PC, Biswas T, Grabiner MD: Age-related changes in spatial and temporal gait variables, *Arch Phys Med Rehabil* 82:31–35, 2001.

82. Gross MT, Foxworth JL: The role of foot orthoses as an intervention for patellofemoral pain, *J Orthop Sports Phys Ther* 33:661–670, 2003.

83. Gupta SD, Bobbert MF, Kistemaker DA: The metabolic cost of walking in healthy young and older adults – a systematic review and meta analysis, *Sci Rep* 9:1–10, 2019.

84. Han S, Kim RS, Harris JD, et al.: The envelope of active hip motion in different sporting, recreational, and daily-living activities: a systematic review, *Gait Posture* 71:227–233, 2019.

85. Hansen EA, Risgaard Kristensen LA, Moller Nielsen A, et al.: The role of stride frequency for walk-to-run transition in humans, *Sci Rep* 7:2010–2017, 2018.

86. Heiden TL, Sanderson DJ, Inglis JT, et al.: Adaptations to normal human gait on potentially slippery surfaces: the effects of awareness and prior slip experience, *Gait Posture* 24:237–246, 2006.

87. Hillman SJ, Stansfield BW, Richardson AM, et al.: Development of temporal and distance parameters of gait in normal children, *Gait Posture* 29:81–85, 2009.

88. Ho KY, Blanchette MG, Powers CM: The influence of heel height on patellofemoral joint kinetics, *Gait Posture* 36:271–275, 2012.

89. Hofmann CL, Okita N, Sharkey NA: Experimental evidence supporting isometric functioning of the extrinsic toe flexors during gait, *Clin Biomech* 28:686–691, 2013.

90. Hollman JH, Kovash FM, Kubik JJ, et al.: Age-related differences in spatiotemporal markers of gait stability during dual task walking, *Gait Posture* 26:113–119, 2007.

91. Holm I, Tveter AT, Fredriksen PM, et al.: A normative sample of gait and hopping on one leg parameters in children 7-12 years of age, *Gait Posture* 29:317–321, 2009.

92. Ijmker T, Lamoth CJC: Gait and cognition: the relationship between gait stability and variability with executive function in persons with and without dementia, *Gait Posture* 35:126–130, 2012.

93. Inman VT, Ralston HJ, Todd F: Human locomotion. In Rose J, Gamble JG, editors: *Human walking*, ed 2, Philadelphia, 1994, Williams & Wilkins.

94. Inman VT, Ralston HJ, Todd F: *Human walking*, Baltimore, 1981, Williams & Wilkins.

95. Ishikawa M, Pakaslahti J, Komi PV: Medial gastrocnemius muscle behavior during human running and walking, *Gait Posture* 25:380–384, 2007.

96. Ito T, Noritake K, Ito Y, et al.: Three-dimensional gait analysis of lower extremity gait parameters in Japanese children aged 6 to 12 years, *Sci Rep* 12:7822–7833, 2022.

97. Ivanenko YP, Poppele RE, Lacquaniti F: Motor control programs and walking, *Neuroscientist* 12:339–348, 2006.

98. Jeng B, Cederberg KLJ, Lai B, et al.: Oxygen cost of over-ground walking in persons with mild-moderate Parkinson's disease, *Gait Posture* 82:1–5, 2020.

99. Kanko RM, Laende EK, Davis EM, et al.: Concurrent assessment of gait kinematics using marker-based and markerless motion capture, *J Biomech* 127:110665–110667, 2021.

100. Kato T, Taniguchi A, Akima H, et al.: Effect of hip angle on neuromuscular activation of the adductor longus and adductor magnus muscles during isometric hip flexion and extension, *Eur J Appl Physiol* 119(7):1611–1617, 2019.

101. Kavanagh JJ, Morrison S, Barrett RS: Lumbar and cervical erector spinae fatigue elicit compensatory postural responses to assist in maintaining head stability during walking, *J Appl Physiol* 101:1118–1126, 2006.

102. Keller TS, Weisberger AM, Ray JL, et al.: Relationship between vertical ground reaction force and speed during walking, slow jogging, and running, *Clin Biomech* 11:253–259, 1996.

103. Kelly LA, Farris DJ, Cresswell AG, et al.: Intrinsic foot muscles contribute to elastic energy storage and return in the human foot, *J Appl Physiol* 126(1):231–238, 2019.

104. Kepple TM, Siegel KL, Stanhope SJ: Relative contributions of the lower extremity joint moments to forward progression and support during gait, *Gait Posture* 6:1, 1997.

105. Kerrigan DC, Croce UD, Marciello M, et al.: A refined view of the determinants of gait: significance of heel rise, *Arch Phys Med Rehabil* 81:1077, 2000.

106. Kerrigan DC, Riley PO, Lelas JL, et al.: Quantification of pelvic rotation as a determinant of gait, *Arch Phys Med Rehabil* 82:217–220, 2001.

107. Khamis S, Carmeli E: Relationship and significance of gait deviations associated with lim length discrepancy: a systematic review, *Gait Posture* 57:115–123, 2017.

108. Kiernan D, O'Sullivan R, Malone A, et al.: Pathological movements of the pelvis and trunk during gait in children with cerebral palsy: a cross-sectional study with 3-dimensoianl kinematics and lower lumbar spinal loading, *Phys Ther* 98:86–94, 2018.

109. Kim Y, Lee KM, Koo S: Joint moments and contact forces in the foot during walking, *J Biomech* 74:79–85, 2018.

110. Knutson LM, Soderberg GL: EMG: use and interpretation in gait. In Craik RL, Oatis CA, editors: *Gait analysis: theory and application*, St Louis, 1995, Mosby.

111. Komistek RD, Stiehl JB, Dennis DA, et al.: Mathematical model of the lower extremity joint reaction forces using Kane's method of dynamics, *J Biomech* 31:185, 1998.

112. Koussou A, Desailly E, Dumas R: Contribution of passive moments to inter-segmental moments during gait: a systematic review, *J Biomech* 122:1–12, 2021.

113. Kressig RW, Gregor RJ, Oliver A, et al.: Temporal and spatial features of gait in older adults transitioning to frailty, *Gait Posture* 20:30–35, 2004.

114. Kuhtz-Buschbeck JP, Jing B: Activity of upper limb muscles during human walking, *J Electromyogr Kinesiol* 22:199–206, 2012.

115. Kung SM, Fink PW, Legg SJ, et al.: What factors determine the preferred gait transition speed in humans? A review of the triggering mechanisms, *Hum Mov Sci* 57:1–12, 2018.

116. Kuo AD, Donelan JM: Dynamic principles of gait and their clinical implications, *Phys Ther* 90:157–174, 2010.

117. Kuo AD: The six determinants of gait and the inverted pendulum analogy: a dynamic walking perspective, *Hum Mov Sci* 26:617–656, 2007.

118. Kutzner I, Heinlein B, Graichen F, et al.: Loading of the knee joint during ergometer cycling: telemetric in vivo data, *J Orthop Sports Phys Ther* 42(12):1032–1038, 2012.

119. Lacquaniti F, Ivanenko YP, Zago M: Development of human locomotion, *Curr Opin Neurobiol* 22:822–828, 2012.

120. Lafortune MA, Cavanagh PR, Sommer III HJ, et al.: Three-dimensional kinematics of the human knee during walking, *J Biomech* 25:347, 1992.

121. Lay AN, Hass CJ, Nichols TR, et al.: The effect of sloped surfaces on locomotion: an electromyographic analysis, *J Biomech* 40:1276–1285, 2007.

122. Lee DV, Harris SL: Linking gait dynamics to mechanical cost of legged locomotion, *Front Robot AI* 5:111–122, 2018.

123. Lerner-Frankiel MB, Vargas S, Brown MB, et al.: Functional community ambulation: what are your criteria? *Clin Manage* 6:12, 1990.

124. Levinger P, Murley GS, Barton CJ, et al.: A comparison of foot kinematics in people with normal- and flat-arched feet using the Oxford foot model, *Gait Posture* 32:519–523, 2010.

125. Lewek MD, Osborn AJ, Wutzke CJ: The influence of mechanically and physiologically imposed stiff-knee gait patterns on the energy cost of walking, *Arch Phys Med Rehabil* 93:123–128, 2012.

126. Li M, Venalainen MS, Chandra SS, et al.: Discrete element and finite element methods provide similar estimations for hip joint contact mechanics during walking gait, *J Biomech* 115:110163–110174, 2021.

127. Liang BW, Wu WH, Meijer OG, et al.: Pelvic step: the contribution of horizontal pelvis rotation to step length in young healthy adults walking on a treadmill, *Gait Posture* 39:105–110, 2014.

128. Lim YP, Lin YC, Pandy MG: Lower-limb muscle function in healthy young and older adults across a range of walking speeds, *Gait Posture* 94:124–130, 2022.

129. Lin YC, Gfoehler M, Pandy MG: Quantitative evaluation of the major determinants of human gait, *J Biomech* 47:1324–1331, 2014.

130. Liu MQ, Anderson FC, Schwartz MH, et al.: Muscle contributions to support and progression over a range of walking speeds, *J Biomech* 41:3243–3252, 2008.

131. Lockart TE, Spaulding JM, Park SH: Age-related slip avoidance strategy while walking over a known slippery surface, *Gait Posture* 26:142–149, 2007.

132. Magalhaes FA, Fonseca ST, Araujo VL, et al.: Midfoot passive stiffness affects foot and ankle kinematics and kinetics during the propulsive phase of walking, *J Biomech* 119:110328–110335, 2021.

133. Magnusson SP, Hansen P, Aagaard P, et al.: Differential strain patterns of the human gastrocnemius aponeurosis and free tendon, in vivo, *Acta Physiol Scand* 177:185–195, 2003.

134. Magnusson SP, Narici MV, Maganaris CN, et al.: Human tendon behavior and adaptation, in vivo, *J Physiol* 586:71–81, 2008.

135. Mahaffey R, Le Warne M, Blandford L, et al.: Age-related changes in three-dimensional foot motion during barefoot walking in children aged between 7 and 11 years old, *Gait Posture* 95:38–43, 2022.

136. Maharaj JN, Cresswell AG, Lichtwark GA: Subtalar joint pronation and energy absorption requirements during walking are related to tibialis posterior tendinous tissue strain, *Sci Rep* 7(1):17958, 2017.

137. Maharaj JN, Cresswell AG, Lichtwark GA: Tibialis anterior tendinous tissue plays a key role in energy absorption during human walking, *J Exp Biol* 222(Pt 11):04, 2019.

138. Marchetti GF, Whitney SL, Blatt PJ, et al.: Temporal and spatial characteristics of gait during performance of the dynamic gait index in people with and people without balance or vestibular disorders, *Phys Ther* 88:640–651, 2008.

139. Marey EJ: De la measure dans les different acts de la locomotion, *C R de L'Acad des Sci de Paris* 97:820–825, 1883.
140. Marey EJ: *La machine animal*, Paris, 1873, Librairie Germer Baillière.
141. Marey EJ: *Movement*, London, 1895, W. Heinemann.
142. Masatoshi K, Yoshitaka I, Nobuhiro K: Relationship between forward propulsion and foot motion during gait in healthy young adults, *J Biomech* 121:1–8, 2021.
143. Massaad F, Lejeune TM, Detrembleur C: The up and down bobbing of human walking: a compromise between muscle work and efficiency, *J Physiol* 582(2):789–799, 2007.
144. McGinley JL, Baker R, Wolfe R, et al.: The reliability of the three-dimensional kinematic gait measurements: a systematic review, *Gait Posture* 29:360–369, 2009.
145. Menz HB, Latt MD, Tiedemann A, et al.: Reliability of the GAITRite walkway system for the quantification of temporo-spatial parameters of gait in young and older people, *Gait Posture* 20:20–25, 2004.
146. Menz HB, Lord SR, Fitzpatrick RC: Acceleration patterns of the head and pelvis when walking on level and irregular surfaces, *Gait Posture* 18:35–46, 2003.
147. Meyns P, Bruijn SM, Duysens J: The how and why of arm swing during human walking, *Gait Posture* 38:555–562, 2013.
148. Michalina B, Ida W, Katarzyna K, et al.: Mechanisms of compensation in the gait of patients with drop foot, *Clin BioMech* 42:14–19, 2017.
149. Mills PM, Barrett RS, Morrison S: Toe clearance variability during walking in young and elderly men, *Gait Posture* 28:101–107, 2008.
150. Mizner RL, Kawaguchi JK, Chmieleski TL: Muscle strength in the lower extremity does not predict postinstruction improvements in the landing patterns of female athletes, *J Orthop Sports Phys Ther* 38:353–361, 2008.
151. Moe-Nilssen R, Helbostad JL: Spatiotemporal gait parameters for older adults-an interactive model adjusting reference data for gender, age, and body height, *Gait Posture* 82:220–226, 2020.
152. Moisan G, Mainville C, Descarreaux M, et al.: Kinematic, kinetic and electromyographic differences between young adults with and without chronic ankle instability during walking, *J Electromyogr Kinesiol* 51:102399–102407, 2020.
153. Moissenet F, Cheze L, Dumas R: A 3D lower limb musculoskeletal model for simultaneous estimation of musculo-tendon, joint contact, ligament and bone forces during gait, *J Biomech* 47:50–58, 2014.
154. Molen HH: *Problems on the evaluation of gait*, Amsterdam, 1973, Free University.
155. Murley GS, Buldt AK, Trump PJ, et al.: Tibialis posterior EMG activity during barefoot walking in people with neutral foot posture, *J Electromyogr Kinesiol* 19:e69, 2009.
156. Murley GS, Landorf KB, Menz HB, et al.: Effect of foot posture, foot orthoses and footwear on lower limb muscle activity during walking and running: a systematic review, *Gait Posture* 29:172–187, 2009.
157. Murley GS, Menz HB, Landorf KB: Electromyographic patterns of tibialis posterior and related muscles when walking at different speeds, *Gait Posture* 39:1080–1085, 2014.
158. Murley GS, Menz HB, Landorf KB: Foot posture influences the electromyographic activity of selected lower limb muscles during gait, *J Foot Ankle Res* 2:35, 2009.
159. Murray MP, Gore DR, Clarkson BH: Walking patterns of patients with unilateral hip pain due to osteoarthritis and avascular necrosis, *J Bone Joint Surg Am* 53:259, 1971.
160. Murray MP, Guten GN, Mollinger LA, et al.: Kinematic and electromyographic patterns of Olympic race walkers, *Am J Sports Med* 11:68, 1983.
161. Murray MP, Kory R, Sepic S: Walking patterns of normal women, *Arch Phys Med Rehabil* 51:637, 1979.
162. Murray MP, Kory RC, Clarkson BH, et al.: Comparison of free and fast speed walking patterns of normal men, *Am J Phys Med* 45:8, 1966.
163. Murray MP, Sepic SB, Barnard EJ: Patterns of sagittal rotation of the upper limbs in walking: study of normal men during free and fast speed walking, *Phys Ther* 47:272, 1967.
164. Muybridge E: *Animal locomotion*, Philadelphia, 1887, University of Pennsylvania Press.
165. Muybridge E: *Human and animal locomotion*, New York, 1979, Dover.
166. Nardon M, Ruzzante F, O'Donnell L, et al.: Energetics of walking in individuals with cerebral palsy and typical development, across severity and age: a systematic review and meta-analysis, *Gait Posture* 90:388–407, 2021.
167. Neal BS, Barton CJ, Gallie R, et al.: Runners with patellofemoral pain have altered biomechanics which targeted interventions can modify: a systematic review and meta-analysis, *Gait Posture* 45:69–82, 2016.
168. Nene A, Byrne C, Hermens H: Is rectus femoris really a part of quadriceps? Assessment of rectus femoris function during gait in able-bodied adults, *Gait Posture* 20:1–13, 2004.
169. Neptune RR, Sasaki K, Kautz SA: The effect of walking speed on muscle function and mechanical energetics, *Gait Posture* 28:135–143, 2008.
170. Nielsen JB: How we walk: central control of muscle activity during human walking, *Neuroscientist* 9:195–204, 2003.
171. Novacheck TF: The biomechanics of running, *Gait Posture* 7:77–95, 1998.
172. Ortega JD, Farley CT: Minimizing center of mass vertical movement increases metabolic cost in walking, *J Appl Physiol* 99:2099–2107, 2005.
173. Ota S, Ueda M, Aimoto K, et al.: Acute influence of restricted ankle dorsiflexion angle on knee mechanics during gait, *Knee* 21:669–675, 2014.
174. Pandy MG, Andriacchi TP: Muscle and joint function in human locomotion, *Annu Rev Biomed Eng* 12:401–433, 2010.
175. Park J: Synthesis of natural arm swing motion in human bipedal walking, *J Biomech* 41:1417–1426, 2008.
176. Patla A: A framework for understanding mobility problems in the elderly. In Craik RL, Oatis CA, editors: *Gait analysis: theory and application*, St Louis, 1995, Mosby.
177. Pederson DR, Brand RA, Davy DT: Pelvic muscle and acetabular contact forces during gait, *J Biomech* 30:959, 1997.
178. Perry J, Burnfield JM: *Gait analysis: normal and pathological function*, ed 2, Thorofare, NJ, 2010, SLACK incorporated.
179. Perry J: *Gait analysis: normal and pathological function*, Thorofare, NJ, 1992, Slack.
180. Phan CB, Shin G, Lee KM, et al.: Skeletal kinematics of the midtarsal joint during walking: midtarsal joint locking revisited, *J Biomech* 95:109287–109295, 2019.
181. Picouleau A, Orsoni N, Hardy J, et al.: Analysis of the effects of arthrodesis of the hallux metatarsophalangeal joint on gait cycle: results of a GAITRite treadmill test, *Int Orthop* 44:2167–2176, 2020.
182. Powers CM: The influence of abnormal hip mechanics on knee injury: a biomechanical perspective, *J Orthop Sports Phys Ther* 40:42–51, 2010.
183. Prins MR, Cornelisse LE, Meijer OG, et al.: Axial pelvis range of motion affects thorax-pelvis timing during gait, *J Biomech* 95:109308–109317, 2019.
184. Quinlan S, Yan AF, Sinclair P, et al.: The evidence for improving balance by strengthening the toe flexor muscles: a systematic review, *Gait Posture* 81:56–66, 2020.
185. Rajagopal A, Dembia CL, DeMers MS, et al.: Full-body musculoskeletal model for muscle-driven simulation of human gait, *IEEE Trans Biomed Eng* 63:2068–2079, 2016.
186. Rajan RA, Kerr M, Evans H, et al.: A prospective clinical and biomechanical analysis of feet following first metatarsophalangeal joint replacement, *Gait Posture* 89:211–216, 2021.
187. Ralston HJ: Effects of immobilization of various body segments on energy cost of human locomotion, *Ergon Suppl* 53, 1965.
188. Rawal YR, Singer JC: The influence of net ground reaction force orientation on mediolateral stability during walking, *Gait Posture* 90:73–79, 2021.
189. Reischl SF, Powers CM, Rao S, et al.: Relationship between foot pronation and rotation of the tibia and femur during walking, *Foot Ankle Int* 20:513, 1999.
190. Requiao LF, Nadeau S, Milot MH, et al.: Quantification of level of effort at the plantarflexors and hip extensors and flexor muscles in healthy subjects walking at different cadences, *J Electromyogr Kinesiol* 15:393–405, 2005.
191. Roelker SA, Kautz SA, Neptune RR: Muscle contributions to mediolateral and anteroposterior foot placement during walking, *J Biomech* 95:109310–109317, 2019.
192. Romkes J, Bracht-Schweizer K: The effect of walking speed on upper body kinematics during gait in healthy subjects, *Gait Posture* 54:304–310, 2017.
193. Rose J, Ralston HJ, Gamble JG: Energetics of walking. In Rose J, Gamble JG, editors: *Human walking*, ed 2, Philadelphia, 1994, Williams & Wilkins.
194. Rosenblatt NJ, Hurt CP, Latash ML, et al.: An apparent contradiction: increasing variability to achieve greater precision? *Exp Brain Res* 232:403–413, 2014.
195. Row E, Beauchamp MK, Wilson JA: Age and sex differences in normative gait patterns, *Gait Posture* 88:109–115, 2021.
196. Rowe E, Beauchamp MK, Astephen Wilson J: Age and sex differences in normative gait patterns, *Gait Posture* 88:109–115, 2021.
197. Rozumalski A, Schwartz MH, Wervey R, et al.: The in vivo three-dimensional motion of the human lumbar spine during gait, *Gait Posture* 25:378–384, 2008.
198. Rudisch J, Jollenbeck T, Vogt L, et al.: Agreement and consistency of five different clinical gait analysis systems in the assessment of spatiotemporal gait parameters, *Gait Posture* 85:55–64, 2021.
199. Russell DM, Apatoczky DT: Walking at the preferred stride frequency minimizes muscle activity, *Gait Posture* 45:181–186, 2016.
200. Saibene F, Minetti AE: Biomechanical and physiological aspects of legged locomotion in humans, *Eur J Appl Physiol* 88:297–316, 2003.
201. Salbach NM, O'Brien KK, Brooks D, et al.: Reference values for standardized tests of walking speed and distance: a systematic review, *Gait Posture* 41:341–360, 2015.
202. Sasaki K, Neptune RR: Muscle mechanical work and elastic energy utilization during walking and running near the preferred gait transition speed, *Gait Posture* 23:383–390, 2006.
203. Saunders JB, Inman VT, Eberhart HD: The major determinants in normal and pathological gait, *J Bone Joint Surg Am* 35:543, 1953.
204. Saxby DJ, Modenese L, Bryant AL, et al.: Tibiofemoral contact forces during walking, running and sidestepping, *Gait Posture* 49:78–85, 2016.
205. Schache AG, Baker R, Vaughan CL: Differences in lower limb transverse plane joint moments during gait when expressed in two alternative reference frames, *J Biomech* 40:9–19, 2007.
206. Schache AG, Baker R: On the expression of joint moments during gait, *Gait Posture* 25:440–452, 2007.
207. Scott SH, Winter DA: Internal forces of chronic running injury sites, *Med Sci Sports Exerc* 22:357, 1990.
208. Semciw AI, Freeman M, Kunstler BE, et al.: Quadratus femoris: an EMG investigation during walking and running, *J Biomech* 48:3433–3439, 2015.
209. Semciw AI, Green RA, Murley GS, et al.: Gluteus minimus: an intramuscular EMG investigation of anterior and posterior segments during gait, *Gait Posture* 39:822–826, 2014.
210. Semciw AI, Pizzari T, Murley GS, et al.: Gluteus medius: an intramuscular EMG investigation of anterior, middle and posterior segments during gait, *J Electromyogr Kinesiol* 23:858–864, 2013.

211. Sethi D, Bharti S, Prakash C: A comprehensive survey on gait analysis: history, parameters, approaches, pose estimation, and future work, *Art Int Med* 129:102314, 2022.

212. Shiavi R: Electromyographic patterns in adult locomotion: a comprehensive review, *J Rehabil* 22:85, 1985.

213. Shumway-Cook A, Woollacott MH: *Motor control: translating research into clinical practice*, Philadelphia, 2006, Lippincott, Williams & Wilkins.

214. Simonsen EB, Dyhre-Poulsen P, Voigt M, et al.: Bone-on-bone forces during loaded and unloaded walking, *Acta Anat* 152:133, 1995.

215. Sloot LH, Malheiros S, Truijen S, et al.: Decline in gait propulsion in older adults over age decades, *Gait Posture* 90:475–482, 2021.

216. Souza RB, Powers CM: Differences in hip kinematics, muscle strength, and muscle activation between subjects with and without patellofemoral pain, *J Orthop Sports Phys Ther* 39:12–19, 2009.

217. Sritharan P, Lin YC, Pandy MG: Muscles that do not cross the knee contribute to the knee adduction moment and tibiofemoral compartment loading during gait, *J Orthop Res* 30:1586–1595, 2012.

218. Stansfield BW, Hillman SJ, Hazlewood ME, et al.: Normalisation of gait data in children, *Gait Posture* 17:81–87, 2003.

219. Stansfield BW, Nicol AC: Hip joint contact forces in normal subjects and subjects with total hip prostheses: walking and stair and ramp negotiation, *Clin Biomech* 17:130–139, 2002.

220. States RA, Krzak JJ, Salem Y, et al.: Instrumented gait analysis for management of gait disorders in children with cerebral palsy: a scoping review, *Gait Posture* 90:1–8, 2021.

221. Stauffer RN, Chao EYS, Brewster RC: Force and motion analysis of the normal, diseased and prosthetic ankle joint, *Clin Orthop Relat Res* 127:189, 1977.

222. Steele KM, DeMers MS, Schwartz MH, et al.: Compressive tibiofemoral joint force during crouch gait, *Gait Posture* 35:556–560, 2012.

223. Steffi Shih HJ, Gordon J, Kulig K: Trunk control during gait: walking with wide and narrow step widths present distinct challenges, *J Biomech* 114:110135–111044, 2021.

224. Stephenson JL, Lamontagne A, De Serres S: The coordination of upper and lower limb movements during gait in healthy and stroke individuals, *Gait Posture* 29:11–16, 2009.

225. Stewart C, Postans N, Schwartz MH, et al.: An exploration of the function of the triceps surae during normal gait using functional electrical stimulation, *Gait Posture* 26:482–488, 2007.

226. Stimpson KH, Heitkamp LN, Horne JS, et al.: Effects of walking speed on the step-by-step control of step width, *J Biomech* 68:78–83, 2018.

227. Sudarsky L: An overview of neurological diseases causing gait disorder. In Spivack BS, editor: *Evaluation and management of gait disorders*, New York, 1995, Marcel Dekker.

228. Sutherland DH: The evolution of clinical gait analysis. Part I: kinesiological EMG, *Gait Posture* 14:61–70, 2001.

229. Tan AM, Weizman Y, Van Netten JJ, et al.: Comparing the applicability of temporal gait symmetry, variability and laterality in bilateral gait conditions: a feasibility study of healthy individuals and people with diabetic neuropathy, *Clin BioMech* 91:105530–105539, 2022.

230. Taylor SJ, Walker PS, Perry JS, et al.: The forces in the distal femur and the knee during walking and other activities measured by telemetry, *J Arthroplasty* 13:428, 1998.

231. Tecchio P, Zamparo P, Nardello F, et al.: Achilles tendon mechanical properties during walking and running are underestimated when its curvature is not accounted for, *J Biomech* 137:1–7, 2022.

232. Terrier P, Reynard F: Effect of age on the variability and stability of gait: a cross-sectional treadmill study in healthy individuals between 20 and 69 years of age, *Gait Posture* 41:170–174, 2015.

233. Tesio L, Rota V: The motion of body center of mass during walking: a review oriented to clinical applications, *Front Neurol* 10:999–1021, 2019.

234. Teufl W, Taetz B, Miezal M, et al.: Automated detection and explainability of pathological gait patterns using a one-class support vector machine trained on inertial measurement unit based gait data, *Clin Biomech* 89:105452–105459, 2021.

235. Thambyah A, Hee HT, Das S, et al.: Gait adaptations in patients with longstanding hip fusion, *J Orthop Surg* 11:154–158, 2003.

236. Thomas SA, Vega D, Arellano CJ: Do humans exploit the metabolic and mechanical benefits of arm swing across slow to fast walking speeds? *J Biomech* 115:110181–110188, 2021.

237. Toyohara R, Kurosawa D, Hammer N, et al.: Finite element analysis of load transition on sacroiliac joint during bipedal walking, *Sci Rep* 10:13683–13694, 2020.

238. Van Criekinge T, Saeys W, Hallemans A, et al.: Age-related differences in muscle activity patterns during walking in healthy individuals, *J Electromyogr Kinesiol* 41:124–131, 2018.

239. van der Krogt MM, Delp SL, Schwartz MH: How robust is human gait to muscle weakness, *Gait Posture* 36:113–119, 2012.

240. van Gelder LMA, Barnes A, Wheat JS, et al.: The use of biofeedback for gait retraining: a mapping review, *Clin Biomech* 59:159–166, 2018.

241. van Gent RN, Siem D, van Middelkoop M, et al.: Incidence and determinants of lower extremity running injuries in long distance runners: a systematic review, *Br J Sports Med* 41:469–480, 2007.

242. van Hedel HJA, Tomatis L, Muller R: Modulating of leg muscle activity and gait kinematics by walking speed and bodyweight unloading, *Gait Posture* 24:35–45, 2006.

243. Vierordt KH: *Das gehen des menschen in gesunden und kranken zuständen nach selbstregistrirenden methoden dargestellt*, Tubingen, Germany, 1881, Laupp.

244. Voigt M, Hansen EA: The puzzle of the walk-to-run transition in humans, *Gait Posture* 86:319–326, 2021.

245. Voss S, Joyce J, Biskis A, et al.: Normative database of spatiotemporal gait parameters using inertial sensors in typically developing children and young adults, *Gait Posture* 80:206–213, 2020.

246. Watanabe K, Kitaoka HB, Fujii T, et al.: Posterior tibial tendon dysfunction and flatfoot: analysis with simulated walking, *Gait Posture* 37(2):264–268, 2013.

247. Waters RL, Barnes G, Husserl T, et al.: Comparable energy expenditure after arthrodesis of the hip and ankle, *J Bone Joint Surg Am* 70:1032, 1988.

248. Weber W, Weber E: *Mechanics of the human walking apparatus, translation by maquet P, Furlong R*, Berlin, Germany, 1991, Springer-Verlag (Original work published in 1894.).

249. Weber W, Weber E: *Mechanik der menschlichen gewerkzeuge. [Mechanics of the human walking apparatus]*, Berlin, Germany, 1894, Springer-Verlag.

250. Weber W, Weber E: *The mechanics of human motion*, Gottingen, Germany, 1836, Dieterischen Buchhandlung.

251. Wesseling M, de Groote F, Meyer C, et al.: Gait alterations to effectively reduce hip contact forces, *J Orthop Res* 33:1094–1102, 2015.

252. Whittington B, Silder A, Heiderscheit B, et al.: The contribution of passive-elastic mechanisms to lower extremity joint kinetics during human walking, *Gait Posture* 27:628–634, 2008.

253. Wille CM, Lenhart RL, Wang S, et al.: Ability of sagittal kinematic variables to estimate ground reaction forces and joint kinetics in running, *J Ortho Sports Phys Ther* 44:825–830, 2014.

254. Williams G, Widnall J, Evans P, et al.: Could failure of the spring ligament complex be the driving force behind the development of the adult flatfoot deformity? *J Foot Ankle Surg* 53(2):152–155, 2014.

255. Willson JD, Kernozek TW, Arndt RL, et al.: Gluteal muscle activation during running in females with and without patellofemoral pain syndrome, *Clin BioMech* 26:735–740, 2011.

256. Winter DA, Eng JJ, Ishac M: Three-dimensional moments, powers and work in normal gait: implications for clinical assessments. In Harris GF, Smith PA, editors: *Human motion analysis: current applications and future directions*, New York, 1996, IEEE Press.

257. Winter DA: *The biomechanics and motor control of human gait: normal, elderly and pathological*, ed 2, Waterloo, Canada, 1991, University of Waterloo Press.

258. Wong DWC, Lam WK, Lee WCC: Gait asymmetry and variability in older adults duirng long-distance walking: implications for gait instability, *Clin BioMech* 72:37–43, 2020.

259. Wren TAL, Tucker CA, Rethlefsen SA, et al.: Clinical efficacy of instrumented gait analysis: systematic review 2020 update, *Gait Posture* 80:274–279, 2020.

260. Youdas JW, Hollman JH, Aalbers MJ, et al.: Agreement between the GAITRite walkway system and a stopwatch-footfall count method for measurement of temporal and spatial gait parameters, *Arch Phys Med Rehabil* 87:1648–1652, 2006.

261. Zarrugh MY, Todd FN, Ralston HJ: Optimization of energy expenditure during level walking, *Eur J Appl Physiol* 33:293, 1974.

STUDY QUESTIONS

1. At what points in the gait (walking) cycle is the potential energy (A) greatest and (B) least?
2. At 10% into the gait cycle, describe the position and direction of rotation of the hip, knee, and ankle with respect to the sagittal plane.
3. (A) Describe the rotation at the ankle between 5% and 40% of the gait cycle with respect to the sagittal plane. (B) Describe the type of muscle activation (eccentric, isometric, concentric) of the ankle plantar flexor and dorsiflexor muscles within the context of the kinematics described in part A.
4. Between about 30% and 50% of the gait cycle, a person with a tight or short heel cord (Achilles tendon) often makes kinematic compensations within the ankle and foot as a way to allow continued forward rotation of the leg relative to the ground. Describe a kinematic compensation that may allow this, including the specific joint(s) where it may occur.
5. At what points in the gait (walking) cycle are the vertical ground reaction forces (A) greatest and (B) least?
6. (A) For 0% to about 50% of the gait cycle, describe the kinematics of the hip joint in the horizontal plane. (B) Using Figure 15.29A as a guide, discuss a possible role of the gluteus minimus and the gluteus medius muscles during these kinematics.
7. Describe kinematic strategies typically used to optimize the vertical and medial-lateral displacements of the center of mass of the body during walking.
8. During about 5% to 20% of the gait cycle, correlate the functional association between the frontal plane kinematics at the stance hip with the type of muscle activation of the gluteus medius.
9. What are the two basic kinematic mechanisms used to increase walking speed?
10. (A) From about 30% to 50% of the gait cycle, describe the likely position and direction of movement of the subtalar joint in the frontal plane. Use frontal plane movements of inversion and eversion (of the calcaneus) as a reference for your description. (B) Using Figure 15.29B as a guide, explain the most likely role of the tibialis posterior muscle in controlling these kinematics.
11. What is one likely role of the adductor longus muscle at 60% to 75% of the gait cycle?
12. Describe the changes that typically occur in gait in aged persons. What natural protection may these changes provide?
13. At what point in the gait (walking) cycle are the (A) semitendinosus and (B) gastrocnemius most likely at their greatest length?
14. Figure 15.40 shows the primary mechanics associated with the production of a varus torque at the knee through most of stance phase. Which tissues at the knee are capable of limiting this torque?
15. Using Figure 15.35A,B,D, explain the exchange of mechanical energy for sagittal plane motion of the hip (Fig. 15.35C) for the transition from stance to swing phase (35%–60% of the gait cycle).
16. Weakness of the ankle dorsiflexor muscles is associated with some very typical gait deviations. Contrast gait deviations at the ankle and foot that may likely occur in persons with the three following levels of dorsiflexion weakness: (A) mild (30% loss of strength or 4/5 based on the standard manual muscle testing scale), (B) moderate (greater than 50% loss of strength or 3–/5 strength), or (C) severe (80%–90% loss of strength or 2/5 strength).
17. Referring to Figure 15.42, explain the virtual lack of energy (power) generation or absorption during 10% to 30% of the gait cycle despite the presence of an increasing plantar flexion torque. As part of the explanation, contrast this virtual lack of energy exchange between 10% and 30% of the cycle to (A) the small energy absorption observed from 0% to 8% of the gait cycle and (B) the significant energy generation present from 45% to 60% of the gait cycle.

Answers to the study questions can be found in the accompanying enhanced eBook version included with the print purchase of this textbook.

Additional Video Educational Content

- Kinematic and Electromyographic Analysis of Walking and Running: An individual walks and runs on a treadmill as surface EMG-driven light bulbs indicate selected muscular activation

- Visual Clinical Evaluation of Walking— Sagittal Plane: Elements of a systematic gait evaluation are provided

- Visual Clinical Evaluation of Walking— Frontal Plane: Elements of a systematic gait evaluation are provided
- Hip Abductor Muscle Deficient Gait: Without and with a cane held in contralateral hand

ALL VIDEOS in this chapter are available in the accompanying enhanced eBook version included with the print purchase of this textbook.

Chapter

16

Kinesiology of Running

BRYAN C. HEIDERSCHEIT, PT, PhD, FAPTA
GUY G. SIMONEAU, PT, PhD, FAPTA

CHAPTER AT A GLANCE

This chapter provides a description of the fundamental kinesiologic characteristics of running. Unless indicated otherwise, the information provided refers to individuals with a normal and mature running pattern, running on level surfaces at a steady average speed for distance running, and using a rearfoot strike pattern. Although this chapter provides enough details to be read independently of the rest of this textbook, Chapters 12 through 15 will facilitate an even greater understanding of running.

SPATIAL AND TEMPORAL DESCRIPTORS

Stride Cycle

The fundamental unit for running is the *stride cycle,* which consists of all motions and events taking place between two consecutive foot-ground contacts of the same foot. Unlike walking, where the heel of the foot makes initial contact with the ground, during running, initial contact can occur at the rearfoot, midfoot, or forefoot and is frequently referred to as foot strike.

Spatial and Temporal Descriptors of Running

- Stride cycle
- Stride length
- Stride time
- Step length
- Step time
- Stride frequency
- Stride rate
- Step width
- Base of gait
- Foot angle
- Running speed
- Running pace

The spatial and temporal descriptors of the running stride cycle are defined in the same manner as walking. For example, the distance and time between successive ground contacts with the same foot are termed the *stride length* and *stride time,* respectively; *step length* and *step time* refer to successive contacts made between opposite feet. Stride length and time change with running speed, such that stride length will increase and stride time will decrease with progressively faster running speed. Another variable, *stride frequency,* is simply the inverse of stride time and reflects the number of strides per second. Most runners will report this value on a per minute basis and use the term *stride rate* (or *step rate* if referring to the number of steps per minute). Although individuals who are taller, longer legged, or heavier may tend to prefer a longer stride length at a given running speed, investigations have consistently shown that these and other anthropometric variables have a weak ($r < 0.40$) correlation to stride length.[25,27]

Step width is the medial-lateral distance between the locations of the feet when in contact with the ground, while *base of gait* describes the medial-lateral distance between the placement of the foot during the middle of stance relative to the body's line of gravity.[28,130] As one progresses from walking to running to sprinting, step width and base of gait gradually decrease, eventually becoming less than zero and reflective of a crossover gait pattern (i.e., the foot crosses the midline of the body). A related measure, *foot angle* or *angle of toe-out,* is the amount of foot abduction relative to the line of progression. Measurements show that foot angle is variable between individuals and across running speeds, with averages for running ranging between 4 and 9 degrees compared with 5 and 7 degrees for walking.[28]

Running speed is a common measure of performance, typically measured in meters per second (m/sec) or miles per hour (mph). *Running pace,* the inverse of speed, is typically measured in minutes per mile (min/mile) or minutes per kilometer (min/km). Among runners and coaches, running pace is more routinely used. Although typical walking speeds are generally less than 2.5 m/sec, running can occur across a much greater speed range, from 2.5 m/sec to greater than 10 m/sec. Not surprisingly, the kinematics and kinetics of running will vary greatly with speed, as well as other factors such as age and sex.

Stance and Swing Phases

The running stride cycle is comprised of two phases: *stance,* when the reference foot is in contact with the ground, and *swing,* when the reference foot is in the air. The stance phase of running is commonly cited as occupying about 40% of the stride cycle with the swing phase comprising the remaining duration;[101] however, as running speed increases, the stance phase portion progressively decreases. For example, at a running speed of 2.25 m/sec (8.1 km/hr), the stance phase accounts for approximately 37% of the stride cycle, but when running speed is increased to 4.50 m/sec (16.2 km/hr), the stance phase only occupies approximately 28% of the stride cycle.[48] Stance phase may only comprise 22% of the stride cycle at maximum running speeds among world class sprinters.[81] Review Fig. 15.52 in Chapter 15 to see the relationship between the duration of stance phase and running speed.

Unlike walking, the running stride cycle does *not* have a period of double-limb support. Only one limb at most is in contact with the ground at any instant during running. Also, in contrast with walking, there are two periods during the stride cycle when neither limb is in contact with the ground. These periods of *float* (or *flight*) occur after one limb has pushed off the ground and before the other limb has made initial contact. Float must be present for the movement to be characterized as running. The increase in swing phase duration that accompanies an increase in running speed is primarily due to greater time spent in float.

SUBDIVISIONS OF STANCE AND SWING PHASES

The *events* defined for the running stride cycle include initial contact, mid stance, heel off, toe off, and mid swing (Fig. 16.1 and Table 16.1). *Initial contact* is the instant the foot contacts the ground, thereby defining 0% of the stride cycle. *Mid stance* occurs when the body's center of mass (located anterior to the sacrum) is directly over the support limb, or when the knees are side by side. This occurs at about 20% of the stride cycle or 50% of stance phase.[54] *Heel off* and *toe off* occur at about 30% and 40% of the stride cycle, respectively, varying greatly with running speed. *Mid swing* occurs at the middle of the swing phase, roughly 70% of the stride cycle,

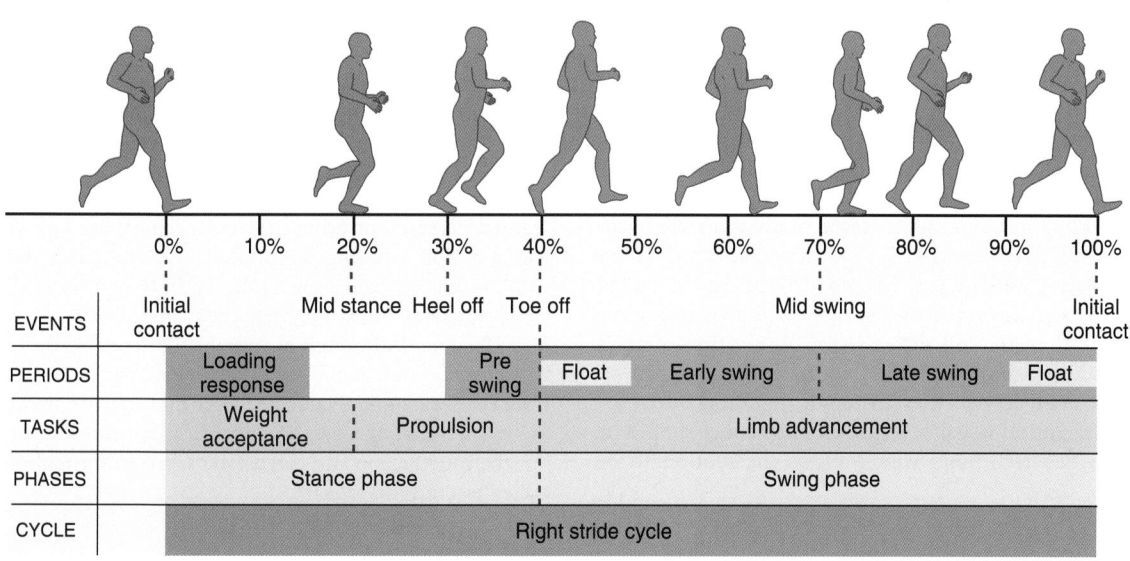

FIGURE 16.1 Terminology used to describe the events and periods of the running stride cycle.

TABLE 16.1 Common Terminology Defining the Subdivisions of the Running Stride Cycle

Phases	Events	Percentage of Stride Cycle	Events of Opposite Limb	Phases of Opposite Limb
Stance	Initial contact	0		Swing
		10		
	Mid stance	20	Mid swing	
	Heel off	30		
Swing	Toe off	40		
		50	Initial contact	Stance
		60		
	Mid swing	70	Mid stance	
		80	Heel off	
		90	Toe off	Swing
Stance	Initial contact	100		

when the knee of the swing limb passes next to the knee of the contralateral stance limb.

The *periods* of the running stride cycle include loading response, pre swing, early swing, and late swing (see Fig. 16.1). *Loading response* occupies the first 15% of the stride cycle, between initial contact and the point of maximum knee flexion. During this period, the limb must gradually accept and absorb the weight of the body. At the end of loading response, the body's center of mass reaches its lowest vertical position. *Pre swing* is from heel off to toe off, when the muscles of the lower limb generate mechanical energy for propulsion. *Early swing* refers to the first half of swing phase, from toe off to mid swing. *Late swing* is the remainder of swing phase, from mid swing to the subsequent initial contact.

Periods of Running Stride Cycle
- Loading response
- Pre swing
- Early swing
- Late swing

JOINT KINEMATICS

There are many similarities in joint motion between walking and running. In general, the overall kinematic pattern is the same, while the magnitude and timing of motion differs. These differences are largely due to the increase in locomotion speed, from a slow jog to a full sprint. The sophisticated motion analysis techniques used to objectively measure running kinematics are similar to those used during walking (see Chapter 15). In the absence of this technology, which is typically the case for most clinical settings, clinicians often rely on direct visual observation of their patients to evaluate running characteristics. Because the lower extremity joint angular velocities are quite high and often key areas of interest, clinical visual observation of a runner should be made from a video recording, which allows the motion to be slowed down.

Unlike walking, where the vast majority of people make initial contact with the ground using their heels, running has more variability in that regard. The part of the foot that initially contacts the ground is termed *foot strike* and can occur in three specific manners: *rearfoot strike, midfoot strike,* and *forefoot strike.* The location of the center of pressure on the foot or shoe at initial contact characterizes the specific foot strike.[26] In the absence of center of pressure data, however, foot strike can be determined by visual inspection of high-speed video.[2,77] Interestingly, it appears that many runners are unable to accurately self-assess their own foot strike pattern, especially those who incorrectly assume they are first striking the ground with their midfoot or forefoot.[49]

The type of foot strike can substantially influence the lower extremity joint kinematics during running. For example, a runner who uses a forefoot strike will have greater ankle plantar flexion and knee flexion at initial contact compared with rearfoot strike. Because a rearfoot strike is present in 88% to 95% of distance runners,[1,73] the following description of joint kinematics will assume this favored foot strike pattern, unless otherwise noted.

Sagittal Plane Kinematics

TRUNK

While running, sagittal plane angular motion occurs throughout the entire trunk,[79] although the medial-lateral axis of rotation is typically assumed to pass through the lumbosacral junction. Described as trunk flexion and extension, the angle of the trunk is defined relative to a vertical plane as opposed to another body segment. Neutral position (0 degrees) coincides with vertical, with trunk flexion referring to rotation in the anterior direction, and trunk extension indicating a rotation in the posterior direction.

Throughout the stride cycle the trunk flexes and extends about 5 to 10 degrees, although on average it remains within a range of 2 to 13 degrees of flexion. Trunk flexion is least at initial contact and reaches its maximum value just after mid stance. As running speed increases, the trunk assumes a more flexed position at initial contact, but the total flexion and extension excursion throughout the stride cycle does not increase.[120]

PELVIS

Pelvic rotation in the sagittal plane, commonly referred to as *tilt*, occurs in the anterior and posterior directions (Fig. 16.2A). The direction of rotation of a point on the iliac crests defines the direction of the tilt. Similar to the trunk, the angle for the pelvis is defined relative to a vertical plane. Two oscillations of motion occur during a running stride cycle, with a total motion amplitude of approximately

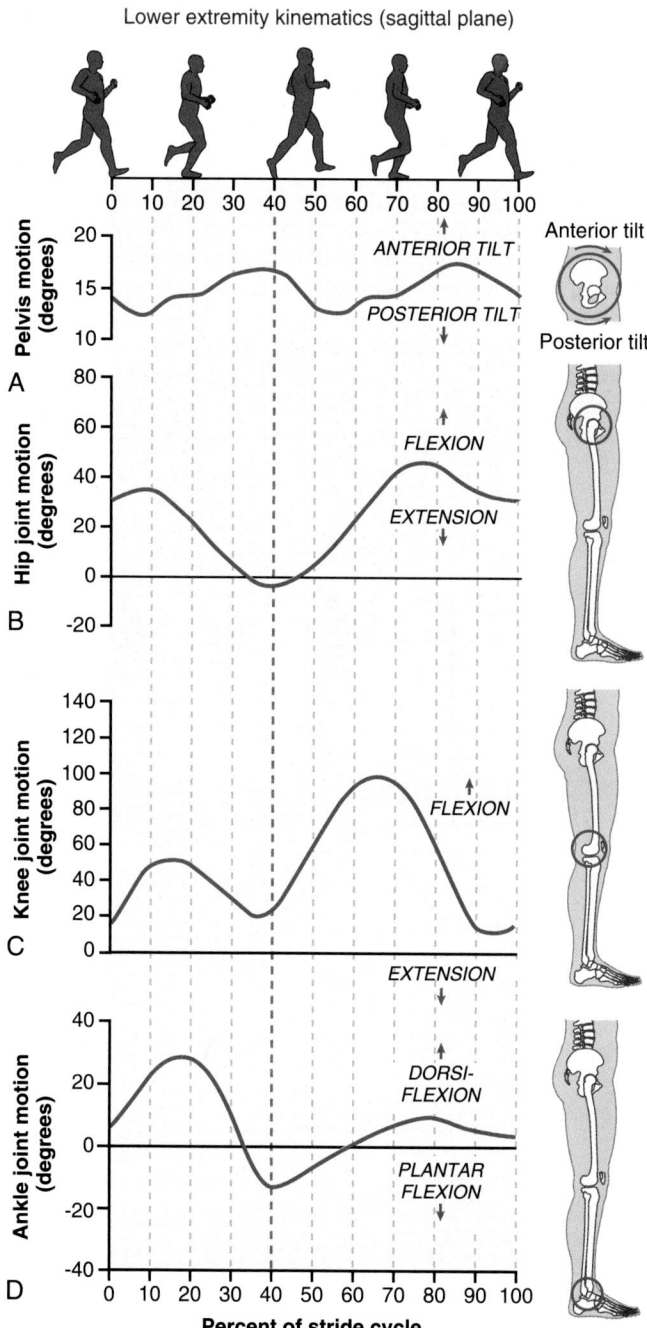

FIGURE 16.2 Sagittal plane angular rotations of the pelvis (A), hip (B), knee (C), and ankle (D) during the running stride cycle. The angle of the pelvis is defined relative to the vertical plane, not another body segment, whereas the remainder of measurements are joint angles defined as the relative relationship between adjacent segments or bones. (Data are a compilation from the literature and original sources.[31,45,54,122])

5 degrees.[79] Throughout the running stride cycle, the pelvis demonstrates an average anterior tilt position of 15 to 20 degrees,[120] which is greater than the 11 degrees of anterior tilt present during standing. Following initial contact, the pelvis posteriorly tilts until about 10% of the stride cycle, after which the pelvis anteriorly tilts, reaching a maximum at toe off. This motion cycle is repeated during the swing phase secondary to the demands placed on the pelvis from the contralateral limb during its stance phase.

HIP

The hip is flexed about 35 degrees at initial contact, and this flexion is maintained or slightly increased during the initial 10% of the stride cycle (see Fig. 16.2B and Video 16.1). After this initial period of flexion, the hip extends throughout the remainder of stance, reaching a maximum of 0 to 5 degrees of hip extension near toe off. The hip flexes during early swing to advance the limb forward, and then reverses into extension before the next initial contact to minimize loss of running speed. Although peak hip flexion increases with increases in lower range running speeds, it does not increase with speeds greater than 80% of maximum sprinting effort.

Based on casual visual observation, the position of the thigh may suggest the occurrence of greater hip extension than just described; however, this would be an inaccurate assessment. Sagittal plane rotation of the hip is defined by the position of the thigh relative to the pelvis. As such, the position of anterior-posterior tilt of the pelvis will affect the hip angle. A good example of this is near toe off, when the pelvis is at maximum anterior tilt, resulting in less true hip extension than what is apparent just from the position of the thigh relative to the vertical.

KNEE

The knee displays a bimodal pattern of motion during the stride cycle, one during stance and one during swing phase (see Fig. 16.2C). The knee is flexed between 10 and 20 degrees at initial contact, reaching a maximum flexion angle of 45 to 50 degrees near mid stance. This knee flexion during loading response plays an important role in decelerating the descent of the body's center of mass. The knee extends throughout the second half of stance, reaching a minimum flexion angle of 20 degrees slightly before toe off. This motion pattern repeats during swing phase but involves a much greater maximum flexion angle of 100 to 120 degrees that occurs near mid swing (70% of the gait cycle). This amount of knee flexion during swing phase reduces the limb's mass moment of inertia by bringing the center of mass of the lower leg and foot closer to the hip's axis of rotation. In doing so, the energy required to advance the swing limb is reduced.

ANKLE

In keeping with the assumption of a rearfoot strike, the ankle (talocrural) joint is positioned in 0 to 5 degrees of dorsiflexion at initial contact (see Fig. 16.2D). (As traditionally described, a 90-degree shank-foot angle is considered 0 degrees of dorsiflexion.) The ankle then dorsiflexes to a maximum of 30 degrees near mid stance, as a result of the tibia advancing over the foot fixed to the ground. Throughout pre swing, the ankle plantar flexes to generate power for propulsion, reaching a maximum of 10 to 20 degrees of plantar flexion just after toe off. Throughout early swing, the ankle dorsiflexes at a slow angular velocity followed by gradual plantar flexion to reposition the foot in only slight dorsiflexion at subsequent initial contact.

FIRST METATARSOPHALANGEAL JOINT

Motion at the first metatarsophalangeal (MTP) joint is difficult to measure during running because of the movement speed and the obscurity that results from the use of footwear. Nonetheless, attempts have been made to quantify this motion.[86,144] At initial contact, the first MTP joint is extended 10 degrees but returns to a neutral position until heel off. After heel off, the first MTP joint gradually extends to commonly reach 30 degrees of extension just before toe off, with greater extension occurring with faster running speeds or when accelerating. Throughout the swing phase, the first MTP joint assumes a relatively neutral position.

Despite running having a greater stride length than walking, less extension of the first MTP joint is required at toe off (review Chapter 15). This may seem counterintuitive but is likely explained by the corresponding position of the knee and ankle. The knee flexion angle at toe off is greater during walking (35 degrees) compared with running (20–25 degrees), with similar hip extension and ankle plantar flexion angles. The lesser knee flexion at toe off during running, compared with walking, will require less extension of the first MTP.

Frontal Plane Kinematics

TRUNK

Trunk rotation in the frontal plane, typically referred to as lateral flexion, is assumed to occur about an anterior-posterior axis located at the lumbosacral junction. Measured relative to a vertical plane, the total amplitude of frontal plane trunk motion while running is approximately 10 degrees, with 5 degrees in each direction.[120] Maximum lateral flexion coincides with ipsilateral initial foot contact.

PELVIS

Rotation or lateral tilt of the pelvis in the frontal plane is measured relative to the horizontal plane with neutral (0 degrees) occurring when the left and right iliac crests are level. The pelvis laterally tilts approximately 10 degrees in the frontal plane during a running stride cycle (Fig. 16.3A).[79] At initial contact, the iliac crest on the stance limb is slightly elevated relative to the contralateral iliac crest, with this position commonly referred to as contralateral tilt; that is, the pelvis is laterally tilted toward the contralateral (swing) side. Contralateral tilt increases during loading response, reaching a maximum position just before mid stance, after which the direction of rotation reverses. The pelvis laterally tilts toward the stance limb (ipsilateral tilt), reaching a maximum position at toe off. This motion cycle repeats during the swing phase because of the demands placed on the pelvis from the contralateral limb during its stance phase.

HIP

At initial contact, the hip is positioned in slight adduction and continues to adduct until reaching a maximum value (8–10 degrees) immediately before mid stance (see Fig. 16.3B and Video 16.2).

Maximum hip adduction is approximately 3 degrees more among females than males[45,121] and tends to increase with running speed.[32] During the remainder of stance, the hip abducts and remains so during early swing, returning to an adducted position during late swing and subsequent initial contact.

The movement of the pelvis largely contributes to the motion of the hip in the frontal plane during running, and this is clearly evident in the timing of the peaks. For example, peak hip adduction and contralateral tilt of the pelvis occur synchronously near mid stance. Likewise, frontal plane rotations of the hip that occur during swing phase coincide with those of the pelvis in response to the contralateral stance limb. While similar patterns and timing of motion are present, the greater amplitude of motion at the hip, compared with the pelvis, indicates that frontal plane motion of the femur is also present during running.

Much attention has been paid to the frontal plane kinematics of the hip during stance phase in regard to running-related injuries of the lower extremities. In particular, excessive (greater than ≈12 degrees) peak hip adduction during the stance phase of running has been associated with a greater risk of developing patellofemoral joint pain.[99] Of interest, runners with patellofemoral joint pain have been taught to reduce their excessive hip adduction during running, resulting in a substantial reduction in their symptoms.[100] This reduction in excessive hip adduction can be achieved through either better control of pelvic or femoral motion, or both.

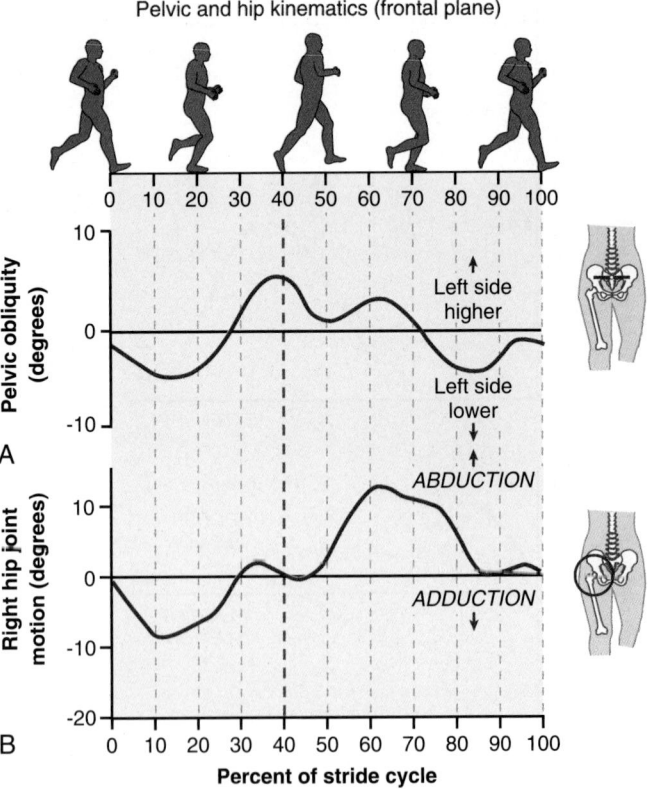

FIGURE 16.3 Frontal plane angular rotations of the pelvis (A) and hip (B) during a running stride cycle. During loading response on the right limb, the left side of the pelvis becomes lower than the right side, creating an oblique alignment that is commonly termed contralateral tilt. Because hip joint rotation is partially defined by motion at the pelvis, this contralateral tilt will contribute to the corresponding hip adduction of the stance limb. (Data are a compilation from the literature and original sources.[54,122])

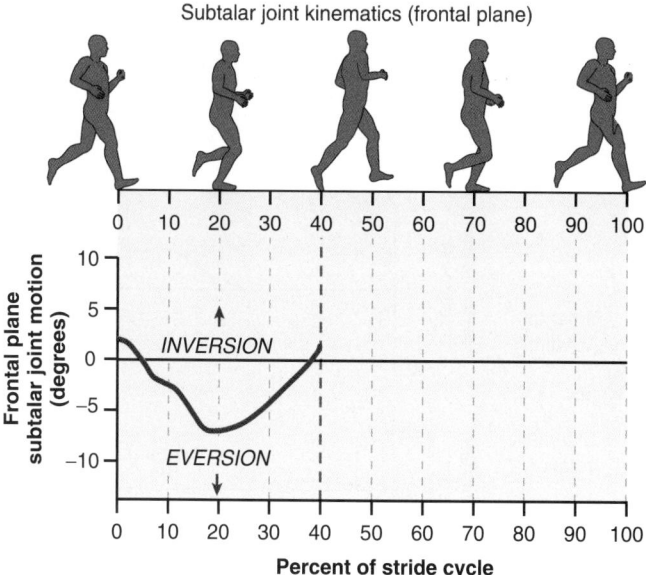

Subtalar joint kinematics (frontal plane)

FIGURE 16.4 Motion of the subtalar joint during stance phase as determined by the frontal plane orientation of the calcaneus relative to the lower leg. Rearfoot eversion is commonly used as a surrogate measure of subtalar joint pronation. (Data are a compilation from the literature and original sources.[28,84,113])

KNEE

Motion of the knee in the frontal plane during running is minimal, inconsistent, and difficult to assign a direction. Joint kinematics derived from pins inserted into the femur and tibia have revealed a total frontal plane motion of about 5 degrees during the stance phase.[114] Several studies have attempted to define frontal plane motion at the knee using skin-mounted reflective markers;[45,83,109] however, caution should be used when interpreting these data because there is poor agreement between skin and bone marker derived knee joint motion in this plane.[114]

SUBTALAR JOINT

Consistent with Chapter 15, frontal plane motion of eversion and inversion at the subtalar joint is considered to be representative of the more global motions of foot pronation and supination, respectively. At the time of initial contact, the position of the subtalar joint varies considerably across individuals, ranging from 5 degrees of inversion to 10 degrees of eversion.[83,113] Despite the variation in position at initial contact, a common pattern of motion is nevertheless present throughout stance phase (Fig. 16.4). The subtalar joint everts during initial stance, reaching peak eversion at 16% of the stride cycle (40% of stance phase). Peak eversion angle can range from 5 to 20 degrees and is largely related to the position of the subtalar joint at initial contact, such that *total* excursion from initial contact to peak eversion is about 10 degrees.[83] During the remainder of stance phase, the subtalar joint inverts to reach a similar position to that of initial contact at toe off.

Horizontal Plane Kinematics

TRUNK

While considering the trunk as a rigid single segment may be appropriate when measuring sagittal and frontal plane motions during

Is Treadmill Running Different Than Running Over Ground?

Assessing an individual's running mechanics, using video cameras or other technology, is typically done during either treadmill or over ground running. In a clinical setting, the choice between the two is often determined based on practicality and feasibility. The primary advantage for performing an over ground analysis is *ecological validity.* That is, most runners run the majority of their distance over ground and not on a treadmill, making over ground running the more natural setting. This is an important consideration, because the analysis needs to capture the runner's typical running mechanics to determine whether these mechanics may be contributing to injury. However, several logistical issues make the analysis of over ground running mechanics challenging, including maintenance of a constant running speed; location of the runner relative to the camera to prevent perspective and parallax errors; and capture of a sufficient number of stride cycles to represent the runner's typical mechanics. Although the use of a treadmill can address all of these issues, additional factors need to be considered such as the runner being comfortable on a treadmill; sufficient stiffness of the treadmill deck to mimic over ground running; and adequate motor power to ensure a constant speed of the treadmill belt. Although it is often assumed that biomechanics are dramatically different when running on a treadmill compared with over ground, if the prior list of factors is addressed, the differences are generally minor.[116]

running, it is not for horizontal plane motions. The amplitude of horizontal plane motions is much less in the lower portion than in the upper portion of the trunk. This is due, in part, to the differing restrictions inherent to the apophyseal joints in the lumbar and thoracic regions (review Chapter 9). Furthermore, horizontal plane motions of the lower trunk are more constrained by the pelvis and lower limb, both of which move opposite to the directions of motion of the trunk and upper limb. As such, horizontal motions of the lower and upper regions of the trunk are often measured separately.

Horizontal plane rotation of the lower trunk (i.e., lumbar spine) demonstrates one sinusoidal oscillation for each running stride cycle, with equal rotation to the left and right. Maximum rotation to the right occurs just before initial contact of the right limb, with continuous rotation to the left occurring throughout stance phase.[122] Maximum rotation to the left is achieved immediately after toe off of the right limb, with right rotation occurring throughout swing phase. The total amplitude of motion is approximately 20 degrees, with about 10 degrees in each direction. However, this amplitude of motion as measured using skin markers may be an overestimate; motion amplitude values acquired with pins surgically attached to bone indicate the total magnitude to be approximately 5 degrees.[79] Thus, the total horizontal plane rotation required of the lower trunk during running is well within the physiologic limits expected at the lumbar spine. Horizontal plane motion of the upper trunk (i.e., thoracic spine) displays the same pattern of motion as the lower trunk but with three times more total amplitude of motion.[79]

PELVIS

The horizontal plane rotation of the pelvis is largely out of phase with that of the trunk. At initial contact of the right limb, the left anterior-superior iliac spine (ASIS) is forward of the right ASIS and continues to rotate forward, reaching a maximum just before mid stance. Relative to the right limb, the pelvis is rotating clockwise as viewed from above, or more commonly termed external rotation of the pelvis (Fig. 16.5A). The pelvis then internally rotates through the remainder of stance phase, achieving a neutral position at toe off. Maximum internal rotation (i.e., left ASIS moves backward relative to the right ASIS) occurs near mid swing, which corresponds to mid stance on the contralateral limb. The pelvis rotates 10 to 15 degrees in the horizontal plane, with equal amounts of internal and external rotation.[122]

The position of the pelvis at initial contact when running is quite different than its position when walking, and this contrast is worth highlighting. Because of double-limb support during walking, the pelvis is *internally* rotated (the contralateral ASIS located posterior to the ASIS of the limb making initial contact) at foot contact to effectively create a longer step length. During running, however, the pelvis is no longer required to act as a pivot point to extend the step length, because the contralateral limb is not fixed to the earth. Instead, at initial contact, the pelvis is *externally* rotated (contralateral ASIS located anterior to the ASIS of the limb making initial contact) with the purposes of minimizing a loss of running speed and aiding advancement of the swing limb.[120]

HIP

Estimates of horizontal plane rotation of the hip tend to vary across studies and between individuals; however, some general conclusions can be made. First, the total amplitude of hip motion across the stride cycle is approximately 10 degrees (see Fig. 16.5B). Second, several direction changes of small amplitude occur primarily during the swing phase, the functional relevance of which is not known. Finally, despite these frequent oscillations, the average hip rotation angle across the entire stride cycle is near 0 degrees or neutral.

The horizontal plane rotation of the hip during loading response appears to be the most variable. Some studies have suggested the hip is externally rotated at initial contact and internally rotates throughout loading response,[121] whereas others have observed the hip to be internally rotated at initial contact with minimal subsequent rotation occurring during loading response.[32,45]

KNEE

Similar to knee motion in the frontal plane, precise measurements of knee motion in the horizontal plane while running require markers affixed directly to the femur and tibia. Such measures have demonstrated that the knee internally rotates 5 to 10 degrees during the initial half of stance phase, with a similar magnitude of external rotation during the latter half of stance.[114] Although the pattern is generally consistent across individuals, the magnitude of motion can vary substantially, with some runners showing no appreciable motion.[45,114]

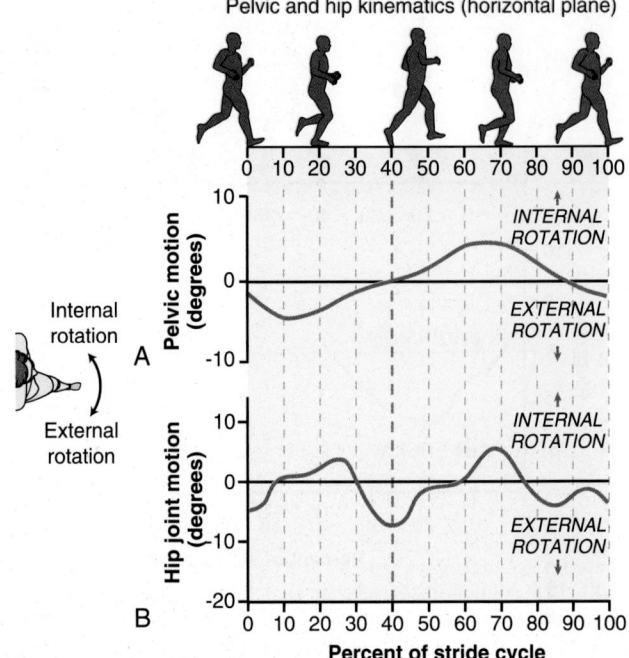

FIGURE 16.5 Horizontal plane angular rotations of the pelvis (A) and hip (B) during a running stride cycle. (Data are a compilation from the literature and original sources.[45,54,122])

Upper Extremity

Arm swing of the upper extremities during running provides important metabolic and biomechanical benefits. For instance, running without arm swing increases the rate of metabolic energy consumption by at least 3% compared with running with arm swing.[7] In the absence of arm swing, increased horizontal plane rotation of the pelvis, by up to 100%,[7] is needed to offset the angular momentum of the lower limbs. The greater trunk muscle activity required to control this increase in pelvic rotation, in turn, carries a metabolic cost.

SHOULDER

Similar to walking, shoulder motion in the sagittal plane while running is sinusoidal and out of phase with the hip. Thus throughout stance phase the shoulder is flexing while the ipsilateral hip is extending, with the opposite pattern occurring during swing phase. At initial contact, the shoulder is extended approximately 40 degrees and then progressively flexes during stance phase to approximately 10 degrees of flexion near toe off. The shoulder then returns to 40 degrees of extension during swing phase in preparation for the subsequent initial contact. The magnitude of shoulder motion is quite variable across individuals and is influenced by the running stride length. That is, the longer the stride length, the greater the shoulder motion.

ELBOW

Throughout the running stride cycle, the elbows are held near 90 degrees of flexion. Some motion may occur but is generally less than 30 degrees. By keeping the elbow flexed, the upper extremity's center of mass is located closer to the medial-lateral axis of the shoulder joint, thereby reducing the limb's mass moment of inertia.

CENTER OF MASS

Displacement of the Center of Mass

Similar to walking, the center of mass (CoM) of the body moves in vertical and side-to-side directions while running, although the timing and magnitude of the movements are quite different. In the vertical direction, the CoM is at its minimum height at mid stance of running, and at its maximum height during the middle of the float portion of early swing. This is quite different than walking, where the CoM is at its maximal height at mid stance and at its minimum height at the midpoint of double-limb support. Total vertical displacement of the CoM during running ranges from 5 to 10 cm, varying considerably with running speed, stride rate, and experience.[52,54,90,142]

The side-to-side movement of the CoM is largely reflective of the step width (i.e., greater side-to-side movement with greater step width). During running, step width is near zero, resulting in minimal side-to-side movement of the CoM.[5] Unlike walking, this suggests minimal need for active control of lateral balance during running.[6]

> **Displacement of the Center of Mass**
> - Total vertical displacement: 5 to 10 cm
> - Total side-to-side displacement: near 0 cm

Potential and Kinetic Energy Considerations

The vertical displacement of the body's CoM during running results in distinctly different mechanical energy fluctuations compared with walking. While running, the potential energy (reflective of the vertical position of the body's CoM) is at a minimum at mid stance and at a maximum at mid float during early swing. Similarly, the kinetic energy during running (predominantly a function of the body's vertical velocity) is also at a minimum at mid stance with its maximum occurring near mid float of early swing. Thus, potential energy and kinetic energy are *in-phase* during running: an arrangement that is only 5% effective at conserving the mechanical energy required to lift and accelerate the CoM.[43] Instead, the running body relies more on the storage and release of energy in elastic tissues, such as tendons, to effectively conserve mechanical energy.

ENERGY EXPENDITURE

The relationship between metabolic energy (as measured by oxygen consumption relative to body mass) and speed is uniquely different for running than for walking. When expressed relative to distance traveled (mL/kg/m), a U-shaped relationship exists between walking speed and energy expenditure, thereby allowing an optimum walking speed to be identified (refer to Fig. 15.26). During running, however, the energy cost to run a given distance is remarkably similar regardless of the speed, indicating a maintained economy of movement. It is unknown exactly how this is achieved, although several factors have been suggested including adjustments in stride length or cadence and sources of mechanical power.[24,27]

Running economy, defined as the metabolic energy demand for a given submaximal running speed (and measured by the rate of steady-state oxygen consumption), is highly variable across individuals. Even among trained runners with similar levels of aerobic fitness, running economy varies about 20% when running at the same speed.[142] Although factors such as age, sex, and environment can contribute to this variation,[89] a substantial portion of variation is believed to be a result of differences in body structure and running mechanics. For example, heavier individuals may have greater running economy per unit of body mass (mL/kg/min) than lighter individuals.[141] Similarly, individuals with less mass concentrated toward the distal lower limbs are likely to have greater running economy, because less muscular work is required to accelerate the lower limbs.[94]

Running mechanics associated with reduced running economy include excessive vertical displacement of the body's CoM,[142] excessive arm movement,[142] and increased posteriorly directed ground reaction forces during the initial half of stance phase.[72] Although runners routinely consider these factors during training, their associations to running economy tend to be moderate at best and are not consistently observed across studies. Furthermore, sagittal plane motions of the hip, knee, and ankle during the stance cycle do not have a clear relationship to running economy.[72] The variability in running economy between individuals does not appear to be explained by a small subset of biomechanical factors, but likely involves the interaction of many.[142] It is also important to remember that the majority of studies that investigated the energy cost of running involve well-trained or elite runners from a rather homogeneous pool of individuals.[118] Thus, these findings may have limited generalizability to the more diverse population of recreational runners.

MUSCLE ACTIVITY

All muscles of the lower extremity and trunk are active to varying amounts during portions of the running stride cycle. Measuring a muscle's activity with electromyography (EMG) gives clues of the muscle's role in controlling the corresponding kinematics (review topic of EMG in Chapter 3). Electromyographic electrodes placed on the skin surface are routinely used to record the activity of large, superficial muscles, whereas intramuscular (fine-wire) electrodes are needed to assess the activity of deeper muscles. The latter approach is technically challenging, which explains the paucity of EMG data in the literature for many of the deep muscles (e.g., hip deep external rotators); however, this should not be interpreted as an indication of their relative unimportance to running. On the contrary, these deep muscles likely play an important synergistic role with the larger more superficial muscles, helping to stabilize and control motion of the trunk and lower extremity joints.

Electromyography allows the activity pattern of muscles to be determined across a stride cycle. The EMG data indicate when a muscle is "on" and "off" (duration) and its relative level of activation (neural drive) throughout the stride cycle. Similar to data related to walking, the reference standard used to define a muscle's relative activation is most often its maximum EMG signal intensity during the running stride cycle. Figs. 16.6A and 16.6B use this reference for each muscle's illustrated EMG signal. Although the intensity of the muscle's activity can be determined, this does not necessarily equate to the amount of muscle force. During movements such as running, complex neuromusculoskeletal computer models are needed to estimate muscle force, where EMG is only one of the commonly used measurements input into these models.

For many human movements, a muscle's activation period corresponds almost exactly with a particular joint movement. However, while running, a muscle often becomes active well before its primary intended function. For example, muscles that are eccentrically active during loading response commonly become active during late swing (80%–100% of the stride cycle). Given the considerable magnitude and rate of loading during initial contact, this preceding muscle activity allows the muscle to be more responsive to the impending demands.[72] The muscle's increased activity before initial contact allows for its force production (and corresponding joint torque and power absorption) to reach a greater level sooner than if the muscle did not activate until initial contact. This is an excellent example of the neuromuscular system developing a pattern of activation specific to the demands of the task. Throughout this entire section on Muscle Activity the reader is strongly encouraged to consult the EMG tracings contained in Fig. 16.6A and Fig. 16.6B.

Trunk

During running, muscles of the trunk have similar roles as during walking, but higher angular velocities, greater potentially destabilizing ground reaction forces, and greater rate and depth of breathing all require higher magnitudes of activation.

ERECTOR SPINAE

The erector spinae that cross the lower thoracic and upper lumbar regions have a biphasic activation pattern, with each burst corresponding to initial contact of each limb (Fig. 16.6A).[22,119] These two bursts of activity control the forward angular momentum of the trunk relative to the pelvis as the foot contacts the unyielding ground. The right and left erector spinae show simultaneous activity.

RECTUS ABDOMINIS

The rectus abdominis displays two distinct periods of activity, although both being of relatively low amplitude. The first period precedes initial contact and lasts until 20% of the stride cycle. The second period occurs from 40% to 70% of the stride cycle, which corresponds to the initial half of stance phase of the contralateral limb.[22] Considering the low level of activity and existing forward momentum of the trunk, it is unlikely that the rectus abdominis is responsible for the prevailing flexed posture of the trunk occurring at this time. Instead, the rectus abdominis activity is thought to be synergistic with the deeper abdominal muscles (such as internal oblique and transversus abdominis) to control and stabilize trunk motion in the horizontal plane and provide support for the abdominal viscera.[61]

Hip

HIP EXTENSORS

The *gluteus maximus* is active before initial contact to initiate hip extension and prepare for loading response. The muscle exhibits its greatest EMG signal early in the period of loading response, peaking between 5% and 10% of the stride cycle.[33,40] The gluteus maximus is briefly active eccentrically following initial contact to decelerate the downward velocity of the body. The muscle becomes concentrically active until mid stance (20% of the stride cycle) to support the

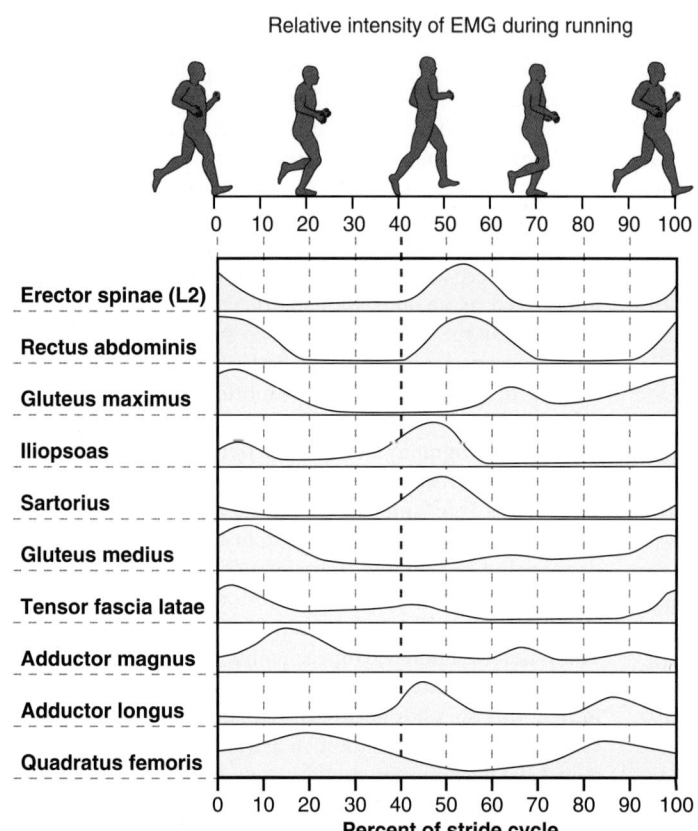

Relative intensity of EMG during running

FIGURE 16.6 (A, B) An electromyographic (EMG) illustration of the relative intensity of muscle activation during running. Different running speeds were used across the studies (2.9 m/sec to 4.62 m/sec), which may influence the magnitude of activity but have minimal effect on the pattern of activity. As such, the Y axis depicts the relative intensity of muscle activation for each muscle as a proportion of the maximum value obtained during the stride cycle. Based on this scaling, while all muscles nearly fill the full vertical scale of their graph, in reality, some muscles, such as the rectus abdominis, are actually only minimally active. Due to this method of scaling the Y axis, it is not possible to compare actual EMG intensities of different muscles across the running stride. (EMG data are obtained from a compilation of several sources, including Cappellini et al, 2006[22]; Chumanov et al, 2012[33]; Semciw et al, 2015[126]; Gazendam and Hof, 2007[48]; Reber et al, 1993[112]; and Andersson et al, 1997.[3] The general patterns of muscle activity are consistent with data reported in other studies.[40,53,88,138])

Figure continued on page 11

body and produce hip extension.[53] Perhaps seeming counterintuitive, the gluteus maximus is virtually inactive throughout the remainder of stance during the time of propulsion—a function driven primarily by the ankle plantar flexors. The gluteus maximus continues mostly inactive during early swing, then becomes eccentrically active again during late swing to decelerate hip flexion before initiating hip extension.[22,33,53,75]

The magnitude of gluteus maximus activity increases substantially during swing phase with running speed, which corresponds to the increased eccentric demands placed on the muscle to decelerate the advancing limb. In particular, peak forces required of the gluteus maximus during the swing phase have been estimated to increase by a factor of 3 when running speed increases from 3.5 m/sec to 7.0 m/sec and by a factor of 6 when speed increases to 9.0 m/sec.[40] Thus, the contributions of the gluteus maximus are much more significant at running speeds more commonly associated with sprinting than distance running.

Altered activity of the gluteus maximus during running is often associated with common running-related injuries, notably patellofemoral joint pain (see Clinical Connection 16.1). However, at present, the EMG literature fails to uncover a pattern of muscle activity that is consistent for individuals with and without injury.[12]

The *adductor magnus* shows a peak activity near mid stance. Given its favorable biomechanics for generating an extension torque when the hip is flexed (review Chapter 12), the adductor magnus is likely active to augment hip extension torque.[48,88]

The *hamstring muscles* (i.e., biceps femoris, semimembranosus, and semitendinosus) are also active before initial contact and remain active until about 30% of the stride cycle.[22,33,40,127] However, the relative contribution of these muscles to overall hip extension during this portion of the stride cycle is about half as much as the contribution from the gluteus maximus.[40] The hamstrings remain virtually inactive until 70% of the stride cycle, reaching an overall peak activity at 85% to 90% of the stride cycle. This burst of eccentric activity is the primary contributor to decelerating hip flexion before initiating hip extension before the subsequent initial contact.[40]

HIP FLEXORS

The *iliopsoas* is active primarily before and after toe off, corresponding to 30% to 60% of the stride cycle.[22] Through toe off, the iliopsoas is eccentrically active, immediately followed by concentric activity just after toe off and into early swing.[75] This pattern of eccentric activation immediately preceding a concentric contraction is termed a "stretch-shortening" cycle and results in an enhanced force of contraction attributable to the combined effects of stretch reflex and elastic energy storage within the tendon.[71,110,131] Peak activity of the iliopsoas occurs just after toe off, corresponding to the muscle's estimated peak force, initiating hip flexion and accelerating the limb forward.[75] As running speed increases, the magnitude of activity and associated force output of the iliopsoas also increases within this period.[3,40]

The *rectus femoris* and *sartorius* assist with hip flexion during early swing.[3] However, because these muscles cross multiple joints, their total contribution to running may be more complex.[75]

HIP ABDUCTORS

The *gluteus medius* activation pattern during running is quite similar to that of the gluteus maximus. That is, the muscle is active before initial contact to prepare for loading response and remains active through most of stance phase.[33,40] The muscle is eccentrically active during loading response to control hip adduction (review Fig. 16.3),

reaching peak activity by 10% of the stride cycle, after which the gluteus medius is concentrically active to produce hip abduction during the remainder of its active period in stance. This period of activity during stance phase corresponds to substantial force production by the gluteus medius and has been estimated to exceed the forces of any other muscle crossing the hip.[75] The muscle remains inactive for the last part of stance phase and through swing until 80% of the stride cycle when a gradual increase in activity is observed in preparation for the subsequent foot contact.

The EMG patterns of the *gluteus minimus* during running are largely similar to that of the gluteus medius.[102] Interestingly, the anterior portion of the gluteus minimus has a second burst of activity during early swing, which likely contributes to hip flexion and hip joint stabilization.[102] Activity patterns of the *tensor fasciae latae* during running obtained by intramuscular electrodes reveal a low level of activity from the muscle from 0% to 60% of the stride cycle.[3] Being a primary hip abductor (review Chapter 12), the tensor fascia latae is likely assisting the gluteus medius and minimus in controlling frontal plane mechanics of the stance limb.

HIP ADDUCTORS AND ROTATORS

Limited EMG information is available for the adductor and rotator muscles of the hip while running. The adductor magnus and longus generally show low-level activity throughout much of the stride cycle. The *adductor magnus* shows a primary peak activity near mid stance, likely to assist with hip extension.[48] Conversely, the *adductor longus* displays its peak activity during early swing, most likely to assist with initiating hip flexion.[22]

The *quadratus femoris*, a deep external rotator, is also generally active through the stride cycle but displays two distinct bursts of activity during stance phase and late swing.[126] Regarded as an important hip external rotator,[62] this muscle likely acts eccentrically to control hip internal rotation during the loading response, as well as to stabilize the femoral head within the acetabulum throughout the stance phase. During the late swing phase, the role of the quadratus femoris is to provide joint stability while the larger hip extensors (e.g., hamstrings) produce substantial extension torques.

Knee

KNEE EXTENSORS

All four heads of the quadriceps (i.e., *rectus femoris, vastus lateralis, vastus intermedius,* and *vastus medialis*) display a burst of activity that precedes initial contact and lasts until 20% of the stride cycle (Fig. 16.6B).[33,88] These muscles are most active, however, during the loading response to eccentrically control knee flexion and support the body's CoM (review Fig. 16.2C).[53,88] The rectus femoris shows a second burst of activity from 40% to 60% of the stride cycle to aid in hip flexion. At 80% of the stride cycle, all four components of the quadriceps become active in preparation for foot contact with the ground.

KNEE FLEXORS

Each of the hamstring muscles shows a similar activation pattern across the running stride cycle.[22,33,88] The hamstrings display a low-to-moderate level of activity throughout the stance phase, as they contribute to hip extension. During early swing, the muscles are essentially inactive with a second and larger burst of activity beginning at 70% and peaking near 90% of the stride cycle.

Relative intensity of EMG during running

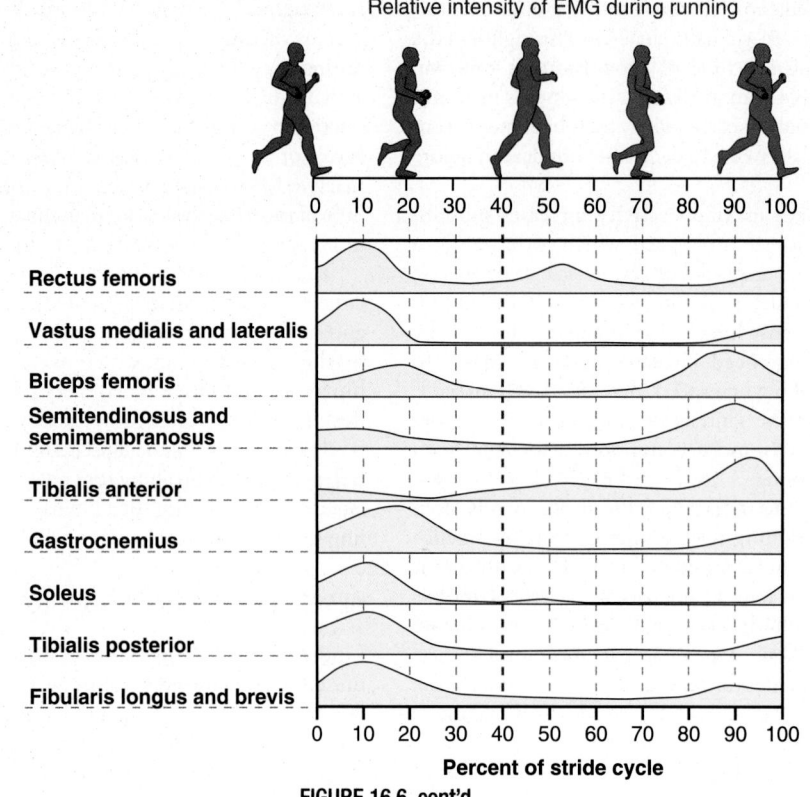

FIGURE 16.6. cont'd.

The primary purpose of this second period of activity is to decelerate knee extension, thereby properly positioning the limb for the impending foot contact with the ground. It is during this part of the stride cycle that the hamstring muscles are most susceptible to a strain injury, especially during high-speed running.[56] The high inertial loads placed on the muscles combined with having to operate in a lengthened position, a combination of hip flexion and knee extension, are responsible for this increased injury risk (see Clinical Connection 16.2).[29]

Ankle-and-Foot

TIBIALIS ANTERIOR

A low level of activity from the tibialis anterior is evident immediately after initial contact to control the lowering of the forefoot to the ground.[33,48] The magnitude of this activity will be greatest in runners using a rearfoot strike because of the increased angle of the foot relative to the ground. The tibialis anterior is most active during swing phase. A small burst of concentric activity occurs during early swing to initiate ankle dorsiflexion after toe off and enable the foot to clear the ground as the limb swings forward. Despite minimal ankle motion, peak activity of the tibialis anterior is present during late swing. This activity is simultaneous with that of the ankle plantar flexors and is present to stiffen the ankle joint in anticipation of the subsequent initial contact.

GASTROCNEMIUS AND SOLEUS

The gastrocnemius and soleus muscles display a nearly identical pattern of activity. Both muscles are active before initial contact and

reach a peak near mid stance.[33] The soleus appears to reach its peak activity slightly before the gastrocnemius.[22,40,53] From 10% to 20% of the stride cycle, these muscles are functioning eccentrically to control ankle dorsiflexion as the tibia rotates over the foot that is fixed on the ground. From mid stance until toe off, the gastrocnemius and soleus are active concentrically to rapidly plantar flex the ankle during pre swing and propel the body forward. Both muscles remain inactive throughout the swing phase until just before the subsequent foot contact.

If a runner uses a forefoot strike, the previous pattern of activity is essentially the same with the exception of a greater level of activity of both muscles immediately before and following initial contact. With a forefoot strike, the force of the ground causes the ankle to rapidly dorsiflex. The ankle plantar flexors therefore naturally respond eccentrically at initial contact, resulting in greater total load incurred by these muscles during each stride, potentially increasing their risk of injury, as well as the injury risk to the Achilles tendon.

TIBIALIS POSTERIOR

Given the anatomic location and depth of this muscle, intramuscular electrodes are required to accurately assess its EMG signal intensity. The few studies that have investigated the activity of the tibialis posterior during running have shown that it remains active essentially throughout the entire stance phase.[104,112] Similar to many other muscles of the lower leg and ankle, the tibialis posterior becomes active just *before* initial contact. This timing ensures that the muscle has adequate time to reach its peak activation by 10% to 20% of the stride cycle. This period of activity coincides with subtalar joint eversion, indicating that the tibialis posterior is active eccentrically during the initial half of stance phase to control foot eversion. From mid stance through toe off, the muscle switches to a concentric activation to initiate subtalar joint inversion in conjunction with the windlass mechanism resulting from extension of the first MTP joint (see Fig. 14.40A). The tibialis posterior is electrically quiet throughout the swing phase, until just before the subsequent foot contact.

FIBULARIS MUSCLES

Similar to the tibialis posterior, the fibularis (peroneus) longus and brevis are active throughout late swing and the entire stance phase.[13,112] Peak activity occurs near 15% of the stride cycle, near the time of peak subtalar joint eversion. As the fibularis muscles are primary foot evertors, it would seem that these muscles may be functioning concentrically to *produce* subtalar joint eversion. However, because the ground reaction force at this point in the running cycle is producing an external eversion torque at the subtalar joint, the need for additional muscle-induced eversion torque is questionable. Therefore it seems plausible that during early stance the fibularis muscles are acting synergistically with the tibialis posterior to provide medial-lateral stability to the subtalar joint, while also contributing to control the rate of ankle dorsiflexion.

KINETICS

Ground Reaction Forces

During the stance phase, the ground exerts forces onto the runner through the foot. These ground reaction forces (GRFs) have been postulated to be associated with many running-related injuries and have therefore long been a primary consideration in the design of running shoes. These forces act on and are directed toward the body's CoM. By convention, the GRFs are expressed along three orthogonal axes: vertical, anterior-posterior, and medial-lateral.

VERTICAL FORCES

The vertical ground reaction force is the largest, reaching an overall peak near 20% of the stride cycle, with a magnitude of approximately 2.5 times body weight (Fig. 16.7C and Video 16.3). This overall peak, termed *active peak,* is associated with the end of the loading response. The magnitude of active peak exceeds body weight as a result of the ground decelerating the downward movement of the body. Before active peak, an additional smaller peak of about 1.5 times body weight is commonly present, often termed *impact peak.* Impact peak, typically reaching about 60% of active peak, occurs at approximately 5% of the stride cycle.

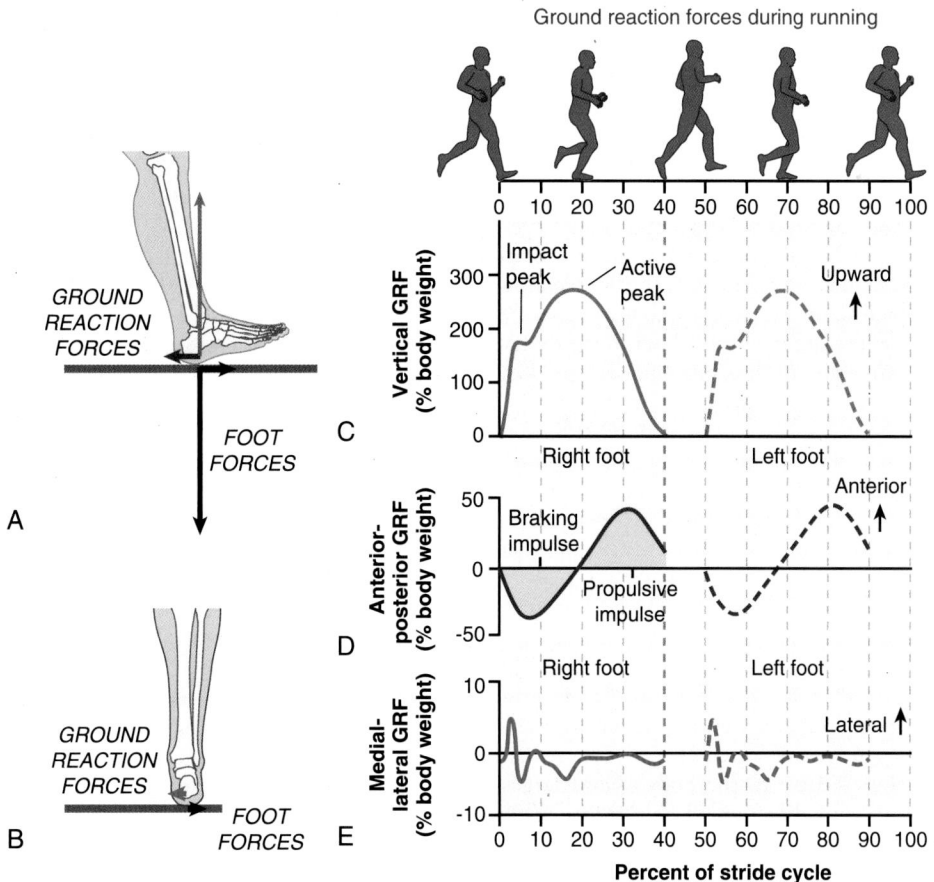

FIGURE 16.7 Ground reaction forces (GRFs) during running. Panel A illustrates the vertical *(orange arrow)* and anterior-posterior GRFs *(red arrow)* and the corresponding foot forces *(black arrows)* at 5% of the stride cycle. Panel B illustrates the medial-lateral forces at 5% of the stride cycle. Panels C–E show the GRFs for a stride cycle. Dashed lines are forces present during stance phase of the left limb.

The impact peak imparts an immediate distal-to-proximal compression force from the leg to the head.[35] This impact force is characterized by its magnitude, as well as its rate of development (loading rate). Impact forces increase when running downhill, with a slower step rate (cadence), and with a pronounced rearfoot strike.[36,44,50,54] High impact forces are commonly believed to be associated with overuse injuries in runners, such as stress fractures of the tibia and metatarsals.[63] However, a closer look at the literature suggests that it may not be the peak magnitude of the impact that is most damaging, but rather the magnitude of the *rate* of loading (i.e., the slope of the vertical force).[147] As a matter of fact, typical vertical impact forces experienced by runners may have a beneficial physiologic effect by providing a stimulus for cartilage and bone growth. These forces are usually injurious only when combined with additional factors such as abnormal running kinematics, prolonged running duration, or insufficient rest.[35]

Vertical Ground Reaction Forces
- Impact peak: initial peak vertical force occurring near 5% of the stride cycle
- Active peak: overall peak vertical force occurring near 20% of the stride cycle

---

ANTERIOR-POSTERIOR FORCES

The anterior-posterior component of the GRF is considerably smaller than the vertical component (Fig. 16.7D and Video 16.3). During the first half of stance phase, it is directed posteriorly, with the area under the force-time curve referred to as the *braking impulse*. This posteriorly directed force and corresponding impulse decelerate the CoM and slow its forward progression. The magnitudes of the peak posterior force and braking impulse are largely influenced by running speed, as well as by the horizontal distance between the foot at initial contact and the CoM. The farther ahead the foot is relative to the CoM, the greater the braking impulse.[140] For this reason, many runners place their foot closer to their CoM at initial contact as a way to reduce the braking impulse. One effective way to do this is to run with a reduced stride length.

From mid stance to toe off, the anterior-posterior GRF is directed anteriorly and serves to propel the body into swing phase *(propulsive impulse)*. When running at a constant velocity on level ground (0 degree inclination), the propulsive impulse will in theory equal the braking impulse. If one attempts to accelerate or run uphill, then the propulsive impulse needs to exceed the braking impulse.

MEDIAL-LATERAL FORCES

The medial-lateral component of the GRF is the smallest in magnitude (i.e., less than 10% of body weight) and the most variable between individuals (Fig. 16.7E and Video 16.4).[26] The medial-lateral location of the foot relative to the body's CoM largely determines the magnitude and direction of this force. While running, the foot is placed nearly directly under the CoM due, in part, to the lack of double-limb support.[28] Similar to walking, a laterally directed GRF is present during the initial 5% of the stride cycle to resist the medial velocity of the foot at initial contact. Unlike walking, however, individuals run with a narrower step width, such that the foot is placed directly under the body's CoM and may even cross over to the opposite side. This narrow step width is commonly observed at fast running speeds including sprinting. When the foot is located under the CoM, the direction of the GRF will oscillate between medial and lateral during the stance phase. The minimal side-to-side movement of the CoM during running suggests a limited need for the active control of lateral balance.[6,28] A narrow step width during running minimizes the torque generated about the anterior-posterior axis of the body's CoM, thereby reducing the muscular effort required to counteract this external torque.

Path of the Center of Pressure

The type of foot strike influences the path of the center of pressure (CoP) under the foot during stance phase.[28] For runners who employ a rearfoot strike, the path of the CoP is very similar to that of walking (refer to Fig. 15.32). The path begins on the posterior-lateral aspect of the plantar surface of the heel at initial contact, and then quickly progresses anteriorly along the midline of the foot into the metatarsal region by 5% of the stride cycle.[17] During the remainder of stance, the CoP path continues anteriorly but at a slower rate, with a slight shift toward the medial aspect of the forefoot throughout the second half of stance and into toe off.

The path of the CoP differs when midfoot and forefoot strike patterns are used because these patterns do not involve the rearfoot contacting the ground.[17,28] Instead, the CoP typically starts near the lateral aspect of the plantar surface of the fifth metatarsal. Then, the CoP rapidly progresses toward the midline of the foot, to structures (i.e., bones, ligaments) better designed to handle the increasing GRFs. Not surprisingly, during the remainder of stance, the CoP largely follows the same path as described for a rearfoot strike.

Joint Torques and Powers

The same underlying principles regarding internal joint torques and powers during walking described in Chapter 15 apply to running. In brief, internal torques predominantly result from muscle-generated forces and provide insight into the role of these muscles in controlling a joint during running. Joint powers (the product of internal torque and joint angular velocity) reflect the rate of energy generation or absorption by muscles crossing a joint and indicate the type of muscle activation (i.e., concentric, eccentric). The area under the power curves reflects the amount of mechanical work performed at the joint over a specified time period, with negative work referring to eccentric activity and positive work to concentric activity. Also, realize that although the torques described and illustrated in the section are considered "internal" (i.e., generated by muscle and connective tissues), the modifier internal will not always be used.

Joint torques and powers provide considerable insights into the biomechanics of running, especially when used in combination with joint kinematics and EMG data. It is worth reminding that joint torque and power do not reflect the contribution and function of *individual* muscles, but all of the muscles (and other connective tissues) crossing the joint of interest. Determining individual contributions requires complex neuromusculoskeletal models that often involve data on muscle excitations, activation dynamics, musculotendon contraction mechanics, and segmental accelerations.[40,53,106,135]

SPECIAL FOCUS 16.2

What Is the Right Running Shoe for Me?

Running footwear has been traditionally prescribed based on the static foot posture of the individual. That is, individuals with a neutral or high medial longitudinal arch are advised to use a cushioned/neutral shoe; those with a moderately low arch are advised to use stability-type shoes; and those with an excessively low arch are advised to use motion control shoes. However, the clinical appropriateness of this algorithm has been challenged based on a lack of scientific evidence.[115] Indeed, a randomized controlled trial concluded that the current convention for prescribing running footwear is not appropriate.[117] Specifically, the study found that runners with neutral foot types may benefit more from a stability category shoe than a neutral shoe, because less running-related pain and fewer missed training days were reported for those using the stability shoe. Further, the study was unable to support the use of motion control shoes in runners with highly pronated feet, i.e., those with excessively low medial longitudinal arches.

Large-scale studies involving branches of the United States military have provided further evidence to question current running shoe prescription procedures.[67-70] In these studies, recruits were randomly assigned to wear either a shoe type matched to their static foot posture (cushioned/neutral shoes for high arches; stability shoes for medium arches; motion control shoes for low arches) or a stability shoe regardless of foot posture. No differences in injury rates were reported between the groups during the subsequent 12 weeks of basic training.

These prospective studies provide strong indication that prescribing running shoes based on foot posture has little influence on injury risk. Thus, if the goal is the prevention of running injuries, this extremely common selection strategy is flawed. While no validated algorithm yet exists to determine the appropriate shoe for an individual that will minimize injury risk while maintaining or improving performance, many have suggested that a runner's perception of comfort may be an important determinant.[91-93,96,98] That is, the shoe that an individual identifies as being comfortable to wear during running should possess the biomechanical features that are relevant to that person. For individuals with running-related injuries, there is no strong evidence either supporting or contradicting the commonly used clinical approach of shoe type prescription based on foot posture, and therefore this approach may still need to be considered.

HIP

In the *sagittal plane,* an extension torque is present at the hip during the initial 30% of the stride cycle primarily to provide vertical support to the body's CoM and to extend the hip (Fig. 16.8 and Video 16.5).[11] The initial portion of this torque (0%–10% of the stride cycle) is associated with power absorption, indicating the eccentric activation of the hip extensors to decelerate the brief hip flexion that occurs immediately after initial contact. The remainder of the extension torque (10%–30% stride cycle) involves power generation and a concentric activation of the hip extensors to extend the hip, therefore contributing to propulsion of the body.

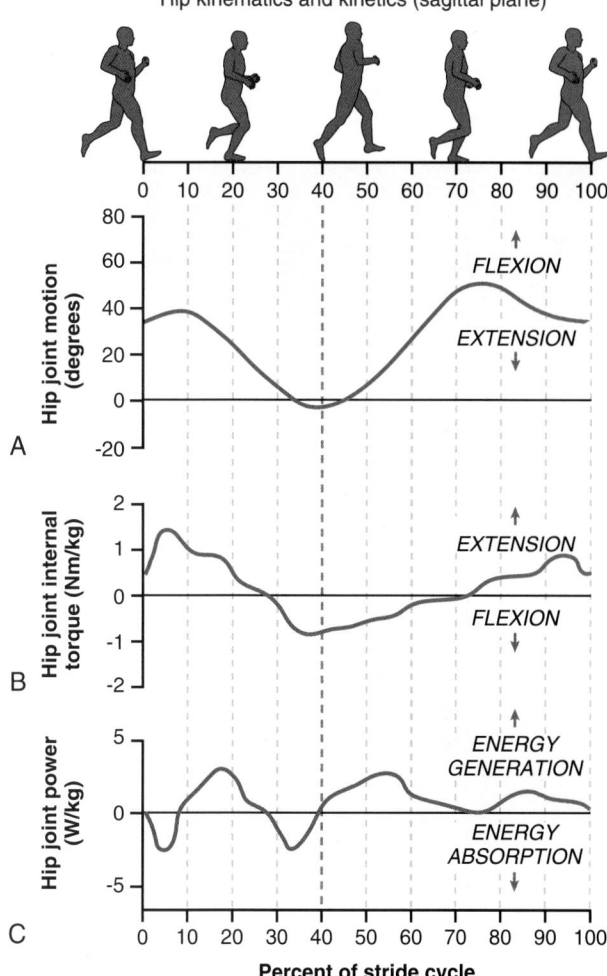

FIGURE 16.8 Sagittal plane hip motion (A), internal torques (B), and powers (C) for a running stride cycle. Torque and power values are normalized to body mass. (Data are a compilation from the literature and original sources.[54,123])

During pre swing and early swing, a hip flexion torque is present that is similarly comprised of a period of power absorption preceding power generation. The power absorption during pre swing reflects the deceleration of hip extension attributable to the eccentric activation of the hip flexors, as well as the passive tension generated by other connective tissues located about the hip. Immediately after toe off and throughout early swing, concentric activity of the hip flexors is associated with power generation needed to advance the limb forward. During late swing, a hip extension torque is needed to decelerate hip flexion and initiate hip extension in preparation for the imminent foot contact.

In the frontal plane, a large hip abduction torque is present throughout the stance phase, reaching a single peak near mid stance (Fig. 16.9 and Video 16.6). Power absorption is present during the initial portion of this torque, indicating eccentric activity of the hip abductors to decelerate and control hip adduction and the associated lowering of the contralateral side of the pelvis. The remainder of this torque involves the concentric activity of the hip abductors to raise the contralateral side of the pelvis and abduct the hip. Throughout swing phase, frontal plane hip torque and power are essentially zero.

Hip kinematics and kinetics (frontal plane)

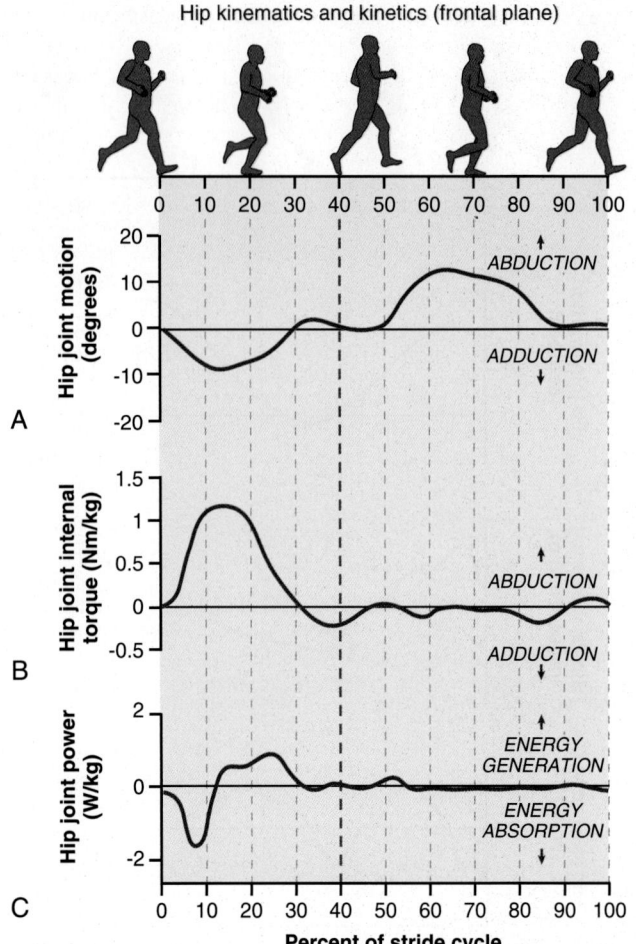

FIGURE 16.9 Frontal plane hip motion (A), internal torques (B), and powers (C) for a running stride cycle. Torque and power values are normalized to body mass. (Data are a compilation from the literature and original sources.[54,99,123])

Hip kinematics and kinetics (horizontal plane)

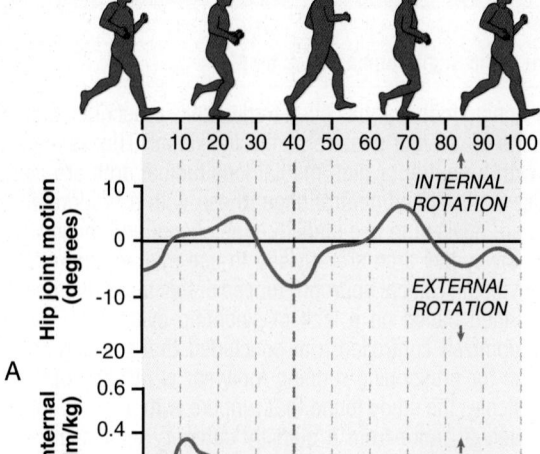

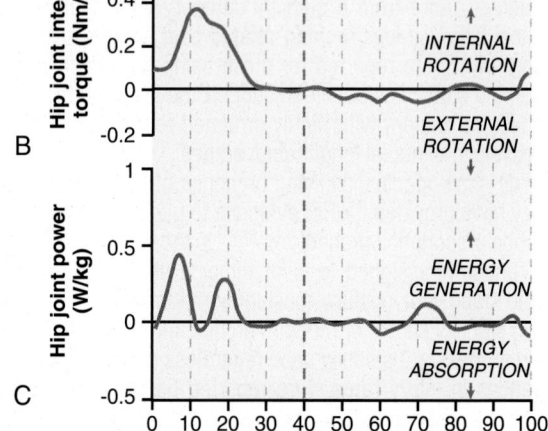

FIGURE 16.10 Horizontal plane hip motion (A), internal torques (B), and powers (C) for a running stride cycle. Torque and power values are normalized to body mass. (Data are a compilation from the literature and original sources.[54,123])

In the horizontal plane, an internal rotation torque is present at the hip during the initial 30% of the stride cycle (Fig. 16.10).[45,65,116,123,128] The peak magnitude of this internal torque is relatively small, less than 30% of the torques produced in the sagittal and frontal planes. Power generation is present, indicating concentric activity of the hip internal rotators to advance the contralateral side of the pelvis forward. As with the frontal plane, horizontal plane hip torque and power are essentially zero throughout pre swing and all of swing phase. Reported hip horizontal plane data are quite variable between publications, largely because of their small magnitudes, difficulty in accurately measuring kinematics, and the method of data processing.[23,40,45,54]

KNEE

In the sagittal plane, a very brief flexion torque is present at the knee for the initial 5% of the stride cycle and is associated with power generation (Fig. 16.11 and Video 16.5). This indicates the knee flexors are concentrically active during and immediately following initial contact, likely to ensure the knee is positioned in flexion for impact shock absorption. A much larger knee extension torque dominates the majority of stance phase, from 5% to 30% of the stride cycle. During loading response, this extension torque is associated with considerable power absorption to control knee flexion,

and has been suggested as a source of chronic knee pain and patellofemoral joint pain in distance runners.[54] Knee extension torque dictates the magnitude of patellofemoral joint loading: as the extension torque increases, so do the patellofemoral joint contact force and stress.[74,76] Running retraining strategies have been suggested to reduce the knee extension torque in runners with chronic knee pain by altering associated kinematic factors. Specifically, a shorter stride length, less peak knee flexion during stance, or an increase in average trunk flexion angle have each been recommended to reduce the demands on the quadriceps and resulting patellofemoral joint stress.[54,76,133]

From the end of loading response until the start of pre swing, the knee extensors are concentrically active to extend the knee and vertically support the CoM. During swing phase, a small extension torque is present at the knee during early swing to decelerate knee flexion, while a more prominent flexion torque occurs during late swing primarily to decelerate and control the amount of knee extension. At the very end of late swing, this same flexion torque generates power to position the knee for the subsequent foot contact.

In the *frontal plane,* an (internal) abduction torque is generally present at the knee during stance phase. This torque is required to balance the (external) adduction torque, as a result of the GRF passing medial to the knee (Video 16.7). The power curve is variable throughout stance, oscillating between generation and absorption, and is relatively small in magnitude because of the minimal frontal plane motion available at the knee. Despite the peak magnitude of the knee abduction torque being only about 30% of the peak sagittal plane torque, it has been associated with patellofemoral joint pain in runners.[129] Running with a slight increase in step width can reduce the knee abduction torque and thereby potentially reduce symptoms in runners with patellofemoral pain.[18] During the swing phase, frontal plane torques and powers remain near zero.

In the *horizontal plane,* knee joint torques and powers are quite small and variable. Generally, an external rotation torque is present throughout stance phase and is associated with a power curve that remains near zero.[45,85]

ANKLE-AND-FOOT

In the *sagittal plane,* a plantar flexion torque is present throughout the stance phase of running (Fig. 16.12 and Video 16.5). Until mid stance, the plantar flexors are eccentrically active to control the tibia advancing over the foot. During the second half of stance phase, the plantar flexors display concentric activity and are a major source of power generation used for forward propulsion. Of the total power generated during the second half of stance phase, 55% comes from the ankle compared with 35% from the knee and 10% from the hip.[54] During early swing, a small dorsiflexion torque is present to initiate ankle dorsiflexion after toe off and enable the foot to clear the ground as the limb swings forward. Throughout the remainder of swing phase, the ankle joint torque and power remain near zero.

Although Fig. 16.12B shows no dorsiflexion torque typically occurring during loading response, some persons will demonstrate a small dorsiflexion torque immediately following initial contact to control the lowering of the forefoot to the ground. This fairly atypical kinetic response tends to occur in runners who use a rearfoot strike with initial contact occurring at the most posterior aspect of the foot. Despite its relatively small magnitude, this dorsiflexion torque has been associated with *anterior exertional compartment syndrome* in runners. Removing this dorsiflexion torque by changing to a forefoot strike can reduce symptoms in runners with this condition.[37]

In the *frontal* and *transverse planes,* the torques and powers of the ankle-and-foot region are very small and variable during running. In the frontal plane, this variability may be related to the convention by which torques are defined and thereby calculated.[103] Nonetheless, a small inversion torque is typically present during the initial half of stance phase, with the subtalar joint invertors being eccentrically active to control subtalar joint eversion. The horizontal plane kinetics are rarely reported across the ankle-and-foot.

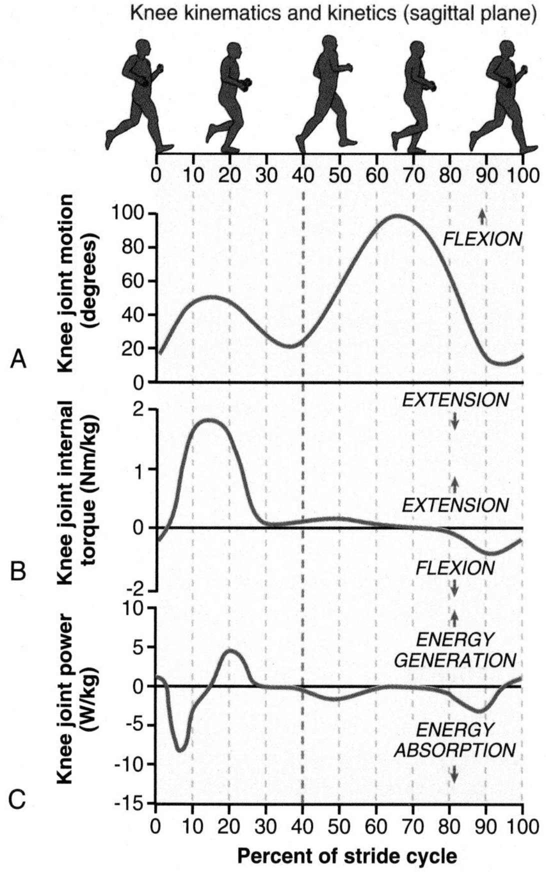

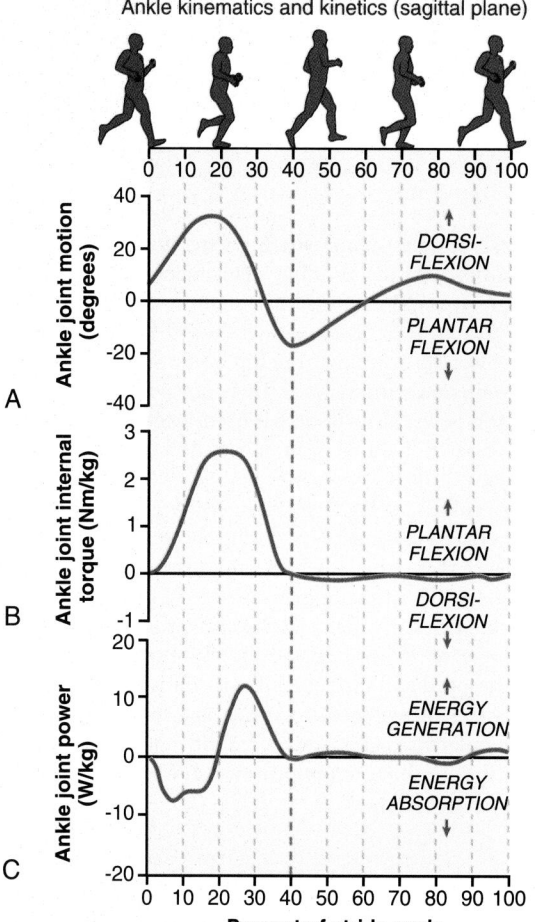

FIGURE 16.11 Sagittal plane knee motion (A), internal torques (B), and powers (C) for a running stride cycle. Torque and power values are normalized to body mass. (Data are a compilation from the literature and original sources.[14,54])

FIGURE 16.12 Sagittal plane ankle motion (A), internal torques (B), and powers (C) for a running stride cycle. Torque and power values are normalized to body mass. (Data are a compilation from the literature and original sources.[14,20,54])

FACTORS AFFECTING RUNNING MECHANICS

Age

Older and younger runners show consistent differences in running mechanics. The most common difference is the reduction in preferred running speed.[34] However, when older and younger runners are asked to run at the same speed, several biomechanical differences persist. For example, older male runners aged 55 to 65 years run with shorter steps and a higher step rate compared with their younger (20–35 years) counterparts.[21] The same differences were observed in runners aged 60 to 69 years, in addition to reductions in float time and vertical displacement of the body's CoM in that older group.[64] Despite these differences in spatiotemporal characteristics, older runners display a greater vertical GRF impact peak and loading rate, and a greater active peak, which suggests a loss of shock-absorbing capacity and a potential increase in susceptibility to lower extremity injuries.[21,64,78]

Although the knee joint torques are generally similar in magnitude between age groups, older runners consistently show a reduction in peak ankle plantar flexion torque and power generation at the ankle. Not surprisingly, injuries involving the calf muscles and Achilles tendon are quite common among older runners. A substantial increase in the knee (external) adduction torque among older female runners has also been observed, suggestive of an increased risk for development of medial knee osteoarthritis or similar conditions.[78] The cause of these age-related effects is unknown, but may be associated with changes in tissue properties, neuromuscular capacity, or metabolic cost.

Sex

In general, females demonstrate greater frontal and horizontal plane motions during running than males. Specifically, females exhibit greater peak hip internal rotation and adduction,[32,45] as well as greater peak knee abduction.[45,80] Females also display greater power absorption at the hip in the frontal and horizontal planes compared with males.[45] This increase in nonsagittal plane motion and power absorption has been suggested to contribute to the risk of patellofemoral joint pain and iliotibial band syndrome in females.

Gluteus maximus EMG signal intensity in females (normalized to the average muscle activity during the stride cycle) is approximately twice that of males when running at the same speed.[32] Furthermore, females display a greater increase in gluteus medius and vastus lateralis activity than males as either running speed or surface incline increases.[32] The sex-specific response of these muscles to changes in speed and surface incline is consistent with the concept that as task challenge increases, males and females utilize different neuromuscular strategies. Sex-related differences in neuromuscular action may contribute to performance and injury risk, and remain an active area of study.

Speed

Speed has a substantial influence on both the kinematics and the kinetics of running. As running speed increases, both stride length and stride frequency increase.[19,25] A greater change is observed in stride length at speeds more common to distance running (2 m/sec to 5 m/sec), while changes in stride frequency occur predominantly during high-speed running and sprinting (7.0 m/sec to 9.0 m/sec).[124] The amount of time that the foot is in contact with the ground decreases as running speed increases, reflective of an increase in muscular-based stiffness throughout the lower extremity. [4,44]

The GRFs increase with running speed, with the largest increases frequently observed at submaximal speeds.[14] For example, the vertical GRF increases by 15% from 40% to 60% of maximum speed, while only a 3% increase occurs from 60% to 100% of maximum speed.[19] Sagittal plane joint torques show a similar relationship to running speed: the greatest increases in knee and ankle torques during stance occur when increasing from one submaximal speed (40%) to another (60%).[123] Musculoskeletal models indicate that, during slow to medium speed running, the gastrocnemius and soleus are responsible for a substantial portion of the vertical GRF and nearly all of the anterior propulsive impulse from the anterior-posterior GRF. However, as running speed approaches maximum, swing phase joint torques continue to increase substantially, especially hip flexion during early swing and hip extension and knee flexion during terminal swing.[124] Thus, sprinting requires considerable power from the iliopsoas, gluteus maximus, and hamstrings.

Surface Incline

Compared with level ground running, vertical GRF impact peak and loading rate increase when running downhill and decrease when running uphill. For example, *impact peak* increased by 32% when running on a surface declined 6 degrees and decreased 22% when running on a surface inclined 6 degrees.[50] This is attributed, in part, to a change in foot strike, with a midfoot landing becoming more likely during running on surfaces inclined more than 3 degrees. The *active peak* of the vertical GRF, however, appears to remain constant across surface inclinations, at least up to a 9-degree incline/decline.

The GRFs generated parallel to the running surface, in particular in the anterior-posterior direction, demonstrate a greater susceptibility to change with incline. As one might expect, the braking impulse increases with downhill running, whereas the propulsive impulse increases with uphill running. Running on a 9-degree decline more than doubles the braking impulse of running on a level surface, whereas a 9-degree incline requires a 65% increase in the propulsive impulse to maintain a constant running speed.[50] The increase in braking impulse during *downhill* running is greater than the corresponding reduction in propulsive impulse. During *uphill* running, however, the reduction in braking impulse is nearly identical to the increase in propulsive impulse.

The combination of increased vertical GRF impact peak and loading rate, as well as braking impulse, suggests that downhill running increases the risk of injury. Therefore it is generally advised that downhill running be avoided for several weeks when returning to running following an injury, such as a tibial stress fracture.

Surface Stiffness

It is typically assumed that vertical GRF impact peak is reduced when running on a more compliant surface such as grass. However, impact peaks are generally similar when running on surfaces with differing mechanical properties.[38,97] This is largely due to corresponding adjustments in joint mechanics to compensate for the surface stiffness. In general, a less stiff lower extremity posture at initial contact will be used when running on a stiff surface.[47] For example, when running on a stiff surface (e.g., asphalt), the runner may adopt greater knee flexion at initial contact to reduce the stiffness of the lower extremity. Another common kinematic adjustment may include using a midfoot or forefoot strike rather than a rearfoot strike. Although there appears to be a substantial individualized response as to how joint angles and torques are adjusted for surface stiffness,[38] the movement of the CoM and the ground contact time remain unaffected.[47] The ability to quickly modulate the stiffness of the lower extremity enables runners to run similarly on a variety of surfaces.[46]

SYNOPSIS

Running is a complex, coordinated movement that requires sophisticated integration of neuromuscular function across the entire body. With a fairly simple goal of moving forward faster, successful running requires just enough muscle activity to control and produce joint motion in all three planes, but not so much as to be metabolically excessive. In this chapter, the kinesiology of running is explored to provide the reader with the details and insights to begin to understand how this is accomplished.

During running, each limb spends more time in the air than it does on the ground, with swing phase comprising about 60% or more of the running stride cycle. As running speed increases, so does the duration of swing phase, primarily because of an increase in the time spent in float. This portion of the swing phase (i.e., float) when both limbs are off the ground is the key differentiating feature to determine whether someone is running or just walking fast.

Initial contact with the ground during running can occur at the rearfoot, midfoot, or forefoot, with the point of contact largely influencing the subsequent joint kinematics of the lower extremity, most notably at the knee and ankle. In short, a forefoot strike involves more knee flexion and ankle plantar flexion at initial contact compared with a rearfoot strike. This chapter emphasizes a rearfoot strike because it is most common, and describes the joint rotations of the hip, knee, and ankle in all three cardinal planes of motion throughout the stride cycle. Corresponding kinematics of the trunk, pelvis, and upper extremities are also described.

The coordinated joint rotations help control the displacement of the body's CoM. During running, the CoM has a minimum height at mid stance and a maximum height during the middle of float in early swing. This results in the potential energy and kinetic energy being *in-phase;* therefore the conservation of mechanical energy relies more on the springlike properties of tissues, such as the Achilles tendon. Unlike walking, the metabolic energy cost to run a given distance is quite similar regardless of speed. Although the mechanism for this economy of movement is unknown, adjustments in joint kinematics, sources of mechanical power, and changes in muscle activity are potential factors.

Several muscles are active eccentrically during part or all of the loading response period of the running stride cycle to decelerate the CoM and associated joint motions. For example, the gluteus maximus, vastus medialis, vastus lateralis, gastrocnemius, and soleus all function in this manner. The eccentric activity of the ankle plantar flexors and the associated lengthening of the Achilles tendon result in energy storage that is subsequently released during the concentric activity of these same muscles during the second half of stance phase. This pattern of eccentric activity preceding concentric activity, or power absorption preceding power generation, is frequent during running and results in force enhancement during the concentric muscle action and improved muscle performance. For example, the iliopsoas is eccentrically active before toe off and then concentrically active during early swing to first decelerate hip extension and then initiate hip flexion and advance the limb forward. Similarly, the hamstring muscles are eccentrically active during the first part of late swing (75%–90% of the stride cycle) to decelerate knee flexion, and then concentrically active during the remainder of swing to position the limb for the subsequent initial contact. Having an appreciation and understanding of this level of detail is essential to effectively diagnose and treat movement impairments and associated pathomechanics.

Running is one of the most popular exercise activities throughout the world and is a movement integral to a number of sports. Although running can provide very valuable health benefits to multiple body systems, the yearly incidence of musculoskeletal injuries related to running ranges from 26% to 92% and is a continual area of study by clinicians and researchers.[137] One factor that can contribute to an increased risk of injury and delay or prevent recovery is an individual's running mechanics. As such, understanding running mechanics is essential in the successful management of individuals with running-related injuries. Knowledge of the typical GRFs, joint kinematics and kinetics, and muscle activity patterns enables the clinician to infer the type and extent of tissue loading, as well as how these factors relate to injury risk and recovery. It also provides a basis for comparison when performing a clinical analysis of an individual's running mechanics.

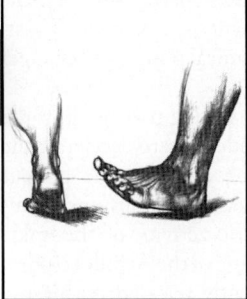

ADDITIONAL CLINICAL CONNECTIONS

CONTENTS

CLINICAL CONNECTION 16.1
Why Is Patellofemoral Joint Pain So Common among Distance Runners?

Approximately 50% of all running-related injuries occur at the knee, with nearly half of those involving the patellofemoral joint.[132] Although several risk factors for patellofemoral joint pain have been suggested,[137,139] the inability of the lower extremity joints to adequately control the loads applied during loading response is often identified.[54,58,100]

Assessment of running mechanics in someone with patellofemoral joint pain may reveal the use of an excessive stride length or a dynamic knee valgus alignment (resulting from excessive hip adduction and internal rotation), both of which are associated with increased loading of the joint.[54,100] Because static knee alignment measurements such as the Q-angle fail to produce a strong correlation with dynamic knee valgus,[55,107] the primary contributing factor appears to be altered neuromuscular control. For example, individuals with patellofemoral pain have shown a combination of delayed onset and shorter duration of gluteus medius muscle activity during running compared with those without patellofemoral pain; no difference in the amplitude of muscle activity was observed.[143] These findings support clinically held notions that reduced activation of the hip abductors is biomechanically associated with reduced control of hip and therefore knee motion (Chapter 13).

Conservative treatment programs for patellofemoral joint pain in runners focus on resistance training for the hip musculature, in particular the hip abductors. Doing so results in a greater reduction in pain and improvement in function than if these exercises are omitted.[10,39,66,95,136] Movement control exercises to encourage proper joint kinematics are also an integral aspect to recovery, because strength training alone may not be sufficient to alter abnormal running mechanics.[59,145]

Running mechanics retraining using biofeedback is an emerging intervention for the treatment of patellofemoral joint pain in runners.[58] Real-time feedback of hip motion has produced improvements in running biomechanics and more importantly led to near-resolution of symptoms.[100] For example, viewing hip frontal plane kinematics while running enabled individuals with patellofemoral pain to reduce peak hip adduction during stance phase, hopefully facilitating a more lasting change in their motor control pattern.[146] Additional retraining strategies have focused on other measures that can reduce patellofemoral joint force during loading response. Running with a 10% increase in step rate effectively reduces the peak patellofemoral joint force encountered during stance phase by 14%.[76] This reduced joint force and corresponding knee joint power absorption primarily arises from altered muscular coordination that reduces the amount of knee flexion at mid stance. Running with a slight increase in trunk flexion can have a similar effect as the GRF moment arm at the knee is reduced.[133]

The clinical management of patellofemoral joint pain among runners has evolved in recent decades, due in large part to our greater understanding of the kinesiology of running. Integrating this knowledge into clinical practice enables the development of more effective strategies for achieving symptom resolution.

ADDITIONAL CLINICAL CONNECTIONS

Hamstring strain injuries are among the most common injuries in sports involving high-speed running and have a recurrence rate as high as 30%.[42,51,105] Accordingly, for the purposes of prevention and rehabilitation, there has been growing interest in determining the biomechanical components of sprinting that are most associated with this injury.

Because of the rapid speed of sprinting, it is very difficult to determine through casual observation exactly when in the sprint cycle hamstring injuries most often occur. Precise analysis, however, shows that during high-speed running, hamstring strain injuries most likely occur during late swing, at a time when the elongated muscles are subjected to large tensional strain.[31] Interestingly, decades earlier, it was proposed that the hamstrings were most vulnerable to injury in early stance.[82] The prevailing thought at the time was that during early stance, the muscles were subjected to large loads due, in part, to the sudden and large ground reaction forces. More recent biomechanical simulation of sprinting, however, shows that the biarticular hamstrings are actually shortening (rather than being rapidly elongated) throughout the stance phase, and that the loads placed on the muscles during this time remain relatively constant as a sprinting athlete approaches maximal running speed.[29] Therefore it appears that other biomechanical factors play a significant role in the mechanics of strain-induced hamstring injury, specifically acting during late swing.[31,106] Throughout late swing, neither limb is in contact with the ground (i.e., float with no ground contact forces); however, the hamstrings are active *and* rapidly lengthening, therefore absorbing energy to decelerate the limb in preparation for foot contact.[29] Importantly, the amount of kinetic energy absorbed in the limb has been shown to be proportional to the running speed squared, such that the negative work done (energy absorbed) by the hamstrings increases substantially with running speed (Fig. 16.13).[30]

Late swing, when large eccentric muscular demands are placed on the hamstrings, is also the time during the running stride when the hamstrings are near their maximal elongation. It is noteworthy that the greatest muscle-tendon unit stretch is incurred by the long head of the biceps femoris,[29] which may explain why it is the most often injured hamstring muscle[41] during high-speed running. Therefore in late swing of high-speed running, the hamstrings undergo an eccentric action as they reach peak stretch just prior to foot strike,[134] a combination of mechanical factors that could potentially lead to a strain injury of the muscle fascicles

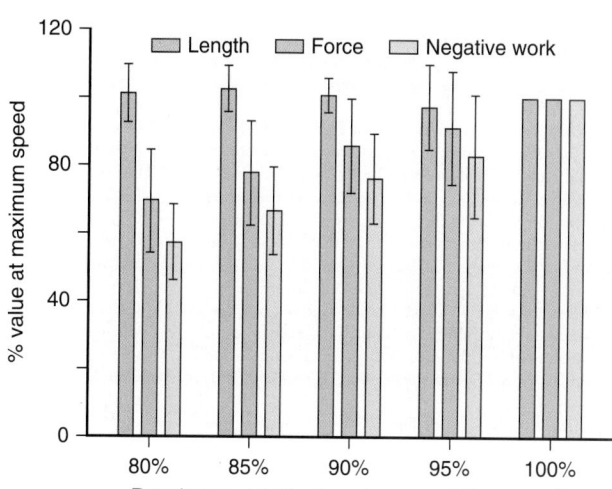

FIGURE 16.13 Biceps femoris long head length, force, and negative work relative to 100% sprinting speed during late swing phase of running. Peak length is similar across all speeds, while force and negative work increase significantly with speed. Negative work increased to the largest extent as speed increased from 80% to maximum sprinting speed. (From Chumanov ES, Heiderscheit BC, Thelen DG: The effect of speed and influence of individual muscles on hamstring mechanics during the swing phase of sprinting. *J Biomech* 40:3555-62, 2007)

and adjacent tendons. The argument for late swing being the most vulnerable time for hamstring injury has been further strengthened by findings from two independent case studies of biomechanical data collected while running athletes actually incurred acute hamstring strain injuries.[56,125] Despite distinctly different experimental conditions, both studies came to the same conclusion: that the stimulus for the injury most likely occurred in the late swing phase.

Understanding the biomechanical state of the hamstring muscle at the time of injury informs the development of targeted injury prevention and recovery strategies. That is, exercise interventions for preventing and managing hamstring strain injuries should involve eccentric activation of the hamstring muscles.[15,16,57,60] To this end, there is evidence demonstrating that not only are eccentric exercises effective in reducing hamstring strain injury incidence,[8,9,108,111] but that they are also likely to be more effective than concentric exercises.[87]

REFERENCES

1. Almeida MO, Davis IS, Lopes AD: Biomechanical differences of foot-strike patterns during running: a systematic review with meta-analysis, *J Orthop Sports Phys Ther* 45:738–755, 2015.
2. Altman AR, Davis IS: A kinematic method for foot-strike pattern detection in barefoot and shod runners, *Gait Posture* 35:298–300, 2012.
3. Andersson EA, Nilsson J, Thorstensson A: Intramuscular EMG from the hip flexor muscles during human locomotion, *Acta Physiol Scand* 161:361–370, 1997.
4. Arampatzis A, Bruggemann GP, Metzler V: The effect of speed on leg stiffness and joint kinetics in human running, *J Biomech* 32:1349–1353, 1999.
5. Arellano CJ, Kram R: The effects of step width and arm swing on energetic cost and lateral balance during running, *J Biomech* 44:1291–1295, 2011.
6. Arellano CJ, Kram R: The energetic cost of maintaining lateral balance during human running, *J Appl Physiol* 112:427–434, 2012.
7. Arellano CJ, Kram R: The metabolic cost of human running: is swinging the arms worth it? *J Exp Biol* 217:2456–2461, 2014.
8. Arnason A, Andersen TE, Holme I, et al.: Prevention of hamstring strains in elite soccer: an intervention study, *Scand J Med Sci Sports* 18:40–48, 2008.
9. Askling C, Karlsson J, Thorstensson A: Hamstring injury occurrence in elite soccer players after preseason strength training with eccentric overload, *Scand J Med Sci Sports* 13:244–250, 2003.
10. Baldon Rde M, Serrao FV, Scattone Silva R, et al.: Effects of functional stabilization training on pain, function, and lower extremity biomechanics in women with patellofemoral pain: a randomized clinical trial, *J Orthop Sports Phys Ther* 44:240–251, 2014. –A248.
11. Bartlett JL, Sumner B, Ellis RG, et al.: Activity and functions of the human gluteal muscles in walking, running, sprinting, and climbing, *Am J Phys Anthropol* 153:124–131, 2014.
12. Barton CJ, Lack S, Malliaras P, et al.: Gluteal muscle activity and patellofemoral pain syndrome: a systematic review, *Br J Sports Med* 47:207–214, 2013.
13. Baur H, Hirschmuller A, Cassel M, et al.: Gender-specific neuromuscular activity of the M. peroneus longus in healthy runners—A descriptive laboratory study, *Clin Biomech (Bristol, Avon)* 25:938–943, 2010.
14. Belli A, Kyrolainen H, Komi PV: Moment and power of lower limb joints in running, *Int J Sports Med* 23:136–141, 2002.
15. Bourne MN, Timmins RG, Opar DA, et al.: An evidence-based framework for strengthening exercises to prevent hamstring injury, *Sports Med* 48:251–267, 2018.
16. Bourne MN, Williams MD, Opar DA, et al.: Impact of exercise selection on hamstring muscle activation, *Br J Sports Med* 51:1021–1028, 2017.
17. Breine B, Malcolm P, Frederick EC, et al.: Relationship between running speed and initial foot contact patterns, *Med Sci Sports Exerc* 46:1595–1603, 2014.
18. Brindle RA, Milner CE, Zhang S, et al.: Changing step width alters lower extremity biomechanics during running, *Gait Posture* 39:124–128, 2014.
19. Brughelli M, Cronin J, Chaouachi A: Effects of running velocity on running kinetics and kinematics, *J Strength Cond Res* 25:933–939, 2011.
20. Buczek FL, Cavanagh PR: Stance phase knee and ankle kinematics and kinetics during level and downhill running, *Med Sci Sports Exerc* 22:669–677, 1990.
21. Bus SA: Ground reaction forces and kinematics in distance running in older-aged men, *Med Sci Sports Exerc* 35:1167–1175, 2003.
22. Cappellini G, Ivanenko YP, Poppele RE, et al.: Motor patterns in human walking and running, *J Neurophysiol* 95:3426–3437, 2006.
23. Cappozzo A, Catani F, Leardini A, et al.: Position and orientation in space of bones during movement: experimental artefacts, *Clin Biomech (Bristol, Avon)* 11:90–100, 1996.

24. Cavagna GA, Kaneko M: Mechanical work and efficiency in level walking and running, *J Physiol* 268:467–481, 1977.
25. Cavanagh PR, Kram R: Stride length in distance running: velocity, body dimensions, and added mass effects, *Med Sci Sports Exerc* 21:467–479, 1989.
26. Cavanagh PR, Lafortune MA: Ground reaction forces in distance running, *J Biomech* 13:397–406, 1980.
27. Cavanagh PR, Williams KR: The effect of stride length variation on oxygen uptake during distance running, *Med Sci Sports Exerc* 14:30–35, 1982.
28. Cavanagh PR: The biomechanics of lower extremity action in distance running, *Foot Ankle* 7:197–217, 1987.
29. Chumanov ES, Heiderscheit BC, Thelen DG: Hamstring musculotendon dynamics during stance and swing phases of high-speed running, *Med Sci Sports Exerc* 43:525–532, 2011.
30. Chumanov ES, Heiderscheit BC, Thelen DG: The effect of speed and influence of individual muscles on hamstring mechanics during the swing phase of sprinting, *J Biomech* 40:3555–3562, 2007.
31. Chumanov ES, Schache AG, Heiderscheit BC, et al.: Hamstrings are most susceptible to injury during the late swing phase of sprinting, *Br J Sports Med* 46:90, 2012.
32. Chumanov ES, Wall-Scheffler C, Heiderscheit BC: Gender differences in walking and running on level and inclined surfaces, *Clin Biomech (Bristol, Avon)* 23:1260–1268, 2008.
33. Chumanov ES, Wille CM, Michalski MP, et al.: Changes in muscle activation patterns when running step rate is increased, *Gait Posture* 36:231–235, 2012.
34. Conoboy P, Dyson R: Effect of aging on the stride pattern of veteran marathon runners, *Br J Sports Med* 40:601–604, 2006.
35. Derrick TR: The effects of knee contact angle on impact forces and accelerations, *Med Sci Sports Exerc* 36:832–837, 2004.
36. Dicharry J: Kinematics and kinetics of gait: from lab to clinic, *Clin Sports Med* 29:347–364, 2010.
37. Diebal AR, Gregory R, Alitz C, et al.: Forefoot running improves pain and disability associated with chronic exertional compartment syndrome, *Am J Sports Med* 40:1060–1067, 2012.
38. Dixon SJ, Collop AC, Batt ME: Surface effects on ground reaction forces and lower extremity kinematics in running, *Med Sci Sports Exerc* 32:1919–1926, 2000.
39. Dolak KL, Silkman C, Medina McKeon J, et al.: Hip strengthening prior to functional exercises reduces pain sooner than quadriceps strengthening in females with patellofemoral pain syndrome: a randomized clinical trial, *J Orthop Sports Phys Ther* 41:560–570, 2011.
40. Dorn TW, Schache AG, Pandy MG: Muscular strategy shift in human running: dependence of running speed on hip and ankle muscle performance, *J Exp Biol* 215:1944–1956, 2012.
41. Ekstrand J, Healy JC, Walden M, et al.: Hamstring muscle injuries in professional football: the correlation of MRI findings with return to play, *Br J Sports Med* 46:112–117, 2012.
42. Ekstrand J, Walden M, Hagglund M: Hamstring injuries have increased by 4% annually in men's professional football, since 2001: a 13-year longitudinal analysis of the UEFA Elite Club injury study, *Br J Sports Med* 50:731–737, 2016.
43. Farley CT, Ferris DP: Biomechanics of walking and running: center of mass movements to muscle action, *Exerc Sport Sci Rev* 26:253–285, 1998.
44. Farley CT, Gonzalez O: Leg stiffness and stride frequency in human running, *J Biomech* 29:181–186, 1996.
45. Ferber R, Davis IM, Williams 3rd DS: Gender differences in lower extremity mechanics during running, *Clin Biomech (Bristol, Avon)* 18:350–357, 2003.
46. Ferris DP, Liang K, Farley CT: Runners adjust leg stiffness for their first step on a new running surface, *J Biomech* 32:787–794, 1999.

47. Ferris DP, Louie M, Farley CT: Running in the real world: adjusting leg stiffness for different surfaces, *Proc Biol Sci* 265:989–994, 1998.
48. Gazendam MG, Hof AL: Averaged EMG profiles in jogging and running at different speeds, *Gait Posture* 25:604–614, 2007.
49. Goss DL, Lewek M, Yu B, et al.: Lower extremity biomechanics and self-reported foot-strike patterns among runners in traditional and minimalist shoes, *J Athl Train* 50:603–611, 2015.
50. Gottschall JS, Kram R: Ground reaction forces during downhill and uphill running, *J Biomech* 38:445–452, 2005.
51. Hallen A, Ekstrand J: Return to play following muscle injuries in professional footballers, *J Sports Sci* 32:1229–1236, 2014.
52. Halvorsen K, Eriksson M, Gullstrand L: Acute effects of reducing vertical displacement and step frequency on running economy, *J Strength Cond Res* 26:2065–2070, 2012.
53. Hamner SR, Seth A, Delp SL: Muscle contributions to propulsion and support during running, *J Biomech* 43:2709–2716, 2010.
54. Heiderscheit BC, Chumanov ES, Michalski MP, et al.: Effects of step rate manipulation on joint mechanics during running, *Med Sci Sports Exerc* 43:296–302, 2011.
55. Heiderscheit BC, Hamill J, Caldwell GE: Influence of Q-angle on lower-extremity running kinematics, *J Orthop Sports Phys Ther* 30:271–278, 2000.
56. Heiderscheit BC, Hoerth DM, Chumanov ES, et al.: Identifying the time of occurrence of a hamstring strain injury during treadmill running: a case study, *Clin Biomech (Bristol, Avon)* 20:1072–1078, 2005.
57. Heiderscheit BC, Sherry MA, Silder A, et al.: Hamstring strain injuries: recommendations for diagnosis, rehabilitation, and injury prevention, *J Orthop Sports Phys Ther* 40:67–81, 2010.
58. Heiderscheit BC: Gait retraining for runners: in search of the ideal, *J Orthop Sports Phys Ther* 41:909–910, 2011.
59. Heiderscheit BC: Lower extremity injuries: is it just about hip strength? *J Orthop Sports Phys Ther* 40:39–41, 2010.
60. Hickey JT, Opar DA, Weiss LJ, et al.: Hamstring strain injury rehabilitation, *J Athl Train* 57:125–135, 2022.
61. Hodges P, Kaigle Holm A, Holm S, et al.: Intervertebral stiffness of the spine is increased by evoked contraction of transversus abdominis and the diaphragm: in vivo porcine studies, *Spine* 28:2594–2601, 2003.
62. Hodges PW, McLean L, Hodder J: Insight into the function of the obturator internus muscle in humans: observations with development and validation of an electromyography recording technique, *J Electromyogr Kinesiol* 24:489–496, 2014.
63. Hreljac A: Impact and overuse injuries in runners, *Med Sci Sports Exerc* 36:845–849, 2004.
64. Karamanidis K, Arampatzis A, Bruggemann GP: Adaptational phenomena and mechanical responses during running: effect of surface, aging and task experience, *Eur J Appl Physiol* 98:284–298, 2006.
65. Kerrigan DC, Franz JR, Keenan GS, et al.: The effect of running shoes on lower extremity joint torques, *PM R* 1:1058–1063, 2009.
66. Khayambashi K, Fallah A, Movahedi A, et al.: Posterolateral hip muscle strengthening versus quadriceps strengthening for patellofemoral pain: a comparative control trial, *Arch Phys Med Rehabil* 95:900–907, 2014.
67. Knapik JJ, Brosch LC, Venuto M, et al.: Effect on injuries of assigning shoes based on foot shape in air force basic training, *Am J Prev Med* 38:S197–S211, 2010.
68. Knapik JJ, Swedler DI, Grier TL, et al.: Injury reduction effectiveness of selecting running shoes based on plantar shape, *J Strength Cond Res* 23:685–697, 2009.
69. Knapik JJ, Trone DW, Swedler DI, et al.: Injury reduction effectiveness of assigning running shoes based on plantar shape in marine corps basic training, *Am J Sports Med* 38:1759–1767, 2010.

70. Knapik JJ, Trone DW, Tchandja J, et al.: Injury-reduction effectiveness of prescribing running shoes on the basis of foot arch height: summary of military investigations, *J Orthop Sports Phys Ther* 44:805–812, 2014.

71. Komi PV: Stretch-shortening cycle: a powerful model to study normal and fatigued muscle, *J Biomech* 33:1197–1206, 2000.

72. Kyrolainen H, Belli A, Komi PV: Biomechanical factors affecting running economy, *Med Sci Sports Exerc* 33:1330–1337, 2001.

73. Larson P, Higgins E, Kaminski J, et al.: Foot strike patterns of recreational and sub-elite runners in a long-distance road race, *J Sports Sci* 29:1665–1673, 2011.

74. Lenhart RL, Smith CR, Vignos MF, et al.: Influence of step rate and quadriceps load distribution on patellofemoral cartilage contact pressures during running, *J Biomech* 48:2871–2878, 2015.

75. Lenhart RL, Thelen DG, Heiderscheit BC: Hip muscle loads during running at various step rates, *J Orthop Sports Phys Ther* 44:766–774, 2014. A1-4.

76. Lenhart RL, Thelen DG, Wille CM, et al.: Increasing running step rate reduces patellofemoral joint forces, *Med Sci Sports Exerc* 46:557–564, 2014.

77. Lieberman DE, Castillo ER, Otarola-Castillo E, et al.: Variation in foot strike patterns among habitually barefoot and shod runners in Kenya, *PLoS ONE* 10:e0131354, 2015.

78. Lilley K, Dixon S, Stiles V: A biomechanical comparison of the running gait of mature and young females, *Gait Posture* 33:496–500, 2011.

79. MacWilliams BA, Rozumalski A, Swanson AN, et al.: Three-dimensional lumbar spine vertebral motion during running using indwelling bone pins, *Spine* 39:E1560–E1565, 2014.

80. Malinzak RA, Colby SM, Kirkendall DT, et al.: A comparison of knee joint motion patterns between men and women in selected athletic tasks, *Clin Biomech (Bristol, Avon)* 16:438–445, 2001.

81. Mann RA, Hagy J: Biomechanics of walking, running, and sprinting, *Am J Sports Med* 8:345–350, 1980.

82. Mann RV: A kinetic analysis of sprinting, *Med Sci Sports Exerc* 13:325–328, 1981.

83. McClay I, Manal K: A comparison of three-dimensional lower extremity kinematics during running between excessive pronators and normals, *Clin Biomech (Bristol, Avon)* 13:195–203, 1998.

84. McClay I, Manal K: The influence of foot abduction on differences between two-dimensional and three-dimensional rearfoot motion, *Foot Ankle Int* 19:26–31, 1998.

85. McClay I, Manal K: Three-dimensional kinetic analysis of running: significance of secondary planes of motion, *Med Sci Sports Exerc* 31:1629–1637, 1999.

86. Milner CE, Brindle RA: Reliability and minimal detectable difference in multisegment foot kinematics during shod walking and running, *Gait Posture* 43:192–197, 2016.

87. Mjolsnes R, Arnason A, Osthagen T, et al.: A 10-week randomized trial comparing eccentric vs. concentric hamstring strength training in well-trained soccer players, *Scand J Med Sci Sports* 14:311–317, 2004.

88. Montgomery 3rd WH, Pink M, Perry J: Electromyographic analysis of hip and knee musculature during running, *Am J Sports Med* 22:272–278, 1994.

89. Morgan DW, Martin PE, Krahenbuhl GS: Factors affecting running economy, *Sports Med* 7:310–330, 1989.

90. Morin JB, Samozino P, Millet GY: Changes in running kinematics, kinetics, and spring-mass behavior over a 24-h run, *Med Sci Sports Exerc* 43:829–836, 2011.

91. Mundermann A, Nigg BM, Humble RN, et al.: Orthotic comfort is related to kinematics, kinetics, and EMG in recreational runners, *Med Sci Sports Exerc* 35:1710–1719, 2003.

92. Mundermann A, Nigg BM, Stefanyshyn DJ, et al.: Development of a reliable method to assess footwear comfort during running, *Gait Posture* 16:38–45, 2002.

93. Mundermann A, Stefanyshyn DJ, Nigg BM: Relationship between footwear comfort of shoe inserts and anthropometric and sensory factors, *Med Sci Sports Exerc* 33:1939–1945, 2001.

94. Myers MJ, Steudel K: Effect of limb mass and its distribution on the energetic cost of running, *J Exp Biol* 116:363–373, 1985.

95. Nakagawa TH, Muniz TB, Baldon Rde M, et al.: The effect of additional strengthening of hip abductor and lateral rotator muscles in patellofemoral pain syndrome: a randomized controlled pilot study, *Clin Rehabil* 22:1051–1060, 2008.

96. Nigg BM, Baltich J, Hoerzer S, et al.: Running shoes and running injuries: mythbusting and a proposal for two new paradigms: 'preferred movement path' and 'comfort filter', *Br J Sports Med* 49:1290–1294, 2015.

97. Nigg BM, Yeadon MR: Biomechanical aspects of playing surfaces, *J Sports Sci* 5:117–145, 1987.

98. Nigg BM: The role of impact forces and foot pronation: a new paradigm, *Clin J Sport Med* 11(2–9), 2001.

99. Noehren B, Hamill J, Davis I: Prospective evidence for a hip etiology in patellofemoral pain, *Med Sci Sports Exerc* 45:1120–1124, 2013.

100. Noehren B, Scholz J, Davis I: The effect of real-time gait retraining on hip kinematics, pain and function in subjects with patellofemoral pain syndrome, *Br J Sports Med* 45:691–696, 2011.

101. Novacheck TF: The biomechanics of running, *Gait Posture* 7:77–95, 1998.

102. Nunes GS, Pizzari T, Neate R, et al.: Gluteal muscle activity during running in asymptomatic people, *Gait Posture* 80:268–273, 2020.

103. O'Connor KM, Hamill J: Frontal plane moments do not accurately reflect ankle dynamics during running, *J Appl Biomech* 21:85–95, 2005.

104. O'Connor KM, Hamill J: The role of selected extrinsic foot muscles during running, *Clin Biomech (Bristol, Avon)* 19:71–77, 2004.

105. Orchard J, Best TM, Verrall GM: Return to play following muscle strains, *Clin J Sport Med* 15:436–441, 2005.

106. Pandy MG, Andriacchi TP: Muscle and joint function in human locomotion, *Annu Rev Biomed Eng* 12:401–433, 2010.

107. Park SK, Stefanyshyn DJ: Greater Q angle may not be a risk factor of patellofemoral pain syndrome, *Clin Biomech (Bristol, Avon)* 26:392–396, 2011.

108. Petersen J, Thorborg K, Nielsen MB, et al.: Preventive effect of eccentric training on acute hamstring injuries in men's soccer: a cluster-randomized controlled trial, *Am J Sports Med* 39:2296–2303, 2011.

109. Phinyomark A, Osis S, Hettinga BA, et al.: Kinematic gait patterns in healthy runners: a hierarchical cluster analysis, *J Biomech* 48:3897–3904, 2015.

110. Rassier DE: The mechanisms of the residual force enhancement after stretch of skeletal muscle: non-uniformity in half-sarcomeres and stiffness of titin, *Proc Biol Sci* 279:2705–2713, 2012.

111. Raya-Gonzalez J, Castillo D, Clemente FM: Injury prevention of hamstring injuries through exercise interventions, *J Sports Med Phys Fitness* 61:1242–1251, 2021.

112. Reber L, Perry J, Pink M: Muscular control of the ankle in running, *Am J Sports Med* 21:805–810, 1993. discussion 810.

113. Reinschmidt C, van Den Bogert AJ, Murphy N, et al.: Tibiocalcaneal motion during running, measured with external and bone marker, *Clin Biomech (Bristol, Avon)* 12(8–16), 1997.

114. Reinschmidt C, van den Bogert AJ, Nigg BM, et al.: Effect of skin movement on the analysis of skeletal knee joint motion during running, *J Biomech* 30:729–732, 1997.

115. Richards CE, Magin PJ, Callister R: Is your prescription of distance running shoes evidence-based? *Br J Sports Med* 43:159–162, 2009.

116. Riley PO, Dicharry J, Franz J, et al.: A kinematics and kinetic comparison of overground and treadmill running, *Med Sci Sports Exerc* 40:1093–1100, 2008.

117. Ryan MB, Valiant GA, McDonald K, et al.: The effect of three different levels of footwear stability on pain outcomes in women runners: a randomised control trial, *Br J Sports Med* 45:715–721, 2011.

118. Saunders PU, Pyne DB, Telford RD, et al.: Factors affecting running economy in trained distance runners, *Sports Med* 34:465–485, 2004.

119. Saunders SW, Schache A, Rath D, et al.: Changes in three dimensional lumbo-pelvic kinematics and trunk muscle activity with speed and mode of locomotion, *Clin Biomech (Bristol, Avon)* 20:784–793, 2005.

120. Schache AG, Bennell KL, Blanch PD, et al.: The coordinated movement of the lumbo-pelvic-hip complex during running: a literature review, *Gait Posture* 10:30–47, 1999.

121. Schache AG, Blanch P, Rath D, et al.: Differences between the sexes in the three-dimensional angular rotations of the lumbo-pelvic-hip complex during treadmill running, *J Sports Sci* 21:105–118, 2003.

122. Schache AG, Blanch P, Rath D, et al.: Three-dimensional angular kinematics of the lumbar spine and pelvis during running, *Hum Mov Sci* 21:273–293, 2002.

123. Schache AG, Blanch PD, Dorn TW, et al.: Effect of running speed on lower limb joint kinetics, *Med Sci Sports Exerc* 43:1260–1271, 2011.

124. Schache AG, Dorn TW, Williams GP, et al.: Lower-limb muscular strategies for increasing running speed, *J Orthop Sports Phys Ther* 44:813–824, 2014.

125. Schache AG, Wrigley TV, Baker R, et al.: Biomechanical response to hamstring muscle strain injury, *Gait Posture* 29:332–338, 2009.

126. Semciw AI, Freeman M, Kunstler BE, et al.: Quadratus femoris: an EMG investigation during walking and running, *J Biomech* 48:3433–3439, 2015.

127. Silder A, Thelen DG, Heiderscheit BC: Effects of prior hamstring strain injury on strength, flexibility, and running mechanics, *Clin Biomech (Bristol, Avon)* 25:681–686, 2010.

128. Snyder KR, Earl JE, O'Connor KM, et al.: Resistance training is accompanied by increases in hip strength and changes in lower extremity biomechanics during running, *Clin Biomech (Bristol, Avon)* 24:26–34, 2009.

129. Stefanyshyn DJ, Stergiou P, Lun VM, et al.: Knee angular impulse as a predictor of patellofemoral pain in runners, *Am J Sports Med* 34:1844–1851, 2006.

130. Stiffler-Joachim MR, Wille C, Kliethermes S, et al.: Factors influencing base of gait during running: consideration of sex, speed, kinematics, and anthropometrics, *J Athl Train* 55:1300–1306, 2020.

131. Taube W, Leukel C, Gollhofer A: How neurons make us jump: the neural control of stretch-shortening cycle movements, *Exerc Sport Sci Rev* 40:106–115, 2012.

132. Taunton JE, Ryan MB, Clement DB, et al.: A retrospective case-control analysis of 2002 running injuries, *Br J Sports Med* 36:95–101, 2002.

133. Teng HL, Powers CM: Sagittal plane trunk posture influences patellofemoral joint stress during running, *J Orthop Sports Phys Ther* 44:785–792, 2014.

134. Thelen DG, Chumanov ES, Hoerth DM, et al.: Hamstring muscle kinematics during treadmill sprinting, *Med Sci Sports Exerc* 37:108–114, 2005.

135. Thelen DG, Chumanov ES, Sherry MA, et al.: Neuromusculoskeletal models provide insights into the mechanisms and rehabilitation of hamstring strains, *Exerc Sport Sci Rev* 34:135–141, 2006.

136. van der Heijden RA, Lankhorst NE, van Linschoten R, et al.: Exercise for treating patellofemoral pain syndrome, *Cochrane Database Syst Rev (Online)*(1):CD010387, 2015.

137. van Gent RN, Siem D, van Middelkoop M, et al.: Incidence and determinants of lower extremity running injuries in long distance runners: a systematic review, *Br J Sports Med* 41:469–480, 2007; discussion 480.

138. Wall-Scheffler CM, Chumanov E, Steudel-Numbers K, et al.: Electromyography activity across gait and incline: the impact of muscular activity on human morphology, *Am J Phys Anthropol* 143:601–611, 2010.

139. Wen DY, Puffer JC, Schmalzried TP: Lower extremity alignment and risk of overuse injuries in runners, *Med Sci Sports Exerc* 29:1291–1298, 1997.

140. Wille CM, Lenhart RL, Wang S, et al.: Ability of sagittal kinematic variables to estimate ground reaction forces and joint kinetics in running, *J Orthop Sports Phys Ther* 44:825–830, 2014.

141. Williams KR, Cavanagh PR, Ziff JL: Biomechanical studies of elite female distance runners, *Int J Sports Med* 8(Suppl 2):107, 1987.

142. Williams KR, Cavanagh PR: Relationship between distance running mechanics, running economy, and performance, *J Appl Physiol* 63:1236–1245, 1987.

143. Willson JD, Kernozek TW, Arndt RL, et al.: Gluteal muscle activation during running in females with and without patellofemoral pain syndrome, *Clin Biomech (Bristol, Avon)* 26:735–740, 2011.

144. Willwacher S, Konig M, Potthast W, et al.: Does specific footwear facilitate energy storage and return at the metatarsophalangeal joint in running? *J Appl Biomech* 29:583–592, 2013.

145. Willy RW, Davis IS: The effect of a hip-strengthening program on mechanics during running and during a single-leg squat, *J Orthop Sports Phys Ther* 41:625–632, 2011.

146. Willy RW, Scholz JP, Davis IS: Mirror gait retraining for the treatment of patellofemoral pain in female runners, *Clin Biomech (Bristol, Avon)* 27:1045–1051, 2012.

147. Zadpoor AA, Nikooyan AA: The relationship between lower-extremity stress fractures and the ground reaction force: a systematic review, *Clin Biomech (Bristol, Avon)* 26(23–28), 2011.

STUDY QUESTIONS

1. Using Figures 16.1, 16.6, and 16.8, describe the mechanical power generated or absorbed by the hip flexor muscles between pre swing and early swing of the stride cycle (specifically, between about 30 and 50 degrees of the stride cycle).

2. Describe how the vertical ground reaction forces change as running speed increases.

3. What common changes in spatiotemporal variables are present in runners over the age of 55 years compared with young adult runners?

4. How do joint kinematics during running differ between males and females?

5. Define and contrast braking impulse and propulsive impulse during running.

6. How can running be distinguished from "speed" walking?

7. Considering the differences in the path of the center of pressure between the three foot strikes, which foot strike(s) is/are more likely to have a greater risk of a metatarsal injury?

8. Using Figures 16.8, 16.11, and 16.12, which joint (hip, knee, or ankle) generates the greatest amount of energy in the sagittal plane during the stance phase of running?

9. Based on Figure 16.6A, the gluteus medius peak activity occurs during loading response. Using Figure 16.9, describe the muscle's functional role during this portion of the running stride cycle.

10. Using Figure 16.7, compare the active peak and impact peak of the vertical ground reaction force.

11. When is the body's center of mass the highest during the running stride cycle, and when is it the lowest? Compare this with when the body's center of mass is highest and lowest during walking.

12. Explain how the combined sagittal plane kinematics at the hip-and-knee during the 40% to 70% period of the running stride cycle influence metabolic efficiency.

13. What is the role of the semitendinosus and semimembranosus (medial hamstring muscles) at the knee during the late swing period of running?

14. Which spatial and temporal descriptors of running are most directly associated with an increase in running speed?

15. Using Figures 16.6B and 16.11 as guides, what can you infer about the type of activation (eccentric, concentric, etc.) and function of the rectus femoris at the knee from 0% to 35% of the running stride cycle?

16. How does the magnitude of horizontal plane rotation differ within the upper and lower trunk while running? What factors could account for this difference?

Answers to the study questions are available in the accompanying enhanced eBook version included with the print purchase of this textbook.

Additional Video Educational Content

- Visual Clinical Evaluation of Running (sagittal plane): Elements of a systematic running evaluation are provided

- Visual Clinical Evaluation of Running (frontal plane): Elements of a systematic running evaluation are provided

All videos in this chapter are available in the accompanying enhanced eBook version included with the print purchase of this textbook

APPENDIX
IV

Reference Materials for Muscle Attachments and Innervations, Muscle Cross-Sectional Areas, and Dermatomes of the Lower Extremity

Part A: Spinal Nerve Root Innervations of the Muscles of the Lower Extremity

| | Spinal Nerve Root | | | | | | | |
| | Lumbar | | | | | Sacral | | |
Muscle	L¹	L²	L³	L⁴	L⁵	S¹	S²	S³
Psoas minor	X							
Psoas major	*X*	X	X	*X*				
Iliacus		X	X	*X*				
Pectineus		X	X	*X*				
Sartorius		X	X					
Quadriceps		*X*	X	*X*				
Adductor brevis		X	X	*X*				
Adductor longus		X	X	*X*				
Gracilis		X	X	*X*				
Obturator externus			X	X				
Adductor magnus		*X*	X	X	X	*X*		
Gluteus medius				X	X	X		
Gluteus minimus				X	X	X		
Tensor fasciae latae				X	X	X		
Gluteus maximus					X	X	*X*	
Piriformis				X	X	X	*X*	
Gemellus superior					X	X	X	
Obturator internus					X	X	X	
Gemellus inferior				X	X	X		
Quadratus femoris				X	X	X		
Biceps (long head)					*X*	X	*X*	
Semitendinosus				*X*	X	X	X	
Semimembranosus				*X*	X	X	*X*	
Biceps (short head)					X	X	*X*	
Tibialis anterior				X	X			
Extensor hallucis longus				*X*	X	X		
Extensor digitorum longus				*X*	X	X		
Fibularis tertius				*X*	X	X		
Extensor digitorum brevis				*X*	X	X		
Fibularis longus				*X*	X	X		
Fibularis brevis				*X*	X	X		
Plantaris				*X*	X	X		
Gastrocnemius						X	X	
Popliteus				X	X	X		
Soleus					*X*	*X*	X	
Tibialis posterior				*X*	X	*X*		
Flexor digitorum longus					X	X	X	
Flexor hallucis longus					*X*	X	X	
Flexor digitorum brevis					*X*	X	X	
Abductor hallucis					*X*	X	X	
Flexor hallucis brevis					*X*	X	X	
Lumbrical I					*X*	X	X	
Abductor digiti minimi						*X*	X	X
Quadratus plantae						*X*	X	X
Flexor digiti minimi						*X*	X	X
Adductor hallucis						*X*	X	X
Plantar interossei							X	X
Dorsal interossei							X	X
Lumbricals II, III, IV						*X*	X	X

Data based on two primary references: Standring S: *Gray's anatomy: the anatomical basis of clinical practice,* ed 42, St Louis, 2021, Elsevier; Kendall FP, McCreary EK, Provance PG, et al: *Muscles: testing and function with posture and pain,* ed 5, Philadelphia, 2005, Lippincott Williams & Wilkins.

X, minor-to-moderate distribution; **X,** major distribution.

Part B: Key Muscles for Testing the Function of Spinal Nerve Roots (L^2 to S^3)

The table shows the key muscles typically used to test the function of individual spinal nerve roots of the lumbosacral plexus (L^2 to S^3). Reduced strength in a key muscle may indicate an injury to or a pathologic process within the associated spinal nerve root. Significant overlap exists in muscle innervation.

Key Muscles	Primary Nerve Root	Sample Test Movements
Iliopsoas	L^2	Hip flexion
Adductor longus	L^2	Hip adduction
Quadriceps	L^3	Knee extension
Tibialis anterior	L^4	Ankle dorsiflexion
Extensor hallucis longus	L^5	Toe extension
Gluteus medius	L^5	Hip abduction
Gluteus maximus	S^1	Hip extension with knee flexed
Semitendinosus	S^1	Knee flexion and internal rotation
Gastrocnemius	S^1	Ankle plantar flexion
Flexor hallucis longus	S^2	Flexion of the great toe
Dorsal and plantar interossei	S^3	Abduction and adduction of the toes

Part C: Dermatomes of the Lower Extremity

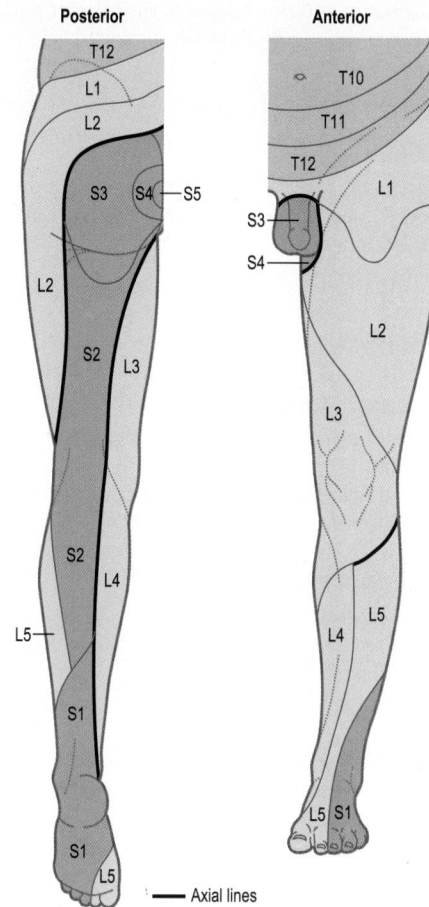

FIGURE IV.1   Dermatomes of the lower extremity. *L^1*, first lumbar nerve root; *S^1*, first sacral nerve root; and so on. (From O'Brien M: Aids in the Examination of the Peripheral Nervous System, 5th ed, Elsevier, Saunders, copyright 2010.)

Part D: Attachments and Innervation of the Muscles of the Lower Extremity

HIP AND KNEE MUSCULATURE

ADDUCTOR BREVIS
Proximal attachment: anterior surface of the inferior pubic ramus
Distal attachment: near and along the proximal one-third of the linea aspera of the femur
Innervation: obturator nerve

ADDUCTOR LONGUS
Proximal attachment: anterior surface of the body of the pubis
Distal attachment: near and along the middle one-third of the linea aspera of the femur
Innervation: obturator nerve

ADDUCTOR MAGNUS
Anterior Head
Proximal attachment: ischial ramus
Distal attachment (horizontal fibers): extreme proximal end of linea aspera of femur
Distal attachment (oblique fibers): entire linea aspera of the femur
Innervation: obturator nerve

Posterior (Extensor) Head
Proximal attachment: ischial tuberosity
Distal attachment: adductor tubercle of the femur
Innervation: tibial portion of sciatic nerve

ARTICULARIS GENU
Proximal attachment: anterior surface of the distal femoral shaft
Distal attachments: proximal capsule and synovial membrane of the knee
Innervation: femoral nerve

BICEPS FEMORIS
Long Head
Proximal attachments: from a common tendon with the semitendinosus; originating from a medial impression on the posterior surface of the ischial tuberosity and part of the sacrotuberous ligament
Distal attachment: head of the fibula; secondary attachments include the lateral collateral ligament, capsule of the proximal tibiofibular joint, and lateral side of the lateral condyle of the tibia
Innervation: tibial portion of the sciatic nerve

Short Head
Proximal attachment: lateral lip of the linea aspera below the gluteal tuberosity
Distal attachment: head of the fibula
Innervation: common fibular (peroneal) portion of the sciatic nerve

GEMELLUS INFERIOR
Proximal attachment: upper part of the ischial tuberosity
Distal attachment: blends with the tendon of the obturator internus
Innervation: nerve to the quadratus femoris and gemellus inferior

GEMELLUS SUPERIOR
Proximal attachment: dorsal surface of the ischial spine
Distal attachment: blends with the tendon of the obturator internus
Innervation: nerve to the obturator internus and gemellus superior

GLUTEUS MAXIMUS
Proximal attachments: outer ilium (immediately posterior to the posterior gluteal line), thoracolumbar fascia, parts of sacrotuberous and sacroiliac ligaments, posterior surface of lower sacrum, and coccyx
Distal attachments: gluteal tuberosity and iliotibial band
Innervation: inferior gluteal nerve

GLUTEUS MEDIUS
Proximal attachment: outer surface of the ilium, above the anterior gluteal line
Distal attachment: superior-posterior and lateral facets of the greater trochanter
Innervation: superior gluteal nerve

GLUTEUS MINIMUS
Proximal attachment: outer surface of the ilium between the anterior and inferior gluteal lines, as far posterior as the greater sciatic notch
Distal attachments: anterior facet of the greater trochanter and portion of capsule of the hip joint
Innervation: superior gluteal nerve

GRACILIS
Proximal attachments: anterior aspect of lower body of pubis and inferior ramus of pubis
Distal attachment: proximal medial surface of the tibia just posterior to the upper end of the attachment of the sartorius
Innervation: obturator nerve

ILIOCAPSULARIS
Proximal attachments: inferior border of the anterior-inferior iliac spine and from the anterior-medial hip capsule
Distal attachment: just distal to the lesser trochanter of the femur
Innervation: femoral nerve

ILIOPSOAS
Psoas Major
Proximal attachments: transverse processes and lateral bodies of the last thoracic and all lumbar vertebrae including the intervertebral discs
Distal attachment: lesser trochanter of the femur

Iliacus
Proximal attachments: superior two-thirds of the iliac fossa, inner lip of the iliac crest, and small region of the sacrum across the sacroiliac joint
Distal attachment: lesser trochanter of the femur (via psoas major tendon); small area of the femur just anterior and inferior to the lesser trochanter.
Innervation of iliopsoas: femoral nerve (psoas major also receives branches from L^1)

ILIOCAPSULARIS
Proximal attachments: anterior-medial capsule of the hip joint and part of anterior-inferior iliac spine
Distal attachment: lesser trochanter of the femur
Innervation: branches from femoral nerve

OBTURATOR EXTERNUS
Proximal attachments: external surface of the obturator membrane and surrounding external surfaces of the inferior pubic ramus and ischial ramus

Distal attachment: medial surface of the greater trochanter at the trochanteric fossa

Innervation: obturator nerve

OBTURATOR INTERNUS

Proximal attachments: internal side of the obturator membrane and the bone surrounding the obturator foramen; bony attachments extend superiorly and slightly posteriorly on the ischium (within the pelvis) towards the greater sciatic notch

Distal attachment: medial surface of the greater trochanter just anterior and superior to the trochanteric fossa

Innervation: nerve to the obturator internus and gemellus superior

PECTINEUS

Proximal attachment: pectineal line (pecten pubis) on superior pubic ramus; part of hip capsule

Distal attachment: pectineal line on the posterior surface of the femur

Innervation: femoral nerve and occasionally a branch from the obturator nerve

PIRIFORMIS

Proximal attachment: anterior side of the sacrum between the sacral foramina; blends partially with the capsule of the sacroiliac joint

Distal attachment: apex of the greater trochanter

Innervation: Superior gluteal nerve; secondary innervation through ventral rami of S^1 and S^2

POPLITEUS

Proximal attachment: by an intracapsular tendon that attaches to the lateral aspect of the lateral femoral condyle; secondary attachments include the lateral meniscus and the head of the fibula via the popliteofibular ligament

Distal attachments: posterior surface of the proximal tibia above the soleal line

Innervation: tibial nerve

PSOAS MINOR

Proximal attachments: transverse processes and lateral bodies of the last thoracic and the first lumbar vertebra including the intervertebral disc

Distal attachment: bony pelvic attachment: inner pelvic brim, just medial to the acetabulum and iliopubic eminence; fascial attachment: tendon blends with iliac fascia that covers the iliopsoas muscle; some tendinous fibers attach into fascia covering obturator internus muscle

Innervation: branches from L^1

QUADRATUS FEMORIS

Proximal attachment: lateral surface of the ischial tuberosity just anterior to the attachments of the semimembranosus

Distal attachment: quadrate tubercle (middle of intertrochanteric crest)

Innervation: nerve to the quadratus femoris and gemellus inferior

RECTUS FEMORIS

Proximal attachments: straight tendon—anterior-inferior iliac spine; reflected tendon—groove around the superior rim of the acetabulum and into the anterior capsule of the hip joint

Distal attachment: base of the patella and, via the patellar tendon, the tibial tuberosity

Innervation: femoral nerve

SARTORIUS

Proximal attachment: anterior-superior iliac spine

Distal attachment: along a line on the proximal medial surface of the tibia

Innervation: femoral nerve

SEMIMEMBRANOSUS

Proximal attachment: lateral impression on the posterior surface of the ischial tuberosity

Distal attachments: posterior aspect of the medial condyle of the tibia; secondary attachments include the medial collateral ligament, fascia covering the popliteus, oblique popliteal ligament, and both lateral and medial menisci

Innervation: tibial portion of the sciatic nerve

SEMITENDINOSUS

Proximal attachments: from a common tendon with the long head of the biceps femoris originating from a medial impression on the posterior surface of the ischial tuberosity and part of the sacrotuberous ligament

Distal attachment: proximal medial surface of the tibia, just posterior to the lower end of the attachment of the sartorius

Innervation: tibial portion of the sciatic nerve

TENSOR FASCIAE LATAE

Proximal attachment: outer surface of the iliac crest just posterior to the anterior-superior iliac spine

Distal attachment: proximal one-third of the iliotibial band of the fascia lata

Innervation: superior gluteal nerve

VASTUS INTERMEDIUS

Proximal attachment: anterior-lateral regions of the upper two-thirds of the femoral shaft

Distal attachments: lateral base of the patella and, via the patellar tendon, the tibial tuberosity

Innervation: femoral nerve

VASTUS LATERALIS

Proximal attachments: upper region of intertrochanteric line, anterior and inferior border of the greater trochanter, lateral region of the gluteal tuberosity, and lateral aspects of the femoral shaft alongside the lateral lip of the linea aspera

Distal attachments: lateral capsule of the knee, base of the patella, and, via the patellar tendon, the tibial tuberosity

Innervation: femoral nerve

VASTUS MEDIALIS

Proximal attachments: lower region of intertrochanteric line, medial aspects of the femoral shaft along the medial lip of linea aspera as far distal as the proximal medial supracondylar line, and into fibers of the adductor magnus

Distal attachments: medial capsule of the knee, base of the patella, and, via the patellar tendon, the tibial tuberosity

Innervation: femoral nerve

ANKLE AND FOOT MUSCULATURE

EXTENSOR DIGITORUM LONGUS

Proximal attachments: lateral condyle of tibia, proximal two-thirds of the medial surface of the fibula, and adjacent interosseous membrane

Distal attachments: by four tendons that attach to the proximal base of the dorsal surface of the middle and distal phalanges via the dorsal digital expansion

Innervation: deep branch of the fibular (peroneal) nerve

EXTENSOR HALLUCIS LONGUS

Proximal attachments: middle section of the medial surface of the fibula and adjacent interosseous membrane

Distal attachments: dorsal base of the distal phalanx of the great toe

Innervation: deep branch of the fibular nerve

FIBULARIS (PERONEUS) BREVIS

Proximal attachment: middle to near-distal aspect of the lateral surface of the fibula

Distal attachment: styloid process of the fifth metatarsal

Innervation: superficial branch of the fibular nerve

FIBULARIS (PERONEUS) LONGUS

Proximal attachments: lateral condyle of tibia; head and proximal two-thirds of the lateral surface of the fibula

Distal attachment: lateral surface of the medial cuneiform and lateral side of the base of the first metatarsal bone

Innervation: superficial branch of the fibular nerve

FIBULARIS (PERONEUS) TERTIUS

Proximal attachments: distal one-third of the medial surface of the fibula and adjacent interosseous membrane

Distal attachment: dorsal surface of the base of the fifth metatarsal

Innervation: deep branch of the fibular nerve

FLEXOR DIGITORUM LONGUS

Proximal attachments: posterior surface of the middle one-third of the tibia just medial to the proximal attachment of the tibialis posterior

Distal attachments: by four separate tendons to the base of the distal phalanx of the four lesser toes

Innervation: tibial nerve

FLEXOR HALLUCIS LONGUS

Proximal attachment: distal two-thirds of most of the posterior surface of the fibula

Distal attachment: plantar surface of the base of the distal phalanx of the great toe

Innervation: tibial nerve

GASTROCNEMIUS

Proximal attachments: by two separate heads from the posterior aspect of the lateral and medial femoral condyle

Distal attachment: calcaneal tuberosity via the Achilles tendon

Innervation: tibial nerve

PLANTARIS

Proximal attachments: most inferior part of lateral supracondylar line of the femur and oblique popliteal ligament of the knee

Distal attachment: joins the medial aspect of the Achilles tendon to insert on the calcaneal tuberosity

Innervation: tibial nerve

SOLEUS

Proximal attachments: posterior surface of the fibula head and proximal one-third of its shaft and from the posterior side of the tibia near the soleal line

Distal attachment: calcaneal tuberosity via the Achilles tendon

Innervation: tibial nerve

TIBIALIS ANTERIOR

Proximal attachments: lateral condyle and proximal two-thirds of the lateral surface of the tibia and the interosseous membrane

Distal attachment: medial and plantar aspects of the medial cuneiform and the base of the first metatarsal

Innervation: deep branch of the fibular nerve

TIBIALIS POSTERIOR

Proximal attachments: proximal two-thirds of the posterior surface of the tibia and fibula and adjacent interosseous membrane

Distal attachment: tendon attaches to every tarsal bone but the talus, plus the bases of the second through the fourth metatarsal bones; main insertion is on the navicular tuberosity and the medial cuneiform bone

Innervation: tibial nerve

INTRINSIC MUSCLES OF THE FOOT

EXTENSOR DIGITORUM BREVIS

Proximal attachment: lateral-distal aspect of the calcaneus just proximal to the calcaneocuboid joint

Distal attachments: usually by four tendons: one to the dorsal surface of the great toe, and the other three join the tendons of the extensor digitorum longus of the second through fourth toes

Innervation: deep branch of the fibular nerve

LAYER 1

ABDUCTOR DIGITI MINIMI

Proximal attachments: lateral process and lateral edge of the medial process of the calcaneal tuberosity, plantar aponeurosis, and plantar surface of the base of the fifth metatarsal bone with flexor digiti minimi

Distal attachment: lateral side of the proximal phalanx of the fifth toe, sharing an attachment with the flexor digiti minimi

Innervation: lateral plantar nerve

ABDUCTOR HALLUCIS

Proximal attachments: flexor retinaculum, medial process of the calcaneus and plantar fascia

Distal attachment: medial side of the base of the proximal phalanx of the hallux, sharing an attachment with the medial tendon of the flexor hallucis brevis

Innervation: medial plantar nerve

FLEXOR DIGITORUM BREVIS

Proximal attachments: medial process of calcaneal tuberosity and central part of the plantar fascia

Distal attachments: each of four tendons splits and inserts on the sides of the plantar aspect of the base of the middle phalanx of the lesser toes

Innervation: medial plantar nerve

LAYER 2

LUMBRICALS

Proximal attachments: from the tendons of the flexor digitorum longus muscle

Distal attachments: each muscle crosses the medial side of each metatarsophalangeal joint to insert into the dorsal digital expansion of the four lesser toes

Innervation: to second toe—medial plantar nerve; to third through fifth toes—lateral plantar nerve

QUADRATUS PLANTAE

Proximal attachments: by two heads from the medial and lateral aspect of the plantar surface of the calcaneus, distal to the calcaneal tuberosity

Distal attachment: lateral border of the flexor digitorum longus common tendon

Innervation: lateral plantar nerve

LAYER 3

ADDUCTOR HALLUCIS

Proximal Attachment

Oblique head: plantar aspect of the base of the second through fourth metatarsals and the fibrous sheath of the fibularis longus tendon

Transverse head: plantar aspect of the ligaments that support the metatarsophalangeal joints of the third through fifth toes

Distal attachments: both heads converge to insert on the lateral base of the proximal phalanx of the great toe along with the lateral tendon of the flexor hallucis brevis

Innervation: lateral plantar nerve

FLEXOR DIGITI MINIMI

Proximal attachments: plantar surface of the base of the fifth metatarsal bone and fibrous sheath covering the tendon of the fibularis longus

Distal attachment: lateral surface of the base of the proximal phalanx of the fifth toe blending with the tendon of the abductor digiti minimi

Innervation: lateral plantar nerve

FLEXOR HALLUCIS BREVIS

Proximal attachments: plantar surface of the cuboid and lateral cuneiform bones, and on parts of the tendon of the tibialis posterior muscle

Distal attachments: by two tendons in which the lateral tendon attaches to the lateral base of the proximal phalanx of the great toe with the adductor hallucis, and the medial tendon attaches to the medial base of the proximal phalanx of the great toe with the abductor hallucis; a pair of sesamoid bones is located within the tendons of this muscle

Innervation: medial plantar nerve

LAYER 4

DORSAL INTEROSSEI

Proximal Attachments

First: adjacent sides of the first and second metatarsals

Second: adjacent sides of the second and third metatarsals

Third: adjacent sides of the third and fourth metatarsals

Fourth: adjacent sides of the fourth and fifth metatarsals

Distal Attachments*

First: medial side of the base of the proximal phalanx of the second toe

Second: lateral side of the base of the proximal phalanx of the second toe

Third: lateral side of the base of the proximal phalanx of the third toe

Fourth: lateral side of the base of the proximal phalanx of the fourth toe

Innervation: lateral plantar nerve

PLANTAR INTEROSSEI

Proximal Attachments

First: medial side of the third metatarsal

Second: medial side of the fourth metatarsal

Third: medial side of the fifth metatarsal

Distal Attachments*

First: medial side of the proximal phalanx of the third toe

Second: medial side of the proximal phalanx of the fourth toe

Third: medial side of the proximal phalanx of the fifth toe

Innervation: lateral plantar nerve

---

* Attaches into the dorsal digital expansion of the toes.

Part E: Physiologic Cross-Sectional Areas of Selected Muscles of the Lower Extremity

Physiologic Cross-Sectional Areas (PCSAs) of a Sample of Adult Human Lower Extremity Muscles*

Muscle	PCSA (cm²) (Mean ± SD)
Hip and Knee Musculature	
Psoas major	7.7 ± 2.3[1]
Psoas minor	0.5 ± 0.3[2]
Iliacus	9.9 ± 3.4[1]
Sartorius	1.9 ± 0.7[1]
Gluteus maximus	33.4 ± 8.8[1]
Gluteus medius	33.8 ± 14.4[1]
Gluteus minimus	8.3 ± 0.5[3]
Piriformis	2.2 ± 0.2[3]
Gemellus superior	0.7 ± 0.1[3]
Obturator internus	3.8 ± 0.3[3]
Gemellus inferior	1.0 ± 0.1[3]
Quadratus femoris	3.8 ± 0.4[3]
Obturator externus	4.5 ± 0.2[3]
Pectineus	2.3 ± 0.2[3]
Adductor brevis	5.0 ± 2.1[1]
Adductor longus	6.5 ± 2.2[1]
Gracilis	2.2 ± 0.8[1]
Adductor magnus	20.5 ± 7.8[1]
Rectus femoris	13.5 ± 5.0[1]
Vastus intermedius	16.7 ± 6.9[1]
Vastus lateralis	35.1 ± 16.1[1]
Vastus medialis	20.6 ± 7.2[1]
Biceps femoris (long head)	11.3 ± 4.8[1]
Biceps femoris (short head)	5.1 ± 1.7[1]
Semitendinosus	4.8 ± 2.0[1]
Semimembranosus	18.4 ± 7.5[1]
Ankle and Foot Musculature	
Tibialis anterior	10.9 ± 3.0[1]
Extensor hallucis longus	2.7 ± 1.5[1]
Extensor digitorum longus	5.6 ± 1.7[1]
Fibularis longus	10.4 ± 3.8[1]
Fibularis brevis	4.9 ± 2.0[1]
Gastrocnemius (lateral head)	9.7 ± 3.3[1]
Gastrocnemius (medial head)	21.1 ± 5.7[1]
Soleus	51.8 ± 14.9[1]
Tibialis posterior	14.4 ± 4.9[1]
Flexor digitorum longus	4.4 ± 2.0[1]
Flexor hallucis longus	1.9 ± 2.7[1]

*Muscles are listed in a general proximal to distal order. Data are from three sources (see superscripts and references below). Due to different methodologies, caution is required when comparing data across studies.

[1]Ward SR, Eng CM, Smallwood LH, et al: Are current measurements of lower extremity muscle architecture accurate? *Clin Orthop Relat Res* 467:1074–1082, 2009.

[2]Neumann DA, Garceau LR: A proposed novel function of the psoas minor revealed through cadaver dissection, *Clin Anat* 28:243–252, 2015.

[3]Parvaresh KC, Chang C, Patel A, et al: Architecture of the short external rotator muscles of the hip. *BMC Musculoskeletal Disorders* 20(1):611, 2019.

Part F: Attachments, Innervation, and Actions of the Muscles of the Pelvic Floor

The muscles that arise from within the "true" pelvis (i.e., that part of the pelvis inferior to the sacral promontory and superior pubic rami) can be conveniently divided into two groups: (1) *muscles of*

the lower extremity (piriformis and obturator internus), which form the walls of the true pelvis, and (2) *muscles of the pelvic floor*. The muscles of the pelvic floor (also referred to as the pelvic diaphragm) include the three parts of the levator ani (pubococcygeus, puborectalis, iliococcygeus) and the ischiococcygeus (also known as the coccygeus) (Fig. IV.2).

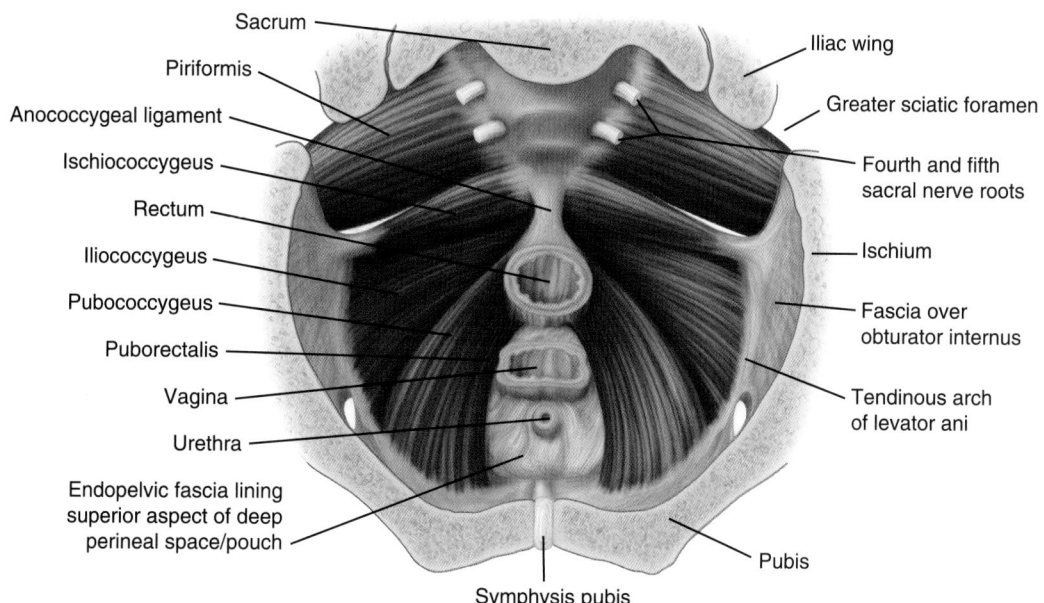

FIGURE IV.2   Muscles of the pelvic floor (pelvic diaphragm); female, viewed from above. Note how the levator ani (pubococcygeus, puborectalis, iliococcygeus) and ischiococcygeus form a continuous sling, designed to support the pelvic organs. Also note the fascia over the obturator internus, serving as a lateral attachment for much of the levator ani. (From Standring S: *British Gray's anatomy: the anatomical basis of clinical practice,* ed 41, 2016, Elsevier, Ltd. [Fig. 63.3].)

Attachments, Innervation, and Actions of Muscles of the Pelvic Floor*

Muscle	Lateral Attachment	Midline Attachment	Innervation	Function

Levator ani
  Pubococcygeus
  Puborectalis
  Iliococcygeus
	From a line that connects the posterior surface of the pubis, obturator internus fascia, tendinous arch, and ischial spine	Anteriorly to the superior surface of the perineal membrane (horizontal fascia extending between right and left ischiopubic rami); posteriorly to the muscles' contralateral partner, distal rectum/anal canal, and anococcygeal ligament	Ventral ramus of S^4, and the inferior rectal branch of the pudendal nerve (S^{2-4})	Contributes to the formation of the pelvic floor, which supports the pelvic organs. Maintains an anorectal angle that functions as a "pinch valve" for bowel continence.
				Relaxes to allow passage of urine or stool.
				Reinforces the external anal sphincter and vaginal sphincter.
				When active with abdominal muscles and the diaphragm, increases intra-abdominal pressure.

Ischiococcygeus (coccygeus): a combined muscle and ligament	Ischial spine and pelvic side of sacrospinous ligament	Lateral margin of the coccyx and adjacent caudal sacrum	Ventral rami of S^{3-4}	Contributes to the formation of the pelvic floor. Assists the levator ani in providing urine and bowel continence.

*This table summarizes general attachments, innervation, and actions of these muscles. For a more detailed account of this material and the associated muscles of the perineum, the reader should consult the following sources: Standring S: *Gray's anatomy: the anatomical basis of clinical practice,* ed 41, St Louis, 2015, Elsevier; Drake RL, Vogl W, Mitchell AWM: *Gray's anatomy for students,* St Louis, 2005, Churchill Livingstone. Acknowledgments to Brenda L. Neumann for reviewing this material.

INDEX

Note: Page numbers followed by *f* indicate figures; *t*, tables and *b*, boxes.

Proteoglycans
  aging and, 46
  in articular cartilage, 38–39
  in bone, 42
  nucleus pulposus and, 351–352
  type II collagen in, 351–352
  vertebral endplate and, 353
Proteoglycan side unit, 36
Protraction
  of craniocervical region, 362
  of cranium, 362f
  of scapulothoracic joint, 131, 131f, 138, 138f, 155b, 158, 158f
  of SC, 134, 138f
Protrusion, mandible, 457, 458f, 459
Proximal drift, of radius, 195
Proximal end of the radius, 217
Proximal end of the ulna, 217
Proximal femur, 494f
  angle of inclination of, 496, 496f
  compact bone of, 43f
  internal structure of, 498, 498f
  pincer-type deformity of, 540b–543b
  rotation of, 496–497
  shape of, 496–498
Proximal humerus, retroversion of, 176b
Proximal interphalangeal joints (PIP)
  arthrokinematics of, 279
  of fingers, flexion of, 279, 279f
  flexor digitorum superficialis and, 282
  oblique retinacular ligaments of, 289, 298f
  of toes, 642
Proximal-on-distal kinematics, 6
Proximal phalanges, 274
  finger MCP and, 274
Proximal pole, of scaphoid, 228
Proximal radio-ulnar joint, 184f, 187
  arthrokinematics at, 208–210
  connective tissue of, 196–197
  dislocation of, 197f, 197b
  forearm pronation and supination and, 201
  pronation at, 200
  sensory nerves of, 204
  supination at, 199
Proximal tibia, 553–554
Proximal tibiofibular joint, 617–618
Proximal-to-mid humerus, 128–130
Proximal transverse arch, 266, 267f
Proximal ulna, 185, 187f
Proximal-ulnar joint, 193–194
Psoas major, 417, 512–513, 512f
  line of force on, 418f
  lumbosacral junction and, function of, 417–418
Psoas minor, 512–513, 512f–513f
Pterygoid fossa, 452–453
Pubic crest, 493
Pubic symphysis, 493
  fibrocartilage of, 40
  rectus abdominis and, 415
Pubic tubercle, 493
Pubis, 493, 493b

Pubofemoral ligament, 501, 502f
Pulled-elbow syndrome, 197f, 197b
Push off, in gait cycle, 676

Q
Q-angle. *See* Quadriceps angle
Quadrate ligament, 197
Quadrate tubercle, 496
Quadratus femoris, 516
  nerve to, 509
  in running, 731
  as short external rotator, 529
Quadratus lumborum, 418, 418f
Quadratus plantae, 654
Quadriceps, 513
  external torque on, 100f, 574–578
  in gait cycle, 693
  knee menisci and, 559
  line of force, 597f
  muscle action of, 574–578
  patella and, 577, 577f
    lateral pull of, 580
  patellar tracking and, 579, 579f
  resistance training and, 100f
  tibial tuberosity and, 553–554
Quadriceps angle (Q-angle), 579
  excessive genu valgum and, 581
  internal rotation of tibia and, 582
  local factors and, 580
  of women, 582
Quadriceps femoris, 572
Quadriceps tendon, 573, 578
Quiet expiration, 468
Quiet inspiration, muscles of, 470–474
Quiet ventilation, 467

R
RA. *See* Rheumatoid arthritis
Radial collateral ligament, 190, 232
  of finger MCP, 274f
Radial deviation
  of fingers, 290
  of wrist, 238–239, 239f, 247b, 248f
    function of, 247–249
Radial fossa, 184
Radial head, 187
  compression fracture of, 193
  fovea of, 193
  fracture of, 190f
Radial neck, 187
Radial nerve, 203, 222b, 242, 280–281
  around humerus, 222b
  supinator muscle and, 213f
Radial notch, 185
Radial synovial sheath, 284f
Radial (bicipital) tuberosity, 187
Radiate ligaments, 468
  of costocorporeal joint, 367
Radiculopathy, 365b
  McKenzie exercises for, 375
Radiocarpal joint, 226, 231, 231f
Radioscaphocapitate ligament, 232

Radio-ulnar joint
  arthrokinematics of, 202, 202f
  distal, 183, 184f, 195–196, 196f
    arthrokinematics at, 208–211
    connective tissue of, 197
    intra-articular discs in, 5
    pronation at, 200
    pronator quadratus muscle and, 217f
    sensory nerves of, 204
    stabilizers of, 198b
    supination at, 199
    ulnar head rotation and, 202
  proximal, 184f, 187
    arthrokinematics at, 208–210
    connective tissue of, 196–197
    dislocation of, 197f, 197b
    forearm pronation and, 201
    forearm supination and, 201
    pronation at, 200
    sensory nerves of, 204
    supination at, 199
  TFCC and, 234
Radius, 183, 184f, 185–187, 186f–187f
  central band and, 194–195
  distal articular surface of, 228
  distal end of, 217
  distracting force on, 195, 195f
  forearm pronation and supination and, 201–202
  fractures of, 194–195, 228
  osteologic features of, 187b
  positive ulnar variance and, 253b–255b
  proximal drift of, 195
  proximal end of, 217
  styloid process of, 226, 228
  translation of, 198
Rami, mandible, 452
Range of motion. *See specific body parts and joints*
Rate coding, 64
  for motor nerves, 67–68
Raw EMG, 70
Rays, of foot, 616
Rearfoot, 611–612
  in gait loading phase, 635
  strike, in running, 724
Recruitment, of motor nerves, 65–67
Rectus abdominis, 414
  gait cycle, 691–692
  muscle action of, 415–416
  in running, 730
Rectus capitis anterior, 425, 425f
Rectus capitis lateralis, 425, 425f
Rectus capitis posterior, head posture and, 428f
Rectus femoris, 513, 573
  in running, 731
  therapeutic stretch of, 536b, 537f
Rectus sheaths, 413–414
Recurrent meningeal nerves, 405
"Red zone," of knee, 559
Regular dense connective tissue, 36
Relative motion, 6